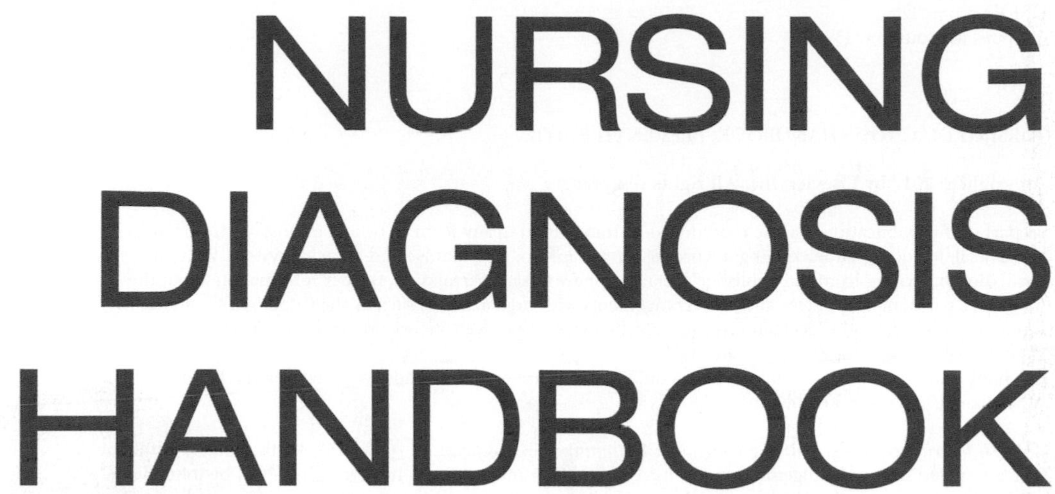

NURSING DIAGNOSIS HANDBOOK

AN EVIDENCE-BASED GUIDE TO PLANNING CARE

Eleventh Edition

Betty J. Ackley, MSN, EdS, RN
Gail B. Ladwig, MSN, RN
Mary Beth Flynn Makic, PhD, RN, CNS, CCNS, FAAN

ELSEVIER

ELSEVIER

3251 Riverport Lane
St. Louis, Missouri 63043

NURSING DIAGNOSIS HANDBOOK, ELEVENTH EDITION ISBN: 978-0-323-32224-9

NANDA International, Inc. Nursing Diagnoses: Definitions & Classifications 2015-2017, Tenth Edition. Edited by T. Heather Herdman and Shigemi Kamitsuru. 2014 NANDA International, Inc. Published 2014 by John Wiley & Sons, Ltd. Companion website: www.wiley.com/go/nursingdiagnoses. In order to make safe and effective judgments using NANDA-I diagnoses it is essential that nurses refer to the definitions and defining characteristics of the diagnoses listed in this work.

Notices

Knowledge and best practice in this field are constantly changing. As new research and experience broaden our understanding, changes in research methods, professional practices, or medical treatment may become necessary.

Practitioners and researchers must always rely on their own experience and knowledge in evaluating and using any information, methods, compounds, or experiments described herein. In using such information or methods they should be mindful of their own safety and the safety of others, including parties for whom they have a professional responsibility.

With respect to any drug or pharmaceutical products identified, readers are advised to check the most current information provided (i) on procedures featured or (ii) by the manufacturer of each product to be administered, to verify the recommended dose or formula, the method and duration of administration, and contraindications. It is the responsibility of practitioners, relying on their own experience and knowledge of their patients, to make diagnoses, to determine dosages and the best treatment for each individual patient, and to take all appropriate safety precautions.

To the fullest extent of the law, neither the Publisher nor the authors, contributors, or editors, assume any liability for any injury and/or damage to persons or property as a matter of products liability, negligence or otherwise, or from any use or operation of any methods, products, instructions, or ideas contained in the material herein.

Previous editions copyrighted 2014, 2011, 2008, 2006, 2004, 2002, 1999, 1997, 1995, 1993.

Library of Congress Cataloging-in-Publication Data

Names: Ackley, Betty J., editor. | Ladwig, Gail B., editor. | Makic, Mary Beth Flynn, editor.
Title: Nursing diagnosis handbook : an evidence-based guide to planning care / [edited by] Betty J. Ackley, Gail B. Ladwig, Mary Beth Flynn Makic.
Description: Eleventh edition. | St. Louis, Missouri : Elsevier, [2017] | Includes bibliographical references and index.
Identifiers: LCCN 2015042558 | ISBN 9780323322249 (pbk. : alk. paper)
Subjects: | MESH: Nursing Diagnosis—Handbooks. | Evidence-Based Nursing—methods—Handbooks. | Patient Care Planning—Handbooks.
Classification: LCC RT48.6 | NLM WY 49 | DDC 616.07/5—dc23
LC record available at http://lccn.loc.gov/2015042558

Content Strategist: Sandra Clark
Content Development Specialist: Jennifer Wade
Publishing Services Manager: Jeff Patterson
Book Production Specialist: Carol O'Connell
Production Manager: Andrea Villamero
Design Direction: Paula Catalano

Printed in Canada

Last digit is the print number: 9 8 7 6 5 4 3

In Memory of Betty J. Ackley

Dreams

Dreams come
Dreams go
Whispers, shouts, images
Dreams come
Dreams go
*Follow, follow**

Betty believed in dreams. This textbook was our dream. We set out to write the best nursing diagnosis textbook ever. Our book is now in 1400 nursing programs. It has been high on Amazon's best seller list. I think her dream is realized. From a handout to students to an international publication. Thank you, dear friend Betty.

Betty passed away in December 2014 at her home with her husband (Dale) and daughter (Dawn) present.

Betty fought a gallant battle with pancreatic cancer for nine months. She loved life, her family, and the profession of nursing. She was an active member of NANDA-I for more than two decades. She was also Professor Emeritus, Jackson Community College (Jackson, Michigan). Betty was an instructor at Jackson Community College for 34 years and was named Faculty of the Year.

Betty provided presentations on nursing diagnosis in Japan and across the United States. She wrote a column on nursing diagnosis for a Japanese journal, *Expert Nurse*. Betty was known for her work as a co-author of several textbooks on diagnoses, outcomes, and interventions. She served on several NANDA-I committees over the years, the most recent of which was as Chair of the most recent nominating committee. She recruited one of the strongest slates of nominees that NANDA-I has had in many years, due to her tireless efforts.

Betty will be remembered as a very giving person. She had an ability to help others in their time of need and provide comfort and direction for them. She was a certified instructor in aerobics, spinning, Zumba, and Pilates. For years she loved to run, and she finished two Detroit Marathons. Her passion included gardening, traveling, authoring this textbook, and watching her two grandchildren grow.

The following is a quote from Betty's husband:

> *Betty saw a need and was able to help fill that need by working to complete this book and see it through to publication. She was very proud of each edition of this book. She always strived to make each edition as good as it could be.*
>
> *Betty was a loving daughter, grandmother, mother, and wife. She cared about people and was always helping everyone to be their very best. This book will continue to be her way of giving to the profession she loved. Nursing gave a lot to Betty, and she returned the love of nursing by writing the most helpful book she could write.*

Dale Ackley

Also Dedicated to

Jerry Ladwig, my wonderful husband, who, after 51 years, is still supportive and helpful—he has been "my right-hand man" in every revision of this book. Also to my very special children, their spouses, and all of my grandchildren: Jerry, Kathy, Alexandra, Elizabeth, and Benjamin Ladwig; Christine, John, Sean, Ciara, and Bridget McMahon; Jennifer, Jim, Abby, Katelyn, Blake, and Connor Martin; Amy, Scott, Ford, and Vaughn Bertram—the greatest family anyone could ever hope for.

Gail B. Ladwig

My husband, Zlatko, and children, Alexander and Erik, whose unconditional love and support are ever present in my life. To my parents and sisters for always encouraging me to follow my passion. To Gail, for her incredible mentorship, guidance, and encouragement this past year. And finally to Betty, for believing in me and providing me with an opportunity to more fully contribute to this amazing textbook in support of nurses and the patients and families we serve.

Mary Beth Flynn Makic

---

*Gail Ladwig, 2015

About the Authors

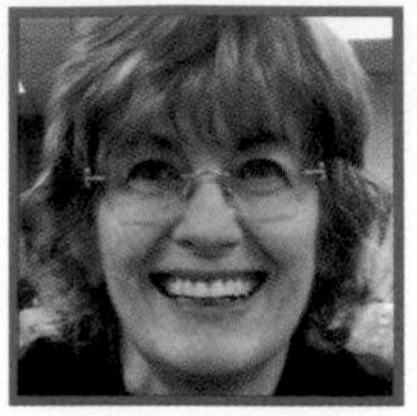

Betty Ackley worked in nursing for 40 years in many capacities. She was a staff nurse on a CCU unit, medical ICU unit, respiratory ICU unit, intensive care unit, and step-down unit. She worked on a gynecological surgery floor and on an orthopedic floor, and spent many years working in oncology. She also was in management and nursing education in a hospital, and she spent 31 years as a professor of nursing at Jackson Community College. At the college she taught medical-surgical nursing, critical care nursing, fundamentals of nursing, nursing leadership, and nutrition. In addition she served as a nursing consultant for nursing continuing education at the college. In 1996 she began the online learning program at Jackson Community College, offering an online course in nutrition. In 2000, Betty was named Faculty of the Year at her college.

Betty presented conferences nationally and internationally in the areas of nursing diagnosis, nursing process, online learning, and evidence-based nursing. She wrote NCLEX-RN questions for the national licensure examination four times and was an expert in the area of testing and NCLEX preparation.

Betty obtained her BSN from Michigan State University, MS in nursing from the University of Michigan, and education specialist degree from Michigan State University.

Betty is co-author of *Nursing Diagnosis: Guide to Planning Care,* which has been a successful text for 20 years, and co-author for four editions of *Mosby's Guide to Nursing Diagnosis*. She was also a lead co-author/editor of *Evidence-Based Nursing Care Guidelines: Medical-Surgical Interventions*. This text is designed to help nurses easily find and use evidence to provide excellence in nursing care. The text was published in 2008 and was named AJN book of the year.

Her free time was spent exercising, especially teaching Zumba and Pilates, and also taking spinning classes, kick boxing, and keeping moving. She taught classes in Total Control, a program to help women with urinary incontinence. In addition, she loved to travel, read, garden, spend time with her grandchildren, and learn anything new!

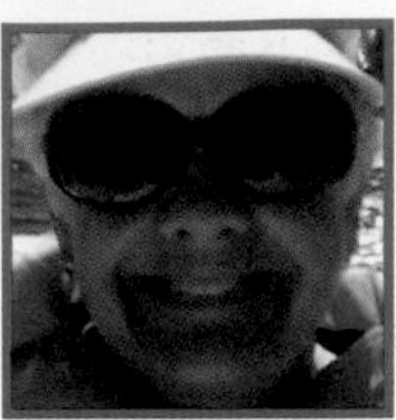

Gail Ladwig is a professor emeritus of Jackson Community College. During her tenure, she served 4 years as the Department Chairperson of Nursing and as a nurse consultant for Continuing Education. She was instrumental in starting a BSN transfer program with the University of Michigan.

Gail has taught classroom and clinical at JCC in fundamentals, med-surg, mental health, and a transfer course for BSN students. In addition, she has taught online courses in pharmacology, as well as a hybrid course (partially online) for BSN transfer students. She has also taught an online course in pathophysiology for the Medical University of South Carolina.

She worked as a staff nurse in medical-surgical nursing and intensive care for more than 20 years prior to beginning her teaching career. She was a certified critical-care nurse for several years and has a master's degree in Psychiatric Mental Health Nursing from Wayne State University. Her master's research was published in the *International Journal of Addictions*.

She has presented nationally and internationally, including Paris, Tokyo, and Puerto Rico, on many topics, including nursing diagnosis, computerized care planning, and holistic nursing topics.

Gail is co-author of *Nursing Diagnosis: Guide to Planning Care,* which has been a very successful text for more than 20 years, and she has been co-author for all editions of *Mosby's Guide to Nursing Diagnosis,* now in its fifth edition. She is also a co-author/editor of *Evidence-Based Nursing Care Guidelines: Medical-Surgical Interventions*. This text was published in 2008 and was named AJN book of the year.

Gail has been an active member and supporter of NANDA-I for many, many years.

Gail is the mother of 4 children and grandmother of 12 and loves to spend time with her grandchildren. She has been married to her husband Jerry for 51 years and is passionate about her family and the profession of nursing.

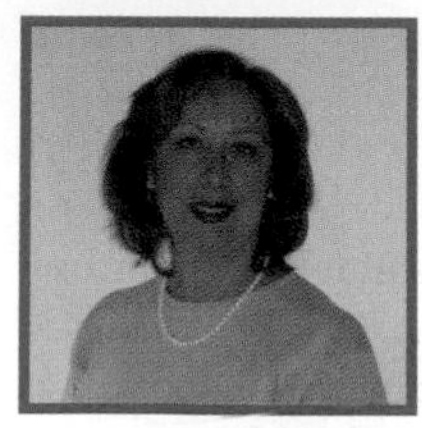

Mary Beth Flynn Makic is an associate professor at the University of Colorado, College of Nursing, Aurora, Colorado. At the college she teaches in the undergraduate and graduate programs. She is co-director of the Clinical Nurse Specialist graduate degree program at the College of Nursing. She has worked predominately in critical care for 30 years. Mary Beth is best known for her publications and presentations, regionally and nationally, as an expert on evidence-based practice in nursing. Her practice expertise and research focuses on the care of the trauma, general surgical, and burn injured patient populations; acute wound healing; pressure ulcer prevention; and hospital-acquired conditions (HACs). She is passionate about nurses' understanding and translating current best evidence into practice to optimize patient and family outcomes. She is co-author of *Trauma Nursing: from Resuscitation through Rehabilitation* and a section editor of *American Association of Critical Care Nurses Procedure Manual for Critical Care.* She is actively involved in several professional nursing and interprofessional organizations.

Contributors

[†]Betty J. Ackley, MSN, EdS, RN
President and Owner, The Betty Ackley, LLC;
Consultant in Nursing Process, Evidence-Based Nursing, and Pilates
Jackson, Michigan

Michelle Acorn, DNP, NP PHC/adult, BA, BScN/PHCNP, MN/ACNP, ENC(C), GNC(C), CAP, CGP
Lead NP
Lakeridge Health
Whitby, Ontario;
Primary Health Care NP, Global Health Coordinator
Nursing Department
University of Toronto
Toronto, Ontario
Canada

Keith A. Anderson, MSW, PhD
Associate Professor
School of Social Work
University of Montana
Missoula, Montana

Amanda Andrews, MA, Ed, BSc, DN, RN, HEA Fellow
Program Lead
Education for Health Group
Warwick
United Kingdom

Jessica Bibbo, MA
Human Development and Family Science
University of Missouri
Columbia, Missouri

Kathaleen C. Bloom, PhD, CNM
Professor and Associate Director
Undergraduate Programs
School of Nursing
University of North Florida
Jacksonville, Florida

Lina Daou Boudiab, MSN, RN
VA Nursing Academic Partnership Faculty
Nursing Services
Aleda E. Lutz Veterans Affairs Medical Center
Saginaw, Michigan

Lisa Burkhart, PhD, RN, ANEF
Associate Professor
Marcella Niehoff School of Nursing
Loyola University
Chicago, Illinois

Melodie Cannon, DNP, MSc/FNP, BHScN, RN(EC), NP-PHC, CEN, GNC(C)
Nurse Practitioner
Internal Medicine/Emergency Department
Rouge Valley Health System
Toronto, Ontario
Canada;
Adjunct Lecturer
Lawrence S. Bloomberg Faculty of Nursing
University of Toronto, Ontario
Canada

Stacey M. Carroll, PhD, ANP-BC
Nursing Department
Rush University College of Nursing
Chicago, Illinois;
School of Nursing
Anna Maria College
Paxton, Massachusetts

Stephanie C. Christensen, PhD, CCC-SLP
Senior Lecturer
Health Sciences
Northern Arizona University
Flagstaff, Arizona

June M. Como, EdD, RN, CNS
Assistant Professor–Nursing
School of Health Sciences
Graduate and Clinical Doctorate in Nursing Programs Coordinator
College of Staten Island—City University of New York
Staten Island, New York

Maureen F. Cooney, DNP, FNP-BC
Pain Management Nurse Practitioner
Westchester Medical Center
Valhalla, New York;
Adjunct Associate Professor
Pace University
College of Health Professions
Lienhard School of Nursing
New York, New York

[†]Deceased.

Ruth M. Curchoe, RN, BSN, MSN, CIC
Independent Consultant, Infection Prevention
Rochester, New York

Mary Alice DeWys, RN, BS, CIMI
Infant Development and Feeding Specialist
Grand Valley University Preemie Development Assessment Team
President of Hassle Free Feeding Program Division of Harmony Through Touch
Grand Rapids, Michigan

Susan M. Dirkes, RN, MS, CCRN
Staff Nurse, Consultant
Intensive Care
University of Michigan Health System
Ann Arbor, Michigan

Roberta Dobrzanski, MSN, RN
Academic Instructional Staff
College of Nursing
University of Wisconsin Oshkosh
Oshkosh, Wisconsin

Julianne E. Doubet, BSN, RN, CEN, NREMT-P
Certified Emergency Nurse
Pre-Hospital Care Educator
Mason, Ohio

Lorraine Duggan, MSN, ACNP-BC
United Health Group–Optum Clinical
Stroudsburg, Pennsylvania

Shelly Eisbach, PhD, RN, PMHNP-BC
Consulting Associate
Duke University School of Nursing
Durham, North Carolina

Dawn Fairlie, ANP, FNP, GNP, DNS(c)
Faculty
College of Staten Island
The City University of New York
Staten Island, New York

Arlene T. Farren, RN, PhD, AOCN, CTN-A
Associate Professor
College of Staten Island
The City University of New York
Staten Island, New York

Debora Yvonne Fields, RN, BSN, MA, LICDC, CCMC
Cleveland, Ohio

Noelle L. Fields, PhD, LCSW
Assistant Professor
School of Social Work
The University of Texas at Arlington
Arlington, Texas

Vanessa Flannery, MSN, PHCNS-BC, CNE
Associate Professor
Nursing Department
Morehead State University
Morehead, Kentucky

Shari D. Froelich, DNP, MSN, MSBA, ANP, BC, ACHPN, PMHNP, BC
Nurse Practitioner
Alcona Health Center
Alpena, Michigan

Tracy P. George, DNP, APRN-BC, CNE
Instructor
Nursing Department
Francis Marion University
Florence, South Carolina

Susanne W. Gibbons, PhD, C-ANP/GNP
Assistant Professor
Daniel K. Inouye Graduate School of Nursing
Uniformed Services University of the Health Sciences
Bethesda, Maryland

Barbara A. Given, PhD, RN, FAAN
University Distinguished Professor
College of Nursing
Michigan State University
East Lansing, Michigan

Mila W. Grady, MSN, RN
Lecturer
College of Nursing
University of Iowa
Iowa City, Iowa

Pauline McKinney Green, PhD, RN, CNE
Professor Emeritus
Graduate Nursing
Howard University College of Nursing and Allied Health Sciences
Washington, DC

Sherry A. Greenberg, PhD, RN, GNP-BC
Program Director, Advanced Certificate in Gerontology
Adjunct Clinical Assistant Professor of Nursing
The Hartford Institute for Geriatric Nursing
NYU College of Nursing
New York, New York

Dianne Frances Hayward, RN, MSN, WHNP
Women's Health Nurse Practitioner
Nursing Education
University of Michigan, Flint
Flint, Michigan;
Oakland Community College
Waterford, Michigan

Paula D. Hopper, MSN, RN, CNE
Professor of Nursing, Emeritus
Jackson College;
Lecturer
Eastern Michigan University
Jackson, Michigan

Wendie A. Howland, MN, RN-BC, CRRN, CCM, CNLCP, LNCC
Life Care Planner, Legal Nurse Consultant
Howland Health Consulting, Inc.
Pocasset, Massachusetts

Rebecca Johnson, PhD, RN, FAAN, FNAP
Millsap Professor of Gerontological Nursing
MU Sinclair School of Nursing;
Professor & Director
Research Center for Human Animal Interaction
MU College of Veterinary Medicine
University of Missouri
Columbia, Missouri

Nicole Jones, MSN, FNP-BC
Family Nurse Practitioner, Adjunct Professor of Nursing
Department of Advanced Nursing
Northern Kentucky University
Highland Heights, Kentucky

Jane M. Kendall, RN, BS, CHT
Holistic Health Consultant
Hilton Head, South Carolina

Katharine Kolcaba, PhD, RN
Professor Emeritus
Nursing Department
The University of Akron
Akron, Ohio

Gail B. Ladwig, MSN, RN
Professor Emeritus
Jackson Community College
Jackson, Michigan
Consultant in Guided Imagery, Healing Touch, and Nursing Diangosis
Hilton Head, South Carolina

Mary Beth Flynn Makic, PhD, RN, CNS, CCNS, FAAN
Associate Professor
University of Colorado College of Nursing
Aurora, Colorado

Mary P. Mancuso, MA, Counseling Psychology
Professional Research Assistant & Patient Education Development Assistant
University of Colorado Hospital
Aurora, Colorado

Victoria K. Marshall, RN, BSN
Graduate Research Assistant
College of Nursing
Michigan State University
East Lansing, Michigan

Marina Martinez-Kratz, MS, RN, CNE
Professor of Nursing
Nursing Department
Jackson College
Jackson, Michigan

Ruth McCaffrey, DNP, ARNP, FNP-BC, GNP-BC, FAAN
Sharon Raddock Distinguished Professor
Christine E. Lynn College of Nursing
Florida Atlantic University
Boca Raton, Florida

Graham J. McDougall, Jr., PhD, RN, FAAN, FGSA
Professor, Martha Saxon Endowed Chair
Capstone College of Nursing
University of Alabama
Tuscaloosa, Alabama

Laura Mcilvoy, PhD, RN, CCRN, CNRN
Associate Professor
School of Nursing
Indiana University Southeast
New Albany, Indiana

Marsha McKenzie, MA Ed, BSN, RN
Associate Dean of Academic Affairs
Big Sandy Community and Technical College
Prestonsburg, Kentucky

Annie Muller, DNP, APN-BC
Assistant Professor of Nursing
Francis Marion Univeristy
Florence, South Carolina

Katherina Nikzad-Terhune, PhD, LCSW
Therapist
Beaumont Behavior Health;
Adjunct Professor
College of Social Work
University of Kentucky
Lexington, Kentucky

Barbara J. Olinzock, MSN, EdD, RN
Assistant Professor in Nursing
School of Nursing
Brooks College of Health
University of North Florida
Jacksonville, Florida

Wolter Paans, MSc, PhD, RN
Professor in Nursing Diagnostics
Hanze University of Applied Sciences
Groningen, The Netherlands

Margaret Elizabeth Padnos, RN, AB, BSN, MA
Independent Nurse Consultant/Poet and Essayist
Holland, Michigan

Chris Pasero, MS, RN-BC, FAAN
Pain Management Educator and Clinical Consultant
Rio Rancho, New Mexico

Kathleen L. Patusky, MA, PhD, RN, CNS
Assistant Professor
School of Nursing
Rutgers University
Newark, New Jersey

Sherry H. Pomeroy, PhD, RN
Associate Professor
School of Nursing
D'Youville College;
Professor Emeritus
School of Nursing
University at Buffalo, The State University of New York
Buffalo, New York

Ann Will Poteet, MS, RN, CNS
Clinical Nurse Specialist
College of Nursing
University of Colorado
Aurora, Colorado

Lori M. Rhudy, PhD, RN, CNRN, ACNS-BC
Clinical Associate Professor
School of Nursing
University of Minnesota;
Clinical Nurse Researcher
Mayo Clinic
Rochester, Minnesota

Mary Jane Roth, RN, BSN, MA
Nurse Clinician
Outpatient Psychiatry
Ann Arbor Veterans Medical Center
Ann Arbor, Michigan

Paula Riess Sherwood, RN, PhD, CNRN, FAAN
Professor and Vice Chair of Research
Acute and Tertiary Care Department
School of Nursing
University of Pittsburgh
Pittsburgh, Pennsylvania

Debra Siela, PhD, RN, CCNS, ACNS-BC, CCRN-K, CNE, RRT
Associate Professor of Nursing
School of Nursing
Ball University
Muncie, Indiana

Kimberly Silvey, MSN, RN
Minimum Data Set Coordinator
Signature Healthcare
Lexington, Kentucky

A.B. St. Aubyn, BSc (Hons), RGN, RM, RHV, DPS:N (CHS), MSc, PGCert (Education), HEA Fellow
Senior Lecturer
Faculty of Health, Education, and Life Sciences
Birmingham City University
Birmingham, United Kingdom

Andrea G. Steiner, MS, RD, LD, CNSC
Clinical Dietitian
Houston, Texas

Elaine E. Steinke, PhD, APRN, CNS-BC, FAHA, FAAN
Professor
School of Nursing
Wichita State University
Wichita, Kansas

Laura May Struble, PhD, GNP-BC
Clinical Assistant Professor
School of Nursing
University of Michigan
Ann Arbor, Michigan

Denise Sullivan, MSN, ANP-BC
Adult Nurse Practitioner, Anesthesiology/Pain Management Service
Jacobi Medical Center
Bronx, New York

Dennis C. Tanner, PhD
Professor of Health Sciences
Program in Speech-Language Sciences and Technology
Department of Health Sciences
Northern Arizona University
Flagstaff, Arizona

Janelle M. Tipton, MSN, RN, AOCN
Oncology Clinical Nurse Specialist; Manager, Outpatient Infusion Center
Eleanor N. Dana Cancer Center
University of Toledo Medical Center
Toledo, Ohio

William J. Trees, DNP, FNP-BC, CNP, RN
Nurse Practitioner
Occupational Medicine
Trihealth, Good Samaritan Hospital;
Clinical Faculty
Advance Nursing Studies
Northern Kentucky University;
Adjunct Faculty
College of Nursing
University of Cincinnati
Cincinnati, Ohio

Barbara Baele Vincensi, PhD, RN, FNP
Assistant Professor of Nursing
Hope College
Holland, Michigan

Kerstin West-Wilson, RNC, IBCLC, BA Biology, BSN, MS Nutrition, Safe Kids NRP Car Seat Certified, BLS Instructor
NICU Discharge Nurse and Lactation Consultant
Henry Zarro Neonatal Intensive Care Unit at the Children's Hospital at Saint Francis
Saint Francis Health System
Tulsa, Oklahoma

Barbara J. Wheeler, RN, BN, MN, IBCLC
Clinical Specialist and Lactation Consultant
Women and Child Program
St. Boniface Hospital;
Instructor II
Faculty of Health Sciences
College of Nursing
University of Manitoba;
Professional Affiliate
Manitoba Centre for Nursing and Health Research
Winnipeg, Manitoba
Canada

Suzanne White, MSN, RN, PHCNS-BC
Assistant Professor of Nursing
Morehead State University
Morehead, Kentucky

Linda S. Williams, RN, MSN
Professor of Nursing
Jackson College
Jackson, Michigan

David Wilson, MS, RNC
Staff Nurse
Children's Hospital at Saint Francis
Tulsa, Oklahoma

Ruth A. Wittmann-Price, PhD, RN, CNS, CNE, CHSE, ANEF, FAAN
Professor and Chairperson, Department of Nursing
Francis Marion University
Florence, South Carolina

Melody Zanotti, RN
Strongsville, Ohio

Karen Zulkowski, DNS, RN
Associate Professor
Nursing Department
Montana State University—Bozeman
Bozeman, Montana

Reviewers

Debbie Bomgaars, RN, BSN, MSN, PhD
Associate Professor of Nursing
Chair of the Department of Nursing
Dordt College
Sioux Center, Iowa

Anna M. Bruch, RN, MSN
Nursing Professor
Illinois Valley Community College
Ogelsby, Illinois

Ruth A. Chaplen, RN, DNP, ACNS-BC, AOCN
Assistant Professor, Clinical
Wayne State University
Detroit, Michigan

Marianne Curia, PhD, MSN, RN
Assistant Professor
University of St. Francis
Joliet, Illinois

Annie Marie Graf, MSN, RN
Advanced Medical Surgical Nursing Lead Faculty
Georgia Southern University
Statesboro, Georgia

Jean Herrmann, MSN, CNRN, RN
Professor, Junior Level Coordinator
Augustana College
Sioux Falls, South Dakota

Jorie L. Kulczak, RN, MSN
Associate Professor
Joliet Junior College
Joliet, Illinois

Marianne F. Moore, PhD, CNM, RN
Assistant Professor
Sam Houston State University
Huntsville, Texas

Laurie J. Palmer, MS, RN, AOCN
Chairperson, Professor
Monroe Community College
Rochester, New York

Charnelle Parmelee, RN, MSN-Nursing Education
Associate Professor of Nursing
Western New Mexico University
Silver City, New Mexico

JoAnne M. Pearce, MS, RN
Assistant Professor
Director of Nursing of Programs (ADRN/PN)
College of Technology
Idaho State University
Pocatello, Idaho

Jane E. Ransom, PhD, RN
Associate Professor
University of Toledo College of Nursing
Toledo, Ohio

Barbara Voshall, DNP
Professor of Nursing
School of Nursing
Graceland University
Lamoni, Iowa

Kim Webb, MN, RN
Adjunct Nursing Instructor
Ponca City, Oklahoma

Preface

Nursing Diagnosis Handbook: An Evidence-Based Guide to Planning Care is a convenient reference to help the practicing nurse or nursing student make a nursing diagnosis and write a care plan with ease and confidence. This handbook helps nurses correlate nursing diagnoses with known information about clients on the basis of assessment findings; established medical, surgical, or psychiatric diagnoses; and the current treatment plan.

Making a nursing diagnosis and planning care are complex processes that involve diagnostic reasoning and critical thinking skills. Nursing students and practicing nurses cannot possibly memorize the extensive list of defining characteristics, related factors, and risk factors for the 235 diagnoses approved by NANDA-International. There are two additional diagnoses that the authors think are significant: Hearing Loss and Vision Loss. These diagnoses are contained in Appendix E. This book correlates suggested nursing diagnoses with what nurses know about clients and offers a care plan for each nursing diagnosis.

Section I, Nursing Process, Clinical Reasoning, Nursing Diagnosis, and Evidence-Based Nursing, is divided into two parts. Part A includes an overview of the nursing process. This section provides information on how to make a nursing diagnosis and directions on how to plan nursing care. It also includes information on using clinical reasoning skills and eliciting the "client's story." Part B includes advanced nursing concepts: Concept mapping, QSEN (Quality and Safety Education for Nurses), Evidence-based nursing care, Quality nursing care, Patient-centered care, Safety, Informatics in nursing, Team/collaborative work with multidisciplinary team, and Root cause thinking.

In **Section II, Guide to Nursing Diagnoses,** the nurse can look up symptoms and problems and their suggested nursing diagnoses for more than 1450 client symptoms; medical, surgical, and psychiatric diagnoses; diagnostic procedures; surgical interventions; and clinical states.

In **Section III, Guide to Planning Care,** the nurse can find care plans for all nursing diagnoses suggested in Section II. We have included the suggested nursing outcomes from the Nursing Outcomes Classification (NOC) and interventions from the Nursing Interventions Classification (NIC) by the Iowa Intervention Project. We believe this work is a significant addition to the nursing process to further define nursing practice with standardized language.

Scientific rationales based on research are included for most of the interventions. This is done to make the evidence base of nursing practice apparent to the nursing student and practicing nurse.

New special features of the eleventh edition of *Nursing Diagnosis Handbook: An Evidence-Based Guide to Planning Care* include the following:

- Labeling of classic older research studies that are still relevant as Classic Evidence Based (CEB)
- Twenty-six new nursing diagnoses recently approved by NANDA-I, along with retiring seven nursing diagnoses: Disturbed energy field, Adult failure to thrive, Readiness for enhanced immunization status, Imbalanced nutrition: more than body requirements, Risk for imbalanced nutrition: more than body requirements, Impaired environmental interpretation syndrome, and Delayed growth and development
- Five revisions of nursing diagnoses made by NANDA-I in existing nursing diagnoses
  - **Old diagnosis:** Ineffective Self-Health management
    Revised diagnosis: Ineffective Health management
  - **Old diagnosis:** Readiness for enhanced Self-Health management
    Revised diagnosis: Readiness for enhanced Health management
  - **Old diagnosis:** Ineffective family Therapeutic Regimen Management
    Revised diagnosis: Ineffective family Health management
  - **Old diagnosis:** Impaired individual Resilience
    Revised diagnosis: Impaired Resilience
  - **Old diagnosis:** Risk for compromised Resilience
    Revised diagnosis: Risk for impaired Resilience
- Further addition of pediatric and critical care interventions to appropriate care plans
- An associated Evolve Online Course Management System that includes a care plan constructor, critical thinking case studies, Nursing Interventions Classification (NIC) and Nursing Outcomes Classification (NOC) labels, PowerPoint slides, and review questions for the NCLEX-RN® exam
- Appendixes for Nursing Diagnoses Arranged by Maslow's Hierarchy of Needs, Nursing Diagnoses Arranged by Gordon's Functional Health Patterns, Motivational Interviewing for Nurses, Wellness-Oriented Diagnostic Categories, and Nursing Care Plans for Hearing Loss and Vision Loss

The following features of *Nursing Diagnosis Handbook: A Guide to Planning Care* are also available:

- Suggested nursing diagnoses for more than 1450 clinical entities, including signs and symptoms, medical diagnoses, surgeries, maternal-child disorders, mental health disorders, and geriatric disorders

- Labeling of nursing research as EBN (Evidence-Based Nursing) and clinical research as EB (Evidence-Based) to identify the source of evidence-based rationales
- An Evolve Online Courseware System with the Ackley-Ladwig Care Plan Constructor that helps the student or nurse write a nursing care plan
- Rationales for nursing interventions that are for the most part based on nursing research
- Nursing references identified for each care plan
- A complete list of NOC outcomes on the Evolve website
- A complete list of NIC interventions on the Evolve website
- Nursing care plans that contain many holistic interventions
- Care plans written by leading national nursing experts from throughout the United States, along with international contributors, who together represent all of the major nursing specialties and have extensive experience with nursing diagnoses and the nursing process. Care plans written by experts include:
  - **Caregiver Role Strain** and **Fatigue** by Dr. Barbara A. Given and Dr. Paula Riess Sherwood
  - Care plans for **Spirituality** by Dr. Lisa Burkhart
  - Care plans for **Religiosity** by Dr. Lisa Burkhart
  - **Impaired Memory** by Dr. Graham J. McDougall, Jr.
  - **Decreased Intracranial adaptive capacity** and **Risk for ineffective Cerebral tissue perfusion** by Dr. Laura Mcilvoy
  - **Unilateral Neglect** by Dr. Lori M. Rhudy
  - **Anxiety, Death Anxiety,** and **Fear** by Dr. Ruth McCaffrey
  - **Impaired Comfort** by Dr. Katharine Kolcaba
  - **Risk for Infection** and **Ineffective Protection** by Ruth M. Curchoe
  - **Readiness for enhanced Communication** and **Impaired verbal Communication** by Dr. Stacey M. Carroll
  - **Sexual dysfunction** and **Ineffective Sexuality pattern** by Dr. Elaine E. Steinke
- A format that facilitates analyzing signs and symptoms by the process already known by nurses, which involves using defining characteristics of nursing diagnoses to make a diagnosis
- Use of NANDA-I terminology and approved diagnoses
- An alphabetical format for Sections II and III, which allows rapid access to information
- Nursing care plans for all nursing diagnoses listed in Section II
- Specific geriatric interventions in appropriate plans of care
- Specific client/family teaching interventions in each plan of care
- Information on culturally competent nursing care included where appropriate
- Inclusion of commonly used abbreviations (e.g., AIDS, MI, CHF) and cross-references to the complete term in Section II

We acknowledge the work of NANDA-I, which is used extensively throughout this text. In some rare cases, the authors and contributors have modified the NANDA-I work to increase ease of use. The original NANDA-I work can be found in *NANDA-I Nursing Diagnoses: Definitions & Classification 2015-2017.* Several contributors are the original submitters/authors of the nursing diagnoses established by NANDA-I. These contributors include the following:

Lisa Burkhart, PhD, RN, ANEF
Impaired Religiosity; Risk for impaired Religiosity; Readiness for enhanced Religiosity; Spiritual distress; Readiness for enhanced Spiritual well-being

Katharine Kolcaba, PhD, RN
Impaired Comfort

Shelly Eisbach, PhD, PMHNP-BC, RN
Risk for compromised Resilience; Impaired individual Resilience; Readiness for enhanced Resilience

David Wilson, MS, RNC
Neonatal Jaundice

Susanne W. Gibbons, PhD, C-ANP/GNP
Self-Neglect

Ruth A. Wittmann-Price, PhD, RN, CNS, CNE, CHSE, ANEF, FAAN
Impaired emancipated Decision-Making, Readiness for enhanced emancipated Decision-Making, Risk for impaired emancipated Decision-Making

Wolter Paans, MSCc, PhD, RN
Labile Emotional Control

We and the consultants and contributors trust that nurses will find this eleventh edition of *Nursing Diagnosis Handbook: An Evidence-Based Guide to Planning Care* a valuable tool that simplifies the process of identifying appropriate nursing diagnoses for clients and planning for their care, thus allowing nurses more time to provide evidence-based care that speeds each client's recovery.

Betty J. Ackley
Gail B. Ladwig
Mary Beth Flynn Makic

Acknowledgments

We would like to thank the following people at Elsevier: Sandy E. Clark, Senior Content Strategist, who supported us with this eleventh edition of the text with intelligence and kindness; Jennifer Wade, Content Development Specialist, who was a continual source of support; a special thank you to Carol O'Connell for project management of this edition; and to Melanie Cole for her support.

We acknowledge with gratitude nurses and student nurses, who are always an inspiration for us to provide fresh and accurate material. We are honored that they continue to value this text and to use it in their studies and practice.

Care has been taken to confirm the accuracy of information presented in this book. However, the authors, editors, and publisher cannot accept any responsibility for consequences resulting from errors or omissions of the information in this book and make no warranty, express or implied, with respect to its contents. The reader should use practices suggested in this book in accordance with agency policies and professional standards. Every effort has been made to ensure the accuracy of the information presented in this text.

We hope you find this text useful in your nursing practice.

Betty J. Ackley
(Betty was very involved in planning and contributed much until she passed away)
Gail B. Ladwig
Mary Beth Flynn Makic

How to Use *Nursing Diagnosis Handbook: An Evidence-Based Guide to Planning Care*

STEP 1: ASSESS

Following the guidelines in Section I, begin to formulate your nursing diagnosis by gathering and documenting the objective and subjective information about the client.

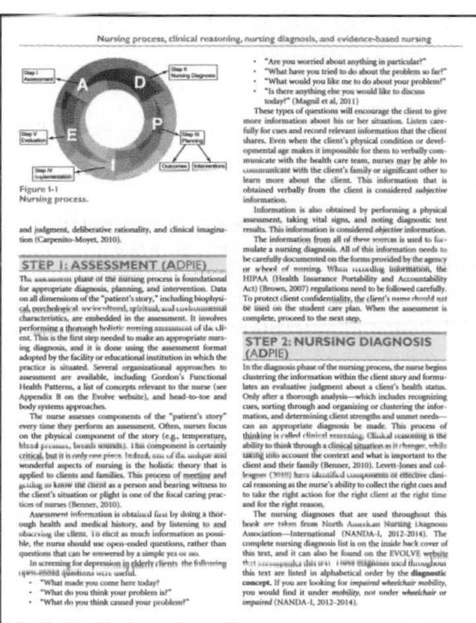

STEP 2: DIAGNOSE

Turn to Section II, Guide to Nursing Diagnoses, and locate the client's symptoms, clinical state, medical or psychiatric diagnoses, and anticipated or prescribed diagnostic studies or surgical interventions (listed in alphabetical order). Note suggestions for appropriate nursing diagnoses.

Then use Section III, Guide to Planning Care, to evaluate each suggested nursing diagnosis and "related to" etiology statement. Section III is a listing of care plans according to NANDA-I, arranged alphabetically by diagnostic concept, for each nursing diagnosis referred to in Section II. Determine the appropriateness of each nursing diagnosis by comparing the Defining Characteristics and/or Risk Factors to the client data collected.

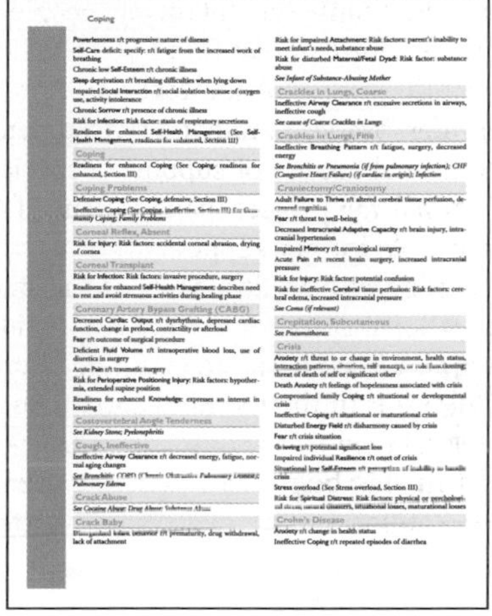

STEP 3: DETERMINE OUTCOMES

Use Section III, Guide to Planning Care, to find appropriate outcomes for the client. Use either the NOC outcomes with the associated rating scales or Client Outcomes as desired.

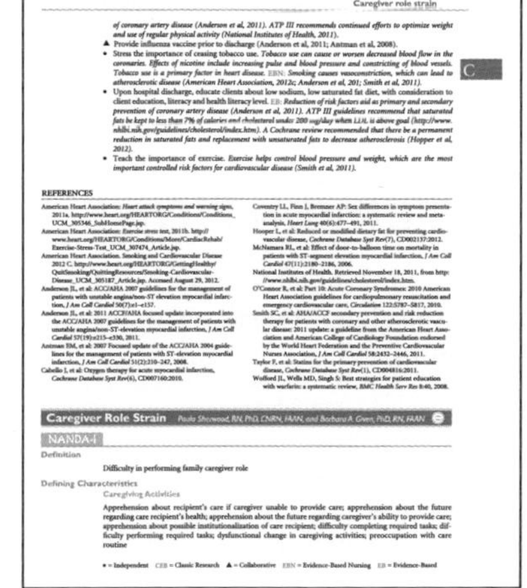

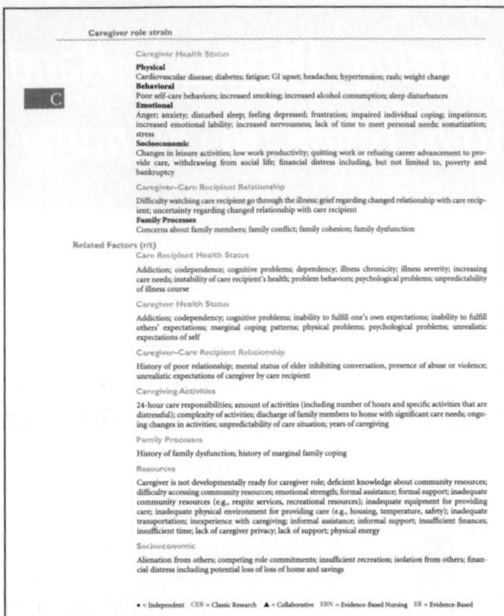

Caregiver role strain

C

Caregiver Health Status

Physical
Cardiovascular disease; diabetes; fatigue; GI upset; headaches; hypertension; rash; weight change
Behavioral
Poor self-care behaviors; increased smoking; increased alcohol consumption; sleep disturbances
Emotional
Anger; anxiety; disturbed sleep; feeling depressed; frustration; impaired individual coping; impatience; increased emotional lability; increased nervousness; lack of time to meet personal needs; somatization; stress
Socioeconomic
Changes in leisure activities; low work productivity; quitting work or refusing career advancement to provide care, withdrawing from social life; financial distress including, but not limited to, poverty and bankruptcy

Caregiver–Care Recipient Relationship

Difficulty watching care recipient go through the illness; grief regarding changed relationship with care recipient; uncertainty regarding changed relationship with care recipient
Family Processes
Concerns about family members; family conflict; family cohesion; family dysfunction

Related Factors (r/t)

Care Recipient Health Status

Addiction; codependence; cognitive problems; dependency; illness chronicity; illness severity; increasing care needs; instability of care recipient's health; problem behaviors; psychological problems; unpredictability of illness course

Caregiver Health Status

Addiction; codependency; cognitive problems; inability to fulfill one's own expectations; inability to fulfill others' expectations; marginal coping patterns; physical problems; psychological problems; unrealistic expectations of self

Caregiver–Care Recipient Relationship

History of poor relationship; mental status of elder inhibiting conversation, presence of abuse or violence; unrealistic expectations of caregiver by care recipient

Caregiving Activities

24-hour care responsibilities; amount of activities (including number of hours and specific activities that are distressful); complexity of activities; discharge of family members to home with significant care needs; ongoing changes in activities; unpredictability of care situation; years of caregiving

Family Processes

History of family dysfunction; history of marginal family coping

Resources

Caregiver is not developmentally ready for caregiver role; deficient knowledge about community resources; difficulty accessing community resources; emotional strength; formal assistance; formal support; inadequate community resources (e.g., respite services, recreational resources); inadequate equipment for providing care; inadequate physical environment for providing care (e.g., housing, temperature, safety); inadequate transportation; inexperience with caregiving; informal assistance; informal support; insufficient finances; insufficient time; lack of caregiver privacy; lack of support; physical energy

Socioeconomic

Alienation from others; competing role commitments; insufficient recreation; isolation from others; financial distress including potential loss of loss of home and savings

• = Independent CEB = Classic Research ▲ = Collaborative EBN = Evidence-Based Nursing EB = Evidence-Based

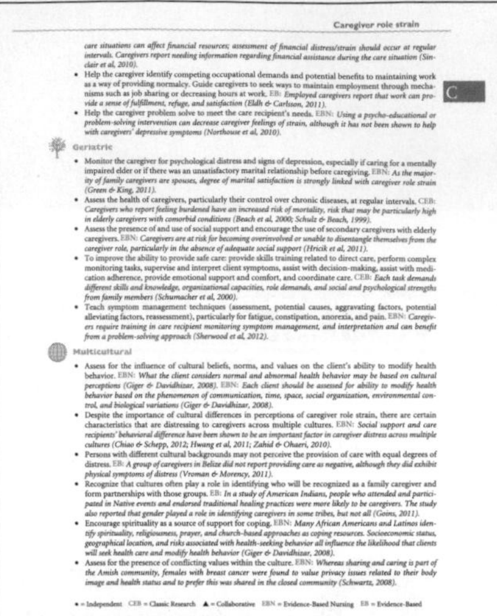

Caregiver role strain

C

care situations can affect financial resources; assessment of financial distress/strain should occur at regular intervals. Caregivers report needing information regarding financial assistance during the care situation (Sinclair et al, 2010).

- Help the caregiver identify competing occupational demands and potential benefits to maintaining work as a way of providing normalcy. Guide caregivers to seek ways to maintain employment through mechanisms such as job sharing or decreasing hours at work. EB: *Employed caregivers report that work can provide a sense of fulfillment, refuge, and satisfaction (Eldh & Carlsson, 2011).*
- Help the caregiver problem solve to meet the care recipient's needs. EBN: *Using a psycho-educational or problem-solving intervention can decrease caregiver feelings of strain, although it has not been shown to help with caregivers' depressive symptoms (Northouse et al, 2010).*

Geriatric

- Monitor the caregiver for psychological distress and signs of depression, especially if caring for a mentally impaired elder or if there was an unsatisfactory marital relationship before caregiving. EBN: *As the majority of family caregivers are spouses, degree of marital satisfaction is strongly linked with caregiver role strain (Green & King, 2011).*
- Assess the health of caregivers, particularly their control over chronic diseases, at regular intervals. CEB: *Caregivers who report feeling burdened have an increased risk of mortality, risk that may be particularly high in elderly caregivers with comorbid conditions (Beach et al, 2000; Schulz & Beach, 1999).*
- Assess the presence of and use of social support and encourage the use of secondary caregivers with elderly caregivers. EBN: *Caregivers are at risk for becoming overinvolved or unable to disentangle themselves from the caregiver role, particularly in the absence of adequate social support (Hrcik et al, 2011).*
- To improve the ability to provide safe care: provide skills training related to direct care, perform complex monitoring tasks, supervise and interpret client symptoms, assist with decision-making, assist with medication adherence, provide emotional support and comfort, and coordinate care. CEB: *Each task demands different skills and knowledge, organizational capacities, role demands, and social and psychological strengths from family members (Schumacher et al, 2000).*
- Teach symptom management techniques (assessment, potential causes, aggravating factors, potential alleviating factors, reassessment), particularly for fatigue, constipation, anorexia, and pain. EBN: *Caregivers require training in care recipient monitoring symptom management, and interpretation and can benefit from a problem-solving approach (Sherwood et al, 2012).*

Multicultural

- Assess for the influence of cultural beliefs, norms, and values on the client's ability to modify health behavior. EBN: *What the client considers normal and abnormal health behavior may be based on cultural perceptions (Giger & Davidhizar, 2008).* EBN: *Each client should be assessed for ability to modify health behavior based on the phenomenon of communication, time, space, social organization, environmental control, and biological variations (Giger & Davidhizar, 2008).*
- Despite the importance of cultural differences in perceptions of caregiver role strain, there are certain characteristics that are distressing to caregivers across multiple cultures. EBN: *Social support and care recipients' behavioral difference have been shown to be an important factor in caregiver distress across multiple cultures (Chiao & Schepp, 2012; Hwang et al, 2011; Zahid & Ohaeri, 2010).*
- Persons with different cultural backgrounds may not perceive the provision of care with equal degrees of distress. EB: *A group of caregivers in Belize did not report providing care as negative, although they did exhibit physical symptoms of distress (Vroman & Morency, 2011).*
- Recognize that cultures often play a role in identifying who will be recognized as a family caregiver and form partnerships with those groups. EB: *In a study of American Indians, people who attended and participated in Native events and endorsed traditional healing practices were more likely to be caregivers. The study also reported that gender played a role in identifying caregivers in some tribes, but not all (Goins, 2011).*
- Encourage spirituality as a source of support for coping. EBN: *Many African Americans and Latinos identify spirituality, religiousness, prayer, and church-based approaches as coping resources. Socioeconomic status, geographical location, and risks associated with health-seeking behavior all influence the likelihood that clients will seek health care and modify health behavior (Giger & Davidhizar, 2008).*
- Assess for the presence of conflicting values within the culture. EBN: *Whereas sharing and caring is part of the Amish community, females with breast cancer were found to value privacy issues related to their body image and health status and to prefer this was shared in the closed community (Schwartz, 2008).*

• = Independent CEB = Classic Research ▲ = Collaborative EBN = Evidence-Based Nursing EB = Evidence-Based

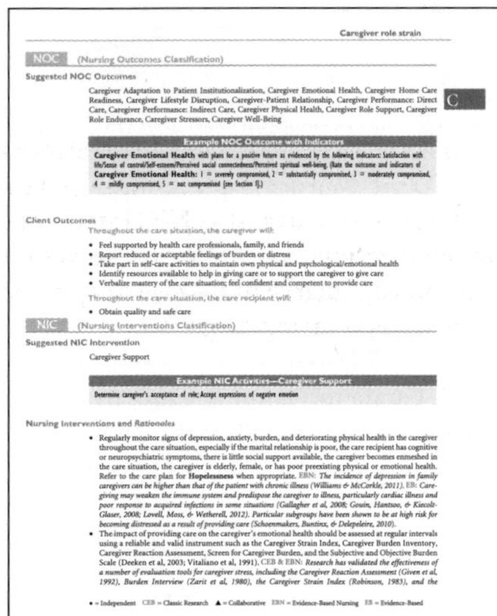

Caregiver role strain

NOC (Nursing Outcomes Classification)

Suggested NOC Outcomes

Caregiver Adaptation to Patient Institutionalization, Caregiver Emotional Health, Caregiver Home Care Readiness, Caregiver Lifestyle Disruption, Caregiver-Patient Relationship, Caregiver Performance: Direct Care, Caregiver Performance: Indirect Care, Caregiver Physical Health, Caregiver Role Support, Caregiver Role Endurance, Caregiver Stressors, Caregiver Well-Being

C

Example NOC Outcome with Indicators

Caregiver Emotional Health with plans for a positive future as evidenced by the following indicators: Satisfaction with life/Sense of control/Self-esteem/Perceived social connectedness/Perceived spiritual well-being (Rate the outcome and indicators of **Caregiver Emotional Health:** 1 = severely compromised, 2 = substantially compromised, 3 = moderately compromised, 4 = mildly compromised, 5 = not compromised [see Section I].)

Client Outcomes

Throughout the care situation, the caregiver will:

- Feel supported by health care professionals, family, and friends
- Report reduced or acceptable feelings of burden or distress
- Take part in self-care activities to maintain own physical and psychological/emotional health
- Identify resources available to help in giving care or to support the caregiver to give care
- Verbalize mastery of the care situation; feel confident and competent to provide care

Throughout the care situation, the care recipient will:

- Obtain quality and safe care

NIC (Nursing Interventions Classification)

Suggested NIC Intervention

Caregiver Support

Example NIC Activities—Caregiver Support

Determine caregiver's acceptance of role; Accept expressions of negative emotion

Nursing Interventions and Rationales

- Regularly monitor signs of depression, anxiety, burden, and deteriorating physical health in the caregiver throughout the care situation, especially if the marital relationship is poor, the care recipient has cognitive or neuropsychiatric symptoms, there is little social support available, the caregiver becomes enmeshed in the care situation, the caregiver is elderly, female, or has poor preexisting physical or emotional health. Refer to the care plan for **Hopelessness** when appropriate. EBN: *The incidence of depression in family caregivers can be higher than that of the patient with chronic illness (Williams & McCorkle, 2011).* EB: *Caregiving may weaken the immune system and predispose the caregiver to illness, particularly cardiac illness and poor response to acquired infections in some situations (Gallagher et al, 2008; Gouin, Hantsoo, & Kiecolt-Glaser, 2008; Lovell, Moss, & Wetherell, 2012). Particular subgroups have been shown to be at high risk for becoming distressed as a result of providing care (Schoenmakers, Buntinx, & Delepeleire, 2010).*
- The impact of providing care on the caregiver's emotional health should be assessed at regular intervals using a reliable and valid instrument such as the Caregiver Strain Index, Caregiver Burden Inventory, Caregiver Reaction Assessment, Screen for Caregiver Burden, and the Subjective and Objective Burden Scale (Deeken et al, 2003; Vitaliano et al, 1991). CEB & EBN: *Research has validated the effectiveness of a number of evaluation tools for caregiver stress, including the Caregiver Reaction Assessment (Given et al, 1992), Burden Interview (Zarit et al, 1980), the Caregiver Strain Index (Robinson, 1983), and the*

• = Independent CEB = Classic Research ▲ = Collaborative EBN = Evidence-Based Nursing EB = Evidence-Based

PLAN INTERVENTIONS

Use Section III, Guide to Planning Care, to find appropriate interventions for the client. Use the Nursing Interventions as found in that section.

GIVE NURSING CARE

Administer nursing care following the plan of care based on the interventions.

EVALUATE NURSING CARE

Evaluate nursing care administered using either the NOC outcomes or Client Outcomes. If the outcomes were not met, and the nursing interventions were not effective, reassess the client and determine if the appropriate nursing diagnoses were made.

DOCUMENT

Document all of the previous steps using the format provided in the clinical setting.

Contents

SECTION

I Nursing Process, Clinical Reasoning, Nursing Diagnosis, and Evidence-Based Nursing

Betty J. Ackley, MSN, EdS, RN, Gail B. Ladwig, MSN, RN, Mary Beth Flynn Makic, PhD, RN, CNS, CCNS, FAAN, and Marina Martinez-Kratz, MS, RN, CNE

Section I is divided into two parts. Part A includes an overview of the nursing process. This section provides information on how to make a nursing diagnosis and directions on how to plan nursing care. It also includes information on using clinical reasoning skills and eliciting the "patient's story." Part B includes advanced nursing concepts.

Part A: The Nursing Process: Using Clinical Reasoning Skills to Determine Nursing Diagnosis and Plan Care

1. **A**ssessing: performing a nursing assessment
2. **D**iagnosing: making nursing diagnoses
3. **P**lanning: formulating and writing outcome statements and determining appropriate nursing interventions based on appropriate best evidence (research)
4. **I**mplementing care
5. **E**valuating the outcomes and the nursing care that has been implemented. Make necessary revisions in care interventions as needed

Part B: Advanced Nursing Concepts

- Concept mapping
- QSEN (Quality and Safety Education for Nurses)
- Evidence-based nursing care
- Quality nursing care
- Patient-centered care
- Safety
- Informatics in nursing
- Team/collaborative work with interprofessional team

PART A The Nursing Process: Using Clinical Reasoning Skills to Determine Nursing Diagnoses and Plan Care

The primary goals of nursing are to (1) determine client/family responses to human problems, level of wellness, and need for assistance; (2) provide physical care, emotional care, teaching, guidance, and counseling; and (3) implement interventions aimed at prevention and assisting the client to meet his or her own needs and health-related goals. The nurse must always focus on assisting clients and families to their highest level of functioning and self-care. The care that is provided should be structured in a way that allows clients the ability to influence their health care and accomplish their self-efficacy goals. The nursing process, which is a problem-solving approach to the identification and treatment of client problems, provides a framework for assisting clients and families to their optimal level of functioning. The nursing process involves five dynamic and fluid phases: **assessment, diagnosis, planning, implementation,** and **evaluation.** Within each of these phases, the client and family story is embedded and is used as a foundation for knowledge, judgment, and actions brought to the client care experience. A description of the "patient's story" and each aspect of the nursing process follow.

THE "PATIENT'S STORY"

The "patient's story" is a term used to describe objective and subjective information about the client that describes who the client is as a person in addition to their usual medical history. Specific aspects of the story include physiological, psychological, and family characteristics; available resources; environmental and social context; knowledge; and motivation. Care is influenced, and often driven, by what the client states—verbally or through their physiologic state. The "patient's story" is fluid and must be shared and understood throughout the client's health care experience.

There are multiple sources for obtaining the patient's story. The primary source for eliciting this story is through communicating directly with the client and the client's family. It is important to understand how the illness (or wellness) state has affected the client physiologically, psychologically, and spiritually. The client's perception of his or her health state is important to understand and may have an impact on subsequent interventions. At times, clients will be unable to tell their story verbally, but there is still much they can communicate through their physical state. The client's family (as the client defines them) is a valuable source of information and can provide a rich perspective on the client. Other valuable sources of the "patient's story" include the client's health record. Every time a piece of information is added to the health record, it becomes a part of the "patient's story." All nursing care is driven by the client's story. The nurse must have a clear understanding of the story to effectively complete the nursing process. Understanding the full story also provides an avenue for identifying mutual goals with the client and family aimed at improving client outcomes and goals.

Note: The "patient's story" is terminology that is used to describe a holistic assessment of information about the client, with the client's and the family's input as much as possible. In this text, we use the term "patient's story" in quotes whenever we refer to the specific process. In all other places, we use the term *client* in place of the word *patient*; we think labeling the person as a client is more respectful and empowering for the person. *Client* is also the term that is used in the National Council Licensure Examination (NCLEX-RN) test plan (National Council of State Boards of Nursing, 2013).

Understanding the "patient's story" is critically important, in that psychological, socioeconomic, and spiritual characteristics play a significant role in the client's ability and desire to access health care. Also knowing and understanding the "patient's story" is an integral first step in giving client-centered care. In today's health care world, the focus is on the client, which leads to increased satisfaction with care. Improving the client's health care experience is part of the Affordable Care Act and is tied to reimbursement through value-based purchasing of care: "participating hospitals are paid for inpatient acute care services based on the quality of care, not just quantity of services they provide" (Centers for Medicare & Medicaid Services, 2014).

THE NURSING PROCESS

The nursing process is an organizing framework for professional nursing practice, a critical thinking process for the nurse to use to give the best care possible to the client. It is very similar to the steps used in scientific reasoning and problem solving. This section is designed to help the nursing student learn how to use this thinking process, the nursing process. Key components of the process include the steps listed below. An easy, convenient way to remember the steps of the nursing process is to use an acronym, **ADPIE** (Figure I-1):

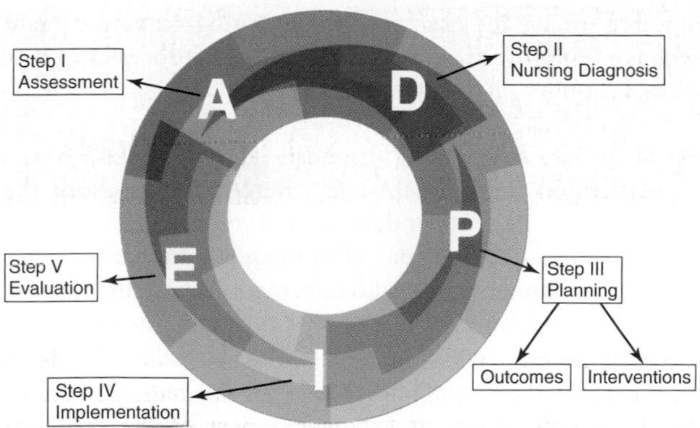

Figure 1-1
Nursing process.

1. **Assess**: perform a nursing assessment
2. **Diagnose**: make nursing diagnoses
3. **Plan**: formulate and write outcome/goal statements and determine appropriate nursing interventions based on the client's reality and evidence (research)
4. **Implement** care
5. **Evaluate** the outcomes and the nursing care that has been implemented. Make necessary revisions in care interventions as needed.

The following is an overview and practical application of the steps of the nursing process. The steps are listed in the usual order in which they are performed.

STEP 1: ASSESSMENT (ADPIE)

The assessment phase of the nursing process is foundational for appropriate diagnosis, planning, and intervention. Data on all dimensions of the "patient's story," including biophysical, psychological, sociocultural, spiritual, and environmental characteristics, are embedded in the assessment. It involves performing a thorough holistic nursing assessment of the client. This is the first step needed to make an appropriate nursing diagnosis, and it is done using the assessment format adopted by the facility or educational institution in which the practice is situated.

The nurse assesses components of the "patient's story" every time an assessment is performed. Often, nurses focus on the physical component of the story (e.g., temperature, blood pressure, breath sounds). This component is certainly critical, but it is only one piece. Indeed, one of the unique and wonderful aspects of nursing is the holistic theory that is applied to clients and families. Clients are active partners in the healing process. Nurses must increasingly develop the skills and systems to incorporate client preferences into care (Hess & Markee, 2014). "The challenge facing the nation, and the opportunity afforded by the Affordable Care Act, is to move from a culture of sickness to a culture of care and then to a culture of health" (Institute of Medicine, 2013). Assessment information is obtained first by completing a thorough health and medical history, and by listening to and observing the client. To elicit as much information as possible, the nurse should use open-ended questions, rather than questions that can be answered with a simple "yes" or "no."

In screening for depression in older clients, the following open-ended questions are useful (Lusk & Fater, 2013):

- What made you come here today?
- What do you think your problem is?
- What do you think caused your problem?
- Are you worried about anything in particular?
- What have you tried to do about the problem so far?
- What would you like me to do about your problem?
- Is there anything else you would like to discuss today?

These types of questions will encourage the client to give more information about his or her situation. Listen carefully for cues and record relevant information that the client shares. Even when the client's physical condition or developmental age makes it impossible for them to verbally communicate with the health care team, nurses may be able to communicate with the client's family or significant other to learn more about the client. This information that is obtained verbally from the client is considered *subjective* information.

Information is also obtained by performing a physical assessment, taking vital signs, and noting diagnostic test results. This information is considered *objective* information.

The information from all of these sources is used to formulate a nursing diagnosis. All of this information needs to be carefully documented on the forms provided by the agency or school of nursing. When recording information, the HIPAA (Health Insurance Portability and Accountability Act) (Foster, 2012) regulations need to be followed carefully. To protect client confidentiality, the client's name should *not* be used on the student care plan. When the assessment is complete, proceed to the next step.

STEP 2: NURSING DIAGNOSIS (ADPIE)

In the diagnosis phase of the nursing process, the nurse begins clustering the information within the client story and formulates an evaluative judgment about a client's health status. Only after a thorough analysis—which includes recognizing cues, sorting through and organizing or clustering the information, and determining client strengths and unmet needs—can an appropriate diagnosis be made. This process of thinking is called *clinical reasoning*. Clinical reasoning is a cognitive process that uses formal and informal thinking strategies to gather and analyze client information, evaluate the significance of this information, and determine the value of alternative actions (Benner, 2010). Benner (2010) describes this cognitive process as "thinking like a nurse." Watson and Rebair (2014) referred to "noticing" as a precursor to clinical reasoning. By noticing the nurse can preempt possible risks or support subtle changes toward recovery. Noticing can be the activity that stimulates nursing action before words are exchanged, preempting need. The nurse synthesizes the evidence while also knowing the client as part of clinical reasoning that informs client specific diagnoses (Cappelletti, Engel, & Prentice, 2014).

The nursing diagnoses that are used throughout this book are taken from North American Nursing Diagnosis Association—International (Herdman & Kamitsuru, 2014). The complete nursing diagnosis list is on the inside front cover of this text, and it can also be found on the EVOLVE website that accompanies this text. The diagnoses used throughout this text are listed in alphabetical order by the **diagnostic concept.** For example, *impaired wheelchair mobility* is found under *mobility*, not under *wheelchair* or *impaired* (Herdman & Kamitsuru, 2014).

The holistic assessment of the client helps determine the type of diagnosis that follows. For example, if during the assessment a client is noted to have unsteady gait and balance disturbance and states, "I'm concerned I will fall while walking down my stairs," but has not fallen previously, then the client would be identified as having a "risk" nursing diagnosis.

Once the diagnosis is determined, the next step is to determine related factors and defining characteristics. The process for formulating a nursing diagnosis with related factors and defining characteristics follows. A client may have many nursing and medical diagnoses, and determining the priority with which each should be addressed requires clinical reasoning and application of knowledge.

Formulating a Nursing Diagnosis with Related Factors and Defining Characteristics

A working nursing diagnosis may have two or three parts. The two-part system consists of the nursing diagnosis and the "related to" (r/t) statement: "Related factors are factors that appear to show some type of patterned relationship with the nursing diagnosis: such factors may be described as antecedent to, associated with, relating to, contributing to, or abetting" (Herdman & Kamitsuru, 2014).

The two-part system is often used when the defining characteristics, or signs and symptoms identified in the assessment, may be obvious to those caring for the client.

The three-part system consists of the nursing diagnosis, the r/t statement, and the defining characteristics, which are "observable cues/inferences that cluster as manifestations of an actual or wellness nursing diagnosis" (Herdman & Kamitsuru, 2014).

Some nurses refer to the three-part diagnostic statement as the **PES system**:

P (problem)—The nursing diagnosis label: a concise term or phrase that represents a pattern of related cues. The nursing diagnosis is taken from the official NANDA-I list.

E (etiology)—"Related to" (r/t) phrase or etiology: related cause or contributor to the problem.

S (symptoms)—Defining characteristics phrase: symptoms that the nurse identified in the assessment.

Here we use the example of a beginning nursing student who is attempting to understand the nursing process and how to make a nursing diagnosis:

Problem: Use the nursing diagnosis label deficient **Knowledge** from the NANDA-I list. Remember to check the definition: "Absence or deficiency of cognitive information related to a specific topic" (Herdman & Kamitsuru, 2014).

Etiology: r/t unfamiliarity with information about the nursing process and nursing diagnosis. At this point the beginning nurse would not be familiar with available resources regarding the nursing process.

Symptoms: Defining characteristics, as evidenced by (aeb) verbalization of lack of understanding: "I don't understand this, and I really don't know how to make a nursing diagnosis."

When using the **PES** system, look at the **S** first, then formulate the three-part statement. (You would have gotten the S, symptoms, which are defining characteristics, from your assessment.)

Therefore, the three-part nursing diagnosis is: deficient **Knowledge** r/t unfamiliarity with information about the nursing process and nursing diagnosis aeb verbalization of lack of understanding.

Types of Nursing Diagnoses

There are three different types of nursing diagnoses.

Problem-Focused Diagnosis. "A clinical judgment concerning an undesirable human response to a health condition/process that exists in an individual, family, group or community" (Herdman & Kamitsuru, 2014, p 22).

"Related factors are an integral part of all problem-focused diagnoses. They are etiologies, circumstances, facts or influences that have some type of relationship with the nursing diagnosis" (Herdman & Kamitsuru, 2014, p 26).

Example of a Problem-Focused Nursing Diagnosis. Overweight related to excessive intake in relation to metabolic needs, concentrating food intake at the end of the day aeb weight 20% over ideal for height and frame. Note: This is a three-part nursing diagnosis.

Risk Nursing Diagnosis. Risk nursing diagnosis is a "clinical judgment concerning the vulnerability of an individual, family, group, or community for developing an undesirable human response to health conditions/life processes" (Herdman & Kamitsuru, 2014, p 22). "The risk diagnosis is supported by risk factors that increase the vulnerability of a client, family, group, or community to an unhealthy event" (Herdman & Kamitsuru, 2014, p 26). Defining characteristics and related factors are observable cues and circumstances or influences that have some type of relationship with the nursing diagnosis that may contribute to a health problem. Identification of related factors allows nursing interventions to be implemented to address the underlying cause of a nursing diagnosis (Herdman & Kamitsuru, 2014, p 26).

Example of a Risk Nursing Diagnosis. Risk for **Overweight:** Risk factor: concentrating food at the end of the day. Note: This is a two-part nursing diagnosis.

Health Promotion Nursing Diagnosis. A clinical judgment concerning motivation and desire to increase well-being and to actualize human health potential that may be expressed by a readiness to enhance specific health behaviors or health state. Health promotion responses may exist in an individual, family, group, or community (Herdman & Kamitsuru, 2014, p 22). Health promotion is different from prevention in that health promotion focuses on being as healthy as possible, as opposed to preventing a disease or problem. The difference between health promotion and disease prevention is that the reason for the health behavior should always be a positive one. *With a health promotion diagnosis, the outcomes and interventions should be focused on enhancing health.*

Example of a Health Promotion Nursing Diagnosis. Readiness for enhanced **Nutrition** aeb expresses willingness to change eating pattern and eat healthier foods. Note: This is a two-part nursing diagnosis.

Application and Examples of Making a Nursing Diagnosis

When the assessment is complete, identify common patterns/symptoms of response *to actual or potential health problems from the assessment* and select an appropriate nursing diagnosis label using clinical reasoning skills. Use the steps with Case Study 1. (The same steps can be followed using an actual client assessment in the clinical setting or in a student assessment.)

A. Highlight or underline the relevant symptoms (defining characteristics). As you review your assessment information, ask: Is this normal? Is this an ideal situation? Is this a problem for the client? You may go back and validate information with the client.

B. Make a list of the symptoms (underlined or highlighted information).

C. Cluster similar symptoms.

D. Analyze/interpret the symptoms. (What do these symptoms mean or represent when they are together?)

E. Select a nursing diagnosis label from the NANDA-I list that fits the appropriate defining characteristics and nursing diagnosis definition.

Case Study 1—An Older Client with Breathing Problems

A. Underline the Symptoms (Defining Characteristics)

A 73-year-old man has been admitted to the unit with a diagnosis of chronic obstructive pulmonary disease (COPD). He states that he has "difficulty breathing when walking short distances." He also states that his "heart feels like it is racing" (heart rate is 110 beats per minute) at the same time. He states that he is "tired all the time," and while talking to you about his story, he is continually wringing his hands and looking out the window.

B. List the Symptoms (Subjective and Objective)

"Difficulty breathing when walking short distances"; "heart feels like it is racing"; heart rate is 110 beats per minute; "tired all the time"; continually wringing his hands and looking out the window.

C. Cluster Similar Symptoms

"Difficulty breathing when walking short distances"
"Heart feels like it is racing"; heart rate = 110 bpm
"Tired all the time"
Continually wringing his hands
Looking out the window

D. Analyze

Interpret the *Subjective Symptoms* (What the Client Has Stated)

- "Difficulty breathing when walking short distances" = exertional discomfort: a defining characteristic of **Activity** intolerance
- "Heart feels like it is racing" = abnormal heart rate response to activity: a defining characteristic of **Activity** intolerance
- "Tired all the time" = verbal report of weakness: a defining characteristic of **Activity** intolerance

Interpret the *Objective Symptoms* (Observable Information)

- Continually wringing his hands = extraneous movement, hand/arm movements: a defining characteristic of **Anxiety**
- Looking out the window = poor eye contact, glancing about: a defining characteristic of **Anxiety**
- Heart rate = 110 beats per minute

E. Select the Nursing Diagnosis Label

In Section II, look up *dyspnea (difficulty breathing)* or *dysrhythmia (abnormal heart rate or rhythm)*, chosen because they are high priority, and you will find the nursing diagnosis **Activity** intolerance listed with these symptoms. Is this diagnosis appropriate for this client?

To validate that the diagnosis **Activity** intolerance is appropriate for the client, turn to Section III and read the NANDA-I definition of the nursing diagnosis **Activity** intolerance: "Insufficient physiological or psychological energy to endure or complete required or desired daily activities" (Herdman & Kamitsuru, 2014, p 225). When reading the definition, ask, "Does this definition describe the symptoms demonstrated by the client?" "Is any more assessment information needed?" "Should I take his blood pressure or take an apical pulse rate?" If the appropriate nursing diagnosis has been selected, the definition should describe the condition that has been observed.

The client may also have defining characteristics for this particular diagnosis. Are the client symptoms that you identified in the list of defining characteristics (e.g., verbal report of fatigue, abnormal heart rate response to activity, exertional dyspnea)?

Another way to use this text and to help validate the diagnosis is to look up the client's medical diagnosis in Section II. This client has a medical diagnosis of COPD. Is Activity Intolerance listed with this medical diagnosis? Consider whether the nursing diagnosis makes sense given the client's medical diagnosis (in this case, COPD). There may be times when a nursing diagnosis is not directly linked to a medical diagnosis (e.g., ineffective **Coping**) but is nevertheless appropriate given nursing's holistic approach to the client/family.

The process of identifying significant symptoms, clustering or grouping them into logical patterns, and then choosing an appropriate nursing diagnosis involves diagnostic reasoning (critical thinking) skills that must be learned in the process of becoming a nurse. This text serves as a tool to help the learner in this process.

"Related to" Phrase or Etiology

The second part of the nursing diagnosis is the "related to" (r/t) phrase. Related factors are those that appear to show some type of patterned relationship with the nursing diagnosis. Such factors may be described as antecedent to, associated with, related to, contributing to, or abetting. Pathophysiological and psychosocial changes, such as developmental age and cultural and environmental situations, may be causative or contributing factors.

Often, a nursing diagnosis is complementary to a medical diagnosis and vice versa. Ideally the etiology (r/t statement), or cause, of the nursing diagnosis is something that can be treated independently by a nurse. When this is the case, the diagnosis is identified as an independent nursing diagnosis.

If medical intervention is also necessary, it might be identified as a collaborative nursing diagnosis. A carefully written, individualized r/t statement enables the nurse to plan nursing interventions and refer for diagnostic procedures, medical treatments, pharmaceutical interventions, and other interventions that will assist the client/family in accomplishing goals and return to a state of optimum health. Diagnoses and treatments provided by the multidisciplinary team all contribute to the client/family outcome. The coordinated effort of the team can only improve outcomes for the client/family and decrease duplication of effort and frustration among the health care team and the client/family.

The etiology is *not* the medical diagnosis. It may be the underlying issue contributing to the nursing diagnosis, but a medical diagnosis is *not* something the nurse can treat independently, without health care provider orders. In the case of the man with COPD, think about what happens when someone has COPD. How does this affect the client? What is happening to him because of this diagnosis?

For each suggested nursing diagnosis, the nurse should refer to the statements listed under the heading "Related Factors (r/t)" in Section III. These r/t factors may or may not be appropriate for the individual client. If they are not appropriate, the nurse should develop and write an r/t statement that is appropriate for the client. For the client from Case Study 1, a two-part statement could be made here:

Problem = Activity Intolerance
Etiology = r/t imbalance between oxygen supply and demand

It was already determined that the client had **Activity** intolerance. With the respiratory symptoms identified from the assessment, imbalance between oxygen supply and demand is appropriate.

Defining Characteristics Phrase

The defining characteristics phrase is the third part of the three-part diagnostic system, and it consists of the signs and symptoms that have been gathered during the assessment phase. The phrase "as evidenced by" (aeb) may be used to connect the etiology (r/t) with the defining characteristics. The use of identifying defining characteristics is similar to the process that the health care provider uses when making a medical diagnosis. For example, the health care provider who observes the following signs and symptoms—diminished inspiratory and expiratory capacity of the lungs, complaints of dyspnea on exertion, difficulty in inhaling and exhaling deeply, and sometimes chronic cough—may make the medical diagnosis of COPD. This same process is used to identify the nursing diagnosis of **Activity** intolerance.

Put It All Together: Writing the Three-Part Nursing Diagnosis Statement

Problem—Choose the label (nursing diagnosis) using the guidelines explained previously. A list of nursing diagnosis labels can be found in Section II and on the inside front cover.

Etiology—Write an r/t phrase (etiology). These can be found in Section II.

Symptoms—Write the defining characteristics (signs and symptoms), or the "as evidenced by" (aeb) list. A list of the signs and symptoms associated with each nursing diagnosis can be found in Section III.

Case Study 1—73-Year-Old Male Client with COPD (Continued)

Using the information from the earlier case study/example, the nursing diagnostic statement would be as follows:

Problem—**Activity** intolerance
Etiology—r/t imbalance between oxygen supply and demand
Symptoms—Verbal reports of fatigue, exertional dyspnea ("difficulty breathing when walking"), and abnormal heart rate response to activity ("racing heart"), heart rate 110 beats per minute.

Therefore, the nursing diagnostic statement for the client with COPD is **Activity** intolerance r/t imbalance between oxygen supply and demand aeb verbal reports of fatigue, exertional dyspnea, and abnormal heart rate in response to activity.

Consider a second case study:

Case Study 2—Woman with Insomnia

As before, the nurse always begins with an assessment. To make the nursing diagnosis, the nurse follows the steps below.

A. Underline the Symptoms

A 45-year-old woman comes to the clinic and asks for medication to help her sleep. She states that she is worrying too much and adds, "It takes me about an hour to get to sleep, and it is very hard to fall asleep. I feel like I can't do anything because I am so tired. My job has become very stressful because of a new boss and too much work."

B. List the Symptoms (Subjective and Objective)

Asks for medication to help her sleep; states she is worrying about too much; "It takes me about an hour to get to sleep"; "it is very hard to fall asleep"; "I feel like I can't do anything because I am so tired"; "My job has become very stressful because of a new boss and too much work."

C. Cluster Similar Symptoms

Asks for medication to help her sleep
"It takes me about an hour to get to sleep."
"It is very hard to fall asleep."
"I feel like I can't do anything because I am so tired."
"I am worrying too much."
"My job is stressful."
"Too much work."

D. Analyze/Interpret the Symptoms

Subjective Symptoms

- Asks for medication to help her sleep; "It takes me about an hour to get to sleep"; "it is very hard to fall asleep"; "I feel like I can't do anything because I am so tired." (All defining characteristics = verbal complaints of difficulty with sleeping.)
- States she is worrying too much (anxiety): "My job is stressful."

Objective Symptoms

- None

E. Select a Nursing Diagnosis with Related Factors and Defining Characteristics

Look up "sleep" in Section II. Listed under the heading "**Sleep** pattern, disturbed" in Section II is the following information:

Insomnia (nursing diagnosis) r/t anxiety and stress

This client states she is worrying too much, which may indicate anxiety; she also recently has increased job stress.

Look up **Insomnia** in Section III. Check the definition: "A disruption in amount and quality of sleep that impairs functioning" (Herdman & Kamitsuru, 2014). Does this describe the client in the case study? What are the related factors? What are the symptoms? Write the diagnostic statement:

Problem—**Insomnia**
Etiology—r/t anxiety, stress
Symptoms—Difficulty falling asleep, "I am so tired, I can't do anything."

The nursing diagnostic statement is written in this format: **Insomnia** r/t anxiety and stress aeb (as evidenced by) difficulty falling asleep.

Note: There are more than 30 case studies available for both student and faculty use on the Evolve website that accompanies this text.

After the diagnostic statement is written, proceed to the next step: planning.

STEP 3: PLANNING (ADPIE)

The planning phase of the nursing process includes the identification of priorities, as well as the determination of appropriate client-specific outcomes and interventions. The nurse in collaboration with the client and family (as applicable) and the rest of the health care team must determine the urgency of the identified problems and prioritize client needs. *Mutual goal setting,* along with *symptom pattern recognition* and *triggers,* helps prioritize interventions and determine which interventions are going to provide the greatest impact. *Symptom pattern recognition* and/or *triggers* is a process of identifying symptoms that clients have related to their illness, understanding which symptom patterns require intervention, and identifying the associated timeframe to intervene effectively. For example, a client with heart failure is noted to gain 5 pounds overnight. Coupling this symptom with other symptoms of edema and shortness of breath while walking can be referred to as "symptom pattern recognition"—in this case, that the client is retaining fluid. The nurse, and often the client/family, recognize these symptoms as an immediate *cause* and that more action/intervention is needed to avoid a potential adverse outcome.

Nursing diagnoses should be prioritized first by immediate needs based on ABC (airway, breathing, and circulation). The highest priority should also be determined by using Maslow's hierarchy of needs. In this hierarchy, priority is given to immediate problems that may be life-threatening (thus ABC). For example, ineffective **Airway** clearance, as evidenced by the symptoms of increased secretions and increased use of inhaler related to asthma, creates an immediate cause compared to the nursing diagnosis of **Anxiety,** a love and belonging or security need, which makes it a lesser priority than ineffective **Airway** clearance. Refer to Appendix A, Nursing Diagnoses Arranged by Maslow's Hierarchy of Needs, for assistance in prioritizing nursing diagnoses.

The planning phase should be done—whenever possible—with the client/family and the multidisciplinary team to maximize efforts and understanding, and increase compliance with the proposed plan and outcomes. For a successful plan of care, measurable goals and outcomes, including nursing interventions, must be identified.

SMART Outcomes

When writing outcome statements, it can be helpful to use the acronym SMART, which means the outcome must be:

Specific
Measurable
Attainable
Realistic
Timed

The SMART acronym is used in business, education, and health care settings. This method assists the nurse in identifying patient outcomes more effectively.

Once priorities are established, outcomes for the client can be easily identified. Client-specific outcomes are determined based on the mutually set goals. Outcomes refer to the measurable degree of the client's response. The client's response/outcome may be intentional and favorable, such as leaving the hospital 2 days after surgery without any complications. The client's outcome can be negative and unintentional, such as demonstrating a surgical site infection. Generally, outcomes are described in relation to the client's response to interventions, for example, the client's cough becomes more productive after the client begins using the controlled coughing technique.

Based on the "patient's story," the nursing assessment, the mutual goals and outcomes identified by the caregiving team and the client/family, and the clinical reasoning that the nurse uses to prioritize his or her work, the nurse then decides what interventions to employ. Based on the nurse's clinical judgment and knowledge, nursing interventions are defined as *all treatments that a nurse performs to enhance client outcomes.*

The selection of appropriate, effective interventions can be individualized to meet the mutual goals established by the client/family. It is then the nurse's education, experience, and skill that allow them to select and carry out interventions to meet that mutual goal.

Outcomes

After the appropriate priority setting of the nursing diagnoses and interventions is determined, outcomes are developed or examined and decided upon. This text includes standardized Nursing Outcomes Classification (NOC) outcomes written by a large team of University of Iowa College of Nursing faculty and students in conjunction with clinicians from a variety of settings (Moorhead et al, 2013). "Nursing-sensitive outcome (NOC) is an individual, family or community state, behavior or perception that is measured along a continuum in response to nursing interventions. The outcomes are stated as concepts that reflect a client, caregiver, family, or community state, perception of behavior rather than as expected goals" (Moorhead et al, 2013).

It is very important for the nurse to *involve* the client and/or family in determining appropriate outcomes. The use of outcomes information creates a continuous feedback loop that is essential to ensuring evidence-based care and the best possible client outcomes, not only for the patient care experience, but also for improving the population's health and reducing health care costs (Weston & Roberts, 2013). The minimum requirements for rating an outcome are when the outcome is selected (i.e., the baseline measure) and when care is completed (i.e., the discharge summary). This may be sufficient in short-stay, acute-care settings. Depending on how rapidly the client's condition is expected to change, some settings may evaluate once a day or once a shift. Community agencies may evaluate every visit or every other visit, for example. Because measurement times are not standardized, they can be individualized for the client and the setting (Moorhead et al, 2013).

Development of appropriate outcomes can be done one of two ways: using the NOC list or developing an appropriate outcome statement, both of which are included in Section III. There are suggested outcome statements for each nursing diagnosis in this text that can be used as written or modified as necessary to meet the needs of the client.

The Evolve website includes a list of additional NOC outcomes. The use of NOC outcomes can be helpful to the nurse because they contain a five-point, Likert-type rating scale that can be used to evaluate progress toward achieving the outcome. In this text, the rating scale is listed, along with some of the more common indicators; for example, see the rating scale for the outcome **Sleep** (Table I-1).

Because the NOC outcomes are specific, they enhance the nursing process by helping the nurse measure and record the outcomes before and after interventions have been performed. The nurse can choose to have clients rate their own progress using the Likert-type rating scale. This involvement can help increase client motivation to progress *toward* outcomes.

After client outcomes are selected or written, and *discussed* with a client, the nurse plans nursing care with the client and establishes a means that will help the client achieve the selected outcomes. The usual means are nursing interventions.

Interventions

Interventions are like roadmaps directing the best ways to provide nursing care. The more clearly a nurse writes an intervention, the easier it will be to complete the journey and arrive at the destination of desired client outcomes.

Section III includes suggested interventions for each nursing diagnosis. The interventions are identified as

TABLE I-1

Example NOC Outcome

Sleep—0004

Domain—Functional Health (I) Care Recipient:

Class—Energy Maintenance (A) Data Source:

Scale(s)—Severely compromised to Not compromised (a) and Severe to None (n)
Definition: Natural periodic suspension of consciousness during which the body is restored.
Outcome Target Rating: Maintain at________ Increase to __________

	Sleep Overall Rating	Severely Compromised 1	Substantially Compromised 2	Moderately Compromised 3	Mildly Compromised 4	Not Compromised 5	
INDICATORS:							
000401	Hours of sleep	1	2	3	4	5	NA
000402	Observed hours of sleep	1	2	3	4	5	
000403	Sleep pattern	1	2	3	4	5	NA
000404	Sleep quality	1	2	3	4	5	NA
000405	Sleep efficiency	1	2	3	4	5	NA
000407	Sleep routine	1	2	3	4	5	NA
000418	Sleeps through the night consistently	1	2	3	4	5	NA
000408	Feelings of rejuvenation after sleep	1	2	3	4	5	NA
000410	Wakeful at appropriate times	1	2	3	4	5	NA
000419	Comfortable bed	1	2	3	4	5	NA
000420	Comfortable temperature in room	1	2	3	4	5	NA
000411	Electroencephalogram findings	1	2	3	4	5	NA
000412	Electromyogram findings	1	2	3	4	5	NA
000413	Electrooculogram findings	1	2	3	4	5	NA
		Severe	**Substantial**	**Moderate**	**Mild**	**None**	
000421	Difficulty getting to sleep	1	2	3	4	5	NA
000406	Interrupted sleep	1	2	3	4	5	NA
000409	Inappropriate napping	1	2	3	4	5	NA
000416	Sleep apnea	1	2	3	4	5	NA
000417	Dependence on sleep aids	1	2	3	4	5	NA
000422	Nightmares	1	2	3	4	5	NA
000423	Nocturia	1	2	3	4	5	NA
000424	Snoring	1	2	3	4	5	NA
000425	Pain	1	2	3	4	5	NA

Adapted from Moorhead S, Johnson, M, Maas ML, & Swanson E. (Eds.). (2013). *Nursing outcomes classification (NOC)* (5th ed.). St Louis: Elsevier.

independent (autonomous actions that are initiated by the nurse in response to a nursing diagnosis) or collaborative (actions that the nurse performs in collaboration with other health care professionals, and that may require a health care provider's order and may be in response to both medical and nursing diagnoses). The nurse may choose the interventions appropriate for the client and individualize them accordingly, or determine additional interventions.

This text also contains several suggested Nursing Interventions Classification (NIC) interventions for each nursing diagnosis to help the reader see how NIC is used along with NOC and nursing diagnoses. The NIC interventions are a comprehensive, standardized classification of treatments that nurses perform. The classification includes both physiological and psychosocial interventions, and covers all nursing specialties. A list of NIC interventions is included on the Evolve website. For more information about NIC interventions, refer to the NIC text (Bulechek et al, 2013).

Putting It All Together—Recording the Care Plan

The nurse must document the actual care plan, including prioritized nursing diagnostic statements, outcomes, and interventions. This may be done electronically or in writing. To ensure continuity of care, the plan must be documented and shared with all health care personnel caring for the client. This text provides rationales, most of which are research based, to validate that the interventions are appropriate and workable.

The Evolve website includes an electronic care plan constructor that can be easily accessed, updated, and individualized. Many agencies are using electronic records, and this is an ideal resource. See the inside front cover of this text for information regarding access to the Evolve website, or go to http://evolve.elsevier.com/Ackley/NDH.

STEP 4: IMPLEMENTATION (ADPIE)

The implementation phase includes the "carrying out" of the specific, individualized, jointly agreed upon interventions in the plan of care. Often, the interventions implemented are focused on *symptom management*, which is alleviating symptoms. Typically, nursing care does not involve "curing" the medical condition causing the symptom. Rather, nursing care focuses on caring for the client/family so they can function at their highest level.

The implementation phase of the nursing process is the point at which you actually give nursing care. You perform the interventions that have been individualized to the client. All the hard work you put into the previous steps (ADP) can now be actualized to assist the client. As the interventions are performed, make sure that they are appropriate for the client. Consider that the client who was having difficulty breathing was also older. He may need extra time to carry out any activity. Check the rationale or research that is provided to determine why the intervention is being used. The evidence should support the individualized actions that you are implementing.

Client outcomes are achieved by the performance of the nursing interventions in collaboration with other disciplines and the client/family. During this phase, the nurse continues to assess the client to determine whether the interventions are effective and the desired outcomes are met.

STEP 5: EVALUATION (ADPIE)

The final phase of the nursing process is evaluation. Evaluation occurs not only at the end of the nursing process, but throughout the process. Evaluation of an intervention is, in essence, another nursing assessment; hence the dynamic feature of the nursing process. The nurse reassesses the client, taking into consideration where the client was before the intervention (i.e., baseline) and where the client is after the intervention. Nurses are also in a great place (at the bedside) to evaluate how clients respond to other, multidisciplinary interventions, and their assessment of the client's response is valuable to determine whether the client's plan of care needs to be altered or not. For example, the client may receive 2 mg of morphine intravenously for pain (a pharmaceutical intervention to treat pain), and the nurse is the member of the health care team who can best assess how the client responded to that medication. Did the client receive relief from pain? Did the client develop any side effects? The nurse's documented evaluation of the client's response will be very helpful to the entire health care team.

The client/family can often tell the nurse how the intervention helped or did not help. This reassessment requires the nurse to revisit the mutual outcomes/goals set earlier and ask, "Are we moving toward that goal, or does the goal seem unreachable after the intervention?" If the outcomes were not met, the nurse begins again with assessment and determines the reason they were not met. Consider the **SMART** acronym and Case Study 1. Were the outcomes **S**pecific? Were the outcomes **M**easurable? Did the client's heart rate decrease? Did the client indicate that it was easier to breathe when walking from his bed to the bathroom? Were the outcomes **A**ttainable and **R**ealistic? Did he still report "being tired"? Did you allow adequate **T**ime for a positive outcome? Also ask yourself whether you identified the correct nursing diagnosis. Should the interventions be changed? At this point, the nurse can look up any new symptoms or conditions that have been identified and adjust the care plan as needed. Decisions about implementing additional interventions may be necessary; if so, they should be made in collaboration with the client/family if possible.

In some instances, the client/family/nurse triad will establish new, achievable goals and continue to cycle through the nursing process until the mutual goals are achieved.

Another important part of the evaluation phase is documentation. The nurse should use the facility's tool for documentation and record the nursing activity that was performed as well as the results of the nursing interventions. Many facilities use problem-oriented charting, in which the nurse evaluates the care and client outcomes as part of charting. Documentation is also necessary for legal reasons, because in a legal dispute, *if it wasn't charted/recorded, it wasn't done.*

Many health care providers use critical pathways or care maps to plan nursing care. The use of nursing diagnoses should be an integral part of any critical pathway/care map to ensure that nursing care needs are being assessed and appropriate nursing interventions are planned and implemented.

PART B Advanced Nursing Process Concepts

Conceptual Mapping and the Nursing Process

Conceptual mapping is an active learning strategy that promotes critical thinking and clinical judgment, and helps increase clinical competency (Jamison & Lis, 2014; George et al, 2014). The process involves developing a diagram or pictorial representation of newly generated ideas. A concept map begins with a central theme or concept, and then related information is diagrammed radiating from the center theme. A concept map can be used to diagram the critical thinking strategy involved in using the nursing process.

Start with a blank sheet of paper; the client should be at the center of the paper. The next step involves linking to the person, via lines, the symptoms (defining characteristics) from the assessment to help determine the appropriate nursing diagnosis.

Figure I-2 is an example of how a concept map can be used to begin the nursing diagnostic process.

After the symptoms are visualized, similar ones can be put together to formulate a nursing diagnosis using another concept map (Figure I-3).

The central theme in this concept map is the nursing diagnosis: **Activity** intolerance, with the defining characteristics/client symptoms as concepts that lead to and support the nursing diagnosis. The conceptual map can then be used as a method for determining outcomes and interventions as desired. The nursing process is a thinking process. Using conceptual mapping is a method to help the nurse or nursing student think more effectively about the client.

Quality and Safety Education for Nurses

The Quality and Safety Education for Nurses (QSEN, 2014) project represents the nursing profession's response to the five health care competencies articulated by the Institute of Medicine (2013). The QSEN project defined those five competencies for nursing and also added the competency of safety. The objective of the QSEN project is to provide nurses with the knowledge, skills, and attitudes critical to improve the quality and safety of health care systems.

The following are the competencies that were identified.

Patient-Centered Care

The QSEN project defines patient-centered care as the ability to "recognize the patient or designee as the source of control and full partner in providing compassionate and coordinated

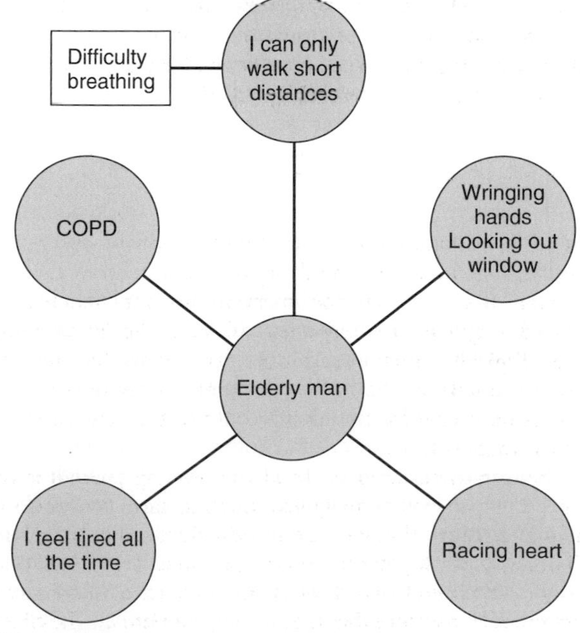

Figure I-2
Example of a concept map.

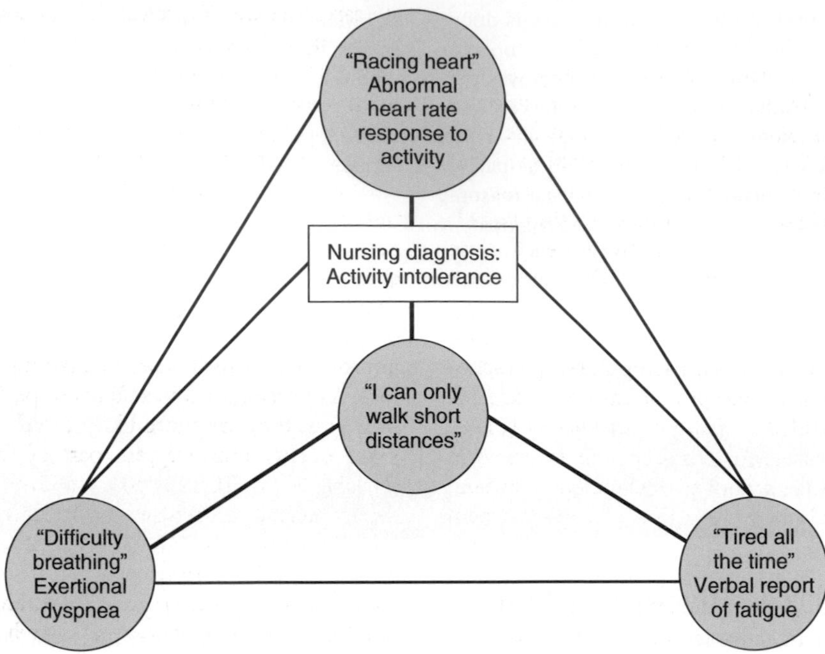

Figure I-3
Formulating a nursing diagnosis using a concept map.

care based on respect for patient's preferences, values, and needs" (QSEN, 2014).

Patient-centered care begins with the nurse learning as much as possible about the client, including their "patient's story" as explained in Part A of this text. The nursing process using nursing diagnosis is intrinsically all about patient-centered care. Here the client/family is a full partner in the entire process, including assessment, nursing diagnosis selection, outcomes, interventions, and evaluation. This competency is about giving care with the client and family in control as they are able, not giving care to them where the nurse is in complete control. The client, family, nurse, health care provider, and other health care workers form a team to partner with the client and family in every way possible.

Client education needs to be centered around the needs of the client, with behavior-changing techniques such as use of motivational interviewing to accomplish the defined goals. At present, too often new health information is given to clients in the form of a lecture, handout, admonishment, or direction where the client is powerless. Motivational interviewing is based on reinforcement of the client's present thoughts and motivations on behavior change, and on respect for the client as an individual (Miller & Rollnick, 2013). This technique has been used for almost 30 years and has an extensive research base showing effectiveness. To learn more about motivational interviewing, refer to the appendix.

Addressing the unique cultural needs of clients is another example of patient-centered care. Nurses who are culturally competent base care planning on cultural awareness and assessments that enables them to identify client values, beliefs, and preferences. Cultural awareness can ensure safe and quality outcomes for all clients by assisting clients to become "safety allies" who can alert professionals to their preferences and deviations from their usual routines (Sherwood & Zomorodi, 2014). This text provides the addition of multicultural interventions that reflect the client's cultural preferences, values, and needs.

Patient-centered care can help nurses change attitudes toward clients, especially when caring for older clients (Pope, 2012). Caring for the retired school teacher who raised four children can be different from just caring for the client woman in Room 234 who has her call light on frequently and is incontinent of urine at too-frequent intervals.

Teamwork and Collaboration

Teamwork and collaboration are defined by the QSEN project as the ability to "function effectively within nursing and interprofessional teams, fostering open communication, mutual respect, and shared decision-making to achieve quality client care" (QSEN, 2014). Interprofessional collaboration has the potential to shift the attitudes and perceptions of health care providers so there is an increased awareness of each other's roles, values, and disciplinary knowledge (Wilson et al, 2014). The need for collaboration by health care professionals is a reality of contemporary health care practice and is written into this text. Collaborative interventions are designated with a triangular symbol Δ. In addition, many nursing interventions are referrals to other health care personnel to best meet the client's needs.

Evidence-Based Practice

Evidence-based practice is defined by the QSEN project as "integrat[ing] best current evidence with clinical expertise and client/family preferences and values for delivery of optimal health care" (QSEN, 2014). It is well established that evidence-based practice results in higher quality care for clients than care that is based on traditional nursing knowledge (Makic et al, 2014). Now it is imperative for each nurse and nursing student to develop clinical inquiry skills, which means the nurse continually questions whether care is being given in the best way possible based on research evidence when possible (Blazeck et al, 2011). Basing nursing practice on evidence or research is a concept that has been added to the nursing process, entitled *evidence-based nursing* (EBN). EBN is a systematic process that uses current evidence in making decisions about the care of clients, including evaluation of quality and applicability of existing research, client preferences, clinical expertise, and available health care resources (Melnyk & Fineout-Overholt, 2011). To determine the best way of giving care, use of evidence-based practice is needed. To make this happen, nurses need ready access to the evidence.

This text includes evidence (research)-based rationales whenever possible. The research ranges along a continuum from a case study about a single client to a systematic review performed by experts that gives quality information to guide nursing care. Every attempt has been made to supply the most current research for the nursing interventions. In Section III, the abbreviation **EBN** is used when interventions have a scientific rationale supported by nursing research. The abbreviation **EB** is used when interventions have a scientific rationale supported by research that has been obtained from disciplines other than nursing. **CEB** is used as a heading for classic research that has not been replicated or is older. It may be either nursing research or research from other disciplines. Many times the **CEB**-labeled research will be the most important studies that have been done on that nursing issue or intervention.

When using **EBN,** it is vitally important that the client's concerns and individual situations be taken into consideration. The nurse must always use critical thinking when applying evidence-based guidelines to any particular nursing situation. Each client is unique in his or her needs and capabilities. To improve outcomes, clinicians and clients should collaborate to formulate a treatment plan that incorporates both evidence-based data and client preferences within the context of each client's specific clinical situation (Muhrer, 2012). This text includes both research and the nursing process. By integrating these concepts, it assists the nurse in increasing the use of evidence-based interventions in the clinical setting.

Quality Improvement

Quality improvement has been used for many years, with processes in place to ensure that the client receives appropriate care. The QSEN project defines quality improvement as the ability to "use data to monitor the outcomes of care processes and use improvement methods to design and test changes to continuously improve the quality and safety of health care systems" (QSEN, 2014). QSEN resources supporting quality improvement initiatives are available at their website (http://qsen.org/competencies/quality-improvement-resources-2/). As with EBP, quality improvement initiatives need to critically examine research in supporting process changes. Research is the basis upon which best practice should be supported (Odom, 2013). It is essential for nurses to participate in the work of quality and performance improvement, which is key to attaining excellence in nursing care. As nurses are educated about performance and quality measures, they are more likely to value these activities and make quality improvement part of their nursing practice (Nelson, 2014). There is potential overlap of work in quality departments and EBN/research departments. These authors hope that the measurement of quality and quality departments in health care collaborate closely with EBN departments so that quality measurement always include relevant nursing research/evidence to effectively improve the practice of nursing.

Safety

Safety is the competency that QSEN added to the five competencies identified by the Institute of Medicine. QSEN defines safety as "minimiz[ing] risk of harm to clients and providers through both system effectiveness and individual performance" (QSEN, 2014).

Client safety is a priority when health care is delivered. Nurses are required to adhere to established standards of care as a guideline for providing safe client care. Internal standards of care are policies and procedures established by health care institutions and are based on the most relevant and current evidence. External standards of care are established by regulatory agencies (e.g., The Joint Commission), professional organizations (e.g., the American Nurses Association), and health care organizations.

Client safety was identified as a priority of care by The Joint Commission through the launch of National Patient Safety Goals in 2002. The Joint Commission (2014) has established standards for improving client safety that include the need for increased handwashing, better client identification before receiving medications or treatments, and protection of suicidal clients from self-harm. Many of these safety standards have been incorporated into the care plans in this text. A safety icon is used to designate specific safety nursing interventions in this text.

Informatics

QSEN defines informatics as the nurse's ability to "use information and technology to communicate, manage knowledge, mitigate error, and support decision making" (QSEN, 2014). Informatics is now a critical part of the nurse's professional role, and every nurse must be computer literate (TIGER,

2014). Key computer proficiencies for nursing practice should include basic computer system and desktop skills, the ability to search for client information, communication using email, ability to search electronic health care databases, and use of technology for client education, client documentation, and client monitoring (Gracie, 2011; Tiger, 2014).

In addition to computer literacy, nurses must also acquire informatic knowledge that addresses client privacy and the security of health care information as it applies to the use of technology (Foster, 2012; TIGER, 2014). Because nurses document on the electronic medical record and use smartphones for access to information on medications, diagnoses, and treatments, there are constant threats to client confidentiality.

Nurses also use clinical decision support systems in many facilities that contain order sets tailored for conditions or types of clients. These systems include information vital to nurses and also may provide alerts about potentially dangerous situations that should *not* be ignored when giving client care.

Nurses need access to technology to effectively bring evidence to the client bedside, because evidence is constantly evolving and books are often out of date before they are published. Use of informatics is integral to use of EBN practice as explained previously.

EBN, safety initiatives, informatics, patient-centered care, teamwork, and quality work together in a synergistic manner lead to excellence in nursing care. Quality care needs to be more than safe; the care should result in the best outcome possible for the client. For this to happen, the client should receive care that is based on evidence of the effectiveness of the care.

The nursing process is continually evolving. This text is all about *thinking* for the nurse to help the client in any way possible. Our goal is to present state-of-the art information to help the nurse and nursing student provide the best care possible.

REFERENCES

Benner, P. (2010). *Educating nurses: a call for radical transformation* (p. 2010). San Francisco: Jossey-Bass.

Blazeck, A., Klem, M. L., & Miller, T. (2011). Building evidence-based practice into the foundations of practice. *Nurse Educator, 36*(3), 124–127.

Bulechek, G., et al. (2013). *Nursing interventions classification (NIC)* (6th ed.). St Louis: Mosby/Elsevier.

Cappelletti, A., Engel, J. E., & Prentice, D. (2014). Systematic review of clinical judgment and reasoning in nursing. *Journal of Nursing Education, 53*(8), 453–458.

Centers for Medicare and Medicaid Services: *CMS issues final rule for the first year of hospital value-based purchasing program.* (2014). At: <https://www.cms.gov/Medicare/Quality-Initiatives-Patient-Assessment-Instruments/hospital-value-based-purchasing/index.html?redirect=/hospital-value-based-purchasing/> Accessed January 31, 2015.

Foster, C. (2012). Advocates of privacy. HIPPA 101. *Washington Nurse, 42*(3), 37.

George, A., et al. (2014). Concept mapping. *Holistic Nursing Practice, 28*(1), 43–47.

Gracie, D. (2011). Nursing informatics competencies and baccalaureate nursing students. *ANIA-CARING Newslett, 26*(2), 7–10.

Herdman, T. H., & Kamitsuru, S. (Eds.), (2014). *NANDA International Nursing Diagnoses: Definitions & Classification, 2015–2017.* Oxford: Wiley Blackwell.

Hess, D., & Markee, D. (2014). Holistic nursing and the patient protection and affordable health care act. *New Mexico Nurse, 59*(1), 10–11.

Institute of Medicine (IOM) (2013). *Population health implications of the Affordable Care Act: Workshop summary.* Washington, DC: The National Academies Press.

Jamison, T., & Lis, G. A. (2014). Engaging the learning by bridging the gap between theory and clinical competence. *N Clinics of North America, 49*(1), 69–80.

The Joint Commission: *National Patient Safety Goals.* (2014). Retrieved from <http://www.jointcommission.org/hap_2014_npsgs/> Accessed June 18, 2015.

Lusk, J. M., & Fater, K. (2013). A concept analysis of patient-centered care. *Nursing Forum, 48*(2), 89–98.

Makic, M. B., Rauen, C., Watson, R., et al. (2014). Examining the evidence to guide practice: challenging practice habits. *Critical Care Nursing, 34*(2), 28–45.

Melnyk, B., & Fineout-Overholt, E. (2011). *Evidence-based practice in nursing & healthcare: A guide to best practice.* Philadelphia: Lippincott Williams & Wilkins.

Miller, W. R., & Rollnick, S. (2013). *Motivational interviewing: helping people change* (3rd ed.). New York: Guilford Press.

Moorhead, S. (Ed.), (2013). *Nursing outcomes classification (NOC)* (5th ed.). St Louis: Elsevier.

Muhrer, J. (2012). Making evidence-based health care relevant for patients. *Journal of Nurse Practitioners, 8*(1), 51–55.

National Council of State Boards of Nursing (2013). *NCLEX-RN Examination, Detailed test plan.* Retrieved from <www.ncsbn.org/2013_NCLEX_RN_Detailed_Test_Plan_Educator.pdf> Accessed June 18, 2015.

Nelson, A. M. (2014). Best practice in nursing: a concept analysis. *International Journal of Nursing Studies, 51*(11), 1507–1516.

Odom-Forren, J. (2013). Research: the foundation for evidence. *Journal of Perianesthesia Nursing, 28*(6), 331–332.

Pope, T. (2012). How person-centered care can improve nurses' attitudes to hospitalized older patients. *Nursing Older People, 24*(1), 32–36.

Quality and Safety Education for Nurses (QSEN). (2014). Retrieved from <qsen.org/competencies/pre-licensure-ksas/> Accessed June 18, 2015.

Sherwood, G., & Zomorodi, M. (2014). A new mindset for quality and safety: the QSEN competencies redefine nurses' roles in practice. *Nephrology Nursing Journal, 41*(1), 15–22, 72.

Technology Informatics Guiding Education Reform (TIGER) (2014). *The TIGER Initiative: informatics competencies for every practicing nurse: recommendations from the TIGER Collaborative.* Retrieved from <http://www.thetigerinitiative.org/default.aspx> Accessed June 18, 2015.

Watson, F., & Rebair, A. (2014). The art of noticing: essential to nursing practice. *British Journal of Nursing, 23*(10), 514–517.

Weston, M., & Roberts, D. (2013). "The influence of quality improvement efforts on patient outcomes and nursing work: a perspective from chief nursing officers at three large health systems" OJIN. *The Online Journal of Issues in Nursing, 18*(3), Manuscript 2.

Wilson, L., Callender, B., Hall, T. L., et al. (2014). Identifying global health competencies to prepare 21st century global health professionals: report from the global health competency subcommittee of the consortium of universities for global health. *Journal of Law, Medicine & Ethics, 42*, 26–31.

SECTION

II

Guide to Nursing Diagnosis

Betty J. Ackley, MSN, EdS, RN, Gail B. Ladwig, MSN, RN,
Mary Beth Flynn Makic, PhD, RN, CNS, CCNS, FAAN, and Melody Zanotti, RN

Section II is an alphabetical listing of client symptoms, client problems, medical diagnoses, psychosocial diagnoses, and clinical states. Each of these will have a list of possible nursing diagnoses. You may use this section to find suggestions for nursing diagnoses for your client.

- Assess the client using the format provided by the clinical setting.
- Locate the client's symptoms, problems, clinical state, diagnoses, surgeries, and diagnostic testing in the alphabetical listing contained in this section.
- Note suggestions given for appropriate nursing diagnoses.
- Evaluate the suggested nursing diagnoses to determine whether they are appropriate for the client and have information that was found in the assessment.
- Use Section III (which contains an alphabetized list of all NANDA-I approved nursing diagnoses) to validate this information and check the definition, related factors, and defining characteristics. Determine whether the nursing diagnosis you have selected is appropriate for the client.

A

A

Abdominal Distention

Constipation r/t decreased activity, decreased fluid intake, decreased fiber intake, pathological process

Dysfunctional **Gastrointestinal** motility r/t decreased perfusion of intestines, medication effect

Nausea r/t irritation of gastrointestinal tract

Imbalanced **Nutrition:** less than body requirements r/t nausea, vomiting

Acute **Pain** r/t retention of air, gastrointestinal secretions

Delayed **Surgical** recovery r/t retention of gas, secretions

Abdominal Hysterectomy

See Hysterectomy

Abdominal Pain

Dysfunctional **Gastrointestinal** motility r/t decreased perfusion, medication effect

Acute **Pain** r/t injury, pathological process

Abdominal Surgery

Constipation r/t decreased activity, decreased fluid intake, anesthesia, opioids

Dysfunctional **Gastrointestinal** motility r/t medication or anesthesia effect, trauma from surgery

Imbalanced **Nutrition:** less than body requirements r/t high metabolic needs, decreased ability to ingest or digest food

Acute **Pain** r/t surgical procedure

Ineffective peripheral **Tissue Perfusion** r/t immobility, abdominal surgery

Risk for delayed **Surgical** recovery r/t extensive surgical procedure

Risk for **Infection:** Risk factor: invasive procedure

Readiness for enhanced **Knowledge:** expresses an interest in learning

See Surgery, Perioperative Care; Surgery, Postoperative Care; Surgery, Preoperative Care

Abdominal Trauma

Disturbed **Body Image** r/t scarring, change in body function, need for temporary colostomy

Ineffective **Breathing** pattern r/t abdominal distention, pain

Deficient **Fluid** volume r/t hemorrhage, active fluid volume loss

Dysfunctional **Gastrointestinal** motility r/t decreased perfusion

Acute **Pain** r/t abdominal trauma

Risk for **Bleeding:** Risk factor: trauma and possible contusion/rupture of abdominal organs

Risk for **Infection:** Risk factor: possible perforation of abdominal structures

Ablation, Radiofrequency Catheter

Fear r/t invasive procedure

Risk for decreased **Cardiac** tissue perfusion: Risk factor: catheterization of heart

Abortion, Induced

Compromised family **Coping** r/t unresolved feelings about decision

Acute **Pain** r/t surgical intervention

Chronic low **Self-Esteem** r/t feelings of guilt

Chronic **Sorrow** r/t loss of potential child

Risk for **Bleeding:** Risk factor: trauma from abortion

Risk for delayed **Development:** Risk factors: unplanned or unwanted pregnancy

Risk for **Infection:** Risk factors: open uterine blood vessels, dilated cervix

Risk for **Post-Trauma** syndrome: Risk factor: psychological trauma of abortion

Risk for **Spiritual** distress: Risk factor: perceived moral implications of decision

Readiness for enhanced **Knowledge:** expresses an interest in learning

Abortion, Spontaneous

Disturbed **Body Image** r/t perceived inability to carry pregnancy, produce child

Disabled family **Coping** r/t unresolved feelings about loss

Ineffective **Coping** r/t personal vulnerability

Interrupted **Family** processes r/t unmet expectations for pregnancy and childbirth

Fear r/t implications for future pregnancies

Grieving r/t loss of fetus

Acute **Pain** r/t uterine contractions, surgical intervention

Situational low **Self-Esteem** r/t feelings about loss of fetus

Chronic **Sorrow** r/t loss of potential child

Risk for **Bleeding:** Risk factor: trauma from abortion

Risk for **Infection:** Risk factors: septic or incomplete abortion of products of conception, open uterine blood vessels, dilated cervix

Risk for **Post-Trauma** syndrome: Risk factor: psychological trauma of abortion

Risk for **Spiritual** distress: Risk factor: loss of fetus

Readiness for enhanced **Knowledge:** expresses an interest in learning

Abruptio Placentae <36 Weeks

Anxiety r/t unknown outcome, change in birth plans

Death **Anxiety** r/t unknown outcome, hemorrhage, or pain

Interrupted **Family** processes r/t unmet expectations for pregnancy and childbirth

Fear r/t threat to well-being of self and fetus

Impaired **Gas** exchange: placental r/t decreased uteroplacental area

Acute **Pain** r/t irritable uterus, hypertonic uterus

Impaired **Tissue** integrity: maternal r/t possible uterine rupture

Risk for **Bleeding:** Risk factor: separation of placenta from uterus causing bleeding

Risk for disproportionate **Growth:** Risk factor: uteroplacental insufficiency

Risk for **Infection:** Risk factor: partial separation of placenta

Risk for disturbed **Maternal–Fetal** dyad: Risk factors: trauma of process, lack of energy of mother

Risk for **Shock:** Risk factor: separation of placenta from uterus

Readiness for enhanced **Knowledge:** expresses an interest in learning

Abscess Formation

Ineffective **Protection** r/t inadequate nutrition, abnormal blood profile, drug therapy, depressed immune function

Impaired **Tissue** integrity r/t altered circulation, nutritional deficit or excess

Readiness for enhanced **Knowledge:** expresses an interest in learning

Abuse, Child

See Child Abuse

Abuse, Spouse, Parent, or Significant Other

Anxiety r/t threat to self-concept, situational crisis of abuse

Caregiver Role Strain r/t chronic illness, self-care deficits, lack of respite care, extent of caregiving required

Impaired verbal **Communication** r/t psychological barriers of fear

Compromised family **Coping** r/t abusive patterns

Defensive **Coping** r/t low self-esteem

Dysfunctional **Family** processes r/t inadequate coping skills

Insomnia r/t psychological stress

Post-Trauma syndrome r/t history of abuse

Powerlessness r/t lifestyle of helplessness

Chronic low **Self-Esteem** r/t negative family interactions

Risk for impaired emancipated **Decision-Making:** Risk factor: inability to verbalize needs and wants

Risk for self-directed **Violence:** Risk factor: history of abuse

Accessory Muscle Use (to Breathe)

Ineffective **Breathing** pattern (See **Breathing** pattern, ineffective, Section III)

See Asthma; Bronchitis; COPD (Chronic Obstructive Pulmonary Disease); Respiratory Infections, Acute Childhood

Accident Prone

Frail Elderly syndrome r/t history of falls

Acute **Confusion** r/t altered level of consciousness

Ineffective **Coping** r/t personal vulnerability, situational crises

Ineffective **Impulse** control (See **Impulse** control, ineffective, Section III)

Risk for **Injury:** Risk factor: history of accidents

Achalasia

Ineffective **Coping** r/t chronic disease

Acute **Pain** r/t stasis of food in esophagus

Impaired **Swallowing** r/t neuromuscular impairment

Risk for **Aspiration:** Risk factor: nocturnal regurgitation

Acid-Base Imbalances

Risk for **Electrolyte** imbalance: Risk factors: renal dysfunction, diarrhea, treatment-related side effects (e.g., medications, drains)

Acidosis, Metabolic

Acute **Confusion** r/t acid-base imbalance, associated electrolyte imbalance

Impaired **Memory** r/t effect of metabolic acidosis on brain function

Imbalanced **Nutrition:** less than body requirements r/t inability to ingest, absorb nutrients

Risk for **Electrolyte** imbalance: Risk factor: effect of metabolic acidosis on renal function

Risk for **Injury:** Risk factors: disorientation, weakness, stupor

Risk for decreased **Cardiac** tissue perfusion: Risk factor: dysrhythmias from hyperkalemia

Risk for **Shock:** Risk factors: abnormal metabolic state, presence of acid state impairing function, decreased tissue perfusion

Acidosis, Respiratory

Activity intolerance r/t imbalance between oxygen supply and demand

Impaired **Gas** exchange r/t ventilation-perfusion imbalance

Impaired **Memory** r/t hypoxia

Risk for decreased **Cardiac** tissue perfusion: Risk factor: dysrhythmias associated with respiratory acidosis

Acne

Disturbed **Body Image** r/t biophysical changes associated with skin disorder

Ineffective **Health** management r/t insufficient knowledge of therapeutic regimen

Impaired **Skin** integrity r/t hormonal changes (adolescence, menstrual cycle)

ACS (Acute Coronary Syndrome)

See MI (Myocardial Infarction)

Acquired Immunodeficiency Syndrome

See AIDS (Acquired Immunodeficiency Syndrome)

Acromegaly

Activity intolerance (See **Activity** intolerance, Section III)

Ineffective **Airway** clearance r/t airway obstruction by enlarged tongue

Disturbed **Body Image** r/t changes in body function and appearance

A

Impaired physical **Mobility** r/t joint pain

Risk for decreased **Cardiac** tissue perfusion: Risk factor: increased atherosclerosis from abnormal health status

Risk for unstable blood **Glucose** level: Risk factor: abnormal physical health status

Sexual dysfunction r/t changes in hormonal secretions

Risk for **Overweight:** Risk factor: energy expenditure less than energy intake

Activity Intolerance, Potential to Develop

Activity intolerance (See **Activity** intolerance, Section III)

Acute Abdominal Pain

Deficient **Fluid** volume r/t air and fluids trapped in bowel, inability to drink

Acute **Pain** r/t pathological process

Risk for dysfunctional **Gastrointestinal** motility: Risk factor: ineffective gastrointestinal tissue perfusion

See Abdominal Pain

Acute Alcohol Intoxication

Ineffective **Breathing** pattern r/t depression of the respiratory center from excessive alcohol intake

Acute **Confusion** r/t central nervous system depression

Dysfunctional **Family** processes r/t abuse of alcohol

Risk for **Aspiration:** Risk factor: depressed reflexes with acute vomiting

Risk for **Infection:** Risk factor: impaired immune system from malnutrition associated with chronic excessive alcohol intake

Risk for **Injury:** Risk factor: chemical (alcohol)

Acute Back Pain

Anxiety r/t situational crisis, back injury

Constipation r/t decreased activity, effect of pain medication

Ineffective **Coping** r/t situational crisis, back injury

Impaired physical **Mobility** r/t pain

Acute **Pain** r/t back injury

Readiness for enhanced **Knowledge:** expresses an interest in learning

Acute Confusion

See Confusion, Acute

Acute Coronary Syndrome

Decreased **Cardiac** output r/t cardiac disorder

Risk for decreased **Cardiac** tissue perfusion (See **Cardiac** tissue perfusion, risk for decreased, Section III)

Acute Lymphocytic Leukemia (ALL)

See Cancer; Chemotherapy; Child with Chronic Condition; Leukemia

Acute Renal Failure/Acute Kidney Failure

See Kidney Failure

Acute Respiratory Distress Syndrome

See ARDS (Acute Respiratory Distress Syndrome)

Adams-Stokes Syndrome

See Dysrhythmia

Addiction

See Alcoholism; Drug Abuse

Addison's Disease

Activity intolerance r/t weakness, fatigue

Disturbed **Body Image** r/t increased skin pigmentation

Deficient **Fluid** volume r/t failure of regulatory mechanisms

Imbalanced **Nutrition:** less than body requirements r/t chronic illness

Risk for **Injury:** Risk factor: weakness

Readiness for enhanced **Knowledge:** expresses an interest in learning

Adenoidectomy

Acute **Pain** r/t surgical incision

Ineffective **Airway** clearance r/t hesitation or reluctance to cough as a result of pain, fear

Nausea r/t anesthesia effects, drainage from surgery

Acute **Pain** r/t surgical incision

Risk for **Aspiration:** Risk factors: postoperative drainage, impaired swallowing

Risk for **Bleeding:** Risk factor: surgical incision

Risk for deficient **Fluid** volume: Risk factors: decreased intake as a result of painful swallowing, effects of anesthesia

Risk for imbalanced **Nutrition:** less than body requirements: Risk factor: reluctance to swallow

Readiness for enhanced **Knowledge:** expresses an interest in learning

Adhesions, Lysis of

See Abdominal Surgery

Adjustment Disorder

Anxiety r/t inability to cope with psychosocial stressor

Labile **Emotional Control** r/t emotional disturbance

Risk-prone **Health** behavior r/t assault to self-esteem

Disturbed personal **Identity** r/t psychosocial stressor (specific to individual)

Situational low **Self-Esteem** r/t change in role function

Impaired **Social** interaction r/t absence of significant others or peers

Adjustment Impairment

Risk-prone **Health** behavior (See **Health** behavior, risk-prone, Section III)

Adolescent, Pregnant

Anxiety r/t situational and maturational crisis, pregnancy

Disturbed **Body Image** r/t pregnancy superimposed on developing body

Decisional Conflict: keeping child versus giving up child versus abortion r/t lack of experience with decision-making,

A

interference with decision-making, multiple or divergent sources of information, lack of support system

Disabled family **Coping** r/t highly ambivalent family relationships, chronically unresolved feelings of guilt, anger, despair

Ineffective **Coping** r/t situational and maturational crisis, personal vulnerability

Ineffective **Denial** r/t fear of consequences of pregnancy becoming known

Interrupted **Family** processes r/t unmet expectations for adolescent, situational crisis

Fear r/t labor and delivery

Deficient **Knowledge** r/t pregnancy, infant growth and development, parenting

Imbalanced **Nutrition:** less than body requirements r/t lack of knowledge of nutritional needs during pregnancy and as growing adolescent

Ineffective **Role** performance r/t pregnancy

Situational low **Self-Esteem** r/t feelings of shame and guilt about becoming or being pregnant

Impaired **Social** interaction r/t self-concept disturbance

Social isolation r/t absence of supportive significant others

Risk for impaired **Attachment:** Risk factor: anxiety associated with the parent role

Risk for delayed **Development:** Risk factor: unplanned or unwanted pregnancy

Risk for urge urinary **Incontinence:** Risk factor: pressure on bladder by growing uterus

Risk for disturbed **Maternal–Fetal** dyad: Risk factors: immaturity, substance use

Risk for impaired **Parenting:** Risk factors: adolescent parent, unplanned or unwanted pregnancy, single parent

Readiness for enhanced **Childbearing** process: reports appropriate prenatal lifestyle

Readiness for enhanced **Knowledge:** expresses an interest in learning

Adoption, Giving Child Up for

Decisional Conflict r/t unclear personal values or beliefs, perceived threat to value system, support system deficit

Ineffective **Coping** r/t stress of loss of child

Interrupted **Family** processes r/t conflict within family regarding relinquishment of child

Grieving r/t loss of child, loss of role of parent

Insomnia r/t depression or trauma of relinquishment of child

Social isolation r/t making choice that goes against values of significant others

Chronic **Sorrow** r/t loss of relationship with child

Risk for **Spiritual** distress: Risk factor: perceived moral implications of decision

Readiness for enhanced **Spiritual** well-being: harmony with self regarding final decision

Adrenocortical Insufficiency

Deficient **Fluid** volume r/t insufficient ability to reabsorb water

Ineffective **Protection** r/t inability to tolerate stress

Delayed **Surgical** recovery r/t inability to respond to stress

Risk for **Shock:** Risk factors: deficient fluid volume, decreased cortisol to initiate stress response to insult to body

See Addison's Disease; Shock, Hypovolemic

Advance Directives

Death **Anxiety** r/t planning for end-of-life health decisions

Decisional Conflict r/t unclear personal values or beliefs, perceived threat to value system, support system deficit

Grieving r/t possible loss of self, significant other

Readiness for enhanced **Spiritual** well-being: harmonious interconnectedness with self, others, higher power, God

Affective Disorders

See Depression (Major Depressive Disorder); Dysthymic Disorder; Manic Disorder, Bipolar I; SAD (Seasonal Affective Disorder)

Age-Related Macular Degeneration

See Macular Degeneration

Aggressive Behavior

Fear r/t real or imagined threat to own well-being

Risk for other-directed **Violence** (See **Violence,** other-directed, risk for, Section III)

Aging

Death **Anxiety** r/t fear of unknown, loss of self, impact on significant others

Impaired **Dentition** r/t ineffective oral hygiene

Risk for **Frail Elderly** syndrome: Risk factors: >70 years, activity intolerance, impaired vision

Grieving r/t multiple losses, impending death

Ineffective **Health** management r/t powerlessness

Hearing Loss r/t exposure to loud noises, aging

Functional urinary **Incontinence** r/t impaired vision, impaired cognition, neuromuscular limitations, altered environmental factors

Impaired **Resilience** r/t aging, multiple losses

Sleep deprivation r/t aging-related sleep-stage shifts

Ineffective **Thermoregulation** r/t aging

Vision Loss r/t aging *(see care plan in Appendix)*

Risk for **Caregiver Role Strain:** Risk factor: inability to handle increasing needs of significant other

Risk for Impaired emancipated **Decision-Making:** Risk factor: inability to process information regarding health care decisions

Risk for **Injury:** Risk factors: vision loss, hearing loss, decreased balance, decreased sensation in feet

Risk for **Loneliness:** Risk factors: inadequate support system, role transition, health alterations, depression, fatigue

A

Readiness for enhanced community **Coping:** providing social support and other resources identified as needed for elderly client

Readiness for enhanced family **Coping:** ability to gratify needs, address adaptive tasks

Readiness for enhanced **Health** management: knowledge about medication, nutrition, exercise, coping strategies

Readiness for enhanced **Knowledge:** specify need to improve health

Readiness for enhanced **Nutrition:** need to improve health

Readiness for enhanced **Relationship:** demonstrates understanding of partner's insufficient function

Readiness for enhanced **Sleep:** need to improve sleep

Readiness for enhanced **Spiritual** well-being: one's experience of life's meaning, harmony with self, others, higher power, God, environment

Readiness for enhanced **Urinary** elimination: need to improve health

Agitation

Acute **Confusion** r/t side effects of medication, hypoxia, decreased cerebral perfusion, alcohol abuse or withdrawal, substance abuse or withdrawal, sensory deprivation or overload

Sleep deprivation r/t sustained inadequate sleep hygiene, sundown syndrome

Agoraphobia

Anxiety r/t real or perceived threat to physical integrity

Ineffective **Coping** r/t inadequate support systems

Fear r/t leaving home, going out in public places

Impaired **Social** interaction r/t disturbance in self-concept

Social isolation r/t altered thought process

Agranulocytosis

Delayed **Surgical** recovery r/t abnormal blood profile

Risk for **Infection:** Risk factor: abnormal blood profile

Readiness for enhanced **Knowledge:** expresses an interest in learning

AIDS (Acquired Immunodeficiency Syndrome)

Death **Anxiety** r/t fear of premature death

Disturbed **Body Image** r/t chronic contagious illness, cachexia

Caregiver Role Strain r/t unpredictable illness course, presence of situation stressors

Diarrhea r/t inflammatory bowel changes

Interrupted **Family** processes r/t distress about diagnosis of human immunodeficiency virus (HIV) infection

Fatigue r/t disease process, stress, decreased nutritional intake

Fear r/t powerlessness, threat to well-being

Grieving: family/parental r/t potential or impending death of loved one

Grieving: individual r/t loss of physical and psychosocial well-being

Hopelessness r/t deteriorating physical condition

Imbalanced **Nutrition:** less than body requirements r/t decreased ability to eat and absorb nutrients as a result of anorexia, nausea, diarrhea; oral candidiasis

Chronic **Pain** r/t tissue inflammation and destruction

Impaired **Resilience** r/t chronic illness

Situational low **Self-Esteem** r/t crisis of chronic contagious illness

Ineffective **Sexuality** pattern r/t possible transmission of disease

Social isolation r/t self-concept disturbance, therapeutic isolation

Chronic **Sorrow** r/t chronic illness

Spiritual distress r/t challenged beliefs or moral system

Risk for deficient **Fluid** volume: Risk factors: diarrhea, vomiting, fever, bleeding

Risk for **Infection:** Risk factor: inadequate immune system

Risk for **Loneliness:** Risk factor: social isolation

Risk for impaired **Oral Mucous Membrane:** Risk factor: immunological deficit

Risk for impaired **Skin** integrity: Risk factors: immunological deficit, diarrhea

Risk for **Spiritual** distress: Risk factor: physical illness

Readiness for enhanced **Knowledge:** expresses an interest in learning

See AIDS, Child; Cancer; Pneumonia

AIDS Dementia

Chronic **Confusion** r/t viral invasion of nervous system

See Dementia

AIDS, Child

Impaired **Parenting** r/t congenital acquisition of infection secondary to intravenous (IV) drug use, multiple sexual partners, history of contaminated blood transfusion

See AIDS (Acquired Immunodeficiency Syndrome); Child with Chronic Condition; Hospitalized Child; Terminally Ill Child, Adolescent; Terminally Ill Child, Infant/Toddler; Terminally Ill Child, Preschool Child; Terminally Ill Child, School-Age Child/Preadolescent; Terminally Ill Child/Death of Child, Parent

Airway Obstruction/Secretions

Ineffective **Airway** clearance (See **Airway** clearance, ineffective, Section III)

Alcohol Withdrawal

Anxiety r/t situational crisis, withdrawal

Acute **Confusion** r/t effects of alcohol withdrawal

Ineffective **Coping** r/t personal vulnerability

Dysfunctional **Family** processes r/t abuse of alcohol

Insomnia r/t effect of alcohol withdrawal, anxiety

Imbalanced **Nutrition:** less than body requirements r/t poor dietary habits

Chronic low **Self-Esteem** r/t repeated unmet expectations

Risk for deficient **Fluid** volume: Risk factors: excessive diaphoresis, agitation, decreased fluid intake

Risk for other-directed **Violence:** Risk factor: substance withdrawal

Risk for self-directed **Violence:** Risk factor: substance withdrawal

Readiness for enhanced **Knowledge:** expresses an interest in learning

Alcoholism

Anxiety r/t loss of control

Risk-prone **Health** behavior r/t lack of motivation to change behaviors, addiction

Acute **Confusion** r/t alcohol abuse

Chronic **Confusion** r/t neurological effects of chronic alcohol intake

Defensive **Coping** r/t denial of reality of addiction

Disabled family **Coping** r/t codependency issues due to alcoholism

Ineffective **Coping** r/t use of alcohol to cope with life events

Labile **Emotional Control** r/t substance abuse

Ineffective **Denial** r/t refusal to acknowledge addiction

Dysfunctional **Family** processes r/t alcohol abuse

Impaired **Home** maintenance r/t memory deficits, fatigue

Insomnia r/t irritability, nightmares, tremors

Impaired **Memory** r/t alcohol abuse

Self-Neglect r/t effects of alcohol abuse

Imbalanced **Nutrition:** less than body requirements r/t anorexia, inappropriate diet with increased carbohydrates

Powerlessness r/t alcohol addiction

Ineffective **Protection** r/t malnutrition, sleep deprivation

Chronic low **Self-Esteem** r/t failure at life events

Social isolation r/t unacceptable social behavior, values

Risk for **Injury:** Risk factor: alteration in sensory or perceptual function

Risk for **Loneliness:** Risk factor: unacceptable social behavior

Risk for other-directed **Violence:** Risk factors: reactions to substances used, impulsive behavior, disorientation, impaired judgment

Risk for self-directed **Violence:** Risk factors: reactions to substances used, impulsive behavior, disorientation, impaired judgment

Alcoholism, Dysfunctional Family Processes

Dysfunctional **Family** processes (See **Family** processes, dysfunctional, Section III)

Alkalosis

See Metabolic Alkalosis

ALL (Acute Lymphocytic Leukemia)

See Cancer; Chemotherapy; Child with Chronic Condition; Leukemia

Allergies

Latex Allergy response r/t hypersensitivity to natural rubber latex

Risk for **Allergy** response: Risk factors: chemical factors, dander, environmental substances, foods, insect stings, medications

Risk for **Latex Allergy** response: Risk factor: repeated exposure to products containing latex

Readiness for enhanced **Knowledge:** expresses an interest in learning

Alopecia

Disturbed **Body Image** r/t loss of hair, change in appearance

Readiness for enhanced **Knowledge:** expresses an interest in learning

Altered Mental Status

See Confusion, Acute; Confusion, Chronic; Memory Deficit

ALS (Amyotrophic Lateral Sclerosis)

See Amyotrophic Lateral Sclerosis (ALS)

Alzheimer's Disease

Caregiver role strain r/t duration and extent of caregiving required

Chronic **Confusion** r/t loss of cognitive function

Compromised family **Coping** r/t interrupted family processes

Frail Elderly syndrome r/t alteration in cognitive functioning

Impaired **Home** maintenance r/t impaired cognitive function, inadequate support systems

Hopelessness r/t deteriorating condition

Insomnia r/t neurological impairment, daytime naps

Impaired **Memory** r/t neurological disturbance

Impaired physical **Mobility** r/t severe neurological dysfunction

Self-Neglect r/t loss of cognitive function

Powerlessness r/t deteriorating condition

Self-Care deficit: specify r/t loss of cognitive function, psychological impairment

Social isolation r/t fear of disclosure of memory loss

Wandering r/t cognitive impairment, frustration, physiological state

Risk for chronic functional **Constipation:** Risk factor: impaired cognitive functioning

Risk for **Injury:** Risk factor: confusion

Risk for **Loneliness:** Risk factor: potential social isolation

Risk for **Relocation** stress syndrome: Risk factors: impaired psychosocial health, decreased health status

Risk for other-directed **Violence:** Risk factors: frustration, fear, anger, loss of cognitive function

Readiness for enhanced **Knowledge:** Caregiver: expresses an interest in learning

See Dementia

AMD (Age-Related Macular Degeneration)

See Macular Degeneration

A

A

Amenorrhea

Imbalanced **Nutrition:** less than body requirements r/t inadequate food intake

See Sexuality, Adolescent

AMI (Acute Myocardial Infarction)

See MI (Myocardial Infarction)

Amnesia

Acute **Confusion** r/t alcohol abuse, delirium, dementia, drug abuse

Dysfunctional **Family** processes r/t alcohol abuse, inadequate coping skills

Impaired **Memory** r/t excessive environmental disturbance, neurological disturbance

Post-Trauma syndrome r/t history of abuse, catastrophic illness, disaster, accident

Amniocentesis

Anxiety r/t threat to self and fetus, unknown future

Decisional Conflict r/t choice of treatment pending results of test

Risk for **Infection:** Risk factor: invasive procedure

Amnionitis

See Chorioamnionitis

Amniotic Membrane Rupture

See Premature Rupture of Membranes

Amputation

Disturbed **Body Image** r/t negative effects of amputation, response from others

Grieving r/t loss of body part, future lifestyle changes

Impaired physical **Mobility** r/t musculoskeletal impairment, limited movement

Acute **Pain** r/t surgery, phantom limb sensation

Chronic **Pain** r/t surgery, phantom limb sensation

Ineffective peripheral **Tissue Perfusion** r/t impaired arterial circulation

Impaired **Skin** integrity r/t poor healing, prosthesis rubbing

Risk for **Bleeding:** Risk factor: vulnerable surgical site

Risk for Impaired **Tissue** integrity: Risk factor: mechanical factors impacting site

Readiness for enhanced **Knowledge:** expresses an interest in learning

Amyotrophic Lateral Sclerosis (ALS)

Death **Anxiety** r/t impending progressive loss of function leading to death

Ineffective **Breathing** pattern r/t compromised muscles of respiration

Impaired verbal **Communication** r/t weakness of muscles of speech, deficient knowledge of ways to compensate and alternative communication devices

Decisional Conflict: ventilator therapy r/t unclear personal values or beliefs, lack of relevant information

Impaired **Resilience** r/t perceived vulnerability

Chronic **Sorrow** r/t chronic illness

Impaired **Swallowing** r/t weakness of muscles involved in swallowing

Impaired spontaneous **Ventilation** r/t weakness of muscles of respiration

Risk for **Aspiration:** Risk factor: impaired swallowing

Risk for **Spiritual** distress: Risk factor: chronic debilitating condition

See Neurologic Disorders

Anal Fistula

See Hemorrhoidectomy

Anaphylactic Shock

Deficient **Fluid** volume r/t compromised regulatory mechanism

Ineffective **Airway** clearance r/t laryngeal edema, bronchospasm

Latex Allergy response r/t abnormal immune mechanism response

Impaired spontaneous **Ventilation** r/t acute airway obstruction from anaphylaxis process

Anaphylaxis Prevention

Risk for **Allergy** response (See **Allergy** response, risk for, Section III)

Anasarca

Excess **Fluid** volume r/t excessive fluid intake, cardiac/renal dysfunction, loss of plasma proteins

Risk for impaired **Skin** integrity: Risk factor: impaired circulation to skin from edema

See Anasarca

Anemia

Anxiety r/t cause of disease

Impaired **Comfort** r/t feelings of always being cold from decreased hemoglobin and decreased metabolism

Fatigue r/t decreased oxygen supply to the body, increased cardiac workload

Impaired **Memory** r/t change in cognition from decreased oxygen supply to the body

Delayed **Surgical** recovery r/t decreased oxygen supply to body, increased cardiac workload

Risk for **Bleeding** (See **Bleeding,** risk for, Section III)

Risk for **Injury:** Risk factor: alteration in peripheral sensory perception

Readiness for enhanced **Knowledge:** expresses an interest in learning

Anemia, in Pregnancy

Anxiety r/t concerns about health of self and fetus

Fatigue r/t decreased oxygen supply to the body, increased cardiac workload

Risk for delayed **Development:** Risk factor: reduction in the oxygen-carrying capacity of blood

Risk for **Infection:** Risk factor: reduction in oxygen-carrying capacity of blood

Risk for disturbed **Maternal–Fetal** dyad: Risk factor: compromised oxygen transport

Readiness for enhanced **Knowledge:** expresses an interest in learning

Anemia, Sickle Cell

See Anemia; Sickle Cell Anemia/Crisis

Anencephaly

See Neural Tube Defects

Aneurysm, Abdominal Surgery

Risk for deficient **Fluid** volume: Risk factor: hemorrhage r/t potential abnormal blood loss

Risk for **Infection:** Risk factor: invasive procedure

Risk for ineffective **Gastrointestinal** perfusion (See **Gastrointestinal** perfusion, ineffective, risk for, Section III)

Risk for ineffective **Renal** perfusion: Risk factor: prolonged ischemia of kidneys

See Abdominal Surgery

Aneurysm, Cerebral

See Craniectomy/Craniotomy; Subarachnoid Hemorrhage

Anger

Anxiety r/t situational crisis

Defensive **Coping** r/t inability to acknowledge responsibility for actions and results of actions

Labile **Emotional Control** r/t stressors

Fear r/t environmental stressor, hospitalization

Grieving r/t significant loss

Risk-prone **Health** behavior r/t assault to self-esteem, disability requiring change in lifestyle, inadequate support system

Powerlessness r/t health care environment

Risk for compromised **Human Dignity:** Risk factors: inadequate participation in decision-making, perceived dehumanizing treatment, perceived humiliation, exposure of the body, cultural incongruity

Risk for **Post-Trauma** syndrome: Risk factor: inadequate social support

Risk for other-directed **Violence:** Risk factors: history of violence, rage reaction

Risk for self-directed **Violence:** Risk factors: history of violence, history of abuse, rage reaction

Angina

Activity intolerance r/t acute pain, dysrhythmias

Anxiety r/t situational crisis

Decreased **Cardiac** output r/t myocardial ischemia, medication effect, dysrhythmia

Ineffective **Coping** r/t personal vulnerability to situational crisis of new diagnosis, deteriorating health

Ineffective **Denial** r/t deficient knowledge of need to seek help with symptoms

Grieving r/t pain, loss of health

Acute **Pain** r/t myocardial ischemia

Ineffective **Sexuality** pattern r/t disease process, medications, loss of libido

Readiness for enhanced **Knowledge:** expresses an interest in learning

Angiocardiography (Cardiac Catheterization)

See Cardiac Catheterization

Angioplasty, Coronary

Fear r/t possible outcome of interventional procedure

Ineffective peripheral **Tissue Perfusion** r/t vasospasm, hematoma formation

Risk for **Bleeding:** Risk factors: possible damage to coronary artery, hematoma formation

Risk for decreased **Cardiac** tissue perfusion: Risk factors: ventricular ischemia, dysrhythmias

Readiness for enhanced **Knowledge:** expresses an interest in learning

Anomaly, Fetal/Newborn (Parent Dealing with)

Anxiety r/t threat to role functioning, situational crisis

Decisional Conflict: interventions for fetus or newborn r/t lack of relevant information, spiritual distress, threat to value system

Disabled family **Coping** r/t chronically unresolved feelings about loss of perfect baby

Ineffective **Coping** r/t personal vulnerability in situational crisis

Interrupted **Family** processes r/t unmet expectations for perfect baby, lack of adequate support systems

Fear r/t real or imagined threat to baby, implications for future pregnancies, powerlessness

Grieving r/t loss of ideal child

Hopelessness r/t long-term stress, deteriorating physical condition of child, lost spiritual belief

Deficient **Knowledge** r/t limited exposure to situation

Impaired **Parenting** r/t interruption of bonding process

Powerlessness r/t complication threatening fetus or newborn

Parental **Role** conflict r/t separation from newborn, intimidation with invasive or restrictive modalities, specialized care center policies

Situational low **Self-Esteem** r/t perceived inability to produce a perfect child

Social isolation r/t alterations in child's physical appearance, altered state of wellness

Chronic **Sorrow** r/t loss of ideal child, inadequate bereavement support

A

Spiritual distress r/t test of spiritual beliefs

Risk for impaired **Attachment:** Risk factor: ill infant unable to effectively initiate parental contact as result of altered behavioral organization

Risk for disorganized **Infant** behavior: Risk factor: congenital disorder

Risk for impaired **Parenting:** Risk factors: interruption of bonding process; unrealistic expectations for self, infant, or partner; perceived threat to own emotional survival; severe stress; lack of knowledge

Risk for **Spiritual** distress: Risk factor: lack of normal child to raise and carry on family name

Anorectal Abscess

Disturbed **Body Image** r/t odor and drainage from rectal area

Acute **Pain** r/t inflammation of perirectal area

Risk for **Constipation:** Risk factor: fear of painful elimination

Readiness for enhanced **Knowledge:** expresses an interest in learning

Anorexia

Deficient **Fluid** volume r/t inability to drink

Imbalanced **Nutrition:** less than body requirements r/t loss of appetite, nausea, vomiting, laxative abuse

Delayed **Surgical** recovery r/t inadequate nutritional intake

Risk for delayed **Surgical** recovery: Risk factor: inadequate nutritional intake

Anorexia Nervosa

Activity intolerance r/t fatigue, weakness

Disturbed **Body Image** r/t misconception of actual body appearance

Constipation r/t lack of adequate food, fiber, and fluid intake

Defensive **Coping** r/t psychological impairment, eating disorder

Disabled family **Coping** r/t highly ambivalent family relationships

Ineffective **Denial** r/t fear of consequences of therapy, possible weight gain

Diarrhea r/t laxative abuse

Interrupted **Family** processes r/t situational crisis

Ineffective family **Health** management r/t family conflict, excessive demands on family associated with complexity of condition and treatment

Imbalanced **Nutrition:** less than body requirements r/t inadequate food intake, excessive exercise

Chronic low **Self-Esteem** r/t repeated unmet expectations

Ineffective **Sexuality** pattern r/t loss of libido from malnutrition

Risk for **Infection:** Risk factor: malnutrition resulting in depressed immune system

Risk for **Spiritual** distress: Risk factor: low self-esteem

See Maturational Issues, Adolescent

Anosmia (Smell, Loss of Ability to)

Imbalanced **Nutrition:** less than body requirements r/t loss of appetite associated with loss of smell

Antepartum Period

See Pregnancy, Normal; Prenatal Care, Normal

Anterior Repair, Anterior Colporrhaphy

Urinary Retention r/t edema of urinary structures

Risk for urge urinary **Incontinence:** Risk factor: trauma to bladder

Readiness for enhanced **Knowledge:** expresses an interest in learning

See Vaginal Hysterectomy

Anticoagulant Therapy

Risk for **Bleeding:** Risk factor: altered clotting function from anticoagulant

Risk for deficient **Fluid** volume: hemorrhage: Risk factor: altered clotting mechanism

Readiness for enhanced **Knowledge:** expresses an interest in learning

Antisocial Personality Disorder

Defensive **Coping** r/t excessive use of projection

Ineffective **Coping** r/t frequently violating the norms and rules of society

Labile **Emotional Control** r/t psychiatric disorder

Hopelessness r/t abandonment

Impaired **Social** interaction r/t sociocultural conflict, chemical dependence, inability to form relationships

Spiritual distress r/t separation from religious or cultural ties

Ineffective **Health** management r/t excessive demands on family

Risk for **Loneliness:** Risk factor: inability to interact appropriately with others

Risk for impaired **Parenting:** Risk factors: inability to function as parent or guardian, emotional instability

Risk for **Self-Mutilation:** Risk factors: self-hatred, depersonalization

Risk for other-directed **Violence:** Risk factor: history of violence, altered thought patterns

Anuria

See Kidney Failure

Anxiety

See **Anxiety,** Section III

Anxiety Disorder

Ineffective **Activity** planning r/t unrealistic perception of events

Anxiety r/t unmet security and safety needs

Death **Anxiety** r/t fears of unknown, powerlessness

Decisional Conflict r/t low self-esteem, fear of making a mistake

Defensive **Coping** r/t overwhelming feelings of dread

Disabled family **Coping** r/t ritualistic behavior, actions

Ineffective **Coping** r/t inability to express feelings appropriately

Ineffective **Denial** r/t overwhelming feelings of hopelessness, fear, threat to self

Insomnia r/t psychological impairment, emotional instability

Impaired **Mood** regulation r/t functional impairment, impaired social functioning, alteration in sleep pattern

Labile **Emotional Control** r/t emotional instability

Powerlessness r/t lifestyle of helplessness

Self-Care deficit r/t ritualistic behavior, activities

Sleep deprivation r/t prolonged psychological discomfort

Risk for **Spiritual** distress: Risk factor: psychological distress

Readiness for enhanced **Knowledge:** expresses an interest in learning

Aortic Aneurysm Repair (Abdominal Surgery)

See Abdominal Surgery; Aneurysm, Abdominal Surgery

Aortic Valvular Stenosis

See Congenital Heart Disease/Cardiac Anomalies

Aphasia

Anxiety r/t situational crisis of aphasia

Impaired verbal **Communication** r/t decrease in circulation to brain

Ineffective **Coping** r/t loss of speech

Ineffective **Health** maintenance r/t deficient knowledge regarding information on aphasia and alternative communication techniques

Aplastic Anemia

Activity intolerance r/t imbalance between oxygen supply and demand

Fear r/t ability to live with serious disease

Risk for **Bleeding:** Risk factor: inadequate clotting factors

Risk for **Infection:** Risk factor: inadequate immune function

Readiness for enhanced **Knowledge:** expresses an interest in learning

Apnea in Infancy

See Premature Infant (Child); Premature Infant (Parent); SIDS (Sudden Infant Death Syndrome)

Apneustic Respirations

Ineffective **Breathing** pattern r/t perception or cognitive impairment, neurological impairment

See Apneustic Respirations

Appendectomy

Deficient **Fluid** volume r/t fluid restriction, hypermetabolic state, nausea, vomiting

Acute **Pain** r/t surgical incision

Delayed **Surgical** recovery r/t rupture of appendix

Risk for **Infection:** Risk factors: perforation or rupture of appendix, surgical incision, peritonitis

Readiness for enhanced **Knowledge:** expresses an interest in learning

See Hospitalized Child; Surgery, Postoperative Care

Appendicitis

Deficient **Fluid** volume r/t anorexia, nausea, vomiting

Acute **Pain** r/t inflammation

Risk for **Infection:** Risk factor: possible perforation of appendix

Readiness for enhanced **Knowledge:** expresses an interest in learning

Apprehension

Anxiety r/t threat to self-concept, threat to health status, situational crisis

Death **Anxiety** r/t apprehension over loss of self, consequences to significant others

ARDS (Acute Respiratory Distress Syndrome)

Ineffective **Airway** clearance r/t excessive tracheobronchial secretions

Death **Anxiety** r/t seriousness of physical disease

Impaired **Gas** exchange r/t damage to alveolar capillary membrane, change in lung compliance

Impaired spontaneous **Ventilation** r/t damage to alveolar capillary membrane

See Ventilated Client, Mechanically

Arrhythmia

See Dysrhythmia

Arterial Insufficiency

Ineffective peripheral **Tissue Perfusion** r/t interruption of arterial flow

Delayed **Surgical** recovery r/t ineffective tissue perfusion

Arthritis

Activity intolerance r/t chronic pain, fatigue, weakness

Disturbed **Body Image** r/t ineffective coping with joint abnormalities

Impaired physical **Mobility** r/t joint impairment

Chronic **Pain** r/t progression of joint deterioration

Self-Care deficit: specify r/t pain with movement, damage to joints

Readiness for enhanced **Knowledge:** expresses an interest in learning

See JRA (Juvenile Rheumatoid Arthritis)

Arthrocentesis

Acute **Pain** r/t invasive procedure

Arthroplasty (Total Hip Replacement)

See Total Joint Replacement (Total Hip/Total Knee/Shoulder); Surgery, Perioperative; Surgery, Postoperative Care; Surgery, Preoperative Care

A

Arthroscopy

Impaired physical **Mobility** r/t surgical trauma of knee

Readiness for enhanced **Knowledge:** expresses an interest in learning

Ascites

Ineffective **Breathing** pattern r/t increased abdominal girth

Imbalanced **Nutrition:** less than body requirements r/t loss of appetite

Chronic **Pain** r/t altered body function

Readiness for enhanced **Knowledge:** expresses an interest in learning

See Ascites; Cancer; Cirrhosis

Asperger's Syndrome

Ineffective **Relationship** r/t poor communication skills, lack of empathy

See Autism

Asphyxia, Birth

Ineffective **Breathing** pattern r/t depression of breathing reflex secondary to anoxia

Ineffective **Coping** r/t uncertainty of child outcome

Fear (parental) r/t concern over safety of infant

Impaired **Gas** exchange r/t poor placental perfusion, lack of initiation of breathing by newborn

Grieving r/t loss of perfect child, concern of loss of future abilities

Impaired spontaneous **Ventilation** r/t brain injury

Risk for impaired **Attachment:** Risk factors: ill infant who is unable to initiate parental contact, hospitalization in critical care environment

Risk for delayed **Development:** Risk factor: lack of oxygen to brain

Risk for disproportionate **Growth:** Risk factor: lack of oxygen to brain

Risk for disorganized **Infant** behavior: Risk factor: lack of oxygen to brain

Risk for **Injury:** Risk factor: lack of oxygen to brain

Risk for ineffective **Cerebral** tissue perfusion: Risk factor: poor placental perfusion or cord compression resulting in lack of oxygen to brain

Aspiration, Danger of

Risk for **Aspiration** (See **Aspiration,** risk for, Section III)

Assault Victim

Post-Trauma syndrome r/t assault

Rape-Trauma syndrome r/t rape

Impaired **Resilience** r/t frightening experience, post-trauma stress response

Risk for **Post-Trauma** syndrome: Risk factors: perception of event, inadequate social support, unsupportive environment, diminished ego strength, duration of event

Risk for **Spiritual** distress: Risk factors: physical, psychological stress

Assaultive Client

Risk for **Injury:** Risk factors: confused thought process, impaired judgment

Risk for other-directed **Violence:** Risk factors: paranoid ideation, anger

Asthma

Activity intolerance r/t fatigue, energy shift to meet muscle needs for breathing to overcome airway obstruction

Ineffective **Airway** clearance r/t tracheobronchial narrowing, excessive secretions

Anxiety r/t inability to breathe effectively, fear of suffocation

Disturbed **Body Image** r/t decreased participation in physical activities

Ineffective **Breathing** pattern r/t anxiety

Ineffective **Coping** r/t personal vulnerability to situational crisis

Ineffective **Health** management (See **Health** management, ineffective, in Section III)

Impaired **Home** maintenance r/t deficient knowledge regarding control of environmental triggers

Sleep deprivation r/t ineffective breathing pattern, cough

Readiness for enhanced **Health** management (See **Health** management, readiness for enhanced, in Section III)

Readiness for enhanced **Knowledge:** expresses an interest in learning

See Child with Chronic Condition; Hospitalized Child

Ataxia

Anxiety r/t change in health status

Disturbed **Body Image** r/t staggering gait

Impaired physical **Mobility** r/t neuromuscular impairment

Risk for **Falls:** Risk factors: gait alteration, instability

Atelectasis

Ineffective **Breathing** pattern r/t loss of functional lung tissue, depression of respiratory function or hypoventilation because of pain

Impaired **Gas** exchange r/t decreased alveolar-capillary surface

Anxiety r/t alteration in respiratory pattern

See Atelectasis

Atherosclerosis

See MI (Myocardial Infarction); CVA (Cerebrovascular Accident); Peripheral Vascular Disease (PVD)

Athlete's Foot

Impaired **Skin** integrity r/t effects of fungal agent

Readiness for enhanced **Knowledge:** expresses an interest in learning

See Itching; Pruritus

ATN (Acute Tubular Necrosis)

See Kidney Failure

Atrial Fibrillation

See Dysrhythmia

Atrial Septal Defect

See Congenital Heart Disease/Cardiac Anomalies

Attention Deficit Disorder

Risk-prone **Health** behavior r/t intense emotional state

Disabled family **Coping** r/t significant person with chronically unexpressed feelings of guilt, anxiety, hostility, and despair

Ineffective **Impulse** control r/t (See **Impulse** control, ineffective, Section III)

Chronic low **Self-Esteem** r/t difficulty in participating in expected activities, poor school performance

Social isolation r/t unacceptable social behavior

Risk for delayed **Development:** Risk factor: behavior disorders

Risk for **Falls:** Risk factor: rapid non-thinking behavior

Risk for **Loneliness:** Risk factor: social isolation

Risk for impaired **Parenting:** Risk factor: lack of knowledge of factors contributing to child's behavior

Risk for **Spiritual** distress: Risk factor: poor relationships

Auditory Problems

See Hearing Impairment

Autism

Impaired verbal **Communication** r/t speech and language delays

Compromised family **Coping** r/t parental guilt over etiology of disease, inability to accept or adapt to child's condition, inability to help child and other family members seek treatment

Disturbed personal **Identity** r/t inability to distinguish between self and environment, inability to identify own body as separate from those of other people, inability to integrate concept of self

Self-Neglect r/t impaired socialization

Impaired **Social** interaction r/t communication barriers, inability to relate to others, failure to develop peer relationships

Risk for delayed **Development:** Risk factor: autism

Risk for **Loneliness:** Risk factor: difficulty developing relationships with other people

Risk for **Self-Mutilation:** Risk factor: autistic state

Risk for other-directed **Violence:** Risk factors: frequent destructive rages toward others secondary to extreme response to changes in routine, fear of harmless things

Risk for self-directed **Violence:** Risk factors: frequent destructive rages toward self, secondary to extreme response to changes in routine, fear of harmless things

See Child with Chronic Condition

Autonomic Dysreflexia

Autonomic Dysreflexia r/t bladder distention, bowel distention, noxious stimuli

Risk for **Autonomic Dysreflexia:** Risk factors: bladder distention, bowel distention, noxious stimuli

Autonomic Hyperreflexia

See Autonomic Dysreflexia

B

Baby Care

Readiness for enhanced **Childbearing** process: demonstrates appropriate feeding and baby care techniques, along with attachment to infant and providing a safe environment

Anxiety r/t situational crisis, back injury

Ineffective **Coping** r/t situational crisis, back injury

Impaired physical **Mobility** r/t pain

Acute **Pain** r/t back injury

Chronic **Pain** r/t back injury

Risk for **Constipation:** Risk factors: decreased activity, side effect of pain medication

Risk for **Disuse** syndrome: Risk factor: severe pain

Readiness for enhanced **Knowledge:** expresses an interest in learning

Bacteremia

Risk for **Infection:** Risk factor: compromised immune system

Risk for **Shock:** Risk factor: development of systemic inflammatory response from presence of bacteria in bloodstream

See Infection; Infection, Potential for

Barrel Chest

See Aging (if appropriate); COPD (Chronic Obstructive Pulmonary Disease)

Bathing/Hygiene Problems

Impaired **Mobility** r/t chronic physically limiting condition

Self-Neglect (See **Self-Neglect,** Section III)

Bathing **Self-Care** deficit (See **Self-Care** deficit, bathing, Section III)

Battered Child Syndrome

Dysfunctional **Family** processes r/t inadequate coping skills

Sleep deprivation r/t prolonged psychological discomfort

Chronic **Sorrow** r/t situational crises

Risk for **Post-Trauma** syndrome: Risk factors: physical abuse, incest, rape, molestation

Risk for **Self-Mutilation:** Risk factors: feelings of rejection, dysfunctional family

Risk for **Suicide:** Risk factor: childhood abuse

See Child Abuse

Battered Person

See Abuse, Spouse, Parent, or Significant Other

Bedbugs, Infestation

Impaired **Home** maintenance r/t deficient knowledge regarding prevention of bedbug infestation

Impaired **Skin** integrity r/t bites of bedbugs

See Itching; Pruritus

Bed Mobility, Impaired

Impaired bed **Mobility** (See **Mobility,** bed, impaired, Section III)

Bed Rest, Prolonged

Deficient **Diversional** activity r/t prolonged bed rest

Impaired bed **Mobility** r/t neuromuscular impairment

Social isolation r/t prolonged bed rest

Risk for chronic functional **Constipation:** Risk factor: insufficient physical activity

Risk for **Disuse** syndrome: Risk factor: prolonged immobility

Risk for **Frail Elderly** syndrome: Risk factor: prolonged immobility

Risk for **Loneliness:** Risk factor: prolonged bed rest

Risk for **Overweight:** Risk factor: energy expenditure below energy intake

Risk for **Pressure** ulcer: Risk factor: prolonged immobility

Bedsores

See Pressure Ulcer

Bedwetting

Ineffective **Health** maintenance r/t unachieved developmental level, neuromuscular immaturity, diseases of the urinary system

Bell's Palsy

Disturbed **Body Image** r/t loss of motor control on one side of face

Imbalanced **Nutrition:** less than body requirements r/t difficulty with chewing

Acute **Pain** r/t inflammation of facial nerve

Risk for **Injury** (eye): Risk factors: decreased tears, decreased blinking of eye

Readiness for enhanced **Knowledge:** expresses an interest in learning

Benign Prostatic Hypertrophy

See BPH (Benign Prostatic Hypertrophy); Prostatic Hypertrophy

Bereavement

Grieving r/t loss of significant person

Insomnia r/t grief

Risk for complicated **Grieving:** Risk factor: emotional instability, lack of social support

Risk for **Spiritual** distress: Risk factor: death of a loved one

Biliary Atresia

Anxiety r/t surgical intervention, possible liver transplantation

Impaired **Comfort** r/t inflammation of skin, itching

Imbalanced **Nutrition:** less than body requirements r/t decreased absorption of fat and fat-soluble vitamins, poor feeding

Risk for **Bleeding:** Risk factors: vitamin K deficiency, altered clotting mechanisms

Risk for ineffective **Breathing** pattern: Risk factors: enlarged liver, development of ascites

Risk for impaired **Skin** integrity: Risk factor: pruritus

See Child with Chronic Condition; Cirrhosis (as complication); Hospitalized Child; Terminally Ill: Child, Adolescent; Infant/Toddler; Preschool Child; School-Age Child/Preadolescent; Death of Child, Parent

Biliary Calculus

See Cholelithiasis

Biliary Obstruction

See Jaundice

Bilirubin Elevation in Neonate

Neonatal **Jaundice** (See **Jaundice,** Neonatal, Section III)

Biopsy

Fear r/t outcome of biopsy

Readiness for enhanced **Knowledge:** expresses an interest in learning

Bioterrorism

Contamination r/t exposure to bioterrorism

Risk for **Infection:** Risk factor: exposure to harmful biological agent

Risk for **Post-Trauma** syndrome: Risk factor: perception of event of bioterrorism

Bipolar Disorder I (Most Recent Episode, Depressed or Manic)

Ineffective **Activity** planning r/t unrealistic perception of events

Fatigue r/t psychological demands

Risk-prone **Health** behavior r/t low state of optimism

Ineffective **Health** maintenance r/t lack of ability to make good judgments regarding ways to obtain help

Self-Care deficit: specify r/t depression, cognitive impairment

Chronic low **Self-Esteem** r/t repeated unmet expectations

Social isolation r/t ineffective coping

Risk for complicated **Grieving:** Risk factor: lack of previous resolution of former grieving response

Risk for **Loneliness:** Risk factors: stress, conflict

Risk for **Spiritual** distress: Risk factor: mental illness

Risk for **Suicide:** Risk factors: psychiatric disorder, poor support system

See Depression (Major Depressive Disorder); Manic Disorder, Bipolar I

Birth Asphyxia

See Asphyxia, Birth

Birth Control

See Contraceptive Method

Bladder Cancer

Urinary Retention r/t clots obstructing urethra

See Cancer; TURP (Transurethral Resection of the Prostate)

Bladder Distention

Urinary Retention r/t high urethral pressure caused by weak detrusor, inhibition of reflex arc, blockage, strong sphincter

Bladder Training

Disturbed **Body Image** r/t difficulty maintaining control of urinary elimination

Functional urinary **Incontinence** r/t altered environment; sensory, cognitive, mobility deficit

Stress urinary **Incontinence** r/t degenerative change in pelvic muscles and structural supports

Urge urinary **Incontinence** r/t decreased bladder capacity, increased urine concentration, overdistention of bladder

Readiness for enhanced **Knowledge:** expresses an interest in learning

Bladder Training, Child

See Toilet Training

Bleeding Tendency

Risk for **Bleeding** (See **Bleeding**, risk for, Section III)

Risk for delayed **Surgical** recovery: Risk factor: bleeding tendency

Blepharoplasty

Disturbed **Body Image** r/t effects of surgery

Readiness for enhanced **Knowledge:** expresses an interest in learning

Blindness

Interrupted **Family** processes r/t shift in health status of family member (change in visual acuity)

Impaired **Home** maintenance r/t decreased vision

Ineffective **Role** performance r/t alteration in health status (change in visual acuity)

Self-Care deficit: specify r/t inability to see to be able to perform activities of daily living

Vision Loss r/t impaired sensory reception, transmission, or integration (*see care plan in Appendix*)

Risk for delayed **Development:** Risk factor: vision impairment

Risk for **Injury:** Risk factor: sensory dysfunction

Readiness for enhanced **Knowledge:** expresses an interest in learning

See Vision Impairment

Blood Disorder

Ineffective **Protection** r/t abnormal blood profile

Risk for **Bleeding:** Risk factor: abnormal blood profile

See ITP (Idiopathic Thrombocytopenic Purpura), Hemophilia, Lacerations, Shock, Hypovolemic

Blood Pressure Alteration

See Hypotension; HTN (Hypertension)

Blood Sugar Control

Risk for unstable blood **Glucose** level (See **Glucose** level, blood, unstable, risk for, Section III)

Blood Transfusion

Anxiety r/t possibility of harm from transfusion

See Anemia

Body Dysmorphic Disorder

Anxiety r/t perceived defect of body

Disturbed **Body Image** r/t overinvolvement in physical appearance

Chronic low **Self-Esteem** r/t lack of self valuing because of perceived body defects

Social isolation r/t distancing self from others because of perceived self body defects

Risk for **Suicide:** Risk factor: perceived defects of body affecting self-valuing and hopes

Body Image Change

Disturbed **Body Image** (See **Body Image,** disturbed, Section III)

Body Temperature, Altered

Ineffective **Thermoregulation** (See **Thermoregulation,** ineffective, Section III)

Bone Marrow Biopsy

Fear r/t unknown outcome of results of biopsy

Acute **Pain** r/t bone marrow aspiration

Readiness for enhanced **Knowledge:** expresses an interest in learning

See disease necessitating bone marrow biopsy (e.g., Leukemia)

Borderline Personality Disorder

Ineffective **Activity** planning r/t unrealistic perception of events

Anxiety r/t perceived threat to self-concept

Defensive **Coping** r/t difficulty with relationships, inability to accept blame for own behavior

Ineffective **Coping** r/t use of maladjusted defense mechanisms (e.g., projection, denial)

Powerlessness r/t lifestyle of helplessness

Social isolation r/t immature interests

Ineffective family **Health** management r/t manipulative behavior of client

Risk for **Caregiver Role Strain:** Risk factors: inability of care receiver to accept criticism, care receiver taking advantage of others to meet own needs or having unreasonable expectations

Risk for **Self-Mutilation:** Risk factors: ineffective coping, feelings of self-hatred

Risk for **Spiritual** distress: Risk factor: poor relationships associated with abnormal behaviors

Risk for self-directed **Violence:** Risk factors: feelings of need to punish self, manipulative behavior

Boredom

Deficient **Diversional** activity r/t environmental lack of diversional activity

Impaired **Mood** regulation r/t emotional instability

Social isolation r/t altered state of wellness

Botulism

Deficient **Fluid** volume r/t profuse diarrhea

Readiness for enhanced **Knowledge:** expresses an interest in learning

Bowel Incontinence

Bowel **Incontinence** r/t decreased awareness of need to defecate, loss of sphincter control, fecal impaction

Readiness for enhanced **Knowledge:** expresses an interest in learning

Bowel Obstruction

Constipation r/t decreased motility, intestinal obstruction

Deficient **Fluid** volume r/t inadequate fluid volume intake, fluid loss in bowel

Imbalanced **Nutrition:** less than body requirements r/t nausea, vomiting

Acute **Pain** r/t pressure from distended abdomen

Bowel Resection

See Abdominal Surgery

Bowel Sounds, Absent or Diminished

Constipation r/t decreased or absent peristalsis

Deficient **Fluid** volume r/t inability to ingest fluids, loss of fluids in bowel

Delayed **Surgical** recovery r/t inability to obtain adequate nutritional status

Risk for dysfunctional **Gastrointestinal** motility (See **Gastrointestinal** motility, dysfunctional, risk for, Section III)

Bowel Sounds, Hyperactive

Diarrhea r/t increased gastrointestinal motility

Bowel Training

Bowel **Incontinence** r/t loss of control of rectal sphincter

Readiness for enhanced **Knowledge:** expresses an interest in learning

Bowel Training, Child

See Toilet Training

BPH (Benign Prostatic Hypertrophy)

Ineffective **Health** maintenance r/t deficient knowledge regarding self-care with prostatic hypertrophy

Insomnia r/t nocturia

Urinary Retention r/t obstruction of urethra

Risk for urge urinary **Incontinence:** Risk factors: detrusor muscle instability with impaired contractility, involuntary sphincter relaxation

Risk for **Infection:** Risk factors: urinary residual after voiding, bacterial invasion of bladder

Readiness for enhanced **Knowledge:** expresses an interest in learning

See Prostatic Hypertrophy

Bradycardia

Decreased **Cardiac** output r/t slow heart rate supplying inadequate amount of blood for body function

Risk for ineffective **Cerebral** tissue perfusion: Risk factors: decreased cardiac output secondary to bradycardia, vagal response

Readiness for enhanced **Knowledge:** expresses an interest in learning

Bradypnea

Ineffective **Breathing** pattern r/t neuromuscular impairment, pain, musculoskeletal impairment, perception or cognitive impairment, anxiety, fatigue or decreased energy, effects of drugs

See Sleep apnea (See **Airway** clearance, ineffective, Section III)

Brain Injury

See Intracranial Pressure, Increased

Brain Surgery

See Craniectomy/Craniotomy

Brain Tumor

Acute **Confusion** r/t pressure from tumor

Fear r/t threat to well-being

Grieving r/t potential loss of physiosocial-psychosocial well-being

Decreased **Intracranial** adaptive capacity r/t presence of brain tumor

Acute **Pain** r/t pressure from tumor

Vision Loss r/t tumor growth compressing optic nerve and/or brain tissue

Risk for **Injury:** Risk factors: sensory-perceptual alterations, weakness

Risk for **Hyperthermia:** Risk factor: loss of thermoregulation with hypothalamic dysfunction

See Cancer; Chemotherapy; Child with Chronic Condition; Craniectomy/Craniotomy; Hospitalized Child; Radiation Therapy; Terminally Ill Child, Adolescent; Terminally Ill Child, Infant/Toddler; Terminally Ill Child, Preschool Child; Terminally Ill Child, School-Age Child/Preadolescent; Terminally Ill Child/Death of Child, Parent

Braxton Hicks Contractions

Activity intolerance r/t increased contractions with increased gestation

Anxiety r/t uncertainty about beginning labor

Fatigue r/t lack of sleep

Stress urinary **Incontinence** r/t increased pressure on bladder with contractions

Insomnia r/t contractions when lying down

Ineffective **Sexuality** pattern r/t fear of contractions associated with loss of infant

Breast Biopsy

Fear r/t potential for diagnosis of cancer

Risk for **Spiritual** distress: Risk factor: fear of diagnosis of cancer

Readiness for enhanced **Knowledge:** expresses an interest in learning

Breast Cancer

Death **Anxiety** r/t diagnosis of cancer

Ineffective **Coping** r/t treatment, prognosis

Fear r/t diagnosis of cancer

Sexual dysfunction r/t loss of body part, partner's reaction to loss

Chronic **Sorrow** r/t diagnosis of cancer, loss of body integrity

Risk for **Spiritual** distress: Risk factor: fear of diagnosis of cancer

Readiness for enhanced **Knowledge:** expresses an interest in learning

See Cancer; Chemotherapy; Mastectomy; Radiation Therapy

Breast Examination, Self

See SBE (Self-Breast Examination)

Breast Lumps

Fear r/t potential for diagnosis of cancer

Readiness for enhanced **Knowledge:** expresses an interest in learning

Breast Pumping

Risk for **Infection:** Risk factors: possible contaminated breast pump, incomplete emptying of breast

Risk for impaired **Skin** integrity: Risk factor: high suction

Readiness for enhanced **Knowledge:** expresses an interest in learning

Breastfeeding, Effective

Readiness for enhanced **Breastfeeding** (See **Breastfeeding,** readiness for enhanced, Section III)

Breastfeeding, Ineffective

Ineffective **Breastfeeding** (See **Breastfeeding,** ineffective, Section III)

See Infant Feeding Pattern, Ineffective; Painful Breasts, Engorgement; Painful Breasts, Sore Nipples

Breastfeeding, Interrupted

Interrupted **Breastfeeding** (See **Breastfeeding,** interrupted, Section III)

Breast Milk, Insufficient

Insufficient **Breast Milk** (See **Breast Milk,** insufficient, Section III)

Breath Sounds, Decreased or Absent

See Atelectasis; Pneumothorax

Breathing Pattern Alteration

Ineffective **Breathing** pattern r/t neuromuscular impairment, pain, musculoskeletal impairment, perception or cognitive impairment, anxiety, decreased energy or fatigue

Breech Birth

Fear: maternal r/t danger to infant, self

Impaired **Gas** exchange: fetal r/t compressed umbilical cord

Risk for **Aspiration:** fetal: Risk factor: birth of body before head

Risk for delayed **Development:** Risk factor: compressed umbilical cord

Risk for impaired **Tissue** integrity: fetal: Risk factor: difficult birth

Risk for impaired **Tissue** integrity: maternal: Risk factor: difficult birth

Bronchitis

Ineffective **Airway** clearance r/t excessive thickened mucus secretion

Readiness for enhanced **Health** management: wishes to stop smoking

Readiness for enhanced **Knowledge:** expresses an interest in learning

Bronchopulmonary Dysplasia

Activity intolerance r/t imbalance between oxygen supply and demand

Excess **Fluid** volume r/t sodium and water retention

Imbalanced **Nutrition:** less than body requirements r/t poor feeding, increased caloric needs as a result of increased work of breathing

See Child with Chronic Condition; Hospitalized Child; Respiratory Conditions of the Neonate

Bronchoscopy

Risk for **Aspiration:** Risk factor: temporary loss of gag reflex

Risk for **Injury:** Risk factors: complication of pneumothorax, laryngeal edema, hemorrhage (if biopsy done)

Bruits, Carotid

Risk for ineffective **Cerebral** tissue perfusion: Risk factors: interruption of carotid blood flow to brain

Bryant's Traction

See Traction and Casts

Buck's Traction

See Traction and Casts

Buerger's Disease

See Peripheral Vascular Disease (PVD)

Bulimia

Disturbed **Body Image** r/t misperception about actual appearance, body weight

Compromised family **Coping** r/t chronically unresolved feelings of guilt, anger, hostility

Defensive **Coping** r/t eating disorder

Diarrhea r/t laxative abuse

Fear r/t food ingestion, weight gain

Imbalanced **Nutrition:** less than body requirements r/t induced vomiting, excessive exercise, laxative abuse

Powerlessness r/t urge to purge self after eating

Chronic low **Self-Esteem** r/t lack of positive feedback

See Maturational Issues, Adolescent

Bunion

Readiness for enhanced **Knowledge:** expresses an interest in learning

Bunionectomy

Impaired physical **Mobility** r/t sore foot

Impaired **Walking** r/t pain associated with surgery

Risk for **Infection:** Risk factors: surgical incision, advanced age

Readiness for enhanced **Knowledge:** expresses an interest in learning

Burn Risk

Risk for **Thermal** injury (See **Thermal** injury, risk for, Section III)

Burns

Anxiety r/t burn injury, treatments

Disturbed **Body Image** r/t altered physical appearance

Deficient **Diversional** activity r/t long-term hospitalization

Fear r/t pain from treatments, possible permanent disfigurement

Deficient **Fluid** volume r/t loss of protective skin

Grieving r/t loss of bodily function, loss of future hopes and plans

Hypothermia r/t impaired skin integrity

Impaired physical **Mobility** r/t pain, musculoskeletal impairment, contracture formation

Imbalanced **Nutrition:** less than body requirements r/t increased metabolic needs, anorexia, protein and fluid loss

Acute **Pain** r/t burn injury, treatments

Chronic **Pain** r/t burn injury, treatments

Ineffective peripheral **Tissue Perfusion** r/t circumferential burns, impaired arterial/venous circulation

Post-Trauma syndrome r/t life-threatening event

Impaired **Skin** integrity r/t injury of skin

Delayed **Surgical** recovery r/t ineffective tissue perfusion

Risk for ineffective **Airway** clearance: Risk factors: potential tracheobronchial obstruction, edema

Risk for deficient **Fluid** volume: Risk factors: loss from skin surface, fluid shift

Risk for **Infection:** Risk factors: loss of intact skin, trauma, invasive sites

Risk for **Peripheral Neurovascular** dysfunction: Risk factor: eschar formation with circumferential burn

Risk for **Post-Trauma** syndrome: Risk factors: perception, duration of event that caused burns

Readiness for enhanced **Knowledge:** expresses an interest in learning

See Hospitalized Child; Safety, Childhood

Bursitis

Impaired physical **Mobility** r/t inflammation in joint

Acute **Pain** r/t inflammation in joint

Bypass Graft

See Coronary Artery Bypass Grafting (CABG)

C

CABG (Coronary Artery Bypass Grafting)

See Coronary Artery Bypass Grafting (CABG)

Cachexia

Frail Elderly syndrome r/t fatigue, feeding self-care deficit

Imbalanced **Nutrition:** less than body requirements r/t inability to ingest food because of physiological factors

Risk for **Infection:** Risk factor: inadequate nutrition

Calcium Alteration

See Hypercalcemia; Hypocalcemia

Cancer

Activity intolerance r/t side effects of treatment, weakness from cancer

Death **Anxiety** r/t unresolved issues regarding dying

Disturbed **Body Image** r/t side effects of treatment, cachexia

Decisional Conflict r/t selection of treatment choices, continuation or discontinuation of treatment, "do not resuscitate" decision

Constipation r/t side effects of medication, altered nutrition, decreased activity

Compromised family **Coping** r/t prolonged disease or disability progression that exhausts supportive ability of significant others

Ineffective **Coping** r/t personal vulnerability in situational crisis, terminal illness

Ineffective **Denial** r/t complicated grieving process

Fear r/t serious threat to well-being

Grieving r/t potential loss of significant others, high risk for infertility

Ineffective **Health** maintenance r/t deficient knowledge regarding prescribed treatment

Hopelessness r/t loss of control, terminal illness

Insomnia r/t anxiety, pain

Impaired physical **Mobility** r/t weakness, neuromusculoskeletal impairment, pain

Imbalanced **Nutrition:** less than body requirements r/t loss of appetite, difficulty swallowing, side effects of chemotherapy, obstruction by tumor

Impaired **Oral Mucous Membrane** r/t chemotherapy, effects of radiation, oral pH changes, decreased oral secretions

Chronic **Pain** r/t metastatic cancer

Powerlessness r/t treatment, progression of disease

Ineffective **Protection** r/t cancer suppressing immune system

Ineffective **Role** performance r/t change in physical capacity, inability to resume prior role

Self-Care deficit: specify r/t pain, intolerance to activity, decreased strength

Impaired **Skin** integrity r/t immunological deficit, immobility

Social isolation r/t hospitalization, lifestyle changes

Chronic **Sorrow** r/t chronic illness of cancer

Spiritual distress r/t test of spiritual beliefs

Risk for **Bleeding:** Risk factor: bone marrow depression from chemotherapy

Risk for **Disuse** syndrome: Risk factors: immobility, fatigue

Risk for impaired **Home** maintenance: Risk factor: lack of familiarity with community resources

Risk for **Infection:** Risk factor: inadequate immune system

Risk for compromised **Resilience:** Risk factors: multiple stressors, pain, chronic illness

Risk for **Spiritual** distress: Risk factor: physical illness of cancer

Readiness for enhanced **Knowledge:** expresses an interest in learning

Readiness for enhanced **Spiritual** well-being: desire for harmony with self, others, higher power, God, when faced with serious illness

See Chemotherapy; Child with Chronic Condition; Hospitalized Child; Leukemia; Radiation Therapy; Terminally Ill Child, Adolescent; Terminally Ill Child, Infant/Toddler; Terminally Ill Child, Preschool Child; Terminally Ill Child, School-Age Child/Preadolescent; Terminally Ill Child/Death of Child, Parent

Candidiasis, Oral

Readiness for enhanced **Knowledge:** expresses an interest in learning

Impaired **Oral Mucous Membrane** r/t overgrowth of infectious agent, depressed immune function

Acute **Pain** r/t oral condition

Capillary Refill Time, Prolonged

Impaired **Gas** exchange r/t ventilation perfusion imbalance

Ineffective peripheral **Tissue Perfusion** r/t interruption of arterial flow

See Shock, Hypovolemic

Carbon Monoxide Poisoning

See Smoke Inhalation

Cardiac Arrest

Post-Trauma syndrome r/t experiencing serious life event

See Dysrhythmia, MI

Cardiac Catheterization

Fear r/t invasive procedure, uncertainty of outcome of procedure

Risk for **Injury:** hematoma: Risk factor: invasive procedure

Risk for decreased **Cardiac** tissue perfusion: Risk factors: ventricular ischemia, dysrhythmia

Risk for **Peripheral Neurovascular** dysfunction: Risk factor: vascular obstruction

Risk for Impaired **Tissue** integrity: Risk factor: invasive procedure

Readiness for enhanced **Knowledge:** expresses an interest in learning postprocedure care, treatment, and prevention of coronary artery disease

Cardiac Disorders

Decreased **Cardiac** output r/t cardiac disorder

Risk for decreased **Cardiac** tissue perfusion: Risk factor: cardiac disorder

See specific cardiac disorder

Cardiac Disorders in Pregnancy

Activity intolerance r/t cardiac pathophysiology, increased demand for cardiac output because of pregnancy, weakness, fatigue

Death **Anxiety** r/t potential danger of condition

Compromised family **Coping** r/t prolonged hospitalization or maternal incapacitation that exhausts supportive capacity of significant others

Ineffective **Coping** r/t personal vulnerability

Interrupted **Family** processes r/t hospitalization, maternal incapacitation, changes in roles

Fatigue r/t physiological, psychological, and emotional demands

Fear r/t potential maternal effects, potential poor fetal or maternal outcome

Powerlessness r/t illness-related regimen

Ineffective **Role** performance r/t changes in lifestyle, expectations from disease process with superimposed pregnancy

Situational low **Self-Esteem** r/t situational crisis, pregnancy

Social isolation r/t limitations of activity, bed rest or hospitalization, separation from family and friends

Risk for decreased **Cardiac** tissue perfusion: Risk factor: strain on compromised heart from work of pregnancy, delivery

Risk for delayed **Development:** Risk factor: poor maternal oxygenation

Risk for deficient **Fluid** volume: Risk factor: sudden changes in circulation after delivery of placenta

Risk for excess **Fluid** volume: Risk factors: compromised regulatory mechanism with increased afterload, preload, circulating blood volume

Risk for impaired **Gas** exchange: Risk factor: pulmonary edema

Risk for disproportionate **Growth:** Risk factor: poor maternal oxygenation

Risk for disturbed **Maternal–Fetal** dyad: Risk factor: compromised oxygen transport

Risk for compromised **Resilience:** Risk factors: multiple stressors, fear

Risk for **Spiritual** distress: Risk factor: fear of diagnosis for self and infant

Readiness for enhanced **Knowledge:** expresses an interest in learning

Cardiac Dysrhythmia

See Dysrhythmia

Cardiac Output, Decreased

Decreased **Cardiac** output r/t cardiac dysfunction

Decreased **Cardiac** output (See **Cardiac** output, decreased, Section III)

Oliguria r/t cardiac dysfunction

Risk for decreased **Cardiac** output (See **Cardiac** output, risk for decreased, Section III)

Cardiac Tamponade

Decreased **Cardiac** output r/t fluid in pericardial sac

See Pericarditis

Cardiogenic Shock

See Shock, Cardiogenic

Cardiovascular Function: Risk for Impaired

Risk for Impaired **Cardiovascular** Function (See impaired **Cardiovascular** function, risk for, Section III)

Caregiver Role Strain

Caregiver Role Strain (See **Caregiver Role Strain,** Section III)

Risk for compromised **Resilience:** Risk factor: stress of prolonged caregiving

Carious Teeth

See Cavities in Teeth

Carotid Endarterectomy

Fear r/t surgery in vital area

Risk for ineffective **Airway** clearance: Risk factor: hematoma compressing trachea

Risk for **Bleeding:** Risk factor: possible hematoma formation, trauma to region

Risk for ineffective **Cerebral** tissue perfusion: Risk factors: hemorrhage, clot formation

Readiness for enhanced **Knowledge:** expresses an interest in learning

Carpal Tunnel Syndrome

Impaired physical **Mobility** r/t neuromuscular impairment

Chronic **Pain** r/t unrelieved pressure on median nerve

Self-Care deficit: bathing, dressing, feeding r/t pain

Carpopedal Spasm

See Hypocalcemia

Casts

Deficient **Diversional** activity r/t physical limitations from cast

Impaired physical **Mobility** r/t limb immobilization

Self-Care deficit: bathing, dressing, feeding r/t presence of cast(s) on upper extremities

Self-Care deficit: toileting r/t presence of cast(s) on lower extremities

Impaired **Walking** r/t cast(s) on lower extremities, fracture of bones

Risk for **Peripheral Neurovascular** dysfunction: Risk factors: mechanical compression from cast, trauma from fracture

Risk for impaired **Skin** integrity: Risk factor: unrelieved pressure on skin from cast

Readiness for enhanced **Knowledge:** expresses an interest in learning

See Traction and Casts

Cataract Extraction

Anxiety r/t threat of permanent vision loss, surgical procedure

Vision Loss r/t edema from surgery (*see care plan in Appendix*)

Risk for **Injury:** Risk factors: increased intraocular pressure, accommodation to new visual field

Readiness for enhanced **Knowledge:** expresses an interest in learning

See Vision Impairment

Cataracts

Vision Loss r/t impaired sensory input (*see care plan in Appendix*)

See Vision Impairment

Catatonic Schizophrenia

Impaired verbal **Communication** r/t cognitive impairment

Impaired **Memory** r/t cognitive impairment

Impaired physical **Mobility** r/t cognitive impairment, maintenance of rigid posture, inappropriate or bizarre postures

Imbalanced **Nutrition:** less than body requirements r/t decrease in outside stimulation, loss of perception of hunger, resistance to instructions to eat

Social isolation r/t inability to communicate, immobility

See Schizophrenia

Catheterization, Urinary

Risk for **Infection:** Risk factor: invasive procedure

Readiness for enhanced **Knowledge:** expresses an interest in learning

Cavities in Teeth

Impaired **Dentition** r/t ineffective oral hygiene, barriers to self-care, economic barriers to professional care, nutritional deficits, dietary habits

Celiac Disease

Diarrhea r/t malabsorption of food, immune effects of gluten on gastrointestinal system

Imbalanced **Nutrition:** less than body requirements r/t malabsorption due to immune effects of gluten

Readiness for enhanced **Knowledge:** expresses an interest in learning

Cellulitis

Acute **Pain** r/t inflammatory changes in tissues from infection

Impaired **Tissue** integrity r/t inflammatory process damaging skin and underlying tissue

Ineffective peripheral **Tissue Perfusion** r/t edema of extremities

Risk for **Vascular Trauma:** Risk factor: infusion of antibiotics

Readiness for enhanced **Knowledge:** expresses an interest in learning

Cellulitis, Periorbital

Acute **Pain** r/t edema and inflammation of skin/tissues

Impaired **Skin** integrity r/t inflammation or infection of skin, tissues

Vision Loss r/t decreased visual field secondary to edema of eyelids (*see care plan in Appendix*)

Readiness for enhanced **Knowledge:** expresses an interest in learning

See Hospitalized Child

Central Line Insertion

Risk for **Infection:** Risk factor: invasive procedure

Risk for **Vascular Trauma** (See **Vascular Trauma**, risk for, Section III)

Readiness for enhanced **Knowledge:** expresses an interest in learning

Cerebral Aneurysm

See Craniectomy/Craniotomy; Intracranial Pressure, Increased; Subarachnoid Hemorrhage

Cerebral Palsy

Impaired verbal **Communication** r/t impaired ability to articulate or speak words because of facial muscle involvement

Deficient **Diversional** activity r/t physical impairments, limitations on ability to participate in recreational activities

Impaired physical **Mobility** r/t spasticity, neuromuscular impairment or weakness

Imbalanced **Nutrition:** less than body requirements r/t spasticity, feeding or swallowing difficulties

Self-Care deficit: specify r/t neuromuscular impairments, sensory deficits

Impaired **Social** interaction r/t impaired communication skills, limited physical activity, perceived differences from peers

Chronic **Sorrow** r/t presence of chronic disability

Risk for **Falls:** Risk factor: impaired physical mobility

Risk for **Injury:** Risk factors: muscle weakness, inability to control spasticity

Risk for impaired **Parenting:** Risk factor: caring for child with overwhelming needs resulting from chronic change in health status

Risk for **Spiritual** distress: Risk factor: psychological stress associated with chronic illness

See Child with Chronic Condition

Cerebral Perfusion

Risk for ineffective **Cerebral** tissue perfusion (See **Cerebral** tissue perfusion, ineffective, risk for, Section III)

Cerebrovascular Accident (CVA)

See CVA (Cerebrovascular Accident)

Cervicitis

Ineffective **Health** maintenance r/t deficient knowledge regarding care and prevention of condition

Ineffective **Sexuality** pattern r/t abstinence during acute stage

Risk for **Infection:** Risk factors: spread of infection, recurrence of infection

Cesarean Delivery

Disturbed **Body Image** r/t surgery, unmet expectations for childbirth

Interrupted **Family** processes r/t unmet expectations for childbirth

Fear r/t perceived threat to own well-being, outcome of birth

Impaired physical **Mobility** r/t pain

Acute **Pain** r/t surgical incision

Ineffective **Role** performance r/t unmet expectations for childbirth

Situational low **Self-Esteem** r/t inability to deliver child vaginally

Risk for **Bleeding:** Risk factor: surgery

Risk for imbalanced **Fluid** volume: Risk factors: loss of blood, fluid shifts

Risk for **Infection:** Risk factor: surgical incision

Risk for **Urinary Retention:** Risk factor: regional anesthesia

Readiness for enhanced **Childbearing** process: a pattern of preparing for, maintaining, and strengthening care of newborn

Readiness for enhanced **Knowledge:** expresses an interest in learning

Chemical Dependence

See Alcoholism; Drug Abuse; Cocaine Abuse; Substance Abuse

Chemotherapy

Death **Anxiety** r/t chemotherapy not accomplishing desired results

Disturbed **Body Image** r/t loss of weight, loss of hair

Fatigue r/t disease process, anemia, drug effects

Nausea r/t effects of chemotherapy

Imbalanced **Nutrition:** less than body requirements r/t side effects of chemotherapy

Impaired **Oral Mucous Membrane** r/t effects of chemotherapy

Ineffective **Protection** r/t suppressed immune system, decreased platelets

C

Risk for **Bleeding:** Risk factors: tumor eroding blood vessel, stress effects on gastrointestinal system

Risk for **Infection:** Risk factor: immunosuppression

Risk for **Vascular Trauma:** Risk factor: infusion of irritating medications

Readiness for enhanced **Knowledge:** expresses an interest in learning

See Cancer

Chest Pain

Fear r/t potential threat of death

Acute **Pain** r/t myocardial injury, ischemia

Risk for decreased **Cardiac** tissue perfusion: Risk factor: ventricular ischemia

See Angina; MI (Myocardial Infarction)

Chest Tubes

Ineffective **Breathing** pattern r/t asymmetrical lung expansion secondary to pain

Impaired **Gas** exchange r/t decreased functional lung tissue

Acute **Pain** r/t presence of chest tubes, injury

Risk for **Injury:** Risk factor: presence of invasive chest tube

Cheyne-Stokes Respiration

Ineffective **Breathing** pattern r/t critical illness

See Heart Failure

CHF (Congestive Heart Failure)

See Heart Failure

Chickenpox

See Communicable Diseases, Childhood

Child Abuse

Interrupted **Family** processes r/t inadequate coping skills

Fear r/t threat of punishment for perceived wrongdoing

Insomnia r/t hypervigilance, fear

Imbalanced **Nutrition:** less than body requirements r/t inadequate caretaking

Acute **Pain** r/t physical injuries

Impaired **Parenting** r/t psychological impairment, physical or emotional abuse of parent, substance abuse, unrealistic expectations of child

Post-Trauma syndrome r/t physical abuse, incest, rape, molestation

Chronic low **Self-Esteem** r/t lack of positive feedback, excessive negative feedback

Impaired **Skin** integrity r/t altered nutritional state, physical abuse

Social isolation: family imposed r/t fear of disclosure of family dysfunction and abuse

Risk for delayed **Development:** Risk factors: shaken baby syndrome, abuse

Risk for disproportionate **Growth:** Risk factor: abuse

Risk for **Poisoning:** Risk factors: inadequate safeguards, lack of proper safety precautions, accessibility of illicit substances because of impaired home maintenance

Risk for **Suffocation:** Risk factors: unattended child, unsafe environment

Risk for **Trauma:** Risk factors: inadequate precautions, cognitive or emotional difficulties

Childbearing Problems

Ineffective **Childbearing** process (See **Childbearing** process, ineffective, Section III)

Risk for ineffective **Childbearing** process: See **Childbearing** process, risk for ineffective, Section III)

Child Neglect

See Child Abuse; Failure to Thrive, Nonorganic

Child with Chronic Condition

Activity intolerance r/t fatigue associated with chronic illness

Compromised family **Coping** r/t prolonged overconcern for child; distortion of reality regarding child's health problem, including extreme denial about its existence or severity

Disabled family **Coping** r/t prolonged disease or disability progression that exhausts supportive capacity of significant others

Ineffective **Coping:** child r/t situational or maturational crises

Decisional Conflict r/t treatment options, conflicting values

Deficient **Diversional** activity r/t immobility, monotonous environment, frequent or lengthy treatments, reluctance to participate, self-imposed social isolation

Interrupted **Family** processes r/t intermittent situational crisis of illness, disease, hospitalization

Ineffective **Health** maintenance r/t exhausting family resources (finances, physical energy, support systems)

Impaired **Home** maintenance r/t overtaxed family members (e.g., exhausted, anxious)

Hopelessness: child r/t prolonged activity restriction, long-term stress, lack of involvement in or passively allowing care as a result of parental overprotection

Insomnia: child or parent r/t time-intensive treatments, exacerbation of condition, 24-hour care needs

Deficient **Knowledge** r/t knowledge or skill acquisition regarding health practices, acceptance of limitations, promotion of maximal potential of child, self-actualization of rest of family

Imbalanced **Nutrition:** less than body requirements r/t anorexia, fatigue from physical exertion

Risk for **Overweight** r/t effects of steroid medications on appetite

Chronic **Pain** r/t physical, biological, chemical, or psychological factors

Powerlessness: child r/t health care environment, illness-related regimen, lifestyle of learned helplessness

Parental **Role** conflict r/t separation from child as a result of chronic illness, home care of child with special needs, interruptions of family life resulting from home care regimen

Chronic low **Self-Esteem** r/t actual or perceived differences; peer acceptance; decreased ability to participate in physical, school, and social activities

Ineffective **Sexuality** pattern: parental r/t disrupted relationship with sexual partner

Impaired **Social** interaction r/t developmental lag or delay, perceived differences

Social isolation: family r/t actual or perceived social stigmatization, complex care requirements

Chronic **Sorrow** r/t developmental stages and missed opportunities or milestones that bring comparisons with social or personal norms, unending caregiving as reminder of loss

Risk for delayed **Development:** Risk factor: chronic illness

Risk for disproportionate **Growth:** Risk factor: chronic illness

Risk for **Infection:** Risk factor: debilitating physical condition

Risk for impaired **Parenting:** Risk factors: impaired or disrupted bonding, caring for child with perceived overwhelming care needs

Readiness for enhanced family **Coping:** impact of crisis on family values, priorities, goals, or relationships; changes in family choices to optimize wellness

Childbirth

Readiness for enhanced **Childbearing** process (See **Childbearing** process, readiness for enhanced, Section III)

See Labor, Normal; Postpartum, Normal Care

Chills

Hyperthermia r/t infectious process

Chlamydia Infection

See STD (Sexually Transmitted Disease)

Chloasma

Disturbed **Body Image** r/t change in skin color

Choking or Coughing with Eating

Impaired **Swallowing** r/t neuromuscular impairment

Risk for **Aspiration:** Risk factors: depressed cough and gag reflexes

Cholecystectomy

Imbalanced **Nutrition:** less than body requirements r/t high metabolic needs, decreased ability to digest fatty foods

Acute **Pain** r/t trauma from surgery

Risk for deficient **Fluid** volume: Risk factors: restricted intake, nausea, vomiting

Readiness for enhanced **Knowledge:** expresses an interest in learning

See Abdominal Surgery

Cholelithiasis

Nausea r/t obstruction of bile

Imbalanced **Nutrition:** less than body requirements r/t anorexia, nausea, vomiting

Acute **Pain** r/t obstruction of bile flow, inflammation in gallbladder

Readiness for enhanced **Knowledge:** expresses an interest in learning

Chorioamnionitis

Anxiety r/t threat to self and infant

Grieving r/t guilt about potential loss of ideal pregnancy and birth

Hyperthermia r/t infectious process

Situational low **Self-Esteem** r/t guilt about threat to infant's health

Risk for **Infection:** Risk factors: infection transmission from mother to fetus; infection in fetal environment

Chronic Confusion

See Confusion, Chronic

Chronic Functional Constipation

(See **Constipation,** chronic functional, section III)

(See **Constipation,** chronic functional, risk for, section III)

Chronic Lymphocytic Leukemia

See Cancer; Chemotherapy; Leukemia

Chronic Obstructive Pulmonary Disease (COPD)

See COPD (Chronic Obstructive Pulmonary Disease)

Chronic Pain

See Pain, Chronic

Chronic Renal Failure (Chronic kidney disease)

See Renal Failure

Chvostek's Sign

See Hypocalcemia

Circumcision

Acute **Pain** r/t surgical intervention

Risk for **Bleeding:** Risk factor: surgical trauma

Risk for **Infection:** Risk factor: surgical wound

Readiness for enhanced **Knowledge:** parent: expresses an interest in learning

Cirrhosis

Chronic **Confusion** r/t chronic organic disorder with increased ammonia levels, substance abuse

Defensive **Coping** r/t inability to accept responsibility to stop substance abuse

Fatigue r/t malnutrition

Ineffective **Health** maintenance r/t deficient knowledge regarding correlation between lifestyle habits and disease process

Nausea r/t irritation to gastrointestinal system

Imbalanced **Nutrition:** less than body requirements r/t loss of appetite, nausea, vomiting

Chronic **Pain** r/t liver enlargement

Chronic low **Self-Esteem** r/t chronic illness

C

Chronic **Sorrow** r/t presence of chronic illness

Risk for **Bleeding:** Risk factors: impaired blood coagulation, bleeding from portal hypertension

Risk for **Injury:** Risk factors: substance intoxication, potential delirium tremens

Risk for impaired **Oral Mucous Membrane:** Risk factors: altered nutrition, inadequate oral care

Risk for impaired **Skin** integrity: Risk factors: altered nutritional state, altered metabolic state

Cleft Lip/Cleft Palate

Ineffective **Airway** clearance r/t common feeding and breathing passage, postoperative laryngeal, incisional edema

Ineffective **Breastfeeding** r/t infant anomaly

Impaired verbal **Communication** r/t inadequate palate function, possible hearing loss from infected eustachian tubes

Fear: parental r/t special care needs, surgery

Grieving r/t loss of perfect child

Ineffective infant **Feeding** pattern r/t cleft lip, cleft palate

Impaired physical **Mobility** r/t imposed restricted activity, use of elbow restraints

Impaired **Oral Mucous Membrane** r/t surgical correction

Acute **Pain** r/t surgical correction, elbow restraints

Impaired **Skin** integrity r/t incomplete joining of lip, palate ridges

Chronic **Sorrow** r/t birth of child with congenital defect

Risk for **Aspiration:** Risk factor: common feeding and breathing passage

Risk for disturbed **Body Image:** Risk factors: disfigurement, speech impediment

Risk for delayed **Development:** Risk factor: inadequate nutrition resulting from difficulty feeding

Risk for deficient **Fluid** volume: Risk factor: inability to take liquids in usual manner

Risk for disproportionate **Growth:** Risk factor: inability to feed with normal techniques

Risk for **Infection:** Risk factors: invasive procedure, disruption of eustachian tube development, aspiration

Readiness for enhanced **Knowledge:** parent: expresses an interest in learning

Clotting Disorder

Fear r/t threat to well-being

Risk for **Bleeding:** Risk factor: impaired clotting

Readiness for enhanced **Knowledge:** expresses an interest in learning

See Anticoagulant Therapy; DIC (Disseminated Intravascular Coagulation); Hemophilia

Cocaine Abuse

Ineffective **Breathing** pattern r/t drug effect on respiratory center

Chronic **Confusion** r/t excessive stimulation of nervous system by cocaine

Ineffective **Coping** r/t inability to deal with life stresses

Risk for decreased **Cardiac** tissue perfusion r/t increase in sympathetic response in the body damaging the heart

See Drug Abuse; Substance Abuse

Cocaine Baby

See Crack Baby; Infant of Substance-Abusing Mother

Codependency

Caregiver Role Strain r/t codependency

Impaired verbal **Communication** r/t psychological barriers

Ineffective **Coping** r/t inadequate support systems

Decisional Conflict r/t support system deficit

Ineffective **Denial** r/t unmet self-needs

Powerlessness r/t lifestyle of helplessness

Cold, Viral

Readiness for enhanced **Comfort** (See **Comfort**, readiness for enhanced, Section III)

Readiness for enhanced **Knowledge:** expresses an interest in learning

Colectomy

Constipation r/t decreased activity, decreased fluid intake

Imbalanced **Nutrition:** less than body requirements r/t high metabolic needs, decreased ability to ingest or digest food

Acute **Pain** r/t recent surgery

Risk for **Infection:** Risk factor: invasive procedure

Readiness for enhanced **Knowledge:** expresses an interest in learning

See Abdominal Surgery

Colitis

Diarrhea r/t inflammation in colon

Deficient **Fluid** volume r/t frequent stools

Acute **Pain** r/t inflammation in colon

Readiness for enhanced **Knowledge:** expresses an interest in learning

See Crohn's Disease; Inflammatory Bowel Disease (Child and Adult)

Collagen Disease

See specific disease (e.g., lupus erythematosus; JRA [juvenile rheumatoid arthritis]); Congenital Heart Disease/Cardiac Anomalies

Colostomy

Disturbed **Body Image** r/t presence of stoma, daily care of fecal material

Ineffective **Sexuality** pattern r/t altered body image, self-concept

Social isolation r/t anxiety about appearance of stoma and possible leakage of stool

Risk for **Constipation:** Risk factor: inappropriate diet

Risk for **Diarrhea:** Risk factor: inappropriate diet

Risk for impaired **Skin** integrity: Risk factor: irritation from bowel contents

Readiness for enhanced **Knowledge:** expresses an interest in learning

Colporrhaphy, Anterior

See Vaginal Hysterectomy

Coma

Death **Anxiety:** significant others r/t unknown outcome of coma state

Interrupted **Family** processes r/t illness or disability of family member

Functional urinary **Incontinence** r/t presence of comatose state

Self-Care deficit: r/t neuromuscular impairment

Ineffective family **Health** management r/t complexity of therapeutic regimen

Risk for **Aspiration:** Risk factors: impaired swallowing, loss of cough or gag reflex

Risk for **Disuse** syndrome: Risk factor: altered level of consciousness impairing mobility

Risk for **Hypothermia:** Risk factors: Inactivity, possible pharmaceutical agents, possible hypothalamic injury

Risk for **Injury:** Risk factor: potential seizure activity

Risk for corneal **Injury:** Risk factor: suppressed corneal reflex

Risk for urinary tract **Injury:** Risk factor: long-term use of urinary catheter

Risk for impaired **Oral Mucous Membrane:** Risk factors: dry mouth, inability to do own mouth care

Risk for **Pressure** ulcer: Risk factor: prolonged immobility

Risk for impaired **Skin** integrity: Risk factor: immobility

Risk for **Spiritual** distress: significant others: Risk factors: loss of ability to relate to loved one, unknown outcome of coma

Risk for impaired **Tissue** integrity: Risk factor: impaired physical mobility

See Head Injury, Subarachnoid Hemorrhage, Increased Intracranial Pressure

Comfort, Loss of

Impaired **Comfort** (See **Comfort,** impaired, Section III)

Readiness for enhanced **Comfort** (See **Comfort,** readiness for enhanced, Section III)

Communicable Diseases, Childhood (e.g., Measles, Mumps, Rubella, Chickenpox, Scabies, Lice, Impetigo)

Impaired **Comfort** r/t pruritus, inflammation or infection of skin, subdermal organisms

Deficient **Diversional** activity r/t imposed isolation from peers, disruption in usual play activities, fatigue, activity intolerance

Ineffective **Health** maintenance r/t nonadherence to appropriate immunization schedules, lack of prevention of transmission of infection

Acute **Pain** r/t impaired skin integrity, edema

Risk for **Infection:** transmission to others: Risk factor: contagious organisms

See Meningitis/Encephalitis; Respiratory Infections, Acute Childhood; Reye's Syndrome

Communication

Readiness for enhanced **Communication** (See **Communication**, readiness for enhanced, Section III)

Communication Problems

Impaired verbal **Communication** (See **Communication**, verbal, impaired, Section III)

Community Coping

Ineffective community **Coping** (See **Coping**, community, ineffective, Section III)

Readiness for enhanced community **Coping:** community sense of power to manage stressors, social supports available, resources available for problem solving

Community Health Problems

Deficient community **Health** (See **Health,** deficient, community, Section III)

Compartment Syndrome

Fear r/t possible loss of limb, damage to limb

Acute **Pain** r/t pressure in compromised body part

Ineffective peripheral **Tissue Perfusion** r/t increased pressure within compartment

Compulsion

See OCD (Obsessive-Compulsive Disorder)

Conduction Disorders (Cardiac)

See Dysrhythmia

Confusion, Acute

Acute **Confusion** r/t older than 70 years of age with hospitalization, alcohol abuse, delirium, dementia, drug abuse

Frail Elderly syndrome r/t impaired memory

Confusion, Chronic

Chronic **Confusion** r/t dementia, Korsakoff's psychosis, multi-infarct dementia, cerebrovascular accident, head injury

Frail Elderly syndrome r/t impaired memory

Impaired **Memory** r/t fluid and electrolyte imbalance, neurological disturbances, excessive environmental disturbances, anemia, acute or chronic hypoxia, decreased cardiac output

Impaired **Mood** regulation r/t emotional instability

See Alzheimer's Disease; Dementia

Confusion, Possible

Risk for acute **Confusion:** Risk factor (See **Confusion,** acute, risk for, Section III)

Congenital Heart Disease/Cardiac Anomalies

Activity intolerance r/t fatigue, generalized weakness, lack of adequate oxygenation

C

Ineffective **Breathing** pattern r/t pulmonary vascular disease

Decreased **Cardiac** output r/t cardiac dysfunction

Excess **Fluid** volume r/t cardiac dysfunction, side effects of medication

Impaired **Gas** exchange r/t cardiac dysfunction, pulmonary congestion

Imbalanced **Nutrition:** less than body requirements r/t fatigue, generalized weakness, inability of infant to suck and feed, increased caloric requirements

Risk for delayed **Development:** Risk factor: inadequate oxygen and nutrients to tissues

Risk for deficient **Fluid** volume: Risk factor: side effects of diuretics

Risk for disproportionate **Growth:** Risk factor: inadequate oxygen and nutrients to tissues

Risk for disorganized **Infant** behavior: Risk factor: invasive procedures

Risk for **Poisoning:** Risk factor: potential toxicity of cardiac medications

Risk for ineffective **Thermoregulation:** Risk factor: neonatal age

See Child with Chronic Condition; Hospitalized Child

Congestive Heart Failure (CHF)/Heart Failure (HF)

See CHF (Congestive Heart Failure)

Conjunctivitis

Acute **Pain** r/t inflammatory process

Vision Loss r/t change in visual acuity resulting from inflammation

Consciousness, Altered Level of

Acute **Confusion** r/t alcohol abuse, delirium, dementia, drug abuse, head injury

Chronic **Confusion** r/t multi-infarct dementia, Korsakoff's psychosis, head injury, cerebrovascular accident, neurological deficit, **Frail Elderly** syndrome

Functional urinary **Incontinence** r/t neurological dysfunction

Decreased **Intracranial** adaptive capacity r/t brain injury

Impaired **Memory** r/t neurological disturbances

Self-Care deficit: specify r/t neuromuscular impairment

Risk for **Aspiration:** Risk factors: impaired swallowing, loss of cough or gag reflex

Risk for **Disuse** syndrome: Risk factor: impaired mobility resulting from altered level of consciousness

Risk for **Falls:** Risk factor: diminished mental status

Risk for impaired **Oral Mucous Membrane:** Risk factors: dry mouth, interrupted oral care

Risk for ineffective **Cerebral** tissue perfusion: Risk factors: increased intracranial pressure, altered cerebral perfusion

Risk for impaired **Skin** integrity: Risk factor: immobility

See Coma, Head Injury, Subarachnoid Hemorrhage, Increased Intracranial Pressure

Constipation

Constipation (See **Constipation,** Section III)

Constipation, Chronic Functional

Constipation (See **Constipation,** chronic functional, Section III)

Constipation, Perceived

Perceived **Constipation** (See perceived **Constipation,** Section III)

Constipation, Risk for

Risk for **Constipation** (See **Constipation,** risk for, Section III)

Risk for chronic functional **Constipation** (See **Constipation,** chronic functional, risk for, Section III)

Contamination

Contamination (See **Contamination,** Section III)

Risk for **Contamination** (See **Contamination,** risk for, Section III)

Continent Ileostomy (Kock Pouch)

Ineffective **Coping** r/t stress of disease, exacerbations caused by stress

Imbalanced **Nutrition:** less than body requirements r/t malabsorption from disease process

Risk for **Injury:** Risk factors: failure of valve, stomal cyanosis, intestinal obstruction

Readiness for enhanced **Knowledge:** expresses an interest in learning

See Abdominal Surgery, Crohn's Disease

Contraceptive Method

Decisional Conflict: method of contraception r/t unclear personal values or beliefs, lack of experience or interference with decision-making, lack of relevant information, support system deficit

Ineffective **Sexuality** pattern r/t fear of pregnancy

Readiness for enhanced **Health** management: requesting information about available and appropriate birth control methods

Convulsions

Anxiety r/t concern over controlling convulsions

Impaired **Memory** r/t neurological disturbance

Risk for **Aspiration:** Risk factor: impaired swallowing

Risk for delayed **Development:** Risk factor: seizures

Risk for **Injury:** Risk factor: seizure activity

Readiness for enhanced **Knowledge:** expresses an interest in learning

See Seizure Disorders, Adult; Seizure Disorders, Childhood

COPD (Chronic Obstructive Pulmonary Disease)

Activity intolerance r/t imbalance between oxygen supply and demand

Ineffective **Airway** clearance r/t bronchoconstriction, increased mucus, ineffective cough, infection

Anxiety r/t breathlessness, change in health status

Death **Anxiety** r/t seriousness of medical condition, difficulty being able to "catch breath," feeling of suffocation

Interrupted **Family** processes r/t role changes

Impaired **Gas** exchange r/t ventilation-perfusion inequality

Ineffective **Health** management (See **Health** management, ineffective, Section III)

Imbalanced **Nutrition:** less than body requirements r/t decreased intake because of dyspnea, unpleasant taste in mouth left by medications, increased need for calories from work of breathing

Powerlessness r/t progressive nature of disease

Self-Care deficit: r/t fatigue from the increased work of breathing

Chronic low **Self-Esteem** r/t chronic illness

Sleep deprivation r/t breathing difficulties when lying down

Impaired **Social** interaction r/t social isolation because of oxygen use, activity intolerance

Chronic **Sorrow** r/t presence of chronic illness

Risk for **Infection:** Risk factor: stasis of respiratory secretions

Readiness for enhanced **Health** management (See **Health** management, readiness for enhanced, Section III)

Coping

Readiness for enhanced **Coping** (See **Coping,** readiness for enhanced, Section III)

Coping Problems

Compromised family **Coping** (see **Coping,** compromised family, Section III)

Defensive **Coping** (See **Coping,** defensive, Section III)

Disabled family **Coping** (See **Coping,** disabled family, Section III)

Ineffective **Coping** (See **Coping,** ineffective, Section III)

Ineffective community **Coping** (see **Coping,** ineffective community, Section III)

Corneal Injury

Risk for corneal **Injury** (See corneal **Injury,** risk for, Section III)

Corneal Reflex, Absent

Risk for **Injury:** Risk factors: accidental corneal abrasion, drying of cornea

Corneal Transplant

Risk for **Infection:** Risk factors: invasive procedure, surgery

Readiness for enhanced **Health** management: describes need to rest and avoid strenuous activities during healing phase

Coronary Artery Bypass Grafting (CABG)

Decreased **Cardiac** output r/t dysrhythmia, depressed cardiac function, change in preload, contractility or afterload

Fear r/t outcome of surgical procedure

Deficient **Fluid** volume r/t intraoperative blood loss, use of diuretics in surgery

Acute **Pain** r/t traumatic surgery

Risk for **Perioperative Positioning** injury: Risk factors: hypothermia, extended supine position

Risk for Impaired **Tissue** integrity: Risk Factor: surgical procedure

Readiness for enhanced **Knowledge:** expresses an interest in learning

Costovertebral Angle Tenderness

See Kidney Stone; Pyelonephritis

Cough, Ineffective

Ineffective **Airway** clearance r/t decreased energy, fatigue, normal aging changes

See Bronchitis; COPD (Chronic Obstructive Pulmonary Disease); Pulmonary Edema

Crack Abuse

See Cocaine Abuse; Drug Abuse; Substance Abuse

Crack Baby

Disorganized **Infant** behavior r/t prematurity, drug withdrawal, lack of attachment

Risk for impaired **Attachment:** Risk factors: parent's inability to meet infant's needs, substance abuse

Risk for disturbed **Maternal–Fetal** dyad: Risk factor: substance abuse

See Infant of Substance-Abusing Mother

Crackles in Lungs, Coarse

Ineffective **Airway** clearance r/t excessive secretions in airways, ineffective cough

See Heart Failure, Pneumonia, Pulmonary Edema

Crackles in Lungs, Fine

Ineffective **Breathing** pattern r/t fatigue, surgery, decreased energy

See Bronchitis or Pneumonia (if from pulmonary infection); CHF (Congestive Heart Failure) (if cardiac in origin); Infection

Craniectomy/Craniotomy

Frail Elderly syndrome r/t alteration in cognition

Fear r/t threat to well-being

Decreased **Intracranial** adaptive capacity r/t brain injury, intracranial hypertension

Impaired **Memory** r/t neurological surgery

Acute **Pain** r/t recent brain surgery, increased intracranial pressure

Risk for ineffective **Cerebral** tissue perfusion: Risk factors: cerebral edema, increased intracranial pressure

Risk for **Injury:** Risk factor: potential confusion

See Coma (if relevant)

Crepitation, Subcutaneous

See Pneumothorax

C

Crisis

Anxiety r/t threat to or change in environment, health status, interaction patterns, situation, self-concept, or role functioning; threat of death of self or significant other

Death **Anxiety** r/t feelings of hopelessness associated with crisis

Compromised family **Coping** r/t situational or developmental crisis

Ineffective **Coping** r/t situational or maturational crisis

Fear r/t crisis situation

Grieving r/t potential significant loss

Impaired individual **Resilience** r/t onset of crisis

Situational low **Self-Esteem** r/t perception of inability to handle crisis

Stress overload (See **Stress** overload, Section III)

Risk for **Spiritual** distress: Risk factors: physical or psychological stress, natural disasters, situational losses, maturational losses

Crohn's Disease

Anxiety r/t change in health status

Ineffective **Coping** r/t repeated episodes of diarrhea

Diarrhea r/t inflammatory process

Ineffective **Health** maintenance r/t deficient knowledge regarding management of disease

Imbalanced **Nutrition:** less than body requirements r/t diarrhea, altered ability to digest and absorb food

Acute **Pain** r/t increased peristalsis

Powerlessness r/t chronic disease

Risk for deficient **Fluid** volume: Risk factor: abnormal fluid loss with diarrhea

Croup

See Respiratory Infections, Acute Childhood

Cryosurgery for Retinal Detachment

See Retinal Detachment

Cushing's Syndrome

Activity intolerance r/t fatigue, weakness

Disturbed **Body Image** r/t change in appearance from disease process

Excess **Fluid** volume r/t failure of regulatory mechanisms

Sexual dysfunction r/t loss of libido

Impaired **Skin** integrity r/t thin vulnerable skin from effects of increased cortisol

Risk for **Infection:** Risk factor: suppression of immune system caused by increased cortisol levels

Risk for **Injury:** Risk factors: decreased muscle strength, brittle bones

Readiness for enhanced **Knowledge:** expresses an interest in learning

Cuts (Wounds)

See Lacerations

CVA (Cerebrovascular Accident)

Anxiety r/t situational crisis, change in physical or emotional condition

Disturbed **Body Image** r/t chronic illness, paralysis

Caregiver Role Strain r/t cognitive problems of care receiver, need for significant home care

Impaired verbal **Communication** r/t pressure damage, decreased circulation to brain in speech center informational sources

Chronic **Confusion** r/t neurological changes

Constipation r/t decreased activity

Ineffective **Coping** r/t disability

Interrupted **Family** processes r/t illness, disability of family member

Frail Elderly syndrome r/t alteration in cognitive functioning

Grieving r/t loss of health

Impaired **Home** maintenance r/t neurological disease affecting ability to perform activities of daily living

Functional urinary **Incontinence** r/t neurological dysfunction

Reflex urinary **Incontinence** r/t loss of feeling to void

Impaired **Memory** r/t neurological disturbances

Impaired physical **Mobility** r/t loss of balance and coordination

Unilateral Neglect r/t disturbed perception from neurological damage

Self-Care deficit: specify r/t decreased strength and endurance, paralysis

Impaired **Social** interaction r/t limited physical mobility, limited ability to communicate

Impaired **Swallowing** r/t neuromuscular dysfunction

Impaired **Transfer Ability** r/t limited physical mobility

Vision Loss r/t pressure damage to visual centers in the brain (*see care plan in Appendix*)

Impaired **Walking** r/t loss of balance and coordination

Risk for **Aspiration:** Risk factors: impaired swallowing, loss of gag reflex

Risk for chronic functional **Constipation:** Risk factor: immobility

Risk for **Disuse** syndrome: Risk factor: paralysis

Risk for **Falls:** Risk factor: paralysis, decreased balance

Risk for **Injury:** Risk factors: vision loss, decreased tissue perfusion with loss of sensation

Risk for ineffective **Cerebral** tissue perfusion: Risk factor: clot, emboli, or hemorrhage from cerebral vessel

Risk for impaired **Skin** integrity: Risk factor: immobility

Readiness for enhanced **Knowledge:** expresses an interest in learning

Cyanosis, Central with Cyanosis of Oral Mucous Membranes

Impaired **Gas** exchange r/t alveolar-capillary membrane changes

Cyanosis, Peripheral with Cyanosis of Nail Beds

Ineffective peripheral **Tissue Perfusion** r/t interruption of arterial flow, severe vasoconstriction, cold temperatures

Cystic Fibrosis

Activity intolerance r/t imbalance between oxygen supply and demand

Ineffective **Airway** clearance r/t increased production of thick mucus

Anxiety r/t dyspnea, oxygen deprivation

Disturbed **Body Image** r/t changes in physical appearance, treatment of chronic lung disease (clubbing, barrel chest, home oxygen therapy)

Impaired **Gas** exchange r/t ventilation-perfusion imbalance

Impaired **Home** maintenance r/t extensive daily treatment, medications necessary for health

Imbalanced **Nutrition:** less than body requirements r/t anorexia; decreased absorption of nutrients, fat; increased work of breathing

Chronic **Sorrow** r/t presence of chronic disease

Risk for **Caregiver Role Strain:** Risk factors: illness severity of care receiver, unpredictable course of illness

Risk for deficient **Fluid** volume: Risk factors: decreased fluid intake, increased work of breathing

Risk for **Infection:** Risk factors: thick, tenacious mucus; harboring of bacterial organisms; immunocompromised state

Risk for **Spiritual** distress: Risk factor: presence of chronic disease

See Child with Chronic Condition; Hospitalized Child; Terminally Ill Child, Adolescent; Terminally Ill Child, Infant/Toddler; Terminally Ill Child, Preschool Child; Terminally Ill Child, School-Age Child/Preadolescent; Terminally Ill Child/Death of Child, Parent

Cystitis

Acute **Pain:** dysuria r/t inflammatory process in bladder and urethra

Impaired **Urinary** elimination: frequency r/t urinary tract infection

Urge urinary **Incontinence:** Risk factor: infection in bladder

Readiness for enhanced **Knowledge:** expresses an interest in learning

Cystocele

Stress urinary **Incontinence** r/t prolapsed bladder

Readiness for enhanced **Knowledge:** expresses an interest in learning

Cystoscopy

Urinary Retention r/t edema in urethra obstructing flow of urine

Risk for **Infection:** Risk factor: invasive procedure

Readiness for enhanced **Knowledge:** expresses an interest in learning

D

Deafness

Impaired verbal **Communication** r/t impaired hearing

Hearing Loss r/t alteration in sensory reception, transmission, integration

Risk for delayed **Development:** Risk factor: impaired hearing

Risk for **Injury:** Risk factor: alteration in sensory perception

Death

Risk for **Sudden Infant Death** syndrome (SIDS) (See **Sudden Infant Death** syndrome, risk for, Section III)

Death, Oncoming

Death **Anxiety** r/t unresolved issues surrounding dying

Compromised family **Coping** r/t client's inability to provide support to family

Ineffective **Coping** r/t personal vulnerability

Fear r/t threat of death

Grieving r/t loss of significant other

Powerlessness r/t effects of illness, oncoming death

Social isolation r/t altered state of wellness

Spiritual distress r/t intense suffering

Readiness for enhanced **Spiritual** well-being: desire of client and family to be in harmony with each other and higher power, God

See Terminally Ill Child, Adolescent; Terminally Ill Child, Infant/Toddler; Terminally Ill Child, Preschool Child; Terminally Ill Child, School-Age Child/Preadolescent; Terminally Ill Child/Death of Child, Parent

Decisions, Difficulty Making

Decisional Conflict r/t support system deficit, perceived threat to value system, multiple or divergent sources of information, lack of relevant information, unclear personal values or beliefs

Readiness for enhanced **Decision-Making** (See **Decision-Making,** readiness for enhanced, Section III)

Decubitus Ulcer

See Pressure Ulcer

Deep Vein Thrombosis (DVT)

See DVT (Deep Vein Thrombosis)

Defensive Behavior

Defensive **Coping** r/t nonacceptance of blame, denial of problems or weakness

Ineffective **Denial** r/t inability to face situation realistically

Dehiscence, Abdominal

Fear r/t threat of death, severe dysfunction

Acute **Pain** r/t stretching of abdominal wall

Impaired **Skin** integrity r/t altered circulation, malnutrition, opening in incision

Delayed **Surgical** recovery r/t altered circulation, malnutrition, opening in incision

Impaired **Tissue** integrity r/t exposure of abdominal contents to external environment

Risk for deficient **Fluid** volume: Risk factor: altered circulation associated with opening of wound and exposure of abdominal contents

Risk for **Infection:** Risk factors: loss of skin integrity, open surgical wound

Dehydration

Deficient **Fluid** volume r/t active fluid volume loss

Impaired **Oral Mucous Membrane** r/t decreased salivation, fluid deficit

Risk for chronic functional **Constipation:** Risk factor: decreased fluid volume

Risk for imbalanced body **Temperature:** Risk factor: hyperthermia due to sensible water loss

See Burns, Heat Stroke, Vomiting, Diarrhea

Delirium

Acute **Confusion** r/t effects of medication, response to hospitalization, alcohol abuse, substance abuse, sensory deprivation or overload, infection, polypharmacy

Impaired **Memory** r/t delirium

Sleep deprivation r/t sustained inadequate sleep hygiene

Risk for **Injury:** Risk factor: altered level of consciousness

Delirium Tremens (DT)

See Alcohol Withdrawal

Delivery

See Labor, Normal

Delusions

Impaired verbal **Communication** r/t psychological impairment, delusional thinking

Acute **Confusion** r/t alcohol abuse, delirium, dementia, drug abuse

Ineffective **Coping** r/t distortion and insecurity of life events

Fear r/t content of intrusive thoughts

Risk for other-directed **Violence:** Risk factor: delusional thinking

Risk for self-directed **Violence:** Risk factor: delusional thinking

Dementia

Chronic **Confusion** r/t neurological dysfunction

Interrupted **Family** processes r/t disability of family member

Frail Elderly syndrome r/t alteration in cognitive functioning

Impaired **Home** maintenance r/t inadequate support system, neurological dysfunction

Imbalanced **Nutrition:** less than body requirements r/t neurological impairment

Functional urinary **Incontinence** r/t neurological dysfunction

Insomnia r/t neurological impairment, naps during the day

Impaired physical **Mobility** r/t alteration in cognitive function

Self-Neglect r/t cognitive impairment

Self-Care deficit: specify r/t psychological or neuromuscular impairment

Chronic **Sorrow:** Significant other r/t chronic long-standing disability, loss of mental function

Impaired **Swallowing** r/t neuromuscular changes associated with long-standing dementia

Risk for **Caregiver Role Strain:** Risk factors: number of caregiving tasks, duration of caregiving required

Risk for Chronic Functional **Constipation:** Risk factor: decreased fluid intake

Risk for **Falls:** Risk factor: diminished mental status

Risk for **Frail Elderly** syndrome: Risk factors: cognitive impairment

Risk for **Injury:** Risk factors: confusion, decreased muscle coordination

Risk for impaired **Skin** integrity: Risk factors: altered nutritional status, immobility

Denial of Health Status

Ineffective **Denial** r/t lack of perception about the health status effects of illness

Ineffective **Health** management r/t denial of seriousness of health situation

Dental Caries

Impaired **Dentition** r/t ineffective oral hygiene, barriers to self-care, economic barriers to professional care, nutritional deficits, dietary habits

Ineffective **Health** maintenance r/t lack of knowledge regarding prevention of dental disease

Depression (Major Depressive Disorder)

Death **Anxiety** r/t feelings of lack of self-worth

Constipation r/t inactivity, decreased fluid intake

Fatigue r/t psychological demands

Ineffective **Health** maintenance r/t lack of ability to make good judgments regarding ways to obtain help

Hopelessness r/t feeling of abandonment, long-term stress

Impaired **Mood** Regulation r/t emotional instability

Insomnia r/t inactivity

Self-Neglect r/t depression, cognitive impairment

Powerlessness r/t pattern of helplessness

Chronic low **Self-Esteem** r/t repeated unmet expectations

Sexual dysfunction r/t loss of sexual desire

Social isolation r/t ineffective coping

Chronic **Sorrow** r/t unresolved grief

Risk for complicated **Grieving:** Risk factor: lack of previous resolution of former grieving response

Risk for **Suicide:** Risk factor: grieving, hopelessness

Dermatitis

Anxiety r/t situational crisis imposed by illness

Impaired **Comfort** r/t itching

Impaired **Skin** integrity r/t side effect of medication, allergic reaction

Readiness for enhanced **Knowledge:** expresses an interest in learning

See Itching

Despondency

Hopelessness r/t long-term stress

See Depression (Major Depressive Disorder)

Destructive Behavior Toward Others

Risk-prone **Health** behavior r/t intense emotional state

Ineffective **Coping** r/t situational crises, maturational crises, disturbance in pattern of appraisal of threat

Risk for other-directed **Violence** (See **Violence,** other-directed, risk for, Section III)

Developmental Concerns

Risk for delayed **Development** (See **Development,** delayed, risk for, Section III)

See Growth and Development Lag

Diabetes in Pregnancy

See Gestational Diabetes (Diabetes in Pregnancy)

Diabetes Insipidus

Deficient **Fluid** volume r/t inability to conserve fluid

Ineffective **Health** maintenance r/t deficient knowledge regarding care of disease, importance of medications

Diabetes Mellitus

Ineffective **Health** maintenance r/t complexity of therapeutic regimen

Ineffective **Health** management (See **Health** management, ineffective, Section III)

Imbalanced **Nutrition:** less than body requirements r/t inability to use glucose (type 1 [insulin-dependent] diabetes)

Risk for **Overweight** r/t excessive intake of nutrients (type 2 diabetes)

Ineffective peripheral **Tissue** perfusion r/t impaired arterial circulation

Powerlessness r/t perceived lack of personal control

Sexual dysfunction r/t neuropathy associated with disease

Vision Loss r/t ineffective tissue perfusion of retina

Risk for unstable blood **Glucose** level (See **Glucose** level, blood, unstable, risk for, Section III)

Risk for **Infection:** Risk factors: hyperglycemia, impaired healing, circulatory changes

Risk for **Injury:** Risk factors: hypoglycemia or hyperglycemia from failure to consume adequate calories, failure to take insulin

Risk for dysfunctional **Gastrointestinal** motility: Risk factor: complication of diabetes

Risk for impaired **Skin** integrity: Risk factor: loss of pain perception in extremities

Risk for delayed **Surgical** recovery: Risk factor: impaired healing due to circulatory changes

Readiness for enhanced **Health** management (See **Health** management, readiness for enhanced, Section III)

Readiness for enhanced **Knowledge:** expresses an interest in learning

See Hyperglycemia; Hypoglycemia

Diabetes Mellitus, Juvenile (IDDM Type 1)

Risk-prone **Health** behavior r/t inadequate comprehension, inadequate social support, low self-efficacy, impaired adjustment attributable to adolescent maturational crises

Disturbed **Body Image** r/t imposed deviations from biophysical and psychosocial norm, perceived differences from peers

Impaired **Comfort** r/t insulin injections, peripheral blood glucose testing

Ineffective **Health** maintenance r/t (See **Health** maintenance, ineffective, Section III)

Imbalanced **Nutrition:** less than body requirements r/t inability of body to adequately metabolize and use glucose and nutrients, increased caloric needs of child to promote growth and physical activity participation with peers

Readiness for enhanced **Knowledge:** expresses an interest in learning

See Diabetes Mellitus; Child with Chronic Condition; Hospitalized Child

Diabetic Coma

Acute **Confusion** r/t hyperglycemia, presence of excessive metabolic acids

Deficient **Fluid** volume r/t hyperglycemia resulting in polyuria

Ineffective **Health** management r/t lack of understanding of preventive measures, adequate blood sugar control

Risk for unstable blood **Glucose** level (See **Glucose** level, blood, unstable, risk for, Section III)

Risk for **Infection:** Risk factors: hyperglycemia, changes in vascular system

See Diabetes Mellitus

Diabetic Ketoacidosis

See Ketoacidosis, Diabetic

Diabetic Retinopathy

Grieving r/t loss of vision

Ineffective **Health** maintenance r/t deficient knowledge regarding preserving vision with treatment if possible, use of low-vision aids

Vision Loss r/t change in sensory reception

See Vision Impairment; Blindness

Dialysis

See Hemodialysis; Peritoneal Dialysis

D

Diaphragmatic Hernia

See Hiatal Hernia

Diarrhea

Diarrhea r/t infection, change in diet, gastrointestinal disorders, stress, medication effect, impaction

Deficient **Fluid** volume r/t excessive loss of fluids in liquid stools

Risk for **Electrolyte** imbalance: Risk factor: effect of loss of electrolytes from frequent stools

DIC (Disseminated Intravascular Coagulation)

Fear r/t threat to well-being

Deficient **Fluid** volume: hemorrhage r/t depletion of clotting factors

Risk for **Bleeding:** Risk factors: microclotting within vascular system, depleted clotting factors

Risk for ineffective **Gastrointestinal** perfusion (See **Gastrointestinal** perfusion, ineffective, risk for, Section III)

Digitalis Toxicity

Decreased **Cardiac** output r/t drug toxicity affecting cardiac rhythm, rate

Ineffective **Health** management r/t deficient knowledge regarding action, appropriate method of administration of digitalis

Dignity, Loss of

Risk for compromised **Human Dignity** (See **Human Dignity**, compromised, risk for, Section III)

Dilation and Curettage (D&C)

Acute **Pain** r/t uterine contractions

Risk for **Bleeding:** Risk factor: surgical procedure

Risk for **Infection:** Risk factor: surgical procedure

Risk for ineffective **Sexuality** pattern: Risk factors: painful coitus, fear associated with surgery on genital area

Readiness for enhanced **Knowledge:** expresses an interest in learning

Dirty Body (for Prolonged Period)

Self-Neglect r/t mental illness, substance abuse, cognitive impairment

Discharge Planning

Impaired **Home Maintenance** r/t family member's disease or injury interfering with home maintenance

Deficient **Knowledge** r/t lack of exposure to information for home care

Relocation stress syndrome: Risk factors: insufficient predeparture counseling, insufficient support system, unpredictability of experience

Readiness for enhanced **Knowledge:** expresses an interest in learning

Discomforts of Pregnancy

Disturbed **Body Image** r/t pregnancy-induced body changes

Impaired **Comfort** r/t enlarged abdomen, swollen feet

Fatigue r/t hormonal, metabolic, body changes

Stress urinary **Incontinence** r/t enlarged uterus, fetal movement

Insomnia r/t psychological stress, fetal movement, muscular cramping, urinary frequency, shortness of breath

Nausea r/t hormone effect

Acute **Pain:** headache r/t hormonal changes of pregnancy

Acute **Pain:** leg cramps r/t nerve compression, calcium/phosphorus/potassium imbalance

Risk for **Constipation:** Risk factors: decreased intestinal motility, inadequate fiber in diet

Risk for **Injury:** Risk factors: faintness and/or syncope caused by vasomotor lability or postural hypotension, venous stasis in lower extremities

Dislocation of Joint

Acute **Pain** r/t dislocation of a joint

Self-Care deficit: r/t inability to use a joint

Risk for **Injury:** Risk factor: unstable joint

Dissecting Aneurysm

Fear r/t threat to well-being

See Abdominal Surgery; Aneurysm, Abdominal Surgery

Disseminated Intravascular Coagulation (DIC)

See DIC (Disseminated Intravascular Coagulation)

Dissociative Identity Disorder (Not Otherwise Specified)

Anxiety r/t psychosocial stress

Ineffective **Coping** r/t personal vulnerability in crisis of accurate self-perception

Disturbed personal **Identity** r/t inability to distinguish self caused by multiple personality disorder, depersonalization, disturbance in memory

Impaired **Memory** r/t altered state of consciousness

See Multiple Personality Disorder (Dissociative Identity Disorder)

Distress

Anxiety r/t situational crises, maturational crises

Death **Anxiety** r/t denial of one's own mortality or impending death

Disuse Syndrome, Potential to Develop

Risk for **Disuse** syndrome: Risk factors: paralysis, mechanical immobilization, prescribed immobilization, severe pain, altered level of consciousness

Diversional Activity, Lack of

Deficient **Diversional** activity r/t environmental lack of diversional activity as in frequent hospitalizations, lengthy treatments

Diverticulitis

Constipation r/t dietary deficiency of fiber and roughage

Diarrhea r/t increased intestinal motility caused by inflammation

Deficient **Knowledge** r/t diet needed to control disease, medication regimen

Imbalanced **Nutrition:** less than body requirements r/t loss of appetite

Acute **Pain** r/t inflammation of bowel

Risk for deficient **Fluid Volume:** Risk factor: diarrhea

Dizziness

Decreased **Cardiac** output r/t alteration in heart rate and rhythm, altered stroke volume

Deficient **Knowledge** r/t actions to take to prevent or modify dizziness and prevent falls

Impaired physical **Mobility** r/t dizziness

Risk for **Falls:** Risk factor: difficulty maintaining balance

Risk for ineffective **Cerebral** tissue perfusion: Risk factor: interruption of cerebral arterial blood flow

Domestic Violence

Impaired verbal **Communication** r/t psychological barriers of fear

Compromised family **Coping** r/t abusive patterns

Defensive **Coping** r/t low self-esteem

Dysfunctional **Family** processes r/t inadequate coping skills

Fear r/t threat to self-concept, situational crisis of abuse

Insomnia r/t psychological stress

Post-Trauma syndrome r/t history of abuse

Powerlessness r/t lifestyle of helplessness

Situational low **Self-Esteem** r/t negative family interactions

Risk for compromised **Resilience:** Risk factor: effects of abuse

Risk for other-directed **Violence:** Risk factor: history of abuse

Down Syndrome

See Child with Chronic Condition; Intellectual Disability

Dress Self (Inability to)

Dressing **Self-Care** deficit r/t intolerance to activity, decreased strength and endurance, pain, discomfort, perceptual or cognitive impairment, neuromuscular impairment, musculoskeletal impairment, depression, severe anxiety

Dribbling of Urine

Overflow urinary **Incontinence** r/t degenerative changes in pelvic muscles and urinary structures

Stress urinary **Incontinence** r/t degenerative changes in pelvic muscles and urinary structures

Drooling

Impaired **Swallowing** r/t neuromuscular impairment, mechanical obstruction

Risk for **Aspiration:** Risk factor: impaired swallowing

Dropout from School

Impaired individual **Resilience** (See **Resilience,** individual, impaired, Section III)

Anxiety r/t conflict about life goals

Ineffective **Coping** r/t inadequate resources

Drug Abuse

Anxiety r/t threat to self-concept, lack of control of drug use

Risk-prone **Health** behavior r/t addiction

Ineffective **Coping** r/t situational crisis

Ineffective **Denial** r/t use of drugs affecting quality of own life and that of significant others

Insomnia r/t effects of drugs

Imbalanced **Nutrition:** less than body requirements r/t poor eating habits

Powerlessness r/t feeling unable to change patterns of drug abuse

Impaired individual **Resilience** (See **Resilience,** individual, impaired, Section III)

Sexual dysfunction r/t actions and side effects of drug abuse

Sleep deprivation r/t prolonged psychological discomfort

Impaired **Social** interaction r/t disturbed thought processes from drug abuse

Spiritual distress r/t separation from religious, cultural ties

Risk for **Injury:** Risk factors: hallucinations, drug effects

Risk for other-directed **Violence:** Risk factor: poor impulse control

See Cocaine Abuse; Substance Abuse

Drug Withdrawal

Anxiety r/t physiological withdrawal

Acute **Confusion** r/t effects of substance withdrawal

Ineffective **Coping** r/t situational crisis, withdrawal

Insomnia r/t effects of medication/substance withdrawal

Imbalanced **Nutrition:** less than body requirements r/t poor eating habits

Risk for other-directed **Violence:** Risk factors: poor impulse control, hallucinations

Risk for self-directed **Violence:** Risk factors: poor impulse control, hallucinations

See Drug Abuse

Dry Eye

Risk for dry **Eye:** Risk factors: (See dry **Eye,** risk for, Section III)

Risk for Corneal **Injury:** Risk factor: suppressed corneal reflex

Readiness for enhanced **Knowledge:** expresses an interest in learning

See Conjunctivitis; Keratoconjunctivitis Sicca

DT (Delirium Tremens)

See Alcohol Withdrawal

DVT (Deep Vein Thrombosis)

Constipation r/t inactivity, bed rest

Impaired physical **Mobility** r/t pain in extremity

Acute **Pain** r/t vascular inflammation, edema

Ineffective peripheral **Tissue** perfusion r/t deficient knowledge of aggravating factors

Delayed **Surgical** recovery r/t impaired physical mobility

Readiness for enhanced **Knowledge:** expresses an interest in learning

Risk for imbalanced body **Temperature:** Risk factor: inactivity

See Anticoagulant Therapy

Dying Client

See Terminally Ill Adult; Terminally Ill Adolescent; Terminally Ill Child, Infant/Toddler; Terminally Ill Child, Preschool Child; Terminally Ill Child, School-Age Child/Preadolescent; Terminally Ill Child/Death of Child, Parent

Dysfunctional Eating Pattern

Imbalanced **Nutrition:** less than body requirements r/t psychological factors

Risk for **Overweight:** Risk factor: psychological factors

See Anorexia Nervosa; Bulimia; Maturational Issues, Adolescent; Obesity

Dysfunctional Family Unit

See Family Problems

Dysfunctional Ventilatory Weaning

Dysfunctional **Ventilatory** weaning response r/t physical, psychological, situational factors

Dysmenorrhea

Nausea r/t prostaglandin effect

Acute **Pain** r/t cramping from hormonal effects

Readiness for enhanced **Knowledge:** expresses an interest in learning

Dyspareunia

Sexual **Dysfunction** r/t lack of lubrication during intercourse, alteration in reproductive organ function

Dyspepsia

Anxiety r/t pressures of personal role

Acute **Pain** r/t gastrointestinal disease, consumption of irritating foods

Readiness for enhanced **Knowledge:** expresses an interest in learning

Dysphagia

Impaired **Swallowing** r/t neuromuscular impairment

Risk for **Aspiration:** Risk factor: loss of gag or cough reflex

Dysphasia

Impaired verbal **Communication** r/t decrease in circulation to brain

Impaired social **Interaction** r/t difficulty in communicating

Dyspnea

Activity intolerance r/t imbalance between oxygen supply and demand

Ineffective **Breathing** pattern r/t compromised cardiac or pulmonary function, decreased lung expansion, neurological impairment affecting respiratory center, extreme anxiety

Fear r/t threat to state of well-being, potential death

Impaired **Gas** exchange r/t alveolar-capillary damage

Insomnia r/t difficulty breathing, positioning required for effective breathing

Sleep deprivation r/t ineffective breathing pattern

Dysrhythmia

Activity intolerance r/t decreased cardiac output

Decreased **Cardiac** output r/t alteration in heart rate, rhythm

Fear r/t threat of death, change in health status

Risk for ineffective **Cerebral** tissue perfusion: Risk factor: decreased blood supply to the brain from dysrhythmia

Readiness for enhanced **Knowledge:** expresses an interest in learning

Dysthymic Disorder

Ineffective **Coping** r/t impaired social interaction

Ineffective **Health** maintenance r/t inability to make good judgments regarding ways to obtain help

Insomnia r/t anxious thoughts

Chronic low **Self-Esteem** r/t repeated unmet expectations

Ineffective **Sexuality** pattern r/t loss of sexual desire

Social Isolation r/t ineffective coping

See Depression (Major Depressive Disorder)

Dystocia

Anxiety r/t difficult labor, deficient knowledge regarding normal labor pattern

Ineffective **Coping** r/t situational crisis

Fatigue r/t prolonged labor

Grieving r/t loss of ideal labor experience

Acute **Pain** r/t difficult labor, medical interventions

Powerlessness r/t perceived inability to control outcome of labor

Risk for **Bleeding:** Risk factor: hemorrhage secondary to uterine atony

Risk for ineffective **Cerebral** tissue perfusion (fetal): Risk factor: difficult labor and birth

Risk for delayed **Development** (Infant): Risk factor: difficult labor and birth

Risk for disproportionate **Growth:** Risk factor: difficult labor and birth

Risk for **Infection:** Risk factor: prolonged rupture of membranes

Risk for impaired **Tissue** integrity (maternal and fetal): Risk factor: difficult labor

Dysuria

Impaired **Urinary** elimination r/t infection/inflammation of the urinary tract

Risk for urge urinary **Incontinence:** Risk factor: detrusor hyperreflexia from infection in the urinary tract

Acute **Pain** r/t infection/inflammation of the urinary tract

E

ECMO (Extracorporeal Membrane Oxygenator)

Death **Anxiety** r/t emergency condition, hemorrhage

Decreased **Cardiac** output r/t altered contractility of the heart

Impaired **Gas** exchange (See **Gas** exchange, impaired, Section III)

See Respiratory Conditions of the Neonate

E. coli Infection

Fear r/t serious illness, unknown outcome

Deficient **Knowledge** r/t how to prevent disease; care of self with serious illness

See Gastroenteritis; Gastroenteritis, Child; Hospitalized Child

Ear Surgery

Acute **Pain** r/t edema in ears from surgery

Hearing Loss r/t invasive surgery of ears, dressings

Risk for delayed **Development:** Risk factor: hearing impairment

Risk for **Falls:** Risk factor: dizziness from excessive stimuli to vestibular apparatus

Readiness for enhanced **Knowledge:** expresses an interest in learning

See Hospitalized Child

Earache

Acute **Pain** r/t trauma, edema, infection

Hearing Loss r/t altered sensory reception, transmission

Ebola Virus Disease

Fear r/t serious threat to well-being

Ineffective **Health** maintenance r/t knowledge deficit regarding transmission, symptoms, and treatment

Social isolation r/t fear of incurable disease

Deficient **Fluid** volume r/t active fluid loss, vomiting, diarrhea, and failure of regulatory mechanisms

Risk for **Infection:** Risk factor: lack of knowledge concerning transmission of disease

Eclampsia

Interrupted **Family** processes r/t unmet expectations for pregnancy and childbirth

Fear r/t threat of well-being to self and fetus

Risk for **Aspiration:** Risk factor: seizure activity

Risk for ineffective **Cerebral** tissue perfusion: fetal: Risk factor: uteroplacental insufficiency

Risk for delayed **Development:** Risk factor: uteroplacental insufficiency

Risk for excess **Fluid** volume: Risk factor: decreased urine output as a result of renal dysfunction

Risk for disproportionate **Growth:** Risk factor: uteroplacental insufficiency

ECT (Electroconvulsive Therapy)

Decisional Conflict r/t lack of relevant information

Fear r/t real or imagined threat to well-being

Impaired **Memory** r/t effects of treatment

See Depression (Major Depressive Disorder)

Ectopic Pregnancy

Death **Anxiety** r/t emergency condition, hemorrhage

Disturbed **Body Image** r/t negative feelings about body and reproductive functioning

Fear r/t threat to self, surgery, implications for future pregnancy

Acute **Pain** r/t stretching or rupture of implantation site

Ineffective **Role** performance r/t loss of pregnancy

Situational low **Self-Esteem** r/t loss of pregnancy, inability to carry pregnancy to term

Chronic **Sorrow** r/t loss of pregnancy, potential loss of fertility

Risk for **Bleeding:** Risk factor: possible rupture of implantation site, surgical trauma

Risk for ineffective **Coping:** Risk factor: loss of pregnancy

Risk for interrupted **Family** processes: Risk factor: situational crisis

Risk for **Infection:** Risk factors: traumatized tissue, surgical procedure

Risk for **Spiritual** distress: Risk factor: grief process

Eczema

Disturbed **Body Image** r/t change in appearance from inflamed skin

Impaired **Comfort:** pruritus r/t inflammation of skin

Impaired **Skin** integrity r/t side effect of medication, allergic reaction

Readiness for enhanced **Knowledge:** expresses an interest in learning

ED (Erectile Dysfunction)

See Erectile Dysfunction (ED); Impotence

Edema

Excess **Fluid** volume r/t excessive fluid intake, cardiac dysfunction, renal dysfunction, loss of plasma proteins

Ineffective **Health** maintenance r/t deficient knowledge regarding treatment of edema

Risk for impaired **Skin** integrity: Risk factors: impaired circulation, fragility of skin

See Heart Failure, Kidney Failure

Elder Abuse

See Abuse, Spouse, Parent, or Significant Other

E

Elderly

See Aging; Frail Elderly Syndrome

Electroconvulsive Therapy

See ECT (Electroconvulsive Therapy)

Electrolyte Imbalance

Risk for **Electrolyte** imbalance (See **Electrolyte** imbalance, risk for, Section III)

Emancipated Decision-Making, Impaired

Risk for impaired emancipated **Decision-Making:** Risk factor: inability or unwillingness to verbalize needs and wants

Readiness for enhanced emancipated **Decision-Making**

Emaciated Person

Frail Elderly syndrome r/t living alone, malnutrition, alteration in cognitive functioning

Imbalanced **Nutrition:** less than body requirements r/t inability to ingest food, digest food, absorb nutrients because of biological, psychological, economic factors

Embolectomy

Fear r/t threat of great bodily harm from embolus

Ineffective peripheral **Tissue Perfusion** r/t presence of embolus

Risk for **Bleeding:** Risk factors: postoperative complication, surgical area

See Surgery, Postoperative Care

Emboli

See Pulmonary Embolism

Embolism in Leg or Arm

Ineffective peripheral **Tissue Perfusion** r/t arterial obstruction from clot

See Deep Vein Thrombosis

Emesis

Nausea (See **Nausea,** Section III)

See Vomiting

Emotional Problems

See Coping Problems

Empathy

Readiness for enhanced community **Coping:** social supports, being available for problem solving

Readiness for enhanced family **Coping:** basic needs met, desire to move to higher level of health

Readiness for enhanced **Spiritual Well-Being:** desire to establish interconnectedness through spirituality

Emphysema

See COPD (Chronic Obstructive Pulmonary Disease)

Emptiness

Social isolation r/t inability to engage in satisfying personal relationships

Chronic **Sorrow** r/t unresolved grief

Spiritual distress r/t separation from religious or cultural ties

Encephalitis

See Meningitis/Encephalitis

Endocardial Cushion Defect

See Congenital Heart Disease/Cardiac Anomalies

Endocarditis

Activity intolerance r/t reduced cardiac reserve, prescribed bed rest

Decreased **Cardiac** output r/t inflammation of lining of heart and change in structure of valve leaflets, increased myocardial workload

Risk for imbalanced **Nutrition:** less than body requirements: Risk factors: fever, hypermetabolic state associated with fever

Risk for ineffective **Cerebral** tissue perfusion: Risk factor: possible presence of emboli in cerebral circulation

Risk for ineffective peripheral **Tissue** perfusion: Risk factor: possible presence of emboli in peripheral circulation

Readiness for enhanced **Knowledge:** expresses an interest in learning

Endometriosis

Grieving r/t possible infertility

Nausea r/t prostaglandin effect

Acute **Pain** r/t onset of menses with distention of endometrial tissue

Sexual dysfunction r/t painful intercourse

Readiness for enhanced **Knowledge:** expresses an interest in learning

Endometritis

Anxiety r/t, fear of unknown

Ineffective **Thermoregulation** r/t infectious process

Acute **Pain** r/t infectious process in reproductive tract

Readiness for enhanced **Knowledge:** expresses an interest in learning

Enuresis

Ineffective **Health** maintenance r/t unachieved developmental task, neuromuscular immaturity, diseases of urinary system

See Toilet Training

Environmental Interpretation Problems

(See chronic **Confusion**)

Epididymitis

Anxiety r/t situational crisis, pain, threat to future fertility

Acute **Pain** r/t inflammation in scrotal sac

Ineffective **Sexuality** pattern r/t edema of epididymis and testes

Readiness for enhanced **Knowledge:** expresses an interest in learning

Epiglottitis

See Respiratory Infections, Acute Childhood (Croup, Epiglottis, Pertussis, Pneumonia, Respiratory Syncytial Virus)

Epilepsy

Anxiety r/t threat to role functioning

Ineffective **Health** management r/t deficient knowledge regarding seizure control

Impaired **Memory** r/t seizure activity

Risk for **Aspiration:** Risk factors: impaired swallowing, excessive secretions

Risk for delayed **Development:** Risk factor: seizure disorder

Risk for **Injury:** Risk factor: environmental factors during seizure

Readiness for enhanced **Knowledge:** expresses an interest in learning

See Seizure Disorders, Adult; Seizure Disorders, Childhood

Episiotomy

Anxiety r/t fear of pain

Disturbed **Body Image** r/t fear of resuming sexual relations

Impaired physical **Mobility** r/t pain, swelling, tissue trauma

Acute **Pain** r/t tissue trauma

Sexual dysfunction r/t altered body structure, tissue trauma

Impaired **Skin** integrity r/t perineal incision

Risk for **Infection:** Risk factor: tissue trauma

Epistaxis

Fear r/t large amount of blood loss

Risk for deficient **Fluid** volume: Risk factor: excessive blood loss

Epstein-Barr Virus

See Mononucleosis

Erectile Dysfunction (ED)

Situational low **Self-Esteem** r/t physiological crisis, inability to practice usual sexual activity

Sexual dysfunction r/t altered body function

Readiness for enhanced **Knowledge:** information regarding treatment for erectile dysfunction

See Impotence

Esophageal Varices

Fear r/t threat of death from hematemesis

Risk for **Bleeding:** Risk factor: portal hypertension, distended variceal vessels that can easily rupture

See Cirrhosis

Esophagitis

Acute **Pain** r/t inflammation of esophagus

Readiness for enhanced **Knowledge:** expresses an interest in learning

ETOH Withdrawal

See Alcohol Withdrawal

Evisceration

See Dehiscence, Abdominal

Exhaustion

Impaired individual **Resilience** (See **Resilience,** individual, impaired, Section III)

Disturbed **Sleep** pattern (See **Sleep** pattern, disturbed, Section III)

Exposure to Hot or Cold Environment

Hyperthermia r/t exposure to hot environment, abnormal reaction to anesthetics

Hypothermia r/t exposure to cold environment

Risk for imbalanced **Body** temperature: Risk factors: extremes of environmental temperature; inappropriate clothing for environmental temperature

External Fixation

Disturbed **Body Image** r/t trauma, change to affected part

Risk for **Infection:** Risk factor: presence of pins inserted into bone

See Fracture

Extracorporeal Membrane Oxygenator (ECMO)

See ECMO (Extracorporeal Membrane Oxygenator)

Eye Discomfort

Risk for dry **Eye** (See **Eye,** dry, risk for, Section III)

Risk for corneal **Injury:** Risk factors: exposure of the eyeball, blinking less than five times per minute

Eye Surgery

Anxiety r/t possible loss of vision

Self-Care deficit: specify r/t impaired vision

Vision Loss r/t surgical procedure, eye pathology

Risk for **Injury:** Risk factor: impaired vision

Readiness for enhanced **Knowledge:** expresses an interest in learning

See Hospitalized Child; Vision Impairment

F

Failure to Thrive, Child

Disorganized **Infant** behavior (See **Infant** behavior, disorganized, Section III)

Insomnia r/t inconsistency of caretaker; lack of quiet, consistent environment

Imbalanced **Nutrition:** less than body requirements r/t inadequate type or amounts of food for infant or child, inappropriate feeding techniques

Impaired **Parenting** r/t lack of parenting skills, inadequate role modeling

Chronic low **Self-Esteem:** parental r/t feelings of inadequacy, support system deficiencies, inadequate role model

Social isolation r/t limited support systems, self-imposed situation

Risk for impaired **Attachment:** Risk factor: inability of parents to meet infant's needs

Risk for delayed **Development** (See **Development,** delayed, risk for, Section III)

Risk for disproportionate **Growth** (See **Growth,** disproportionate, risk for, Section III)

Falls, Risk for

Risk for **Falls** (See **Falls,** risk for, Section III)

F

Family Problems

Compromised family **Coping** (See **Coping,** family, compromised, Section III)

Disabled family **Coping** (See **Coping,** family, disabled, Section III)

Interrupted **Family Processes** r/t situation transition and/or crises, developmental transition and/or crises

Ineffective family **Health** management (See family **Health** management, ineffective, Section III)

Readiness for enhanced family **Coping:** needs sufficiently gratified, adaptive tasks effectively addressed to enable goals of self-actualization to surface

Family Process

Dysfunctional **Family** processes (See **Family** processes, dysfunctional, Section III)

Interrupted **Family** processes (See **Family** processes, interrupted, Section III)

Readiness for enhanced **Family** processes (See **Family** processes, readiness for enhanced, Section III)

Readiness for enhanced **Relationship** (See **Relationship,** readiness for enhanced, Section III)

Fatigue

Fatigue (See **Fatigue,** Section III)

Fear

Death **Anxiety** r/t fear of death

Fear r/t identifiable physical or psychological threat to person

Febrile Seizures

See Seizure Disorders, Childhood (Epilepsy, Febrile Seizures, Infantile Spasms)

Fecal Impaction

See Impaction of Stool

(See **Constipation,** Section III)

(See **Constipation**, chronic functional, Section III)

Fecal Incontinence

Bowel **Incontinence** r/t neurological impairment, gastrointestinal disorders, anorectal trauma, weakened perineal muscles

Feeding Problems, Newborn

Ineffective **Breastfeeding** (See **Breastfeeding,** ineffective, Section III)

Insufficient **Breastfeeding** (See **Breastfeeding,** insufficient, Section III)

Disorganized **Infant** behavior r/t prematurity, immature neurological system

Ineffective infant **Feeding** pattern r/t prematurity, neurological impairment or delay, oral hypersensitivity, prolonged nothing-by-mouth status

Impaired **Swallowing** r/t prematurity

Risk for delayed **Development:** Risk factor: inadequate nutrition

Risk for deficient **Fluid** volume: Risk factor: inability to take in adequate amount of fluids

Risk for disproportionate **Growth:** Risk factor: feeding problems

Femoral Popliteal Bypass

Anxiety r/t threat to or change in health status

Acute **Pain** r/t surgical trauma, edema in surgical area

Ineffective peripheral **Tissue Perfusion** r/t impaired arterial circulation

Risk for **Bleeding:** Risk factor: surgery on arteries

Risk for **Infection:** Risk factor: invasive procedure

Fetal Alcohol Syndrome

See Infant of Substance-Abusing Mother

Fetal Distress/Nonreassuring Fetal Heart Rate Pattern

Fear r/t threat to fetus

Ineffective peripheral **Tissue Perfusion:** fetal r/t interruption of umbilical cord blood flow

Fever

Ineffective **Thermoregulation** r/t infectious process

Risk for Imbalanced body **Temperature:** Risk factors: acute brain injury; pharmaceutical agent

Fibrocystic Breast Disease

See Breast Lumps

Filthy Home Environment

Impaired **Home** maintenance (See **Home** maintenance, impaired, Section III)

Self-Neglect r/t mental illness, substance abuse, cognitive impairment

Financial Crisis in the Home Environment

Impaired **Home** maintenance r/t insufficient finances

Fistulectomy

See Hemorrhoidectomy

Flail Chest

Ineffective **Breathing** pattern r/t chest trauma

Fear r/t difficulty breathing

Impaired **Gas** exchange r/t loss of effective lung function

Impaired spontaneous **Ventilation** r/t paradoxical respirations

Flashbacks

Post-Trauma syndrome r/t catastrophic event

Flat Affect

Hopelessness r/t prolonged activity restriction creating isolation, failing or deteriorating physiological condition, long-term stress, abandonment, lost belief in transcendent values or higher power or God

Risk for **Loneliness:** Risk factors: social isolation, lack of interest in surroundings

See Depression (Major Depressive Disorder); Dysthymic Disorder

Flesh-Eating Bacteria (Necrotizing Fasciitis)

See Necrotizing Fasciitis (Flesh-Eating Bacteria)

Fluid Balance

Readiness for enhanced **Fluid** balance (See **Fluid** balance, readiness for enhanced, Section III)

Fluid Volume Deficit

Deficient **Fluid** volume r/t active fluid loss, vomiting, diarrhea, failure of regulatory mechanisms

Risk for **Shock:** Risk factors: hypovolemia, sepsis, systemic inflammatory response syndrome (SIRS)

Fluid Volume Excess

Excess **Fluid** volume r/t compromised regulatory mechanism, excess sodium intake

Fluid Volume Imbalance, Risk for

Risk for imbalanced **Fluid** volume: Risk factor: major invasive surgeries

Food Allergies

Diarrhea r/t immune effects of offending food on gastrointestinal system

Risk for **Allergy** response: Risk factor: specific foods

Readiness for enhanced **Knowledge:** expresses an interest in learning

See Anaphylactic Shock if relevant

Foodborne Illness

Diarrhea r/t infectious material in gastrointestinal tract

Deficient **Fluid** volume r/t active fluid loss from vomiting and diarrhea

Deficient **Knowledge** r/t care of self with serious illness, prevention of further incidences of foodborne illness

Nausea r/t contamination irritating stomach

Risk for dysfunctional **Gastrointestinal** motility: Risk factor: contaminated food

See Gastroenteritis; Gastroenteritis, Child; Hospitalized Child; E. coli *Infection*

Food Intolerance

Risk for dysfunctional **Gastrointestinal** motility: Risk factor: food intolerance

Foreign Body Aspiration

Ineffective **Airway** clearance r/t obstruction of airway

Ineffective **Health** maintenance r/t parental deficient knowledge regarding high-risk items

Risk for **Suffocation:** Risk factor: inhalation of small objects

See Safety, Childhood

Formula Feeding of Infant

Grieving: maternal r/t loss of desired breastfeeding experience

Risk for **Constipation:** infant: Risk factor: iron-fortified formula

Risk for **Infection:** infant: Risk factors: lack of passive maternal immunity, supine feeding position, contamination of formula

Readiness for enhanced **Knowledge:** expresses an interest in learning

Fracture

Deficient **Diversional** activity r/t immobility

Impaired physical **Mobility** r/t limb immobilization

Acute **Pain** r/t muscle spasm, edema, trauma

Post-Trauma syndrome r/t catastrophic event

Impaired **Walking** r/t limb immobility

Risk for ineffective peripheral **Tissue Perfusion:** Risk factors: immobility, presence of cast

Risk for **Peripheral Neurovascular** dysfunction: Risk factors: mechanical compression, treatment of fracture

Risk for impaired **Skin** integrity: Risk factors: immobility, presence of cast

Readiness for enhanced **Knowledge:** expresses an interest in learning

Fractured Hip

See Hip Fracture

Frail Elderly Syndrome

Activity intolerance r/t sensory changes

Risk for **Frail Elderly** syndrome (see **Frail Elderly** syndrome, risk for, Section III)

Risk for **Injury:** Risk factors: impaired vision, impaired gait

Risk for **Powerlessness:** Risk factor: inability to maintain independence

Frequency of Urination

Stress urinary **Incontinence** r/t degenerative change in pelvic muscles and structural support

Urge urinary **Incontinence** r/t decreased bladder capacity, irritation of bladder stretch receptors causing spasm, alcohol, caffeine, increased fluids, increased urine concentration, overdistended bladder

Impaired **Urinary** elimination r/t urinary tract infection

Urinary retention r/t high urethral pressure caused by weak detrusor, inhibition of reflex arc, strong sphincter, blockage

Friendship

Readiness for enhanced **Relationship:** expresses desire to enhance communication between partners

G

Frostbite

Acute **Pain** r/t decreased circulation from prolonged exposure to cold

Ineffective peripheral **Tissue Perfusion** r/t damage to extremities from prolonged exposure to cold

Impaired **Tissue** integrity r/t freezing of skin and tissues

See Hypothermia

Frothy Sputum

See CHF (Congestive Heart Failure); Pulmonary Edema; Seizure Disorders, Adult; Seizure Disorders, Childhood (Epilepsy, Febrile Seizures, Infantile Spasms)

Fusion, Lumbar

Anxiety r/t fear of surgical procedure, possible recurring problems

Impaired physical **Mobility** r/t limitations from surgical procedure, presence of brace

Acute **Pain** r/t discomfort at bone donor site, surgical operation

Risk for **Injury:** Risk factor: improper body mechanics

Risk for **Perioperative Positioning** injury: Risk factor: immobilization during surgery

Readiness for enhanced **Knowledge:** expresses an interest in learning

G

Gag Reflex, Depressed or Absent

Impaired **Swallowing** r/t neuromuscular impairment

Risk for **Aspiration:** Risk factors: depressed cough or gag reflex

Gallop Rhythm

Decreased **Cardiac** output r/t decreased contractility of heart

Gallstones

See Cholelithiasis

Gang Member

Impaired individual **Resilience** (See **Resilience,** individual, impaired, Section III)

Gangrene

Fear r/t possible loss of extremity

Ineffective peripheral **Tissue** perfusion r/t obstruction of arterial flow

See Diabetes Mellitus, Peripheral Vascular Disease

Gas Exchange, Impaired

Impaired **Gas** exchange r/t ventilation-perfusion imbalance

Gastric Ulcer

See GI Bleed (Gastrointestinal Bleeding); Ulcer, Peptic (Duodenal or Gastric)

Gastritis

Imbalanced **Nutrition:** less than body requirements r/t vomiting, inadequate intestinal absorption of nutrients, restricted dietary regimen

Acute **Pain** r/t inflammation of gastric mucosa

Risk for deficient **Fluid** volume: Risk factors: excessive loss from gastrointestinal tract from vomiting, decreased intake

Gastroenteritis

Diarrhea r/t infectious process involving intestinal tract

Deficient **Fluid** volume r/t excessive loss from gastrointestinal tract from diarrhea, vomiting

Nausea r/t irritation to gastrointestinal system

Imbalanced **Nutrition:** less than body requirements r/t vomiting, inadequate intestinal absorption of nutrients, restricted dietary intake

Acute **Pain** r/t increased peristalsis causing cramping

Risk for **Electrolyte** imbalance: Risk factor: loss of gastrointestinal fluids high in electrolytes

Readiness for enhanced **Knowledge:** expresses an interest in learning

See Gastroenteritis, Child

Gastroenteritis, Child

Impaired **Skin** integrity: diaper rash r/t acidic excretions on perineal tissues

Readiness for enhanced **Knowledge:** expresses an interest in learning

Acute **Pain** r/t increased peristalsis causing cramping

See Gastroenteritis; Hospitalized Child

Gastroesophageal Reflux (GERD)

Ineffective **Airway** clearance r/t reflux of gastric contents into esophagus and tracheal or bronchial tree

Ineffective **Health** maintenance r/t deficient knowledge regarding anti-reflux regimen (e.g., positioning, change in diet)

Acute **Pain** r/t irritation of esophagus from gastric acids

Risk for **Aspiration:** Risk factor: entry of gastric contents in tracheal or bronchial tree

Gastroesophageal Reflux, Child

Ineffective **Airway** clearance r/t reflux of gastric contents into esophagus and tracheal or bronchial tree

Anxiety: parental r/t possible need for surgical intervention

Deficient **Fluid** volume r/t persistent vomiting

Imbalanced **Nutrition:** less than body requirements r/t poor feeding, vomiting

Risk for **Aspiration:** Risk factor: entry of gastric contents in tracheal or bronchial tree

Risk for impaired **Parenting:** Risk factors: disruption in bonding as a result of irritable or inconsolable infant; lack of sleep for parents

Readiness for enhanced **Knowledge:** expresses an interest in learning

See Child with Chronic Condition; Hospitalized Child

Gastrointestinal Bleeding (GI Bleed)

See GI Bleed (Gastrointestinal Bleeding)

Gastrointestinal Hemorrhage

See GI Bleed (Gastrointestinal Bleeding)

Gastrointestinal Surgery

Risk for **Injury:** Risk factor: inadvertent insertion of nasogastric tube through gastric incision line

Risk for ineffective **Gastrointestinal** perfusion (See **Gastrointestinal** perfusion, ineffective, risk for, Section III)

See Abdominal Surgery

Gastroschisis/Omphalocele

Ineffective **Airway** clearance r/t complications of anesthetic effects

Impaired **Gas** exchange r/t effects of anesthesia, subsequent atelectasis

Grieving r/t threatened loss of infant, loss of perfect birth or infant because of serious medical condition

Risk for deficient **Fluid** volume: Risk factors: inability to feed because of condition, subsequent electrolyte imbalance

Risk for **Infection:** Risk factor: disrupted skin integrity with exposure of abdominal contents

Risk for **Injury:** Risk factors: disrupted skin integrity, ineffective protection

Gastrostomy

Risk for impaired **Skin** integrity: Risk factor: presence of gastric contents on skin

See Tube Feeding

Genital Herpes

See Herpes Simplex II

Genital Warts

See STD (Sexually Transmitted Disease)

GERD

See Gastroesophageal Reflux (GERD)

Gestational Diabetes (Diabetes in Pregnancy)

Anxiety r/t threat to self and/or fetus

Impaired **Nutrition:** less than body requirements r/t decreased insulin production and glucose uptake in cells

Risk for **Overweight:** fetal: r/t excessive glucose uptake

Impaired **Nutrition:** more than body requirements: fetal r/t excessive glucose uptake

Risk for delayed **Development:** fetal: Risk factor: endocrine disorder of mother

Risk for unstable blood **Glucose:** Risk factor: excessive intake of carbohydrates

Risk for disproportionate **Growth:** fetal: Risk factor: endocrine disorder of mother

Risk for disturbed **Maternal–Fetal** dyad: Risk factor: impaired glucose metabolism

Risk for impaired **Tissue** integrity: fetal: Risk factors: large infant, congenital defects, birth injury

Risk for impaired **Tissue** integrity: maternal: Risk factor: delivery of large infant

Readiness for enhanced **Knowledge:** expresses an interest in learning

See Diabetes Mellitus

GI Bleed (Gastrointestinal Bleeding)

Fatigue r/t loss of circulating blood volume, decreased ability to transport oxygen

Fear r/t threat to well-being, potential death

Deficient **Fluid** volume r/t gastrointestinal bleeding, hemorrhage

Imbalanced **Nutrition:** less than body requirements r/t nausea, vomiting

Acute **Pain** r/t irritated mucosa from acid secretion

Risk for ineffective **Coping:** Risk factors: personal vulnerability in crisis, bleeding, hospitalization

Readiness for enhanced **Knowledge:** expresses an interest in learning

Gingivitis

Impaired **Oral Mucous Membrane** r/t ineffective oral hygiene

Glaucoma

Deficient **Knowledge** r/t treatment and self-care for disease

Vision Loss r/t untreated increased intraocular pressure *(see care plan in Appendix)*

See Vision Impairment

Glomerulonephritis

Excess **Fluid** volume r/t renal impairment

Imbalanced **Nutrition:** less than body requirements r/t anorexia, restrictive diet

Acute **Pain** r/t edema of kidney

Readiness for enhanced **Knowledge:** expresses an interest in learning

Gluten Allergy

See Celiac Disease

Gonorrhea

Acute **Pain** r/t inflammation of reproductive organs

Risk for **Infection:** Risk factor: spread of organism throughout reproductive organs

Readiness for enhanced **Knowledge:** expresses an interest in learning

See STD (Sexually Transmitted Disease)

Gout

Impaired physical **Mobility** r/t musculoskeletal impairment

Chronic **Pain** r/t inflammation of affected joint

Readiness for enhanced **Knowledge:** expresses an interest in learning

H

Grandiosity

Defensive **Coping** r/t inaccurate perception of self and abilities

Grand Mal Seizure

See Seizure Disorders, Adult; Seizure Disorders, Childhood (Epilepsy, Febrile Seizures, Infantile Spasms)

Grandparents Raising Grandchildren

Anxiety r/t change in role status

Decisional Conflict r/t support system deficit

Parental **Role** conflict r/t change in parental role

Compromised family **Coping** r/t family role changes

Interrupted **Family** processes r/t family roles shift

Ineffective **Role** performance r/t role transition, aging

Ineffective family **Health** management r/t excessive demands on individual or family

Risk for impaired **Parenting:** Risk factor: role strain

Risk for **Powerlessness:** Risk factors: role strain, situational crisis, aging

Risk for **Spiritual** distress: Risk factor: life change

Readiness for enhanced **Parenting:** physical and emotional needs of children are met

Graves' Disease

See Hyperthyroidism

Grieving

Grieving r/t anticipated or actual significant loss, change in life status, style, or function

Grieving, Complicated

Complicated **Grieving** r/t expected or sudden death of a significant other with whom there was a volatile relationship, emotional instability, lack of social support

Risk for complicated **Grieving:** Risk factors: death of a significant other with whom there was a volatile relationship, emotional instability, lack of social support

Groom Self (Inability to)

Bathing **Self-Care** deficit (See **Self-Care** deficit, bathing, Section III)

Dressing **Self-Care** deficit (See **Self-Care** deficit, dressing, Section III)

Growth and Development Lag

Risk for disproportionate **Growth** (See **Growth,** disproportionate, risk for, Section III)

Guillain-Barré Syndrome

Impaired **Spontaneous Ventilation** r/t weak respiratory muscles

Risk for **Aspiration** r/t ineffective cough; depressed gag reflex

See Neurologic Disorders

Guilt

Grieving r/t potential loss of significant person, animal, prized material possession, change in life role

Impaired individual **Resilience** (See **Resilience,** individual, impaired, Section III)

Situational low **Self-Esteem** r/t unmet expectations of self

Risk for complicated **Grieving:** Risk factors: actual loss of significant person, animal, prized material possession, change in life role

Risk for **Post-Trauma** syndrome: Risk factor: exaggerated sense of responsibility for traumatic event

Readiness for enhanced **Spiritual** well-being: desire to be in harmony with self, others, higher power or God

H

H1N1

See Influenza

Hair Loss

Disturbed **Body Image** r/t psychological reaction to loss of hair

Imbalanced **Nutrition:** less than body requirements r/t inability to ingest food because of biological, psychological, economic factors

Halitosis

Impaired **Dentition** r/t ineffective oral hygiene

Impaired **Oral Mucous Membrane** r/t ineffective oral hygiene

Hallucinations

Anxiety r/t threat to self-concept

Acute **Confusion** r/t alcohol abuse, delirium, dementia, mental illness, drug abuse

Ineffective **Coping** r/t distortion and insecurity of life events

Risk for **Self-Mutilation:** Risk factor: command hallucinations

Risk for other-directed **Violence:** Risk factors: catatonic excitement, manic excitement, rage or panic reactions, response to violent internal stimuli

Risk for self-directed **Violence:** Risk factors: catatonic excitement, manic excitement, rage or panic reactions, response to violent internal stimuli

Head Injury

Ineffective **Breathing** pattern r/t pressure damage to breathing center in brainstem

Acute **Confusion** r/t increased intracranial pressure

Decreased **Intracranial** adaptive capacity r/t increased intracranial pressure

Risk for ineffective **Cerebral** tissue perfusion: Risk factors: effects of increased intracranial pressure, trauma to brain

Vision Loss r/t pressure damage to sensory centers in brain (*see care plan in Appendix*)

See Neurologic Disorders

Headache

Acute **Pain** r/t lack of knowledge of pain control techniques or methods to prevent headaches

Ineffective **Health** management r/t lack of knowledge, identification, elimination of aggravating factors

Health Behavior, Risk-Prone

Risk-prone **Health** behavior: Risk factors (See **Health** behavior, risk-prone, Section III)

Health Maintenance Problems

Ineffective **Health** maintenance (See **Health** maintenance, ineffective, Section III)

Ineffective **Health** management (See **Health** management, ineffective, Section III)

Health-Seeking Person

Readiness for enhanced **Health** management (See **Health** management, readiness for enhanced, Section III)

Hearing Impairment

Impaired verbal **Communication** r/t inability to hear own voice

Hearing Loss (See **Hearing Loss,** Section III)

Social isolation r/t difficulty with communication

Heart Attack

See MI (Myocardial Infarction)

Heartburn

Nausea r/t gastrointestinal irritation

Acute **Pain:** heartburn r/t inflammation of stomach and esophagus

Risk for imbalanced **Nutrition:** less than body requirements: Risk factor: pain after eating

Readiness for enhanced **Knowledge:** expresses an interest in learning

See Gastroesophageal Reflux (GERD)

Heart Failure

Activity intolerance r/t weakness, fatigue

Decreased **Cardiac** output r/t impaired cardiac function, increased preload, decreased contractility, increased afterload

Constipation r/t activity intolerance

Fatigue r/t disease process with decreased cardiac output

Fear r/t threat to one's own well-being

Excess **Fluid** volume r/t impaired excretion of sodium and water

Impaired **Gas** exchange r/t excessive fluid in interstitial space of lungs

Powerlessness r/t illness-related regimen

Risk for **Shock** (cardiogenic): Risk factors: decreased contractility of heart, increased afterload

Readiness for enhanced **Health** management (See **Health** management, readiness for enhanced, Section III)

See Child with Chronic Condition; Congenital Heart Disease/Cardiac Anomalies; Hospitalized Child

Heart Surgery

See Coronary Artery Bypass Grafting (CABG)

Heat Stroke

Deficient **Fluid** volume r/t profuse diaphoresis from high environmental temperature

Hyperthermia r/t vigorous activity, high environmental temperature, inappropriate clothing

Hematemesis

See GI Bleed (Gastrointestinal Bleeding)

Hematuria

See Kidney Stone; UTI (Urinary Tract Infection)

Hemianopia

Anxiety r/t change in vision

Unilateral Neglect r/t effects of disturbed perceptual abilities

Visual Loss r/t impaired sensory reception, transmission, integration

Risk for **Injury:** Risk factor: disturbed sensory perception

Hemiplegia

Anxiety r/t change in health status

Disturbed **Body Image** r/t functional loss of one side of body

Impaired physical **Mobility** r/t loss of neurological control of involved extremities

Self-Care deficit: specify: r/t neuromuscular impairment

Impaired **Sitting** r/t partial paralysis

Impaired **Standing** r/t partial paralysis

Impaired **Transfer** ability r/t partial paralysis

Unilateral Neglect r/t effects of disturbed perceptual abilities

Impaired **Walking** r/t loss of neurological control of involved extremities

Risk for **Falls:** Risk factor: impaired mobility

Risk for impaired **Skin** integrity: Risk factors: alteration in sensation, immobility; pressure over bony prominence

See CVA (Cerebrovascular Accident)

Hemodialysis

Ineffective **Coping** r/t situational crisis

Interrupted **Family** processes r/t changes in role responsibilities as a result of therapy regimen

Excess **Fluid** volume r/t renal disease with minimal urine output

Powerlessness r/t treatment regimen

Risk for **Caregiver Role Strain:** Risk factor: complexity of care receiver treatment

Risk for **Electrolyte** imbalance: Risk factor: effect of metabolic state on kidney function

Risk for deficient **Fluid** volume: Risk factor: excessive removal of fluid during dialysis

Risk for **Infection:** Risk factors: exposure to blood products, risk for developing hepatitis B or C, impaired immune system

Risk for **Injury:** Risk factors: clotting of blood access, abnormal surface for blood flow

Risk for impaired **Tissue** integrity: Risk factor: mechanical factor associated with fistula formation

Readiness for enhanced **Knowledge:** expresses an interest in learning

See Renal Failure; Renal Failure, Child with Chronic Condition

Hemodynamic Monitoring

Risk for **Infection:** Risk factor: invasive procedure

Risk for **Injury:** Risk factors: inadvertent wedging of catheter, dislodgment of catheter, disconnection of catheter

Risk for impaired **Tissue** integrity: Risk factor: invasive procedure

See Shock; Cardiogenic, Hypovolemic, Septic, Systemic Inflammatory Response Syndrome (SIRS)

Hemolytic Uremic Syndrome

Fatigue r/t decreased red blood cells

Fear r/t serious condition with unknown outcome

Deficient **Fluid** volume r/t vomiting, diarrhea

Nausea r/t effects of uremia

Risk for **Injury:** Risk factors: decreased platelet count, seizure activity

Risk for impaired **Skin** integrity: Risk factor: diarrhea

See Hospitalized Child; Renal Failure, Acute/Chronic, Child

Hemophilia

Fear r/t high risk for AIDS infection from contaminated blood products

Impaired physical **Mobility** r/t pain from acute bleeds, imposed activity restrictions, joint pain

Acute **Pain** r/t bleeding into body tissues

Risk for **Bleeding:** Risk factors: deficient clotting factors, child's developmental level, age-appropriate play, inappropriate use of toys or sports equipment

Readiness for enhanced **Knowledge:** expresses an interest in learning

See Child with Chronic Condition; Hospitalized Child; Maturational Issues, Adolescent

Hemoptysis

Fear r/t serious threat to well-being

Risk for ineffective **Airway** clearance: Risk factor: obstruction of airway with blood and mucus

Risk for deficient **Fluid** volume: Risk factor: excessive loss of blood

Hemorrhage

Fear r/t threat to well-being

Deficient **Fluid** volume r/t massive blood loss

See Hypovolemic Shock

Hemorrhoidectomy

Anxiety r/t embarrassment, need for privacy

Constipation r/t fear of pain with defecation

Acute **Pain** r/t surgical procedure

Urinary Retention r/t pain, anesthetic effect

Risk for **Bleeding:** Risk factors: inadequate clotting, trauma from surgery

Readiness for enhanced **Knowledge:** expresses an interest in learning

Hemorrhoids

Impaired **Comfort** r/t itching in rectal area

Constipation r/t painful defecation, poor bowel habits

Impaired **Sitting** r/t pain and pressure

Readiness for enhanced **Knowledge:** expresses an interest in learning

Hemothorax

Deficient **Fluid** volume r/t blood in pleural space

See Pneumothorax

Hepatitis

Activity intolerance r/t weakness or fatigue caused by infection

Deficient **Diversional** activity r/t isolation

Fatigue r/t infectious process, altered body chemistry

Imbalanced **Nutrition:** less than body requirements r/t anorexia, impaired use of proteins and carbohydrates

Acute **Pain** r/t edema of liver, bile irritating skin

Social isolation r/t treatment-imposed isolation

Risk for deficient **Fluid** volume: Risk factor: excessive loss of fluids from vomiting and diarrhea

Readiness for enhanced **Knowledge:** expresses an interest in learning

Hernia

See Hiatal Hernia; Inguinal Hernia Repair

Herniated Disk

See Low Back Pain

Herniorrhaphy

See Inguinal Hernia Repair

Herpes in Pregnancy

Fear r/t threat to fetus, impending surgery

Situational low **Self-Esteem** r/t threat to fetus as a result of disease process

Risk for **Infection** (infant): Risk factors: transplacental transfer during primary herpes, exposure to active herpes during birth process

See Herpes Simplex II

Herpes Simplex I

Impaired **Oral Mucous Membrane** r/t inflammatory changes in mouth

Herpes Simplex II

Ineffective **Health** maintenance r/t deficient knowledge regarding treatment, prevention, spread of disease

Acute **Pain** r/t active herpes lesion

Situational low **Self-Esteem** r/t expressions of shame or guilt

Sexual dysfunction r/t disease process

Impaired **Tissue** integrity r/t active herpes lesion

Impaired **Urinary** elimination r/t pain with urination

Herpes Zoster

See Shingles

HHNS (Hyperosmolar Hyperglycemic Nonketotic Syndrome)

See Hyperosmolar Hyperglycemic Nonketotic Syndrome (HHNS)

Hiatal Hernia

Ineffective **Health** maintenance r/t deficient knowledge regarding care of disease

Nausea r/t effects of gastric contents in esophagus

Imbalanced **Nutrition:** less than body requirements r/t pain after eating

Acute **Pain** r/t gastroesophageal reflux

Hip Fracture

Acute **Confusion** r/t sensory overload, sensory deprivation, medication side effects, advanced age, pain

Constipation r/t immobility, opioids, anesthesia

Fear r/t outcome of treatment, future mobility, present helplessness

Impaired physical **Mobility** r/t surgical incision, temporary absence of weight bearing, pain when walking

Acute **Pain** r/t injury, surgical procedure, movement

Powerlessness r/t health care environment

Self-Care deficit: specify r/t musculoskeletal impairment

Impaired **Transfer** ability r/t immobilization of hip

Impaired **Walking** r/t temporary absence of weight bearing

Risk for **Bleeding:** Risk factors: postoperative complication, surgical blood loss

Risk for **Infection:** Risk factor: invasive procedure

Risk for **Injury:** Risk factors: activities such as greater than 90-degree flexion of hips that can result in dislodged prosthesis, unsteadiness when ambulating

Risk for **Perioperative Positioning** injury: Risk factors: immobilization, muscle weakness, emaciation

Risk for **Peripheral Neurovascular** dysfunction: Risk factors: trauma, vascular obstruction, fracture

Risk for impaired **Skin** integrity: Risk factor: immobility

Hip Replacement

See Total Joint Replacement (Total Hip/Total Knee/Shoulder)

Hirschsprung's Disease

Constipation: bowel obstruction r/t inhibited peristalsis as a result of congenital absence of parasympathetic ganglion cells in distal colon

Grieving r/t loss of perfect child, birth of child with congenital defect even though child expected to be normal within 2 years

Imbalanced **Nutrition:** less than body requirements r/t anorexia, pain from distended colon

Acute **Pain** r/t distended colon, incisional postoperative pain

Impaired **Skin** integrity r/t stoma, potential skin care problems associated with stoma

Readiness for enhanced **Knowledge:** expresses an interest in learning

See Hospitalized Child

Hirsutism

Disturbed **Body Image** r/t excessive hair

Hitting Behavior

Acute **Confusion** r/t dementia, alcohol abuse, drug abuse, delirium

Risk for other-directed **Violence** (See **Violence,** other-directed, risk for, Section III)

HIV (Human Immunodeficiency Virus)

Fear r/t possible death

Ineffective **Protection** r/t depressed immune system

See AIDS (Acquired Immunodeficiency Syndrome)

Hodgkin's Disease

See Anemia; Cancer; Chemotherapy

Homelessness

Impaired **Home** maintenance r/t impaired cognitive or emotional functioning, inadequate support system, insufficient finances

Home Maintenance Problems

Impaired **Home** maintenance (See **Home** maintenance, impaired, Section III)

Self-Neglect r/t mental illness, substance abuse, cognitive impairment

Powerlessness r/t interpersonal interactions

Risk for **Trauma:** Risk factor: being in high-crime neighborhood

Hope

Readiness for enhanced **Hope** (See **Hope,** readiness for enhanced, Section III)

Hopelessness

Hopelessness (See **Hopelessness,** Section III)

Hospitalized Child

Activity intolerance r/t fatigue associated with acute illness

Anxiety: separation (child) r/t familiar surroundings and separation from family and friends

Compromised family **Coping** r/t possible prolonged hospitalization that exhausts supportive capacity of significant people

Ineffective **Coping:** parent r/t possible guilt regarding hospitalization of child, parental inadequacies

Deficient **Diversional** activity r/t immobility, monotonous environment, frequent or lengthy treatments, reluctance to participate, therapeutic isolation, separation from peers

Interrupted **Family** processes r/t situational crisis of illness, disease, hospitalization

Fear r/t deficient knowledge or maturational level with fear of unknown, mutilation, painful procedures, surgery

Hopelessness: child r/t prolonged activity restriction, uncertain prognosis

Insomnia: child or parent r/t 24-hour care needs of hospitalization

Acute **Pain** r/t treatments, diagnostic or therapeutic procedures, disease process

Powerlessness: child r/t health care environment, illness-related regimen

Risk for impaired **Attachment:** Risk factor: separation

Risk for delayed **Development:** regression: Risk factors: disruption of normal routine, unfamiliar environment or caregivers, developmental vulnerability of young children

Risk for **Injury:** Risk factors: unfamiliar environment, developmental age, lack of parental knowledge regarding safety (e.g., side rails, IV site/pole)

Risk for imbalanced **Nutrition:** less than body requirements: Risk factors: anorexia, absence of familiar foods, cultural preferences

Readiness for enhanced family **Coping:** impact of crisis on family values, priorities, goals, relationships in family

See Child with Chronic Condition

Hostile Behavior

Risk for other-directed **Violence:** Risk factor: antisocial personality disorder

HTN (Hypertension)

Ineffective **Health** management (See **Health** management, ineffective, Section III)

Readiness for enhanced **Health** management (See **Health** management, readiness for enhanced, Section III)

Risk for **Overweight:** Risk factor: lack of knowledge of relationship between diet and disease process

Human Immunodeficiency Virus (HIV)

See AIDS (Acquired Immunodeficiency Syndrome); HIV (Human Immunodeficiency Virus)

Humiliating Experience

Risk for compromised **Human Dignity** (See **Human Dignity,** compromised, risk for, Section III)

Huntington's Disease

Decisional Conflict r/t whether to have children

See Neurologic Disorders

Hydrocele

Acute **Pain** r/t severely enlarged hydrocele

Ineffective **Sexuality** pattern r/t recent surgery on area of scrotum

Hydrocephalus

Decisional Conflict r/t unclear or conflicting values regarding selection of treatment modality

Interrupted **Family** processes r/t situational crisis

Imbalanced **Nutrition:** less than body requirements r/t inadequate intake as a result of anorexia, nausea, vomiting, feeding difficulties

Risk for delayed **Development:** Risk factor: sequelae of increased intracranial pressure

Risk for disproportionate **Growth:** Risk factor: sequelae of increased intracranial pressure

Risk for **Infection:** Risk factor: sequelae of invasive procedure (shunt placement)

Risk for ineffective **Cerebral** tissue perfusion: Risk factors: interrupted flow, hypervolemia of cerebral ventricles

Risk for **Falls:** Risk factors: acute illness, alteration in cognitive functioning

See Normal Pressure Hydrocephalus (NPH); Child with Chronic Condition; Hospitalized Child; Mental Retardation (if appropriate); Premature Infant (Child); Premature Infant (Parent)

Hygiene, Inability to Provide Own

Frail Elderly syndrome r/t living alone

Self-Neglect (See **Self-Neglect,** Section III)

Bathing **Self-Care** deficit (See **Self-Care** deficit, bathing, Section III)

Hyperactive Syndrome

Decisional Conflict r/t multiple or divergent sources of information regarding education, nutrition, medication regimens; willingness to change own food habits; limited resources

Parental **Role** conflict: when siblings present r/t increased attention toward hyperactive child

Compromised family **Coping** r/t unsuccessful strategies to control excessive activity, behaviors, frustration, anger

Ineffective **Impulse** control r/t disorder of development, environment that might cause frustration or irritation

Ineffective **Role** performance: parent r/t stressors associated with dealing with hyperactive child, perceived or projected blame for causes of child's behavior, unmet needs for support or care, lack of energy to provide for those needs

Chronic low **Self-Esteem** r/t inability to achieve socially acceptable behaviors; frustration; frequent reprimands, punishment, or scolding for uncontrolled activity and behaviors; mood fluctuations and restlessness; inability to succeed academically; lack of peer support

Impaired **Social** interaction r/t impulsive and overactive behaviors, concomitant emotional difficulties, distractibility and excitability

Risk for delayed **Development:** Risk factor: behavior disorders

Risk for impaired **Parenting:** Risk factor: disruptive or uncontrollable behaviors of child

Risk for other-directed **Violence:** parent or child: Risk factors: frustration with disruptive behavior, anger, unsuccessful relationships

Hyperbilirubinemia (Infant)

Anxiety: parent r/t threat to infant, unknown future

Parental **Role** conflict r/t interruption of family life because of care regimen

Neonatal **Jaundice** r/t abnormal breakdown of red blood cells following birth

Imbalanced **Nutrition:** less than body requirements (infant) r/t disinterest in feeding because of jaundice-related lethargy

Risk for disproportionate **Growth:** infant: Risk factor: disinterest in feeding because of jaundice-related lethargy

Risk for imbalanced body **Temperature:** infant: Risk factor: phototherapy

Risk for **Injury:** infant: Risk factors: kernicterus, phototherapy lights

Hypercalcemia

Decreased **Cardiac** output r/t bradydysrhythmia

Impaired physical **Mobility** r/t decreased muscle tone

Imbalanced **Nutrition:** less than body requirements r/t gastro intestinal manifestations of hypercalcemia (nausea, anorexia, ileus)

Risk for **Disuse** syndrome: Risk factor: comatose state impairing mobility

Hypercapnia

Fear r/t difficulty breathing

Impaired **Gas** exchange r/t ventilation-perfusion imbalance, retention of carbon dioxide

See ARDS, COPD, Sleep Apnea,

Hyperemesis Gravidarum

Anxiety r/t threat to self and infant, hospitalization

Deficient **Fluid** volume r/t excessive vomiting

Impaired **Home** maintenance r/t chronic nausea, inability to function

Nausea r/t hormonal changes of pregnancy

Imbalanced **Nutrition:** less than body requirements r/t excessive vomiting

Powerlessness r/t health care regimen

Social isolation r/t hospitalization

Risk for **Electrolyte** imbalance: Risk factor: vomiting

Hyperglycemia

Ineffective **Health** management r/t complexity of therapeutic regimen, decisional conflicts, economic difficulties, unsupportive family, insufficient cues to action, deficient knowledge, mistrust, lack of acknowledgment of seriousness of condition

Risk for unstable blood **Glucose** level (See **Glucose** level, blood, unstable, risk for, Section III)

See Diabetes Mellitus

Hyperkalemia

Risk for **Activity** intolerance: Risk factor: muscle weakness

Risk for decreased **Cardiac** tissue perfusion: Risk factor: abnormal electrolyte level affecting heart rate and rhythm

Risk for excess **Fluid** volume: Risk factor: untreated renal failure

Hypernatremia

Risk for deficient **Fluid** volume: Risk factors: abnormal water loss, inadequate water intake

Hyperosmolar Hyperglycemic Nonketotic Syndrome (HHNS)

Acute **Confusion** r/t dehydration, electrolyte imbalance

Deficient **Fluid** volume r/t polyuria, hyperglycemia, inadequate fluid intake

Risk for **Electrolyte** imbalance: Risk factor: effect of metabolic state on kidney function

Risk for **Injury:** seizures: Risk factors: hyperosmolar state, electrolyte imbalance

See Diabetes Mellitus; Diabetes Mellitus, Juvenile (IDDM Type 1)

Hyperphosphatemia

Deficient **Knowledge** r/t dietary changes needed to control phosphate levels

See Renal Failure

Hypersensitivity to Slight Criticism

Defensive **Coping** r/t situational crisis, psychological impairment, substance abuse

Hypertension (HTN)

See HTN (Hypertension)

Risk for decreased **Cardiac** output: Risk factors: decreased contractility and altered conductivity associated with myocardial damage

Risk for impaired **Cardiovascular** function: Risk factors: obesity, inadequate physical activity and failure to alter diet

Hyperthermia

Hyperthermia (See **Hyperthermia,** Section III)

Hyperthyroidism

Anxiety r/t increased stimulation, loss of control

Diarrhea r/t increased gastric motility

Insomnia r/t anxiety, excessive sympathetic discharge

Imbalanced **Nutrition:** less than body requirements r/t increased metabolic rate, increased gastrointestinal activity

Risk for **Injury:** eye damage: Risk factor: protruding eyes without sufficient lubrication

Readiness for enhanced **Knowledge:** expresses an interest in learning

Hyperventilation

Ineffective **Breathing** pattern r/t anxiety, acid-base imbalance

See Anxiety Disorder, Dyspnea, Heart Failure

Hypocalcemia

Activity intolerance r/t neuromuscular irritability

Ineffective **Breathing** pattern r/t laryngospasm

Imbalanced **Nutrition:** less than body requirements r/t effects of vitamin D deficiency, renal failure, malabsorption, laxative use

Hypoglycemia

Acute **Confusion** r/t insufficient blood glucose to brain

Ineffective **Health** management r/t deficient knowledge regarding disease process, self-care

Imbalanced **Nutrition:** less than body requirements r/t imbalance of glucose and insulin level

Risk for unstable blood **Glucose** level (See **Glucose** level, blood, unstable, risk for, Section III)

See Diabetes Mellitus; Diabetes Mellitus, Juvenile (IDDM Type 1)

Hypokalemia

Activity intolerance r/t muscle weakness

Risk for decreased **Cardiac** tissue perfusion: Risk factor: possible dysrhythmia from electrolyte imbalance

Hypomagnesemia

Imbalanced **Nutrition:** less than body requirements r/t deficient knowledge of nutrition, alcoholism

See Alcoholism

Hypomania

Insomnia r/t psychological stimulus

See Manic Disorder, Bipolar I

Hyponatremia

Acute **Confusion** r/t electrolyte imbalance

Excess **Fluid** volume r/t excessive intake of hypotonic fluids

Risk for **Injury:** Risk factors: seizures, new onset of confusion

Hypoplastic Left Lung

See Congenital Heart Disease/Cardiac Anomalies

Hypotension

Decreased **Cardiac** output r/t decreased preload, decreased contractility

Risk for deficient **Fluid** volume: Risk factor: excessive fluid loss

Risk for ineffective **Cerebral** tissue perfusion: Risk factors: hypovolemia, decreased contractility, decreased afterload

Risk for ineffective **Gastrointestinal** perfusion (See **Gastrointestinal** perfusion, ineffective, risk for, Section III)

Risk for ineffective **Renal** perfusion: Risk factor: prolonged ischemia of kidneys

Risk for **Shock** (See **Shock,** risk for, Section III)

See Dehydration, Heart Failure, MI

Hypothermia

Hypothermia (See **Hypothermia,** Section III)

Risk for **Hypothermia** (see **Hypothermia,** risk for, Section III)

Hypothyroidism

Activity intolerance r/t muscular stiffness, shortness of breath on exertion

Constipation r/t decreased gastric motility

Impaired **Gas** exchange r/t respiratory depression

Impaired **Skin** integrity r/t edema, dry or scaly skin

Risk for **Overweight:** Risk factor: decreased metabolic process

Hypovolemic Shock

See Shock, Hypovolemic

Hypoxia

Acute **Confusion** r/t decreased oxygen supply to brain

Fear r/t breathlessness

Impaired **Gas** exchange r/t altered oxygen supply, inability to transport oxygen

Risk for **Shock** (See **Shock,** risk for, Section III)

Hysterectomy

Constipation r/t opioids, anesthesia, bowel manipulation during surgery

Ineffective **Coping** r/t situational crisis of surgery

Grieving r/t change in body image, loss of reproductive status

Acute **Pain** r/t surgical injury

Sexual dysfunction r/t disturbance in self-concept

Urinary retention r/t edema in area, anesthesia, opioids, pain

Risk for **Bleeding:** Risk factor: surgical procedure

Risk for **Constipation:** Risk factors: opioids, anesthesia, bowel manipulation during surgery

Risk for ineffective peripheral **Tissue** perfusion: Risk factor: deficient knowledge of aggravating factors

Readiness for enhanced **Knowledge:** Expresses an interest in learning

See Surgery, Perioperative; Surgery, Preoperative; Surgery, Postoperative

I

IBS (Irritable Bowel Syndrome)

Constipation r/t low-residue diet, stress

Diarrhea r/t increased motility of intestines associated with disease process, stress

Ineffective **Health** management r/t deficient knowledge, powerlessness

Chronic **Pain** r/t spasms, increased motility of bowel

Risk for **Electrolyte** imbalance: Risk factor: diarrhea

Readiness for enhanced **Health** management: expresses desire to manage illness and prevent onset of symptoms

ICD (Implantable Cardioverter/Defibrillator)

Anxiety r/t possible dysrhythmia, threat of death

Decreased **Cardiac** output r/t possible dysrhythmia

Readiness for enhanced **Knowledge:** expresses an interest in learning

IDDM (Insulin-Dependent Diabetes)

See Diabetes Mellitus

Identity Disturbance/Problems

Disturbed personal **Identity** r/t situational crisis, psychological impairment, chronic illness, pain

Risk for disturbed personal **Identity** (See **Identity**, personal, risk for disturbed in Section III)

Idiopathic Thrombocytopenic Purpura (ITP)

See ITP (Idiopathic Thrombocytopenic Purpura)

Ileal Conduit

Disturbed **Body Image** r/t presence of stoma

Ineffective **Health** management r/t new skills required to care for appliance and self

Ineffective **Sexuality** pattern r/t altered body function and structure

Social isolation r/t alteration in physical appearance, fear of accidental spill of urine

Risk for **Latex Allergy** response: Risk factor: repeated exposures to latex associated with treatment and management of disease

Risk for impaired **Skin** integrity: Risk factor: difficulty obtaining tight seal of appliance

Readiness for enhanced **Knowledge:** expresses an interest in learning

Ileostomy

Disturbed **Body Image** r/t presence of stoma

Diarrhea r/t dietary changes, alteration in intestinal motility

Deficient **Knowledge** r/t limited practice of stoma care, dietary modifications

Ineffective **Sexuality** pattern r/t altered body function and structure

Social isolation r/t alteration in physical appearance, fear of accidental spill of ostomy contents

Risk for impaired **Skin** integrity: Risk factors: difficulty obtaining tight seal of appliance, caustic drainage

Readiness for enhanced **Knowledge:** expresses an interest in learning

Ileus

Deficient **Fluid** volume r/t loss of fluids from vomiting, fluids trapped in bowel

Dysfunctional **Gastrointestinal** motility r/t effects of surgery, decreased perfusion of intestines, medication effect, immobility

Nausea r/t gastrointestinal irritation

Acute **Pain** r/t pressure, abdominal distention

Readiness for enhanced **Knowledge:** expresses an interest in learning

Immobility

Ineffective **Breathing** pattern r/t inability to deep breathe in supine position

Acute **Confusion:** elderly r/t sensory deprivation from immobility

Constipation r/t immobility

Risk for **Frail Elderly** syndrome: Risk factors: low physical activity, bed rest

Impaired physical **Mobility** r/t medically imposed bed rest

Ineffective peripheral **Tissue Perfusion** r/t interruption of venous flow

Powerlessness r/t forced immobility from health care environment

Impaired **Walking** r/t limited physical mobility, deconditioning of body

Risk for **Disuse** syndrome: Risk factor: immobilization

Risk for impaired **Skin** integrity: Risk factors: pressure over bony prominences, shearing forces when moved; pressure from devices

Risk for Impaired **Tissue** Integrity: Risk factors: mechanical factors from pressure over bony prominences, shearing forces when moved; pressure from devices

Risk for **Overweight:** Risk factor: energy expenditure less than energy intake

Readiness for enhanced **Knowledge:** expresses an interest in learning

Immunization

See Readiness for enhanced **Health** management, Section III

Immunosuppression

Risk for **Infection:** Risk factors: immunosuppression; exposure to disease outbreak

Impaired **Social** interaction r/t therapeutic isolation

Impaction of Stool

Constipation r/t decreased fluid intake, less than adequate amounts of fiber and bulk-forming foods in diet, medication effect, or immobility

Imperforate Anus

Anxiety r/t ability to care for newborn

Deficient **Knowledge** r/t home care for newborn

Impaired **Skin** integrity r/t pruritus

Impaired Sitting

Impaired physical **Mobility** r/t musculoskeletal, cognitive, or neuromuscular disorder

Impaired Standing

Activity intolerance r/t insufficient physiological or psychological energy

Powerlessness r/t loss of function

Impetigo

Impaired **Skin** integrity r/t infectious disease

Readiness for enhanced **Knowledge:** expresses an interest in learning

See Communicable Diseases, Childhood

Implantable Cardioverter/Defibrillator (ICD)

See ICD (Implantable Cardioverter/Defibrillator)

Impotence

Situational low **Self-Esteem** r/t physiological crisis, inability to practice usual sexual activity

Sexual dysfunction r/t altered body function

Readiness for enhanced **Knowledge:** treatment information for erectile dysfunction

I

See Erectile Dysfunction (ED)

Impulsiveness

Ineffective **Impulse** control r/t (See **Impulse** control, ineffective in Section III)

Inactivity

Activity intolerance r/t imbalance between oxygen supply and demand, sedentary lifestyle, weakness, immobility

Hopelessness r/t deteriorating physiological condition, long-term stress, social isolation

Impaired physical **Mobility** r/t intolerance to activity, decreased strength and endurance, depression, severe anxiety, musculoskeletal impairment, perceptual or cognitive impairment, neuromuscular impairment, pain, discomfort

Risk for **Constipation:** Risk factor: insufficient physical activity

Incompetent Cervix

See Premature Dilation of the Cervix (Incompetent Cervix)

Incontinence of Stool

Disturbed **Body Image** r/t inability to control elimination of stool

Bowel **Incontinence** r/t decreased awareness of need to defecate, loss of sphincter control

Toileting **Self-Care** deficit r/t cognitive impairment, neuromuscular impairment, perceptual impairment, weakness

Situational low **Self-Esteem** r/t inability to control elimination of stool

Risk for impaired **Skin** integrity: Risk factor: presence of stool

Incontinence of Urine

Functional urinary **Incontinence** r/t altered environment; sensory, cognitive, or mobility deficits

Overflow urinary **Incontinence** r/t relaxation of pelvic muscles and changes in urinary structures

Reflex urinary **Incontinence** r/t neurological impairment

Stress urinary **Incontinence** (See **Incontinence,** urinary, stress, Section III)

Urge urinary **Incontinence** (See **Incontinence,** urinary, urge, Section III)

Toileting **Self-Care** deficit r/t cognitive impairment

Situational low **Self-Esteem** r/t inability to control passage of urine

Risk for impaired **Skin** integrity: Risk factor: presence of urine on perineal skin

Indigestion

Nausea r/t gastrointestinal irritation

Imbalanced **Nutrition:** less than body requirements r/t discomfort when eating

Induction of Labor

Anxiety r/t medical interventions, powerlessness

Decisional Conflict r/t perceived threat to idealized birth

Ineffective **Coping** r/t situational crisis of medical intervention in birthing process

Acute **Pain** r/t contractions

Situational low **Self-Esteem** r/t inability to carry out normal labor

Risk for **Injury:** maternal and fetal: Risk factors: hypertonic uterus, potential prematurity of newborn

Readiness for enhanced **Family** processes: family support during induction of labor

Infant Apnea

See Premature Infant (Child); Respiratory Conditions of the Neonate; SIDS (Sudden Infant Death Syndrome)

Infant Behavior

Disorganized **Infant** behavior r/t pain, oral/motor problems, feeding intolerance, environmental overstimulation, lack of containment or boundaries, prematurity, invasive or painful procedures

Risk for disorganized **Infant** behavior: Risk factors: pain, oral/motor problems, environmental overstimulation, lack of containment or boundaries

Readiness for enhanced organized **Infant** behavior: stable physiologic measures, use of some self-regulatory measures

Infant Care

Readiness for enhanced **Childbearing** process: a pattern of preparing for, maintaining, and strengthening care of newborn infant

Infant Feeding Pattern, Ineffective

Ineffective infant **Feeding** pattern r/t prematurity, neurological impairment or delay, oral hypersensitivity, prolonged nothing-by-mouth order

Infant of Diabetic Mother

Decreased **Cardiac** output r/t cardiomegaly

Deficient **Fluid** volume r/t increased urinary excretion and osmotic diuresis

Imbalanced **Nutrition:** less than body requirements r/t hypotonia, lethargy, poor sucking, postnatal metabolic changes from hyperglycemia to hypoglycemia and hyperinsulinism

Risk for delayed **Development:** Risk factor: prolonged and severe postnatal hypoglycemia

Risk for impaired **Gas** exchange: Risk factors: increased incidence of cardiomegaly, prematurity

Risk for unstable blood **Glucose** level: Risk factor: metabolic change from hyperglycemia to hypoglycemia and hyperinsulinism

Risk for disproportionate **Growth:** Risk factor: prolonged and severe postnatal hypoglycemia

Risk for disturbed **Maternal–Fetal** dyad: Risk factor: impaired glucose metabolism

See Premature Infant (Child); Respiratory Conditions of the Neonate

Infant of Substance-Abusing Mother (Fetal Alcohol Syndrome, Crack Baby, Other Drug Withdrawal Infants)

Ineffective **Airway** clearance r/t pooling of secretions from the lack of adequate cough reflex, effects of viral or bacterial lower airway infection as a result of altered protective state

Interrupted **Breastfeeding** r/t use of drugs or alcohol by mother

Diarrhea r/t effects of withdrawal, increased peristalsis from hyperirritability

Ineffective infant **Feeding** pattern r/t uncoordinated or ineffective sucking reflex

Disorganized **Infant** behavior r/t exposure and or withdrawal from toxic substances (alcohol and drugs)

Ineffective **Childbearing** process r/t inconsistent prenatal health visits, suboptimal maternal nutrition, substance abuse

Insomnia r/t hyperirritability or hypersensitivity to environmental stimuli

Imbalanced **Nutrition:** less than body requirements r/t feeding problems; uncoordinated or ineffective suck and swallow; effects of diarrhea, vomiting, or colic associated with maternal substance abuse

Impaired **Parenting** r/t impaired or absent attachment behaviors, inadequate support systems

Risk for delayed **Development:** Risk factor: substance abuse

Risk for disproportionate **Growth:** Risk factor: substance abuse

Risk for **Infection:** skin, meningeal, respiratory: Risk factor: stress effects of withdrawal

See Cerebral Palsy; Child with Chronic Condition; Crack Baby; Failure to Thrive, Nonorganic; Hospitalized Child; Hyperactive Syndrome; Premature Infant (Child); SIDS (Sudden Infant Death Syndrome)

Infantile Polyarteritis

See Kawasaki Disease

Infection

Hyperthermia r/t increased metabolic rate

Ineffective **Protection** r/t inadequate nutrition, abnormal blood profiles, drug therapies, treatments

Impaired **Social** interaction r/t therapeutic isolation

Risk for **Vascular Trauma:** Risk factor: infusion of antibiotics

Infection, Potential for

Risk for **Infection** (See **Infection,** risk for, Section III)

Infertility

Ineffective **Health** management r/t deficient knowledge about infertility

Powerlessness r/t infertility

Chronic **Sorrow** r/t inability to conceive a child

Spiritual distress r/t inability to conceive a child

Inflammatory Bowel Disease (Child and Adult)

Ineffective **Coping** r/t repeated episodes of diarrhea

Diarrhea r/t effects of inflammatory changes of the bowel

Deficient **Fluid** volume r/t frequent and loose stools

Imbalanced **Nutrition:** less than body requirements r/t anorexia, decreased absorption of nutrients from gastrointestinal tract

Acute **Pain** r/t abdominal cramping and anal irritation

Impaired **Skin** integrity r/t frequent stools, development of anal fissures

Social isolation r/t diarrhea

See Child with Chronic Condition; Crohn's Disease; Hospitalized Child; Maturational Issues, Adolescent

Influenza

Deficient **Fluid** volume r/t inadequate fluid intake

Ineffective **Health** management r/t lack of knowledge regarding preventive immunizations

Ineffective **Thermoregulation** r/t infectious process

Acute **Pain** r/t inflammatory changes in joints

Readiness for enhanced **Knowledge:** information to prevent or treat influenza

Inguinal Hernia Repair

Impaired physical **Mobility** r/t pain at surgical site and fear of causing hernia to rupture

Acute **Pain** r/t surgical procedure

Urinary retention r/t possible edema at surgical site

Risk for **Infection:** Risk factor: surgical procedure

Injury

Risk for **Falls:** Risk factors: orthostatic hypotension, impaired physical mobility, diminished mental status

Risk for **Injury:** Risk factor: environmental conditions interacting with client's adaptive and defensive resources

Risk for corneal **Injury:** Risk factors: blinking less than five times per minute, mechanical ventilation, pharmaceutical agent, prolonged hospitalization

Risk for **Thermal** injury: Risk factors: cognitive impairment, inadequate supervision, developmental level

Risk for urinary tract **Injury:** Risk factor: inflammation and/or infection from long-term use of urinary catheter

Insanity

See Mental Illness, Psychosis

Insomnia

(See **Insomnia,** Section III)

Insulin Shock

See Hypoglycemia

Intellectual Disability

Impaired verbal **Communication** r/t developmental delay

Interrupted **Family** processes r/t crisis of diagnosis and situational transition

Grieving r/t loss of perfect child, birth of child with congenital defect or subsequent head injury

Deficient community **Health** r/t lack of programs to address developmental deficiencies

Impaired **Home** maintenance r/t insufficient support systems

Self-Neglect r/t learning disability

Self-Care deficit: bathing, dressing, feeding, toileting r/t perceptual or cognitive impairment

Self-Mutilation r/t inability to express tension verbally

Social isolation r/t delay in accomplishing developmental tasks

Spiritual distress r/t chronic condition of child with special needs

Stress overload r/t intense, repeated stressor (chronic condition)

Impaired **Swallowing** r/t neuromuscular impairment

Risk for ineffective **Activity** planning r/t inability to process information

Risk for delayed **Development:** Risk factor: cognitive or perceptual impairment

Risk for disproportionate **Growth:** Risk factor: mental retardation

Risk for impaired **Religiosity:** Risk factor: social isolation

Risk for **Self-Mutilation:** Risk factors: separation anxiety, depersonalization

Readiness for enhanced family **Coping:** adaptation and acceptance of child's condition and needs

See Child with Chronic Condition; Safety, Childhood

Intermittent Claudication

Deficient **Knowledge** r/t lack of knowledge of cause and treatment of peripheral vascular diseases

Acute **Pain** r/t decreased circulation to extremities with activity

Ineffective peripheral **Tissue Perfusion** r/t interruption of arterial flow

Risk for **Injury:** Risk factor: tissue hypoxia

Readiness for enhanced **Knowledge:** prevention of pain and impaired circulation

See Peripheral Vascular Disease (PVD)

Internal Cardioverter/Defibrillator (ICD)

See ICD (Implantable Cardioverter/Defibrillator)

Internal Fixation

Impaired **Walking** r/t repair of fracture

Risk for **Infection:** Risk factors: traumatized tissue, broken skin

See Fracture

Interstitial Cystitis

Acute **Pain** r/t inflammatory process

Impaired **Urinary** elimination r/t inflammation of bladder

Risk for **Infection:** Risk factor: suppressed inflammatory response

Readiness for enhanced **Knowledge:** expresses an interest in learning

Intervertebral Disk Excision

See Laminectomy

Intestinal Obstruction

See Ileus, Bowel Obstruction

Intestinal Perforation

See Peritonitis

Intoxication

Anxiety r/t loss of control of actions

Acute **Confusion** r/t alcohol abuse

Ineffective **Coping** r/t use of mind-altering substances as a means of coping

Impaired **Memory** r/t effects of alcohol on mind

Risk for **Aspiration:** Risk factors: diminished mental status, vomiting

Risk for **Falls:** Risk factor: diminished mental status

Risk for other-directed **Violence:** Risk factor: inability to control thoughts and actions

Intraaortic Balloon Counterpulsation

Anxiety r/t device providing cardiovascular assistance

Decreased **Cardiac** output r/t heart dysfunction needing counterpulsation

Compromised family **Coping** r/t seriousness of significant other's medical condition

Impaired physical **Mobility** r/t restriction of movement because of mechanical device

Risk for **Peripheral Neurovascular** dysfunction: Risk factors: vascular obstruction of balloon catheter, thrombus formation, emboli, edema

Risk for **Infection:** Risk factor: invasive procedure

Risk for impaired **Tissue** integrity: Risk factor: invasive procedure

Intracranial Pressure, Increased

Ineffective **Breathing** pattern r/t pressure damage to breathing center in brainstem

Acute **Confusion** r/t increased intracranial pressure

Decreased **Intracranial** adaptive capacity r/t sustained increase in intracranial pressure

Impaired **Memory** r/t neurological disturbance

Vision Loss r/t pressure damage to sensory centers in brain

Risk for ineffective **Cerebral** tissue perfusion: Risk factors: body position, cerebral vessel circulation deficits

See Head Injury, Subarachnoid Hemorrhage

Intrauterine Growth Retardation

Anxiety: maternal r/t threat to fetus

Ineffective **Coping:** maternal r/t situational crisis, threat to fetus

Impaired **Gas** exchange r/t insufficient placental perfusion

Imbalanced **Nutrition:** less than body requirements r/t insufficient placenta

Situational low **Self-Esteem:** maternal r/t guilt about threat to fetus

Spiritual distress r/t unknown outcome of fetus

Risk for **Powerlessness:** Risk factor: unknown outcome of fetus

Intravenous Therapy

Risk for **Vascular Trauma:** Risk factor: infusion of irritating chemicals

Intubation, Endotracheal or Nasogastric

Disturbed **Body Image** r/t altered appearance with mechanical devices

Impaired verbal **Communication** r/t endotracheal tube

Imbalanced **Nutrition:** less than body requirements r/t inability to ingest food because of the presence of tubes

Impaired **Oral Mucous Membrane** r/t presence of tubes

Acute **Pain** r/t presence of tube

Iodine Reaction with Diagnostic Testing

Risk for adverse reaction to iodinated **Contrast Media** (See reaction to iodinated **Contrast Media**, risk for adverse, Section III)

Irregular Pulse

See Dysrhythmia

Irritable Bowel Syndrome (IBS)

See IBS (Irritable Bowel Syndrome)

Isolation

Impaired individual **Resilience** (See **Resilience,** individual, impaired, Section III)

Social isolation (See **Social** isolation, Section III)

Itching

Impaired **Comfort** r/t inflammation of skin causing itching

Risk for impaired **Skin** integrity: Risk factor: scratching, dry skin

ITP (Idiopathic Thrombocytopenic Purpura)

Deficient **Diversional** activity r/t activity restrictions, safety precautions

Ineffective **Protection** r/t decreased platelet count

Risk for **Bleeding:** Risk factors: decreased platelet count, developmental level, age-appropriate play

See Hospitalized Child

J

Jaundice

Imbalanced **Nutrition,** less than body requirements r/t decreased appetite with liver disorder

Risk for **Bleeding:** Risk factor: impaired liver function

Risk for impaired **Liver** function: Risk factors: possible viral infection, medication effect

Risk for impaired **Skin** integrity: Risk factors: pruritus, itching

See Cirrhosis; Hepatitis

Jaundice, Neonatal

Neonatal **Jaundice** (See **Jaundice,** neonatal, Section III)

Risk for ineffective **Gastrointestinal** perfusion: Risk factor: liver dysfunction

Readiness for enhanced **Health** management (parents): expresses desire to manage treatment: assessment of jaundice when infant is discharged from the hospital, when to call the physician, and possible preventive measures such as frequent breastfeeding

See Hyperbilirubinemia

Jaw Pain and Heart Attacks

See Angina; Chest Pain; MI (Myocardial Infarction)

Jaw Surgery

Deficient **Knowledge** r/t emergency care for wired jaws (e.g., cutting bands and wires), oral care

Imbalanced **Nutrition:** less than body requirements r/t jaws wired closed, difficulty eating

Acute **Pain** r/t surgical procedure

Impaired **Swallowing** r/t edema from surgery

Risk for **Aspiration:** Risk factor: wired jaws

Jittery

Anxiety r/t unconscious conflict about essential values and goals, threat to or change in health status

Death **Anxiety** r/t unresolved issues relating to end of life

Risk for **Post-Trauma** syndrome: Risk factors: occupation, survivor's role in event, inadequate social support

Jock Itch

Ineffective **Health** management r/t prevention and treatment of disorder

Impaired **Skin** integrity r/t moisture and irritating or tight-fitting clothing

See Itching

Joint Dislocation

See Dislocation of Joint

Joint Pain

See Arthritis; Bursitis; JRA (Juvenile Rheumatoid Arthritis); Osteoarthritis; Rheumatoid Arthritis

Joint Replacement

Risk for **Peripheral Neurovascular** dysfunction: Risk factor: orthopedic surgery

Risk for impaired **Tissue** integrity: Risk factor: invasive procedure

See Total Joint Replacement (Total Hip/Total Knee/Shoulder)

JRA (Juvenile Rheumatoid Arthritis)

Impaired **Comfort** r/t altered health status

Fatigue r/t chronic inflammatory disease

Impaired physical **Mobility** r/t pain, restricted joint movement

Acute **Pain** r/t swollen or inflamed joints, restricted movement, physical therapy

Self-Care deficit: feeding, bathing, dressing, toileting r/t restricted joint movement, pain

Risk for compromised **Human Dignity:** Risk factors: perceived intrusion by clinicians, invasion of privacy

Risk for **Injury:** Risk factors: impaired physical mobility, splints, adaptive devices, increased bleeding potential from antiinflammatory medications

Risk for compromised **Resilience:** Risk factor: chronic condition

Risk for situational low **Self-Esteem:** Risk factor: disturbed body image

Risk for impaired **Skin** integrity: Risk factors: splints, adaptive devices

See Child with Chronic Condition; Hospitalized Child

K

Kaposi's Sarcoma

Risk for complicated **Grieving:** Risk factor: loss of social support

Risk for impaired **Religiosity:** Risk factors: illness/hospitalization, ineffective coping

Risk for impaired **Resilience:** Risk factor: serious illness

See AIDS (Acquired Immunodeficiency Syndrome)

Kawasaki Disease

Anxiety: parental r/t progression of disease, complications of arthritis, and cardiac involvement

Impaired **Comfort** r/t altered health status

Hyperthermia r/t inflammatory disease process

Imbalanced **Nutrition:** less than body requirements r/t impaired oral mucous membranes

Impaired **Oral Mucous Membrane** r/t inflamed mouth and pharynx; swollen lips that become dry, cracked, fissured

Acute **Pain** r/t enlarged lymph nodes; erythematous skin rash that progresses to desquamation, peeling, denuding of skin

Impaired **Skin** integrity r/t inflammatory skin changes

Risk for imbalanced **Fluid** volume: Risk factor: hypovolemia

Risk for decreased **Cardiac** tissue perfusion: Risk factor: cardiac involvement

See Hospitalized Child

Keloids

Disturbed **Body Image** r/t presence of scar tissue at site of a healed skin injury

Readiness for enhanced **Health** management: desire to have information to manage condition

Keratoconjunctivitis Sicca (Dry Eye Syndrome)

Risk for dry **Eye:** Risk factors: aging, staring at a computer screen for long intervals

Risk for **Infection:** Risk factor: dry eyes that are more vulnerable to infection

Risk for corneal **Injury:** Risk factors: dry eye; exposure of the eyeball

Vision Loss r/t dry eye resulting in film or obstruction of vision *(see care plan in Appendix)*

See Conjunctivitis

Keratoplasty

See Corneal Transplant

Ketoacidosis, Alcoholic

See Alcohol Withdrawal; Alcoholism

Ketoacidosis, Diabetic

Deficient **Fluid** volume r/t excess excretion of urine, nausea, vomiting, increased respiration

Impaired **Memory** r/t fluid and electrolyte imbalance

Imbalanced **Nutrition:** less than body requirements r/t body's inability to use nutrients

Risk for unstable blood **Glucose** level: Risk factor: deficient knowledge of diabetes management (e.g., action plan)

Risk for **Powerlessness:** Risk factor: illness-related regimen

Risk for impaired **Resilience:** Risk factor: complications of disease

See Diabetes Mellitus

Keyhole Heart Surgery

See MIDCAB (Minimally Invasive Direct Coronary Artery Bypass)

Kidney Disease Screening

Risk for ineffective **Renal** perfusion: Risk factors: hypovolemia, hypertension, alteration in metabolism

Readiness for enhanced **Health** management: seeks information for screening

Kidney Failure

Activity intolerance r/t effects of anemia, heart failure

Death **Anxiety** r/t unknown outcome of disease

Decreased **Cardiac** output r/t effects of heart failure, elevated potassium levels interfering with conduction system

Impaired **Comfort** r/t pruritus

Ineffective **Coping** r/t depression resulting from chronic disease

Fatigue r/t effects of chronic uremia and anemia

Excess **Fluid** volume r/t decreased urine output, sodium retention, inappropriate fluid intake

Ineffective **Health** management r/t complexity of health care regimen, inadequate number of cues to action, perceived barriers, powerlessness

Imbalanced **Nutrition:** less than body requirements r/t anorexia, nausea, vomiting, altered taste sensation, dietary restrictions

Impaired **Oral Mucous Membrane** r/t irritation from nitrogenous waste products

Chronic **Sorrow** r/t chronic illness

Spiritual distress r/t dealing with chronic illness

Impaired **Urinary** elimination r/t effects of disease, need for dialysis

Risk for **Electrolyte** imbalance: Risk factor: renal dysfunction

Risk for **Infection:** Risk factor: altered immune functioning

Risk for **Injury:** Risk factors: bone changes, neuropathy, muscle weakness

Risk for impaired **Oral Mucous Membrane:** Risk factors: dehydration, effects of uremia

Risk for **Powerlessness:** Risk factor: chronic illness

Risk for **Sepsis:** Risk factor: infection

Kidney Failure Acute/Chronic, Child

Disturbed **Body Image** r/t growth retardation, bone changes, visibility of dialysis access devices (shunt, fistula), edema

Deficient **Diversional Activity** r/t immobility during dialysis

See Child with Chronic Condition; Hospitalized Child

Kidney Failure, Nonoliguric

Anxiety r/t change in health status

Risk for deficient **Fluid** volume: Risk factor: loss of large volumes of urine

See Kidney Failure

Kidney Stone

Acute **Pain** r/t obstruction from kidney calculi

Impaired **Urinary** elimination: urgency and frequency r/t anatomical obstruction, irritation caused by stone

Risk for **Infection:** Risk factor: obstruction of urinary tract with stasis of urine

Readiness for enhanced **Knowledge:** expresses an interest in learning about prevention of stones

Kidney Transplantation, Donor

Impaired emancipated **Decision-Making** r/t harvesting of kidney from traumatized donor

Moral Distress r/t conflict among decision makers, end-of-life decisions, time constraints for decision-making

Spiritual distress r/t grieving from loss of significant person

Readiness for enhanced **Communication:** expressing thoughts and feelings about situation

Readiness for enhanced family **Coping:** decision to allow organ donation

Readiness for enhanced emancipated **Decision-Making:** expresses desire to enhance understanding and meaning of choices

Readiness for enhanced **Resilience:** decision to donate organs

Readiness for enhanced **Spirituality:** inner peace resulting from allowance of organ donation

See Nephrectomy

Kidney Transplantation, Recipient

Anxiety r/t possible rejection, procedure

Ineffective **Health** maintenance r/t long-term home treatment after transplantation, diet, signs of rejection, use of medications

Deficient **Knowledge** r/t specific nutritional needs, possible paralytic ileus, fluid or sodium restrictions

Impaired **Urinary** elimination r/t possible impaired renal function

Risk for **Bleeding:** Risk factor: surgical procedure

Risk for **Infection:** Risk factor: use of immunosuppressive therapy to control rejection

Risk for ineffective **Renal** perfusion: Risk factor: transplanted kidney

Risk for **Shock:** Risk factor: possible hypovolemia

Risk for **Spiritual** distress: Risk factor: obtaining transplanted kidney from someone's traumatic loss

Readiness for enhanced **Spiritual** well-being: acceptance of situation

Kidney Transplant

Ineffective **Protection** r/t immunosuppressive therapy

Risk for ineffective **Renal** perfusion: Risk factor: complications from transplant procedure

Readiness for enhanced **Decision-making:** expresses desire to enhance understanding of choices

Readiness for enhanced **Family** processes: adapting to life without dialysis

Readiness for enhanced **Health** management: desire to manage the treatment and prevention of complications after transplantation

Readiness for enhanced **Spiritual** well-being: heightened coping, living without dialysis

See Kidney Failure, Kidney Transplantation, Donor; Kidney Transplantation, Recipient; Nephrectomy; Perioperative Care; Surgery, Postoperative Care; Surgery, Preoperative Care

Kidney Tumor

See Wilms' Tumor

Kissing Disease

See Mononucleosis

Knee Replacement

See Total Joint Replacement (Total Hip/Total Knee/Shoulder)

Knowledge

Readiness for enhanced **Knowledge** (See **Knowledge,** readiness for enhanced, Section III)

Knowledge, Deficient

Ineffective **Health** maintenance r/t lack of or significant alteration in communication skills (written, verbal, and/or gestural)

Deficient **Knowledge** (See **Knowledge,** deficient, Section III)

Readiness for enhanced **Knowledge** (See **Knowledge,** readiness for enhanced, Section III)

Kock Pouch

See Continent Ileostomy (Kock Pouch)

Korsakoff's Syndrome

Acute **Confusion** r/t alcohol abuse

Dysfunctional **Family** processes r/t alcoholism as possible cause of syndrome

Impaired **Memory** r/t neurological changes associated with excessive alcohol intake

Self-Neglect r/t cognitive impairment from chronic alcohol abuse

Risk for **Falls:** Risk factor: cognitive impairment from chronic alcohol abuse

Risk for **Injury:** Risk factors: sensory dysfunction, lack of coordination when ambulating from chronic alcohol abuse

Risk for impaired **Liver** function: Risk factor: substance abuse (alcohol)

Risk for imbalanced **Nutrition:** less than body requirements: Risk factor: lack of adequate balanced intake from chronic alcohol abuse

L

Labor, Induction of

See Induction of Labor

Labor, Normal

Anxiety r/t fear of the unknown, situational crisis

Impaired **Comfort** r/t labor

Fatigue r/t childbirth

Deficient **Knowledge** r/t lack of preparation for labor

Labor **Pain** r/t uterine contractions, stretching of cervix and birth canal

Impaired **Tissue** integrity r/t passage of infant through birth canal, episiotomy

Risk for ineffective **Childbearing** process (See **Childbearing** process, Section III)

Risk for **Falls:** Risk factors: excessive loss or shift in intravascular fluid volume, orthostatic hypotension

Risk for deficient **Fluid** volume: Risk factor: excessive loss of blood

Risk for **Infection:** Risk factors: multiple vaginal examinations, tissue trauma, prolonged rupture of membranes

Risk for **Injury:** fetal: Risk factor: hypoxia

Risk for **Post-Trauma** syndrome: Risk factors: trauma or violence associated with labor pains, medical or surgical interventions, history of sexual abuse

Readiness for enhanced **Childbearing** process: responds appropriately, is proactive, bonds with infant, uses support systems

Readiness for enhanced family **Coping:** significant other provides support during labor

Readiness for enhanced **Health** management: prenatal care and childbirth education birth process

Readiness for enhanced **Power:** expresses readiness to enhance participation in choices regarding treatment during labor

Labor Pain

Labor **Pain** r/t uterine contractions, stretching of cervix and birth canal

Labyrinthitis

Ineffective **Health** management r/t delay in seeking treatment for respiratory and ear infections

Risk for **Injury** r/t dizziness

Readiness for enhanced **Health** management: management of episodes

See Ménière's Disease

Lacerations

Readiness for enhanced **Health** management: appropriate care of injury

Risk for **Infection:** Risk factor: broken skin

Risk for **Trauma:** Risk factor: children playing with dangerous objects

Lactation

See Breastfeeding, Ineffective; Breastfeeding, Interrupted; Breastfeeding, Readiness for Enhanced

Lactic Acidosis

Decreased **Cardiac** output r/t altered heart rate/rhythm, preload, and contractility

Risk for **Electrolyte** imbalance: Risk factor: impaired regulatory mechanism

Risk for decreased **Cardiac** tissue perfusion: Risk factor: hypoxia

See Ketoacidosis, Diabetes Mellitus

Lactose Intolerance

Readiness for enhanced **Knowledge:** interest in identifying lactose intolerance, treatment, and substitutes for milk products

See Abdominal Distention; Diarrhea

Laminectomy

Anxiety r/t change in health status, surgical procedure

Impaired **Comfort** r/t surgical procedure

Deficient **Knowledge** r/t appropriate postoperative and postdischarge activities

Impaired physical **Mobility** r/t neuromuscular impairment

Acute **Pain** r/t localized inflammation and edema

Urinary retention r/t competing sensory impulses, effects of opioids or anesthesia

Risk for **Bleeding:** Risk factor: surgery

Risk for **Infection:** Risk factor: invasive procedure, surgery

Risk for **Perioperative Positioning** injury: Risk factor: prone position

See Surgery, Perioperative; Surgery, Postoperative; Surgery, Preoperative

Language Impairment

See Speech Disorders

Laparoscopic Laser Cholecystectomy

See Cholecystectomy; Laser Surgery

Laparoscopy

Urge urinary **Incontinence** r/t pressure on the bladder from gas

Acute **Pain:** shoulder r/t gas irritating the diaphragm

Risk for ineffective **Gastrointestinal** perfusion: Risk factor: complications from procedure

Laparotomy

See Abdominal Surgery

Large Bowel Resection

See Abdominal Surgery

Laryngectomy

Ineffective **Airway** clearance r/t surgical removal of glottis, decreased humidification

Death **Anxiety** r/t unknown results of surgery

Disturbed **Body Image** r/t change in body structure and function

Impaired **Comfort** r/t surgery

Impaired verbal **Communication** r/t removal of larynx

Interrupted **Family** processes r/t surgery, serious condition of family member, difficulty communicating

Grieving r/t loss of voice, fear of death

Ineffective **Health** management r/t deficient knowledge regarding self-care with laryngectomy

Imbalanced **Nutrition:** less than body requirements r/t absence of oral feeding, difficulty swallowing, increased need for fluids

Impaired **Oral Mucous Membrane** r/t absence of oral feeding

Chronic **Sorrow** r/t change in body image

Impaired **Swallowing** r/t edema, laryngectomy tube

Risk for **Electrolyte** imbalance: Risk factor: fluid imbalance

Risk for complicated **Grieving:** Risk factors: loss, major life event

Risk for compromised **Human Dignity:** Risk factor: inability to communicate

Risk for **Infection:** Risk factors: invasive procedure, surgery

Risk for **Powerlessness:** Risk factors: chronic illness, change in communication

Risk for impaired **Resilience:** Risk factor: change in health status

Risk for situational low **Self-Esteem:** Risk factor: disturbed body image

Laser Surgery

Impaired **Comfort** r/t surgery

Constipation r/t laser intervention in vulval and perianal areas

Deficient **Knowledge** r/t preoperative and postoperative care associated with laser procedure

Acute **Pain** r/t heat from laser

Risk for **Bleeding:** Risk factor: surgery

Risk for **Infection:** Risk factor: delayed heating reaction of tissue exposed to laser

Risk for **Injury:** Risk factor: accidental exposure to laser beam

LASIK Eye Surgery (Laser-Assisted in Situ Keratomileusis)

Impaired **Comfort** r/t surgery

Decisional Conflict r/t decision to have surgery

Risk for **Infection:** Risk factor: invasive procedure/surgery

Readiness for enhanced **Health** management: surgical procedure preoperative and postoperative teaching and expectations

Latex Allergy

Latex Allergy response (See **Latex Allergy** response, Section III)

Risk for **Latex Allergy** response (See **Latex Allergy** response, risk for, Section III)

Readiness for enhanced **Knowledge:** prevention and treatment of exposure to latex products

Laxative Abuse

Perceived **Constipation** r/t health belief, faulty appraisal, impaired thought processes

Lead Poisoning

Contamination r/t flaking, peeling paint in presence of young children

Impaired **Home** maintenance r/t presence of lead paint

Risk for delayed **Development:** Risk factor: lead poisoning

Left Heart Catheterization

See Cardiac Catheterization

Legionnaires' Disease

Contamination r/t contaminated water in air-conditioning systems

See Pneumonia

Lens Implant

See Cataract Extraction; Vision Impairment

Lethargy/Listlessness

Frail Elderly syndrome r/t alteration in cognitive function

Fatigue r/t decreased metabolic energy production

Insomnia r/t internal or external stressors

Risk for ineffective **Cerebral** tissue perfusion: Risk factor: carbon dioxide retention and/or lack of oxygen supply to brain

Leukemia

Ineffective **Protection** r/t abnormal blood profile

Fatigue r/t abnormal blood profile and/or side effects of chemotherapy treatment

Risk for imbalanced **Fluid** volume: Risk factors: nausea, vomiting, bleeding, side effects of treatment

Risk for **Infection:** Risk factor: ineffective immune system

Risk for impaired **Resilience:** Risk factor: serious illness

See Cancer; Chemotherapy

Leukopenia

Ineffective **Protection** r/t leukopenia

Risk for **Infection:** Risk factor: low white blood cell count

Level of Consciousness, Decreased

See Confusion, Acute; Confusion, Chronic

L

Lice

Impaired **Comfort** r/t inflammation, pruritus

Readiness for enhanced **Health** management: preventing and treating infestation

Impaired **Home** maintenance r/t close unsanitary, overcrowded conditions

Self-Neglect r/t lifestyle

See Communicable Diseases, Childhood

Lifestyle, Sedentary

Sedentary lifestyle (See **Sedentary** lifestyle, Section III)

Risk for ineffective peripheral **Tissue Perfusion:** Risk factor: lack of movement

Lightheadedness

See Dizziness; Vertigo

Limb Reattachment Procedures

Anxiety r/t unknown outcome of reattachment procedure, use and appearance of limb

Disturbed **Body Image** r/t unpredictability of function and appearance of reattached body part

Grieving r/t unknown outcome of reattachment procedure

Spiritual distress r/t anxiety about condition

Stress overload r/t multiple coexisting stressors, physical demands

Risk for **Bleeding:** Risk factor: severed vessels

Risk for **Perioperative Positioning** injury: Risk factor: immobilization

Risk for **Peripheral Neurovascular** dysfunction: Risk factors: trauma, orthopedic and neurovascular surgery, compression of nerves and blood vessels

Risk for **Powerlessness:** Risk factor: unknown outcome of procedure

Risk for impaired **Religiosity:** Risk factors: suffering, hospitalization

See Surgery, Postoperative Care

Liposuction

Disturbed **Body Image** r/t dissatisfaction with unwanted fat deposits in body

Risk for impaired **Resilience:** Risk factor: body image disturbance

Readiness for enhanced **Decision-Making:** expresses desire to make decision regarding liposuction

Readiness for enhanced **Self-Concept:** satisfaction with new body image

See Surgery, Perioperative Care; Surgery, Postoperative Care; Surgery, Preoperative Care

Lithotripsy

Readiness for enhanced **Health** management: expresses desire for information related to procedure and aftercare and prevention of stones

See Kidney Stone

Liver Biopsy

Anxiety r/t procedure and results

Risk for deficient **Fluid** volume: Risk factor: hemorrhage from biopsy site

Risk for **Infection:** Risk factor: invasive procedure

Risk for **Powerlessness:** Risk factor: inability to control outcome of procedure

Liver Cancer

Risk for **Bleeding:** Risk factor: liver dysfunction

Risk for **Falls:** Risk factor: confusion associated with liver dysfunction

Risk for ineffective **Gastrointestinal** perfusion: Risk factor: liver dysfunction

Risk for impaired **Liver** function: Risk factor: disease process

Risk for impaired **Resilience:** Risk factor: serious illness

See Cancer; Chemotherapy; Radiation Therapy

Liver Disease

See Cirrhosis; Hepatitis

Liver Function

Risk for impaired **Liver** function (See **Liver** function, impaired, risk for, Section III)

Liver Transplant

Impaired **Comfort** r/t surgical pain

Decisional Conflict r/t acceptance of donor liver

Ineffective **Protection** r/t immunosuppressive therapy

Risk for impaired **Liver** function: Risk factors: possible rejection, infection

Readiness for enhanced **Family** processes: change in physical needs of family member

Readiness for enhanced **Health** management: desire to manage the treatment and prevention of complications after transplantation

Readiness for enhanced **Spiritual** well-being: heightened coping

See Surgery, Perioperative Care; Surgery, Postoperative Care; Surgery, Preoperative Care

Living Will

Moral Distress r/t end-of-life decisions

Readiness for enhanced **Decision-Making:** expresses desire to enhance understanding of choices for decision making

Readiness for enhanced **Relationship:** shares information with others

Readiness for enhanced **Religiosity:** request to meet with religious leaders or facilitators

Readiness for enhanced **Resilience:** uses effective communication

Readiness for enhanced **Spiritual** well-being: acceptance of and preparation for end of life

See Advance Directives

Lobectomy

See Thoracotomy

Loneliness

Spiritual distress r/t loneliness, social alienation

Risk for **Loneliness** (See **Loneliness,** risk for, Section III)

Risk for impaired **Religiosity:** Risk factor: lack of social interaction

Readiness for enhanced **Hope:** expresses desire to enhance interconnectedness with others

Readiness for enhanced **Relationship:** expresses satisfaction with complementary relationship between partners

Loose Stools (Bowel Movements)

Diarrhea r/t increased gastric motility

Risk for dysfunctional **Gastrointestinal** motility (See **Gastrointestinal** motility, dysfunctional, risk for, Section III)

See Diarrhea

Loss of Bladder Control

See Incontinence of Urine

Loss of Bowel Control

See Incontinence of Stool

Lou Gehrig's Disease

See Amyotrophic Lateral Sclerosis (ALS)

Low Back Pain

Impaired **Comfort** r/t back pain

Ineffective **Health** maintenance r/t deficient knowledge regarding self-care with back pain

Impaired physical **Mobility** r/t back pain

Chronic **Pain** r/t degenerative processes, musculotendinous strain, injury, inflammation, congenital deformities

Urinary Retention r/t possible spinal cord compression

Risk for **Powerlessness:** Risk factor: living with chronic pain

Readiness for enhanced **Health** management: expresses desire for information to manage pain

Low Blood Pressure

See Hypotension

Low Blood Sugar

See Hypoglycemia

Lower GI Bleeding

See GI Bleed (Gastrointestinal Bleeding)

Lumbar Puncture

Anxiety r/t invasive procedure and unknown results

Deficient **Knowledge** r/t information about procedure

Acute **Pain** r/t possible loss of cerebrospinal fluid

Risk for ineffective **Cerebral** tissue perfusion: Risk factor: treatment-related side effects

Risk for **Infection:** Risk factor: invasive procedure

Lumpectomy

Decisional Conflict r/t treatment choices

Readiness for enhanced **Knowledge:** preoperative and postoperative care

Readiness for enhanced **Spiritual** well-being: hope of benign diagnosis

See Cancer

Lung Cancer

See Cancer; Chemotherapy; Radiation Therapy; Thoracotomy

Lung Surgery

See Thoracotomy

Lupus Erythematosus

Disturbed **Body Image** r/t change in skin, rash, lesions, ulcers, mottled erythema

Fatigue r/t increased metabolic requirements

Ineffective **Health** maintenance r/t deficient knowledge regarding medication, diet, activity

Acute **Pain** r/t inflammatory process

Powerlessness r/t unpredictability of course of disease

Impaired **Religiosity** r/t ineffective coping with disease

Chronic **Sorrow** r/t presence of chronic illness

Spiritual distress r/t chronicity of disease, unknown etiology

Risk for decreased **Cardiac** tissue perfusion: Risk factor: altered circulation

Risk for impaired **Resilience:** Risk factor: chronic disease

Risk for impaired **Skin** integrity: Risk factors: chronic inflammation, edema, altered circulation

Lyme Disease

Impaired **Comfort** r/t inflammation

Fatigue r/t increased energy requirements

Deficient **Knowledge** r/t lack of information concerning disease, prevention, treatment

Acute **Pain** r/t inflammation of joints, urticaria, rash

Risk for decreased **Cardiac** output: Risk factor: dysrhythmia

Risk for **Powerlessness:** Risk factor: possible chronic condition

Lymphedema

Disturbed **Body Image** r/t change in appearance of body part with edema

Excess **Fluid** volume r/t compromised regulatory system; inflammation, obstruction, or removal of lymph glands

Deficient **Knowledge** r/t management of condition

Risk for **Infection**: Risk factors: abnormal lymphatic system allowing stasis of fluids with decreased resistance to infection

Risk for situational low **Self-Esteem:** Risk factor: disturbed body image

Lymphoma

See Cancer

M

Macular Degeneration

Ineffective **Coping** r/t visual loss

Compromised family **Coping** r/t deteriorating vision of family member

Risk-prone **Health** behavior r/t deteriorating vision while trying to maintain usual lifestyle

Hopelessness r/t deteriorating vision

Sedentary lifestyle r/t visual loss

Self-Neglect r/t change in vision

Social isolation r/t inability to drive because of visual changes

Vision Loss r/t impaired visual function

Risk for **Falls:** Risk factor: visual difficulties

Risk for **Injury:** Risk factor: inability to distinguish traffic lights and safety signs

Risk for **Powerlessness:** Risk factor: deteriorating vision

Risk for impaired **Religiosity:** Risk factor: possible lack of transportation to church

Risk for impaired **Resilience:** Risk factor: changing vision

Readiness for enhanced **Health** management: appropriate choices of daily activities for meeting the goals of a treatment program

Magnetic Resonance Imaging (MRI)

See MRI (Magnetic Resonance Imaging)

Major Depressive Disorder

See Depression (Major Depressive Disorder)

Malabsorption Syndrome

Diarrhea r/t lactose intolerance, gluten sensitivity, resection of small bowel

Dysfunctional **Gastrointestinal** motility r/t disease state

Deficient **Knowledge** r/t lack of information about diet and nutrition

Imbalanced **Nutrition:** less than body requirements r/t inability of body to absorb nutrients because of physiological factors

Risk for **Electrolyte** imbalance: Risk factors: hypovolemia, hyponatremia, hypokalemia

Risk for imbalanced **Fluid** volume: Risk factors: diarrhea, hypovolemia

Risk for disproportionate **Growth:** Risk factor: malnutrition from malabsorption

See Abdominal Distention

Maladaptive Behavior

See Crisis; Post-Trauma Syndrome; Suicide Attempt

Malaise

See Fatigue

Malaria

Contamination r/t geographic area

Risk for **Contamination:** Risk factors: increased environmental exposure (not wearing protective clothing, not using insecticide or repellant on skin and in room in areas where infected mosquitoes are present); inadequate defense mechanisms (inappropriate use of prophylactic regimen)

Risk for impaired **Liver** function: Risk factor: complications of disease

Readiness for enhanced community **Coping:** uses resources available for problem solving

Readiness for enhanced **Health** management: expresses desire to enhance immunization status /vaccination status

Readiness for enhanced **Resilience:** immunization status

See Anemia

Male Infertility

See Erectile Dysfunction (ED); Infertility

Malignancy

See Cancer

Malignant Hypertension (Arteriolar Nephrosclerosis)

Decreased **Cardiac** output r/t altered afterload, altered contractility

Fatigue r/t disease state, increased blood pressure

Excess **Fluid** volume r/t decreased kidney function

Risk for ineffective **Cerebral** tissue perfusion: Risk factor: elevated blood pressure damaging cerebral vessels

Risk for acute **Confusion:** Risk factors: increased blood urea nitrogen or creatinine levels

Risk for imbalanced **Fluid** volume: Risk factors: hypertension, altered kidney function

Risk for ineffective **Renal** perfusion: Risk factor: elevated blood pressure damaging the kidney

Readiness for enhanced **Health** management: expresses desire to manage the illness, high blood pressure

Malignant Hyperthermia

Hyperthermia r/t anesthesia reaction associated with inherited condition

Risk for ineffective **Renal** perfusion: Risk factors: hyperthermia and muscle destruction (rhabdomyolysis)

Readiness for enhanced **Health** management: knowledge of risk factors

Malnutrition

Insufficient **Breast Milk** r/t (See **Breast Milk,** insufficient, Section III)

Frail Elderly syndrome r/t undetected malnutrition

Deficient **Knowledge** r/t misinformation about normal nutrition, social isolation, lack of food preparation facilities

Imbalanced **Nutrition:** less than body requirements r/t inability to ingest food, digest food, or absorb nutrients because of biological, psychological, or economic factors; institutionalization (i.e., lack of menu choices)

Ineffective **Protection** r/t inadequate nutrition

Ineffective **Health** management r/t inadequate nutrition

Self-Neglect r/t inadequate nutrition

Risk for disproportionate **Growth:** Risk factor: malnutrition

Risk for **Powerlessness:** Risk factor: possible inability to provide adequate nutrition

Mammography

Readiness for enhanced **Health** management: follows guidelines for screening

Readiness for enhanced **Resilience:** responsibility for self-care

Manic Disorder, Bipolar I

Anxiety r/t change in role function

Ineffective **Coping** r/t situational crisis

Ineffective **Denial** r/t fear of inability to control behavior

Interrupted **Family** processes r/t family member's illness

Risk-prone **Health** behavior r/t low self-efficacy

Ineffective **Health** management r/t unpredictability of client, excessive demands on family, chronic illness, social support deficit

Impaired **Home** maintenance r/t altered psychological state, inability to concentrate

Disturbed personal **Identity** r/t manic state

Insomnia r/t constant anxious thoughts

Imbalanced **Nutrition:** less than body requirements r/t lack of time and motivation to eat, constant movement

Impaired individual **Resilience** r/t psychological disorder

Ineffective **Role** performance r/t impaired social interactions

Self-Neglect r/t manic state

Sleep deprivation r/t hyperagitated state

Risk for ineffective **Activity** planning r/t inability to process information

Risk for **Caregiver Role Strain:** Risk factor: unpredictability of condition

Risk for imbalanced **Fluid** volume: Risk factor: hypovolemia

Risk for **Powerlessness:** Risk factor: inability to control changes in mood

Risk for **Spiritual** distress: Risk factor: depression

Risk for **Suicide:** Risk factor: bipolar disorder

Risk for self-directed **Violence:** Risk factors: hallucinations, delusions

Risk for other-directed **Violence:** Risk factor: pathologic intoxication

Readiness for enhanced **Hope:** expresses desire to enhance problem-solving goals

Manipulative Behavior

Defensive **Coping** r/t superior attitude toward others

Ineffective **Coping** r/t inappropriate use of defense mechanisms

Self-Mutilation r/t use of manipulation to obtain nurturing relationship with others

Self-Neglect r/t maintaining control

Impaired **Social** interaction r/t self-concept disturbance

Risk for **Loneliness:** Risk factor: inability to interact appropriately with others

Risk for situational low **Self-Esteem:** Risk factor: history of learned helplessness

Risk for **Self-Mutilation:** Risk factor: inability to cope with increased psychological or physiological tension in healthy manner

Marfan Syndrome

Decreased **Cardiac** output r/t dilation of the aortic root, dissection or rupture of the aorta

Risk for decreased **Cardiac** tissue perfusion: Risk factor: heart-related complications from Marfan syndrome

Readiness for enhanced **Health** management: describes reduction of risk factors

See Mitral Valve Prolapse; Scoliosis

Mastectomy

Disturbed **Body Image** r/t loss of sexually significant body part

Impaired **Comfort** r/t altered body image; difficult diagnosis

Death **Anxiety** r/t threat of mortality associated with breast cancer

Fatigue r/t increased metabolic requirements

Fear r/t change in body image, prognosis

Deficient **Knowledge** r/t self-care activities

Nausea r/t chemotherapy

Acute **Pain** r/t surgical procedure

Sexual dysfunction r/t change in body image, fear of loss of femininity

Chronic **Sorrow** r/t disturbed body image, unknown long-term health status

Spiritual distress r/t change in body image

Risk for **Infection:** Risk factors: surgical procedure, broken skin

Risk for impaired physical **Mobility:** Risk factors: nerve or muscle damage, pain

Risk for **Post-Trauma** syndrome: Risk factors: loss of body part, surgical wounds

Risk for **Powerlessness:** Risk factor: fear of unknown outcome of procedure

Risk for impaired **Resilience:** Risk factor: altered body image

See Cancer; Modified Radical Mastectomy; Surgery, Perioperative; Surgery, Postoperative; Surgery, Preoperative

Mastitis

Anxiety r/t threat to self, concern over safety of milk for infant

Ineffective **Breastfeeding** r/t breast pain, conflicting advice from health care providers

Deficient **Knowledge** r/t antibiotic regimen, comfort measures

Acute **Pain** r/t infectious disease process, swelling of breast tissue

Ineffective **Role** performance r/t change in capacity to function in expected role

M

Maternal Infection

Ineffective **Protection** r/t invasive procedures, traumatized tissue

See Postpartum, Normal Care

Maturational Issues, Adolescent

Ineffective **Coping** r/t maturational crises

Risk-prone **Health** behavior r/t inadequate comprehension, negative attitude toward health care

Interrupted **Family** processes r/t developmental crises of adolescence resulting from challenge of parental authority and values, situational crises from change in parental marital status

Deficient **Knowledge:** potential for enhanced health maintenance r/t information misinterpretation, lack of education regarding age-related factors

Impaired **Social** interaction r/t ineffective, unsuccessful, or dysfunctional interaction with peers

Social isolation r/t perceived alteration in physical appearance, social values not accepted by dominant peer group

Risk for Ineffective **Activity** planning: Risk factor: unrealistic perception of personal competencies

Risk for disturbed personal **Identity:** Risk factor: maturational issues

Risk for **Injury:** Risk factor: thrill-seeking behaviors

Risk for chronic low **Self-Esteem:** Risk factor: lack of sense of belonging in peer group

Risk for situational low **Self-Esteem:** Risk factor: developmental changes

Readiness for enhanced **Communication:** expressing willingness to communicate with parental figures

Readiness for enhanced **Relationship:** expresses desire to enhance communication with parental figures

See Sexuality, Adolescent; Substance Abuse (if relevant)

Maze III Procedure

See Dysrhythmia; Open Heart Surgery

MD (Muscular Dystrophy)

See Muscular Dystrophy (MD)

Measles (Rubeola)

See Communicable Diseases, Childhood

Meconium Aspiration

See Respiratory Conditions of the Neonate

Meconium Delayed

Risk for neonatal **Jaundice:** Risk factor: delayed meconium

Melanoma

Disturbed **Body Image** r/t altered pigmentation, surgical incision

Fear r/t threat to well-being

Ineffective **Health** maintenance r/t deficient knowledge regarding self-care and treatment of melanoma

Acute **Pain** r/t surgical incision

Chronic **Sorrow** r/t disturbed body image, unknown long-term health status

Readiness for enhanced **Health** management: describes reduction of risk factors; protection from sunlight's ultraviolet rays

See Cancer

Melena

Fear r/t presence of blood in feces

Risk for imbalanced **Fluid** volume: Risk factor: hemorrhage

See GI Bleed (Gastrointestinal Bleeding)

Memory Deficit

Impaired **Memory** (See **Memory,** impaired, Section III)

Ménière's Disease

Risk for **Injury:** Risk factor: symptoms of disease

Readiness for enhanced **Health** management: expresses desire to manage illness

See Dizziness; Nausea; Vertigo

Meningitis/Encephalitis

Ineffective **Airway** clearance r/t seizure activity

Impaired **Comfort** r/t altered health status

Excess **Fluid** volume r/t increased intracranial pressure, syndrome of inappropriate secretion of antidiuretic hormone

Decreased **Intracranial** adaptive capacity r/t sustained increase in intracranial pressure

Impaired **Mobility** r/t neuromuscular or central nervous system insult

Acute **Pain** r/t biological injury

Risk for **Aspiration:** Risk factor: seizure activity

Risk for acute **Confusion:** Risk factor: infection of brain

Risk for **Falls:** Risk factors: neuromuscular dysfunction and confusion

Risk for **Injury:** Risk factor: seizure activity

Risk for impaired **Resilience:** Risk factor: illness

Risk for **Shock:** Risk factor: infection

Risk for ineffective **Cerebral** tissue perfusion: Risk factors: cerebral tissue edema and inflammation of meninges, increased intracranial pressure; infection

See Hospitalized Child

Meningocele

See Neural Tube Defects

Menopause

Impaired **Comfort** r/t symptoms associated with menopause

Insomnia r/t hormonal shifts

Impaired **Memory** r/t change in hormonal levels

Sexual dysfunction r/t menopausal changes

Ineffective **Sexuality** pattern r/t altered body structure, lack of lubrication, lack of knowledge of artificial lubrication

Ineffective **Thermoregulation** r/t changes in hormonal levels

Risk for urge urinary **Incontinence:** Risk factor: changes in hormonal levels affecting bladder function

Risk for **Overweight:** Risk factor: change in metabolic rate caused by fluctuating hormone levels

Risk for **Powerlessness:** Risk factor: changes associated with menopause

Risk for impaired **Resilience:** Risk factor: menopause

Risk for situational low **Self-Esteem:** Risk factors: developmental changes, menopause

Readiness for enhanced **Health** management: verbalized desire to manage menopause

Readiness for enhanced **Self-Care:** expresses satisfaction with body image

Readiness for enhanced **Spiritual** well-being: desire for harmony of mind, body, and spirit

Menorrhagia

Fear r/t loss of large amounts of blood

Risk for deficient **Fluid** volume: Risk factor: excessive loss of menstrual blood

Mental Illness

Defensive **Coping** r/t psychological impairment, substance abuse

Ineffective **Coping** r/t situational crisis, coping with mental illness

Compromised family **Coping** r/t lack of available support from client

Disabled family **Coping** r/t chronically unexpressed feelings of guilt, anxiety, hostility, or despair

Ineffective **Denial** r/t refusal to acknowledge abuse problem, fear of the social stigma of disease

Risk-prone **Health** behavior r/t low self-efficacy

Disturbed personal **Identity** r/t psychoses

Ineffective **Relationship** r/t effects of mental illness in partner relationship

Chronic **Sorrow** r/t presence of mental illness

Stress overload r/t multiple coexisting stressors

Ineffective family **Health** management r/t chronicity of condition, unpredictability of client, unknown prognosis

Risk for **Loneliness:** Risk factor: social isolation

Risk for **Powerlessness:** Risk factor: lifestyle of helplessness

Risk for impaired **Resilience:** Risk factor: chronic illness

Risk for chronic low **Self-Esteem:** Risk factor: presence of mental illness/repeated negative reinforcement

Metabolic Acidosis

See Ketoacidosis, Alcoholic; Ketoacidosis, Diabetic; Risk for Shock; Risk for Sepsis

Metabolic Alkalosis

Deficient **Fluid** volume r/t fluid volume loss, vomiting, gastric suctioning, failure of regulatory mechanisms

Metastasis

See Cancer

Methicillin-Resistant *Staphylococcus aureus* (MRSA)

See MRSA (Methicillin-Resistant Staphylococcus aureus*)*

MI (Myocardial Infarction)

Activity intolerance r/t imbalance between oxygen supply and demand

Anxiety r/t threat of death, possible change in role status

Death **Anxiety** r/t seriousness of medical condition

Constipation r/t decreased peristalsis from decreased physical activity, medication effect, change in diet

Ineffective family **Coping** r/t spouse or significant other's fear of partner loss

Ineffective **Denial** r/t fear, deficient knowledge about heart disease

Interrupted **Family** processes r/t crisis, role change

Fear r/t threat to well-being

Ineffective **Health** maintenance r/t deficient knowledge regarding self-care and treatment

Acute **Pain** r/t myocardial tissue damage from inadequate blood supply

Situational low **Self-Esteem** r/t crisis of MI

Ineffective **Sexuality** pattern r/t fear of chest pain, possibility of heart damage

Risk for **Powerlessness:** Risk factor: acute illness

Risk for **Shock:** Risk factors: hypotension, myocardial dysfunction, hypoxia

Risk for **Spiritual** distress: Risk factor: physical illness

Risk for decreased **Cardiac** output: Risk factors: alteration in heart rate, rhythm, and contractility

Risk for decreased **Cardiac** tissue perfusion: Risk factors: coronary artery spasm, hypertension, hypotension, hypoxia

Readiness for enhanced **Knowledge:** expresses an interest in learning about condition

See Angioplasty (Coronary); Coronary Artery Bypass Grafting (CABG)

MIDCAB (Minimally Invasive Direct Coronary Artery Bypass)

Risk for **Bleeding:** Risk factor: surgery

Readiness for enhanced **Health** management: preoperative and postoperative care associated with surgery

Risk for **Infection:** Risk factor: surgical procedure

See Angioplasty, Coronary; Coronary Artery Bypass Grafting (CABG)

Midlife Crisis

Ineffective **Coping** r/t inability to deal with changes associated with aging

Powerlessness r/t lack of control over life situation

Spiritual distress r/t questioning beliefs or value system

Risk for disturbed personal **Identity**

Risk for chronic low **Self-Esteem:** Risk factor: ineffective coping with loss

Readiness for enhanced **Relationship:** meets goals for lifestyle change

Readiness for enhanced **Spiritual** well-being: desire to find purpose and meaning to life

Migraine Headache

Ineffective **Health** maintenance r/t deficient knowledge regarding prevention and treatment of headaches

Readiness for enhanced **Health** management: expresses desire to manage illness

Acute **Pain:** headache r/t vasodilation of cerebral and extracerebral vessels

Risk for impaired **Resilience:** Risk factors: chronic illness, disabling pain

Milk Intolerance

See Lactose Intolerance

Minimally Invasive Direct Coronary Bypass (MIDCAB)

See MIDCAB (Minimally Invasive Direct Coronary Artery Bypass)

Miscarriage

See Pregnancy Loss

Mitral Stenosis

Activity intolerance r/t imbalance between oxygen supply and demand

Anxiety r/t possible worsening of symptoms, activity intolerance, fatigue

Decreased **Cardiac** output r/t incompetent heart valves, abnormal forward or backward blood flow, flow into a dilated chamber, flow through an abnormal passage between chambers

Fatigue r/t reduced cardiac output

Ineffective **Health** maintenance r/t deficient knowledge regarding self-care with disorder

Risk for decreased **Cardiac** tissue perfusion: Risk factor: incompetent heart valve

Risk for **Infection:** Risk factors: invasive procedure, risk for endocarditis

Mitral Valve Prolapse

Anxiety r/t symptoms of condition: palpitations, chest pain

Fatigue r/t abnormal catecholamine regulation, decreased intravascular volume

Fear r/t lack of knowledge about mitral valve prolapse, feelings of having heart attack

Ineffective **Health** maintenance r/t deficient knowledge regarding methods to relieve pain and treat dysrhythmia and shortness of breath, need for prophylactic antibiotics before invasive procedures

Acute **Pain** r/t mitral valve regurgitation

Risk for ineffective **Cerebral** tissue perfusion: Risk factor: postural hypotension

Risk for **Infection:** Risk factor: invasive procedures

Risk for **Powerlessness:** Risk factor: unpredictability of onset of symptoms

Readiness for enhanced **Knowledge:** expresses interest in learning about condition

Mobility, Impaired Bed

Impaired bed **Mobility** (See **Mobility,** bed, impaired, Section III)

Mobility, Impaired Physical

Impaired physical **Mobility** (See **Mobility,** physical, impaired, Section III)

Risk for **Falls:** Risk factor: impaired physical mobility

Mobility, Impaired Wheelchair

Impaired wheelchair **Mobility** (See **Mobility,** wheelchair, impaired, Section III)

Modified Radical Mastectomy

Impaired emancipated **Decision-Making**

Readiness for enhanced **Communication:** willingness to enhance communication

See Mastectomy

Mononucleosis

Activity intolerance r/t generalized weakness

Impaired **Comfort** r/t sore throat, muscle aches

Fatigue r/t disease state, stress

Ineffective **Health** maintenance r/t deficient knowledge concerning transmission and treatment of disease

Acute **Pain** r/t enlargement of lymph nodes, oropharyngeal edema

Impaired **Swallowing** r/t enlargement of lymph nodes, oropharyngeal edema

Risk for **Injury:** Risk factor: possible rupture of spleen

Risk for **Loneliness:** Risk factor: social isolation

Mood Disorders

Caregiver Role Strain r/t overwhelming needs of care receiver, unpredictability of mood alterations

Labile **Emotional Control** r/t (See Labile **Emotional Control,** Section III)

Risk-prone **Health** behavior r/t hopelessness, altered locus of control

Impaired **Mood** regulation r/t (See **Mood** regulation, impaired, Section III)

Self-Neglect r/t inability to care for self

Social isolation r/t alterations in mental status

Risk for situational low **Self-Esteem:** Risk factor: unpredictable changes in mood

Readiness for enhanced **Communication:** expresses feelings

See specific disorder: Depression (Major Depressive Disorder); Dysthymic Disorder; Hypomania; Manic Disorder, Bipolar I

Moon Face

Disturbed **Body Image** r/t change in appearance from disease and medication(s)

Risk for situational low **Self-Esteem:** Risk factor: change in body image

See Cushing's Syndrome

Moral/Ethical Dilemmas

Impaired emancipated **Decision-Making** r/t questioning personal values and belief, which alter decision

Moral Distress r/t conflicting information guiding moral or ethical decision-making

Risk for **Powerlessness:** Risk factor: lack of knowledge to make a decision

Risk for **Spiritual** distress: Risk factor: moral or ethical crisis

Readiness for enhanced emancipated **Decision-Making:** expresses desire to enhance congruency of decisions with personal values and goals

Readiness for enhanced **Religiosity:** requests assistance in expanding religious options

Readiness for enhanced **Resilience:** vulnerable state

Readiness for enhanced **Spiritual** well-being: request for interaction with others regarding difficult decisions

Morning Sickness

See Hyperemesis Gravidarum; Pregnancy, Normal

Motion Sickness

See Labyrinthitis

Mottling of Peripheral Skin

Ineffective peripheral **Tissue Perfusion** r/t interruption of arterial flow, decreased circulating blood volume

Risk for **Shock:** Risk factor: inadequate circulation to perfuse body

Mourning

See Grieving

Mouth Lesions

See Mucous Membrane, Impaired Oral

MRI (Magnetic Resonance Imaging)

Anxiety r/t fear of being in closed spaces

Readiness for enhanced **Health** management: describes reduction of risk factors associated with exam

Deficient **Knowledge** r/t unfamiliarity with information resources; exam information

Readiness for enhanced **Knowledge:** expresses interest in learning about exam

MRSA (Methicillin-Resistant *Staphylococcus aureus*)

Impaired **Skin** integrity r/t infection

Delayed **Surgical** recovery r/t infection

Ineffective **Thermoregulation** r/t severe infection stimulating immune system

Impaired **Tissue** integrity r/t wound, infection

Risk for **Loneliness:** Risk factor: physical isolation

Risk for impaired **Resilience:** Risk factor: illness

Risk for **Shock:** Risk factor: sepsis

Mucocutaneous Lymph Node Syndrome

See Kawasaki Disease

Mucous Membrane, Impaired Oral

Impaired **Oral Mucous Membrane** (See **Oral Mucous Membrane,** impaired, Section III)

Multi-Infarct Dementia

See Dementia

Multiple Gestations

Anxiety r/t uncertain outcome of pregnancy

Death **Anxiety** r/t maternal complications associated with multiple gestations

Insufficient **Breast Milk** r/t multiple births

Ineffective **Childbearing** process r/t unavailable support system

Fatigue r/t physiological demands of a multifetal pregnancy and/or care of more than one infant

Impaired **Home** maintenance r/t fatigue

Stress urinary **Incontinence** r/t increased pelvic pressure

Insomnia r/t impairment of normal sleep pattern; parental responsibilities

Deficient **Knowledge** r/t caring for more than one infant

Neonatal **Jaundice** r/t feeding pattern not well established

Deficient **Knowledge** r/t caring for more than one infant

Imbalanced **Nutrition:** less than body requirements r/t physiological demands of a multifetal pregnancy

Stress overload r/t multiple coexisting stressors, family demands

Impaired **Walking** r/t increased uterine size

Risk for ineffective **Breastfeeding:** Risk factors: lack of support, physical demands of feeding more than one infant

Risk for delayed **Development:** fetus: Risk factor: multiple gestations

Risk for disproportionate **Growth:** fetus: Risk factor: multiple gestations

Risk for neonatal **Jaundice:** Risk factors: abnormal weight loss, prematurity, feeding pattern not well-established

Readiness for enhanced **Childbearing** process: demonstrates appropriate care for infants and mother

Readiness for enhanced **Family** processes: family adapting to change with more than one infant

Multiple Personality Disorder (Dissociative Identity Disorder)

Anxiety r/t loss of control of behavior and feelings

Disturbed **Body Image** r/t psychosocial changes

Defensive **Coping** r/t unresolved past traumatic events, severe anxiety

Ineffective **Coping** r/t history of abuse

Hopelessness r/t long-term stress

Disturbed personal **Identity** r/t severe child abuse

Chronic low **Self-Esteem** r/t rejection, failure

Risk for **Self-Mutilation:** Risk factor: need to act out to relieve stress

Readiness for enhanced **Communication:** willingness to discuss problems associated with condition

See Dissociative Identity Disorder (Not Otherwise Specified)

Multiple Sclerosis (MS)

Ineffective **Activity** planning r/t unrealistic perception of personal competence

Ineffective **Airway** clearance r/t decreased energy or fatigue

Impaired physical **Mobility** r/t neuromuscular impairment

Self-Neglect r/t functional impairment

Powerlessness r/t progressive nature of disease

Self-Care deficit: specify r/t neuromuscular impairment

Sexual dysfunction r/t biopsychosocial alteration of sexuality

Chronic **Sorrow** r/t loss of physical ability

Spiritual distress r/t perceived hopelessness of diagnosis

Urinary Retention r/t inhibition of the reflex arc

Risk for **Disuse** syndrome: Risk factor: physical immobility

Risk for **Injury:** Risk factors: altered mobility, sensory dysfunction

Risk for imbalanced **Nutrition:** less than body requirements: Risk factors: impaired swallowing, depression

Risk for **Powerlessness:** Risk factor: chronic illness

Risk for impaired **Religiosity:** Risk factor: illness

Risk for **Thermal Injury:** Risk factor: neuromuscular impairment

Readiness for enhanced **Health** management: expresses a desire to manage condition

Readiness for enhanced **Self-Care:** expresses desire to enhance knowledge of strategies and responsibility for self-care

Readiness for enhanced **Spiritual** well-being: struggling with chronic debilitating condition

See Neurologic Disorders

Mumps

See Communicable Diseases, Childhood

Murmurs

Decreased **Cardiac** output r/t altered preload/afterload

Risk for decreased **Cardiac** tissue perfusion: Risk factor: incompetent valve

Risk for **Fatigue:** Risk factor: decreased cardiac output

Muscular Atrophy/Weakness

Risk for **Disuse** syndrome: Risk factor: impaired physical mobility

Risk for **Falls:** Risk factor: impaired physical mobility

Muscular Dystrophy (MD)

Activity intolerance r/t fatigue, muscle weakness

Ineffective **Activity** planning r/t unrealistic perception of personal competence

Ineffective **Airway** clearance r/t muscle weakness and decreased ability to cough

Constipation r/t immobility

Fatigue r/t increased energy requirements to perform activities of daily living

Impaired physical **Mobility** r/t muscle weakness and development of contractures

Imbalanced **Nutrition:** less than body requirements r/t impaired swallowing or chewing

Self-Care deficit: feeding, bathing, dressing, toileting r/t muscle weakness and fatigue

Self-Neglect r/t functional impairment

Impaired **Transfer** ability r/t muscle weakness

Impaired **Walking** r/t muscle weakness

Risk for **Aspiration:** Risk factor: impaired swallowing

Risk for decreased **Cardiac** tissue perfusion: Risk factor: hypoxia associated with cardiomyopathy

Risk for **Disuse** syndrome: Risk factor: complications of immobility

Risk for **Falls:** Risk factor: muscle weakness

Risk for **Infection:** Risk factor: pooling of pulmonary secretions as a result of immobility and muscle weakness

Risk for **Injury:** Risk factors: muscle weakness and unsteady gait

Risk for **Overweight:** Risk factor: inactivity

Risk for **Powerlessness:** Risk factor: chronic condition

Risk for impaired **Religiosity:** Risk factor: illness

Risk for impaired **Resilience:** Risk factor: chronic illness

Risk for situational low **Self-Esteem:** Risk factor: presence of chronic condition

Readiness for enhanced **Self-Concept:** acceptance of strength and abilities

Risk for impaired **Skin** integrity: Risk factors: immobility, braces, or adaptive devices

See Child with Chronic Condition; Hospitalized Child

MVC (Motor Vehicle Crash)

See Fracture; Head Injury; Injury; Pneumothorax

Myasthenia Gravis

Ineffective **Airway** clearance r/t decreased ability to cough and swallow

Interrupted **Family** processes r/t crisis of dealing with diagnosis

Fatigue r/t paresthesia, aching muscles, weakness of muscles

Impaired physical **Mobility** r/t defective transmission of nerve impulses at the neuromuscular junction

Imbalanced **Nutrition:** less than body requirements r/t difficulty eating and swallowing

Impaired **Swallowing** r/t neuromuscular impairment

Risk for **Caregiver Role Strain:** Risk factors: severity of illness of client, overwhelming needs of client

Risk for impaired **Religiosity:** Risk factor: illness

Risk for impaired **Resilience:** Risk factor: new diagnosis of chronic, serious illness

Readiness for enhanced **Spiritual** well-being: heightened coping with serious illness

See Neurologic Disorders

Mycoplasma Pneumonia

See Pneumonia

Myelocele

See Neural Tube Defects

Myelomeningocele

See Neural Tube Defects

Myocardial Infarction (MI)

See MI (Myocardial Infarction)

Myocarditis

Activity intolerance r/t reduced cardiac reserve and prescribed bed rest

Decreased **Cardiac** output r/t altered preload/afterload

Deficient **Knowledge** r/t treatment of disease

Risk for decreased **Cardiac** tissue perfusion: Risk factors: hypoxia, hypovolemia, cardiac tamponade

Readiness for enhanced **Knowledge:** treatment of disease

See Heart Failure, if appropriate

Myringotomy

Fear r/t hospitalization, surgical procedure

Ineffective **Health** maintenance r/t deficient knowledge regarding care after surgery

Acute **Pain** r/t surgical procedure

Risk for **Infection:** Risk factor: invasive procedure

See Ear Surgery

Myxedema

See Hypothyroidism

N

Narcissistic Personality Disorder

Defensive **Coping** r/t grandiose sense of self

Impaired emancipated **Decision-Making** r/t lack of realistic problem-solving skills

Interrupted **Family** processes r/t taking advantage of others to achieve own goals

Risk-prone **Health** behavior r/t low self-efficacy

Disturbed personal **Identity** r/t psychological impairment

Ineffective **Relationship** r/t lack of mutual support/respect between partners

Impaired individual **Resilience** r/t psychological disorders

Impaired **Social** interaction r/t self-concept disturbance

Risk for **Loneliness:** Risk factors: emotional deprivation, social isolation

Narcolepsy

Anxiety r/t fear of lack of control over falling asleep

Disturbed **Sleep** pattern r/t uncontrollable desire to sleep

Risk for **Trauma:** Risk factor: falling asleep during potentially dangerous activity

Readiness for enhanced **Sleep:** expresses willingness to enhance sleep

Narcotic Use

See Opiate Use (preferred terminology)

Nasogastric Suction

Impaired **Oral Mucous Membrane** r/t presence of nasogastric tube

Risk for **Electrolyte** imbalance: Risk factor: loss of gastrointestinal fluids that contain electrolytes

Risk for imbalanced **Fluid** volume: Risk factor: loss of gastrointestinal fluids without adequate replacement

Risk for dysfunctional **Gastrointestinal** motility: Risk factor: decreased intestinal motility

Nausea

Nausea (See **Nausea,** Section III)

Near-Drowning

Ineffective **Airway** clearance r/t aspiration of fluid

Aspiration r/t aspiration of fluid into lungs

Fear: parental r/t possible death of child, possible permanent and debilitating sequelae

Impaired **Gas** exchange r/t laryngospasm, holding breath, aspiration, inflammation

Grieving r/t potential death of child, unknown sequelae, guilt about accident

Ineffective **Health** maintenance r/t parental deficient knowledge regarding safety measures appropriate for age

Hypothermia r/t central nervous system injury, prolonged submersion in cold water

Risk for delayed **Development:** Risk factors: hypoxemia, cerebral anoxia

Risk for disproportionate **Growth:** Risk factor: exposure to violence

Risk for complicated **Grieving:** Risk factors: potential death of child, unknown sequelae, guilt about accident

Risk for **Infection:** Risk factors: aspiration, invasive monitoring

Risk for ineffective **Cerebral** tissue perfusion: Risk factor: hypoxia

Readiness for enhanced **Spiritual** well-being: struggle with survival of life-threatening situation

See Child with Chronic Condition; Hospitalized Child; Safety, Childhood; Terminally Ill Child/Death of Child, Parent

N

Nearsightedness

Readiness for enhanced **Health** management: need for correction of myopia

Nearsightedness; Corneal Surgery

See LASIK Eye Surgery (Laser-Assisted in Situ Keratomileusis)

Neck Vein Distention

Decreased **Cardiac** output r/t decreased contractility of heart resulting in increased preload

Excess **Fluid** volume r/t excess fluid intake, compromised regulatory mechanisms

See Congestive Heart Failure; Heart Failure

Necrosis, Kidney Tubular; Necrosis, Acute Tubular

See Kidney Failure

Necrotizing Enterocolitis

Ineffective **Breathing** pattern r/t abdominal distention, hypoxia

Diarrhea r/t infection

Deficient **Fluid** volume r/t vomiting, gastrointestinal bleeding

Neonatal **Jaundice** r/t feeding pattern not well-established

Imbalanced **Nutrition:** less than body requirements r/t decreased ability to absorb nutrients, decreased perfusion to gastrointestinal tract

Risk for dysfunctional **Gastrointestinal** motility: Risk factor: infection

Risk for ineffective **Gastrointestinal** perfusion: Risk factors: shunting of blood away from mesenteric circulation and toward vital organs as a result of perinatal stress, hypoxia

Risk for **Infection:** Risk factors: bacterial invasion of gastrointestinal tract, invasive procedures

See Hospitalized Child; Premature Infant (Child)

Negative Feelings About Self

Chronic low **Self-Esteem** r/t long-standing negative self-evaluation

Self-Neglect r/t negative feelings

Readiness for enhanced **Self-Concept:** expresses willingness to enhance self-concept

Neglect, Unilateral

Unilateral Neglect (See **Unilateral Neglect,** Section III)

Neglectful Care of Family Member

Caregiver Role Strain r/t overwhelming care demands of family member, lack of social or financial support

Disabled family **Coping** r/t highly ambivalent family relationships, lack of respite care

Interrupted **Family** processes r/t situational transition or crisis

Deficient **Knowledge** r/t care needs

Impaired individual **Resilience** r/t vulnerability from neglect

Risk for compromised **Human Dignity:** Risk factor: inadequate participation in decision-making

Neonatal Jaundice

Neonatal **Jaundice** (See neonatal **Jaundice,** Section III)

Neonate

Readiness for enhanced **Childbearing** process: appropriate care of newborn

See Newborn, Normal; Newborn, Postmature; Newborn, Small for Gestational Age (SGA)

Neoplasm

Fear r/t possible malignancy

See Cancer

Nephrectomy

Anxiety r/t surgical recovery, prognosis

Ineffective **Breathing** pattern r/t location of surgical incision

Constipation r/t lack of return of peristalsis

Acute **Pain** r/t incisional discomfort

Spiritual distress r/t chronic illness

Risk for **Bleeding:** Risk factor: surgery

Risk for imbalanced **Fluid** volume: Risk factors: vascular losses, decreased intake

Risk for **Infection:** Risk factors: invasive procedure, lack of deep breathing because of location of surgical incision

Risk for ineffective **Renal** perfusion: Risk factor: kidney disease

Nephrostomy, Percutaneous

Acute **Pain** r/t invasive procedure

Impaired **Urinary** elimination r/t nephrostomy tube

Risk for **Infection:** Risk factor: invasive procedure

Nephrotic Syndrome

Activity intolerance r/t generalized edema

Disturbed **Body Image** r/t edematous appearance and side effects of steroid therapy

Excess **Fluid** volume r/t edema resulting from oncotic fluid shift caused by serum protein loss and kidney retention of salt and water

Imbalanced **Nutrition:** less than body requirements r/t anorexia, protein loss

Imbalanced **Nutrition:** more than body requirements r/t increased appetite attributable to steroid therapy

Social isolation r/t edematous appearance

Risk for **Infection:** Risk factor: altered immune mechanisms caused by disease and effects of steroids

Risk for ineffective **Renal** perfusion: Risk factor: kidney disease

Risk for impaired **Skin** integrity: Risk factor: edema

See Child with Chronic Condition; Hospitalized Child

Neural Tube Defects (Meningocele, Myelomeningocele, Spina Bifida, Anencephaly)

Chronic functional **Constipation** r/t immobility or less than adequate mobility

Grieving r/t loss of perfect child, birth of child with congenital defect

Reflex urinary **Incontinence** r/t neurogenic impairment

Total urinary **Incontinence** r/t neurogenic impairment

Urge urinary **Incontinence** r/t neurogenic impairment

Impaired **Mobility** r/t neuromuscular impairment

Chronic low **Self-Esteem** r/t perceived differences, decreased ability to participate in physical and social activities at school

Impaired **Skin** integrity r/t incontinence

Risk for delayed **Development:** Risk factor: inadequate nutrition

Risk for disproportionate **Growth:** Risk factor: congenital disorder

Risk for **Latex Allergy** response: Risk factor: multiple exposures to latex products

Risk for imbalanced **Nutrition:** more than body requirements: Risk factors: diminished, limited, or impaired physical activity

Risk for **Powerlessness:** Risk factor: debilitating disease

Risk for impaired **Skin** integrity: lower extremities: Risk factor: decreased sensory perception

Readiness for enhanced family **Coping:** effective adaptive response by family members

Readiness for enhanced **Family** processes: family supports each other

See Child with Chronic Condition; Premature Infant (Child)

Neuralgia

See Trigeminal Neuralgia

Neuritis (Peripheral Neuropathy)

Activity intolerance r/t pain with movement

Ineffective **Health** maintenance r/t deficient knowledge regarding self-care with neuritis

Acute **Pain** r/t stimulation of affected nerve endings, inflammation of sensory nerves

See Neuropathy, Peripheral

Neurogenic Bladder

Reflex urinary **Incontinence** r/t neurological impairment

Urinary Retention r/t interruption in the lateral spinal tracts

Risk for **Latex Allergy** response: Risk factor: repeated exposures to latex associated with possible repeated catheterizations

Neurologic Disorders

Ineffective **Airway** clearance r/t perceptual or cognitive impairment, decreased energy, fatigue

Acute **Confusion** r/t dementia, alcohol abuse, drug abuse, delirium

Ineffective **Coping** r/t disability requiring change in lifestyle

Interrupted **Family** processes r/t situational crisis, illness, or disability of family member

Grieving r/t loss of usual body functioning

Impaired **Home** maintenance r/t client's or family member's disease

Risk for corneal **Injury:** Risk factor: lack of spontaneous blink reflex

Impaired **Memory** r/t neurological disturbance

Impaired physical **Mobility** r/t neuromuscular impairment

Imbalanced **Nutrition:** less than body requirements r/t impaired swallowing, depression, difficulty feeding self

Powerlessness r/t progressive nature of disease

Self-Care deficit: specify r/t neuromuscular dysfunction

Sexual dysfunction r/t biopsychosocial alteration of sexuality

Social isolation r/t altered state of wellness

Impaired **Swallowing** r/t neuromuscular dysfunction

Risk for **Disuse** syndrome: Risk factors: physical immobility, neuromuscular dysfunction

Risk for **Injury:** Risk factors: altered mobility, sensory dysfunction, cognitive impairment

Risk for ineffective **Cerebral** tissue perfusion: Risk factor: cerebral disease/injury

Risk for impaired **Religiosity:** Risk factor: life transition

Risk for impaired **Skin** integrity: Risk factors: altered sensation, altered mental status, paralysis

See specific condition: Alcohol Withdrawal; Amyotrophic Lateral Sclerosis (ALS); CVA (Cerebrovascular Accident); Delirium; Dementia; Guillain-Barré Syndrome; Head Injury; Huntington's Disease; Spinal Cord Injury; Myasthenia Gravis; Muscular Dystrophy; Parkinson's Disease

N

Neuropathy, Peripheral

Chronic **Pain** r/t damage to nerves in the peripheral nervous system as a result of medication side effects, vitamin deficiency, or diabetes

Ineffective **Thermoregulation** r/t decreased ability to regulate body temperature

Risk for **Injury:** Risk factors: lack of muscle control, decreased sensation

Risk for impaired **Skin** integrity: Risk factor: poor perfusion

Risk for **Thermal** Injury r/t nerve damage

See Peripheral Vascular Disease (PVD)

Neurosurgery

See Craniectomy/Craniotomy

Newborn, Normal

Breastfeeding r/t normal oral structure and gestational age greater than 34 weeks

Ineffective **Thermoregulation** r/t immaturity of neuroendocrine system

Risk for **Sudden Infant Death** syndrome: Risk factors: lack of knowledge regarding infant sleeping in prone or side-lying position, prenatal or postnatal infant smoke exposure, infant overheating or overwrapping, loose articles in the sleep environment

N

Risk for **Infection:** Risk factors: open umbilical stump, immature immune system

Risk for **Injury:** Risk factors: immaturity, need for caretaking

Readiness for enhanced **Childbearing** process: appropriate care of newborn

Readiness for enhanced organized **Infant** behavior: demonstrates adaptive response to pain

Readiness for enhanced **Parenting:** providing emotional and physical needs of infant

Newborn, Postmature

Hypothermia r/t depleted stores of subcutaneous fat

Impaired **Skin** integrity r/t cracked and peeling skin as a result of decreased vernix

Risk for ineffective **Airway** clearance: Risk factor: meconium aspiration

Risk for unstable blood **Glucose** level: Risk factor: depleted glycogen stores

Newborn, Small for Gestational Age (SGA)

Neonatal **Jaundice** r/t neonate age and difficulty feeding

Imbalanced **Nutrition:** less than body requirements r/t history of placental insufficiency

Ineffective **Thermoregulation** r/t decreased brown fat, subcutaneous fat

Risk for delayed **Development:** Risk factor: history of placental insufficiency

Risk for disproportionate **Growth:** Risk factor: history of placental insufficiency

Risk for **Injury:** Risk factors: hypoglycemia, perinatal asphyxia, meconium aspiration

Risk for **Sudden Infant Death** syndrome: Risk factor: low birth weight

Nicotine Addiction

Risk-prone **Health** behavior r/t smoking

Ineffective **Health** maintenance r/t lack of ability to make a judgment about smoking cessation

Risk for impaired **Skin** integrity: Risk factor: poor tissue perfusion associated with nicotine

Powerlessness r/t perceived lack of control over ability to give up nicotine

Readiness for enhanced emancipated **Decision-Making:** expresses desire to enhance understanding and meaning of choices

Readiness for enhanced **Health** management: expresses desire to learn measures to stop smoking

NIDDM (Non-Insulin-Dependent Diabetes Mellitus)

Readiness for enhanced **Health** management: expresses desire for information on exercise and diet to manage diabetes

See Diabetes Mellitus

Nightmares

Post-Trauma syndrome r/t disaster, war, epidemic, rape, assault, torture, catastrophic illness, or accident

Nipple Soreness

Impaired **Comfort** r/t physical condition

See Painful Breasts; Sore Nipples, Breastfeeding

Nocturia

Urge urinary **Incontinence** r/t decreased bladder capacity, irritation of bladder stretch receptors causing spasm, alcohol, caffeine, increased fluids, increased urine concentration, overdistention of bladder

Impaired **Urinary** elimination r/t sensory motor impairment, urinary tract infection

Risk for **Powerlessness:** Risk factor: inability to control nighttime voiding

Nocturnal Myoclonus

See Restless Leg Syndrome; Stress

Nocturnal Paroxysmal Dyspnea

See PND (Paroxysmal Nocturnal Dyspnea)

Noncompliance

Ineffective **Health** management (See **Health** management, ineffective, Section III)

Non–Insulin-Dependent Diabetes Mellitus (NIDDM)

See Diabetes Mellitus

Normal Pressure Hydrocephalus (NPH)

Impaired verbal **Communication** r/t obstruction of flow of cerebrospinal fluid affecting speech

Acute **Confusion** r/t increased intracranial pressure caused by obstruction to flow of cerebrospinal fluid

Impaired **Memory** r/t neurological disturbance

Risk for ineffective **Cerebral** tissue perfusion: Risk factor: fluid pressing on the brain

Risk for **Falls:** Risk factor: unsteady gait as a result of obstruction of cerebrospinal fluid

Norovirus

See Viral Gastroenteritis

NSTEMI (non-ST-elevation myocardial infarction)

See MI (Myocardial Infarction)

Nursing

See Breastfeeding, Effective; Breastfeeding, Ineffective; Breastfeeding, Interrupted

Nutrition

Readiness for enhanced **Nutrition**. (See **Nutrition,** readiness for enhanced, Section III)

Nutrition, Imbalanced

Imbalanced **Nutrition:** less than body requirements (See **Nutrition:** less than body requirements, imbalanced, Section III)

Obesity (See **Obesity,** Section III)

Overweight (See **Overweight,** Section III)

Risk for **Overweight** (See **Overweight,** risk for, Section III)

O

Obesity

Disturbed **Body Image** r/t eating disorder, excess weight

Risk-prone **Health** behavior: r/t negative attitude toward health care

Obesity (See **Obesity,** Section III)

Chronic low **Self-Esteem** r/t ineffective coping, overeating

Risk for ineffective peripheral **Tissue Perfusion:** Risk factor: sedentary lifestyle

Readiness for enhanced **Nutrition:** expresses willingness to enhance nutrition

OBS (Organic Brain Syndrome)

See Organic Mental Disorders; Dementia

Obsessive-Compulsive Disorder (OCD)

See OCD (Obsessive-Compulsive Disorder)

Obstruction, Bowel

See Bowel Obstruction

Obstructive Sleep Apnea

Insomnia r/t blocked airway

Obesity r/t excessive intake related to metabolic need

See PND (Paroxysmal Nocturnal Dyspnea)

OCD (Obsessive-Compulsive Disorder)

Ineffective **Activity** planning r/t unrealistic perception of events

Anxiety r/t threat to self-concept, unmet needs

Impaired emancipated **Decision-Making** r/t inability to make a decision for fear of reprisal

Disabled family **Coping** r/t family process being disrupted by client's ritualistic activities

Ineffective **Coping** r/t expression of feelings in an unacceptable way, ritualistic behavior

Risk-prone **Health** behavior r/t inadequate comprehension associated with repetitive thoughts

Powerlessness r/t unrelenting repetitive thoughts to perform irrational activities

Impaired individual **Resilience** r/t psychological disorder

Risk for situational low **Self-Esteem:** Risk factor: inability to control repetitive thoughts and actions

ODD (Oppositional Defiant Disorder)

Anxiety r/t feelings of anger and hostility toward authority figures

Ineffective **Coping** r/t lack of self-control or perceived lack of self-control

Disabled **Family** coping r/t feelings of anger, hostility; defiant behavior toward authority figures

Risk-prone **Health** behavior r/t multiple stressors associated with condition

Ineffective **Impulse** control r/t anger/compunction to engage in disruptive behaviors

Chronic or situational low **Self-Esteem** r/t poor self-control and disruptive behaviors

Impaired **Social** interaction r/t being touchy or easily annoyed, blaming others for own mistakes, constant trouble in school

Social isolation r/t unaccepted social behavior

Ineffective family **Health** management r/t difficulty in limit setting and managing oppositional behaviors

Risk for ineffective **Activity** planning: Risk factors: unrealistic perception of events, hedonism, insufficient social support

Risk for impaired **Parenting:** Risk factors: children's difficult behaviors and inability to set limits

Risk for **Powerlessness:** Risk factor: inability to deal with difficult behaviors

Risk for **Spiritual** distress: Risk factors: anxiety and stress in dealing with difficult behaviors

Risk for other-directed **Violence:** Risk factors: history of violence, threats of violence against others, history of antisocial behavior, history of indirect violence

Older Adult

See Aging

Oliguria

Deficient **Fluid** volume r/t active fluid loss, failure of regulatory mechanism, inadequate intake

See Cardiac Output, Decreased; Kidney Failure; Shock, Hypovolemic

Omphalocele

See Gastroschisis/Omphalocele

Oophorectomy

Risk for ineffective **Sexuality** pattern: Risk factor: altered body function

See Surgery, Perioperative; Surgery, Postoperative; Surgery, Preoperative

OPCAB (Off-Pump Coronary Artery Bypass)

See Angioplasty, Coronary; Coronary Artery Bypass Grafting (CABG)

Open Heart Surgery

Risk for decreased **Cardiac** tissue perfusion: Risk factor: cardiac surgery

See Coronary Artery Bypass Grafting (CABG); Dysrhythmia

Open Reduction of Fracture with Internal Fixation (Femur)

Anxiety r/t outcome of corrective procedure

Impaired physical **Mobility** r/t postoperative position, abduction of leg, avoidance of acute flexion

Powerlessness r/t loss of control, unanticipated change in lifestyle

Risk for **Infection:** Risk factor: surgical procedure

Risk for **Perioperative Positioning** injury: Risk factor: immobilization

Risk for **Peripheral Neurovascular** dysfunction: Risk factors: mechanical compression, orthopedic surgery, immobilization

See Surgery, Postoperative Care

Opiate Use

Chronic **Pain** syndrome r/t prolonged use of opiates

Risk for **Constipation:** Risk factor: effects of opiates on peristalsis

See Drug Abuse; Drug Withdrawal

Opportunistic Infection

Delayed **Surgical** recovery r/t abnormal blood profiles, impaired healing

Risk for **Infection:** Risk factor: abnormal blood profiles

See AIDS (Acquired Immunodeficiency Syndrome); HIV (Human Immunodeficiency Virus)

Oppositional Defiant Disorder (ODD)

See ODD (Oppositional Defiant Disorder)

Oral Mucous Membrane, Impaired

Impaired **Oral Mucous Membrane** (See **Oral Mucous Membrane,** impaired, Section III)

Oral Thrush

See Candidiasis, Oral

Orchitis

Readiness for enhanced **Health** management: follows recommendations for mumps vaccination

See Epididymitis

Organic Mental Disorders

Frail Elderly syndrome r/t alteration in cognitive function

Impaired **Social** interaction r/t disturbed thought processes

Risk for disturbed personal **Identity:** Risk factor: delusions/fluctuating perceptions of stimuli

Risk for **Infection:** Risk factor: surgical procedure

See Dementia

Orthopedic Traction

Ineffective **Role** performance r/t limited physical mobility

Impaired **Social** interaction r/t limited physical mobility

Impaired **Transfer** ability r/t limited physical mobility

Risk for impaired **Religiosity:** Risk factor: immobility

See Traction and Casts

Orthopnea

Ineffective **Breathing** pattern r/t inability to breathe with head of bed flat

Decreased **Cardiac** output r/t inability of heart to meet demands of body

Orthostatic Hypotension

See Dizziness

Osteoarthritis

Acute **Pain** r/t movement

Impaired **Walking** r/t inflammation and damage to joints

See Arthritis

Osteomyelitis

Deficient **Diversional** activity r/t prolonged immobilization, hospitalization

Fear: parental r/t concern regarding possible growth plate damage caused by infection, concern that infection may become chronic

Ineffective **Health** maintenance r/t continued immobility at home, possible extensive casts, continued antibiotics

Impaired physical **Mobility** r/t imposed immobility as a result of infected area

Acute **Pain** r/t inflammation in affected extremity

Ineffective **Thermoregulation** r/t infectious process

Risk for **Constipation:** Risk factor: immobility

Risk for **Infection:** Risk factor: inadequate primary and secondary defenses

Risk for impaired **Skin** integrity: Risk factor: irritation from splint or cast

See Hospitalized Child

Osteoporosis

Deficient **Knowledge** r/t diet, exercise, need to abstain from alcohol and nicotine

Impaired physical **Mobility** r/t pain, skeletal changes

Imbalanced **Nutrition:** less than body requirements r/t inadequate intake of calcium and vitamin D

Acute **Pain** r/t fracture, muscle spasms

Risk for **Injury:** fracture: Risk factors: lack of activity, risk of falling resulting from environmental hazards, neuromuscular disorders, diminished senses, cardiovascular responses to drugs

Risk for **Powerlessness:** Risk factor: debilitating disease

Readiness for enhanced **Health** management: expresses desire to manage the treatment of illness and prevent complications

Ostomy

See Child with Chronic Condition; Colostomy; Ileal Conduit; Ileostomy

Otitis Media

Acute **Pain** r/t inflammation, infectious process

Risk for delayed **Development:** speech and language: Risk factor: frequent otitis media

Risk for **Infection:** Risk factors: eustachian tube obstruction, traumatic eardrum perforation, infectious disease process

Readiness for enhanced **Knowledge:** information on treatment and prevention of disease

Ovarian Carcinoma

Death **Anxiety** r/t unknown outcome, possible poor prognosis

Fear r/t unknown outcome, possible poor prognosis

Ineffective **Health Maintenance** r/t deficient knowledge regarding self-care, treatment of condition

Readiness for enhanced **Family Processes:** family functioning meets needs of client

Readiness for enhanced **Resilience:** participates in support groups

See Chemotherapy; Hysterectomy; Radiation Therapy

P

Pacemaker

Anxiety r/t change in health status, presence of pacemaker

Death **Anxiety** r/t worry over possible malfunction of pacemaker

Deficient **Knowledge** r/t self-care program, when to seek medical attention

Acute **Pain** r/t surgical procedure

Risk for **Bleeding:** Risk factor: surgery

Risk for decreased **Cardiac** tissue perfusion: Risk factor: pacemaker malfunction

Risk for **Infection:** Risk factors: invasive procedure, presence of foreign body (catheter and generator)

Risk for **Powerlessness:** Risk factor: presence of electronic device to stimulate heart

Readiness for enhanced **Health** management: appropriate health care management of pacemaker

Paget's Disease

Disturbed **Body Image** r/t possible enlarged head, bowed tibias, kyphosis

Deficient **Knowledge** r/t appropriate diet high in protein and calcium, mild exercise

Chronic **Sorrow** r/t chronic condition with altered body image

Risk for **Trauma:** fracture: Risk factor: excessive bone destruction

Pain, Acute

Acute **Pain** (See **Pain,** acute, Section III)

Pain, Chronic

Chronic **Pain** (See **Pain,** chronic, Section III)

Painful Breasts, Engorgement

Acute **Pain** r/t distention of breast tissue

Ineffective **Role** performance r/t change in physical capacity to assume role of breastfeeding mother

Impaired **Tissue** integrity r/t excessive fluid in breast tissues

Risk for ineffective **Breastfeeding:** Risk factors: pain, infant's inability to latch on to engorged breast

Risk for **Infection:** Risk factor: milk stasis

Painful Breasts, Sore Nipples

Insufficient **Breast Milk** r/t long breastfeeding time/pain response

Ineffective **Breastfeeding** r/t pain

Acute **Pain** r/t cracked nipples

Ineffective **Role** performance r/t change in physical capacity to assume role of breastfeeding mother

Impaired **Skin** integrity r/t mechanical factors involved in suckling, breastfeeding management

Risk for **Infection:** Risk factor: break in skin

Pallor of Extremities

Ineffective peripheral **Tissue Perfusion** r/t interruption of vascular flow

See Shock; Peripheral Vascular disease (PVD)

Palpitations (Heart Palpitations)

See Dysrhythmia

Pancreatic Cancer

Death **Anxiety** r/t possible poor prognosis of disease process

Ineffective family **Coping** r/t poor prognosis

Fear r/t poor prognosis of the disease

Grieving r/t shortened life span

Deficient **Knowledge** r/t disease-induced diabetes, home management

Spiritual distress r/t poor prognosis

Risk for impaired **Liver** function: Risk factor: complications from underlying disease

See Cancer; Chemotherapy; Radiation Therapy; Surgery, Perioperative; Surgery, Postoperative; Surgery, Preoperative

Pancreatitis

Ineffective **Breathing** pattern r/t splinting from severe pain, disease process and inflammation

Ineffective **Denial** r/t ineffective coping, alcohol use

Diarrhea r/t decrease in pancreatic secretions resulting in steatorrhea

Deficient **Fluid** volume r/t vomiting, decreased fluid intake, fever, diaphoresis, fluid shifts

Ineffective **Health** maintenance r/t deficient knowledge concerning diet, alcohol use, medication

Nausea r/t irritation of gastrointestinal system

Imbalanced **Nutrition:** less than body requirements r/t inadequate dietary intake, increased nutritional needs as a result of acute illness, increased metabolic needs caused by increased body temperature, disease process

Acute **Pain** r/t irritation and edema of the inflamed pancreas

Chronic **Sorrow** r/t chronic illness

Readiness for enhanced **Comfort:** expresses desire to enhance comfort

P

Panic Disorder (Panic Attacks)

Ineffective **Activity** planning r/t unrealistic perception of events

Anxiety r/t situational crisis

Ineffective **Coping** r/t personal vulnerability

Risk-prone **Health** behavior r/t low self-efficacy

Disturbed personal **Identity** r/t situational crisis

Post-Trauma syndrome r/t previous catastrophic event

Social isolation r/t fear of lack of control

Risk for **Loneliness:** Risk factor: inability to socially interact because of fear of losing control

Risk for **Post-Trauma** syndrome: Risk factors: perception of the event, diminished ego strength

Risk for **Powerlessness:** Risk factor: ineffective coping skills

Readiness for enhanced **Coping:** seeks problem-oriented and emotion-oriented strategies to manage condition

See Anxiety; Anxiety Disorder

Paralysis

Disturbed **Body Image** r/t biophysical changes, loss of movement, immobility

Impaired **Comfort** r/t prolonged immobility

Constipation r/t effects of spinal cord disruption, inadequate fiber in diet

Ineffective **Health** maintenance r/t deficient knowledge regarding self-care with paralysis

Impaired **Home** maintenance r/t physical disability

Reflex urinary **Incontinence** r/t neurological impairment

Impaired physical **Mobility** r/t neuromuscular impairment

Impaired wheelchair **Mobility** r/t neuromuscular impairment

Self-Neglect r/t functional impairment

Powerlessness r/t illness-related regimen

Self-Care deficit: specify r/t neuromuscular impairment

Sexual dysfunction r/t loss of sensation, biopsychosocial alteration

Chronic **Sorrow** r/t loss of physical mobility

Impaired **Transfer** ability r/t paralysis

Risk for **Autonomic Dysreflexia:** Risk factor: cause of paralysis

Risk for **Disuse** syndrome: Risk factor: paralysis

Risk for **Falls:** Risk factor: paralysis

Risk for **Injury:** Risk factors: altered mobility, sensory dysfunction

Risk for **Latex Allergy** response: Risk factor: possible repeated urinary catheterizations

Risk for **Post-Trauma** syndrome: Risk factor: event causing paralysis

Risk for impaired **Religiosity:** Risk factors: immobility, possible lack of transportation

Risk for impaired **Resilience:** Risk factor: chronic disability

Risk for situational low **Self-Esteem:** Risk factor: change in body image and function

Risk for impaired **Skin** integrity: Risk factors: altered circulation, altered sensation, immobility

Readiness for enhanced **Self-Care:** expresses desire to enhance knowledge and responsibility for strategies for self-care

See Child with Chronic Condition; Hemiplegia; Hospitalized Child; Neural Tube Defects; Spinal Cord Injury

Paralytic Ileus

Constipation r/t decreased gastrointestinal motility

Deficient **Fluid** volume r/t loss of fluids from vomiting, retention of fluid in bowel

Dysfunctional **Gastrointestinal** motility r/t recent abdominal surgery, electrolyte imbalance

Nausea r/t gastrointestinal irritation

Acute **Pain** r/t pressure, abdominal distention, presence of nasogastric tube

See Bowel Obstruction

Paranoid Personality Disorder

Ineffective **Activity** planning r/t unrealistic perception of events

Anxiety r/t uncontrollable intrusive, suspicious thoughts

Risk-prone **Health** behavior r/t intense emotional state

Disturbed personal **Identity** r/t difficulty with reality testing

Impaired individual **Resilience** r/t psychological disorder

Chronic low **Self-Esteem** r/t inability to trust others

Social isolation r/t inappropriate social skills

Risk for **Loneliness:** Risk factor: social isolation

Risk for other-directed **Violence:** Risk factor: being suspicious of others and their actions

Paraplegia

See Spinal Cord Injury

Parathyroidectomy

Anxiety r/t surgery

Risk for ineffective **Airway** clearance: Risk factors: edema or hematoma formation, airway obstruction

Risk for **Bleeding:** Risk factor: surgery

Risk for impaired verbal **Communication:** Risk factors: possible laryngeal damage, edema

Risk for **Infection:** Risk factor: surgical procedure

See Hypocalcemia

Parent Attachment

Risk for impaired **Attachment** (See **Attachment,** impaired, risk for, Section III)

Readiness for enhanced **Childbearing** process: demonstrates appropriate care of newborn

See Parental Role Conflict

Parental Role Conflict

Parental **Role** conflict (See **Role** conflict, parental, Section III)

Ineffective **Relationship** r/t unrealistic expectations

Chronic **Sorrow** r/t difficult parent–child relationship

Risk for **Spiritual** distress: Risk factor: altered relationships

Readiness for enhanced **Parenting:** willingness to enhance parenting

Parenting

Readiness for enhanced **Parenting** (See **Parenting,** readiness for enhanced, Section III)

Parenting, Impaired

Impaired **Parenting** (See **Parenting,** impaired, Section III)

Chronic **Sorrow** r/t difficult parent–child relationship

Risk for **Spiritual** distress: Risk factor: altered relationships

Parenting, Risk for Impaired

Risk for impaired **Parenting** (See **Parenting,** impaired, risk for, Section III)

See Parenting, Impaired

Paresthesia

Risk for **Injury:** Risk factors: inability to feel temperature changes, pain

Risk for impaired **Skin** integrity: Risk factor: impaired sensation

Risk for **Thermal** injury: Risk factor: neuromuscular impairment

Parkinson's Disease

Impaired verbal **Communication** r/t decreased speech volume, slowness of speech, impaired facial muscles

Constipation r/t weakness of muscles, lack of exercise, inadequate fluid intake, decreased autonomic nervous system activity

Frail Elderly syndrome r/t chronic illness

Imbalanced **Nutrition:** less than body requirements r/t tremor, slowness in eating, difficulty in chewing and swallowing

Chronic **Sorrow** r/t loss of physical capacity

Risk for **Injury:** Risk factors: tremors, slow reactions, altered gait

See Neurologic Disorders

Paroxysmal Nocturnal Dyspnea (PND)

See PND (Paroxysmal Nocturnal Dyspnea)

Patent Ductus Arteriosus (PDA)

See Congenital Heart Disease/Cardiac Anomalies

Patient-Controlled Analgesia (PCA)

See PCA (Patient-Controlled Analgesia)

Patient Education

Deficient **Knowledge** r/t lack of exposure to information misinterpretation, unfamiliarity with information resources to manage illness

Readiness for enhanced emancipated **Decision-Making:** expresses desire to enhance understanding of choices for decision-making

Readiness for enhanced **Knowledge** (specify): interest in learning

Readiness for enhanced **Health** management: expresses desire for information to manage the illness

PCA (Patient-Controlled Analgesia)

Deficient **Knowledge** r/t self-care of pain control

Nausea r/t side effects of medication

Risk for **Injury:** Risk factors: possible complications associated with PCA

Risk for **Vascular Trauma:** Risk factors: insertion site and length of insertion time

Readiness for enhanced **Knowledge:** appropriate management of PCA

Pectus Excavatum

See Marfan Syndrome

Pediculosis

See Lice

PEG (Percutaneous Endoscopic Gastrostomy)

See Tube Feeding

Pelvic Inflammatory Disease (PID)

See PID (Pelvic Inflammatory Disease)

Penile Prosthesis

Ineffective **Sexuality** pattern r/t use of penile prosthesis

Risk for **Infection:** Risk factor: invasive surgical procedure

Risk for situational low **Self-Esteem:** Risk factor: ineffective sexuality pattern

Readiness for enhanced **Health** management: seeks information regarding care and use of prosthesis

See Erectile Dysfunction (ED); Impotence

Peptic Ulcer

See Ulcer, Peptic (Duodenal or Gastric)

Percutaneous Transluminal Coronary Angioplasty (PTCA)

See Angioplasty, Coronary

Pericardial Friction Rub

Decreased **Cardiac** output

Acute Pain r/t inflammation, effusion

Risk for decreased **Cardiac** tissue perfusion: Risk factors: inflammation in pericardial sac, fluid accumulation compressing heart

Pericarditis

Activity intolerance r/t reduced cardiac reserve, prescribed bed rest

Decreased **Cardiac** output r/t impaired cardiac function from inflammation of pericardial sac

Risk for decreased **Cardiac** tissue perfusion: Risk factor: inflammation in pericardial sac

P

Deficient **Knowledge** r/t unfamiliarity with information sources

Risk for imbalanced **Nutrition:** less than body requirements: Risk factors: fever, hypermetabolic state associated with fever

Acute **Pain** r/t biological injury, inflammation

Periodontal Disease

Risk for impaired **Oral Mucous Membranes** (See **Oral Mucous Membranes,** impaired, risk for, Section III)

Perioperative Hypothermia

Risk for **Perioperative Hypothermia** (See **Perioperative Hypothermia,** risk for, Section III)

Perioperative Positioning

Risk for **Perioperative Positioning** injury (See **Perioperative Positioning** injury, risk for, Section III)

Peripheral Neuropathy

See Neuropathy, Peripheral

Peripheral Neurovascular Dysfunction

Risk for **Peripheral Neurovascular** dysfunction (See **Peripheral Neurovascular** dysfunction, risk for, Section III)

See Neuropathy, Peripheral; Peripheral Vascular Disease (PVD)

Peripheral Vascular Disease (PVD)

Ineffective **Health** maintenance r/t deficient knowledge regarding self-care and treatment of disease

Chronic **Pain:** intermittent claudication r/t ischemia

Ineffective peripheral **Tissue Perfusion** r/t disease process

Risk for **Falls:** Risk factor: altered mobility

Risk for **Injury:** Risk factors: tissue hypoxia, altered mobility, altered sensation

Risk for **Peripheral Neurovascular** dysfunction: Risk factor: possible vascular obstruction

Risk for impaired **Tissue** integrity: Risk factor: altered circulation or sensation

Readiness for enhanced **Health** management: self-care and treatment of disease

See Neuropathy, Peripheral; Peripheral Neurovascular Dysfunction

Peritoneal Dialysis

Ineffective **Breathing** pattern r/t pressure from dialysate

Impaired **Comfort** r/t instillation of dialysate, temperature of dialysate

Impaired **Home** maintenance r/t complex home treatment of client

Deficient **Knowledge** r/t treatment procedure, self-care with peritoneal dialysis

Chronic **Sorrow** r/t chronic disability

Risk for ineffective **Coping:** Risk factor: disability requiring change in lifestyle

Risk for unstable blood **Glucose** level: Risk factors: increased concentrations of glucose in dialysate, ineffective medication management

Risk for imbalanced **Fluid** volume: Risk factor: medical procedure

Risk for **Infection:** peritoneal: Risk factors: invasive procedure, presence of catheter, dialysate

Risk for **Powerlessness:** Risk factors: chronic condition and care involved

See Child with Chronic Condition; Hemodialysis; Hospitalized Child; Kidney Failure; Kidney Failure, Acute/Chronic, Child

Peritonitis

Ineffective **Breathing** pattern r/t pain, increased abdominal pressure

Constipation r/t decreased oral intake, decrease of peristalsis

Deficient **Fluid** volume r/t retention of fluid in bowel with loss of circulating blood volume

Nausea r/t gastrointestinal irritation

Imbalanced **Nutrition:** less than body requirements r/t nausea, vomiting

Acute **Pain** r/t inflammation and infection of gastrointestinal system

Risk for dysfunctional **Gastrointestinal** motility: Risk factor: gastrointestinal disease

Pernicious Anemia

Diarrhea r/t malabsorption of nutrients

Fatigue r/t imbalanced nutrition: less than body requirements

Impaired **Memory** r/t lack of adequate red blood cells

Nausea r/t altered oral mucous membrane; sore tongue, bleeding gums

Imbalanced **Nutrition:** less than body requirements r/t lack of appetite associated with nausea and altered oral mucous membrane

Impaired **Oral Mucous Membrane** r/t vitamin deficiency; inability to absorb vitamin B_{12} associated with lack of intrinsic factor

Risk for **Falls:** Risk factors: dizziness, lightheadedness

Risk for **Peripheral Neurovascular** dysfunction: Risk factor: anemia

Persistent Fetal Circulation

See Congenital Heart Disease/Cardiac Anomalies

Personal Identity Problems

Disturbed personal **Identity** (See **Identity,** personal, disturbed, Section III)

Risk for disturbed personal **Identity** (See disturbed personal **Identity,** risk for, Section III)

Personality Disorder

Ineffective **Activity** planning r/t unrealistic perception of events

Impaired individual **Resilience** r/t psychological disorder

See specific disorder: Antisocial Personality Disorder; Borderline Personality Disorder; OCD (Obsessive-Compulsive Disorder); Paranoid Personality Disorder

Pertussis (Whooping Cough)

Risk for impaired emancipated **Decision-Making** r/t whether to administer usual childhood vaccinations

See Respiratory Infections, Acute Childhood

Pesticide Contamination

Contamination r/t use of environmental contaminants; pesticides

Risk for **Allergy** response r/t repeated exposure to pesticides

Risk for disproportionate **Growth:** Risk factor: environmental contamination

Petechiae

See Anticoagulant Therapy; Clotting Disorder; DIC (Disseminated Intravascular Coagulation); Hemophilia

Petit Mal Seizure

Readiness for enhanced **Health** management: wears medical alert bracelet; limits hazardous activities such as driving, swimming, working at heights, operating equipment

See Epilepsy

Pharyngitis

See Sore Throat

Phenylketonuria (PKU)

See PKU (Phenylketonuria)

Pheochromocytoma

Anxiety r/t symptoms from increased catecholamines—headache, palpitations, sweating, nervousness, nausea, vomiting, syncope

Ineffective **Health** maintenance r/t deficient knowledge regarding treatment and self-care

Insomnia r/t high levels of catecholamines

Nausea r/t increased catecholamines

Risk for decreased **Cardiac** tissue perfusion: Risk factor: hypertension

See Surgery, Perioperative; Surgery, Postoperative; Surgery, Preoperative

Phlebitis

See Thrombophlebitis

Phobia (Specific)

Fear r/t presence or anticipation of specific object or situation

Powerlessness r/t anxiety about encountering unknown or known entity

Impaired individual **Resilience** r/t psychological disorder

Readiness for enhanced **Power:** expresses readiness to enhance identification of choices that can be made for change

See Anxiety; Anxiety Disorder; Panic Disorder (Panic Attacks)

Photosensitivity

Ineffective **Health** maintenance r/t deficient knowledge regarding medications inducing photosensitivity

Risk for dry **Eye:** Risk factors: pharmaceutical agents, sunlight exposure

Risk for impaired **Skin** integrity: Risk factor: exposure to sun

Physical Abuse

See Abuse, Child; Abuse, Spouse, Parent, or Significant Other

Pica

Anxiety r/t stress

Imbalanced **Nutrition:** less than body requirements r/t eating nonnutritive substances

Impaired **Parenting** r/t lack of supervision, food deprivation

Risk for **Constipation:** Risk factor: presence of undigestible materials in gastrointestinal tract

Risk for dysfunctional **Gastrointestinal** motility: Risk factor: abnormal eating behavior

Risk for **Infection:** Risk factor: ingestion of infectious agents via contaminated substances

Risk for **Poisoning:** Risk factor: ingestion of substances containing lead

See Anemia

PID (Pelvic Inflammatory Disease)

Ineffective **Health** maintenance r/t deficient knowledge regarding self-care, treatment of disease

Acute **Pain** r/t biological injury; inflammation, edema, congestion of pelvic tissues

Ineffective **Sexuality** pattern r/t medically imposed abstinence from sexual activities until acute infection subsides, change in reproductive potential

Risk for **Infection:** Risk factors: insufficient knowledge to avoid exposure to pathogens; proper hygiene, nutrition, other health habits

See Maturational Issues, Adolescent; STD (Sexually Transmitted Disease)

PIH (Pregnancy-Induced Hypertension/ Preeclampsia)

Anxiety r/t fear of the unknown, threat to self and infant, change in role functioning

Death **Anxiety** r/t threat of preeclampsia

Deficient **Diversional** activity r/t bed rest

Interrupted **Family** processes r/t situational crisis

Impaired **Home** maintenance r/t bed rest

Deficient **Knowledge** r/t lack of experience with situation

Impaired physical **Mobility** r/t medically prescribed limitations

Impaired **Parenting** r/t prescribed bed rest

Powerlessness r/t complication threatening pregnancy, medically prescribed limitations

Ineffective **Role** performance r/t change in physical capacity to assume role of pregnant woman or resume other roles

Situational low **Self-Esteem** r/t loss of idealized pregnancy

Impaired **Social** interaction r/t imposed bed rest

Risk for imbalanced **Fluid** volume: Risk factors: hypertension, altered kidney function

Risk for **Injury:** fetal: Risk factors: decreased uteroplacental perfusion, seizures

Risk for **Injury:** maternal: Risk factors: vasospasm, high blood pressure

Readiness for enhanced **Knowledge:** exhibits desire for information on managing condition

Piloerection

Hypothermia r/t exposure to cold environment

Pimples

See Acne

Pink Eye

See Conjunctivitis

Pinworms

Impaired **Comfort** r/t itching

Impaired **Home** maintenance r/t inadequate cleaning of bed linen and toilet seats

Insomnia r/t discomfort

Readiness for enhanced **Health** management: proper handwashing; short, clean fingernails; avoiding hand, mouth, nose contact with unwashed hands; appropriate cleaning of bed linen and toilet seats

Pituitary Tumor, Benign

See Cushing's Disease

PKU (Phenylketonuria)

Risk for delayed **Development:** Risk factors: not following strict dietary program; eating foods extremely low in phenylalanine; avoiding eggs, milk, any foods containing aspartame (e.g., NutraSweet)

Readiness for enhanced **Health** management: testing for PKU and following prescribed dietary regimen

Placenta Abruptio

Death **Anxiety** r/t threat of mortality associated with bleeding

Fear r/t threat to self and fetus

Ineffective **Health** maintenance r/t deficient knowledge regarding treatment and control of hypertension associated with placenta abruptio

Acute **Pain:** abdominal/back r/t premature separation of placenta before delivery

Risk for **Bleeding:** Risk factor: placenta abruptio

Risk for deficient **Fluid** volume: Risk factor: maternal blood loss

Risk for **Powerlessness:** Risk factors: complications of pregnancy and unknown outcome

Risk for **Shock:** Risk factor: hypovolemia

Risk for **Spiritual** distress: Risk factor: fear from unknown outcome of pregnancy

Placenta Previa

Death **Anxiety** r/t threat of mortality associated with bleeding

Disturbed **Body Image** r/t negative feelings about body and reproductive ability, feelings of helplessness

Ineffective **Coping** r/t threat to self and fetus

Deficient **Diversional** activity r/t long-term hospitalization

Interrupted **Family** processes r/t maternal bed rest, hospitalization

Fear r/t threat to self and fetus, unknown future

Impaired **Home** maintenance r/t maternal bed rest, hospitalization

Impaired physical **Mobility** r/t medical protocol, maternal bed rest

Ineffective **Role** performance r/t maternal bed rest, hospitalization

Situational low **Self-Esteem** r/t situational crisis

Spiritual distress r/t inability to participate in usual religious rituals, situational crisis

Risk for **Bleeding:** Risk factor: placenta previa

Risk for **Constipation:** Risk factors: bed rest, pregnancy

Risk for deficient **Fluid** volume: Risk factor: maternal blood loss

Risk for imbalanced **Fluid** volume: Risk factor: maternal blood loss

Risk for **Injury:** fetal and maternal: Risk factors: threat to uteroplacental perfusion, hemorrhage

Risk for disturbed **Maternal–Fetal** dyad: Risk factor: complication of pregnancy

Risk for impaired **Parenting:** Risk factors: maternal bed rest, hospitalization

Risk for ineffective peripheral **Tissue Perfusion:** placental: Risk factors: dilation of cervix, loss of placental implantation site

Risk for **Powerlessness:** Risk factors: complications of pregnancy, unknown outcome

Risk for **Shock:** Risk factor: hypovolemia

Plantar Fasciitis

Impaired **Comfort** r/t inflamed structures of feet

Impaired physical **Mobility** r/t discomfort

Acute **Pain** r/t inflammation

Chronic **Pain** r/t inflammation

Pleural Effusion

Ineffective **Breathing** pattern r/t pain

Excess **Fluid** volume r/t compromised regulatory mechanisms; heart, liver, or kidney failure

Acute **Pain** r/t inflammation, fluid accumulation

Pleural Friction Rub

Ineffective **Breathing** pattern r/t pain

Acute **Pain** r/t inflammation, fluid accumulation

Pleural Tap

See Pleural Effusion

Pleurisy

Ineffective **Breathing** pattern r/t pain

Impaired **Gas** exchange r/t ventilation perfusion imbalance

Acute **Pain** r/t pressure on pleural nerve endings associated with fluid accumulation or inflammation

Impaired **Walking** r/t activity intolerance, inability to "catch breath"

Risk for ineffective **Airway** clearance: Risk factors: increased secretions, ineffective cough because of pain

Risk for **Infection:** Risk factor: exposure to pathogens

PMS (Premenstrual Tension Syndrome)

Fatigue r/t hormonal changes

Excess **Fluid** volume r/t alterations of hormonal levels inducing fluid retention

Deficient **Knowledge** r/t methods to deal with and prevent syndrome

Acute **Pain** r/t hormonal stimulation of gastrointestinal structures

Risk for **Powerlessness:** Risk factors: lack of knowledge and ability to deal with symptoms

Risk for impaired **Resilience:** Risk factor: PMS symptoms

Readiness for enhanced **Communication:** willingness to express thoughts and feelings about PMS

Readiness for enhanced **Health** management: desire for information to manage and prevent symptoms

PND (Paroxysmal Nocturnal Dyspnea)

Anxiety r/t inability to breathe during sleep

Ineffective **Breathing** pattern r/t increase in carbon dioxide levels, decrease in oxygen levels

Insomnia r/t suffocating feeling from fluid in lungs on awakening from sleep

Sleep deprivation r/t inability to breathe during sleep

Risk for decreased **Cardiac** tissue perfusion: Risk factor: hypoxia

Risk for **Powerlessness:** Risk factor: inability to control nocturnal dyspnea

Readiness for enhanced **Sleep:** expresses willingness to learn measures to enhance sleep

Pneumonectomy

See Thoracotomy

Pneumonia

Activity intolerance r/t imbalance between oxygen supply and demand

Ineffective **Airway** clearance r/t inflammation and presence of secretions

Impaired **Gas** exchange r/t decreased functional lung tissue

Ineffective **Health** management r/t deficient knowledge regarding self-care and treatment of disease

Imbalanced **Nutrition:** less than body requirements r/t loss of appetite

Impaired **Oral Mucous Membrane** r/t dry mouth from mouth breathing, decreased fluid intake

Ineffective **Thermoregulation** r/t infectious process

Risk for acute **Confusion:** Risk factors: underlying illness, hypoxia

Risk for deficient **Fluid** volume: Risk factor: inadequate intake of fluids

Risk for **Vascular Trauma:** Risk factor: irritation from intravenous antibiotics

See Respiratory Infections, Acute Childhood

Pneumothorax

Fear r/t threat to own well-being, difficulty breathing

Impaired **Gas** exchange r/t ventilation-perfusion imbalance, decreased functional lung tissue

Acute **Pain** r/t recent injury, coughing, deep breathing

Risk for **Injury:** Risk factor: possible complications associated with closed chest drainage system

See Chest Tubes

Poisoning, Risk for

Risk for **Poisoning** (See **Poisoning,** risk for, Section III)

Poliomyelitis

See Paralysis

Polydipsia

Readiness for enhanced **Fluid** balance: excessive thirst gone when diabetes is controlled

See Diabetes Mellitus

Polyphagia

Readiness for enhanced **Nutrition:** knowledge of appropriate diet for diabetes

See Diabetes Mellitus

Polyuria

Readiness for enhanced **Urinary** elimination: willingness to learn measures to enhance urinary elimination

See Diabetes Mellitus

Postoperative Care

See Surgery, Postoperative

Postpartum Depression

Anxiety r/t new responsibilities of parenting

Disturbed **Body Image** r/t normal postpartum recovery

Ineffective **Childbearing** process r/t depression/lack of support system

Ineffective **Coping** r/t hormonal changes

Fatigue r/t childbirth, postpartum state, crying child

Risk-prone **Health** behavior r/t lack of support systems

Impaired **Home** maintenance r/t fatigue, care of newborn

Hopelessness r/t stress, exhaustion

Deficient **Knowledge** r/t lifestyle changes

Impaired **Parenting** r/t hormone-induced depression

Ineffective **Role** performance r/t new responsibilities of parenting

Sexual dysfunction r/t fear of another pregnancy, postpartum pain, lochia flow

Sleep deprivation r/t environmental stimulation of newborn

Impaired **Social** interaction r/t change in role functioning

Risk for disturbed personal **Identity** r/t role change/depression/inability to cope

Risk for situational low **Self-Esteem:** Risk factor: decreased power over feelings of sadness

Risk for **Spiritual** distress: Risk factors: altered relationships, social isolation

Readiness for enhanced **Hope:** expresses desire to enhance hope and interconnectedness with others

See Depression (Major Depressive Disorder)

Postpartum Hemorrhage

Activity intolerance r/t anemia from loss of blood

Death **Anxiety** r/t threat of mortality associated with bleeding

Disturbed **Body Image** r/t loss of ideal childbirth

Insufficient **Breast Milk** r/t fluid volume depletion

Interrupted **Breastfeeding** r/t separation from infant for medical treatment

Decreased **Cardiac** output r/t hypovolemia

Fear r/t threat to self, unknown future

Deficient **Fluid** volume r/t uterine atony, loss of blood

Impaired **Home** maintenance r/t lack of stamina

Deficient **Knowledge** r/t lack of exposure to situation

Acute **Pain** r/t nursing and medical interventions to control bleeding

Ineffective peripheral **Tissue Perfusion** r/t hypovolemia

Risk for **Bleeding:** Risk factor: postpartum complications

Risk for impaired **Childbearing:** Risk factor: postpartum complication

Risk for imbalanced **Fluid** volume: Risk factor: maternal blood loss

Risk for **Infection:** Risk factors: loss of blood, depressed immunity

Risk for impaired **Parenting:** Risk factor: weakened maternal condition

Risk for **Powerlessness:** Risk factor: acute illness

Risk for **Shock:** Risk factor: hypovolemia

Postpartum, Normal Care

Anxiety r/t change in role functioning, parenting

Effective **Breastfeeding** r/t basic breastfeeding knowledge, support of partner and health care provider

Fatigue r/t childbirth, new responsibilities of parenting, body changes

Acute **Pain** r/t episiotomy, lacerations, bruising, breast engorgement, headache, sore nipples, epidural or intravenous site, hemorrhoids

Sexual dysfunction r/t recent childbirth

Impaired **Tissue** integrity r/t episiotomy, lacerations

Sleep deprivation r/t care of infant

Impaired **Urinary** elimination r/t effects of anesthesia, tissue trauma

Risk for **Constipation:** Risk factors: hormonal effects on smooth muscles, fear of straining with defecation, effects of anesthesia

Risk for **Infection:** Risk factors: tissue trauma, blood loss

Readiness for enhanced family **Coping:** adaptation to new family member

Readiness for enhanced **Hope:** desire to increase hope

Readiness for enhanced **Parenting:** expresses willingness to enhance parenting skills

Post-Trauma Syndrome

Post-Trauma syndrome (See **Post-Trauma** syndrome, Section III)

Post-Trauma Syndrome, Risk for

Risk for **Post-Trauma** syndrome (See **Post-Trauma** syndrome, risk for, Section III)

Post-Traumatic Stress Disorder (PTSD)

See PTSD (Post-Traumatic Stress Disorder)

Potassium, Increase/Decrease

See Hyperkalemia; Hypokalemia

Power/Powerlessness

Powerlessness (See **Powerlessness,** Section III)

Risk for **Powerlessness** (See **Powerlessness,** risk for, Section III)

Readiness for enhanced **Power** (See **Power,** readiness for enhanced, Section III)

Preeclampsia

See PIH (Pregnancy-Induced Hypertension/Preeclampsia)

Pregnancy, Cardiac Disorders

See Cardiac Disorders in Pregnancy

Pregnancy-Induced Hypertension/ Preeclampsia (PIH)

See PIH (Pregnancy-Induced Hypertension/Preeclampsia)

Pregnancy Loss

Anxiety r/t threat to role functioning, health status, situational crisis

Compromised family **Coping** r/t lack of support by significant other because of personal suffering

Ineffective **Coping** r/t situational crisis

Grieving r/t loss of pregnancy, fetus, or child

Acute **Pain** r/t surgical intervention

Ineffective **Role** performance r/t inability to assume parenting role

Ineffective **Sexuality** pattern r/t self-esteem disturbance resulting from pregnancy loss and anxiety about future pregnancies

Chronic **Sorrow** r/t loss of a fetus or child

Spiritual distress r/t intense suffering from loss of child

Risk for deficient **Fluid** volume: Risk factor: blood loss

Risk for complicated **Grieving:** Risk factor: loss of pregnancy

Risk for **Infection:** Risk factor: retained products of conception

Risk for **Powerlessness:** Risk factor: situational crisis

Risk for ineffective **Relationship:** Risk factor: poor communication skills in dealing with the loss

Risk for **Spiritual** distress: Risk factor: intense suffering

Readiness for enhanced **Communication:** willingness to express feelings and thoughts about loss

Readiness for enhanced **Hope:** expresses desire to enhance hope

Readiness for enhanced **Spiritual** well-being: desire for acceptance of loss

Pregnancy, Normal

Anxiety r/t unknown future, threat to self secondary to pain of labor

Disturbed **Body Image** r/t altered body function and appearance

Interrupted **Family** processes r/t developmental transition of pregnancy

Fatigue r/t increased energy demands

Fear r/t labor and delivery

Deficient **Knowledge** r/t primiparity

Nausea r/t hormonal changes of pregnancy

Imbalanced **Nutrition:** less than body requirements r/t growing fetus, nausea

Imbalanced **Nutrition:** more than body requirements r/t deficient knowledge regarding nutritional needs of pregnancy

Sleep deprivation r/t uncomfortable pregnancy state

Impaired **Urinary** elimination r/t frequency caused by increased pelvic pressure and hormonal stimulation

Risk for **Constipation:** Risk factor: pregnancy

Risk for **Sexual** dysfunction: Risk factors: altered body function, self-concept, body image with pregnancy

Readiness for enhanced **Childbearing** process: appropriate prenatal care

Readiness for enhanced family **Coping:** satisfying partner relationship, attention to gratification of needs, effective adaptation to developmental tasks of pregnancy

Readiness for enhanced **Family** processes: family adapts to change

Readiness for enhanced **Health** management: seeks information for prenatal self care

Readiness for enhanced **Nutrition:** desire for knowledge of appropriate nutrition during pregnancy

Readiness for enhanced **Parenting:** expresses willingness to enhance parenting skills

Readiness for enhanced **Relationship:** meeting developmental goals associated with pregnancy

Readiness for enhanced **Spiritual** well-being: new role as parent

See Discomforts of Pregnancy

Premature Dilation of the Cervix (Incompetent Cervix)

Ineffective **Activity** planning r/t unrealistic perception of events

Ineffective **Coping** r/t bed rest, threat to fetus

Deficient **Diversional** activity r/t bed rest

Fear r/t potential loss of infant

Grieving r/t potential loss of infant

Deficient **Knowledge** r/t treatment regimen, prognosis for pregnancy

Impaired physical **Mobility** r/t imposed bed rest to prevent preterm birth

Powerlessness r/t inability to control outcome of pregnancy

Ineffective **Role** performance r/t inability to continue usual patterns of responsibility

Situational low **Self-Esteem** r/t inability to complete normal pregnancy

Sexual dysfunction r/t fear of harm to fetus

Impaired **Social** interaction r/t bed rest

Risk for **Infection:** Risk factor: invasive procedures to prevent preterm birth

Risk for **Injury:** fetal: Risk factors: preterm birth, use of anesthetics

Risk for **Injury:** maternal: Risk factor: surgical procedures to prevent preterm birth (e.g., cerclage)

P

Risk for impaired **Resilience:** Risk factor: complication of pregnancy

Risk for **Spiritual** distress: Risk factors: physical/psychological stress

Premature Infant (Child)

Insufficient **Breast Milk** r/t ineffective sucking, latching on of the infant

Impaired **Gas** exchange r/t effects of cardiopulmonary insufficiency

Disorganized **Infant** behavior r/t prematurity

Insomnia r/t noisy and noxious intensive care environment

Neonatal **Jaundice** r/t infant experiences difficulty making transition to extrauterine life

Imbalanced **Nutrition:** less than body requirements r/t delayed or understimulated rooting reflex, easy fatigue during feeding, diminished endurance

Impaired **Swallowing** r/t decreased or absent gag reflex, fatigue

Ineffective **Thermoregulation** r/t large body surface/weight ratio, immaturity of thermal regulation, state of prematurity

Risk for delayed **Development:** Risk factor: prematurity

Risk for disproportionate **Growth:** Risk factor: prematurity

Risk for **Infection:** Risk factors: inadequate, immature, or undeveloped acquired immune response

Risk for **Injury:** Risk factor: prolonged mechanical ventilation, retinopathy of prematurity (ROP) secondary to 100% oxygen environment

Risk for neonatal **Jaundice:** Risk factor: late preterm birth

P

Readiness for enhanced organized **Infant** behavior: use of some self-regulatory measures

Premature Infant (Parent)

Ineffective **Breastfeeding** r/t disrupted establishment of effective pattern secondary to prematurity or insufficient opportunities

Decisional Conflict r/t support system deficit, multiple sources of information

Compromised family **Coping** r/t disrupted family roles and disorganization, prolonged condition exhausting supportive capacity of significant persons

Grieving r/t loss of perfect child possibly leading to complicated grieving

Complicated **Grieving** (prolonged) r/t unresolved conflicts

Parental **Role** conflict r/t expressed concerns, expressed inability to care for child's physical, emotional, or developmental needs

Chronic **Sorrow** r/t threat of loss of a child, prolonged hospitalization

Spiritual distress r/t challenged belief or value systems regarding moral or ethical implications of treatment plans

Risk for impaired **Attachment:** Risk factors: separation, physical barriers, lack of privacy

Risk for disturbed **Maternal–Fetal** dyad: Risk factor: complication of pregnancy

Risk for **Powerlessness:** Risk factor: inability to control situation

Risk for impaired **Resilience:** Risk factor: premature infant

Risk for **Spiritual** distress: Risk factor: challenged belief or value systems regarding moral or ethical implications of treatment plans

Readiness for enhanced **Family** process: adaptation to change associated with premature infant

See Child with Chronic Condition; Hospitalized Child

Premature Rupture of Membranes

Anxiety r/t threat to infant's health status

Disturbed **Body Image** r/t inability to carry pregnancy to term

Ineffective **Coping** r/t situational crisis

Grieving r/t potential loss of infant

Situational low **Self-Esteem** r/t inability to carry pregnancy to term

Risk for ineffective **Childbearing** process: Risk factor: complication of pregnancy

Risk for **Infection:** Risk factor: rupture of membranes

Risk for **Injury:** fetal: Risk factor: risk of premature birth

Premenstrual Tension Syndrome (PMS)

See PMS (Premenstrual Tension Syndrome)

Prenatal Care, Normal

Readiness for enhanced **Childbearing** process: appropriate prenatal lifestyle

Readiness for enhanced **Knowledge:** appropriate prenatal care

Readiness for enhanced **Spiritual** well-being: new role as parent

See Pregnancy, Normal

Prenatal Testing

Anxiety r/t unknown outcome, delayed test results

Acute **Pain** r/t invasive procedures

Risk for **Infection:** Risk factor: invasive procedures during amniocentesis or chorionic villus sampling

Risk for **Injury:** fetal r/t invasive procedures

Preoperative Teaching

See Surgery, Preoperative Care

Pressure Ulcer

Impaired bed **Mobility** r/t intolerance to activity, pain, cognitive impairment, depression, severe anxiety, severity of illness

Imbalanced **Nutrition:** less than body requirements r/t limited access to food, inability to absorb nutrients because of biological factors, anorexia

Acute **Pain** r/t tissue destruction, exposure of nerves

Impaired **Skin** integrity: stage I or II pressure ulcer r/t physical immobility, mechanical factors, altered circulation, skin irritants, excessive moisture

Impaired **Tissue** integrity: stage III or IV pressure ulcer r/t altered circulation, impaired physical mobility, excessive moisture

Risk for **Infection:** Risk factors: physical immobility, mechanical factors (shearing forces, pressure, restraint, altered circulation, skin irritants, excessive moisture, open wound)

Risk for **Pressure** ulcer (See **Pressure** ulcer, risk for, Section III)

Preterm Labor

Anxiety r/t threat to fetus, change in role functioning, change in environment and interaction patterns, use of tocolytic drugs

Ineffective **Coping** r/t situational crisis, preterm labor

Deficient **Diversional** activity r/t long-term hospitalization

Grieving r/t loss of idealized pregnancy, potential loss of fetus

Impaired **Home** maintenance r/t medical restrictions

Impaired physical **Mobility** r/t medically imposed restrictions

Ineffective **Role** performance r/t inability to carry out normal roles secondary to bed rest or hospitalization, change in expected course of pregnancy

Situational low **Self-Esteem** r/t threatened ability to carry pregnancy to term

Sexual dysfunction r/t actual or perceived limitation imposed by preterm labor and/or prescribed treatment, separation from partner because of hospitalization

Sleep deprivation r/t change in usual pattern secondary to contractions, hospitalization, treatment regimen

Impaired **Social** interaction r/t prolonged bed rest or hospitalization

Risk for **Injury:** fetal: Risk factors: premature birth, immature body systems

Risk for **Injury:** maternal: Risk factor: use of tocolytic drugs

Risk for **Powerlessness:** Risk factor: lack of control over preterm labor

Risk for **Vascular Trauma:** Risk factor: intravenous medication

Readiness for enhanced **Childbearing** process: appropriate prenatal lifestyle

Readiness for enhanced **Comfort:** expresses desire to enhance relaxation

Readiness for enhanced **Communication:** willingness to discuss thoughts and feelings about situation

Problem-Solving Dysfunction

Defensive **Coping** r/t situational crisis

Impaired Emancipated **Decision-Making** r/t problem solving dysfunction

Risk for chronic low **Self-Esteem:** Risk factor: repeated failures

Readiness for enhanced **Communication:** willing to share ideas with others

Readiness for enhanced **Relationship:** shares information and ideas between partners

Readiness for enhanced **Resilience:** identifies available resources

Readiness for enhanced **Spiritual** well-being: desires to draw on inner strength and find meaning and purpose to life

Projection

Anxiety r/t threat to self-concept

Defensive **Coping** r/t inability to acknowledge that own behavior may be a problem, blaming others

Chronic low **Self-Esteem** r/t failure

Impaired **Social** interaction r/t self-concept disturbance, confrontational communication style

Risk for **Loneliness:** Risk factor: blaming others for problems

See Paranoid Personality Disorder

Prolapsed Umbilical Cord

Fear r/t threat to fetus, impending surgery

Ineffective peripheral **Tissue Perfusion:** fetal r/t interruption in umbilical blood flow

Risk for ineffective **Cerebral** tissue perfusion: fetal: Risk factor: cord compression

Risk for **Injury:** maternal: Risk factor: emergency surgery

Prostatectomy

See TURP (Transurethral Resection of the Prostate)

Prostatic Hypertrophy

Ineffective **Health** maintenance r/t deficient knowledge regarding self-care and prevention of complications

Sleep deprivation r/t nocturia

Urinary Retention r/t obstruction

Risk for **Infection:** Risk factors: urinary residual after voiding, bacterial invasion of bladder

See BPH (Benign Prostatic Hypertrophy)

P

Prostatitis

Impaired **Comfort** r/t inflammation

Ineffective **Health** maintenance r/t deficient knowledge regarding treatment

Urge urinary **Incontinence** r/t irritation of bladder

Ineffective **Protection** r/t depressed immune system

Pruritus

Impaired **Comfort** r/t itching

Deficient **Knowledge** r/t methods to treat and prevent itching

Risk for impaired **Skin** integrity: Risk factor: scratching from pruritus

Psoriasis

Disturbed **Body Image** r/t lesions on body

Impaired **Comfort** r/t irritated skin

Ineffective **Health** maintenance r/t deficient knowledge regarding treatment modalities

Powerlessness r/t lack of control over condition with frequent exacerbations and remissions

Impaired **Skin** integrity r/t lesions on body

Psychosis

Ineffective **Activity** planning r/t compromised ability to process information

Ineffective **Health** maintenance r/t cognitive impairment, ineffective individual and family coping

Self-Neglect r/t mental disorder

Impaired individual **Resilience** r/t psychological disorder

Situational low **Self-Esteem** r/t excessive use of defense mechanisms (e.g., projection, denial, rationalization)

Risk for disturbed personal **Identity:** Risk factor: psychosis

Impaired **Mood** regulation r/t psychosis

Risk for **Post-Trauma** syndrome: Risk factor: diminished ego strength

See Schizophrenia

PTCA (Percutaneous Transluminal Coronary Angioplasty)

See Angioplasty, Coronary

PTSD (Posttraumatic Stress Disorder)

Anxiety r/t exposure to internal or external cues that symbolize or resemble an aspect of the traumatic event

Chronic **Sorrow** r/t chronic disability (e.g., physical, mental)

Death **Anxiety** r/t psychological stress associated with traumatic event

Ineffective **Breathing** pattern r/t hyperventilation associated with anxiety

Ineffective **Coping** r/t extreme anxiety

Ineffective **Impulse** control r/t thinking of initial trauma experience

Insomnia r/t recurring nightmares

Post-Trauma syndrome r/t exposure to a traumatic event

Sleep deprivation r/t nightmares interrupting sleep associated with traumatic event

Spiritual distress r/t feelings of detachment or estrangement from others

Risk for impaired **Resilience:** Risk factor: chronicity of existing crisis

Risk for **Powerlessness:** Risk factors: flashbacks, reliving event

Risk for ineffective **Relationship:** Risk factor: stressful life events

Risk for self- or other-directed **Violence:** Risk factors: fear of self or others

Readiness for enhanced **Comfort:** expresses desire to enhance relaxation

Readiness for enhanced **Communication:** willingness to express feelings and thoughts

Readiness for enhanced **Spiritual** well-being: desire for harmony after stressful event

Pulmonary Edema

Anxiety r/t fear of suffocation

Ineffective **Airway** clearance r/t presence of tracheobronchial secretions

Decreased **Cardiac** output r/t increased preload, infective forward perfusion

Impaired **Gas** exchange r/t extravasation of extravascular fluid in lung tissues and alveoli

Ineffective **Health** maintenance r/t deficient knowledge regarding treatment regimen

Sleep deprivation r/t inability to breathe

Risk for acute **Confusion:** Risk factor: hypoxia

See Heart Failure

Pulmonary Embolism

Anxiety r/t fear of suffocation

Decreased **Cardiac** output r/t right ventricular failure secondary to obstructed pulmonary artery

Fear r/t severe pain, possible death

Impaired **Gas** exchange r/t altered blood flow to alveoli secondary to embolus

Deficient **Knowledge** r/t activities to prevent embolism, self-care after diagnosis of embolism

Acute **Pain** r/t biological injury, lack of oxygen to cells

Ineffective peripheral **Tissue Perfusion** r/t deep vein thrombus formation

See Anticoagulant Therapy

Pulmonary Stenosis

See Congenital Heart Disease/Cardiac Anomalies

Pulse Deficit

Risk for Decreased **Cardiac** output r/t dysrhythmia

See Dysrhythmia

Pulse Oximetry

Readiness for enhanced **Knowledge:** information about treatment regimen

See Hypoxia

Pulse Pressure, Increased

See Intracranial Pressure, Increased

Pulse Pressure, Narrowed

See Shock, Hypovolemic

Pulses, Absent or Diminished Peripheral

Ineffective peripheral **Tissue Perfusion** r/t interruption of arterial flow

Risk for **Peripheral Neurovascular** dysfunction: Risk factors: fractures, mechanical compression, orthopedic surgery trauma, immobilization, burns, vascular obstruction

Purpura

See Clotting Disorder

Pyelonephritis

Ineffective **Health** maintenance r/t deficient knowledge regarding self-care, treatment of disease, prevention of further urinary tract infections

Acute **Pain** r/t inflammation and irritation of urinary tract

Disturbed **Sleep** pattern r/t urinary frequency

Impaired **Urinary** elimination r/t irritation of urinary tract

Risk for ineffective **Renal** perfusion: Risk factor: infection

Pyloric Stenosis

Imbalanced **Nutrition:** less than body requirements r/t vomiting secondary to pyloric sphincter obstruction

Acute **Pain** r/t abdominal fullness

Risk for decreased **Fluid** volume: Risk factors: vomiting, dehydration

See Hospitalized Child

Pyloromyotomy (Pyloric Stenosis Repair)

See Surgery Preoperative, Perioperative, Postoperative

R

RA (Rheumatoid Arthritis)

See Rheumatoid Arthritis (RA)

Rabies

Ineffective **Health** maintenance r/t deficient knowledge regarding care of wound, isolation, and observation of infected animal

Acute **Pain** r/t multiple immunization injections

Risk for ineffective **Cerebral** tissue perfusion: Risk factor: rabies virus

Radial Nerve Dysfunction

Acute **Pain** r/t trauma to hand or arm

See Neuropathy, Peripheral

Radiation Therapy

Activity intolerance r/t fatigue from possible anemia

Disturbed **Body Image** r/t change in appearance, hair loss

Diarrhea r/t irradiation effects

Fatigue r/t malnutrition from lack of appetite, nausea, and vomiting; side effect of radiation

Deficient **Knowledge** r/t what to expect with radiation therapy, how to do self-care

Nausea r/t side effects of radiation

Imbalanced **Nutrition:** less than body requirements r/t anorexia, nausea, vomiting, irradiation of areas of pharynx and esophagus

Impaired **Oral Mucous Membrane** r/t irradiation effects

Ineffective **Protection** r/t suppression of bone marrow

Risk for impaired **Oral Mucous Membranes:** Risk factor: Radiation treatments

Risk for **Powerlessness:** Risk factors: medical treatment and possible side effects

Risk for impaired **Resilience:** Risk factor: radiation treatment

Risk for impaired **Skin** integrity: Risk factor: irradiation effects

Risk for **Spiritual** distress: Risk factors: radiation treatment, prognosis

Radical Neck Dissection

See Laryngectomy

Rage

Risk-prone **Health** behavior r/t multiple stressors

Labile Emotional Control r/t psychiatric disorders and mood disorders

Impaired individual **Resilience** r/t poor impulse control

Stress overload r/t multiple coexisting stressors

Risk for **Self-Mutilation:** Risk factor: command hallucinations

Risk for **Suicide:** Risk factor: desire to kill self

Risk for other-directed **Violence:** Risk factors: panic state, manic excitement, organic brain syndrome

Rape-Trauma Syndrome

Rape-Trauma syndrome (See **Rape-Trauma** syndrome, Section III)

Chronic **Sorrow** r/t forced loss of virginity

Risk for ineffective **Childbearing** process r/t to trauma and violence

Risk for **Post-Trauma** syndrome: Risk factor: trauma or violence associated with rape

Risk for **Powerlessness:** Risk factor: inability to control thoughts about incident

Risk for ineffective **Relationship** r/t to trauma and violence

Risk for chronic low **Self-Esteem** r/t perceived lack of respect from others/feeling violated

Risk for **Spiritual** distress: Risk factor: forced loss of virginity

Rash

Impaired **Comfort** r/t pruritus

Impaired **Skin** integrity r/t mechanical trauma

Risk for **Infection:** Risk factors: traumatized tissue, broken skin

Risk for **Latex Allergy** response: Risk factor: allergy to products associated with latex

Rationalization

Defensive **Coping** r/t situational crisis, inability to accept blame for consequences of own behavior

Ineffective **Denial** r/t fear of consequences, actual or perceived loss

Impaired individual **Resilience** r/t psychological disturbance

Risk for **Post-Trauma** syndrome: Risk factor: survivor's role in event

Readiness for enhanced **Communication:** expresses desire to share thoughts and feelings

Readiness for enhanced **Spiritual** well-being: possibility of seeking harmony with self, others, higher power, God

Rats, Rodents in Home

Impaired **Home** maintenance r/t lack of knowledge, insufficient finances

Risk for **Allergy** response r/t repeated exposure to environmental contamination

See Filthy Home Environment

Raynaud's Disease

Deficient **Knowledge** r/t lack of information about disease process, possible complications, self-care needs regarding disease process and medication

Ineffective peripheral **Tissue Perfusion** r/t transient reduction of blood flow

Acute **Pain** r/t transient reduction in blood flow

RDS (Respiratory Distress Syndrome)

See Respiratory Conditions of the Neonate

Rectal Fullness

Chronic functional **Constipation** r/t decreased activity level, decreased fluid intake, inadequate fiber in diet, decreased peristalsis, side effects of antidepressant or antipsychotic therapy

Risk for chronic functional **Constipation:** Risk factor: habitual denial of or ignoring urge to defecate

Rectal Lump

See Hemorrhoids

Rectal Pain/Bleeding

Chronic functional **Constipation** r/t pain on defecation

Deficient **Knowledge** r/t possible causes of rectal bleeding, pain, treatment modalities

Acute **Pain** r/t pressure of defecation

Risk for **Bleeding:** Risk factor: rectal disease

R

Rectal Surgery

See Hemorrhoidectomy

Rectocele Repair

Chronic functional **Constipation** r/t painful defecation

Ineffective **Health** maintenance r/t deficient knowledge of postoperative care of surgical site, dietary measures, exercise to prevent constipation

Acute **Pain** r/t surgical procedure

Urinary retention r/t edema from surgery

Risk for **Bleeding:** Risk factor: surgery

Risk for **Infection:** Risk factors: surgical procedure, possible contamination of area with feces

Reflex Incontinence

Reflex urinary **Incontinence** (See **Incontinence,** urinary, reflex, Section III)

Regression

Anxiety r/t threat to or change in health status

Defensive **Coping** r/t denial of obvious problems, weaknesses

Self-Neglect r/t functional impairment

Powerlessness r/t health care environment

Impaired individual **Resilience** r/t psychological disturbance

Ineffective **Role** performance r/t powerlessness over health status

See Hospitalized Child; Separation Anxiety

Regretful

Anxiety r/t situational or maturational crises

Death **Anxiety** r/t feelings of not having accomplished goals in life

Risk for **Spiritual** distress: Risk factor: inability to forgive

Rehabilitation

Ineffective **Coping** r/t loss of normal function

Impaired physical **Mobility** r/t injury, surgery, psychosocial condition warranting rehabilitation

Self-Care deficit: specify r/t impaired physical mobility

Risk for **Falls:** Risk factor: physical deconditioning

Readiness for enhanced **Comfort:** expresses desire to enhance feeling of comfort

Readiness for enhanced **Self-Concept:** accepts strengths and limitations

Readiness for enhanced **Health Management:** expresses desire to manage rehabilitation

Relationship

Ineffective **Relationship** (See ineffective **Relationship,** Section III)

Readiness for enhanced **Relationship** (See Risk for enhanced **Relationship** see Section III)

Relaxation Techniques

Anxiety r/t situational crisis

Readiness for enhanced **Comfort:** expresses desire to enhance relaxation

Readiness for enhanced **Health** management: desire to manage illness

Readiness for enhanced **Religiosity:** requests religious materials or experiences

Readiness for enhanced **Resilience:** desire to enhance resilience

Readiness for enhanced **Self-Concept:** willingness to enhance self-concept

Readiness for enhanced **Spiritual** well-being: seeking comfort from higher power

Religiosity

Impaired **Religiosity** (See **Religiosity,** impaired, Section III)

Risk for impaired **Religiosity** (See **Religiosity,** impaired, risk for, Section III)

Readiness for enhanced **Religiosity** (See **Religiosity,** readiness for enhanced, Section III)

Religious Concerns

Spiritual distress r/t separation from religious or cultural ties

Risk for impaired **Religiosity:** Risk factors: ineffective support, coping, caregiving

Risk for **Spiritual** distress: Risk factors: physical or psychological stress

Readiness for enhanced **Spiritual** well-being: desire for increased spirituality

Relocation Stress Syndrome

Relocation stress syndrome (See **Relocation** stress syndrome, Section III)

Risk for **Relocation** stress syndrome (See **Relocation** stress syndrome, risk for, Section III)

Respiratory Acidosis

See Acidosis, Respiratory

Respiratory Conditions of the Neonate (Respiratory Distress Syndrome [RDS], Meconium Aspiration, Diaphragmatic Hernia)

Ineffective **Airway** clearance r/t sequelae of attempts to breathe in utero resulting in meconium aspiration

Fatigue r/t increased energy requirements and metabolic demands

Impaired **Gas** exchange r/t decreased surfactant, immature lung tissue

Dysfunctional **Ventilator** weaning response r/t immature respiratory system

Risk for **Infection:** Risk factors: tissue destruction or irritation as a result of aspiration of meconium fluid

See Bronchopulmonary Dysplasia; Hospitalized Child; Premature Infant, Child

Respiratory Distress

See Dyspnea

Respiratory Distress Syndrome (RDS)

See Respiratory Conditions of the Neonate

Respiratory Infections, Acute Childhood (Croup, Epiglottitis, Pertussis, Pneumonia, Respiratory Syncytial Virus)

Activity intolerance r/t generalized weakness, dyspnea, fatigue, poor oxygenation

Ineffective **Airway** clearance r/t excess tracheobronchial secretions

Ineffective **Breathing** pattern r/t inflamed bronchial passages, coughing

Fear r/t oxygen deprivation, difficulty breathing

Deficient **Fluid** volume r/t insensible losses (fever, diaphoresis), inadequate oral fluid intake

Impaired **Gas** exchange r/t insufficient oxygenation as a result of inflammation or edema of epiglottis, larynx, bronchial passages

Imbalanced **Nutrition:** less than body requirements r/t anorexia, fatigue, generalized weakness, poor sucking and breathing coordination, dyspnea

Ineffective **Thermoregulation** r/t infectious process

Risk for **Aspiration:** Risk factors: inability to coordinate breathing, coughing, sucking

Risk for **Infection:** transmission to others: Risk factor: virulent infectious organisms

Risk for **Injury** (to pregnant others): Risk factors: exposure to aerosolized medications (e.g., ribavirin, pentamidine), resultant potential fetal toxicity

Risk for **Suffocation:** Risk factors: inflammation of larynx, epiglottis

See Hospitalized Child

Respiratory Syncytial Virus

See Respiratory Infections, Acute Childhood

Restless Leg Syndrome

Disturbed **Sleep** pattern r/t leg discomfort during sleep relieved by frequent leg movement

Chronic **Pain** r/t leg discomfort

See Stress

Retarded Growth and Development

See Growth and Development Lag

Retching

Nausea r/t chemotherapy, postsurgical anesthesia, irritation to gastrointestinal system, stimulation of neuropharmacological mechanisms

Imbalanced **Nutrition:** less than body requirements r/t inability to ingest food

Risk for **Fatigue:** Risk factor: stress of retching, muscle contractions

Retinal Detachment

Anxiety r/t change in vision, threat of loss of vision

Deficient **Knowledge** r/t symptoms, need for early intervention to prevent permanent damage

Vision Loss r/t impaired visual acuity

Risk for impaired **Home** maintenance: Risk factors: postoperative care, activity limitations, care of affected eye

Risk for impaired **Resilience:** Risk factor: possible loss of vision

See Vision Impairment

Retinopathy, Diabetic

See Diabetic Retinopathy

Retinopathy of Prematurity (ROP)

Risk for **Injury:** Risk factors: prolonged mechanical ventilation, ROP secondary to 100% oxygen environment

See Retinal Detachment

Rh Factor Incompatibility

Anxiety r/t unknown outcome of pregnancy

Neonatal **Jaundice** r/t Rh factor incompatibility

Deficient **Knowledge** r/t treatment regimen from lack of experience with situation

Powerlessness r/t perceived lack of control over outcome of pregnancy

Risk for **Injury:** fetal: Risk factors: intrauterine destruction of red blood cells, transfusions

Risk for neonatal **Jaundice** r/t Rh factor incompatibility

Readiness for enhanced **Health** management: prenatal care, compliance with diagnostic and treatment regimen

Rhabdomyolysis

Ineffective **Coping** r/t seriousness of condition

Impaired physical **Mobility** r/t myalgia and muscle weakness

Risk for deficient **Fluid** volume: Risk factor: reduced blood flow to kidneys

Risk for ineffective **Renal** perfusion: Risk factor: possible kidney failure from obstruction of kidney

Risk for **Shock:** Risk factor: hypovolemia

Readiness for enhanced **Health** management: seeks information to avoid condition

See Kidney Failure

Rheumatic Fever

See Endocarditis

Rheumatoid Arthritis (RA)

Imbalanced **Nutrition:** less than body requirements r/t loss of appetite

Chronic **Pain** r/t joint inflammation

Risk for impaired **Resilience:** Risk factor: chronic, painful, progressive disease

See Arthritis; JRA (Juvenile Rheumatoid Arthritis)

Rib Fracture

Ineffective **Breathing** pattern r/t fractured ribs

Acute **Pain** r/t movement, deep breathing

Impaired **Gas** exchange r/t ventilation-perfusion imbalance, decreased depth of ventilation

Ridicule of Others

Defensive **Coping** r/t situational crisis, psychological impairment, substance abuse

Risk for **Post-Trauma** syndrome: Risk factor: perception of event

Ringworm of Body

Impaired **Comfort** r/t pruritus

Impaired **Skin** integrity r/t presence of macules associated with fungus

See Itching; Pruritus

Ringworm of Nails

Disturbed **Body Image** r/t appearance of nails, removed nails

Ringworm of Scalp

Disturbed **Body Image** r/t possible hair loss (alopecia)

See Itching; Pruritus

Roaches, Invasion of Home with

Impaired **Home** maintenance r/t lack of knowledge, insufficient finances

See Filthy Home Environment

Role Performance, Altered

Ineffective **Role** performance (See **Role** performance, ineffective, Section III)

ROP (Retinopathy of Prematurity)

See Retinopathy of Prematurity (ROP)

RSV (Respiratory Syncytial Virus)

See Respiratory Infection, Acute Childhood

Rubella

See Communicable Diseases, Childhood

Rubor of Extremities

Ineffective peripheral **Tissue Perfusion** r/t interruption of arterial flow

See Peripheral Vascular Disease (PVD)

Ruptured Disk

See Low Back Pain

S

SAD (Seasonal Affective Disorder)

Readiness for enhanced **Resilience:** uses SAD lights during winter months

See Depression (Major Depressive Disorder)

Sadness

Complicated **Grieving** r/t actual or perceived loss

Impaired **Mood** regulation r/t chronic illness (See **Mood** regulation, impaired, Section III)

Spiritual distress r/t intense suffering

Risk for **Powerlessness:** Risk factor: actual or perceived loss

Risk for **Spiritual** distress: Risk factor: loss of loved one

Readiness for enhanced **Communication:** willingness to share feelings and thoughts

Readiness for enhanced **Spiritual** well-being: desire for harmony after actual or perceived loss

See Depression (Major Depressive Disorder); Major Depressive Disorder

Safe Sex

Readiness for enhanced **Health** management: takes appropriate precautions during sexual activity to keep from contracting sexually transmitted disease

See Sexuality, Adolescent; STD (Sexually Transmitted Disease)

Safety, Childhood

Deficient **Knowledge:** potential for enhanced health maintenance r/t parental knowledge and skill acquisition regarding appropriate safety measures

Risk for **Aspiration** (See **Aspiration,** risk for, Section III)

Risk for **Injury:** Risk factors: developmental age, altered home maintenance

Risk for impaired **Parenting:** Risk factors: lack of available and effective role model, lack of knowledge, misinformation from other family members (old wives' tales)

Risk for **Poisoning:** Risk factors: use of lead-based paint; presence of asbestos or radon gas; drugs not locked in cabinet; household products left in accessible area (bleach, detergent, drain cleaners, household cleaners); alcohol and perfume within reach of child; presence of poisonous plants; atmospheric pollutants

Risk for **Thermal** injury: Risk factor: inadequate supervision

Readiness for enhanced **Childbearing** process: expresses appropriate knowledge for care of child

Salmonella

Impaired **Home** maintenance r/t improper preparation or storage of food, lack of safety measures when caring for pet reptile

Risk for **Shock:** Risk factors: hypovolemia, diarrhea, sepsis

Readiness for enhanced **Health** management: avoiding improperly prepared or stored food, wearing gloves when handling pet reptiles or their feces

See Gastroenteritis; Gastroenteritis, Child

Salpingectomy

Decisional Conflict r/t sterilization procedure

Grieving r/t possible loss from tubal pregnancy

Risk for impaired **Urinary** elimination: Risk factor: trauma to ureter during surgery

See Hysterectomy; Surgery, Perioperative Care; Surgery, Postoperative Care; Surgery, Preoperative Care

Sarcoidosis

Anxiety r/t change in health status

Impaired **Gas** exchange r/t ventilation-perfusion imbalance

Ineffective **Health** maintenance r/t deficient knowledge regarding home care and medication regimen

Acute **Pain** r/t possible disease affecting joints

Ineffective **Protection** r/t immune disorder

Risk for decreased **Cardiac** tissue perfusion: Risk factor: dysrhythmias

Risk for impaired **Skin** integrity: Risk factor: immunological disorder

SARS (Severe Acute Respiratory Syndrome)

Risk for **Infection:** Risk factor: increased environmental exposure (travelers in close proximity to infected persons, traveling when a fever is present)

Readiness for enhanced **Knowledge:** information regarding travel and precautions to avoid exposure to SARS

See Pneumonia

SBE (Self-Breast Examination)

Readiness for enhanced **Health** management: desires to have information about SBE

Readiness for enhanced **Knowledge:** self-breast examination

Scabies

See Communicable Diseases, Childhood

Scared

Anxiety r/t threat of death, threat to or change in health status

Death **Anxiety** r/t unresolved issues surrounding end-of-life decisions

Fear r/t hospitalization, real or imagined threat to own well-being

Impaired individual **Resilience** r/t violence

Readiness for enhanced **Communication:** willingness to share thoughts and feelings

Schizophrenia

Ineffective **Activity** planning r/t compromised ability to process information

Anxiety r/t unconscious conflict with reality

Impaired verbal **Communication** r/t psychosis, disorientation, inaccurate perception, hallucinations, delusions

Ineffective **Coping** r/t inadequate support systems, unrealistic perceptions, inadequate coping skills, disturbed thought processes, impaired communication

Deficient **Diversional** activity r/t social isolation, possible regression

Interrupted **Family** processes r/t inability to express feelings, impaired communication

Fear r/t altered contact with reality

Ineffective **Health** maintenance r/t cognitive impairment, ineffective individual and family coping, lack of material resources

Ineffective family **Health** management r/t chronicity and unpredictability of condition

Impaired **Home** maintenance r/t impaired cognitive or emotional functioning, insufficient finances, inadequate support systems

Hopelessness r/t long-term stress from chronic mental illness

Disturbed personal **Identity** r/t psychiatric disorder

Impaired **Memory** r/t psychosocial condition

Imbalanced **Nutrition:** less than body requirements r/t fear of eating, lack of awareness of hunger, disinterest toward food

Impaired individual **Resilience** r/t psychological disorder

Self-Care deficit: specify r/t loss of contact with reality, impairment of perception

Self-Neglect r/t psychosis

Sleep deprivation r/t intrusive thoughts, nightmares

Impaired **Social** interaction r/t impaired communication patterns, self-concept disturbance, disturbed thought processes

Social isolation r/t lack of trust, regression, delusional thinking, repressed fears

Chronic **Sorrow** r/t chronic mental illness

Spiritual distress r/t loneliness, social alienation

Risk for **Caregiver Role Strain:** Risk factors: bizarre behavior of client, chronicity of condition

Risk for compromised **Human Dignity:** Risk factor: stigmatizing label

Risk for **Loneliness:** Risk factor: inability to interact socially

Risk for **Post-Trauma** syndrome: Risk factor: diminished ego strength

Risk for **Powerlessness:** Risk factor: intrusive, distorted thinking

Risk for impaired **Religiosity:** Risk factors: ineffective coping, lack of security

Risk for **Suicide:** Risk factor: psychiatric illness

Risk for self-directed **Violence:** Risk factors: lack of trust, panic, hallucinations, delusional thinking

Risk for other-directed **Violence:** Risk factor: psychotic disorder

Readiness for enhanced **Hope:** expresses desire to enhance interconnectedness with others and problem-solve to meet goals

Readiness for enhanced **Power:** expresses willingness to enhance participation in choices for daily living and health and enhance knowledge for participation in change

Sciatica

See Neuropathy, Peripheral

Scoliosis

Risk-prone **Health** behavior r/t lack of developmental maturity to comprehend long-term consequences of noncompliance with treatment procedures

Disturbed **Body Image** r/t use of therapeutic braces, postsurgery scars, restricted physical activity

Impaired **Comfort** r/t altered health status and body image

Impaired **Gas** exchange r/t restricted lung expansion as a result of severe presurgery curvature of spine, immobilization

Ineffective **Health** maintenance r/t deficient knowledge regarding treatment modalities, restrictions, home care, postoperative activities

Impaired physical **Mobility** r/t restricted movement, dyspnea caused by severe curvature of spine

Acute **Pain** r/t musculoskeletal restrictions, surgery, reambulation with cast or spinal rod

Impaired **Skin** integrity r/t braces, casts, surgical correction

Chronic **Sorrow** r/t chronic disability

Risk for **Infection:** Risk factor: surgical incision

Risk for **Perioperative Positioning** injury: Risk factor: prone position

Risk for impaired **Resilience:** Risk factor: chronic condition

Readiness for enhanced **Health** management: desires knowledge regarding treatment for condition

See Hospitalized Child; Maturational Issues, Adolescent

S

Sedentary Lifestyle

Activity intolerance r/t sedentary lifestyle

Sedentary lifestyle (See **Sedentary** lifestyle, Section III)

Obesity (See **Obesity,** Section III)

Overweight (See **Overweight,** Section III)

Risk for **Overweight** (See **Overweight,** Section III)

Risk for ineffective peripheral **Tissue Perfusion:** Risk factor: insufficient knowledge of aggravating factors (e.g., immobility, obesity)

Readiness for enhanced **Coping:** seeking knowledge of new strategies to adjust to sedentary lifestyle

Seizure Disorders, Adult

Acute **Confusion** r/t postseizure state

Social isolation r/t unpredictability of seizures, community-imposed stigma

Risk for ineffective **Airway** clearance: Risk factor: accumulation of secretions during seizure

Risk for **Falls:** Risk factor: uncontrolled seizure activity

Risk for **Powerlessness:** Risk factor: possible seizure

Risk for impaired **Resilience:** Risk factor: chronic illness

Readiness for enhanced **Knowledge:** anticonvulsive therapy

Readiness for enhanced **Self-Care:** expresses desire to enhance knowledge and responsibility for self-care

See Epilepsy

Seizure Disorders, Childhood (Epilepsy, Febrile Seizures, Infantile Spasms)

Ineffective **Health** maintenance r/t lack of knowledge regarding anticonvulsive therapy, fever reduction (febrile seizures)

Social isolation r/t unpredictability of seizures, community-imposed stigma

Risk for ineffective **Airway** clearance: Risk factor: accumulation of secretions during seizure

Risk for delayed **Development:** Risk factors: effects of seizure disorder, parental overprotection

Risk for disproportionate **Growth:** Risk factors: congenital disorder, malnutrition

Risk for **Falls:** Risk factor: possible seizure

Risk for **Injury:** Risk factors: uncontrolled movements during seizure, falls, drowsiness caused by anticonvulsants

See Epilepsy

Self-Breast Examination (SBE)

See SBE (Self-Breast Examination)

Self-Care

Readiness for enhanced **Self-Care** (See **Self-Care,** readiness for enhanced, Section III)

Self-Care Deficit, Bathing

Bathing **Self-Care** deficit (See **Self-Care** deficit, bathing, Section III)

Self-Care Deficit, Dressing

Dressing **Self-Care** deficit (See **Self-Care** deficit, dressing, Section III)

Self-Care Deficit, Feeding

Feeding **Self-Care** deficit (See **Self-Care** deficit, feeding, Section III)

Self-Care Deficit, Toileting

Toileting **Self-Care** deficit (See **Self-Care** deficit, toileting, Section III)

Self-Concept

Readiness for enhanced **Self-Concept** (See **Self-Concept,** readiness for enhanced, Section III)

Self-Destructive Behavior

Post-Trauma syndrome r/t unresolved feelings from traumatic event

Risk for **Self-Mutilation:** Risk factors: feelings of depression, rejection, self-hatred, depersonalization; command hallucinations

Risk for **Suicide:** Risk factor: history of self-destructive behavior

Risk for self-directed **Violence:** Risk factors: panic state, history of child abuse, toxic reaction to medication

Self-Esteem, Chronic Low

Chronic low **Self-Esteem** (See **Self-Esteem,** low, chronic, Section III)

Risk for disturbed personal **Identity:** Risk factor: chronic low self-esteem

Self-Esteem, Situational Low

Situational low **Self-Esteem** (See **Self-Esteem,** low, situational, Section III)

Risk for situational low **Self-Esteem** (See **Self-Esteem,** low, situational, risk for, Section III)

Self-Mutilation

Ineffective **Impulse** control r/t ineffective management of anxiety

Self-Mutilation (See **Self-Mutilation,** Section III)

Risk for **Self-Mutilation** (See **Self-Mutilation,** risk for, Section III)

Senile Dementia

Ineffective **Relationship** r/t cognitive changes in one partner

Sedentary lifestyle r/t lack of interest in movement

See Dementia

Separation Anxiety

Ineffective **Coping** r/t maturational and situational crises, vulnerability related to developmental age, hospitalization, separation from family and familiar surroundings, multiple caregivers

Insomnia r/t separation for significant others

Risk for impaired **Attachment:** Risk factor: separation

See Hospitalized Child

Sepsis, Child

Impaired **Gas** exchange r/t pulmonary inflammation associated with disease process

Imbalanced **Nutrition:** less than body requirements r/t anorexia, generalized weakness, poor sucking reflex

Delayed **Surgical** recovery r/t presence of infection

Ineffective **Thermoregulation** r/t infectious process, septic shock

Ineffective peripheral **Tissue Perfusion** r/t arterial or venous blood flow exchange problems, septic shock

Risk for deficient **Fluid** volume: Risk factor: inflammation leading to decreased systemic vascular resistance

Risk for impaired **Skin** integrity: Risk factor: desquamation caused by disseminated intravascular coagulation

See Hospitalized Child; Premature Infant, Child

Septicemia

Imbalanced **Nutrition:** less than body requirements r/t anorexia, generalized weakness

Ineffective peripheral **Tissue Perfusion** r/t decreased systemic vascular resistance

Risk for deficient **Fluid** volume: Risk factors: vasodilation of peripheral vessels, leaking of capillaries

Risk for **Shock:** Risk factors: hypotension, hypovolemia

See Sepsis, Child; Shock, Septic

Severe Acute Respiratory Syndrome (SARS)

See SARS (Severe Acute Respiratory Syndrome); Pneumonia

Sexual Dysfunction

Sexual dysfunction (See **Sexual** dysfunction, Section III)

Ineffective **Relationship** r/t reported sexual dissatisfaction between partners

Chronic **Sorrow** r/t loss of ideal sexual experience, altered relationships

Risk for chronic low **Self-Esteem**

See Erectile Dysfunction (ED)

Sexuality, Adolescent

Disturbed **Body Image** r/t anxiety caused by unachieved developmental milestone (puberty) or deficient knowledge regarding reproductive maturation with expressed concerns regarding lack of growth of secondary sex characteristics

Impaired emancipated **Decision-Making:** sexual activity r/t undefined personal values or beliefs, multiple or divergent sources of information, lack of relevant information

Ineffective **Impulse** control r/t denial of consequences of actions

Deficient **Knowledge:** potential for enhanced health maintenance r/t multiple or divergent sources of information or lack of relevant information regarding sexual transmission of disease, contraception, prevention of toxic shock syndrome

See Maturational Issues, Adolescent

Sexuality Pattern, Ineffective

Ineffective **Sexuality** pattern (See **Sexuality** pattern, ineffective, Section III)

Sexually Transmitted Disease (STD)

See STD (Sexually Transmitted Disease)

Shaken Baby Syndrome

Decreased intracranial **Adaptive** capacity r/t brain injury

Impaired **Parenting** r/t stress, history of being abusive

Impaired individual **Resilience** r/t poor impulse control

Stress overload r/t intense repeated family stressors, family violence

Risk for other-directed **Violence:** Risk factors: history of violence against others, perinatal complications

See Child Abuse; Suspected Child Abuse and Neglect (SCAN), Child; Suspected Child Abuse and Neglect (SCAN), Parent

Shakiness

Anxiety r/t situational or maturational crisis, threat of death

Shame

Situational low **Self-Esteem** r/t inability to deal with past traumatic events, blaming of self for events not in one's control

Shingles

Acute **Pain** r/t vesicular eruption along the nerves

Ineffective **Protection** r/t abnormal blood profiles

Social isolation r/t altered state of wellness, contagiousness of disease

Risk for **Infection:** Risk factor: tissue destruction

See Itching

Shivering

S

Impaired **Comfort** r/t altered health status

Fear r/t serious threat to health status

Hypothermia r/t exposure to cool environment

Ineffective **Thermoregulation** r/t serious infectious process resulting in immune response of fever

See Shock, Septic

Shock, Cardiogenic

Decreased **Cardiac** output r/t decreased myocardial contractility, dysrhythmia

Shock, Hypovolemic

Deficient **Fluid** volume r/t abnormal loss of fluid, trauma, third spacing

Shock, Septic

Deficient **Fluid** volume r/t abnormal loss of intravascular fluid, pooling of blood in peripheral circulation, overwhelming inflammatory response

Ineffective **Protection** r/t inadequately functioning immune system

See Sepsis, Child; Septicemia

Shoulder Repair

Self-Care deficit: bathing, dressing, feeding r/t immobilization of affected shoulder

Risk for **Perioperative Positioning** injury: Risk factor: immobility

See Surgery, Preoperative; Surgery, Perioperative; Surgery, Postoperative; Total Joint Replacement (Total Hip/Total Knee/Shoulder)

Sickle Cell Anemia/Crisis

Activity intolerance r/t fatigue, effects of chronic anemia

Deficient **Fluid** volume r/t decreased intake, increased fluid requirements during sickle cell crisis, decreased ability of kidneys to concentrate urine

Impaired physical **Mobility** r/t pain, fatigue

Acute **Pain** r/t viscous blood, tissue hypoxia

Ineffective peripheral **Tissue Perfusion** r/t effects of red cell sickling, infarction of tissues

Risk for decreased **Cardiac** tissue perfusion: Risk factors: effects of red cell sickling, infarction of tissues

Risk for disproportionate **Growth:** Risk factor: chronic illness

Risk for **Infection:** Risk factor: alterations in splenic function

Risk for impaired **Resilience:** Risk factor: chronic illness

Risk for ineffective cerebral **Tissue** perfusion: Risk factors: effects of red cell sickling, infarction of tissues

Risk for ineffective **Gastrointestinal** perfusion: Risk factors: coagulopathy, sickle cell anemia.

See Child with Chronic Condition; Hospitalized Child

SIDS (Sudden Infant Death Syndrome)

Anxiety: parental worry r/t life-threatening event

Interrupted **Family** processes r/t stress as a result of special care needs of infant with apnea

Grieving r/t potential loss of infant

Insomnia: parental/infant r/t home apnea monitoring

Deficient **Knowledge:** potential for enhanced health maintenance r/t knowledge or skill acquisition of cardiopulmonary resuscitation and home apnea monitoring

Impaired **Resilience** r/t sudden loss

Risk for **Sudden Infant Death** syndrome (See **Sudden Infant Death** syndrome, risk for, Section III)

Risk for **Powerlessness:** Risk factor: unanticipated life-threatening event

See Terminally Ill Child/Death of Child, Parent

Sitting Problems

Impaired **Sitting** (See **Sitting,** impaired, Section III)

Situational Crisis

Ineffective **Coping** r/t situational crisis

Interrupted **Family** processes r/t situational crisis

Risk for ineffective **Activity** planning: Risk factor: inability to process information

Risk for disturbed personal **Identity:** Risk factor: situational crisis

Readiness for enhanced **Communication:** willingness to share feelings and thoughts

Readiness for enhanced **Religiosity:** requests religious material and/or experiences

Readiness for enhanced **Resilience:** desire to enhance resilience

Readiness for enhanced **Spiritual** well-being: desire for harmony following crisis

SJS (Stevens-Johnson Syndrome)

See Stevens-Johnson Syndrome (SJS)

Skin Cancer

Ineffective **Health** maintenance r/t deficient knowledge regarding self-care with skin cancer

Ineffective **Protection** r/t weakened immune system

Impaired **Tissue** integrity r/t abnormal cell growth in skin, treatment of skin cancer

Readiness for enhanced **Health** management: follows preventive measures

Readiness for enhanced **Knowledge:** self-care to prevent and treat skin cancer

Skin Disorders

Impaired **Skin** integrity (See **Skin** integrity, impaired, Section III)

Skin Turgor, Change in Elasticity

Deficient **Fluid** volume r/t active fluid loss

Sleep

Readiness for enhanced **Sleep** (See **Sleep,** readiness for enhanced, Section III)

Sleep Apnea

Ineffective **Breathing** pattern r/t obesity, substance abuse, enlarged tonsils, smoking, or neurological pathology such as a brain tumor

Sleep Deprivation

Fatigue r/t lack of sleep

Sleep deprivation (See **Sleep** deprivation, Section III)

Sleep Problems

Insomnia (See **Insomnia,** Section III)

Sleep Pattern, Disturbed, Parent/Child

Insomnia: child r/t anxiety or fear

Insomnia: parent r/t parental responsibilities, stress

See Suspected Child Abuse and Neglect (SCAN), Child and Parent

Slurring of Speech

Impaired verbal **Communication** r/t decrease in circulation to brain, brain tumor, anatomical defect, cleft palate

Situational low **Self-Esteem** r/t speech impairment

See Communication Problems

Small Bowel Resection

See Abdominal Surgery

Smell, Loss of Ability to

Risk for **Injury:** Risk factors: inability to detect gas fumes, smoke smells

See Anosmia

Smoke Inhalation

Ineffective **Airway** clearance r/t smoke inhalation

Impaired **Gas** exchange r/t ventilation-perfusion imbalance

Risk for acute **Confusion:** Risk factor: decreased oxygen supply

Risk for **Infection:** Risk factors: inflammation, ineffective airway clearance, pneumonia

Risk for **Poisoning:** Risk factor: exposure to carbon monoxide

Readiness for enhanced **Health** management: functioning smoke detectors and carbon monoxide detectors in home and work, escape route planned and reviewed

See Atelectasis; Burns; Pneumonia

Smoking Behavior

Insufficient **Breast Milk** r/t smoking

Risk-prone **Health** behavior r/t smoking

Ineffective **Health** maintenance r/t denial of effects of smoking, lack of effective support for smoking withdrawal

Readiness for enhanced **Knowledge:** expresses interest in smoking cessation

Risk for dry **Eye:** Risk factor: smoking

Risk for ineffective peripheral **Tissue Perfusion:** Risk factor: effect of nicotine

Risk for **Thermal** injury: Risk factor: unsafe smoking behavior

Social Interaction, Impaired

Impaired **Social** interaction (See **Social** interaction, impaired, Section III)

Social Isolation

Social isolation (See **Social** isolation, Section III)

Sociopathic Personality

See Antisocial Personality Disorder

Sodium, Decrease/Increase

See Hyponatremia; Hypernatremia

Somatization Disorder

Anxiety r/t unresolved conflicts channeled into physical complaints or conditions

Ineffective **Coping** r/t lack of insight into underlying conflicts

Ineffective **Denial** r/t displaced psychological stress to physical symptoms

Nausea r/t anxiety

Chronic **Pain** r/t unexpressed anger, multiple physical disorders, depression

Impaired individual **Resilience** r/t possible psychological disorders

Sore Nipples, Breastfeeding

Ineffective **Breastfeeding** r/t deficient knowledge regarding correct feeding procedure

See Painful Breasts, Sore Nipples

Sore Throat

Impaired **Comfort** r/t sore throat

Deficient **Knowledge** r/t treatment, relief of discomfort

Impaired **Oral Mucous Membrane** r/t inflammation or infection of oral cavity

Impaired **Swallowing** r/t irritation of oropharyngeal cavity

Sorrow

Grieving r/t loss of significant person, object, or role

Chronic **Sorrow** (See **Sorrow,** chronic, Section III)

Readiness for enhanced **Communication:** expresses thoughts and feelings

Readiness for enhanced **Spiritual** well-being: desire to find purpose and meaning of loss

Spastic Colon

See IBS (Irritable Bowel Syndrome)

Speech Disorders

Anxiety r/t difficulty with communication

Impaired verbal **Communication** r/t anatomical defect, cleft palate, psychological barriers, decrease in circulation to brain

Spina Bifida

See Neural Tube Defects

Spinal Cord Injury

Deficient **Diversional** activity r/t long-term hospitalization, frequent lengthy treatments

Fear r/t powerlessness over loss of body function

Complicated **Grieving** r/t loss of usual body function

Sedentary lifestyle r/t lack of resources or interest

Impaired wheelchair **Mobility** r/t neuromuscular impairment

Impaired **Standing** r/t spinal cord injury

Urinary Retention r/t inhibition of reflex arc

Risk for **Latex Allergy** response: Risk factor: continuous or intermittent catheterization

Risk for **Autonomic Dysreflexia:** Risk factors: bladder or bowel distention, skin irritation, deficient knowledge of patient and caregiver

Risk for ineffective **Breathing** pattern: Risk factor: neuromuscular impairment

Risk for **Infection:** Risk factors: chronic disease, stasis of body fluids

Risk for **Loneliness:** Risk factor: physical immobility

Risk for **Powerlessness:** Risk factor: loss of function

Risk for **Pressure** ulcer: Risk factor: immobility and decreased sensation

See Child with Chronic Condition; Hospitalized Child; Neural Tube Defects; Paralysis

Spinal Fusion

Impaired bed **Mobility** r/t impaired ability to turn side to side while keeping spine in proper alignment

Impaired physical **Mobility** r/t musculoskeletal impairment associated with surgery, possible back brace

Readiness for enhanced **Knowledge:** expresses interest in information associated with surgery

See Acute Back; Back Pain; Scoliosis; Surgery, Preoperative Care; Surgery, Perioperative Care; Surgery, Postoperative Care

Spiritual Distress

Spiritual distress (See **Spiritual** distress, Section III)

Risk for chronic low **Self-Esteem:** Risk factor: unresolved spiritual issues

Risk for **Spiritual** distress (See **Spiritual** distress, risk for, Section III)

Spiritual Well-Being

Readiness for enhanced **Spiritual** well-being (See **Spiritual** well-being, readiness for enhanced, Section III)

Splenectomy

See Abdominal Surgery

Sprains

Acute **Pain** r/t physical injury

Impaired physical **Mobility** r/t injury

Impaired **Walking** r/t injury

Standing Problems

Impaired **Standing** (see Impaired **Standing,** Section III)

Stapedectomy

Hearing Loss r/t edema from surgery

Acute **Pain** r/t headache

Risk for **Falls:** Risk factor: dizziness

Risk for **Infection:** Risk factor: invasive procedure

Stasis Ulcer

Impaired **Tissue** integrity r/t chronic venous congestion

Risk for **Infection:** Risk factor: open wound

See CHF (Congestive Heart Failure); Varicose Veins

STD (Sexually Transmitted Disease)

Impaired **Comfort** r/t infection

Fear r/t altered body function, risk for social isolation, fear of incurable illness

Ineffective **Health** maintenance r/t deficient knowledge regarding transmission, symptoms, treatment of STD

Ineffective **Sexuality** pattern r/t illness, altered body function, need for abstinence to heal

Social isolation r/t fear of contracting or spreading disease

Risk for **Infection:** spread of infection: Risk factor: lack of knowledge concerning transmission of disease

Readiness for enhanced **Knowledge:** seeks information regarding prevention and treatment of STDs

See Maturational Issues, Adolescent; PID (Pelvic Inflammatory Disease)

STEMI (ST-Elevation Myocardial Infarction)

See MI (Myocardial Infarction)

Stent (Coronary Artery Stent)

Risk for **Injury:** Risk factor: complications associated with stent placement

Risk for decreased **Cardiac** tissue perfusion: Risk factor: possible restenosis

Risk for **Vascular Trauma:** Risk factors: insertion site, catheter width

Readiness for enhanced **Decision-Making:** expresses desire to enhance risk-benefit analysis, understanding and meaning of choices, and decisions regarding treatment

See Angioplasty, Coronary; Cardiac Catheterization

Sterilization Surgery

Decisional Conflict r/t multiple or divergent sources of information, unclear personal values or beliefs

See Surgery, Preoperative Care; Surgery, Perioperative Care; Surgery, Postoperative Care; Tubal Ligation; Vasectomy

Stertorous Respirations

Ineffective **Airway** clearance r/t pharyngeal obstruction

Stevens-Johnson Syndrome (SJS)

Impaired **Oral Mucous Membrane** r/t immunocompromised condition associated with allergic medication reaction

Acute **Pain** r/t painful skin lesions and painful mucosa lesions

Impaired **Skin** integrity r/t allergic medication reaction

Risk for deficient **Fluid** volume: Risk factors: factors affecting fluid needs (hypermetabolic state, fever), excessive losses through normal routes (vomiting and diarrhea)

Risk for **Infection:** Risk factor: sloughing skin

Risk for impaired **Liver** function: Risk factor: impaired immune response

Stillbirth

See Pregnancy Loss

Stoma

See Colostomy; Ileostomy

Stomatitis

Impaired **Oral Mucous Membrane** r/t pathological conditions of oral cavity; side effects of chemotherapy

Risk for impaired **Oral Mucous Membranes** (See impaired **Oral Mucous Membranes,** risk for, Section III)

Stone, Kidney

See Kidney Stone

Stool, Hard/Dry

Chronic functional **Constipation** r/t inadequate fluid intake, inadequate fiber intake, decreased activity level, decreased gastric motility

Straining with Defecation

Chronic functional **Constipation** r/t less than adequate fluid intake, less than adequate dietary intake

Risk for decreased **Cardiac** output: Risk factor: vagal stimulation with dysrhythmia resulting from Valsalva maneuver

Strep Throat

Risk for **Infection:** Risk factor: exposure to pathogen

See Sore Throat

Stress

Anxiety r/t feelings of helplessness, feelings of being threatened

Ineffective **Coping** r/t ineffective use of problem-solving process, feelings of apprehension or helplessness

Fear r/t powerlessness over feelings

Stress overload r/t intense or multiple stressors

Readiness for enhanced **Communication:** shows willingness to share thoughts and feelings

Readiness for enhanced **Spiritual** well-being: expresses desire for harmony and peace in stressful situation

See Anxiety

Stress Urinary Incontinence

Stress urinary **Incontinence** r/t degenerative change in pelvic muscles

Stridor

Ineffective **Airway** clearance r/t obstruction, tracheobronchial infection, trauma

Stroke

See CVA (Cerebrovascular Accident)

Stuttering

Anxiety r/t impaired verbal communication

Impaired verbal **Communication** r/t anxiety, psychological problems

Subarachnoid Hemorrhage

Acute **Pain:** headache r/t irritation of meninges from blood, increased intracranial pressure

Risk for ineffective **Cerebral** tissue perfusion: Risk factor: bleeding from cerebral vessel

See Intracranial Pressure, Increased

Substance Abuse

Compromised family **Coping** r/t codependency issues

Defensive **Coping** r/t substance abuse

Disabled family **Coping** r/t differing coping styles between support persons

Ineffective **Coping** r/t use of substances to cope with life events

Ineffective **Denial** r/t refusal to acknowledge substance abuse problem

Dysfunctional **Family** processes r/t substance abuse

Deficient community **Health** r/t prevention and control of illegal substances in community

Ineffective **Impulse** control r/t addictive process

Ineffective **Relationship** r/t inability for well-balanced collaboration between partners

Insomnia r/t irritability, nightmares, tremors

Risk for impaired **Attachment:** Risk factor: substance abuse

Risk for disturbed personal **Identity:** Risk factor: ingestion/inhalation of toxic chemicals

Risk for chronic low **Self-Esteem:** Risk factors: perceived lack of respect from others, repeated failures, repeated negative reinforcement

Risk for **Thermal** injury: Risk factor: intoxication with drugs or alcohol

Risk for **Vascular Trauma:** Risk factor: chemical irritant self injected into veins

Risk for self-directed **Violence:** Risk factors: reactions to substances used, impulsive behavior, disorientation, impaired judgment

Risk for other-directed **Violence:** Risk factor: access to weapon

Readiness for enhanced **Coping:** seeking social support and knowledge of new strategies

Readiness for enhanced **Self-Concept:** accepting strengths and limitations

See Alcoholism; Drug Abuse; Maturational Issues, Adolescent

Substance Abuse, Adolescent

S

See Alcohol Withdrawal; Maturational Issues, Adolescent; Substance Abuse

Substance Abuse in Pregnancy

Ineffective **Childbearing** process r/t substance abuse

Defensive **Coping** r/t denial of situation, differing value system

Ineffective **Health** management r/t addiction

Deficient **Knowledge** r/t lack of exposure to information regarding effects of substance abuse in pregnancy

Risk for impaired **Attachment:** Risk factors: substance abuse, inability of parent to meet infant's or own personal needs

Risk for **Infection:** Risk factors: intravenous drug use, lifestyle

Risk for **Injury:** fetal: Risk factor: effects of drugs on fetal growth and development

Risk for **Injury:** maternal: Risk factor: drug or alcohol use

Risk for impaired **Parenting:** Risk factor: lack of ability to meet infant's needs due to addiction with use of alcohol or drugs

See Alcoholism; Drug Abuse; Substance Abuse

Sucking Reflex

Effective **Breastfeeding** r/t regular and sustained sucking and swallowing at breast

Sudden Infant Death Syndrome (SIDS)

See SIDS (Sudden Infant Death Syndrome)

Suffocation, Risk for

Risk for **Suffocation** (See **Suffocation,** risk for, Section III)

Suicide Attempt

Risk-prone **Health** behavior r/t low self-efficacy

Ineffective **Coping** r/t anger, complicated grieving

Hopelessness r/t perceived or actual loss, substance abuse, low self-concept, inadequate support systems

Ineffective **Impulse** control r/t inability to modulate stress, anxiety

Post-Trauma syndrome r/t history of traumatic events, abuse, rape, incest, war, torture

Impaired individual **Resilience** r/t poor impulse control

Situational low **Self-Esteem** r/t guilt, inability to trust, feelings of worthlessness or rejection

Social isolation r/t inability to engage in satisfying personal relationships

Spiritual distress r/t hopelessness, despair

Risk for **Post-Trauma** syndrome: Risk factor: survivor's role in suicide attempt

Risk for **Suicide** (See **Suicide,** risk for, Section III)

Readiness for enhanced **Communication:** willingness to share thoughts and feelings

Readiness for enhanced **Spiritual** well-being: desire for harmony and inner strength to help redefine purpose for life

See Violent Behavior

Support System, Inadequate

Readiness for enhanced family **Coping:** ability to adapt to tasks associated with care, support of significant other during health crisis

Readiness for enhanced **Family** processes: activities support the growth of family members

Readiness for enhanced **Parenting:** children or other dependent person(s) expressing satisfaction with home environment

Suppression of Labor

See Preterm Labor; Tocolytic Therapy

Surgery, Perioperative Care

Risk for imbalanced **Fluid** volume: Risk factor: surgery

Risk for **Perioperative Hypothermia:** Risk factors: inadequate covering of client, cold surgical room

Risk for **Perioperative Positioning** injury: Risk factors: predisposing condition, prolonged surgery

Surgery, Postoperative Care

Activity intolerance r/t pain, surgical procedure

Anxiety r/t change in health status, hospital environment

Deficient **Knowledge** r/t postoperative expectations, lifestyle changes

Nausea r/t manipulation of gastrointestinal tract, postsurgical anesthesia

Imbalanced **Nutrition:** less than body requirements r/t anorexia, nausea, vomiting, decreased peristalsis

Ineffective peripheral **Tissue Perfusion** r/t hypovolemia, circulatory stasis, obesity, prolonged immobility, decreased coughing, decreased deep breathing

Acute **Pain** r/t inflammation or injury in surgical area

Delayed **Surgical** recovery r/t extensive surgical procedure, postoperative surgical infection

Urinary retention r/t anesthesia, pain, fear, unfamiliar surroundings, client's position

Risk for **Bleeding:** Risk factor: surgical procedure

Risk for ineffective **Breathing** pattern: Risk factors: pain, location of incision, effects of anesthesia or opioids

Risk for **Constipation:** Risk factors: decreased activity, decreased food or fluid intake, anesthesia, pain medication

Risk for imbalanced **Fluid** volume: Risk factors: hypermetabolic state, fluid loss during surgery, presence of indwelling tubes, fluids used to distend organ structures being absorbed into body

Risk for **Infection:** Risk factors: invasive procedure, pain, anesthesia, location of incision, weakened cough as a result of aging

Surgery, Preoperative Care

Anxiety r/t threat to or change in health status, situational crisis, fear of the unknown

Insomnia r/t anxiety about upcoming surgery

Deficient **Knowledge** r/t preoperative procedures, postoperative expectations

Readiness for enhanced **Knowledge:** shows understanding of preoperative and postoperative expectations for self-care

Surgical Recovery, Delayed

Delayed **Surgical** recovery (See **Surgical** recovery, delayed, Section III)

Risk for delayed **Surgical** recovery (See **Surgical** recovery, delayed, risk for, Section III)

Suspected Child Abuse and Neglect (SCAN), Child

Ineffective **Activity** planning r/t lack of family support

Anxiety: child r/t threat of punishment for perceived wrongdoing

Deficient community **Health** r/t inadequate reporting and follow-up of SCAN

Disturbed personal **Identity** r/t dysfunctional family processes

Rape-Trauma syndrome r/t altered lifestyle because of abuse, changes in residence

Risk for impaired **Resilience:** Risk factor: adverse situation

Readiness for enhanced community **Coping:** obtaining resources to prevent child abuse, neglect

See Child Abuse; Hospitalized Child; Maturational Issues, Adolescent

Suspected Child Abuse and Neglect (SCAN), Parent

Disabled family **Coping** r/t dysfunctional family, underdeveloped nurturing parental role, lack of parental support systems or role models

Dysfunctional **Family** processes r/t inadequate coping skills

Ineffective **Health** maintenance r/t deficient knowledge of parenting skills as result of unachieved developmental tasks

Impaired **Home** maintenance r/t disorganization, parental dysfunction, neglect of safe and nurturing environment

Ineffective **Impulse** control r/t projection of anger, frustration onto child

Impaired **Parenting** r/t unrealistic expectations of child; lack of effective role model; unmet social, emotional, or maturational needs of parents; interruption in bonding process

Impaired individual **Resilience** r/t poor impulse control

Chronic low **Self-Esteem** r/t lack of successful parenting experiences

Risk for other-directed **Violence:** parent to child: Risk factors: inadequate coping mechanisms, unresolved stressors, unachieved maturational level by parent

Suspicion

Disturbed personal **Identity** r/t psychiatric disorder

Powerlessness r/t repetitive paranoid thinking

Impaired **Social** interaction r/t disturbed thought processes, paranoid delusions, hallucinations

Risk for self-directed **Violence:** Risk factor: inability to trust

Risk for other-directed **Violence:** Risk factor: impulsiveness

Swallowing Difficulties

Impaired **Swallowing** (See **Swallowing,** impaired, Section III)

Swine Flu (H1N1)

See Influenza

Syncope

Anxiety r/t fear of falling

Impaired physical **Mobility** r/t fear of falling

Ineffective **Health** management r/t lack of knowledge in how to prevent syncope

Social isolation r/t fear of falling

Risk for decreased **Cardiac** output: Risk factor: dysrhythmia

Risk for **Falls:** Risk factor: syncope

Risk for **Injury:** Risk factors: altered sensory perception, transient loss of consciousness, risk for falls

Risk for ineffective **Cerebral** tissue perfusion: Risk factor: interruption of blood flow

Syphilis

See STD (Sexually Transmitted Disease)

Systemic Lupus Erythematosus

See Lupus Erythematosus

T

T & A (Tonsillectomy and Adenoidectomy)

Ineffective **Airway** clearance r/t hesitation or reluctance to cough because of pain

Deficient **Knowledge:** potential for enhanced health maintenance r/t insufficient knowledge regarding postoperative nutritional and rest requirements, signs and symptoms of complications, positioning

Nausea r/t gastric irritation, pharmaceuticals, anesthesia

Acute **Pain** r/t surgical incision

Risk for **Aspiration:** Risk factors: postoperative drainage and impaired swallowing

Risk for deficient **Fluid** volume: Risk factors: decreased intake because of painful swallowing, effects of anesthesia (nausea, vomiting), hemorrhage

Risk for imbalanced **Nutrition:** less than body requirements: Risk factors: hesitation or reluctance to swallow

Tachycardia

See Dysrhythmia

Tachypnea

Ineffective **Breathing** pattern r/t pain, anxiety, hypoxia

See cause of Tachypnea

Tardive Dyskinesia

Ineffective **Health** management r/t complexity of therapeutic regimen or medication

Deficient **Knowledge** r/t cognitive limitation in assimilating information relating to side effects associated with neuroleptic medications

Risk for **Injury:** Risk factor: drug-induced abnormal body movements

T

Taste Abnormality

Frail Elderly syndrome r/t chronic illness

TB (Pulmonary Tuberculosis)

Ineffective **Airway** clearance r/t increased secretions, excessive mucus

Ineffective **Breathing** pattern r/t decreased energy, fatigue

Fatigue r/t disease state

Impaired **Gas** exchange r/t disease process

Ineffective **Health** management r/t deficient knowledge of prevention and treatment regimen

Impaired **Home** maintenance management r/t client or family member with disease

Ineffective **Thermoregulation** r/t presence of infection

Risk for **Infection:** Risk factor: insufficient knowledge regarding avoidance of exposure to pathogens

Readiness for enhanced **Health** management: takes medications according to prescribed protocol for prevention and treatment

TBI (Traumatic Brain Injury)

Interrupted **Family** processes r/t traumatic injury to family member

Chronic **Sorrow** r/t change in health status and functional ability

Risk for **Post-Trauma** syndrome: Risk factor: perception of event causing TBI

Risk for impaired **Religiosity:** Risk factor: impaired physical mobility

Risk for impaired **Resilience:** Risk factor: crisis of injury

See Head Injury; Neurologic Disorders

TD (Traveler's Diarrhea)

Diarrhea r/t travel with exposure to different bacteria, viruses

Risk for deficient **Fluid** volume: Risk factors: excessive loss of fluids, diarrhea

Risk for **Infection:** Risk factors: insufficient knowledge regarding avoidance of exposure to pathogens (water supply, iced drinks, local cheeses, ice cream, undercooked meat, fish and shellfish, uncooked vegetables, unclean eating utensils, improper handwashing)

Temperature, Decreased

Hypothermia r/t exposure to cold environment

Temperature, High

Hyperthermia r/t neurological damage, disease condition with high temperature, excessive heat, inflammatory response

Temperature Regulation, Impaired

Ineffective **Thermoregulation** r/t trauma, illness, cerebral injury

TEN (Toxic Epidermal Necrolysis)

See Toxic Epidermal Necrolysis (TEN)

Tension

Anxiety r/t threat to or change in health status, situational crisis

Readiness for enhanced **Communication:** expresses willingness to share feelings and thoughts

See Stress

Terminally Ill Adult

Death **Anxiety** r/t unresolved issues relating to death and dying

Risk for **Spiritual** distress: Risk factor: impending death

Readiness for enhanced **Religiosity:** requests religious material and/or experiences

Readiness for enhanced **Spiritual** well-being: desire to achieve harmony of mind, body, spirit

See Terminally Ill Child/Death of Child, Parent

Terminally Ill Child, Adolescent

Disturbed **Body Image** r/t effects of terminal disease, already critical feelings of group identity and self-image

Ineffective **Coping** r/t inability to establish personal and peer identity because of the threat of being different or not being healthy, inability to achieve maturational tasks

Impaired **Social** interaction r/t forced separation from peers

See Child with Chronic Condition; Hospitalized Child, Terminally Ill Child/Death of Child, Parent

Terminally Ill Child, Infant/Toddler

Ineffective **Coping** r/t separation from parents and familiar environment from inability to understand dying process

See Child with Chronic Condition, Terminally Ill Child/Death of Child, Parent

Terminally Ill Child, Preschool Child

Fear r/t perceived punishment, bodily harm, feelings of guilt caused by magical thinking (i.e., believing that thoughts cause events)

See Child with Chronic Condition, Terminally Ill Child/Death of Child, Parent

Terminally Ill Child, School-Age Child/Preadolescent

Fear r/t perceived punishment, body mutilation, feelings of guilt

See Child with Chronic Condition, Terminally Ill Child/Death of Child, Parent

Terminally Ill Child/Death of Child, Parent

Compromised family **Coping** r/t inability or unwillingness to discuss impending death and feelings with child or support child through terminal stages of illness

Decisional Conflict r/t continuation or discontinuation of treatment, do-not-resuscitate decision, ethical issues regarding organ donation

Ineffective **Denial** r/t complicated grieving

Interrupted **Family** processes r/t situational crisis

Grieving r/t death of child

Hopelessness r/t overwhelming stresses caused by terminal illness

Insomnia r/t grieving process

Impaired **Parenting** r/t risk for overprotection of surviving siblings

Powerlessness r/t inability to alter course of events

Impaired **Social** interaction r/t complicated grieving

Social isolation: imposed by others r/t feelings of inadequacy in providing support to grieving parents

Social isolation: self-imposed r/t unresolved grief, perceived inadequate parenting skills

Spiritual distress r/t sudden and unexpected death, prolonged suffering before death, questioning the death of youth, questioning the meaning of one's own existence

Risk for complicated **Grieving:** Risk factors: prolonged, unresolved, obstructed progression through stages of grief and mourning

Risk for impaired **Resilience:** Risk factor: impending death

Readiness for enhanced family **Coping:** impact of crisis on family values, priorities, goals, or relationships; expressed interest or desire to attach meaning to child's life and death

Tetralogy of Fallot

See Congenital Heart Disease/Cardiac Anomalies

Tetraplegia

Autonomic dysreflexia r/t bladder or bowel distention, skin irritation, infection, deficient knowledge of patient and caregiver

Grieving r/t loss of previous functioning

Powerlessness r/t inability to perform previous activities

Impaired **Sitting** r/t paralysis of extremities

Impaired spontaneous **Ventilation** r/t loss of innervation of respiratory muscles, respiratory muscle fatigue

Risk for **Aspiration:** Risk factor: inadequate ability to protect airway from neurological damage

Risk for **Infection:** Risk factor: urinary stasis

Risk for impaired **Skin** integrity: Risk factor: physical immobilization and decreased sensation

Risk for ineffective **Thermoregulation:** Risk factors: inability to move to increase temperature, possible presence of infection to increase temperature

Thermoregulation, Ineffective

Ineffective **Thermoregulation** (See **Thermoregulation,** ineffective, Section III)

Thoracentesis

See Pleural Effusion

Thoracotomy

Activity intolerance r/t pain, imbalance between oxygen supply and demand, presence of chest tubes

Ineffective **Airway** clearance r/t drowsiness, pain with breathing and coughing

Ineffective **Breathing** pattern r/t decreased energy, fatigue, pain

Deficient **Knowledge** r/t self-care, effective breathing exercises, pain relief

Acute **Pain** r/t surgical procedure, coughing, deep breathing

Risk for **Bleeding:** Risk factor: surgery

Risk for **Infection:** Risk factor: invasive procedure

Risk for **Injury:** Risk factor: disruption of closed-chest drainage system

Risk for **Perioperative Positioning** injury: Risk factors: lateral positioning, immobility

Risk for **Vascular Trauma:** Risk factors: chemical irritant; antibiotics

Thought Disorders

See Schizophrenia

Thrombocytopenic Purpura

See ITP (Idiopathic Thrombocytopenic Purpura)

Thrombophlebitis

See DVT

Thyroidectomy

Risk for ineffective **Airway** clearance r/t edema or hematoma formation, airway obstruction

Risk for impaired verbal **Communication:** Risk factors: edema, pain, vocal cord or laryngeal nerve damage

Risk for **Injury:** Risk factor: possible parathyroid damage or removal

See Surgery, Preoperative Care; Surgery, Perioperative Care; Surgery, Postoperative Care

TIA (Transient Ischemic Attack)

Acute **Confusion** r/t hypoxia

Readiness for enhanced **Health** management: obtains knowledge regarding treatment prevention of inadequate oxygenation

See Syncope

Tic Disorder

See Tourette's Syndrome (TS)

Tinea Capitis

Impaired **Comfort** r/t inflammation from skin irritation

See Ringworm of Scalp

Tinea Corporis

See Ringworm of Body

Tinea Cruris

See Jock Itch; Itching; Pruritus

Tinea Pedis

See Athlete's Foot; Itching; Pruritus

Tinea Unguium (Onychomycosis)

See Ringworm of Nails

Tinnitus

Ineffective **Health** maintenance r/t deficient knowledge regarding self-care with tinnitus

T

Hearing Loss r/t ringing in ears obscuring hearing

Tissue Damage, Corneal

Risk for corneal **Injury** (See corneal **Injury,** risk for, Section III)

Tissue Damage, Integumentary

Impaired **Tissue** integrity (See **Tissue** integrity, impaired, Section III)

Risk for impaired **Tissue** integrity (See **Tissue** integrity, impaired, risk for, Section III)

Tissue Perfusion, Peripheral

Ineffective peripheral **Tissue Perfusion** (See **Tissue Perfusion,** peripheral, ineffective, Section III)

Risk for ineffective peripheral **Tissue Perfusion** (See **Tissue Perfusion,** peripheral, ineffective, risk for, Section III)

Toileting Problems

Toileting **Self-Care** deficit r/t impaired transfer ability, impaired mobility status, intolerance of activity, neuromuscular impairment, cognitive impairment

Impaired **Transfer** ability r/t neuromuscular deficits

Toilet Training

Deficient **Knowledge:** parent r/t signs of child's readiness for training

Risk for **Constipation:** Risk factor: withholding stool

Risk for **Infection:** Risk factor: withholding urination

Tonsillectomy and Adenoidectomy (T & A)

See T & A (Tonsillectomy and Adenoidectomy)

Toothache

Impaired **Dentition** r/t ineffective oral hygiene, barriers to self-care, economic barriers to professional care, nutritional deficits, lack of knowledge regarding dental health

Acute **Pain** r/t inflammation, infection

Total Anomalous Pulmonary Venous Return

See Congenital Heart Disease/Cardiac Anomalies

Total Joint Replacement (Total Hip/Total Knee/Shoulder)

Disturbed **Body Image** r/t large scar, presence of prosthesis

Impaired physical **Mobility** r/t musculoskeletal impairment, surgery, prosthesis

Risk for **Injury:** neurovascular: Risk factors: altered peripheral tissue perfusion, impaired mobility, prosthesis

Risk for **Peripheral Neurovascular** dysfunction r/t immobilization, surgical procedure

Ineffective peripheral **Tissue** perfusion r/t surgery

See Surgery, Preoperative Care; Surgery, Perioperative Care; Surgery, Postoperative Care

Total Parenteral Nutrition (TPN)

See TPN (Total Parenteral Nutrition)

Tourette's Syndrome (TS)

Hopelessness r/t inability to control behavior

Impaired individual **Resilience** r/t uncontrollable behavior

Risk for situational low **Self-Esteem:** Risk factors: uncontrollable behavior, motor and phonic tics

See Attention Deficit Disorder

Toxemia

See PIH (Pregnancy-Induced Hypertension/Preeclampsia)

Toxic Epidermal Necrolysis (TEN) (Erythema Multiforme)

Death **Anxiety** r/t uncertainty of prognosis

See Stevens-Johnson Syndrome (SJS)

TPN (Total Parenteral Nutrition)

Imbalanced **Nutrition:** less than body requirements r/t inability to digest food or absorb nutrients as a result of biological or psychological factors

Risk for **Electrolyte** imbalance: Risk factor: need for regulation of electrolytes in TPN fluids

Risk for excess **Fluid** volume: Risk factor: rapid administration of TPN

Risk for unstable blood **Glucose** level: Risk factor: high glucose levels in TPN to be regulated according to blood glucose levels

Risk for **Infection:** Risk factors: concentrated glucose solution, invasive administration of fluids

Risk for **Vascular Trauma:** Risk factors: insertion site, length of treatment time

Tracheoesophageal Fistula

Ineffective **Airway** clearance r/t aspiration of feeding because of inability to swallow

Imbalanced **Nutrition:** less than body requirements r/t difficulties swallowing

Risk for **Aspiration:** Risk factor: common passage of air and food

Risk for **Vascular Trauma:** Risk factors: venous medications and site

See Respiratory Conditions of the Neonate; Hospitalized Child

Tracheostomy

Ineffective **Airway** clearance r/t increased secretions, mucous plugs

Anxiety r/t impaired verbal communication, ineffective airway clearance

Disturbed **Body Image** r/t abnormal opening in neck

Impaired verbal **Communication** r/t presence of mechanical airway

Deficient **Knowledge** r/t self-care, home maintenance management

Acute **Pain** r/t edema, surgical procedure

Risk for **Aspiration:** Risk factor: presence of tracheostomy

Risk for **Bleeding:** Risk factor: surgical incision

Risk for **Infection:** Risk factors: invasive procedure, pooling of secretions

Traction and Casts

Constipation r/t immobility

Deficient **Diversional** activity r/t immobility

Impaired physical **Mobility** r/t imposed restrictions on activity because of bone or joint disease injury

Acute **Pain** r/t immobility, injury, or disease

Self-Care deficit: feeding, dressing, bathing, toileting r/t degree of impaired physical mobility, body area affected by traction or cast

Impaired **Transfer** ability r/t presence of traction, casts

Risk for **Disuse** syndrome: Risk factor: mechanical immobilization

See Casts

Transfer Ability

Impaired **Transfer** ability (See **Transfer** ability, impaired, Section III)

Transient Ischemic Attack (TIA)

See TIA (Transient Ischemic Attack)

Transposition of Great Vessels

See Congenital Heart Disease/Cardiac Anomalies

Transurethral Resection of the Prostate (TURP)

See TURP (Transurethral Resection of the Prostate)

Trauma in Pregnancy

Anxiety r/t threat to self or fetus, unknown outcome

Deficient **Knowledge** r/t lack of exposure to situation

Acute **Pain** r/t trauma

Impaired **Skin** integrity r/t trauma

Risk for **Bleeding:** Risk factor: trauma

Risk for deficient **Fluid** volume: Risk factor: fluid loss

Risk for **Infection:** Risk factor: traumatized tissue

Risk for **Injury:** fetal: Risk factor: premature separation of placenta

Risk for disturbed **Maternal–Fetal** dyad: Risk factor: complication of pregnancy

Trauma, Risk for

Risk for **Trauma** (See **Trauma,** risk for, Section III)

Traumatic Brain Injury (TBI)

See TBI (Traumatic Brain Injury); Intracranial Pressure, Increased

Traumatic Event

Post-Trauma syndrome r/t previously experienced trauma

Traveler's Diarrhea (TD)

See TD (Traveler's Diarrhea)

Trembling of Hands

Fear r/t threat to or change in health status, threat of death, situational crisis

Tricuspid Atresia

See Congenital Heart Disease/Cardiac Anomalies

Trigeminal Neuralgia

Ineffective **Health** management r/t deficient knowledge regarding prevention of stimuli that trigger pain

Imbalanced **Nutrition:** less than body requirements r/t pain when chewing

Acute **Pain** r/t irritation of trigeminal nerve

Risk for corneal **Injury:** Risk factor: possible decreased corneal sensation

Truncus Arteriosus

See Congenital Heart Disease/Cardiac Anomalies

TS (Tourette's Syndrome)

See Tourette's Syndrome (TS)

TSE (Testicular Self-Examination)

Readiness for enhanced **Health** management: seeks information regarding self-examination

Tubal Ligation

Decisional Conflict r/t tubal sterilization

See Laparoscopy

Tube Feeding

Risk for **Aspiration:** Risk factors: improperly administered feeding, improper placement of tube, improper positioning of client during and after feeding, excessive residual feeding or lack of digestion, altered gag reflex

Risk for deficient **Fluid** volume: Risk factor: inadequate water administration with concentrated feeding

Risk for imbalanced **Nutrition:** less than body requirements: Risk factors: intolerance to tube feeding, inadequate calorie replacement to meet metabolic needs

Tuberculosis (TB)

See TB (Pulmonary Tuberculosis)

TURP (Transurethral Resection of the Prostate)

Deficient **Knowledge** r/t postoperative self-care, home maintenance management

Acute **Pain** r/t incision, irritation from catheter, bladder spasms, kidney infection

Urinary retention r/t obstruction of urethra or catheter with clots

Risk for **Bleeding:** Risk factor: surgery

Risk for deficient **Fluid** volume: Risk factors: fluid loss, possible bleeding

Risk for urge urinary **Incontinence:** Risk factor: edema from surgical procedure

Risk for **Infection:** Risk factors: invasive procedure, route for bacteria entry

U

U

Ulcer, Peptic (Duodenal or Gastric)

Fatigue r/t loss of blood, chronic illness

Ineffective **Health** maintenance r/t lack of knowledge regarding health practices to prevent ulcer formation

Nausea r/t gastrointestinal irritation

Acute **Pain** r/t irritated mucosa from acid secretion

Risk for ineffective **Gastrointestinal** perfusion: Risk factor: ulcer

See GI Bleed (Gastrointestinal Bleeding)

Ulcerative Colitis

See Inflammatory Bowel Disease (Child and Adult)

Ulcers, Stasis

See Stasis Ulcer

Unilateral Neglect of One Side of Body

Unilateral Neglect (See **Unilateral Neglect,** Section III)

Unsanitary Living Conditions

Impaired **Home** maintenance r/t impaired cognitive or emotional functioning, lack of knowledge, insufficient finances, addiction

Risk for **Allergy** response: Risk factor: exposure to environmental contaminants

Urgency to Urinate

Urge urinary **Incontinence** (See **Incontinence,** urinary, urge, Section III)

Risk for urge urinary **Incontinence** (See **Incontinence,** urinary, urge, risk for, Section III)

Urinary Catheter

Risk for urinary tract **Injury:** Risk factors: confused client, long-term use of catheter, large retention balloon or catheter, perirectal burn injured client

Urinary Diversion

See Ileal Conduit

Urinary Elimination, Impaired

Impaired **Urinary** elimination (See **Urinary** elimination, impaired, Section III)

Urinary Incontinence

See Incontinence of Urine

Urinary Retention

Urinary Retention (See **Urinary Retention,** Section III)

Urinary Tract Infection (UTI)

See UTI (Urinary Tract Infection)

Urolithiasis

See Kidney Stone

Uterine Atony in Labor

See Dystocia

Uterine Atony in Postpartum

See Postpartum Hemorrhage

Uterine Bleeding

See Hemorrhage; Postpartum Hemorrhage; Shock, Hypovolemic

UTI (Urinary Tract Infection)

Ineffective **Health** maintenance r/t deficient knowledge regarding methods to treat and prevent UTIs, prolonged use of indwelling urinary catheter

Acute **Pain:** dysuria r/t inflammatory process in bladder

Impaired **Urinary** elimination: frequency r/t urinary tract infection

Risk for urge urinary **Incontinence:** Risk factor: hyperreflexia from cystitis

Risk for ineffective **Renal** perfusion: Risk factor: infection

V

VAD (Ventricular Assist Device)

See Ventricular Assist Device (VAD)

Vaginal Hysterectomy

Urinary retention r/t edema at surgical site

Risk for urge urinary **Incontinence:** Risk factors: edema, congestion of pelvic tissues

Risk for **Infection:** Risk factor: surgical site

Risk for **Perioperative Positioning** injury: Risk factor: lithotomy position

Vaginitis

Impaired **Comfort** r/t pruritus, itching

Ineffective **Health** maintenance r/t deficient knowledge regarding self-care with vaginitis

Ineffective **Sexuality** pattern r/t abstinence during acute stage, pain

Vagotomy

See Abdominal Surgery

Value System Conflict

Decisional Conflict r/t unclear personal values or beliefs

Spiritual distress r/t challenged value system

Readiness for enhanced **Spiritual** well-being: desire for harmony with self, others, higher power, God

Varicose Veins

Ineffective **Health** maintenance r/t deficient knowledge regarding health care practices, prevention, treatment regimen

Chronic **Pain** r/t impaired circulation

Ineffective peripheral **Tissue Perfusion** r/t venous stasis

Risk for impaired **Tissue** integrity: Risk factor: altered peripheral tissue perfusion

Vascular Dementia (Formerly Called Multiinfarct Dementia)

See Dementia

Vascular Obstruction, Peripheral

Anxiety r/t lack of circulation to body part

Acute **Pain** r/t vascular obstruction

Ineffective peripheral **Tissue Perfusion** r/t interruption of circulatory flow

Risk for **Peripheral Neurovascular** dysfunction: Risk factor: vascular obstruction

Vasectomy

Decisional Conflict r/t surgery as method of permanent sterilization

Venereal Disease

See STD (Sexually Transmitted Disease)

Ventilated Client, Mechanically

Ineffective **Airway** clearance r/t increased secretions, decreased cough and gag reflex

Ineffective **Breathing** pattern r/t decreased energy and fatigue as a result of possible altered nutrition: less than body requirements, neurological disease or damage

Impaired verbal **Communication** r/t presence of endotracheal tube, inability to phonate

Fear r/t inability to breathe on own, difficulty communicating

Impaired **Gas** exchange r/t ventilation-perfusion imbalance

Powerlessness r/t health treatment regimen

Social isolation r/t impaired mobility, ventilator dependence

Impaired spontaneous **Ventilation** r/t metabolic factors, respiratory muscle fatigue

Dysfunctional **Ventilatory** weaning response r/t psychological, situational, physiological factors

Risk for **Falls:** Risk factors: impaired mobility, decreased muscle strength

Risk for **Infection:** Risk factors: presence of endotracheal tube, pooled secretions

Risk for pressure **Ulcer:** Risk factor: decreased mobility

Risk for impaired **Resilience:** Risk factor: illness

See Child with Chronic Condition; Hospitalized Child; Respiratory Conditions of the Neonate

Ventricular Assist Device (VAD)

Anxiety r/t possible failure of device

Risk for **Infection:** Risk factor: device insertion site

Risk for **Vascular Trauma:** Risk factor: insertion site

Readiness for enhanced **Decision-Making:** expresses desire to enhance the understanding of the meaning of choices regarding implanting a ventricular assist device

See Open Heart Surgery

Ventricular Fibrillation

See Dysrhythmia

Vertigo

See Syncope

Violent Behavior

Risk for other-directed **Violence** (See **Violence,** other-directed, risk for, Section III)

Risk for self-directed **Violence** (See **Violence,** self-directed, risk for, Section III)

Viral Gastroenteritis

Diarrhea r/t infectious process, Norovirus

Deficient **Fluid** volume r/t vomiting, diarrhea

Ineffective **Health** management r/t inadequate handwashing

See Gastroenteritis, Child

Vision Impairment

Fear r/t loss of sight

Social isolation r/t altered state of wellness, inability to see

Vision Loss r/t impaired visual function; integration; reception; and or transmission

Risk for impaired **Resilience:** Risk factor: presence of new crisis

See Blindness; Cataracts; Glaucoma

Vomiting

Nausea r/t chemotherapy, postsurgical anesthesia, irritation to the gastrointestinal system, stimulation of neuropharmacological mechanisms

Imbalanced **Nutrition:** less than body requirements r/t inability to ingest food

Risk for **Electrolyte** imbalance: Risk factor: vomiting

VTE (Venous Thromboembolism)

See DVT (Deep Vein Thrombosis)

W

Walking Impairment

Impaired **Walking** (See **Walking,** impaired, Section III)

Wandering

Wandering (See **Wandering,** Section III)

Weakness

Fatigue r/t decreased or increased metabolic energy production

Risk for **Falls:** Risk factor: weakness

Weight Gain

Overweight (See **Overweight,** Section III)

Weight Loss

Imbalanced **Nutrition:** less than body requirements r/t inability to ingest food because of biological, psychological, economic factors

Wellness-Seeking Behavior

Readiness for enhanced **Health** management: expresses desire for increased control of health practice

Wernicke-Korsakoff Syndrome

See Korsakoff's Syndrome

W

West Nile Virus

See Meningitis/Encephalitis

Wheelchair Use Problems

Impaired wheelchair **Mobility** (See **Mobility,** wheelchair, impaired, Section III)

Wheezing

Ineffective **Airway** clearance r/t tracheobronchial obstructions, secretions

Wilms' Tumor

Chronic functional **Constipation** r/t obstruction associated with presence of tumor

Acute **Pain** r/t pressure from tumor

See Chemotherapy; Hospitalized Child; Radiation Therapy; Surgery, Preoperative Care; Surgery, Perioperative Care; Surgery, Postoperative Care

Withdrawal from Alcohol

See Alcohol Withdrawal

Withdrawal from Drugs

See Drug Withdrawal

Wound Debridement

Acute **Pain** r/t debridement of wound

Impaired **Tissue** integrity r/t debridement, open wound

Risk for **Infection:** Risk factors: open wound, presence of bacteria

Wound Dehiscence, Evisceration

Fear r/t client fear of body parts "falling out," surgical procedure not going as planned

Disturbed **Body Image** r/t change in body structure and wound appearance

Imbalanced **Nutrition:** less than body requirements r/t inability to digest nutrients, need for increased protein for healing

Risk for deficient **Fluid** volume: Risk factors: inability to ingest nutrients, obstruction, fluid loss

Risk for **Injury:** Risk factor: exposed abdominal contents

Risk for delayed **Surgical** recovery: Risk factors: separation of wound, exposure of abdominal contents

Wound Infection

Disturbed **Body Image** r/t open wound

Imbalanced **Nutrition:** less than body requirements r/t biological factors, infection, fever

Ineffective **Thermoregulation** r/t infection in wound resulting in fever

Impaired **Tissue** integrity r/t wound, presence of infection

Risk for imbalanced **Fluid** volume: Risk factor: increased metabolic rate

Risk for **Infection:** spread of: Risk factor: imbalanced nutrition: less than body requirements

Risk for delayed **Surgical** recovery: Risk factor: presence of infection

Wounds, Open

See Lacerations

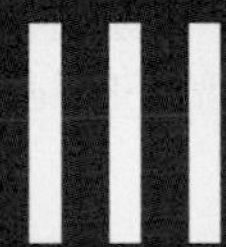

SECTION

III Guide to Planning Care

Section III is a collection of NANDA-I nursing diagnosis care plans. The care plans are arranged alphabetically by diagnostic concept. They contain definitions, defining characteristics, and related factors if appropriate. Risk Diagnoses, however, only contain "risk factors." Care plans include suggested outcomes and interventions for all nursing diagnoses.

MAKING AN ACCURATE NURSING DIAGNOSIS

Verify the accuracy of the previously suggested nursing diagnoses (from Section II) or from alphabetized list (inside back cover) for the client.

STEPS

- Read the definition for the suggested nursing diagnosis and determine if it is appropriate.
- Compare the Defining Characteristics with the symptoms that were identified from the client data collected.

or

- Compare the Risk Factors with the factors that were identified from the client data collected.

WRITING OUTCOMES STATEMENTS AND NURSING INTERVENTIONS

After selecting the appropriate nursing diagnosis, use this section to write outcomes and interventions:

STEPS

- Use the Client Outcomes/Nursing Interventions as written by the authors and contributors (select ones that are appropriate for your client).

or

- Use the NOC/NIC outcomes and interventions (as appropriate for your client).
- Read the rationales; the majority of rationales are based on nursing or clinical research that validates the efficacy of the interventions. Every attempt has been made to utilize current references; however, some significant research has not been replicated. Important research studies that are older than 5 years are included because they are the only evidence available. They are designated as **CEB** (Classic Evidence-Based).

Following these steps, you will be able to write an evidence-based nursing care plan.

- Follow this care plan to administer nursing care to the client.
- Document all steps and evaluate and update the care plan as needed.

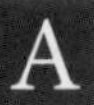

Activity intolerance

Lorraine Duggan, MSN, ACNP-BC

NANDA-I

Definition

Insufficient physiological or psychological energy to endure or complete required or desired daily activities

Defining Characteristics

Abnormal blood pressure response to activity; abnormal heart rate response to activity; ECG change (e.g., arrhythmia, conduction abnormality, ischemia); exertional discomfort; exertional dyspnea; fatigue; generalized weakness

Related Factors (r/t)

Bed rest; generalized weakness; imbalance between oxygen supply/demand; immobility; sedentary lifestyle

NOC (Nursing Outcomes Classification)

Suggested NOC Outcomes

Activity Tolerance; Endurance; Energy Conservation; Self-Care: Instrumental Activities of Daily Living (IADLs)

Example NOC Outcome with Indicators

Activity Tolerance as evidenced by the following indicators: Oxygen saturation with activity/Pulse rate with activity/Respiratory rate with activity/Blood pressure with activity/Electrocardiogram findings/Skin color/Walking distance. (Rate the outcome and indicators of **Activity Tolerance:** 1 = severely compromised, 2 = substantially compromised, 3 = moderately compromised, 4 = mildly compromised, 5 = not compromised [see Section I].)

Client Outcomes

Client Will (Specify Time Frame)

- Participate in prescribed physical activity with appropriate changes in heart rate, blood pressure, and breathing rate; maintain monitor patterns (rhythm and ST segment) within normal limits
- State symptoms of adverse effects of exercise and report onset of symptoms immediately
- Maintain normal skin color; skin is warm and dry with activity
- Verbalize an understanding of the need to gradually increase activity based on testing, tolerance, and symptoms
- Demonstrate increased tolerance to activity

NIC (Nursing Interventions Classification)

Suggested NIC Interventions

Activity Therapy; Energy Management; Exercise Therapy: Ambulation

Example NIC Activities—Energy Management

Monitor cardiorespiratory response to activity; Monitor location and nature of discomfort or pain during movement/activity

Nursing Interventions and *Rationales*

- Determine cause of Activity intolerance (see Related Factors) and determine whether cause is physical, psychological, or motivational. QSEN: *As nurses we are called upon to assure higher levels of safety and quality for our clients by our governments, professional organizations, and hospital administrations. It is essential that we implement evidence-based nursing care strategies to reduce avoidable errors in care so that clinical outcomes improve (Vollman, 2013).*

- If mainly on bed rest, minimize cardiovascular deconditioning by positioning the client in an upright position several times daily if possible. CEB: *With bed rest there is a shift of fluids from the extremities to the thoracic cavity from the loss of gravitational stress. Positioning in an upright position helps maintain optimal fluid distribution and maintain orthostatic tolerance (Perme & Chandrashekar, 2009).*
- Assess the client daily for appropriateness of activity and bed rest orders. Mobilize the client as soon as possible. EB: *Mobilization is a cost-effective and simple method of maintaining stable cardiovascular parameters (i.e., blood pressure, heart rate), countering orthostatic intolerance, and reducing the risk of secondary problems in clients during long-term immobilization (Wieser, 2014).*
- If the client is mostly immobile, consider use of a transfer chair: a chair that becomes a stretcher. CEB: *Using a transfer chair where the client is pulled onto a flat surface and then seated upright in the chair can help previously immobile clients get out of bed (Perme & Chandrashekar, 2009).*
- When appropriate, gradually increase activity, allowing the client to assist with positioning, transferring, and self-care as able. Progress the client from sitting in bed to dangling, to standing, to ambulation. Always have the client dangle at the bedside before standing to evaluate for postural hypotension. EB: *A reduction in plasma volume associated with bed rest impacts the physiological responses of autonomic control of circulation (Dorantes-Mendez et al, 2013).*
- When getting a client up, observe for symptoms of intolerance such as nausea, pallor, dizziness, visual dimming, and impaired consciousness, as well as changes in vital signs; manual blood pressure monitoring is best. *When an adult rises to the standing position, blood pools in the lower extremities; symptoms of central nervous system hypoperfusion may occur, including feelings of weakness, nausea, headache, lightheadedness, dizziness, blurred vision, fatigue, tremulousness, palpitations, and impaired cognition.* EBN: *Automatic devices cannot reliably detect or rule out orthostatic hypotension, indicating that nurses need to use manual devices to take accurate postural blood pressures for optimal client care (Dind et al, 2011).*
- If the client has symptoms of postural hypotension, such as dizziness, lightheadedness, or pallor, take precautions, such as dangling the client and applying leg compression stockings before the client stands. EB: *Put graduated compression stockings on the client or use lower limb compression bandaging, if ordered, to return blood to the heart and brain. Have the client dangle at the side of the bed with legs hanging over the edge of the bed, flexing and extending the feet several times after sitting up, then standing slowly with someone holding the client. If the client becomes lightheaded or dizzy, return him to bed immediately (Tibaldi et al, 2014).*
- Perform range-of-motion (ROM) exercises if the client is unable to tolerate activity or is mostly immobile. See care plan for Risk for **Disuse** syndrome.
- Monitor and record the client's ability to tolerate activity: note pulse rate, blood pressure, respiratory pattern, dyspnea, use of accessory muscles, and skin color before, during, and after the activity. If the following signs and symptoms of cardiac decompensation develop, activity should be stopped immediately:
  - Onset of chest discomfort or pain
  - Dyspnea
  - Palpitations
  - Excessive fatigue
  - Lightheadedness, confusion, ataxia, pallor, cyanosis, nausea, or any peripheral circulatory insufficiency
  - Dysrhythmia
  - Exercise hypotension
  - Excessive rise in blood pressure
  - Inappropriate bradycardia
  - Increased heart rate
  - Decreased oxygen saturation

The above are symptoms of intolerance to activity and continuation of activity may result in client harm (Goldman, 2011).

▲ Instruct the client to stop the activity immediately and report to the health care provider if the client is experiencing the following symptoms: new or worsened intensity or increased frequency of discomfort; tightness or pressure in chest, back, neck, jaw, shoulders, and/or arms; palpitations; dizziness; weakness; unusual and extreme fatigue; excessive air hunger. *Pulse rate and arterial blood oxygenation indicate cardiac/exercise tolerance; pulse oximetry identifies hypoxia (Goldman, 2011).*

- Observe and document skin integrity several times a day. ***Activity** intolerance, if resulting in immobility, may lead to pressure ulcers. Mechanical pressure, moisture, friction, and shearing forces all predispose to their development.* Refer to the care plan Risk for impaired **Skin** integrity.
- Assess for constipation. If present, refer to care plan for **Constipation.** ***Activity** intolerance is associated with increased risk of **Constipation.***
- ▲ Refer the client to physical therapy to help increase activity levels and strength.
- ▲ Consider a dietitian referral to assess nutritional needs related to **Activity** intolerance; provide nutrition as indicated. If the client is unable to eat food, use enteral or parenteral feedings as needed.
- Recognize that malnutrition causes significant morbidity due to the loss of lean body mass.
- Provide emotional support and encouragement to the client to gradually increase activity. Work with the client to set mutual goals that increase activity levels. Fear of breathlessness, pain, or falling may decrease willingness to increase activity. EB: *In clients with Parkinson's disease, motivations for exercising included hope that exercise would slow the disease or prevent a decline in function, feeling better with exercise, belief that exercise is beneficial, and encouragement from family members (Ene et al, 2011).*
- ▲ Observe for pain before activity. If possible, treat pain before activity and ensure that the client is not heavily sedated. *Pain restricts the client from achieving a maximal activity level and is often exacerbated by movement.*
- ▲ Obtain any necessary assistive devices or equipment needed before ambulating the client (e.g., walkers, canes, crutches, portable oxygen).
- ▲ Use a gait walking belt when ambulating the client. CEB: *Gait belts improve the caregiver's grasp, reducing the incidence of injuries in clients and nurses (Nelson et al, 2003).*
- ▲ *Use evidence-based practices for safe client handling to reduce the risk of injury for both clients and health care workers (Elnitsky et al, 2014).*

Activity Intolerance Due to Respiratory Disease

- If the client is able to walk and has chronic obstructive pulmonary disease (COPD), use the traditional 6-minute walk distance to evaluate ability to walk.
- ▲ Ensure that the chronic pulmonary client has oxygen saturation testing with exercise. Use supplemental oxygen to keep oxygen saturation 90% or above or as prescribed with activity. *Oxygen therapy can improve exercise ability and long-term administration of oxygen can increase survival in clients with COPD (Gold Report, 2012).*
- Monitor a respiratory client's response to activity by observing for symptoms of respiratory intolerance, such as increased dyspnea, loss of ability to control breathing rhythmically, use of accessory muscles, nasal flaring, appearance of facial distress, and skin tone changes such as pallor and cyanosis.
- Instruct and assist the client with COPD in using conscious, controlled breathing techniques during exercise, including pursed-lip breathing, and inspiratory muscle use.
- ▲ Evaluate the client's nutritional status. Refer to a dietitian if indicated. Use nutritional supplements to increase nutritional level if needed.
- ▲ For the client in the intensive care unit, consider mobilizing the client with passive exercise. EBN: *Nurses should consider incorporating at least 20 minutes of passive exercise early in the plan of care for critically ill clients treated with mechanical ventilation so that opportunities to improve client outcomes are not missed (Amidei & Sole, 2013).*
- ▲ Refer the COPD client to a pulmonary rehabilitation program. EB: *Pulmonary rehabilitation is a highly effective and safe intervention to reduce hospital admissions and mortality and to improve health-related quality of life in clients with COPD who have recently suffered an exacerbation (Puhan et al, 2009).*

Activity Intolerance Due to Cardiovascular Disease

- If the client is able to walk and has heart failure, consider use of the 6-minute walk test to determine physical ability.
- Allow for periods of rest before and after planned exertion periods such as meals, baths, treatments, and physical activity.
- ▲ Refer to a heart failure program or cardiac rehabilitation program for education, evaluation, and guided support to increase activity and rebuild life. EB: *Exercise-based cardiac rehabilitation is effective in reducing total and cardiovascular mortality and hospital admissions (Heran et al, 2011).*
- ▲ Refer to a community support program that includes support of significant others.

A

▲ EB: *Contemporary studies now suggest that behavior change and multifactorial risk factor modification—especially smoking cessation and more intensive measures to control hyperlipidemia with diet, drugs, and exercise—may slow, halt, or even reverse (albeit modestly) the otherwise inexorable progression of atherosclerotic CHD (Spring, 2013).*
- See care plan for Decreased **Cardiac** output for further interventions.

Pediatric

- Focus interview questions toward exercise tolerance specifically including any history of asthma exacerbations. EB: *Cardiopulmonary deconditioning should be considered as an important differential diagnosis for breathlessness among obese adolescents. Some of these children may need pulmonary rehabilitation if difficulty breathing is the perceived reason for not exercising (Shim et al, 2013).*

Geriatric

- Slow the pace of care. Allow the client extra time to carry out physical activities. *Slow gait in older adults may be related to fear of falling, decreased strength in muscles, reduced balance or visual acuity, knee flexion contractures, and foot pain.* QSEN: *Older patients with chronic cardiac conditions are more vulnerable to falls and injuries. Cardiovascular conditions, prevalent in older people, are also the frequent cause of potentially harmful fall injuries in this group. The need to identify the fall risk-related factors that cluster with arrhythmia and syncope is relevant, in that it will potentially reduce patients' risk for falls and fall injuries (Belita et al, 2013).*
- *Encourage families to help/allow an older client to be independent in whatever activities possible.* EB: *Physical activity and cognitive exercise may improve memory and executive functions in older people with mild cognitive impairment (Teixeira et al, 2012).*

▲ Assess for swaying, poor balance, weakness, and fear of falling while older clients stand/walk. Refer to physical therapy if appropriate. CEB: *Fear of falling and repeat falling is common in the older population. Balance rehabilitation provides individualized treatment for persons with various deficits associated with balance (Studer, 2008).* Refer to the care plan for Risk for **Falls** and Impaired **Walking**.

▲ Initiate ambulation by simply ambulating a patient a few steps from bed to chair, once a health care provider's out-of-bed order is obtained. EBN: *Lack of ambulation and deconditioning effects of bed rest are one of the most predictable causes of loss of independent ambulation in hospitalized older persons. Nurses have been identified as the professional most capable of promoting walking independence in the hospital setting (Doherty-King & Bowers, 2013).*

▲ Evaluate medications the client is taking to see if they could be causing **Activity** intolerance. EB: *Medications such as beta-blockers; lipid lowering agents, which can damage muscle; antipsychotics, which have a common side effect of orthostatic hypotension; some antihypertensives; and lowering the blood pressure to normal in older adults can result in decreased functioning (Society, 2012).*

▲ If heart disease is causing **Activity** intolerance, refer the client for cardiac rehabilitation.

▲ Refer the disabled older client to physical therapy for functional training including gait training, stepping, and sit-to-stand exercises, or for strength training. CEB: *A Cochrane review found that progressive resistance strength training to improve function is effective in older clients (Liu & Latham, 2009).*

Home Care

▲ Begin discharge planning as soon as possible with the case manager or social worker to assess the need for home support systems and the need for community or home health services. EB: *Home-based exercise appears more effective in increasing daily ambulatory activity in the community setting than supervised exercise in clients with intermittent claudication (Gardner et al, 2011).*

▲ Assess the home environment for factors that contribute to decreased activity tolerance such as stairs or distance to the bathroom. Refer the client for occupational therapy, if needed, to assist the client in restructuring the home and ADL patterns. *During hospitalization, clients and families often estimate energy requirements at home inaccurately because the hospital's availability of staff support distorts the level of care that will be needed.*

▲ Refer the client for physical therapy for strength training and possible weight training to regain strength, increase endurance, and improve balance. If the client is homebound, the physical therapist can also initiate cardiac rehabilitation.

- Encourage progress with positive feedback. *The client's experience should be validated within expected norms. Recognition of progress enhances motivation.*

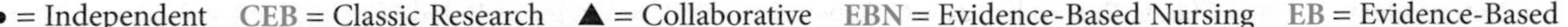

A

- Teach the client/family the importance of and methods for setting priorities for activities, especially those having a high energy demand (e.g., home/family events). Instruct in realistic expectations.
- Encourage routine low-level exercise periods such as a daily short walk or chair exercises. EB: *Older adults participating in low levels of regular exercise can establish and maintain a home-based exercise program that yields immediate and long-term physical and affective benefits (Teri et al, 2011).*
- Provide the client/family with resources such as senior centers, exercise classes, educational and recreational programs, and volunteer opportunities that can aid in promoting socialization and appropriate activity. *Social isolation can be an outcome of and contribute to **Activity** intolerance.* EB: *Community-based resistance training and dietary modifications can improve body composition, muscle strength, and physical function in overweight and obese older adults (Straight et al, 2011).*
- Instruct the client and family in the importance of maintaining proper nutrition.
- Instruct the client in use of dietary supplements as indicated. *Illness may suppress appetite, leading to inadequate nutrition.*

▲ Refer to medical social services as necessary to assist the family in adjusting to major changes in patterns of living because of **Activity** intolerance.

▲ Assess the need for long-term supports for optimal activity tolerance of priority activities (e.g., assistive devices, oxygen, medication, catheters, massage), especially for a hospice client. Evaluate intermittently.

▲ Refer to home health aide services to support the client and family through changing levels of activity tolerance. Introduce aide support early. Instruct the aide to promote independence in activity as tolerated.

- Allow terminally ill clients and their families to guide care. Control by the client or family respects their autonomy and promotes effective coping.
- Provide increased attention to comfort and dignity of the terminally ill client in care planning. *Interventions should be provided as much for psychological effect as for physiological support. For example, oxygen may be more valuable as a support to the client's psychological comfort than as a booster of oxygen saturation.*

▲ Institute case management of frail elderly to support continued independent living.

Client/Family Teaching and Discharge Planning

- Instruct the client on techniques for avoiding **Activity** intolerance, such as controlled breathing techniques.
- Teach the client techniques to decrease dizziness from postural hypotension when standing up.
- Help client with energy conservation and work simplification techniques in ADLs.
- Describe to the client the symptoms of **Activity** intolerance, including which symptoms to report to the physician.
- Explain to the client how to use assistive devices, oxygen, or medications before or during activity.
- Help the client set up an activity log to record exercise and exercise tolerance.

REFERENCES

Amidei, C., & Sole, M. (2013). Physiological responses to passive exercise in adults receiving mechanical ventilation. *American Journal of Critical Care, 22,* 337–348.

Belita, L., Ford, P., & Kirkpatrick, H. (2013). The development of an assessment and intervention falls guide for older hospitalized adults with cardiac conditions. *European Journal of Cardiovascular Nursing, 12,* 302–309.

Dind, A., et al. (2011). The inaccuracy of automatic devices taking postural measurements in the emergency department. *International Journal of Nursing Practice, 17,* 525–533.

Doherty-King, B., & Bowers, B. (2013). Attributing the responsibility for ambulating patients: a qualitative study. *International Journal of Nursing Studies, 50,* 1240–1246.

Dorantes-Mendez, G., Baselli, G., Arbeille, P., et al. (2013). *Comparison of Baroreflex Sensitivity Gain During Mild Lower Body Negative Pressure in Presence and Absence of Long Duration Bed Rest. Computing in Cardiology Conference,* (pp. 763–766). Milan, Italy.

Elnitsky, C. A., et al. (2014). Implications in the use of patient safety in the use of safe patient handling equipment: a national survey. *International Journal of Nursing Studies, 51*(12), 1624–1633.

Ene, H., McRae, C., & Schenkman, M. (2011). Attitudes toward exercise following participation in an exercise intervention study. *Journal of Neurologic Physical Therapy, 35,* 34–40.

Gardner, A., et al. (2011). Efficacy of quantified home-based exercise and supervised exercise in patients with intermittent claudication: a randomized controlled trial. *Circulation, 123,* 491–498.

Global Initiative for Chronic Obstructive Lung Disease (GOLD Report). (2012, August 2). *Guidelines Global Strategy for Diagnosis Management.* Retrieved from GoldCOPD <www.goldcopd.org>.

Goldman, L. (2011). *Goldman Cecil's Medicine.* St. Louis: Saunders.

Heran, B., et al. (2011). Exercise-Based Cardiac Rehabilitation for Coronary Heart Disease. *Cochrane Database System Review.* Retrieved from Database System Review.

Liu, C., & Latham, N.K. (2009). Progressive resistance strength training for improving physical function in older adults. *Cochrane Database System Review.*

Nelson, A., et al. (2003). Safe patient handling and movement. *American Journal of Nursing*, 32.

Perme, C., & Chandrashekar, R. (2009). Early mobility and walking program for patients in intensive care units: creating a standard of care. *American Journal of Critical Care*, *18*, 212–221.

Puhan, M., et al. (2009). Pulmonary rehabilitation following exacerbations of chronic obstructive pulmonary disease. *Cochrane Database System Review*, (1), CD005305.

Shim, Y., Burnette, A., Lucas, S., et al. (2013). Physical deconditioning as a cause of breathlessness among obese adolescents with a diagnosis of asthma. *PLoS ONE*, *8*(4), e61022.

Society, A. G. (2012, August 2). *Beers Criteria*. Retrieved from American Geriatrics <http://www.americangeriatrics.org>.

Spring, B. E. (2013, October 7). *Better Population Health through Behavior Change in Adults: A Call to Action*. Retrieved from Circulation <http://circ.ahajournals.org>.

Straight, C., et al. (2011). Effects of resistance training and dietary changes on physical function and body composition in overweight and obese older adults. *Journal of Physical Activity and Health*, Epub.

Studer, M. (2008). Keep it moving: advances in gait training techniques help clients reduce balance issues. *Rehabilitation Management*, *21*, 10–15.

Teixeira, C., et al. (2012). Non-pharmacological interventions on cognitive functions in older people with mild cognitive impairment. *Archives of Gerontological Geriatrics*, *54*, 175–180.

Teri, L., et al. (2011). A randomized controlled clinical trial of the seattle protocol for activity in older adults. *Journal of the American Geriatric Society*, *59*, 1188–1196.

Tibaldi, M., Brescianini, A., Sciarrillo, I., et al. (2014). Prevalence and clinical implications of orthostatic hypotension in elderly. *Hypertension*, *3*, 155.

Vollman, K. (2013). Interventional patient hygiene: discussion of the issues and a proposed model for implementation of the nursing care basics. *Intensive and Critical Care Nursing*, *29*, 250–255.

Wieser, M. G. (2014). Cardiovascular control and stabilization via inclination and mobilization during bed rest. *Medical & Biological Engineering and Computing*, *52*, 53–64.

Risk for Activity intolerance

Betty J. Ackley, MSN, EdS, RN, and Mary Beth Flynn Makic, PhD, RN, CNS, CCNS, FAAN

NANDA-I

Definition

Vulnerable to insufficient physiological or psychological energy to endure or complete required or desired daily activities, which may compromise health

Risk Factors

Circulatory problems; History of previous intolerance; Inexperience with an activity; Physical deconditioning; Respiratory condition

NIC, NOC, Client Outcomes, Nursing Interventions, Client/Family Teaching and Discharge Planning, *Rationales*, and References

Refer to care plan for **Activity** intolerance.

Ineffective Activity planning

Annie Muller, DNP, APN-BC, and Gail B. Ladwig, MSN, RN

NANDA-I

Definition

Inability to prepare for a set of actions fixed in time and under certain conditions

Defining Characteristics

Absence of plan; excessive anxiety about a task to be undertaken; insufficient organizational skills; insufficient resources (e.g., financial social, knowledge); pattern of failure; pattern of procrastination; unmet goals for chosen activity; worry about a task to be undertaken

Related Factors

Flight behavior when faced with proposed solution; hedonism; insufficient information processing ability; insufficient social support; unrealistic perception of event; unrealistic perception of personal abilities

NOC Outcomes (Nursing Outcomes Classification)

Suggested NOC Outcomes

Cognition; Cognition Orientation; Concentration; Decision-Making; Information Processing; Memory

Example NOC Outcome with Indicators

Cognition as evidenced by the following indicators: Communication clear and appropriate for age/Comprehension of the meaning of situations/Information processing/Alternatives weighed when making decisions. (Rate the outcome and indicators of **Cognition:** 1 = severely compromised, 2 = substantially compromised, 3 = moderately compromised, 4 = mildly compromised, 5 = not compromised [see Section I].)

Patient Outcomes

Patient Will (Specify Time Frame)

- Verbalize need for self-directed activity
- Choose the health care option that fits his or her lifestyle within an appropriate amount of time that allows enactment of the choice
- Describe how the chosen option fits into current lifestyle before or after the decision has been made
- Verbalize the need for a behavioral change to improve physical activity

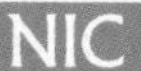

NIC Interventions (Nursing Interventions Classification)

Suggested NIC Interventions

Anxiety Reduction; Behavior Management; Behavior Modification; Calming Technique; Coping Enhancement; Decision-Making Support; Life Skills Enhancement; Planning Assistance; Sequence Guidance

Example NIC Activities—Coping Enhancement

Assist client in developing an objective appraisal of the event; Explore with client previous methods of dealing with life problems

Nursing Interventions and *Rationales*

- Ask the client how he or she perceives the situation in order to gather his personal vision of the problem and how they envisage their self-involvement. Specify the goals. *Clients and caregivers may have different priorities on what is important (Junius-Walker et al, 2011).*
  - Identify the informational needs of the client: understanding of the client's state of health, supervision of client's treatment if he or she is receiving treatment, diet, and important telephone numbers. EBN: *This study of clients with stage 4 chronic kidney disease validated the need for an individual assessment to determine the unique informational needs of each person (Lewis et al, 2010).*
  - Tackle the client's fears and worries and encourage him to make a cognitive reconstruction. Use "desire thinking." Drill and repeat: "I can change false ideas that make me believe that I am unable to carry out (achieve) my plan." EBN: *Desire thinking is a voluntary cognitive process involving verbal and imaginal elaboration of a desired target. Recent research has highlighted the role of desire thinking in the maintenance of addictive, eating, and impulse control disorders (Caselli & Spada, 2011).*
- Client verbalizes need for behavioral change for improved physical activity. EB: *This study reflects how combining planning and coping planning of a client's self-worth can be beneficial in promoting an exercise program for those individuals who lack self-esteem (Kroon et al, 2014).*
- Encourage clients to verbalize the need for physical activity to help reduce role overload. EB: *This study demonstrated the need for planning activities for those individuals who were experiencing a role overload in life to allow them time for leisure activities (Lovell & Butler, 2015).*
- ▲ Determine as fairly as possible the success factors needed for the planning and success of the project: financial resources; the family situation; prior medical, psychiatric, and psychosocial conditions; material resources; and the ability to manage stress. EBN: *Discussions identifying resources help to handle past resources, the functional solutions of everyday life, favorable changes, exceptions and differences in everyday*

life, the availability of support, and the prospects of future. By noting and providing feedback to families, the nurse offers families a new perspective on themselves (Häggman-Laitila et al, 2010).

A

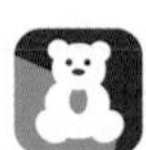

Pediatric

- Begin activity planning in preschool-aged children of working parents. EB: *This study focused on the inactivity of migrant workers' preschool-aged children and the need to have a more structured and planned activity for the migrant worker. The focus was on the child because not much is known and very little research has been done. Also, there is a wide disparity of health in this population. The results showed very little physical activity was encouraged by parents and there was a great need for intervention to help with developing future healthy lifestyle for reducing potential long-term health problems (Grzywacz et al, 2014).*
- Establish a contract. EBN: *This study of adolescents with type 1 diabetes indicated that behavioral contracts may be an important adjunct to reduce nagging and improve outcomes with behavioral changes (Carroll et al, 2011).*
- Provide support to the schools for physical activities in all venues of schools. EB: *Depending on the location of the school and the available resources, schools may promote a physical activity program that is beneficial and available to the student. Schools with few resources have limited staff available, which can be a barrier to promoting a healthy lifestyle to the adolescent student. (Hobin et al, 2013).*

Geriatric

- Plan activities for older clients. EB: *In a study of stroke clients, it was found that physical activity may improve quality of life, physical function, and self-worth (Walter et al, 2015).*
- Plan activities for older clients with impaired mental function. EB: *In this study, it was found that clients with impaired mental function are often limited in their ability to become involved with planned physical activity; therefore, staff are needed to intervene and assist with the planned activity (Koring et al, 2012).*

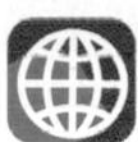

Multicultural

- Provide literature and information in the appropriate language for the client who speaks little to no English. EB: *This study was able to show those clients who did not speak English fluently were not adequately prepared or educated to the needs for physical activity. Nor were they well represented in the study to show that culture was represented in understanding about cognitive health and risks of Alzheimer's disease (Rose et al, 2013).*
- Preplanning educational programs for the culturally diverse population needs to be developed. EB: *Low level of preplanning and poor organization of physical activities for the culturally diverse causes a loss of participation by those involved due to lack of understanding the concepts involved (Jeong et al, 2015).*

Home Care

- Have a preplanned activity exercise for the home client with a debilitating musculoskeletal disease to help improve functional status. EB: *This study showed an improvement for those clients who were homebound due to a musculoskeletal disorder, thereby improving their personal commitment to exercise for increasing their functional ability by gaining some muscle strength and range of motion (Hideyuki & Hitoshi, 2014).*
- Assess the home environment for barriers that can impact the client's motivation to be a participant in the activity planned. EB: *The research study done on homebound older adults showed that the client knew and understood the need for planned physical activity, but were not motivated to participate because they thought their age was a barrier. The idea is to teach the older client; while age may be a factor in some types of activity planning or exercise, there are many ways to adapt to the activity that can be accommodating to the client's ability (Burton et al, 2013).*
- For additional interventions, refer to care plans **Anxiety,** Readiness for enhanced family **Coping,** Readiness for enhanced **Decision-Making, Fear,** Readiness for enhanced **Hope,** Readiness for enhanced **Power,** Readiness for enhanced **Spiritual** well-being, and Readiness for enhanced **Health** management.

REFERENCES

Burton, E., Lewin, G., & Boldy, D. (2013). Barriers and motivators to being physically active for older home care patients. *Physical & Occupational Therapy in Geriatrics, 31*(1), 21–35.

Carroll, A. E., et al. (2011). Contracting and monitoring relationships for adolescents with type 1 diabetes: a pilot study. *Diabetes Tech Therapeut, 13*(5), 543–549.

A

Caselli, G., & Spada, M. M. (2011). The Desire Thinking Questionnaire: development and psychometric properties. *Addictive Behaviors*, *36*(11), 1061–1067.

Grzywacz, J. G., Suerken, C. K., Zapata-Roblyer, M. I., et al. (2014). Physical activity of preschool-aged Latino children in farm-worker families. *American Journal of Health Behavior*, *38*(5), 717–725.

Häggman-Laitila, A., Tanninen, H., & Pietilä, A. (2010). Effectiveness of resource-enhancing family-oriented intervention. *Journal of Clinical Nursing*, *19*(17/18), 2500–2510.

Hideyuki, N., & Hitoshi, T. (2014). Effects of home exercise on physical function and activity in home care patients with Parkinson's disease. *Journal of Physical Therapy Science*, *26*(11), 1701–1706.

Hobin, E. P., Leatherdale, S., Manske, S., et al. (2013). Are environmental influences on physical activity distinct for urban, suburban, and rural schools? A multilevel study among secondary school students in Ontario, Canada. *Journal of School Health*, *83*(5), 357–367.

Jeong, S., Ohr, S., Pich, J., et al. (2015). Planning ahead among community-dwelling older people from culturally and linguistically diverse background: a cross-sectional survey. *Journal of Clinical Nursing*, *24*(1/2), 244–255.

Junius-Walker, U., et al. (2011). Health and treatment priorities of older patients and their general practitioners: a cross-sectional study. *Qual Primary Care*, *19*, 67–76.

Koring, M., Richert, J., Parchau, L., et al. (2012). A combined planning and self-efficacy intervention to promote physical activity: A multiple mediation analysis. *Psychology, Health & Medicine*, *17*(4), 488–498.

Kroon, F. P., van der Burg, L. R., Buchbinder, R., et al. (2014). Self-management education programmes for osteoarthritis. *The Cochrane Library.*

Lewis, A. L., Stabler, K. A., & Welch, J. L. (2010). Perceived informational needs, problems, or concerns among patients with stage 4 chronic kidney disease. *Nephrology Nursing Journal: Journal of the American Nephrology Nurses' Association*, *37*(2), 143–149.

Lovell, G. P., & Butler, F. R. (2015). Physical activity behavior and role overload in mothers. *Health Care for Women International*, *36*(3), 342–355.

Rose, I. D., Friedman, D. B., Marquez, D. X., et al. (2013). What are older Latinos told about physical activity and cognition? A content analysis of a top-circulating magazine. *Journal of Aging & Health*, *25*(7), 1143–1158.

Walter, T., Hale, L., & Smith, C. (2015). Blue prescription: A single subject design intervention to enable physical therapy for people with stroke. *International Journal of Therapy & Rehabilitation*, *22*(2), 87–95.

Risk for Ineffective Activity planning *Gail B. Ladwig, MSN, RN*

NANDA-I

Definition

Vulnerable to an inability to prepare for a set of actions fixed in time and under certain conditions, which may compromise health

Risk Factors

Flight behavior when faced with proposed solution; hedonism; insufficient information processing ability; insufficient social support; pattern of procrastination; unrealistic perception of event; unrealistic perception of personal abilities

NOC, NIC, Client Outcomes, Nursing Interventions, Client/Family Teaching and Discharge Planning, *Rationales,* and References

Refer to ineffective **Activity** planning.

Ineffective Airway clearance *Debra Siela, PhD, RN, CCNS, ACNS-BC, CCRN-K, CNE, RRT*

NANDA-I

Definition

Inability to clear secretions or obstructions from the respiratory tract to maintain a clear airway

Defining Characteristics

Absent cough; adventitious breath sounds; alteration in respiratory pattern; alteration in respiratory rate; cyanosis; difficulty verbalizing; diminished breath sounds; dyspnea; excessive sputum; ineffective cough; orthopnea; restlessness; wide-eyed look

Related Factors (r/t)

Environmental

Exposure to smoke; second-hand smoke; smoking

A

Obstructed Airway

Airway spasm; chronic obstructive pulmonary disease; exudate in the alveoli; excessive mucus; foreign body in airway; hyperplasia of bronchial walls; presence of artificial airway; retained secretions

Physiological

Allergic airways; asthma; infection; neuromuscular impairment

NOC (Nursing Outcomes Classification)

Suggested NOC Outcomes

Aspiration Prevention; Respiratory Status: Airway Patency, Gas Exchange, Ventilation

Example NOC Outcome with Indicators

Respiratory Status: Ventilation as evidenced by the following indicators: Respiratory rate/Respiratory rhythm/Depth of inspiration/Chest expansion symmetrical/Ease of breathing/Tidal volume/Vital capacity (Rate each indicator of **Respiratory Status: Ventilation:** 1 = severe deviation from normal range, 2 = substantial deviation from normal range, 3 = moderate deviation from normal range, 4 = mild deviation from normal range, 5 = no deviation from normal range [see Section I].)

Client Outcomes

Client Will (Specify Time Frame)

- Demonstrate effective coughing and clear breath sounds
- Maintain a patent airway at all times
- Explain methods useful to enhance secretion removal
- Explain the significance of changes in sputum to include color, character, amount, and odor
- Identify and avoid specific factors that inhibit effective airway clearance

NIC (Nursing Interventions Classification)

Suggested NIC Interventions

Airway Management; Airway Suctioning; Cough Enhancement

Example NIC Activities—Airway Management

Instruct how to cough effectively; Auscultate breath sounds, noting areas of decreased or absent ventilation and presence of adventitious sounds

Nursing Interventions and *Rationales*

- Auscultate breath sounds every 1 to 4 hours. *Breath sounds are normally clear or scattered fine crackles at bases, which clear with deep breathing. The presence of coarse crackles during late inspiration indicates fluid in the airway; wheezing indicates an airway obstruction (Fauci et al, 2008).*
- Monitor respiratory patterns, including rate, depth, and effort. *A normal respiratory rate for an adult without dyspnea is 12 to 16 breaths per minute (Bickley & Szilagyi, 2012). With secretions in the airway, the respiratory rate will increase.*
- Monitor blood gas values and pulse oxygen saturation levels as available. An oxygen saturation of less than 90% (normal: 95% to 100%) or a partial pressure of oxygen of less than 80 mm Hg (normal: 80 to 100 mm Hg) indicates significant oxygenation problems (Schultz, 2011).

▲ Administer oxygen as ordered. *Oxygen administration has been shown to correct hypoxemia (Wong & Elliott, 2009).*

- Position the client to optimize respiration (e.g., head of bed elevated 30 to 45 degrees). *An upright position allows for maximal lung expansion; lying flat causes abdominal organs to shift toward the chest, which crowds the lungs and makes it more difficult to breathe.* EB: *In a mechanically ventilated client, there is a decreased incidence of ventilator-associated pneumonia if the client is positioned at a 30- to 45-degree semi-recumbent position rather than a supine position* (Siela, 2010; Bell, 2011; Johanna Briggs Institute, 2014).

A

- • Help the client deep breathe and perform controlled coughing. Have the client inhale deeply, hold breath for several seconds, and cough two or three times with mouth open while tightening the upper abdominal muscles. CEB: *Controlled coughing uses the diaphragmatic muscles, making the cough more forceful and effective (Gosselink et al, 2008).*
- • If the client has obstructive lung disease, such as chronic obstructive pulmonary disease (COPD), cystic fibrosis, or bronchiectasis, consider helping the client use the forced expiratory technique, the "huff cough." The client does a series of coughs while saying the word "huff." *This technique prevents the glottis from closing during the cough and is effective in clearing secretions (Bhowmik et al, 2009; Gosselink et al, 2008; GOLD, 2015).*
- ▲ Encourage the client to use an incentive spirometer. Recognize that controlled coughing and deep breathing may be just as effective as incentive spirometry (Gosselink et al, 2008).
- • Encourage activity and ambulation as tolerated. If the client cannot be ambulated, turn the client from side to side at least every 2 hours. *Body movement helps mobilize secretions.* (See interventions for impaired **Gas** exchange for further information on positioning a respiratory patient.)
- • Encourage fluid intake of up to 2500 mL/day within cardiac or renal reserve. *Fluids help minimize mucosal drying and maximize ciliary action to move secretions.*
- ▲ Administer medications such as bronchodilators or inhaled steroids as ordered. Watch for side effects such as tachycardia or anxiety with bronchodilators, or inflamed pharynx with inhaled steroids. *Bronchodilators decrease airway resistance, improve the efficiency of respiratory movements, improve exercise tolerance, and can reduce symptoms of dyspnea on exertion (Barnett, 2008). Pharmacologic therapy in COPD is used to reduce symptoms, reduce the frequency and severity of exacerbation, and improve health strategies and exercise tolerance (GOLD, 2015).*
- ▲ Provide percussion, vibration, and oscillation as appropriate (Gosselink et al, 2008).
- • Observe sputum, noting color, odor, and volume. *Normal sputum is clear or gray and minimal; abnormal sputum is green, yellow, or bloody; malodorous; and often copious. The presence of purulent sputum during a COPD exacerbation can be sufficient indication for starting empirical antibiotic treatment. Notify health care provider of purulent sputum (GOLD, 2015).*

Critical Care

- ▲ In intubated patients, body positioning and mobilization may optimize airway secretion clearance. An early mobility and walking program can promote weaning from ventilator support as a patient's overall strength and endurance improve (Gosselink et al, 2008; Perme & Chandrashekar, 2009).
- ▲ *Early mobility and physical rehabilitation can reduce muscle weakness, mechanical ventilation duration, intensive care unit stay, and hospital stay (Mendez-Tellez & Needham, 2012; Spruit et al, 2013). The Awakening and Breathing Coordination, Delirium Monitoring and Management, and Early Mobility (ABCDE) bundle has criteria to determine when patients are candidates for early mobility (Balas et al, 2012).* An early mobility and walking program can promote weaning from ventilator support as a patient's overall strength and endurance improve (Gosselink et al, 2008; Perme & Chandrashekar, 2009).
- • If the client is intubated and is stable, consider getting the client up to sit at the edge of the bed, transfer to a chair, or walk as appropriate, if an effective interdisciplinary team is developed to keep the client safe. *For every week of bedrest, muscle strength can decrease 20%; early ambulation also helped patients develop a positive outlook (Perme & Chandrashekar, 2009).*
- ▲ If the client is intubated, consider use of kinetic therapy, using a kinetic bed that slowly moves the client with 40-degree turns. *Rotational therapy may decrease the incidence of pulmonary complications in high-risk patients with increasing ventilator support requirements, who are at risk for ventilator-associated pneumonia, and with clinical indications for acute lung injury or acute respiratory distress syndrome with worsening $Pa{O_2}:FI{O_2}$ ratio, presence of fluffy infiltrates via chest radiograph concomitant with pulmonary edema, and refractory hypoxemia (Bein et al, 2012).*
- • Reposition the client as needed. Use rotational or kinetic bed therapy in clients for whom side-to-side turning is contraindicated or difficult. EBN: *Changing position frequently decreases the incidence of atelectasis, pooling of secretions, and resultant pneumonia (Burns, 2011).* EB/EBN: *Continuous, lateral rotational therapy has been shown to improve oxygenation and decrease the incidence of VAP (Burns, 2011).*
- • When suctioning an endotracheal tube or tracheostomy tube for a client on a ventilator, do the following:

- Explain the process of suctioning beforehand and ensure the client is not in pain or overly anxious. *Suctioning can be a frightening experience; an explanation along with adequate pain relief or needed sedation can reduce stress, anxiety, and pain (Chulay & Seckel, 2011).*
- Hyperoxygenate before and between endotracheal suction sessions. *Studies have demonstrated that hyperoxygenation may help prevent oxygen desaturation in a suctioned client (Chulay & Seckel, 2011; Pedersen et al, 2009; Siela, 2010).*
- Suction for less than 15 seconds. *Studies demonstrated that because of a drop in the partial pressure of oxygen with suctioning, that preferably no more than 10 seconds be used actually suctioning, with the entire procedure taking 15 seconds (Chulay & Seckel, 2011; Pedersen et al, 2009).*
- Use a closed, in-line suction system. Closed in-line suctioning has minimal effects on heart rate, respiratory rate, tidal volume, and oxygen saturation (Chulay & Seckel, 2011; Seymour et al, 2009).
- Avoid saline instillation during suctioning. EBN: *Repeated studies have demonstrated that saline instillation before suctioning has an adverse effect on oxygen saturation in both adults and children (Chulay & Seckel, 2011; Rauen et al, 2008; Pederson et al, 2009; Siela, 2010).*
- *Use of a subglottic suctioning endotracheal tube reduces the incidence of ventilator-associated pneumonia (VAP) or ventilator-associated complications (Hass et al, 2014).*
- *Use of nonstick endotracheal tubes can reduce the formation of biofilm and hence VAP (Haas et al, 2014).*
- Document results of coughing and suctioning, particularly client tolerance and secretion characteristics such as color, odor, and volume (Chulay & Seckel, 2011).

Pediatric

- Educate parents about the risk factors for ineffective airway clearance such as foreign body ingestion and passive smoke exposure.
- See the care plan Risk for **Suffocation** for more interventions on choking. EB: *Passive smoke exposure significantly increases the risk of respiratory infections in children (Chatzimicael et al, 2008).*
- Educate children and parents on the importance of adherence to peak expiratory flow monitoring for asthma self-management.
- Educate parents and other caregivers that cough and cold medication bought over the counter are not safe for a child younger than 2 unless specifically ordered by a health care provider. *Over-the-counter cold and cough medications are no longer recommended for children younger than age 2 unless recommended by a health care provider. Minimal data exist to support their effectiveness, and overuse can cause harm (Woo, 2008).*

Geriatric

- Encourage ambulation as tolerated without causing exhaustion. *Immobility is often harmful to older adults because it decreases ventilation and increases stasis of secretions, leading to atelectasis or pneumonia.*
- Actively encourage older adults to deep breathe and cough. *Cough reflexes are blunted, and coughing is decreased in older adults.*
- Ensure adequate hydration within cardiac and renal reserves. *Older adults are prone to dehydration and therefore more viscous secretions, because they frequently use diuretics or laxatives and forget to drink adequate amounts of water.*

Home Care

- Some of the above interventions may be adapted for home care use.
- ▲ Begin discharge planning as soon as possible with case manager or social worker to assess need for home support systems, assistive devices, and community or home health services.
- Assess home environment for factors that exacerbate airway clearance problems (e.g., presence of allergens, lack of adequate humidity in air, poor air flow, stressful family relationships).
- Assess affective climate within family and family support system. *Problems with respiratory function and resulting anxiety can provoke anger and frustration in the client. Feelings may be displaced onto caregiver and require intervention to ensure continued caregiver support.* Refer to care plan for **Caregiver Role Strain.**
- Refer to GOLD guidelines for management of home care and indications of hospital admission criteria. http://www.goldcopd.org/.

- When respiratory procedures are being implemented, explain equipment and procedures to family members and caregivers, and provide needed emotional support. *Family members assuming responsibility for respiratory monitoring often find this stressful. They may not have been able to assimilate fully any instructions provided by hospital staff.*
- When electrically based equipment for respiratory support is being implemented, evaluate home environment for electrical safety, proper grounding, and so on. Ensure that notification is sent to the local utility company, the emergency medical team, and police and fire departments.
- Provide family with support for care of a client with chronic or terminal illness. *Breathing difficulty can provoke extreme anxiety, which can interfere with the client's ability or willingness to adhere to the treatment plan.*
- Refer to care plan for **Anxiety.** *Witnessing breathing difficulties and facing concerns of dealing with chronic or terminal illness can create fear in caregiver. Fear inhibits effective coping.* Refer to care plan for **Powerlessness.**
- Instruct the client to avoid exposure to persons with upper respiratory infections, to avoid crowds of people, and wash hands after each exposure to groups of people, or public places.

▲ Determine client adherence to medical regimen. Instruct the client and family in importance of reporting effectiveness of current medications to health care provider. *Inappropriate use of medications (too much or too little) can influence amount of respiratory secretions.*

- Teach the client when and how to use inhalant or nebulizer treatments at home.
- Teach the client/family importance of maintaining regimen and having "as-needed" drugs easily accessible at all times. *Success in avoiding emergency or institutional care may rest solely on medication compliance or availability.*
- Instruct the client and family in the importance of maintaining proper nutrition, adequate fluids, rest, and behavioral pacing for energy conservation and rehabilitation.
- Instruct in use of dietary supplements as indicated. *Illness may suppress appetite, leading to inadequate nutrition. Supplements will allow clients to eat with minimal energy consumption.*
- Identify an emergency plan, including criteria for use. *Ineffective airway clearance can be life-threatening.*

▲ Refer for home health aide services for assistance with activities of daily living (ADLs). *Clients with decreased oxygenation and copious respiratory secretions are often unable to maintain energy for ADLs.*

▲ Assess family for role changes and coping skills. Refer to medical social services as necessary. *Clients with decreased oxygenation are unable to maintain role activities and therefore experience frustration and anger, which may pose a threat to family integrity. Family counseling to adapt to role changes may be needed.*

▲ For the client dying at home with a terminal illness, if the "death rattle" is present with gurgling, rattling, or crackling sounds in the airway with each breath, recognize that anticholinergic medications can often help control symptoms, if given early in the process. *Anticholinergic medications can help decrease the accumulation of secretions, but do not decrease existing secretions. This medication must be administered early in the process to be effective (Hipp & Letizia, 2009; Fielding & Long, 2014).*

▲ For the client with a death rattle, nursing care includes turning to mobilize secretions, keeping the head of the bed elevated for postural drainage of secretions, and avoiding suctioning. *Suctioning is a distressing and painful event for clients and families, and is rarely effective in decreasing the death rattle (Hipp & Letizia, 2009; Fielding & Long, 2014).*

Client/Family Teaching and Discharge Planning

▲ Teach the importance of not smoking. Refer to a smoking cessation program, and encourage clients who relapse to keep trying to quit. Ensure that the client receives appropriate medications to support smoking cessation from the primary health care provider. EB: *A systemic review of research demonstrated that the combination of medications and an intensive, prolonged counseling program supporting smoking cessation were effective in promoting long-term abstinence from smoking (Fiore et al, 2008). A Cochrane review found that use of the antidepressant medications increased the rate of smoking withdrawal two to three times more than smoking withdrawal without use of medications (Hughes et al, 2014).*

▲ Teach the client how to use a flutter clearance device if ordered, which vibrates to loosen mucus and gives positive pressure to keep airways open (Bhowmik et al, 2009; Gosselink et al, 2008). CEB: *A study demonstrated that use of the mucus clearance device had improved exercise performance compared with COPD clients who use a sham device (Wolkove et al, 2004). A Cochrane review found that there was no clear evidence that oscillation was more or less effective than other forms of physiotherapy for airway clearance in cystic fibrosis (Morrison & Agnew, 2009).*

▲ Teach the client how to use peak expiratory flow rate (PEFR) meter if ordered and when to seek medical attention if PEFR reading drops. Also teach how to use metered dose inhalers and self-administer inhaled corticosteroids as ordered following precautions to decrease side effects.

- Teach the client how to deep breathe and cough effectively. CEB: *Controlled coughing uses the diaphragmatic muscles, making the cough more forceful and effective (Gosselink et al, 2008).*
- Teach the client/family to identify and avoid specific factors that exacerbate ineffective airway clearance, including known allergens and especially smoking (if relevant) or exposure to secondhand smoke.
- Educate the client and family about the significance of changes in sputum characteristics, including color, character, amount, and odor. *With this knowledge, the client and family can identify early the signs of infection and seek treatment before acute illness occurs.*
- Teach the client/family the importance of taking antibiotics as prescribed, consuming all tablets until the prescription has run out. *Taking the entire course of antibiotics helps eradicate bacterial infection, which decreases lingering, chronic infection.*
- Teach the family of the dying client in hospice with a death rattle that rarely are clients aware of the fluid that has accumulated, and help them find evidence of comfort in the client's nonverbal behavior (Hipp & Letizia, 2009; Fielding & Long, 2014).

REFERENCES

Balas, M. C., Vasilevskis, E. E., Burke, W. J., et al. (2012). Critical care nurses' role in implementing the "ABCDE Bundle" into practice. *Critical Care Nurse, 32*(2), 35–38, 40–48.

Barnett, M. (2008). Nursing management of chronic obstructive pulmonary disease. *British Journal of Nursing, 17*(21), 1314–1318.

Bein, T., Zimmermann, M., Schiewe-Laggartner, F., et al. (2012). Continuous lateral rotation therapy and systematic inflammatory response in posttraumatic acute lung injury: Results from a prospective randomized study. *Injury, 43*, 1893–1897.

Bell, L. (2011). AACN Practice Alert-Prevention of Aspiration. *American Association of Critical Care Nurses*. Retrieved from <http://www.aacn.org/wd/practice/docs/practicealerts/prevention-aspiration-practice-alert.pdf?menu=aboutus>.

Bhowmik, A., Chahal, K., & Austin, G. (2009). Improving mucociliary clearance in chronic obstructive pulmonary disease. *Respiratory Medicine, 103*(4), 496–502.

Bickley, L. S., & Szilagyi, P. (2012). *Bate's Guide to physical examination* (p. 11). Philadelphia: Lippincott, Williams and Wilkins.

Burns, S. M. (2011). Invasive Mechanical Ventilation (Through an artificial airway): volume and pressure modes. In D. J. Lynn-McHale (Ed.), *AACN Procedure Manual for Critical Care* (6th ed.). Philadelphia: Saunders Elsevier.

Chatzimicael, A., Tsalkidis, A., & Cassimos, D. (2008). Effect of passive smoking on lung function and respiratory infection. *Indian Journal of Pediatrics, 75*(4), 335–340.

Chulay, M., & Seckel, M. (2011). Suctioning: Endotracheal tube or tracheostomy tube. In D. J. Lynn-McHale (Ed.), *AACN Procedure Manual for Critical Care* (6th ed.). Philadelphia: Saunders Elsevier.

Fauci, A., Braunwald, E., & Kasper, D. L. (2008). *Harrison's principles of internal medicine* (17th ed.). New York: McGraw-Hill.

Fielding, F., & Long, C. O. (2014). The death rattle dilemma. *J of Hospice & Palliative Nursing, 16*(8). Retrieved <http://www.medscape.com/viewarticle/834898>.

Fiore, M. C., Jaen, C. R., & Baker, T. B. (2008). *Treating tobacco use and dependence clinical practice guideline 2008 update*. Rockville MD: U.S. Department of Health and Human Services, Public Health Service.

GOLD. Global strategy for the diagnosis, management, and prevention of COPD (revised 2015), *Global Initiative for Chronic Obstructive Lung Disease*. http://www.goldcopd.org/uploads/users/files/GOLD_Report_2015_Apr2.pdf. Retrieved April 23, 2015.

Gosselink, R., Bott, J., Johnson, M., et al. (2008). Physiotherapy for adult patients with critical illness: recommendations of the European respiratory society and European society of critical care medicine task force on physiotherapy for critically ill patients. *Intensive Care Medicine, 34*(7), 1188–1199.

Haas, C. F., Eakin, R. M., Konkle, M. A., et al. (2014). Endotracheal tubes: old and new. *Respiratory Care, 59*(6), 933–955.

Hipp, B., & Letizia, M. J. (2009). Understanding and responding to the death rattle in dying patients. *Medsurg Nursing, 18*(1), 17–21.

Hughes, J. R., Stead, L. F., Hartmann-Boyce, J., et al. (2014). Antidepressants for smoking cessation. *Cochrane Database of Systematic Reviews*, 2014, (1), Art. No.: CD000031.

Joanna Briggs Institute (2014). *Ventilator-associated pneumonia prevention*.

Mendez-Tellez, P. A., & Needham, D. M. (2012). Early physical rehabilitation in the ICU and ventilator liberation. *Respiratory Care, 57*(10), 1663–1669.

Morrison, L., & Agnew, J. (2009). Oscillating devices for airway clearance in people with cystic fibrosis. *Cochrane Database Systematic Review*, (1), CD006842.

Pedersen, C. M., Rosendahl-Nielsen, M., Hjermind, J., et al. (2009). Endotracheal suctioning of the adult intubated patient—what is the evidence? *Intensive and Critical Care Nursing, 25*(1), 21–30.

Perme, C., & Chandrashekar, R. (2009). Early mobility and walking program for patients in intensive care units: creating a standard of care. *American Journal of Critical Care, 18*(3), 212–220.

Rauen, C. A., Chulay, M., Bridges, E., et al. (2008). Seven evidence-based practice habits: putting some sacred cows out to pasture. *Critical Care Nurse, 28*(2), 98–123.

Schultz, S. (2011). Oxygen saturation monitoring with pulse oximetry. In E. Lynn-McHale Weigand (Ed.), *AACN Procedure Manual for Critical Care* (6th ed.). Phildelphia, PA: Saunders Elsevier.

Seymour, C., Cross, B., & Cooke, C. (2009). Physiologic impact of closed-system endotracheal suctioning in spontaneously breathing patients receiving mechanical ventilation. *Respiratory Care, 54*(3), 367–374.

Siela, D. (2010). Evaluation standards for management of artificial airways. *Critical Care Nurse, 30*(4), 76–78.

Spruit, M. A., Singh, S. J., Garvey, C., et al. (2013). An official American Thoracic Society/European Respiratory Society Statement: Key concepts and advances in pulmonary rehabilitation.

A

American Journal of Respiratory and Critical Care Medicine, 188(8), e13–e64.

Wolkove, N., et al. (2004). A randomized trial to evaluate the sustained efficacy of a mucus clearance device in ambulatory patients with chronic obstructive pulmonary disease. *Canadian Respiratory Journal: Journal of the Canadian Thoracic Society, 11*(8), 567–572.

Wong, M., & Elliott, M. (2009). The use of medical orders in acute care oxygen therapy. *British Journal of Nursing, 18*(8), 462–464.

Woo, T. (2008). Pharmacology of cough and cold medicines. *Journal of Pediatric Health Care, 22*(2), 73–79.

Risk for Allergy response

Gail B. Ladwig, MSN, RN, and Marina Martinez-Kratz, MS, RN, CNE

NANDA-I

Definition

Vulnerable to exaggerated immune response or reaction to substances which may compromise health

Risk Factors

Allergy to insect sting; exposure to allergen (e.g., pharmaceutical agent); exposure to environmental allergen (e.g., dander, dust, mold, pollen); exposure to toxic chemical; food allergy (e.g., avocado, banana, chestnut, kiwi, peanut, shellfish, mushroom, tropical fruit); repeated exposure to allergen-producing environmental substance

NOC Outcomes (Nursing Outcomes Classification)

Suggested NOC Outcomes

Allergic Response: Systemic; Immune Hypersensitivity Response; Knowledge: Health Behavior, Risk Control, Risk Detection; Tissue Integrity: Skin and Mucous Membranes

Example NOC Outcome with Indicators

Immune Hypersensitivity Response as evidenced by the following indicators: Respiratory, cardiac, gastrointestinal, renal and neurological function status IER/Free of allergic reactions. (Rate each indicator of **Immune Hypersensitivity Response:** 1 = not controlled, 2 = slightly controlled, 3 = moderately controlled, 4 = well controlled, 5 = very well controlled [see Section I].) IER, In expected range.

Client Outcomes

Client Will (Specify Time Frame)

- State risk factors for allergies
- Demonstrate knowledge of plan to treat allergic reaction

NIC Interventions (Nursing Interventions Classification)

Suggested NIC Interventions

Allergy Management; Environmental Risk Protection

Example NIC Activity

Place an allergy band on client

Nursing Interventions and *Rationales*

- A careful history is important in detecting allergens and avoidance of allergen. EB: *Spice allergy is rare but spices are widely used and may be in cosmetics. The diagnoses depend on a good history and well-designed testing; treatment is strict avoidance (Chen & Bahna, 2011). Food allergy is among the most common of the allergic disorders. If food allergy or lactose intolerance is suspected, workup should include a detailed allergy-focused clinical history to determine whether the adverse reaction is typically an immediate*

(IgE-mediated) or more delayed-type (non–IgE-mediated) allergic reaction, or whether it may be lactose intolerance, a form of nonallergic hypersensitivity (Waddell, 2011).

- • Obtain a precise history of allergies, as well as medications taken and foods ingested before surgery. EBN: *A thorough nursing assessment of allergies supports and improves the plan of care by identifying the patient's risk factors (Cochico, 2012).*
- ▲ Teach the client about correct use of the injectable epinephrine and have the client do a return demonstration. EB: *Recent research on the correct use of the injectable epinephrine showed that 84% of the patients were unable to do correctly (Bonds et al, 2015).*
- ▲ Carefully assess the client for allergies. Below is information that is important for clients with allergies. Refer for immediate treatment if anaphylaxis is suspected.

Causes

Common allergens include animal dander; bee stings or stings from other insects; foods, especially nuts, fish, and shellfish; insect bites; medications; plants; pollens

Symptoms

Common symptoms of a mild allergic reaction include hives (especially over the neck and face), itching, nasal congestion, rashes, watery, red eyes

Symptoms of a moderate or severe reaction include cramps or pain in the abdomen, chest discomfort or tightness, diarrhea, difficulty breathing, difficulty swallowing, dizziness or lightheadedness, fear or feeling of apprehension or anxiety, flushing or redness of the face, nausea and vomiting, palpitations, swelling of the face, eyes, or tongue, weakness, wheezing, unconsciousness

First Aid

For a mild to moderate reaction: Calm and reassure the person having the reaction, because anxiety can worsen symptoms.

1. Try to identify the allergen and have the person avoid further contact with it. If the allergic reaction is from a bee sting, scrape the stinger off the skin with something firm (e.g., fingernail or plastic credit card). Do not use tweezers; squeezing the stinger will release more venom.
2. Apply cool compresses and over-the-counter hydrocortisone cream for itchy rash.
3. Watch for signs of increasing distress.
4. Get medical help. For a mild reaction, a health care provider may recommend over-the-counter medications (e.g., antihistamines).

For a Severe Allergic Reaction (Anaphylaxis)

1. Check the person's airway, breathing, and circulation (the ABCs of Basic Life Support). A warning sign of dangerous throat swelling is a very hoarse or whispered voice, or coarse sounds when the person is breathing in air. If necessary, begin rescue breathing and cardiopulmonary resuscitation.
2. Call 911.
3. Calm and reassure the person.
4. If the allergic reaction is from a bee sting, scrape the stinger off the skin with something firm (e.g., fingernail or plastic credit card). Do not use tweezers; squeezing the stinger will release more venom.
5. If the person has emergency allergy medication on hand, help the person take or inject the medication. Avoid oral medication if the person is having difficulty breathing.
6. Take steps to prevent shock. Have the person lie flat, raise the person's feet about 12 inches, and cover him or her with a coat or blanket. Do NOT place the person in this position if a head, neck, back, or leg injury is suspected or if it causes discomfort.

Do NOT

- Do NOT assume that any allergy shots the person has already received will provide complete protection.
- Do NOT place a pillow under the person's head if he or she is having trouble breathing. This can block the airways.
- Do NOT give the person anything by mouth if the person is having trouble breathing.

When to Contact a Medical Professional

Call for immediate medical emergency assistance if:

- The person is having a severe allergic reaction—always call 911. Do not wait to see if the reaction is getting worse.
- The person has a history of severe allergic reactions (check for a medical ID tag).

Prevention

Avoid triggers such as foods and medications that have caused an allergic reaction (even a mild one) in the past. Ask detailed questions about ingredients when you are eating away from home. Carefully examine ingredient labels.

- If you have a child who is allergic to certain foods, introduce one new food at a time in small amounts so you can recognize an allergic reaction.
- People who know that they have had serious allergic reactions should wear a medical ID tag.
- Preoperative patients should be closely assessed for allergies to soybeans and eggs. EBN: *Allergies to soybeans and eggs contraindicate the use of propofol, a short-acting hypnotic commonly used in anesthesia (Cochico, 2012).*

▲ If you have a history of serious allergic reactions, carry emergency medications (e.g., a chewable form of diphenhydramine and injectable epinephrine or a bee sting kit) according to your health care provider's instructions.

- Do not use your injectable epinephrine on anyone else. They may have a condition (e.g., a heart problem) that could be negatively affected by this drug. EB: *Although first-time exposure may only produce a mild reaction, repeated exposures may lead to more serious reactions. Once a person has had an exposure or an allergic reaction (is sensitized), even a very limited exposure to a very small amount of allergen can trigger a severe reaction. Most severe allergic reactions occur within seconds or minutes after exposure to the allergen. However, some reactions can occur after several hours, particularly if the allergen causes a reaction after it has been eaten. In very rare cases, reactions develop after 24 hours.*
- *Anaphylaxis is a sudden and severe allergic reaction that occurs within minutes of exposure. Immediate medical attention is needed for this condition. Without treatment, anaphylaxis can get worse very quickly and lead to death within 15 minutes (Medline Plus, 2012).*

▲ Refer the client for skin testing to confirm IgE-mediated allergic response. EB: *Identifying clients who are less sensitive is important, so that they can be started on immunotherapy. An informal survey of low-reacting clients treated with immunotherapy showed a high degree of success (Boyles & John, 2011). Allergy testing serves to confirm an allergic trigger suspected on the basis of history (Sicherer & Wood, 2012).*

- See care plans for **Latex Allergy** response and Risk for **Latex Allergy** response.

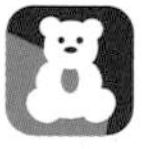

Pediatric

▲ Teach parents and children with allergies to peanuts and tree nuts to avoid them and to identify them. EB: *Dietary avoidance is the primary management of these allergies and requires the ability to identify peanuts or tree nuts. Treatment of nut allergies with dietary avoidance should include education for both adults and children on identification of peanuts and tree nuts (Hostetler et al, 2012).*

▲ Teach parents and children with asthma about modifiable risk factors, which include allergy triggers. EB: *Attention to these allergy triggers will improve asthma control and reduce the burden of disease (Schatz, 2012).*

▲ Counsel parents to limit infant exposure to traffic-related air pollution. EB: *Recent research demonstrates that higher traffic-related air pollution exposure during infancy was associated with higher hyperactivity scores in children (Newman et al, 2013).*

▲ Suspect FPIES (food protein-induced enterocolitis syndrome) in formula-fed infants with repetitive emesis, diarrhea, dehydration, and lethargy 1 to 5 hours after ingesting the offending food (the most common are cow's milk, soy, and rice). Remove the offending food. EB: *Early recognition of FPIES and removal of the offending food is important to prevent misdiagnosis and mismanagement of symptoms from other causes. Close follow-up is required to determine when foods may be added back into the diet. FPIES typically occurs before 6 months of age. Diagnosis is made by history and physician-supervised oral food challenges (Leonard & Nowak-Wegrzyn, 2011).*

▲ Children should be screened for seafood allergies and avoid seafood and any foods containing seafood if an allergy is detected. EB: *Seafood allergy is now a leading cause of anaphylaxis in both the United States and Australia. This study confirmed a seafood as common and important cause of food allergy in Australian children, presenting with a high rate of anaphylaxis (Turner et al, 2011).*

REFERENCES

Bonds, R. S., Asawa, A., & Ghazi, A. I. (2015). Misuse of medical devices: a persistent problem in self-management of asthma and allergic disease. *Annals of Allergy, Asthma and Immunology*, *114*(1), 74–76.e2.

Boyles, J. H., Jr., & John, H. (2011). A comparison of techniques for evaluating IgE-mediated allergies. *ENT: Ear Nose Throat J*, *90*(4), 164–169.

Chen, J. L., & Bahna, S. (2011). Spice allergy. *Annals of Allergy, Asthma and Immunology*, *107*(3), 191–199.

Cochico, S. G. (2012). Propofol allergy: assessing for patient risks. *AORN Journal*, *96*(4), 398–408.

Hostetler, T. L., et al. (2012). The ability of adults and children to visually identify peanuts and tree nuts. *Annals of Allergy, Asthma and Immunology*, *108*(1), 25–29.

Leonard, S. A., & Nowak-Wegrzyn, A. (2011). Food protein-induced enterocolitis syndrome: an update on natural history and review of management. *Annals of Allergy, Asthma and Immunology*, *107*(2), 95–100.

Medline Plus. *Allergic reactions: causes, symptoms, first aid, prevention.* Retrieved May 2012 from <http://www.nlm.nih.gov/medlineplus/ency/article/000005.htm>.

Newman, N. C., Ryan, P., LeMasters, G., et al. (2013). Traffic-Related Air Pollution Exposure in the First Year of Life and Behavioral Scores at 7 Years of Age. *Environmental Health Perspectives*, *121*(6), 731–737.

Schatz, M. (2012). Predictors of asthma control: what can we modify? *Current Opinion In Allergy & Clinical Immunology*, *12*(3), 263–268.

Sicherer, S., & Wood, R. (2012). Allergy testing in childhood: using allergen-specific IgE tests. *Pediatrics*, *129*(1), 193–197.

Turner, P., et al. (2011). Seafood allergy in children: a descriptive study. *Annals of Allergy, Asthma and Immunology*, *106*(6), 494–501.

Waddell, L. (2011). Living with food allergy. *The Journal of Family Health Care*, *21*(4), 21–28.

Anxiety

Ruth McCaffrey, DNP, ARNP, FNP-BC, GNP-BC, FAAN

NANDA-I

Definition

Vague, uneasy feeling of discomfort or dread accompanied by an autonomic response (the source often nonspecific or unknown to the individual); a feeling of apprehension caused by anticipation of danger. It is an alerting sign that warns of impending danger and enables the individual to take measures to deal with threat

Defining Characteristics

Behavioral

Decrease in productivity; extraneous movement; fidgeting; glancing about; hypervigilance; insomnia; poor eye contact; restlessness; scanning behavior; worry about change in life event

Affective

Anguish; apprehensiveness; distress; fear; feelings of inadequacy; helplessness; increase in wariness; irritability; jitteriness; overexcitement; rattled; regretful; self-focused; uncertain; worried

Physiological

Facial tension; hand tremors; increased perspiration; increased tension; shakiness; trembling; voice quivering

Sympathetic

Alteration in respiratory pattern; anorexia; brisk reflexes; cardiovascular excitation; diarrhea; dry mouth; facial flushing; heart palpitations; increase in blood pressure; increase in heart rate; increase in respiratory rate; pupil dilation; superficial vasoconstriction; twitching; weakness

Parasympathetic

Abdominal pain; alteration in sleep pattern; decrease in heart rate; decreased blood pressure; diarrhea; faintness; fatigue; nausea; tingling in extremities; urinary frequency; urinary hesitancy; urinary urgency

Cognitive

Alteration in attention; alteration in concentration; awareness of physiological symptoms; blocking of thoughts; confusion; decrease in perceptual field; diminished ability to learn; diminished ability to problem solve; fear; forgetfulness; preoccupation; rumination; tendency to blame others

A

Related Factors (r/t)

Conflict about life goals; exposure to toxin; family history of anxiety; heredity; interpersonal contagion; interpersonal transmission; major change (e.g., economic status, environment, health status, role function, role status); maturational crisis; situational crisis; stressors; substance abuse; threat of death; threat to current status; unmet needs; value conflict

NOC (Nursing Outcomes Classification)

Suggested NOC Outcomes

Aggression Self-Restraint; Anxiety Level; Anxiety Self-Control; Coping; Impulse Self-Control

Example NOC Outcome with Indicators

Anxiety Self-Control as evidenced by the following indicators: Eliminates precursors of anxiety/Monitors physical manifestations of anxiety/Controls anxiety response (Rate the outcome and indicators of **Anxiety Self-Control:** 1 = never demonstrated, 2 = rarely demonstrated, 3 = sometimes demonstrated, 4 = often demonstrated, 5 = consistently demonstrated [see Section I].)

Client Outcomes

Client Will (Specify Time Frame)

- Identify and verbalize symptoms of anxiety
- Identify, verbalize, and demonstrate techniques to control anxiety
- Verbalize absence of or decrease in subjective distress
- Have vital signs that reflect baseline or decreased sympathetic stimulation
- Have posture, facial expressions, gestures, and activity levels that reflect decreased distress
- Demonstrate improved concentration and accuracy of thoughts
- Demonstrate return of basic problem-solving skills
- Demonstrate increased external focus
- Demonstrate some ability to reassure self

NIC (Nursing Interventions Classification)

Suggested NIC Intervention

Anxiety Reduction

Example NIC Activities—Anxiety Reduction

Use calm, reassuring approach; Explain all procedures, including sensations likely to be experienced during the procedure

Nursing Interventions and *Rationales*

- Assess the client's level of anxiety and physical reactions to anxiety (e.g., tachycardia, tachypnea, nonverbal expressions of anxiety). Consider using the Hamilton Anxiety Scale, which grades 14 symptoms on a scale of 0 (not present) to 4 (very severe). Symptoms evaluated are mood, tension, fear, insomnia, concentration, worry, depressed mood, somatic complaints, and cardiovascular, respiratory, gastrointestinal, genitourinary, autonomic, and behavioral symptoms. EBN: *Generalized anxiety disorder (GAD) is the most common anxiety with a 12-month prevalence of 3.1% in population-based survey and between 5.3% and 7.6% among patients who visit primary care offices. The highest rate of GAD (7.7%) occurs in persons 45 to 49 years of age, and the lowest rate (3.6%) occurs in persons 60 years and older. Women are almost twice as likely as men to be diagnosed with GAD over their lifetime (Kavan et al, 2009).*
- Rule out withdrawal from alcohol, sedatives, or smoking as the cause of anxiety. EB: *Military personnel sent to war zones have higher levels of depression that are often exacerbated by alcohol and sedative use (Gale et al, 2010). When withdrawing from either sedatives or alcohol, participants in this study demonstrated elevated levels of anxiety and nervousness (McCabe et al, 2011).*
- Use empathy to encourage the client to interpret the anxiety symptoms as normal. EBN: *The way a nurse interacts with a client influences his/her quality of life. Providing psychological and social support can reduce*

A

the symptoms and problems associated with anxiety (Wagner & Bear, 2009). In another study, patients undergoing couples therapy felt significantly more trust and responded with more success to those therapists who provided empathetic and compassionate responses and suggestions (Benson et al, 2012).

- If irrational thoughts or fears are present, offer the client accurate information and encourage him or her to talk about the meaning of the events contributing to the anxiety. EBN: *In one study providing cancer patients with accurate information about their disease, prognosis and outcomes significantly reduced their anxiety and increased empowerment (Lauzier et al, 2014).*
- Encourage the client to use positive self-talk. EBN: *Reducing negative self-talk and increasing positive self-talk can be beneficial for all types of anxiety (Hill, 2010). One research study showed that self-talk strengthens both actual behavior performance and prospective behavioral intentions (Dolcos & Albarracin, 2014).*
- Intervene when possible to remove sources of anxiety. EBN: *Removing or reducing sources of stress and anxiety among clients has been shown to decrease hypertension and comorbid conditions (Lobjanidze et al, 2010).*
- Explain all activities, procedures, and issues that involve the client; use nonmedical terms and calm, slow speech. Do this in advance of procedures when possible, and validate the client's understanding. EBN: *In one study, preoperative information reduced the anxiety of clients undergoing surgery under regional anesthesia (Jiala et al, 2010).*

▲ Use massage therapy to reduce anxiety. EBN: *Massage was shown to be an excellent method for reducing anxiety (Labrique-Walusis et al, 2010).*

▲ Consider massage therapy for preoperative clients. EBN: *Patients were highly satisfied with massage, and no major barriers to implementing massage therapy were identified. Massage therapy may be an important component of the healing experience for patients after cardiovascular surgery (Sutshall et al, 2010).*

- Use therapeutic touch and healing touch techniques. EBN: *One study showed that Reiki therapeutic touch reduced anxiety and pain (Sagkal, et al, 2013).*
- Use guided imagery to decrease anxiety. EBN: *Anxiety was decreased with the use of guided imagery during an intervention for postoperative pain (Thomas & Sethares, 2010).*
- Suggest yoga to the client. EB: *Yoga and massage lessened anxiety in burn patients (Parlak et al, 2010). Seven days' intensive residential yoga program reduces pain, anxiety, and depression, and improves spinal mobility in lower back pain (Tekur et al, 2012).*
- Provide clients with a means to listen to music of their choice or audiotapes. EBN: *Music can provide an effective method of reducing potentially harmful physiological responses arising from anxiety (Korhan et al, 2011). Among ICU patients receiving acute ventilatory support for respiratory failure, patient directed music resulted in greater reduction in anxiety compared with usual care, but not compared with NCH (noise cancelling headphones). Concurrently, patient directed music resulted in greater reduction in sedation frequency compared with usual care (Chlan et al, 2013).*

Pediatric

- The above interventions may be adapted for the pediatric client.

Geriatric

▲ Monitor the client for depression. Use appropriate interventions and referrals. EB: *GAD is a common and disabling disorder in later life that is highly comorbid with mood, anxiety, and personality disorders; psychiatric comorbidity is associated with an increased risk for medical conditions in this population. Considering that late-life GAD is associated with impaired quality of life but low levels of professional help-seeking, increased effort is needed to help individuals with this disorder to access effective treatments (Mackenzie et al, 2011).*

- Older adults report less worry than younger adults. EB: *Generalized anxiety disorder is a common diagnosis in older adults (Heinz et al, 2011).*
- Observe for adverse changes if antianxiety drugs are taken. EB: *Older adults are notably vulnerable to adverse drug reactions, particularly during unexpected hospitalizations (Bilyeu et al, 2011).*
- Mindfulness meditation is successful in mediating anxiety. EBN: *Mediation analyses indicated that mindfulness fully mediated changes in acute anxiety symptoms, and partially mediated changes in worry and trait anxiety. These researchers concluded that mindful based stress reduction exercises are an effective treatment for anxiety disorders and related symptoms (Vollestad et al, 2011).*

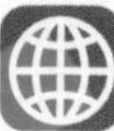

Multicultural

- Assess for the presence of culture-bound anxiety states. EBN: *Prevalence and expression of social anxiety/seasonal affective disorder (SAD) depends on the particular culture. Asian cultures typically show the lowest rates, whereas Russian and United States samples show the highest rates, of SAD (Hoffman et al, 2010).*
- Identify how anxiety is manifested in the culturally diverse client. EBN: *Clinical presentation of anxiety disorders, with respect to symptom presentation and the interpretation of symptoms, varies across cultures. A difference in catastrophic cognitions about anxiety symptoms across cultures is hypothesized to be a key aspect of cross-cultural variation in the anxiety disorders (Marques et al, 2011).*
- For diverse clients experiencing preoperative anxiety, provide music of their choice. EBN: *This exploratory study demonstrated the positive impact of live music as a holistic patient intervention directed toward reducing pain, anxiety, and muscle tension during the preoperative, intraoperative, and postoperative periods (Sand-Jecklin & Emerson, 2010).*

Home Care

- The above interventions may be adapted for home care use.
- ▲ Assess for suicidal ideation. Implement emergency plan as indicated. EBN: *Suicidal ideation may occur in response to co-occurring depression or a sense of hopelessness over severe anxiety symptoms or once antidepressant medications have been started (Mitchell et al, 2009).* See care plan for Risk for **Suicide.**
- Assess for influence of anxiety on medical regimen. EBN: *Anxiety can affect a patient's ability to complete their medical regimen as prescribed, including taking medications, exercise, diet, and follow up therapies (Hynninen et al, 2010).*
- Assess for presence of depression. EBN: *Clinician report generally had the most favorable sensitivity and specificity for measuring depressive symptoms and treatment recommendations, respectively (Henry et al, 2014).*
- Assist family to be supportive of the client in the face of anxiety symptoms. EBN: *Supporting the formal and information caregivers of a patient with anxiety as well as the patient may improve overall patient outcomes and allows the family to fully understand the problems the patient is experiencing (Kang et al, 2011).*
- ▲ Consider referral for the prescription of antianxiety or antidepressant medications for clients who have panic disorder (PD) or other anxiety-related psychiatric disorders. EBN: *The use of antidepressants, especially SSRI medications, is effective in many cases of anxiety (Katzman, 2009).*
- ▲ Assist the client/family to institute medication regimen appropriately. Instruct in side effects, importance of taking medications as ordered, and effects to report immediately to health care provider. EBN: *Patient interviews revealed that patients' values and beliefs, barriers to treatment, and prior medication-taking behavior were of primary importance in understanding medication discontinuance (Garavalia et al, 2011).*
- ▲ Refer for psychiatric home health care services for client reassurance and implementation of a therapeutic regimen. EBN: *Providing home health services for patients with anxiety increases self efficacy and reduces symptoms of anxiety, stress, and depression (Shelby et al, 2009).*

Client/Family Teaching and Discharge Planning

- ▲ Teach use of appropriate community resources in emergency situations (e.g., suicidal thoughts), such as hotlines, emergency departments, law enforcement, and judicial systems. EB: *Identification and sharing of best practices associated with emergency and community services would provide an opportunity for improvement in care for families dealing with anxiety and depression (Weiss et al, 2012).*
- Teach the client/family the symptoms of anxiety. EBN: *Teach families to have a general understanding of what is happening to the patient with anxiety and help them to accept assistance to overcome their anxiety (Smith et al, 2011).*
- Teach the client techniques to self-manage anxiety. EBN: *Computerized self-help treatments have been shown to be a less-intensive, cost-effective way to deliver empirically validated treatments for a variety of psychological problems (Newman et al, 2011).*
- Teach the client to visualize or fantasize about the absence of anxiety or pain, successful experience of the situation, resolution of conflict, or outcome of procedure. EBN: *Use of guided imagery has been useful for reducing anxiety (Tyron & McKay, 2009).*

- Teach relationship between a healthy physical and emotional lifestyle and a realistic mental attitude. EBN: *Some aspects of healthy lifestyle for anxiety disorders include identifying unhealthy relationships, building a strong support system, and adopting general healthy lifestyle habits (Smith et al, 2011).*

REFERENCES

Benson, L., McGinn, M., & Christensen, A. (2012). Common principals of couples therapy. *Behavior Therapy, 43*(1), 25–35.

Bilyeu, K., et al. (2011). Cultivating quality: reducing the use of potentially inappropriate medications in older adults. *The American Journal of Nursing, 111*(1), 47–52.

Chlan, L., Weinert, C., Heiderscheidt, A., et al. (2013). Effects of patient-directed music intervention on anxiety and sedative exposure in critically ill patients receiving mechanical ventilatory support: a randomized clinical trial. *Journal of the American Medical Association, 309*(22), 2335–2544.

Dolcos, S., & Albarracin, D. (2014). The inner speech of behavioral regulation: Intentions and task performance strengthen when you talk to yourself as a You. *European Journal of Social Psychology, 44*(6), 636–642.

Gale, C., Wilson, J., & Deary, I. (2010). Globus sensation and psychopathology in men: the Vietnam experience. *Psychosomat Med, 71*(9), 1026–1031.

Garavalia, L., et al. (2011). Medication discussion question: developing a guide to facilitate patient-clinician communication about heart medications. *The Journal of Cardiovascular Nursing, 26*(4), E12–E29.

Heinz, A., Mann, K., Weinberger, D. R., et al. (2011). Sooner or later: age at onset of generalized anxiety disorder in older adults. *Depression and Anxiety, 29*(1), 39–46.

Henry, S. G., Feng, B., Franks, P., et al. (2014). Methods for assessing patient–clinician communication about depression in primary care: what you see depends on how you look. *Health Services Research.*

Hill, J. (2010) *Less perfection, less stress.* Retrieved November 6, 2011, from <http://thestressreliefhandbook.com/2010/02/less-perfection-less-stress>.

Hoffman, A., Asnaani, A., & Hinton, D. (2010). Cultural aspects of social anxiety and social anxiety disorder. *Depression and Anxiety, 27*(2), 1117–1127.

Hynninen, M., Bjerke, N., Pallesen, S., et al. (2010). A randomized controlled trial of cognitive behavioral therapy for anxiety and depression in COPD. *Respiratory Medicine, 104*(7), 986–994.

Jiala, H. A., French, J. L., Foxall, G. L., et al. (2010). Effect of preoperative multimedia information on perioperative anxiety in patients undergoing procedures under regional anaesthesia. *British Journal of Anesthesia, 104*(3), 369–374.

Kang, X., Li, Z., & Nolan, M. (2011). Informal caregivers' experiences of caring for patients with chronic heart failure: systematic review and metasynthesis of qualitative studies. *The Journal of Cardiovascular Nursing, 26*(5), 386–394.

Katzman, M. (2009). Current considerations in the treatment of generalized anxiety disorder. *CNS Drugs, 23*(2), 103–120.

Kavan, M., Elsasser, G., & Barone, E. (2009). General anxiety disorder assessment and management. *American Family Physician, 79*(9), 785–791.

Korhan, E. A., Khorshid, L., & Uyar, M. (2011). The effect of music therapy on physiological signs of anxiety in patients receiving mechanical ventilatory support. *Journal of Clinical Nursing, 20*, 1026–1034.

Labrique-Walusis, F., Keister, K., & Russell, A. (2010). Massage therapy for stress management: Implications for nursing practice. *Orthopaedic Nursing, 29*(4), 254–257.

Lauzier, S., Campbell, H. S., Livingston, P. M., et al. (2014). Indicators for evaluating cancer organizations' support services: Performance and associations with empowerment. *Cancer.*

Lobjanidze, N., et al. (2010). Interaction between depression-anxiety disorders and hypertension. *J Hypertension, 28*, e94.

McCabe, S., et al. (2011). Medical misuse of controlled medications among adolescents. *Archives of Pediatrics and Adolescent Medicine, 165*(8), 729–735.

Mackenzie, C., Reynolds, K., Chou, K., et al. (2011). Prevalence and correlates of generalized anxiety disorder in a national sample of older adults. *The American Journal of Geriatric Psychiatry, 19*(4), 305–314.

Marques, L., Robinaugh, D., LaBlanc, N., et al. (2011). Cross-cultural variations in the prevalence and presentation of anxiety disorders. *Review of Neurotherapeutics, 11*(2), 313–322.

Mitchell, A., et al. (2009). Depression, anxiety and quality of life in suicide survivors. *Archives of Psychiatric Nursing, 23*(1), 2–10.

Newman, M., Szkodny, L., Llera, S., et al. (2011). A review of technology-assisted self-help and minimal contact therapies for anxiety and depression: Is human contact necessary for therapeutic efficacy? *Clinical Psychology Review, 31*(1), 89–103.

Parlak, G., Polat, S., & Nuran, A. (2010). Itching, pain, and anxiety levels are reduced with massage therapy and yoga stretching in burned adolescents. *Journal of Burn Care and Research, 31*(3), 429–432.

Sagkal, T., Eser, I., & Uyar, M. (2013). The effect of reiki touch therapy on pain and anxiety. *Complementary Medicine, 3*(4), 141–146.

Sand-Jecklin, K., & Emerson, H. (2010). The impact of a live therapeutic music intervention on patients' experience of pain, anxiety, and muscle tension. *Holistic Nursing Practice, 24*(1), 7–15.

Shelby, R., et al. (2009). Pain catastrophizing in patients with noncardiac chest pain: relationships with pain, anxiety, and disability. *Psychosomat Med, 71*(8), 861–868.

Smith, M., Jaffe-Gill, E., & Segal, J. (2011). *Generalized anxiety disorder (GAD): symptoms, treatment, and self-help.* Accessed July 25, 2012, at <http://helpguide.org/mental/generalized_anxiety_disorder.htm>.

Sutshall, B., Wentworth, S., Engen, L., et al. (2010). Effect of massage therapy on pain, anxiety, and tension after cardiac surgery: A randomized study. *Complementary Therapies in Clinical Practice, 16*(2), 70–75.

Tekur, P., Nagarathna, R., Chametcha, S., et al. (2012). A comprehensive yoga programs improves pain, anxiety and depression in chronic low back pain patients more than exercise: An RCT. *Complementary Therapies in Medicine, 20*(3), 107–119.

Thomas, K., & Sethares, K. (2010). Is guided imagery effective in reducing pain and anxiety in the postoperative total joint arthroplasty patient? *Orthopaedic Nursing, 29*(6), 393–399.

Tyron, W., & McKay, D. (2009). Memory modification as an outcome variable in anxiety disorder treatment. *Journal of Anxiety Disorders, 23*(4), 546–556.

Vollestad, J., Silversten, V., & Nielson, G. (2011). Mindfulness-based stress reduction for patients with anxiety disorders: Evaluation in a randomized controlled trial. *Behaviour Research and Therapy, 49*(4), 281–288.

Wagner, D., & Bear, M. (2009). Patient satisfaction with nursing care: a concept analysis within a nursing framework. *Journal of Advanced Nursing, 65*(3), 692–701.

Weiss, A., Chang, G., Rauch, S., et al. (2012). Patient- and practice-related determinants of emergency department length of stay for patients with psychiatric illness. *Annals of Emergency Medicine, 60*(2), 162–171.

Death Anxiety

Ruth McCaffrey, DNP, ARNP, FNP-BC, GNP-BC, FAAN

NANDA-I

Definition

Vague uneasy feeling of discomfort or dread generated by perceptions of a real or imagined threat to one's existence

Defining Characteristics

Concern about strain on the caregiver; deep sadness; fear of developing terminal illness; fear of loss of mental abilities when dying; fear of pain related to dying; fear of premature death; fear of prolonged dying process; fear of suffering related to dying; fear of the dying process; negative thoughts related to death and dying; powerlessness; worried about the impact of one's death on significant other

Related Factors (r/t)

Anticipation of adverse consequences of anesthesia; anticipation of impact of death on others; anticipation of pain; anticipation of suffering; confronting the reality of terminal disease; discussions on topic of death; experiencing dying process; near-death experience; nonacceptance of own mortality; observations related to death; perceived imminence of death; uncertainty about encountering a higher power; uncertainty about life after death; uncertainty about the existence of a higher power; uncertainty of prognosis

NOC (Nursing Outcomes Classification)

Suggested NOC Outcomes

Dignified Life Closure; Fear; Self-Control; Health Beliefs: Perceived Threat

Example NOC Outcome with Indicators

Dignified Life Closure as evidenced by the following indicators: Expresses readiness for death/Resolves important issues/Shares feelings about dying/Discusses spiritual concerns. (Rate the outcome and indicators of **Dignified Life Closure:** 1 = never demonstrated, 2 = rarely demonstrated, 3 = sometimes demonstrated, 4 = often demonstrated, 5 = consistently demonstrated [see Section I].)

Client Outcomes

Client Will (Specify Time Frame)

- State concerns about impact of death on others
- Express feelings associated with dying
- Seek help in dealing with feelings
- Discuss realistic goals
- Use prayer or other religious practice for comfort

NIC (Nursing Interventions Classification)

Suggested NIC Interventions

Dying Care; Grief Work Facilitation; Spiritual Support

Example NIC Activities—Dying Care

Communicate willingness to discuss death; Support client and family through stages of grief

Nursing Interventions and *Rationales*

- ▲ Assess the psychosocial maturity of the individual. EB: *In a large study, females scored higher on death anxiety than males. Additional tests reported that life satisfaction, an altering consciousness coping style, and avoidance coping was significantly related to risk for developing a stress-related illness when faced with the death of a loved one (Moore, 2013).*
- ▲ Assess clients for pain and provide pain relief measures. EBN: *Providing pain management and pain relief measures is the factor that most improves dying clients' quality of life at the end of life. Pain management should be a first priority for care providers during this time (Zhang et al, 2012).*
- • Assess client for fears related to death. EBN: *Unbearable suffering is the outcome of an intensive process associated with death anxiety. According to clients, hopelessness is an essential element of unbearable suffering. Physical issues and feelings of loss may cause suffering during this time. Personality characteristics and biographical aspects greatly influence the burden of suffering. Unbearable suffering that accompanies death anxiety can only be understood in the continuum of the client's perspectives of the past and present, and expectations of the future (Dees et al, 2011).*
- • Assist clients with life planning: consider and redefine main life goals, focus on areas of strength and/or goals that will provide satisfaction, adopt realistic goals, and recognize those that are impossible to achieve. EB: *Advance planning improves end of life care and client and family satisfaction, and reduces stress, anxiety, and depression in surviving relatives (Detering et al, 2010).*
- • Assist clients with life review and reminiscence. EB: *When challenges emerged, the participants implemented "the search to find an acceptable and satisfying completion to this life," engaging family members, friends, and the hospice team in an effort to relieve discomfort and regain a degree of control (McSherry, 2011).*
- • Provide music of the client's choosing. EBN: *Traditionally, music has played an important role in human culture and has had a powerful influence on human behavior. Music has a unique capacity for immersing an individual to such a degree that the closeness can be felt and painful aloneness may be alleviated (Chi & Young, 2011).*
- • Provide social support for families, understanding what is most important to families who are caring for clients at the end of life. EBN: *When nurses make the intensive care unit a comfortable place for the dying patients and their loved ones, we also make the patients' deaths comfortable for us (Millner et al, 2009).*
- • Encourage clients to pray. EBN: *Mindfulness and prayer allow for a step back from thoughts, increased coping for those who are dying, and their families (Monroe et al, 2012).*

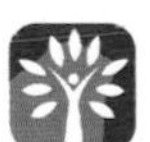

Geriatric

- • Carefully assess older adults for issues regarding death anxiety. EB: *Older adults in this study and review were more fearful for others than of the dying process. Women were more afraid of death of loved ones and of the consequences of their own death on those loved ones than were men (Azaiza et al, 2011).*
- • Provide back massage for clients who have anxiety regarding issues such as death. EBN: *Back massage significantly reduced anxiety in the study population. Systolic BP decreased to a greater degree in the male participants, particularly in those with greater levels of anxiety and higher systolic BP (Chen et al, 2013).*
- • Refer to care plan for **Grieving.**

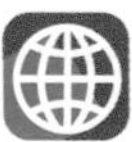

Multicultural

- • Assist clients to identify with their culture and its values. EB/EBN: *Christians scored significantly lower for death anxiety than both nonreligious and Muslim groups, and Muslims scored significantly higher than the nonreligious group (Gareth & McAdie, 2009).*
- • Refer to care plans for **Anxiety** and **Grieving.**

Home Care

- • The above interventions may be adapted for home care.
- • Identify times and places when anxiety is greatest. Provide for psychological support at those times, using such strategies as personal contact, telephone contact, diversionary activities, or therapeutic self. EBN: *Participants across conditions reported similar levels of anxiety, suggesting that promoting an interest in sustained contact can be accomplished without reducing anxiety, but rather by shielding individuals from the negative effects of anxiety during social interactions (Stern & West, 2014).*

A

- Support religious beliefs; encourage the client to participate in services and activities of choice. EBN: *Enhancing the psychosocial and spiritual well-being of cancer patients can reduce their death anxiety and promote better quality of life (Shukla & Rishi, 2014).*
- ▲ Refer to medical social services or mental health services, including support groups as appropriate (e.g., anticipatory grieving groups from hospice, visiting volunteers of hospice). EB: *Preparatory grief was found to reduce emotional stress. Experience with hospice focused on the intense preoccupation with the dying, loneliness, tearfulness, cognitive dysfunction, irritability, anger, and social withdrawal. This study found that talking mobilizes strength to cope with the situation (Asa & Agneta, 2012).*
- Encourage the client to verbalize feelings to family/caregivers, counselors, and self. Identify the client's preferences for end-of-life care; provide assistance in honoring preferences as much as practicable. EB: *Music may be an effective tool for reviewing one's life, through which a client moves toward acceptance of death by giving meaning to his or her life. Near the end of life, prescriptive music may be used during bedside vigils to accompany the client in the transition from life to death (Black & Thompson, 2012).*
- ▲ Assist the client in making contact with death-related planning organizations, if appropriate, such as the Cremation Society and funeral homes. EB: *Advanced care planning is important to older clients. However, when clients are not accepting of death or if death is outside of the client's understanding, it can be difficult to work on advanced care planning. Nurses should explore whether the client accepts dying as a likely outcome and assess the client's fears of dying and need for control before attempting any planning (Piers et al, 2013).*
- Refer to care plan for **Powerlessness.**

Client/Family Teaching and Discharge Planning

- Promote more effective communication to family members engaged in the caregiving role. Encourage them to talk to their loved one about areas of concern. Both caregivers and care receivers often avoid discussing areas of concern. EBN: *Encouraging loved ones to discuss their wishes and areas of concern will assist the family during the grieving process; they will know the wishes of the dying family member and can carry them out as much as possible (Webb & Guarino, 2011).*
- Allow family members to be physically close to their dying loved one, giving them permission, instruction, and opportunities to touch. Keep family members informed. EBN: *A novel approach at one VA hospital was to use Skype as a tool for client and family/friend communication. This was especially useful when clinical symptoms, functional status, financial concerns, and geographic limitations prohibited in-person visits. It was very satisfying to both family/friends and clients (Brecher, 2012).*

REFERENCES

Asa, J., & Agneta, G. (2012). Anticipatory grief among close relatives of patients at hospice and palliative care wards. *American Journal of Hospice and Palliative Care, 30*, 29–34.

Azaiza, F., et al. (2011). Death and dying anxiety among bereaved and nonbereaved elderly parents. *Death Studies, 35*(7), 610–624.

Black, B. P., & Thompson, P. P. (2012). Music as a therapeutic resource in end of life care. *Journal of Hospice and Palliative Care, 14*(2), 118–125.

Brecher, D. B. (2012). The use of Skype in a community hospital palliative medicine consultation service. *Journal of Palliative Medicine, 16*(1), 110–112.

Chen, W., Liu, L., Yeh, S., et al. (2013). Effect of back massage intervention on anxiety, comfort, and physiologic responses in patients with congestive heart failure. *The Journal of Alternative and Complementary Medicine*, May, *19*(5), 464–470.

Chi, G., & Young, A. (2011). Selection of music for relaxation and alleviating pain: literature review. *Holistic Nursing Practice, 25*(3), 127–135.

Dees, M., Vernooji, M., Dekkers, W., et al. (2011). Unbearable suffering: a qualitative study on the perspectives of patients who request assistance in dying. *Journal of Medical Ethics, 37*, 727–734.

Detering, K. M., Hancock, A. D., Reade, M. C., et al. (2010). The impact of advance care planning on end of life care in elderly patients: randomized controlled trial. *British Medical Journal, 340*, c1345.

Gareth, J. M., & McAdie, T. (2009). Are personality, well-being and death anxiety related to religious affiliation? *Ment Health Relig Cult, 12*(2), 115–120.

McSherry, C. (2011). The inner life at the end of life. *J Hospice Palliat Care, 13*(2), 112–120.

Millner, P., Paskiewicz, S., & Kautz, D. (2009). A comfortable place to say good-bye. *Dimen Crit Care Nurs, 28*(1), 13–17.

Moore, G. (2013). *The relationship between religious orientation, coping style, and psychological health on death anxiety and life satisfaction.* Bachelors Final Year Project, Dublin Business School found online at <http://esource.dbs.ie/handle/10788/1604?show=full>.

Monroe, N., Lynch, C., Losasso, V., et al. (2012). Mindfulness to Reduce Psychosocial Stress. *Mindfulness, 3*(1), 22–29.

Piers, R., Eechoud, I., VanCamp, S., et al. (2013). Advance Care Planning in terminally ill and frail older persons. *Patient Education and Counseling, 90*(3), 323–329.

Shukla, P., & Rishi, P. (2014). A correlational study of psychosocial & spiritual well being and death anxiety among advanced stage cancer patients. *American Journal of Applied Psychology, 2*(3), 59–65.

Stern, C., & West, T. (2014). Circumventing anxiety during interpersonal encounters to promote interest in contact:

An implementation intention approach. *Journal of Experimental Psychology, 50*, 82–93.

Webb, J., & Guarino, A. (2011). Life after death of a loved one: long term distress among surrogate decision makers. *J Hospice Palliat Care, 13*(6), 378–386.

Zhang, B., Nilsson, M., & Prigerson, H. (2012). Factors important to patients' quality of life at the end of life. *Archives of Internal Medicine, 172*(15), 1133–1142.

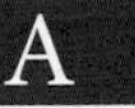

Risk for Aspiration *Debra Siela, PhD, RN, CCNS, ACNS-BC, CCRN-K, CNE, RRT*

NANDA-I

Definition

Vulnerable to entry of gastrointestinal secretions, oropharyngeal secretions, solids, or fluids to the tracheobronchial passages, which may compromise health

Risk Factors

Barrier to elevating upper body; decrease in gastrointestinal motility; decrease in level of consciousness; delayed gastric emptying; depressed gag reflex; enteral feedings; facial surgery; facial trauma; impaired ability to swallow; incompetent lower esophageal sphincter; increase in gastric residual; increase in intragastric pressure; ineffective cough; neck surgery; neck trauma; oral surgery; oral trauma; presence of oral/nasal tube (e.g., tracheal, feeding); treatment regimen; wired jaw

NOC (Nursing Outcomes Classification)

Suggested NOC Outcomes

Aspiration Prevention; Respiratory Status: Ventilation; Swallowing Status

Example NOC Outcome with Indicators

Aspiration Prevention as evidenced by the following indicators: Avoids risk factors/Maintains oral hygiene/Positions self upright for eating and drinking/Selects foods according to swallowing ability/Selects foods and fluid of proper consistency/Remains upright for 30 minutes after eating. (Rate the outcome and indicators of **Aspiration Prevention:** 1 = never demonstrated, 2 = rarely demonstrated, 3 = sometimes demonstrated, 4 = often demonstrated, 5 = continually demonstrated [see Section I].)

Client Outcomes

Client Will (Specify Time Frame)

- Maintain patent airway and clear lung sounds
- Swallow and digest oral, nasogastric, or gastric feeding without aspiration

NIC (Nursing Interventions Classification)

Suggested NIC Interventions

Aspiration Precautions

Example NIC Activities—Airway Management

Monitor level of consciousness, cough reflex, gag reflex, and swallowing ability; Check nasogastric or gastrostomy residual before feeding

Nursing Interventions and *Rationales*

- Monitor respiratory rate, depth, and effort. Note any signs of aspiration such as dyspnea, cough, cyanosis, wheezing, hoarseness, foul-smelling sputum, or fever. If new onset of symptoms, perform oral suction and notify provider immediately. CEB/EB: *Signs of aspiration should be detected as soon as possible to prevent further aspiration and to initiate treatment that can be lifesaving (Buckley & Cabrera, 2011;*

A

Swaminathan et al, 2015). Because of laryngeal pooling and residue in clients with dysphagia, silent aspiration may occur (Metheny, 2011b).

- Auscultate lung sounds frequently and before and after feedings; note any new onset of crackles or wheezing. CEB: *With decreased symptoms of pneumonia, an increased respiratory rate and/or crackles may be the first sign of pneumonia (Metheny, 2011b).*
- Take vital signs frequently, noting onset of a fever, increased respiratory rate, and increased heart rate.
- Before initiating oral feeding, check client's gag reflex and ability to swallow by feeling the laryngeal prominence as the client attempts to swallow (Rees, 2013). If client is having problems swallowing, see nursing interventions for Impaired **Swallowing.**
- If client needs to be fed, feed slowly and allow adequate time for chewing and swallowing. CEB: *Slowed feeding allows time for more deliberate swallowing, reducing aspiration (Rees, 2013).*
- When feeding client, watch for signs of impaired swallowing or aspiration, including coughing, choking, and spitting food.
- Have suction machine available when feeding high-risk clients. If aspiration does occur, suction immediately. *A client with aspiration needs immediate suctioning and may need further lifesaving interventions such as intubation and mechanical ventilation (Rees, 2013).*
- Keep the head of the bed (HOB) elevated at 30 to 45 degrees, preferably with the client sitting up in a chair at 90 degrees when feeding. Keep head elevated for an hour after eating. EBP: *Decreased gastric reflux occurs at both 30- and 45-degree HOB elevation. Thus, gastric fed patients should be maintained at the highest HOB elevation that is comfortable to prevent aspiration (Metheny & Franz, 2013).*
- Note presence of nausea, vomiting, or diarrhea. Treat nausea promptly with antiemetics.
- If the client shows symptoms of nausea and vomiting, position on side. *The side-lying position can help the client expel the vomitus and decrease the risk for aspiration (Chard, 2013).*
- Assess the abdomen and listen to bowel sounds frequently, noting if they are decreased, absent, or hyperactive. *Decreased or absent bowel sounds can indicate an ileus with possible vomiting and aspiration; increased high-pitched bowel sounds can indicate a mechanical bowel obstruction with possible vomiting and aspiration (Longo et al, 2012).*
- Note new onset of abdominal distention or increased rigidity of abdomen. EB: *Abdominal distention or rigidity can be associated with paralytic or mechanical obstruction and an increased likelihood of vomiting and aspiration (Longo et al, 2012).*
- If client has a tracheostomy, ask for referral to speech pathologist for swallowing studies before attempting to feed. EB: *There is an increased risk for aspiration when tracheostomy tubes are in place, and inflating the cuff does not prevent aspiration (Rees, 2013).*
- Provide meticulous oral care including brushing of teeth at least two times per day. *Good oral care can prevent bacterial or fungal contamination of the mouth, which can be aspirated.* EB: *Research has shown that excellent dental care/oral care can be effective in preventing hospital-acquired (or extended care-acquired) pneumonia (Munro, 2014).*
- Sedation agents can reduce cough and gag reflexes as well as interfere with the client's ability to manage oropharyngeal secretions. EB: *Using the smallest effective level of sedation may help reduce risk of aspiration (Bell, 2011; Barr et al, 2013).*

Enteral Feedings

- Insert nasogastric feeding tube using the internal nares to distal-lower esophageal-sphincter distance, an updated version of the Hanson method. The ear-to-nose-to-xiphoid-process is often inaccurate. CEB: *A study demonstrated that the revised Hanson's method was more accurate in predicting the correct distance than the traditional method (Ellett et al, 2011).*
- *Verification of gastric tube placement should initially be obtained by radiography. Other methods of assessing proper gastric tube placement include capnography, aspirate assessment, tube markings, and pH tests. Auscultation should not be used to assess gastric tube placement (Bell, 2011; Amirlak et al, 2012; Williams et al, 2014).*
- Tape the feeding tube securely to the nose using a skin protectant under the tape. EBN: *A research study found that insertion of the feeding tube into the small intestine and keeping the HOB position elevated to at least 30 degrees reduced the incidence of aspiration and aspiration-related pneumonia drastically in critically ill clients (Metheny et al, 2010). Another study found that aspiration and pneumonia were reduced by feeding the clients in the mid-duodenum or farther in the small intestine (Metheny et al, 2011).*

- Check to make sure the initial nasogastric feeding tube placement was confirmed by x-ray, with the openings of the tube in the stomach, not the esophagus or lungs. This is especially important if a small-bore feeding tube is used, although larger tubes used for feedings or medication administration should be verified by radiography also. *Radiographic verification of placement remains the gold standard for determining safe placement of feeding tubes (Guenter, 2010; Bell, 2011; Metheny et al, 2012a; Williams et al, 2014).*
- After radiographic verification of correct placement of the tube or the intestines, mark the tube's exit site clearly with tape or a permanent marker (Simons & Abdallah, 2012).
- Measure and record the length of the tube that is outside of the body at defined intervals to help ensure correct placement. *Note the length of the tube outside of the body; it is possible for a tube to slide out and be in the esophagus, without obvious disruption of the tape (Bankhead et al, 2009).*
- Note the placement of the tube on any chest or abdominal radiographs that are obtained for the client. *Acutely ill clients receive frequent x-ray examinations. These are available for the nurse to determine continued correct placement of the nasogastric tube (Bell, 2011; Simons & Abdallah, 2012). When using electromagnetic feed tube placement, radiographic confirmation of tube position is preferred due to the variance of the ability of clinicians to place the tube (Metheny & Meert, 2014).*
- Check the pH of the aspirate. *If the pH reading is 4 or less, the tube is probably in the stomach. Recognize that the pH may not indicate correct placement if the client is receiving continuous tube feedings, is receiving a hydrogen ion blocker or proton pump inhibitor, has blood in the aspirate, or is receiving antacids (Bell, 2011; Simons & Abdallah, 2012).*
- Use a number of determinants for verification of correct placement before each feeding or every 4 hours if the client is on continuous feeding. Measure length of tube outside the body, and review recent x-ray results, check pH of aspirate if relevant, and characteristic appearance of aspirate. If findings do not ensure correct placement of the tube, obtain a radiograph to verify placement. Do not rely on the air insufflation method to assess correct tube placement. CEB/EBN: *The ausculatory air insufflation method is not reliable for differentiating between gastric or respiratory placement; the "whooshing" sound can be heard even if the tube is incorrectly placed in the lung (Bell, 2011; Simons & Abdallah, 2012; Williams et al, 2014).*
- *Capnography (CO_2 sensor) may be used to assess proper tube placement (Gilbert & Burns, 2012; Williams et al, 2014).*
- Follow unit policy regarding checking for gastric residual volume during continuous feedings or before feedings, and holding feedings if increased residual is present. CEB/EBN: *There is little evidence to support the use of measurement of gastric residual volume, and the practice may or may not be effective in preventing aspiration (Makic et al, 2011). It is still done at intervals (Metheny et al, 2012b; Bell, 2011) especially if there is a question of tube feeding intolerance. The practice of holding tube feedings if there is increased residual reduces the amount of calories given to the client. If the client has a small-bore feeding tube, it is difficult to check gastric residual volume and may be inaccurate. It is unclear if aspiration for residual volumes helps reduce the risk of aspiration (Metheny et al, 2012b); practice guidelines suggest continuing to feed the patient until the residual is greater than 500 mL (Canadian Clinical Practice Guidelines, 2013; Elke et al, 2015).*
- Follow unit protocol regarding returning or discarding gastric residual volume. At this time there is not a definitive research base to guide practice. CEB/EBN: *A study of the effectiveness of either returning gastric residual volumes to the client or discarding them resulted in inconclusive findings and more research is needed in the area (Williams & Leslie, 2010).*
- Do not use glucose testing to determine correct placement of enteral tube, and to identify aspirated enteral feeding. *Glucose was found in tracheal secretions of clients who were not receiving enteral feedings (Guenter, 2010).*
- Do not use blue dye to tint enteral feedings (Guenter, 2010). *The presence of blue and green skin and urine and serum discoloration from use of blue dye has been associated with the death of clients. The U.S. Food and Drug Administration (2009) has reported at least 12 deaths from the use of blue dye in enteral feedings.*
- During enteral feedings, position client with HOB elevated 30 to 45 degrees (Bell, 2011; Schallom et al, 2015). CEB: *A study of mechanically ventilated clients receiving tube feedings demonstrated that there was an increase of the presence of pepsin (from gastric contents) in pulmonary secretions if the client was in a flat position versus being positioned with head elevated (Metheny & Franz, 2013). Generally do not turn off the tube feeding when repositioning clients. Stopping the tube feeding during repositioning is counterproductive because the client receives less nutrition and the rate of emptying of the stomach is slow. If it is imperative*

to keep the HOB elevated, consider use of reverse Trendelenburg (head higher than feet) when repositioning (Metheny, 2011a).

- Take actions to prevent inadvertent misconnections with enteral feeding tubes into intravenous (IV) lines or other harmful connections. Safety actions that should be taken to prevent misconnections include:
  - Trace tubing back to origin. Recheck connections at time of client transfer and at change of shift.
  - Label all tubing.
  - Use oral syringes for medications through the enteral feeding; **do not use IV syringes.**
  - Teach nonprofessional personnel "Do Not Reconnect" if a line becomes dislodged; rather, find the nurse instead of taking the chance of plugging the tube into the wrong place. *Enteral feeding tube lines have been inadvertently plugged into IV peripheral catheters, peritoneal dialysis catheters, central lines, medical gas tubing, and tracheostomies, resulting in death in some cases (Guenter, 2010).*

Critical Care

- Recognize that critically ill clients are at an increased risk for aspiration because of severe illness and interventions that compromise the gag reflex. *Predisposing causes of aspiration include sedation, endotracheal intubation and mechanical ventilation, neurological disorders, altered level of consciousness, hemodynamic instability, and sepsis (Makic et al, 2011).*
- Recognize that intolerance to feeding as defined by increased gastric residual is more common early in the feeding process. EB: *A study found that feeding intolerance in critical care clients happened commonly in the first 5 days of feeding, and feeding intolerance was associated with increased length of both critical care and hospital length of stay (O'Connor et al, 2011).*
- *Maintain endotracheal cuff pressures at an appropriate level to prevent leakage of secretions around the cuff (Bell, 2011).*
- *Pepsin and amylase are biomarkers of microaspiration of gastric contents in tracheal aspirate. Amylase presence is a better biomarker of aspiration of oral contents in the tracheal aspirate. Both pepsin and amylase were present in tracheal aspirate of critically ill patients even with backrest elevation of 30 degrees. HOB elevation is inversely related to the presence of pepsin (Sole et al, 2014).*

Geriatric

- Carefully check older client's gag reflex and ability to swallow before feeding. *A slowed rate of swallowing is common in older adults (Rees, 2013).*
- Watch for signs of aspiration pneumonia in older adults with cerebrovascular accidents, even if there are no apparent signs of difficulty swallowing or of aspiration. *Bedside evaluation for swallow and aspiration can be inaccurate.* EB: *Silent aspiration can occur in the older population (Metheny, 2011b).*
- Recognize that older adults with aspiration pneumonia have fewer symptoms than younger people; repeat cases of pneumonia in older adults are generally associated with aspiration (Eisenstadt, 2010). *Aspiration pneumonia can be undiagnosed in older adults because of decreased symptoms; sometimes the only obvious symptom may be new onset of delirium (Metheny, 2011b).*
- Use central nervous system depressants cautiously; older clients may have an increased incidence of aspiration with altered levels of consciousness. *Older clients have altered metabolism, distribution, and excretion of drugs. Many medications can interfere with the swallowing reflex, including antipsychotic drugs, proton pump inhibitors, and angiotensin-converting enzyme inhibitors (van der Maarel-Wierink et al, 2011).*
- Keep an older, mostly bedridden client sitting upright for 45 minutes to 1 hour after meals.
- Recommend to families that enteral feedings may or may not be indicated for clients with advanced dementia. Instead, if possible use hand-feeding assistance, modified food consistency as needed, and feeding favorite foods for comfort (Sorrell, 2010). EB/CEB: *Research has demonstrated that tube feedings in this population do not prevent malnutrition or aspiration, improve survival, reduce infections, or result in other positive outcomes (Teno et al, 2010).*

Home Care

- The above interventions may be adapted for home care use.
- For clients at high risk for aspiration, obtain complete information from the discharging institution regarding institutional management.
- Assess the client and family for willingness and cognitive ability to learn and cope with swallowing, feeding, and related disorders.

- Assess caregiver understanding and reinforce teaching regarding positioning and assessment of the client for possible aspiration.
- Provide the client with emotional support in dealing with fears of aspiration. *Fear of choking can provoke extreme anxiety, which can interfere with the client's ability or willingness to adhere to the treatment plan.* Refer to care plan for **Anxiety.**
- Establish emergency and contingency plans for care of the client. *Clinical safety of the client between visits is a primary goal of home care nursing.*
- Have a speech and occupational therapist assess the client's swallowing ability and other physiological factors and recommend strategies for working with the client in the home (e.g., pureeing foods served to the client; providing adequate adaptive equipment for independence in eating). *Successful strategies allow the client to remain part of the family.*
- Obtain suction equipment for the home as necessary.
- Teach caregivers safe, effective use of suctioning devices. Inform the client and family that only individuals instructed in suctioning should perform the procedure.
- Institute case management of frail elderly to support continued independent living.

Client/Family Teaching and Discharge Planning

- Teach the client and family signs of aspiration and precautions to prevent aspiration.
- Teach the client and family how to safely administer tube feeding.
- Teach the family about proper client positioning to facilitate feeding and reduce risk of aspiration.
- Verify client family/caregiver knowledge about feeding, aspiration precautions, and signs of aspiration.

REFERENCES

Amirlak, B., et al. (2012). Pneumothorax following feeding tube placement: Precaution and treatment. *Acta Medica Iranica*, *50*(5), 355–358.

Bankhead, R., Boullata, J., Brantley, S., et al. (2009). A A.S.P.E.N. enteral nutrition practice recommendations. *Journal of Parenteral Enteral Nutrition*, *33*(2), 122–167.

Barr, J., Fraser, G. L., Puntillo, K., et al. (2013). Clinical practice guidelines for the management of pain, agitation, and delirium in adult patients in the intensive care unit. *Critical Care Medicine*, *41*(1), 263–306.

Bell, L. (2011). AACN Practice Alert-Prevention of Aspiration. *American Association of Critical Care Nurses*. Retrieved from <http://www.aacn.org/wd/practice/docs/practicealerts/prevention-aspiration-practice-alert.pdf?menu=aboutus>.

Buckley, L., & Cabrera, G. (2011). Pneumonia aspiration (anaerobic). *CINAHL Information Systems*.

Canadian Clinical Practice Guidelines (2013). *Strategies to optimize the delivery of EN: Use of and threshold for gastric residual volumes*. Retrieved from <http://www.criticalcarenutrition.com/docs/cpgs2012/5.5.pdf>.

Chard, R. (2013). Care of postoperative patients. In D. Ignatavicius & M. L. Workman (Eds.), *(2013). Medical-Surgical Nursing: Patient-Centered Collaborative Care* (7th ed., pp. 284–301). St. Louis, MO: W.B. Saunders Company.

Eisenstadt, E. S. (2010). Dysphagia and aspiration pneumonia in older adults. *Journal of American Academy Nursing Practitioners*, *22*(1), 17–22.

Elke, G., Felbinger, T. W., & Heyland, D. K. (2015). Gastric residual volume in critically ill patients: A dead marker or still alive? *Nutrition in Clinical Practice*, *30*(1), 59–71.

Ellett, M. L., Cohen, M. D., Perkins, S. M., et al. (2011). Predicting the insertion length for gastric tube placement in neonates. *Journal of Obstetric, Gynecologic, & Neonatal Nurses*, *40*(4), 412–421.

Gilbert, R. T., & Burns, S. M. (2012). Increasing the safety of blind gastric tube placement in pediatric patients. *Journal of Pediatric Nursing*, *27*(5), 528–532.

Guenter, P. (2010). Safe practices for enteral nutrition in critically ill patients. *Critical Care Nurse Clinics of North America*, *22*(2), 197–208.

Longo, D., et al. (2012). *Harrison's principles of internal medicine* (18th ed.). New York: McGraw-Hill.

Makic, M. B. F., VonRueden, K. T., Rauen, C. A., et al. (2011). Evidence-based practice habits: Putting more sacred cows out to pasture. *Critical Care Nurse*, *31*(2), 38–62.

Metheny, N. A. (2011a). Turning tube feeding off while repositioning patients in bed: ask the experts. *Critical Care Nurse*, *31*(2), 96–97.

Metheny, N. A. (2011b). Preventing aspiration in older adults with dysphagia. *Med-Surg Matters*, *20*(5), 6–7.

Metheny, N. A., Davis-Jackson, J., & Stewart, B. (2010). Effectiveness of an aspiration risk-reduction protocol. *Nursing Research*, *59*(1), 18–25.

Metheny, N. A., & Frantz, R. A. (2013). Head-of-bed elevation in critically ill patients: A review. *Critical Care Nurse*, *33*(3), 53–67.

Metheny, N. A., & Meert, K. L. (2014). Effectiveness of an electromagnetic feeding tube placement device in detecting inadvertent respiratory placement. *American Journal of Critical Care*, *23*(3), 240–248.

Metheny, N. A., Mills, A. C., & Stewart, B. J. (2012b). Monitoring for intolerance to gastric tube feedings: A national survey. *American Journal of Critical Care*, *21*(2), e33–e40.

Metheny, N. A., Stewart, B. J., & McClave, S. A. (2011). Relationship between feeding tube site and respiratory outcomes. *Journal of Parenteral and Enteral Nutrition*, *35*(3), 346–355.

Metheny, N. A., Stewart, B. J., & Mills, A. C. (2012a). Blind insertion of feeding tubes in intensive care units: A national survey. *American Journal of Critical Care*, *21*(5), 352–360.

Munro, C. L. (2014). Oral Health: Something to smile about! *American Journal of Critical Care*, *23*(4), 282–289.

O'Connor, S., Rivett, J., Deane, A., et al. (2011). Nasogastric feeding intolerance in the critically ill—a prospective observational study. *Australian Critical Care*, *24*(1), 22.

Rees, H. C. (2013). Care of patients requiring oxygen therapy or tracheostomy. In D. Ignatavicius & M. L. Workman (Eds.), *(2013). Medical-Surgical Nursing: Patient-Centered Collaborative Care* (7th ed., pp. 562–580). St. Louis, MO: W.B. Saunders Company.

Schallom, M., Dykeman, B., Kirby, J., et al. (2015). Head-of-Bed elevation and early outcomes of gastric reflux, aspiration, and pressure ulcers: A feasibility study. *American Journal of Critical Care, 24*(1), 57–66.

Simons, S. R., & Abdallah, L. M. (2012). Bedside assessment of enteral tube placement aligning practice with evidence. *American Journal of Nursing, 112*(2), 40–48.

Sole, M. L., Conrad, J., Bennett, M., et al. (2014). Pepsin and amylase in oral and tracheal secretions: A pilot study. *American Journal of Critical Care, 23*(4), 334–338.

Sorrell, J. (2010). Use of feeding tubes in patients with advanced dementia. *J Psychosoc Nurs, 48*(5), 15–18.

Swaminathan, A., Stearns, D. A., Varkey, A. B., et al. (2015). Aspiration pneumonitis and pneumonia. *Medscape*. Retrieved <http://emedicine.medscape.com/article/296198-overview#aw2aab6b2>.

Teno, J. M., Mitchell, S. L., Gozalo, P. L., et al. (2010). Hospital characteristics associated with feeding tube placement in nursing home residents with advanced cognitive impairment. *Journal of American Medical Association, 303*, 544–550.

U.S. Food and Drug Administration (USFDA). (2009). *Reports of blue dye discoloration and death in patients receiving enteral feedings tinted with the dye, FD & C Blue no. 1.*FDA Public Health Advisory. Accessed April 27, 2015 from <http://www.fda.gov/ForIndustry/ColorAdditives/ColorAdditivesinSpecificProducts/InMedicalDevices/ucm142395.htm>.

van derMaarel-Wierink, C., Vanobbergen, J. N. O., Bronkhorst, E. M., et al. (2011). Risk factors for aspiration pneumonia in frail older people: a systematic review. *Journal of American Medical Directors Association, 12*(5), 344–354.

Williams, T., & Leslie, G. (2010). Should gastric aspirate be discarded or retained when gastric residual volume is removed from gastric tubes? *Australian Critical Care, 23*(4), 215–217.

Williams, T. A., et al. (2014). Frequency of aspirating gastric tubes for patients receiving enteral nutrition in the ICU: A randomized controlled trial. *JPEN, 38*(7), 809–816.

Risk for impaired Attachment

Mary Alice DeWys, RN, BS, CIMI, and Margaret Elizabeth Padnos, RN, AB, BSN, MA

NANDA-I

Definition

Vulnerable to disruption of the interactive process between parent/significant other and child that fosters the development of a protective and nurturing reciprocal relationship

Risk Factors

Anxiety; child's illness prevents effective initiation of parental contact; disorganized infant behavior; inability of parent to meet personal needs; insufficient privacy; parental conflict resulting from disorganized infant behavior; parent-child separation; physical barrier (e.g., infant in isolette); prematurity; substance abuse

NOC (Nursing Outcomes Classification)

Suggested NOC Outcomes

Parent-Infant Attachment; Parenting Performance

Example NOC Outcomes with Indicators

Holds infant close, touches, strokes, pats infant, responds to infant cues, holds infant for feeding, vocalizes to infant. (Rate the outcome and indicators of appropriate parent and infant behaviors that demonstrate an enduring affectionate bond: 1 = never demonstrated, 2 = rarely demonstrated, 3 = sometimes demonstrated, 4 = often demonstrated, 5 = consistently demonstrated [see Section I].)

Client Outcomes

Parent(s)/Caregiver(s) Will (Specify Time Frame)

- Be willing to consider pumping breast milk (and storing appropriately) or breastfeeding, if feasible
- Demonstrate behaviors that indicate secure attachment to infant/child
- Provide a safe environment, free of physical hazards
- Provide nurturing environment sensitive to infant/child's need for nutrition/feeding, sleeping, comfort, and social play
- Read and respond contingently to infant/child's distress
- Support infant's self-regulation capabilities, intervening when needed
- Engage in mutually satisfying interactions that provide opportunities for attachment

- Give infant nurturing sensory experiences (e.g., holding, cuddling, stroking, rocking)
- Demonstrate an awareness of developmentally appropriate activities that are pleasurable, emotionally supportive, and growth fostering
- Avoid physical and emotional abuse and/or neglect as retribution for parent's perception of infant/child's misbehavior
- State appropriate community resources and support services

NIC (Nursing Interventions Classification)

Suggested NIC Interventions

Anticipatory Guidance; Attachment Process; Attachment Promotion; Coping Enhancement; Developmental Care; Parent Education: Infant

Example NIC Activities—Anticipatory Guidance

Instruct about normal development and behavior, as appropriate; Provide a ready reference for the client (e.g., educational materials, pamphlets), as appropriate.

Nursing Interventions and *Rationales*

- Establish a trusting relationship with parent/caregiver. EBN: *"Overall, the research indicates that health care professionals urgently need to address the concerns of parents (N = 600) and their emotional reactions, be positive with communication exchanges, encourage parents to seek help, enhance parents' capability to positively explore the sources of social support and fully mobilize all social forces to ease psychological pressure" (Kong et al, 2013).*
- Support mothers of preterm infants in providing pumped breast milk to their babies until they are ready for oral feedings and transitioning from gavage to breast. EBN: *A Turkish study found stimulation with breast milk odor effective in decreasing length of transition of preterm infants from gavage to oral feeding and associated with shorter length of hospital stay (Yildiz et al, 2011).*
- Identify factors related to postpartum depression (PPD)/major depression and offer appropriate interventions/referrals. EB: *An Australian study of nulliparous women (N = 1507) highlights the need to "integrate concern for physical health with initiatives to address psychological well-being" for extreme tiredness, lower back pain, breast problems, urinary incontinence, perineal pain, constipation, hemorrhoids, and cesarean wound pain (Woolhouse et al, 2014).* EBN: *Because a mother's unpreparedness for premature childbirth may predispose her to "multiple and continuous waves of emotional responses, which will consequently lead to decline in performance ... and mental irritation," more attention should be given to support these mothers as the main caregivers of their infants (Valizadeh et al, 2014).*
- Identify eating disorders/comorbid factors related to depression and offer appropriate interventions/referrals. CEB: *Combined psychological stressors of new motherhood and body image concerns of pregnancy may predispose exacerbation of eating disorder symptoms and development of postpartum mood disorders, in which mothers can be nonresponsive, inconsistent, or rejecting of the infant (Astrachan-Fletcher et al, 2008).* EBN: *Even though they may have prioritized food before their children's need—or in the words of one participant (N = 9), "food comes before anything," overall, mothers juggled the competing demands of their eating disorder with their children's needs" (Stitt & Reupert, 2014).*
- Nurture parents so that they in turn can nurture their infant/child. EBN: *The principles of family-centered care (FCC)—respect, honoring diversity, supporting parents' choice, tailoring practice to individual family needs—help families feel supported in helping achieve the best outcome for their child at all levels of care (Gephart & McGrath, 2012).*
- Offer parents opportunities to verbalize their childhood fears associated with attachment. CEB: *"Parental lack of resolution concerning loss or trauma has been proposed to result in atypical parenting behaviors, which may have a disorganizing effect on the parent-child relationship" (Bernier & Meins, 2008).*
- Suggest journaling or scrapbooking as a way for parents of hospitalized infants to cope with stress and emotions. EB: *Beyond the obvious value of providing lifetime family mementoes, taking digital photos and writing journal notes have been found (1) to give a sense of parental empowerment, (2) to reduce maternal psychological distress, (3) to facilitate parent-infant bonding, (4) to reaffirm mutual trust between parents and staff (Subhani & Kanwal, 2012).*

- Offer parent-to-parent support to parents of infants in the neonatal intensive care unit (NICU). EBN: *In one neonatal unit, parent-support volunteers collaborated with staff to create an innovative educational and psychosocial support program specifically targeting* teen parents *in order to help them increase engagement with their hospitalized infants and their caregiving confidence (Walsh & Goser, 2013).*
- Encourage parents of hospitalized infants to "personalize the baby" by bringing in clothing, pictures of themselves, toys, and tapes of their voices. CEB: *These actions help parents claim the infant as their own and support families' confidence/competence in caring for their infants at their own pace (Lawhon, 2002).*
- Encourage physical closeness using skin-to-skin experiences as appropriate. EB: *Because kangaroo mother care (KMC) provides proven health benefits to high-risk infants, involves parents in their care, and humanizes the NICU experience/environment, it is a commonly recognized model of care for very preterm infants as well as infants who "are not so preterm and not so tiny babies who are transferred from or admitted to the NICU (Davanzo et al, 2013).*
- Plan ways for parents to interact/assist with infant/child caregiving. EB: *The COPE program (Creating Opportunities for Family Empowerment), an audiotaped educational program, has been effective in (1) teaching parents how to engage with and care for their hospitalized infant and (2) reducing maternal stress (Gooding et al, 2011). "In the beginning, having parents lay hands on their infant is enough to develop a bond and connection"; in time, wiping their infant's mouth and helping with diaper changes "facilitate the parents' participation in care" (Zimmerman & Bauersachs, 2012).*
- Educate parents about the importance of the infant-caregiver relationship as a foundation for the development of the infant's self-regulation capacities. EB: *Both contingent responsiveness and emotional-affective support model socialization practices and allow parents to support management of infant arousal states (Lynn et al, 2011).*
- Assist parents in developing new caregiving competencies and/or revising/extending old ones. CEB: *Five caregiving domains are identified: (1) being with infant, (2) knowing infant as a person, (3) giving care, (4) communicating/engaging with others regarding infant/parent needs, (5) problem-solving/decision-making/learning (Pridham et al, 1998).*
- Educate parents in reading/responding sensitively to their infant's unique "body language" (behavior cues) that communicate approach ("I'm ready to play"), avoidance/stress ("I'm unhappy. I need a change."), and self-calming ("I'm helping myself"). CEBN: *Mothers with lower competence and more technology-dependent children may perceive their children as more vulnerable and their cues as harder to read (Holditch-Davis et al, 2011).*
- Educate and support parents' ability to relieve infant/child's stress/distress. CEBN: *In facilitated tucking by parents (FTP), a parent holds the infant in a side-lying, fetal position and offers skin-to-skin contact with the hands during a stressful/painful situation (Axelin et al, 2010).* EB: *Controlled music stimulation appears safe and effective in ameliorating pain/stress in premature infants after undergoing heel-sticks (Tramo et al, 2011).*
- Guide parents in adapting their behaviors/activities with infant/child cues and changing needs. EB: *"For patterns of positive communication to lead to successful regulation of affect, the caregiver must be receptive to the infant's cues, appropriately responsive, and motivated to foster further opportunities for interactions" (Lynn et al, 2011).*
- Attend to both parents and infant/child to strengthen high-quality interactions. CEB: *A mother's behavioral and brain responses to her infant's cues may be important predictors of infant development; in cases of maternal depression or substance abuse, an infant's smiling face may fail to elicit positive caregiving (Strathearn et al, 2008).* EB: *"Positive facial expressions from one's own infant may play a particularly important role in eliciting maternal responses and strengthening the mother-infant bond" (Strathearn & Kim, 2013).*
- Assist parents with providing pleasurable sensory learning experiences (i.e., sight, sound, movement, touch, and body awareness). EB: *A Finnish study found that, when combined with kangaroo care, music therapy helped parents of preterm infants (N = 61) feel more relaxed and able to focus on "being together with the infant" in a "calm space" in which they were able to exclude disturbing and stressful sounds, as well as stress and anxiety" (Teckenberg-Jansson et al, 2011).*
- Encourage physical closeness using skin-to-skin experiences as appropriate. EB: *When intermittent KMC is not deemed appropriate, parents must be taught alternative ways to minimize negative effects of separation from their baby (e.g., gentle containing touch, proprioceptive sense stimulation, face-to-face visual contact, talking, reading, singing soothing lullabies, and olfactory stimulation (Davanzo et al, 2013).*

A

- Encourage parents and caregivers to massage their infants and children. CEB: *Preliminary studies suggest that infant massage combined with kinesthetic stimulation may have positive effects on preterm infants: greater weight gain, improved bone mineralization, earlier hospital discharge, and more optimal behavioral and motor responses compared to controls (Massaro et al, 2009).* EB: *A study of preterm and low-birth-weight infants who received massage reported the following results: greater alert and daytime activity in the first month of life; less awakening during sleep, and less crying in the second and third months; significantly greater weight gain at 2 and 3 months of age compared to infants who did not receive massage (Karbasi et al, 2014).*
- Identify mothers who may need assistance in enhancing maternal role attainment (MRA). CEBN: *"Mothers with more illness-related distress and less alert infants, and unmarried and less educated mothers may need interventions to enhance MRA" (Miles et al, 2011).*
- Recognize that fathers, compared to mothers, may have different starting points in the attachment process in the NICU as nurses encourage parents to have early skin-to-skin contact. CEBN: *One study showed that after giving birth prematurely, mothers felt powerless, experiencing the immediate postnatal period as surreal and strange. Fathers, however, experienced the birth as a shock but were ready to become immediately involved (Fegran et al, 2008).* CEB: *Specific experiences (e.g., receiving information consistently, speaking to a male health care provider may help fathers regain a sense of control to help them fulfill their various roles as protectors/partners/breadwinners (Arockiasamy et al, 2008).* EB: *A study conducted in an Irish NICU raises awareness of the need for health care professionals to consider the unique perspective of fathers regarding (1) "feeling like a second parent" because the primary focus is on the mother and infant and (2) viewing information sharing as a "double-edged sword" with both positive and negative effects (Hollywood & Hollywood, 2011).*

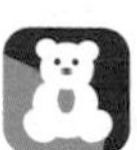

Pediatric

- Recognize and support infant/child's capacity for self-regulation and intervene when appropriate. CEB: *Infants must learn to take in sensory information while simultaneously managing not to become overaroused and overwhelmed by stimuli (DeGangi & Breinbauer, 1997; Greenspan, 1992).*
- Provide lyrical, soothing music in nursery and home that is age-appropriate (i.e., corrected, in the case of premature infants) and contingent with state/behavioral cues. EBN: *"Before adopting an intervention such as music for use in the NICU, nurses should (1) consider the parents' viewpoints about their preferences (e.g., recorded, classical, lullabies, mother's humming/singing) and (2) offer guidance as needed regarding the individual infant's response to musical stimuli" (Pölkki et al, 2012).*
- Recognize and support infant/child's attention capabilities. CEB: *"The ability to take an interest in the sights, sounds, and sensations of the world" is a significant developmental milestone (Greenspan & Wieder, 1998).*
- Encourage opportunities for mutually satisfying interactions between infant and parent. CEB: *The process of attachment involves communication and synchronous and rhythmic patterns of interaction (Rossetti, 1999).*
- Encourage opportunities for physical closeness. CEB: *Despite overwhelming evidence provided by this comprehensive literature review regarding benefits of infant massage (e.g., increased weight gain and bone density), "preterm infant massage is only practiced in 38% of NICUs (Field et al, 2010).* EB: A Finnish study *proposes "that repeated combination of music therapy and kangaroo care may be more beneficial for preterm infants than KC alone" in terms of beneficial physiological outcomes (e.g., increased oxygen saturation) and parent reports of feeling calm and relaxed (Teckenberg-Jansson et al, 2011).*

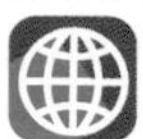

Multicultural

- Provide culturally sensitive parent support to non–English-speaking mothers and families. CEBN: *In a study contrasting NICU norms in Christchurch, New Zealand, and Tokyo, Japan, areas of difference in parental support needs included (1) establishment of oral feeding, (2) nursing care–related decision-making, (3) parental information/involvement early in hospitalization, (4) visiting regulations, and (5) Western-based interventions (Ichijima, 2009).* EB: *Congruent parent-to-parent matching is an important way to help non-Anglophone mothers mobilize their strengths; cope with feelings of loss, guilt, helplessness, and anxiety; and increase access to services (Ardal et al, 2011).*
- Discuss cultural norms with families to provide care that is appropriate for enhancing attachment with the infant/child. EB: *Recognition of the NICU norms that may hinder parent-staff communication is important in nursing practice (Ichijima et al, 2011).*

A

- Promote the attachment process in women who have abused substances by providing a culturally based, women-centered treatment environment. CEB: *Pregnant/postpartum Asian/Pacific Islander women identified provisions for the newborn, infant health care, parent education, and infant-mother bonding as conducive to their treatment (Morelli et al, 2001).*
- Promote attachment process/development of maternal sensitivity in incarcerated women. EB: *By creating a simple and uncomplicated plan for an incarcerated mother to pump and store her breast milk, "nurses have the opportunity to change the mothering experience" as they promote maternal-infant attachment and improve health for mother and infant (Allen & Baker, 2013).*
- Empower family members to draw on personal strengths in which multiple worldviews/values are recognized, incorporated, and negotiated. CEBN: *According to a Thai study of NICU parents, the need to be strong, to be there, and to care for infants emerged as main themes in parents' stories (Sitanon, 2009).* EBN: *A study by Heidari et al (2012) found that "having a premature infant with anomalies is viewed as a family flaw," carrying with it the "stigma of shame."*
- Encourage positive involvement and relationship development between children and fathers. EB: *A study by Kadivar and Mozafarinia (2013) confirmed that using the HUG Your Baby DVD and family-friendly instructional program with NICU fathers increased their knowledge of infant behavior and is likely to boost their confidence, promote the parent-child relationship, and strengthen the family unit (Kadivar & Mozafarinia, 2013).*

Home Care

- The above interventions may be adapted for home care use.
- Assess quality of interaction between parent and infant/child. CEB: *In a study regarding effectiveness of home visiting by paraprofessionals/nurses, outcomes of nurse visitations in particular included more responsive mother-child interaction, less emotional vulnerability in response to fear stimuli among infants, greater infant emotional vitality in response to joy/anger stimuli, and less likelihood of language delays (Olds et al, 2002).*
- Use "interaction coaching" (i.e., teaching mother to let the infant lead) so that the mother will match her interaction style to the baby's cues. EBN: *Although delivery of personalized interventions is labor intensive, and testing ways to provide targeted interventions in order to promote sensitive, responsive maternal-infant interactions is challenging, these are supported by current research (Mayberry & Horowitz, 2011).*

▲ Provide supportive care for infants and children whose parents have been deployed during wartime. EB: *Given the stressful task facing returning service members (i.e., reintegrating themselves into families "whose internal rhythms have changed and where children have taken on new roles"), the authors advocate for strengthening community support services and adopting public health education measures that reduce the stigma of seeking treatment for post-traumatic stress disorder (Lester & Flake, 2013).*

- Encourage custodial grandparents to utilize support groups available for caregivers of children. *A strengths-based support group for caregiving grandmothers recommended five interventions adaptable to nursing practice: (1) disseminate health information regarding chronic conditions (e.g., diabetes, heart disease, high cholesterol, arthritis, migraines, ocular hypertension); (2) expand practical information regarding social service, financial and legal resources; (3) explore spiritual and religious connections that could serve as sources of psychological well-being and sustenance; (4) provide socioemotional support to help manage mental health issues; (5) utilize youth "lock-ins" and outings to give needed breaks from childcare responsibilities (Collins, 2011).* EB: *The Family Child Care Network Impact Study found that relationship-based network supports delivered by specially trained staff were associated with higher quality caregiving by childcare providers (Bromer & Bibbs, 2011).*

REFERENCES

Allen, D., & Baker, B. (2013). Supporting mothering through breastfeeding for incarcerated women. *Journal of Obstetrical & Gynecological Nursing, 42*(Suppl. 1), S103.

Ardal, F., Sulman, J., & Fuller-Thompson, E. (2011). Support like a walking stick: parent-buddy matching for language and culture in the NICU. *Neonat Netw, 30*(2), 89–98.

Arockiasamy, V., Holsti, L., & Albersheim, S. (2008). Fathers' experience in the neonatal intensive care unit: a search for control. *Pediatrics, 121*(2), e215–e222.

Astrachan-Fletcher, E., Veldhuis, C., Lively, N., et al. (2008). The reciprocal effects of eating disorders and the postpartum period: a review of the literature and recommendations for clinical care. *Journal of Women's Health, 17*(2), 227–239.

Axelin, A., Lehtonen, L., Pelander, T., et al. (2010). Mothers' different styles of involvement in preterm infant pain care. *Journal of Obstetrical & Gynecological Nursing, 39*(4), 415–424.

Bernier, A., & Meins, E. (2008). A threshold approach to understanding the origins of attachment disorganization. *Developmental Psychology, 44*(4), 969–982.

Bromer, J., & Bibbs, T. (2011). Improving support services for family child care through relationship-based training. *Zero to Three, 31*(5), 22–29.

Collins, W. L. (2011). A strengths-based support group to empower African-American grandmothers raising grandchildren. *Social Work and Christianity, 38*(4), 453–466.

Davanzo, R., Pierpaolo, B., Travan, L., et al. (2013). Intermittent kangaroo mother care: a NICU protocol. *Journal of Human Lactation, 29*(3), 332–338.

DeGangi, G. A., & Breinbauer, C. (1997). The symptomatology of infants and toddlers with regulatory disorders. *Journal of Developmental Learning Disabilities, 1*(1), 183–215.

Fegran, L., Helseth, S., & Fagermoen, M. S. (2008). A comparison of mothers' and fathers' experiences of the attachment process in a neonatal intensive care unit. *Journal of Clinical Nursing, 17*(6), 810–816.

Field, T., Diego, M., & Hernandez-Reif, M. (2010). Preterm infant massage therapy research: A review. *Infant Behavior and Development, 33*(2), 115–124.

Gephart, S. M., & McGrath, J. M. (2012). Family-centered care of the surgical neonate. *Newborn and Infant Nursing Reviews, 12*(1), 5–7.

Gooding, J. S., Cooper, L. G., Blaine, A. I., et al. (2011). Family support and family-centered care in the neonatal intensive care unit: Origins, advances, impact. *Seminars in Perinatology, 35*(1), 20 28.

Greenspan, S. I. (1992). *Infancy and early childhood: the practice of clinical assessment and intervention with emotional and developmental challenges*. Madison, CT: International Universities Press.

Greenspan, S. I., & Wieder, S. (1998). *The child with special needs: encouraging intellectual and emotional growth*. Reading, MA: Perseus Books.

Heidari, H., Hasanpour, M., & Fooladi, M. (2012). The Iranian parents of premature infants in NICU experience stigma of shame. *Medical Archives, 66*(1), 35–40.

Holditch-Davis, D., Miles, M. S., Burchinal, M. R., et al. (2011). Maternal role attainment with medically fragile infants: part 2. Relationship to the quality of parenting. *Research Nursing Health, 34*(1), 35–48.

Hollywood, M., & Hollywood, E. (2011). The lived experiences of fathers of a premature baby on a neonatal intensive care unit. *Journal of Neonatal Nursing, 17*, 32–40.

Ichijima, E. (2009). *Nursing roles in parental support: a cross-cultural comparison between neonatal intensive care units in New Zealand and Japan*. Canterbury, UK: University of Canterbury.

Ichijima, E., Kirk, R., & Hornblow, A. (2011). Parental support in neonatal intensive care units: a cross-cultural comparison between New Zealand and Japan. *Journal of Pediatric Nursing, 26*(3), 206–215.

Kadivar, M., & Mozafarinia, S. M. (2013). Supporting fathers in a NICU: Effects of the HUG your baby program on fathers' understanding of preterm infant behavior. *Journal of Perinatal Education, 22*(2), 113–119.

Karbasi, S. S., Golestan, M., & Fallah, R. (2014). Effect of massage therapy on sleep behavior in low birth weight infants. *Iranian Journal of Pediatrics, 24*(S2), S47.

Kong, L.-P., Cui, Y., Qiu, Y.-F., et al. (2013). Anxiety and depression in parents of sick neonates: a hospital-based study. *Journal of Clinical Nursing, 22*, 1163–1172.

Lawhon, G. (2002). Integrated nursing care: vital issues important in the humane care of the newborn. *Seminars in Neonatology, 7*, 441–446.

Lester, P., & Flake, E. (2013). How wartime military service affects children and families. *The Future of Children, 23*(2).

Lynn, L. N., Cuskelly, M., O.'Callaghan, M. J., et al. (2011). Self-regulation: a new perspective on learning problems experienced by children born extremely preterm. *Australian Journal of Educational and Developmental Psychology, 11*, 1–10.

Massaro, A. N., Hammad, T. A., Jazzo, B., et al. (2009). Massage with kinesthetic stimulation improves weight gain in preterm infants. *J Perinat, 29*(5), 352–357.

Mayberry, L., & Horowitz, J. A. (2011). Postpartum depression. In J. J. Fitzpatrick & M. Kazer (Eds.), *Encyclopedia of Nursing Research* (3rd ed.). New York: Springer.

Miles, M. S., Holditch-Davis, D., Burchinal, M. R., et al. (2011). Maternal role attainment with medically fragile infants: part 1. Measurement and correlates during the first year of life. *Research in Nursing and Health, 34*(1), 20–34.

Morelli, P. T., Fong, R., & Oliveira, J. (2001). Culturally competent substance abuse treatment for Asian/Pacific Islander women. *Journal of Human Behavior Soc Environment, 3*(3/4), 263.

Olds, D. L., et al. (2002). Home visiting by paraprofessionals and by nurses: a randomized, controlled trial. *Pediatrics, 110*(3), 486–496.

Pölkki, T. 1., Korhonen, A., & Laukkala, H. (2012). Expectations associated with the use of music in neonatal intensive care: a survey from the viewpoint of parents. *Journal for Specialists in Pediatric Nursing, 17*(4), 321–328.

Pridham, K. F., Schulte, H. D., Limbo, R., et al. (1998). Guided participation and development of care-giving competencies for families of low-birth-weight infants. *Journal of Advanced Nursing, 28*(5), 948–958.

Rossetti, L. M. (1999). *Infant-toddler Assessment*. Boston: Little, Brown and Company.

Sitanon, T. (2009). *Thai parents' experiences of parenting preterm infants during hospitalization in the neonatal intensive care unit*, unpublished doctoral dissertation. University of Washington, School of Nursing.

Subhani, M. T., & Kanwal, I. (2012). Digital scrapbooking as a standard of care in neonatal intensive care units: Initial experience. *Neonatal Network, 31*(3), 162–168.

Stitt, N., & Reupert, A. (2014). Mothers with an eating disorder: 'food comes before anything.' *Journal of Psychiatric & Mental Health Nursing, 21*(6), 509–517.

Strathearn, L., & Kim, S. (2013). Mothers' amygdala response to positive or negative infant affect is modulated by personal relevance. *Frontiers in Neuroscience, 7*, 176.

Strathearn, L., Li, J., Fonagy, P., et al. (2008). What's in a smile? Maternal brain responses to infant facial cues. *Pediatrics, 122*(1), 40–51, Jul.

Teckenberg-Jansson, P., Huotilainen, M., Pölkki, T., et al. (2011). Rapid effects of neonatal music therapy combined with kangaroo care on prematurely-born infants. *Nordic Journal of Music Therapy, 20*(1), 22–42.

Tramo, M. J., Lense, M., Van Ness, C., et al. (2011). Effects of music on physiological and behavioral indices of acute pain and stress in premature infants: clinical trial and literature review. *Music Med, 3*(2), 72–83.

Valizadeh, L., Zamanzadeh, V., Mohammadi, E., et al. (2014). Continuous and multiple waves of emotional responses: Mother's experience with a premature infant. *Iran Journal of Nurse Midwifery, 19*(4), 340–348.

Walsh, J., & Goser, L. (2013). Development of an innovative NICU teen parent support program: One unit's experience. *Journal of Perinatal & Neonatal Nursing, 27*(2), 176–183.

Woolhouse, H., Gartland, D., Perlen, S., et al. (2014). Physical health after childbirth and maternal depression in the first 12 months post partum: Results of an Australian nulliparous pregnancy cohort study. *Midwifery, 20*, 378–384.

Yildiz, A., Arikan, D., Gözüm, S., et al. (2011). The effect of the odor of breast milk on the time needed for transition from gavage to total oral feeding in preterm infants. *Journal of Nursing Scholarship, 43*(3), 265–273, 2011.

Zimmerman, K., & Bauersachs, C. (2012). *International Journal of Childbirth Education, 27*(1), 50–53.

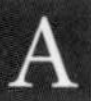

Autonomic Dysreflexia *Mary Beth Flynn Makic, PhD, RN, CNS, CCNS, FAAN*

NANDA-I

Definition

Life-threatening, uninhibited sympathetic response of the nervous system to a noxious stimulus after a spinal cord injury at T7 or above

Defining Characteristics

Blurred vision; bradycardia; chest pain; chilling; conjunctival congestion; diaphoresis (above the injury); headache (diffuse pain in different areas of the head and not confined to any nerve distribution area); Horner's syndrome; metallic taste in mouth; nasal congestion; pallor (below injury); paresthesia; paroxysmal hypertension; pilomotor reflex; red blotches on skin (above the injury); tachycardia

Related Factors

Bladder distention; bowel distention; insufficient caregiver knowledge of disease process; insufficient knowledge of disease process; skin irritation

NOC (Nursing Outcomes Classification)

Suggested NOC Outcomes

Neurological Status; Neurological Status: Autonomic; Vital Signs

Example NOC Outcome with Indicators

Neurological Status: Autonomic as evidenced by the following indicators: Systolic blood pressure/Diastolic blood pressure/Apical heart rate/Perspiration response pattern/Goose bumps response pattern/Pupil reactivity/Peripheral tissue perfusion. (Rate each indicator of **Neurological Status: Autonomic:** 1 = severely compromised, 2 = substantially compromised, 3 = moderately compromised, 4 = mildly compromised, 5 = not compromised [see Section I].)

Client Outcomes

Client Will (Specify Time Frame)

- Maintain normal vital signs
- Remain free of dysreflexia symptoms
- Explain symptoms, prevention, and treatment of dysreflexia

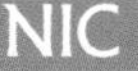

NIC (Nursing Interventions Classification)

Suggested NIC Intervention

Dysreflexia Management

Example NIC Activities—Dysreflexia Management

Identify and minimize stimuli that may precipitate dysreflexia; Monitor for signs and symptoms of autonomic dysreflexia

Nursing Interventions and *Rationales*

- Monitor the client for symptoms of dysreflexia, particularly those with high-level and more extensive spinal cord injuries. See Defining Characteristics. EB: *Autonomic dysreflexia (AD) occurs in up to 90% of clients with high level spinal cord injury (Cragg & Krassioukov, 2013). Because most clients are asymptomatic, it is important to recognize risk factors for AD, such as higher and more complete injuries and injuries related to trauma (Huang et al, 2011).*
- ▲ Collaborate with providers and caregivers to identify the cause of dysreflexia. AD is triggered by a stimulus from below the level of injury. The most common triggers are distention of the bladder, kidney stones,

kink in urinary catheter, urinary tract infection, fecal impaction, pressure ulcer, ingrown toenail, menstruation, hemorrhoids, invasive testing, and sexual intercourse (Cragg & Krassioukov, 2013; Wan & Krassioukov, 2014). **EB:** *Health care practitioners and caregivers should assess for conditions that place the client at risk for AD. Clients with upper thoracic and cervical injuries often have lower resting blood pressure, thus elevated blood pressure with AD may be less obvious, necessitating the importance of always assessing the condition (Jackson & Acland, 2011; Cragg & Krassioukov, 2013).*

▲ If symptoms of dysreflexia are present, place client in high Fowler's position, remove all support hoses or binders, loosen clothing, and immediately determine the noxious stimulus causing the response. If blood pressure cannot be decreased within 1 minute, notify the provider emergently (i.e., STAT). **EB:** *These steps promote venous pooling, decrease venous return, and decrease blood pressure. The client should be rapidly evaluated by both the health care provider and nurse to find the possible cause (Jackson & Acland, 2011; Furlan, 2013; Urden et al, 2013).* To determine the stimulus for dysreflexia:
  - ❍ First, assess bladder function. Check for distention, and if present catheterize the client using an anesthetic jelly as a lubricant. Do not use the Valsalva maneuver or Crede's method to empty the bladder. Ensure existing catheter patency. Also assess for signs of urinary tract infection. **EB:** *AD is commonly associated with bowel or bladder dysfunction in persons with a spinal cord injury (Furusawa et al, 2011; Cragg & Krassioukov, 2013).*
  - ❍ Second, assess bowel function. Numb the bowel area with a topical anesthetic as ordered and gently check for impaction. **EB:** *For clients who require manual removal of stool, pretreatment with lidocaine cream may decrease the flow of impulses from the bowel and lower blood pressure during removal (Urden et al, 2013; Faaborg et al, 2014).*
  - ❍ Third, assess the skin, looking for any points of pressure and ingrown toenails.

▲ Initiate antihypertensive therapy as soon as ordered and monitor for cardiac dysrhythmias. **EB:** *Due to the large amount of sympathetic discharge following AD, clients in hypertensive crisis are at risk for arrhythmias, myocardial infarction, and cerebral hemorrhage (Furlan, 2013; Wan & Krassioukov, 2014).*

▲ Be careful not to increase noxious sensory stimuli during assessment for cause of AD. If numbing agent is ordered, use it on anus and 1 inch of rectum before attempting to remove a fecal impaction. If necessary to replace an obstructed catheter, use an anesthetic jelly as ordered during the insertion. **EB:** *Increased noxious sensory stimuli can exacerbate the abnormal response and worsen the client's prognosis (Urden et al, 2013).*

• Monitor vital signs every 3 to 5 minutes during acute event; continue to monitor vital signs after event is resolved (e.g., symptoms resolve and vital signs return to baseline, usually up to 2 hours post event). **EB:** *It is possible for the client to develop rebound hypotension after the acute event because of the use of antihypertensive medications, or symptoms of dysreflexia may reoccur (Urden et al, 2013; Furlan, 2013).*

• Watch for complications of dysreflexia, including signs of cerebral hemorrhage, seizures, cardiac dysfunction, or intraocular hemorrhage. **EB:** *Extremely high blood pressure can cause intracranial hemorrhage, myocardial injury and dysfunction, and death (Wan & Krassioukov, 2014).*

• Accurately and completely record any incidences of dysreflexia; especially note the precipitating stimuli. *It is imperative to determine noxious stimuli that precipitated AD and whether the condition is persistent, requiring the client to take medications routinely or implement different interventions to prevent repeat incidences (Cragg & Krassioukov, 2013).*

• Use the following interventions to prevent dysreflexia:
  - ❍ Ensure that drainage from an indwelling catheter is good and that bladder is not distended. Assess the client frequently for signs and symptoms of urinary tract infection.
  - ❍ Ensure a regular pattern of defecation to prevent fecal impaction. **EB:** *AD is commonly associated with bowel dysfunction in persons with a spinal cord injury (Wan & Krassioukov, 2014). A recent study found that bowel management with transanal irrigation was less traumatic than bowel management by digital rectal evacuation (Faaborg et al, 2014).*
  - ❍ Frequently change position of client to relieve pressure and prevent formation of pressure ulcers.

▲ If ordered, apply an anesthetic agent to any wound below the level of injury before performing wound care. **EB:** *Stimuli that would cause pain in persons without spinal cord injury can lead to AD (Furlan 2013; Urden et al, 2013).*

▲ Because episodes can recur, notify all health care team members of the possibility of a dysreflexia episode. All health care personnel working with the client should be aware of the condition and how to treat it.

▲ For female clients with spinal cord injury, assess the client for AD during menstrual cycle. If the client becomes pregnant, collaborate with obstetrical health care practitioners to monitor for signs and

symptoms of dysreflexia. EB: *Autonomic dysreflexia may signal the onset of labor or be a sign of preterm labor. Women undergoing cesarean section should be carefully monitored intraoperatively and postoperatively (Walsh et al, 2010).*

Home Care

- The above interventions may be adapted for home care use.
- Provide the client and caregiver with written information on common causes of AD and initial treatment. *An AD card is available from the SCI-INFO-PAGES online resource for clients with quadriplegia and paraplegia (http://www.sci-info-pages.com/ad.html) as well as from the Christopher and Dana Reeve Foundation (http://www.christopherreeve.org/site/c.mtKZKgMWKwG/b.7717499/k.D633/Autonomic_Dysreflexia_AD_Card__Send_to_a_Friend/apps/ka/ecard/choosecard.asp).*
- Provide resources to the client with any known proclivity toward dysreflexia to wear a medical alert bracelet and carry a medical alert wallet card when not in a safe environment (i.e., not with someone who knows client has the condition and can respond appropriately).
- ▲ Establish an emergency plan: obtain provider orders for medications to be used in situations in which first aid does not work and plans to identify potential stimuli. EB: *Medication administered immediately can reverse early stage dysreflexia. Notify health care provider of emergency (Craig Hospital, 2013). If orders have not been obtained or client does not have emergency medications, contact emergency medical services.*
- When episode of dysreflexia is resolved, monitor blood pressure every 30 to 60 minutes for next 2 hours or admit to institution for observation. EB: *Autonomic dysreflexia can have a profound effect on vasculature, leading to chronic cardiovascular dysfunction (Furlan, 2013).*

Client/Family Teaching and Discharge Planning

- Teach recognition of the earliest symptoms of dysreflexia, the actions that should be taken when they occur, and the need to obtain help immediately. Give client a written card describing signs and symptoms of AD and initial actions. CEB: *Clients and caregivers at risk for not understanding the key elements of AD occurrence and management are clients with nontraumatic etiologies, those with T5 or lower injuries, those in the youngest age group at injury, and those who had a shorter duration of injury (Schottler et al, 2009). Clients have reported knowledge gaps regarding AD and having symptoms of AD but not recognizing the condition (McGillivray et al, 2009).*
- Teach steps to prevent dysreflexia episodes: care of bladder, bowel, and skin and prevention of other forms of noxious stimuli (e.g., not wearing clothing that is too tight, nail care). Discuss the potential impact of sexual intercourse and pregnancy on autonomic dysreflexia. EB: *Autonomic dysreflexia may be triggered by ejaculation and sperm retrieval for men (McGuire et al, 2011).*

REFERENCES

Christopher and Dana Reeve Foundation. *Paralysis Resource Center, AD Card.* Retrieved June 15, 2015 <http://www.christopherreeve.org/site/c.mtKZKgMWKwG/b.7717499/k.D633/Autonomic_Dysreflexia_AD_Card__Send_to_a_Friend/apps/ka/ecard/choosecard.asp>.

Craig Hospital. (2013). *Autonomic Dysreflexia.* Retrieved April 11, 2015 <http://craighospital.hostworks.net/repository/documents/HeathInfo/PDFs/765.AutonomicDysreflexia.pdf>.

Cragg, J., & Krassioukov, A. (2013). Autonomic dysreflexia: Five things to know about. *CMAJ.*

Faaborg, P. M., Christensen, P., Krassioukov, A., et al. (2014). Autonomic dysreflexia during bowel evacuation procedures and bladder filling in subjects with spinal cord injury. *Spinal Cord, 52,* 494–498.

Furlan, J. C. (2013). Autonomic dysreflexia: A clinical emergency. *J Trauma Acute Care Surg, 75*(3), 496–500.

Furusawa, K., et al. (2011). Incidence of symptomatic autonomic dysreflexia varies according to the bowel and bladder management techniques in patients with spinal cord injury. *Spinal Cord, 49*(1), 49–54.

Huang, Y. H., et al. (2011). Autonomic dysreflexia during urodynamic examinations in patients with suprasacral spinal cord injury. *Archives of Physical Medicine and Rehabilitation, 92*(9), 1450–1454.

Jackson, C. R., & Acland, R. (2011). Knowledge of autonomic dysreflexia in the emergency department. *Emergency Medicine Journal, 28*(10), 866–869.

McGillivray, C. F., Hitzig, S. L., Craven, B. C., et al. (2009). Evaluating knowledge of autonomic dysreflexia among individuals with spinal cord injury and their families. *The Journal of Spinal Cord Medicine, 32*(1), 54–62.

McGuire, C., et al. (2011). Electroejaculatory stimulation for male infertility secondary to spinal cord injury. *Urology, 77*(1), 83–87.

Schottler, J., et al. (2009). Patient and caregiver knowledge of autonomic dysreflexia among youth with spinal cord injury. *Spinal Cord, 47*(9), 681–686.

Quadriplegic, Paraplegic & Caregiver Resources. SCI-INFO-PAGES. (2015). *Autonomic Dysreflexia.* Retrieved April 11, 2015 <http://www.sci-info-pages.com/ad.html>.

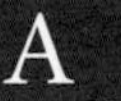

Urden, L. D., Stacy, K. M., & Lough, M. E. (2013). *Critical Care Nursing 7th ed., Nursing Management Plan: Autonomic dysreflexia.* St. Louis, MO: Elsevier, Mosby.

Walsh, P., Grange, C., & Beale, N. (2010). Anaesthetic management of an obstetric patient with idiopathic acute transverse myelitis. *International Journal of Obstetric Anesthesia, 18*(1), 98–101.

Wan, D., & Krassioukov, A. (2014). Life-threatening outcomes associated with autonomic dysreflexia: A clinical review. *The Journal of Spinal Cord Medicine, 37*(1), 1–9.

Risk for Autonomic Dysreflexia

Betty J. Ackley, MSN, EdS, RN, and Mary Beth Flynn Makic, PhD, RN, CNS, CCNS, FAAN

NANDA-I

Definition

Vulnerable to life-threatening, uninhibited response of the sympathetic nervous system after spinal shock in an individual with spinal cord injury or lesion at T6 or above (has been demonstrated in clients with injuries at T7 and T8), which may compromise health

Risk Factors

Cardiopulmonary Stimuli

Deep vein thrombosis; pulmonary emboli

Gastrointestinal Stimuli

Bowel distention; constipation; difficult passage of feces; digital stimulation; enemas; esophageal reflux disease; fecal impaction; gallstones; gastric ulcer; gastrointestinal system pathology; hemorrhoids; suppositories

Musculoskeletal-Integumentary Stimuli

Cutaneous stimulations (e.g., pressure ulcer, ingrown toenail, dressings, burns, rash); fracture; heterotrophic bone; pressure over bony prominence; pressure over genitalia; range-of-motion exercises; spasm; sunburn; wound

Neurological Stimuli

Irritating stimuli below level of injury; painful stimuli below level of injury

Regulatory Stimuli

Extremes of environmental temperature; temperature fluctuations

Reproductive Stimuli

Ejaculation; labor and delivery period; menstruation; ovarian cyst; pregnancy; sexual intercourse

Situational Stimuli

Constrictive clothing (e.g., straps, stockings, shoes); pharmaceutical agent; positioning; substance withdrawal (e.g., narcotic, opiate); surgical procedure

Urological Stimuli

Bladder distention; bladder spasm; cystitis; detrusor sphincter dyssynergia; epididymitis; instrumentation; renal calculi; surgical procedure; urethritis; urinary catheterization; urinary tract infection

NIC, NOC, Client Outcomes, Nursing Interventions, Client/Family Teaching and Discharge Planning, *Rationales,* and References

Refer to care plan for **Autonomic Dysreflexia.**

Risk for Bleeding

June M. Como, EdD, RN, CNS

B

NANDA-I

Definition

Vulnerable to a decrease in blood volume, which may compromise health

Risk Factors

Aneurysm; circumcision; disseminated intravascular coagulopathy; gastrointestinal condition (e.g., ulcer, polyps, varices); history of falls; impaired liver function (e.g., cirrhosis, hepatitis); inherent coagulopathy (e.g., thrombocytopenia); insufficient knowledge of bleeding precautions; postpartum complications (e.g., uterine atony, retained placenta); pregnancy complications (e.g., premature rupture of membranes, placenta previa/abruption, multiple gestation); trauma; treatment regimen

NOC (Nursing Outcomes Classification)

Suggested NOC Outcomes

Blood Coagulation; Blood Loss Severity; Circulation Status; Fall Prevention Behavior; Gastrointestinal Function; Knowledge: Personal Safety, Maternal Status, Physical Injury Severity, Risk Control, Safe Home Environment, Vital Signs

Example NOC Outcome with Indicators

Blood Coagulation as evidenced by the following indicators: Clot formation, International normalized ratio (INR), Hemoglobin (HGB), Platelet Count, Bleeding, Bruising, Hematuria, Hematemesis. (Rate the outcome and indicators of **Blood Coagulation:** 1 = severe deviation from normal range, 2 = substantial deviation from normal range, 3 = moderate deviation from normal range, 4 = mild deviation from normal range, 5 = no deviation from normal range.)

Client Outcomes

Client Will (Specify Time Frame)

- Discuss precautions to prevent bleeding complications
- Explain actions that should be taken if bleeding happens
- Maintain adherence to agreed upon anticoagulant medication and lab work regimens
- Monitor for signs and symptoms of bleeding
- Maintain a mean arterial pressure above 70 mm Hg, a heart rate between 60 and 100 bpm with a normal rhythm, and urine output greater than 0.5 mL/kg/hr
- Maintain warm, dry skin

NIC (Nursing Interventions Classification)

Suggested NIC Interventions

Admission Care; Bleeding Precautions; Bleeding Reduction; Blood Product Administration; Circumcision Care; Fluid Management; Health Screening; Hemorrhage Control; Neurologic Monitoring; Postpartum Care; Risk Identification; Teaching: Disease Process; Teaching: Prescribed Medication; Oxygen Therapy; Shock Prevention; Surveillance; Vital Signs Monitoring

Example NIC Activities—Bleeding Precautions

Monitor the client closely for hemorrhage; Monitor coagulation studies; Monitor orthostatic vital signs, including blood pressure; Instruct the client and/or family on signs of bleeding and appropriate actions in case bleeding occurs

Nursing Interventions and *Rationales*

- Perform admission risk assessment for falls and for signs of bleeding. Safety precautions should be implemented for all at risk clients. EBN: *Upon client admission to any health care facility, nurses should assess for fall risk factors that could increase the risk of bleeding (Holmes, 2011).*

- Monitor the client closely for hemorrhage, especially in those at increased risk for bleeding. Watch for any signs of bleeding, including bleeding of the gums, blood in sputum, emesis, urine or stool, bleeding from a wound, bleeding into the skin with petechiae, and purpura. EB: *Clients at increased risk for bleeding may include older individuals (>60 years of age), individuals with active gastroduodenal ulcer, intrapartum and postpartum women, previous bleeding episode, hypertension, labile INRs, low platelet count, active malignancy, renal or liver failure, intensive care unit stay, drug or alcohol use, coadministration of antiplatelets and nonsteroidal antiinflammatory drugs (NSAIDs), and antithrombotic and anticoagulant therapies (Hastings-Tolsma et al, 2013; Chen et al, 2011; Chua et al, 2011; Decousus et al, 2011). Individuals who take selective serotonin reuptake inhibitors (SSRIs) with or without a history of gastrointestinal bleeding may be at increased risk for bleeding especially if also taking NSAIDs or low-dose aspirin (Lanbos et al, 2011; Andrade et al, 2010). Use of aspirin and clopidogrel in the treatment of clients with image verified "small" subcortical strokes demonstrated higher rates of bleeding when compared with treatment with aspirin alone (Stiles, 2011).*
- If bleeding develops, apply pressure over the site or appropriate artery as needed. Apply pressure dressing if indicated. EB: *Nonpharmacological means, such as application of pressure, may reduce bleeding (Makris et al, 2013; Matteucci et al, 2011).*

▲ Collaborate on an appropriate bleeding management plan, including nonpharmacological and pharmacological measures to stop bleeding based on the antithrombotic used. EB: *Recommendations for bleeding risk prevention and management carefully weigh the risks and benefits of nonpharmacological and pharmacological interventions (Makris et al, 2013).*

▲ Monitor coagulation studies, including prothrombin time, INR, activated partial thromboplastin time (aPTT), fibrinogen, fibrin degradation/split products, and platelet counts as appropriate. EB: *New oral anticoagulants often have no requirement for routine coagulation studies; however, vigilance is still warranted in that risk for bleeding without benefit of reversal agents exists (Levy, 2014; Siegal & Crowther, 2013). INR is the preferred method to evaluate warfarin therapy, typically at least 16 hours after the last dose is administered. Dose adjustments will not result in a steady state INR value for up to 3 weeks (ICSI, 2011).* CEB: *The aPTT is most commonly used to assess unfractionated heparin (UH) therapy but some clients may require additional testing to assess for heparin resistance (Russo, 2011). Replacement of UH with low-molecular-weight heparin and other new anticoagulants may be forthcoming but UH is still a drug of choice because of its ability to rapidly reverse effect with protamine sulfate (Lehman & Frank, 2009).*

- Assess vital signs at frequent intervals to assess for physiological evidence of bleeding, such as tachycardia, tachypnea, and hypotension. Symptoms may include dizziness, shortness of breath, and fatigue. EB: *Carefully assess for compensatory changes associated with bleeding, including increased heart rate and respiratory rate. Initially blood pressure may be stable, before beginning to decrease. Assess for orthostatic blood pressure changes (drop in systolic by >20 mm Hg and/or a drop in diastolic by >10 mm Hg in 3 minutes) by taking blood pressure with the client in lying, sitting, and standing positions (Matteucci et al, 2011; Urden et al, 2009). Prospective identification of clients at risk for massive transfusion is an imprecise science (Vandromme et al, 2011), although higher shock index (≥0.9) has been associated with increased bleeding risk (Olaussen et al, 2014).*

▲ Monitor all medications for potential to increase bleeding, including aspirin, NSAIDs, SSRIs, and complementary and alternative therapies such as coenzyme Q10 and ginger. EB: *Antiplatelet medications can increase the risk of bleeding in high-risk clients (ICSI, 2011). Ginger, when taken with medicines that slow clotting, may increase the chances for bruising and bleeding (Medline Plus, 2011).* CEB: *In a study of adults receiving warfarin, coenzyme Q10 and ginger appeared to increase the risk of bleeding (Shalansky et al, 2007).*

Consensus on Delivery of Inpatient Anticoagulant Therapy 2013

▲ **QSEN:** Systems-based process should be used for the management of inpatient anticoagulant therapy (Nutescu et al, 2013).

▲ **QSEN:** Multidisciplinary involvement that is accountable and provides leadership should be incorporated (Nutescu et al, 2013).

▲ **QSEN:** Seamless integration of anticoagulant system with all client resources including electronic health records (Nutescu et al, 2013;Villanueva et al, 2013).

▲ **QSEN:** Evidence-based standards, periodically reviewed, should be used to ensure appropriate use of anticoagulant therapies in all situations (Nutescu et al, 2013).

▲ **QSEN:** Competency based education for all multidisciplinary personnel engaged in anticoagulant management (Nutescu et al, 2013).
▲ **QSEN:** Ensure safe and effective use of therapies during care transitions and discharge through appropriate client education (Nutescu et al, 2013).
▲ **QSEN:** Ensure safe care transitions and maintenance of prescribed anticoagulants (Nutescu et al, 2013).
▲ **QSEN:** Measure quality indicators and assess client outcomes with a focus on quality improvement (Nutescu et al, 2013).

Safety Guidelines for Anticoagulant Administration: Joint Commission National Patient Safety Goals

Follow approved protocol for anticoagulant administration:

- Use prepackaged medications and prefilled or premixed parenteral therapy as ordered
- Check laboratory tests (i.e., INR) before administration
- Use programmable pumps when using parenteral administration
- Ensure appropriate education for client/family and all staff concerning anticoagulants used
- Notify dietary services when warfarin is prescribed (to reduce vitamin K in diet)
- Monitor for any symptoms of bleeding before administration. EB: *Standard defined protocols can decrease errors in administration (Joint Commission, 2011).*
- Anticoagulation therapy is complex. EBN: *Nurses have an integral role in medication management through the education of clients (Howland, 2012).* EB: *Medication reconciliation techniques and predischarge education employed by pharmacists in an emergency department setting demonstrated enhanced accuracy of preadmission medication listings, resulting in a reduction in readmission rates (Gardella et al, 2012).* CEB: *Risk of bleeding is reduced in clients who receive appropriate education in anticoagulant therapy use (Metlay et al, 2008).*

▲ Before administering anticoagulants, assess the clotting profile of the client. If the client is on warfarin, assess the INR. Hold the medication if the INR is outside of the recommended parameters and notify the health care provider or advanced practice nurse. EB: *Target INR for warfarin is between 2 and 3 for nonvalvular atrial fibrillation and between 2.5 and 3.5 for valvular atrial fibrillation. Risk for bleeding is increased when INR is >4 and risk for thromboembolism increases when INR is <1.7. A 2% to 4% risk for bleeding remains in individuals within therapeutic range of INR. Dose adjustments of 15% usually change the INR level by 1 (ICSI, 2011). A safety advisory was issued by the Australian regulatory authority for the anticoagulant dabigatran (Pradaxa) due to an increase in the number of bleeding-related adverse events (Hughes, 2011).*

▲ Recognize that vitamin K for vitamin K antagonists (e.g., warfarin, phenprocoumon, Sinthrome, and phenindione) may be given orally or intravenously as ordered for INR levels greater than 5. In some circumstances, pro-hemostatic therapies may be warranted (tranexamic acid, desmopressin, fresh frozen plasma, cryoprecipitate, platelet transfusion, fibrinogen concentrate, prothrombin complex concentrate, activated prothrombin complex concentrate and/or recombinant factor VIIa) if serious or life-threatening bleeding occurs (Makris et al, 2013). EB: *With INR levels above 5, it is recommended to give vitamin K rather than withholding the warfarin; administration of vitamin K is by oral or intravenous route, because subcutaneous and intramuscular routes result in erratic absorption (ICSI, 2011).*

▲ Manage fluid resuscitation and volume expansion as ordered. EB: *A Cochrane systematic review including 86 trials and more than 5000 subjects suggests that there is no evidence that any one colloidal solution is safer or more effective than any other (Bunn & Trivedi, 2012). Prehospital administration of plasma may mitigate trauma-induced coagulopathy (Moore et al, 2014).* CEB: *Blood products (including human albumin), non–blood products or combinations can be used to restore circulating blood volume in individuals at risk for blood losses from trauma, burns, or surgery. Administration of albumin over normal sterile saline does not alter survival rates (Alderson et al, 2004).*

▲ Consider use of permissive hypotension and restrictive transfusion strategies when treating bleeding episodes. EB: *Hypotensive resuscitation (permissive hypotension), which maintains effective although low mean arterial pressures, may allow adequate perfusion without disruption of coagulation mechanisms, although additional research is warranted (Gourgiotis et al, 2013). A study of 921 subjects with upper gastrointestinal bleeding suggests that restrictive strategies (transfusing when hemoglobin level fell to below 7 g per deciliter) improved survival (P = .02) and resulted in fewer adverse events (P = .02) (Villanueva, 2013).*

▲ Consider discussing the coadministration of a proton-pump inhibitor alongside traditional NSAIDs, or with the use of a cyclo-oxygenase 2 inhibitor with the prescriber. EB: *Risk of NSAID-related bleeding may be reduced with the use of a proton-pump inhibitor or cyclo-oxygenase 2 inhibitor (van Soest et al, 2012; Chua et al, 2011; Rahme & Bernatsky, 2011; Wu et al, 2011).*

- Ensure adequate nurse staffing to provide a high level of surveillance capability. EBN/QSEN: *A key component in surveillance is monitoring; additional research is warranted in this area to identify new technologies and processes to optimize surveillance (Henneman et al, 2012).* CEB: *The size and mix of nurse staffing in hospitals has been demonstrated to have a direct impact on client outcomes. Lower levels of nurse staffing have been associated with higher rates of poor client outcomes, including those outcomes caused by gastrointestinal bleeding and "failure to rescue" (Needleman et al, 2002).*

B

Pediatric

▲ Recognize that prophylactic vitamin K administration should be used in neonates for vitamin K deficiency bleeding (VKDB). EB: *A dose of 0.5 to 1 mg vitamin K remains a standard administration for neonates to avoid VKDB and associated problems (Lippi & Franchini, 2011).*

▲ Recognize warning signs of VKDB, including minimal bleeds, evidence of cholestasis (icteric sclera, dark urine, irritability), and failure to thrive. EB: *Signs of classic VKDB may be mild and include delayed or difficulty feeding or bruising in 24 hours to 1 week, whereas late VKDB associated with breastfeeding may occur at 2 to 12 weeks (Lippi & Franchini, 2011).*

▲ Use caution in administering NSAIDs in children. CEB: *A study of children aged 2 months to 16 years found that although upper gastrointestinal bleeding is rare, one third of the cases seen were attributable to exposure to NSAIDs at doses used for analgesia or antipyretic purposes (Grimaldi-Bensouda et al, 2010).* EB: *A Cochrane review of 15 trials including about 1000 children found insufficient evidence to exclude an increase in bleeding risk after using NSAIDs, although the findings supported use of NSAIDs to reduce emesis (Lewis et al, 2013).*

▲ Monitor children and adolescents for potential bleeding after trauma. EB: *Trauma in children aged 1 through 12 years has been associated with early coagulopathy and subsequent bleeding (Christiaans et al, 2014).* CEB: *Children and adolescents who take SSRIs need to be closely monitored because the potential for bleeding exists across age groups (Andrade et al, 2010).*

▲ Closely monitor children after cardiac surgery for excessive blood loss. EB: *In a study of 182 children aged from neonate to older than 3 years, postoperative blood loss was found to be significantly associated with age (P = .003) and presence of cyanotic disease (P = .01) (Faraoni & Van der Linden, 2014).*

Client/Family Teaching and Discharge Planning

- Teach client and family or significant others about any anticoagulant medications prescribed, including when to take, how often to have lab tests done, signs of bleeding to report, dietary restrictions needed, and precautions to be followed. Instruct the client to report any adverse side effects to his or her health care provider. *Medication teaching includes the drug name, purpose, administration instructions (e.g., with or without food), necessary lab tests, and any side effects to be aware of. Provision of such information using clear communication principles and an understanding of the client's health literacy level may facilitate appropriate adherence to the therapeutic regimen by enhancing knowledge base (Joint Commission, 2011; National Institutes of Health [NIH], 2011).*
- Instruct the client and family on disease process and rationale for care. When clients and their family members have sufficient understanding of their disease process they can participate more fully in care and healthy behaviors. Knowledge empowers clients and family members, allowing them to be active participants in their care. CEBN: *Use of written and verbal education enhances client retention of information needed when managing potent medications (Nurit et al, 2009).*
- Provide client and family or significant others with both oral and written educational materials that meet the standards of client education and health literacy. EB: *The use of clear communication, materials written at a fifth grade level, and the teach-back method enhance the client's ability to understand important health-related information and improves self-care safety (NIH, 2011).*

REFERENCES

Alderson, P., et al. (2004). Human albumin solution for resuscitation and volume expansion in critically ill patients. *Cochrane Database of Systematic Reviews*, (4), CD001208.

Andrade, C., et al. (2010). Serotonin reuptake inhibitor antidepressants and abnormal bleeding: a review for clinicians and a reconsideration of mechanisms. *Journal of Clinical Psychology, 71*, 1565–1575.

B

Bunn, F., & Trivedi, D. (2012). Colloid solutions for fluid resuscitation. *Cochrane Database of Systematic Reviews.*

Chen, W., et al. (2011). Association between CHADS2 risk factors and anticoagulation-related bleeding: a systematic literature review. *Mayo Clinic Proceedings, 86*, 509–521.

Christiaans, S. C., Duhachek-Stapelman, A. L., Russell, R. T., et al. (2014). Coagulopathy After Severe Pediatric Trauma. *Shock (Augusta, Ga.), 41*, 476–490.

Chua, S., et al. (2011). Gastrointestinal bleeding and outcomes after percutaneous coronary intervention for ST-segment elevation myocardial infarction. *American Journal of Critical Care, 20*, 218–225.

Decousus, H., et al. (2011). Factors at admission associated with bleeding risk in medical patients: findings from the IMPROVE investigators. *Chest, 139*, 69–79.

Faraoni, D., & Van der Linden, P. (2014). Factors affecting postoperative blood loss in children undergoing cardiac surgery. *Journal of Cardiothoracic Surgery, 9*, 32.

Gardella, J. E., Cardwell, T. B., & Nnadi, M. (2012). Improving medication safety with accurate preadmission medication lists and postdischarge education. *Joint Commission Journal on Quality & Patient Safety, 38*, 452–458.

Gourgiotis, S., Gemenetzis, G., Kocher, H. M., et al. (2013). Permissive hypotension in bleeding trauma patients: helpful or not and when? *Critical Care Nurse, 33*, 18–25.

Grimaldi-Bensouda, L., et al. (2010). Clinical features and risk factors for upper gastrointestinal bleeding in children: a case-crossover study. *European Journal of Clinical Pharmacology, 6*, 831–837.

Hastings-Tolsma, M., Bernard, R., Brody, M., et al. (2013). Chorioamnionitis: Prevention and management. *Maternal Child Health, 38*, 206–212.

Henneman, E. A., Gawlinski, A., & Giuliano, K. K. (2012). Surveillance: a strategy for improving patient safety in acute and critical care units. *Critical Care Nurse, 32*, e9–e18.

Holmes, S. (2011). Risk for bleeding. In B. Ackley & G. Ladwig (Eds.), *Nursing diagnosis handbook* (ed. 9). St Louis, MO: Mosby.

Howland, R. H. (2012). Effective medication management. *Journal of Psychosocial Nursing and Mental Health Services, 50*, 13–15.

Hughes, S. (2011). Dabigatran: Australia issues bleeding warning. *Heartwire*, From: <http://www.medscape.com/viewarticle/751161_print>. Retrieved October 9, 2011.

Institute for Clinical Systems Improvement (ICSI) (2011). *Antithrombotic therapy supplement*, Bloomington, MN: ICSI.

Joint Commission (2011). *Hospital national patient safety goals*. From: <http://www.jointcommission.org/hap_2011_npsgs/>. Retrieved October 10, 2011.

Lanbos, C., Dasgupta, K., Nedjar, H., et al. (2011). Risk of bleeding associated with combined use of selective serotonin reuptake inhibitors and antiplatelet therapy following acute myocardial infarction. *Canadian Medical Association Journal, 183*, 1835–1843.

Lehman, C., & Frank, E. (2009). Laboratory monitoring of heparin therapy: partial thromboplastin time or anti-Xa assay? *Labmed, 40*(1), 47–51.

Levy, J. H. (2014). Pharmacology and safety of new oral anticoagulants: the challenge of bleeding persists. *Clinics in Laboratory Medicine, 34*, 443–452.

Lewis, S., Nicholson, A., Cardwell ME, et al. (2013). Nonsteroidal anti-inflammatory drugs and perioperative bleeding in paediatric tonsillectomy. *Cochrane Database of Systematic Reviews.*

Lippi, G., & Franchini, M. (2011). Vitamin K in neonates: facts and myths. *Blood Transfusion, 9*, 4–9.

Makris, M., Van Veen, J. J., Tait, C. R., et al. (2013). Guideline on the management of bleeding in patients on antithrombotic agents. *British Journal of Haematology, 160*, 35–46.

Matteucci, R., Schub, T., & Pravikoff, D. (2011). Shock, hypovolemic. *CINAHL nursing guide*. Nursing Reference Center.

Medline Plus. (2011). Ginger. *MedLine Plus*, 11. <http://www.nlm.nih.gov/medlineplus/druginfo/natural/961.html>. Retrieved: November 11, 2011.

Metlay, J., et al. (2008). Patient reported receipt of medication instructions for warfarin is associated with reduced risk of serious bleeding events. *J Gen Intern Med, 23*(10), 1589–1594.

Moore, E. E., Chin, T. L., Chapman, M. C., et al. (2014). Plasma first in the field for postinjury hemorrhagic shock. *Shock (Augusta, Ga.), 41*, 35–38.

National Institutes of Health (NIH) (2011). *Clear communication: An NIH health literacy initiative*. From: <http://www.nih.gov/clearcommunication/plainlanguage.htm>. Retrieved August 3, 2012.

Needleman, J., et al. (2002). Nurse staffing and quality of care in hospitals in the United States. *Policy Politics & Nursing Practice, 3*, 306–308.

Nurit, P., et al. (2009). Evaluation of a nursing intervention project to promote patient medication education. *Journal of Clinics in Nursing, 18*, 2530–2536.

Nutescu, E. A., Wittkowsky, A. K., Burnett, A., et al. (2013). Delivery of optimized inpatient anticoagulation therapy: consensus statement from the anticoagulation forum. *Annals of Pharmacotherapy, 47*, 714–724.

Olaussen, A., Blackburn, T., Mitra, B., et al. (2014). Review article: shock index for prediction of critical bleeding post-trauma: a systematic review. *Emergency Medicine Australasia, 26*, 223–228.

Rahme, E., & Bernatsky, S. (2011). NSAIDs and risk of lower gastrointestinal bleeding. *Lancet, 376*, 7.

Russo, W. (2011). Laboratory monitoring of heparin therapy. *UTMB Health*, 11. Retrieved November 12, 2011, <http://www.utmb.edu/lsg/hem/HEPARIN_THERAPY.htm>.

Shalansky, S., et al. (2007). Risk of warfarin-related bleeding events and supratherapeutic international normalized ratios associated with complementary and alternative medicine: a longitudinal analysis. *Pharmacotherapy, 27*, 1237–1247.

Siegal, D. M., & Crowther, M. A. (2013). Acute management of bleeding in patients on novel oral anticoagulants. *European Heart Journal, 34*, 489–498b.

Stiles, S. (2011). Clopidogrel-aspirin arm halted in SPS3 stroke trial. *Heartwire*, 10. Retrieved October 7, 2011, <http://www.medscape.com/viewarticle/751011_print>.

Urden, L., Stacy, K., & Lough, M. (2009). *Thelan's critical care nursing: diagnosis and management* (ed. 6). Philadelphia, PA: Mosby.

Vandromme, M., et al. (2011). Prospective identification of patients at risk for massive transfusion: an imprecise endeavor. *American Surgeon, 77*, 155–161.

van Soest, E. M., Valkhoff, V. E., Mazzaglia, G., et al. (2012). Suboptimal gastroprotective coverage of NSAID use and the risk of upper gastrointestinal complications. *Gastroenterology, 140*, S–45.

Villanueva, C., Colomo, A., Bosch, A., et al. (2013). Transfusion strategies for acute upper gastrointestinal bleeding. *New England Journal of Medicine, 368*, 11–21.

Wu, H., et al. (2011). Pantoprazole for the prevention of gastrointestinal bleeding in high-risk patients with acute coronary syndromes. *Journal of Critical Care, 26*, 434.e1–434.e6.

Disturbed Body Image *Gail B. Ladwig, MSN, RN, and Marsha McKenzie, MA Ed, BSN, RN*

B

NANDA-I

Definition

Confusion in mental picture of one's physical self

Defining Characteristics

Absence of body part; alteration in body function; alteration in body structure; alteration in view of one's body (e.g., appearance, structure, function); avoids looking at one's body; avoids touching one's body; behavior of acknowledging one's body; behavior of monitoring one's body; change in ability to estimate spatial relationship of body to environment; change in lifestyle; change in social involvement; depersonalization of body part by use of impersonal pronouns; depersonalization of loss by use of impersonal pronouns; emphasis on remaining strengths; extension of body boundary (e.g., includes external object); fear of reaction by others; focus on past appearance; focus on past function; focus on previous strength; heightened achievement; hiding of body part; negative feeling about body; nonverbal response to change in body (e.g., appearance, structure, function); nonverbal response to perceived change in body (e.g., appearance, structure, function); overexposure of body part; perceptions that reflect an altered view of one's body appearance; personalization of body part by name; personalization of loss by name; preoccupation with change; preoccupation with loss; refusal to acknowledge change; trauma to nonfunctioning body part

Related Factors (r/t)

Alteration in body function (due to, for example, anomaly, disease, medication, pregnancy, radiation, surgery, trauma); alteration in cognitive functioning; alteration in self perception; cultural incongruence; developmental transition; illness; impaired psychosocial functioning; injury; spiritual incongruence; surgical procedure; trauma; treatment regimen

NOC (Nursing Outcomes Classification)

Suggested NOC Outcomes

Body Image; Self-Esteem; Acceptance Health Status: Coping, Identity

Example NOC Outcome with Indicators

Body Image as evidenced by the following indicators: Congruence between body reality, body ideal, and body presentation/Satisfaction with body appearance/Adjustment to changes in physical appearance. (Rate the outcome and indicators of **Body Image:** 1 = never positive, 2 = rarely positive, 3 = sometimes positive, 4 = often positive, 5 = consistently positive [see Section I].)

Client Outcomes

Client Will (Specify Time Frame)

- Demonstrate adaptation to changes in physical appearance or body function as evidenced by adjustment to lifestyle change
- Identify and change irrational beliefs and expectations regarding body size or function
- Recognize health-destructive behaviors and demonstrate willingness to adhere to treatments or methods that will promote health
- Verbalize congruence between body reality and body perception
- Describe, touch, or observe affected body part
- Demonstrate social involvement rather than avoidance and use adaptive coping and/or social skills
- Use cognitive strategies or other coping skills to improve perception of body image and enhance functioning
- Use strategies to enhance appearance (e.g., wig, clothing)

NIC (Nursing Interventions Classification)

B

Suggested NIC Interventions

Body Image Enhancement; Eating Disorder Management; Referral; Self-Awareness Enhancement; Self-Esteem Enhancement; Support Group Weight Gain Assistance

Example NIC Activities—Body Image Enhancement

Determine client's body image expectations based on developmental stage; Assist client to identify actions that will enhance appearance

Nursing Interventions and *Rationales*

- • Incorporate psychosocial questions related to body image as part of nursing assessment to identify clients at risk for body image disturbance (e.g., body builders; cancer survivors; clients with eating disorders, burns, skin disorders, polycystic ovary disease; or those with stomas/ostomies/colostomies or other disfiguring conditions). CEB: *Assessment of psychosocial issues can help identify clients at risk for body image concerns as a result of a disfiguring condition (Borwell, 2009). Nurses, caring for clients during their hospital stay, are in the ideal position to assess how they are emotionally adapting to having a disfigurement (Bowers, 2008).*
- ▲ Discuss treatment options and outcomes for women diagnosed with breast cancer. Be prepared to explore options of lumpectomy vs. mastectomy and the potential for reconstructive surgery. Include cosmetic and appliance options available to mitigate effects of mastectomy and/or chemotherapy, such as wigs and customized mastectomy bras. EB: *Disturbance of body image has a relationship to the extent of the surgical procedure and the perceived ability to mitigate these body alterations (Rosenberg et al, 2013).*
- • Discuss individual emphasis placed on body image before mastectomy. Be aware of increased psychosocial distress for women who maintain great emphasis on personal appearance. EB: *A study of 46 women undergoing mastectomy found higher rates of depression and psychological distress in women with a history of high body maintenance and appearance ideals (Arroyo & Lopez, 2011).*
- ▲ Assess for history of childhood maltreatment in clients suffering from body dissatisfaction, anorexia, or other eating disorders and make appropriate psychosocial referrals if indicated. EB: *The results from this study indicate specific forms of childhood maltreatment (emotional and sexual abuse) are significantly associated with body dissatisfaction, depressive symptoms, and eating disorders (Dunkley et al, 2010).*
- ▲ Assess for body dysmorphic disorder (BDD) (pathological preoccupation with muscularity and leanness; occurs more often in males than in females), and refer to psychiatry or other appropriate provider. EB: *BDD is a prevalent and disabling preoccupation with a slight or imagined defect in appearance. Results from the small number of available randomized controlled trials suggest that serotonin reuptake inhibitors and cognitive behavioral therapy (CBT) may be useful in treating clients with BDD (Ipser et al, 2009; Phillips, 2010).*
- ▲ Determine if body image impairment is actual or perceived and extent to which it affects the social actions and behaviors through the use of assessment tools such as Assessment of the Attitudinal Component of Body Image in Children or the Measures of Body Satisfaction and Related Concepts in Adolescents and Adults. EB: *Perceived defects or alterations in appearance do not necessarily reflect actual observed changes and psychosocial distress must be determined through individual assessment (Bolton et al, 2010).*
- • Assess for lipodystrophy (an abnormal redistribution of adipose tissue) in clients receiving antiretroviral therapy for HIV/AIDS. This condition is common and can be a source of distress to clients. EBN: *Lipodystrophy is often an unavoidable side effect of antiretroviral therapy. Clients suffering from this syndrome are often ignored when expressing concerns about body changes. Nurses are uniquely qualified to assess these clients as well as provide education and psychosocial support (Gagnon & Holmes, 2011).*
- • Discuss expectations for weight loss and anticipated body changes with clients planning to undergo bariatric surgery for morbid obesity. Assist the client in identifying realistic goals. EB: *Morbidly obese clients often set unrealistic goals for ideal body weight and appearance following bariatric surgery. Guidance is necessary to help them understand limitations of the surgery (Munoz et al, 2010).*

B

▲ Use cognitive-behavioral therapy (CBT) to assist the client to express his emotions and feelings. EBN: *This study of clients with bulimia used CBT and helped the clients to disentangle themselves regarding body image and weight (Huang & Hsieh, 2010).*
• Provide education and support for clients receiving treatments or medications that have the potential to alter body image. Discuss alternatives if available. EBN: *Men receiving androgen-deprivation therapy as a treatment for prostate cancer may be at greater risk for body image dissatisfaction (Harrington et al, 2009).*
• Take cues from clients regarding their readiness to look at a wound (ask if the client has seen the wound yet) and use clients' questions or comments as way to teach about wound care and healing. CEB: *Tailoring interventions to individual clients and reading their nonverbal cues likely contribute to their ability to heal emotionally from impact of wound on body image (Birdsall & Weinberg, 2001).*
▲ Encourage clients to participate in regular aerobic and/or nonaerobic exercise when feasible. CEB: *Participants of this study demonstrated higher levels of body satisfaction following the very first exercise session (Vocks et al, 2009).*
▲ Provide client with a list of appropriate community support groups (e.g., Reach to Recovery, Ostomy Association). EB: *This study of three different cancer groups (a group for women with metastatic cancer, a colorectal cancer support group, and a group for Chinese cancer clients) showed their perceived benefits were similar; the groups provided information, acceptance, and understanding (Bell et al, 2010).*

Pediatric

Many of the above interventions are appropriate for the pediatric client.

▲ Refer parents of children with eating disorders to a support group. EB: *Parents indicated that support groups assisted them in understanding eating disorder symptoms and treatment and in supporting their child struggling with an eating disorder. Additionally, the group was a source of emotional support. Results suggest that inclusion of a parent support group in the outpatient treatment of children and adolescents with eating disorders has important implications for parents (Pasold et al, 2010).*
▲ When caring for teenagers, be aware of the impact of acne vulgaris on quality of life. The impact was proportional to the severity of acne. Assess for symptoms of social withdrawal, limited eye contact, and expressions of low self esteem. Educate teens on skin care and hygiene, and assist with referrals to a dermatologist when needed. EB: *Research performed by Tasoula et al (2012) showed that feelings of unworthiness attributable to negative appraisal by peers were present in half of subjects with acne in their study.*
▲ Refer families of children with severe facial burns for psychosocial support. EB: *Severe facial burn influences health-related quality of life in children. Additional psychosocial support is suggested to enhance recovery for clients with severe face burns and their families during the years following injury (Stubbs et al, 2011).*
▲ Assess family dynamics and refer parents of adolescents with anorexia or other eating disorders to professional family counseling if indicated. EB: *This study indicated that when adolescents' basic psychological needs are met, they are less likely to worry about the adequacy of body appearance and engage in unhealthy weight control behaviors. Parenting practices such as lack of emotional support or demanding conformity have negative impacts on adolescents suffering from eating disorders (Thøgersen-Ntoumani et al, 2010).*

Geriatric

• Focus on remaining abilities. Have client make a list of strengths. CEB: *Results from unstructured interviews with women aged 61 to 92 years regarding their perceptions and feelings about their aging bodies suggest that women exhibit the internalization of ageist beauty norms, even as they assert that health is more important to them than physical attractiveness and comment on the "naturalness" of the aging process (Hurd, 2000).*
• Encourage regular exercise for older adults. EB: *Research done by Mortensen et al (2012) supports the importance of physical activity to preserve functioning in older adults.*

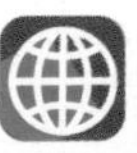

Multicultural

• Assess for the influence of cultural beliefs, regional norms, and values on the client's body image. EB: *A study of young adults living in Hawaii and Australia demonstrated a tolerance for body sizes that are significantly larger than the body mass index size considered healthy (Knight et al, 2010).* EBN: *Each client*

B

should be assessed for body image based on the phenomenon of communication, time, space, social organization, environmental control, and biological variations (Giger & Davidhizar, 2008). EB: *A study of Muslim women found that the strength of their religious faith was inversely related to body dissatisfaction (Mussap, 2009).*

- Acknowledge that body image disturbances can affect all individuals regardless of culture, race, or ethnicity. EB: *Results in this study suggest that gender and cultural differences in body image among adolescents are significant (Ceballos & Czyzewska, 2010). Body image disorders are becoming increasingly prevalent in developing non-Western countries such as China (Xu et al, 2010).*

Home Care

- The above interventions may be adapted for home care use.
- Assess client's level of social support. Social support is one of the determinants of the client's recovery and emotional health. CEB: *Females who perceived they have good social support were found to adapt better to changes in body image after stoma surgery (Brown & Randle, 2005).*
- Assess family/caregiver level of acceptance of client's body changes. CEB: *Family members' expressions and reactions were found to impact women's coping, and negative reactions in particular increased the women's level of anxiety (Brown & Randle, 2005).*
- Encourage clients to discuss concerns related to sexuality and provide support or information as indicated. Many conditions that affect body image also affect sexuality. CEB: *Brown & Randle (2005) found that clients (particularly females) with stomas often believe they are less sexually attractive after surgery, even though their sexual partner may not share that view. However, clients who underwent urostomy surgery often experienced a decrease in sexual functioning.*
- Teach all aspects of care. Involve clients and caregivers in self-care as soon as possible. Do this in stages if clients still have difficulty looking at or touching changed body part. EB: *Prostate cancer clients need interventions that assist them to manage the effects of their disease. Programs need to include spouses because they also are negatively affected by the disease and can influence client outcomes (Kershaw et al, 2008).*

Client/Family Teaching and Discharge Planning

- Teach appropriate care of surgical site (e.g., mastectomy site, amputation site, ostomy site). CEB: *Integration of a cosmetic program into the routine nursing care for oral cancer clients is highly recommended. This study confirmed that cosmetic rehabilitation had positive effects on the body image of oral cancer clients (Huang & Liu, 2008).*
- Encourage significant others to offer support. CEB: *Clients with heart failure in this study managed depressive symptoms that affect health-related quality of life by engaging in activities such as exercise and reading, and by using positive thinking, spirituality, and social support. Helping clients find enhanced social support is important (Dekker et al, 2009).*

▲ Refer clients who are having difficulty with personal acceptance, personal and social body image disruption, sexual concerns, reduced self-care skills, and management of surgical complications to an interdisciplinary team or specialist (e.g., ostomy nurse) if available. CEB: *There is sufficient research-based evidence to conclude that intestinal ostomy surgery exerts a clinically relevant impact on health-related quality of life and that nursing interventions can ameliorate this effect (Pittman et al, 2009).*

REFERENCES

Arroyo, J. M. G., & López, M. L. D. (2011). Psychological problems derived from mastectomy: a qualitative study. *International Journal of Surgical Oncology, 2011*, 132461.

Bell, K., et al. (2010). Is there an "ideal cancer" support group? Key findings from a qualitative study of three groups. *Journal of Psychosocial Oncology, 28*(4), 432–449.

Birdsall, C., & Weinberg, K. (2001). Adult clients looking at their burn injuries for the first time. *The Journal of Burn Care and Rehabilitation, 22*(5), 360–364.

Bolton, M. A., Lobben, I., & Stern, T. A. (2010). The impact of body image on patient care. *Primary Care Companion to the Journal of Clinical Psychiatry, 12*(2), PCC.10r00947.

Borwell, B. (2009). Rehabilitation and stoma care: addressing the psychological needs. *British Journal of Nursing (Mark Allen Publishing), 18*(4), S20-2–S24-5.

Bowers, B. (2008). Providing effective support for patients facing disfiguring surgery. *British Journal of Nursing (Mark Allen Publishing), 17*(2), 94–98.

Brown, H., & Randle, J. (2005). Living with a stoma: a review of the literature. *Journal of Clinical Nursing, 14*(1), 74–81.

Ceballos, N., & Czyzewska, M. (2010). Body image in Hispanic/Latino vs. European American adolescents: implications for treatment and prevention of obesity in underserved populations. *Journal of Health Care for the Poor and Underserved, 21*(3), 823–838.

Dekker, R. L., et al. (2009). Living with depressive symptoms: patients with heart failure. *American Journal of Critical Care*, *18*(4), 310–318.

Dunkley, D. M., Masheb, R. M., & Grilo, C. M. (2010). Childhood maltreatment, depressive symptoms, body dissatisfaction in patients with binge eating disorder: the mediating role of self-criticism. *The International Journal of Eating Disorders*, *43*(3), 274–281.

Gagnon, M., & Holmes, D. (2011). Bodies in mutation: understanding lipodystrophy among women living with HIV/AIDS. *Research and Theory for Nursing Practice*, *25*(1), 23–39.

Giger, J., & Davidhizar, R. (2008). *Transcultural nursing: assessment and intervention* (ed. 4). St Louis: Mosby.

Harrington, J. M., Jones, E. G., & Badger, T. (2009). Body image perceptions in men with prostate cancer. *Oncology Nursing Forum*, *36*(2), 167–172.

Huang, C., & Hsieh, C. (2010). Treating bulimia nervosa: a nurse's experience using cognitive behavior therapy [Chinese]. *Hu Li Za Zhi the Journal of Nursing*, *57*(Suppl. 2), 29–34.

Huang, S., & Liu, H. E. (2008). Effectiveness of cosmetic rehabilitation on the body image of oral cancer patients in Taiwan. *Supportive Care in Cancer*, *16*(9), 981–986.

Hurd, L. C. (2000). Older women's body image and embodied experience: an exploration. *Journal of Women and Aging*, *12*(3–4), 77–97.

Ipser, J. C., Sander, C., & Stein, D. J. (2009). Pharmacotherapy and psychotherapy for body dysmorphic disorder. *Cochrane Database of Systematic Reviews*, (1), CD005332.

Kershaw, T. S., et al. (2008). Longitudinal analysis of a model to predict quality of life in prostate cancer patients and their spouses. *Annals of Behavioral Medicine: A Publication of the Society of Behavioral Medicine*, *36*(2), 117–128.

Knight, T., Latner, J. D., & Illingworth, D. (2010). Tolerance of larger body sizes by young adults living in Australia and Hawaii. *Eating Disorders*, *18*, 425–434.

Mortensen, S. P., Nyberg, M., Winding, K., et al. (2012). Lifelong physical activity preserves functional sympatholysis and purinergic signalling in the ageing human leg. *The Journal of Physiology*, *590*(Pt. 23), 6227–6236.

Munoz, D., et al. (2010). Changes in desired body shape after bariatric surgery. *Eating Disorders*, *18*, 347–354.

Mussap, A. J. (2009). Strength of faith and body image in Muslim and non-Muslim women. *Mental Health, Religion & Culture*, *12*(2), 121–127.

Pasold, T. L., Boateng, B. A., & Portilla, M. G. (2010). The use of a parent support group in the outpatient treatment of children and adolescents with eating disorders. *Eating Disorders*, *18*(4), 318–332.

Phillips, K. A. (2010). Body dysmorphic disorder. *Dialogues in Clinical Neuroscience*, *12*(2), 221–232.

Pittman, J., Kozell, K., & Gray, M. (2009). Should WOC nurses measure health-related quality of life in patients undergoing intestinal ostomy surgery? *Journal of Wound, Ostomy, and Continence Nursing*, *36*(3), 254–265.

Rosenberg, S. M., Tamimi, R. M., Gelber, S., et al. (2013). Body image in recently diagnosed young women with early breast cancer. *Psycho-Oncology*, *22*(8), 1849–1855.

Stubbs, T. K., et al. (2011). Psychosocial impact of childhood face burns: a multicenter, prospective, longitudinal study of 390 children and adolescents. *Burns: Journal of the International Society for Burn Injuries*, *37*(3), 387–394.

Tasoula, E., Gregoriou, S., Chalikias, J., et al. (2012). The impact of acne vulgaris on quality of life and psychic health in young adolescents in Greece. Results of a population survey. *Anais Brasileiros de Dermatologia*, *87*(6), 862–869.

Thøgersen-Ntoumani, C., Ntoumanis, N., & Mikitaras, N. (2010). Unhealthy weight control behaviors in adolescent girls: a process model based on self-determination theory. *Psychology and Health*, *25*(5), 535–550.

Vocks, S., et al. (2009). Effects of a physical exercise session on state body image: the influence of pre-experimental body dissatisfaction and concerns about weight and shape. *Psychology and Health*, *24*(6), 713–729.

Xu, X., et al. (2010). Body dissatisfaction, engagement in body change behaviors and sociocultural influences on body image among Chinese adolescents. *Body Image*, *7*(2), 156–164.

Insufficient Breast Milk

Kerstin West-Wilson, RNC, IBCLC, and David Wilson, MS, RNC

NANDA-I

Definition

Low production of maternal breast milk

Defining Characteristics

Infant

Constipation; frequent crying; frequently seeks to suckle at breast; prolonged breastfeeding time; suckling time at breast appears unsatisfactory; voids small amounts of concentrated urine; weight gain less than 500 g in a month

Mother

Absence of milk production with nipple stimulation; delay in milk production; expresses breast milk less than prescribed volume

Related Factors

Infant

Ineffective latching on to breast; ineffective sucking reflex; insufficient opportunity for suckling at the breast; insufficient suckling time at breast; rejection of breast

B

Mother

Alcohol consumption; insufficient fluid volume; malnutrition; pregnancy; smoking; treatment regimen

NOC (Nursing Outcomes Classification)

Suggested NOC Outcomes

Breastfeeding Establishment: Infant, Maternal; Breastfeeding Maintenance; Anxiety Self-control; Parent-Infant Attachment

Example NOC Outcome with Indicators

Breastfeeding Establishment: as evidenced by the following indicators: Proper alignment/latch on/areolar compression/suck reflex/Nursing minimum of 15 minutes per breast/Urinations and stools appropriate for age/Weight gain appropriated for age. (Rate the outcome and indicators of **Breastfeeding Establishment:** 1 = not adequate, 2 = slightly adequate, 3 = moderately adequate, 4 = substantially adequate, 5 = totally adequate [see Section I].)

Client Outcomes

Client Will (Specify Time Frame)

- State knowledge of indicators of adequate milk supply
- State and demonstrate measures to ensure adequate milk supply

NIC (Nursing Interventions Classification)

Suggested NIC Interventions

Lactation Counseling; Lactation Suppression; Kangaroo Care; Parent Education: Infant

Example NIC Activities—Lactation Counseling

Correct misconceptions, misinformation, and inaccuracies about breastfeeding; Provide educational material, as needed; Encourage attendance at breastfeeding classes and support groups for "perceived insufficient milk supply" (Gatti, 2008).

Nursing Interventions and *Rationales*

- Provide lactation support at all phases of lactation (Neifert & Bunick, 2013; Nielsen et al, 2011).
- *Communicate routine advice to mothers without making them feel pressured or guilty and nurses should be aware of "how" they give routine instructions (Flaherman et al, 2012).*
- Initiate skin-to-skin contact at birth and undisturbed contact for the first hour following birth; the mother should be encouraged to watch the baby, not the clock. *These behaviors are associated with an abundant milk supply (Noonan, 2011; Parker et al, 2013).*
- Encourage postpartum women to start breastfeeding based on infant need as early as possible and reduce formula use to increase breastfeeding frequency. Use nonnarcotic analgesics as early as possible. EBN: *These interventions are suggested to decrease early weaning in this study of women who had cesarean deliveries and perceived insufficient milk supply (Lin et al, 2011; Chantry, 2014; Gatti, 2008; Kent et al, 2013; Lou et al, 2014; Nielsen et al, 2011).*
- Provide suggestions for mothers on how to increase milk production and how to determine whether there is insufficient milk supply. EBN: *Teach mothers how to determine low intake of breast milk by checking baby's wet diapers (fewer than 6 to 8) and monitoring the frequency and amount of baby's bowel movements. Provide suggestions to women on how to increase milk production, such as improving latch-on, increasing frequency of feedings, offering both breasts during each breastfeeding session, and drinking enough fluids (Yen-Ju & McGrath, 2011; Gatti, 2008; Ndikom et al, 2014).*
- Instruct mothers that breastfeeding frequency, sucking times, and amounts are variable and normal. Assist mothers in optimal milk removal frequency. EBN: *Breastfeeding rates may be affected by a maternal perception of insufficient milk production and less than optimal milk removal frequency (Kent et al, 2012; Kent et al, 2013).*

▲ Consider the use of medication for mothers of preterm infants with insufficient expressed breast milk. EBN: *Breast milk remains the optimal form of enteral nutrition for term and preterm infants until up to 6 months postnatal age. In these studies there was modest improvement in expressing breast milk (EBM) values with the use of a galactogogue medication (Donovan & Buchanan, 2012).*

▲ *Need to be more cautious with recommending galactagogues.*

▲ *Not in the scope of practice for IBLC lactation consultants to recommend galactagogues (Academy of Breastfeeding Medicine Protocol Committee, 2011; Donovan & Buchanan, 2012).*

B

Pediatric

- Provide individualized follow-up with extra home visits or outpatient visits for teen mothers within the first few days after hospital discharge and encourage schools to be more compatible with breastfeeding. *Adolescent mothers in the United States are much less likely to imitate breastfeeding than older mothers. This study indicated that these interventions may be helpful for teens who desire to breastfeed (Tucker et al, 2011).*

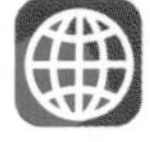

Multicultural

- Provide information and support to mothers on benefits of breastfeeding at antenatal visits. EB: *A study of mothers of infants in Bhaktapur, Nepal, found that, although proper breastfeeding is the most cost-effective intervention for reducing childhood morbidity and mortality, adherence to breastfeeding recommendations in developing countries is not satisfactory. Although many mothers instituted breastfeeding within 1 hour of delivery, continuation for up to 6 months was not common. Very few mothers received any information on breastfeeding during the antenatal visit (Ulak et al, 2012; Neifert & Bunik, 2013; Sultana et al, 2013).*
- Refer to care plans Interrupted **Breastfeeding** and Readiness for enhanced **Breastfeeding** for additional interventions.

REFERENCES

Academy of Breastfeeding Medicine Protocol Committee, ABM Clinical Protocol #9. (2011). Use of galactagogues in initiating or augmenting the rate of maternal milk secretion (First Revision January 2011). *Breastfeeding Medicine*, 6(1), 41–49.

Chantry, C. J. (2014). In-hospital formula use increases early breastfeeding cessation among first-time mothers intending to exclusively breastfeed. *Journal of Pediatrics*, *164*(6), 1339–1348.

Donovan, T. J., & Buchanan, K. (2012). Medications for increasing milk supply in mothers expressing breastmilk for their preterm hospitalised infants. *Cochrane Database of Systematic Reviews*, (3), CD005544.

Flaherman, V. J., et al. (2012). Maternal experience of interactions with providers among mothers with milk supply concern. *Clinical Pediatrics*, *51*(8), 778–784.

Gatti, L. (2008). Maternal perceptions of insufficient milk supply in breastfeeding. *Journal of Nursing Scholarship*, *40*(4), 355–363.

Kent, J., Prime, D., & Garbin, C. (2012). Principles for maintaining or increasing breast milk production. *Journal of Obstetric, Gynecologic, and Neonatal Nursing*, *41*(1), 114–121.

Kent, J. C., et al. (2013). Longitudinal changes in breastfeeding patterns from 1 to 6 months of lactation. *Breastfeeding Medicine*, *8*(4), 401–407.

Lin, S. Y., et al. (2011). Factors related to milk supply perception in women who underwent cesarean section. *The Journal of Nursing Research*, *19*(2), 94–101.

Lou, Z., et al. (2014). Maternal reported indicators and causes of insufficient milk supply. *Journal of Human Lactation*, (on line publication).

Ndikom, C. M., et al. (2014). Extra fluids for breastfeeding mothers for increasing milk production. *Cochrane Database of Systematic Reviews*, (6).

Neifert, M., & Bunik, M. (2013). Overcoming clinical barriers to exclusive breastfeeding. *Pediatric Clinics of North America*, *60*, 115–145.

Nielsen, S., et al. (2011). Adequacy of milk intake during exclusive breastfeeding: a longitudinal study. *Pediatrics*, *128*(4), 907–914.

Noonan, M. (2011). Breastfeeding: is my baby getting enough milk? *British Journal of Midwifery*, *19*(2), 82–89.

Parker, L. A., et al. (2013). Strategies for increased milk volume in mothers of VLBW infants. *The American Journal of Maternal Child Nursing*, *38*(6), 385–390.

Sultana, A., et al. (2013). Clinical update and treatment of lactation insufficiency. *Medical Journal of Islamic World Academy of Sciences*, *21*(1), 19–28.

Tucker, C. M., Wilson, E. K., & Samandari, G. (2011). Infant feeding experiences among teen mothers in North Carolina: findings from a mixed-methods study. *International Breastfeeding Journal*, *6*, 14.

Ulak, M., et al. (2012). Infant feeding practices in Bhaktapur, Nepal: a cross-sectional, health facility based survey. *International Breastfeeding Journal*, *7*(1), 1–8.

Yen-Ju, H., & McGrath, J. (2011). Predicting breastfeeding duration related to maternal attitudes in a Taiwanese sample. *The Journal of Perinatal Education: An ASPO*, *20*(4), 188–199.

Ineffective Breastfeeding

Barbara J. Wheeler, RN, BN, MN, IBCLC

B

NANDA-I

Definition

Difficulty providing milk to an infant or young child directly from the breasts, which may compromise nutritional status of the infant/child

Defining Characteristics

Inadequate infant stooling; infant arching at breast; infant crying at breast; infant crying within first hour after breastfeeding; infant fussing within 1 hour of breastfeeding; infant inability to latch on to maternal breast correctly; infant resisting latching on to breast; infant unresponsive to other comfort measures; insufficient infant weight gain; insufficient emptying of each breast per feeding; insufficient signs of oxytocin release; perceived inadequate milk supply; sore nipples persisting beyond first week; sustained infant weight loss; unsustained suckling at the breast

Related Factors (r/t)

Delayed lactogenesis II; inadequate milk supply; insufficient family support; insufficient opportunity for suckling at breast; insufficient parental knowledge regarding breastfeeding techniques; insufficient parental knowledge regarding importance of breastfeeding; interrupted breastfeeding ; maternal ambivalence; maternal anxiety; maternal breast anomaly; maternal fatigue; maternal obesity; maternal pain; oropharyngeal defect; pacifier use; poor infant sucking reflex; prematurity; previous breast surgery; previous history of breastfeeding failure; short maternity leave; supplemental feedings with artificial nipple

NOC (Nursing Outcomes Classification)

Suggested NOC Outcomes and Example

Refer to care plan for Readiness for enhanced **Breastfeeding.**

Client Outcomes

Client Will (Specify Time Frame)

- Achieve effective breastfeeding (dyad)
- Verbalize/demonstrate techniques to manage breastfeeding problems (mother)
- Manifest signs of adequate intake at the breast (infant)
- Manifest positive self-esteem in relation to the infant feeding process (mother)
- Explain alternative method of infant feeding if unable to continue exclusive breastfeeding (mother)

NIC (Nursing Interventions Classification)

Suggested NIC Interventions and Example

Refer to care plan Readiness for enhanced **Breastfeeding.**

Nursing Interventions and *Rationales*

- Identify women with risk factors for lower breastfeeding initiation and continuation rates (lack of information, inadequate family and social support) as well as factors contributing to ineffective breastfeeding as early as possible in the perinatal experience. EBN: *Nurses are well positioned to provide accurate information and support the development of breastfeeding skills, which facilitates breastfeeding confidence and success (Neifert & Bunik, 2013).*
- Provide time for clients to express expectations and concerns, and provide emotional support as needed. EBN: *Lactation consultants, nurses, and peers play a key role in the establishment and continuation of breastfeeding (Neifert & Bunik, 2013).*
- Encourage skin-to-skin holding, beginning immediately after delivery. EB: *Skin-to-skin holding is associated with improved milk supply, early initiation of breastfeeding, and improved breastfeeding duration (Moore et al, 2012).*

B

- Use valid and reliable tools to measure breastfeeding performance and to predict early discontinuance of breastfeeding whenever possible/feasible. CEB: *Ho and McGrath (2010) compared and contrasted the clinical usefulness and psychometric properties of seven self-report instruments and found that they each contribute to our understanding of breastfeeding in various ways. The Breastfeeding Self-Efficacy Scale has demonstrated an ability to predict breastfeeding success or failure, thus providing opportunity for focused education and support for mothers who need it (Dennis, 2003).*
- Promote comfort and relaxation to reduce pain and anxiety. CEB: *Discomfort and increased tension are factors associated with reduced let-down reflex and premature discontinuance of breastfeeding. Anxiety and fear are associated with decreased milk production (Mezzacappa & Katkin, 2002).*
- Avoid supplemental feedings. EB: *A correlation exists between hospital staff providing formula and/or water supplements and failure to succeed with exclusive breastfeeding (Kaikini & Hyrkas, 2014).*
- Teach mother to observe for infant behavioral cues and responses to breastfeeding. EBN: *Monitor and assess the mom and baby for several breastfeeding sessions. Teaching mother will build her confidence and knowledge base, which facilitates successful breastfeeding (Noonan, 2011).*

▲ Provide necessary equipment/instruction/assistance for milk expression as needed. EBN: *Expressing breast milk by hand may be more effective in the removal of milk, particularly in the immediate postpartum period, than the use of electric pumps (Flaherman et al, 2012).*

▲ Provide referrals and resources: lactation consultants, nurse and peer support programs, community organizations, and written and electronic sources of information. EBN: *Systematic reviews support the use of professionals with special skills in breastfeeding, peer support programs, and written and electronic information to promote continued breastfeeding (Neifert & Bunik, 2013).*

- See care plan for Readiness for enhanced **Breastfeeding.**

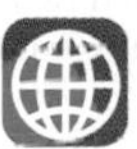

Multicultural

- Assess whether the client's cultural beliefs about breastfeeding are contributing to ineffective breastfeeding. CEB: *Some cultures may add semisolid food within the first month of life as a result of concerns that the infant is not getting enough to eat and the perception that "big is healthy" (Higgins, 2000).* EBN: *Some traditional cultures, including the Turkish, consider colostrum unsuitable to feed the newborn, thus formula may be required to prevent hypoglycemia and dehydration (Demirtas, 2012).*
- Assess the influence of family support on the decision to continue or discontinue breastfeeding. EB: *Family members' impressions and ideas about breastfeeding influence breastfeeding initiation and duration (Odom et al, 2014).*
- Provide traditional ethnic foods for breastfeeding mothers. CEB: *One barrier to breastfeeding is a lack of hospital foods that allow women to follow a traditional diet postpartum. After a staff training program on breastfeeding, and the creation of a Cambodian menu, initiation rates increased significantly more in Cambodians than in non-Cambodians. Postintervention, there was no significant difference between breastfeeding initiation rates among Cambodian women (66.7%) compared with non-Cambodians (68.9%) (Galvin et al, 2008).*
- See care plan for Readiness for enhanced **Breastfeeding.**

Home Care

- The above interventions may be adapted for home care use.
- Provide anticipatory guidance in relation to home management of breastfeeding. EB: *The two most common problems experienced by breastfeeding women are nipple and/or breast pain and low (or perceived low) milk supply; these problems may be preventable with anticipatory guidance (Amir, 2014). For mothers returning to the workforce, longer maternity leaves and regularly pumping milk during the workday are associated with longer breastfeeding duration (Neifert & Bunik, 2013).*

▲ Investigate availability of and refer to public health department, hospital home follow-up breastfeeding program, or other postdischarge support. EBN: *Postdischarge follow-up has been associated with improved breastfeeding duration (Mejdoubi et al, 2014).*

- See care plan for Risk for impaired **Attachment.**

Client/Family Teaching and Discharge Planning

- Instruct the client on maternal breastfeeding behaviors/techniques (preparation for, positioning, initiation of/promoting latch-on, burping, completion of session, and frequency of feeding). Consider use of a video. EBN: *Assess breastfeeding mothers to determine knowledge deficits and provide teaching.*

B

Assisting with breastfeeding and addressing the mother's concerns facilitate breastfeeding success (Neifert & Bunik, 2013).

- Teach the client self-care measures for the breastfeeding woman (e.g., breast care, management of breast/nipple discomfort, nutrition/fluid, rest/activity). CEB: *Painful nipples, mastitis, adequate hydration, and fatigue are some of the problems a breastfeeding woman may experience (Ladewig et al, 2010).*
- Provide information regarding infant cues and behaviors related to breastfeeding and appropriate maternal responses (e.g., cues that the infant is ready to feed, behaviors during feeding that contribute to effective breastfeeding, measures of infant feeding adequacy). *Improved knowledge base and ongoing support to learn psychomotor skills facilitates effective breastfeeding (Neifert & Bunik, 2013).*
- Provide education to partner/family/significant others as needed. EBN/EB: *Family members' impressions and ideas about breastfeeding influence breastfeeding initiation and duration (Odom et al, 2014).*

REFERENCES

See Readiness for enhanced **Breastfeeding** for additional references.

Amir, L. H. (2014). Managing common breastfeeding problems in the community. *British Medical Journal, 348*, g2954.

Demirtas, B. (2012). Strategies to support breastfeeding: a review. *International Nursing Review, 59*, 474–481.

Dennis, C. L. (2003). The breastfeeding self-efficacy scale: psychometric assessment of the short form. *Journal of Obstetric, Gynecologic, & Neonatal Nursing, 32*(6), 734–744.

Flaherman, V. J., Gay, B., Scott, C., et al. (2012). Randomised trial comparing hand expression with breast pumping for mothers of term newborns feeding poorly. *Archives of Disease in Childhood. Fetal and Neonatal Edition, 97,* F19–F23.

Galvin, S., et al. (2008). A practical intervention to increase breastfeeding initiation among Cambodian women in the U.S. *Maternal and Child Health Journal, 12*(4), 545–547.

Higgins, B. (2000). Puerto Rican cultural beliefs: influence on infant feeding practices in western New York. *Journal of Transcultural Nursing, 11*(1), 19–30.

Ho, Y. J., & McGrath, J. M. (2010). A review of the psychometric properties of breastfeeding assessment tools. *Journal of Obstetric, Gynecologic, and Neonatal Nursing, 39*(4), 386–400.

Kaikini, K. L., & Hyrkas, K. (2014). Mothers' intention to breastfeed and hospital practices on breastfeeding: a longitudinal study at 6 months after birth on predictors of breastfeeding in a cohort of mothers from a large northern New England Medical Centre. *Journal of Obstetric, Gynecologic, and Neonatal Nursing, 43*, S78.

Ladewig, A. P., London, M. L., & Davidson, M. R. (2010). Breastfeeding nutrition and newborn nutrition. In M. Davidson, M. London, & P. Ladewig (Eds.), *Contemporary maternal-newborn nursing care* (ed. 7). Upper Saddle River, NJ: Pearson.

Mejdoubi, J., van den Heijkant, S. C. C. M., van Leerdam, F. J. M., et al. (2014). Effects of nurse home visitation on cigarette smoking, pregnancy outcomes, and breastfeeding: a randomized controlled trial. *Midwifery, 30*, 688–695.

Mezzacappa, E. S., & Katkin, E. S. (2002). Breast-feeding is associated with reduced perceived stress and negative mood in mothers. *Health Psychology, 21*(2), 187–193.

Moore, E. R., Anderson, G. C., Bergman, N., et al. (2012). Early skin-to-skin contact for mothers and their healthy newborn infants. *Cochrane Database Systematic Reviews*, (5), CD003519.

Neifert, M., & Bunik, M. (2013). Overcoming clinical barriers to exclusive breastfeeding. *Pediatric Clinics of North America, 60*, 115–145.

Noonan, M. (2011). Breastfeeding: Is my baby getting enough milk? *British Journal of Midwifery, 19*(2), 82–89.

Odom, E. C., Li, R., Scanlong, K. S., et al. (2014). Association of family and health care provider opinion on infant feeding with mother's breastfeeding decision. *Journal of the Academy of Nutrition and Dietetics, 114*(8), 1203–1207.

Interrupted Breastfeeding

Barbara J. Wheeler, RN, BN, MN, IBCLC

NANDA-I

Definition

Break in the continuity of providing milk to an infant or young child directly from the breasts, which may compromise breastfeeding success and/or nutritional status of the infant/child.

Defining Characteristics

Nonexclusive breastfeeding

Related Factors (r/t)

Contraindications to breastfeeding (e.g., pharmaceutical agents); hospitalization of child; infant illness; maternal employment; maternal illness; maternal infant separation; need to abruptly wean infant; prematurity

B

NOC (Nursing Outcomes Classification)

Suggested NOC Outcomes

Breastfeeding Maintenance; Knowledge: Breastfeeding; Parent-Infant Attachment

Example NOC Outcome with Indicators

Breastfeeding Maintenance as evidenced by the following indicators: Infant's growth and development in normal range/Ability to safely collect and store breast milk/Awareness that breastfeeding can continue beyond infancy/Knowledge of benefits from continued breastfeeding. (Rate the outcome and indicators of **Breastfeeding Maintenance: Infant:** 1 = not adequate, 2 = slightly adequate, 3 = moderately adequate, 4 = substantially adequate, 5 = totally adequate [see Section I].)

Client Outcomes

Client Will (Specify Time Frame)

Infant

- Receive mother's breast milk if not contraindicated by maternal conditions (e.g., certain drugs, infections) or infant conditions (e.g., galactosemia)

Maternal

- Maintain lactation
- Achieve effective breastfeeding or satisfaction with the breastfeeding experience
- Demonstrate effective methods of breast milk collection and storage

NIC (Nursing Interventions Classification)

Suggested NIC Interventions

Bottle Feeding; Emotional Support; Lactation Counseling

Example NIC Activities—Lactation Counseling

Instruct patient to contact lactation consultant to assist in determining status of milk supply (i.e., whether insufficiency is perceived or actual); Encourage employers to provide opportunities for and private facilities for lactating mothers to pump and store breast milk during the work day

Nursing Interventions and *Rationales*

- Discuss and provide support for mother's desire/intention to begin or resume breastfeeding. EB: *Mothers who perceived that care providers favored exclusive breastfeeding achieved significantly higher rates of exclusive breastfeeding at 1 and 3 months, as compared with those who perceived care providers were neutral about the method of infant feeding (Ramakrishnan et al, 2014).* EBN: *Breastfeeding rates are improved when hospitals have written breastfeeding policies and when staff has enhanced education regarding breastfeeding knowledge, attitudes, and skills (Li et al, 2014).*
- Clarify that interruption in breastfeeding is truly necessary. (Expert recommendation): *Mothers are sometimes inappropriately advised to discontinue breastfeeding (Sachs & AAP Committee on Drugs, 2013). When there is a question of possible contraindication to breastfeeding, a discussion of potential risks versus probable, known benefits of breastfeeding must be held with mother and family (Lawrence, 2013).*
- Provide anticipatory guidance to the mother/family regarding potential duration of the interruption when possible/feasible. Reassure mother/family that measures to sustain or restart lactation and promote parent-infant attachment can make it possible to resume breastfeeding when the condition/situation requiring interruption is resolved. EB: *Mothers who had never breastfed, and those who had stopped, were successful in establishing or reestablishing breastfeeding with the help of lactation support (Nyati et al, 2014).*
- Reassure the mother/family that the infant will benefit from any amount of breast milk provided. EBN: *One of the most common reasons mothers supplement or stop breastfeeding is their perception of the baby not getting milk and/or enough milk (Noonan, 2011).*

B

- Assess mother's concerns, and observe mother performing psychomotor skills (expression, storage, alternative feeding, skin to skin care, and/or breastfeeding) and assist as needed. EBN: *Individualized support and instruction improves likelihood of breastfeeding success (Demirtas, 2012).*
- Collaborate with mother/family/health care providers (as needed) to develop a plan for skin-to-skin contact. EBN: *Skin-to-skin contact between mothers and newborns results in improved rates of exclusive breastfeeding (Brown et al, 2014).*
- Collaborate with the mother/family/health care provider/employer (as needed) to develop a plan for expression/pumping of breast milk and/or infant feeding. EB: *Workplaces whose environments include supervisor or peer support, space (not in the bathroom) in which to pump, a fridge, rental pump, and on-site daycare were associated with improved duration of exclusive breastfeeding (Bai & Wunderlich, 2013).*
- Monitor for signs indicating infant's ability to breastfeed and interest in breastfeeding. EBN: *Teach the mother to recognize and respond to her baby's feeding cues and signs that her breasts are filling (Noonan, 2011).*

▲ Use supplementation only as medically indicated. EBN: *A correlation exists between hospital staff providing formula and/or water supplements and failure to succeed with breastfeeding (Kaikini & Hyrkas, 2014).*

- Provide anticipatory guidance for common problems associated with interrupted breastfeeding (e.g., incomplete emptying of milk glands, diminishing milk supply, infant difficulty with resuming breastfeeding, or infant refusal of alternative feeding method). EBN: *Emotional support, as well as information regarding how to prevent and respond to breastfeeding problems, contributes to promotion of exclusive breastfeeding (Neifert & Bunik, 2013).*

▲ Initiate follow-up and make appropriate referrals.

- Assist the client to accept and learn an alternative method of infant feeding if effective breastfeeding is not achieved. CEB: *If it is clear that breastfeeding cannot be achieved after the interruption and an alternative feeding method must be instituted, the mother needs support and education (Mozingo et al, 2000).*
- See care plans for Readiness for enhanced **Breastfeeding** and Ineffective **Breastfeeding.**

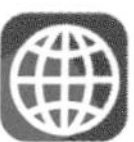

Multicultural

- Teach culturally appropriate techniques for maintaining lactation. CEB: *The Oketani method of breast massage is used by Japanese and other Asian women. Oketani breast massage improved quality of human milk by increasing total solids, lipids, casein concentration, and gross energy (Foda et al, 2004). Some traditional cultures, including the Turkish, consider colostrum unsuitable to feed the newborn, thus formula may be required to prevent hypoglycemia and dehydration (Demirtas, 2012).*
- See care plans for Readiness for enhanced **Breastfeeding** and Ineffective **Breastfeeding.**

Home Care

- The above interventions may be adapted for home care use.

Client/Family Teaching and Discharge Planning

- Teach mother effective methods to express breast milk. EBN: *Expressing breast milk by hand may be more effective in the removal of milk, particularly in the immediate postpartum period, than the use of electric pumps (Flaherman et al, 2012).*
- Teach mother/parents about skin-to-skin care. EBN: *Skin-to-skin care promotes attachment, facilitates improved milk production, and contributes to improved rate and duration of breastfeeding (Brown et al, 2014).*
- Instruct mother on safe breast milk handling techniques. EB: *Breastfeeding mothers can retain the high quality of breast milk and the health of their infant by using safe preparation guidelines and storage methods (CDC, 2014).*
- See care plans for Readiness for enhanced **Breastfeeding** and Ineffective **Breastfeeding.**

REFERENCES

See readiness for enhanced **Breastfeeding** for additional references.

Bai, Y., & Wunderlich, S. M. (2013). Lactation accommodation in the workplace and duration of exclusive breastfeeding. *Journal of Midwifery & Women's Health*, *58*(6), 690–696.

Brown, P. A., Kaiser, K. L., & Nailon, R. E. (2014). Integrating quality improvement and translational research models to increase exclusive breastfeeding. *Journal of Obstetric, Gynecologic, and Neonatal Nursing*, *43*, 545–553.

Centers for Disease Control and Prevention (CDC) (2014). *Proper Handling and Storage of Human Milk.* U.S. Department of Health and Human Services, CDC. From: <http://www.cdc.gov/breastfeeding/recommendations/handling_breastmilk.htm>. Retrieved 30 October 2014.

Demirtas, B. (2012). Strategies to support breastfeeding: a review. *International Nursing Review, 59*, 474–481.

Flaherman, V. J., Gay, B., Scott, C., et al. (2012). Randomised trial comparing hand expression with breast pumping for mothers of term newborns feeding poorly. *Archives of Disease in Childhood. Fetal and Neonatal Edition, 97*, F19–F23.

Foda, M. I., et al. (2004). Composition of milk obtained from unmassaged versus massaged breasts of lactating mothers. *Journal of Pediatric Gastroenterology and Nutrition, 38*(5), 484–487.

Kaikini, K. L., & Hyrkas, K. (2014). Mothers' intentions to breastfeed and hospital practices on breastfeeding: a longitudinal study at 6 months after birth on predictors of breastfeeding in a cohort of mothers from a large northern New England Medical Centre. *Journal of Obstetric, Gynecologic, and Neonatal Nursing, 43*, S78.

Lawrence, R. M. (2013). Circumstances when breastfeeding is contraindicated. *Pediatrics Clinics of North America, 60*(1), 295–318.

Li, C. M., Li, R., Ashley, C. G., et al. (2014). Associations of hospital staff training and policies with early breastfeeding practices. *Journal of Human Lactation, 30*(1), 88–96.

Mozingo, J. N., et al. (2000). "It wasn't working." Women's experiences with short-term breastfeeding. *MCN. the American Journal of Maternal Child Nursing, 25*(3), 120–126.

Neifert, M., & Bunik, M. (2013). Overcoming clinical barriers to exclusive breastfeeding. *Pediatric Clinics of North America, 60*, 115–145.

Noonan, M. (2011). Breastfeeding: Is my baby getting enough milk? *British Journal of Midwifery, 19*(2), 82–89.

Nyati, M., Kim, H. Y., Goga, A., et al. (2014). Support for relactation among mothers of HIV-infected children: a pilot study in Soweto. *Breastfeeding Medicine*, At: <http://www-ncbi-nlm-nih-gov.proxy2.lib.umanitoba.ca/pubmed/25188674>; epub ahead of print. Accessed 30 October 2014.

Ramakrishnan, R., Oberg, C. M., & Kirby, R. S. (2014). The association between maternal perception of obstetric and pediatric care providers' attitudes and exclusive breastfeeding outcomes. *Journal of Human Lactation, 30*(1), 80–87.

Sachs, H. C., & AAP Committee on Drugs. (2013). The transfer of drugs and therapeutics into human breast milk: an update on selected topics. *Pediatrics, 132*(3), e796–e809.

Readiness for enhanced Breastfeeding

Barbara J. Wheeler, RN, BN, MN, IBCLC

NANDA-I

Definition

A pattern of providing milk to an infant or young child directly from the breasts, which may be strengthened

Defining Characteristics

Mother expresses desire to enhance ability to provide breast milk for child's nutritional needs; mother expresses desire to enhance ability to exclusively breastfeed

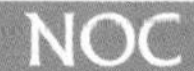

NOC (Nursing Outcomes Classification)

Suggested NOC Outcomes

Breastfeeding Establishment: Infant, Maternal; Breastfeeding Maintenance

Example NOC Outcome with Indicators

Breastfeeding Establishment: Infant as evidenced by the following indicators: Proper alignment and latch-on/Proper areolar grasp/Proper areolar compression/Correct suck and tongue placement/Audible swallow/Nursing a minimum of 5 to 10 minutes per breast/Minimum eight feedings per day/Urinations per day appropriate for age/Weight gain appropriate for age. (Rate the outcome and indicators of **Breastfeeding Establishment: Infant:** 1 = not adequate, 2 = slightly adequate, 3 = moderately adequate, 4 = substantially adequate, 5 = totally adequate [see Section I].)

Client Outcomes

Client Will (Specify Time Frame)

- Maintain effective breastfeeding without supplementation with formula
- Maintain normal growth patterns (infant)
- Verbalize satisfaction with breastfeeding process (mother)

NIC (Nursing Interventions Classification)

B

Suggested NIC Interventions

Lactation Counseling

Example NIC Activities—Lactation Counseling

Provide information about psychological and physiological benefits of breastfeeding; Provide mother the opportunity to breastfeed after birth, when possible

Nursing Interventions and *Rationales*

- Encourage expectant mothers to learn about breastfeeding before and during pregnancy. EBN: *Systematic reviews have identified that health education, particularly individualized education, significantly increases breastfeeding initiation rates (Neifert & Bunik, 2013).*
- Encourage and facilitate early skin-to-skin contact (position includes contact of the naked baby with the mother's bare chest). EB: *Skin-to-skin holding is associated with improved milk supply, early initiation of breastfeeding, and improved breastfeeding duration (Moore et al, 2012).*
- Encourage rooming-in and breastfeeding on demand. EBN: *Mothers who room-in with their infants have greater percentages of exclusive breastfeeding when released from the hospital (Neifert & Bunik, 2013).*
- Monitor the breastfeeding process and identify opportunities to enhance knowledge and experience regarding breastfeeding. EB: *While mothers and babies are in the hospital it is essential that hospital personnel support their effort to learn to breastfeed (CDC, 2011).*
- Give encouragement/positive feedback related to breastfeeding mother-infant interactions. CEB: *Positive feedback builds confidence. The Breastfeeding Self-Efficacy Scale, which measures maternal breastfeeding confidence, has demonstrated higher self-efficacy (confidence) is associated with longer duration of breastfeeding (Dennis, 2003).*
- Discuss prevention and treatment of common breastfeeding problems, such as nipple pain and/or trauma. EB: *Common problems experienced by breastfeeding women may be preventable with anticipatory guidance, or successfully managed with prompt assistance from a health care provider (Amir, 2014).*
- Teach mother to observe for infant behavioral cues and responses to breastfeeding. EBN: *Monitor and assess the mom and baby for several breastfeeding sessions. Teaching mother will build her confidence and knowledge base, which facilitates successful breastfeeding (Noonan, 2011).*
- Identify current support-person network and opportunities for continued breastfeeding support. EB: *Family members' impressions and ideas about breastfeeding influence breastfeeding initiation and duration (Odom et al, 2014).*
- Avoid supplemental bottle feedings and do not provide samples of formula on discharge. EB: *A correlation exists between hospital staff providing formula and/or water supplements and failure to succeed with exclusive breastfeeding (Kaikini & Hyrkas, 2014).*

▲ Provide follow-up contact; as available provide home visits and/or peer counseling. EBN: *Systematic reviews support the use of professionals with special skills in breastfeeding and peer support programs to promote continued breastfeeding (Neifert & Bunik, 2013).*

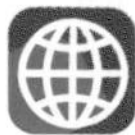

Multicultural

- Assess for the influence of cultural beliefs, norms, and values on current breastfeeding practices. CEB: *The Hispanic mother may believe stress and anger make bad milk, which makes a breastfeeding infant ill. Some Hispanic women neutralize the bowel when weaning from breast to bottle by feeding only anise tea for 24 hours (Gonzalez et al, 2008).* EBN: *Some traditional cultures, including the Turkish, consider colostrum unsuitable to feed the newborn, thus formula may be required to prevent hypoglycemia and dehydration (Demirtas, 2012).*

Home Care

- The above interventions may be adapted for home care use.

Client/Family Teaching and Discharge Planning

- Include the partner and other family members in education about breastfeeding. EB: *Family members' impressions and ideas about breastfeeding influence breastfeeding initiation and duration (Odom et al, 2014).*
- Teach the client the importance of maternal nutrition. EB: *Consumption or avoidance of specific foods or drinks is generally not necessary. Breastfeeding mothers should consume 450 to 500 calories more than nonpregnant, nonnursing women. Adequate intake of DHA is important with an average daily intake of 200 to 300 mg (the amount ingested with consumption of one to two portions of fish per week) recommended (AAP, 2012).*
- Teach mother about the infant's subtle hunger cues (e.g., rooting, sucking, mouthing, hand-to-mouth, hand-to-hand activity) and encourage her to breastfeed whenever signs are apparent. EB: *Evidence-based practice guidelines support the teaching/reinforcement of these skills as important to effective breastfeeding (Holmes et al, 2013).*
- Review guidelines for frequency (at least every 2 to 3 hours, or 8 to 12 feedings per 24 hours) and duration (until suckling and swallowing slow down and satiety is reached) of feeding times. EB: *In the first few days, frequent and regular stimulation of the breasts is important to establish an adequate milk supply; after breastfeeding is established, feeding lasts until the breasts are drained (Holmes et al, 2013).*
- Provide information about common infant behaviors related to breastfeeding, and appropriate maternal responses. EBN: *Improved knowledge base and ongoing support to learn psychomotor skills facilitates effective breastfeeding (Neifert & Bunik, 2013).*

▲ Provide referrals and resources: lactation consultants, nurse and peer support programs, community organizations, and written and electronic sources of information. EBN: *Systematic reviews support the use of professionals with special skills in breastfeeding, peer support programs, and written and electronic information to promote continued breastfeeding (Neifert & Bunik, 2013).*

REFERENCES

American Academy of Pediatrics (AAP), Section on Breastfeeding. (2012). Breastfeeding and the use of human milk. *Pediatrics*, *129*(3), e827–e841.

Amir, L. H. (2014). Managing common breastfeeding problems in the community. *British Medical Journal*, *348*, g2954.

Centers for Disease Control and Prevention (CDC) (2011). *Breastfeeding report card-United States*. Atlanta, GA: U.S. Department of Health and Human Services, CDC. <http://www.cdc.gov/breastfeeding/data/reportcard.htm>.

Demirtas, B. (2012). Strategies to support breastfeeding: a review. *International Nursing Review*, *59*, 474–481.

Dennis, C. L. (2003). The breastfeeding self-efficacy scale: psychometric assessment of the short form. *Journal of Obstetric, Gynecologic, & Neonatal Nursing*, *32*(6), 734–744.

Gonzalez, E., Owens, D., & Esperat, C. (2008). Mexican Americans. In J. Giger & R. Davidhizar (Eds.), *Transcultural nursing: assessment and intervention*. St Louis: Mosby.

Holmes, A. V., McLeod, A. Y., Bunik, M., et al. (2013). Clinical Protocol # 5: Peripartum breastfeeding management for the healthy mother and infant at term. *Breastfeeding Medicine*, *8*(6), 469–473.

Kaikini, K. L., & Hyrkas, K. (2014). Mothers' intention to breastfeed and hospital practices on breastfeeding: a longitudinal study at 6 months after birth on predictors of breastfeeding in a cohort of mothers from a large northern New England Medical Centre. *Journal of Obstetric, Gynecologic, and Neonatal Nursing*, *43*, S78.

Moore, E. R., Anderson, G. C., Bergman, N., et al. (2012). Early skin-to-skin contact for mothers and their healthy newborn infants. *Cochrane Database Systematic Reviews*, (5), CD003519.

Neifert, M., & Bunik, M. (2013). Overcoming clinical barriers to exclusive breastfeeding. *Pediatric Clinics of North America*, *60*, 115–145.

Noonan, M. (2011). Breastfeeding: Is my baby getting enough milk? *British Journal of Midwifery*, *19*(2), 82–89.

Odom, E. C., Li, R., Scanlong, K. S., et al. (2014). Association of family and health care provider opinion on infant feeding with mother's breastfeeding decision. *Journal of the Academy of Nutrition and Dietetics*, *114*(8), 1203–1207.

Ineffective Breathing pattern

Debra Siela, PhD, RN, CCNS, ACNS-BC, CCRN-K, CNE, RRT

NANDA-I

Definition

Inspiration and/or expiration that does not provide adequate ventilation

B

Defining Characteristics

Abnormal breathing pattern (e.g., rate, rhythm, depth); altered chest excursion; bradypnea; decrease in expiratory pressure; decrease in inspiratory pressure; decrease in minute ventilation; decrease in vital capacity; dyspnea; increase in anterior-posterior chest diameter; nasal flaring; orthopnea; prolonged expiration phase; pursed-lip breathing; tachypnea; use of accessory muscles to breathe; use of three-point position

Related Factors (r/t)

Anxiety; body position that inhibits lung expansion; bony deformity; chest wall deformity; fatigue; chest wall deformity; fatigue; hyperventilation; hypoventilation syndrome; musculoskeletal impairment; neurological immaturity; neurological impairment (e.g., positive electroencephalogram, head trauma, seizure disorders); neuromuscular impairment; obesity; pain; respiratory muscle fatigue; spinal cord injury

NOC (Nursing Outcomes Classification)

Suggested NOC Outcomes

Respiratory Status: Airway Patency, Ventilation; Vital Signs

Example NOC Outcome with Indicators

Respiratory Status: Ventilation as evidenced by the following indicators: Respiratory rate/Moves sputum out of airway/Adventitious breath sounds not present/Shortness of breath not present/Auscultated breath sounds/Auscultated vocalization/Chest x-ray findings (Rate each indicator of **Respiratory Status: Ventilation:** 1 = severe deviation from normal range, 2 = substantial deviation from normal range, 3 = moderate deviation from normal range, 4 = mild deviation from normal range, 5 = no deviation from normal range [see Section I].)

Client Outcomes

Client Will (Specify Time Frame)

- Demonstrate a breathing pattern that supports blood gas results within the client's normal parameters
- Report ability to breathe comfortably
- Demonstrate ability to perform pursed-lip breathing and controlled breathing
- Identify and avoid specific factors that exacerbate episodes of ineffective breathing patterns

NIC (Nursing Interventions Classification)

Suggested NIC Interventions

Airway Management; Respiratory Monitoring

Example NIC Activities—Airway Management

Encourage slow, deep breathing, turning, and coughing; Monitor respiratory and oxygenation status as appropriate

Nursing Interventions and *Rationales*

- Monitor respiratory rate, depth, and ease of respiration. *Normal respiratory rate is 10 to 20 breaths/min in the adult (Jarvis, 2015).* EBN: *When the respiratory rate exceeds 30 breaths/min, along with other physiological measures, a study demonstrated that a significant physiological alteration existed (Hagle, 2008).*
- Note pattern of respiration. If client is dyspneic, note what seems to cause the dyspnea, the way in which the client deals with the condition, and how the dyspnea resolves or gets worse. EBN: *Ask the patient if they are short of breath (Campbell, 2011). Use a tool such as the Respiratory Distress Observation Scale (RDOS) for assessing acutely ill or critically ill patients in respiratory distress who cannot self-report dyspnea (Campbell et al, 2010).*
- Note amount of anxiety associated with the dyspnea. *A normal respiratory pattern is regular in a healthy adult. To assess dyspnea, it is important to consider all of its dimensions, including antecedents, mediators, reactions, and outcomes.*
- Attempt to determine if client's dyspnea is physiological or psychological in cause. *The evaluation of a client with dyspnea continues to be dependent on a thorough history and physical examination. In the client*

with acute worsening of chronic breathlessness, the health care provider must be attuned to the possibility of a new pathophysiological derangement superimposed on a known disorder. Instruments or sections of instruments pertaining to dyspnea should be classified as addressing domains of sensory-perceptual experience, affective distress, or symptom/disease impact or burden (Parshall et al, 2012). EB: *Maximal respiratory work is less unpleasant than moderately intense air hunger, and unpleasantness of dyspnea can vary independently from perceived intensity, consistent with pain. Separate dimensions should be measured (Banzett et al, 2008). A study found that when the cause was psychological (medically unexplained dyspnea), there was affective dyspnea, anxiety, and tingling in the extremities. Whereas, when the dyspnea was physiological, there was associated wheezing, cough, sputum, and palpitations (Han et al, 2008).*

- The rapidity of which the onset of dyspnea is noted is also an indicator of the severity of the pathological condition (Croucher, 2014).

Psychological Dyspnea—Hyperventilation

- Monitor for symptoms of hyperventilation including rapid respiratory rate, sighing breaths, lightheadedness, numbness and tingling of hands and feet, palpitations, and sometimes chest pain (Bickley & Szilagyi, 2012).
- Assess cause of hyperventilation by asking client about current emotions and psychological state.
- Ask the client to breathe with you to slow down respiratory rate. *Maintain eye contact and give reassurance. By making the client aware of respirations and giving support, the client may gain control of the breathing rate.*

▲ Consider having the client breathe in and out of a paper bag as tolerated. *This simple treatment helps associated symptoms of hyperventilation including helping to retain carbon dioxide, which will decrease associated symptoms of hyperventilation (Bickley & Szilagyi, 2012).*

▲ If client has chronic problems with hyperventilation, numbness and tingling in extremities, dizziness, and other signs of panic attacks, refer for counseling.

Physiological Dyspnea

▲ Ensure that client in acute dyspneic state has received any ordered medications, oxygen, and any other treatment needed.

- *Determine intensity, unpleasantness, or distress of dyspnea using a rating scale such as an intensity focused modified Borg scale or visual analogue scale (Parshall et al, 2012).*
- *Note client description of the quality of breathing discomfort, such as chest tightness, air hunger, inability to breathe deeply, urge to breathe, starved for air, feeling of suffocation (Parshall et al, 2012).*
- Note use of accessory muscles, nasal flaring, retractions, irritability, confusion, or lethargy. *These symptoms signal increasing respiratory difficulty (Campbell, 2011).*
- Observe color of tongue, oral mucosa, and skin for signs of cyanosis. *In central cyanosis, both the skin and mucous membranes are affected due to seriously impaired pulmonary function from unventilated or underventilated alveoli. Peripheral cyanosis (skin only) usually indicates vasoconstriction or obstruction to blood flow (Loscalzo, 2013).*
- Auscultate breath sounds, noting decreased or absent sounds, crackles, or wheezes. *These abnormal lung sounds can indicate a respiratory pathology associated with an altered breathing pattern (Croucher, 2014).*
- *Assess for hemodynamic stability for the client with acute dyspnea. Rapid evaluation for impending respiratory failure is essential and includes fragmented speech, tripod positioning, diaphoresis, cyanosis, Pao_2 less than 50 mm Hg, $Paco_2$ greater than 70, and use of accessory muscles. Hypotension along with dyspnea indicates threat of cardiopulmonary collapse (Croucher, 2014).*

▲ Monitor oxygen saturation continuously using pulse oximetry. Note blood gas results as available. *An oxygen saturation of less than 90% (normal: 95% to 100%) or a partial pressure of oxygen of less than 80 mm Hg (normal: 80 to 100 mm Hg) indicates significant oxygenation problems.*

- Using touch on the shoulder, coach the client to slow respiratory rate, demonstrating slower respirations, making eye contact with the client, and communicating in a calm, supportive fashion. *The nurse's presence, reassurance, and help in controlling the client's breathing can be beneficial in decreasing anxiety.* EB: *Anxiety is an important indicator of severity of client's disease with chronic obstructive pulmonary disease (COPD) (Campbell et al, 2011).*
- Support the client in using pursed-lip and controlled breathing techniques. *Pursed-lip breathing may relieve dyspnea in advanced COPD (Pashall et al, 2012). Pursed-lip breathing results in increased use of intercostal muscles, decreased respiratory rate, increased tidal volume, and improved oxygen saturation levels*

(Faager et al, 2008). EBN: *A systematic review found pursed-lip breathing effective in decreasing dyspnea (Carrieri-Kohlman & Donesky-Cuenco, 2008).*

- If the client is acutely dyspneic, consider having the client lean forward over a bedside table, resting elbows on the table if tolerated. *Leaning forward can help decrease dyspnea, possibly because gastric pressure allows better contraction of the diaphragm (Langer et al, 2009). This is called the tripod position and is used during times of distress, including when walking.*
- Position the client in an upright or semi-Fowler's position. *Most patients will have optimal vital capacity, oxygenation, and reduced dyspnea when upright with arms elevated on pillows or a bedside table (Campbell, 2011).* See Nursing Interventions and *Rationales* for Impaired **Gas** exchange for further information on positioning.
- ▲ Administer oxygen as ordered. *Oxygen administration has been shown to correct hypoxemia, which causes dyspnea (Wong & Elliott, 2009; Campbell, 2011). But, supplemental oxygen may not relieve all dyspnea (Parshall et al, 2012).*
- *Mechanical ventilation, invasive or noninvasive, is a reliable means of reducing dyspnea associated with respiratory failure (Campbell, 2011).*
- *Opioids may be used for both acute and terminal dyspnea, considering careful safe dosing for relief and side effect of constipation (Campbell, 2011; Parshall et al, 2012).*
- Increase client's activity to walking three times per day as tolerated. Assist the client to use oxygen during activity as needed. See Nursing Interventions and *Rationales* for **Activity** intolerance. Walking 20 minutes per day is recommended for those unable to be in a structured program (GOLD, 2015). *Supervised exercise has been shown to decrease dyspnea and increase tolerance to activity (GOLD, 2015).*
- Schedule rest periods before and after activity. *Respiratory clients with dyspnea are easily exhausted and need additional rest. Nurses coordinate all patient care and are integral to ensuring spacing of activity to minimize or prevent dyspnea (Campbell, 2011).*
- ▲ Evaluate the client's nutritional status. Refer to a dietitian if needed. Use nutritional supplements to increase nutritional level if needed. *Improved nutrition may help increase inspiratory muscle function and decrease dyspnea.* CEB: *A study found that almost half of a group of clients with COPD were malnourished, which can lead to an exacerbation of the disease (Odencrants et al, 2008).*
- Provide small, frequent feedings. *Small feedings are given to avoid compromising ventilatory effort and to conserve energy. Clients with dyspnea often do not eat sufficient amounts of food because their priority is breathing.*
- Offer a fan to move the air in the environment. EBN: *A systematic review found that the movement of cool air on the face can be effective in relieving dyspnea in pulmonary clients (Carrieri-Kohlman & Donesky-Cuenco, 2008).* EBP: *Handheld fans can significantly reduce dyspnea in clients with chronic breathlessness (Galbraith et al, 2010).*
- Encourage the client to take deep breaths at prescribed intervals and do controlled coughing.
- Help the client with chronic respiratory disease to evaluate dyspnea experience to determine whether previous incidences of dyspnea were similar and to recognize that the client survived those incidences. Encourage the client to be self-reliant if possible, use problem-solving skills, and maximize use of social support. *The focus of attention on sensations of breathlessness has an impact on judgment used to determine the intensity of the sensation (Campbell et al, 2011).*
- See Ineffective **Airway** clearance if client has a problem with increased respiratory secretions.
- ▲ Refer the client with COPD for pulmonary rehabilitation. EB: *A Cochrane study found pulmonary rehabilitation programs highly effective and safe for a client who has an exacerbation of COPD (Puhan et al, 2009). Among the beneficial effects of pulmonary rehabilitation are a reduction in exertional dyspnea during exercise and improved exercise tolerance, as well as decreases in self-reported dyspnea with activity (Parshall et al, 2012). Appropriately resourced home-based exercise training has proven effective in reducing dyspnea and increasing exercise performance activity in the context of pulmonary rehabilitation (Spruit et al, 2013). Pulmonary rehabilitation benefits for COPD patients include reduction of the perceived intensity of breathlessness (GOLD, 2015).*

Geriatric

- Assess respiratory systems in older adults with the understanding that inspiratory muscles weaken, resulting in a slight barrel chest. Expiratory muscles work harder with use of accessory muscles (Martin-Plank, 2014).

- Encourage ambulation as tolerated. *Immobility is harmful to older adults because it decreases ventilation and increases stasis of secretions (Thomas, 2009).*
- Encourage older clients to sit upright or stand and to avoid lying down for prolonged periods during the day. *Thoracic aging results in decreased lung expansion; an erect position fosters maximal lung expansion (Thomas, 2009).*

Home Care

- The above interventions may be adapted for home care use.
- Work with the client to determine what strategies are most helpful during times of dyspnea. Educate and empower the client to self-manage the disease associated with impaired gas exchange. EBN/EB: *A study found that use of oxygen, self-use of medication, and breathing fresh air were most helpful in dealing with dyspnea (Thomas, 2009). Evidence-based reviews have found that self-management offers clients with COPD effective options for managing the illness, leading to more positive outcomes (Kaptein et al, 2008).*
- Assist the client and family with identifying other factors that precipitate or exacerbate episodes of ineffective breathing patterns (i.e., stress, allergens, stairs, activities that have high energy requirements). *Awareness of precipitating factors helps clients avoid them and decreases risk of ineffective breathing episodes (Campbell et al, 2011).*
- Assess client knowledge of and compliance with medication regimen. *Client/family may need repetition of instructions received at hospital discharge, and may require reiteration as fear of a recent crisis decreases. Fear interferes with the ability to assimilate new information.*
- ▲ Refer the client for telemonitoring with a pulmonologist as appropriate, with use of an electronic spirometer or an electronic peak flowmeter. EB: *A systematic review of home telemonitoring for conditions such as COPD, asthma, and lung transplantation found that use of telemonitoring resulted in early detection of deterioration of clients' respiratory status, and positive client receptiveness to the approach (Jaana et al, 2009).*
- Teach the client and family the importance of maintaining the therapeutic regimen and having as-needed drugs easily accessible at all times. *Appropriate and timely use of medications can decrease the risk of exacerbating ineffective breathing. The 2015 GOLD Report states that bronchodilator medications are central to management of dyspnea (GOLD, 2015).*
- Provide the client with emotional support in dealing with symptoms of respiratory difficulty. Provide family with support for care of a client with chronic or terminal illness. Refer to care plan for **Anxiety.** *Witnessing breathing difficulties and facing concerns of dealing with chronic or terminal illness can create fear in caregiver. Fear inhibits effective coping (Campbell et al, 2011).*
- When respiratory procedures (e.g., apneic monitoring for an infant) are being implemented, explain equipment and procedures to family members, and provide needed emotional support. *Family members assuming responsibility for respiratory monitoring often find this stressful. They may not have been able to assimilate fully any instructions provided by hospital staff (Martin-Plank et al, 2014).*
- When electrically based equipment for respiratory support is being implemented, evaluate home environment for electrical safety, such as proper grounding. Ensure that notification is sent to the local utility company, the emergency medical team, police and fire departments. *Notification is important to provide for priority service.*
- Refer to GOLD guidelines for management of home care and indications of hospital admission criteria.
- Support clients' efforts at self-care. Ensure they have all the information they need to participate in care.
- Identify an emergency plan including when to call your health care provider or 911. *Having a ready emergency plan reassures the client and promotes client safety.*
- ▲ Refer to occupational therapy for evaluation and teaching of energy conservation techniques (Langer et al, 2009).
- ▲ Refer to home health aide services as needed to support energy conservation. *Energy conservation decreases the risk of exacerbating ineffective breathing (Langer et al, 2009).*
- ▲ Institute case management of frail elderly to support continued independent living (Martin-Plank et al, 2014).

B

Client/Family Teaching and Discharge Planning

- Teach pursed-lip and controlled breathing techniques. EB: *Studies have demonstrated that pursed-lip breathing was effective in decreasing breathlessness and improving respiratory function (Faager et al, 2008). Pursed-lip breathing may relieve dyspnea in advanced COPD (Parshall et al, 2012).*
- Teach about dosage, actions, and side effects of medications. *Inhaled steroids and bronchodilators can have undesirable side effects, especially when taken in inappropriate doses.*
- Using a pre-recorded tape, teach client progressive muscle relaxation techniques. EB: *Relaxation therapy can help reduce dyspnea and anxiety (Langer et al, 2009). Benefits of pulmonary rehabilitation include reduction of anxiety and depression associated with COPD (GOLD, 2015).*
- Teach the client to identify and avoid specific factors that exacerbate ineffective breathing patterns, such as exposure to other sources of air pollution, especially smoking. If client smokes, refer to the smoking cessation section in the impaired **Gas** exchange care plan.

REFERENCES

Banzett, R., Pedersen, S., Schwartzstein, R., et al. (2008). The affective dimension of laboratory dyspnea. *American Journal of Respiratory and Critical Care Medicine, 177*, 1384–1390.

Bickley, L. S., & Szilagyi, P. (2012). *Bate's guide to physical examination* (ed. 11). Philadelphia: Lippincott.

Campbell, M. L. (2011). Dyspnea. *AACN Advanced Critical Care, 22*(3), 257–264.

Campbell, M. L., Templin, T., & Walch, J. A. (2010). A respiratory distress observation scale for patients unable to self-report dyspnea. *Journal of Palliative Medicine, 13*(3), 285–290.

Carrieri-Kohlman, V., & Donesky-Cuenco, D. (2008). Dyspnea management. An EBP guideline. In B. Ackley, G. Ladwig, & B. A. Swann (Eds.), *Evidence-based nursing care guidelines: medical-surgical Interventions*. Philadelphia: Mosby Elsevier.

Croucher, B. (2014). The challenge of diagnosing dyspnea. *AACN Advanced Critical Care, 25*(3), 284–290.

Faager, G., Stahle, A., & Larsen, F. F. (2008). Influence of spontaneous pursed lips breathing on walking endurance and oxygen saturation in patients with moderate to severe chronic obstructive pulmonary disease. *Clinical Rehabilitation, 22*(8), 675–683.

Galbraith, S., Fagan, P., Perkins, P., et al. (2010). Does the use of a handheld fan improve chronic dyspnea? A randomized controlled crossover trial. *Journal of Pain and Symptom Management, 39*, 831–838.

GOLD Global strategy for the diagnosis, management, and prevention of COPD (revised 2015), *Global Initiative for Chronic Obstructive Lung Disease*. <http://www.goldcopd.org/uploads/users/files/GOLD_Report_2015_Apr2.pdf>. Retrieved April 23, 2015.

Hagle, M. (2008). Vital signs monitoring. An EBP guideline. In B. Ackley, G. Ladwig, & B. A. Swann (Eds.), *Evidence-based nursing care guidelines: medical-surgical interventions*. Philadelphia: Mosby.

Han, J., Zhu, Y., Li, S., et al. (2008). The language of medically unexplained dyspnea. *Chest, 133*(4), 961–968.

Jaana, M., Paré, G., & Sicotte, C. (2009). Home telemonitoring for respiratory conditions: a systematic review. *American Journal of Managed Care, 15*(5), 313–320.

Jarvis, C. (2015). General Survey, Measurement, Vital Signs. In C. Jarvis (Ed.), *Physical Examination & Health Assessment* (ed. 7). St. Louis: Saunders Elsevier.

Kaptein, A. A., Scharloo, M., & Fischer, M. J. (2008). 50 years of psychological research on patients with COPD—road to ruin or highway to heaven? *Respiratory Medicine, 103*(1), 3–11.

Langer, D., Hendriks, E., & Burtin, C. (2009). A clinical practice guideline for physiotherapists treating patients with chronic obstructive pulmonary disease based on a systematic review of available evidence. *Clinical Rehabilitation, 23*(5), 445–462.

Loscalzo, J. (2013). Hypoxia and cyanosis. In J. Loscalzo (Ed.), *Harrison's pulmonary and critical care medicine* (ed. 2, pp. 21–25). New York: McGraw Hill Education Medical.

Martin-Plank, L. (2014). Chest Disorders. In L. Kennedy-Malone, K. R. Fletcher, & L. Martin-Plank (Eds.), *Advanced Practice Nursing in the Care of Older Adults*. Philadelphia: F.A. Davis Company.

Odencrants, S., Ehnfors, M., & Ehrenbert, A. (2008). Nutritional status and patient characteristics for hospitalized older patients with chronic obstructive pulmonary disease. *Journal of Clinical Nursing, 17*(13), 1771–1778.

Parshall, M. B., Schwartzstein, R. M., Adams, L., et al. (2012). An official American Thoracic Society statement: update on the mechanisms, assessment, and management of dyspnea. *American Journal of Respiratory and Critical Care Medicine, 185*(4), 435–452.

Puhan, M., Scharplatz, M., & Troosters, T. (2009). Pulmonary rehabilitation following exacerbations of chronic obstructive pulmonary disease. *Cochrane Database Systematic Review*, (1), CD005305.

Spruit, M. A., Singh, S. J., Garvey, C., et al. (2013). An official American Thoracic Society/European Respiratory Society Statement: Key concepts and advances in pulmonary rehabilitation. *American Journal of Respiratory and Critical Care Medicine, 188*(8), e13–e64.

Thomas, L. (2009). Effective dyspnea management strategies identified by elders with end-stage chronic obstructive pulmonary disease. *Applied Nursing Research, 22*(2), 79–85.

Wong, M., & Elliott, M. (2009). The use of medical orders in acute care oxygen therapy. *British Journal of Nursing, 18*(8), 462–464.

Decreased Cardiac output *Ann Will Poteet, MS, RN, CNS*

NANDA-I

Definition

Inadequate blood pumped by the heart to meet the metabolic demands of the body

Defining Characteristics

Altered Heart Rate/Rhythm

Bradycardia, electrocardiogram change (e.g., arrhythmia, conduction abnormality, ischemia)

Altered Preload

Decreased central venous pressure (CVP); Decrease in pulmonary artery wedge pressure (PAWP); edema; fatigue; heart murmur; increase in CVP; increase in PAWP; jugular vein distention; weight gain

Altered Afterload

Abnormal skin color (e.g., pale, dusky, cyanosis); alteration in blood pressure; clammy skin; decrease in peripheral pulses; decrease in pulmonary vascular resistance (PVR); decrease in systemic vascular resistance (SVR); dyspnea; increase in PVR; increase in SVR; oliguria, prolonged capillary refill

Altered Contractility

Adventitious breath sounds; coughing; decreased cardiac index; decrease in ejection fraction; decrease in left ventricular stroke work index; decrease in stroke volume index; orthopnea; paroxysmal nocturnal dyspnea; presence of S3 heart sound; presence of S4 heart sound

Behavioral/Emotional

Anxiety; restlessness

Related Factors (r/t)

Alteration in heart rate; alteration in heart rhythm; altered afterload, altered contractility; altered preload; altered stroke volume

NOC (Nursing Outcomes Classification)

Suggested NOC Outcomes

Cardiac Pump Effectiveness; Circulation Status; Tissue Perfusion: Abdominal Organs, Peripheral; Vital Signs

Example NOC Outcome with Indicators

Cardiac Pump Effectiveness as evidenced by the following indicators: Blood pressure/Heart rate/Cardiac index/Ejection fraction/Activity tolerance/Peripheral pulses/Neck vein distention not present/Heart rhythm/Heart sounds/Angina not present/Peripheral edema not present/Pulmonary edema not present. (Rate the outcome and indicators of **Cardiac Pump Effectiveness:** 1 = severe deviation from normal range, 2 = substantial deviation from normal range, 3 = moderate deviation from normal range, 4 = mild deviation from normal range, 5 = no deviation from normal range [see Section I].)

Client Outcomes

Client Will (Specify Time Frame)

- Demonstrate adequate cardiac output as evidenced by blood pressure, pulse rate and rhythm within normal parameters for client; strong peripheral pulses; maintained level of mentation, lack of chest discomfort or dyspnea, and adequate urinary output; an ability to tolerate activity without symptoms of dyspnea, syncope, or chest pain
- Remain free of side effects from the medications used to achieve adequate cardiac output
- Explain actions and precautions to prevent primary or secondary cardiac disease

NIC (Nursing Interventions Classification)

Suggested NIC Interventions

C

Cardiac Care; Cardiac Care: Acute

Example NIC Activities—Cardiac Care

Evaluate chest pain (e.g., intensity, location, radiation, duration, and precipitating and alleviating factors); Document cardiac dysrhythmias

Nursing Interventions and *Rationales*

- Recognize primary characteristics of decreased cardiac output as fatigue, dyspnea, edema, orthopnea, paroxysmal nocturnal dyspnea, and increased CVP. Recognize secondary characteristics of decreased cardiac output as weight gain, hepatomegaly, jugular venous distention, palpitations, lung crackles, oliguria, coughing, clammy skin, and skin color changes. EBN: *A nursing study to validate characteristics of the nursing diagnosis decreased cardiac output in a clinical environment identified and categorized related client characteristics that were present as primary or secondary (Martins et al, 2010).*
- Monitor and report presence and degree of symptoms including dyspnea at rest or with reduced exercise capacity, orthopnea, paroxysmal nocturnal dyspnea, nocturnal cough, distended abdomen, fatigue, or weakness. Monitor and report signs including jugular vein distention, S3 gallop, rales, positive hepatojugular reflux, ascites, laterally displaced or pronounced point of maximal impact, heart murmurs, narrow pulse pressure, cool extremities, tachycardia with pulsus alternans, and irregular heartbeat. EB: *These are symptoms and signs consistent with heart failure (HF) and decreased cardiac output (Yancy et al, 2013).* EB: *In a study of primary care clients, breathlessness during exercise, limitations in physical activity, and orthopnea were the three most significant symptoms most often associated with HF (Devroey & Van Casteren, 2011).*
- Monitor orthostatic blood pressures and daily weights. EB: *These interventions assess for fluid volume status (Yancy et al, 2013).*
- Recognize that decreased cardiac output can occur in a number of noncardiac disorders such as septic shock and hypovolemia. Expect variation in orders for differential diagnoses related to decreased cardiac output, because orders will be distinct to address the primary cause of the altered cardiac output.
- Obtain a thorough history. EB: *It is important to assess for cardiac and noncardiac disorders and/or behaviors that might accelerate the progression of HF symptoms, such as high sodium diet, excess fluid intake, or missed medication doses (Yancy et al, 2013).*

▲ Monitor pulse oximetry and administer oxygen as needed per health care provider's order. Supplemental oxygen increases oxygen availability to the myocardium and can relieve symptoms of hypoxemia. Resting hypoxia or oxygen desaturation may indicate fluid overload or concurrent pulmonary disease.

- Place client in semi-Fowler's or high Fowler's position with legs down or in a position of comfort. Elevating the head of the bed and legs in down position may decrease the work of breathing and may also decrease venous return and preload.
- During acute events, ensure client remains on short-term bed rest or maintains activity level that does not compromise cardiac output.
- Provide a restful environment by minimizing controllable stressors and unnecessary disturbances. Reducing stressors decreases cardiac workload and oxygen demand.

▲ Apply graduated compression stockings or intermittent sequential pneumatic compression (ISPC) leg sleeves as ordered. Ensure proper fit by measuring accurately. Remove stocking at least twice a day, then reapply. Assess the condition of the extremities frequently. Graduated compression stockings may be contraindicated in clients with peripheral arterial disease (Kahn et al, 2012). EB: *A study that assessed effects of ISPC on healthy adults found that there were significant increases in cardiac output, stroke volume, and ejection fraction due to increased preload and decreased afterload (Bickel et al, 2011);* EB: *A Cochrane review that assessed use of knee-length graduated compression stockings versus thigh-length graduated compression stockings found no difference in effectiveness. Type of stocking should be determined by patient preference, cost, and ease of use (Sajid et al, 2012).* EB: *Graduated compression stockings, alone or used in conjunction with other prevention modalities, help promote venous return and reduce the risk of deep vein thrombosis in hospitalized clients (Sachdeva et al, 2014).*

▲ Check blood pressure, pulse, and condition before administering cardiac medications such as angiotensin-converting enzyme inhibitors, angiotensin receptor blockers, digoxin, and beta-blockers. Notify health care provider if heart rate or blood pressure is low before holding medications. It is important that the nurse evaluate how well the client is tolerating current medications before administering cardiac medications; do not hold medications without health care provider input. The health care provider may decide to have medications administered even though the blood pressure or pulse rate has lowered.

• Observe for and report chest pain or discomfort; note location, radiation, severity, quality, duration, and associated manifestations such as nausea, indigestion, or diaphoresis; also note precipitating and relieving factors. Chest pain/discomfort may indicate an inadequate blood supply to the heart, which can further compromise cardiac output. EB: *Clients with decreased cardiac output may present with myocardial ischemia. Those with myocardial ischemia may present with decreased cardiac output and HF (Amsterdam et al, 2014; Yancy et al, 2013).*

▲ If chest pain is present, refer to the interventions in risk for Decreased **Cardiac** tissue perfusion care plan.

• Recognize the effect of sleep disordered breathing in HF and that sleep disorders are common in patients with HF (Yancy et al, 2013). EB: *Central sleep apnea is recognized as an independent risk factor for worsening HF and reduced survival in patients with HF. The pathological effects of sleep apnea that contribute to worsening cardiac function include sympathetic nervous system stimulation, systemic inflammation, oxidative stress, and endothelial dysfunction (Costanzo et al, 2015).*

• Administer continuous positive airway pressure (CPAP) or supplemental oxygen at night as ordered for management of suspected or diagnosed sleep apnea. EB: *Both CPAP and nocturnal oxygen supplementation have been shown to reduce episodes of sleep apnea, reduce sympathetic nervous system stimulation, and improve cardiac function (Costanzo et al, 2015).*

▲ Closely monitor fluid intake, including intravenous lines. Maintain fluid restriction if ordered. In clients with decreased cardiac output, poorly functioning ventricles may not tolerate increased fluid volumes. EB: *Fluid restriction along with sodium restriction can enhance volume management with diuretics, and in some patients can improve outcomes (Yancy et al, 2013).*

• Monitor intake and output (I&O). If client is acutely ill, measure hourly urine output and note decreases in output. Decreased cardiac output results in decreased perfusion of the kidneys, with a resulting decrease in urine output. EB: *Clinical practice guidelines cite that monitoring I&Os is useful for monitoring effects of HF treatment, including diuretic therapy (Yancy et al, 2013).*

▲ Note results of initial diagnostic studies, including electrocardiography, echocardiography, and chest radiography. EB: *Clinical practice guidelines suggest that chest radiography, echocardiography, and electrocardiogram are recommended in the initial assessment of HF (Yancy et al, 2013).*

▲ Note results of further diagnostic imaging studies such as radionuclide imaging, stress echocardiography, cardiac catheterization, or magnetic resonance imaging (MRI). EB: *Clinical practice guidelines state that radionuclide and MRI are useful studies when assessing left ventricular ejection fraction and volume if echocardiography is not sufficient (Yancy et al, 2013).*

▲ Review laboratory data as needed including arterial blood gases, complete blood count, serum electrolytes (sodium, potassium, magnesium, calcium), blood urea nitrogen, creatinine, urinalysis, glucose, fasting lipid profile, liver function tests, thyroid stimulating hormone, B-type natriuretic peptide (BNP assay), or N-terminal pro-B-type natriuretic peptide (NTpro-BNP). Routine blood work can provide insight into the etiology of HF and extent of decompensation. EB: *Clinical practice guidelines recommend that BNP or NTpro-BNP assay should be measured in clients when the cause of HF is not known, and to determine prognosis or disease severity in chronic or acute decompensated HF (Yancy et al, 2013).*

• Gradually increase activity when the client's condition is stabilized by encouraging slower paced activities, or shorter periods of activity, with frequent rest periods following exercise prescription; observe for symptoms of intolerance. Take blood pressure and pulse before and after activity and note changes. Activity of the cardiac client should be closely monitored. See **Activity** intolerance.

▲ Serve small, frequent, sodium-restricted, low saturated fat meals. Sodium-restricted diets help decrease fluid volume excess. Low saturated fat diets help decrease atherosclerosis, which can cause coronary artery disease. Clients with cardiac disease tolerate smaller meals better because they require less cardiac output to digest (Hooper et al, 2012). EB: *Excess sodium can contribute to elevation of blood pressure, renal impairment, ventricular hypertrophy, diastolic dysfunction, and fibrosis of coronary arteries (Whelton et al, 2012).* EB: *A study that compared cardiac event-free survival between clients who ingested more or less than 3 g of dietary sodium daily found that those who were NYHA class III or IV clients benefited the most from dietary intake less than 3 g daily (Lennie et al, 2011);* EBN: *A study that compared HF symptoms with*

C

dietary sodium intake found that those with sodium intake greater than 3 g per day had more HF symptoms (Son et al, 2011).

- ▲ Monitor bowel function. Provide stool softeners as ordered. Caution client not to strain when defecating. Decreased activity, pain medication, and diuretics can cause constipation. EBN: *Clients with HF have autonomic dysfunction, which places them at risk for reduced mean arterial blood pressure and reduced cerebral blood flow. Autonomic challenges, such as the Valsalva maneuver, can put the HF client at risk for hypoperfusion, ischemia, and stroke (Serber et al, 2014).*
- • Weigh the client at the same time daily (after voiding). Daily weight is a good indicator of fluid balance. Use the same scale if possible when weighing clients for consistency. Increased weight and severity of symptoms can signal decreased cardiac function with retention of fluids. EB: *Clinical practice guidelines state that weighing at the same time daily is useful to assess effects of diuretic therapy (Yancy et al, 2013).*
- ▲ Provide influenza and pneumococcal vaccines as needed before client discharge for those who have yet to receive those inoculations (Centers for Disease Control, 2015).
- • Assess for presence of anxiety and refer for treatment if present. See Nursing Interventions and *Rationales* for **Anxiety** to facilitate reduction of anxiety in clients and family. EB: *A study that assessed the relationship between anxiety and incidence of death, emergency department visits, or hospitalizations found that those with higher anxiety had significantly worse outcomes than those with lower anxiety (De Jong et al, 2011).*
- ▲ Assess for presence of depression and refer for treatment if needed. EB: *Depression is common in clients with HF, and it has been found that individuals with depressive symptoms have poorer quality of life, use health care services more frequently, have poorer self-care, and have worse clinical outcomes (Yancy et al, 2013).* EBN: *A study on combined depression and level of perceived social support found that depressive symptoms were an independent predictor of increased morbidity and mortality, and those with lower perceived social support had 2.1 times higher risk of events than nondepressed clients with high perceived social support (Chung et al, 2011).*
- ▲ Refer to a cardiac rehabilitation program for education and monitored exercise. EB: *Exercise training or regular physical activity is recommended for HF patients. Cardiac rehabilitation can improve quality of life and functional capacity, and decrease mortality (Arena et al, 2012; Smith et al, 2011; Yancy et al, 2013). A systematic review of outcomes of exercise based interventions in clients with systolic HF found that hospitalizations and those for systolic HF were reduced for clients in an exercise program and quality of life was improved (Taylor et al, 2014). In a study to assess effects of exercise in HF clients, exercise tolerance and left ventricular ejection fraction increased with exercise training (Alves et al, 2012).*
- ▲ Refer to an HF program for education, evaluation, and guided support to increase activity and rebuild quality of life. Support for the HF client should be patient-centered, culturally sensitive, and include family and social support. EB: *Multidisciplinary systems of care that are designed to support clients with HF can improve outcomes (Arena et al, 2012; Weintraub et al, 2010; Yancy et al, 2013).* CEB: *A study assessing the 6-month outcomes of a nurse practitioner-coordinated HF center found that readmissions, length of stay, and cost per case were all significantly reduced, while quality of life was significantly improved (Crowther et al, 2002).*

Critically Ill

- ▲ Observe for symptoms of cardiogenic shock, including impaired mentation, hypotension, decreased peripheral pulses, cold clammy skin, signs of pulmonary congestion, and decreased organ function. If present, notify health care provider immediately. Cardiogenic shock is a state of circulatory failure from loss of cardiac function associated with inadequate organ perfusion and a high mortality rate. EB: *Critical cardiogenic shock presents with severe hypotension, increasing inotropic and vasopressor support, organ hypoperfusion, and worsening acidosis and lactate levels (Yancy et al, 2013).*
- ▲ If shock is present, monitor hemodynamic parameters for an increase in pulmonary wedge pressure, an increase in systemic vascular resistance, or a decrease in stroke volume, cardiac output, and cardiac index. EB: *Hemodynamic monitoring with a pulmonary artery catheter can be beneficial in patients with respiratory distress, impaired systemic perfusion, and dependence on intravenous inotropic support, and when clinical assessment is inadequate or severe symptoms persist despite recommended therapies (Yancy et al, 2013).*
- ▲ Titrate inotropic and vasoactive medications within defined parameters to maintain contractility, preload, and afterload per health care provider's order. By following parameters, the nurse ensures maintenance of a delicate balance of medications that stimulate the heart to increase contractility, while maintaining

adequate perfusion of the body. EB: *Clinical practice guidelines recommend that intravenous inotropic drugs might be reasonable for HF clients presenting with low blood pressure and low cardiac output to maintain systemic perfusion and preserve end-organ performance (Yancy et al, 2013; Weintraub et al, 2010).*

▲ Identify significant fluid overload and initiate intravenous diuretics as ordered. Monitor I&Os, daily weight, and vital signs, as well as signs and symptoms of congestion. Watch laboratory data, including serum electrolytes, creatinine, and urea nitrogen. EB: *Intravenous loop diuretics should be initiated in the HF client who presents with significant fluid overload as either intermittent boluses or continuous infusion to reduce morbidity (Yancy et al, 2013).*

C

▲ When using pulmonary arterial catheter technology, be sure to appropriately level and zero the equipment, use minimal tubing, maintain system patency, perform square wave testing, position the client appropriately, and consider correlation to respiratory and cardiac cycles when assessing waveforms and integrating data into client assessment. EB: *Clinical practice guidelines recommend that invasive hemodynamic monitoring can be useful in acute HF with persistent symptoms when therapy is refractory, fluid status is unclear, systolic pressures are low, renal function is worsening, vasoactive agents are required, or when considering advanced device therapy or transplantation (Yancy et al, 2013).*

▲ Observe for worsening signs and symptoms of decreased cardiac output when using positive pressure ventilation. EB: *Positive pressure ventilation and mechanical ventilation are associated with a decrease in preload and cardiac output (Lukacsovitis et al, 2012; Yucel et al, 2011).*

▲ Recognize that clients with cardiogenic pulmonary edema may have noninvasive positive pressure ventilation ordered. EB: *Clinical practice guidelines for HF state that continuous positive airway pressure improves daily functional capacity and quality of life for those with HF and obstructive sleep apnea and is reasonable for clients with refractory HF not responding to other medical therapies (Costanzo et al, 2015; Yancy et al, 2013).*

▲ Monitor client for signs and symptoms of fluid and electrolyte imbalance when clients are receiving ultrafiltration or continuous renal replacement therapy (CRRT). Clients with refractory HF may have ultrafiltration or CRRT ordered as a mechanical method to remove excess fluid volume. EB: *Clinical practice guidelines cite that ultrafiltration is reasonable for clients with obvious volume overload and congestion, and refractory congestion not responsive to medical therapy (Yancy et al, 2013).*

• Recognize that hypoperfusion from low cardiac output can lead to altered mental status and decreased cognition. CEB: *A study that assessed an association among cardiac index and neuropsychological ischemia found that decreased cardiac function, even with normal cardiac index, was associated with accelerated brain aging (Jefferson et al, 2010).*

• Recognize that clients with severe HF may undergo additional therapies, such as internal pacemaker or defibrillator placement, and/or placement of a ventricular assist device (VAD). EB: *The use of VADs is a reasonable treatment as a bridge to recovery, transplant, or decision making in selected HF clients with reduced ejection fraction and profound hemodynamic compromise (Yancy et al, 2013).*

Geriatric

• Recognize that older clients may demonstrate fatigue and depression as signs of HF and decreased cardiac output.

▲ If the client has heart disease causing activity intolerance, refer for cardiac rehabilitation. EB: *Cardiac rehabilitation can positively affect an individual's overall health outcome, especially in the older population, due to increased frailty and functional limitations (Arena et al, 2012).* EBN: *A study that assessed clients' acceptance of a cardiac rehabilitation program found knowledge and perceived quality of life had increased significantly, and anxiety and depression had been reduced at the end of the program and at 6-month follow-up (Muschalla et al, 2011).*

▲ Recognize that edema can present differently in the older population. EB: *In the older population, lower extremity edema is often related to peripheral causes, such as dependency, rather than cardiac causes (Yancy et al, 2013).*

▲ Recognize that blood pressure control is beneficial for older clients to reduce the risk of worsening HF. EB: *Hypertension treatment is particularly beneficial in the older population, and control of both systolic and diastolic hypertension has been shown to reduce the risk of incident HF (Yancy et al, 2013).*

▲ Recognize that renal function is not always accurately represented by serum creatinine in the older population due to less muscle mass (Yancy et al, 2013).

▲ Observe for side effects from cardiac medications. Older adults can have difficulty with metabolism and excretion of medications due to decreased function of the liver and kidneys; therefore, toxic side effects

C

are more common. EB: *Older adults are at increased risk for digoxin toxicity, especially at larger doses, due to lower body mass and impaired renal function (Yancy et al, 2013).*

- ▲ Older adults may require more frequent visits, closer monitoring of medication dose changes, and more gradual increases in medications, due to changes in the metabolism of medications and impaired renal function (Yancy et al, 2013).
- ▲ As older adults approach end of life, clinicians should help to facilitate a comprehensive plan of care that incorporates the patient and family's values, goals, and preferences (Allen et al, 2012).

Home Care

- Some of the above interventions may be adapted for home care use. Home care agencies may use specialized staff and methods to care for chronic HF clients. CEB: *A study assessing HF outcomes over a 10-year period between a multidisciplinary home care intervention and usual care found significantly improved survival and prolonged event-free survival and was both cost- and time-effective (Ingles et al, 2006).*
- Assess for fatigue and weakness frequently. Assess home environment for safety, as well as resources/obstacles to energy conservation.
- Help family adapt daily living patterns to establish life changes that will maintain improved cardiac functioning in the client. Take the client's perspective into consideration and use a holistic approach in assessing and responding to client planning for the future.
- Assist client to recognize and exercise power in using self-care management to adjust to health change. Refer to care plan for **Powerlessness.**
- ▲ Refer to medical social services, cardiac rehabilitation, telemonitoring and case management as necessary for assistance with home-care, access to resources, and counseling about the impact of severe or chronic cardiac diseases. EB: *Access to systems that promote care coordination is essential for successful care of the HF client. Good communication and documentation between services, health care providers, and transitions of care is essential to ensure improved outcomes in HF clients (Albert et al, 2015; Smith et al, 2011; Yancy et al, 2013).*
- ▲ As the client chooses, refer to palliative care for care, which can begin earlier in the care of the HF client. Palliative care can be used to increase comfort and quality of life in the HF client before end-of-life care (Buck & Zambroski, 2012). EB: *Palliative care should address quality of life, ongoing symptom control, preferences about end-of-life, psychosocial distress, and caregiver support (Yancy et al, 2013).*
- ▲ If the client's condition warrants, refer to hospice. EB: *The palliative care and HF teams are best suited to determine when end-of-life care is appropriate for the patient and family (Yancy et al, 2013).* CEB: *The multidisciplinary hospice team can reduce hospital readmission, increase functional capacity, and improve quality of life in end-stage HF (Coviello et al, 2002).*

Client/Family Teaching and Discharge Planning

- Begin discharge planning as soon as possible upon admission to the emergency department (ED) if appropriate with a case manager or social worker to assess home support systems and the need for community or home health services. EB: *Discharge planning should include adherence to the treatment plan, medication management, follow-up with health care providers and care coordination, dietary and physical activities, cardiac rehabilitation, and secondary prevention recommendations (Albert et al, 2015; Yancy et al, 2013).*
- Discharge education should be comprehensive, evidence based, culturally sensitive, and include both the client and family (Yancy et al, 2013).
- Teach client about any medications prescribed. Medication teaching includes the drug name, its purpose, administration instructions, such as taking it with or without food, and any side effects to be aware of. Instruct the client to report any adverse side effects to his/her health care provider.
- Teach the importance of performing and recording daily weights upon arising for the day, and to report weight gain. Ask if client has a scale at home; if not, assist in getting one. EB: *Clinical practice guidelines suggest that daily weight monitoring leads to early recognition of excess fluid retention, which, when reported, can be offset with additional medication to avoid hospitalization from heart failure decompensation (Yancy et al, 2013).*
- Teach the types and progression patterns of worsening heart failure symptoms, when to call a health care provider for help, and when to go to the hospital for urgent care (Yancy et al, 2013).
- Stress the importance of ceasing tobacco use. EB: *Tobacco use can cause or worsen decreased blood flow in the coronaries, as well as cause vasoconstriction, which can lead to atherosclerotic disease. Effects of*

nicotine include increasing pulse and blood pressure and constricting of blood vessels. Tobacco use is a primary factor in heart disease. (American Heart Association, 2014; Smith et al, 2011).

- ▲ Individuals should be screened for electronic cigarette use (e-cigarette). EB: *While more studies are needed regarding the health effects of e-cigarette use, the American Heart Association recommends that all health care providers educate their patients regarding the long-term use of e-cigarettes given the known toxicities present in e-cigarettes, as well as the presence of nicotine in most types of e-cigarettes (Bhatnagar et al, 2014).*
- • Upon hospital discharge, educate clients about low sodium, low saturated fat diet, with consideration to client education, literacy, and health literacy level. EB: *Excess sodium intake is directly related to elevated blood pressure (Whelton et al, 2012). A Cochrane review recommended that there be a permanent reduction in dietary saturated fats and replacement with unsaturated fats to reduce the risk of cardiovascular disease (Hooper et al, 2012).*
- • Instruct client and family on the importance of regular follow-up care with health care providers. EB: *Post discharge support can significantly reduce hospital readmissions and improve health care outcomes, quality of life, and costs (Hernandez et al, 2010; Yancy et al, 2013).*
- ▲ Teach stress reduction (e.g., imagery, controlled breathing, and muscle relaxation techniques). CEB: *A study that assessed effects of relaxation or exercise in heart failure clients versus controls found that those who participated in regular relaxation therapy or exercise training reported greater improvements in psychological outcomes, with the relaxation group significantly improving depression and the exercise training group more improving fatigue (Yu et al, 2007).*
- • Discuss advance directives with the HF client, including resuscitation preferences. EB: Evidence suggests that advance directives can help to reduce overall health care costs, reduce in-hospital deaths, and increase hospice use (Yancy et al, 2013).
- • Patients should be provided with education regarding the influenza vaccine and pneumococcal vaccine prior to discharge. EB: *The influenza vaccine is recommended for all adults, and the pneumococcal vaccine is recommended for individuals greater than 65 years old and for individuals who are at high risk for cardiovascular disease (Centers for Disease Control, 2015).*
- • Teach the importance of physical activity as tolerated. EB: *Exercise helps control blood pressure and weight, which are the most important controlled risk factors for cardiovascular disease. Individuals should engage in aerobic physical activity of moderate to vigorous intensity, three to four times per week (Eckel et al, 2013).*

REFERENCES

Albert, N. M., Barnason, S., Deswal, A., et al. (2015). Transitions of care in heart failure: a scientific statement from the American Heart Association. *Circulatory Heart Failure*, *8*, 384–409.

Allen, L. A., Stevenson, L. W., Grady, K. L., et al. (2012). Decision making in advanced heart failure: a scientific statement from the American Heart Association. *Circulation*, *125*, 1928–1952.

Alves, A. J., et al. (2012). Exercise training improves diastolic function in heart failure patients. *Medicine and Science in Sports and Exercise*, *44*(5), 776–785.

American Heart Association. (2014). *Smoking & cardiovascular disease (heart disease)*. Retrieved from: <http://www.heart.org/HEARTORG/GettingHealthy/QuitSmoking/-/HEARTORG/GettingHealthy/QuitSmoking/QuittingResources/Smoking-Cardiovascular-Disease_UCM_305187_Article.jsp>.

Amsterdam, E. A., Wenger, N. K., Brindis, R. G., et al. (2014). AHA/ACC guideline for the management of patients with non-ST elevation acute coronary syndromes: a report of the American College of Cardiology/American Heart Association Task Force on Practice Guidelines. *Circulation*, *23*(30), e344–e426.

Arena, R., Williams, M., Forman, D. E., et al. (2012). Increasing referral and participation rates to outpatient cardiac rehabilitation: the valuable role of healthcare professionals in the inpatient and home health settings: a science advisory from the American Heart Association. *Circulation*, *125*, 1321–1329.

Bhatnagar, A., Whitsel, L. P., Ribisl, K. M., et al. (2014). Electronic cigarettes: a policy statement from the American Heart Association. *Circulation*, *130*, 1418–1436.

Bickel, A., et al. (2011). The physiological impact of intermittent sequential pneumatic compression (ISPC) leg sleeves on cardiac activity. *American Journal of Surgery*, *202*, 15–22.

Buck, H. G., & Zambroski, C. H. (2012). Upstreaming palliative care for patients with heart failure. *Journal of Cardiovascular Nursing*, *27*(2), 147–153.

Centers for Disease Control. (Updated 2015). *Adult immunization schedules*. Retrieved from: <http://www.cdc.gov/vaccines/schedules/hcp/adult.html>.

Chung, M. L., et al. (2011). Depressive symptoms and poor social support have a synergistic effect on event-free survival in patients with heart failure. *Heart and Lung: The Journal of Critical Care*, *40*(6), 492–501.

Costanzo, M. R., Khayat, R., Ponikowski, P., et al. (2015). Mechanisms and clinical consequences of untreated central sleep apnea in heart failure. *Journal of American Colleges of Cardiology*, *65*(1), 72–84.

Coviello, J. S., Hricz, L., & Masulli, P. S. (2002). Client challenge: accomplishing quality of life in end-stage heart failure: a hospice multidisciplinary approach. *Home Healthcare Nurse*, *20*, 195–198.

Crowther, M., et al. (2002). Evidence-based development of a hospital-based heart failure center. *Reflections on Nursing Leadership*, *28*(2), 32–33.

De Jong, M. J., et al. (2011). Linkages between anxiety and outcomes in heart failure. *Heart and Lung: The Journal of Critical Care*, *40*(5), 393–404.

Devroey, D., & Van Casteren, V. (2011). Signs for early diagnosis of heart failure in primary health care. *Vascular Health Risk Management*, *7*, 591–596.

Eckel, R. H., Jakicic, J. M., Ard, J. D., et al. (2013). 2013 AHA/ACC guideline on lifestyle management to reduce cardiovascular risk: a report of the American College of Cardiology/American Heart Association Task Force on Practice Guidelines. *Circulation, 129*(Suppl. 2), S76–S99.

Hernandez, A. F., et al. (2010). Relationship between early physician follow-up and 30-day readmission among Medicare beneficiaries hospitalized for heart failure. *JAMA: The Journal of the American Medical Association, 303*(17), 1716–1722.

Hooper, L., Summerbell, C. D., Thompson, R., et al. (2012). Reduced or modified dietary fat for preventing cardiovascular disease (review). *The Cochrane Library*, (Issue 5). Retrieved from: <http://onlinelibrary.wiley.com.hsl-ezproxy.ucdenver.edu/doi/10.1002/14651858.CD002137.pub3/pdf>.

Ingles, S. C., et al. (2006). Extending the horizon in chronic heart failure: effects of multidisciplinary, home-based intervention relative to usual care. *Circulation, 114*(23), 2466–2473.

Jefferson, A. L., et al. (2010). Cardiac index is associated with brain aging: the Framingham Heart study. *Circulation, 122*(7), 690–697.

Kahn, S., et al. (2012). *Antithrombotic therapy and prevention of thrombosis*, ed 9, American College of Chest Physician Evidence-Based Clinical Practice Guidelines Online Only Articles. *Chest, 141*(Suppl. 2), e195S–e226S.

Lennie, T. A., et al. (2011). Three gram sodium intake is associated with longer event-free survival only in patients with advanced heart failure. *Journal of Cardiac Failure, 17*(4), 325–330.

Lukacsovitis, J., Carlussi, A., & Hill, N. (2012). Physiological changes during low and high intensity non-invasive ventilation. *European Respiratory Journal, 39*(4), 869–875.

Martins, Q. C., Alita, G., & Rabelo, E. R. (2010). Decreased cardiac output: clinical validation in patients with decompensated heart failure. *International Journal of Nursing Terminology Classification, 21*(4), 156–165.

Muschalla, B., Glatz, J., & Karger, G. (2011). Cardiac rehabilitation with a structured education programme for patients with chronic heart failure-illness-related knowledge, mental wellbeing and acceptance in participants. *Rehabilitation, 50*(2), 103–110.

Sachdeva, A., Dalton, M., Amaragiri, S. V., et al. (2014). Graduated compression stockings for prevention of deep vein thrombosis. *The Cochrane Library*, (Issue 12). Retrieved from: <http://onlinelibrary.wiley.com.hsl-ezproxy.ucdenver.edu/doi/10.1002/14651858.CD001484.pub3/abstract>.

Sajid, M. S., Desai, M., Morris, R. W., et al. (2012). Knee length versus thigh length graduated compression stockings for prevention of deep vein thrombosis in postoperative surgical patients: review. *The Cochrane Library*, (Issue 5). Retrieved from: <http://onlinelibrary.wiley.com.hsl-ezproxy.ucdenver.edu/doi/10.1002/14651858.CD007162.pub2/abstract>.

Serber, S. L., Rinsky, B., Kumar, R., et al. (2014). Cerebral blood flow velocity and vasomotor reactivity during autonomic challenges in heart failure. *Nursing Research, 63*(3), 194–202.

Smith, S. C., Benjamin, E. J., Bonow, R. O., et al. (2011). AHA/ACCF secondary prevention and risk reduction therapy for patient with coronary and other atherosclerotic vascular disease: 2011 update: a guideline from the American Heart Association and American College of Cardiology Foundation. *Circulation, 124*, 2458–2473.

Son, Y. J., Lee, Y., & Song, E. K. (2011). Adherence to a sodium-restricted diet is associated with lower symptom burden and longer cardiac event-free survival in patients with heart failure. *Journal of Clinical Nursing, 20*(21/22), 3029–3038.

Taylor, R. S., Sagar, V. A., Davies, E. J., et al. (2014). Exercise based rehabilitation for heart failure. *The Cochrane Library*, (Issue 4). Retrieved from: <http://onlinelibrary.wiley.com.hsl-ezproxy.ucdenver.edu/doi/10.1002/14651858.CD003331.pub4/abstract>.

Weintraub, N. L., Collins, S. P., Pang, P. S., et al. (2010). Acute heart failure syndromes: emergency department presentation, treatment, and disposition: current approaches and future aims: a scientific statement from the American Heart Association. *Circulation, 122*, 1975–1996.

Whelton, P. K., Appel, L. J., Sacco, R. L., et al. (2012). Sodium, blood pressure, and cardiovascular disease: further evidence supporting the American Heart Association sodium reduction recommendations. *Circulation, 126*, 2880–2889.

Yancy, C. W., Jessup, M., Bozkurt, B., et al. (2013). ACCF/AHA guideline for the management of heart failure: a report of the American College of Cardiology Foundation/American Heart Association Task Force on Practice Guidelines. *Circulation, 128*, e240–e327.

Yu, D. S., et al. (2007). Non-pharmacological interventions in older people with heart failure: effects of exercise training and relaxation therapy. *Gerontology, 53*(2), 74–81.

Yucel, S., et al. (2011). Nursing diagnoses in patients having mechanical ventilation support in a respiratory intensive care unit in Turkey. *International Journal of Nursing Practice, 17*(5), 502–508.

Risk for decreased Cardiac output

Mary Beth Flynn Makic, PhD, RN, CNS, CCNS, FAAN, and Ann Will Poteet, MS, RN, CNS

NANDA-I

Definition

Vulnerable to inadequate blood pumped by the heart to meet metabolic demands of the body, which may compromise health

Risk Factors

Alteration in heart rate; alteration in heart rhythm; alteration in afterload; altered contractility; altered preload; altered stroke volume

NIC, NOC, Client Outcomes, Nursing Interventions, Client/Family Teaching and Discharge Planning, *Rationales*, and References

Refer to care plan for Decreased **Cardiac** output.

Risk for decreased Cardiac tissue perfusion

Ann Will Poteet, MS, RN, CNS

NANDA-I

Definition

Vulnerable to a decrease in cardiac (coronary) circulation, which may compromise health

Risk Factors

Cardiac tamponade; cardiovascular surgery; coronary artery spasm; diabetes mellitus; family history of cardiovascular disease; hyperlipidemia; hypertension; hypovolemia; hypoxemia; hypoxia; increase in C-reactive protein; insufficient knowledge about modifiable risk factors (e.g., smoking, sedentary lifestyle, obesity); pharmaceutical agent; substance abuse

NOC (Nursing Outcomes Classification)

Suggested NOC Outcomes

Cardiac Pump Effectiveness; Circulation Status; Tissue Perfusion: Cardiac; Tissue Perfusion: Cellular; Vital Signs

Example NOC Outcome with Indicators

Tissue Perfusion: Cardiac as evidenced by the following indicators: Angina/Arrhythmia/Tachycardia/Bradycardia/Nausea/Vomiting/Profuse diaphoresis. (Rate the outcome and indicators of **Tissue Perfusion: Cardiac:** 1 = severe, 2 = substantial, 3 = moderate, 4 = mild, 5 = none [see Section I].)

Client Outcomes

Client Will (Specify Time Frame)

- Maintain vital signs within normal range
- Retain an asymptomatic cardiac rhythm (have absence of arrhythmias, tachycardia, or bradycardia)
- Be free from chest and radiated discomfort as well as associated symptoms related to acute coronary syndromes (ACSs)
- Deny nausea and be free of vomiting
- Have skin that is dry and of normal temperature

NIC (Nursing Interventions Classification)

Suggested NIC Interventions

Cardiac Care; Cardiac Precautions; Embolus Precautions; Dysrhythmia Management; Vital Signs Monitoring; Shock Management: Cardiac

Example NIC Activity—Cardiac Precautions

Avoid causing intense emotional situations; Avoid overheating or chilling the client; Provide small frequent meals; Substitute artificial salt and limit sodium intake if appropriate; Promote effective techniques for reducing stress; Restrict smoking

Nursing Interventions and *Rationales*

- Be aware that the primary cause of ACS—unstable angina (UA), non–ST-elevation myocardial infarction (NSTEMI), and ST-elevation myocardial infarction (STEMI)—is an imbalance between myocardial oxygen consumption and demand that is associated with partially or fully occlusive thrombus development in coronary arteries (Amsterdam et al, 2014).
- Assess for symptoms of coronary hypoperfusion and possible ACS, including chest discomfort (pressure, tightness, crushing, squeezing, dullness, or achiness), with or without radiation (or originating) in the retrosternum, back, neck, jaw, shoulder, or arm discomfort or numbness; shortness of breath (SOB); associated diaphoresis; abdominal pain; dizziness, lightheadedness, loss of consciousness, or unexplained

C

fatigue; nausea or vomiting with chest discomfort, heartburn, or indigestion; associated anxiety. EB: *These symptoms are signs of decreased cardiac perfusion and ACS such as UA, NSTEMI, or STEMI, as well as other cardiovascular disorders such as aortic aneurysm, valve disorders, and pericarditis. A physical assessment will aid in assessment of the extent, location, and presence of, and complications resulting from a myocardial infarction (MI). It will promote rapid triage and treatment. It is also important to assess whether the client had a prior stroke, heart failure, or other cardiovascular disorder. It is important to note that certain psychiatric disorders (somatoform disorders, panic attack, anxiety disorders) can mimic ACS, but are typically noncardiac causes of chest pain (Amsterdam et al, 2014).*

- • Consider atypical presentations of ACS for women, older adults, and individuals with diabetes mellitus, impaired renal function, and dementia. EB/CEB: *Women, older adults, and individuals with diabetes mellitus, impaired renal function, and dementia may present with atypical findings (Amsterdam et al, 2014; Mieres et al, 2014). A systematic review of differences showed that women had significantly less chest discomfort and were more likely to present with fatigue, neck pain, syncope, nausea, right arm pain, dizziness, and jaw pain (Coventry et al, 2011).*
- • Review the client's medical, surgical, social, and familial history. EB: *A medical history must be concise and detailed to determine the possibility of ACSs and to help determine the possible cause of cardiac symptoms and pathology (Amsterdam et al, 2014).*
- • Perform physical assessments for both CAD and noncoronary findings related to decreased coronary perfusion, including vital signs, pulse oximetry, equal blood pressure in both arms, heart rate, respiratory rate, and pulse oximetry. Check bilateral pulses for quality and regularity. Report tachycardia, bradycardia, hypotension or hypertension, pulsus alternans or pulsus paradoxus, tachypnea, or abnormal pulse oximetry reading. Assess cardiac rhythm for arrhythmias; skin and mucous membrane color, temperature, and dryness; and capillary refill. Assess neck veins for elevated central venous pressure, cyanosis, and pericardial or pleural friction rub. Examine client for cardiac S_4 gallop, new heart murmur, lung crackles, altered mentation, pain on abdominal palpation, decreased bowel sounds, or decreased urinary output. EB: *These indicators help assess for cardiac and noncardiac etiologies of symptoms and differential diagnoses (Amsterdam et al, 2014).*
- ▲ Administer supplemental oxygen as ordered and needed for clients presenting with ACS, respiratory distress, or other high-risk features of hypoxemia to maintain a Po_2 of at least 90%. EB: *American Heart Association guidelines for emergency cardiovascular care during ACS recommend administering oxygen for breathlessness, hypoxemia, signs of heart failure, or if signs of shock are present, and the need for oxygen should be guided by noninvasive monitoring of oxygen saturation. There is limited evidence to support or refute the use of high-flow or low-flow supplemental oxygen if a normal oxygen level (>90%) is present (Amsterdam et al, 2014; O'Connor et al, 2010).* EB: *A Cochrane review found there was limited evidence to support or refute the use of routine supplemental oxygen with ACS, recommending further studies (Cabello et al, 2013).*
- ▲ Use continuous pulse oximetry as ordered. EB: *Prevention and treatment of hypoxemia includes maintaining arterial oxygen saturation over 90% (Amsterdam et al, 2014).*
- ▲ Insert one or more large-bore intravenous catheters to keep the vein open. Routinely assess saline locks for patency. Clients who come to the hospital with possible decrease in coronary perfusion or ACS may have intravenous fluids and medications ordered routinely or emergently to maintain or restore adequate cardiac function and rhythm.
- ▲ Observe the cardiac monitor for hemodynamically significant arrhythmias, ST depressions or elevations, T-wave inversions and/or q-waves as signs of ischemia or injury. Report abnormal findings. EB: *Arrhythmias and electrocardiogram (ECG) changes indicate myocardial ischemia, injury, and/or infarction. Note that left ventricular hypertrophy, ventricular pacing, and bundle branch blocks can mask signs of ischemia or injury (Amsterdam et al, 2014).*
- • Have emergency equipment and defibrillation capability nearby and be prepared to defibrillate immediately if ventricular tachycardia with clinical deterioration or ventricular fibrillation occurs. EB: *Life-threatening ventricular arrhythmias require defibrillation (Hazinski et al, 2010).*
- ▲ Perform a 12-lead ECG as ordered, to be interpreted within 10 minutes of emergency department arrival and during episodes of chest discomfort or angina equivalent. EB: *A 12-lead ECG should be performed within 10 minutes of emergency department arrival for all clients who are having chest discomfort. ECGs are used to identify the area of ischemia or injury, such as ST depressions or elevations, new left-bundle branch block, T-wave inversions, and/or q waves, and to guide treatment (Amsterdam et al, 2014).*

C

- ▲ Administer nonenteric coated aspirin as ordered, as soon as possible after presentation and for maintenance. EB: *Aspirin has been shown to prevent platelet clumping, aggregation, and activation that leads to thrombus formation, which in coronary arteries leads to ACSs. Contraindications include active peptic ulcer disease, bleeding disorders, and aspirin allergy (Amsterdam et al, 2014; O'Gara et al, 2013).*
- ▲ Administer nitroglycerin tablets sublingually as ordered, every 5 minutes until the chest pain is resolved while also monitoring the blood pressure for hypotension, for a maximum of three doses as ordered. Administer nitroglycerin paste or intravenous preparations as ordered. EB: *Nitroglycerin causes coronary arterial and venous dilation, and at higher doses peripheral arterial dilation, thus reducing preload and afterload and decreasing myocardial oxygen demand while increasing oxygen delivery (Amsterdam et al, 2014).*
- • Do not administer nitroglycerin preparations to individuals with hypotension, or individuals who have received phosphodiesterase type 5 inhibitors, such as sildenafil, tadalafil, or vardenafil, in the last 24 hours (48 hours for long-acting preparations). EB: *Synergistic effect causes marked exaggerated and prolonged vasodilation/hypotension (Amsterdam et al, 2014).*
- ▲ Administer morphine intravenously as ordered every 5 to 30 minutes until pain is relieved while monitoring blood pressure when nitroglycerin alone does not relieve chest discomfort. EB: *Morphine has potent analgesic and antianxiolytic effects and causes mild reductions in blood pressure and heart rate that reduce myocardial oxygen consumption. Hypotension and respiratory depression are the most serious complications of morphine use, and naloxone may be administered as ordered for morphine overdose (Amsterdam et al, 2014).*
- ▲ Assess and report abnormal lab work results of cardiac enzymes, specifically troponin I or T, B-type natriuretic peptide, chemistries, hematology, coagulation studies, arterial blood gases, finger stick blood sugar, elevated C-reactive protein, or drug screen. EB: *Abnormalities can identify the cause of the decreased perfusion and identify complications related to the decreased perfusion such as anemia, hypovolemia, coagulopathy, drug abuse, hyperglycemia, kidney (renal) failure, and heart failure. Markedly elevated cardiac enzymes are usually indicative of an MI, and the cardiac enzymes can also help determine short- and long-term prognosis (Amsterdam et al, 2014).*
- • Assess for individual risk factors for coronary artery disease, such as hypertension, dyslipidemia, cigarette smoking, diabetes mellitus, or family history of heart disease. Other risk factors including sedentary lifestyle, obesity, or cocaine or amphetamine use. Note age and gender as risk factors. EB: *Certain conditions place clients at higher risk for decreased cardiac tissue perfusion (Amsterdam et al, 2014; Mieres et al, 2014).*
- ▲ Administer additional heart medications as ordered, including beta blockers, calcium channel blockers, angiotensin-converting enzyme inhibitors, angiotensin II receptor blockers, aldosterone antagonists, antiplatelet agents, and anticoagulants. Always check blood pressure and pulse rate before administering these medications. If the blood pressure or pulse rate is low, contact the health care provider to establish whether the medication should be withheld. Also check platelet counts, renal function, and coagulation studies as ordered to assess proper effects of these agents. EB: *These medications are useful to optimize cardiac and kidney function, including blood pressure, heart rate, myocardial oxygen demand, intravascular fluid volume, and cardiac rhythm (Amsterdam et al, 2014).*
- ▲ Administer lipid-lowering therapy as ordered. EB: *Use of statin drugs has been shown to reduce an individual's risk of recurrent MI, stroke, and coronary heart disease mortality, especially with high-intensity statins that lower low-density lipoprotein cholesterol levels (Amsterdam et al, 2014, Stone et al, 2013). A systematic review of statin use in primary prevention of cardiovascular disease showed reductions in all-cause mortality, major vascular events, and revascularizations (Taylor et al, 2014).*
- ▲ Prepare client with education, withholding of meals and/or medications, and intravenous access for early invasive therapy with cardiac catheterization, reperfusion therapy, and possible percutaneous coronary intervention in individuals with refractory angina or hemodynamic or electrical instability, and first medical contact to device time of less than 90 minutes if STEMI is suspected. EB: *First medical contact to device time of less than 90 minutes was associated with improved client outcomes (Amsterdam et al, 2014; O'Gara et al, 2013).*
- ▲ Prepare clients with education, withholding of meals and/or medications, and intravenous access for noninvasive cardiac diagnostic procedures such as 2D echocardiogram, exercise, or pharmacological stress test, and cardiac computed tomography scan as ordered. EB: *Clients suspected of decreased coronary perfusion should receive these diagnostic procedures as appropriate to evaluate for coronary artery disease (Amsterdam et al, 2014; Fletcher et al, 2013; Mieres et al, 2014).*

▲ Request a referral to a cardiac rehabilitation program. EB: *Cardiac rehabilitation programs are designed to limit the physiological and psychological effects of cardiac disease, reduce the risk for sudden cardiac death and reinfarction, control symptoms and stabilize or reverse the process of plaque formation, and enhance psychosocial and vocational status of clients (Amsterdam et al, 2014).*

Geriatric

- Consider atypical presentations of possible ACS in older adults. CEB: *Older adults may present with atypical signs and symptoms such as weakness, stroke, syncope, or change in mental status (Amsterdam et al, 2014).*

▲ Ask the prescriber about possible reduced dosage of medications for older clients, considering weight, creatinine clearance, and glomerular filtration rate. EB: *Older clients can have reduced pharmacokinetics and pharmacodynamics, including reduced muscle mass, reduced renal and hepatic function, and reduced volume of distribution that can alter drug dosing, efficacy, and safety, as well as some drug-drug interactions (Amsterdam et al, 2014; Stone et al, 2013).*

- Consider issues such as quality of life, palliative care, end-of-life care, and differences in sociocultural aspects for clients and families when supporting them in decisions regarding aggressiveness of care. Ask about living wills, as well as medical and durable power of attorney. EB: *Management decisions, including decisions regarding invasive treatment, should be client-centered and take into account client preferences and goals, comorbidities, cognitive and functional status, and life expectancy (Amsterdam et al, 2014).*

Client/Family Teaching and Discharge Planning

▲ Client and family education regarding a multidisciplinary plan of care should start early. Special attention to client and family education should occur during transitions of care. EB: *It is important to provide the client and family with a comprehensive plan of care and education materials that are evidence-based to assist with client compliance and to potentially reduce hospital readmissions related to ACS. The plan of care should take into consideration the client's psychosocial and socioeconomic status, access to care, risk for depression and/or social isolation, and health care disparities (Amsterdam et al, 2014).*

- Teach the client and family to call 911 for symptoms of new angina, existing angina unresponsive to rest and sublingual nitroglycerin tablets, or heart attack, or if an individual becomes unresponsive. EB/CEB: *Morbidity and mortality from MI can be reduced significantly when symptoms are recognized and emergency medical services activated, shortening time to definitive treatment (Hazinski et al, 2010).*
- Upon discharge, instruct clients about symptoms of ischemia, when to cease activity, when to use sublingual nitroglycerin, and when to call 911. EB/CEB: *Degree and extent of myocardial ischemia is related to duration of time with inadequate supply of oxygen-rich blood (Hazinski et al, 2010).*
- Teach client about any medications prescribed. Medication teaching includes the drug name, its purpose, administration instructions such as taking it with or without food, and any side effects to be aware of. Instruct the client to report any adverse side effects to the health care provider.
- Upon hospital discharge, educate clients and significant others about discharge medications, including nitroglycerin sublingual tablets or spray, with written, easy to understand, culturally sensitive information. EB: *Clients and significant others need to be prepared to act quickly and decisively to relieve ischemic discomfort (Amsterdam et al, 2014).*
- Provide client education related to risk factors for decreased cardiac tissue perfusion, such as hypertension, hypercholesterolemia, diabetes mellitus, tobacco use, advanced age, and gender (female). EB: *Those with two or more risk factors should have a 10-year risk screening for development of symptomatic coronary heart disease. Client education is a vital part of nursing care for the client. Start with the client's base level of understanding and use that as a foundation for further education. It is important to factor in cultural and/or religious beliefs in the education provided (Amsterdam et al, 2014; Eckel et al, 2013; Goff et al, 2013).*
- Instruct the client on antiplatelet and anticoagulation therapy, and about signs of bleeding, need for ongoing medication compliance, and international normalized ratio monitoring. EB: *Special attention and education should be provided to older individuals, because they are at greater risk for bleeding (Amsterdam et al, 2014).*
- After discharge, continue education and support for client blood pressure and diabetes control, weight management, and resumption of physical activity. EB: *Reducing risk factors acts as secondary prevention of coronary artery disease (Amsterdam et al, 2014; Eckel et al, 2013).*

▲ Clients should be provided with education regarding the influenza vaccine and pneumococcal vaccine before hospital discharge. EB: *The influenza vaccine is recommended for all adults, and the pneumococcal vaccine is recommended for individuals older than 65 years and for individuals who are at high risk for cardiovascular disease (Amsterdam et al, 2014; Centers for Disease Control, 2014).*

▲ Stress the importance of ceasing tobacco use. EB: *Tobacco use can cause or worsen decreased blood flow in the coronaries, as well as cause vasoconstriction, which can lead to atherosclerotic disease. Effects of nicotine include increasing pulse and blood pressure and constricting blood vessels. Tobacco use is a primary factor in heart disease (American Heart Association, 2014; Amsterdam et al, 2014).*

▲ Individuals should be screened for electronic cigarette use (e-cigarette). EB: *While more studies are needed regarding the health effects of e-cigarette use, the American Heart Association recommends that all health care providers educate their clients regarding the long-term use of e-cigarettes given the known toxicities present in e-cigarettes, as well as the presence of nicotine in most types of e-cigarettes (Bhatnagar et al, 2014).*

▲ Upon hospital discharge, educate clients about a low sodium, low saturated fat diet, with consideration to client education, literacy, and health literacy level. EB: *Reducing risk factors acts as secondary prevention of coronary artery disease (Amsterdam et al, 2014; Eckel et al, 2013). A Cochrane review recommended that there be a permanent reduction in dietary saturated fats and replacement with unsaturated fats to reduce the risk of cardiovascular disease (Hopper et al, 2012).*

• Teach the importance of physical activity. EB: *Exercise helps control blood pressure and weight, which are the most important controlled risk factors for cardiovascular disease. Individuals should engage in aerobic physical activity of moderate to vigorous intensity, three to four times per week (Amsterdam et al, 2014; Eckel et al, 2013).*

REFERENCES

American Heart Association. (2014). *Smoking & cardiovascular disease (heart disease)*. Retrieved from: <http://www.heart.org/HEARTORG/GettingHealthy/QuitSmoking/-/HEARTORG/GettingHealthy/QuitSmoking/QuittingResources/Smoking-Cardiovascular-Disease_UCM_305187_Article.jsp>.

Amsterdam, E. A., Wenger, N. K., Brindis, R. G., et al. (2014). AHA/ACC guideline for the management of patients with non-ST elevation acute coronary syndromes: a report of the American College of Cardiology/American Heart Association Task Force on Practice Guidelines. *Circulation*, *23*(30), e344–e426.

Bhatnagar, A., Whitsel, L. P., Ribisl, K. M., et al. (2014). Electronic cigarettes: a policy statement from the American Heart Association. *Circulation*, *130*, 1418–1436.

Cabello, J. B., Burls, A., Emparanza, J. I., et al. (2013). *Oxygen therapy for acute myocardial infarction. The Cochrane Library*, (Issue 8). Retrieved from: <http://onlinelibrary.wiley.com.hsl-ezproxy.ucdenver.edu/doi/10.1002/14651858.CD007160.pub3/pdf>.

Centers for Disease Control and Prevention (2014). *Influenza*. <http://www.cdc.gov/flu/about/season/flu-season-2015-2016.htm>.

Coventry, L. L., Finn, J., & Bremner, A. P. (2011). Sex differences in symptom presentation in acute myocardial infarction: a systematic review and meta-analysis. *Heart and Lung: The Journal of Critical Care*, *40*(6), 477–491.

Eckel, R. H., Jakicic, J. M., Ard, J. D., et al. (2013). 2013 AHA/ACC guideline on lifestyle management to reduce cardiovascular risk: a report of the American College of Cardiology/American Heart Association Task Force on Practice Guidelines. *Circulation*, *129*(Suppl. 2), S76–S99.

Fletcher, G. F., Ades, P. A., Kligfield, P., et al. (2013). Exercise standards for testing and training: a scientific statement from the American Heart Association. *Circulation*, *128*, 873–934.

Goff, D. C., Lloyd-Jones, D. M., Bennett, G., et al. (2013). 2013 ACC/AHA guideline on the assessment of cardiovascular risk: a report of American College of Cardiology/American Heart Association Task Force on Practice Guidelines. *Circulation*, *129*(Suppl. 2), S49–S73.

Hazinski, M. F., et al. (2010). Executive summary: 2010 international consensus on cardiopulmonary resuscitation and emergency cardiovascular care science with treatment recommendations. *Curculation*, *122*(Suppl.), S250–S275.

Hooper, L., Summerbell, C. D., Thompson, R., et al. (2012). Reduced or modified dietary fat for preventing cardiovascular disease (review). *The Cochrane Library*, (Issue 5). Retrieved from: <http://onlinelibrary.wiley.com.hsl-czproxy.ucdenver.edu/doi/10.1002/14651858.CD002137.pub3/pdf>.

Mieres, J. H., Gulati, M., Bairey Merz, N., et al. (2014). Role of noninvasive testing in the clinical evaluation of women with suspected ischemic heart disease: a consensus statement from the American Heart Association. *Circulation*, *130*, 350–379.

O'Connor, R. E., Bossaert, L., Arntz, H. R., et al. (2010). Part 9: acute coronary syndromes: 2010 international consensus on cardiopulmonary resuscitation and emergency cardiovascular care science with treatment recommendations. *Circulation*, *122*(Suppl. 2), S422–S465.

O'Gara, P. T., et al. (2013). 2013 ACCF/AHA guideline for the management of ST-elevation myocardial infarction: executive summary: a report of the American College of Cardiology Foundation/American Heart Association Task Force on Practice Guidelines. *Circulation*, *127*(4), 529–555.

Stone, N. J., Robinson, J. G., Lichtenstein, A. H., et al. (2013). 2013 ACC/AHA guideline on the treatment of blood cholesterol to reduce atherosclerotic cardiovascular risk in adults: a report of the American College of Cardiology/American Heart Association Task Force on Practice Guidelines. *Circulation*, *129*(Suppl. 2), S1–S45.

Taylor, F., Huffman, M. D., Macedo, A. F., et al. (2014). Statins for the primary prevention of cardiovascular disease. *The Cochrane Library*, (Issue 1). Retrieved from: <http://onlinelibrary.wiley.com.hsl-ezproxy.ucdenver.edu/doi/10.1002/14651858.CD004816.pub5/pdf>.

Risk for impaired Cardiovascular function

Mary Beth Flynn Makic, PhD, RN, CNS, CCNS, FAAN, and Ann Will Poteet, MS, RN, CNS

NANDA-I

Definition

Vulnerable to internal or external causes that can damage one or more vital organs and the circulatory system itself

Risk Factors

Age older than 65 years; diabetes mellitus; dyslipidemia; family history of cardiovascular disease; history of cardiovascular disease; hypertension; insufficient knowledge of modifiable risk factors; obesity; pharmaceutical agent; sedentary lifestyle; smoking

NOC, NIC, Client Outcomes, Nursing Interventions, Client/Family Teaching and Discharge Planning, *Rationales,* and References

Refer to care plan for Decreased **Cardiac** output, Risk for decreased **Cardiac** tissue perfusion, and **Sedentary** lifestyle.

Caregiver Role Strain

Paula Riess Sherwood, RN, PhD, CNRN, FAAN, and Barbara A. Given, PhD, RN, FAAN

NANDA-I

Definition

Difficulty in performing family/significant other caregiver role

Defining Characteristics

Caregiving Activities

Apprehension about future ability to provide care; apprehension about the future health of receiver; apprehension about possible institutionalization of care receiver; apprehension about well-being of care receiver if unable to provide care; difficulty completing required tasks; difficulty performing required tasks; dysfunctional change in caregiving activities; preoccupation with care routine

Caregiver Health Status: Physiological

Cardiovascular disease; diabetes mellitus; fatigue; gastrointestinal distress; headache; hypertension; rash; weight change

Caregiver Health Status: Emotional

Alteration in sleep pattern; anger; depression; emotional vacillation; frustration; impatience; ineffective coping strategies; insufficient time to meet personal needs; nervousness; somatization; stressors

Caregiver Health Status: Socioeconomic

Changes in leisure activities; low work productivity; refusal of career advancement; social isolation

Caregiver-Care Receiver Relationship

Difficulty watching care receiver with illness; grieving of changes with care recipient; uncertainty about changes in relationship with care receiver

Family Processes

Concerns about family members; family conflict

Related Factors (r/t)

Care Recipient Health Status

Alteration in cognitive functioning; chronic illness; codependency; dependency; illness severity; increase in care needs; problematic behavior; psychiatric disorder; substance abuse; unpredictability of illness trajectory; unstable health condition

Caregiver Health Status

Alteration in cognitive functioning; codependency; ineffective coping strategies; insufficient fulfillment of others' expectations insufficient fulfillment of self-expectations; physical conditions; substance abuse; unrealistic self-expectations

Caregiver-Care Receiver Relationship

Abusive relationship; care receiver's condition inhibits conversation; pattern of ineffective relationships; unrealistic care receiver expectations; violent relationship

Caregiving Activities

Around-the-clock care responsibilities; change in nature care of activities; complexity of care activities; duration of caregiving; excessive caregiving activities; recent discharge home with significant care needs; unpredictability of care situation

Family Processes

Pattern of family dysfunction; pattern of ineffective family coping

Resources

Caregiver not developmentally ready for caregiver role; difficulty accessing assistance; difficulty accessing community resources; difficulty accessing support; financial crisis (e.g., debt, insufficient finances); inexperience with caregiving; insufficient assistance; insufficient caregiver privacy; insufficient community resources (e.g., respite services, recreation, social support); insufficient emotional resilience; insufficient equipment for providing care; insufficient knowledge about community resources; insufficient physical environment for providing care; insufficient time; insufficient transportation

Socioeconomic

Alienation; competing role commitments; insufficient recreation; social isolation

NOC (Nursing Outcomes Classification)

Suggested NOC Outcomes

Caregiver Adaptation to Patient Institutionalization; Caregiver Emotional Health; Caregiver Home Care Readiness; Caregiver Lifestyle Disruption; Caregiver-Patient Relationship; Caregiver Performance: Direct Care; Caregiver Performance: Indirect Care; Caregiver Physical Health; Caregiver Role Support; Caregiver Role Endurance; Caregiver Stressors; Caregiver Well-Being

Example NOC Outcome with Indicators

Caregiver Emotional Health with plans for a positive future as evidenced by the following indicators: Satisfaction with life/Sense of control/Self-esteem/Perceived social connectedness/Perceived spiritual well-being. (Rate the outcome and indicators of **Caregiver Emotional Health:** 1 = severely compromised, 2 = substantially compromised, 3 = moderately compromised, 4 = mildly compromised, 5 = not compromised [see Section I].)

Client Outcomes

Throughout the Care Situation, the Caregiver Will

- Feel supported by health care professionals, family, and friends; Report reduced or acceptable feelings of burden or distress; Take part in self-care activities to maintain own physical and psychological/emotional health; Identify resources available to help in giving care or to support the caregiver to give care; Verbalize mastery of the care situation; Feel confident and competent to provide care;
- Ask for help

Throughout the Care Situation, the Care Recipient Will

- Obtain quality and safe care

NIC (Nursing Interventions Classification)

Suggested NIC Intervention

C

Caregiver Support

Example NIC Activities—Caregiver Support

Determine caregiver's acceptance of role; Accept expressions of negative emotion

Nursing Interventions and *Rationales*

- Regularly monitor signs of depression, anxiety, burden, and deteriorating physical health in the caregiver throughout the care situation, especially if the relationship is poor, the care recipient has cognitive or neuropsychiatric symptoms, there is little social support available, the caregiver becomes enmeshed in the care situation, the caregiver is older, female, or has poor preexisting physical or emotional health. Refer to the care plan for **Hopelessness** when appropriate. EBN: *High levels of distress in caregivers are linked to multiple variables (van der Lee et al, 2014).* EB: *Caregiving may weaken the immune system and predispose the caregiver to illness, particularly cardiac illness and poor response to acquired infections (Fonareva & Oken, 2014; Lovell et al, 2012).*
- The impact of providing care on the caregiver's emotional health should be assessed at regular intervals using a reliable and valid instrument such as the Caregiver Strain Risk Index, which was validated with caregivers of clients with diagnosed Parkinson's disease. EBN: *Family caregivers face potential strain in caring for persons with Parkinson's disease because of the unpredictability of symptom presentation. The Caregiver Strain Risk Screen (CSRS) was developed and tested for initial validation. The 28-item CSRS demonstrated acceptable validity and reliability in measuring caregiver strain (Abendroth, 2015). Caregiver assessment should be done at regular intervals throughout the care trajectory (Adelman et al, 2014).*
- Identify potential caregiver resources such as mastery, social support, optimism, and positive aspects of care. EB/EBN: *Research has shown that caregivers can have simultaneous positive and negative responses to providing care. Positive responses may help buffer the negative effects of providing care on caregivers' emotional health and may also increase the effectiveness of interventions to reduce strain (Kruithof et al, 2011).*
- Screen for caregiver role strain at the onset of the care situation, at regular intervals throughout the care situation, and with changes in care recipient status and care transitions, including institutionalization. EB/EBN: *Care situations that last for several months or years can cause wear and tear that exhaust caregivers' coping mechanisms and available resources, and that may continue after the care recipient has been institutionalized (Paun & Farran, 2011). In addition, changes in the care recipient's health status necessitate new skills and monitoring from the caregiver and affect the caregiver's ability to continue to provide care (Given et al, 2011). Providing caregiver support throughout the care situation may decrease care recipient institutionalization (Matsuzawa et al, 2011).*
- Watch for caregivers who become enmeshed in the care situation. EBN: *Caregivers are at risk for becoming overinvolved or unable to disentangle themselves from the caregiver role, particularly in the absence of adequate social support (Hricik et al, 2011).*
- Arrange for intervals of respite care for the caregiver; encourage use if available. EB: *Respite care provides time away from the care situation and may help alleviate some caregiver distress (Maayan et al, 2014).*
- Regularly monitor social support for the caregiver and help the caregiver identify and use appropriate support systems for varying times in the care situation. EBN: *Lower levels of perceived support can cause caregivers to feel abandoned and increase their distress (Hwang et al, 2011).*
- Encourage the caregiver to grieve over changes in the care recipient's condition and give the caregiver permission to share angry feelings in a safe environment. Refer to nursing interventions for **Grieving**. EB: *Caregivers grieve the loss of personhood of their loved one, especially when dementia is involved (Kramer et al, 2011).*
- Help the caregiver find personal time to meet his or her needs, learn stress management techniques, schedule regular health screenings, and schedule regular respite time. EB: *Due to increased risk for poor physical health as a result of providing care, caregivers must feel empowered to maintain self-care activities (Merluzzi et al, 2011). Interventions to provide support for family caregivers have shown improvements in caregiver health (Basu et al, 2013).*

C

- Encourage the caregiver to talk about feelings, concerns, uncertainties, and fears. Support groups can be used to gain mutual and educational support. EBN: *Support groups can improve depressive symptoms and burden, particularly for female caregivers (Chien et al, 2011).* EB: *Social support groups can be effective over the Internet, using forums such as Facebook (Bender et al, 2011).*
- Observe for any evidence of caregiver or care recipient violence or abuse, particularly verbal abuse; if evidence is present, speak with the caregiver and care recipient separately. EB/CEB: *Caregiver violence is possible and screening should be done at regular intervals (Hoover & Polson, 2014).*

▲ Involve the family in care transitions; use a multidisciplinary team to provide medical and social services for instruction and planning specific to the care situation. EBN: *Family members need education specific to their situation beyond what is traditionally provided at discharge; this educational approach should be proactive and anticipate potential problems in the home (Loupis & Faux, 2013).*

▲ Encourage regular communication with the care recipient and with the health care team. EB: *There can be a large discrepancy between what the health care professional feels he or she has communicated and what the caregiver reports hearing (Molinuevo et al, 2011).*

- Help caregiver assess his or her financial resources (services reimbursed by insurance, available support through community and religious organizations) and the impact of providing care on his or her financial status. EB/EBN: *Better physical and mental health outcomes were common for caregivers and non-caregivers who reported having more resources (e.g., higher income, better preparedness for future financial need, higher satisfaction with transportation and housing, and no limitation of usual daily activities) (Ahn et al, 2012).*
- Help the caregiver identify competing occupational demands and potential benefits to maintaining work as a way of providing normalcy. Guide caregivers to seek ways to maintain employment through mechanisms such as job sharing or decreasing hours at work. EB: *Employed caregivers report that work can provide a sense of fulfillment, refuge, and satisfaction (Eldh & Carlsson, 2011).*
- Help the caregiver problem solve to meet the care recipient's needs. EBN: *Interventions that teach caregivers problem-solving skills have been shown to positively influence caregivers' psychosocial well-being (Cheng et al, 2014).*

Geriatric

- Monitor the caregiver for psychological distress and signs of depression, especially if caring for a mentally impaired older adult or if there was an unsatisfactory marital relationship before caregiving. EBN: *As the majority of family caregivers are spouses, degree of marital satisfaction is strongly linked with caregiver role strain (Green & King, 2011).*
- Assess the health of caregivers, particularly their control over chronic diseases, at regular intervals. CEB: *Caregivers with high levels of depressive symptoms have demonstrated poor health and increased health care utilization and cost (Zhu et al, 2014).*
- Assess the presence of and use of social support and encourage the use of secondary caregivers with older caregivers. EBN: *Social support has been shown to be an integral part of maintaining caregiver health (Quinn et al, 2014).*
- To improve the ability to provide safe care: provide skills training related to direct care, perform complex monitoring tasks, supervise and interpret client symptoms, assist with decision-making, assist with medication adherence, provide emotional support and comfort, and coordinate care. CEB: *Each task demands different skills and knowledge, and caregivers show a desire to master these skills (Moon & Adams, 2013).*
- Teach symptom management techniques (assessment, potential causes, aggravating factors, potential alleviating factors, reassessment), particularly for fatigue, constipation, anorexia, and pain. EBN: *Caregivers require training in care recipient monitoring symptom management and interpretation, and can benefit from a problem-solving approach (Sherwood et al, 2012).*

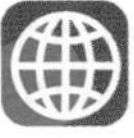

Multicultural

- Assess for the influence of cultural beliefs, norms, and values on the client's ability to modify health behavior. EBN: *What the client considers normal and abnormal health behavior may be based on cultural perceptions (Giger, 2014).* EBN: *Each client should be assessed for ability to modify health behavior based on the phenomenon of communication, time, space, social organization, environmental control, and biological variations (Giger, 2014).*
- Despite the importance of cultural differences in perceptions of caregiver role strain, there are certain characteristics that are distressing to caregivers across multiple cultures. EBN: *Social support and care*

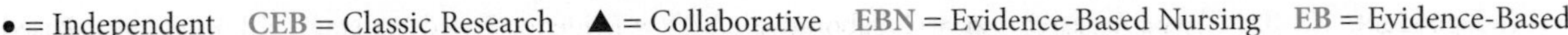

C

recipients' behavioral difference have been shown to be an important factor in caregiver distress across multiple cultures (Chiao & Schepp, 2012; Hwang et al, 2011; Zahid & Ohaeri, 2010).

- Persons with different cultural backgrounds may not perceive the provision of care with equal degrees of distress. EB: *A group of caregivers in Belize did not report providing care as negative, although they did exhibit physical symptoms of distress (Vroman & Morency, 2011).*
- Recognize that cultures often play a role in identifying who will be recognized as a family caregiver and form partnerships with those groups. EB: *In a study of American Indians, people who attended and participated in Native events and endorsed traditional healing practices were more likely to be caregivers. The study also reported that gender played a role in identifying caregivers in some tribes, but not all (Goins et al, 2011).*
- Encourage spirituality as a source of support for coping. EBN: *Many African Americans and Latinos identify spirituality, religiousness, prayer, and church-based approaches as coping resources. Socioeconomic status, geographical location, and risks associated with health-seeking behavior all influence the likelihood that clients will seek health care and modify health behavior (Giger, 2014).*
- Assess for the presence of conflicting values within the culture. EBN: *Whereas sharing and caring is part of the Amish community, females with breast cancer were found to value privacy issues related to their body image and health status and to prefer this was shared in the closed community (Schwartz, 2008).*
- Recognize that different cultures value and use caregiving resources in different ways. CEB: *When Korean and Caucasian American caregivers were compared, there was more family support in Korean caregivers while Caucasian Americans were more likely to use formal support (Kong, 2007).*

Home Care

- Assess the client and caregiver at every visit for quality of relationship, and for the quality of caring that exists. EB: *Quality of the caregiver-care recipient relationship and the impact of the care situation on that relationship can be an important source of distress or support for the caregiver (van der Lee et al, 2014). Chronic illness, especially dementia, can represent a gradual and devastating loss of the marital relationship as it existed formerly.*
- Assess preexisting strengths and weaknesses the caregiver brings to the situation, as well as current responses, depression, and fatigue levels. EB/EBN: *Caregivers' personality type, mastery, self-efficacy, optimism, and social support have all been linked to the amount of distress the caregiver will perceive as a result of providing care (Adelman et al, 2014).*

▲ Refer the client to home health aide services for assistance with activities of daily living and light housekeeping. Allow the caregiver to gain confidence in the respite provider. *Home health aide services can provide physical relief and respite for the caregiver.* EB: *The need for caregiver respite has been linked with the number of hours per week spent providing care (Hughes et al, 2014).*

Client/Family Teaching and Discharge Planning

- Identify client and caregiver factors that necessitate the use of formal home care services, that may affect provision of care, or that need to be addressed before the client can be safely discharged from home care. EBN: *Although home care resources can be useful in decreasing caregiver distress, they are not used with regularity across client populations. Health care practitioners should assess for the need for support resources prior to discharge and at routine intervals throughout the care situation, tailoring community resources to individual caregiver needs (Greene et al, 2011). Interventions prior to discharge may include medication management, medication reconciliation, identification of medical red flags, identification of community-based resources, and specific caregiver concerns about home care (Hendrix et al, 2011).*
- Collaborate with the caregiver and discuss the care needs of the client, disease processes, medications, and what to expect; use a variety of instructional techniques (e.g., explanations, demonstrations, visual aids) until the caregiver is able to express a degree of comfort with care delivery. EB: *Knowledge and confidence are separate concepts. Self-assurance in caregiving will decrease the amount of distress the caregiver perceives as a result of providing care (Giovannetti et al, 2012; Ostwald et al, 2014) and may improve the quality of care provided.*
- Assess family caregiving skill. The identification of caregiver difficulty with any of a core set of processes highlights areas for intervention. CEB: *The ability to engage effectively and smoothly in nine processes has been identified as constituting family caregiving skill: monitoring client behavior, interpreting changes accurately, making decisions, taking action, making adjustment to care, accessing resources, providing hands-on care, working together with the ill person, and negotiating the health care system (Schumacher et al, 2000).*

EB: *Caregiver skills training has been shown to improve caregiver knowledge and skills and may be reimbursable within governmental health care plans (Gitlin et al, 2010).*

- Discharge care should be individualized to specific caregiver needs and care situations, and enable them to be prepared. EBN: *Interventions implemented by advanced practice nurses have been successful in preventing negative outcomes (Bradway et al, 2012; Stone, 2014).*
- Assess the caregiver's need for information such as information on symptom management, disease progression, specific skills, and available support. EBN: *Caregiver interventions should be individualized to meet specific caregiver needs (Greene et al, 2011; Hendrix et al, 2011). Multicomponent strategies to provide education, support, counseling, and linkage to community resources to ease transitions from the hospital to the home can improve caregiver health and coping (Ostwald et al, 2014).*
- Teach the caregiver warning signs for burnout, depression, and anxiety. Help them identify a resource in case they begin to feel overwhelmed.
- Teach the caregiver methods for managing disruptive behavioral symptoms if present. Refer to the care plan for Chronic **Confusion.** CEB: *Behavioral interventions that consist of nine to 12 sessions over several months have been shown to be as effective as pharmacological interventions to control behavioral problems in the care recipient (Brodaty & Arasaratnam, 2012).*
- Teach the caregiver how to provide the care needed and put a plan in place for monitoring the care provided.
- Provide ongoing support and evaluation of care skills as the care situation and care demands change.
- Provide information regarding the care recipient's diagnosis, treatment regimen, and expected course of illness.

▲ Refer to counseling or support groups to assist in adjusting to the caregiver role and periodically evaluate not only the caregiver's emotional response to care but the safety of the care delivered to the care recipient.

REFERENCES

Abendroth, M. (2015). Development and initial validation of a Parkinson's disease caregiver strain risk screen. *Journal of Nursing Measurement*, *23*(1), 4–21.

Adelman, R. D., et al. (2014). Caregiver burden: A clinical review. *JAMA: The Journal of the American Medical Association*, *311*(10), 1052–1060.

Ahn, S., Hochhalter, A. K., Moudouni, D. K., et al. (2012). Self-reported physical and mental health of older adults: The roles of caregiving and resources. *Maturitas*, *71*(1), 62–69.

Basu, R., Hochhalter, A. K., & Stevens, A. B. (2013). The impact of the REACH II intervention on caregivers' perceived health. *Journal of Applied Gerontology*.

Bender, J. L., Jimenez-Marroquin, M. C., & Jadad, A. R. (2011). Seeking support on Facebook: a content analysis of breast cancer groups. *Journal of Medical Internet Research*, *13*(1), e16.

Bradway, C., et al. (2012). A qualitative analysis of an advanced practice nurse-directed transitional care model intervention. *The Gerontologist*, *52*(3), 394–407.

Brodaty, H., & Arasaratnam, C. (2012). Meta-analysis of nonpharmacological interventions for neuropsychiatric syptoms of dementia. *The American Journal of Psychiatry*, *169*(9), 946–953.

Cheng, H. Y., Chair, S. Y., & Chau, J. P. (2014). The effectiveness of psychosocial interventions for stroke family caregivers and stroke survivors. *Patient Education and Counseling*, *95*(1), 30–44.

Chien, L. Y., et al. (2011). Caregiver support groups in patients with dementia: a meta-analysis. *International Journal of Geriatric Psychiatry*, *26*(10), 1089–1098.

Chiao, C. Y., & Schepp, K. G. (2012). The impact of foreign caregiving on depression among older people in Taiwan: model testing. *Journal of Advanced Nursing*, *68*(5), 1090–1099.

Eldh, A. C., & Carlsson, E. (2011). Seeking a balance between employment and the care of an ageing parent. *Scandinavian Journal of Caring Sciences*, *25*(2), 285–293.

Fonareva, I., & Oken, B. S. (2014). Physiological and functional consequences of caregiving for relatives with dementia. *International Psychogeriatrics*, *26*(5), 725–747.

Giger, J. (2014). *Transcultural nursing: Assessment and Intervention* (6th ed., Kindle Edition). St Louis: Mosby.

Giovannetti, E. R., et al. (2012). Difficulty assisting with health care tasks among caregivers of multimorbid older adults. *Journal of General Internal Medicine*, *27*(1), 37–44.

Gitlin, L. N., Jacobs, M., & Earland, T. V. (2010). Translation of a dementia caregiver intervention for delivery in homecare as a reimbursable Medicare service: outcomes and lessons learned. *The Gerontologist*, *50*(6), 847–854.

Given, B. A., Sherwood, P., & Given, C. W. (2011). Support for caregivers of cancer patients: transition after active treatment. *Cancer Epidemiology, Biomarkers and Prevention: A Publication of the American Association for Cancer Research, Cosponsored by the American Society of Preventive Oncology*, *20*(10), 2015–2021.

Goins, R. T., et al. (2011). Adult caregiving among American Indians: the role of cultural factors. *The Gerontologist*, *51*(3), 310–320.

Green, T. L., & King, K. M. (2011). Relationships between biophysical and psychosocial outcomes following minor stroke. *Canadian Journal of Neuroscience Nursing*, *33*(2), 15–23.

Greene, A., et al. (2011). Can assessing caregiver needs and activating community networks improve caregiver-defined outcomes? A single-blind, quasi-experimental pilot study: community facilitator pilot. *Palliative Medicine*, *26*(7), 917–923.

Hendrix, C. C., et al. (2011). Pilot study: individualized training for caregivers of hospitalized older veterans. *Nursing Research*, *60*(6), 436–441.

Hoover, R. M., & Polson, M. (2014). Detecting elder abuse and neglect: Assessment and intervention. *American Family Physician*, *89*(6), 453–460.

Hricik, A., et al. (2011). Changes in caregiver perceptions over time in response to providing care for a loved one with a primary malignant brain tumor. *Oncology Nursing Forum, 38*(2), 149–155.

Hughes, T. B., et al. (2014). Correlates of objective and subjective measures of caregiver burden among dementia caregivers: Influence of unmet patient and caregiver dementia-related care needs. *International Psychogeriatrics, 26*(11), 1875–1883.

Hwang, B., et al. (2011). Caregiving for patients with heart failure. *American Journal of Critical Care, 20*(6), 431–442.

Kong, E. H. (2007). The influence of culture on the experiences of Korean, Korean American, and Caucasian-American family caregivers of frail older adults: a literature review. *Taehan Kanho Hakhoe chi, 37*(2), 213–220.

Kramer, B. J., et al. (2011). Complicated grief symptoms in caregivers of persons with lung cancer. *Omega, 62*(3), 201–220.

Kruithof, W. J., Visser-Meily, J. M., & Post, M. W. (2011). Positive caregiving experiences are associated with life satisfaction in spouses of stroke survivors. *Journal of Stroke and Cerebrovascular Diseases*, [Epub ahead of print].

Loupis, Y. M., & Faux, S. G. (2013). Family conferences in stroke rehabilitation: A literature review. *Journal of Stroke and Cerebrovascular Diseases, 22*(6), 883–893.

Lovell, B., Moss, M., & Wetherell, M. (2012). The psychosocial, endocrine and immune consequences of caring for a child with autism or ADHD. *Psychoneuroendocrinology, 37*(4), 534–542.

Maayan, N., Soares-Weiser, K., & Lee, H. (2014). Respite care for people with dementia and their carers. *Cochrane Database of Systematic Reviews.*

Matsuzawa, T., et al. (2011). Predictive factors for hospitalized and institutionalized caregiving of the aged patients with diabetes mellitus in Japan. *The Kobe Journal of Medical Sciences, 56*(4), E173–E183.

Merluzzi, T. V., et al. (2011). Assessment of self-efficacy for caregiving: the critical role of self-care in caregiver stress and burden. *Palliative and Supportive Care, 9*(1), 15–24.

Molinuevo, J. L., & Hernandez, B. (2011). TRACE: Assessment of the information provided by the medical specialist on Alzheimer's disease and that retained by the patient caregivers. *Neurologia (Barcelona, Spain)*, [Epub ahead of print].

Moon, H., & Adams, K. B. (2013). The effectiveness of dyadic interventions for people with dementia and their caregivers. *Dementia (Basel, Switzerland), 12*(6), 821–839.

Ostwald, S. K., Godwin, K. M., Cron, S. G., et al. (2014). Home-based psychoeducational and mailed information programs for stroke-caregiving dyads post-discharge: A randomized trial. *Disability and Rehabilitation, 36*(1), 55–62.

Paun, O., & Farran, C. J. (2011). Chronic grief management for dementia caregivers in transition. *Journal of Gerontological Nursing, 37*(12), 28–35.

Quinn, K., Murray, C., & Malone, C. (2014). Spousal experiences of coping with and adapting to caregiving for a partner who has a stroke: A meta-analysis of qualitative research. *Disability and Rehabilitation, 36*(3), 185–198.

Schumacher, K. L., Stewart, B. J., Archbold, P. G., et al. (2000). Family caregiving skill: development of the concept. *Research in Nursing and Health, 23*(3), 191–203.

Schwartz, K. (2008). Breast cancer and health care beliefs, values, and practices of Amish women. *Dissertation Abstracts, 29*(1), 587.

Sherwood, P. R., et al. (2012). The impact of a problem-solving intervention on increasing caregiver assistance and improving caregiver health. *Supportive Care in Cancer, 20*(9), 1937–1947.

Stone, K. (2014). Enhancing preparedness and satisfaction of caregivers of patients discharged from an inpatient rehabilitation facility using an interactive website. *Rehabilitation Nursing, 39*(2), 76–85.

Van der Lee, J., et al. (2014). Multivariate models of subjective caregiver burden in dementia: A systematic review. *Ageing Research Reviews, 15*, 76–93.

Vroman, K., & Morency, J. (2011). "I do the best I can": caregivers' perceptions of informal caregiving for older adults in Belize. *International Journal of Aging and Human Development, 72*(1), 1–25.

Zahid, M. A., & Ohaeri, J. U. (2010). Relationship of family caregiver burden with quality of care and psychopathology in a sample of Arab subjects with schizophrenia. *BMC Psychiatry, 10*, 71.

Zhu, C. W., et al. (2014). Health-care use and cost in dementia caregivers: Longitudinal results from the Predictors Caregiver Study. *Alzheimer's & Dementia*, [Epub ahead of print].

Risk for Caregiver Role Strain *Jane M. Kendall, RN, BS, CHT*

NANDA-I

Definition

Vulnerable to difficulty in performing the family/significant other caregiver role, which may compromise health

Risk Factors

Alteration in cognitive functioning in care receiver; care receiver discharged home with significant needs; care receiver exhibits bizarre behavior; care receiver exhibits deviant behavior; caregiver health impairment; caregiver isolation; caregiver not developmentally ready for caregiver role; caregiver's competing role commitments; caregiving task complexity; codependency; congenital disorder; developmental delay; developmental delay of caregiver; excessive caregiving activities; exposure to violence; extended duration of caregiving required family isolation; female caregiver; illness severity of care receiver; inadequate physical environment for providing care; ineffective caregiver coping pattern; ineffective family adaptation; experience with caregiving; instability in care receiver's health; insufficient caregiver recreation; insufficient respite for caregiver;

partner as caregiver; pattern of family dysfunction prior to the caregiving situation; pattern of ineffective relationship between caregiver and care receiver; prematurity; presence of abuse (e.g., physical, psychological, sexual); psychological disorder in caregiver; psychological disorder in care receiver; stressors; substance abuse; unpredictability of illness trajectory

NIC, NOC, Client Outcomes, Nursing Interventions, Client/Family Teaching, *Rationales*, and References

Refer to care plan for **Caregiver Role Strain.**

Risk for ineffective Cerebral tissue perfusion

Laura Mcilvoy, PhD, RN, CCRN, CNRN

NANDA-I

Definition

Vulnerable to a decrease in cerebral tissue circulation, which may compromise health

Risk Factors

Abnormal partial thromboplastin time; abnormal prothrombin time; akinetic left ventricular wall segment; aortic atherosclerosis; arterial dissection; atrial fibrillation; atrial myxoma; brain injury (e.g., cerebrovascular impairment, neurological illness, trauma, tumor); brain neoplasm; carotid stenosis; cerebral aneurysm; coagulopathy (e.g., sickle cell anemia); dilated cardiomyopathy; disseminated intravascular coagulopathy; embolism; hypercholesterolemia; hypertension; infective endocarditis; mechanical prosthetic valve; mitral stenosis; pharmaceutical agent; recent myocardial infarction; sick sinus syndrome; substance abuse; treatment regimen

NOC (Nursing Outcomes Classification)

Suggested NOC Outcomes

Acute Confusion Level; Tissue Perfusion: Cerebral; Agitation Level; Neurological Status; Cognition; Seizure Control; Motor Strength

Example NOC Outcome with Indicators

Tissue Perfusion: Cerebral as evidenced by the following indicators: Headache/Restlessness/Listlessness/Agitation/Vomiting/Fever/Impaired Cognition/Decreased level of consciousness/Motor weakness/Dysphagia/Slurred speech. (Rate the outcome and indicators of **Tissue Perfusion: Cerebral:** 1 = severe, 2 = substantial, 3 = moderate, 4 = mild, 5 = none [see Section I].)

Client Outcomes

Client Will (Specify Time Frame)

- State absence of headache
- Demonstrate appropriate orientation to person, place, time, and situation
- Demonstrate ability to follow simple commands
- Demonstrate equal bilateral motor strength
- Demonstrate adequate swallowing ability

NIC (Nursing Interventions Classification)

Suggested NIC Interventions

Medication Management; Neurologic Monitoring; Positioning: Neurologic; Cerebral Perfusion Promotion; Fall Prevention; Cognitive Stimulation; Environmental Management: Safety

Example NIC Activities—Neurological Monitoring

Monitor pupillary size, shape, symmetry, and reactivity; Monitor level of consciousness; Monitor level of orientation; Monitor trend of Glasgow Coma Scale; Monitor facial symmetry; Note complaint of headache

C

Nursing Interventions and *Rationales*

- To decrease risk of reduced cerebral perfusion related to stroke or transient ischemic attack:
  - Obtain a family history of hypertension and stroke to identify persons who may be at increased risk of stroke. EB: *A positive family history of stroke increases risk of stroke by approximately 30% (Goldstein et al, 2011).*
  - Monitor blood pressure (BP) regularly, because hypertension is a major risk factor for both ischemic and hemorrhagic stroke. EB: *Systolic BP should be treated to a goal of less than 140 mm Hg and diastolic BP to less than 90 mm Hg, while clients with diabetes or renal disease have a BP goal of less than 130/80 mm Hg (Goldstein et al, 2011).*
  - Teach hypertensive clients the importance of taking their health care provider-ordered antihypertensive agent to prevent stroke. EB: *Treatment of hypertension in adults with diabetes with an angiotensin converting enzyme inhibitor (ACEI) or an angiotensin receptor blockers (ARB) is useful (Goldstein et al, 2011).*
  - Stress smoking cessation at every encounter with clients, using multimodal techniques to aid in quitting, such as counseling, nicotine replacement, and oral smoking cessation medications. EB: *Epidemiological studies show a consistent and overwhelming relationship between smoking and both ischemic and hemorrhagic stroke (Goldstein et al, 2011).*
  - Teach clients who experience a transient ischemic attack (TIA) that they are at increased risk for a stroke. EB: *The 90-day risk for stroke after a TIA is as high as 17%, with the greatest risk occurring in the first week (Furie et al, 2011).*
  - Screen clients 65 years of age and older for atrial fibrillation with pulse assessment. EB: *Atrial fibrillation is associated with a fivefold increase in stroke. Systematic pulse assessment in primary care setting resulted in a 60% increase in the detection of atrial fibrillation (Goldstein et al, 2011).*
  - Call 911 or activate the rapid response team of a hospital immediately when clients display symptoms of stroke as determined by the Cincinnati Stroke Scale (F: facial drooping; A: arm drift on one side; S: speech slurred), being careful to note the time of symptom appearance. Additional symptoms of stroke include sudden numbness/weakness of face, arm or leg, especially on one side, sudden confusion, trouble speaking or understanding, sudden difficulty seeing with one or both eyes, sudden trouble walking, dizziness, loss of balance or coordination, or sudden severe headache (National Stroke Association, 2012). EB: *The Cincinnati Stroke Scale (derived from the NIH Stroke Scale) is used to identify clients having a stroke who may be candidates for thrombolytic therapy (Jauch et al, 2013). EMS activation results in faster health care provider assessment, computed tomography, and neurological evaluation, which facilitates administering thrombolytics to eligible stroke victims within the required 3-hour time period (Jauch et al, 2013).*
  - Use clinical practice guidelines for glycemic control and BP targets to guide the care of clients with diabetes who have had a stroke or TIA. EB: *The American Stroke Association recommends that evidence-based guidelines be used in the care of clients with diabetes. Good glycemic control has been associated with decreased incidence of strokes (Furie et al, 2011; Handelsman et al, 2011).*
  - Maintain head of bed less than 30 degrees in the acute phase (<72 hours of symptom onset) of ischemic stroke. EB: *Cortical cerebral blood flow is decreased when head of bed is elevated from 0 degrees to 30 degrees in clients with acute ischemic stroke (Favilla et al, 2014).*
  - Head of bed may be elevated to sitting position without detrimental effect to cerebral blood flow in clients with ischemic stroke or subarachnoid hemorrhagic at 72 hours after symptom onset. EB: *Head of bed elevation of 45 degrees and 70 degrees in the subacute phase of ischemic stroke resulted in minor changes in cerebral blood flow velocities (Aries et al, 2013).* EB: *Cerebral blood flow had no significant changes in head of bed elevations from 0 degree to 90 degrees in clients with subarachnoid hemorrhage at day 3, 7, and 10 (Kung et al, 2013).*
  - Administer oral nimodipine as prescribed by the healthcare provider after subarachnoid hemorrhagic strokes for 21 days. EB: *Nimodipine, a calcium channel blocker, has been shown by multiple randomized clinical trials to improve outcome by limiting delayed cerebral ischemia after subarachnoid hemorrhage strokes (Diringer et al, 2011).*

▲ To decrease risk of reduced cerebral perfusion pressure (CPP): Cerebral perfusion pressure = Mean arterial pressure − intracranial pressure (CPP = MAP − ICP): See care plan for Decreased **Intracranial** adaptive capacity.
  - Maintain euvolemia. CEB: *Infusing intravenous fluids to sustain normal circulating volume helps maintain normal cerebral blood flow (Bullock et al, 2001).*

▲ To treat decreased CPP:
- ❍ Clients with subarachnoid hemorrhagic stroke experiencing delayed cerebral ischemia, as evidenced by declining neurological exam, should undergo a trial of induced hypertension. EB: *Hypertension increased cerebral blood flow and produced neurological improvement in the majority of clients (Diringer et al, 2011).*
- ❍ Administer phenylephrine infusion to raise MAP per collaborative protocol. EB: *Phenylephrine was more effective than dopamine in raising MAP and more effective than norepinephrine in raising CPP in severely injured clients with traumatic brain injury (Sookplung et al, 2011).*

C

REFERENCES

Aries, M. J., Elting, J. W., Stewart, R., et al. (2013). Cerebral blood flow velocity changes during upright positioning in bed after acute stroke: an observational study. *British Medical Journal Open*, *3*, 1–4. Retrieved from: <http://dx.doi.org/10.1136/bmjopen-2013-002960>.

Bullock, R., Chestnut, R., & Clifton, G. (2001). Management and prognosis of severe traumatic brain injury. *Journal of Neurotrauma*, *17*(6&7), 451–627.

Diringer, M. N., Bleck, T. P., Claude, H. J., et al. (2011). Critical care management of patients following aneurysmal subarachnoid hemorrhage: recommendations from the Neurocritical Care Society's Multidisciplinary Consensus Conference. *Neurocritical Care*, *15*(2), 211–240.

Favilla, C. G., Mesquita, R. C., Mullen, M., et al. (2014). Optical bedside monitoring of cerebral blood flow in acute ischemic stroke patients during head-of-bed manipulation. *Stroke; a Journal of Cerebral Circulation*, *45*, 1269–1274.

Furie, K. L., Kasner, S. E., Adams, R. J., et al. (2011). Guidelines for the prevention of stroke in patients with stroke or transient ischemic attack: a guideline for healthcare professionals from the AHA/ASA. *Stroke; a Journal of Cerebral Circulation*, *42*, 227–276.

Goldstein, L. B., Bushnell, C. D., Adams, R. J., et al. (2011). Guidelines for the primary prevention of stroke: a guideline for healthcare professionals from AHA/ASA. *Stroke; a Journal of Cerebral Circulation*, *42*, 517–584.

Handelsman, Y., Mechanick, J. I., Blonde, L., et al. (2011). American Association of Clinical Endocrinologist medical guidelines for clinical practice for developing a diabetes mellitus comprehensive care plan. *Endocrine Practice*, *17*(Suppl. 2), 1–53.

Jauch, E. C., Saver, J. L., Adams, H. P., et al. (2013). Guidelines for the early management of patients with acute ischemic stroke: A guideline for healthcare professionals from the AHA/ASA. *Stroke; a Journal of Cerebral Circulation*, *44*, 870–947.

Kung, D. K., Chalouhi, N., Jabbour, P. M., et al. (2013). Cerebral blood flow dynamics and head-of-bed changes in the setting of subarachnoid hemorrhage. *BioMed Research International*, *2013*, 1–4. Retrieved from: <http://dx.doi.org/10.1155/2013/640638>.

National Stroke Association. (2012). *Recognizing Stroke*. <http://www.stroke.org/understand-stroke/recognizing-stroke>.

Sookplung, P., Siriussawakul, A., Malakouti, A., et al. (2011). Vasopressor use and effect on blood pressure after severe adult traumatic brain injury. *Neurocritical Care*, *15*(1), 46–54.

Ineffective Childbearing process

Dianne Frances Hayward, RN, MSN, WHNP

NANDA-I

Definition

Pregnancy and childbirth process and care of the newborn that does not match the environmental context, norms, and expectations

Definition

During Pregnancy

Inadequate prenatal care; inadequate prenatal lifestyle (e.g., elimination, exercise, nutrition personal hygiene, sleep); inadequate preparation of newborn care items; inadequate preparation of the home environment; ineffective management of unpleasant symptoms in pregnancy; insufficient access of support system; insufficient respect for unborn baby; unrealistic birth plan

During Labor and Delivery

Decrease in proactivity during labor and delivery; inadequate lifestyle for stage of labor (e.g., elimination, exercise, nutrition, personal hygiene, sleep); inappropriate response to onset of labor; insufficient access or support system; insufficient attachment behavior

After Birth

Inadequate baby care techniques; inadequate postpartum lifestyle (e.g., elimination, exercise, nutrition personal hygiene, sleep); inappropriate baby feeding techniques; inappropriate breast care; insufficient access of support system; insufficient attachment behavior; unsafe environment for infant

C

Related Factors

Domestic violence; inconsistent prenatal heath visits; insufficient knowledge of childbearing process; inadequate maternal nutrition; insufficient parental role model; insufficient prenatal care; insufficient support system; low maternal confidence; maternal powerlessness; maternal psychological distress; substance abuse; unplanned pregnancy; unrealistic birth plan; unsafe environment; unwanted pregnancy

NOC Nursing Outcomes Classification

Suggested NOC Outcomes

Fetal Status: Antepartum, Intrapartum; Maternal Status: Antepartum, Intrapartum; Depression Level; Family Resiliency; Knowledge: Substance Use Control; Social Support; Spiritual Support

Example NOC Outcome with Indicators

Maternal Status: Antepartum as evidenced by the following indicators: Emotional attachment to fetus/Coping with discomforts of pregnancy/Mood lability/Has realistic birth plan/Has support system. (Rate each indicator of **Maternal Status: Antepartum:** 1 = severe deviation from normal range, 2 = substantial deviation from normal range, 3 = moderate deviation from normal range, 4 = mild deviation from normal range, 5 = no deviation from normal range [see Section I].)

Client Outcomes

Client Will (Specify Time Frame)

Antepartum

- Obtain early prenatal care in the first trimester and maintain regular visits
- Obtain knowledge level needed for appropriate care of oneself during pregnancy including good nutrition and psychological health
- Understand the risks of substance abuse and resources available
- Feel empowered to seek social and spiritual support for emotional well-being during pregnancy
- Use support systems for labor and emotional support
- Develop a realistic birth plan, taking into account any high-risk pregnancy issues
- Understand the labor and delivery process and comfort measures to manage labor pain

Postpartum

- Use a safe environment for self and infant
- Obtain knowledge to provide appropriate newborn care and postpartum care of self
- Obtain knowledge to develop appropriate bonding and parenting skills

NIC (Nursing Interventions Classification)

Suggested NIC Interventions

High-Risk Pregnancy Care; Intrapartal Care

Example NIC Activities—High-Risk Pregnancy Care

Instruct patient on importance of receiving regular prenatal care and to follow plan of care by taking prescribed medications and following nutrition guidelines; Encourage identification of psychosocial/psychological issues and substance use and appropriate treatment and referrals as needed

Nursing Interventions and *Rationales*

- Encourage early prenatal care and regular prenatal visits. EB/EBN: *Women who attended for less than four visits or started care late were at risk for a poorer outcome. Culture must also be assessed to provide appropriate prenatal care (Beeckman et al, 2013; Lewallen, 2011).* EBN: *A study compared outcomes of infants born to women who received Medicaid and prenatal care coordination (PNCC) services versus women who received Medicaid but did not receive PNCC. Women who received PNCC services resulted in delivery of fewer low-birth-weight infants, fewer preterm infants, and fewer infants transferred to the neonatal intensive care unit. PNCC is an effective strategy for preventing adverse birth outcomes (Van Dijk et al, 2011).*

▲ Identify any high-risk factors that may require additional surveillance, such as preterm labor, hypertensive disorders of pregnancy, diabetes, depression, other chronic medical conditions, presence of fetal anomalies, or other high-risk factors. EB: *Timely and accurate antenatal screening is believed to be an important factor in preventing preterm birth, screening for gestational diabetes, preeclampsia, intrauterine growth restriction, and depression, to mention a few. Finding and treating problems early improves outcome (Beeckman et al, 2013).*

▲ Assess and screen for signs and symptoms of depression during pregnancy and in the postpartum period including history of depression or postpartum depression, poor prenatal care, poor weight gain, hygiene issues, sleep problems, substance abuse, and preterm labor. If depression is present, refer for behavioral-cognitive counseling, and/or medication (postpartum period only). Both counseling and medication are considered relatively equal to help with depression. EB/EBN: *Screen pregnant women using a tool like the Patient Health Questionnaire (PHQ-9) for depression risk identification. When comprehensive screening is not included during antepartum care, there is less likelihood that significant information will be revealed. Subsequently, undiagnosed clinical depression in pregnancy may lead to serious perinatal complications such as inadequate maternal weight gain, preterm birth, and low infant birth weight (Breedlove & Fryzelka, 2011; Sidebottom et al, 2012; Rollans et al, 2013).*

▲ Observe for signs of alcohol use and counsel women to stop drinking during pregnancy. Give appropriate referral for treatment if needed. EB: *Alcohol is teratogenic, and prenatal exposure may result in growth impairment, facial abnormalities, central nervous system and/or intellectual impairment, and behavioral disorders. Evidence suggests women's past pregnancy, current drinking behavior, and attitude toward alcohol use in pregnancy were the strongest predictors of alcohol consumption in pregnancy (Barclay, 2011; Peadon et al, 2011).*

▲ Obtain a smoking history and counsel women to stop smoking for the safety of the baby. Give appropriate referral to smoking cessation program if needed. CEB: *Tobacco smoking in pregnancy remains one of the few preventable factors associated with pregnancy complications. Use the 5As (tobacco cessation interventions) to treat tobacco use and dependence in pregnant women. According to the USDHHS Clinical Practice Guidelines, health care professionals should at every contact (1) ask if a woman is a tobacco user, (2) advise her to quit, (3) assess her willingness to quit, (4) assist with the quit attempt (such as counseling, medication), and (5) arrange for follow-up (telephone support 1-800-QUIT-NOW). The evidence is compelling, even a minimal (less than 3 minute) intervention can make a difference in motivation to quit smoking (USDHHS, 2008).*

▲ Monitor for substance abuse with recreational drugs. Refer to drug treatment program as needed. Refer opiate-dependent women to methadone clinics to improve maternal and fetal pregnancy outcomes. EBN: *The drug addict is obsessed by the drug of choice because of a change in the pathophysiology of the brain. Treating addiction as a chronic disease instead of a moral weakness is more supportive to women who abuse drugs. It is important to involve a pregnant woman in a treatment program like a methadone clinic to help to stabilize the maternal–fetal dyad. Methadone prevents withdrawal symptoms and eliminates drug craving. Methadone blocks the euphoric effects of illegal self-administered narcotics. It also supports stable maternal opioid levels to protect the fetus from repeated occurrences of withdrawal and decreases the risk for sexually transmitted infections by decreasing drug-seeking behaviors such as prostitution. When a woman makes the decision to enroll in a methadone treatment program, she is taking a significant step toward recovery (Maguire, 2014).*

▲ Monitor for psychosocial issues including lack of social support system, loneliness, depression, lack of confidence, maternal powerlessness, domestic violence, and socioeconomic problems. CEB: *A study that compared psychosocial assessment versus routine care for pregnant women concluded that the health care providers who assessed psychosocial factors were more likely to identify psychosocial concerns, including family violence, and to rate the level of concern as high. In two trials, women identified they did not want to feel so alone, be judged, or be misunderstood, and they wanted to feel an increased sense of their own worth. Social support interventions can improve health. The use of doulas or labor coaches can provide assistance in addressing social-psychological issues and socioeconomic disparities (Austin et al, 2008; Gentry et al, 2010; Small et al, 2011).*

▲ Monitor for signs of domestic violence. Refer to a community program for abused women that provides safe shelter as needed. EB: *Women who were involved in intimate partner violence were more likely to experience negative outcomes such as preterm delivery and delivery of low-birth-weight infants (Shneyderman & Kiely, 2013). Women enduring domestic violence are often in denial. Pregnancy and immediately postpartum are highly vulnerable times for mothers and their infants to experience domestic violence. These women also need to be assessed regularly because they may not be ready to seek help at first. This may be the only time a pregnant victim of domestic violence comes in contact with a health care provider who can assess for the abuse and take action to resolve it (Menezes Cooper, 2013).*

- Provide antenatal education to increase the woman's knowledge needed to make informed choices during pregnancy, labor, and delivery and to promote a healthy lifestyle. EB: *Antenatal classes must be interesting enough to maintain attention, relevant to the attendees, and understandable. The parents should feel empowered that the decisions they make about maternity care and parenthood are made with up-to-date evidence-based information and fit into their lifestyle. O'Sullivan et al (2014) found that class sizes tended to be too large to include class participation. They also reported educators sometimes just focused on maternity care and not on parenthood, healthy lifestyle, and changing relationships. Although resources are available, the educators reported their facility had limited educational resources.*
- Encourage expectant parents to prepare a realistic birth plan in order to prepare for the physical and emotional aspects of the birth process and to plan ahead for how they want various situations handled. CEB: *The degree of satisfaction the mothers have with the birth of their baby is increased when they have made an individualized birth plan and the medical team and parents are able to follow it (Sato & Umeno, 2011).*
- Encourage good nutritional intake during pregnancy to facilitate proper growth and development of the fetus. Women should consume an additional 300 calories per day during pregnancy, take a multimicronutrient supplement containing at least 400 μg folic acid, and achieve a total weight gain of 25 to 30 lb. EB: *A healthy, varied diet (e.g., Choosemyplate.gov) is of vital importance for optimal birth outcome, including taking a multivitamin with folic acid from before conception to at least the twelfth week of pregnancy, as well as a vitamin D supplement throughout pregnancy. Many women are not following the guidelines and there are concerns for these vulnerable groups (USDA, 2014; Williamson & Wyness, 2013). Inadequate levels of key nutrients during crucial periods of fetal development may lead to changes within fetal tissues, predisposing the infant to chronic illnesses and conditions in later life (Procter & Campbell, 2014).*

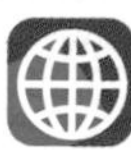

Multicultural

- ▲ Provide for a translator if needed. EB: *The health care industry must recognize that providing translators for language assistance is an important tool for improving quality of care, saving lives, and avoiding costly and dangerous medical errors. Although costly, the American health care industry needs to comply with federal and state laws as well as accreditation standards by being prepared to provide care in at least 100 different languages (Rivers & Rivers, 2013).*
- ▲ Provide depression screening for clients of all ethnicities. EB: *Race and ethnicity are important risk factors for antenatal depression. A study found that non-Hispanic white women, black women, and Asian/Pacific Islander women had an increased risk for antenatal depression. The prevalence of antenatal depression was 15.3% in black women, 6.9% in Latinas, and 3.6% in non-Hispanic white women (Gavin et al, 2011).* EB: *Screening Latina women for depression, 20.4% were positive for depressive symptoms and 36.7% reported psychosocial issues such as intimate partner violence and substance abuse while pregnant (Connelly et al, 2013).* CEB: *Women who are depressed are at risk for unhealthy behaviors such as using tobacco, alcohol, and or drugs. They either sleep too much or not enough, their hygiene suffers, and they are less likely to attend prenatal visits. Maternal levels of corticosteroids and catecholamine are increased, which directly affect the growth and development of the fetus. Maternal depression may also affect bonding (Bowen & Muhajarine, 2006).*
- Perform a cultural assessment and provide obstetrical care that is culturally appropriate to ensure a safe and satisfying childbearing experience. EBN: *Just because a woman is a part of a certain culture, it is not safe to assume she follows all the beliefs of that culture. Asking about what she needs and expects is vital. Nurses must acknowledge that the maternity health care system has a unique culture that may clash with the cultures of many of our clients. Women not accustomed to this culture of potential risk in prenatal care, childbirth, and neonatal care may be frightened, overwhelmed, or made to feel guilty if they are not willing to undergo some of the expected interventions (Lewallen, 2011).*

REFERENCES

Austin, M. P., Priest, S. R., & Sullivan, E. A. (2008). Antenatal psychosocial assessment for reducing perinatal mental health morbidity. *Cochrane Database of Systematic Reviews*, (4), CD005124.

Barclay, L. (2011). ACOG calls for alcohol screen annually and at prenatal visit. *Obstetrics and Gynecology*, *18*, 383–388.

Beeckman, K., Louckx, F., Downe, S., et al. (2013). The relationship between antenatal care and preterm birth: the importance of content of care. *European Journal of Public Health*, *23*(3), 366–371.

Bowen, A., & Muhajarine, N. (2006). Antenatal depression: nurses who understand the prevalence, signs and symptoms, and risk factors associated with antenatal depression (AD) can play a valuable role in identifying AD and preventing the sequelae in pregnant women and their families. *Canadian Nurse*, *102*(9), 27–30.

Breedlove, G., & Fryzelka, D. (2011). Depression screening during pregnancy. *Journal of Midwifery and Women's Health*, *56*(1), 18–25.

Connelly, C. D., Hazen, A. L., Baker-Ericzén, M. J., et al. (2013). Is screening for depression in the perinatal period enough? The co-occurrence of depression, substance abuse, and intimate partner violence in culturally diverse pregnant women. *Journal of Women's Health* (15409996), *22*(10), 844–852.

Gavin, A. R., Melville, J. L., Rue, T., et al. (2011). Racial differences in the prevalence of antenatal depression. *General Hospital Psychiatry*, *33*(2), 87–93.

Gentry, Q., Nolte, K., Gonzalez, A., et al. (2010). "Going beyond the call of doula": A grounded theory analysis of the diverse roles community-based doulas play in the lives of pregnant and parenting adolescent mothers. *Journal of Perinatal Education*, *19*(4), 24–40.

Lewallen, L. P. (2011). The importance of culture in childbearing. *Journal of Obstetric, Gynecologic, and Neonatal Nursing: JOGNN/NAACOG*, *40*, 4–8.

Maguire, D. (2014). Drug addiction in pregnancy: Disease not moral failure. *Neonatal Network*, *33*(1), 11–18.

Menezes Cooper, T. (2013). Domestic Violence and Pregnancy: A Literature Review. *International Journal of Childbirth Education*, *28*(3), 30–33.

O'Sullivan, C., O'Connell, R., & Devane, D. (2014). A descriptive survey of the educational preparation and practices of antenatal educators in Ireland. *Journal of Perinatal Education*, *23*(1), 33–40.

Peadon, E., Payne, J., Henley, N., et al. (2011). Attitudes and behaviour predict women's intention to drink alcohol during pregnancy: the challenge for health professionals. *BMC Public Health*, *11*, 584.

Procter, S. B., & Campbell, C. G. (2014). Position of the Academy of Nutrition and Dietetics: Nutrition and lifestyle for a healthy pregnancy outcome. *Journal of The Academy of Nutrition & Dietetics*, *114*(7), 1099–1103.

Rivers, K., & Rivers, D. L. (2013). Foreign language difficulties in American healthcare: The challenges of medical translation regulation and remuneration. *National Social Science Proceedings*, *52*(1), 150–160.

Rollans, M., Schmied, V., Kemp, L., et al. (2013). 'We just ask some questions…' the process of antenatal psychosocial assessment by midwives. *Midwifery*, *29*(8), 935–942.

Sato, S., & Umeno, Y. (2011). The relationship between the recognition of postpartum mothers' birth plan and the degree of satisfaction with delivery. *Journal of Japan Academy of Midwifery*, *25*(1), 27–35.

Shneyderman, Y., & Kiely, M. (2013). Intimate partner violence during pregnancy: victim or perpetrator? Does it make a difference? *BJOG: An International Journal Of Obstetrics & Gynaecology*, *120*(11), 1375–1385.

Sidebottom, A., Harrison, P., Godecker, A., et al. (2012). Validation of the Patient Health Questionnaire (PHQ)-9 for prenatal depression screening. *Archives Of Women's Mental Health*, *15*(5), 367–374.

Small, R., Taft, A. J., & Brown, S. J. (2011). The power of social connection and support in improving health: lessons from social support interventions with childbearing women. *BMC Public Health*, *11*, S4.

US Department of Agriculture, (USDA). (2014). *Nutritional needs during pregnancy. Choosemyplate.gov/pregnancy.* Retrieved from: <http://www.choosemyplate.gov/pregnancy-breastfeeding/pregnancy-nutritional-needs.html>.

U.S. Department of Health and Human Services (USDHHS). (2008). *Treating tobacco use and dependence: clinical practice guideline 2008 update. Pregnant smokers.* Retrieved from: <http://www.ahrq.gov/clinic/tobacco/treating_tobacco_use08.pdf>.

Van Dijk, J. W., Anderko, L., & Stetzer, F. (2011). The impact of prenatal care coordination on birth outcomes. *J Obstet Gynecol Neonat Nurs*, *40*, 98–108.

Williamson, C., & Wyness, L. (2013). Nutritional requirements in pregnancy and use of dietary supplements. *Community Practitioner*, *86*(8), 44–47.

C

Readiness for enhanced Childbearing process

Gail B. Ladwig, MSN, RN, and Dianne Frances Hayward, RN, MSN, WHNP

NANDA-I

Definition

A pattern of preparing for and maintaining a healthy pregnancy, childbirth process, and care of newborn for ensuring well-being that can be strengthened

Defining Characteristics

During Pregnancy

Expresses desire to enhance knowledge of childbearing process; expresses desire to enhance management of unpleasant pregnancy symptoms; expresses desire to enhance prenatal lifestyle (e.g., elimination, exercise, nutrition, personal hygiene, sleep); expresses desire to enhance preparation for newborn

C

During Labor and Delivery

Expresses desire to enhance lifestyle appropriate for stage of labor (e.g., elimination, exercise, nutrition, personal hygiene, sleep); expresses desire to enhance proactivity during labor and delivery

After Birth

Expresses desire to enhance attachment behavior; expresses desire to enhance baby care techniques; expresses desire to enhance baby feeding techniques; expresses desire to enhance breast care; expresses desire to enhance environmental safety for the baby; expresses desire to enhance postpartum lifestyle (e.g., elimination, exercise, nutrition, personal hygiene, sleep); expresses desire to enhance use of support system

NOC (Nursing Outcomes Classification)

Suggested NOC Outcomes

Knowledge: Pregnancy; Knowledge: Infant Care; Knowledge: Postpartum Maternal Health

Example NOC Outcome with Indicators

Knowledge: Pregnancy as evidenced by client conveying understanding of the following indicators: Importance of frequent prenatal care/Importance of prenatal education/Benefits of regular exercise/Healthy nutritional practices/Anatomic and physiological changes with pregnancy/Psychological changes associated with pregnancy/Birthing options/Effective labor techniques/ Signs and symptoms of labor. (Rate the outcome and indicators of **Knowledge: Pregnancy:** 1 = no knowledge, 2 = limited knowledge, 3 = moderate knowledge, 4 = substantial knowledge, 5 = extensive knowledge [see Section I].)

Client Outcomes

Client Will (Specify Time Frame)

During Pregnancy
- State importance of frequent prenatal care/education
- State knowledge of anatomic, physiological, psychological changes with pregnancy
- Report appropriate lifestyle choices prenatal: Activity and exercise/healthy nutritional practices

During Labor and Delivery
- Report appropriate lifestyle choices during labor
- State knowledge of birthing options, signs and symptoms of labor, and effective labor techniques

After Birth
- Report appropriate lifestyle choices postpartum
- State normal physical sensations following delivery
- State knowledge of recommended nutrient intake, strategies to balance activity and rest, appropriate exercise, time frame for resumption of sexual activity, strategies to manage stress
- List strategies to bond with infant
- State knowledge of proper handling and positioning of infant/infant safety
- State knowledge of feeding technique and bathing of infant

NIC (Nursing Interventions Classification)

Suggested NIC Interventions

Prenatal Care; Intrapartal Care; Postpartal Care; Attachment Promotion; Infant Care: Newborn

Example NIC Activities—Prenatal Care

Encourage prenatal class attendance; Discuss nutritional needs and concerns (e.g., balanced diet, folic acid, food safety, and supplements); Discuss activity level with client (e.g., appropriate exercise, activities to avoid, and importance of rest); Discuss importance of participating in prenatal care throughout entire pregnancy while encouraging involvement of client's partner or other family member

Nursing Interventions and *Rationales*

Refer to care plans: Risk for impaired **Attachment;** Readiness for enhanced **Breastfeeding;** Readiness for enhanced family **Coping;** Readiness for enhanced **Family** processes; Risk for disproportionate **Growth;** Readiness for enhanced **Nutrition;** Readiness for enhanced **Parenting;** Ineffective **Role** performance.

C

Prenatal Care

- ▲ Ensure that pregnant clients have an adequate diet and take multi-micronutrient supplements containing at least 400 micrograms of folic acid during pregnancy. EB: *A healthy, varied diet (i.e., Choosemyplate.gov) is of vital importance for optimal birth outcome, and this includes taking a folic acid supplement from before conception to the 12th week of pregnancy, as well as a vitamin D supplement throughout pregnancy; many women are not following these guidelines and there are concerns for vulnerable groups (USDA, 2014; Williamson & Wyness, 2013).*
- • Encourage pregnant clients to include enriched cereal grain products in their diets. EB: *Folate is a B vitamin that helps prevent neural tube defects, serious abnormalities of the brain and spinal cord. Fortified cereals are great sources of folic acid. (Mayo Clinic, 2014).* CEB: *The number of pregnancies affected by neural tube defects greatly decreased in the United States after the fortification of cereal grain products with folic acid was mandated (CDC, 2010).*
- • Assess smoking status of pregnant clients and offer effective smoking-cessation interventions. EB: *Prenatal smoking prevalence remains high in the United States. It is one of the most significant modifiable risk factors for adverse infant outcomes (e.g., low birth weight, preterm birth [preterm], and sudden infant death syndrome). To reduce prenatal smoking prevalence, efforts should focus on delivering evidence-based cessation interventions (Tong et al, 2011; Batech et al, 2013; USDHHS Clinical Practice Guidelines, 2008).*
- • Also see Risk for disturbed **Maternal–Fetal** dyad for USDHHS guidelines.
- ▲ Assess for signs of depression and make appropriate referral: inadequate weight gain, underutilization of prenatal care, increased substance use, and premature birth. Past personal or family history of depression, single, poor health functioning, and alcohol use. EBN: *Social and emotional health problems associated with depression in the perinatal period can lead to poor outcomes for women, their infants, and their families (Rollans et al, 2013).*
- • Discuss breastfeeding with a pregnant client, including all the benefits both to the infant and the mother EB: *Pregnant women need information about overcoming potential breastfeeding problems and the physiology of breastfeeding. Interventions designed to promote breastfeeding confidence need to be directed to primiparas and women with a lack of breastfeeding knowledge (Laanterä et al, 2012).*

Intrapartal Care

- • Encourage psychosocial support during labor, especially by the father of the baby or the woman's mother if possible. EB: *When a husband provides continuous support during his wife's labor, his presence is considered effective in reducing her dissatisfaction with the childbirth process. According to Lacerda et al (2014), the ideal companion is someone with whom the client has a bond and is trusted. The father of the child ranked first, followed by the mother of the postpartum woman.* EBN: *The key to promoting a normal birth and reducing medical interventions is high-quality continuous support. This support increases a woman's perception of a positive birth experience, fosters a positive adaptation to motherhood, and reduces the risk for posttraumatic stress disorder and other postpartum mental health problems (Ross-Davie & Cheyne, 2014; Sapkota et al, 2013).*
- • Consider using aromatherapy during labor. EB: *Aromatherapy has been used in childbirth to reduce anxiety and pain (Horowitz, 2011).*
- • Provide massage and relaxation techniques during labor. EB: *There is some evidence to suggest that relaxation and massage may improve management of labor pain, with few adverse effects. These interventions relieved pain and improved satisfaction with pain and childbirth experience when compared with placebo or standard care. Relaxation was associated with fewer assisted vaginal births (Jones et al, 2012).*
- • Offer the client in labor a clear liquid diet and water if allowed. EB: *There is insufficient evidence to make conclusions about the relationship between fasting times for clear liquids and the risk for emesis, reflux, or pulmonary aspiration during labor. Although there is some disagreement, the majority of experts agree that oral intake of clear liquids during labor does not lead to increased maternal complications (ACOG, 2013).*

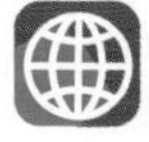

Multicultural

Prenatal

- • Assess the client's beliefs and concerns about prenatal care. Provide culturally appropriate prenatal care for clients. EBN: *Most Samoan women attended their first antenatal appointment in their first trimester of pregnancy. Fewer attended antenatal care later in pregnancy (fifteenth week or after). Samoan women*

C

viewed pregnancy as wellness. Most participants did not relate to the content of mainstream antenatal classes because they were not culturally appropriate (Tanuvasa et al, 2013; Torres et al, 2012).

▲ Refer the client to a centering pregnancy group (8 to 10 women of similar gestational age receive group prenatal care after initial obstetrical visit) or group prenatal care. EB: *Group prenatal care appears to have created a benefit to the women, not just with their birth experiences, but also with the psychological and social aspects of this life change (Risisky et al, 2013).*

Intrapartal

- Assess client's beliefs and concerns about labor. Consider the client's culture when assisting in labor and delivery. EBN: *A culturally appropriate OB/GYN service has input from the community, provides options, and respects choices (Simmonds et al, 2012). According to van Dijk et al (2013), most clients of these services desired the option of culturally appropriate care but typically did not receive it.*

Postpartal

- Assess client's beliefs and concerns about the postpartum period. Provide culturally appropriate health and nutrition information and guidance on contemporary postpartum practices and take away common misconceptions about traditional dietary and health behaviors (e.g., fruit and vegetables should be restricted because of cold nature). Encourage a balanced diet and discourage unhealthy hygiene taboos. EB: *Many cultures practice food taboos surrounding pregnancy with consequent depletion of vital nutrients, which can be detrimental to both the mother and fetus (Oni & Tukur, 2012).* EBN: *In some cultures, women refuse to bathe and wash their hair after childbirth and during the postpartum period. The influence of beliefs and taboos offers health risks for the postpartum woman and newborn. In contrast, beliefs and taboos that do not offer health risks should not be countered because they contribute to the well-being of postpartum women (Trettene & Manci, 2012).*

Home Care

Prenatal

▲ Involve pregnant drug users in drug treatment programs that include coordinated interventions in several areas: drug use, infectious diseases, mental health, personal and social welfare, and gynecological/obstetric care. EBN: *The drug addict is obsessed by the drug of choice because of a change in the pathophysiology of the brain. Treating addiction as a chronic disease instead of a moral weakness will be more supportive to women who abuse drugs. It is important to involve a pregnant woman in a treatment program like a methadone clinic to help to stabilize the maternal–fetal dyad. Methadone prevents withdrawal symptoms and eliminates drug craving. Methadone blocks the euphoric effects of illegal self-administered narcotics. It also supports stable maternal opioid levels to protect the fetus from repeated occurrences of withdrawal and decreases the risk for STIs (sexually transmitted infections) by decreasing drug-seeking behaviors such as prostitution. When a woman makes the decision to enroll in a methadone treatment program, she is taking a significant step toward recovery (Maguire, 2014).*

Postpartal

- Provide video conferencing to support new parents. EBN: *Parents viewed videoconferencing as a possible chance to obtain extra support after returning home with their newborns (Lindberg, 2013).*
- Consider reflexology for postpartum women to improve sleep quality. EBN: *A systematic review and meta-analysis indicates that foot reflexology is a useful nursing intervention to relieve fatigue and to promote sleep (Lee et al, 2011).*

Client/Family Teaching and Discharge Planning

Prenatal

- Provide dietary and lifestyle counseling as part of prenatal care to pregnant women. EB: *A healthy prepregnancy weight, appropriate weight gain, physical activity during pregnancy, intake of a wide variety of foods, appropriate vitamin and mineral supplementation, avoidance of alcohol and other harmful substances, regular prenatal visits, and safe food handling are all components leading to a healthy pregnancy outcome. Pregnancy is a crucial period and maternal nutrition and lifestyle choices are major influences on mother and infant/child health. Healthy lifestyle changes are the key to the health of the next generation (Procter & Campbell, 2014).*

- Provide the following information in parenting classes via DVD and Internet: support mechanisms, information and antenatal education, breastfeeding, practical baby care, and relationship changes. Include fathers in the parenting classes. EB: *Most fathers, expectant and experienced, felt there were not enough resources to support their education, spaces to support their involvement, or recognition of their experiences and feelings about pregnancy, labor, birth, and fathering. As the findings from the St. George and Fletcher (2011) study indicate, receiving encouragement and education that supports involved fathers is welcomed by many men. Although fathers' contribution to their children's well-being varies across cultures and roles, the effect of a father's positive involvement reaches far into the future of the child's social, emotional, and cognitive well-being.*
- Provide group prenatal care to families in the military. EB: *A 3-year randomized clinical trial was conducted to examine differences in perinatal health behaviors, perinatal and infant health outcomes, and family health outcomes for women receiving group prenatal care (GPC) when compared with those receiving individual prenatal care. Women in GPC were almost 6 times more likely to receive adequate prenatal care than women in individual prenatal care and were considerably more satisfied with their care (Kennedy et al, 2011).*

Postpartal

- Encourage physical activity in postpartum women, after being cleared by health care provider; provide telephone counseling, teach postpartum women that exercise may reduce anxiety and depression, encourage to download phone apps that help track exercise like Fitbit or Pedometer Master. EBN: *Exercise during the postpartum period is important for healthy weight loss and decreasing anxiety (Lewis et al, 2011).* EB: *Research on anxiety, depression, and exercise shows that the psychological and physical benefits of exercise can help reduce anxiety and improve mood (Mayo Clinic Staff, 2014).*

▲ Provide breastfeeding mothers contact information for a lactation consultant, phone numbers and website information for La Leche League (http://www.lalecheleague.org), and local breastfeeding support groups. EB: *Problems with breastfeeding are encountered in up to 80% of mother–infant dyads. In Western societies, the difficulties decrease the breastfeeding rate within the first months considerably. Dealing with the problems of breastfeeding efficiently requires a profound understanding of its physiology, as well as of its psychological, cultural, and social factors (Bergmann et al, 2014).*

- Teach mothers of young children principles of a healthy lifestyle: Substitute foods high in saturated fat with foods moderate in polyunsaturated fatty acids (PUFAs) such as avocados, tuna, walnuts, and olive oil. Include lean protein, fruits and vegetables, and complex carbohydrates. It is also important to increase physical activity. EB: *Parents are the most important influence on their child. Parents can do many things to help their children develop healthy eating habits for life. Offering a variety of foods helps children get the nutrients they need from every food group. They will also be more likely to try new foods and to like more foods (USDA, 2011). It is not recommended to feed children a low-fat diet but to make sure fats are good fats (PUFAs).* EBN: *Omega 3 PUFAs are required for very early brain development, and that need continues throughout life. These essential fatty acids are crucial in cell functioning. Humans are not able to synthesize omega 3 PUFAs; therefore, they must be included in the daily diet (Helvig & Decker, 2014).*

REFERENCES

ACOG Committee Opinion No. 441: Oral intake during labor (2009 reaffirmed 2013). *Obstetrics & Gynecology, 114*(3), 714.

Batech, M., Tonstad, S., Job, J., et al. (2013). Estimating the impact of smoking cessation during pregnancy: The San Bernardino County experience. *Journal of Community Health, 38*, 838–846.

Bergmann, R. L., Bergmann, K. E., von Weizsäcker, K., et al. (2014). Breastfeeding is natural but not always easy: Intervention for common medical problems of breastfeeding mothers—a review of the scientific evidence. *Journal of Perinatal Medicine, 42*(1), 9–18.

Centers for Disease Control and Prevention (CDC). (2010). CDC grand rounds: Additional opportunities to prevent neural tube defects with folic acid fortification. *MMWR. Morbidity and Mortality Weekly Report, 59*(31), 980–984.

Helvig, A., & Decker, M. (2014). Omega 3 fatty acids and the brain: Implications for nursing practice. *British Journal of Neuroscience Nursing, 10*(1), 29–37.

Horowitz, S. (2011). Aromatherapy: current and emerging applications. *Alternative and Complementary Therapies, 17*(1), 26–31.

Jones, L., Othman, M., Dowswell, T., et al. (2012). Pain management for women in labour: An overview of systematic reviews. *Cochrane Database of Systematic Reviews*, 14;3:CD009234.

Kennedy, H., Farrell, T., Paden, R., et al. (2011). A randomized clinical trial of group prenatal care in two military settings. *Military Medicine, 176*(10), 1169–1177.

Laanterä, S., Pietilä, A., Ekström, A., et al. (2012). Confidence in breastfeeding among pregnant women. *Western Journal of Nursing Research*, *34*(7), 933–951.

de Lacerda, A. B., da Silva, R. R., & Davim, R. B. (2014). Women's perception about the companion during labor. *Journal of Nursing: UFPE Online*, *8*(8), 2710–2715. Available from: CINAHL Complete, Ipswich, MA.

Lee, J., Han, M., Chung, Y., et al. (2011). Effects of foot reflexology on fatigue, sleep and pain: A systematic review and meta-analysis. *Journal of Korean Academy of Nursing*, *41*(6), 821–833.

Lewis, B. A., Martinson, B. C., Sherwood, N. E., et al. (2011). A pilot study evaluating a telephone-based exercise intervention for pregnant and postpartum women. *Journal Midwifery Womens Health*, *56*(2), 127–131.

Lindberg, B. (2013). Access to videoconferencing in providing support to parents of preterm infants: Ascertaining parental views. *Journal of Neonatal Nursing*, *19*(5), 259–265.

Maguire, D. (2014). Drug addiction in pregnancy: Disease not moral failure. *Neonatal Network*, *33*(1), 11–18.

Mayo Clinic. (2014). *Drugs and supplements: Folate*. This evidence-based monograph was prepared by *The Natural Standard Research Collaboration* <www.naturalstandard.com>.

Mayo Clinic Staff. (2014). Depression and anxiety: Exercise eases symptoms. *Mayo Foundation for Medical Education and Research*. Retrieved from: <http://www.mayoclinic.org/diseases-conditions/depression/in-depth/depression-and-exercise/art-20046495>.

Oni, O. A. 1., & Tukur, J. (2012). Identifying pregnant women who would adhere to food taboos in a rural community: A community-based study. *African Journal of Reproductive Health*, *16*(3), 68–76.

Procter, S. B., & Campbell, C. G. (2014). Position of the Academy of Nutrition and Dietetics: Nutrition and lifestyle for a healthy pregnancy outcome. *Journal of The Academy Of Nutrition & Dietetics*, *114*(7), 1099–1103.

Rollans, M., Schmied, V., Kemp, L., et al. (2013). "We just ask some questions..." the process of antenatal psychosocial assessment by midwives. *Midwifery*, *29*(8), 935–942.

Risisky, D., Asghar, S., Chaffee, M., et al. (2013). Women's perceptions using the centering pregnancy model of group prenatal care. *Journal of Perinatal Education*, *22*(3), 136–144.

Ross-Davie, M., & Cheyne, H. (2014). Intrapartum support: what do women want? A literature review. *Evidence Based Midwifery*, *12*(2), 52–58.

Sapkota, S., Kobayashi, T., & Takase, M. (2013). Impact on perceived postnatal support, maternal anxiety and symptoms of depression in new mothers in Nepal when their husbands provide continuous support during labour. *Midwifery*, *29*(11), 1264–1271.

Simmonds, D. M., West, L., Porter, J., et al. (2012). The role of support person for Ngaanyatjarra women during pregnancy and birth. *Women and Birth: Journal of the Australian College of Midwives*, *25*(2), 79–85.

St. George, J. M., & Fletcher, R. J. (2011). Fathers online: Learning about fatherhood through the Internet. *The Journal of Perinatal Education: An ASPO*, *20*(3), 154–162.

Tanuvasa, A., Cumming, J., Churchward, M., et al. (2013). Samoan women's attitudes towards antenatal and midwifery care. *British Journal of Midwifery*, *21*(10), 710–721.

Tong, V., Dietz, P., England, L., et al. (2011). Age and racial/ethnic disparities in prepregnancy smoking among women who delivered live births. *Preventing Chronic Disease*, *8*(6), A121.

Torres, M. E., Smithwick, J., Luchok, K. J., et al. (2012). Reducing maternal and child health disparities among Latino immigrants in South Carolina through a tailored, culturally appropriate and participant-driven initiative. *Californian Journal of Health Promotion*, *10*(2), 1–14.

Trettene, A., & Manci, M. (2012). Influence of beliefs and taboos in the puerperal period: Performance of the nurse [Portuguese]. *Revista Nursing*, *15*(169), 315–320.

US Department of Agriculture, (USDA). (2011). Be a healthy role model for children: 10 tips for setting good examples. *Choosemyplate.gov*. Retrieved from: <www.choosemyplate.gov/food-groups/downloads/TenTips/DGTipsheet12BeAHealthyRoleModel>.

US Department of Agriculture, (USDA). (2014). Nutritional needs during pregnancy. *Choosemyplate.gov/pregnancy*. Retrieved from: <http://www.choosemyplate.gov/pregnancy-breastfeeding/pregnancy-nutritional-needs.html>.

U.S. Department of Health and Human Services (USDHHS). (2008). Treating tobacco use and dependence: Clinical practice guideline 2008 update. *Pregnant smokers*. Retrieved from: <http://www.ahrq.gov/clinic/tobacco/treating_tobacco_use08.pdf>.

van Dijk, M., Ruiz, M. J., Letona, D., et al. (2013). Ensuring intercultural maternal health care for Mayan women in Guatemala: a qualitative assessment. *Culture, Health & Sexuality*, *15*, S365–S382.

Williamson, C., & Wyness, L. (2013). Nutritional requirements in pregnancy and use of dietary supplements. *Community Practitioner*, *86*(8), 44–47.

Risk for ineffective Childbearing process *Jane M. Kendall, RN, BS, CHT*

NANDA-I

Definition

Vulnerable to not matching environmental context, norms and expectations of pregnancy, childbirth process, and the care of the newborn

Risk Factors

Domestic violence; inconsistent prenatal health visits; insufficient cognitive readiness for parenting; insufficient knowledge of childbearing process; inadequate maternal nutrition; insufficient parental role model; insufficient prenatal care; insufficient support system; low maternal confidence; maternal powerlessness; maternal psychological distress; substance abuse; unplanned pregnancy; unrealistic birth plan; unwanted pregnancy

NOC, NIC, Client Outcomes, Nursing Interventions, Client/Family Teaching, *Rationales*, and References

Refer to care plan for Ineffective **Childbearing** process.

Impaired Comfort *Katharine Kolcaba, PhD, RN*

NANDA-I

Definition

Perceived lack of ease, relief, and transcendence in physical, psychospiritual, environmental, cultural and/or social dimensions

Defining Characteristics

Alteration in sleep pattern; anxiety; crying; discontent with situation; distressing symptoms; fear feeling cold; feeling hot; feeling of discomfort; feeling of hunger; inability to relax; irritability; itching; moaning; restlessness; sighing; uneasy in situation

Related Factors (r/t)

Illness-related symptoms; insufficient environmental control; insufficient privacy; insufficient resources (e.g., financial, social, knowledge); insufficient situational control; noxious environmental stimuli; treatment regimen

NOC (Nursing Outcomes Classification)

Suggested NOC Outcomes

Client Satisfaction; Symptom Control; Comfort Status; Coping; Hope; Pain and/or Anxiety Management; Personal Well-Being; Spiritual Health

Example NOC Outcomes with Indicators

Comfort Status as evidenced by the following indicators: Physical and psychological well-being/Symptom control/Enhanced comfort. (Rate the outcome and indicators of **Comfort Status:** 1 = severely compromised, 2 = substantially compromised, 3 = moderately compromised, 4 = mildly compromised, 5 = not compromised [see Section I].)

Client Outcomes

Client Will (Specify Time Frame)

- Provide evidence for improved comfort compared to baseline
- Identify strategies, with or without significant others, to improve and/or maintain acceptable comfort level
- Perform appropriate interventions, with or without significant others, as needed to improve and/or maintain acceptable comfort level
- Evaluate the effectiveness of strategies to maintain/and or reach an acceptable comfort level
- Maintain an acceptable level of comfort when possible

NIC (Nursing Interventions Classification)

Suggested NIC Interventions

Calming Techniques; Massage; Healing Touch; Still Point Induction; Heat/Cold Application; Hope Inspiration; Humor; Meditation Facilitation; Music Therapy; Pain Management; Presence; Progressive Muscle Relaxation; Spiritual Growth Facilitation; Distraction

Example NIC Activities—Hope Inspiration

Assist the client/significant others to identify areas of hope in life; Help expand spiritual self; Involve the client actively in own care

C

Nursing Interventions and *Rationales*

- Assess client's understanding of ranking his or her comfort level. CEB: *Performing accurate comfort measurements is essential for providing evidence about which strategies and interventions are effective (Kolcaba, 2003).*
- Ask about client's current level of comfort. This is the first step in helping clients achieve improved comfort. CEB: *It is important for nurses to address detractors from comfort (Kolcaba, 2003). Sources of assessment data to determine level of comfort can be subjective, objective, primary, or secondary (Kolcaba, 2014).*
- Comfort is a holistic state under which pain management is included. CEB: *Management of discomforts, however, can be better managed, and with fewer analgesics, by also addressing other comfort needs such as anxiety, insufficient information, social isolation, and financial difficulties (Kolcaba, 2003).* CEB: *One randomized study (N = 53) found that female breast cancer clients undergoing radiation therapy rated their overall comfort as being greater than the sum of the hypothesized components of comfort, which provided evidence for the theory of the holistic nature of comfort (Kolcaba, 2014).*
- Assist clients to understand how to rate their current state of holistic comfort, using the institution's preferred method of documentation. CEB: *Documentation of comfort pre-nursing and post-nursing interactions is essential to demonstrate efficacy of nursing activities (Kolcaba et al, 2014).*
- Enhance feelings of trust between the client and the health care provider. To attain the highest comfort level, clients must be able to trust their nurse. CEB: *This randomized design (N = 31) demonstrated the importance of promoting open relationships with clients, which helps to acknowledge their individuality. Knowing the client/significant others is essential in the provision of optimum palliative and terminal care (Kolcaba, 2014).*
- Manipulate the environment as necessary to improve comfort. CEB: *Addressing clients' environmental preferences or needs enhances holistic comfort (Kolcaba, 2003).* CEB: *In two experimental studies, the protocol included that all clients be asked about preferences for light, furnishings, body position, television settings, and so on (Dowd et al, 2007).*
- Encourage early mobilization and provide routine position changes. Range of motion and weight bearing decrease physical discomforts and disability associated with bed rest. CEB: *Before hand massage, positions of comfort were assured to maximize the effect of the intervention (Kolcaba et al in Kolcaba, 2000).*
- Provide simple massage. Massage has many therapeutic effects, including improved relaxation, circulation, and well-being. EBN: *Several quantitative studies support the efficacy of simple massage for enhancing holistic comfort (Townsend et al, 2014; Kolcaba et al in Kolcaba, 2000).*
- Provide healing touch, which is well-suited for clients who cannot tolerate more stimulating interventions. CEB: *Inform the client of options for control of discomfort such as meditation and guided imagery, and provide these interventions if appropriate (Dowd et al, 2007).*
- Use empathy as a response to a client's negative emotions. EBN: *An evaluation interaction analysis found that an accurate empathic response to a client's expressions of negative emotions can contribute to comfort (Eide et al, 2011).*
- Encourage clients to use relaxation techniques to reduce pain, anxiety, depression, and fatigue. EBN: *In a quantitative study with 22 participants, the effects of traditional massage and cranial still point induction were statistically significant in improving comfort and decreasing chronic pain (Townsend et al, 2014).*

Geriatric

- Use hand massage for older adults. Most older adults respond well to touch and the health care provider's presence. Lines of communication open naturally during hand massage. CEB: *In an experiment (N = 60), the effects of hand massage on comfort of nursing home residents was found to be significant immediately after the massage compared to residents who did not receive hand massage (Kolcaba et al in Kolcaba, 2014).*
- Discomfort from cold can be treated with warmed blankets. There are physiological dangers associated with hypothermia. EBN: *A study (N = 126) found significantly increased comfort and decreased anxiety in clients who used self-controlled warming gowns (Wagner et al, 2006, in Kolcaba, 2014).*
- Use complementary therapies such as doll therapy in clients with dementia to increase comfort and reduce stress. EBN: *In a review of the literature, doll therapy reduced panic, anxiety, and aggression while improving the dining experience and social interaction (Mitchell & O'Donnell, 2013).*
- Address any unmet physical, psychological, emotional, spiritual, and environmental needs when attempting to mediate the behavior of an older client with dementia. EBN: *A case study demonstrated that all*

possible causes for demented older clients' behavior must be considered to maximize comfort (Gallagher & Long, 2011).

- Provide simple massage. CEB: *Simple massage addresses four contexts of holistic comfort (Kolcaba, 2003).* CEB: *A prospective study (N = 52) found that providing massage to nursing home residents with dementia was effective in controlling agitation (Holliday-Welsh et al, 2009).*

C

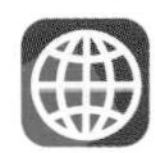

Multicultural

- Identify and clarify cultural language used to describe pain and other discomforts. Expressions of pain and discomfort vary across cultures. CEB: *Clients may interchange words meaning discomfort and pain, may not admit to having pain, may refer to minor discomforts as pain, or may not discuss nonpainful discomforts at all (Kolcaba, 2003).*
- Assess skin for ashy or yellow-brown appearance. CEB: *Black skin appears ashy and brown skin appears yellow-brown when clients have pallor sometimes associated with discomfort (Peters, 2007).*
- Use soap sparingly if the skin is dry. Black skin tends to be dry, and soap exacerbates this condition.
- Encourage and allow clients to practice their own cultural beliefs and recognize the impact that different cultures have on a client's belief about health care, comforting measures, and decision-making. *Hindus believe in reincarnation, which gives them comfort during the dying process. Hindus also believe that physical suffering can lead to spiritual growth (Thrane, 2010).*
- Assess for cultural and religious beliefs when providing care. EB: *In a hermeneutic phenomenological study in six medical-surgical wards in Iran (N = 22), it was found that family members play an important role in the comfort of the client. It was also found that caregivers should allow clients to follow religious and traditional principles to facilitate comfort despite physical constraints (Yousefi et al, 2009).*

Client/Family Teaching and Discharge Planning

- Teach techniques to use when the client is uncomfortable, including relaxation techniques, guided imagery, hand massage, and music therapy. CEB: *Interventions such as progressive muscle relaxation training, guided imagery, and music therapy can effectively decrease the perception of uncomfortable sensations, including pain (Kolcaba, 2003).* CEB: *Families want to learn how to provide comfort measures to their loved ones who are uncomfortable (Kolcaba et al, 2004, in Kolcaba, 2014).*
- At end of life, the dying client is comforted by having a companion. EBN: *A grounded theory study demonstrated the importance of teaching the family of a dying client how to accompany the client on his or her final journey, sharing stories, thoughts, doubts, feelings, and emotions (Martins & Basto, 2011).*
- Instruct the client and family about prescribed medications and complementary therapies that improve comfort (Kolcaba, 2003).
- Teach the client to follow up with the health care provider if discomfort persists. There are many avenues for enhancing comfort (Kolcaba, 2003).
- Encourage clients to use the Internet as a means of providing education to complement medical care for those who may be homebound or unable to attend face-to-face education. CEB: *In a randomized trial with intervention (N = 41), it was found that the Internet was an effective mode for delivering self-care education to older clients with chronic pain (Berman et al, 2009).*

Mental Health

- Encourage clients to use guided imagery techniques. Guided imagery helps distract clients from stressful situations and facilitates relaxation. CEB: *A quasi-experimental study (N = 60) found that clients who listened to a guided imagery compact disk once a day for 10 days had improved comfort and decreased depression, anxiety, and stress over time (Apùstolo & Kolcaba, 2009, in Kolcaba, 2014).*
- Provide psychospiritual support and a comforting environment to enhance comfort during emotional crises. EBN: *A case study demonstrates the importance of reducing stimuli in the environment of clients with dementia (Gallagher & Long, 2011).* CEB: *In a cross-sectional descriptive study (N = 98), it was found that cancer clients had lower comfort levels relating to psychospiritual and environmental comfort than to physical and sociocultural comfort. Improvements in psychospiritual and environmental support will enhance overall comfort (Kim & Kwon, 2007).*
- When nurses attend to the comfort of perioperative clients, the clients' sense of hope for a full recovery increases. EBN: *In a quantitative study with 191 participants, direct and significant relationships were observed between comfort and hope (Seyedfatemi et al, 2014).*

- Providing music and verbal relaxation therapy enhances holistic comfort by reducing anxiety. EBN: *A literature review found that music and verbal relaxation therapy provided reduced chemotherapy-induced anxiety (Lin et al, 2011).*
- Caregivers should not hesitate to use humor when caring for their clients. CEB: *Analysis of two studies found that humor can be comforting and can contribute to a positive experience for both client and caregiver (Kinsman-Dean & Major, 2008).*

REFERENCES

Berman, R., Iris, M., Bode, R., et al. (2009). The effectiveness of an online mind-body intervention for older adults with chronic pain. *The Journal of Pain, 10*(1), 68–79.

Dowd, T., et al. (2007). Comparison of healing touch and coaching on stress and comfort in young college students. *Holistic Nursing Practice, 21*(4), 194–202.

Eide, H., Sibbern, T., & Johannessen, T. (2011). Empathic accuracy of nurses' immediate response to fibromyalgia patients' expressions of negative emotions: an evaluation using interaction analysis. *Journal of Advanced Nursing, 67*(6), 1242–1253.

Gallagher, M., & Long, D. O. (2011). Demystifying behaviors, addressing pain, and maximizing comfort research and practice: partners in care. *J Hospice Palliat Nurs, 13*(2), 71–78.

Holliday-Welsh, D., Gessert, C., & Renier, C. (2009). Massage in the management of agitation in nursing home residents with cognitive impairment. *Geriatric Nursing (New York, N.Y.), 30*(2), 108–117.

Kim, K. S., & Kwon, S. H. (2007). Comfort and quality of life of cancer patients. *Asian Nursing Research, 1*, 125–135.

Kinsman-Dean, R. A., & Major, J. E. (2008). From critical care to comfort care: the sustaining value of humour. *Journal of Clinical Nursing, 17*, 1088–1095.

Kolcaba, K. (2003). *Comfort theory and practice: a holistic vision for health care*. New York: Springer.

Kolcaba, K. (2014). *TheComfortLine.com*. Retrieved Nov 15 from: <www.TheComfortLine.com>.

Lin, M. F., et al. (2011). A randomized controlled trial of the effect of music therapy and verbal relaxation on chemotherapy-induced anxiety. *Journal of Clinical Nursing, 20*, 988–999.

Martins, C., & Basto, M. (2011). Relieving the suffering of end-of-life patients: A Grounded Theory study. *Journal of Hospice and Palliative Nursing, 13*(3), 161–171.

Mitchell, G., & O'Donnell, H. (2013). The therapeutic use of doll therapy in dementia. *The British Journal of Nursing, 22*(6), 329–334.

Peters, J. (2007). Examining and describing skin conditions. *The Journal of Practical Nursing, 34*(8), 39–40, 43, 45.

Seyedfatemi, N., Rafi, F., Rezaei, M., et al. (2014). Comfort and hope in the preanesthesia stage in patients undergoing surgery. *Journal of Perianesthesia Nursing, 29*(3), 213–220.

Thrane, S. (2010). Hindu end of life. *Journal of Hospice and Palliative Nursing, 12*(6), 337–342.

Townsend, C., Bonham, E., Chase, L., et al. (2014). A comparison of still point induction to massage therapy in reducing pain and increasing comfort in chronic pain. *Holistic Nursing Practice, 28*(2), 78–84.

Wagner, D., Byrne, M., & Kolcaba, K. (2006). Effect of comfort warming on preoperative patients. *AORN Journal, 84*(3), 1–13.

Yousefi, H., et al. (2009). Comfort as a basic need in hospitalized patients in Iran: hermeneutic phenomenology study. *Journal of Clinical Nursing, 65*(9), 1891–1898.

Readiness for enhanced Comfort

Lina Daou Boudiab, MSN, RN

NANDA-I

Definition

A pattern of ease, relief, and transcendence in physical, psychospiritual, environmental, and/or social dimensions that is sufficient for well-being and can be strengthened

Defining Characteristics

Expresses desire to enhance comfort; expresses desire to enhance feelings of contentment; expresses desire to enhance relaxation; expresses desire to enhance resolution of complaints

NOC Outcomes (Nursing Outcomes Classification)

Suggested NOC Outcomes

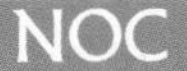

Client Satisfaction: Caring; Symptom Control; Comfort Status; Coping; Hope; Motivation; Pain Control; Participation in Health Care Decisions; Spiritual Health

Example NOC Outcomes with Indicators

Comfort Status as evidenced by the following indicators: Physical well-being/Symptom control/Psychological well-being. (Rate the outcome and indicators of **Comfort Level:** 1 = not at all satisfied, 2 = somewhat satisfied, 3 = moderately satisfied, 4 = very satisfied, 5 = completely satisfied [see Section I].)

Client Outcomes

Client Will (Specify Time Frame)

- Assess current level of comfort as acceptable
- Express the need to achieve an enhanced level of comfort
- Identify strategies to enhance comfort
- Perform appropriate interventions as needed for increased comfort
- Evaluate the effectiveness of interventions at regular intervals
- Maintain an enhanced level of comfort when possible

NIC Interventions (Nursing Interventions Classification)

Suggested NIC Interventions

Calming Technique; Cutaneous Stimulation; Environmental Management; Comfort; Heat/Cold Application; Hope Inspiration; Humor; Meditation Facilitation; Music Therapy; Pain Management; Presence; Simple Guided Imagery; Simple Massage; Simple Relaxation Therapy; Spiritual Growth Facilitation; Therapeutic Play; Therapeutic Touch; Touch; Distraction

Example NIC Activities—Spiritual Growth Facilitation

Assist the client with identifying barriers and attitudes that hinder growth or self-discovery; Assist the client to explore beliefs as related to healing of the body, mind, and spirit; Model healthy relating and reasoning skills

Nursing Interventions and *Rationales*

- Assess clients' comfort needs and current level of comfort in various contexts, as outlined in Kolcaba's (2003) Comfort theory and practice: physical, psychospiritual, sociocultural, and environmental. CEB: *Assessing comfort needs helps develop holistic, client-centered comfort interventions, while establishing a baseline helps evaluate their effectiveness by comparing comfort levels after each intervention to the previous baseline (Kolcaba, 2003).*
- Educate clients about the various contexts of comfort and help them understand that enhanced comfort is a desirable, positive, and achievable goal. CEB: *Human beings strive to have their basic comfort needs met, with comfort being more than just the absence of pain (Kolcaba, 2003). Having clients view comfort more holistically may be especially helpful when total relief and ease of symptoms may not be achievable, and the goal of health care becomes helping clients transcend their comfort needs (Kolcaba, 2003).*
- Enhance feelings of trust between the client and the health care provider in order to maintain an effective and therapeutic relationship. CEB: *To attain the highest comfort level, a client must be able to trust the nurse (Hupcey et al, 2000).* EBN: *Trust is an essential element in the nurse-client relationship that is fostered through caring attitudes, availability, respect, empathy, sensitivity to client needs, competence, and good communication (Dinç & Gastmans, 2013).*
- Maintain an open and effective communication with clients and keep them informed about their health, their plan of care, and their environment. EBN: *Evidence suggests that sharing of information genuinely and empathetically with adult oncology clients and encouraging them to ask questions strengthen the nurse-client relationship and empower clients to reach out to nurses for emotional support (Joanna Briggs Institute, 2011), and it enhances their psychospiritual comfort.* EBN: *Communicating to hospitalized cardiothoracic clients the source of sounds heard or expected to be heard around the unit, such as alarms, staff conversations, and rolling carts alleviated their anxiety and enhanced relaxation (Mackrill et al, 2013), hence promoting their environmental comfort.*
- Implement comfort rounds that regularly assess for clients' comfort needs. EBN: *Regular 1-hour or 2-hour rounds that address pain, positioning, personal needs, and environment were found to increase client satisfaction, decrease call light usage, and promote safety by decreasing fall rates (Ciccu-Moore et al, 2014; Chu, 2014).*
- Collaborate with other health care professionals, such as health care providers, pharmacists, social workers, chaplains, occupational and physical therapists, dietitians, among others, in planning interventions that address comfort needs in various contexts: physical, psychospiritual, sociocultural, and environmental.

- Educate clients about and encourage the use of various integrative therapies and modalities to provide options that enhance comfort, beyond the traditional plan of care. Institute of Medicine (IOM) AND PAIN—Examples of such modalities are listed below:
  - Therapeutic massage and touch therapy. **EBN:** *Massage and touch therapy have been found to promote comfort in clients with dementia by decreasing anxiety and agitation (Battaglini, 2014). There is evidence to support recommending massage to clients with subacute and chronic back pain, mechanical neck pain, and labor pain, as well as to decrease anxiety and blood pressure and to improve quality of life in clients with HIV/AIDS (D'Arcy, 2014). Furthermore, case studies on using the M-technique (M standing for manual), a structured light stroking technique, seemed to decrease agitation and pain in palliative care clients and promote their and their families' comfort (Roberts & Campbell, 2011).*
  - Guided imagery. **EBN:** *Guided imagery was also effective in improving chronic tension headaches and body pain, as well as promoting overall mental health and energy level (Read, 2013).*
  - Mindfulness and mindfulness-based interventions such as mindfulness-based stress reduction (MBSR), mantra repetition (silent repetition of a sacred word), mindfulness meditation, and mindful breathing and walking, among others. Since the original research by Kabat-Zinn, founder of MBSR, and colleagues established the effectiveness of mindfulness in helping clients manage chronic pain and improving body image and other symptoms, including anxiety and depression (Kabat-Zinn, Lipworth, & Burney, 1985), mindfulness-based interventions have been used to promote physical and psychospiritual comfort. **EB:** *A study of MBSR in cancer clients concluded that mindfulness promotes a sense of calmness, inner peace, and personal and spiritual growth (Labellea et al, 2014), while a small randomized controlled trial found MBSR to be effective in treating chronic insomnia (Gross et al, 2011).* **EBN:** *Mantra repetition is found to decrease posttraumatic stress disorder (PTSD) symptoms and increase sense of well-being in veterans, when added to their traditional PTSD treatment plan (Bormann et al, 2014).*
  - Energy therapy or biofield therapy such as healing touch, therapeutic touch, and reiki. Biofield therapy seems to be promising in promoting comfort and relaxation, but more sound and systematic research is needed to build a strong body of evidence. **EBN/EB:** *Healing touch has been found effective as an adjunct therapy in relieving anxiety and depression (Harlow, 2013), as well as symptoms of PTSD when coupled with guided imagery in returning active military exposed to combat (Jain et al, 2012).* **EBN:** *Biofield therapy strengthens the immune system, decreases stress, and allows the body to heal. It can be integrated in the care of cancer clients in various settings for relaxation and symptom management, as well as in those with musculoskeletal and joint pain, agitation and dementia, and other chronic conditions (Gonella et al, 2014).*
  - Acupuncture and auricular acupuncture. **EB:** *There is strong evidence that acupuncture is effective in alleviating nausea and vomiting, headache, and back and neck pain (Rathnayake, 2014). A study of acupuncture in women in later stages of pregnancy concluded that the modality decreased low back and pelvic pain and increased function (Pennick & Liddle, 2013), while another found that it improved pain and stiffness in clients with fibromyalgia (Deare et al, 2013).* **EB:** *The National Acupuncture Detox Association five-point ear acupuncture protocol has been effective in reducing cravings and withdrawal symptoms associated with substance abuse. Growing research suggests it may be promising as well for pain relief, promotion of comfort and relaxation, and decrease in PTSD symptoms in veterans.*
  - Aromatherapy
  - Music
  - Other mind-body therapies. **EB:** *The most common therapies used were meditation, imagery, and yoga. Research demonstrating the connection between the mind and body has therefore increased interest in the potential use of these therapies (Wolsko et al, 2004).* **EBN:** *Meditation has been shown to reduce anxiety, relieve pain, decrease depression, enhance mood and self-esteem, decrease stress, and generally improve clinical symptoms (Bonadonna, 2003). A review of clinical trials for meditation and massage used in end of life found that there was a significant relationship between meditation and pain reduction in the two studies that assessed pain (Lafferty et al, 2006).*
- Foster and instill hope in clients whenever possible. **EBN:** *A study of clients undergoing surgery in the preanesthesia stage found a strong correlation between hope and comfort (Seyedfatemi et al, 2014).* See the care plan for **Hopelessness.**
- Provide opportunities for and enhance spiritual care activities. The need for comfort and reassurance may be perceived as spiritual needs. To meet these needs, nurses engaged in interaction when they comforted and assured clients. Participants also identified absolution as a spiritual need, and there is evidence

that forgiveness may bring one feelings of joy, peace, and elation, and a sense of renewed self-worth (Narayanasomy et al, 2004). Individuals who practiced spiritual meditation were found to have a greater increase in pain tolerance (Wachholtz & Pargament, 2008).

▲ Enhance social support and family involvement. EBN: *Methods to help terminally ill clients and their families transition from cure to comfort care included spending an increased amount of time with one's family, appointing one close friend to act as a contact person for other friends, and establishing an email listserv for updates of a client's status and care (Duggleby & Berry, 2005).* Promote participation in creative arts and activity programs. CEBN: *A creative arts program for caregivers of cancer clients was shown to decrease anxiety, and positive emotions were expressed (Walsh et al, 2004). The use of an individualized music protocol program by older women was shown to promote and maintain sleep (Johnson, 2003).*

▲ Encourage clients to use health information technology (HIT) as needed. Client services can now include management of medications, symptoms, emotional support, health education, and health information (Moody, 2005). EBN: *In this study, clients experienced significantly lower dimensions of pain and discomfort with nursing intervention via telephone (Franzen et al, 2009).*

- Evaluate the effectiveness of all interventions at regular intervals and adjust therapies as necessary. It is important for nurses to determine comfort and pain management goals because comfort goals will change with circumstances. Ask questions and ask them frequently, such as, "How is your comfort?" Establish guidelines for frequency of assessment and document responses, noting whether goals are being met (Kolcaba, 2003). EB: *A comprehensive palliative care project was conducted at 11 sites. The interdisciplinary review process built trust, endorsed creativity, and ultimately resulted in better meeting the needs of clients, families, and the community (London et al, 2005). Evaluation must be planned for, ongoing, and systematic. Evaluation demonstrates caring and responsibility on the part of the nurse (Wilkinson & VanLeuven, 2007).*

Geriatric

- Refer to above interventions for geriatric interventions.

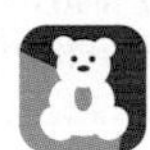

Pediatric

- Assess and evaluate child's level of comfort at frequent intervals. Comfort needs should be individually assessed and planned for. With assessment of pain in children, it is best to use input from the parents or a primary care provider. Use only accepted scales for standardized pain assessment (Remke & Chrastek, 2007).
- Skin-to-skin contact (SSC) and selection of the most effective method improves the comfort of newborns during routine blood draws. EB: *Premature infants who received skin-to-skin contact demonstrated a decrease in pain reaction during heel lancing (Castral et al, 2008).*
- Adjust the environment as needed to enhance comfort. Environmental comfort measures include maintaining orderliness; quiet; minimizing furniture; special attention to temperature, light and sound, color, and landscape (Kolcaba & DeMarco, 2005).
- Encourage parental presence whenever possible. The same basic principles for managing pain in adults and children apply to neonates. In addition to other comfort measures, parental presence should be encouraged whenever possible (Pasero, 2004). EBN: *This study reported the effects of co-residence and caregiving on the parents of children dying with AIDS. Although parents who did more caregiving did experience anxiety, insomnia, and fatigue, the caregiving experiences for many parents gave them an opportunity to fulfill their perceived duty as parents before their child died. This in turn resulted in better physical and emotional health outcomes (Kespichayawattana & VanLandingham, 2003).*
- Promote use of alternative comforting strategies such as positioning, presence, massage, spiritual care, music therapy, art therapy, and story-telling to enhance comfort when needed. In addition to oral sucrose, other comfort measures should be used to alleviate pain such as swaddling, skin-to-skin contact with mother, nursing, rocking, and holding (Pasero, 2004). EBN: *Building on the belief that parents are the primary care providers and health care resource for families, the blended infant massage-parenting program is effective for both mother and infant (Porter & Porter, 2004).* EBN: *In this study, focus groups were conducted with Moroccan pediatric oncology nurses and health care providers to better understand how pain management was achieved in children with cancer. When no medication was available to relieve pain, other techniques were used to comfort clients. These included using cold therapy, being present, holding a child's hand, using distraction techniques, playing with the child, story-telling, and encouraging parental engagement activities (McCarthy et al, 2004).* EB: *In a study that examined the effects of music on pain in a pediatric burn unit during nursing procedures, the use of music during procedures reduced pain*

C

(Whitehead-Pleaux et al, 2007). EBN: *A talk-and-touch intervention by the mothers of infants in the preanesthesia care unit found that 62% of the mothers thought that the intervention made a difference in the pain the infant experienced and 73% thought that talk and touch decreased their infant's distress (Rennick et al, 2011).*

- Support the child's spirituality. CEB: *Children are born with an intrinsic spiritual essence that can be enhanced. Spirituality promotes a sense of hope, comfort, and strength and creates a sense of being loved and nurtured by a higher power (Elkins & Cavendish, 2004).*

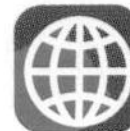

Multicultural

- Identify cultural beliefs, values, lifestyles, practices, and problem-solving strategies when assessing clients. Cultural sensitivity must always be a component of pain assessment. The nurse must remember that pain expression will vary among clients and that variation must also be acknowledged within cultures (Andrews & Boyle, 2003). EBN: *In a qualitative study that identified issues in pain management, cultural beliefs were cited as impediments or barriers to pain management; for example, some Moroccan health care providers thought illness-related pain was inevitable, that suffering was normal, and that it had to be endured, especially by boys (McCarthy et al, 2004).* EBN: *In a qualitative study, Muslim clients, particularly Shiites, expressed feeling more comfortable when they were allowed to practice their religious beliefs (Yousefi et al, 2009).*
- Enhance cultural knowledge by actively seeking out information regarding different cultural and ethnic groups. *Cultural knowledge is the process of actively seeking information about different cultural and ethnic groups such as their world views, health conditions, health practices, use of home remedies or self-medication, barriers to health care, and risk-taking or health-seeking behaviors (Institute of Medicine, 2002).*

▲ Recognize the impact of culture on communication styles and techniques. Communication and culture are closely intertwined, and communication is the way culture is transmitted and preserved. It influences how feelings are expressed, decisions are made, and what verbal and nonverbal expressions are acceptable. *By the age of 5, cultural patterns of communication can be identified in children (Giger & Davidhizar, 2004).*

- Provide culturally competent care to clients from different cultural groups. Cultural competency requires health care providers act appropriately in the context of daily interactions with people who are different from themselves. Health care providers need to honor and respect the beliefs, interpersonal styles, attitudes, and behaviors of others. This level of cultural awareness requires health care providers to refrain from forming stereotypes and judgments based on one's own cultural framework (Institute of Medicine, 2002). EBN: *The findings from a review of two studies of Japanese and American women suggest that although there were common ethical concerns between the two cultures, the cultural context of the underlying values may create very different meanings and result in different nursing practices (Wros et al, 2004).*

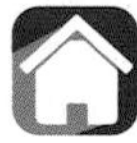

Home Care

- The nursing interventions described for Readiness for enhanced **Comfort** may be used with clients in the home care setting. When needed, adaptations can be made to meet the needs of specific clients, families, and communities.

▲ Make appropriate referrals to other organizations or health care providers as needed to enhance comfort. Referrals should have merit, be practical, timely, individualized, coordinated, and mutually agreed upon by all involved (Hunt, 2005).

▲ Promote an interdisciplinary approach to home care. Members of the interdisciplinary team who provide specialized care to enhance comfort can include the health care provide, physical therapist, occupational therapist, nutritionist, music therapist, and social worker, among others (Stanhope & Lancaster, 2006).

- Evaluate regularly if enhanced comfort is attainable in the home care setting. Home health agencies monitor client outcomes closely. Evaluation is an ongoing process and is essential for the provision of quality care (Stanhope & Lancaster, 2006).
- Use music therapy at home. EBN: *The use of music 30 minutes before peak agitation in clients with dementia demonstrated that their mean pain levels after listening to music were significantly lower than before the music intervention (Park, 2010).*

Client/Family Teaching and Discharge Planning

- Teach client how to regularly assess levels of comfort.
- Instruct client that a variety of interventions may be needed at any given time to enhance comfort.
- Help clients understand that enhanced comfort is an achievable goal.

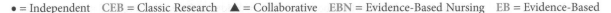

- Teach techniques to enhance comfort as needed.
- ▲ When needed, empower clients to seek out other health professionals as members of the interdisciplinary team to assist with comforting measures and techniques.
- Encourage self-care activities and continued self-evaluation of achieved comfort levels to ensure enhanced comfort is maintained.

C

REFERENCES

Andrews, M., & Boyle, J. (2003). *Transcultural concepts in nursing* (4th ed.). Philadelphia: Lippincott Williams & Wilkins.

Battaglini, E. (2014). Dementia: Massage and Touch. *Joanna Briggs Institute [Evidence Summaries]*. Retrieved from: <www.Joannabriggs.org>.

Bonadonna, R. (2003). Meditation's impact on chronic illness. *Holistic Nursing Practice*, *17*(6), 309–319.

Bormann, J. E., Oman, D., Walter, K. H., et al. (2014). Mindful Attention Increases and Mediates Psychological Outcomes Following Mantram Repetition Practice in Veterans with Posttraumatic Stress Disorder. *Medical Care*, *52*(12 (Suppl. 5)), S13–S18.

Castral, T., et al. (2008). The effects of skin-to-skin contact during acute pain in preterm newborns. *European Journal of Pain*, *12*(4), 464–471.

Chu, V. (2014). Nursing Rounds: Clinician Information. *Joanna Briggs Institute [Evidence Summaries]*. Retrieved from: <www.Joannabriggs.org>.

Ciccu-Moore, R., Grant, F., Niven, B., et al. (2014). Care and comfort rounds: Improving standards. *Nursing Management—UK*, *20*(9), 18–23.

D'Arcy, M. (2014). Massage Therapy: Various Conditions. *Joanna Briggs Institute [Evidence Summaries]*. Retrieved from: <www.Joannabriggs.org>.

Deare, J. C., Zheng, Z., Xue, C. C. L., et al. (2013). Acupuncture for treating fibromyalgia (Review). *The Cochrane Library*. Retrieved from: <http://www.thecochranelibrary.com>.

Dinç, L., & Gastmans, C. (2013). Trust in nurse-patient relationships: a literature review. *Nursing Ethics*, *20*(5), 501–516. [Epub 2013 Feb 20].

Duggleby, W., & Berry, P. (2005). Transitions and shifting goals of care for palliative patients and their families. *Clinical Journal of Oncology Nursing*, *9*(4), 425–428.

Elkins, M., & Cavendish, R. (2004). Developing a plan for pediatric spiritual care. *Holistic Nursing Practice*, *18*(4), 179–184.

Franzen, C., et al. (2009). Injured road users' health-related quality of life after telephone intervention: a randomized controlled trial. *Journal of Clinical Nursing*, *18*(1), 108–116.

Giger, J., & Davidhizar, R. (2004). *Transcultural nursing: assessment and intervention* (4th ed.). St. Louis: Mosby.

Gonella, S., Garrino, L., & Dimonte, G. (2014). Biofield Therapies and Cancer-Related Symptoms: A Review. *Clinical Journal of Oncology Nursing*, *18*(5), 568–576.

Gross, C. R., Kreitzer, M. J., Reilly-Spong, M., et al. (2011). Mindfulness-based stress reduction versus pharmacotherapy for chronic primary insomnia: a randomized controlled clinical trial. *Explore (New York, N.Y.)*, *7*(2), 76–87.

Harlow, C. R. (2013). *A critical analysis of healing touch for symptoms of depression and anxiety*. (Unpublished doctoral dissertation). University of Arizona: Tucson, AZ.

Hunt, R. (2005). *Introduction to community-based nursing* (3rd ed.). Philadelphia: Lippincott.

Hupcey, J. E., Penrod, J., & Morse, J. M. (2000). Establishing and maintaining trust during acute care hospitalizations, including commentary by Robinson CA. *Scholarly Inquiry for Nursing Practice*, *14*(3), 227–248.

Institute of Medicine. (2002). *Speaking of health*. Washington, DC: National Academies Press.

Jain, S., McMahon, G. F., Hasen, P., et al. (2012). Healing Touch with Guided Imagery for PTSD in returning active duty military: a randomized controlled trial. *Military Medicine*, *177*(9), 1015–1021.

Joanna Briggs Institute. (2011). Effective communication between registered nurses and adult oncology patients in inpatient settings. *Best Practice: Evidence-based information sheets for health professionals*, *15*(1), 1–4.

Johnson, J. (2003). The use of music to promote sleep in older women. *Journal of Community Health Nursing*, *20*, 27–35.

Kabat-Zinn, J., Lipworth, L., & Burney, R. (1985). The clinical use of mindfulness meditation for the self-regulation of chronic pain. *Journal of Behavioral Medicine*, *8*(2), 163–190.

Kespichayawattana, J., & VanLandingham, M. (2003). Effects of coresidence and caregiving on health of Thai parents of adult children with AIDS. *Journal of Nursing Scholarship: an Official Publication of Sigma Theta Tau International Honor Society of Nursing/Sigma Theta Tau*, *35*(3), 217–224.

Kolcaba, K. (2003). *Comfort theory and practice*. New York: Springer.

Kolcaba, K., & DeMarco, M. (2005). Comfort theory and application to pediatric nursing. *Pediatric Nursing*, *31*(3), 187–194.

Labellea, L. E., Lawlor-Savagea, L., Campbella, T. S., et al. (2014). Does self-report mindfulness mediate the effect of Mindfulness-Based Stress Reduction (MBSR) on spirituality and posttraumatic growth in cancer patients? *The Journal of Positive Psychology*. Retrieved from: <http://dx.doi.org/10.1080/17439760.2014.927902>.

Lafferty, W., et al. (2006). Evaluating CAM treatment at the end of life: a review of clinical trials for massage and meditation. *Complementary Therapies in Medicine*, *14*(2), 100–112.

London, M., et al. (2005). Evaluation of a comprehensive, adaptable, life-affirming, longitudinal palliative care project. *Journal of Palliative Medicine*, *8*(6), 1214–1225.

Mackrill, J., Cain, R., Jennings, P., et al. (2013). Sound source information to improve cardiothoracic patients' comfort. *British Journal of Nursing*, *22*(7), 387–393.

McCarthy, P., et al. (2004). Managing children's cancer pain in Morocco. *Journal of Nursing Scholarship*, *36*(1), 11–15.

Moody, L. (2005). E-health web portals: delivering holistic healthcare and making home the point of care. *Holistic Nursing Practice*, *19*(4), 156–160.

Narayanasomy, A., et al. (2004). Responses to the spiritual needs of older people. *Journal of Advanced Nursing*, *48*(1), 6–16.

Park, H. (2010). Effects of music on pain for home-dwelling persons with dementia. *Pain Management Nursing*, *11*(3), 141–147.

Pasero, C. (2004). Pain relief for neonates. *The American Journal of Nursing*, *104*(5), 44–47.

Pennick, V., & Liddle, S. D. (2013). Interventions for preventing and treating pelvic and back pain in pregnancy (Review). *The Cochrane Library*. Retrieved from: <http://www.thecochranelibrary.com>.

Porter, L., & Porter, B. (2004). A blended infant massage-parenting enhancement program for recovering substance abusing mothers. *Pediatric Nursing*, *30*(5), 363–401.

Rathnayake, T. (2014). Acupuncture: Effectiveness Review. *Joanna Briggs Institute [Evidence Summaries]*. Retrieved from: <www.Joannabriggs.org>.

Read, S. (2013). Chronic pain: Nursing interventions. *Joanna Briggs Institute [Evidence Summaries]*. Retrieved from: <www.Joannabriggs.org>.

Remke, S., & Chrastek, J. (2007). Improving care in the home for children with palliative care needs. *Home Healthcare Nurse, 25*(1), 45–51.

Rennick, J., et al. (2011). Mothers' experiences of touch and talk nursing intervention to optimise pain management in the PICU: a qualitative study. *Intensive and Critical Care Nursing, 27*(3), 151–157.

Roberts, K., & Campbell, H. (2011). Using the M technique as therapy for patients at the end of life: Two case studies. *International Journal of Palliative Nursing, 17*(3), 114–118.

Seyedfatemi, N., Rafii, F., Rezaei, M., et al. (2014). Comfort and hope in the preanesthesia stage in patients undergoing surgery. *Journal of Perianesthesia Nursing, 29*(3), 213–220.

Stanhope, M., & Lancaster, J. (2006). *Foundation of nursing in the community* (2nd ed.). St. Louis: Mosby.

Wachholtz, A., & Pargament, K. (2008). Migraines and meditation: does spirituality matter? *Journal of Behavioral Medicine, 31*(4), 351–366.

Walsh, S., Martin, S., & Schmidt, L. (2004). Testing the efficacy of a creative-arts intervention with family caregivers of patients with cancer. *Journal of Nursing Scholarship, 36*(3), 214–219.

Whitehead-Pleaux, A. M., et al. (2007). Exploring the effects of music therapy on pediatric pain: phase 1. *Journal of Music Therapy, 46*(3), 217–241.

Wilkinson, J., & VanLeuven, K. (2007). *Fundamentals of nursing*. Philadelphia: FA Davis.

Wolsko, P., et al. (2004). Use of mind-body medical therapies. *Journal of General Internal Medicine, 19*, 43–50.

Wros, P., Doutrich, D., & Izumi, S. (2004). Ethical concerns: comparison of values from two cultures. *Nursing and Health Sciences, 6*(2), 131–140.

Yousefi, H., et al. (2009). Comfort as a basic need in hospitalized patients in Iran: a hermeneutic phenomenology study. *Journal of Advanced Nursing, 65*(9), 1891–1898.

Readiness for enhanced Communication

Stacey M. Carroll, PhD, ANP-BC, and Suzanne White, MSN, RN, PHCNS-BC

NANDA-I

Definition

A pattern of exchanging information and ideas with others that can be strengthened

Defining Characteristics

Expresses desire to enhance communication

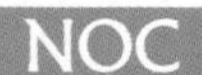

NOC (Nursing Outcomes Classification)

Suggested NOC Outcomes

Communication; Communication: Expressive, Receptive

Example NOC Outcome with Indicators

Communication as evidenced by the following indicators: Use of spoken language/Use of written language/Acknowledgment of messages received/Exchanges messages accurately with others. (Rate the outcome and indicators of **Communication:** 1 = severely compromised, 2 = substantially compromised, 3 = moderately compromised, mildly compromised, 5 = not compromised [see Section I].)

Client Outcomes

Client Will (Specify Time Frame)

- Express willingness to enhance communication
- Demonstrate ability to speak or write a language
- Form words, phrases, and language
- Express thoughts and feelings
- Use and interpret nonverbal cues appropriately
- Express satisfaction with ability to share information and ideas with others

NIC (Nursing Interventions Classification)

Suggested NIC Interventions

Active Listening; Communication Enhancement: Hearing Deficit; Communication Enhancement: Speech Deficit

C

Example NIC Activities—Communication Enhancement: Hearing Deficit

Listen attentively; Allow patient adequate time to process communication and respond; Verify what was said or written using patient's response before continuing

Nursing Interventions and *Rationales*

- • Establish a therapeutic nurse-client relationship: provide appropriate education for the client, demonstrate caring by being present to the client. CEB: *Clients who were nonvocal and ventilated appreciated nursing care that was delivered in an individualized, caring manner (Carroll, 2007).*
- • Assess the client's readiness to communicate, using an individualized approach, and avoid making assumptions regarding the client's preferred communication method. EBN: *Using varied communication approaches improved communication efficiency and client engagement (Radtke et al, 2011).* EB: *Increased numbers of communication methods decreased fear and anger in those who were mechanically ventilated (Khalaila et al, 2011).*
- • Assess the client's literacy level so information can be tailored accordingly. *The Rapid Estimate of Adult Literacy in Medicine—Short Form (REALM SF) provides a quick valid assessment (AHRQ, 2014).*
- • Use these practical guidelines to assist in communication: Listen attentively and provide a comfortable environment for communicating; slow down and listen to the client's story; use augmentative and alternative communication methods (e.g., lip reading, communication boards, writing, body language, and computer/electronic communication devices) as appropriate; repeat instructions if necessary; limit the amount of information given; have the client "teach back" to confirm understanding; avoid asking, "Do you understand?"; be respectful, caring, and sensitive. EB: *Multiple augmentative and alternative communication methods, applied with an individualized and creative approach, aid in facilitating communication (Radtke et al, 2011).*
- ▲ Use interdisciplinary collaboration to ensure continuity of enhanced communication. EB: *Effective interdisciplinary collaboration and follow-up was recommended when working with clients with significant communication impairments after having a stroke (Jones et al, 2013).*
- ▲ Refer couples in maladjusted relationships for psychosocial intervention and social support to strengthen communication; consider nurse specialists. EB: *Being part of a strong dyad may serve as a buffering factor regarding posttraumatic stress related to a cancer diagnosis (Brosseau et al, 2011).*
- • Consider using music to enhance communication between a client who is dying and his or her family. CEB: *In clients with communication difficulties, music therapy resulted in improvement in communication (Leow et al, 2010).*
- • Encourage clients with aphasia to sing. EB: *Participation in a community choir led by a neurologic music therapist resulted in qualitatively identified improvement/changes in communication among clients with aphasia (Tamplin et al, 2013).*
- • See care plan for Impaired verbal **Communication.**

Pediatric

- • All individuals involved in the care and everyday life of children with learning difficulties need to have a collaborative approach to communication. EBN: *Collaboration in tasks requires the formation of personal relationships based on mutual trust and respect (Callery & Milnes, 2012).*
- • See care plan for Impaired verbal **Communication.**

Geriatric

- ▲ Assess for hearing and vision impairments, and make appropriate referrals for hearing aids. EB: *Healthy People 2020 recommends early identification of people with hearing and vision loss (Healthy People 2020, 2014).*

C

- Use touch if culturally acceptable when communicating with older clients and their families. EBN: *Touch has a calming effect on a client who may be frightened due to difficulty with communication (Grossbach et al, 2011).*
- Consider singing during caregiving of clients with dementia. EB: *When professional caregivers sang to clients with dementia during care, enhanced communication and cooperation resulted (Hammar et al, 2011).*
- See care plan for Impaired verbal **Communication.**

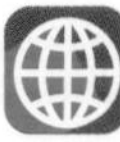

Multicultural

- See care plan for Impaired verbal **Communication.**

Home Care

- The interventions described previously may be used in home care.
- See care plan for Impaired verbal **Communication.**

Client/Family Teaching and Discharge Planning

- See care plan for Impaired verbal **Communication.**

REFERENCES

See impaired verbal **Communication** for additional references.

Agency for Healthcare Research and Quality (AHRQ). (2014). *Health literacy measurement tools*, Retrieved September 10, 2014, from: <http://www.ahrq.gov/professionals/quality-patient-safety/quality-resources/tools/literacy/index.html>.

Brosseau, D. C., McDonald, M. J., & Stephen, J. E. (2011). The moderating effect of relationship quality in partner secondary traumatic stress among couples coping with cancer. *Families, Systems and Health: The Journal of Collaborative Family Healthcare, 29*(2), 114–126.

Callery, P., & Milnes, L. (2012). Communication between nurses, children and their parents in asthma review consultations. *Journal of Clinical Nursing, 21*(11/12), 1641–1650.

Carroll, S. M. (2007). Silent, slow lifeworld: the communication experiences of nonvocal ventilated patients. *Qualitative Health Research, 17*(9), 1165–1177.

Grossbach, I., Stranberg, S., & Chlan, L. (2011). Promoting effective communication for patients receiving mechanical ventilation. *Critical Care Nurse, 31*(3), 46–61.

Hammar, L. M., et al. (2011). Communicating through caregiver singing during morning care situations in dementia care. *Scandinavian Journal of Caring Sciences, 25*, 160–168.

Healthy People 2020. *Hearing and other sensory or communication disorders*, Retrieved September 12, 2014, from: <www.healthypeople.gov/2020/topicsobjectives2020/overviewaspx?topicid=20>.

Jones, C., et al. (2013). Alleviating psychosocial issues for individuals with communication impairments and their families following stroke: a case series of interdisciplinary assessment and intervention. *Neurorehabilitation, 32*(2), 351–358.

Khalaila, R., et al. (2011). Communication difficulties and psychoemotional distress in patients receiving mechanical ventilation. *American Journal of Critical Care, 20*(6), 470–479.

Leow, M., Drury, V., & Hong, P. (2010). The experience and expectations of terminally ill patients receiving music therapy in the palliative setting: a systematic review. *JBI Library of Systematic Reviews, 8*(27), 1088–1111.

Radtke, J. V., et al. (2011). Listening to the voiceless patient: case reports in assisted communication in the intensive care unit. *Journal of Palliative Medicine, 14*(6), 791–795.

Tamplin, J., et al. (2013). "Stroke a Chord": the effect of singing in a community choir on mood and social engagement for people living with aphasia following a stroke. *Neurorehabilitation, 32*(4), 929–941.

Impaired verbal Communication

Stacey M. Carroll, PhD, ANP-BC, and Suzanne White, MSN, RN, PHCNS-BC

NANDA-I

Definition

Decreased, delayed, or absent ability to receive, process, transmit, and/or use a system of symbols

Defining Characteristics

Absence of eye contact; difficulty comprehending communication; difficulty expressing thoughts verbally (e.g., aphasia, dysphasia, apraxia, dyslexia); difficulty forming sentences; difficulty forming words (e.g., aphonia, dyslalia, dysarthria); difficulty in selective attending; difficulty in use of body expressions; difficulty in use of facial expressions; difficulty maintaining communication; difficulty speaking; difficulty verbalizing; disoriented to person; disoriented to place; disoriented to time; does not speak; dyspnea; inability to speak; inability to speak language of caregiver; inability to use body expressions; inability to use facial expressions;

inappropriate verbalization; partial visual deficit; refusal to speak; slurred speech stuttering; total visual deficit

Related Factors (r/t)

Absence of significant other; alteration in development; alteration if perception; alteration in self concept; central nervous system impairment; cultural incongruence; emotional disturbance; environmental barrier; insufficient information; insufficient stimuli; low self-esteem; oropharyngeal defect; physical barrier (e.g., tracheostomy, intubation); physiological condition (e.g., brain tumor, decreased circulation to brain, weakened musculoskeletal system); psychotic disorder; treatment regimen; vulnerability

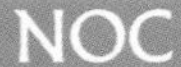

NOC (Nursing Outcomes Classification)

Suggested NOC Outcomes

Communication; Communication: Expressive, Receptive

Example NOC Outcome with Indicators

Communication as evidenced by the following indicators: Use of spoken and written language/Acknowledgment of messages received/Exchanges messages accurately with others. (Rate the outcome and indicators of **Communication:** 1 = severely compromised, 2 = substantially compromised, 3 = moderately compromised, 4 = mildly compromised, 5 = not compromised [see Section I].)

Client Outcomes

Client Will (Specify Time Frame)

- Use effective communication techniques
- Use alternative methods of communication effectively
- Demonstrate congruency of verbal and nonverbal behavior
- Demonstrate understanding even if not able to speak
- Express desire for social interactions

NIC (Nursing Interventions Classification)

Suggested NIC Interventions

Active Listening; Communication Enhancement: Hearing Deficit; Communication Enhancement: Speech Deficit

Example NIC Activities—Communication Enhancement: Hearing Deficit

Listen attentively; Allow client adequate time to process communication and respond; Verify what was said or written using client's response before continuing

Nursing Interventions and *Rationales*

- Use a comprehensive nursing assessment to determine the language spoken, cultural considerations, literacy level, cognitive level, and use of glasses and/or hearing aids. EBN: *Language barriers, low literacy, and lack of understanding are barriers to effective communication (Taylor et al, 2013).*
- Determine client's own perception of communication difficulties and potential solutions when possible. *In clients with aphasia, nurses should avoid making assumptions regarding communication (Borthwick, 2012).* EB: *The Communication Confidence Rating Scale for Aphasia (CCRSA) was found to be an effective tool for assessment of the self-report of communication confidence among clients with aphasia (Babbitt et al, 2011).*
- Involve a familiar person when attempting to communicate with a client who has difficulty with communication, if accepted by the client. EB: *A competent communication partner—family member or not—reduced stress in the client by facilitating effective communication (Laasko et al, 2011).*
- Listen carefully. Validate verbal and nonverbal expressions particularly when dealing with pain and use appropriate scales for pain when appropriate. EB/EBN: *The critical care pain observation tool and the*

C

behavioral pain scale are valid and reliable options for use in clients who are nonverbal (Aust, 2013; Flynn Makic, 2013).

- Use appropriate scales to assess communication and behavior in clients who are nonvocal and mechanically ventilated. EBN: *Although further testing is needed, preliminary research shows that the revised Communication Interaction Behavior Instrument scale has good face validity and shows good interrater reliability for use with older adults who are ventilated and nonvocal (Nilsen et al, 2014).*
- Use therapeutic communication techniques: speak in a well-modulated voice, use simple communication, maintain eye contact at the client's level, get the client's attention before speaking, and show concern for the client. EBN: *Effective communication entails involving clients, being sensitive to client needs, and ensuring client understanding (O'Hagan et al, 2014).*
- Avoid ignoring the client with verbal impairment; be engaged and provide meaningful responses to client concerns. Place call light or bell within reach of client who cannot verbally call for help. *Safety is at risk when communication barriers are present (Giammarino et al, 2012).* EBN: *Ignoring clients was found to be a negative communication strategy (O'Hagan et al, 2014).*
- Use touch as appropriate. *Touch has a calming effect on a client who may be frightened due to difficulty with communication (Grossbach et al, 2011).*
- Use presence: spend time with the client, allow time for responses, and make the call light readily available. *Client-centered care involves respect, communication, and comfort (Bechtold & Fredericks, 2014).*
- Explain all health care procedures. CEBN: *Clients who were nonvocal and ventilated were attuned to everything occurring around them, and they appreciated explanations from the nurse (Carroll, 2007).*
- Be persistent in deciphering what the client is saying, and do not pretend to understand when the message is unclear. *In clients with aphasia, nurses should allow the client extra time to communicate and should not interrupt the client (Borthwick, 2012).* CEBN: *Persons who were nonvocal and ventilated appreciated persistence on the nurses' part with respect to being understood, and found it bothersome when others pretended to understand them (Carroll, 2007).*
- Use an individualized and creative multidisciplinary approach to augmentative and alternative communication (AAC) assistance and other interventions. *Ensure the choice of AAC is driven by clients' communication needs rather than by the device (Light & McNaughton, 2013).* EB: *A combination of high-technology (with voice output) and low-technology options improved communication efficiency (Radtke et al, 2011).* EB: *AAC improved communication among those with intellectual disabilities (Hagan & Thompson, 2014).*
- Use consistent nursing staff for those with communication impairments. CEBN: *Consistent nursing care increased client-nurse communication and decreased client powerlessness (Carroll, 2007).*

▲ Consult communication specialists from various disciplines as appropriate. Speech language pathologists, audiologists, and interpreters provide comprehensive communication assistance for those with impaired communication. *Lip reading therapists (LRTs) are proficient lip readers who determine what a nonvocal client is mouthing and then verbalize the client's words verbatim to others, in order to facilitate communication (Carroll, 2003; Grossbach et al, 2011).* EB: *Lip reading interpreters can assist in meeting nonvocal clients' communication needs (Meltzer et al, 2012).* EB: *Interprofessional communication was found to be important for client safety (Brock et al, 2013).*

▲ When the client is having difficulty communicating, assess and refer for audiology consultation for hearing loss. Suspect hearing loss when:
  - Client frequently complains that people mumble, claims that others' speech is not clear, or client hears only parts of conversations.
  - Client often asks people to repeat what they said.
  - Client's friends or relatives state that client doesn't seem to hear very well, or plays the television or radio too loudly.
  - Client does not laugh at jokes due to missing too much of the story.
  - Client needs to ask others about the details of a meeting that the client attended.
  - Client cannot hear the doorbell or the telephone.
  - Client finds it easier to understand others when facing them, especially in a noisy environment.

- People with hearing loss do not hear sounds clearly. The loss may range from hearing speech sounds faintly or in a distorted way to profound deafness (American Academy of Audiology, 2011).
- When communicating with a client with a hearing loss:
  - Obtain client's attention before speaking and face toward his or her unaffected side or better ear while allowing client to see speaker's face at a reasonably close distance; use gestures as appropriate to aid

in communication. *Correct positioning increases the client's awareness of the interaction and enhances the client's ability to communicate (Alexander Graham Bell Association for the Deaf and Hard of Hearing, 2011; Thiart & Saxby, 2011).* EB: *Gestures are helpful communication tools both for those with hearing loss and those with normal hearing who are faced with environmental noises or other factors impeding hearing (Obermeier et al, 2012).*

C

- ❍ Provide sufficient light and do not stand in front of window. *Light illuminates the speaker's face, making expressions and lip movements clearer; standing in front of a window causes glare, which impedes the client's ability to clearly see the speaker (Alexander Graham Bell Association for the Deaf and Hard of Hearing, 2011; Thiart & Saxby, 2011).*
- ❍ Remove masks if safe to do so, or use see-through masks. Information on see-through masks: www.amphl.org.
- ❍ Reduce background noise whenever possible. *Noise reduction facilitates understanding (Cleveland Clinic, 2012).*
- ❍ Do not raise voice or over-enunciate. *This practice distorts the voice and lips, inhibiting effective lip-reading (Cleveland Clinic, 2012).*
- ❍ Avoid making assumptions about the communication choice of those with hearing loss or voice impairments. CEBN: *After seeking client input, communication rounds or communication care plans can be completed (Happ et al, 2010).*
- ❍ Encourage physical activity among those with hearing loss. EB: *Lower levels of physical activity were found among those with moderate or greater hearing loss (Chen et al, 2014).* EB: *Hearing loss in older adults is associated with frailty (Kamil et al, 2014).*

Pediatric

- • Observe behavioral communication cues in infants. EB: *Reissland et al (2012) studied mothers and infants (N = 50) and found that preverbal infants express pain by crying and with facial and body behaviors, which have to be interpreted by the caregiver.*
- • Identify and define at least two new forms of socially acceptable communication alternatives that may be used by children with significant disabilities. EB: *Pasco and Tohill (2011) conducted a study of nonverbal children with autism spectrum disorder (N = 23) and found that the Picture Exchange Communication System (PECS) may provide valuable predictive information regarding social communication skills.* EB: *Brady et al (2013) investigated a model of language development for nonverbal school-aged children (N = 93) and found the importance of enriching social communication input across home and school environments, as well as assessments of and interventions aimed at improving comprehension, play, visual discrimination, and communication complexity.*
- • Teach children with severe disabilities functional communication skills. EB: *Allen and Marshall (2011) conducted a study involving parent-child interaction therapy (PCIT) (N = 16) for school-aged children with specific language impairment and found that PCIT offered a single block of therapy where the parents' communication and interaction skills are developed to provide the child with an appropriate language-rich environment.*
- ▲ Refer children with primary speech and language delay/disorder for speech and language therapy interventions. EB: *Pasco and Tohill (2011) conducted a study of nonverbal children with autism spectrum disorder (N = 23) and found the assessment of the developmental level of potential PECS users may provide valuable predictive information for speech-and-language therapists and other professionals in relation to the likely degree of progress and in setting realistic and achievable targets.*

Geriatric

- • Carefully assess all clients for hearing difficulty using an audiometer. Healthy People 2020 encourages early identification of people with hearing loss (Healthy People 2020, 2014).
- • Avoid use of "elderspeak." CEB: *Using elderspeak, a speech style similar to baby talk that fails to communicate appropriate respect, increases resistiveness to care in clients with dementia (Williams et al, 2009).*
- • Initiate communication with the client with dementia, and give client time to respond. The responsibility to use a creative approach and take the time to listen and understand clients who have dementia lies with the clinician (Jootun & McGhee, 2011).
- • Encourage the client to wear hearing aids, if appropriate. EB: *Hearing aid usage is low among older adults with hearing loss, despite the benefits of hearing aids (Gopinath et al, 2011).*

C

- Facilitate communication through reminiscing with memory boxes that contain objects, photographs, and writings that have meaning for the client. Reminiscence stimulates memories, thus improving communication (Swann, 2013). CEB: *Collage creation as a means of reminiscence facilitated the conveying of information by older adults with dementia who had difficulty communicating verbally (Stallings, 2010).*
- Continue to find means to communicate even with those who are completely nonverbal. EB: *Spontaneous reciprocal interaction promoted family harmony among nonvocal clients with severe dementia (Walmsley & McCormack, 2014).*

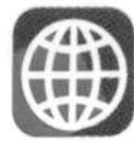

Multicultural

- Nurses should become more sensitive to the meaning of a culture's nonverbal communication modes, such as eye contact, facial expression, touching, and body language. EBN: *Kozlowska and Doboszynska (2012) conducted a study among nurses (N = 95) and found that among nonverbal means of communication in everyday practice, those who participated most frequently used touch, facial expression, and visual contact in a conscious way when delivering care.*
- Assess for the influence of cultural beliefs, norms, and values on the client's communication process. EBN: *In a 2011 study by El-Amouri and O'Neill that aimed to identify cross-cultural communication needs of hospitals, findings suggested that recognition of the importance of cross-cultural communication skills and intercultural literacy in nurse education were of significant importance in providing culturally competent care.*
- Assess personal space needs, acceptable communication styles, acceptable body language, interpretation of eye contact, perception of touch, and use of paraverbal modes when communicating with the client. EB: *A 2011 study by Hasnain et al (N = 27) found that the majority (93.8%) of responding clients reported that their health care provider did not understand their religious or cultural needs.*
- Assess for how language barriers contribute to health disparities among ethnic and racial minorities. EBN: *Taylor et al (2013) found that language barriers were the main obstacle in eliciting an accurate medical history, explaining and gaining pain scores, communicating reasons for client transport delays, arranging appointments by telephone, explaining medication and side effects, or diagnosing and communicating problems (N = 34).*
- Although touch is generally beneficial, there may be times when it may not be advisable due to cultural considerations. CEB/EBN: *Touch is largely culturally defined and conveys various meanings depending on the client's culture (Leininger & McFarland, 2002; Lewis et al, 2011).*
- Modify and tailor the communication approach in keeping with the client's particular culture. *A 2011 study by Fakhr-Movahedi et al conducted among eight Iranian nurses and nine clients suggested that socio-cultural-economic issues between nurses and clients influence nurse-client communication.*
- Use reminiscence therapy as a language intervention. EB: *Issues of culture, language, and aging are challenging. Less engaged residents and clients who are nonverbal, immobile, or who have other occupational performance issues may become engaged in occupations of reminiscence that are rich in personal meaning and relevance (Hodges & Schmidt, 2009).*
- The Office of Minority Health of the U.S. Department of Health and Human Services standards on culturally and linguistically appropriate services (CLAS) in health care should be used as needed. EB: *The National Standards for Culturally and Linguistically Appropriate Services in Health and Health Care (The National CLAS Standards) aim to improve health care quality and advance health equity by establishing a framework for organizations to serve the nation's increasingly diverse communities (CLAS, 2014).*

Home Care

The interventions described previously may be adapted for home care use.

Client/Family Teaching and Discharge Planning

▲ Refer the client to a speech-language pathologist (SLP) or audiologist. Audiological assessment quantifies and qualifies hearing in terms of the degree of hearing loss, the type of hearing loss, and the configuration of the hearing loss. Once a particular hearing loss has been identified, a treatment and management plan can be put into place by an SLP (Baumgartner et al, 2008).

▲ Teach the client and family techniques to increase communication, including the use of communication devices and tactile touch. Incorporate multidisciplinary recommendations. The nurse plays a critical role in individualized communication assessment as clients transition from hospital to home (Cerantola & Happ, 2012). EB: *Recommendations by SLPs were omitted from discharge summaries at a high rate, placing clients at risk for lack of continuity of care (Kind et al, 2011).* EB: *Clients who are mechanically ventilated at home have a long struggle to find effective communication methods (Laasko et al, 2011).*

REFERENCES

Alexander Graham Bell Association for the Deaf and Hard of Hearing. *Communicating with people who have a hearing loss.* Retrieved July 13, 2011, from: <http://agbell.org/NetCommunity/Document.Doc?id=343>.

Allen, J., & Marshall, C. R. (2011). Parent-Child Interaction Therapy (PCIT) in school-aged children with specific language impairment. *International Journal of Language & Communication Disorders, 46*(4), 397–410.

American Academy of Audiology. *How's your hearing?* Retrieved July 13, 2011, from: <http://www.howsyourhearing.org>.

Aust, M. P. (2013). Pain assessment in nonverbal patients. *American Journal of Critical Care, 22*(3), 256.

Babbitt, E. M., et al. (2011). Psychometric properties of the Communication Confidence Rating Scale for Aphasia (CCRSA): phase 2. *Aphasiology, 25*(6/7), 727–735.

Baumgartner, C. A., Bewyer, E., & Bruner, D. (2008). Management of communication and swallowing in intensive care: the role of the speech pathologist. *AACN Advance Critical Care, 19*(4), 433–443.

Bechtold, A., & Fredericks, S. (2014). Key concepts in patient-centered care. *American Nurse Today, 9*(7), 35–36.

Borthwick, S. (2012). Communication impairment in patients following stroke. *Nursing Standard, 26*(19), 35–41.

Brock, D., et al. (2013). Interprofessional education in team communication: working together to improve patient safety. *BMJ Quality & Safety, 22*(5), 414–423.

Brady, N. C., Thiemann-Bourque, K., Fleming, K., et al. (2013). Predicting language outcomes for children learning augmentative and alternative communication: child and environmental factors. *Journal of Speech, Language & Hearing Research, 56*(5), 1595–1612.

Carroll, S. M. (2003). Lip-reading translating for non-vocal ventilated patients. *JAMPHL Online, 1*(2), Retrieved November 26, 2006, from: <www.amphl.org>.

Carroll, S. M. (2007). Silent, slow lifeworld: the communication experiences of nonvocal ventilated patients. *Qualitative Health Research, 17*(9), 1165–1177.

Cerantola, C., & Happ, M. B. (2012). Transitional care for communication impaired older adults: ICU to home. *Geriatric Nursing, 33*(6), 489–492.

Chen, D. S., et al. (2014). Association between hearing impairment and self-reported difficulty in physical functioning. *Journal of the American Geriatrics Society, 62*(5), 850–856.

CLAS (Culturally and Linguistically Appropriate Services), Retrieved October 25, 2014 from: <http://minorityhealth.hhs.gov/omh/browse.aspx?lvl=2&lvlid=53>.

Cleveland Clinic. (2012). *Tips to improve communication when talking to someone with hearing loss.* Retrieved September 10, 2014, from: <http://my.clevelandclinic.org/disorders/hearing_loss/hic-tips-improve-communication-when-talking-someone-hearing-loss.aspx>.

El-Amouri, S., & O'Neill, S. (2011). Supporting cross-cultural communication and culturally competent care in the linguistically and culturally diverse hospital settings of UAE. *Contemporary Nurse: A Journal for the Australian Nursing Profession, 39*(2), 240–255.

Fakhr-Movahedi, A., Salsali, M., Negharandeh, R., et al. (2011). A qualitative content analysis of nurse-patient communication in Iranian nursing. *International Nursing Review, 58*(2), 171–180.

Flynn Makic, M. B. (2013). Pain management in the nonverbal critically ill patient. *Journal of Perianesthesia Nursing, 28*(2), 98–101.

Giammarino, C., et al. (2012). Safety considerations for patients with communication disorders in rehabilitation medicine settings. *Physical Medicine & Rehabilitation Clinics of North America, 23*(2), 343–347.

Gopinath, B., et al. (2011). Incidence and predictors of hearing aid use and ownership among older adults with hearing loss. *Annals of Epidemiology, 21*(7), 497–506.

Grossbach, I., Stranberg, S., & Chlan, L. (2011). Promoting effective communication for patients receiving mechanical ventilation. *Critical Care Nurse, 31*(3), 46–61.

Hagan, L., & Thompson, H. (2014). It's good to talk: Developing the communication skills of an adult with intellectual disability through augmentative and alternative communication. *British Journal of Learning Disabilities, 42*(1), 66–73.

Happ, M. B., et al. (2010). SPEACS-2: intensive care unit "communication rounds" with speech language pathology. *Geriatric Nursing (New York, N.Y.), 31*(3), 170–177.

Hasnain, M., Connell, K. J., Menon, U., et al. (2011). Patient-centered care for Muslim women: provider and patient perspectives. *Journal of Women's Health (15409996), 20*(1), 73–83.

Healthy People 2020. *Hearing and other sensory or communication disorders.* Retrieved September 12, 2014, from: <www.healthypeople.gov/2020/topicsobjectives2020/overviewaspx?topicid=20>.

Hodges, C., & Schmidt, R. (2009). An exploration of reminiscence and post-war European immigrants living in a multicultural aged-care setting in Australia. *Occupational Therapy International, 16*(2), 154–168.

Jootun, D., & McGhee, G. (2011). Effective communication with people who have dementia. *Nursing Standard, 25*(25), 40–46.

Kamil, R. J., Li, L., & Lin, F. R. (2014). Association between hearing impairment and frailty in older adults. *Journal of the American Geriatrics Society, 62*(6), 1186–1188.

Kind, A., et al. (2011). Omission of dysphagia therapies in hospital discharge communications. *Dysphagia, 26*(1), 49–61.

Kozlowska, L., & Doboszynska, A. (2012). Nurses' nonverbal methods of communicating with patients in the terminal phase. *International Journal of Palliative Nursing, 18*(1), 40–46.

Laasko, K., et al. (2011). Communication experience of individuals treated with home ventilation. *International Journal of Language and Communication Disorders, 46*(6), 686–699.

Leininger, M. M., & McFarland, M. R. (2002). *Transcultural nursing: concepts, theories, research and practices* (ed. 3). New York: McGraw-Hill.

Lewis, S. L., et al. (2011). *Medical surgical nursing: assessment and management of clinical problems* (ed. 8). St Louis: Elsevier.

Light, J., & McNaughton, D. (2013). Putting people first: re-thinking the role of technology in augmentative and alternative communication intervention. *AAC: Augmentative & Alternative Communication, 29*(4), 299–309.

Meltzer, E. C., et al. (2012). Lip-reading and the ventilated patient. *Critical Care Medicine, 40*(5), 1529–1531.

Nilsen, M. L., et al. (2014). Adaptation of a communication interaction behavior instrument for use in mechanically ventilated, nonvocal older adults. *Nursing Research, 63*(1), 3–13.

Obermeier, C., Dolk, T., & Gunter, T. C. (2012). The benefit of gestures during communication: evidence from hearing and hearing-impaired individuals. *Cortex; a Journal Devoted to the Study of the Nervous System and Behavior, 48*(7), 857–870.

O'Hagan, S., et al. (2014). What counts as effective communication in nursing? Evidence from nurse educators' and clinicians' feedback on nurse interactions with simulated patients. *Journal of Advanced Nursing*, *70*(6), 1344–1355.
Pasco, G., & Tohill, C. (2011). Predicting progress in Picture Exchange Communication System (PECS) use by children with autism. *International Journal of Language & Communication Disorders*, *46*(1), 120–125.
Radtke, J. V., et al. (2011). Listening to the voiceless patient: case reports in assisted communication in the intensive care unit. *Journal of Palliative Medicine*, *14*(6), 791–795.
Reissland, N., Harvey, H., & Mason, J. (2012). Effects of maternal parity, depression and stress on two-month-old infant expression of pain. *Journal of Reproductive & Infant Psychology*, *30*(4), 363–376.
Stallings, J. W. (2010). Collage as a therapeutic modality for reminiscence in patients with dementia. *Art Therapy*, *37*(3), 136–140.
Swann, J. I. (2013). Dementia and reminiscence: not just a focus on the past. *Nursing & Residential Care*, *15*(12), 790–795.
Taylor, S. P., Nicolle, C., & Maguire, M. (2013). Cross-cultural communication barriers in health care. *Nursing Standard*, *27*(31), 35–43.
Thiart, M., & Saxby, H. *Augmentative and alternative communication manual for nursing personnel*. Retrieved 2011, from: <www.patientprovidercommunication.org>.
Walmsley, B. D., & McCormack, L. (2014). The dance of communication: retaining family membership despite severe non-speech dementia. *Dementia (Basel, Switzerland)*, *13*(5), 626–641.
Williams, K. N., et al. (2009). Elderspeak communication: impact on dementia care. *American Journal of Alzheimer's Disease and Other Dementias*, *24*(1), 11–20.

Acute Confusion

Mila W. Grady, MSN, RN

NANDA-I

Definition

Abrupt onset of reversible disturbances of consciousness, attention, cognition, and perception that develop over a short period of time

Defining Characteristics

Agitation; alteration in cognitive functioning; alteration in level of consciousness; alteration in psychomotor functioning; hallucinations; inability to initiate goal-directed behavior; inability to initiate purposeful behavior; insufficient follow-through with goal directed behavior; insufficient following-through with purposeful behavior; misperception; restlessness

Related Factors (r/t)

Age >60 years; alteration in sleep-wake cycle; delirium; dementia; substance abuse, polypharmacy

NOC (Nursing Outcomes Classification)

Suggested NOC Outcomes

Cognition; Distorted Thought Self-Control; Information Processing

Example NOC Outcome with Indicators

Cognition as evidenced by the following indicators: Communication clear for age/Comprehension of the meaning of situations/Attentiveness/Concentration/Cognitive orientation. (Rate the outcome and indicators of **Cognition:** 1 = severely compromised, 2 = substantially compromised, 3 = moderately compromised, 4 = mildly compromised, 5 = not compromised [see Section I].)

Client Outcomes

Client Will (Specify Time Frame)

- Demonstrate restoration of cognitive status to baseline
- Be oriented to time, place, and person
- Demonstrate appropriate motor behavior
- Maintain functional capacity

NIC (Nursing Interventions Classification)

Suggested NIC Interventions

Delirium Management; Delusion Management

Example NIC Activities—Delirium Management

Inform client of time, place, and person as needed; Provide information slowly and in small doses with frequent rest periods

C

Nursing Interventions and *Rationales*

- Recognize that delirium is characterized by an acute onset, a fluctuating course, inattention, and disordered thinking.
- Identify the three distinct types of delirium: hyperactive (easy to recognize), hypoactive (commonly missed), and mixed (the most commonly occurring). (Downing et al, 2013).
- Hyperactive: delirium characterized by restlessness, agitation, irritability, hypervigilance, hallucinations, and delusions; client may be combative or may attempt to remove tubes, lines
  - Hypoactive: delirium characterized by decreased motor activity, decreased vocalization, detachment, apathy, lethargy, somnolence, reduced awareness of surroundings, and confusion
  - Mixed: delirium characterized by the client fluctuating between periods of hyperactivity and agitation and hypoactivity and sedation. EBN: *Delirium is underrecognized by both medical and nursing staff, particularly the hypoactive form (Cerejeira & Mukaetova-Ladinska, 2011).*
- Obtain an accurate history and perform a mental status examination that includes the following assessment:
  - History from a reliable source that documents an acute and fluctuating change in cognitive function, attention, and behavior from baseline
  - Cognition as evidenced by level of consciousness; orientation to time, person, and place; thought process (thinking may be disorganized, distorted, fragmented, slow, or accelerated with delirium; conversation may be irrelevant or rambling); and content (perceptual disturbances such as visual, auditory or tactile delusions or hallucinations)
  - Level of attention (may be decreased or may fluctuate with delirium; may be unable to focus, shift, or sustain attention; may be easily distracted or may be hypervigilant)
  - Behavior characteristics and level of psychomotor behavior (activity may be increased or decreased and may include restlessness, finger tapping, picking at bedclothes, changing position frequently, spastic movements or tremors, or decreased psychomotor activity such as sluggishness, staring into space, remaining in the same position for prolonged periods)
  - Level of consciousness (may be easily aroused, lethargic, drowsy, difficult to arouse, unarousable, hyperalert, easily startled, overly sensitive to stimuli)
  - Mood and affect (may be paranoid or fearful with delirium; may have rapid mood swings)
  - Insight and judgment (may be impaired)
  - Memory (recent and immediate memory is impaired with delirium; unable to register new information)
  - Language (may have rapid, rambling, slurred, incoherent speech)
  - Altered sleep-wake cycle (insomnia, excessive daytime sleepiness)
  - EB: *Establishing the client's baseline mental status by obtaining an accurate history and performing a brief cognitive assessment observing for key diagnostic criteria are important in the diagnosis of delirium (Inouye et al, 2014).*
- Assess the client's behavior and cognition systematically and continually throughout the day and night; use a validated tool to assess presence of delirium, such as the Confusion Assessment Method (CAM) or Delirium Observation Screening Scale (DOS). EB: *The CAM is accurate, brief, and easy to use (Grover & Kate, 2012); the DOS was found to be a useful screening tool in a small study of verbally active palliative care clients (Detroyer et al, 2014).*
- Recognize that delirium may be superimposed on dementia; the nurse must be aware of the client's baseline cognitive function. EB: *Dementia increases the risk and severity of delirium (Voyer et al, 2011b); delirium superimposed on dementia was a strong predictor of decline in function and resultant institutionalization of older adults admitted to a rehabilitation facility (Morandi et al, 2014).*
- Identify predisposing factors that may precede the development of delirium: dementia, cognitive impairment, functional impairment, visual impairment, alcohol misuse, multiple comorbidities, severe illness, history of transient ischemic attack or stroke, depression, history of delirium, and advanced age (older than 70). EB: *Delirium is a multifactorial syndrome most commonly seen in the intensive care unit (ICU),*

C

palliative care, and postoperative settings; identification of risk factors is important for prevention (Inouye et al, 2014).

- Identify precipitating factors that may precede the development of delirium, especially for individuals with predisposing factors: use of restraints, indwelling bladder catheter, metabolic disturbances, polypharmacy, pain, infection, dehydration, blood loss, constipation, electrolyte imbalances, immobility, general anesthesia, hospital admission for fractures or hip surgery, anticholinergic medications, anxiety, sleep deprivation, lack of use of vision and/or hearing aids, and environmental factors. EB: *Prevention of delirium must be a high priority in light of frequency of occurrence, high treatment costs, longer hospital length of stay, higher rates of functional decline and resultant institutional care, and greater mortality; delirium may persist and lead to long-term cognitive decline (O'Mahoney et al, 2011).* EB: *Interventions to prevent or lessen the length and severity of delirium may be developed when early identification of delirium risk is instituted (van Boogaard et al, 2012).*

▲ Assess for and report possible physiological alterations (e.g., sepsis, hypoglycemia, hypoxia, hypotension, infection, changes in temperature, fluid and electrolyte imbalance, and use of medications with known cognitive and psychotropic side effects). EB: *Systemic disturbances, including immunologic, metabolic, neuroinflammatory, endocrinological, and neurological factors lead to alterations in neurotransmitter synthesis and availability, which leads to delirium (Maldonado, 2013).*

- ❍ Treat the underlying risk factors or the causes of delirium in collaboration with the health care team: establish/maintain normal fluid and electrolyte balance, normal body temperature, normal oxygenation (if the client experiences low oxygen saturation, deliver supplemental oxygen), normal blood glucose levels, and normal blood pressure, and address malnutrition and anemia. EB: *Early recognition of risk factors may help to prevent the negative sequelae of delirium (Fineberg et al, 2013).*

▲ Conduct a medication review and eliminate unnecessary medications; potentially inappropriate medications for older adults at risk for delirium include anticholinergics, benzodiazepines, corticosteroids, H_2 receptor antagonists, sedative hypnotics, tricyclic antidepressants (American Geriatrics Society, 2012). EB: *A software based program that identified potential delirium-causing medications and triggered a medication review and monitoring plan by pharmacists led to a decreased incidence of delirium in long-term care (Clegg et al, 2014); polypharmacy is associated with delirium and a reduction of polypharmacy improves cognition (Van der Cammen et al, 2014).*

- ❍ Communicate client status, cognition, and behavioral manifestations to all necessary health care providers.
- ❍ Monitor for any trends occurring in these manifestations, including laboratory tests. CEB: *Careful monitoring is needed to identify the potential etiologic factors for delirium (Sendelbach & Guthrie, 2009).*

- Identify, evaluate and treat pain quickly and adequately (see care plans for Acute **Pain** or Chronic **Pain**). EB: *Untreated pain is a potential cause of delirium, as is excessive opioid administration (Clegg & Young, 2011).*
- Promote regulation of bowel and bladder function; use bladder scanning to identify retention; avoid prolonged insertion of urinary catheters and remove catheters as soon as possible. EB: *Stool impaction may cause urinary retention, which is associated with delirium (Boddaert et al, 2014).* EB: *Constipation may precipitate delirium (O'Mahoney et al, 2011); urinary catheterization is associated with delirium (Ahmed et al, 2014).*
- Ensure adequate nutritional and fluid intake. EB: *Malnutrition is significantly associated with delirium (Ahmed et al, 2014); attending to correct levels of B vitamins, antioxidants, glucose, water, and lipids may lead to resolution of delirium (Sanford & Flaherty, 2014).*
- Promote early mobilization and rehabilitation in a progressive manner. EB: *Avoiding immobility and promoting early mobilization postoperatively reduces delirium (Butler et al, 2013).* EBN: *Standardized early mobilization protocols promote functional status, prevent complications associated with functional decline, and contribute to greater well-being and/or decreased length of stay for medical-surgical inpatients (Pashikanti & Von Ah, 2012).*
- Promote continuity of care; avoid frequent changes in staff and surroundings. EB: *Changes may contribute to feelings of disorientation and confusion (O'Mahoney et al, 2011).*
- Plan care that allows for an appropriate sleep-wake cycle. Refer to the care plan for **Sleep** deprivation. EB: *Interventions to promote sleep were associated with a decreased incidence of delirium (Patel et al, 2014).*
- Facilitate appropriate sensory input by having clients use aids (e.g., glasses, hearing aids, dentures) as needed; check for impacted ear wax. EB: *Delirium can be addressed with nonpharmacologic interventions, such as decreasing sensory impairment (Javedan & Tulebaev, 2014) or avoiding sensory overload*

for clients with agitation. EB: *Multicomponent interventions, such as encouraging use of vision and hearing aids, may assist in the prevention of delirium in individuals who are not cognitively impaired (Khan et al, 2012).*

- Modulate sensory exposure; eliminate excessive noise, use appropriate lighting based on the time of day, and establish a calm environment. EB: *Noise levels in the hospital, often from staff conversation and other avoidable sources, are higher than recommended and lead to significant sleep loss (Yoder et al, 2012).*
- Provide cognitive stimulation through conversation about current events, viewpoints, relationships and encourage reminiscence or word games. EBN: *Daily cognitive stimulation can prevent cognitive decline and promote cognitive recovery (Cheng et al, 2012).*
- Provide reality orientation, including identifying self by name at each encounter with the client, calling the client by their preferred name, and the gentle use of orientation techniques; when reorientation is not effective, use distraction. EB: *Efforts to reorient may agitate some clients; changing the subject may help calm the client (Flaherty & Little, 2011).*
- Provide clocks and calendars, update dry erase white boards each shift, encourage family to visit regularly and to bring familiar objects from home, such as family photos or an afghan, and gently correct misperceptions. EB: *Persons at risk for delirium should be provided clocks and calendars that are easily visible; family and friends may help with reorientation (O'Mahoney et al, 2011).*
- Use gentle, caring communication; provide reassurance of safety; give simple explanations of procedures.
- Provide supportive nursing care, including meeting basic needs such as feeding, regular toileting, and ensuring adequate hydration; closely observe behaviors that provide clues to what might be distressing the client. Delirious clients are unable to care for themselves due to their confusion (Rubin et al, 2011). EB: *Understanding and anticipating behaviors promotes client comfort and safety (Flaherty & Little, 2011).*

▲ Recognize that delirium is frequently treated with antipsychotic medications or sedatives; if there is no other way to keep the client safe, administer these medications cautiously, as ordered, while monitoring for medication side effects. EB: *Reducing unnecessary medications, pain, stress, sleep deprivation, inflammation and other neurological insults is crucial, because antipsychotics and sedatives may actually prolong the duration of delirium and worsen outcomes (Inouye et al, 2014).*

- ❍ For clients nearing the end of life, for whom delirium may be irreversible, focus on relief of symptoms by increasing supervision, reducing invasive lines and devices that restrict movement, keeping the bed in low position, and placing mats on the floor; support of family, caregivers, and the health care team is also of prime importance. EB: *Nonpharmacologic means should always be used to ameliorate delirium and may be used in conjunction with medication; delirium is distressing to those caring for the client (Irwin et al, 2013).*
- ❍ Choose the appropriate medication and consider the type and reversibility of the delirium; titrate the medication to control the symptoms and minimize side effects. EB: *Pharmacologic means can be rapid, safe, and effective using the lowest effective dose of the appropriate medication based on the type of delirium (Irwin et al, 2013).*

Critical Care

- Recognize admission risk factors for delirium. EB: *ICU clients are at increased risk for delirium due to greater use of sedatives, analgesics, severity of illness, age, infection, multiorgan failure, sleep deprivation, surgery, fracture, restraint use, immobility, tubes, catheters, hypovolemia, polypharmacy, malnutrition, electrolyte imbalance, and stroke (Mistraletti et al, 2012).*
- Obtain an accurate history regarding cognitive impairment and mental health, including history of anxiety and depression, alcohol use, medication use, chronic pain, and use of benzodiazepines. EBN: *An accurate history guides appropriate interventions to maximize neurocognitive status of older adults with complex illnesses in the ICU (Tate & Happ, 2011).*
- Assess level of arousal using the Richmond Agitation Sedation Scale; clients receiving a score of −5 to −4 are comatose and unable to be assessed for delirium. EB: *Establishing level of arousal before using the Confusion Assessment Method for the ICU (CAM-ICU) decreases the incidence of inappropriate "unable to assess" (UTA) ratings on the CAM-ICU; it was found that noncomatose clients were inappropriately determined to be UTA (Swan, 2014).*
- Assess for pain every 2 to 3 hours or more frequently as needed with a standardized assessment tool, which includes either a numerical rating scale or one with behavioral indicators, such as the Behavioral Pain Scale (BPS) or Critical Care Pain Observation Tool (CPOT). EB: *The self-report is the gold standard*

C

for pain assessment (Barr & Pandharipande, 2013); the BPS and CPOT are the most valid and reliable tools to use for adult ICU clients (excluding brain injured) with intact motor function and observable behaviors, who are unable to self-report (Barr et al, 2013). EBN: *Uncontrolled pain is common in the ICU and can contribute to delirium; routine assessment of pain may decrease duration of ventilation and ICU length of stay, and increase client satisfaction (Stites, 2013); clients are less likely to communicate symptoms such as pain when delirious (Tate et al, 2013).*

▲ Incorporate the Awakening and Breathing Coordination, Delirium Monitoring and Management, and Early Mobility (ABCDE) ICU delirium and weakness prevention bundle in conjunction with the interdisciplinary team. EB: *Interdisciplinary communication and daily rounds and staff education facilitate optimal ABCDE bundle implementation (Balas et al, 2013); bundle implementation leads to less delirium, reduced ventilator time, and more time out of bed (Balas et al, 2014).*
  ❍ Assess safety of and implement a spontaneous awakening trial (SAT) using an established protocol. EB: *Daily interruption of sedation may be beneficial when it results in a reduced total dose of sedative administered; minimizing the depth and duration of sedation is beneficial for reducing delirium (Reade & Finfer, 2014).*
  ❍ Assess safety of and implement a spontaneous breathing trial (SBT). EBN: *Implementing SAT/SBT protocols reduces the duration and use of mechanical ventilation, which may lead to decreased complications and does not increase self-extubation (Jones et al, 2014).*
  ❍ Assess sedation and agitation level using a valid and reliable tool; titrate sedation to target sedation level. EB: *Sedatives and analgesics prescribed to improve client-ventilator dyssynchrony and treat anxiety and pain may precipitate delirium (Banerjee et al, 2011); for most clients being ventilated in the ICU, a score of 3-4 on the Riker or a score of −2-0 on the Richmond are appropriate targets (Reade & Finfer, 2014).*
  ❍ Screen for delirium using a reliable and valid monitoring tool once per shift or more often if delirium is present, and recognize that hypoactive delirium is the form most often present in the ICU; communicate and discuss results with the interdisciplinary team. EB: *The CAM-ICU and the Intensive Care Delirium Screening Checklist are the most valid and reliable tools for adult ICU clients (Barr et al, 2013); staff education, discussion of delirium during bedside rounds, and documentation promote successful screening and treatment (Brummel et al, 2013).* EBN: *The hypoactive form of delirium is the most common form seen in the ICU and contributes to the under-recognition of delirium by clinicians (Tate et al, 2013).*
  ❍ Assess safety to begin mobilization; collaborate with physical therapy (PT), occupational therapy (OT), and respiratory therapy (RT) to implement an early mobility plan using a progressive approach. EB: *Early mobilization of stable ICU clients may significantly reduce the length of delirium and length of stay and prevent other complications related to immobility (Hunter et al, 2014).*

- Encourage visits from families and educate families about delirium if it occurs. EB: *Delirium is distressing to clients and families; providing education can alleviate distress (Irwin et al, 2013).* EBN: *Families are most familiar with the client's baseline behavior, assist in the diagnosis of delirium, and by their presence, may help to prevent and ameliorate delirium (Keyser et al, 2012).*
- Promote uninterrupted sleep by grouping cares at night to avoid sleep interruption, offering eye mask, soft music, and earplugs; optimizing room temperature; reducing noise and light after 10 PM; and avoiding excessive daytime napping. EB: *Sleep deprivation and delirium in the ICU may be iatrogenic; engaging clients to keep them more awake during the day may ensure better outcomes (Weinhouse, 2014).* EBN: *Multifaceted approaches are required to promote sleep in the ICU in order to avoid the negative consequences of disrupted sleep (Kamdar et al, 2013).*

Geriatric

- The interventions described previously are relevant to the geriatric client.
- Reorient high-risk clients frequently, answer questions, discuss concerns; use a white board, clock, watch, and calendar, and encourage family members to bring familiar objects from home such as family photos or afghan to assist with orientation. EB: *Environmental factors may be modified to improve outcomes for clients with delirium (McCusker et al, 2013).*
- Provide cognitive stimulation by discussing current events, reading the newspaper, promoting reminiscence, or using games. EB: *Therapeutic activities can minimize cognitive decline (Zaubler et al, 2013).*
- Promote use of glasses, assistive hearing devices, hearing aids, and dentures. CEB: *Sensory impairment is a modifiable risk factor for delirium.*

C

- Provide feeding assistance as needed. See care plan for Imbalanced **Nutrition:** less than body requirements.
- ▲ Determine whether the client is adequately nourished; watch for protein-calorie malnutrition. Consult with health care provider or dietitian as needed. EB: *Malnutrition is significantly associated with delirium (Ahmed et al, 2014); attending to correct levels of B vitamins, antioxidants, glucose, water, and lipids may lead to resolution of delirium (Sanford & Flaherty, 2014).*
- Promote adequate hydration; keep a glass of water within easy reach of the client and offer fluids frequently. EB: *Keeping a glass of water within reach abated dehydration and delirium in the long-term care population (McCusker et al, 2013).*
- Avoid use of restraints; remove all nonessential equipment such as telemetry, blood pressure cuffs, catheters, and intravenous lines as soon as possible. EBN: *In a study of long-term care residents with dementia, the use of physical restraints was the factor most associated with delirium; initiate alternative interventions (Voyer et al, 2011a).*
- Evaluate all medications for potential to cause or exacerbate delirium; potentially inappropriate medications for older adults at risk for delirium include tricyclic antidepressants, anticholinergics, antipsychotics, benzodiazepines, corticosteroids, H_2 receptor antagonists, and sedative hypnotics. EB: *To enhance client safety, medications used for older adults should be routinely assessed for inappropriateness (Morandi et al, 2011).*
- Assess pain frequently and treat pain with the lowest dose of regularly scheduled medication as well as with nonpharmacologic approaches; use client self-report or a validated behavioral pain scale to assess pain accurately. EB: *Uncontrolled pain can lead to delirium (Stites, 2013).*
- ▲ Assess risk for falls and implement fall prevention strategies. EB: *Geriatric syndromes are more common in older adults with delirium discharged to postacute care facilities; proactively addressing risk factors may improve outcomes (Anderson et al, 2012).*
- Recognize that delirium may be superimposed on dementia; determine client's baseline cognitive status. EB: *Dementia increases the risk and severity of delirium (Voyer et al, 2011b); delirium superimposed on dementia was a strong predictor of decline in function and resultant institutionalization of older adults admitted to a rehabilitation facility (Morandi et al, 2014).*
- ▲ Determine whether the client is nourished; watch for protein-calorie malnutrition. Consult with health care provider or dietitian as needed. EB: *Malnutrition is significantly associated with delirium (Ahmed et al, 2014); attending to correct levels of B vitamins, antioxidants, glucose, water, and lipids may lead to resolution of delirium (Sanford & Flaherty, 2014).*
- Explain hospital routines and procedures slowly and in simple terms; repeat information as necessary.
- Provide continuity of care when possible, avoid room changes, and encourage frequent visits from family members or significant others. EB: *Frequent changes may contribute to confusion (O'Mahoney et al, 2011).*
- Educate family members about delirium assessment and strategies to use to prevent and lessen delirium; use the Family Confusion Assessment Method (FAM-CAM) assessment tool to solicit accurate information from caregivers regarding the presence of delirium. EBN: *A small pilot study found that forming a trusting and respectful partnership with family caregivers in delirium prevention impacts family and nurse satisfaction (Rosenbloom & Fick, 2013); the FAM-CAM is a sensitive screening tool to assist in the early diagnosis of delirium in individuals with preexisting dementia (Steis et al, 2012).*
- If clients know that they are not thinking clearly, acknowledge the concern. Fear is frequently experienced by people with delirium. EB: *Confusion is frightening; the memory of the delirium can be distressing to clients and families (Partridge et al, 2013).*

Home Care

- The interventions described previously are relevant to home care use. Assess and monitor for acute changes in cognition and behavior. EB: *Delirium has an acute onset and fluctuating course, and is characterized by disordered thinking and a change in behavior (Downing et al, 2013).*
- Recognize that delirium is reversible but can become chronic if untreated in a multidisciplinary fashion; the client may be discharged from the hospital to home care in a state of undiagnosed delirium. EB: *Complete recovery may be possible with appropriate multidisciplinary care (Wakefield et al, 2014).*
- Avoid preconceptions about the source of acute confusion; assess each occurrence on the basis of available evidence.
- ▲ Institute case management of frail elderly clients to support continued independent living if possible once delirium has resolved.

C

Client/Family Teaching and Discharge Planning

▲ Teach the family to recognize signs of early confusion and seek medical help.

• Counsel the client and family regarding the management of delirium and its sequelae. Increased care requirements at discharge may be needed for clients who have experienced delirium; frailty and delirium can lead to functional decline and institutionalization (Quinlan et al, 2011).

REFERENCES

Ahmed, S., Leurent, B., & Sampson, E. L. (2014). Risk factors for incident delirium among older people in acute hospital medical units: A systematic review and meta-analysis. *Age and Ageing*, *43*(3), 326–333.

American Geriatrics Society. (2012). Beers Criteria Update Expert Panel. (2012). American Geriatrics Society updated Beers Criteria for potentially inappropriate medication use in older adults. *Journal of the American Geriatrics Society*, *60*(4), 616–631.

Anderson, C. P., Ngo, L. H., & Marcantonio, E. R. (2012). Complications in postacute care are associated with persistent delirium. *Journal of the American Geriatrics Society*, *60*(6), 1122–1127.

Balas, M. C., Burke, W. J., & Gannon, D., et al. (2013). Implementing the awakening and breathing coordination, delirium monitoring/management, and early exercise/mobility bundle into everyday care: Opportunities, challenges, and lessons learned for implementing the ICU Pain, Agitation, and Delirium Guidelines. *Critical Care Medicine*, *41*(9 Suppl. 1), S116–S127.

Balas, M. C., Vasilevskis, E. E., & Olsen, K. M., et al. (2014). Effectiveness and safety of the awakening and breathing coordination, delirium monitoring/management, and early exercise/mobility bundle. *Critical Care Medicine*, *42*(5), 1024–1036.

Banerjee, A., Girard, T. D., & Pandharipande, P. (2011). The complex interplay between delirium, sedation, and early mobility during critical illness: Applications in the trauma unit. *Current Opinion in Anesthesiology*, *24*(2), 195–201.

Barr, J., & Pandharipande, P. P. (2013). The pain, agitation, and delirium care bundle: Synergistic benefits of implementing the 2013 Pain, Agitation, and Delirium Guidelines in an integrated and interdisciplinary fashion. *Critical Care Medicine*, *41*(9 Suppl. 1), S99–S115.

Barr, J., Fraser, G. L., & Puntillo, K., et al. (2013). Clinical practice guidelines for the management of pain, agitation, and delirium in adult patients in the intensive care unit. *Critical Care Medicine*, *41*(1), 263–306.

Boddaert, J., Cohen-Bittan, J., & Khiami, F., et al. (2014). Postoperative admission to a dedicated geriatric unit decreases mortality in elderly patients with hip fracture. *PLoS One*, *9*(1), e83795.

Brummel, N. E., Vasilevskis, E. E., & Han, J. H., et al. (2013). Implementing delirium screening in the ICU: Secrets to success. *Critical Care Medicine*, *41*(9), 2196–2208.

Butler, I., Sinclair, L., & Tipping, B. (2013). Current concepts in the management of delirium. *Continuing Medical Education*, *31*(10), 363–366.

Cerejeira, J., & Mukaetova-Ladinska, E. B. (2011). A clinical update on delirium: From early recognition to effective management. *Nursing Research and Practice*, *2011*, 875196.

Cheng, C. M., Chiu, M. J., & Wang, J. H., et al. (2012). Cognitive stimulation during hospitalization improves global cognition of older Taiwanese undergoing elective total knee and hip replacement surgery. *Journal of Advanced Nursing*, *68*(6), 1322–1329.

Clegg, A., & Young, J. B. (2011). Which medications to avoid in people at risk of delirium: A systematic review. *Age and Aging*, *40*(1), 23–29.

Clegg, A., Siddiqi, N., & Heaven, A., et al. (2014). Interventions for preventing delirium in older people in institutional long-term care. *The Cochrane Database of Systematic Reviews*, (1), CD009537, Jan 31.

Detroyer, E., Clement, P. M., & Baeten, N., et al. (2014). Detection of delirium in palliative care unit patients: A prospective descriptive study of the Delirium Observation Screening Scale administered by bedside nurses. *Palliative Medicine*, *28*(1), 79–86.

Downing, L. J., Caprio, T. V., & Lyness, J. M. (2013). Geriatric psychiatry review: Differential diagnosis and treatment of the 3 D's—delirium, dementia, and depression. *Current Psychiatry Reports*, *15*(6), 365.

Fineberg, S. J., Nandyala, S. V., & Marquez-Lara, A., et al. (2013). Incidence and risk factors for postoperative delirium after lumbar spine surgery. *Spine (Phila Pa 1976)*, *38*(20), 1790–1796.

Flaherty, J. H., & Little, M. O. (2011). Matching the environment to patients with delirium: Lessons learned from the delirium room, a restraint-free environment for older hospitalized adults with delirium. *Journal of the American Geriatrics Society*, *59*(Suppl. 2), S295–S300.

Grover, S., & Kate, N. (2012). Assessment scales for delirium: A review. *World Journal of Psychiatry*, *2*(4), 58–70.

Hunter, A., Johnson, L., & Coustasse, A. (2014). Reduction of intensive care unit length of stay: The case of early mobilization. *Health Care Management (Frederick)*, *33*(2), 128–135.

Inouye, S. K., Westendorp, R. G., & Saczynski, J. S. (2014). Delirium in elderly people. *Lancet*, *383*(9920), 911–922.

Irwin, S. A., Pirrello, R. D., & Hirst, J. M., et al. (2013). Clarifying delirium management: Practical, evidenced-based, expert recommendations for clinical practice. *Journal of Palliative Medicine*, *16*(4), 423–435.

Javedan, H., & Tulebaev, S. (2014). Management of common postoperative complications: Delirium. *Clinics in Geriatric Medicine*, *30*(2), 271–278.

Jones, K., Newhouse, R., & Johnson, K., et al. (2014). Achieving quality health outcomes through the implementation of a spontaneous awakening and spontaneous breathing trial protocol. *AACN Advanced Critical Care*, *25*(1), 33–42.

Kamdar, B. B., Yang, J., & King, L. M., et al. (2013). Developing, implementing, and evaluating a multifaceted quality improvement intervention to promote sleep in an ICU. *American Journal of Medical Quality*, [Epub ahead of print]; Nov 22.

Keyser, S. E., Buchanan, D., & Edge, D. (2012). Providing delirium education for family caregivers of older adults. *Journal of Gerontological Nursing*, *38*(8), 24–31.

Khan, B. A., Zawahiri, M., & Campbell, N. L., et al. (2012). Delirium in hospitalized patients: Implications of current evidence on clinical practice and future avenues for research: A systematic evidence review. *Journal of Hospital Medicine*, *7*(7), 580–589.

Koster, S., Hensens, A. G., & Schuurmans, M. J., et al. (2011). Risk factors of delirium after cardiac surgery: A systematic review. *European Journal of Cardiovascular Nursing*, *10*(4), 197–204.

Maldonado, J. R. (2013). Neuropathogenesis of delirium: Review of current etiologic theories and common pathways. *American Journal of Geriatric Psychiatry*, *21*(12), 1190–1222.

McCusker, J., Cole, M. G., & Voyer, P., et al. (2013). Environmental factors predict the severity of delirium symptoms in long-term care residents with and without delirium. *Journal of the American Geriatrics Society*, *61*(4), 502–511.

Mistraletti, G., Pelosi, P., & Mantovani, E. S., et al. (2012). Delirium: Clinical approach and prevention. *Best Practice and Research. Clinical Anaesthesiology*, *26*(3), 311–326.

Morandi, A., Davis, D., & Fick, D. M., et al. (2014). Delirium superimposed on dementia strongly predicts worse outcomes in older rehabilitation inpatients. *Journal of the American Medical Directors Association*, *15*(5), 349–354.

Morandi, A., Vasilevskis, E. E., & Pandharipande, P. P., et al. (2011). Inappropriate medications in elderly ICU survivors: Where to intervene? *Archives of Internal Medicine*, *171*(11), 1032–1034.

O'Mahoney, R., Murthy, L., & Akunne, A., et al. (2011). Synopsis of the National Institute for Health and Clinical Excellence guideline for prevention of delirium. *Annals of Internal Medicine*, *154*(11), 746–751.

Partridge, J. S., Martin, F. C., & Harari, D., et al. (2013). The delirium experience: What is the effect on patients, relatives and staff and what can be done to modify this? *International Journal of Geriatric Psychiatry*, *28*(8), 804–812.

Pashikanti, L., & Von Ah, D. (2012). Impact of early mobilization protocol on the medical-surgical inpatient population: An integrated review of literature. *Clinical Nurse Specialist*, *26*(2), 87–94.

Patel, J., Baldwin, J., & Bunting, P., et al. (2014). The effect of a multicomponent multidisciplinary bundle of interventions on sleep and delirium in medical and surgical intensive care patients. *Anaesthesia*, *69*(6), 540–549.

Quinlan, N., Marcantonio, E. R., & Inouye, S. K., et al. (2011). Vulnerability: The crossroads of frailty and delirium. *Journal of the American Geriatrics Society*, *59*(Suppl. 2), S262–S268.

Reade, M. C., & Finfer, S. (2014). Sedation and delirium in the intensive care unit. *New England Journal of Medicine*, *370*(5), 444–454.

Rosenbloom, D. A., & Fick, D. M. (2013). Nurse/family caregiver intervention for delirium increases delirium knowledge and improves attitudes toward partnership. *Geriatric Nursing*, [Epub ahead of print].

Rubin, F. H., Neal, K., & Fenlon, K., et al. (2011). Sustainability and scalability of the hospital elder life program at a community hospital. *Journal of the American Geriatrics Society*, *59*(2), 359–365.

Sanford, A. M., & Flaherty, J. H. (2014). Do nutrients play a role in delirium? *Current Opinion in Clinical Nutrition and Metabolic Care*, *17*(1), 45–50.

Sendelbach, S., & Guthrie, P. F. (2009). *Acute confusion/delirium evidence-based guideline*. Iowa City, IA: The University of Iowa John A. Hartford Foundation Center of Geriatric Nursing Excellence.

Steis, M. R., Evans, L., & Hirschman, K. B., et al. (2012). Screening for delirium using family caregivers: Convergent validity of the Family Confusion Assessment Method and interviewer-rated Confusion Assessment Method. *Journal of the American Geriatrics Society*, *60*(11), 2121–2126.

Stites, M. (2013). Observational pain scales in critically ill adults. *Critical Care Nursing*, *33*(3), 68–78.

Swan, J. T. (2014). Decreasing inappropriate unable-to-assess ratings for the confusion assessment method for the intensive care unit. *American Journal of Critical Care*, *23*(1), 60–69.

Tate, J. A., & Happ, M. B. (2011). Neurocognitive problems in critically ill older adults: The importance of history. *Geriatric Nursing*, *32*(4), 285–287.

Tate, J. A., Sereika, S., & Divirgilio, D., et al. (2013). Symptom communication during critical illness: The impact of age, delirium, and delirium presentation. *Journal of Gerontological Nursing*, *39*(8), 28–38.

van den Boogaard, M., Pickkers, P., & Slooter, A. J., et al. (2012). Development and validation of PRE-DELIRIC (PREdiction of DELIRium in ICu patients) delirium prediction model for intensive care patients: Observational multicenter study. *British Medical Journal*, *344*, e420.

van der Cammen, T. J., Rajkumar, C., & Onder, G., et al. (2014). Drug cessation in complex older adults: Time for action. *Age and Ageing*, *43*(1), 20–25.

Voyer, P., Richard, S., & Doucet, L., et al. (2011a). Factors associated with delirium severity among older persons with dementia. *Journal of Neuroscience Nursing*, *43*(2), 62–69.

Voyer, P., Richard, S., & Doucet, L., et al. (2011b). Precipitating factors associated with delirium among long-term care residents with dementia. *Applied Nursing Research*, *24*(3), 171–178.

Wakefield, D., Thompson, L., & Bruce, S. (2014). A Lilliputian army under the floorboards: Persistent delirium with complete though prolonged recovery. *BMJ Case Reports*, pii: bcr2013202639.

Weinhouse, G. L. (2014). Delirium and sleep disturbances in the intensive care unit: Can we do better? *Current Opinion in Anaesthesiology*, [epub ahead of print].

Yoder, J. C., Staisiunas, P. G., & Meltzer, D. O., et al. (2012). Noise and sleep among adult medical inpatients: Far from a quiet night. *Archive of Internal Medicine*, *172*(1), 68–70.

Zaubler, T. S., Murphy, K., & Rizzuto, L., et al. (2013). Quality improvement and cost savings with multicomponent delirium interventions: Replication of the Hospital Elder Life Program in a community hospital. *Psychosomatics*, *54*(3), 219–226.

Chronic Confusion *Mila W. Grady, MSN, RN*

NANDA-I

Definition

Irreversible, long-standing, and/or progressive deterioration of intellect and personality characterized by decreased ability to interpret environmental stimuli; decreased capacity for intellectual thought processes; manifested by disturbances of memory, orientation, and behavior

C

Defining Characteristics

Alteration in interpretation; alteration in personality; alteration in response to stimuli; alteration in short-term memory; impaired social functioning; chronic cognitive impairment; normal level of consciousness; organic brain disorder; progressive alteration in cognitive impairment

Related Factors (r/t)

Alzheimer's disease; cerebrovascular accident; Korsakoff's psychosis; multi-infarct dementia

NOC (Nursing Outcomes Classification)

Suggested NOC Outcomes

Cognition; Cognitive Orientation; Distorted Thought Self-Control

Example NOC Outcome with Indicators

Cognition as evidenced by the following indicators: Cognitive orientation/Communicates clearly for age/Comprehends the meaning of situations/Attentiveness/Concentration. (Rate the outcome and indicators of **Cognition:** 1 = severely compromised, 2 = substantially compromised, 3 = moderately compromised, 4 = mildly compromised, 5 = not compromised [see Section I].)

Client Outcomes

Client Will (Specify Time Frame)

- Remain content and free from harm
- Function at maximal cognitive level
- Participate in activities of daily living at the maximum of functional ability
- Have minimal episodes of agitation (agitation occurs in up to 70% of clients with dementia)

NIC (Nursing Interventions Classification)

Suggested NIC Interventions

Dementia Management; Environmental Management; Surveillance: Safety

Example NIC Activities—Dementia Management

Use distraction rather than confrontation to manage behavior; Give one simple direction at a time

Nursing Interventions and *Rationales*

- Determine the client's cognitive level using a screening tool such as the Mini-Mental State Exam (MMSE), Mini-Cog (includes a three-item recall and clock drawing test), or Montreal Cognitive Assessment. *Culture and ethnicity (Struble & Sullivan, 2011), and language and education (Velayudhan et al, 2014) must be taken into account when interpreting the results of cognitive testing; an abnormal score necessitates further evaluation. For older adults with mild cognitive impairment, the Short Test of Mental Status and Montreal Cognitive Assessment are more sensitive diagnostic tools than the MMSE (Petersen, 2011).*
- ▲ In clients who are complaining of memory loss, assess for depression, alcohol use, medication use, problems with sleep, and nutrition status. *These factors may be implicated in memory loss (Struble & Sullivan, 2011).*
- ▲ Recognize that pharmacological treatment to slow the progression of Alzheimer's disease is most effective when used early in the course of the disease. *The U.S. Food and Drug Administration has approved five drugs that slow the progression of symptoms for approximately 6 to 12 months (Thies et al, 2011).*
- If the client is hospitalized, gather information about the client's preadmission cognitive functioning, daily routines and care, and decision-making capacity. Establishing continuity of care lessens risk for hospitalized clients. Informed consent may create a dilemma; decision-making capacity will vary depending on the degree of cognitive impairment (Weitzel et al, 2011). EBN: *Individuals with a history of cognitive dysfunction are at higher risk for acute confusion during acute illness (Voyer et al, 2011a).*
- Assess the client for signs of depression: anxiety, sadness, irritability, agitation, somatic complaints, tension, loss of concentration, insomnia, poor appetite, apathy, flat affect, and withdrawn behavior. EB:

Depression in dementia is common (Enache et al, 2011), and often unrecognized and undertreated. The Cornell Scale for Depression in Dementia and the Montgomery-Asberg Depression Rating Scale may be used for screening purposes in individuals who cannot be interviewed and may enhance recognition of depression in nursing home practice (Leontjevas et al, 2012).

C

- Assess the client for anxiety if he or she reports worry regarding physical or cognitive health; reports feelings of being anxious, short of breath, or dizzy; or exhibits behaviors such as restlessness, irritability, sensitivity to noise, motor tension, fatigue, or disturbed sleep. The Rating Anxiety in Dementia (RAID) scale may be used; this may require caregiver input. Recognize that anxiety is common in dementia, is often undiagnosed, and may significantly impact quality of life. EB: *The RAID scale is a reliable and valid tool for identifying and measuring anxiety in dementia (Snow et al, 2012).*

▲ Recognize that clients with Alzheimer's disease may experience neuropsychiatric symptoms such as apathy, anxiety and depression, delusions, disinhibition, euphoria, hallucinations, agitation, including verbal/vocal behavior, and aggression; nonpharmacological interventions for management should be attempted first. EB: *Neuropsychiatric symptoms are common in individuals with dementia living in nursing homes; agitation and apathy are the most prevalent symptoms (Selbaek et al, 2013). Nonpharmacological and individualized behavioral interventions should be the first approach to treatment; medications should be used selectively and sparingly (Borisovskaya et al, 2014).*

- Obtain information about the client's life history, interests, routines, needs, and preferences from the family or significant others; collaborate with family members to engage in reminiscence. EBN: *Understanding the individual's past and sharing memories enhances communication and client and staff satisfaction (Cooney et al, 2014).*
- Begin each interaction with the client by gaining and maintaining eye contact, identifying yourself, and calling the client by name. Approach the client with a caring, accepting, and empathetic attitude, and speak calmly and slowly. EB: *Specific communication skills training for caregivers improves the well-being and quality of life in individuals with dementia and increases positive interactions (Eggenberger et al, 2013).*
- To enhance communication, use a calm approach, avoid distractions, show interest, keep communication simple, give clear choices and one-step instructions, give the client time with word finding, use repetition and rephrasing, and use gestures, prompts, and cues or visual aids. Listen attentively to understand nonverbal messages, and engage in topics of interest to the client. EB: *These communication techniques assist in focusing attention, incorporate nonverbal means of communication, simplify memory demands, compensate for cognitive slowing, and assist with retrieval and comprehension (Smith et al, 2011).*
- Engage the client in scheduled activities that relate to past interests, experiences, and hobbies and are matched to current preferences and abilities. CEB: *Activities that were once meaningful to the client in terms of self-identity are more likely to result in engagement, even for those with severe cognitive impairment. Residents with current interests in art, music, and pets were more engaged in stimuli that reflected those current interests (Cohen-Mansfield et al, 2010).*
- Promote regular exercise. EB: *Exercise programs can improve the ability to perform activities of daily living (Forbes et al, 2013); a small study demonstrated that a specific walking program for individuals in the later stages of dementia can reduce functional and cognitive decline (Venturelli et al, 2011).*
- Provide opportunities for contact with nature or nature-based stimuli, such as facilitating time spent outdoors or indoor gardening. EBN: *Gardens and horticultural activities stimulate the senses, may improve well-being, and may reduce disruptive behavior in individuals with dementia (Gonzalez & Kirkevold, 2013).*
- Provide animal-assisted therapy to enhance the care environment. EB: *In a study of animal-assisted therapy with a group of clients with severe Alzheimer's disease, animal-assisted therapy was associated with a decrease in sadness and anxiety and an increase in motor activity and positive emotions (Mossello et al, 2011).* EBN: *Centrally located aquariums were found to decrease problematic behaviors in individuals residing in dementia specific units and improved staff satisfaction (Edwards et al, 2014).*
- Break down self-care tasks into simple steps, giving one direction at a time. For example, instead of saying, "Take a shower," say to the client, "Please follow me. Sit down on the bed. Take off your shoes. Now take off your socks." Use gestures when giving directions; allow for adequate time and model the desired action if needed or possible. EB: *Assistance in focusing attention, modeling behavior, and using prompts and cues maximizes communication with individuals with dementia (Smith et al, 2011).*
- Promote engagement in individual client routines and facilitate success by keeping frequently used items in a visible and consistent location. EBN: *Person-centered care environments facilitate the completion of activities of daily living in individuals with dementia and positively impact quality of life (Sjögren et al, 2013).*

C

- Use reminiscence and life review therapeutic interventions for clients in the early to middle stages of dementia; ask questions about the client's past activities and important events and experiences from the past while using photographs, videos, artifacts, music, newspaper clippings, or multimedia technology to stimulate memories. EB: *In a small preliminary study using YouTube videos, it was found that reminiscence and life review may improve well-being and social engagement (O'Rourke et al, 2011); reminiscence positively impacts quality of life in clients with dementia living in long-term care (O'Shea et al, 2014). Memories from childhood or young adulthood are generally intact in the early and middle stages of Alzheimer's (Smith et al, 2011).*
- Engage clients in the middle to late stages of dementia in creative expression through the use of Time Slips story-telling groups or through person-centered art activities. EB: *A small qualitative study demonstrated that Time Slips positively impacted creativity, quality of life, and behavior of clients with dementia and assisted staff to gain a better understanding of residents in the nursing home community (George & Houser, 2014). An exploratory study that used an intergenerational and person-centered arts activity program called Opening Minds through Art demonstrated an improvement in pleasure and engagement for participants using this program versus using a program with traditional arts activities such a scrapbooking and coloring (Sauer et al, 2014).*
- If the client is verbally agitated (repetitive verbalizations, complaints, moaning, muttering, threats, screaming), assess for and address unsatisfied basic needs or environmental factors that may be addressed and redirect the individual. EB: *Disruptive vocalizations may be an indication that the client with dementia has the need for comfort, attention, or more or less stimulation (Bédard et al, 2011); redirection may be an effective nonpharmacological means to reduce vocalizations (Yusupov & Galvin, 2014).*
- Assist clients in wayfinding, monitoring them so that they do not get lost in unfamiliar settings; place cues and familiar objects in the environment. EB: *Living in a familiar environment that provides opportunities for privacy as well as social contact is associated with better quality of life for individuals with dementia (Fleming et al, 2014).*
- For clients who wander, refer to the **Wandering** care plan.
- Promote sleep by promoting daytime activity, creating a restful sleep environment, decreasing waking, and promoting quiet. EB: *Sleep disorders are very common in those with dementia; individuals with Lewy body dementia experience disturbed sleep twice as often as those without Lewy Body dementia (Bliwise et al, 2011).* CEB: *Promoting a dark and quiet nighttime environment, providing a comfortable sleeping temperature for the client, encouraging physical activity, especially in the afternoon, maintaining a consistent schedule of meals and activities, maintaining a bright daytime environment, and facilitating outdoor activity are all methods of improving sleep (Neikrug & Ancoli-Israel, 2010).*
- Provide activities for the client, such as folding, sorting, or stacking activities, arranging flowers, or other hobbies or routines the individual enjoyed before the onset of dementia. CEB: *The purposeful use of activities tailored to an individual's abilities may allow the individual to maintain social roles and feelings of connectedness, express themselves in a positive way, enhance self-identity, reduce frustration, and prevent boredom, resulting in less agitation (Gitlin et al, 2009).* EBN: *A small pilot study demonstrated that volunteers may be trained to engage clients in meaningful individualized activities in order to enhance quality of life (Van der Ploeg et al, 2014).*
- Anticipate and assess for physical stressors such as fatigue, hunger, thirst, constipation, urinary symptoms, and pain. EBN: *Safe function is enhanced through the establishment of consistent routines and anticipation of basic needs (Lavoie-Vaughan, 2014).*

▲ If the client becomes increasingly confused and/or agitated, perform the following steps:
  - ❍ Assess the client for physiological causes, including acute hypoxia, pain, medication effects, malnutrition, and infections such as urinary tract infection, fatigue, electrolyte disturbances, and constipation. *Dementia increases the risk and severity of delirium, which may be precipitated by several factors (Voyer et al, 2011b).*
  - ❍ Assess for psychological causes, including changes in the environment, caregiver, or routine; demands to perform beyond capacity; or multiple competing stimuli, including discomfort. Encourage communication by addressing the client in a calm, gentle tone of voice and by using appropriate body language, facial expressions, and gestures. EB: *Agitated behaviors can be an expression of a need that is not being met; needs assessment is facilitated through methods to enhance communication so that needs may be expressed (Cohen-Mansfield et al, 2014).*
  - ❍ Use music as a nonpharmacological approach to managing agitation. Identify the client's music preferences; interview family members if necessary. EB: *Music therapy may lead to a short-term decrease in*

agitation in individuals with dementia (Vink et al, 2013). EBN: *Using percussion instruments with familiar music was found to be a cost effective method for decreasing anxiety and improving psychological well-being (Sung et al, 2012); both active and passive musical interventions may improve quality of life (Vasionyte & Madison, 2013).*

- ❍ In clients with agitated behaviors, rather than confronting the client, decrease stimuli in the environment or provide gentle stimulation through diversional activities such as quiet music, looking through a photo album with a staff member, or providing the client with textured items to handle. EBN: *Soothing music at mealtimes may improve agitated behavior (Ho et al, 2011); clients with dementia are frequently overstimulated or understimulated, and activities that provide one-to-one attention from staff may decrease agitation (Maseda et al, 2014).*
- ❍ If clients with dementia become more agitated, assess for pain. EBN: *Pain assessment should include the use of a valid and reliable observer-rated tool such as the Pain Assessment in Advanced Dementia Scale (PAINAD); self-report, the gold standard of pain assessment, may be difficult as dementia advances (Lukas et al, 2013).*

C

- ▲ Avoid using restraints if possible. EB: *The use of trunk restraints is associated with higher fall risk for clients with dementia (Luo et al, 2011).*
- ▲ Use as-needed or low-dose regular dosing of psychotropic or antianxiety drugs only as a last resort; start with the lowest possible dose. EB: *Psychotropic medications can cause serious adverse effects such as sedation, cardiovascular symptoms, and falls; use nonpharmacological interventions to reduce their use (Richter et al, 2012).*
- ▲ Avoid the use of anticholinergic medications such as diphenhydramine. Anticholinergic medications have a high side-effect profile that includes disorientation, urinary retention, and excessive drowsiness, especially in those with decreased cognition. EB: *Older adults with dementia are especially sensitive to the side effects of anticholinergics; one study found that 23% of older adults with dementia use anticholinergic medications (Sura et al, 2013).*
- • For interventions on bathing, refer to the geriatric interventions in the care plan for Bathing **Self-Care** deficit.
- • For care of early dementia clients with primarily symptoms of memory loss, see the care plan for Impaired **Memory**.
- • For clients nearing the end of life, consider a hospice referral. EB: *Family members of individuals with dementia reported higher perceptions of the quality of care and quality of dying experience with hospice care (Teno et al, 2011).*
- • For care of clients with self-care deficits, see the appropriate care plan (Feeding **Self-Care** deficit; Dressing **Self-Care** deficit; Toileting **Self-Care** deficit).

Geriatric

NOTE: All interventions are appropriate for geriatric clients.

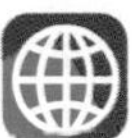

Multicultural

- • Assess for the influence of cultural beliefs, norms, and values on the family's or caregiver's understanding of chronic confusion or dementia; assist the family or caregiver in identifying barriers that would prevent the use of social services or other supportive services that could help reduce the impact of caregiving and refer to social services or other supportive services. EB: *African Americans are at a higher risk for Alzheimer's disease; cultural diversity exists within the older age group of African Americans, influences perceptions of health and knowledge of Alzheimer's disease, and may lead to health disparity (Rovner et al, 2013). Individuals from minority ethnic groups are more cognitively impaired at the time of diagnosis and seek care later in the disease process; a variety of barriers exist for seeking care (Sayegh & Knight, 2013).*
- • Inform the client's family or caregiver of the meaning of and reasons for common behavior observed in clients with dementia. EB: *An understanding of behavior enables the client's family or caregiver to provide the client with a safe environment. Disease expression may vary in different ethnoracial groups; Latinos were found in one study to have more depressive symptoms (Livney et al, 2011).*

Home Care

NOTE: Keeping the client as independent as possible is important. Because community-based care is usually less structured than institutional care, in the home setting the goal of maintaining safety for the client takes on primary importance.

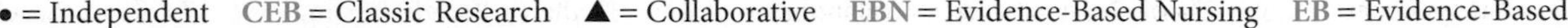

C

- The interventions described previously may be adapted for home care use.
- Provide information to the family and home care client regarding advance directives. *A variety of factors influence the initiation of advance care planning discussions (van der Steen et al, 2014); determining health care preferences and goals in the early stages of dementia is preferable for facilitating optimal end of life care.*
- Assess the client's memory and executive function deficits before assuming the inability to make any medical decisions; driving capacity and financial capacity should be assessed for clients with mild cognitive impairment. *Decisional capacities for informed consent include understanding and demonstrating comprehension of diagnosis and treatment-related information, appreciation of the significance of the information, reasoning regarding alternatives and consequences, and expressing a choice (Weitzel et al, 2011).*
- Assess the home for safety features and client needs for assistive devices. Refer to the interventions for Feeding **Self-Care** deficit, Dressing **Self-Care** deficit, and Bathing **Self-Care** deficit as needed.
- Promote cognitive stimulation and memory training exercises for individuals in the early stages of dementia. EBN: *Cognitive stimulation therapy may positively impact mood, quality of life, and cognitive function (Yamanaka et al, 2013).*
- Provide education and support to the family regarding effective communication, home safety, fall prevention, engagement in meaningful activities, ways to manage cognitive and behavioral changes, and comprehensive health care including screening for depression; be prepared to offer support and information to family members who live at a distance as well. EB: *The need for care, services, and support for individuals in the community with dementia and their caregivers is often unmet; evaluation and diagnosis of dementia, personal and home safety, physical and mental health care, advanced care planning, and legal issues are needs that should be addressed (Black et al, 2013).*
- Use familiar aspects of the environment (smells, music, foods, pictures) to cue the client, capitalizing on habit to remind the client of activities in which the client can participate. CEB: *While clients with dementia are probably unable to learn new activities because of deteriorated explicit memory, preserved implicit memory or habit may be useful in maximizing functional ability (Hong & Song, 2009).*
- Instruct the caregiver to provide a balanced activity schedule that does not stress the client or deprive him or her of stimulation; avoid sustained low- or high-stimulation activity. CEB: *Planned individualized structured activities can prevent agitation (Gitlin et al, 2009).*
- Encourage the caregiver to plan leisure activities that promote cognitive and physical stimulation. EB: *One study that tested the effects of engaging in both tai chi exercises and the game of mahjong found that these activities were beneficial in preserving cognitive function and delayed cognitive decline in some domains of cognitive function (Cheng et al, 2014).*

▲ If the client will require extensive supervision on an ongoing basis, evaluate the client for adult day health care programs. Refer the family to medical social services to assist with this process if necessary. *Day care programs provide safe, structured care for the client and respite for the family, provide care on a sliding scale fee basis, and provide stress relief and respite for the caregiver (Alzheimer's Association, 2014).* EB: *Adult day services use can decrease care-related stressors for the caregiver, which can positively impact the health of the caregiver (Zarit et al, 2013).*

- Encourage the family to include the client in family activities when possible. Reinforce the use of therapeutic communication guidelines (see Client/Family Teaching and Discharge Planning) and sensitivity to the number of people present. *These steps help the client maintain dignity and lead to familial socialization of the client.*
- Assess family caregivers for caregiver stress, loneliness, and depression. Refer to the care plan for **Caregiver Role Strain.**

▲ Refer the client to medical social services as necessary to evaluate financial resources and initiate benefits, and to facilitate access to health care providers and community-based organizations such as support groups and training programs for caregivers. EB: *Comprehensive and coordinated care has the potential to maximize function and independence and reduce caregiver stress while reducing overall costs (Reuben et al, 2013).*

▲ Institute case management for frail elderly clients to support continued independent living.

Client/Family Teaching and Discharge Planning

- In the client's early stages of dementia, provide the caregiver with information on illness processes, needed care, available services, role changes, and importance of advance directives discussion; facilitate family cohesion. EB: *Education provided to caregivers early in the disease trajectory may assist them to anticipate care needs and role changes and to facilitate involving the individual with dementia in care decisions (de Vugt & Verhey, 2013).*

- • Teach the family communication strategies, personal care techniques, mobility enhancement, prevention, recognition and management of anxiety and depression, strategies for handling challenging behaviors and legal and financial considerations. **EBN:** *Clients and caregivers reported overwhelming satisfaction with in-home care delivery provided by a nurse practitioner who addressed dementia care issues proactively (Fortinsky et al, 2014).*
- • Discuss with the family what to expect as the dementia progresses.
- ▲ Counsel the family about resources available regarding end-of-life decisions and legal concerns. **CEB:** *Family members report distress regarding decision-making throughout the course of dementia, having insufficient information, lack of support in having these discussions with family members in the early stages of dementia, role conflict, maintaining the dignity of their family member, family conflict, supporting caregivers throughout the process and assisting them in advocacy is essential (Livingston et al, 2010).*
- ▲ Inform the family that as dementia progresses, hospice care may be available in the home or nursing home in the terminal stages to help the caregiver. **EB:** *Goals for care include appropriate management of delirium and pain, avoidance of polypharmacy, and promotion of quality of life, comfort, and family and caregiver support (Merel et al, 2014).*

C

REFERENCES

Alzheimer's Association. (2014). *Alzheimer's and dementia caregiver center.* Retrieved from: <http://www.alz.org/care/alzheimers-dementia-adult day-centers.asp#cost>.

Bédard, A., Landreville, P., Voyer, P., et al. (2011). Reducing verbal agitation in people with dementia: Evaluation of an intervention based on the satisfaction of basic needs. *Aging and Mental Health, 15*(7), 855–865.

Black, B. S., Johnston, D., Rabins, P. V., et al. (2013). Unmet needs of community-residing persons with dementia and their informal caregivers: Findings from the maximizing independence at home study. *Journal of the American Geriatrics Society, 61*(12), 2087–2095.

Bliwise, D. L., Mercaldo, N. D., Avidan, A. Y., et al. (2011). Sleep disturbance in dementia with Lewy bodies and Alzheimer's disease: A multicenter analysis. *Dementia and Geriatric Cognitive Disorders, 31*(3), 239–246.

Borisovskaya, A., Pascualy, M., & Borson, S. (2014). Cognitive and neuropsychiatric impairments in Alzheimer's Disease: Current treatment strategies. *Current Psychiatry Reports, 16*(9), 470.

Cheng, S. T., Chow, P. K., Song, Y. Q., et al. (2014). Mental and physical activities delay cognitive decline in older persons with dementia. *American Journal of Geriatric Psychiatry, 22*(1), 63–74.

Cohen-Mansfield, J., Thein, K., & Marx, M. S. (2014). Predictors of the impact of nonpharmacologic interventions for agitation in nursing home residents with advanced dementia. *Journal of Clinical Psychiatry, 75*(7), e666–e671.

Cohen-Mansfield, J., Marx, M. S., Thein, K., et al. (2010). The impact of past and present preferences on stimulus engagement in nursing home residents with dementia. *Aging in Mental Health, 14*(1), 67–73.

Cooney, A., Hunter, A., & Murphy, K., et al. (2014). Seeing me through my memories: A grounded theory study on using reminiscence with people with dementia living in long-term care. *Journal of Clinical Nursing,* [epub before print].

de Vugt, M. E., & Verhey, F. R. (2013). The impact of early dementia diagnosis and intervention on informal caregivers. *Progress in Neurobiology, 110*(11), 54–62.

Edwards, N. E., Beck, A. M., & Lim, E. (2014). Influence of aquariums on resident behavior and staff satisfaction in dementia units. *Western Journal of Nursing Research,* [epub ahead of print].

Eggenberger, E., Heimerl, K., & Bennett, M. I. (2013). Communication skills training in dementia care: A systematic review of effectiveness, training content, and didactic methods in different care settings. *International Psychogeriatrics, 25*(3), 345–358.

Enache, D., Winblad, B., & Aarsland, D. (2011). Depression in dementia: Epidemiology, mechanisms, and treatment. *Current Opinion in Psychiatry, 24*(6), 461–472.

Fleming, R., Goodenough, B., Low, L. F., et al. (2014). The relationship between the quality of the built environment and the quality of life of people with dementia in residential care. *Dementia (Basel, Switzerland),* [epub ahead of print].

Forbes, D., Thiessen, E. J., Blake, C. M., et al. (2013). Exercise programs for people with dementia. *Cochrane Database of Systematic Reviews,* (12), Art. No.: CD006489.

Fortinsky, R. H., Delaney, C., Harel, O., et al. (2014). Results and lessons learned from a nurse practitioner-guided dementia care intervention for primary care patients and their family caregivers. *Research in Gerontological Nursing, 7*(3), 126–137.

George, D. R., & Houser, W. S. (2014). "I'm a storyteller!": Exploring the benefits of TimeSlips Creative Expression Program at a nursing home. *American Journal of Alzheimer's Disease and Other Dementias,* [epub ahead of print].

Gitlin, L. N., Winter, L., Vause Earland, T., et al. (2009). The tailored activity program to reduce behavioral symptoms in individuals with dementia: Feasibility, acceptability, and replication potential. *The Gerontologist, 49*(3), 428–439.

Gonzalez, M. T., & Kirkevold, M. (2013). Benefits of sensory garden and horticultural activities in dementia: A modified scoping review. *Journal of Clinical Nursing,* [epub ahead of print].

Hong, G. R., & Song, J. A. (2009). Relationship between familiar environment and wandering behaviour among Korean elders with dementia. *Journal of Clinical Nursing, 18*(9), 1365–1373.

Ho, S.-Y., Lai, H.-L., Jeng, S.-Y., et al. (2011). The effects of researcher-composed music at mealtime on agitation in nursing home residents with dementia. *Archives of Psychiatric Nursing, 25*(6), e49–e55.

Lavoie-Vaughan, N. (2014). A critical analysis and adaptation of a clinical practice guideline for the management of behavioral problems in residents with dementia in long-term care. *Nursing Clinics of North America, 49*(1), 103–113.

Leontjevas, R., Gerritsen, D. L., Vernooij-Dassen, M., et al. (2012). Comparative validation of proxy-based Montgomery-Asberg depression rating scale and Cornell scale for depression in dementia in nursing home residents with dementia. *American Journal of Geriatric Psychiatry*, *20*(11), 985–993.

Livingston, G., Leavey, G., Manela, M., et al. (2010). Making decisions for people with dementia who lack capacity: Qualitative study of family carers in UK. *British Medical Journal*, *341*, c4184.

Livney, M. G., Clark, C. M., Karlawish, J. H., et al. (2011). Ethnoracial differences in the clinical characteristics of Alzheimer's disease at initial presentation at an urban Alzheimer's disease center. *American Journal of Geriatric Psychiatry*, *19*(5), 430–439.

Lukas, A., Barber, J. B., Johnson, P., et al. (2013). Observer-rated pain assessment instruments improve both the detection of pain and the evaluation of pain intensity in people with dementia. *European Journal of Pain*, *17*(10), 1558–1568.

Luo, H., Lin, M., & Castle, N. (2011). Physical restraint use and falls in nursing homes: A comparison between residents with and without dementia. *American Journal of Alzheimer's Disease and Other Dementias*, *26*(1), 44–50.

Maseda, A., Sanchez, A., Marante, M. P., et al. (2014). Multisensory stimulation on mood, behavior, and biomedical parameters in people with dementia: Is it more effective than conventional one-to-one stimulation? *American Journal of Alzheimer's Disease and Other Dementias*, [Epub ahead of print].

Merel, S., DeMers, S., & Vig, E. (2014). Palliative care in advanced dementia. *Clinics of Geriatric Medicine*, *30*(3), 469–492.

Mossello, E., Ridolfi, A., Mello, A. M., et al. (2011). Animal-assisted activity and emotional status of patients with Alzheimer's disease in day care. *International Psychogeriatrics*, *23*(6), 899–905.

Neikrug, A. B., & Ancoli-Israel, S. (2010). Sleep disturbances in nursing homes. *Journal of Nutrition, Health and Aging*, *14*(3), 207–211.

O'Shea, E., Devane, D., Cooney, A., et al. (2014). The impact of reminiscence on the quality of life of residents with dementia in long-stay care. *International Journal of Geriatric Psychiatry*, [epub ahead of print].

O'Rourke, J., Tobin, F., O'Callaghan, S., et al. (2011). You tube: A useful tool for reminiscence therapy in dementia? *Age and Ageing*, *40*(6), 742–744.

Petersen, R. C. (2011). Mild cognitive impairment. *New England Journal of Medicine*, *364*(23), 2227–2234.

Reuben, D. B., Evertson, L. C., Wenger, N. S., et al. (2013). The University of California at Los Angeles Alzheimer's and dementia care program for comprehensive, coordinated, patient-centered care: Preliminary data. *Journal of the American Geriatrics Society*, *61*(12), 2214–2218.

Richter, T., Meyer, G., Möhler, R., et al. (2012). Psychosocial interventions for reducing antipsychotic medication in care home residents. *Cochrane Database Systems Review*, (12), CD008634.

Rovner, B. W., Casten, R. J., & Harris, L. F. (2013). Cultural diversity and views on Alzheimer disease in older African Americans. *Alzheimer's Disease and Associated Disorders*, *27*(2), 133–137.

Sauer, P. E., Fopma-Loy, J., Kinney, J. M., et al. (2014). It makes me feel like myself": Person-centered versus traditional visual arts activities for people with dementia. *Dementia (Basel, Switzerland)*, [epub ahead of print].

Sayegh, P., & Knight, B. G. (2013). Cross-cultural differences in dementia: The sociocultural health belief model. *International Psychogeriatrics*, *25*(4), 517–530.

Selbaek, G., Engedal, K., & Bergh, S. (2013). The prevalence and course of neuropsychiatric symptoms in nursing home patients with dementia: A systematic review. *Journal of the American Medical Directors Association*, *14*(3), 161–169.

Sjögren, K., Lindkvist, M., Sandman, P. O., et al. (2013). Person-centeredness and its association with resident well-being in dementia care units. *Journal of Advanced Nursing*, *69*(10), 2196–2206.

Smith, E. R., Broughton, M., Baker, R., et al. (2011). Memory and communication support in dementia: Research-based strategies for caregivers. *International Psychogeriatrics*, *23*(2), 256–263.

Snow, A. L., Huddleston, C., Robinson, C., et al. (2012). Psychometric properties of a structured interview guide for the rating for anxiety in dementia. *Aging and Mental Health*, *16*(5), 592–602. [Epub 2012 Feb 28].

Struble, L. M., & Sullivan, B. J. (2011). Cognitive health in older adults. *Nurse Practitioner*, *36*(4), 24–34.

Sung, H. C., Lee, W. L., Li, T. L., et al. (2012). A group music intervention using percussion instruments with familiar music to reduce anxiety and agitation of institutionalized older adults with dementia. *International Journal of Geriatric Psychiatry*, *27*(6), 621–627.

Sura, S. D., Carnahan, R. M., Chen, H., et al. (2013). Prevalence and determinants of anticholinergic medication use in elderly dementia patients. *Drugs and Aging*, *30*(10), 837–844.

Teno, J. M., Gozalo, P. L., Lee, I. C., et al. (2011). Does hospice improve quality of care for persons dying from dementia? *Journal of the American Geriatrics Society*, *59*(8), 1531–1536.

Thies, W., Bleiler, L., & Alzheimer's Association. (2011). 2011 Alzheimer's disease facts and figures. *Alzheimer's and Dementia*, *7*(2), 208–244.

Van der Ploeg, E. S., Walker, H., & O'Connor, D. W. (2014). The feasibility of volunteers facilitating personalized activities for nursing home residents with dementia and agitation. *Geriatric Nursing*, *35*(2), 142–146.

van der Steen, J. T., van Soest-Poortvliet, M. C., Hallie-Heierman, M., et al. (2014). Factors associated with initiation of advance care planning in dementia: a systematic review. *Journal of Alzheimer's Disease*, *40*(3), 743–757.

Vasionyte, I., & Madison, G. (2013). Musical intervention for patients with dementia: A meta-analysis. *Journal of Clinical Nursing*, *22*(9–10), 1203–1216.

Velayudhan, L., Ryu, S. H., Raczek, M., et al. (2014). Review of brief cognitive tests for patients with suspected dementia. *International Psychogeriatrics*, *26*(8), 1247–1262.

Venturelli, M., Scarsini, R., & Schena, F. (2011). Six-month walking program changes cognitive and ADL performance in patients with Alzheimer. *American Journal of Alzheimer's Disease and Other Dementia*, *26*(5), 381–388.

Vink, A. C., Zuidersma, M., Boersma, F., et al. (2013). The effect of music therapy compared with general recreational activities in reducing agitation in people with dementia: A randomized controlled trial. *International Journal of Geriatric Psychiatry*, *28*(10), 1031–1038.

Voyer, P., Richard, S., Doucet, L., et al. (2011a). Factors associated with delirium severity among older persons with dementia. *Journal of Neuroscience Nursing*, *43*(2), 62–69.

Voyer, P., Richard, S., Doucet, L., et al. (2011b). Precipitating factors associated with delirium among long-term care residents with dementia. *Applied Nursing Research*, *24*(3), 171–178.

Weitzel, T., Robinson, S., Barnes, M. R., et al. (2011). The special needs of the hospitalized patient with dementia. *Medsurg Nursing*, *20*(1), 13–18.

Yamanaka, K., Kawano, Y., Noguchi, D., et al. (2013). Effects of cognitive stimulation therapy Japanese version (CST-J) for people with dementia: A single-blind, controlled clinical trial. *Aging and Mental Health*, *17*(5), 579–586.

Yusupov, A., & Galvin, J. E. (2014). Vocalization in dementia: A case report and review of the literature. *Case Reports in Neurology*, *6*(1), 126–133.

Zarit, S. H., Kim, K., Femia, E. E., et al. (2013). The effects of adult day services on family caregivers' daily stress, affect, and health: Outcomes from the daily stress and health (DaSH) study. *The Gerontologist*, *54*(4), 570–579.

Risk for acute Confusion *Betty J. Ackley, MSN, EdS, RN*

NANDA-I

Definition

Vulnerable to reversible disturbances of consciousness, attention, cognition, and perception that develop over a short period of time, which may compromise health

Risk Factors

Age ≥ 60 years; alteration in cognitive functioning; alteration in sleep-wake cycle; dehydration; dementia; history of cerebral vascular accident; impaired metabolic functioning (e.g., azotemia, decreased hemoglobin, electrolyte imbalance, increase in blood urea nitrogen/creatinine); impaired mobility; inappropriate use of restraints; infection; male gender; malnutrition; pain; pharmaceutical agent; sensory deprivation; substance abuse; urinary retention

NIC, NOC, Client Outcomes, Nursing Interventions, Client/Family Teaching, *Rationales*, and References

Refer to care plan for Acute **Confusion.**

Constipation *Amanda Andrews, MA, Ed, BSc, DN, RN, HEA Fellow, and A.B. St. Aubyn, BSc (Hons), RGN, RM, RHV, DPS:N (CHS), MSc, PGCert (Education), HEA Fellow*

NANDA-I

Definition

Decrease in normal frequency of defecation accompanied by difficult or incomplete passage of stool and/or passage of excessively hard, dry stool

Defining Characteristics

Abdominal pain; abdominal tenderness with palpable muscle resistance; abdominal tenderness without palpable muscle resistance; anorexia; atypical presentations in older adults (e.g., change in mental status, urinary incontinence, unexplained falls, elevated body temperature); borborygmi; bright red blood with stool; change in bowel pattern; decrease in stool frequency; decrease in stool volume; distended abdomen; fatigue; hard, formed stool; headache; hyperactive bowel sounds; hypoactive bowl sounds; inability to defecate; increase in intra-abdominal pressure; indigestion; liquid stool; pain with defecation; palpable abdominal mass; palpable rectal mass; percussed abdominal dullness; rectal fullness; rectal pressure; severe flatus; soft, paste-like stool in rectum; straining with defecation; vomiting

Related Factors

Functional

Abdominal muscle weakness; average daily physical activity is less than recommended for gender and age; habitually ignores urge to defecate; inadequate toileting habits; irregular defecation habits; recent environmental change

Mechanical

Electrolyte imbalance; hemorrhoids; Hirschsprung's disease; neurological impairment (e.g., positive electroencephalogram, head trauma, seizure disorders); obesity; postsurgical bowel obstruction; pregnancy; prostate enlargement; rectal abscess; rectal anal fissures; rectal anal stricture; rectal prolapsed; rectal ulcer; rectocele; tumors

C

Pharmacological

Laxative abuse; pharmaceutical agent

Physiological

Decrease in gastrointestinal motility; dehydration; eating habit change (e.g., foods, eating times); inadequate dentition; inadequate oral hygiene; insufficient dietary habits; insufficient fiber intake; insufficient fluid intake

Psychological

Confusion; depression; emotional disturbance

NOC (Nursing Outcomes Classification)

Suggested NOC Outcomes

Bowel Elimination; Hydration

Example NOC Outcome with Indicators

Bowel Elimination as evidenced by the following indicators: Elimination pattern/Stool soft and formed/Passage of stool without aids/Ease of stool passage. (Rate each indicator of **Bowel Elimination:** 1 = severely compromised, 2 = substantially compromised, 3 = moderately compromised, 4 = mildly compromised, 5 = not compromised [see Section I].)

Client Outcomes

Client Will (Specify Time Frame)

Maintain passage of soft, formed stool every 1 to 3 days without straining; State relief from discomfort of constipation; Identify measures that prevent or treat constipation

NIC (Nursing Interventions Classification)

Suggested NIC Intervention

Constipation/Impaction Management

Example NIC Activities—Constipation/Impaction Management

Identify factors (e.g., medications, bed rest, and diet) that may cause or contribute to constipation/impaction; Institute a toileting schedule, as appropriate

Nursing Interventions and *Rationales*

- Introduce yourself to the client and any companions, and inform them of your role. Introducing yourself to a client helps establish and develop a therapeutic relationship that recognizes the person within the client and forms the basis for building trust upon which to base the provision of care (Howatson-Jones et al, 2012).
- Gain consent to carry out care before proceeding further with the assessment. Clients have the right of autonomy both legally and morally and therefore should be fully involved in the decision-making process (Avery, 2013).
- Wash hands using a recognized technique. EB: *Performing strict hand-hygiene regimens significantly reduces the incidence of infection with methicillin-resistant* Staphylococcus aureus *and* Clostridium difficile *(Health Protection Agency, 2013).*
- Assess usual pattern of defecation and establish the extent of the constipation problem. EB: *A detailed and accurate assessment of the patient enables the nurse to plan interventions, monitor outcomes, and evaluate care, ensuring no unnecessary treatment is rendered (Matthews, 2011).*
  - Bowel habits
    - Time of day
    - Amount and frequency of stool
    - Consistency of stool (using the Bristol Stool Scale)
    - Bleeding/passing mucus on defecation
    - History of bowel habits and/or laxative use

- ❍ Lifestyle assessment
  - Fiber content in diet
  - Daily fluid intake
  - Exercise patterns
  - Personal remedies for constipation
  - Recently stopped smoking
  - Alcohol consumption/recreational drug use
- ❍ Past medical history
  - Obstetrical/gynecological/urological history and surgeries
  - Diseases that affect bowel motility
  - Bleeding/passing mucous on defecation
  - Current medications
- ❍ Emotional influences
  - Anxiety and depression
  - Long-term defecation issues
  - Stress

- Assess usual pattern of defecation, including time of day, amount and frequency of stool, consistency of stool; history of bowel habits or laxative use; diet, including fiber and fluid intake; exercise patterns; personal remedies for constipation; obstetrical/gynecological history; surgeries; diseases that affect bowel motility; alterations in perianal sensation; present bowel regimen. Individual bowel habits vary and clients with constipation experience a variety of symptoms (Spinzi et al, 2009; Kyle 2011a).
- Consider emotional influences (e.g., depression and anxiety) on defecation. Emotions influence gastrointestinal function, possibly because control of both emotions and gastrointestinal function is located in the limbic system of the brain. Difficulties with defecation often begin in childhood (e.g., during toilet training), and constipation is also associated with sexual and physical abuse, depression, and anxiety (Whitehead et al, 2009). EBN: *In a study, clients with functional constipation were compared to normal controls; subjects with functional constipation had significantly higher anxiety and depression scores (Zhou et al, 2010).*
- Complete a physical examination (palpation for abdominal distention, percussion for dullness, and auscultation for bowel sounds). A physical examination provides positive and negative findings and may provide the diagnosis without the need for further testing. It may also reveal unsuspected findings or confirm normality (Rhoads & Murphy-Jensen, 2014).
- Encourage the client or family to keep a 7-day diary of bowel habits to include time of day, length of time spent on the toilet, consistency, amount and frequency of stool, and any straining (using the Bristol Stool Scale). EB: *Keeping a diary helps establish a patient's bowel pattern and may contribute to the patient's adherence to the proposed care plan (Andrews & Morgan, 2013).*
- Encourage the client or family to keep a 7-day diary of lifestyle issues in relation to bowel habits to include fluid consumption, fiber content in diet, usual bowel stimulus and exercise regimen. EB: *Enabling patients to present their condition in their own words ensures that they feel the health care professionals understand their concerns (Smith, 2012).*
- Use the Bristol Stool Scale to assess stool consistency. *The Bristol Stool Scale is widely used as a more objective measure to describe stool consistency (Tack et al, 2011).*

▲ Review the client's current medications. EB: *Many medications are associated with chronic constipation including opioids, anticholinergics, antidepressants, antihypertensives (e.g., clonidine, calcium channel blockers), antispasmodics, diuretics, anticonvulsants, and psychotropics (Eoff & Lembo, 2008; Spinzi et al, 2009). If clients are suffering from constipation and are taking constipating medications, consult with the health care provider about the possibilities of decreasing the medication dosages or finding an alternative medication that is less constipating (Gallagher et al, 2008; Kyle, 2011b).*

- Discuss with clients already taking opioids (temporarily or long term) that constipation is a common side effect. Advise them to contact their health care provider for a prescription of an appropriate laxative. *The thorough and comprehensive assessment of patients on opioids experiencing constipation will also allow for a bowel function approach for laxative prescribing rather than one based on the opioid dose alone (Andrews & Morgan, 2012).*

▲ Recognize that opioids cause constipation. If the client is receiving temporary opioids (e.g., for acute postoperative pain), request an order for routine stool softeners from the primary care provider, monitor bowel movements, and request a laxative for the client if constipation develops. If the client is receiving around-the-clock opiates (e.g., for palliative care), request an order for Senokot-S and institute a bowel regimen. *Opioids cause constipation because they decrease propulsive movement in the colon and enhance sphincter tone, making it difficult to defecate. Senokot-S is recommended to prevent constipation when opioids are given around the clock (Kyle, 2007).* EB: *In a study of clients with hip fracture who received opioids following surgery, clients who received prophylactic laxatives were less likely to develop constipation than those who did not (Davies et al, 2008).*

▲ If the client is terminally ill and is receiving around-the-clock opioids for palliative care, speak with the prescribing health care provider about ordering methylnaltrexone, a drug that blocks opioid effects on the gastrointestinal tract without interfering with analgesia. *Methylnaltrexone is FDA approved for clients in palliative care when other laxatives are ineffective (Greenwood-Van Meerveld & Standifer, 2008). Methylnaltrexone does not replace, but is given in addition to, the usual laxative regimen (Kyle, 2009).* EB: *In a randomized control trial (RCT) of subjects with opioid-induced constipation, a significantly greater percentage of those who received methylnaltrexone had a bowel movement within 4 hours (without other laxatives) than those who received placebo (Thomas et al, 2008). In a randomized study of clients who took opioids for chronic, nonmalignant pain, those who received subcutaneous methylnaltrexone daily or every other day had significantly more bowel movements than subjects who received placebo (Michna et al, 2011).*

• If new onset of constipation, determine whether the client has recently stopped smoking. *Constipation is common, but usually transient, when people stop smoking (Wilcox et al, 2010).* CEB: *In a survey about perceived effects of various foods and beverages on constipation, cigarettes was the item that was most often perceived to have a laxative effect among smokers in all three groups (Müller-Lissner et al, 2005).*

• Palpate for abdominal distention, percuss for dullness, and auscultate bowel sounds. *In clients with constipation the abdomen is often distended and tender, and stool in the colon produces a dull percussion sound. Bowel sounds will be present.*

▲ Check for impaction; if present, perform digital removal of stool per the health care provider's order. An impaction is hard stool that is too large to move through the sphincter and must be removed manually. Clients with neurogenic bowel dysfunction (e.g., spinal cord injury) commonly require manual evacuation of stool (Coggrave & Norton, 2010).

▲ Advise a fiber intake of 18 to 25 g daily and suggest foodstuffs high in fiber (e.g., prune juice, leafy green vegetables, whole meal bread and pasta). *Fiber creates bulky feces and stretches the bowel wall to stimulate peristalsis, thus shortening bowel transit time (Kyle, 2012).*

• Add fiber gradually to the diet to decrease bloating and flatus. *Larger stools move through the colon faster than smaller stools, and dietary fiber makes stools bigger because it is undigested in the upper intestinal tract. Fiber fermentation by bacteria in the colon produces gas. The effectiveness of water-insoluble fibers (e.g., wheat bran) on bowel function is well supported by research, and there is growing evidence that water-soluble fibers (e.g., psyllium) also promote laxation (Vuksan et al, 2008).* CEB: *The Nurses' Health Study found that women with a median fiber intake of 20 g/day were less likely to experience constipation than those with a median intake of 7 g/day (Dukas et al, 2003). In a study of subjects receiving each of five treatments in a randomized design, the five treatments included (1) bran cereal, (2) bran with corn cereal, (3) bran with psyllium cereal, (4) a cereal blend of 70% glucomannan and 30% xanthan, and (5) the low-fiber control diet. All four cereals produced significantly greater bowel movement than the low-fiber control diet and all were well tolerated (Vuksan et al, 2008). Researchers found that rye bread shortened intestinal transit time, softened the feces, and eased defecation in women with constipation, and that yogurt lessened the bloating and flatulence resulting from rye bread (Hongisto et al, 2006).*

• Use a mixture of bran cereal, applesauce, and prune juice; begin administration in small amounts and gradually increase amount. Keep refrigerated. Always check with the primary care provider before initiating this intervention. It is important that the client also ingest sufficient fluids. CEB: *This bran mixture has been shown to be effective even with short-term use in older clients recovering from acute conditions; however, it has not been tested with an RCT (Joanna Briggs Institute, 2008). Note: Giving fiber without sufficient fluid may result in worsening of constipation. Additional dietary fiber and bulk-forming laxatives are inappropriate for those who have difficulty ingesting adequate fluids, such as clients in palliative care (Kyle, 2007).*

• Provide prune or prune juice daily. Each 100 g of prunes contains about 6 g of fiber, 15 g of sorbitol, and 184 mg of polyphenol; all have laxative effects (Attaluri et al, 2011). CEB: *In a study about the perceived effects of various foods and beverages on stool consistency, more than half of subjects surveyed reported that prunes had a softening effect on their stools (Müller-Lissner et al, 2005). In a randomized study, dried prunes produced significantly more complete spontaneous bowel movements per week than psyllium, and both treatments produced significantly more complete spontaneous bowel movements than at baseline (Attaluri et al, 2011).*

C

- Advise a fluid intake of 1.5 to 2 L of fluid per day (ideally, 6 to 8 glasses of water), unless contraindicated by comorbidities, such as kidney or heart disease. *Water passes into the gut to promote the formation of a softer fecal mass and provides lubrication to prevent a blockage of the gut (Boyle, 2013).*
- ▲ If the client is uncomfortable or in pain due to constipation or has acute or chronic constipation that does not respond to increased fiber, fluid, activity, and appropriate toileting, refer the client to the primary care provider for an evaluation of bowel function and health status. *There can be multiple causes of constipation, such as endocrine disorders (e.g., hypothyroidism), depression, neurological conditions (e.g., multiple sclerosis and Parkinson's disease), anorectal disorders, and Hirschsprung's disease (Eoff & Lembo, 2008).*
- Encourage physical activity within the client's current ability to mobilize. Encourage turning and changing position in bed if immobile. For clients with reduced mobility, encourage knee to chest raises, waist twists, and stretching the arms away from the body. For fully mobile clients, encourage walking and swimming. *Physical activity can help stimulate peristaltic waves in the colon and encourage the transit of feces to the rectum (Rogers, 2013; Andersen et al, 2006).*
- Demonstrate the use of gentle external abdominal massage, using aroma therapy oils, following the direction of colon activity. *Abdominal massage encourages rectal loading by increasing intra-abdominal pressure and in some cases it may elicit rectal waves, which may stimulate the somato-autonomic reflex and enhance bowel sensation (McClurg et al, 2011).*
- Recommend clients establish a regular elimination routine. If required assist clients to the bathroom at the same time every day, being mindful of the need for privacy (closing of bathroom doors). *Establishing a routine allows for the use of the gastrocolic reflex, especially in the morning, which aids defecation (Rogers, 2013).*
- Provide privacy for defecation. If not contraindicated, help the client to the bathroom and close the door. *Bowel elimination is a private act in Western cultures, and a lack of privacy can hinder the defecation urge, thus contributing to constipation (Kyle, 2011a).*
- Help clients onto a bedside commode or toilet so they can either squat or lean forward while sitting. Recognize that it is difficult to impossible to defecate in the lying supine position. Sitting upright allows gravity to aid defecation. **CEB:** *A study of men found that flexing the hip to 90 degrees or more straightens the angle between the anus and the rectum and pulls the anal canal open, decreasing the resistance to the movement of feces from the rectum and the amount of pressure needed to empty the rectum. Hip flexion is greatest when squatting or when leaning forward while sitting (Tagart, 1966). In a study involving volunteers, defecation required significantly less time and was significantly easier when squatting than when sitting (Sikirov, 2003). In another study, researchers found a significant decrease in the ability of subjects to defecate both a water-filled balloon and a silicone device in the lying position versus the sitting position (Rao et al, 2006).*
- Educate the client how to adopt the best posture for defecation. Keep knees slightly higher than hips, keep feet flat on the floor and lean forward putting elbows onto knees. **EB:** *Adopting the correct position to open one's bowels allows the angle of the rectum and anal canal to straighten out. This facilitates an increase in abdominal pressure, which makes defecation more effective (Rogers, 2013).*
- Teach clients of the importance of responding promptly to the urge to defecate. **EB:** *The body's natural "call to stool" should be heeded in that it is a response to the stimulation of nerve endings in the rectum when a stool is present. Ignoring this urge will result in the rectum becoming desensitized to a stool in situ (Coggrave et al, 2014).* **CEB:** *A study of male volunteers determined that the defecation urge can be delayed and that delaying defecation decreased bowel movement frequency, stool weight, and transit time (Klauser et al, 1990).*
- Consider the use of laxatives, suppositories, enemas, and bowel irrigation as required if other more natural interventions are not effective. *Laxative therapies can be used in conjunction with lifestyle changes (while waiting for the lifestyle changes to take effect or if the change is not sufficient in itself) (Marples, 2011).*
- Discourage the use of long-term laxatives and enemas and advise clients to gradually reduce their use if taken regularly. *Long-term use or overuse of laxatives can cause health problems (e.g., electrolyte imbalance) or hide symptoms that may be from a serious medical condition, such as cardiac arrhythmias (Aschenbrenner, 2014).*

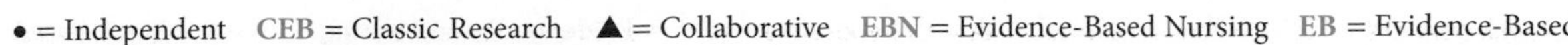

C

Geriatric

- Assess older adults for the presence of factors that contribute to constipation, including dietary fiber and fluid intake (less than 1.5 L/day), physical activity, use of constipating medications, and diseases that are associated with constipation.
- Explain the importance of adequate fiber intake, fluid intake, activity, and established toileting routines to ensure soft, formed stool. EB: *Strong evidence exists for the efficacy of adequate hydration and dietary fiber in the prevention of constipation in older adults; moderate evidence exists for the effectiveness of increased activity for those restricted to bed rest (Joanna Briggs Institute, 2008). In an RCT of older nursing home residents who were chronically ill and regularly used laxatives, those who received an additional 5.1 g of oat bran with their usual diets had significant reductions in laxative use when compared to those who did not (Sturtzel & Elmadfa, 2008).* CEB: *A study involving institutionalized older men with chronic constipation demonstrated that, with use of a bran mixture, clients were able to discontinue use of oral laxatives (Howard et al, 2000).*
- Determine the client's perception of normal bowel elimination and laxative use; promote adherence to a regular schedule. EB: *In a survey in the United States, United Kingdom, Germany, France, Italy, Brazil, and South Korea, older subjects reported more constipation and used laxatives more often than younger subjects (Wald et al, 2008).*
- Explain why straining (Valsalva maneuver) should be avoided. *Excessive straining can cause syncope or cardiac dysrhythmias in susceptible people (Gallagher et al, 2008).*
- Respond quickly to the client's call for assistance with toileting.
- Offer food, fluids, activity, and toileting opportunities to older clients who are cognitively impaired. *Even cognitively impaired individuals who are unable to initiate a request for food, fluids, and so forth may respond when opportunities are offered (Gallagher et al, 2008).* EB: *In an RCT involving nursing home residents, subjects who received the treatment protocol (offering of food, fluid, activity, and toileting opportunities) had significantly more bowel movements than the control group. Both cognitively intact and cognitively impaired subjects benefited from the treatment (Schnelle et al, 2010).*
- Avoid regular use of enemas in older adults. *Enemas can cause fluid and electrolyte imbalances (Gallagher et al, 2008) and damage to the colonic mucosa (Schmelzer et al, 2004). However, judicious enema use may help prevent impactions (Gallagher et al, 2008).*

▲ Use opioids cautiously. Opioids cause constipation (Davies et al, 2008).

- Position the client on the toilet or commode and place a small footstool under the feet. Placing a small footstool helps the client assume a squatting posture to facilitate defecation.

Home Care

- The interventions described previously may be adapted for home care use.
- Take complaints seriously and evaluate claims of constipation in a matter-of-fact manner. Continued constipation can lead to bowel obstruction, a medical emergency. Use of a matter-of-fact manner will limit positive reinforcement of the behavior if actual constipation does not exist. Refer to the care plan for Perceived **Constipation**.
- Assess the self-care management activities the client is already using. CEB: *Many older adults seek solutions to constipation, with laxative use a frequent remedy that creates its own problems (Annells & Koch, 2002).*
- Offer the following treatment recommendations:
  - Acknowledge the client's life-long experience of bowel function; respect beliefs, attitudes, and preferences, and avoid patronizing responses.
  - Make available comprehensive, useful written information about constipation and possible solutions.
  - Make available empathetic and accessible professional care to provide treatment and advice; a multidisciplinary approach (including health care provider, nurse, and pharmacist) should be used.
  - Institute a bowel management program.
  - Consider affordability when suggesting solutions to constipation; discuss cost-effective strategies.
  - Discuss a range of solutions to constipation and allow the client to choose the preferred options.
  - Have orders in place for a suppository and enema as the need may occur. As part of a bowel management program, suppositories or enemas may become necessary.
- Although the use of a bedside commode may be necessitated by the client's condition, allow the client to use the toilet in the bathroom when possible and provide assistance. *Bowel elimination is a private act, and a lack of privacy can contribute to constipation.*

- In older clients, routinely advise consumption of fluids, fruits, and vegetables as part of the diet, and ambulation if the client is able. Introduce a bowel management program at the first sign of constipation. Constipation is a major problem for terminally ill or hospice clients, who may need very high doses of opioids for pain management (Sykes, 2006).

▲ Refer for consideration of the use of polyethylene glycol 3350 (PEG-3350) for constipation. CEB: *In a study of PEG-3350 use for idiopathic constipation, researchers concluded that it appeared to be safe and efficacious when dietary and lifestyle changes were ineffective. Clients reported increased perceived bowel control, with reduced complaints of straining, stool hardness, bloating, and gas (Stoltz et al, 2001). There is good evidence to support the use of PEG for chronic constipation (Ramkumar & Rao, 2005).*

- Advise the client against attempting to remove impacted feces on his or her own. *Older or confused clients in particular may attempt to remove feces and cause rectal damage.*
- When using a bowel program, establish a pattern that is very regular and allows the client to be part of the family unit. Regularity of the program promotes psychological and/or physiological readiness to evacuate stool. Families of home care clients often cannot proceed with normal daily activities until bowel programs are complete.

Client/Family Teaching and Discharge Planning

- Instruct the client on normal bowel function and the need for adequate fluid and fiber intake, activity, and a defined toileting pattern in a bowel program.
- Encourage the client to heed defecation warning signs and develop a regular schedule of defecation by using a stimulus such as a warm drink or prune juice. *Most cases of constipation are mechanical and result from habitual neglect of impulses that signal the appropriate time for defecation.*
- Encourage the client to avoid long-term use of laxatives and enemas and to gradually withdraw from their use if they are used regularly. *Use of stimulant laxatives should be avoided; long-term use can result in dependence on laxative for defecation (Roerig et al, 2010).*
- If not contraindicated, teach the client how to do bent-leg sit-ups to increase abdominal tone; also encourage the client to contract the abdominal muscles frequently throughout the day. Help the client develop a daily exercise program to increase peristalsis.
- Provide client with comprehensive written information about constipation and its management. EB: *Providing patients with well-written, evidence-based information about their condition and treatment can have a beneficial effect on the outcomes of treatment. In addition, patients are more likely to retain important information that will assist them in making informed decisions about their care (Coulter, 2011).*

▲ Collaborate with members of the interprofessional team to provide treatment and advice to clients and caregivers. Team working is a central process in health care organizations. It increases the capacity of teams to absorb and develop new knowledge, which will improve patient health and well-being (Ortega et al, 2013).

- Formalize all advice by providing a bowel management program reiterating the mechanism of normal bowel function and the need for adequate fluid and fiber intake, physical activity, and a defined toileting pattern in an agreed bowel program. EB: *The implementation of an organized bowel management program is effective and significantly reduces hospital admissions in patients with severe idiopathic constipation (Russell et al, 2013).*
- Document all care and advice given in a factual and comprehensive manner. *Good record keeping is an integral part of nursing practice and is essential to the provision of safe and effective care (St. Aubyn & Andrews, 2012).*

REFERENCES

Andersen, C., et al. (2006). The effect of a multidimensional exercise program on symptoms and side-effects in cancer patient undergoing chemotherapy-the use of semi-structured diaries. *European Journal of Oncology Nursing, 10*, 247–262.

Andrews, A., & Morgan, G. (2012). Constipation management in palliative care: treatments and the potential of independent nurse prescribing. *International Journal of Palliative Nursing, 18*(1), 17–22.

Andrews, A., & Morgan, G. (2013). Constipation in palliative care: treatment options and considerations for individual patient management. *International Journal of Palliative Nursing, 19*(6), 226–273.

Annells, M., & Koch, T. (2002). Older people seeking solutions to constipation: the laxative mire. *Journal of Clinical Nursing, 11*, 603.

Aschenbrenner, D. S. (2014). Overuse of certain OTC laxatives may be dangerous. *American Journal of Nursing, 114*(5), 25.

Attaluri, A., et al. (2011). Randomised clinical trial: dried plums (prunes) vs psyllium for constipation. *Alimentary Pharmacology and Therapeutics, 33*, 822–828.

C

Avery, G. (2013). *Law and Ethics in Nursing and Healthcare an Introduction*. London: Sage Publications Inc.
Boyle, J. (2013). Roughage to regulate. *World of Irish Nursing and Midwifery, 21*(7), 53–55.
Coggrave, M. J., & Norton, C. (2010). The need for manual evacuation and oral laxatives in the management of neurogenic bowel dysfunction after spinal cord injury: a randomized controlled trial of a stepwise protocol. *Spinal Cord, 48*, 504–510.
Coggrave, K., Norton, C., & Cody, J. D. (2014). Management of faecal incontinence and constipation in adults with central neurological diseases. *Cochrane Database of Systematic Reviews*, (1), CD002115.
Coulter, A. (2011). *Engaging Patients in Health Care*. Berkshire: McGraw Hill Open University Press.
Davies, E. C., et al. (2008). The use of opioids and laxatives, and incidence of constipation, in patients requiring neck-of-femur (NOF) surgery: a pilot study. *Journal of Clinical Pharmacy and Therapeutics, 33*, 561–566.
Dukas, L., Willett, W. C., & Giovannucci, E. L. (2003). Association between physical activity, fiber intake, and other lifestyle variables and constipation in a study of women. *The American Journal of Gastroenterology, 98*(8), 1790–1796.
Eoff, J. C., & Lembo, A. G. (2008). Optimal treatment of chronic constipation in managed care: review and roundtable discussion. *Journal of Managed Care & Specialty Pharmacy, 14*(9–a), S1–S17.
Gallagher, P. F., O'Mahony, D., & Quigley, M. M. (2008). Management of chronic constipation in the elderly. *Drugs and Aging, 25*(10), 807–821.
Greenwood-Van Meerveld, B., & Standifer, K. M. (2008). Methylnaltrexone in the treatment of opioid-induced constipation. *Clin and experimental gastroenterology, 1*, 49–58.
Health protection Agency. (2013). *Hand Washing Technique*. Available at: <www.hpa.org.uk/Topics/InfectiousDiseases/infectionsAZ/Handwashing>.
Hongisto, S.-M., et al. (2006). A combination of fibre-rich rye bread and yoghurt containing *Lactobacillus GG* improves bowel function in women with self-reported constipation. *European Journal of Clinical Nutrition, 60*, 319–324.
Howard, L. V., West, D., & Ossip-Klein, D. J. (2000). Chronic constipation management for institutionalized older adults. *Geriatric Nursing (New York, N.Y.), 21*(2), 78.
Howatson-Jones, L., Standing, M., & Roberts, S. (Eds.), (2012). *Patient Assessment and Care Planning in Nursing*. London: Sage Publications Inc.
Joanna Briggs Institute. (2008). Management of constipation in older adults. *Australian Nursing Journal (July 1993), 16*(5), 32–35.
Klauser, A. G., et al. (1990). Behavioral modification of colonic function. Can constipation be learned? *Digestive Diseases and Sciences, 35*(10), 1271–1275.
Kyle, G. (2007). Constipation and palliative care-where are we now? *International Journal of Palliative Nursing, 13*(1), 6–16.
Kyle, G. (2009). Methylnaltrexone: a subcutaneous treatment for opioid-induced constipation in palliative care patients. *International Journal of Palliative Nursing, 15*(11), 533–540.
Kyle, G. (2011a). Risk assessment and management tools for constipation. *British Journal of Community Nursing, 16*(5), 224–230.
Kyle, G. (2011b). Managing constipation in adult patients. *Nurse Prescribing, 9*(10), 482–490.
Kyle, G. (2012). The older person: management of constipation. *British Journal of Community Nursing, 15*(2), 60–63.
Matthews, E. (2011). Nursing *Care Planning*. London: Lippincott Williams & Wilkins.
Marples, G. (2011). Diagnosis and management of slow transit constipation in adults. *Nursing Standard, 26*(8), 41–48.
McClurg, D., Hagen, S., & Dickinson, L. (2011). Abdominal massage for the treatment of constipation (Protocol). *Cochrane Database of Systematic Reviews*, (4), *CD009089*.
Michna, E., et al. (2011). Subcutaneous methylnaltrexone for treatment of opioid-induced constipation in patients with chronic, nonmalignant pain: a randomized controlled study. *The Journal of Pain, 12*(5), 554–562.
Müller-Lissner, S. A., et al. (2005). The perceived effect of various foods and beverages on stool consistency. *European Journal of Gastroenterology and Hepatology, 17*, 109–112.
Ortega, A., Sanchez-Manzanares, M., Gil, F., et al. (2013). Enhancing team learning in nursing teams through beliefs about interpersonal contexts. *The Journal of advanced Nursing, 69*(1), 363–370.
Rao, S. S. C., Kavolic, R., & Rao, S. (2006). Influence of body position and stool characteristics on defecation in humans. *The American Journal of Gastroenterology, 206*(101), 2790–2796.
Ramkumar, D., & Rao, S. S. (2005). Efficacy and safety of traditional medical therapies for chronic constipation: systematic review. *The American Journal of Gastroenterology, 100*(4), 936–971.
Rhoads, J., & Murphy-Jensen, M. (2014). *Differential diagnoses for the advanced practice nurse*. NY: Springer Publishing Company.
Roerig, J. L., et al. (2010). Laxative abuse: epidemiology, diagnosis and management. *Drugs, 70*(12), 1487–1503.
Rogers, J. (2013). Management of constipation in the community. *Journal of Community Nursing, 27*(1), 20–24.
Russell, K. W., et al. (2013). *The implementation of an organised bowel management programme is effective and significantly reduces hospital admissions in patients with severe idiopathic constipation*. Available at: <https://aap.confex.com/aap/2013/webprogram/Paper21641.html>.
Schmelzer, M., et al. (2004). Safety and effectiveness of large-volume enema solutions. *Applied Nursing Research, 17*(4), 265–274.
Schnelle, J. F., et al. (2010). A controlled trial of an intervention to improve urinary and fecal incontinence and constipation. *Journal of the American Geriatrics Society, 58*(8), 1504–1511.
Sikirov, D. (2003). Comparison of straining during defecation in three positions: results and implications for human health. *Digestive Diseases and Sciences, 48*(7), 1201–1205.
Smith, G. D. (2012). Diagnosis and assessment of irritable bowel syndrome: current perspectives. *Gastrointestinal Nursing, 10*(2), 39.
Spinzi, G., et al. (2009). Constipation in the elderly. *Drugs and Aging, 26*(6), 469–474.
Stoltz, R., et al. (2001). An efficacy and consumer preference study of polyethylene glycol 3350 for the treatment of constipation in regular laxative users. *Home Health Consult, 8*(2), 21.
Sturtzel, B., & Elmadfa, I. (2008). Intervention with dietary fiber to treat constipation and reduce laxative use in residents of nursing homes. *Annals of Nutrition and Metabolism, 52*(Suppl. 1), 54–56.
St. Aubyn, B., & Andrews, A. (2012). Documentation. In M. Aldridge & S. Wanless (Eds.), *Developing Healthcare Skills through Simulation*. London: Sage Publications Inc.
Sykes, N. P. (2006). The pathogenesis of constipation. *The Journal of Supportive Oncology, 4*(5), 213–218.
Tack, J., et al. (2011). Diagnosis and treatment of chronic constipation-a European perspective. *Neurogastroenterology and Motility, 23*, 697–710.
Tagart, R. E. B. (1966). The anal canal and rectum: their varying relationship and its effect on anal continence. *Diseases of the Colon and Rectum, 9*(6), 449–452.

Thomas, J., et al. (2008). Methylnaltrexone for opioid-induced constipation in advanced illness. *The New England Journal of Medicine, 358*(22), 2332–2343.

Vuksan, V., et al. (2008). Using cereal to increase dietary fiber intake to the recommended level and the effect of fiber on bowel function in healthy persons consuming North American diets. *The American Journal of Clinical Nutrition, 88*, 1256–1262.

Wald, A., et al. (2008). A multinational survey of prevalence and patterns of laxative use among adults with self-defined constipation. *Alimentary Pharmacology and Therapeutics, 28*, 917–930.

Whitehead, W. E., et al. (2009). Conservative and behavioral management of constipation. *Neurogastroenterology and Motility, 21*(Suppl. 2), 55–61.

Wilcox, C. S., et al. (2010). An open-label study of naltrexone and bupropion combination therapy for smoking cessation in overweight and obese subjects. *Addictive Behaviors, 35*(3), 229–234.

Zhou, L., et al. (2010). Functional constipation: implications for nursing interventions. *Journal of Clinical Nursing, 19*, 1838–1843.

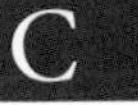

Chronic functional Constipation

Amanda Andrews, MA, Ed, BSc, DN, RN, HEA Fellow, and A.B. St. Aubyn, BSc (Hons), RGN, RM, RHV, DPS:N (CHS), MSc, PGCert (Education), HEA Fellow

NANDA-I

Definition

Infrequent or difficult evacuation of feces, which has been present for at least three of the prior 12 months

Defining Characteristics

Abdominal distention; adult: presence of ≥ 2 of the following symptoms on Rome III classification system; lumpy or hard stools in ≥ 25% defecations; straining during ≥ 25% of defecations; sensation of incomplete evacuation for ≥ 25% of defecations; sensation of anorectal obstruction/blockage for ≥ 25% of defecations; manual maneuvers to facilitate ≥ 25% of defecations (digital manipulation, pelvic floor support); ≤3 evacuations per week.; child: ≤4 years; presence of ≥ 2 criteria on Roman III pediatric classification system for ≥ 1 month; ≤2 defecations per week; ≥1 episode of fecal incontinence per week; stool retentive posturing; painful or hard bowel movements; presence of large fecal mass in the rectum; large diameter stools that may obstruct the toilet; child: ≥4 years: presence of > 2 criteria on Roman III pediatric classification system for ≥ 2 months; ≤2 defecations per week; ≥1 episode of fecal incontinence per week; stool retentive posturing; painful or hard bowel movements; presence of large fecal mass in the rectum; large diameter stools that may obstruct the toilet; fecal impaction; fecal incontinence (in children); leakage of stool with digital stimulation; pain with defecation; palpable abdominal mass; positive fecal occult blood test; prolonged straining; type 1 or 2 on Bristol Stool Chart; amyloidosis; anal fissure; anal stricture; autonomic neuropathy; cerebral vascular accident; chronic intestinal pseudo-obstruction; chronic renal insufficiency; colorectal cancer; dehydration; dementia; depression; dermatomyositis; diabetes mellitus; diet disproportionally high in protein and fat; extraintestinal mass; failure to thrive; habitually ignores urge to defecate; hemorrhoids; Hirschsprung's disease; hypercalcemia; hypothyroidism; impaired mobility; inflammatory bowel disease; insufficient dietary intake; insufficient fluid intake; ischemic stenosis; low caloric intake; low fiber diet; multiple sclerosis; myotonic dystrophy; panhypopituitarism; paraplegia; Parkinson's disease; pelvic floor dysfunction; perineal damage; pharmaceutical agent; polypharmacy; porphyria; postinflammatory stenosis; pregnancy; proctitis; scleroderma; sedentary lifestyle; slow solon transit time; spinal cord injury; surgical stenosis

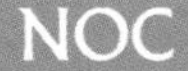

(Nursing Outcomes Classification)

Suggested NOC Outcomes

Example NOC Outcome with Indicators

Bowel Elimination as evidenced by the following indicators: Elimination pattern/Stool soft and formed/Passage of stool without aids/Ease of stool passage. (Rate each indicator of **Bowel Elimination:** 1 = severely compromised, 2 = substantially compromised, 3 = moderately compromised, 4 = mildly compromised, 5 = not compromised [see Section I].)

Client Outcomes

Client Will (Specify Time Frame)

- Maintain passage of soft, formed stool every 1 to 3 days without straining
- State relief from discomfort of constipation
- Identify measures that prevent or treat constipation

C

NIC (Nursing Interventions Classification)

Suggested NIC Intervention

Constipation/Impaction Management

Example NIC Activities—Constipation/Impaction Management

Identify factors (e.g., medications, bed rest, and diet) that may cause or contribute to constipation/impaction; Institute a toileting schedule, as appropriate

Nursing Interventions and *Rationales*

All Client Ages

- Introduce yourself to the client and anyone accompanying him or her and inform them of your role. *Introducing yourself to a client helps establish and develop a therapeutic relationship that recognizes the person within the client and forms the basis for building trust on which to base the provision of care (Howatson-Jones et al, 2012).*
- Gain consent to carry out care before proceeding further with the assessment. *Clients have the right of autonomy both legally and morally and therefore should be fully involved in the decision-making process (Avery, 2013)*
- Wash hands using a recognized technique. *Strict hand-hygiene regimens significantly reduce the incidence of methicillin-resistant Staphylococcus aureus and Clostridium difficile (Health Protection Agency, 2013).*
- Assess usual pattern of defecation and establish the extent of the constipation problem to include:
  - Bowel habits
    - Time of day
    - Amount and frequency of stool
    - Consistency of stool (using the Bristol Stool Scale)
    - Bleeding/passing mucus on defecation
    - History of bowel habits and/or laxative use
    - Assess children younger than 4 years using the Rome III pediatric classification (for at least 1 month)
    - Assess children older than age 4 years using the Rome III pediatric classification (for at least 2 months)
    - Assess adults using the Rome III classification. *Rome III criteria, devised in 2006, specify that clients must be symptomatic with at least two or more of the criteria that are relevant to their specific age range (Leung et al, 2011).*
  - Lifestyle assessment
    - Fiber content in diet
    - Daily fluid intake
    - Exercise patterns
    - Personal remedies for constipation
    - Recently stopped smoking
    - Alcohol consumption/recreational drug use
    - Personal habits related to defecation
  - Past medical history
    - Obstetrical/gynecological/urological history and surgeries
    - Existing anatomical anomalies (e.g., anal fissures, anal strictures and hemorrhoids)
    - Diseases that affect bowel motility (e.g., colorectal cancer, chronic intestinal pseudo-obstruction and Hirschsprung's disease)
    - Bleeding/passing mucus on defecation
    - Current medications
    - *Established algorithms and guidelines recommend that secondary pathology and causes of constipation are identified and firstly excluded before moving on to assessment of diet and lifestyle issues (Tack et al, 2011)*

  - Emotional influences
    - Anxiety and depression
    - Long-term defecation issues
    - Stress
- EB: *A detailed and accurate assessment of the client enables the nurse to plan interventions, monitor outcomes, and evaluate care, ensuring no unnecessary treatment is carried out (Matthews, 2011).*
- Complete a physical assessment (palpation for abdominal distention, percussion for dullness, auscultation for bowel sounds, observation for anal fissures, anal strictures, and hemorrhoids). *A physical examination provides positive and negative findings and may provide the diagnosis without the need for further testing. It may also reveal unsuspected findings or confirm normality (Rhoads & Murphy-Jensen, 2014).*
- Encourage the client or family to keep a 7-day diary of bowel habits to include time of day, length of time spent on the toilet, consistency, amount and frequency of stool, and any straining (using the Bristol Stool Scale). *Keeping a diary helps establish a client's bowel pattern and may contribute to the client's adherence to the proposed care plan (Andrews & Morgan 2013).*
- Encourage the client or family to keep a 7-day diary of lifestyle issues in relation to bowel habits to include fluid consumption, fibre content in diet, usual bowel stimulus and exercise regime. *Enabling clients to present their condition in their own words ensures that they feel the health care professionals understand their concerns (Smith, 2012).*
- Actively encourage the use of reward/star charts with children when establishing regular bowel routines. *Research highlights that children respond better to positive enforcement when learning to manage constipation with regular toileting rather than confrontation about the problem (Afzal et al, 2011).*
- Discuss with clients already taking opioids (temporarily or long term) that constipation is a common side effect. Advise the client to contact their primary health care provider for a prescription of an appropriate laxative. *The thorough and comprehensive assessment of clients on opioids experiencing constipation will also allow for a bowel function approach for laxative prescribing rather than one based on the opioid dose alone (Andrews & Morgan, 2012).*
- Advise a fiber intake of 18 to 25 g of fiber daily and suggest foodstuffs to facilitate this diet (e.g., prune juice, leafy green vegetables, wholemeal bread and pasta). *Fiber creates bulky feces and stretches the bowel wall to stimulate peristalsis, thus shortening bowel transit time (Kyle, 2012).*
- Advise a fluid intake of 1.5 to 2 L of fluid per day (ideally, 6 to 8 glasses of water), unless this is contraindicated by comorbidities such as renal or heart disease. *Water passes into the gut to promote the formation of a softer fecal mass and provides lubrication to prevent a blockage of the gut (Boyle, 2013).*
- Encourage physical activity within the client's current ability to mobilize. Encourage turning and changing position in bed if immobile. For reduced mobility clients, encourage knee to chest raises, waist twists, and stretching the arms away from the body. For fully mobile clients, encourage walking and swimming. *Physical activity can help stimulate peristaltic waves in the colon and encourage the transit of feces to the rectum (Rogers, 2013).*
- Demonstrate the use of gentle external abdominal massage, using aroma therapy oils, following the direction of colon activity. EB: *Abdominal massage encourages rectal loading by increasing intraabdominal pressure and in some cases it may elicit rectal waves that may stimulate the somatoautonomic reflex and enhance bowel sensation (McClurg et al, 2011).*
- Recommend clients establish a regular elimination routine. If required, assist clients to the bathroom at the same time every day, being mindful of the need for privacy (closing of bathroom doors). *Establishing a routine allows for the use of the gastrocolic reflex, especially in the morning, which aids defecation (Rogers, 2013).*
- Educate the client how to adopt the best posture for defecation: keep knees slightly higher than hips, keep feet flat on the floor and lean forward, putting elbows onto knees. *Adopting the correct position to open one's bowels allows the angle of the rectum and anal canal to straighten. This facilitates an increase in abdominal pressure, which makes defecation more effective (Rogers, 2013).*
- Consider the teaching of biofeedback therapy to encourage a "new normal" bowel routine for clients to adopt. EB: *A meta-analysis random control trial concluded that the use of biofeedback therapy in chronic constipation was successful and warranted the time and effort involved in establishing a bowel routine (Enck et al, 2009).*
- Teach clients of the need to respond promptly to the defecation urge. EB: *The body's natural "call to stool" should be heeded because it is a response to the stimulation of nerve endings in the rectum when a stool is*

present. Ignoring this urge results in the rectum becoming desensitized to a stool in situ (Coggrave et al, 2014).

- Consider the use of laxatives, suppositories, enemas, and bowel irrigation as required when other more natural interventions are not effective. EB: *Laxative therapies can be used in conjunction with lifestyle changes (while waiting for the lifestyle changes to take effect or if the change is not sufficient in itself) (Marples, 2011; Kyle, 2011). Bowel irrigation is thought to both stimulate colonic reflex and act as a mechanical bowel washout (Coggrave et al, 2014).*
- Discourage the use of long-term laxatives and enemas, and advise clients to gradually reduce their use if taken regularly. *Long-term use or overuse of laxatives can cause health problems (e.g., electrolyte imbalance) or hide symptoms of a serious medical condition, such as cardiac arrhythmias (Aschenbrenner, 2014).*
- Provide client with comprehensive written information about constipation and its management. EB: *Research shows that providing clients with well-written evidence-based information about their condition and treatment can have a beneficial effect on the outcomes of treatment. In addition clients are more likely to retain important information that will assist them in making informed decisions about their care (Coulter, 2011).*
- Provide written instructions for children about taking their medication and about how the bowel works. *Written clear information provided to children with chronic functional constipation will help them understand and therefore recognize when they are at risk for constipation recurrence (NICE, 2010).*
- Liaise with members of the interprofessional team as appropriate to provide treatment and advice to clients and caregivers. *Team work is a central process in health care organizations. It increases the capacity of teams to absorb and develop new knowledge, which will improve clients' health and well-being (Ortega et al, 2013).*
- Educate the client on the mechanism of normal bowel function and the need for adequate fluid and fiber intake, physical activity, and a defined toileting pattern in an agreed-upon bowel management program. *The implementation of an organized bowel management program is effective and significantly reduces hospital admissions in clients with severe idiopathic constipation (Russell et al, 2013).*
- Document all care and advice given in a factual and comprehensive manner. *Good record keeping is an integral part of nursing practice and is essential to the provision of safe and effective care (St. Aubyn & Andrews, 2012).*

REFERENCES

Andrews, A., & Morgan, G. (2012). Constipation management in palliative care: treatments and the potential of independent nurse prescribing. *International Journal of Palliative Nursing, 18*(1), 17–22.

Andrews, A., & Morgan, G. (2013). Constipation in palliative care: treatment options and considerations for individual patient management. *International Journal of Palliative Nursing, 19*(6), 226–273.

Aschenbrenner, D. S. (2014). Overuse of certain OTC laxatives may be dangerous. *American Journal of Nursing, 114*(5).

Afzal, N. A., Tighe, M. P., & Thomas, M. A. (2011). *Constipation in Children.* Available at: <http://www.biomedcentral.com/content/pdf/1824-7288-37-28.pdf>.

Avery, G. (2013). *Law and Ethics in Nursing and Healthcare an Introduction.* London: Sage Publications Inc.

Boyle, J. (2013). Roughage to regulate. *World of Irish Nursing and Midwifery, 21*(7), 53–55.

Coggrave, K., Norton, C., & Cody, J. D. (2014). Management of faecal incontinence and constipation in adults with central neurological diseases. *Cochrane Database of Systematic Reviews,* (1), CD002115.

Coulter, A. (2011). *Engaging Patients in Health Care.* Berkshire: McGraw Hill Open University press.

Enck, P., Van Dervoort, I. R., & Klosterhalfen, S. (2009). Biofeedback therapy in faecal incontinence and constipation. *Neurogastroentrology Motility, 21*(11), 1131–1141.

Health Protection Agency. (2013). *Ayliffe Hand Washing Technique.* Available at: <www.hpa.org.uk/Topics/InfectiousDiseases/infectionsAZ/Handwashing>.

Howatson-Jones, L., Standing, M., & Roberts, S. (Eds.), (2012). *Patient Assessment and Care Planning in Nursing.* London: Sage Publications Inc.

Kyle, G. (2011). Managing constipation in adult patients. *Nurse Prescribing, 9*(10), 482–490.

Kyle, G. (2012). The older person: Management of Constipation. *British Journal of Community Nursing, 15*(2), 60–63.

Leung, L., Riutta, T., Kotecha, J., et al. (2011). Chronic constipation: an evidence-based review. *The Journal of the American Board of Family Medicine, 24*(4), 436–452.

Matthews, E. (2011). *Nursing Care Planning.* London: Lippincott Williams & Wilkins.

Marples, G. (2011). Diagnosis and management of slow transit constipation in adults. *Nursing Standard, 26*(8), 41–48.

McClurg, D., Hagen, S., & Dickinson, L. (2011). Abdominal massage for the treatment of constipation (Protocol). *Cochrane Database of Systematic Reviews,* (4), CD009089.

Ortega, A., Sanchez-Manzanares, M., Gil, F., et al. (2013). Enhancing team learning in nursing teams through beliefs about interpersonal contexts. *The Journal of advanced Nursing, 69*(1).

Rhoads, J., & Murphy-Jensen, M. (2014). *Differential diagnoses for the advanced practice nurse.* NY: Springer Publishing Company.

Rogers, J. (2013). Management of constipation in the community. *Journal of Community Nursing, 27*(1), 20–24.

Russell, K. W., Zobell, S., Barnhart, D. C., et al. (2013). *The implementation of an organised bowel management programme is effective and significantly reduces hospital admissions in patients with severe idiopathic constipation*. Available at: <https://aap.confex.com/aap/2013/webprogram/Paper21641.html>.

Smith, G. D. (2012). Diagnosis and assessment of irritable bowel syndrome: current perspectives. *Gastrointestinal Nursing, 10*(2).

St. Aubyn, B., & Andrews, A. (2012). Documentation. In M. Aldridge & S. Wanless (Eds.), *Developing Healthcare Skills through Simulation*. London: Sage Publications Inc.

Tack, J., Muller - Lissner, S., Stanghellini, V., et al. (2011). Diagnosis and Treatment of Chronic Constipation—a European Perspective. *Neurogastroentrology Motility, 23*(8), 697–710.

The National Institute for Health and Care Excellence (NICE). (2010). *Constipation in children and young people: Diagnosis and management of idiopathic childhood constipation in primary and secondary care*. Available: <https://www.nice.org.uk/guidance/cg99> Accessed 15.04.22.

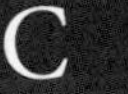

Perceived Constipation

Amanda Andrews, MA, Ed, BSc, DN, RN, HEA Fellow, and A.B. St. Aubyn, BSc (Hons), RGN, RM, RHV, DPS:N (CHS), MSc, PGCert (Education), HEA Fellow

NANDA-I

Definition

Self-diagnosis of constipation combined with abuse of laxatives, enemas, and/or suppositories to ensure a daily bowel movement

Defining Characteristics

Enema abuse; expects a daily bowel movement; expects a daily bowel movement at the same time every day; laxative abuse; suppository abuse

Related Factors

Cultural health believes; family health beliefs; impaired thought process

NOC (Nursing Outcomes Classification)

Suggested NOC Outcomes

Bowel Elimination; Health Beliefs; Health Beliefs: Perceived Threat

Example NOC Outcome with Indicators

Bowel Elimination as evidenced by the following indicators: Elimination pattern/Stool soft and formed/ Passage of stool without aids/Ease of stool passage. (Rate each indicator of **Bowel Elimination:** 1 = severely compromised, 2 = substantially compromised, 3 = moderately compromised, 4 = mildly compromised, 5 = not compromised [see Section I].)

Client Outcomes

Client Will (Specify Time Frame)

- Regularly defecate soft, formed stool without use of aids
- Explain the need to decrease or eliminate the use of stimulant laxatives, suppositories, and enemas
- Identify alternatives to stimulant laxatives, enemas, and suppositories for ensuring defecation
- Explain that defecation does not have to occur every day

NIC (Nursing Interventions Classification)

Suggested NIC Interventions

- Bowel Management; Medication Management

Example NIC Activities—Bowel Management

Note preexistent bowel problems, bowel routine, and use of laxatives; Initiate a bowel training program, as appropriate

Nursing Interventions and *Rationales*

- Introduce yourself to the client and any companions, and inform them of your role. *Introducing yourself to a client helps establish and develop a therapeutic relationship that recognizes the person within the client and forms the bases for building trust upon which to base the provision of care (Howatson-Jones et al, 2012).*

- Gain consent before proceeding further with the assessment. *Clients have the right of autonomy both legally and morally and therefore should be fully involved in the decision-making process (Avery, 2013).*
- Wash hands using a recognized technique. EB: *Performing strict hand-hygiene regimens significantly reduces the incidence of infection with methicillin-resistant* Staphylococcus aureus *and* Clostridium difficile *(Health Protection Agency, 2013).*
- Assess usual pattern of defecation and establish the extent of the perceived constipation problem to include:
    - Bowel Habits
        - Time of day
        - Amount and frequency of stool
        - Consistency of stool (using the Bristol Stool Scale)
        - Bleeding/passing mucus on defecation
        - Patient history of bowel habits and/or laxative use
        - Family history of bowel habits and/or laxative use

      EB: *A detailed and accurate assessment of the patient enables the nurse to plan interventions, monitor outcomes, and evaluate care, ensuring no unnecessary treatment is rendered (Matthews, 2011).*
    - Lifestyle Assessment
        - Fiber content in diet
        - Daily fluid intake
        - Exercise patterns
        - Personal remedies for constipation
        - Cultural remedies for constipation
        - Recently stopped smoking
        - Alcohol consumption/recreational drug use

      EB: *Alcohol has a dehydrating effect on the body. One of the key causes of constipation is dehydration of stools. A lack of water in the bowel leads to hard fecal matter, which is difficult to pass (Derbyshire, 2011).*
    - Past Medical History
        - Obstetrical/gynecological/urological history and surgeries
        - Diseases that affect bowel motility
        - Bleeding/passing mucus on defecation
        - Current medications
    - Emotional Influences
        - Anxiety and depression/psychological disorders
        - History of eating disorders
        - History of physical/or sexual abuse
        - Long-term defecation issues
        - Stress

      EB: *Clients' psychological reactions to the experience of constipation change over time. Anxiety and fear about the anticipated health-related consequences of constipation are often expressed. The absence of a bowel movement or the failure of constipation treatment can lead to anxiety and depression (Dhingra et al, 2012).* EB: *Stress can alter the mucosal immune function of the central nervous system. This causes afferent signals to the gut to be reduced, causing constipation (Drossman, 2011).*
- Encourage the client or family to keep a 7-day diary of bowel habits to include time of day, length of time spent on the toilet, consistency, amount and frequency of stool, and any straining (using the Bristol Stool Scale). EB: *Keeping a diary helps establish a patient's bowel pattern and may contribute to the patient's adherence to the proposed care plan (Andrews & Morgan, 2013).*
- Encourage the client or family to keep a 7-day diary of lifestyle issues in relation to bowel habits to include fluid consumption, fiber content in diet, usual bowel stimulus, and exercise regimen. EB: *Enabling patients to present their condition in their own words ensures that they feel the health care professionals understand their concerns (Smith, 2012).*
- Educate the client that it is not necessary to have a daily bowel movement. EB: *A healthy bowel function can vary from three stools each day to three stools each week. The criteria of choice for establishing a diagnosis of constipation are often the Rome III criteria. The criteria based definition calls for the presence of two or more of the symptom for at least 3 months for a definition of constipation (Leung et al, 2011).*
- Encourage the client to record use of laxatives, suppositories, or enemas, and suggest replacing them with an increase in fluid and fiber intake. EB: *Overtreatment with laxatives can result in iatrogenic diarrhea,*

which can lead to dehydration, delirium, and the false-positive labeling and unnecessary treatment of C. difficile *carriers. This can result in increased morbidity and mortality, and a longer stay in hospital. By improving the assessment and treatment of constipation, patient outcomes should improve, resulting in significant hospital cost savings (Linton, 2014).*

C

- Advise a fiber intake of 18 to 25 g daily and suggest foodstuffs high in fiber (e.g., prune juice, leafy green vegetables, whole meal bread and pasta). *Fiber creates bulky feces and stretches the bowel wall to stimulate peristalsis, thus shortening bowel transit time* (Kyle, 2012). *For further information on use of fiber, please refer to the care plan for* **Constipation.**
- Advise a fluid intake of 1.5 to 2 L of fluid per day (ideally, 6 to 8 glasses of water), unless contraindicated by comorbidities, such as kidney or heart disease. *Water passes into the gut to promote the formation of a softer fecal mass and provides lubrication to prevent a blockage of the gut (Boyle, 2013).*
- Obtain a referral to a dietitian for analysis of the client's diet and fluid intake to provide strategies to improve diet and nutrition.
- Encourage physical activity within the client's current ability to mobilize. Encourage turning and changing position in bed if immobile. For clients with reduced mobility, encourage knee to chest raises, waist twists, and stretching the arms away from the body. For fully mobile clients, encourage walking and swimming. *Physical activity can help stimulate peristaltic waves in the colon and encourage the transit of feces to the rectum (Rogers, 2013).*
- Demonstrate the use of gentle external abdominal massage, using aroma therapy oils, following the direction of colon activity. *Abdominal massage encourages rectal loading by increasing intra-abdominal pressure and in some cases it may elicit rectal waves, which may stimulate the somato-autonomic reflex and enhance bowel sensation (McClurg et al, 2011).*
- Recommend clients establish a regular elimination routine. If required assist clients to the bathroom at the same time every day, being mindful of the need for privacy (closing of bathroom doors). *Establishing a routine allows for the use of the gastrocolic reflex, especially in the morning, which aids defecation (Rogers, 2013).*
- Observe for the presence of an eating disorder, the use of laxatives to control or decrease weight; refer for counseling if needed. *People with eating disorders suffer from constipation and other gastrointestinal symptoms, or use laxatives as part of inducing weight loss (Roerig et al, 2010).* CEB: *Laxative abuse is found in clients with both anorexia and bulimia nervosa and may be associated with worsening of the eating disorder as a form of self-harm (Tozzi et al, 2006).*
- Observe family cultural patterns related to eating and bowel habits. Cultural patterns may control bowel habits.

Client/Family Teaching and Discharge Planning

- Provide education to the client on ways to adopt the best posture for defecation. Keep knees slightly higher than hips, keep feet flat on the floor and lean forward putting elbows onto knees. *Adopting the correct position to open one's bowels allows the angle of the rectum and anal canal to straighten out. This facilitates an increase in abdominal pressure, which makes defecation more effective (Rogers, 2013).*
- Teach clients of the importance of responding promptly to the urge to defecate. EB: *The body's natural "call to stool" should be heeded in that it is a response to the stimulation of nerve endings in the rectum when a stool is present. Ignoring this urge will result in the rectum becoming desensitized to a stool in situ (Coggrave et al, 2014).*
- Discourage the use of long-term laxatives and enemas and explain the potential harmful effects of the continual use of defecation aids such as laxatives and enemas. EB: *"Lazy bowel syndrome" may occur if laxatives are used too frequently, causing the bowel to become dependent on laxatives to stimulate a bowel movement. Overuse of laxatives can also lead to poor absorption of vitamins and other nutrients, and to damage of the gastrointestinal tract (Mayo Foundation for Medical Education and Research, 2011).*
- Advise clients to gradually reduce their use of laxatives, if taken regularly, which may take months to achieve. *Long-term use or overuse of laxatives can cause health problems (e.g., electrolyte imbalance) or hide symptoms that may be from a serious medical condition, such as cardiac arrhythmias (Aschenbrenner, 2014).*
- Provide client with comprehensive written information about constipation and its management. EB: *Providing patients with well-written, evidence-based information about their condition and treatment can have a beneficial effect on the outcomes of treatment. In addition, patients are more likely to retain important information that will assist them in making informed decisions about their care (Coulter, 2011).*

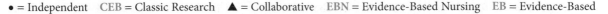

- Collaborate with members of the interprofessional team to provide treatment and advice to clients and caregivers. *Team working is a central process in health care organizations. It increases the capacity of teams to absorb and develop new knowledge, which will improve patient health and well-being (Ortega et al, 2013).*
- Formalize all advice by providing a bowel management program reiterating the mechanism of normal bowel function and the need for adequate fluid and fiber intake, physical activity, and a defined toileting pattern in an agreed bowel program. EB: *The implementation of an organized bowel management program is effective and significantly reduces hospital admissions in patients with severe idiopathic constipation* (Russell et al, 2013).
- Document all care and advice given in a factual and comprehensive manner. *Good record keeping is an integral part of nursing practice and is essential to the provision of safe and effective care (St. Aubyn & Andrews, 2012).*

REFERENCES

Andrews, A., & Morgan, G. (2013). Constipation in palliative care: treatment options and considerations for individual patient management. *International Journal of Palliative Nursing, 19*(6), 226–273.

Aschenbrenner, D. S. (2014). Overuse of certain OTC laxatives may be dangerous. *American Journal of Nursing, 114*(5), 25.

Avery, G. (2013). *Law and Ethics in Nursing and Healthcare: An Introduction.* London: Sage Publications Inc.

Boyle, J. (2013). Roughage to regulate. *World of Irish Nursing and Midwifery, 21*(7), 53–55.

Coggrave, K., Norton, C., & Cody, J. D. (2014). Management of Faecal Incontinence and Constipation in Adults with Central Neurological Diseases. *Cochrane Database of Systematic Reviews,* (1), CD002115.

Coulter, A. (2011). *Engaging Patients in Health Care.* Berkshire: McGraw Hill Open University Press.

Derbyshire, S. (2011). *Dehydration in hospitals.* Available at: <www.naturalhydrationcouncil.org.uk> Accessed 14.09.04.

Dhingra, L., et al. (2012). A Qualitative Study to explore psychological distress an illness burden associated with opioid induced constipation in cancer patients with advanced disease. *Palliative Medicine, 27*(5).

Drossman, D. A. (2011). Abuse, Trauma and GI illness: Is there a link? *American Journal of Gastroenterology, 106*(1).

Health Protection Agency. (2013). *Ayliffe Hand Washing Technique.* Available at: <www.hpa.org.uk/Topics/InfectiousDiseases/infectionsAZ/Handwashing>.

Howatson-Jones, L., Standing, M., & Roberts, S. (Eds.), (2012). *Patient Assessment and Care Planning in Nursing.* London: Sage Publications Inc.

Kyle, G. (2012). The older person: Management of Constipation. *British Journal of Community Nursing, 15*(2), 60–63.

Leung, L., Riutta, T., Kotecha, J., et al. (2011). Chronic Constipation: An Evidence-based Review. *Journal of American Board of Family Medicine, 24*(4).

Linton, A. (2014). *Improving Management of Constipation in an inpatient setting using a care bundle. British medical Journal Quality Improvement Reports.* Available at: <http://qir.bmj.com/content/3/1/u201903.w1002.full> Accesses 14.09.04.

Matthews, E. (2011). *Nursing Care Planning.* London: Lippincott Williams & Wilkins.

Mayo Foundation for Medical Education and Research Mayo Clinic. (2011). *Constipation, Diseases and Condition.* Available at: <www.mayoclinic.com/health/constipation/DS00063/DSECTION=symptoms> Accessed 14.09.04.

McClurg, D., Hagen, S., & Dickinson, L. (2011). Abdominal massage for the treatment of constipation (Protocol). *Cochrane Database of Systematic Reviews,* (4), CD009089.

Ortega, A., Sanchez-Manzanares, M., Gil, F., et al. (2013). Enhancing team learning in nursing teams through beliefs about interpersonal contexts. *The Journal of advanced Nursing, 69*(1), 363–370.

Roerig, J. S., et al. (2010). Laxative abuse: epidemiology, diagnosis and management. *Drugs, 70*(12), 1487–1503.

Rogers, J. (2013). Management of Constipation in the Community. *Journal of Community Nursing, 27*(1), 20–24.

Russell, K. W., et al. (2013). *The implementation of an organised bowel management programme is effective and significantly reduces hospital admissions in patients with severe idiopathic constipation.* Available at: <https://aap.confex.com/aap/2013/webprogram/Paper21641.html>.

Smith, G. D. (2012). Diagnosis and assessment of irritable bowel syndrome: current perspectives. *Gastrointestinal Nursing, 10*(2), 39.

St. Aubyn, B., & Andrews, A. (2012). Documentation. In M. Aldridge & S. Wanless (Eds.), *Developing Healthcare Skills through Simulation.* London: Sage Publications Inc.

Tozzi, F., et al. (2006). Features associated with laxative abuse in individuals with eating disorders. *Psychosomat Medicine, 68*(3), 470–477.

Risk for Constipation *Betty J. Ackley, MSN, EdS, RN*

NANDA-I

Definition

Vulnerable to a decrease in normal frequency of defecation accompanied by difficult or incomplete passage of stool, which may compromise health

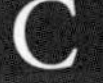

Risk Factors

Functional

Abdominal weakness; average daily physical activity is less than recommended for gender and age; habitually ignores urge to defecate; inadequate toileting habits; irregular defecation habits; recent environmental change

Psychological

Confusion; depression; emotional disturbance

Physiological

Decrease in gastrointestinal motility; dehydration; eating habit change (e.g., foods, eating times); inadequate dentition; inadequate oral hygiene; insufficient dietary habits; insufficient fiber intake; insufficient fluid intake

Pharmacological

Iron salts; laxative abuse; pharmaceutical agent

Mechanical

Electrolyte imbalance; hemorrhoids; Hirschsprung's disease; neurological impairment (e.g., positive electroencephalogram, head trauma, seizure disorders); obesity; postsurgical obstruction; pregnancy; prostate enlargement; rectal abscess; rectal anal fissures; rectal anal stricture; rectal prolapse; rectal ulcer; rectocele; tumor

NIC, NOC, Client Outcomes, Nursing Interventions, Client/Family Teaching, *Rationales,* and References

Refer to care plans for **Constipation.**

Risk for chronic functional Constipation *Mary Beth Flynn Makic, PhD, RN, CNS, CCNS, FAAN*

NANDA-I

Definition

Vulnerable to infrequent or difficult evacuation of feces, which has been present nearly 3 of the prior 12 months, which may compromise health

Risk Factors

Aluminum-containing antacids; antiepileptics; antihypertensives; anti-Parkinsonian agents (anticholinergic or dopaminergic); calcium-channel antagonists; chronic intestinal pseudo-obstruction; decreased food intake; dehydration; depression; diet proportionally high in protein and fat; diuretics; failure to thrive; habitual ignoring of urge to defecate; impaired mobility; low-fiber diet; insufficient fluid intake; inactive lifestyle; iron preparations; low caloric intake; nonsteroidal anti-inflammatories; opioids; polypharmacy; slow colon transit time; tricyclic antidepressants

NIC, NOC, Client Outcomes, Nursing Interventions, Client/Family Teaching and Discharge Planning, *Rationales,* and References

Refer to care plan for Chronic functional **Constipation.**

Contamination *Pauline McKinney Green, PhD, RN, CNE*

NANDA-I

Definition

Exposure to environmental contaminants in doses sufficient to cause adverse health effects

C

Defining Characteristics

Pesticides

Dermatological effects of pesticide exposure; gastrointestinal effects of pesticide exposure; neurological effects of pesticide exposure; pulmonary effects of pesticide exposure; renal effects of pesticide exposure

Chemicals

Dermatological effects of chemical exposure; gastrointestinal effects of chemical exposure; immunological effects of chemical exposure; neurological effects of chemical exposure; pulmonary effects of chemical exposure; renal effects of chemical exposure

Biologicals

Dermatological effects of exposure to biological; gastrointestinal effects of biological exposure; neurological effects of biological exposure; pulmonary effects of biological exposure; renal effects of biological exposure

Pollution

Neurological effects of pollution exposure; pulmonary effects of pollution exposure

Waste

Dermatological effects of waste exposure; gastrointestinal effects of waste exposure; hepatic effects of waste exposure; pulmonary effects of waste exposure

Radiation

Exposure to radioactive material; genetic effects of radiation exposure; immunological effects of radiation exposure; neurological effects of radiation exposure; oncological effects of radiation exposure

Related Factors (r/t)

External

Carpeted flooring; chemical contamination of food; chemical contamination of water; economically disadvantaged; exposure to areas with high contaminant level; exposure to atmospheric pollutants; exposure to bioterrorism; exposure to disaster (natural or man-made); exposure to radiation; flaking, peeling surface in presence of young children (e.g., paint, plaster); household hygiene practices; inadequate breakdown of contaminant; inadequate municipal services (e.g., trash removal, sewage treatment facilities); inadequate protective clothing; inappropriate use of protective clothing; ingestion of contaminated material (e.g., radioactive, food, water); personal hygiene practices; playing where environmental contaminants are used; unprotected exposure to chemical (e.g., arsenic); use of environmental contaminates in the home; use of noxious material in insufficiently ventilated area (e.g., lacquer, paint); use of noxious material without effective protection (e.g., lacquer, paint)

Internal

Age (e.g., children < 5 years, older adults); concomitant exposure; developmental characteristics of children; extremes of age; female gender; gestational age during exposure; inadequate nutrition; preexisting disease; pregnancy; previous exposure to contaminant; smoking

NOC (Nursing Outcomes Classification)

Suggested NOC Outcomes

Community Health Status; Family Physical Environment; Anxiety Level; Fear Level

Example NOC Outcome with Indicators

Community Health Status as evidenced by the following indicators: Evidence of health protection measures/Compliance with environmental health standards/Health status of population. (Rate the outcome and indicators of **Community Health Status:** 1 = poor, 2 = fair, 3 = good, 4 = very good, 5 = excellent [see Section I].)

C

Client Outcomes

Client Will (Specify Time Frame)

- Have minimal health effects associated with contamination
- Cooperate with appropriate decontamination protocol
- Participate in appropriate isolation precautions

Community Will (Specify Time Frame)

- Use health surveillance data system to monitor for contamination incidents
- Use disaster plan to evacuate and triage affected members
- Have minimal health effects associated with contamination
- Employ measures to reduce household environmental risks

NIC (Nursing Interventions Classification)

Suggested NIC Interventions

Triage: Disaster; Infection Control; Anxiety Reduction; Crisis Intervention; Health Education

Example NIC Activities—Triage: Disaster

Initiate appropriate emergency measures, as indicated; Monitor for and treat life-threatening injuries or acute needs

Nursing Interventions and *Rationales*

- ▲ Help individuals cope with contamination incident by doing the following:
  - ❍ Use groups that have survived terrorist attacks as useful resource for victims
  - ❍ Provide accurate information on risks involved, preventive measures, use of antibiotics and vaccines
  - ❍ Assist to deal with feelings of fear, vulnerability, and grief
  - ❍ Encourage individuals to talk to others about their fears
  - ❍ Assist victims to think positively and to move toward the future
- ▲ *In a crisis situation, interventions aimed at supporting an individual's coping help the person deal with feelings of fear, helplessness, and loss of control that are normal reactions in a crisis situation.*
- • Triage, stabilize, transport, and treat affected community members. EB: *Accurate triage and early treatment provide the best chance of survival to affected persons (Veenema, 2013).*
- • Prioritize mental health care for highly vulnerable risk groups or those with special needs (deeply affected groups, women, older persons, children and adolescents, displaced persons—especially those living in shelters, persons with preexisting mental health disorders (including those living in institutions) (Pan American Health Organization, 2012).
- • Collaborate with other agencies (local health department, emergency medical service [EMS], state and federal agencies). *Communication among agencies increases ability to handle crisis efficiently (CDC, 2014a; Veenema, 2013).*
- • Use approved procedures for decontamination of persons, clothing, and equipment. *Victims may first require decontamination before entering health facility to receive care in order to prevent the spread of contamination (U.S. Army Medical Research Institute of Infectious Diseases, 2011).*
- • Use appropriate isolation precautions: universal, airborne, droplet, and contact isolation. *Proper use of isolation precautions prevents cross-contamination by contaminating agents (U.S. Army Medical Research Institute of Infectious Diseases, 2011).* EB: *A study of health care workers' client interactions found transfer of multidrug-resistant bacteria to workers' gowns and gloves increased after client contact with environmental contamination and recommended improved compliance with contact precautions and aggressive environmental cleaning (Morgan et al, 2012).*
- • Monitor individual for therapeutic effects, side effects, and compliance with post-exposure drug therapy. Drug therapy may extend over a long period of time and requires monitoring for compliance as well as for therapeutic and side effects (Veenema, 2013).
- • Perform effective hand washing before and after handling medical charts, entering case notes, touching clients, and performing procedures, especially in intensive care unit environments. EB: *A prospective study to identify and compare the incidence of bacterial contamination of hospital charts found the plastic chart*

covers to be contaminated (63.5% for general wards and 83.2% for special units); chart covers can act as vectors and potential sources of infection (Chen et al, 2014).

- Prevent cross contamination by systematically disinfecting stethoscopes (diaphragm and tubing) after each use. EB: *A study of the contamination level of health care providers' hands and stethoscopes found that the contamination level of the stethoscope is substantial after a single health care provider examination and is comparable to the contamination of parts of the health care provider's hand (Longtin et al, 2014).*
- Complete proper hand washing after touching the client's privacy curtain and before touching the client. EB: *A longitudinal study determined that privacy curtains are contaminated with potentially pathogenic bacteria within 1 week of use; following the correct order for hand washing prevents contact with contaminated surfaces of privacy curtains (Ohl et al, 2012).*

C

Geriatric

- Help the client identify age-related factors that may affect response to contamination incidents.
- Advise older adults to follow public notices related to drinking water. *Contaminated water can harm the health of older persons and those with chronic conditions (CDC, 2014b).*
- Encourage older adults to receive influenza vaccination when it is available, beginning as early as late August and continuing through the end of February. *Flu vaccination protects against influenza and protects those in proximity who are more vulnerable to serious flu illness (CDC, 2013a).*
- Instruct older adults with special needs or chronic conditions to plan for emergencies and keep medications, prescriptions, and special devices on hand (Federal Emergency Management Agency, 2014).

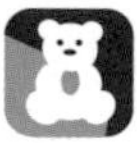

Pediatric

- Provide environmental health hazard information. *Developing children are more vulnerable to environmental toxicants due to greater and longer exposure and particular susceptibility windows (Children's Environmental Health Network, 2013).*
- Reduce risks from exposure to environmental contaminants by identifying the ages and life stages of children. EB: *The World Health Organization recommends coordination of hazard and exposure assessment using children's ages and life stages to accommodate for children's physiology and developmental stage that contribute to opportunities for environmental exposure and contamination (Hubal et al, 2014).*
- Screen newly arrived immigrant and refugee children for elevated blood lead levels secondary to lead hazards in older housing. EB: *Resettlement in areas with older housing stock increases risk for lead poisoning (CDC, 2013b).*
- Be aware that the risk for lead exposure is much higher in many of the countries from which children are adopted than in the United States (CDC, 2014c).
- Use the latest reference level of 5 μg/dL to identify children and environments associated with lead-exposure hazards. EB: *CDC currently recommends using 5 μg/dL as the reference value in place of the previously recommended level of 10 μg/dL; reference values are updated every 4 years based on the most recent population-based blood lead surveys among children (CDC, 2012).*

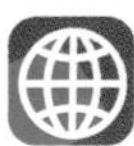

Multicultural

- Ask about use of imported or culture-specific products that contain lead, such as greta and azarcon (Hispanic folk medicine for upset stomach and diarrhea), ghasard (Indian folk medicine tonic), and ba-baw-san (Chinese herbal remedy). *Immigrant children are at increased risk for contamination, particularly from lead, related to exposure to imported culture-specific products (CDC, 2013c).*
- Nurses need to consider the cultural and social factors that impact access to and understanding of the health care system, particularly for groups such as migrant workers who do not have consistent health care providers. EB: *Subtle cultural biases in how nurses approach care can affect outcomes (Holmes, 2011; Hubal et al, 2014).*

Home Care

- Assess current environmental stressors and identify community resources. *Accessing resources decreases stress and increases ability to cope.*
- Recognize that relocated and unemployed individuals/families are at risk for psychological distress. EB: *People who lose their social network are at a very high risk for post-event psychological distress and require appropriate care (Oyama et al, 2012).*

C

- Support policy and program initiatives that provide emergency mental health services following large-scale contamination events. EB: *A study of the utilization of mental health services following a major disaster found community mental health service use increased in the period following the event and that brief interventions were more effective than conventional multisession interventions (Boscarino et al, 2011).*
- Instruct community members concerned about lead in drinking water from plumbing pipes and fixtures to have the water tested by calling the EPA drinking water hotline at 800-426-4791.
- Educate community members to reduce exposure to lead by inquiring about lead-based paint before buying a home or renting an apartment built before 1978; Federal law requires disclosure of known information about lead-based paint (EPA, 2014).
- Instruct individuals and families that food contamination occurs through a variety of mechanisms and that food safety is associated with proper washing of hands and utensils, prompt refrigeration of food, and cooking foods at the correct temperature. EB: *Pathogens can be introduced into food from infected humans who handle food without thoroughly washing their hands, from food that touches surfaces or utensils contaminated by pathogens in raw food, and improper refrigeration or heating of food (CDC, 2013d).*

Client/Family Teaching and Discharge Planning

- Provide truthful information to the person or family affected.
- Discuss signs and symptoms of contamination.
- Explain decontamination protocols.
- Explain need for isolation procedures.
- *Well-managed efforts at communication of contamination information ensure that messages are correctly formulated, transmitted, and received and that they result in meaningful actions.*
- Emphasize the importance of pre- and post-exposure treatment of contamination. *Early treatment decreases associated complications related to contamination (ATSDR, 2014).*
- Provide parents with actionable information to reduce environmental contamination in the home. EBN: *A randomized educational intervention to reduce contamination in the home demonstrated significant reduction in biomarker levels and improved environmental health self-efficacy and precaution adoption (Butterfield et al, 2011).*

REFERENCES

Agency for Toxic Substances and Disease Registry (ATSDR). (2014). *Medical management guideline for parathion.* Retrieved from: <http://www.atsdr.cdc.gov/MMG/MMG.asp?id=1140&tid=246>.

Boscarino, J. A., Adams, R. E., & Figley, C. R. (2011). Mental health service use after the World Trade Center disaster. Utilization trends and comparative effectiveness. *The Journal of Nervous and Mental Diseases, 199,* 91–99.

Butterfield, P. G., Hill, W., & Postma, J. (2011). Effectiveness of a household environmental health intervention delivered by rural public health nurses. *American Journal of Public Health, 101*(Suppl. 1), S262–S270.

Centers for Disease Control & Prevention (CDC). (2012). *CDC response to advisory committee on childhood lead poisoning prevention recommendations in "Low level lead exposure harms children: A renewed call for primary prevention".* Retrieved from: <http://www.cdc.gov/nceh/lead/acc/pp/cdc_response-lead_exposure_recs.pdf>.

Centers for Disease Control & Prevention (CDC). (2013a). *What are the benefits of flu vaccination?* Retrieved from: <http://www.cdc.gov/flu/pdf/freeresources/general/flu-vaccine-benefits.pdf>.

Centers for Disease Control & Prevention (CDC). (2013b). *Lead screening during the domestic medical examination for newly arrived refugees.* Retrieved from: <http://www.cdc.gov/immigrantrefugeehealth.pdf/lead-guidelines.pdf>.

Centers for Disease Control & Prevention (CDC). (2013c). *Folk medicine.* Retrieved from: <http://www.cdc.gov/nceh/lead.tips/folkmedicine.htm>.

Centers for Disease Control & Prevention (CDC). (2013d). *Food safety. Prevention and education.* Retrieved from: <http://www.cdc.gov/foodsafety/prevention.html>.

Centers for Disease Control and Prevention (CDC). (2014a). *Office of Public Health Preparedness and Response.* 2013-2014 national snapshot of public health preparedness. Retrieved from: <http://www.cdc.govphpr/pubs- links/2013/documents/2013_Preparedness_Report_Section3.pdf>.

Centers for Disease Control & Prevention (CDC). (2014b). *Water-related diseases and contamination in public water systems.* Retrieved from: <http://www.cdc.gov/healthywater/drinking/public/water_diseases.html>.

Centers for Disease Control and Prevention (CDC). (2014c). *International adoption and prevention of lead poisoning.* Retrieved from: <http://www.cdc.gov/nceh/lead.tips/adoption.htm>.

Chen, K.-H., Chen, L.-R., & Wang, Y.-K. (2014). Contamination of medical charts: An important source of potential infection in hospitals. *PLoS ONE, 9*(2), e78512.

Children's Environmental Health Network. (2013). *Children's environmental health 101.* Retrieved from: <http://www.cehn,org/resources/ceh101>.

Environmental Protection Agency (EPA). (2014). *Protect your family.* Retrieved from: <http://www2.epa.gov/lead>.

Federal Emergency Management Agency (FEMA). (2014). *Individuals with disabilities or access and functional needs.* Retrieved from: <http://www.cdc.ready.gov/individuals-access-functional-needs>.

Holmes, S. M. (2011). The clinical gaze in the practice of migrant health: Mexican migrants in the United States. *Social Science and Medicine, 74*(6), 873–881.

Hubal, E., de Wet, T., & Du Toit, L. (2014). Identifying important life stages for monitoring and assessing risks from exposures to environmental contaminants: Results of a World Health Organization review. *Regulatory Toxicology and Pharmacology, 69*, 113–124.

Longtin, Y., Schneider, A., & Tschopp, C. (2014). Contamination of stethoscopes and physicians' hands after a physical examination. *Mayo Clinic Proceedings, 89*(3), 291–299.

Morgan, D. J., Rogawski, B. S., & Thom, K. A. (2012). Transfer of multidrug-resistant bacteria to healthcare workers' gloves and gowns after patient contact increases with environmental contamination. *Critical Care Medicine, 40*(4), 1045–1051.

Ohl, M., Schweizer, M., & Graham, M. (2012). Hospital privacy curtains are frequently and rapidly contaminated with potentially pathogenic bacteria. *American Journal of Infection Control, 40*, 904–906.

Oyama, M., Nakamura, K., Suda, Y., et al. (2012). Social network disruption as a major factor associated with psychological distress 3 years after 2004 Niigata-Chuetsu earthquake in Japan. *Environmental Health and Prevention Medicine, 17*, 118–123.

Pan American Health Organization. (2012). *Mental health and psychosocial support in disaster situations in the Caribbean.* Washington, DC: PAHO.

U. S. Army Medical Research Institute of Infectious Diseases. (2011). *USAMRIID's medical management of biological casualties handbook* (7th ed.). Fort Detrick, MD: Author.

Veenema, T. G. (2013). *Disaster nursing and emergency preparedness for chemical, biological and radiological terrorism and other hazards* (3rd ed.). New York: Springer.

Risk for Contamination *Betty J. Ackley, MSN, EdS, RN*

NANDA-I

Definition

Vulnerable to exposure to environmental contaminants, which may compromise health

Risk Factors

External

Carpeted flooring; chemical contamination of food; chemical contamination of water; economically disadvantaged; exposure to areas with high contaminant level; exposure to atmospheric pollutants; exposure to bioterrorism; exposure to disaster (natural or man-made); exposure to radiation; flaking, peeling surface in presence of young children (e.g., paint, plaster); inadequate breakdown of contaminant; inadequate household hygiene practices; inadequate municipal services (e.g., trash removal, sewage treatment facilities); inadequate personal hygiene practices; inadequate protective clothing; inappropriate use of protective clothing; playing where environmental contaminants are used; unprotected exposure to chemical (e.g., arsenic); unprotected exposure to heavy metal (e.g., chromium, lead); use of environmental contaminant in the home; use of noxious material insufficiently ventilated area (e.g., lacquer, paint); use of noxious material without effective protection (e.g., lacquer, paint)

Internal

Concomitant exposure; developmental characteristics of children; extremes of age; female gender; gestational age during exposure; inadequate nutrition; preexisting disease; pregnancy; previous exposure to contaminant; smoking

NIC, NOC, Client Outcomes, Nursing Interventions, Client/Family Teaching, *Rationales*, and References

Refer to care plans for **Contamination.**

Risk for adverse reaction to iodinated Contrast Media
Paula D. Hopper, MSN, RN, CNE, and Betty J. Ackley, MSN, EdS, RN

NANDA-I

Definition

Vulnerable to noxious or unintended reaction associated with the use of iodinated contrast media that can occur within 7 days after contrast agent injection, which may compromise health

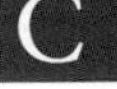

Risk Factors

Anxiety; chronic illness; concurrent use of pharmaceutical agents (e.g., beta blockers, interleukin-2, metformin nephrotoxins); contrast media precipitates adverse event (e.g., iodine concentration, viscosity, ion toxicity); dehydration; extremes of age; fragile vein (e.g., chemotherapy/radiation in limb to be injected, indwelling line for more than 24 hours, axillary lymph node dissection in limb to be injected, distal intravenous [IV] access site); generalized debilitation; history of allergy; history of previous adverse effect from iodinated contrast media; unconsciousness

NOC (Nursing Outcomes Classification)

Suggested NOC Outcomes

Tissue Perfusion: Renal; Kidney Function

Example NOC Outcome with Indicators

Kidney Function as evidenced by 24-hour intake and output balance/Blood urea nitrogen/Serum creatinine/Urine color/Serum electrolytes. (Rate the outcome and indicators of **Kidney Function:** 1 = severely compromised, 2 = substantially compromised, 3 = moderately compromised, 4 = mildly compromised, 5 = not compromised [see Section I].)

Client Outcomes

Client Will (Specify Time Frame)

- Maintain normal blood urea nitrogen and serum creatinine levels
- Maintain urine output of 0.5 mL/kg/hr
- Maintain serum electrolytes (K^+, PO_4, Na^+) within normal limits

NIC (Nursing Interventions Classification)

Suggested NIC Interventions

Fluid/Electrolyte Management; Laboratory Data Interpretation

Example NIC Activities—Fluid/Electrolyte Management

Monitor for serum electrolytes levels, as available; Weigh daily and monitor trends; Monitor vital signs, as appropriate

Nursing Interventions and *Rationales*

Recognize that iodinated contrast media can be harmful to clients in a number of ways, including onset of contrast-induced nephropathy, allergic reactions to the dye, and damage to veins and vascular access devices.

Contrast-Induced Nephropathy (CIN)

Protect clients from contrast media induced nephropathy by taking the following actions:

▲ Assess clients for low body mass index (BMI) or history of heart failure. Low BMI and heart failure are risk factors for CIN (Balemans et al, 2012).

▲ In nondiabetic clients with acute coronary syndrome, assess for presence of hyperglycemia on admission and report to health care provider. "[Index] admission high blood glucose in acute coronary syndrome patients not known to be diabetic is associated with increased incidence of contrast induced nephropathy after percutaneous coronary intervention" (Islam et al, 2013).

• Identify clients who have had multiple doses of iodinated contrast media in less than 24 hours and report to health care provider. *Repeat administration of contrast material may be a risk factor for CIN (American College of Radiology, 2013).*

• Notify the health care provider and the radiology staff if the client has preexisting renal disease. *Clients with preexisting impaired renal function are susceptible to develop acute contrast media–induced nephropathy (Schilcher et al, 2011; Wong et al, 2011).*

▲ Ensure that clients having diagnostic testing with contrast are well hydrated with isotonic IV fluids as ordered before and after the examination. EB: *Incidence of CIN is reduced by IV hydration with isotonic fluids (lactated Ringer's or 0.9% normal saline) before and after IV contrast administration (American*

College of Radiology, 2013). Low incidence of CIN is associated with the use of hydration (Balemans et al, 2012).

- ▲ Verify that a baseline serum creatinine has been drawn from clients at risk for CIN. *A baseline value is important for comparison following the contrast injection (American College of Radiology, 2013).*
- • Recognize that many clients with decreased renal function are not aware of their health status and that a questionnaire checklist administered before testing may not be satisfactory to determine which clients with impaired renal function should receive contrast media carefully or which are not candidates for testing utilizing contrast media. EB: *A study found that use of a preprocedure checklist was not effective in identifying all the clients with a history of chronic kidney disease to protect them from further kidney damage; instead, point-of-care creatinine testing was recommended (Kalisz et al, 2011).*
- • Be vigilant for signs of CIN in clients who have cancer. *Clients with cancer are vulnerable to CIN, especially within 45 days of chemotherapy and in those with hypertension (Cicin et al, 2014).*
- • Monitor the client carefully for symptoms of hypovolemia following use of contrast media, including measuring intake and output, obtaining blood pressure measurements, and assessing for new onset of postural hypotension with dizziness. *Hypovolemia can result following contrast media administration due to the increased osmolarity of the contrast media, resulting in postprocedure diuresis (O'Donovan, 2011).*
- ▲ Monitor for and report signs of acute kidney injury for 48 hours following iodinated contrast administration in clients at risk: absolute serum creatinine increase $\geq$ 0.3 mg/dL, percentage increase in serum creatinine $\geq$ 50%, or urine output reduced to $\leq$ 0.5 mL/kg/hr for at least 6 hours. *These are signs of acute kidney injury (American College of Radiology, 2013).*

Allergic Reaction to Contrast Media

- ▲ Discuss premedication with steroids or diphenhydramine with health care provider for clients who have had previous reactions to contrast media. *Premedication may reduce the incidence of allergic reaction in some clients (American College of Radiology, 2013).*
- ▲ Monitor carefully for symptoms of a reaction, which can be mild, moderate, or severe. Report all symptoms to primary care provider because symptoms can advance rapidly from mild to severe.
  - ❍ *Mild reactions*: Urticaria, pruritus, rhinorrhea, nausea, emesis, diaphoresis, coughing, dizziness
  - ❍ *Moderate reactions*: Persistent emesis, widespread urticaria, headache, edema of the face, laryngeal edema, mild dyspnea, palpitations, tachycardia/bradycardia, hypertension, abdominal cramps
  - ❍ *Severe reactions:* Severe bronchospasm, severe arrhythmias, severe hypotension, pulmonary edema, laryngeal edema, seizures, syncope, death (Wilson, 2011)
  - ❍ *Both allergic and allergic-like (anaphylactoid) reactions can occur. Life-threatening events usually occur within 20 minutes after injection (American College of Radiology, 2013).*

Vein Damage and Damage to Vascular Access Devices

- • Recognize that only vascular access devices labeled "power injectable" can be used to administer power injected contrast media. These include a power port, a power PICC line, and a power central venous catheter (Radiology and Biomedical Imaging, 2014). *A regular vascular access device used for administration of contrast media can rupture from the high pressures used to administer the contrast media.* EB: *A retrospective study of the function of 204 power ports found that they are safe for use with power injections of contrast media (Goltz et al, 2012). The U.S. Food and Drug Administration has received more than 250 adverse event reports in which vascular access devices have ruptured when used with power injectors. The adverse events include rupture and device fragmentation (Earhart & McMahon, 2011).*
- • Reduce the risk of vein and vascular access device damage with the following:
  - ❍ Maintain constant communication with the client during the injection. Discontinue the injection if the client reports pain or the sensation of swelling at the injection site. *These are signs of complications (American College of Radiology, 2013).*
  - ❍ Be vigilant in clients at increased risk of extravasation. *Clients at increased risk include those who cannot communicate such as infants, older adults, or those with altered consciousness; severely ill or debilitated clients; clients with abnormal circulation in the affected limb; clients receiving the injection via a peripheral IV line that has been in place for more than 24 hours or into a vein that has been punctured multiple times; clients with arterial insufficiency or compromised venous or lymphatic drainage in the affected extremity (American College of Radiology, 2013).*
  - ❍ Assess for venous backflow before injecting contrast. *If backflow is not obtained, the catheter may need adjustment (American College of Radiology, 2013).*

- ❍ Directly monitor and palpate the venipuncture site during the first 15 seconds of injection. *A critical step in preventing significant extravasation is direct monitoring of the venipuncture site (American College of Radiology, 2013).*
- • After diagnostic testing using contrast media given intravenously, inspect the IV site used for administration for possible problems, such as extravasation or development of compartment syndrome with excessive amounts of contrast pushed into the tissues under pressure. *The incidence of serious complications associated with the media has increased since advent of use of power or pressure mechanical injectors. Although rare, compartment syndrome can result in infection, loss of use of the affected extremity, necrosis, skin sloughing, amputation, need for skin grafting, paralysis, and death (Wilson, 2011).*

C

Geriatric

- • Screen the older client thoroughly before diagnostic testing utilizing contrast media. *Older adults are more likely to have preexisting renal failure along with other comorbidities and are more vulnerable to development of renal damage (O'Donovan, 2011).*

REFERENCES

American College of Radiology. (2013). *ACR manual on contrast media: version 9* (pp. 38–39). Reston, VA: American College of Radiology.

Balemans, C. E. A., et al. (2012). Epidemiology of contrast material-induced nephropathy in the era of hydration. *Radiology*, *263*(3), 706–713.

Cicin, I., et al. (2014). Incidence of contrast-induced nephropathy in hospitalized patients with cancer. *European Radiology*, *24*(1), 184–190.

Earhart, A., & McMahon, P. (2011). Vascular access and contrast media. *Journal of Infusion Nursing: the Official Publication of the Infusion Nurses Society*, *34*(2), 97–105.

Goltz, J. P., et al. (2012). Totally implantable venous power ports of the forearm and the chest: initial clinical experience with port devices approved for high-pressure injections. *The British Journal of Radiology*, *85*(1019), e966–e972.

Islam, N., et al. (2013). Impact of blood glucose levels on contrast induced nephropathy after percutaneous coronary intervention in patients not known to be diabetic with acute coronary syndrome. *Cardiovascular Journal*, *6*(1), 23–30.

Kalisz, K. R., et al. (2011). Detection of renal dysfunction by point-of-care creatinine testing in patients undergoing peripheral MR angiography. *AJR. American Journal of Roentgenology*, *197*(2), 430–435.

O'Donovan, K. (2011). Preventing contrast-induced nephropathy part 2: preventive strategies. *British Journal of Community Nursing*, *6*(1), 6–10.

Radiology and Biomedical Imaging. (2014). *Patient Care: Vascular access and use of central lines and ports in adults. University of California San Francisco*. Retrieved from: <http://www.radiology.ucsf.edu/patient-care/patient-safety/contrast/iodinated/vascular-access-adults>.

Schilcher, G., et al. (2011). Early detection and intervention using neutrophil gelatinase associated lipocalin (NGAL) may improve renal outcome of acute contrast media induced nephropathy: a randomized controlled trial in patients undergoing intra-arterial angiography (ANTI-CIN Study). *BMC Nephrology*, *17*, 12–39.

Wilson, B. (2011). Contrast media-induced compartment syndrome. *Radiologic Technology*, *83*(1), 63–77.

Wong, P. C., Li, Z., Guo, J., et al. (2011). Pathophysiology of contrast-induced nephropathy. *International Journal of Cardiology*, *158*(2), 186–192.

Compromised family Coping

Katherina Nikzad-Terhune, PhD, LCSW

NANDA-I

Definition

A usually supportive primary person (family member, significant other, or close friend) provides insufficient, ineffective, or compromised support, comfort, assistance, or encouragement that may be needed by the client to manage or master adaptive tasks related to his or her health challenge

Defining Characteristics

Assistive behaviors by support person produce unsatisfactory results; client complaint about support person's response to health problems; client concern about support person's response to health problem; limitation in communication between support person and client; protective behavior by support person incongruent with client's abilities; protective behavior by support person incongruent with client's need for autonomy; support person reports inadequate understanding that interferes with effective behaviors; support person reports insufficient knowledge that interferes with effective behaviors; support person reports preoccupation with own reaction to client's need; support person withdraws from client

Related Factors (r/t)

Coexisting situations affecting the support person; developmental crises experienced by support person; exhaustion of support person's capacity; family disorganization; family role change; insufficient information available to support person; insufficient reciprocal support; insufficient support given by client to support person; insufficient understanding of information by support person; misinformation obtained by support person; preoccupation by support person with concern outside of family; prolonged disease that exhausts capacity of support person; situational crisis faced by support person

NOC (Nursing Outcomes Classification)

Suggested NOC Outcomes

Caregiver Emotional Health; Caregiver-Client Relationship; Family Coping; Family Participation in Professional Care; Family Support During Treatment

Example NOC Outcome with Indicators

Family Coping as evidenced by the following indicators: Confronts family problems/Manages family problems/Reports needs for family assistance. (Rate each indicator of **Family Coping:** 1 = never demonstrated, 2 = rarely demonstrated, 3 = sometimes demonstrated, 4 = often demonstrated, 5 = consistently demonstrated [see Section I].)

Client Outcomes

Family/Significant Person Will (Specify Time Frame)

- Verbalize internal resources to help deal with the situation
- Verbalize knowledge and understanding of illness, disability, or disease
- Provide support and assistance as needed
- Identify need for and seek outside support

NIC (Nursing Interventions Classification)

Suggested NIC Interventions

Caregiver Support; Coping Enhancement; Family Involvement Promotion; Family Mobilization; Family Support; Mutual Goal Setting; Normalization Promotion; Sibling Support

Example NIC Activitis—Family Support

Appraise family's emotional reaction to client's condition; Promote trusting relationship with family

Nursing Interventions and *Rationales*

- Assess the strengths and deficiencies of the family system. EBN: *Thorough and comprehensive assessments offer valuable information regarding how problems evolve within the family context over time, and allow for anticipatory care and guidance to help family members acquire and maintain support and coping strategies (Wright & Leahey, 2012).*
- Establish rapport with families by providing accurate communication. EBN: *Enthusiasm or interest demonstrated by health care professionals helps establish stronger rapport and a therapeutic relationship with clients (Bahrami, 2011).*
- Assist family members to recognize the need for help and teach them how to ask for it.
- Encourage expression of positive thoughts and emotions to help reduce stress. EB: *A comprehensive survey of meta-analyses examining the efficacy of cognitive behavioral therapy (CBT) found it to be a strong evidence-based intervention to use with a variety of complex issues, including stress reduction (Hofmann et al, 2012).*
- Encourage family members to verbalize feelings. Spend time with them, sit down and make eye contact, and offer coffee and other nourishment.

- Incorporate family variables, including dyadic adjustment, into assessment protocols and intervention strategies. EB: *Pereira et al (2012) revealed a positive relationship among dyadic adjustment, psychological morbidity, and family coping in clients and their partners, in that better dyadic adjustment predicted family coping in the client.*
- Provide privacy during family visits. If possible, maintain flexible visiting hours to accommodate more frequent family visits. If possible, arrange staff assignments so the same staff members have contact with the family. Familiarize other staff members with the situation in the absence of the usual staff member. *Providing privacy, maintaining flexible hours, and arranging consistent staff assignments reduces stress, enhances communication, and facilitates the building of trust.*
- Provide education to clients regarding active coping strategies to use in situations involving chronic illnesses. EBN: *Active coping strategies, including planning, giving priority, reappraisal, waiting, and acceptance, were predictive of better quality of life and lower levels of depression and hopelessness in cancer clients (van Laarhoven et al, 2011).*
- Use evidence-based tools to assess for post-intensive care syndrome (e.g., anxiety, acute stress disorder, posttraumatic stress, depression, and complicated grief) in families who have experienced a critical illness. EB: *Prevention strategies for post-intensive care syndrome include adequate communication and involving families in decision-making processes, while treatment strategies include support groups and referrals for treatment (Davidson et al, 2012).*
- Refer the family with ill family members to appropriate resources for assistance as indicated (e.g., counseling, psychotherapy, financial assistance, or spiritual support).

Pediatric

- Provide screening for postpartum depression (PPD) during the prenatal period and during the 6-week postpartum check-up to identify symptoms of depression in mothers. CEB: *The Edinburgh Postnatal Depression Scale (EPDS) is the most widely used screening tool for detecting PPD and has been shown to be effective both prenatally and postnatally for detecting symptoms of depression in women (Cox et al, 1987).*

▲ Consider medication management and psychosocial interventions, including individual therapy, group therapy, support groups, and brief psychotherapy. EB: *These are effective treatment strategies for managing PPD (Miniati et al, 2014; Kleiman & Raskin, 2013).*

▲ Use preventive strategies, such as screening, psychoeducation, postpartum debriefing, and companionship in the delivery room (e.g., community volunteer). EBN: *These strategies play an important role in the prevention of and recovery from PPD (Dennis & Dowswell, 2013).*

- Provide educational and psychosocial interventions, such as coping skills training, in treatment for families and their adolescents who have diabetes. EBN: *Educational and support interventions help improve coping skills for parents of adolescents with diabetes (Konradsdottir & Svavarsdottir, 2011).*
- Provide readily available resources to support parents of children with autism and their families. EBN: *Study findings from Hall (2011) highlighted the association between the low adaptive functioning of the child with autism and increased parental stress, the need for additional family support, and the need for effective coping strategies.*
- Provide family-centered care during neonatal intensive care to encourage family members to play an active role in providing emotional, social, and developmental support. EBN: *When neonatal intensive care unit staff collaborate with parents, families become more involved in decision-making processes and care planning, and are empowered to impact the process of their infant's recovery (Gooding et al, 2011).*
- Provide evidence-based psychological therapies for parents with children with chronic conditions. EB: *Psychological therapies (e.g., cognitive behavioral therapy and problem-solving therapy) that included parents significantly improved child symptoms for painful conditions immediately after treatment (Eccleston et al, 2012).*
- Assist with fostering co-parenting alliances in fragile families. EB: *Providing preventive interventions to support the development of a positive co-parenting alliance between parents who have not made an enduring relationship commitment to one another can help benefit children and families (McHale et al, 2012).*
- Provide options for home-based interventions when severe childhood illnesses make it difficult for children and families to participate in interventions. EBN: *A home-based 12-week cognitive training program for child cancer survivors yielded significant increases in working memory and decreases in parent-rated attention problems following the intervention (Hardy et al, 2011).*

C

Geriatric

▲ Perform a holistic assessment of all needs of informal spousal caregivers. EBN: *Caregiver assessments should be systematic, should take into consideration the caregiver's perspective, and should include follow-up on care coordination and linkages to services (Levine, 2011). Refer caregivers of clients with Alzheimer's disease to a monthly psychoeducational support group (i.e., the Alzheimer's Association), and incorporate nonpharmacological support programs for caregivers.* EB: *Nonpharmacological interventions, such as skill training programs for stress management, in home support, individual or group psychotherapy, and respite programs, demonstrate efficacy in reducing caregiver stress and burden (Gallagher-Thompson et al, 2012).*

▲ Provide caregivers with options for Internet-based support strategies to enhance coping. EB: *Creating bonds between caregivers using online support programs produces beneficial psychological outcomes among caregivers, including improved coping (Namkoong et al, 2012).*

- Assist in finding transportation to enable family members to visit. EB: *If a family member is homebound and unable to visit, encourage alternative contact (e.g., telephone, cards and letters, email) to provide ongoing scheduled progress reports and to help reduce loneliness and isolation. Visually impaired older adults, who experience more limitations with driving, have a higher risk for loneliness (Alma et al, 2011).*
- Assist informal caregivers with reducing unmet needs by helping them obtain the information and education necessary for caring for an older adult with a chronic health condition. EB: *Evidence supports the use of a health information delivery system (e.g., providing information that is proactive, understandable, and individualized) specifically designed to meet the unique needs of informal caregivers of older adults with chronic health conditions (Washington et al, 2011).*

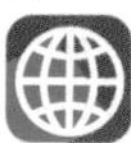

Multicultural

- Acknowledge racial/ethnic differences at the onset of care. EBN: *Accurate cultural knowledge assists in enhancing the ability of health care service providers to identify and understand cultural factors that influence diagnosis, treatment, and illness management, and create warm and trusting relationships with their clients (Higginbottom et al, 2011).*
- Assess for the influence of cultural beliefs, norms, and values on the individual/family/community's perceptions of coping. EB: *Cultural values are a valid predictor of coping when traits are taken into account (Bardi & Guerra, 2011).*
- Use valid and culturally competent assessment tools and procedures when working with families with different racial/ethnic backgrounds. EBN: *The cultural information in nursing models and assessments should encompass health beliefs and practices, communication styles, religious orientation, and the degree of acculturation amongst others (Higginbottom et al, 2011).*
- Provide culturally relevant interventions by understanding and using treatment strategies that are acceptable and effective for a particular culture. EB: *Interventions should be theoretical based and incorporate cultural beliefs within a contextual framework in order for prevention and risk reduction messages to reach targeted at risk populations (Wyatt et al, 2012).*
- Provide opportunities for families to discuss spirituality. EBN: *African American women with breast cancer use more positive religious coping and experience less distress and greater spiritual well-being (Gaston-Johansson et al, 2013).*
- Determine how the family's cultural context impacts their decisions in regard to managing and coping with a child's illness; recognize and validate the cultural context. EBN: *Nurses and other clinicians working with families must include cultural variables when assisting family members with ill children, and demonstrating competency and respect for one's cultural values helps ensure the good of the client as well as client autonomy (Leever, 2011).*

Home Care

- The interventions described previously may be adapted for home care use.
- Assess the reason behind the breakdown of family coping. *Knowledge of the reasons behind compromised coping will assist in identification of appropriate interventions. Refer to the care plan for* **Caregiver Role Strain**.
- During the time of compromised coping, increase visits to ensure the safety of the client, support of the family, and reassurance regarding expectations for prognosis as appropriate. EBN: *When providing care in the home setting, conforming to the norms and values of clients and their families is extremely important for building rapport and ensuring a sense of safety (Lindahl et al, 2011).*

▲ Assess the needs of the caregiver in the home, and intervene to meet needs as appropriate; explore all available resources that may be used to provide adequate home care (e.g., parish nursing as an effective adjunct, home health aide services to relieve the caregiver's fatigue).

▲ Encourage caregivers to attend to their own physical, mental, and spiritual health, and give more specific information about the client's needs and ways to meet them.

▲ Refer the family to medical social services for evaluation and supportive counseling. Serve as an advocate, mentor, and role model for caregiving; provide written information for the care needed by the client.

▲ A positive approach and caring by the nurse and concrete task definition and assignment reinforce positive coping strategies and allow caregivers to feel less guilty when tasks are delegated to multiple caregivers.

▲ When a terminal illness is the precipitating factor for ineffective coping, offer hospice services and support groups as possible resources. EBN: *Research suggests that clients and their families highly value hospice care services and report experiencing beneficial outcomes as a result of using hospice services, including effective pain management and avoiding death in the hospital setting (Candy et al, 2011).*

• Encourage the client and family to discuss changes in daily functioning and routines created by the client's illness, and validate discomfort resulting from changes. *Individuals who live together for a long period tend to become familiar with each other's patterns: for example, meals are expected at certain times or a spouse becomes accustomed to the client's sleep habits.*

• Support positive individual and family coping efforts. *Positive feedback reinforces desired behaviors and supports the family unit.*

▲ If compromised family coping interferes with the ability to support the client's treatment plan, refer for psychiatric home health care services for family counseling and/or Internet-based behavioral interventions. EBN: *Schubart et al (2011) identified two characteristics contributing to Internet interventions that engage users: (1) the intervention targets participants with serious health concerns, and (2) the intervention adapts to individual needs.*

Client/Family Teaching and Discharge Planning

• Assess for and address grief issues that arise in the process, including anticipatory grief. EB: *Research conducted by Garand et al (2012) revealed high levels of anticipatory grief in dementia caregivers, suggesting that this grief reaction may be highest at the earliest stages of Alzheimer's disease caregiving, or when family members begin to provide care assistance to their loved one with mild cognitive impairment.*

▲ Refer women with breast cancer and their family caregivers to support groups and other services that provide assistance with daily coping. Refer women with breast cancer and their family caregivers to support groups, including social network sites and online communities, to provide assistance with daily coping. EB: *Social network sites and online communities present a convenient way to exchange information and support for breast cancer survivors, including awareness, service promotion, client/caregiver support, and fundraising (Bender et al, 2011).*

• Promote individual and family relaxation and stress-reduction strategies. *The immune system weakens in response to stress; persistent relaxation may elicit positive effects on one's immune system (Kang et al, 2011).*

▲ Refer parents to support and education groups to provide opportunities for parents to access support, learn new parenting skills, and ultimately, optimize their relationships with their children after divorce. EB: *Through education, parents can be taught to improve the quality of their parenting, which has been linked to improvements in children's academic functioning and reductions in children's mental health and substance use problems (Sigal et al, 2011).*

• Provide Internet-based resources, including online social networking groups, to enhance social support, bonding, and coping for caregivers. EB: *Perceived bonding through social support yields positive effects on caregivers' problem-focused coping strategies (Namkoong et al, 2012).*

REFERENCES

Alma, M., Van der Mei, S. F., & Feitsma, W. N. (2011). Loneliness and self-management abilities in the visually impaired elderly. *Journal of Aging and Health, 23*, 843–861.

Bahrami, M. (2011). Why differences exist? An interpretive approach to nurses' perceptions of cancer patients' quality of life. *Iranian Journal of Nursing and Midwifery Research, 16*(1), 117–124.

Bardi, A., & Guerra, V. M. (2011). Cultural values predict coping using culture as an individual difference variable in multicultural samples. *Journal of Cross-Cultural Psychology, 42*(6), 908–927.

Bender, J., Jimenez-Marroquin, M., & Jadad, A. R. (2011). Seeking support on Facebook: A content analysis of breast cancer groups. *Journal of Medical Internet Research, 13*(1), e16.

C

Candy, B., Holman, A., Leurent, B., et al. (2011). Hospice care delivered at home, in nursing homes and in dedicated hospice facilities: A systematic review of quantitative and qualitative evidence. *International Journal of Nursing Studies, 48*(1), 121–133.

Cox, J. L., Holden, J. M., & Sagovsky, R. (1987). Detection of postnatal depression: Development of the 10-item Edinburgh Postnatal Depression Scale. *The British Journal of Psychiatry: The Journal of Mental Science, 150*, 782–786.

Davidson, J., Jones, C., & Bienvenu, J. (2012). Family response to critical illness: *Postintensive care syndrome—family. Critical Care Medicine, 40*(2), 618–624.

Dennis, C. L., & Dowswell, T. (2013). Psychosocial and psychological interventions for preventing postpartum depression. *The Cochrane database of Systematic Reviews.*

Eccleston, C., Palermo, T., Fisher, E., et al. (2012). Psychological interventions for parents of children and adolescents with chronic illness. *The Cochrane database of Systematic Reviews*, Advance online publication.

Gallagher-Thompson, D., Tzuang, Y. M., Au, L., et al. (2012). International perspectives on nonpharmacological best practices for dementia family caregivers: A review. *Clinical Gerontologist, 35*(4), 316–355.

Garand, L., Lingler, J. H., & Dew, M. A. (2012). Anticipatory grief in new family caregivers of persons with mild cognitive impairment and dementia. *Alzheimer Disease and Associated Disorders, 26*(2), 159–165.

Gaston-Johansson, F., Haisfield-Wolfe, M. E., Reddick, B., et al. (2013). The relationships among coping strategies, religious coping, and spirituality in African American women with breast cancer receiving chemotherapy. *Oncology Nursing Forum, 40*(2), 120–131.

Gooding, J., Cooper, L., Blaine, A., et al. (2011). Family support and family-centered care in the neonatal intensive care unit: Origins, advances, impact. *Seminars in Perinatology, 35*(1), 20–28.

Hall, H. (2011). The relationships among adaptive behaviors of children with autism, family support, parenting stress, and coping. *Issues in Comprehensive Pediatric Nursing, 34*, 4–25.

Hardy, K., Willard, V., & Bonner, M. (2011). Computerized cognitive training in survivors of childhood cancer: A Pilot Study. *Journal of Pediatric Oncology Nursing, 28*(1), 27–33.

Higginbottom, G., Richter, M. S., Mogale, R. S., et al. (2011). Identification of nursing assessment models/tools validated in clinical practice for use with diverse ethno-cultural groups: An integrative review of the literature. *BMC Nursing, 10*(16), 1–11.

Hofmann, S., Asnaani, A., Vonk, I., et al. (2012). The efficacy of cognitive behavioral therapy: A review of meta-analyses. *Cognitive Therapy and Research, 36*(5), 427–440.

Kang, D. H., McArdle, T., Park, N., et al. (2011). Dose effects of relaxation practice on immune responses in women newly diagnosed with breast cancer: An exploratory study. *Oncology Nursing Forum, 38*(3), E240–E252.

Kleiman, K. R., & Raskin, V. D. (2013). *This isn't what I expected: Overcoming postpartum depression* (2nd ed.). Boston, MA: Da Capo.

Konradsdottir, E., & Svavarsdottir, E. K. (2011). How effective is a short-term educational and support intervention for families of an adolescent with type 1 diabetes? *Journal for Specialists in Pediatric Nursing, 16*(4), 295–304.

Leever, M. (2011). Cultural competence: Reflections on patient autonomy and patient good. *Nursing Ethics, 18*(4), 560–570.

Levine, C. (2011). Supporting family caregivers: The hospital nurse's assessment of family caregiver needs. *American Journal of Nursing, 111*(10), 47–51.

Lindahl, B., Lide'n, E., & Lindblad, B. (2011). A meta-synthesis describing the relationships between patients, informal caregivers and health professionals in home-care settings. *Journal of Clinical Nursing, 20*(3–4), 454–463.

McHale, J., Waller, M., & Pearson, J. (2012). Coparenting interventions for fragile families: What do we know and where do we need to go next? *Family Process, 51*(3), 284–306.

Miniati, M., Callari, A., Calugi, S., et al. (2014). Interpersonal psychotherapy for postpartum depression: A systematic review. *Archives of Women's Mental Health, 17*(4), 257–268.

Namkoong, K., DuBenske, L., Shaw, B., et al. (2012). Creating a bond between caregivers online: Effect on caregivers' coping strategies. *Journal of Health Communication: International Perspectives, 17*(2), 125–140.

Pereira, M., Brito, L., & Smith, T. (2012). Dyadic adjustment, family coping, body image, quality of life and psychological morbidity in patients with psoriasis and their partners. *International Journal of Behavioral Medicine, 19*(3), 260–269.

Schubart, J., Stuckey, H., Ganeshamoorthy, A., et al. (2011). Chronic health conditions and Internet behavioral interventions: A review of factors to enhance user engagement. *Computers, Informatics, Nursing, 29*(2), 81–92.

Sigal, A., Sandler, I., Wolchik, S., et al. (2011). Do parent education programs promote healthy postdivorce parenting? Critical distinctions and a review of the evidence. *Family Court Review, 49*(1), 120–139.

van Laarhoven, H., Schilderman, J., Bleijenberg, G., et al. (2011). Coping, quality of life, depression, and hopelessness in cancer patients in a curative and palliative, end-of-life care setting. *Cancer Nursing, 34*(4), 302–314.

Washington, K., Meadows, S., Elliot, S., et al. (2011). Information needs of informal caregivers of older adults with chronic health conditions. *Patient Education and Counseling, 83*, 37–44.

Wright, L. M., & Leahey, M. (2012). *Nurses and families: A guide to family assessment and intervention.* Philadelphia: FA Davis.

Wyatt, G. E., Williams, J. K., Gupta, A., et al. (2012). Are cultural values and beliefs included in U.S. based HIV interventions? *Preventative Medicine, 55*(5), 362–370.

Defensive Coping

Arlene T. Farren, RN, PhD, AOCN, CTN-A

NANDA-I

Definition

Repeated projection of falsely positive self-evaluation based on a self-protective pattern that defends against underlying perceived threats to positive self-regard

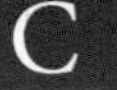

Defining Characteristics

Alteration in reality testing; denial of problems; denial of weaknesses; difficulty establishing relationships; difficulty maintaining relationships; grandiosity; hostile laughter; hypersensitivity to a discourtesy; hypersensitivity to criticism; insufficient follow through with treatment; insufficient participation in treatment; projection of blame; projection of responsibility; rationalization of failures; reality distortion; ridicule of others; superior attitude toward others

Related Factors

Conflict between self-perception and value system; fear of failure; fear of humiliation; fear of repercussions; insufficient confidence in others; insufficient resilience; insufficient self-confidence; insufficient support system; uncertainty unrealistic self-expectations

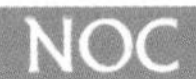

NOC (Nursing Outcomes Classification)

Suggested NOC Outcomes

Coping; Decision-Making; Impulse Self-Control; Information Processing

Example NOC Outcome with Indicators

Coping as evidenced by the following indicators: Identifies effective and ineffective coping patterns/Modifies lifestyle to reduce stress. (Rate the outcome and indicators of **Coping:** 1 = never demonstrated, 2 = rarely demonstrated, 3 = sometimes demonstrated, 4 = often demonstrated, 5 = consistently demonstrated [see Section I].)

Client Outcomes

Client Will (Specify Time Frame)

- Acknowledge need for change in coping style
- Accept responsibility for own behavior
- Establish realistic goals with validation from caregivers
- Solicit caregiver validation in decision-making

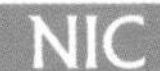

NIC (Nursing Interventions Classification)

Suggested Nursing Interventions

Body Image Enhancement; Complex Relationship Building; Coping Enhancement; Patient Contracting; Resiliency Promotion; Self-Awareness Enhancement; Self-Esteem Enhancement; Socialization Enhancement; Surveillance

Example NIC Activities—Self-Awareness Enhancement

Encourage client to recognize and discuss thoughts and feelings; Assist client in identifying behaviors that are self-destructive

Nursing Interventions and *Rationales*

- Assess for possible symptoms associated with defensive coping: depressive symptoms, excessive self-focused attention, negativism and anxiety, hypertension, posttraumatic stress disorder (e.g., exposure to terrorism), unjust world beliefs. EB: *In a study of coping styles and anxiety in a small sample (N = 47) of persons with chronic low back pain, researchers found evidence of more defensiveness than in the general population. Researchers suggested that individuals with defensive high-anxious coping styles may be at risk for poorer psychological and physical outcomes and recommended assessment of these characteristics and further research to ensure appropriate treatments and improved outcomes (Lewis et al, 2012).* EB: *Defensive reactions were present in a sample of college women (N = 1679) who identified as having experience with childhood abuse or other traumas; researchers concluded that victims' defensive reactions to trauma may contribute to the unique effects of trauma (Bottoms et al, 2012).*

▲ Use cognitive behavioral interventions. EBN: *In a randomized control trial (N = 240), 120 in each group—experimental and control), a nurse-led cognitive behavioral intervention addressed inaccurate thinking and promoted more positive self-regard; the experimental group had improved quality of life, which included physical and psychological health, relief of symptom, and social functioning (Zhuang et al, 2013).*

C

- Ask appropriate questions to assess whether denial (defensive coping) is being used in association with health problems including alcoholism, myocardial infarction (MI), or rheumatoid arthritis. EBN: *In a qualitative study of 28 people after MI, researchers found that those who used negative coping, including denial and defensive coping, did not make the necessary changes toward physical and psychological health and experienced depression; researchers recommended follow-up care including psychoeducational interventions (Salminen-Tuomaala et al, 2012).* EBN: *In a case-based article, Wilson (2013) demonstrates a nurse-provided approach to Screening, Brief Intervention, and Referral to Treatment (SBIRT), an approach recommended by the Substance Abuse and Mental Health Services Administration (2015), in a client requiring a peripherally inserted central catheter for a man with liver disease due to alcoholism.* EB: *In a 5-year prospective study of adults with rheumatoid arthritis (N = 74), researchers found that defensive coping impacted responses to pain and overall health, leading to poorer outcomes (Goulia et al, 2015).*
- Promote interventions with multisensory stimulation environments. EB: *In a review of the literature regarding sharing multisensory body space with others for those with altered bodies, such as amputations or congenital limb absence, researchers concluded that sharing multisensory body space is pertinent and may close the gap between neurology and psychiatry in the treatment of persons with altered bodies (Brugger & Lenggenhager, 2014).*
- Empower the client/caregiver's self-knowledge. EB: *In a qualitative study of adults receiving highly active antiretroviral treatment for HIV and methadone maintenance, participants described tension between negative feelings such as denial and positive feelings of empowerment (Batchelder et al, 2013).*

Geriatric

- ▲ Identify problems with alcohol in older adults with the appropriate tools and make suitable referrals. EB: *Community-dwelling older adults (N = 370) completed the Drinking Motives Questionnaire (DMQ); findings indicated that the most frequent motivation for drinking was social, with enhancement and coping motives, respectively, as the top three motivations (Gilson et al, 2013).* CEB: *Tools such as the Alcohol Use Disorders Identification Test (AUDIT), Michigan Alcohol Screening Test-Geriatric Version (MAST-G), and the Alcohol-Related Problems Survey (ARPS) may have additional use in this population. Brief interventions have been shown to be effective in producing sustained abstinence or reducing levels of consumption, thereby decreasing hazardous and harmful drinking (Culberson, 2006).*
- Encourage exercise for positive coping. EBN: *One research group identified that exercise is known to facilitate maintenance of functional abilities in older adults and tested an intervention to encourage older adults (N = 106) to engage in physical activity/exercise using peer mentors. The researchers found high participation and retention and improved fitness scores in all mentored groups (Dorgo et al, 2013).* EB: *Researchers performed a secondary analysis of data to examine the use of physical activity (PA) in mid and older adults during a smoking cessation attempt (N = 799), the researchers found that physical activity, primarily walking, was used by only a small percent of participants (11.6%); women were more likely to use PA as a coping strategy than men; the researchers recommend further study and approaches that encourage older adults to engage in PA for general health and quality of life (Treviño et al, 2014).*
- Stimulate individual reminiscence therapy. EBN: *Structured reminiscence is an evidence-based, independent nursing intervention that is used with individuals and groups and is used to increase emotional awareness and enhance social interactions in older adults (Stinson & Long, 2014).*
- Stimulate group reminiscence therapy. EBN: *Stinson's structured group reminiscence is a multisession evidence-based approach used with older adults (Stinson & Long, 2014).* EB: *A multimedia intergenerational reminiscence program was tested in a small (N = 26) group of community-dwelling older adults; qualitative data from stories and focus groups indicated the intervention showed promise as a group intergenerational intervention (Chonody & Wang, 2013).*

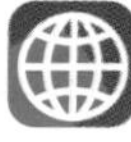

Multicultural

- Acknowledge racial/ethnic differences at the onset of care. EB: *In a qualitative study of white professionals working with racial minority immigrant clients, researchers found that while some professionals reported being comfortable discussing race and cultural differences, some expressed discomfort and difficulty, and others did not perceive race and culture to be a priority; the researchers recommended further attention to cultural competence training in clinical programs (Singer & Tummala-Narra, 2013).*

C

- Assess an individual's sociocultural backgrounds in teaching self-management and self-regulation. EBN: *A systematic review of qualitative evidence related to women's coping with type 2 diabetes indicated that in multiple countries self-management is challenged by the complexities of regimens and women's multiple-caregiving roles; researchers recommended recognition of the coping and emotional factors by health care providers; families, and friends, psychoeducation programs for clients and families, and enhanced support of family and friends (Li et al, 2014).* EB: *In a study of the Cellie Coping Kit for Sickle Cell Disease, researchers provided the intervention to 15 black/African American children aged 6 to 14 years and their health care providers; although the researchers reported strong acceptability, some sociocultural issues like living situation and health literacy did provide challenges to the use of the tool (Marsac et al, 2014).*
- Encourage the client to use spiritual coping mechanisms such as faith and prayer. CEB/EBN: *In a qualitative study of Thai Buddhist and Muslim women's (N = 48) use of religion and spiritual practices related to self-management of type 2 diabetes, researchers found four themes that related to cultural or spiritual practices, including prayer, that helped them cope, despite poor glycemic control (Lundberg & Thrakul, 2013).* EB: *In a study of religion and coping with racial discrimination among African American (N = 2032) and Caribbean blacks (N = 857), researchers found that both groups were similar in their likelihood of using prayer for coping with discrimination (Hayward & Krause, 2015).*
- Encourage spirituality as a source of support for coping. EBN: *In a small (N = 17) pilot study of African American women with breast cancer, women reported high levels of spiritual and positive religious coping (sense of purpose in life) strategies such as prayer; researchers recommended that although the findings of the pilot are not generalizable, spirituality and religious coping need to be explored as core coping mechanisms for African American women with breast cancer (Gaston-Johansson et al, 2013).*

Home Care

▲ Refer the client for programs that teach coping skills. EBN: *In a small pilot study of an intervention with mothers and their children who were exposed to domestic violence, researchers found preliminary evidence that the intervention (a relationally based multi-method program) improved defensive avoidance (Kearney & Cushing, 2012).* EB: *Researchers examining bullying and the association with cultural/family factors, substance use, and depressive symptoms in ninth and tenth grade Hispanic youth (N = 1167) found the stress of acculturation was associated with substance use and depressive symptoms and the need for the development of coping skills in youth; recommendations included school-based programs to teach coping skills (Forster et al, 2013).*

Client/Family Teaching and Discharge Planning

- Teach coping skills to clients and caregivers. EBN: *Teaching and modeling problem-solving skills to mothers with children who were exposed to domestic violence improved defensive avoidance (Kearney & Cushing, 2012).* EBN: *In a trial of a culturally adapted cognitive behavioral therapy intervention to promote coping skills among Chinese Americans with type 2 diabetes, strategies and coping skills that addressed personal, family, and illness specific topics were included; researchers reported enhanced efficacy for self-management (Chesla et al, 2013).*
- Teach reflexive and expressive writing to address emotions. EBN: *Journaling was used in an intervention study to enhance civility among nursing students; researchers found coping improvements in self-controlling and positive reappraisal (Jenkins et al, 2013).* EB: *In a randomized trial of expressive writing in the third person, 44 undergraduates wrote about their deepest thoughts and feelings about a traumatic or very stressful life event; findings included less intrusive thinking in both groups but third-person writers had better outcomes in overall health than did the first-person writers; researchers recommend third-person expressive writing for those recovering from traumatic or highly stressful events (Andersson & Conley, 2013).*

REFERENCES

Refer to ineffective **Coping** for additional references.

Andersson, M. A., & Conley, C. S. (2013). Optimizing the perceived benefits and health outcomes of writing about traumatic life events. *Stress and Health: Journal of the International Society for the Investigation of the Stress*, *29*, 40–49.

Batchelder, A. W., Brisban, M., Litwin, A. H., et al. (2013). "Damaging what wasn't damaged already": Psychological tension and antiretroviral adherence among HIV-infected methadone-maintained drug users. *AIDS Care*, *25*, 1370–1374.

Bottoms, B. L., Najdowski, C. J., Epstein, M. A., et al. (2012). Trauma severity and defensive emotion-regulation reactions as predictors of forgetting childhood trauma. *Journal of Trauma & Dissociation: the official journal of the International Society for the Study of Dissociation (ISSD)*, *13*, 291–310.

Brugger, P., & Lenggenhager, B. (2014). The bodily self and its disorders: Neurological, psychological, and social aspects. *Current Opinion in Neurology*, *27*, 644–652.

Chesla, C. A., Chun, K. M., Kwan, C. M. L., et al. (2013). Testing the efficacy of culturally adapted coping skills training for Chinese American immigrants with type 2 diabetes using community-based participatory research. *Research in Nursing & Health*, *36*, 359–372.

Chonody, J., & Wang, D. (2013). Connecting older adults to the community through multimedia: An intergenerational reminiscence program. *Activities, Adaptation, & Aging*, *37*, 79–93.

Culberson, J. W. (2006). Alcohol use in the elderly: beyond the CAGE. Part 2: Screening instruments and treatment strategies. *Geriatrics*, *61*(11), 20–26.

Dorgo, S., King, G. A., Bader, J. O., et al. (2013). Outcomes of a peer mentor implemented fitness program in older adults: A quasi-randomized controlled trial. *International Journal of Nursing Studies*, *50*, 1156–1165.

Forster, M., Dyal, S. R., Baezconde-Garbanati, L., et al. (2013). Bullying victimization as a mediator of associations between cultural/familial variables, substance use, and depressive symptoms among Hispanic youth. *Ethnicity & Health*, *18*, 415–432.

Gaston-Johansson, F., Haisfield-Wolfe, M. E., Reddick, B., et al. (2013). The relationships among coping strategies, religious coping, and spirituality in African American Women with breast cancer receiving chemotherapy. *Oncology Nursing Forum*, *40*, 120–131.

Gilson, K., Bryant, C., Bei, B., et al. (2013). Validation of the drinking motives questionnaire in older adults. *Addictive Behaviors*, *38*, 2196–2202.

Goulia, P., Voulgari, P. V., Tsifetaki, N., et al. (2015). Sense of coherence and self-sacrificing defense style as predictors of psychological distress and quality of life in rheumatoid arthritis: A 5-year prospective study. *Rheumatology International*, *35*, 691–700.

Hayward, R. D., & Krause, N. (2015). Religion and strategies for coping with racial discrimination among African Americans and Caribbean Blacks. *International Journal of Stress Management*, *22*, 70–91.

Jenkins, S. D., Kerber, C. S., & Woith, W. M. (2013). An intervention to promote civility among nursing students. *Nursing Education Perspectives*, *34*, 95–100.

Kearney, J. A., & Cushing, E. (2012). A multi-modal pilot intervention with violence-exposed mothers in a child psychiatric trauma-focused treatment program. *Issues in Mental Health Nursing*, *33*, 544–552.

Lewis, S. E., Fowler, N. E., Woby, S. R., et al. (2012). Defensive coping styles, anxiety, and chronic low back pain. *Physiotherapy*, *98*(1), 86–88.

Li, J., Drury, V., & Taylor, B. (2014). A systematic review of the experience of older women living and coping with type 2 diabetes. *International Journal of Nursing Practice*, *20*, 126–134.

Lundberg, P. C., & Thrakul, S. (2013). Religion and self-management of Thai Buddhist and Muslim women with type 2 diabetes. *Journal of Clinical Nursing*, *22*, 1907–1916.

Marsac, M. L., Alderfer, M. A., Smith-Whitely, K., et al. (2014). *Clinical Practice in Pediatric Psychology*, *2*, 389–399.

Salminen-Tuomaala, M., Åstedt-Kurki, P., Rekiaro, M., et al. (2012). Coping experiences: A pathway toward different coping orientations four and twelve months after myocardial infarction—A grounded theory approach. *Nursing Research and Practice*, *2012*, Article ID 674783, 9 pages.

Singer, R. R., & Tummala-Narra, P. (2013). White clinicians' perspectives on working with racial minority immigrant clients. *Professional Psychology, Research and Practice*, *44*, 290–298.

Stinson, C., & Long, E. M. (2014). Reminiscence: Improving the quality of life for older adults. *Geriatric Nursing*, *35*, 399–404.

Substance Abuse and Mental Health Services Administration. (2015). *Screening, brief intervention, and referral to treatment (SBIRT)*. Retrieved from: <http://www.samhsa.gov/sbirt> June 2015.

Treviño, L. A., Baker, L., McIntosh, S., et al. (2014). Physical activity as a coping strategy for smoking cessation in mid-life and older adults. *Addictive Behaviors*, *39*, 885–888.

Wilson, K. M. (2013). Integrating procedural care with addiction support: An example from a PICC nurse. *Medsurg Nursing*, *22*, 128–135.

Zhuang, S., An, S., & Zhao, Y. (2013). Effect of cognitive behavioral interventions on the quality of life in Chinese heroin-dependent individuals in detoxification: A randomized controlled trial. *Journal of Clinical Nursing*, *23*, 1239–1248.

Ineffective community Coping *Roberta Dobrzanski, MSN, RN*

NANDA-I

Definition

A pattern of community activities for adaptation and problem solving that is unsatisfactory for meeting the demands or needs of the community

Defining Characteristics

Community does not meet expectations of its members; deficient community participation; elevated community illness rate; excessive community conflict; excessive stress; high incidence of community problems (e.g., homicides, vandalism, terrorism, robbery, abuse, unemployment, poverty, militancy, mental illness); perceived community powerlessness; perceived community vulnerability

Related Factors

Exposure to disaster (natural or man-made); history of disaster (e.g., natural, man-made); inadequate resources for problem solving; insufficient community resources (e.g., respite, recreation, social support); nonexistent community systems

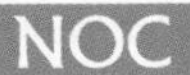 (Nursing Outcomes Classification)

C

Suggested NOC Outcomes

Community Competence; Community Health Status; Community Violence Level

Example NOC Outcome with Indicators

Community Competence as evidenced by the following indicators: Participation rates in community activities/Consideration of common and competing interests among groups when solving community problems/Representation of all segments of the community in problem solving/Effective use of conflict management strategies. (Rate the outcome and indicators of **Community Competence:** 1 = poor, 2 = fair, 3 = good, 4 = very good, 5 = excellent [see Section I].)

Community Outcomes

A Broad Range of Community Members Will (Specify Time Frame)

- Participate in community actions to improve power resources
- Develop improved communication among community members
- Participate in problem solving
- Demonstrate cohesiveness in problem solving
- Develop new strategies for problem solving
- Express power to deal with change and manage problems

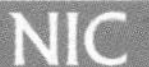 (Nursing Interventions Classification)

Suggested NIC Interventions

Community Health Development; Program Development

Example NIC Activities—Community Health Development

Enhance community support networks; Identify and develop potential community leaders; Unify community members behind a common mission; Ensure that community members maintain control over decision-making

Nursing Interventions and *Rationales*

NOTE: The diagnosis of Ineffective **Coping** does not apply and should not be used when stress is being imposed by external sources or circumstance. If the community is a victim of circumstances, using the nursing diagnosis Ineffective **Coping** is equivalent to blaming the victim. See the care plan for Readiness for enhanced community **Coping.**

▲ Establish a collaborative partnership with the community (see the care plan for Readiness for enhanced community **Coping** for additional references). EBN: *Community activation to promote health encompasses organized efforts in increased community awareness, establishes a general consensus about health problems, coordinates partnerships to change environmentally based health issues, allocates resources across organizations, and promotes citizen participation in positive health outcomes (Pender et al, 2011).*

• Assist the community with team building. EBN: *Health partnerships across various community settings help optimize the health of the community, promote continuity of care, and synergistically use resources to achieve optimal efficiency and enhanced effectiveness (Pender et al, 2011).*

• Participate with community members in the identification of stressors and assessment of distress; for example, observe and participate in faith-based organizations that want to improve community stress management. EBN: *Health programs in faith-based organizations are increasingly forming partnerships with nursing for health promotion programs and make a significant difference in health outcomes (Anderson & McFarlane, 2011).*

▲ Identify the health services and information resources that are currently available in the community. EBN: *Gynecological cancer survivors in Queensland were studied to identify awareness of, utilization of, and factors associated with use of community support services. Seventy-two percent were aware of the primary cancer support organization, Cancer Council Queensland; 74% were aware of booklets; 66% were aware of helplines; 56% were aware of support groups, and 50% were aware of Internet resources. Less than half were aware of other services (Beesley et al, 2010).*

C

- ▲ Consult with community mediation services, for example, the National Association of Community Mediation. EB: *Community mediation services effectively resolve conflicts and encourage stakeholders to exert direct and indirect pressure within the community (Handley & Howell-Moroney, 2010).*
- • Work with community members to increase awareness of ineffective coping behaviors (e.g., conflicts that prevent community members from working together, anger and hate that paralyze the community, health risk behaviors of adolescents). EBN: *Problem solving is essential for effective coping. Community members in partnership with health care providers can modify behaviors that interfere with problem solving (Anderson & McFarlane, 2011).*
- • Provide support to the community and help community members identify and mobilize additional supports. EBN: *Often people need help mobilizing supports that are available (Pender et al, 2011).*
- • Advocate for the community in multiple arenas (e.g., television, newspapers, and governmental agencies). EBN: *Advocacy is a specific form of caring that enhances power resources for community coping (Anderson & McFarlane, 2011).*
- • Write grant proposals to help community members obtain funds for programs that reduce stress or improve coping. EBN: *The programs that are necessary may be expensive, and often funds may not be available without the assistance of public or privately funded grants (Anderson & McFarlane, 2011).*
- • Work with members of the community to identify and develop coping strategies that promote a sense of power (e.g., obtaining sources for funding, collaborating with other communities). EBN: *A first step in power enhancement is for the community to identify and develop its own coping strategies (Anderson & McFarlane, 2011).*
- • Protect children from exposure to community conflicts. EB: *McKelvey et al (2011) examined the extent to which community violence impacts 18-year-old adolescents' psychosocial outcomes and found that the effects of community violence differ based on gender and family conflict in the home during childhood, influencing adolescent depression, anxiety, risk taking, and antisocial behavior.*

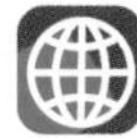

Multicultural

- • Acknowledge the stressors unique to racial/ethnic communities. EBN: *Understanding ethnic interpretations and cultural determinants that contribute to clients' stress assists the nurse in promoting health within a community (Anderson & McFarlane, 2011).*
- • Identify community strengths with community members. EB: *Latino men from three urban housing communities in the southeastern United States identified Latino community strengths and general community strengths as factors that promote health and prevent risk (Rhodes et al, 2009).*
- • Work with members of the community to prioritize and target health goals specific to the community. EB: *Such prioritization and targeting will increase feelings of control over and sense of ownership of programs (Anderson & McFarlane, 2011; Chinn, 2012).*
- • Establish and sustain partnerships with key individuals within communities when developing and implementing programs. EB: *Health partnerships between collaborating parties are a crucial strategy to optimize the health of a community (Pender et al, 2011).*
- • Use mentoring strategies for community members. EB: *In a study of child vaccination in Haiti, it was found that mother's use of traditional healer services was negatively associated with vaccination of their children, underscoring the potential of enlisting the support of traditional healers in promoting child health by mentoring and educating traditional healers in supporting vaccination efforts (Muula et al, 2009).*
- • Use community church settings as a forum for advocacy, teaching, and program implementation. EBN: *Participant and pastor feedback supported the feasibility of ongoing faith-based screening and education programs as one way to reduce risk factors for diabetes, cardiovascular disease, and stroke in Southern rural African Americans (Frank & Grubbs, 2008).*

Community Teaching

- • Teach strategies for stress management.
- • Explain the relationship between enhancing power resources and coping.

REFERENCES

Anderson, E. T., & McFarlane, J. (2011). *Community as partner: theory and practice in nursing* (6th ed.). Philadelphia: Lippincott Williams & Wilkins.

Beesley, V. L., et al. (2010). Gynecological cancer survivors and community support services: referral, awareness, utilization and satisfaction. *Psycho-Oncology*, *19*(1), 54–61.

Chinn, P. L. (2012). *New directions for building community* (8th ed.). Boston: Jones and Bartlett.
Frank, D., & Grubbs, L. (2008). A faith-based screening/education program for diabetes, CVD, and stroke in rural African Americans. *The ABNF Journal: Official Journal of the Association of Black Nursing Faculty in Higher Education, Inc*, *19*(3), 96–101.
Handley, D. M., & Howell-Moroney, M. (2010). Ordering stakeholder relationships and citizen participation: evidence from the community development block grant program. *Public Administration Review*, *70*, 601–609.
McKelvey, L. M., et al. (2011). Growing up in violent communities: do family conflict and gender moderate impacts on adolescents' psychosocial development? *Journal of Abnormal Child Psychology*, *39*, 95–107.
Muula, A. S., et al. (2009). Association between maternal use of traditional healer services and child vaccination coverage in Pont-Sonde, Haiti. *International Journal for Equity in Health*, *8*, 1.
Pender, N. J., Murdaugh, C. L., & Parsons, M. A. (2011). *Health promotion in nursing practice* (6th ed.). Upper Saddle River, NJ: Prentice Hall.
Rhodes, S. D., et al. (2009). Sexual and alcohol risk behaviours of immigrant Latino men in the southeastern USA. *Culture, Health and Sexuality*, *11*(1), 17–34.

C

Ineffective Coping

Arlene T. Farren, RN, PhD, AOCN, CTN-A

NANDA-I

Definition

Inability to form a valid appraisal of the stressors, inadequate choices of practiced responses, and/or inability to use available resources

Defining Characteristics

Alteration in concentration; alteration in sleep pattern; change in communication pattern; destructive behavior toward others; destructive behavior toward self; difficulty organizing information; fatigue; frequent illness; inability to ask for help; inability to attend to information; inability to deal with a situation; inability to meet basic needs; inability to meet role expectation; ineffective coping strategies; insufficient access of social support; insufficient goal directed behavior; insufficient problem resolution; insufficient problem-solving skills; risk taking behavior; substance abuse

Related Factors

Gender differences in coping strategies; high degree of threat; inability to conserve adaptive energies; inaccurate threat appraisal; Inadequate confidence in ability to deal with a situation; inadequate opportunity to prepare for stressor; inadequate resources; ineffective tension release strategies; insufficient sense of control; insufficient social support; maturational crisis; situational crisis; uncertainty

NOC (Nursing Outcomes Classification)

Suggested NOC Outcomes

Coping; Decision-Making; Impulse Self-Control; Information Processing

Example NOC Outcome with Indicators

Coping as evidenced by the following indicators: Identifies effective and ineffective coping patterns/Modifies lifestyle to reduce stress. (Rate the outcome and indicators of **Coping:** 1 = never demonstrated, 2 = rarely demonstrated, 3 = sometimes demonstrated, 4 = often demonstrated, 5 = consistently demonstrated [see Section I].)

Client Outcomes

Client Will (Specify Time Frame)

- Use effective coping strategies
- Use behaviors to decrease stress
- Remain free of destructive behavior toward self or others
- Report decrease in physical symptoms of stress
- Report increase in psychological comfort
- Seek help from a health care professional as appropriate

C

NIC (Nursing Interventions Classification)

Suggested NIC Interventions

Coping Enhancement; Decision-Making Support

Example NIC Activities—Coping Enhancement

Assist the client in developing an objective appraisal of the event; Explore with the client previous methods of dealing with life problems

Nursing Interventions and *Rationales*

- Observe for contributing factors of ineffective coping such as poor self-concept, grief, lack of problem-solving skills, lack of support, recent change in life situation, maturational or situational crises. EBN: *Factors predicting caregiver burden among caregivers of individuals with dementia (N = 302) included the number of hours of caregiving, lack of support, co-residence, spousal status, and use of coping strategies (Kim et al, 2012).* EB: *In a large sample (N =758) of people living with HIV, the top three life stressors identified were taking on too many things at once, not having enough money for what is needed, and having a scary experience in childhood that one continues to think about (Gibson et al, 2011).*
- Use verbal and nonverbal therapeutic communication approaches including empathy, active listening, and confrontation to encourage the client and family to express emotions such as sadness, guilt, and anger (within appropriate limits); verbalize fears and concerns; and set goals. EBN: *Active, empathic listening and values clarifying communication techniques are strategies used by neonatal intensive care nurses (N = 25) engaged in a pilot study of a guided family-centered care intervention to support parents' coping strategies (Weis et al, 2014). Likewise, positive health care provider communication techniques were also found to be important for coping with all the phases of the cancer experience (Molina et al, 2014).* Collaborate with the client to identify strengths such as the ability to relate the facts and to recognize the source of stressors. EBN: *Northouse (2012) made recommendations such as identifying strengths in clients and family caregivers to help them cope with cancer based on a program of research.* EB: *Ruddick (2011) describes solution-focused communications as enhancing the identification of strengths and resources for coping.*
- Encourage the client to describe previous stressors and the coping mechanisms used. EB: *Researchers found that fatigue in mothers of children with an autism spectrum disorder due to problematic child behaviors was associated with ineffective coping and maternal stress (Seymour et al, 2013).* Be supportive of coping behaviors; allow the client time to relax. CEBN: *Solari-Twadell (2010) found a selection of nursing interventions used by parish nurses (N = 1161) to provide coping assistance to women including presence, touch, emotional support, and coping enhancement.*
- Provide opportunities for the client to discuss the meaning the situation might have for the client. EBN: *Qualitative researchers in the Netherlands found that adults recently admitted to a nursing home described the meaning of the situation in conflicting ways; some individuals expressed a sense of meaninglessness due to feelings of boredom, loneliness, or lack of hope for improvement, and others expressed a sense of meaning in their lives and their contributions to society, which contributed to their coping capacity and sense of dignity (Oosterveld-Vlug et al, 2014).* EBN: *Elmir (2014) interviewed 21 women who experienced postpartum hemorrhage and emergency hysterectomy and found that all the women found meaning in life that helped them cope with the situation and get on with their lives in the aftermath of the emergency situation.*
- Assist the client to set realistic goals and identify personal skills and knowledge. EB: *In a qualitative study, adults (N = 9) who were able to lose 10% of body weight and maintain the loss for a minimum of 12 months differed from those (N = 9) who were not successful at weight maintenance on factors such as realistic goal setting, self-monitoring, and other effective coping skills (McKee et al, 2013).*
- Provide information regarding care before care is given. EBN: *Family members of intensive care unit clients at risk for dying identified nursing actions such as providing information helped family members to cope (Adams et al, 2014).*
- Discuss changes with the client before making them. EBN/QSEN: *Knobf (2013) discusses the ways being prepared is essential to persons with cancer throughout the survivorship trajectory; it helps to deal with uncertainty, develop awareness of the illness and treatments, and provide client-centered, safe, quality cancer nursing care.* EBN: *When dealing with adults with cancer, the authors assert the importance of informing clients of treatment-related symptoms and toxicities to help clients prepare for the treatment course;*

furthermore, nurses should discuss additional coping strategies to help with managing treatment-related problems (Boucher et al, 2011).

- Provide mental and physical activities within the client's ability (e.g., reading, television, radio, crafts, outings, movies, dinners out, social gatherings, exercise, sports, games). EB/CEBN: *In a pilot study of a nurse-based, in-home transitional care intervention for seriously mentally ill persons, researchers found that one of the factors of importance to community transition was involvement in daily activities (Rose et al, 2007).*
- Discuss the client's and family's power to change a situation or the need to accept a situation. CEBN: *Researchers conducted a controlled trial of a nursing intervention to facilitate older adults' (N = 89) access to community resources to assist them to remain at home. Researchers found the older adults accepted the intervention and had improved health empowerment, purposeful participation in goal attainment, and well-being (Shearer et al, 2010).* EBN: *Following a review of the literature, Knobf (2013) concluded that meeting clients/families' informational and support needs contribute to client empowerment and overall coping ability.*
- Offer instruction regarding alternative coping strategies. EBN: *A Recovery Education program used in inpatient behavioral health units include strategies of cognitive behavioral therapy, mindfulness mediation, and other coping strategies for persons with mental illness (Knutson et al, 2013).* EBN: *A variation of the COPE intervention, a theory-based intervention, was piloted for parents of children with cancer (COPE-PCC), with the small sample (N = 15) suggesting the intervention, which included education, information, and behavior-skill development, facilitated coping for both children and mothers (Peek & Melnyk, 2014).*
- Encourage use of spiritual resources as desired. EBN: *Researchers found that African American women living with HIV use spiritual practices to cope with HIV and ensuing depression, and recommend nurses include spiritual practices in assessments and plans of care (Peltzer et al, 2015).* EB: *In a small randomized control trial of a psychoeducational intervention (45 minute sessions once per week for 3 weeks) to promote problem-solving strategies in college-aged students (N = 25) who were found to be highly neurotic, the researchers found the participants had significant improvement in problem solving at 11 weeks after the intervention (Stillmaker & Kasser, 2013).*
- Encourage use of social support resources. EB: *Researchers found that in genderqueer individuals (N = 64) higher reported social support and the use of more facilitative coping was associated with less anxiety (Budge et al, 2014).*
- ▲ Refer for additional or more intensive therapies as needed. CEBN/EBN/QSEN: *More complex interventions are available to assist with coping, for example, a nurse-delivered intervention for depression in clients with cancer and for persons with mental health issues (Forchuk, 2009; Knutson et al, 2013).*

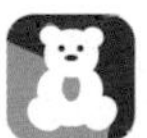

Pediatric

- Monitor the client's risk of harming self or others and intervene appropriately. QSEN: *See care plan for risk for* ***Suicide****.* CEB/QSEN: *Adolescents may use self-harming behaviors as a means of communication or of coping (Murray & Wright, 2006).* EB: *A research team in Italy studied differences in coping strategies of adolescents aged 12 to 20 (N = 1713) and found that adolescents who were in the self-harm group used less help-seeking behaviors and support and used more avoidance coping strategies than adolescents who do not self-harm (Guerreriro et al, 2015).*
- Monitor adolescents for exposure to community violence. EB: *In one study of Latino adolescents (N = 223) in ninth grade, researchers found negative psychological effects of exposure to community violence (Epstein-Ngo et al, 2013).*
- Support adolescent and children's individual coping styles. EBN: *Qualitative researchers found that children (N = 10, ages 7 to 12 years) hospitalized and receiving chemotherapy used coping strategies such as understanding the need for treatment, seeking relief from pain and treatment side effects, seeking pleasure in nourishment, engaging in entertaining/fun activities, staying hopeful for a cure, and support (Sposito et al, 2015).* CEBN: *In a study of coping of 4- to 6-year-olds who were hospitalized, researchers concluded that it was essential to support children's individual coping strategies with information, guidance, and participation in decisions (Salmela et al, 2010).*
- Encourage social support, religion-based coping, and moderate aerobic exercise as appropriate. EB: *Epstein-Ngo and colleagues (2013) identified the use of religion-based coping and seeking social support as the more frequent coping responses in Latino adolescents who were exposed to community violence.* CEB: *Exercise was found to decrease the likelihood of depressive feelings when used as a positive coping strategy for school-aged children with angry feelings (Goodwin, 2006).*

C

Geriatric

- ▲ Assess and report possible physiological alterations (e.g., sepsis, hypoglycemia, hypotension, infection, changes in temperature, fluid and electrolyte imbalances, and use of medications with known cognitive and psychotropic side effects). EBN/QSEN: *Findings from a study on psychotropic medication use and physical and psychological outcomes in older adults in long-term care (N = 419) indicated that older adults receiving psychotropic medications have poorer physical and psychological outcomes and are less likely to engage in functional activities and experience poorer quality of life (Galik & Resnick, 2013).* CEB: *A reversible pathophysiological process may be causing symptoms (Rocchiccioli & Sanford, 2009).*
- • Screen for elder neglect or other forms of elder mistreatment. QSEN/EBN: *The majority of participants in a study of 76 older adults indicated they would not disclose elder abuse to a doctor or nurse; the researchers concluded that screening of community-dwelling older adults for elder abuse is warranted (Ziminski Pickering & Rempusheski, 2014).*
- • Encourage the client to make choices (as appropriate) and participate in planning care and scheduled activities. EBN: *In a small study (N = 20) of older adults with symptomatic myeloma, the majority of participants reported a preference for participation in treatment decisions; the researchers recommended oncology nurses and other health care providers respect the autonomy of clients and their role choices in treatment decision making (Tariman et al, 2014).*
- • Target selected coping mechanisms for older persons based on client features, use, and preferences. EBN: *Older adults described coping processes that they perceived as part of successful aging; researchers found more evidence of gerotranscendence than spirituality and recommended interventions to enhance these factors to improve older adults' quality of life (Troutman-Jordan & Staples, 2014).* EB: *Researchers found that European American adults showed development to early old age toward coping mechanisms that were judged more adaptive; in late old age, the pattern was reversed, which suggests coping in late old age presents challenges (Diehl et al, 2014).*
- • Increase and mobilize support available to older persons by encouraging a variety of mechanisms involving family, friends, peers, and health care providers. CEBN: *Researchers conducted a controlled trial of a nursing intervention to facilitate older adults' (N = 89) access to community resources to assist them to remain at home. Researchers found the older adults accepted the intervention and had improved health empowerment, purposeful participation in goal attainment, and well-being (Shearer et al, 2010).*
- • Actively listen to complaints and concerns. EBN: *One of the most frequently used strategies by nurses in end-of-life care and communication was active and passive listening (Boyd et al, 2011).*
- • Engage the client in reminiscence. EBN: *An evidence-based reminiscence protocol was developed for use with older persons; it is a 12-session structured protocol that includes themes such as firsts, positive memories, and favorite holidays. The developer recommends nurses and other health care workers be trained in the protocol and use it in a variety of settings to enhance/improve quality of life for older adults (Stinson & Long, 2014).*

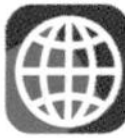

Multicultural

- • Assess for the influence of cultural beliefs, norms, and values on the client's perceptions of effective coping. EBN: *The representation of "strength" influences African American women's conceptualization of depression and coping strategies (Porter & Pacquiao, 2011).*
- • Assess the influence of fatalism and/or passivity on the client's coping behavior. EBN: *Deniz and Ayaz (2014) found that Turkish women (N = 322) with a newborn (aged 0 to 3 months) who had stress due to personal physical self-care, baby care, and social life were likely to adopt an emotion-oriented passive coping style characterized by acceptance of things as they are even though they wanted a different situation.* Assess the influence of cultural conflicts that may affect coping abilities. EBN: *In one ethnographic study, the researcher concluded that in the United States, there are differences between nurses' cultures and those of Syrian Muslims and suggested that improved cultural knowledge can lessen cultural pain and conflicts (Wehbe-Alamah, 2011).*
- • Assess for intergenerational family problems that can overwhelm coping abilities. EB: *Incarcerated (many for long-term sentences) older adults (N = 677) experienced trauma and stress related to lack of contact with and concerns about family; types of coping used were social, cognitive, and spiritual coping (Maschi et al, 2015).* Encourage spirituality as a source of support for coping. EB: *Researchers examined coping strategies in three groups: Caucasian, Korean, and African American older women (N = 343) and found all three groups used religious/spiritual coping (Lee & Mason, 2013).*

- Negotiate with the client with regard to the aspects of coping behavior that will need to be modified. QSEN/EB: *Adolescents in Italy who self-harm used more avoidance coping strategies; researchers recommend enhancing the use of help-seeking behaviors (Guerreriro et al, 2015).*
- Encourage moderate aerobic exercise or other forms of physical activity (as appropriate). EBN/EB: *Global researchers have found that exercise contributes to coping by people with a variety of conditions, such as women living with fibromyalgia in Spain (group-based exercise program) (Beltrán-Carrillo et al, 2013), adults in Germany trying to cope with chronic neck pain (90 minutes of Iyengar yoga once per week for 9 weeks) (Cramer et al, 2013), middle age Europeans as a coping tool for smoking cessation (primarily walking) (Treviño et al, 2014), and in the U.S. for young adults in college experiencing depression (general exercise) (Aselton, 2012).*

C

- Identify which family members the client can count on for support. EBN: *In a study of Irish mothers who experienced the loss of child, participants used formal and self-support in addition to family support which was received from partners, other family members, and friends (Jennings & Nicholl, 2014).*
- Support the inner resources that clients use for coping. EBN: *Self-transcendence is an inner resource for coping and well-being; both self-transcendence and spiritual well-being have been found to be high in a sample of Older Order Amish (N = 134) (Sharpnack et al, 2011).* EBN: *Researchers conducting a large study of Finnish and Swedish older adults' (N = 6119) inner strength and self-rated health found that inner strength was important in changing the relationship between disease and self-rated health; they concluded that interventions to enhance inner strength may support coping with disease in older adults (Viglund et al, 2014).*
- Use an empowerment framework to redefine coping strategies. EBN: *Yang and colleagues (2015) engaged women (N = 68) who were marriage migrants from Asian countries married to Taiwanese men in a health empowerment program (3 hours for eight sessions) using participatory action research; the project resulted in building of social networks, enhanced self-worth, resilience, and improved health literacy.* EB: *In a qualitative study of deaf people in the United States, researchers found that many participants self-identified as members of an ethno-linguistic minority. Both individual and community empowerment strategies were uncovered in the Internet weblog format, such as the value of using American Sign Language, use of humor, and advocating for social justice (Hamill & Stein, 2011).*

Home Care

- The interventions described previously may be adapted for home care use.

▲ **QSEN:** *Assess for suicidal tendencies. Refer for mental health care immediately if indicated.*

▲ **QSEN:** *Identify an emergency plan should the client become suicidal. Ineffective coping can occur in a crisis situation and can lead to suicidal ideation if the client sees no hope for a solution. A suicidal client is not safe in the home environment unless supported by professional help. Refer to the care plan for risk for* **Suicide.**

- Discuss preferred coping strategies of family caregivers. EBN: *One qualitative study of informal caregivers (N = 20) in a home palliative care program identified a variety of coping strategies; support of family and friends was the most cited (Epiphaniou et al, 2012).*
- Encourage the client to participate knowingly in their care. Refer to the care plan for **Powerlessness.** EBN: *Prenatal women (second and third trimester) (N = 21) who participated in a 6-week yoga program had enhanced feelings of power from participating in this 6-week program; participants shared journal entries that indicated through their involvement in the program they were feeling more relaxed, had more strength, and had a better mood (Reis & Alligood, 2014).*

▲ Refer the client and family to support groups. EB: *One mixed method study exploring the role of online and in-person support groups for breast cancer survivors (N = 73) found that 31% of respondents used the online support to assist with unmet needs, provide treatment and symptom management information, they joined online due to lack of access locally, or due to increased stress or uncertainty (Bender et al, 2013).*

▲ If monitoring medication use, contract with the client or solicit assistance from a responsible caregiver. CEB: *Older adults with arthritis identified taking medications as an assertive action coping strategy (Tak, 2006).*

▲ Institute case management for frail elderly clients to support continued independent living. EB: *In a study of one transitional care model for at-risk seniors that included follow-up phone calls and home care visits, hospital readmissions were significantly decreased (61%) and participant quality of life was improved; the researchers concluded that social support, health education, and follow-up are effective home care strategies for at-risk older adults (Watkins et al, 2012).*

Client/Family Teaching and Discharge Planning

- • Teach the client to problem solve. Have the client define the problem and cause, and list the advantages and disadvantages of the options. EB: *Teaching problem-solving skills to clients using a structured approach (1 hour per week for six sessions) has been found to be helpful to those experiencing depression (Erdley et al, 2014). Provide the seriously ill client and his or her family with needed information regarding the condition and treatment.* EBN: *In a qualitative study of former ICU clients, participants shared that information and education for themselves and their families was an important need (Deacon, 2012).*
- • Teach relaxation techniques. EBN: *Based on a review of the literature, the researchers found evidence of the positive effects of a variety of relaxation approaches for persons experiencing mental disorders (Shah et al, 2014).* EB: *A randomized control trial of persons with generalized anxiety disorder (N = 93) indicated that mindfulness meditation improved coping (Hoge et al, 2013).*
- • Work closely with the client to develop appropriate educational tools that address individualized needs. CEB: *Researchers developed a purpose-based information assessment (PIA) tool to evaluate how effective the information met the clients' individual needs; findings included estimates supporting the validity, reliability, and sensitivity of the PIA. Researchers concluded that the PIA can be used to identify strengths and limitations in meeting an individual's information needs (Feldman-Stewart et al, 2007).*
- ▲ Teach the client about available community resources (e.g., therapists, ministers, counselors, self-help groups). EBN: *Researchers concluded from a review of the literature regarding couples surviving prostate cancer that in addition to meeting educational needs, nurses must assess for potential concerns and make recommendations and referrals to assist couples with finding appropriate resources for coping with issues related to their relationship (Galbraith et al, 2011).*

REFERENCES

Adams, J. A., Anderson, R. A., Docherty, S. L., et al. (2014). Nursing strategies to support family members of ICU patients at high risk of dying. *Heart and Lung: The Journal of Critical Care, 43*, 406–415.

Aselton, P. (2012). Sources of stress and coping in American college students who have been diagnosed with depression. *Journal of Child and Adolescent Psyhciatric Nursing: Official Publication of the Association of Child and Adolescent Phyhciatric Nurses, Inc, 25*, 119–123.

Beltrán-Carrillo, V. J., Tortosa-Martínez, J., Jennings, G., et al. (2013). Contributions of a group-based exercise program for coping with fibromyalgia: A qualitative study giving voice to female patients. *Women and Health, 53*, 612–629.

Bender, J. L., Katz, J., Ferris, L. E., et al. (2013). What is the role of online support from the perspective of facilitators of face-to-face support groups? A multi-method study of use of breast cancer online communities. *Patient Education and Counseling, 93*, 472–479.

Boucher, J., Olson, L., & Piperdi, B. (2011). Preemptive management of dermatologic toxicities associated with epidermal growth factor receptor inhibitors. *Clinical Journal of Oncology Nursing, 15*, 501–508.

Boyd, D., et al. (2011). Nurses' perceptions and experiences with end-of-life communication and care. *Oncology Nursing Forum, 38*(3):E229–E239.

Budge, S. L., Rossman, H. K., & Howard, K. A. S. (2014). Coping and psychological distress among queergender individuals: the moderating effect of social support. *Journal of LGBT Issues in Counseling, 8*(1), 95–117.

Cramer, H., Lauche, R., Haller, H., et al. (2013). "I'm more in balance": A qualitative study of yoga for patients with chronic neck pain. *Journal of Alternative and Complementary Medicine (New York, N.Y.), 19*, 536–542.

Deacon, K. S. (2012). Re-building life after ICU: A qualitative study of the patients' perspective. *Intensive & Critical Care Nursing: the Official Journal of the British Association of Critical Care Nurses, 28*, 114–122.

Deniz, E., & Ayaz, S. (2014). Factors causing stress in women with babies 0-3 months old and their coping styles. *Journal of Psychiatric and Mental Health Nursing, 21*, 587–593.

Diehl, M., Chui, H., Hay, E. L., et al. (2014). Change in coping and defense mechanisms across adulthood: Longitudinal findings in a European American sample. *Developmental Psychology, 50*, 634–648.

Elmir, R. (2014). Finding meaning in life following emergency postpartum hysterectomy; What doesn't kill us makes us stronger. *Journal of Midwifery & Women's Health, 59*, 510–515.

Epiphaniou, E., Hamilton, D., Bridger, S., et al. (2012). Adjusting to the caregiving role: The importance of coping and support. *International Journal of Palliative Nursing, 18*, 541–545.

Epstein-Ngo, Q., Maurizi, L. K., Bregman, A., et al. (2013). In response to community violence: Coping strategies and involuntary stress responses among Latino adolescents. *Cultural Diversity and Ethnic Minority Psychology, 19*, 38–49.

Erdley, S. D., Gellis, Z. D., Bogner, H. A., et al. (2014). Problem-solving therapy to improve depression scores among older hemodialysis patients: A pilot randomized trial. *Clinical Nephroology, 82*, 26–33.

Feldman-Stewart, D., Brennestuhl, S., & Brundage, M. D. (2007). A purpose-based evaluation of information for patients: An approach to measuring effectiveness. *Patient Education and Counseling, 65*(3), 311–319.

Forchuk, C. (2009). A nurse-delivered intervention was effective for depression in patients with cancer. *Evidence-Based Nursing, 12*(1), 17.

Galbraith, M. E., Fink, R., & Wilkins, G. G. (2011). Couples surviving prostate cancer: challenges in their lives and relationships. *Seminars in Oncology Nursing, 27*, 300–308.

Galik, E., & Resnick, B. (2013). Psychotropic medication use and association with physical and psychosocial outcomes in nursing home residents. *Journal of Psychiatric and Mental Health Nursing, 20*, 244–252.

Gibson, K., et al. (2011). Mastery and coping moderate the negative effect of acute and chronic stressors on mental health-related quality of life in HIV. *AIDS Patient Care and Stds, 25*(6), 371–381.

Goodwin, R. D. (2006). Association between coping with anger and feelings of depression among youths. *American Journal of Public Health, 96*, 664–669.

Guerreriro, D. F., Figueira, M. L., Cruz, D., et al. (2015). Coping strategies of adolescents who self-harm. *Crisis, 36*(1), 31–37.

Hamill, A. C., & Stein, C. H. (2011). Culture and empowerment in the deaf community: an analysis of internet weblogs. *Journal of Community Applied Social Psychology, 21*, 388–406.

Hoge, E. A., Bui, E., Marques, L., et al. (2013). Randomized controlled trial of mindfulness meditation for generalized anxiety disorder: Effects on anxiety and stress reactivity. *The Journal of Clinical Psychiatry, 74*, 786–792.

Jennings, V., & Nicholl, H. (2014). Bereavement support used by mothers in Ireland following the death of their child from a life-limiting condition. *International Journal of Palliative Nursing, 20*(4), 173–178.

Kim, H., Chang, M., Rose, K., et al. (2012). Predictors of caregiver burden in caregivers of individuals with dementia. *Journal of Advanced Nursing, 68*, 846–855.

Knobf, M. T. (2013). Being prepared: Essential to self-care and quality of life for the person with cancer. *Clinical Journal of Oncology Nursing, 17*, 255–261.

Knutson, M. B., Newberry, S., & Schaper, A. (2013). Recovery education: A tool for psychiatric nurses. *Journal of Psychiatric and Mental Health Nursing, 20*, 874–881.

Lee, H. S., & Mason, D. (2013). Optimism and coping strategies among Caucasian, Korean, and African American older women. *Healthcare for Women International, 34*, 1084–1096.

Maschi, T., Viola, D., & Koskinen, L. (2015). Trauma, stress, and coping among older adults in prison: Towards a human rights and intergenerational family justice action agenda. *Traumatology*, Advanced online publication. <http://dx.doi.org/10.1037/trm0000021>.

McKee, H., Ntoumanis, N., & Smith, B. (2013). Weight maintenance: Self-regulatory factors underpinning success and failure. *Psychology & Health, 10*, 1207–1223.

Molina, Y., Yi, J. C., Martinez-Gutierrez, J., et al. (2014). Resilience among patients across the cancer continuum: Diverse perspectives. *Clinical Journal of Oncology Nursing, 18*, 93–101.

Murray, B. L., & Wright, K. (2006). Integration of a suicide risk assessment and intervention approach: The perspective of youth. *Journal of Psychiatric and Mental Health Nursing, 13*, 157–164.

Northouse, L. L. (2012). Helping patients and family caregivers cope with cancer. *Oncology Nursing Forum, 39*, 500–506.

Oosterveld-Vlug, M. G., Pasman, H. R. W., van Gennip, I. E., et al. (2014). Dignity and the factors that influence it according to nursing home residents: a qualitative interview study. *Journal of Advanced Nursing, 70*, 97–106.

Peek, G., & Melnyk, B. M. (2014). A coping intervention for mothers of children diagnosed with cancer: connecting theory and research. *Applied Nursing Research, 27*, 202–204.

Peltzer, J., Domian, E., & Teel, C. (2015). Living in the everydayness of HIV infection: Experiences of young African-American women. *Medsurg Nursing, 24*, 111–118.

Porter, S. N., & Pacquiao, D. F. (2011). Social and cultural construction of depression among African American women. *UPNAAI Nursing Journal, 7*(1), 13–15, 17–19.

Reis, P. J., & Alligood, M. R. (2014). Prenatal yoga in late pregnancy and optimism, power, and well-being. *Nursing Science Quarterly, 27*, 30–36.

Rocchiccioli, J. T., & Sanford, J. T. (2009). Revisiting geriatric failure to thrive: a complex and compelling clinical condition. *Journal of Gerontology Nursing, 35*(1), 18–24.

Rose, L. E., Gerson, L., & Carbo, C. (2007). Transitional care for seriously mentally ill persons: a pilot study. *Archives of Psychiatric Nursing, 21*, 297–308.

Ruddick, F. (2011). Coping with problems by focusing on solutions. *Mental Health Practice, 14*(8), 28–30.

Salmela, M., Salanterä, S., & Aronen, E. T. (2010). Coping with hospital related fears: experiences of pre-school-aged children. *Journal of Advanced Nursing, 66*, 1222–1231.

Seymour, M., Wood, C., Giallo, R., et al. (2013). Fatigue, stress and coping in mothers of children with an autism spectrum disorder. *Journal of Autism and Developmental Disorders, 43*, 1547–1554.

Shah, L. B., Klainin-Yobas, P., Torres, S., et al. (2014). Efficacy of psychoeducation and relaxation interventions on stress-related variables in people with mental disorders: A literature review. *Archives of Psychiatric Nursing, 28*, 94–101.

Sharpnack, P. A., Quinn-Griffin, M. T., Benders, A. M., et al. (2011). Self-transcendence and spiritual well-being in the Amish. *Journal of Holistic Nursing, 29*, 91–97.

Shearer, B. C., Fleury, J. D., & Belyea, M. (2010). Randomized control trial of the health empowerment intervention: feasibility and impact. *Nursing Research, 59*, 203–211.

Solari-Twadell, P. A. (2010). Providing coping assistance for women with behavioral interventions. *Journal of Obstetric Gynecologic and Neonatal Nursing: JOGNN/NAACOG, 39*, 205–211.

Sposito, A. M. P., Silva-Rodriguez, F. M., Sparapani, V. D., et al. (2015). Coping strategies used by hospitalized children with cancer undergoing chemotherapy. *Journal of Nursing Scholarship, 47*, 143–151.

Stillmaker, J., & Kasser, T. (2013). Instruction in problem-solving skills increases in hedonic balance of highly neurotic individuals. *Cognitive Therapy and Research, 37*, 380–382.

Stinson, C., & Long, E. M. (2014). Reminiscence: Improving quality of life for older adults. *Geriatric Nursing, 35*, 399–404.

Tak, S. H. (2006). An insider perspective of daily stress and coping in elders with arthritis. *Orthopedic Nursing, 25*(2), 27–32.

Tariman, J. D., Doorenbos, A., Schepp, K. G., et al. (2014). Older adults newly diagnosed with symptomatic myeloma and treatment decision making. *Oncology Nursing Forum, 41*, 411–419.

Treviño, L. A., Baker, L., McIntosh, S., et al. (2014). Physical activity as a coping strategy for smoking cessation in mid-life and older adults. *Addictive Behaviors, 39*, 885–888.

Troutman-Jordan, M., & Staples, J. (2014). Successful aging from the viewpoint of older adults. *Research and Theory for Nursing Practice, 28*, 87–104.

Viglund, K., Jonsén, E., Strandberg, G., et al. (2014). Inner strength as a mediator of the relationship between disease and self-rated health among old people. *Journal of Advanced Nursing, 70*, 144–152.

Watkins, L., Hall, C., & Kring, D. (2012). Hospital to home: A transition program for frail older adults. *Professional Case Management, 17*(3), 117–123.

Wehbe-Alamah, H. (2011). The use of Culture Care Theory with Syrian Muslims in the mid-western United States. *Online Journal of Cultural Competence Nursing Healthcare, 1*(3), 1–12.

Weis, J., Zoffmann, V., & Egerod, I. (2014). Improved nurse-parent communication in neonatal intensive care unit: Evaluation and adjustment of an implementation strategy. *Journal of Clinical Nursing, 23*, 3478–3489.

Yang, Y., Wang, H., Lee, F., et al. (2015). Health empowerment among immigrant women in transnational marriages in Taiwan. *Journal of Nursing Scholarhsip: an Official Publication of Sigma Theta Tau International Honor Society of Nursing/Sigma Theta Tau, 47*, 135–142.

Ziminski Pickering, C. E. Z., & Rempusheski, V. F. (2014). Examining barriers to self-reporting of elder physical abuse in community-dwelling older adults. *Geriatric Nursing, 35*, 120–125.

C

Disabled family Coping *Marsha McKenzie, MA Ed, BSN, RN*

NANDA-I

C

Definition

Behavior of primary person (family member, significant other, or close friend) that disables his or her capacities and/or the client's capacities to effectively address tasks essential to either person's adaptation to the health challenge

Defining Characteristics

Abandonment; aggression; agitation; carrying on usual routines without regard for client's needs; client's development of dependence; depression; desertion; disregarding client's needs; distortion of reality regarding client's health problem; family behaviors that are detrimental to well-being; hostility; impaired individualization; impaired restructuring of a meaningful life for self; intolerance; neglectful care of client in regard to basic human needs; neglectful care of client in regard to illness treatment; neglectful relationships with other family members; prolonged overconcern for client; psychosomaticism; rejection; taking on illness signs of client

Related Factors (r/t)

Arbitrary handling of family's resistance to treatment; dissonant coping styles for dealing with adaptive tasks by the significant person and client; dissonant coping styles among significant people; highly ambivalent family relationships; significant person with chronically unexpressed feelings (e.g., guilt, anxiety, hostility, despair)

NOC (Nursing Outcomes Classification)

Suggested NOC Outcomes

Caregiver Well-Being; Family Coping; Family Normalization; Neglect Recovery

Example NOC Outcome with Indicators

Family Normalization as evidenced by the following indicators: Adapts family routines to accommodate needs of affected member/Meets physical and psychosocial needs of family members/Provides activities appropriate to age and ability for affected family member/Uses community support groups. (Rate the outcome and indicators of **Family Normalization:** 1 = never demonstrated, 2 = rarely demonstrated, 3 = sometimes demonstrated, 4 = often demonstrated, 5 = consistently demonstrated [see Section I].)

Client Outcomes

Family/Significant Person Will (Specify Time Frame)

- Identify normal family routines that will need to be adapted
- Participate positively in the client's care within the limits of his or her abilities
- Identify responses that may be harmful
- Acknowledge and accept the need for assistance with circumstances
- Identify appropriate activities for affected family member

NIC (Nursing Interventions Classification)

Suggested NIC Interventions

Family Process Maintenance; Caregiver Support; Family Support; Family Therapy; Respite Care

Example NIC Activities—Family Process Maintenance

Determine typical family processes; Minimize family routine disruption by facilitating family routines and rituals such as private meals together or family discussions for communication and decision-making; Design schedules of home care activities that minimize disruption of family routine

Nursing Interventions and *Rationales*

- Families dealing with life-changing illnesses should be involved with the management process from the outset of treatment. Education and counseling should be provided early and repeatedly as learning and coping needs are reassessed. Caregivers should be invited to attend therapy sessions at an early stage. EBN: *These interventions are effective treatment for stroke victims and families to aid in coping (Gillespie & Campbell, 2011).*
- Assess coping strategies of both the patient and the spouse when managing women with breast cancer and men with prostate cancer. EB: *The findings of Kraemer et al (2011) suggest that active engagement by both the patient and the partner can have salutary effects on patient adjustment. A congruent coping strategy by patient and partner generally predicted better adaptation than did dissimilar coping.* EB: *A study conducted by Lambert et al (2012) concluded that coping with prostate cancer was more effective when both the patient and spouse were assisted with management of the illness.*

▲ Health care practitioners should be prepared to give specific information to families regarding the trajectory of a terminal illness. EB: *This study found that families felt the need to have more specific information and open communication regarding the anticipated course of a terminal illness, especially when young children are involved. Nurses and their colleagues have an important role to play in providing emotional support and in providing referrals to support services (Bugge et al, 2009).*

- Nurses caring for clients with terminal cancer should recognize the need to treat family caregivers as "pseudopatients." EBN: *The burden and stress of caring for a loved one throughout a terminal illness will most likely cause caregivers to need clinical care themselves if inadequate support is not provided during the stressful stages of cancer care (Northfield & Nebauer, 2010).*
- Provide psychosocial intervention for parents dealing with a child who is suffering from a serious illness. Allow time for parents to express feelings. Recognize and validate parent's feelings of anxiety, depression, and stress. EBN: *The diagnosis of childhood cancer has an impact on the entire family. Interventions focused on facilitating parental coping will have a positive impact on the entire family (Peek & Melnyk, 2010).*
- Assess social support of family members caring for survivors of traumatic brain injuries. Facilitate realistic expectations about caregiving. CEB: *Family members providing care following traumatic brain injuries often internalize the survivor's impairments as a sign that they are not masterful caregivers (Hanks et al, 2007).*
- Assist families to identify physical and mental health effects of caregiving. CEB: *Evidence over the last two decades shows that caregiving is a major public health issue. Caregiving has features of a chronic stress experience with high levels of unpredictability and uncontrollability leading to secondary stress in multiple life domains (Schulz & Sherwood, 2008).*
- Assist family members to find professional assistance for primary stressors such as financial issues, insurance coverage, or communicating with professionals.
- Handle dysfunctional family dynamics in an open, transparent, and professional way. Remain neutral when dealing with family conflicts and avoid involvement in long-term prior conflicts. EBN: *Maintaining a neutral, professional position in managing clients and families in an end-of-life care setting is essential (Holst et al, 2009).*
- Respect and promote the spiritual needs of the client and family. EBN: *Spiritual well-being is associated with better mental health and positive coping skills of family caregivers (Yeh & Bull, 2009).*

Pediatric

- Siblings of sick children should be considered at risk for emotional disturbances until a full assessment of the family and social support circumstances proves otherwise. CEB: *Siblings of sick children frequently suffer from anxiety and depression. Socioeconomic status and parental stress are strong predictors of sibling outcomes (O'Brien et al, 2009).*
- Assist parents and children suffering from chronic illness to develop accommodative coping skills (adapting to stressors rather than attempting to change the stressors). EB: *Compas et al (2012) found considerable evidence across chronic childhood illnesses and medical conditions that suggests that secondary control coping, or accommodative coping, is related to better adjustment in children and adolescents.*
- Assess educational level of parents of ill children and construct parent teaching to address educational attainment. EB: *Gage-Bouchard et al (2013) found programs that address educational gaps and teach caregivers planning and active coping skills may be beneficial for parents with lower educational attainment, particularly men.*

C

- Assess parents of children with chronic illness for depression. EB: *Grey et al (2011) note that parental coping with the stress of diabetes is likely to play an important role in child and family adjustment to the disease.*
- Recognize predictors of anger in adolescents: anxiety, depression, exposure to violence, and trait anger. EBN: *A meta-analytic study of predictors of anger in adolescents found these traits can forecast moderate to substantial effects in relation to anger (Mahon et al, 2010).*

Geriatric

- Assess family members who are caring for clients in long-term care facilities for compassion fatigue: symptoms include the inability to disengage from the suffering of the loved one, a growing feeling of hopelessness or despair, sadness or grief, and inattention to personal care or outside responsibilities. Encourage family members to attend to their own physical, emotional, and social needs. Develop relationships of trust with family caregivers, providing them with a sense of confidence in the level of care their loved ones will be receiving in their absence. Promote therapeutic relationships with family members who are assisting with care, allowing for sharing of concerns and emotions. EBN: *This study explored the effects of compassion fatigue in family members caring for loved ones in long-term care facilities, suggesting implications for nursing staff (Perry, 2010).*
- Be aware of age-related deterioration in coping skills. EB: *Diehl et al (2014) found that the defense mechanisms of doubt, displacement, and regression increased after the age of 65 years. Linear age-related decreases were found for the coping mechanism of ego regression and the defense mechanisms of isolation and rationalization.*

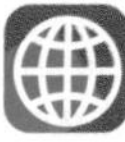

Multicultural

- Health care professionals working with African American adolescents who are coping with parental cancer should be sensitive to the potential for post-traumatic growth. EB: *A qualitative study of African American youths found they are able to attain post-traumatic growth as early as age 11, following the experience of parental cancer. Previous studies of white adolescents found post-traumatic growth only in older adolescents. This study suggests the possibility of a cultural difference in coping abilities found among African American adolescents (Ma et al, 2010).*

Home Care

The interventions described previously may be adapted for home care use.

- Assess for strain in family caregivers. EBN: *Using a tool such as the Modified Caregiver Strain Index gives the nurse information about a caregiver's abilities. It also could identify a need to evaluate the care recipient's living situation (Onega, 2008).* EB: *Williams et al (2010) conducted a study of a significant number of caregivers of Alzheimer's patients at home and found that video-based coping skills training and telephone coaching resulted in improved mental and physical health outcomes as well as reduced medical care costs among caregivers.*

Client/Family Teaching and Discharge Planning

- Involve the client and family in the planning of care as often as possible; mutual goal setting is considered part of "client safety." Major changes in the fifth annual issuance of National Patient Safety Goals include home care, assisted living, and disease-specific care programs in 2009. An expectation is to "encourage patients' active involvement in their own care as a patient safety strategy" (The Joint Commission, 2009).
- Recognize that family decision-makers may need additional psychosocial support services. EBN: *Family members directly responsible for health care decisions are most at risk for psychological stress (Hickman et al, 2010).*
- Educate family members regarding stress management techniques including massage and alternative therapies. EBN: *Education, support, psychotherapy, and respite interventions have demonstrated the greatest effect in reducing caregiver strain and burden. A significant decline was observed in the depression and anxiety scores of caregivers in the treatment group receiving massage therapy (Honea et al, 2008).*

REFERENCES

Bugge, K. E., Helseth, S., & Darbyshire, P. (2009). Parents' experiences of a family support program when a parent has incurable cancer. *Journal of Clinical Nursing, 18*, 3480–3488.

Compas, B. E., Jaser, S. S., Dunn, M. J., et al. (2012). Coping with Chronic Illness in Childhood and Adolescence. *Annual Review of Clinical Psychology, 8*, 455–480.

Diehl, M., Chui, H., Hay, E. L., et al. (2014). Change in coping and defense mechanisms across adulthood: Longitudinal findings in a european-american sample. *Developmental Psychology*, *50*(2), 634–648.

Gage-Bouchard, E. A., Devine, K. A., & Heckler, C. E. (2013). The relationship between socio-demographic characteristics, family environment, and caregiver coping in families of children with cancer. *Journal of Clinical Psychology in Medical Settings*, *20*(4), 478–487.

Gillespie, D., & Campbell, F. (2011). Effects of stroke on family carers and family relationships. *Nursing Standard*, *26*(2), 39–46.

Grey, M., Jaser, S. S., Whittemore, R., et al. (2011). Coping skills training for parents of children with type 1 diabetes: 12-month outcomes. *Nursing Research*, *60*(3), 173–181.

Hanks, R. A., Rapport, L. J., & Vangel, S. (2007). Caregiving appraisal after traumatic brain injury: the effects of functional status, coping style, social support and family functioning. *Neurorehabilitation*, *22*, 43–52.

Hickman, R. L., et al. (2010). Informational coping style and depressive symptoms in family decision makers. *American Journal of Critical Care*, *19*(5), 410–420.

Holst, L., et al. (2009). Dire deadlines: coping with dysfunctional family dynamics in an end-of-life care setting. *International Journal of Palliative Nursing*, *15*(1), 34–41.

Honea, N. J., et al. (2008). Putting evidence into practice: nursing assessment and interventions to reduce family caregiver strain and burden. *Clinical Journal of Oncology Nursing*, *12*(3), 507–516.

The Joint Commission. *National patient safety goals*. (2009). From: <www.jointcommission.org/NR/rdonlyres/DB3D6A66 DA79-412B-97E5-6FC400663127/0/OME_NPSG_Outline.pdf2009> Retrieved March 31, 2009.

Kraemer, L. M., Stanton, A. L., Meyerowitz, B. E., et al. (2011). A longitudinal examination of couples' coping strategies as predictors of adjustment to breast cancer. *Journal of Family Psychology*, *25*(6), 963–972.

Lambert, S. D., Girgis, A., Turner, J., et al. (2012). A pilot randomized controlled trial of the feasibility of a self-directed coping skills intervention for couples facing prostate cancer: Rationale and design. *Health and Quality of Life Outcomes*, *10*, 119.

Ma, K. K., Nino, A., & Jacobs, S. (2010). "It has been a good experience for me": growth experiences among African American youths coping with parental cancer. *Families, Systems & Health*, *28*(3), 274–289.

Mahon, N. E., et al. (2010). A meta-analytic study of predictors of anger in adolescents. *Nursing Research*, *59*(3), 178–184.

Northfield, S., & Nebauer, M. (2010). The caregiving journey for family members of relatives with cancer: how do they cope? *Clinical Journal of Oncology Nursing*, *14*(5), 567–577.

O'Brien, I., Duffy, A., & Nicholl, H. (2009). Impact of childhood chronic illnesses on siblings: a literature review. *British Journal of Nursing (Mark Allen Publishing)*, *18*(22), 1358, 1360–1365.

Onega, L. (2008). Helping those who help others: the modified caregiver strain index. *The American Journal of Nursing*, *108*(9), 62–69.

Peek, G., & Melnyk, B. M. (2010). Coping interventions for parents of children newly diagnosed with cancer: an evidence review with implications for clinical practice and future research. *Pediatric Nursing*, *36*(6), 306–313.

Perry, B. (2010). Family caregivers' compassion fatigue in long-term facilities. *Nursing Older People*, *22*(4), 26–31.

Schulz, R., & Sherwood, P. R. (2008). Physical and mental health effects of family caregiving. *The American Journal of Nursing*, *108*(Suppl. 9), 23–27.

Williams, V. P., Bishop-Fitzpatrick, L., Lane, J. D., et al. (2010). Video-Based Coping Skills (VCS) to Reduce Health Risk and Improve Psychological and Physical Well-being in Alzheimer's Disease Family Caregivers. *Psychosomatic Medicine*, *72*(9), 897–904.

Yeh, P., & Bull, M. (2009). Influences of spiritual well-being and coping on mental health of family caregivers for elders. *Research in Gerontological Nursing*, *2*(3), 173–181.

C

Readiness for enhanced Coping

Arlene T. Farren, RN, PhD, AOCN, CTN-A

NANDA-I

Definition

A pattern of cognitive and behavioral efforts to manage demands related to well-being, which can be strengthened

Defining Characteristics

Awareness of possible environmental change; expresses desire to enhance knowledge of stress management strategies; expresses desire to enhance management of stressors; expresses desire to enhance social support; expresses desire to enhance use of emotion oriented strategies; expresses desire to enhanced use of problem oriented strategies; expresses desire to enhance use of spiritual resource

NOC (Nursing Outcomes Classification)

Suggested NOC Outcomes

Coping; Personal Well-Being; Social Interaction Skills; Quality of life

Example NOC Outcome with Indicators

Coping as evidenced by the following indicators: Identifies effective coping patterns/Uses effective coping strategies. (Rate the outcome and indicators of **Coping:** 1 = never demonstrated, 2 = rarely demonstrated, 3 = sometimes demonstrated, 4 = often demonstrated, 5 = consistently demonstrated [see Section I].)

C

Client Outcomes

Client Will (Specify Time Frame)

- Acknowledge personal power
- State awareness of possible environmental changes that may contribute to decreased coping
- State that stressors are manageable
- Seek new effective coping strategies
- Seek social support for problems associated with coping
- Demonstrate ability to cope, using a broad range of coping strategies
- Use spiritual support of personal choice

NIC (Nursing Interventions Classification)

Suggested NIC Interventions

Coping Enhancement; Health Education; Decision-Making Support

Example NIC Activities—Coping Enhancement

Assist client in developing an objective appraisal of the event; Explore with client previous methods of dealing with life problems

Nursing Interventions and *Rationales*

- Assess and support positive psychological strengths, that is, hope, optimism, self-efficacy, resiliency, and social support. EBN: *Researchers found that army wives (N = 102) who experienced deployment separation from spouses, used support systems as an effective coping strategy (Blank et al, 2012).* EBN: *Based on a systematic review (N = 57 studies) covering the phases of the cancer experience, researchers found resilience and optimism are protective characteristics that contribute to coping and well-being (Molina et al, 2014).*
- Be physically and emotionally present for the client while using a variety of therapeutic communication techniques. EBN: *In a study exploring the experiences and needs of families (N = 20) in one intensive care unit, the researcher found that families need communication of information and prognosis in a manner that reflects caring, compassion, and attention to their supportive needs (Gutierrez, 2012).* EBN: *Adult primary care clients (N = 251) receiving early cancer care identified nurses' use of active listening, providing information, and being present for client-centered care as critical behaviors of oncology nurse navigators (Horner et al, 2013).*
- Empower the client to set realistic goals and to engage in problem solving. EBN: *In a randomized control trial testing the effectiveness of a 16 week Oncology Nurse Navigator (ONN) program compared to standard care to support clients with cancer (N = 251) during early treatment, researchers described the intervention, which included the use of using problem solving and motivational interviewing in the provision of psychosocial support (Horner et al, 2013).* EB: *The use of active problem solving contributed to coping effectiveness in a sample of 434 adults with rheumatoid arthritis (Englbrecht et al, 2012).*
- Encourage expression of positive thoughts and emotions. EBN: *In an intervention study of Turkish family caregivers of adults with mental illness, a family to family support intervention resulted in improvements in self-confidence and optimism in the experimental group (N = 34) following the intervention from baseline and at 3 months while there was no change in the control group (N = 34) at any measurement period (Bademli & Duman, 2014).*
- Encourage the client to use spiritual coping mechanisms such as faith and prayer. EBN: *In a qualitative study of the lived spiritual experiences of those receiving outpatient surgery, clients (N = 7) described their use of spiritual coping and that spiritual care at a time of vulnerability contributed to their well-being (Griffin, 2013).* EBN: *Use of spiritual coping such as praying has been associated with increased psychological well-being and decreased psychological distress in samples of Caucasian and African American early breast cancer survivors (Gaston-Johansson et al, 2013b; Schreiber, 2011).*
- Encourage the client to visit favorite natural settings or to have access to a window or pictures and sounds of nature. EBN: *Research demonstrates that a client's connection to nature can play a crucial role in his/her healing (Morrison, 2011). In a pilot study of an intervention using nature (garden walking) and art, researchers found markedly reduced self-reports of depression in a sample of older adults (McCaffrey et al, 2011).*

- Help the client with serious and chronic conditions such as depression, cancer diagnosis, and chemotherapy treatment to maintain social support networks or assist in building new ones. EBN: *Women with advanced breast cancer (N = 35) receiving high-dose chemotherapy were treated with a comprehensive coping strategy program that included the use of social support and other coping enhancement skills; the treatment group had improved quality of life at 1 year posttreatment (Gaston-Johansson et al, 2013a).*

C

▲ Refer women facing diagnostic and curative breast cancer surgery for psychosocial support. EBN: *In a pilot randomized control trial, a psychoeducation intervention showed promise for increasing overall quality of life and lowering psychological symptom distress in women breast cancer survivors (N = 25) (Park et al, 2012).*

▲ Refer for cognitive-behavioral therapy (CBT) to enhance coping skills. EBN: *Gaston-Johansson et al (2013a) from the Johns Hopkins School of Nursing conducted an intervention study that included cognitive restructuring as part of a comprehensive coping strategies program and found that women with breast cancer in the intervention group (N = 38) had improved well-being and quality of life compared with the control group (N = 35) at 1 year postintervention.* EB: *Another intervention, called the No-Panic CBT Self-Help program, demonstrated that CBT was effective for a wide range of anxiety disorders (Hawkins, 2011).* Refer to the care plans for Readiness for enhanced **Communication** and Readiness for enhanced **Spiritual** well-being.

Pediatric

- Encourage children and adolescents to engage in diversional activities and exercise to promote self-esteem, enhance coping, and prevent behavioral and other physical and psychosocial problems. EBN: *Researchers examining physical activity in children attending school (N = 133) found that enjoyment and self-efficacy were important influences in promoting physical activity in children (Ling et al, 2015).* EBN: *In a qualitative study of hospitalized children (N = 10) receiving chemotherapy for cancer, researchers found that engaging children in entertaining activities and having fun were among positive coping strategies (Spósito et al, 2015).*
- Encourage families of children with chronic illness to try additional coping strategies. EBN: *Families of children with autism (N = 38) participated in a descriptive study examining severity of behaviors and coping strategies; the researchers concluded that early diagnosis and intervention for the children and their families including community social support was needed (Hall, 2012).* EB: *Continued support for parents is necessary when children complete therapy for cancer (Wakefield et al, 2011).*

Geriatric

- Encourage active, meaning-based coping strategies for older adults with chronic illness. EBN: *In a qualitative study of older adults living with HIV (N = 40) residing in an urban environment, researchers uncovered four themes: accessing support, helping one's self as well as others, and tapping into their own spirituality that address successful coping for the participants (DeGrezia & Scrandis, 2015).*
- Consider the use of Web-based and technological resources for older adults in the community. EB: *The results of a mixed method systematic review of 112 articles indicated that approximately 24% of the articles addressed Web-based packages and assistive information technology that assists older adults and their family caregivers with health information, resources for performing tasks safely, engaging in self-management, increasing coping strategies, and other types of support; studies indicated client satisfaction as an outcome (Vedel et al, 2013).*
- Refer the older client to self-help support groups that address health, psychosocial, and/or social support. EB: *In a mixed age sample with more than 50% of the participants older than age 50 years (range 19 to 83 years), Internet-based self-help groups for persons who experienced cancer (N = 350) have been associated with perceived increased coping as well as improved satisfaction with perceived health status (Seckin, 2013).* EB: *Greysen et al (2013) studied social isolation in older veterans and recommended the use of in-person and Internet-based self-help support groups.*

▲ Refer the client with Alzheimer's disease who is terminally ill to hospice. EBN: *Hospice care is encouraged for those with Alzheimer's disease; hospice admission increases as the hours of care and caregiver burden increase (Karikari-Martin et al, 2012).*

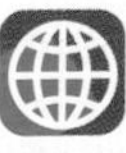

Multicultural

- Assess an individual's sociocultural backgrounds to identify factors that support coping. EBN: *In a qualitative study of native Hawaiian migrants to the mainland United States (N = 41), researchers identified*

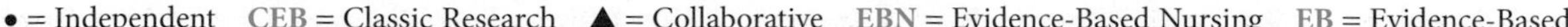

C

themes including nurturing relationships with family and friends that contribute to the participants' perceptions of well-being (Lassetter et al, 2012). EB: *In a study comparing coping strategies used by Caucasian, Korean, and African American older women (N = 343), researchers found there are differences in preferred coping strategies used by the three ethnic groups; the most common strategy used by all three groups was religious/spiritual belief systems (Lee & Mason, 2013).*

- Encourage spirituality as a source of support for coping. EBN: *Religion and spiritual practices were used by Buddhist and Muslim Thai women to cope with type 2 diabetes self-management (Lundberg & Thrakul, 2013).*
- Facilitate positive ethnocultural identity to enhance coping. EB: *Ojeda and Liang (2014) examined coping in Mexican American adolescent men (N = 93) and found that ethnocultural factors such as positive affirmation and view of one's ethnic identity, as well as culture bound characteristics such as caballerismo (positive Latino masculinity), was associated with more effective coping strategies, such as positive reframing, planning, and the use of humor.* EB: *In African American women who self-reported experience with trauma (N = 161), higher self-esteem and well-being were associated with more effective, active coping strategies (Stevens-Watkins et al, 2014).*
- Foster intergenerational support. EB: *A qualitative study explored the phenomena of racism, trauma, and coping in 19 adults of color and identified that intergenerational support contributed to coping in the participants (Lowe et al, 2012).* Refer to the care plan for Ineffective **Coping.**

Home Care

- The interventions described previously may be adapted for home care use.
- Engage both clients and their caregivers as a dyad. EBN: *In a review of a program of research about helping clients and family caregivers cope with cancer, Northouse (2012) relates lessons learned about caring for client and family caregiver dyad; recommendations include identifying strengths, three-way, open communication and alliances, and promoting active coping (vs. avoidant coping).*
- Provide an Internet-based health coach to encourage self-management for clients with chronic conditions such as depression, impaired mobility, and chronic pain. EBN: *Telephone health coaching, along with in-person individual educational sessions and group sessions, was included in a psychoeducation intervention randomized control trial pilot study in women survivors of breast cancer (N = 48); researchers concluded the intervention showed promise to increase overall quality of life and decrease psychological symptom distress (Park et al, 2012).*
- Refer the client to mutual health support groups. EBN: *A review of the literature regarding peer support suggests that peer support has the potential for positive outcomes in individuals in recovery (Repper & Carter, 2011).*
- Refer prostate cancer clients and their spouses to family programs that include family-based interventions of communication, hope, coping, uncertainty, and symptom management. EBN: *Researchers conducted a qualitative study of prostate cancer survivors and their spouses (N = 95) to determine the long-term quality of life effects of treatment at 36 months after treatment; the recommendations included offering counseling to couples following treatment to improve quality of life and assist with managing relationship intimacy (Harden et al, 2013).*

▲ Refer combat veterans and service members directly involved in combat as well as those providing support to combatants, including nurses for mental health services. EBN: *Veterans' transition to home life is deeply embedded in the context of relationships. Nurses can use Swanson's theory of caring to find guidance for ways to provide meaningful support to veterans (Wands, 2011).*

Client/Family Teaching and Discharge Planning

- Teach the client about available community resources (e.g., therapists, ministers, counselors, self-help groups, family education groups). EBN: *Navigators provide community resources on post-discharge follow-up to minimize gaps in care and promote independence in older adults; in this study, readmissions were decreased and participants reported improved quality of life (Watkins et al, 2012).*
- Teach caregivers using a variety of interventions that contribute to coping. EBN: *Researchers conducting a systematic review of 17 articles regarding couples-based intervention for coping with cancer recommended interventions that include skills training, psychoeducational interventions, and client/family support (Li & Loke, 2014).*
- Teach expressive writing, journaling, and education about emotions. EBN: *Journaling was one of the components of an intervention study aimed to promote civility among nursing students; there were*

improvements in coping in the areas of self-controlling, seeking social support, and positive reappraisal after the intervention (Jenkins et al, 2013). EB: *Researchers used a combination of expressive writing with elements of psychoeducation on emotion regulation with adolescents. It demonstrated that this may be an effective preventive tool to improve psychosocial adjustment by establishing functional emotion regulation strategies (Horn et al, 2011).*

REFERENCES

Refer to ineffective **Coping** for additional references.

Bademli, K., & Duman, Z. C. (2014). Effects of a family to family support program on mental health and coping strategies of caregivers of adults with mental illness: A randomized control study. *Archives of Psychiatric Nursing, 28*, 392–398.

Blank, C., Adams, L. A., Kittelson, B., et al. (2012). Coping behaviors used by Army wives during deployment separation and their perceived effectiveness. *Journal of the American Academy of Nurse Practitioners, 24*, 660–668.

DeGrezia, M. G., & Scrandis, D. (2015). Successful coping in urban community-dwelling older adults with HIV. *Journal of the Association of Nurses in Aids Care, 26*(12), 151–163.

Englbrecht, M., Gossec, L., DeLongis, A., et al. (2012). The impact of coping strategies on mental and physical well-being in patients with rheumatoid arthritis. *Seminars in Arthritis & Rheumatism, 41*, 545–555.

Gaston-Johansson, F., Fall-Dickson, J., Nanda, J. P., et al. (2013a). Long-term effect of the self-management comprehensive coping strategies program on quality of life in patients with breast cancer treated with high dose chemotherapy. *Psycho Oncology, 22*, 530–539.

Gaston-Johansson, F., Haisfield-Wolfe, M. E., Reddick, B., et al. (2013b). The relationships among coping strategies, religious coping, and spirituality in African American women with breast cancer receiving chemotherapy. *Oncology Nursing Forum, 40*, 120–131.

Greysen, S. R., Horwitz, L. I., Covinsky, K. E., et al. (2013). Does social isolation predict rehospitalization and mortality among HIV+ and uninfected older veterans? *Journal of the American Geriatric Society, 61*, 1456–1463.

Griffin, A. (2013). The lived spiritual experiences of patients transitioning through outpatient surgery. *AORN Journal, 97*, 243–254.

Gutierrez, K. M. (2012). Experiences and needs of families regarding prognostic communication in an intensive care unit: Supporting families at the end of life. *Critical Care Nursing Quarterly, 35*, 299–313.

Hall, H. R. (2012). Families of children with autism: Behaviors of children, community support, and coping. *Issues in Comprehensive Pediatric Nursing, 35*, 111–131.

Harden, J., Sanda, M. G., Wei, J. T., et al. (2013). Survivorship after prostate cancer treatment: Spouses quality of life at 36 months. *Oncology Nursing Forum, 40*, 567–573.

Hawkins, M. (2011). CBT-based self-help in treating anxiety. *Healthcare Counselling and Psychotherapy Journal*, 1124–1127.

Horn, A. B., Pössel, P., & Hautzinger, M. (2011). Promoting adaptive emotion regulation and coping in adolescence. *Journal of Health Psychology, 16*, 258–273.

Horner, K., Ludman, E. J., McCorkle, R., et al. (2013). An oncology nurse navigator program designed to eliminate gaps in early cancer care. *Clinical Journal of Oncology Nursing, 17*, 43–48.

Jenkins, S. D., Kerber, C. S., & Woith, W. M. (2013). An intervention to promote civility among nursing students. *Nursing Education Perspective, 34*, 95–100.

Karikari-Martin, P., McCann, J. J., Hebert, L. E., et al. (2012). Do community and caregiver factors influence hospice use at the end of life among older adults with Alzheimer disease? *Journal of Hospice and Palliative Nursing, 14*, 225–237.

Lassetter, J. H., Callister, L. C., & Ziyamoto, S. Z. (2012). Perceptions of health and well-being held by native Hawaiian migrants. *Journal of Transcultural Nursing, 23*, 5–13.

Lee, H. S., & Mason, D. (2013). Optimism and coping strategies among Caucasian, Korean, and African American older women. *Healthcare for Women International, 34*, 1084–1096.

Li, Q., & Loke, A. Y. (2014). A systematic review of spousal couple-based intervention studies for couples coping with cancer: direction for the development of interventions. *Psycho-Oncology, 23*, 731–739.

Ling, J., Robbins, L. B., McCarthy, V. L., et al. (2015). Psychosocial determinants of physical activity in children attending afterschool programs: A path analysis. *Nursing Research, 64*, 190–199.

Lowe, S. M., Okubo, Y., & Reilly, M. F. (2012). A qualitative inquiry into racism, trauma, and coping: Implications for supporting victims of racism. *Professional Psychology, Research and Practice, 43*, 190–198.

Lundberg, P. C., & Thrakul, S. (2013). Religion and self-management in Thai Buddhist and Muslim women with type 2 diabetes. *Journal of Clinical Nursing, 22*, 1907–1916.

McCaffrey, R., et al. (2011). Garden walking and art therapy for depression in older adults. *Research Gerontological Nursing, 4*(4), 237–242.

Molina, Y., Yi, J. C., Martinez-Gutierrez, J., et al. (2014). Resilience among patients across the cancer continuum. *Clinical Journal of Oncology Nursing, 18*, 93–101.

Morrison, M. (2011). Healing environments. *PN, 65*(2), 12–13.

Northouse, L. L. (2012). Helping patients and family caregivers cope with cancer. *Oncology Nursing Forum, 39*, 500–506.

Ojeda, L., & Liang, C. T. (2014). Ethnocultural and gendered determinants of coping in Mexican-American adolescent men. *Psychology of Men and Masculinity, 15*, 296–304.

Park, J. H., et al. (2012). Quality of life and symptom experience in breast cancer survivors after participating in a psychoeducational support program: a pilot study. *Cancer Nursing, 35*(1), e34–e41.

Repper, J., & Carter, T. (2011). A review of the literature on peer support in mental health services. *Journal of Mental Health, 20*, 392–411.

Schreiber, J. A. (2011). Image of God: effect of coping and psychospiritual outcomes in early breast cancer survivors. *Oncology Nursing Forum, 38*, 293–301.

Seckin, G. (2013). Satisfaction with health status among cyber patients: Testing a mediation model of electronic coping support. *Behavior and Information Technology, 32*, 91–101.

Sposito, A., Silva-Rodriques, F., Sparapani, V., et al. (2015). Coping strategies used by hospitalized children with cancer undergoing chemotherapy. *Journal of Nursing Scholarship, 47*, 143–151.

Stevens-Watkins, D., Sharma, S., Knighton, J. S., et al. (2014). Examining cultural correlates of active coping among African American female trauma survivors. *Psychological Trauma Theory, Research, Practice, and Policy, 6*, 328–336.

Vedel, I., Akhlaghpour, S., Vaghofi, I., et al. (2013). Health information technology in geriatrics and gerontology: A mixed systematic review. *Journal of American Medical Informatics Association, 20,* 1109–1119.

Wakefield, C. E., et al. (2011). Parental adjustment to the completion of their child's cancer treatment. *Pediatric Blood and Cancer, 56*(4), 524–531.

Wands, L. M. (2011). Caring for veterans return home from Middle Eastern wars. *Nursing Science Quarterly, 24,* 180–186.

Watkins, L., Hall, C., & Kring, D. (2012). Hospital to home: A transitional program for frail older adults. *Professional Case Management, 17,* 117–125.

Readiness for enhanced community Coping

Roberta Dobrzanski, MSN, RN

NANDA-I

Definition

A pattern of community activities for adaptation and problem solving for meeting the demands or needs of the community, which can be strengthened

Defining Characteristics

Expresses desire to enhance availability of community recreation programs; expresses desire to enhance availability of community relaxation programs; expresses desire to enhance communication among community members; expresses desire to enhance communication between aggregates and larger community; expresses desire to enhance community planning for predictable stressors; expresses desire to enhance community resources for managing stressors; expresses desire to enhance community responsibility for stress management; expresses desire to enhance problem solving for identified issue

NOC (Nursing Outcomes Classification)

Suggested NOC Outcomes

Community Competence; Community Health Status

Example NOC Outcome with Indicators

Community Health Status as evidenced by the following indicators: Prevalence of health promotion programs, health status of infants, children, adolescents, adults, elders, participation rates in community health programs. (Rate the outcome and indicators of **Community Health Status:** 1 = poor, 2 = fair, 3 = good, 4 = very good, 5 = excellent [see Section I].)

Community Outcomes

Community Will (Specify Time Frame)

- Develop enhanced coping strategies
- Maintain effective coping strategies for management of stress

NIC (Nursing Interventions Classification)

Suggested NIC Interventions

Environmental Management: Community; Health Policy Monitoring: Program Development

Example NIC Activities—Program Development

Assist the group or community in identifying significant health needs or problems; Identify alternative approaches to address the need(s) or problem(s)

Nursing Interventions and *Rationales*

Note: Interventions depend on the specific aspects of community coping that can be enhanced (e.g., planning for stress management, communication, development of community power, community perceptions of stress, community coping strategies). *Nursing interventions are conducted in collaboration with key members of the community, community/public health nurses, and members of other disciplines (Anderson & McFarlane, 2011).*

- Describe the roles of community/public health nurses in working with healthy communities. EBN: *Nurses at general and specialists' levels (bachelor's and master's degrees) have significant roles in helping communities achieve optimum health, including coping with stress (Chinn, 2012).*
- Help the community obtain funds for additional programs, or identify resources to assist in the funding of additional programs. EBN: *Healthy communities may need additional funding sources to strengthen community resources (Anderson & McFarlane, 2011; Chinn, 2012).*
- Encourage positive attitudes toward the community through the media and other sources. EB: *Negative attitudes or stigmas create additional stress and deficits in social support (Anderson & McFarlane, 2011; Chinn, 2012).*
- Help community members collaborate with one another for power enhancement and coping skills. EBN: *Community members may not have sufficient skills to collaborate for enhanced coping. Health care providers can promote effective collaboration skills (Anderson & McFarlane, 2011; Chinn, 2012).*
- Assist community members with cognitive skills and habits of mind for problem solving. Teach critical thinking and strategizing skills to help open lines of communication and facilitate participation. EBN: *The cognitive skills and habits of mind of critical thinking support problem-solving ability (Rubenfeld & Scheffer, 2010).*
- Demonstrate optimum use of power resources. EBN: *Optimum use of power resources and working for community empowerment supports coping (Chinn, 2012).*
- Reduce poverty whenever possible. EB: *Poverty is a major determinant of poor health, and people living on low income consistently have higher rates of morbidity and mortality due to chronic and acute illness. Therefore, primary health care providers should consider and address income as a distinct risk to health, and researchers should explore these issues with a broader group of primary care providers and people who live in poverty (Bloch, Rozmovits, & Giambrone, 2011).*

▲ Collaborate with community members to improve educational levels within the community. EB: *Patient safety, self-care behaviors, adherence to treatment plans, knowledge of one's medical condition, health care quality, and positive health outcomes are compromised by low health literacy. There is also compromised physical and mental health, as well as greater risk for hospitalization and increased mortality (Evangelista et al, 2010).*

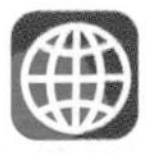

Multicultural

- Refer to care plan for Ineffective community **Coping.**

Client/Family Teaching and Discharge Planning

- Review coping skills, power for coping, and the use of power resources.

REFERENCES

Refer to ineffective community **Coping** for additional references.

Anderson, E., & McFarlane, J. (2011). *Community as partner: theory and practice in nursing* (6th ed.). Philadelphia: Wolters Kluwer/ Lippincott Willams & Wilkins.

Bloch, G., Rozmovits, L., & Giambrone, B. (2011). Barriers to primary care responsiveness to poverty as a risk factor for health. *BMC Family Practice, 12*, 62.

Chinn, P. L. (2012). *New directions for building community* (8th ed.). Boston: Jones and Bartlett.

Evangelista, L. S., et al. (2010). Health literacy and the patient with heart failure-implications for patient care and research: a consensus statement of the Heart Failure Society of America. *Journal of Cardiac Failure, 16*(1), 9–16.

Rubenfeld, M. G., & Scheffer, B. K. (2010). *Critical thinking tactics for nurses: achieving IOM competencies* (2nd ed.). Boston: Jones and Bartlett.

Readiness for enhanced family Coping

Keith A. Anderson, MSW, PhD

NANDA-I

Definition

A pattern of management of adaptive tasks by primary person (family member, significant other, or close friend) involved with the client's health change, which can be strengthened

Defining Characteristics

Expresses desire to acknowledge growth impact of crisis; expresses desire to choose experiences that optimize wellness; expresses desire to enhance connection with others who have experienced a similar situation; expresses desire to enhance enrichment of lifestyle; expresses desire to enhance health promotion

NOC (Nursing Outcomes Classification)

Suggested NOC Outcomes

Family Coping; Health-Seeking Behavior; Participation in Health Care Decisions

Example NOC Outcome with Indicators

Family Coping as evidenced by the following indicators: Confronts and manages family problems/Cares for needs of all family members. (Rate the outcome and indicators of **Family Coping:** 1 = never demonstrated, 2 = rarely demonstrated, 3 = sometimes demonstrated, 4 = often demonstrated, 5 = consistently demonstrated [see Section I].)

Client Outcomes

Client Will (Specify Time Frame)

State a plan indicating coping strengths, abilities, and resources as well as areas for growth and change; Perform tasks and engage resources needed for growth and change; Evaluate changes and continually reevaluate plan for continued growth

NIC Interventions (Nursing Interventions Classification)

Suggested NIC Interventions

Family Integration Promotion; Family Involvement Promotion; Family Support; Mutual Goal Setting

Example NIC Activities—Family Coping

Facilitate communication of concerns and feelings between clients and family or among family members; Provide resources that support and encourage adaptive family coping; Respect and support adaptive coping mechanisms used by family

Nursing Interventions and *Rationales*

▲ Assess the structure, resources, and coping abilities of families and use these assessments in selecting interventions and formulating care plans. EB/EBN: *It is critical to understand the resiliency and coping capabilities of families; the use of established assessment instruments (e.g., Family Assessment Device) can provide insight into family dynamics and the coping styles and resources of family systems (Mansfield et al, 2014; Knapp et al, 2013).*

▲ Acknowledge, assess, and support the spiritual needs and resources of families and clients. EBN: *Spirituality has been found to be an important, yet often overlooked, coping resource for families and clients during illness and recovery (O'Brien, 2014).*

▲ Establish rapport with families and empower their decision-making through effective, accurate, and empathic communication. EBN: *Effective engagement and communication between health care providers and clients' families can help establish rapport, provide timely and desired information to families, and empower families in their caregiving activities and decision-making capacities (Wittenberg-Lyles et al, 2012; Curtis et al, 2013).*

▲ Provide family members with educational and skill-building interventions to alleviate caregiving stress and to facilitate adherence to prescribed plans of care. EBN: *The provision of psychoeducational and supportive interventions may enable family members to gain a sense of control in the caregiving role and to become more comfortable in providing care and making informed decisions (Northouse et al, 2013; Ostlund & Persson, 2014).*

▲ Develop, provide, and encourage family members to use counseling services and interventions. EB/EBN: *Family-centered counseling interventions have been shown to be effective, particularly in situations regarding serious illness and difficult family decisions (Cheng et al, 2014; Hopkinson et al, 2012).*

▲ Identify and refer to support programs that discuss experiences and challenges similar to those faced by the family (e.g., cancer support groups). EB: *While there is wide diversity in the format of support programs, couple and family support approaches can be beneficial and enhance coping (Chambers et al, 2011; Shields et al, 2012).*

▲ Incorporate the use of emerging technologies to increase the reach of interventions to support family coping. EB/EBN: *Emerging computer and Internet-based supportive and educational interventions may hold promise in enhancing family members' well-being and informational needs (Hu et al, 2014; Northouse et al, 2014).*

▲ Refer to Compromised family **Coping** for additional interventions.

Pediatric

▲ Identify and assess the management styles of families and facilitate the use of more effective ways of coping with childhood illness. EB: *Understanding the dominant characteristics of each family's coping styles and resources and helping them to use more effective management styles can result in better family functioning and treatment outcomes (Barrera et al, 2014).*

▲ Provide educational and supportive interventions for families caring for children with illness and disability. EB/EBN: *Providing information, training parents in care management, and offering supportive programs can reduce stress levels in parents and lead to better outcomes for children (Marsac et al, 2012; Tomlinson et al, 2012).*

Geriatric

▲ Encourage family caregivers to participate in counseling and support groups. EB/EBN: *While a wide variety of programs exist, certain counseling and support group programs have been found to be effective in increasing family resourcefulness and lowering caregiver burden, anxiety, depression, and family conflict (Gonzalez et al, 2014; Nichols et al, 2011).*

▲ Provide educational and therapeutic interventions to family caregivers that focus on knowledge and skill building. EB/EBN: *Psychoeducational interventions that are accessible and tailored to individual needs can be highly valued and useful to family caregivers (Boots et al, 2014; Li et al, 2014).*

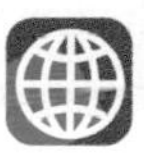

Multicultural

▲ Acknowledge and understand the importance of cultural influences in families and ensure that assessments and assessment tools account for such cultural differences. EB/EBN: *Family coping tends to vary across cultures and may impact the fit, reliability, and validity of existing family functioning and coping assessment tools (Higginbottom et al, 2011; Kuo, 2011).*

▲ Understand and incorporate cultural differences into interventions to enhance the impact of family interventions. EBN: *Tailoring interventions to the customs, beliefs, preferences, and strengths of specific groups may increase effectiveness (Davey et al, 2013; Gray et al, 2014; Dayer-Berenson, 2014).*

REFERENCES

Barrera, M., Hancock, K., Rokeach, A., et al. (2014). Does the use of the revised Psychosocial Assessment Tool (PATrev) result in improved quality of life and psychosocial risk in Canadian families with a child newly diagnosed with cancer? *Psycho-Oncology*, *23*, 165–172.

Boots, L., de Vugt, M., van Knippenberg, R., et al. (2014). A systematic review of internet-based supportive interventions for caregivers of patients with dementia. *International Journal of Geriatric Psychiatry*, *29*, 331–344.

Chambers, S. K., Pinnock, C., Lepore, S. J., et al. (2011). A systematic review of psychosocial interventions for men with prostate cancer and their partners. *Patient Education and Counseling*, *85*, e75–e88.

Cheng, H. Y., Chair, S. Y., & Chau, J. P. (2014). The effectiveness of psychosocial interventions for stroke family caregivers and stroke survivors: A systematic review and meta-analysis. *Patient Education and Counseling*, *95*, 30–44.

Curtis, J. R., Back, A. L., Ford, D. W., et al. (2013). Effect of communication skills training for residents and nurse practitioners on quality of communication with patients with serious illness. *JAMA: The Journal of the American Medical Association*, *310*(21), 2271–2281.

Davey, M. P., Kissil, K., Lynch, L., et al. (2013). A culturally adapted intervention for African-American families coping with parental cancer: Outcomes of a pilot study. *Psycho-Oncology*, *22*(7), 1572–1580.

Dayer-Berenson, L. (2014). *Cultural competencies for nurses: Impact on health and illness*. Burlington, MA: Jones & Bartlett Learning.

Gonzalez, E. W., Polansky, M., Lippa, C. F., et al. (2014). Enhancing resourcefulness to improve outcomes in family caregivers and persons with Alzheimer's disease: A pilot randomized trial. *International Journal of Alzheimer's Disease*, Advance online publication.

Gray, W. N., Szulczewski, L. J., Regan, S. M. P., et al. (2014). Cultural influences in pediatric cancer from diagnosis to cure/end of life. *Journal of Pediatric Oncology Nursing*, *31*(5), 252–271.

Higginbottom, G. M. A., Richter, M. S., Mogale, R. S., et al. (2011). Identification of nursing assessment models/tools validated in clinical use with diverse ethno-cultural groups: an integrative review of the literature. *BMC Nursing*, *10*(16), 1–11.

Hopkinson, J. B., Brown, J. C., Okamoto, I., et al. (2012). The effectiveness of patient-family carer (couple) intervention for the management of symptoms and other health-related problems in people affected by cancer: A systematic literature search and narrative review. *Journal of Pain and Symptom Management*, *43*(1), 111–142.

Hu, C., Kung, S., Rummans, T. A., et al. (2014). Reducing caregiver stress with internet-based interventions: A systematic review of open-label and randomized controlled trials. *Journal of the American Medical Informatics Association*, Advance online publication.

Knapp, S. J., Sole, M. L., & Byers, J. F. (2013). The EPICS Family Bundle and its effects on stress and coping of families of critically ill trauma patients. *Applied Nursing Research*, *26*, 51–57.

Kuo, B. C. H. (2011). Culture's consequences on coping: Theories, evidences, and dimensionalities. *Journal of Cross-Cultural Psychology*, *42*(6), 1084–1100.

Li, R., Cooper, C., Barber, J., et al. (2014). Coping strategies as mediators of the effect of the START (strategies for relatives) intervention on psychological morbidity for family cares of people with dementia in a randomized controlled trial. *Journal of Affective Disorders*, *168*, 298–305.

Mansfield, A. K., Keitner, G. I., & Dealy, J. (2014). The Family Assessment Device: An update. *Family Process*, Advance online publication.

Marsac, M. L., Hildenbrand, A. K., Clawson, K., et al. (2012). Acceptability and feasibility of family use of the Cellie Cancer Coping Kit. *Supportive Care in Cancer*, *20*(12), 3315–3324.

Nichols, L. O., Martindale-Adams, J., & Burns, R. (2011). Translation of a dementia caregiver support program in a health care system—REACH VA. *Archives of Internal Medicine*, *171*(4), 353–359.

Northouse, L. L., Mood, D. W., Schafenacker, A., et al. (2013). Randomized clinical trial of a brief and extensive dyadic interventions for advanced cancer patients and their family caregivers. *Psycho-Oncology*, *22*, 555–563.

Northouse, L. L., Schafenacker, A., Barr, K. L., et al. (2014). A tailored Web-based psychoeducational intervention for cancer patients and their family caregivers. *Cancer Nursing*, *37*(5), 321–330.

O'Brien, M. E. (2014). *Spirituality in nursing: Standing on holy ground* (5th ed.). Burlington, MA: Jones & Bartlett Learning.

Ostlund, U., & Persson, C. (2014). Examining family responses to family systems nursing interventions: An integrative review. *Journal of Family Nursing*, *20*, 259–286.

Shields, C. G., Finley, M. A., Chawla, N., et al. (2012). Couple and family interventions in health problems. *Journal of Marital and Family Therapy*, *38*(1), 265–280.

Tomlinson, P. S., Peden-McAlpine, C., & Sherman, S. (2012). A family systems nursing intervention model for paediatric health crisis. *Journal of Advanced Nursing*, *68*(3), 705–714.

Wittenberg-Lyles, E., Goldsmith, J., Richardson, B., et al. (2012). The practical nurse: A case for COMFORT communication training. *The American Journal of Hospice & Palliative Medicine*, *30*(2), 162–166.

Readiness for enhanced Decision-Making

Dawn Fairlie, ANP, FNP, GNP, DNS(c)

NANDA-I

Definition

A pattern of choosing a course of action for meeting short- and long-term health-related goals, which can be strengthened

Defining Characteristics

Expresses desire to enhance congruency of decisions with sociocultural goal; expresses desire to enhance congruency of decisions with sociocultural value; expresses desire to enhance congruency of decisions with goal; expresses desire to enhance congruency of decisions with values; expresses desire to enhance decision-making; expresses desire to enhance risk-benefit analysis of decisions; expresses desire to enhance understanding of choices for decision-making; expresses desire to enhance understanding of meaning of choices; expresses desire to enhance use of reliable evidence for decisions

NOC (Nursing Outcomes Classification)

Suggested NOC Outcomes

Decision-Making; Participation in Health Care Decisions; Personal Autonomy

Example NOC Outcome with Indicators

Participation in Health Care Decisions as evidenced by the following indicators: Claims decision-making responsibility/Exhibits self-direction in decision-making/Seeks reputable information/Specifies health outcome preferences. (Rate the outcome and indicators of **Participation in Health Care Decisions:** 1 = never demonstrated, 2 = rarely demonstrated, 3 = sometimes demonstrated, 4 = often demonstrated, 5 = consistently demonstrated [see Section I].)

Client Outcomes

Client Will (Specify Time Frame)

- Review treatment options with providers
- Ask questions about the benefits and risks of treatment options
- Communicate decisions about treatment options to providers in relation to personal preferences, values, and goals

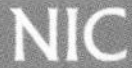

NIC (Nursing Interventions Classification)

Suggested NIC Interventions

Decision-Making Support; Mutual Goal Setting; Support System Enhancement; Values Clarification

Example NIC Activities—Decision-Making Support

Help client identify the advantages and disadvantages of each alternative; Facilitate collaborative decision-making; Help client explain decisions to others, as needed

Nursing Interventions and *Rationales*

- Support and encourage clients and their representatives to engage in health care decisions. EB: *Decisional conflict was assessed using the Decisional Conflict Scale among pregnant women considering antidepressant medication treatment. Although many pregnant women facing decisions regarding the use of antidepressant medication experience decisional conflict, their decisions were facilitated by interpersonal supports and emotional support reduced decisional conflict and facilitated the decision-making process (Walton et al, 2014).* EBN: *Decision aids are intended to help people participate in decisions that involve weighing the benefits and harms of treatment options, often with scientific uncertainty. Stacey et al (2014) concluded that there is high-quality evidence that decision aids improve clients' knowledge regarding options and reduce decisional conflict.*
- Respect personal preferences, values, needs, and rights. EB: *"Denial of this right of autonomy and self-determination may worsen the individual's physical and existential suffering" (Soriano & Lagman, 2012).*
- Determine the degree of participation desired by the client. EB: *"Ultimately, a patient must be able to understand the information given to him, evaluate the consequences of the options presented, deliberate on these options based on his values, communicate this choice, and maintain consistency over time" (Soriano & Lagman, 2012).*
- Provide information that is appropriate, relevant, and timely. EB: *Decisional conflict was assessed using the Decisional Conflict Scale among pregnant women considering antidepressant medication treatment. Although many pregnant women facing decisions regarding the use of antidepressant medication experience decisional conflict, their decisions were facilitated by interpersonal supports and emotional support reduced decisional conflict and facilitated the decision-making process (Walton et al, 2014).*
- Determine the health literacy of clients and their representatives before helping with decision-making. EB: *A randomized trial of a decision aid for coronary heart disease (CHD) adherence was conducted by Sheridan et al (2014), who reported that most participants found the decision aid easy to use and easy to understand. Participants reported improvement in personalization of information and that the decision aid helped them to decide what was important to them.*
- Tailor information to the specific needs of individual clients, according to principles of health literacy. EB: *Ko et al (2014) studied cultural and linguistic adaptation of a multimedia colorectal cancer screening Decision Aid for Spanish-Speaking Latinos. They concluded that new interventions that address the needs of diverse U.S. populations are needed to reduce health disparities. Additionally they noted the importance of adapting English-language health interventions to facilitate communication and decision-making.*
- Motivate clients to be as independent as possible in decision-making. EB: *According to Roberts (2014), national ethics and regulatory standards mandate that individuals must be offered as much choice in the decisional process whereby they make these decisions independently and true to their personal beliefs and values.*
- Identify the client's level of choice in decision-making. EBN: *A study conducted by Feenstra et al (2015) examined incorporating the child's perspective into his or her decision-making process. They found that*

treatment choices can successfully be made by parents together with their child and recommended interventions that successfully meet the needs of all those involved.

- Focus on the positive aspects of decision-making rather than the decisional conflicts. EBN: *Numerous studies conducted during development of the health promotion model show that promotion differs from prevention and requires a positive rather than negative approach (Pender et al, 2011).*
- Design educational interventions for decision support. EBN: *A Cochrane review of decision aids (pamphlets, videos, or Web-based tools) concluded that use of decision aids fosters a positive effect on communication between clients and their health care provider and influenced the time required for the consultation. Additionally, there was an improvement with more detailed decision aids when compared to simpler decision aids, and both were better than usual care (Stacey et al, 2011).*
- Acknowledge the complexity of everyday self-care decisions related to self-management of chronic illnesses. EBN: *In a study of chronically ill community dwelling elders, Bonney (2014) found that this population prefers to learn about prognosis and end of life through conversations with their health care provider and supplementation from written materials. Decision aids can increase knowledge and more education leads to better decision-making.*

Geriatric

- The above interventions may be adapted for geriatric use.
- Facilitate collaborative decision-making. EBN: *A study of the shared decision-making process of persons with dementia identified a broad spectrum of the shared decision-making process. Results indicated that not all persons with dementia are excluded from participating in the decision-making process (Miller et al, 2014).*

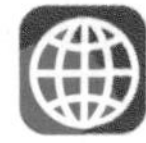

Multicultural

- Use existing decision aids for particular types of decisions or develop decision aids as indicated. EBN: *Decision aids are intended to help people participate in decisions that involve weighing the benefits and harms of treatment options often with scientific uncertainty. Stacey et al (2014) concluded that there is high-quality evidence that decision aids improve clients' knowledge regarding options and reduce decisional conflict.* EB: *Ko et al (2014) studied cultural and linguistic adaptation of a multimedia colorectal cancer screening Decision Aid for Spanish-Speaking Latinos. They concluded that new interventions that address the needs of diverse U.S. populations are needed to reduce health disparities. Additionally they noted the importance of adapting English-language health interventions to facilitate communication and decision-making.*

Home Care

- The above interventions may be adapted for home care use.
- Develop clinical practice guidelines that include shared decision-making. EB: *According to Agoritsas et al (2015), clinical practice guidelines have for the most part been tailored to meet the educational needs of clinicians and seldom support shared decision-making. Furthermore, identifying decisions where shared decision-making is indicated is particularly important. Decision aids can be used with clinical practice guidelines. They recommend the generic production of decision aids from clinical practice guidelines.*

REFERENCES

Agoritsas, T., Heen, A. F., Brandt, L., et al. (2015). Decision aids that really promote shared decision making: the pace quickens. *BMJ (Clinical Research Ed)*, *350*, g7624.

Bonney, L. A. (2014). *Personal characteristics and learning preferences in end-of-life decision making of chronically ill community dwelling elders* (Doctoral dissertation, ILLINOIS STATE UNIVERSITY).

Feenstra, B., Lawson, M. L., Harrison, D., et al. (2015). Decision coaching using the Ottawa family decision guide with parents and their children: a field testing study. *BMC Medical Informatics and Decision Making*, *15*(1), 5.

Ko, L. K., Reuland, D., Jolles, M., et al. (2014). Cultural and linguistic adaptation of a multimedia colorectal cancer screening decision aid for Spanish-speaking Latinos. *Journal of Health Communication*, *19*(2), 192–209.

Miller, L. M., Whitlatch, C. J., & Lyons, K. S. (2014). Shared decision-making in dementia: A review of patient and family carer involvement. *Dementia (Basel, Switzerland)*, 1471301214555542.

Pender, N. J., Murdaugh, C. L., & Parsons, M. A. (2011). *Health promotion in nursing practice* (6th ed.). Upper Saddle River, NJ: Pearson Prentice Hall.

Roberts, L. W. (2014). Informed consent and the capacity for voluntarism. *American Journal of Psychiatry*, *159*, 705–712.

Sheridan, S. L., Draeger, L. B., Pignone, M. P., et al. (2014). The effect of a decision aid intervention on decision making about coronary heart disease risk reduction: secondary analyses of a randomized trial. *BMC Medical Informatics and Decision Making*, *14*(1), 14.

Soriano, M. A., & Lagman, R. (2012). When the patient says no. *The American Journal of Hospice and Palliative Care*, *29*, 401–404.

Stacey, D., Bennett, C. L., Barry, M. J., et al. (2011). Decision aids for people facing health treatment or screening decisions. *Cochrane Database of Systematic Reviews, 10*(10).

Stacey, D., Légaré, F., Col, N. F., et al. (2014). Decision aids for people facing health treatment or screening decisions. *The Cochrane Library*.

Walton, G. D., Ross, L. E., Stewart, D. E., et al. (2014). Decisional conflict among women considering antidepressant medication use in pregnancy. *Archives of women's mental health, 17*(6), 493–501.

Impaired emancipated Decision-Making

Ruth A. Wittmann-Price, PhD, RN, CNS, CNE, CHSE, ANEF, FAAN

NANDA-I

Definition

A process of choosing a health care decision that does not include personal knowledge and/or consideration of social norms, or does not occur in a flexible environment resulting in decisional dissatisfaction

Defining Characteristics

Delay in enacting chosen health care option; distress when listening to others' opinion; excessive concern about what others think is the best decision; excessive fear of what others think about a decision; feeling constrained in describing own opinion; inability to choose a health care option that best fits current lifestyle; limited verbalization about health care option in others' presence

Related Factors

Decrease in understanding of all available health care options; inability to adequately verbalize perceptions about health care options; inadequate time to discuss health care options; insufficient privacy to openly discuss health care options; limited decision-making experience; traditional hierarchical family; traditional hierarchical health care system

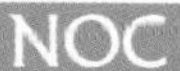

NOC Outcomes (Nursing Outcomes Classification)

Suggested NOC Outcomes

Decision-Making; Self-Esteem; Coping; Health Promotion Behavior; Stress Level; Communication; Self-Care; Participation In Health Care Decisions; Health-Seeking Behavior; Knowledge: Treatment Options; Psychosocial Adjustment

Example NOC Outcome with Indicators

Participation in Health Care Decisions as evidenced by the following indicator: Claims decision making responsibility. (Rate the outcome and indicators of **Participation in Health Care Decisions:** 1 = never demonstrated, 2 = rarely demonstrated, 3 = sometimes demonstrated, 4 = often demonstrated, 5 = consistently demonstrated [see Section I].)

Client Outcomes

Client Will (Specify Time Frame)

- Verbalize option outcomes freely before making a health care decision
- Freely verbalize own opinion with health care providers before making a health care decision
- Choose the health care option that fits his or her lifestyle within an appropriate amount of time that allows enactment of the choice
- Describe how the chosen option fits into his or her current lifestyle before or after the decision has been made
- Verbalizes appropriate concern about others' opinions before making the health care choice
- Remains stress-free when listening to others' opinions before making the health care choice
- Arrives at a decision in a timely manner

NIC Interventions (Nursing Interventions Classification)

Suggested NIC Interventions

Decision-Making Support

D

Example NIC Activities—Emancipated Decision-Making

Assist client in making an emancipated decision about health care options by discussing social norms with the client; Provide a flexible environment; Encourage the client to use personal knowledge

Nursing Interventions and *Rationales*

- Assess client's readiness to openly discussing the decision-making process. EBN: *A qualitative study in China demonstrated that older adults were open to discuss end-of-life care even though traditional and cultural barriers have long been present (Chan & Pang, 2011).*
- Use active listening in a nonjudgmental manner to provide the client with a flexible decision-making environment. CEB: *Listening and hearing clients' stories (N = 12), without labeling them, provides them with a voice which they need to negotiate the health care system (Van Den Tillaart et al, 2009).* EBN: *A correlational study demonstrates that active listening may be enhanced when nurses (N = 31) are aware of their own attitudes on a subject before they engage in a dialogue with a client (Boyd et al, 2011).*
- Use anticipatory guidance by proactively providing the client with information. EB: *Social workers found, through a qualitative, case-based study conducted by interviewing family members, that anticipatory guidance is needed before a decisional crisis occurs (Mamier & Winslow, 2014).* EBN: *Wittmann-Price et al (2011) found in a mixed method study that the majority of pregnant clients (N = 50) reported they had been provided with information prenatally, but not all clients felt they were given enough information at the time of delivery to make an informed choice.*
- Establish a purposeful provider-client relationship. EB: *A qualitative psychology study done by Cook and Loomis (2012) demonstrated that clients (N = 15) should remain as the center focus in the decision-making process in order to maintain control.* EB: *Clients (N = 17) who have fears about diagnosis and treatments were therapeutically treated by establishing a purposeful provider-client relationship in which "listening" was most valued by clients (Nunes et al, 2013).*
- ▲ Refer to counseling as needed. EB: *A qualitative psychology study indicated that a woman's perception of her childbirth experience was interwoven with her feelings of having been provided choices through education and consultation (Cook & Loomis, 2012).* CEB: *Wittmann-Price (2006) demonstrated in a quantitative correlational study that women's (N = 97) decision-making was empowered when they were provided resources and information to arrive at an emancipated choice.*
- Provide decision-making support. EBN: *Support may help guard against oppressive health care practices as demonstrated in a qualitative case study done by Treloar and Gunn (2012) that focused on why women choose to smoke.* EBN: *de Rosenroll et al (2013) found that significant others need their physical and emotional needs met to play a supportive role in decision-making for dialysis clients.*
- Provide a flexible environment by encouraging others to accept client's choice. EBN: *Tully and Ball (2013) interviewed 115 mothers about mode of delivery; participants differentiated health care issues from social issues surrounding childbirth, demonstrating that social issues play a role in the decisional process.* CEB: *Wittmann-Price and Bhattacharya (2008) quantitatively studied pain management decisions for clients in labor (N = 92) and found that a flexible environment was needed in order for the client to make a supported and emancipated decision.*
- Encourage the client to use personal knowledge as part of the decision-making process to increase decisional satisfaction. EBN: *Women can make health care decisions that are right for them if they can use personal knowledge to overcome oppressive social forces (Stepanuk et al, 2013).* CEB: *Using personal knowledge is the best indicator to making an emancipated decision and correlates strongly and positively with satisfaction with the decision (Wittmann-Price, 2006).*

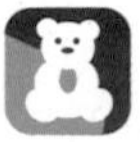

Pediatric

- When able, involve client in health care decision-making when possible. EBN: *Mitchell (2014) studied disabled young adults (N = 10) and found that they viewed health care decisions as important, and each individual "framed" the decision differently, but all included consideration of independence.* EBN: *Kennedy (2014) did a systematic review about pediatric clients ages 4 to 18 years and found that interventional studies (N = 5) indicated communication and education assisted clients to actively participate in the decision-making process.*

- Provide parental information in the decision-making process. EBN: *Three focus groups of parents identified areas of needed information in order to make decisions regarding newborn care (Rothwell et al, 2013).* EBN: *Holland et al (2014) developed a decision support tool in a correlation study (N = 197) to determine clients who need discharge planning and referrals to assist in decisional processes.*

D

Critical Care

- Enhance client decision-making in critical care setting. EBN: *Bridges et al (2013) synthesized 16 studies and found that the conditions of critical care settings appear best suited to forming therapeutic relationships, while nurses working on acute nursing units more often report moral distress resulting from delivering unsatisfactory care due to lack of ability to build a nurse-client relationship.*

Geriatric

- Include geriatric clients in the decisional process. EBN: *Hardin (2012) describes older adults' level of decision-making participation in critical care units and identified that nurses need to assess the clients' preferred level of involvement with decisions before assuming that they prefer not to be involved.* EB: *Isaacs et al (2013) studied older adults (N = 159) requiring outpatient analgesic treatment for a chronic illness and found that being active participants in the pain management decision increased client satisfaction and decreased analgesic use.*
- Include family in the decision making process when needed. EB: *Einterz et al (2012) developed and validated a decision tool to assist surrogate decision-makers for clients with dementia.* EBN: *Kryworuchko et al (2013) did a systematic review of the literature about end-of-life decision-making and found that using shared decision-making trended toward decreasing family member anxiety and decreasing intensive care unit length of stay.*

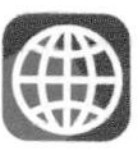

Multicultural

- Consider cultural influences on decision-making. EBN: *Mead et al (2013) did a systematic review of minority clients' decision-making regarding cancer treatment and found that factors that mattered to clients were categorized into themes: being part of the decision-making process; including client, family, and important others; community, and provider factors.* EBN: *Duke (2013) qualitatively studied three diverse cultural groups living in the United States to discuss end-of-life decision-making and found that there were differences in preferences for treatments such as artificial nutrition.*

Home Care

- Use open communication to assist clients to develop health care plans to which they can adhere. EBN: *Cook and Loomis (2012) studied open communication between women and their caregivers and found that it enhanced clients' knowledge and empowers them to implement the decision.* EBN: *Truglio-Londrigan (2013) interviewed 10 homecare nurses about their perception of shared decision-making and recorded four important themes: decision-making needs to begin at the level of the client, providing education for the decision-making process, including the "village" or the significant social piece in the process, and ultimately identifying whose decision it is.*

REFERENCES

Boyd, D., Merkh, K., Rutledge, D. N., et al. (2011). Nurses' perceptions and experiences with end-of-life communication and care. *Oncology Nursing Forum*, *38*(3), E229–E239.

Bridges, J., Nicholson, C., Maben, J., et al. (2013). Capacity for care: Meta-ethnography of acute care nurses' experiences of the nurse-patient relationship. *Journal of Advanced Nursing*, *69*(4), 760–772.

Chan, H. Y. L., & Pang, S. M. C. (2011). Readiness of Chinese frail old age home residents towards end-of-life care decision making. *Journal of Clinical Nursing*, *20*, 1454–1461.

Cook, K., & Loomis, C. (2012). The impact of choice and control on women's childbirth experience. *The Journal of Perinatal Education*, *21*(3), 158–168.

de Rosenroll, A., Higuchi, K. S., Dutton, K. S., et al. (2013). Perspectives of significant others in dialysis modality decision-making: A qualitative study. *Canadian Association of Nephrology Nurses and Technologists*, *23*(4), 17–24.

Duke, G. (2013). Attitudes regarding life-sustaining measures in people born in Japan, China, and Vietnam and living in Texas. *International Journal of Palliative Nursing*, *19*(2), 76–83.

Einterz, S. F., Gilliam, R., Chang, L. F., et al. (2012). Development and testing of a decision aid on goals of care for advanced dementia. *Journal of the American Medical Directors Association, 15*(4), 251–255.

Hardin, S. R. (2012). Care Patients: Participation in Decision Making. *Critical Care Nurse, 32*(6), 43–50.

Holland, D. E., Conlon, P. M., Rohlik, G. M., et al. (2014). Developing and testing a discharge planning decision support tool for hospitalized pediatric patients. *Journal for Specialists in Pediatric Nursing, 19*(2), 149–161.

Isaacs, C. G., Kistler, C., Hunold, K. M., et al. (2013). Shared decision-making in the selection of outpatient analgesics for older individuals in the emergency department. *Journal of the American Geriatric Society, 61*(5), 793–798.

Kennedy, C. (2014). Systematic review summary: Interventions for promoting participation in shared decision making for children with cancer. *Singapore Nursing Journal, 41*(1), 43, 44.

Kryworuchko, J., Hill, E., Murray, M. A., et al. (2013). Interventions for shared decision-making about life support in the intensive care unit: A systematic review. *World View on Evidence-based Nursing, 10*, 3–16.

Mamier, I., & Winslow, B. W. (2014). Divergent views of placement decision-making: A qualitative case study. *Issues in Mental Health Nursing, 35*(1), 13–20.

Mead, E. L., Doorenbos, A. Z., Javid, S. H., et al. (2013). Shared decision-making for cancer care among racial and ethnic minorities: A systematic review. *American Journal of Public Health, 103*(12), e15–e29.

Mitchell, W. A. (2014). Making choices about medical interventions: the experience of disabled young people with degenerative conditions. *Health Expectations, 17*(2), 254–266.

Nunes, J., Ventura, T., Encarnação, R., et al. (2013). What do patients with medically unexplained physical symptoms (MUPS) think? A qualitative study. *Mental Health in Family Medicine, 10*, 67–79.

Rothwell, E., Clark, L., Anderson, R., et al. (2013). Residual newborn screening samples for research: Parental information needs for decision-making. *Journal for Specialists in Pediatric Nursing, 18*, 115–122.

Stepanuk, K. M., Fisher, K. M., Wittmann-Price, R., et al. (2013). Women's decision-making regarding medication use in pregnancy for anxiety and/or depression. *Journal of Advanced Nursing, 69*(11), 2470–2480.

Treloar, D., & Gunn, J. (2012). Caught in the tapestry of tobacco: Why I smoke. *Contemporary Nurse, 41*(1), 51–57.

Truglio-Londrigan, M. (2013). Shared decision-making in home-care from the nurse's perspective: Sitting at the kitchen table—a qualitative descriptive study. *Journal of Clinical Nursing*, (19/20), 2883–2895.

Tully, K. P., & Ball, H. L. (2013). Misrecognition of need: Women's experiences of and explanations for undergoing cesarean delivery. *Social Science and Medicine, 85*, 103–111.

Van Den Tillaart, S., Kurtz, D., & Cash, P. (2009). Powerlessness, marginalized identify, and silencing of health concerns: Voiced realities of women living with a mental health diagnosis. *International Journal of Mental Health Nursing, 18*, 153–163.

Wittmann-Price, R. A., Fliszar, R., & Bhattacharya, A. (2011). Elective cesarean births: Are women making emancipated decisions? *Applied Nursing Research, 24*, 147–152.

Wittmann-Price, R. A., & Bhattacharya, A. (2008). Reexploring the subconcepts of the Wittmann-Price Theory of Emancipated Decision-making in Women's Healthcare. *Advances in Nursing Science, 31*(3), 225–236.

Wittmann-Price, R. A. (2006). Exploring the subconcepts of the Wittmann-Price Theory of Emancipated Decision-making in Women's Health Care. *Journal of Nursing Scholarship, 38*(4), 377–382.

Readiness for enhanced emancipated Decision-Making

Ruth A. Wittmann-Price, PhD, RN, CNS, CNE, CHSE, ANEF, FAAN

NANDA-I

Definition

A process of choosing a health care decision that includes personal knowledge and/or consideration of social norms, which can be strengthened

Defining Characteristics

Expresses desire to enhance ability to choose health care options that best fit current lifestyle; expresses desire to enhance ability to enact chosen health care option; expresses desire to enhance ability to understand all available health care options; expresses desire to enhance ability to verbalize own opinion without constraint; expresses desire to enhance comfort to verbalize health care options in the presence of others; expresses desire to enhance confidence in decision-making; expresses desire to enhance confidence to discuss health care options openly; expresses desire to enhance decision making; expresses desire to enhance privacy to discuss health care options

NOC Outcomes (Nursing Outcomes Classification)

Suggested NOC Outcomes

Decision-Making; Self-Esteem; Coping; Health Promotion Behavior; Stress Level; Communication; Self-Care; Participation in Health Care Decisions; Health-Seeking Behavior; Knowledge: Treatment Options; Psychosocial Adjustment

Example NOC Outcome with Indicators

Participation in Health Care Decisions as evidenced by the following indicator: Claims decision making responsibility. (Rate the outcome and indicators of **Participation in Health Care Decisions:** 1 = never demonstrated, 2 = rarely demonstrated, 3 = sometimes demonstrated, 4 = often demonstrated, 5 = consistently demonstrated [see Section I].)

D

Client Outcomes

Client Will (Specify Time Frame)

- Verbalize option of outcomes freely before making a health care decision
- Freely verbalize own opinion with health care providers before making a health care decision
- Choose the health care option that best fits his or her lifestyle within an appropriate amount of time that allows enactment of the choice
- Describe how the chosen option fits into his or her current lifestyle before or after the decision has been made
- Verbalizes appropriate concern about others' opinions before making the health care choice
- Remains stress-free when listening to others' opinions before making the health care choice
- Arrives at a decision in a timely manner

NIC Interventions (Nursing Interventions Classification)

Suggested NIC Interventions

Decision-Making Support

Example NIC Activities—Emancipated Decision-Making

Assist client in making an emancipated decision about health care options by discussing social norms with the client; Provide a flexible environment; Encourage the client to use personal knowledge

Nursing Interventions and *Rationales*

- Assess client's readiness to choose through active listening. EB: *Greenstein et al (2013) studied active listening skills of health care providers during handoff reports using a "HEAR" checklist and found that active listening is rare with interruptions, being present 98% of the time.* CEB: *Bryant (2009) reviewed literature about active listening and describes four themes present when a health care provider is actively listening to the client, including (1) being present, (2) being interested, (3) having time, and (4) being respectful.*
- Use anticipatory guidance by proactively providing the client with information. (Refer to Impaired emancipated **Decision-Making.**)
- Establish a purposeful provider-client relationship. EB: *Zeidler (2011) studied the services provided by the First Nation group for Aboriginal people and found that open dialogue leads to the development of services that are relevant and responsive to clients' needs and can be accomplished by professionals who engage in a respectful and mutually beneficial collaborative learning process.* EBN: *Woolley et al (2012) implemented relationship-based care on a medical-surgical unit and the unit had positive results, including an increase in client satisfaction, a reduction in falls, fewer hospital acquired pressure ulcers, and decreasing call light use.*
- ▲ Include interdisciplinary health care professionals as needed to increase knowledge of chosen option. EB: *Rainchuso (2013) discusses that the health care practices of oral hygiene in women and infants is predicated on misconceptions and lack of knowledge and evidence demonstrate no detrimental effects of pregnant women receiving routine and restorative care while pregnant.*
- Provide decision-making support. (Refer to Impaired emancipated **Decision-Making.**)
- Continue to provide a flexible environment for client to enact choice. EBN: *Smith and Kirkpatrick (2013) used solution-focused brief therapy in clients with chronic obstructive pulmonary disease to be more supportive of clients by adopting a "not knowing" position while the client is placed in the position of "expert."* EBN: *Webster (2013) used standardized examples to teach therapeutic communication to students; outcome data demonstrated such education increased students' ability to address clients' preferences, values, and beliefs.*

- Encourage the client to use personal knowledge as part of the decision-making process to increase decisional satisfaction. EBN: *Scaffidi et al (2014) found that clients (N = 45) with increased personal knowledge about the risks and benefits of trial of labor after a cesarean delivery were found to be positively associated with deciding to have vaginal delivery instead of cesarean delivery.*

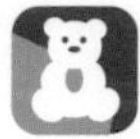

Pediatric

D

- Understand interventions that parents prefer when in the decision-making process. EBN: *Rosales and Allen (2012) describe "optimism bias" in parents who make decisions that are risk-taking for children and underscore the fact that this concept is not yet measurable.*

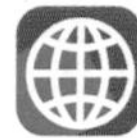

Multicultural

- Use open communication to assist clients to develop health care plans to which they can adhere. EBN: *Vandewark (2014) studied the correlations between knowledge and attitude and found them to be significantly related.* EBN: *Kilanowski (2013) studied Latino migrant farm workers (N = 31) and found that clients preferred comic book–style handouts, games, food replicas, text in English/Spanish, and digital video discs or digital versatile discs, but did not like black-and-white photos or cartoon-like illustrations, concluding that it is important to offer information in colored illustrations, in sizes that mothers may easily carry in purses, and with limited verbiage on a page.*

Home Care

- Optimize self-care personal knowledge for home care. EBN: *Johansson (2013) found that increasing dialysis clients' personal knowledge about home therapies increased their decision-making capacity.* EBN: *Truglio-Londrigan (2013) did a qualitative study involving homecare nurses (N = 13) and found that decisions in the home include assessing "where the client is" on issues of education and significant others, and based on this information the client decides who will be making decisions regarding their care.*
- Refer to care plan Impaired emancipated **Decision-Making** for additional interventions for pediatric, critical care, geriatric, and multicultural care.

REFERENCES

Bryant, L. (2009). The art of active listening. *Practice Nurse*, *37*(6), 49–52.

Greenstein, E. A., Arora, V. M., Staisiunas, P. G., et al. (2013). Characterising physician listening behaviour during hospitalist handoffs using the HEAR checklist. *BMJ Quality & Safety*, *22*(3), 203–209.

Johansson, L. (2013). Shared decision making and patient involvement in choosing home therapies. *Journal of Renal Care*, *39*, 9–15.

Kilanowski, J. F. (2013). Anticipatory guidance preferences of Latina migrant farmworker. *Journal of Pediatric Healthcare*, *27*(3), 164–171.

Smith, S., & Kirkpatrick, P. (2013). Use of solution-focused brief therapy to enhance therapeutic communication in patients with COPD. *Primary Health Care*, *23*(10), 27–32.

Rainchuso, L. (2013). Improving oral health outcomes from pregnancy through infancy. *Journal of Dental Hygiene*, *87*(6), 330–335.

Rosales, P. P., & Allen, P. L. J. (2012). Optimism bias and parental views on unintentional injuries and safety: Improving anticipatory guidance in early childhood. *Pediatric Nursing*, *38*(2), 73–79.

Scaffidi, R. M., Posmontier, B., Bloch, J. R., et al. (2014). The relationship between personal knowledge and decision self-efficacy in choosing trial of labor after cesarean. *Journal of Midwifery & Women's Health*, *59*(3), 246–253.

Truglio-Londrigan, M. (2013). Shared decision-making in home-care from the nurse's perspective: Sitting at the kitchen table—a qualitative descriptive study. *Journal of Clinical Nursing*, *22*(19/20), 2883–2895.

Vandewark, A. C. (2014). Breastfeeding attitudes and knowledge in bachelor of science in nursing candidates. *Journal of Perinatal Education*, *23*(3), 135–141.

Webster, D. (2013). Relationship-based care: Implementing a caring, healing environment. *Journal of Nursing Education*, *52*(11), 645–648.

Woolley, J., Perkins, R., Laird, P., et al. (2012). Relationship-based care: implementing a caring, healing environment. *Medsurg Nursing*, *21*(3), 179–184.

Zeidler, D. (2011). Building a relationship: Perspectives from one First Nations Community. *Canadian Journal of Speech-Language Pathology & Audiology*, *35*(2), 136–143.

Risk for impaired emancipated Decision-Making

Ruth A. Wittmann-Price, PhD, RN, CNS, CNE, CHSE, ANEF, FAAN

NANDA-I

Definition

Vulnerable to the process of choosing a health care decision that does not include personal knowledge and/or considerations of social norms, or does not occur in a flexible environment, resulting in decisional satisfaction

Risk Factors

Inadequate time to discuss health care options; insufficient confidence to openly discuss health care options; insufficient information regarding health care options; insufficient privacy to openly discuss health care options; insufficient self-confidence in decision-making; limited decision-making experience; traditional hierarchical family; traditional hierarchical health care systems

NOC (Nursing Outcomes Classification)

Suggested NOC Outcomes

Decision-Making; Self-Confidence; Coping; Health Promotion Behavior; Stress Level; Communication; Self-Care; Participation in Health Care Decisions; Health-Seeking Behavior; Knowledge; Treatment Options; Psychosocial Adjustment

Example NOC Outcome with Indicators

Participation in Health Care Decisions as evidenced by the following indicator: Claims decision making responsibility. (Rate the outcome and indicators of **Participation in Health Care Decisions:** 1 = never demonstrated, 2 = rarely demonstrated, 3 = sometimes demonstrated, 4 = often demonstrated, 5 = consistently demonstrated [see Section I].)

Client Outcomes

Client Will (Specify Time Frame)

- Verbalize option outcomes freely before making a health care decision in a private setting with whom he or she feels comfortable
- Freely verbalize own opinion with health care providers before making a health care decision
- Discuss how options fit or hinder his or her lifestyle within an appropriate amount of time that allows enactment of the choice
- Discuss concerns about others' opinions before making the health care choice
- Decrease stress about others' opinions by placing options in perspective through informational resources
- Discuss the time frame in which the decision needs to be made

NIC Interventions (Nursing Interventions Classification)

Suggested NIC Interventions

Establish Rapport; Decision-Making Support

Example NIC Activities—Emancipated Decision-Making

Assist client to verbalize and discuss barriers that she or he perceives in making an emancipated decision about health care options; Acknowledge social norms about decision options; Provide a flexible environment that is safe and private for the discussions. Use empathy to understand the client's personal point of view about the options

Nursing Interventions and *Rationales*

- Assess client's vulnerability for an impaired decision-making process. EBN: *Goldberg & Shorten (2014) studied the decision-making perceptions for clients during childbirth and their providers, and observe providers being paternalistic and trying to influence the client's decision while nurses tried to suggest that it was the client's decision.* EBN: *Ebert et al (2014) quantitatively studied socially disadvantaged women and found that they wanted to engage in health care decisions but did not feel safe to engage due to inadequate information, perceived risks in not conforming, and the actions and reactions of nurses when they did seek choices which resulted in a silent compliance.*

D

- Assess the client's experience with decision-making. EB: *Chong et al (2013) interviewed interprofessional providers (N = 31) to learn about perceived barriers for using shared decision-making in mental health care and identified consumers' lack of competence to participate as a frequently cited barrier.* EBN: *Mayer et al (2014) used hermeneutic phenomenology to study women's decisions to seek help for signs of acute myocardial infarction and found that each client was informed by their unique social circumstances and past experiences.*
- Recognize traditional hierarchical family and health care system. EB: *Légaré and Witteman (2013) analyzed barriers to a shared decision-making process and recognize that more health care providers need training in the approach and to better engage the client.* EB: *Dierckx et al (2013) studied shared decision-making* (SDM) *between therapist perception and client preferred level of involvement in 237 consultations and found that SDM was not offered although clients preferred to provide their opinion about the treatment because physical therapists did not often recognize this factor and tended to apply a paternalistic approach.*
- Provide privacy to discuss health care options. EBN: *Jackson and McCulloch (2014) studied older rural women's decision to seek help for heart conditions and found women had difficulty identifying heart attack symptoms and were reluctant to access care because of concerns of maintaining their privacy.* EBN: *Peak et al (2012) explored the experiences of persons with HIV (N = 10) attending an assisted reproductive treatment program and found through interview that disclosure of HIV status and managing confidentiality were a significant challenge related to decision-making for infertility treatment.*
- Allow the client time to choose. EBN: *Cook et al (2014) used a mixed method approach to study the implementation of the nonreport option in Texas regarding sexual assault victims and found significant to reporting was confidentiality processes, storage and shipment of evidence, and the use of the nonreport option.* EB: *Pieterse et al (2013) performed a systematic literature review to identify process theories (N = 4) that guided decision-making practices and found that they encouraged clients to consider all options, discouraged clients from jumping to the first option, included client's values, compared options, and provided time to decide.*

▲ Understand primary care providers' role in the decision-making process. EB: *Uy et al (2014) used a mixed method study involving primary care practices (N = 4) and concluded that in order for clients to experience decisional support interventions that health care provider engagement and financial incentives were important.* EBN: *O'Sullivan and Rae (2014) studied psychiatric clients' perceptions of shared decision-making in relation to medication management and found clients wanted good quality information about medicines and alternative treatments from providers.*

- Provide informational resources. EBN: *Schroy et al (2014) used a cross-sectional survey with providers (N = 42) using a decision aid with clients for colon cancer screening adherence and the majority felt that the tool increased client knowledge, helped clients identify a preferred screening option, improved the quality of decision-making, and saved time.* EB: *Mathew et al (2014) studied client satisfaction with care and maximizing adherence with migraine treatment plans using a cross-sectional survey. The majority of participants (92%) preferred that the decision to prescribe a triptan be a joint decision and clients generally felt health care providers did a good job educating them.*
- Provide encouragement so clients increase their confidence in the decision-making process. EB: *Reeve et al (2013) did a systematic review of the literature (N = 21) to understand why clients do or do not decide on inappropriate medication use and identified the following barriers/enablers: disagreement/agreement with "appropriateness" of cessation, absence/presence of a "process" for cessation, negative/positive "influences" to cease medication, and "fear" of cessation and "dislike" of medications.* EB: *Joseph-Williams et al (2014) did a systematic review of the literature for shared decision-making barriers and found that themes related to clients' knowledge and the power imbalance in the doctor-client relationship and knowledge alone is insufficient and power is more difficult to attain.*

Pediatric

- Understand the parent/guardian's vulnerability when making health care decisions for their children. EB: *Crowe et al (2014) used a questionnaire to discover how parents chose a language mode for their child and found that factors such as family, community, and advice from others were significant.*

- Understand adolescent decision-making processes. EB: *DeBellis et al (2013) studied the decision-making process of adolescents in using cannabis and found that the participants (N = 23) demonstrated distinctly different activation patterns during risky decision-making and reward processing compared to nonusers (N = 18).*
- Refer to care plan Impaired emancipated **Decision-Making** for additional interventions for critical care, geriatric, multicultural care, and home care.

REFERENCES

Chong, W. W., Aslani, P., & Chen, T. F. (2013). Shared decision-making and interprofessional collaboration in mental healthcare: A qualitative study exploring perceptions of barriers and facilitators. *Journal of Interprofessional Care*, *27*(5), 373–379.

Cook, H. L., Busch-Armendariz, N. B., Vohn, S. S., et al. (2014). Giving sexual assault survivors time to decide: An exploration of the use and effects of the nonreport option. *American Journal of Nursing*, *114*(3), 26–36.

Crowe, K., McLeod, S., Mckinnon, D. H., et al. (2014). Speech, sign, or multilingualism for children with hearing loss: Quantitative insights into caregivers' decision making. *Language, Speech & Hearing Services in Schools*, *45*(3), 234–247.

DeBellis, M. D., Wang, L., Bergman, S. R., et al. (2013). Neural mechanisms of risky decision-making and reward response in adolescent onset cannabis use disorder. *Drug and Alcohol Dependence*, *133*(1), 134–145.

Dierckx, K., Deveugele, M., Roosen, P., et al. (2013). Implementation of shared decision making in physical therapy: Observed level of involvement and patient preference. *Physical Therapy*, *93*(10), 1321–1330.

Ebert, L., Bellchambers, H., Ferguson, A., et al. (2014). Socially disadvantaged women's views of barriers to feeling safe to engage in decision-making in maternity care. *Women and Birth: Journal of the Australian College of Midwives*, *27*(2), 132–137.

Goldberg, H. B., & Shorten, A. (2014). Patient and provider perceptions of decision making about use of epidural analgesia during childbirth: A thematic analysis. *Journal of Perinatal Education*, *23*(3), 142–150.

Jackson, M. N. G., & McCulloch, B. J. (2014). 'Heart attack' symptoms and decision-making: The case of older rural women. *Rural and Remote Health*, *14*(2), 1–13.

Joseph-Williams, N., Elwyn, G., & Edwards, A. (2014). Knowledge is not power for patients: A systematic review and thematic synthesis of patient-reported barriers and facilitators to shared decision making. *Patient Education & Counseling*, *94*(3), 291–309.

Légaré, F., & Witteman, H. O. (2013). Shared decision making: Examining key elements and barriers to adoption into routine clinical practice. *Health Affairs*, *32*(2), 276–284.

Mathew, P. G., Pavlovic, J. M., Lettich, A., et al. (2014). Education and decision making at the time of triptan prescribing: Patient expectations vs actual practice. *Headache: The Journal of Head & Face Pain*, *54*(4), 698–708.

Mayer, M., Readers, G. L., & McCallum, J. (2014). An exploration of women's decision trajectories: Seeking professional help for an AMI. *British Journal of Cardiac Nursing*, *9*(7), 351–358.

O'Sullivan, M. J., & Rae, S. (2014). Shared decision making in psychiatric medicines management. *Mental Health Practice*, *17*(8), 16–22.

Peak, S. A., Nowoweiski, S. J., & Giles, M. L. (2012). A qualitative study of HIV serodiscordant patients accessing assisted reproductive treatment. *Journal of Reproductive & Infant Psychology*, *30*(4), 413–422.

Pieterse, A. H., de Vries, M., Kunneman, M., et al. (2013). Theory-informed design of values clarification methods: A cognitive psychological perspective on patient health-related decision making. *Social Science & Medicine*, *77*, 156–163.

Reeve, E., To, J., Hendrix, I., et al. (2013). Patient barriers to and enablers of deprescribing: A systematic review. *Drugs and Aging*, *30*(10), 793–807.

Schroy, P. C., Mylvaganam, S., & Davidson, P. (2014). Provider perspectives on the utility of a colorectal cancer screening decision aid for facilitating shared decision making. *Health Expectations*, *17*(1), 27–35.

Uy, V., May, S. G., Tietbohl, C., et al. (2014). Barriers and facilitators to routine distribution of patient decision support interventions: a preliminary study in community-based primary care settings. *Health Expectations*, *17*(3), 353–364.

Decisional Conflict

Dawn Fairlie, ANP, FNP, GNP, DNS(c)

NANDA-I

Definition

Uncertainty about course of action to be taken when choice among competing actions involves risk, loss, or challenge to values and beliefs

Defining Characteristics

Delay in decision-making; distress while attempting a decision; physical sign of distress (e.g., increase in heart rate, restlessness); physical sign of tension; questioning of moral principle while attempting a decision; questioning of moral rule while attempting a decision; questioning of moral values while attempting a decision; questioning of personal beliefs while attempting a decision; questioning of personal values while attempting a decision; recognizes undesired consequences of actions being considered; self-focused; uncertainty about choices; vacillating among choices

Related Factors (r/t)

Conflict with moral obligation; conflicting information sources; inexperience with decision-making; insufficient information; insufficient support system; interference in decision-making; moral principle supports mutually inconsistent actions; moral rule supports mutually inconsistent actions; moral value supports mutually inconsistent actions; perceived threat to value system; unclear personal beliefs unclear personal values

NOC (Nursing Outcomes Classification)

Suggested NOC Outcomes

Decision-Making; Information Processing; Participation in Health Care Decisions; Personal Autonomy

Example NOC Outcome with Indicators

Decision-Making as evidenced by the following indicators: Identifies relevant information/Identifies alternatives/Identifies potential consequences of each alternative/Identifies needed resources to support each alternative. (Rate the outcome and indicators of **Decision-Making:** 1 = severely compromised, 2 = substantially compromised, 3 = moderately compromised, 4 = mildly compromised, 5 = not compromised [see Section I].)

Client Outcomes

Client Will (Specify Time Frame)

- State the advantages and disadvantages of choices
- Share fears and concerns regarding choices and responses of others
- Seek resources and information necessary for making an informed choice
- Make an informed choice

NIC (Nursing Interventions Classification)

Suggested NIC Intervention

Decision-Making Support

Example NIC Activities—Decision-Making Support

Inform client of alternative views or solutions in a clear and supportive manner; Provide information requested by client

Nursing Interventions and *Rationales*

- Observe for factors causing or contributing to conflict (e.g., value conflicts, fear of outcome, poor problem-solving skills). EBN: *When studying clients with prostate cancer, Chien et al (2014) found that different treatments may cause conflicts in treatment decision-making and that decisional conflict improved over time. Additionally, education level, decision preferences, and psychosocial adjustment were associated with decisional conflict. They concluded that nurses must provide clients with adequate information and psychosocial intervention to reduce decisional conflict.*
- Provide emotional support. EB: *Knops et al (2013) evaluated associations between decisional conflict and emotions and found a decrease in decisional conflict leads to less decision postponing behavior and anxiety.* EB: *Decisional conflict was assessed using the Decisional Conflict Scale (DCS) among pregnant women considering antidepressant medication treatment. Although many pregnant women facing decisions regarding the use of antidepressant medication experience decisional conflict, their decisions were facilitated by interpersonal supports, and emotional support reduced decisional conflict and facilitated the decision-making process (Walton et al, 2014).*
- Use decision aids or computer-based decision aids to assist clients in making decisions. EB: *A Cochrane review of decision aids (pamphlets, videos, or Web-based tools) concluded that use of decision aids fosters a positive effect on communication with health care providers and influenced the time required for the*

consultation. Additionally, there was an improvement with more detailed decision aids when compared to simpler decision aids, and both were better than usual care (Stacey et al, 2011). EB: *A randomized trial of a decision aid for CHD adherence was conducted by Sheridan et al (2014), who reported that most participants found the decision aid easy to use and easy to understand. Participants reported improvement in personalization of information and that the decision aid helped them to decide what was important to them.*

- Initiate health teaching and referrals when needed. EBN: *A prospective cross-sectional study of Australian women with early breast cancer reported that many women experienced post treatment distress requiring referral for psychological assessment and long term support (Budden et al, 2014). They concluded that individualized decision support interventions by nurses can help to identify women at risk and refer them to specialist services.*
- Facilitate communication between the client and family members regarding the final decision; offer support to the person actually making the decision. EBN: *A study of surrogate decision-makers' decisional conflict with end of life decision-making found that surrogates who had discussed end of life preferences with their loved one experienced less decisional conflict than those who had not discussed preferences (Fairlie, 2014).*

Geriatric

- Carefully assess clients with dementia regarding ability to make decisions. EBN: *A study of the shared decision-making process of persons with dementia identified a broad spectrum of the shared decision-making process. Results indicated that not all persons with dementia are excluded from participating in the decision-making process (Miller et al, 2014).*
- Support previous wishes for clients with dementia. EBN: *Educational level, commitment of nursing personnel and organizational culture influences participation in care by clients with dementia. Client participation was described as letting the clients make their own decisions, adjusting the choices, making decisions on behalf of the residents Client participation was regarded as being grounded in the idea that being master of one's own life is essential to the dignity and self-esteem of all people (Helgesen et al, 2014).*
- Discuss the purpose of advance directives such as a living well or medical power of attorney. EB: *A Swedish study compared attitudes and knowledge about the implantable cardioverter defibrillator (ICD) to determine how well HF clients could participate in end-of-life decisions. Whether to deactivate an ICD at end-of-life was queried. Clients with an ICD were not prepared to engage in shared decision-making about their ICD and its use at the end-of-life (Strömberg et al, 2014).* EB: *A systematic review of advance care planning (ACP) interventions that included communication about end-of-life care increased the completion of advance directives was performed by Houben et al (2014). They found that communication about ACP improved concordance between preferences for care and delivered care and may improve other outcomes, such as quality of communication. Additionally, ACP interventions increase the completion of advance directives, occurrence of discussions about ACP, concordance between preferences for care and delivered care, and are likely to improve other outcomes for clients and their loved ones in different adult populations.*

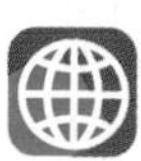

Multicultural

- Assess for the influence of cultural beliefs, norms, and values on the client's decision-making conflict. EB: *A study of two hundred sixty-six parents of children with a life-threatening illness (Knapp et al, 2014) investigated how decisional conflict varies among racial and ethnic subgroups. Analyses suggest that minority parents report less effective decision-making and report less support in decision-making compared to white, non-Hispanic parents and concluded that significant differences exist by race, ethnicity, language. It is important to address these differences when creating clinical care plans, engaging in shared decision-making, and creating interventions to alleviate decisional conflict.* EB: *African American men with prostate cancer were encouraged to discuss screening alternatives with health care providers for informed decision-making (IDM). The intervention significantly promoted IDM among men who reported more education, being married, having financial resources, and younger age (Sultan et al, 2014).*
- Provide support for client's decision-making. EBN: *Decision aids are intended to help people participate in decisions that involve weighing the benefits and harms of treatment options often with scientific uncertainty. Stacey et al (2014) concluded that there is high-quality evidence that decision aids improve client's knowledge regarding options and reduce decisional conflict.*
- Use cross-cultural decision aids when possible to enhance an informed decision-making process. EB: *Ko et al (2014) studied cultural and linguistic adaptation of a multimedia colorectal cancer screening Decision Aid for Spanish-Speaking Latinos. They concluded that new interventions that address the needs of diverse*

U.S. populations are needed to reduce health disparities. Additionally they noted the importance of adapting English-language health interventions to facilitate communication and decision-making.

Home Care

- The interventions described previously may be adapted for home care use.
- ▲ Before providing any home care, assess the client plan for advance directives (living will and power of attorney). If a plan exists, place a copy in the client file. If no plan exists, offer information on advance directives according to agency policy. Refer for assistance in completing advance directives as necessary. Do not witness a living will. *This is a legal requirement of the Consolidated Omnibus Budget Reconciliation Act (COBRA, 2009).*
- Assess the client and family for consensus (or lack thereof) regarding the issue in conflict. EB: *Miller et al (2014) reviewed empirical findings concerning the decision-making process of persons with dementia and their family caregivers and focused on the extent of involvement of persons with decision-making responsibility. They found that some families include persons with dementia in the decision-making, but cautioned that there is a broad view of what shared decision-making in dementia entails.*
- Refer to care plan for **Anxiety** as indicated.

Client/Family Teaching and Discharge Planning

- Instruct the client and family members to provide advance directives in the following areas:
  - Person to contact in an emergency
  - Preference (if any) to die at home or in the hospital
  - Desire to initiate advanced directives, such as a living will or medical power of attorney
  - Desire to donate an organ
  - Funeral arrangements (i.e., burial, cremation)
- ▲ EBN: *Shared decision makers experienced less decisional conflict when they had discussed the client's preferences with the client (Fairlie, 2014).*
- Inform the family of treatment options; encourage and defend self-determination. EB: *Weeks et al (2014) identified three phases of decision-making when clients with cancer consider complementary and alternative medicine (CAM) modalities. They noted that each phase involves different patterns of information-seeking and evaluation. They concluded that treatment choices are guided by beliefs, values, and other social and cultural norms and that clients frequently need help with discussing and prioritizing treatment decisions.*
- Recognize and allow the client to discuss the selection of complementary therapies available, such as spiritual support, relaxation, imagery, exercise, lifestyle changes, diet (e.g., macrobiotic, vegetarian), and nutritional supplementation. EB: *Weeks et al (2014) reported that clients with cancer frequently report anxiety and conflict surrounding CAM treatment. They found that decisions about CAM by clients with cancer is a complex, dynamic, nonlinear process and found increased levels of conflict and anxiety for clients who consider CAM as a part of their cancer care.*
- ▲ Provide the Physician Orders for Life-Sustaining Treatment (POLST) form for clients and families faced with end-of-life choices across the health care continuum. CEB: *The POLST form ensures that end-of-life choices can be implemented in all settings, from the home through the health care continuum. The POLST form was congruent with residents' existing advance directives for health care (Meyers et al, 2004).*

REFERENCES

Budden, L. M., Hayes, B. A., & Buettner, P. G. (2014). Women's decision satisfaction and psychological distress following early breast cancer treatment: a treatment decision support role for nurses. *International Journal of Nursing Practice*, *20*(1), 8–16.

Chien, C. H., Chuang, C. K., Liu, K. L., et al. (2014). Changes in decisional conflict and decisional regret in patients with localised prostate cancer. *Journal of Clinical Nursing*.

COBRA. *The Consolidated Omnibus Budget Reconciliation Act*. Retrieved April 15, 2009, from: <http://www.dol.gov/dol/topic/health-plans/cobra.htm>.

Fairlie, D. (2014). *Does end of life terminology influence decisional conflict in surrogate decision makers?* (Doctoral dissertation, CUNY GRADUATE CENTER).

Helgesen, A. K., Larsson, M., & Athlin, E. (2014). Patient participation in special care units for persons with dementia: A losing principle? *Nursing Ethics*, *21*(1), 108–118. [Epub 2013 Jun 21].

Houben, C. H., Spruit, M. A., Groenen, M. T., et al. (2014). Efficacy of advance care planning: a systematic review and meta-analysis. *Journal of the American Medical Directors Association*, *15*(7), 477–489. [Epub 2014 Mar 2].

Knapp, C., Sberna-Hinojosa, M., Baron-Lee, J., et al. (2014). Does Decisional Conflict Differ Across Race and Ethnicity Groups? A Study of Parents Whose Children Have A Life-Threatening Illness. *Journal of Palliative Medicine*, *17*(5), 559–567.

Knops, A. M., Goossens, A., Ubbink, D. T., et al. (2013). Interpreting Patient Decisional Conflict Scores Behavior and Emotions in

Decisions about Treatment. *Medical Decision Making, 33*(1), 78–84.

Ko, L. K., Reuland, D., Jolles, M., et al. (2014). Cultural and linguistic adaptation of a multimedia colorectal cancer screening decision aid for Spanish-speaking Latinos. *Journal of Health Communication, 19*(2), 192–209.

Meyers, J. L., et al. (2004). Physician orders for life-sustaining treatment form: honoring end-of-life directives for nursing home residents. *Journal of Gerontological Nursing, 30*(9), 37–46.

Miller, L. M., Whitlatch, C. J., & Lyons, K. S. (2014). Shared decision-making in dementia: A review of patient and family carer involvement. *Dementia (Basel, Switzerland)*, 1471301214555542.

Sheridan, S. L., Draeger, L. B., Pignone, M. P., et al. (2014). The effect of a decision aid intervention on decision making about coronary heart disease risk reduction: secondary analyses of a randomized trial. *BMC Medical Informatics and Decision Making, 14*(1), 14.

Stacey, D., Bennett, C. L., Barry, M. J., et al. (2011). Decision aids for people facing health treatment or screening decisions. *Cochrane Database of Systematic Reviews, 10*(10).

Stacey, D., Légaré, F., Col, N. F., et al. (2014). Decision aids for people facing health treatment or screening decisions. *The Cochrane Library*.

Strömberg, A., Thylén, I., & Moser, D. (2014). Shared Decision-Making about End-of-Life Care for Heart Failure Patients with an Implantable Cardioverter Defibrillator: A National Cohort Study. *Journal of Cardiac Failure, 20*(8), S11.

Sultan, D. H., Rivers, B. M., Osongo, B. O., et al. (2014). Affecting African American Men's Prostate Cancer Screening Decision-making through a Mobile Tablet-Mediated Intervention. *Journal of Health Care for the Poor and Underserved, 25*(3), 1262.

Walton, G. D., Ross, L. E., Stewart, D. E., et al. (2014). Decisional conflict among women considering antidepressant medication use in pregnancy. *Archives of women's mental health, 17*(6), 493–501.

Weeks, L., Balneaves, L. G., Paterson, C., et al. (2014). Decision-making about complementary and alternative medicine by cancer patients: integrative literature review. *Open Medicine, 8*(2), e54.

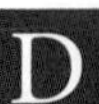

Ineffective Denial

Julianne E. Doubet, BSN, RN, CEN, NREMT-P

NANDA-I

Definition

Conscious or unconscious attempt to disavow the knowledge or meaning of an event to reduce anxiety and/or fear, leading to the detriment of health

Defining Characteristics

Delays seeking health care; denies fear of death; denies fear of invalidism; displaces fear of impact of the condition; displaces source of symptoms; does not admit impact of disease on life; does not perceive relevance of danger; does not perceive relevance of symptoms; inappropriate affect; minimizes symptoms; refusal of health care; use of dismissive gestures when speaking of distressing event; use of dismissive comments when speaking of distressing event; use of treatment not advised by health care professional

Related Factors (r/t)

Anxiety; excessive stress; fear of death; fear of loss of autonomy; fear of separation; ineffective coping strategies; insufficient emotional support insufficient sense of control; perceived inadequacy in dealing with strong emotions; threat of unpleasant reality

NOC (Nursing Outcomes Classification)

Suggested NOC Outcomes

Acceptance: Health Status; Anxiety Self-Control; Health Beliefs: Perceived Threat; Symptom Control

Example NOC Outcome with Indicators

Anxiety Self-Control as evidenced by the following indicators: Eliminates precursors of anxiety/Monitors physical manifestations of anxiety/Controls anxiety response. (Rate the outcome and indicators of **Anxiety Self-Control:** 1 = never demonstrated, 2 = rarely demonstrated, 3 = sometimes demonstrated, 4 = often demonstrated, 5 = consistently demonstrated [see Section I].)

Client Outcomes

Client Will (Specify Time Frame)

- Seek out appropriate health care attention when needed
- Use home remedies only when appropriate

- Display appropriate affect and verbalize fears
- Actively engage in treatment program related to identified "substance" of abuse
- Remain substance-free
- Demonstrate alternate adaptive coping mechanism

NIC (Nursing Interventions Classification)

Suggested NIC Intervention

Anxiety Reduction

Example NIC Activities—Anxiety Reduction

Use a calm, reassuring approach; Stay with the patient to promote safety and reduce fear

Nursing Interventions and *Rationales*

- Assess the client's and family's understanding of the illness, the treatments, and expected outcomes. EBN: *Effective communication between client and health care provider in relation to health promotion, disease prevention, and disease management is key to optimal health outcomes (Heinrich & Karner, 2011).* EB: *Communication difficulties in health care may arise when health care providers concentrate on the client's diseases and its management, but fail to take into consideration the client's lifestyle and feelings about health problems (Gaulden et al, 2012).*
- Allow client time for adjustment to his/her situation. EBN: *Thoughtful contemplation of life expectancy and end-of-life care are vital for clients to ensure their continued optimum quality of life (Walczak et al, 2014).*
- Aid the client in making choices regarding treatment and actively involve him or her in the decision-making process. EBN: *Current focus is on the person as the primary decision-maker in his/her health care and is apropos in relation to the key concept of quality of life, as defined by the person or community and expressed in the nursing theory of Human Becoming (Poirier, 2012).*
- Allow the client to express and use denial as a coping mechanism if appropriate to treatment. EB: *Sirri and Grandi (2012) suggest that those assessing a client who suffers illness denial, should bear in mind that denial may sometimes preclude patients from suffering overwhelming psychological and emotional distress as a result of a life-threatening or stigmatizing diagnosis.*
- Support the client's spiritual coping measures. EBN: *According to Baldacchino et al (2013), spiritual, though not necessarily religious, coping, may enhance adjustment of clients to their chronic illnesses.*
- Develop a trusting, therapeutic relationship with the client/family. EBN: *According to Dinc and Gastmans (2013), in their study of the literature focusing on nurse-patient relationships, nurses' professional expertise and interpersonal caring qualities were essential in developing trust; however, a combination of factors could hamper that trusting relationship.*
- Assist the client in using existing and additional sources of support. EBN: *Health care providers should recognize the individual's needs, including emotional, psychosocial, sexual, and relational, of those who suffer from chronic illness and provide suitable information and support, especially for those who are isolated from the mainstream (Spring et al, 2011).*
- Refer to care plans for Defensive **Coping** and Dysfunctional **Family** processes.

Geriatric

- Allow the client to explain his/her concepts of their health care needs, then use reality-focused techniques whenever possible to provide feedback. EB: *Clients should be made conscious of the fact that primary medical treatment, even when associated with a positive prognosis, does not in and of itself predict how well clients will fare during their lifetime (Linden et al, 2014).*
- Encourage communication among family members. EBN: *This study testifies to the importance of the mutual influences of patient, family, and nurse during a critical illness and supports the inclusion of family in all facets of their loved one's care (Cypress, 2011).*
- Recognize denial and be aware that grieving may prolong denial. EBN: *Nurses should understand the importance of reconciliation in the grief process and provide professional, empathetic care (Gustafsson et al, 2011).*

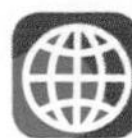

Multicultural

- Assess for the influence of cultural beliefs, norms, and values involved in the client's understanding of and ability to acknowledge health status. EB: *Lee and Mason (2014) suggest that health care practitioners should develop programs that include ethnic- and gender-specific components, which, in turn, will aid older adults in coping with the stress caused by illness.*
- Discuss with the client those aspects of his/her health behavior/lifestyle that will remain unchanged by health status and those aspects of health behavior that need to be modified to improve health status. EBN: *"Culturally sensitive interventions are required to ensure people of culturally and linguistically diverse backgrounds have the appropriate skills to self-manage their complex medical conditions," Williams et al (2014).*
- Assess the role of fatalism in the client's ability to acknowledge health status. EB: *Some minorities, due to cultural factors (e.g., fatalism, medical mistrust), have negative attitudes toward health care interventions: targeting these cultural issues may help reduce undertreatment of minorities (Lin et al, 2014).*

Home Care

- Previously mentioned interventions may be adapted for home care utilization.
- Observe family interaction and roles. Refer the client/family for follow-up if prolonged denial is a risk. EBN: *A study by Benkel et al (2012) indicates that there is a connection between the loved one's understanding of a fatal disease and the caregiver's ability to cope.*
- Encourage communication between family members, particularly when dealing with the loss of a significant person. EBN: *Nurses should offer support and comfort to those who have lost a loved one and through empathetic communication: observe for nonverbal clues and the need for further interventions (Reid et al, 2011).*

Client/Family Teaching and Discharge Planning

- Instruct client and family to recognize the signs and symptoms of recurring illness and the appropriate responses to alteration in client's health status. EBN: *It has been found that patients and their families are commonly confused after hospital emergency department release about aftercare based on their discharge instructions; follow-up phone calls may be of some benefit to address educational needs (Zavala & Shaeffer, 2011).*
- Consider the client's belief in and use of complementary therapies in self-managing his/her disease. EBN: *No matter what other care is provided, nurses should support any program type that genuinely makes a difference for the client and his/her family (Madden, 2014).*
- Teach family members that denial may continue throughout the adjustment to treatment and they should not be confrontational. EB: *Losses come with progressing years and may dictate interpersonal and selfish readjustments to relationships, occupations, and avocations: the use of denial as a defense mechanism may play a significant role in these situations (Clemens, 2014).*

▲ Inform family of available community support resources. EBN: *The nurse will come in contact with family caregivers who are striving to keep their loved one at home, but find that physical, emotional, and monetary burdens necessitate an intervention to tap into targeted support (Schrauf, 2011).*

REFERENCES

See defensive **Coping** for additional references.

Baldacchino, D., Torskenaes, K., Kalfoss, M., et al. (2013). Spiritual coping in rehabilitation—a comparative study: part 2. *British Journal of Nursing, 11*, 402–408.

Benkel, I., Wijk, H., & Molander, U. (2012). Hospital staff opinions concerning loved ones' understanding of the patient's life-limiting disease and the loved ones' need for support. *Journal of Palliative Medicine, 15*(51–55), 2012.

Clemens, N. A. (2014). On letting go: with age comes renunciation. *Journal of Psychiatric Practice, 20*, 370–372.

Cypress, B. (2011). The lived ICU experience of nurses, patients and family members: a phenomenological study with Merleau-Pontian perspective. *Intensive and Critical Care Nursing, 27*, 278–280.

Dinc, L., & Gastmans, C. (2013). Trust in nurse-patient relationships: a literature review. *Nursing Ethics, 20*, 501–516.

Gaulden, C. M., Jorgenson, J., Sadigh, G. I., et al. (2012). Interventions for providers to promote a patient-centered approach in clinical consultations. *Cochrane Data Base of Systemic Reviews, 12*, 12.

Gustafsson, L. K., Wiklund-Gustin, L., & Lindstrom, U. A. (2011). The meaning of reconciliation: women's stories about their experience of reconciliation with suffering from grief. *Scandinavian Journal of Caring Science, 25*, 525–532.

Heinrich, C., & Karner, K. (2011). Ways to optimize understanding health related information: the patients' perspective. *Geriatric Nursing, 32*, 29–38.

Lee, H., & Mason, D. (2014). Cultural and gender differences in coping strategies between Caucasian Americans Korean American older people. *Journal of Cross-cultural Gerontology, 27*.

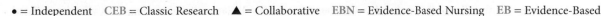

Lin, J. J., Mhango, G., Wall, M. M., et al. (2014). Cultural factors associated with disparities in lung cancer care. *Annals of the American Thoracic Society, 11*, 489–495.

Linden, W., MacKenzie, R., Rnic, K., et al. (2014). Emotional adjustment over 1 year post-diagnosis on patients with cancer: understanding and predicting adjustment trajectories. *Supportive Care in Cancer, 1*.

Madden, R. (2014). A nurse's journey into complimentary therapies. *Nursing News, 38*, 5.

Poirier, P. A. (2012). Human becoming: transcending the now to explore the possibilities in health policy. *Nursing Science Quarterly, 25*, 104–110.

Reid, M., McDowell, J., & Hoskins, R. (2011). Communicating news of a patient's death to relatives. *British Journal of Nursing, 20*, 737–742.

Schrauf, C. (2011). Factors that influence state policies for caregivers of patients with chronic kidney disease and how to impact them. *Nephrology Nursing Journal, 38*, 395–403.

Sirri, L., & Grandi, S. (2012). Illness behavior. *Advances in Psychosomatic Medicine, 32*, 160–181.

Spring, A., Cudney, S., Weinert, C., et al. (2011). Spousal support experiences of rural women living with chronic illness. *Holistic Nursing Practice, 25*, 71–75.

Walczak, A., Buton, P. N., Clayton, J. M., et al. (2014). Discussing prognosis and end of life care in the final year of life: a randomized trial of nurse-led communication support programme for patients. *BMJ Open, 4*, e005745.

Williams, A., Manias, E., Cross, W., et al. (2014). Motivational interviewing to explore culturally and linguistically diverse people's co-morbidity medication self efficacy. *Journal of Clinical Nursing, 30*.

Zavala, S., & Shaffer, C. (2011). Do patients understand discharge instructions? *Journal of Emergency Nursing, 37*, 138–140.

Impaired Dentition

Betty J. Ackley, MSN, EdS, RN

NANDA-I

Definition

Disruption in tooth development/eruption patterns or structural integrity of individual teeth

Defining Characteristics

Abraded teeth; absence of teeth; dental caries; enamel discoloration; erosion of enamel; excessive oral calculus; excessive oral plaque; facial asymmetry; halitosis; incomplete tooth eruption for age; loose tooth; malocclusion; premature loss of primary teeth; root caries; tooth fracture; tooth misalignment; toothache

Related Factors (r/t)

Barriers to self-care, bruxism; chronic vomiting, difficulty accessing dental care; economically disadvantaged; excessive intake of fluoride; excessive use of abrasive oral cleaning agents; genetic predisposition; habitual use of staining substance (e.g., coffee, red wine, tea, tobacco); insufficient dietary habits; insufficient knowledge of dental health; insufficient oral hygiene; malnutrition; oral temperature sensitivity; pharmaceutical agent

NOC (Nursing Outcomes Classification)

Suggested NOC Outcomes

Oral Health

Example NOC Outcome with Indicators

Oral Health as evidenced by the following indicators: Cleanliness of teeth/Cleanliness of gums/Cleanliness of dentures/Tongue integrity/Gum integrity. (Rate the outcome and indicators of **Oral Health:** 1 = severely compromised, 2 = substantially compromised, 3 = moderately compromised, 4 = mildly compromised, 5 = not compromised [see Section I].)

Client Outcomes

Client Will (Specify Time Frame)

- Have clean teeth, healthy pink gums
- Be free of halitosis
- Explain how to perform oral care
- Demonstrate ability to masticate foods without difficulty
- State free of pain in mouth

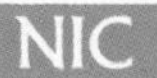

(Nursing Interventions Classification)

Suggested NIC Interventions

Oral Health Maintenance; Oral Health Promotion; Oral Health Restoration

Example NIC Activities—Oral Health Maintenance

Establish a mouth care routine; Arrange for dental check-ups as needed

D

Nursing Interventions and *Rationales*

- ▲ Inspect oral cavity/teeth at least once daily and note any discoloration, presence of debris, amount of plaque buildup, presence of lesions such as white lesions or patches, edema, or bleeding, and intactness of teeth. Refer to a dentist or periodontist as appropriate. *Systematic inspection can identify impending problems. White lesions are often leukoplakia, which is a precursor to squamous cell carcinoma. If the lesion is cancerous, prompt treatment is needed (Engelke & Pravikoff, 2010).*
- If the client is free of bleeding disorders and is able to swallow, encourage the client to brush teeth with a soft toothbrush using fluoride-containing toothpaste at least two times per day. Do not use foam swabs or lemon glycerin swabs to clean the teeth. EB: *Oral bacteria cause caries and periodontal disease. Plaque is a biofilm of bacteria, which often becomes contaminated with antibiotic-resistant bacteria in the hospitalized client (Roberts & Mullany, 2010).* CEB: *The toothbrush is the most important tool for oral care; toothbrushing is the most effective method of reducing plaque and controlling periodontal disease; a nursing study demonstrated that foam swabs are not effective in removing plaque (Pearson & Hutton, 2002). Lemon glycerin swabs dry the oral mucosa and can erode the tooth enamel (Foss-Durant & McAffee, 1997; Meurman et al, 1996; Poland, 1987). Inspect the gingiva for signs of gingivitis. Normally the gums should be pink and firm; gingivitis is likely when the gums are red and loose. Bleeding from the gums in an indication of gingivitis, and the client should see a dentist (Bissett, 2011).*
- Encourage the client to floss the teeth at least once per day if free of a bleeding disorder, or if the client is unable, floss the teeth for the client. EB: *A Cochrane review found that there is some evidence that flossing in addition to toothbrushing reduces gingivitis compared to toothbrushing alone. Also, there is some evidence that flossing plus toothbrushing may be associated with a small reduction in plaque at 1 and 3 months (Sambunjak et al, 2011).*
- Use a rotation-oscillation power toothbrush for removal of dental plaque. EB: *Multiple studies have found a rotation-oscillation power toothbrush more effective than an ultrasonic toothbrush (Biesbrock et al, 2008; He et al, 2008; Williams et al, 2008). A systematic review found that the powered toothbrush was safe to use on both hard and soft dental tissues (Robinson, 2011).*
- Determine the client's mental status and manual dexterity; if the client is unable to care for self, nursing personnel must provide dental hygiene. The nursing diagnosis Bathing **Self-Care** deficit is then applicable.
- If the client is unable to brush own teeth, follow this procedure:

1. Position the client sitting upright or on side.
2. Use a soft bristle baby toothbrush.
3. Use fluoride toothpaste and tap water or saline as a solution.
4. Brush teeth in an up-and-down manner.
5. Suction as needed.

Each client must receive oral care including toothbrushing two times every day to maintain healthy teeth and mouth, and to prevent complications associated with periodontitis (the advanced form of gum disease that can cause tooth loss), which is associated with health problems such as cardiovascular disease, stroke, and bacterial pneumonia (ADA, 2015).

- Monitor the client's nutritional and fluid status to determine if adequate. Recommend the client eat a balanced diet and limit between-meal snacks. *Poor nutrition predisposes clients to dental disease (ADA, 2015).*
- Recommend the client stop or at least decrease intake of soft drinks. *Sugar-containing soft drinks can cause cavities, and the low pH of the drink can cause erosion in teeth (ADA, 2015).* EB: *A study demonstrated a much higher incidence of caries in children who drank soft drinks, as well as increased intake of processed foods (Llena & Forner, 2008).*

- Instruct the client with halitosis to clean the tongue when performing oral hygiene. Brush tongue with a tongue scraper or toothbrush and follow with a mouth rinse. EB: *A Cochrane review found that tongue cleaning was effective for short-term control of halitosis (Van der Sleen et al, 2010).*
- Determine the client's usual method of oral care. Whenever possible, build on the client's existing knowledge base and current practices to develop an individualized plan of care.
- Tell the client to direct the toothbrush at a 45-degree angle toward the tooth surfaces, not horizontally (ADA, 2015).
- Use an antimicrobial mouthwash as ordered or tap water or saline only for a mouth rinse. Avoid the use of hydrogen peroxide, or alcohol-based mouthwashes. *Some antimicrobial mouthwashes have demonstrated effective action in decreasing bacterial counts in plaque and decreasing gingivitis (ADA, 2015).* CEB: *Hydrogen peroxide can cause mucosal damage and is extremely foul tasting to clients (Tombes & Gallucci, 1993).*

▲ Recommend client see a dentist at prescribed intervals, generally two times per year if teeth are in satisfactory condition. *It is important to see a dentist at regular intervals for preventive dental care (ADA, 2015).*

▲ If there are any signs of bleeding when the teeth are brushed, refer the client to a dentist or, if obvious signs of inflamed gums, a periodontist. Bleeding along with halitosis is associated with gingivitis. *Beginning gingivitis can often be reversed with good oral hygiene; with more advanced cases a periodontist may be needed to correct the condition.* If platelet numbers are decreased, or if the client is edentulous, use moistened Toothettes or a specially made very soft toothbrush for oral care. *A regular toothbrush can cause soft tissue injury and bleeding in clients with low numbers of platelets.*

- Recognize that good dental care/oral care can be effective in preventing hospital acquired (or extended care acquired) pneumonia. CEB/EB: *Many references have found that dental/oral care was effective in preventing new onset of pneumonia (Arpin, 2009; Ishikawa et al 2008; Sarin et al, 2008).*
- Provide scrupulous dental care to critically ill clients, including ventilated clients to prevent ventilator-associated pneumonia. EB/EBN: *Numerous studies have demonstrated decreased incidence of ventilator-associated pneumonia with good oral care (Fields, 2008; Panchabhai et al, 2009).*
- If teeth are nonfunctional for chewing, modification of oral intake (e.g., edentulous diet, soft diet) may be necessary. The nursing diagnosis imbalanced **Nutrition:** less than body requirements may apply.
- If the client is unable to swallow, keep suction nearby when providing oral care.
- See care plan for impaired **Oral Mucous Membrane.**

Pregnant Client

- Encourage the expectant mother to eat a healthy, balanced diet that is rich in calcium. The teeth usually start to form in the gums during the second trimester of pregnancy. *To encourage the development of good, strong teeth, expectant mothers should eat a healthy, balanced diet that is rich in calcium (ADA, 2015).*
- Advise the pregnant mother not to smoke. CEB: *Maternal smoking during pregnancy has been associated with increased caries in the teeth of the child (Iida et al, 2007).*
- Advise the expectant mother to practice good care of her teeth, to protect her child's teeth once born. *Dental caries in children are associated with high levels of* Streptococcus mutans. *This bacterium is commonly spread from the mother with infected teeth to the infant by tasting of food and sharing of utensils once the child is born (Kagihara et al, 2009).*

Infant Oral Hygiene

- Gently wipe baby's gums with a clean washcloth or sterile gauze at least once a day. *Wiping gums prevents bacterial buildup in the mouth.*
- Never allow the child to fall asleep with a bottle containing milk, formula, fruit juice, or sweetened liquids. If the child needs a comforter between regular feedings, at night, or during naps, fill a bottle with cool water or give the child a clean pacifier recommended by the dentist or health care provider. Never give child a pacifier dipped in any sweet liquid. Avoid filling child's bottle with liquids such as sugar water and soft drinks. *Decay occurs when sweetened liquids such as milk, formula, and fruit juice are given and are left clinging to an infant's teeth for long periods. Bacteria in the mouth use these sugars as food to produce acids that attack the teeth (ADA, 2015; Kagihara et al, 2009).*

▲ When multiple teeth appear, brush with small toothbrush with small (pea-size) amount of fluoride toothpaste. Recommend that child either use a fluoride gel or fluoride varnish. *Use of topical fluoride (mouth rinses, gels, or varnishes) in addition to toothpaste containing fluoride resulted in a modest reduction of cavity formation versus use of fluoride toothpaste only (Marinho et al, 2003).*

- Advise parents to begin dental visits at 1 year of age. Caries and infection of the first set of teeth have been associated with problems of alignment of permanent teeth, difficulty chewing, problems speaking, sleeping, concentrating, and learning, as well as problems with self-esteem (*Kagihara et al, 2009*).

D

Older Children

▲ Encourage the family to talk with the dentist about dental sealants, which can help prevent cavities in permanent teeth. EB: *A Cochrane review found that use of dental sealants on the molars of children was effective in preventing caries (Ahovuo-Saloranta et al, 2008).*

- Teach to brush teeth twice a day. EB: *Twice daily tooth brushing is a low-cost, effective strategy to reduce the risk of childhood caries (Huebner & Milgrom, 2015).*
- Recommend the child use dental floss to help prevent gum disease. The dentist will give guidelines on when to start using floss.
- Recommend to parents that they not permit the child to smoke or chew tobacco, and stress the importance of setting a good example by not using tobacco products themselves.
- Recommend the child drink fluoridated water when possible. Fluoride in drinking water is one of several available fluoride resources. *The American Dental Association strongly endorses use of fluoridated water, based on scientific research that validates the effectiveness in preventing cavities (ADA, 2015).* EB: *Community water fluoridation remains an effective public health strategy for delivering fluoride to prevent tooth decay and is the most feasible and cost-effective strategy for reaching entire communities (U.S. Department of Health & Human Services Federal Panel on Community Water Fluoridation, 2015).*
- Recommend the child use toothpaste containing fluoride. EB: *A Cochrane study demonstrated that use of fluoride toothpaste was effective in preventing caries in children and adolescents when compared to placebo (Walsh et al, 2010).*

Geriatric

- Provide dentists with accurate medication history to avoid drug interactions and client harm. If the client is taking anticoagulants, the INR should be reviewed before providing dental care.
- Help clients brush own teeth, or provide dental care after breakfast and before bed every day. *If the client lacks dexterity in hands, consider use of a toothbrush by embedding the handle in foam tubing. Also consider use of a powered toothbrush because it has a larger handle (Bissett, 2011).*
- If the client has dementia or delirium and exhibits care-resistant behavior such as fighting, biting, or refusing care, use the following method:

1. Ensure client is in a quiet environment such as own bathroom, sitting or standing at the sink to prime memory for appropriate actions.
2. Approach the client at eye level within his/her range of vision.
3. Approach with a smile, and begin conversation with a touch of the hand and gradually move up.
4. Use mirror-mirror technique, standing behind the client, and brush and floss teeth.
5. Use respectful adult speech, not elderspeak/sing song voice, calling "deary," "honey," or the like. *Elderspeak is a documented trigger for care-resistant behavior (Herman & Williams, 2009).*
6. Promote self-care when client brushes own teeth if possible.
7. Use distractors when needed, singing, talking, reminiscing, or use of a teddy bear.

▲ EBN: *Use of specific techniques can decrease the fear-evoked response to nursing care, and increase the effectiveness of nurses providing oral care to clients (Jablonski et al, 2011).*

▲ Ensure that dentures are removed and cleaned regularly, preferably after every meal and before bedtime. Soak dentures at night in cold water. Dentures left in the mouth at night impede circulation to the palate and predispose the client to oral lesions. EB: *A Cochrane review found a lack of evidence about the effectiveness of the different denture cleaning methods considered including chemical and mechanical methods of cleaning (de Souza et al, 2009).*

▲ Support other caregivers providing oral hygiene. Physical and cognitive impairment in older adults can interfere with the client's ability to perform oral hygiene, and oral hygiene should be provided by a caregiver. If no caregiver is available, the client is prone to dental problems such as dental caries, tooth abscess, tooth fracture, and gingival and periodontal disease.

D

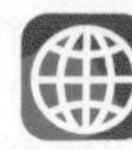

Multicultural

- Assess for the influence of cultural beliefs, norms, and values on the client's understanding of dental care. EBN: *What the client considers normal and abnormal dental care may be based on cultural perceptions (Giger & Davidhizar, 2008).*
- Assess for barriers to access to dental care, such as lack of insurance. *Children from racial minority groups may have significantly more difficulty in accessing dental care (Savage et al, 2004).* CEB: *African Americans and persons of lower socioeconomic status reported more new dental symptoms, were less likely to obtain dental care, and reported more tooth loss (Gilbert et al, 2003).*

Home Care

- Assess client patterns for daily and professional dental care and related patterns (e.g., smoking, nail biting). Assess for environmental influences on dental status (e.g., fluoride).
- Assess client facilities and financial resources for providing dental care. *Lack of appropriate facilities or financial resources is a barrier to positive dental care patterns. Provision for dental care may be missing from health care plans or unavailable to the uninsured.*
- Request dietary log from the client, adding column for type of food (i.e., soft, pureed, regular).
- Observe a typical meal to assess first-hand the impact of impaired dentition on nutrition. *Clients, especially older adults, are often hesitant to admit nutritional changes that may be embarrassing because of poor dentition.*
- Assist the client with accessing financial or other resources to support optimum dental and nutritional status.

Client/Family Teaching and Discharge Planning

- Teach how to inspect the oral cavity and monitor for problems with the teeth and gums.
- Teach how to implement a personal plan of dental hygiene, including appropriate brushing of teeth and tongue and use of dental floss. Utilize motivational interviewing to facilitate increased compliance in dental care. EB: *A study demonstrated improved dental hygiene with decreased amount of plaque when motivational interviewing was used as compared to a usual teaching session on dental care (Godard et al, 2011). A systematic review found motivational interviewing more effective in changing oral health than usual care (Watt, 2010). See Motivational Interviewing in Appendix C.*
- Advise the clients to change their toothbrush every 3 to 4 months, because after that toothbrushes are less effective in removing plaque and are a source of bacterial contamination of the mouth and teeth *(ADA, 2015).*
- Teach the client the value of having an optimal fluoride concentration in drinking water, and to brush teeth twice daily with toothpaste containing fluoride.
- Teach clients of all ages the need to decrease intake of sugary foods and to brush teeth regularly.
- Inform individuals who are considering tongue piercing of the potential complications such as chipping and cracking of teeth and possible trauma to the gingiva. If piercing is done, teach the client how to care for the wound and prevent complications. EB: *A study demonstrated that 74% of adolescents with tongue piercing had complications or alterations (Firoozmand et al, 2009). Another study demonstrated that gingival recession was associated with oral piercing (Slutzkey & Levin, 2008).*

REFERENCES

American Dental Association (ADA). *MouthHealthy: ADA's Award-Winning Consumer Website*, June 12, 2015. Retrieved, from: <http://www.ada.org/en/public-programs/mouthhealthy>.

Ahovuo-Saloranta, A., et al. (2008). Pit and fissure sealants for preventing dental decay in the permanent teeth of children and adolescents. *Cochrane Database of Systematic Reviews*, (4), CD001830.

Arpin, S. (2009). Oral hygiene in elderly people in hospitals and nursing homes. *Evidence-based Dentistry*, *10*(2), 46.

Biesbrock, A. R., Walters, P. A., & Bartizek, R. D. (2008). Plaque removal efficacy of an advanced rotation-oscillation power toothbrush versus a new sonic toothbrush. *American Journal of Dentistry*, *21*(3), 185–188.

Bissett, S. M. (2011). Guide to providing mouth care for older people. *Nursing Older People*, *23*(10), 14–21.

de Souza, R. F., et al. (2009). Interventions for cleaning dentures in adults. *Cochrane Database of Systematic Reviews*, (4), CD007395.

Engelke, A., & Pravikoff, D. *Leukoplakia, oral. Nursing reference center*, Oct 29, 2010, CINAHL nursing guide.

Fields, L. B. (2008). Oral care intervention to reduce incidence of ventilator-associated pneumonia in the neurologic intensive care unit. *The Journal of Neuroscience Nursing: Journal of the American Association of Neuroscience Nurses*, *40*(5), 291–298.

Firoozmand, L. M., Paschotto, D. R., & Almeida, J. D. (2009). Oral piercing complications among teenage students. *Oral Health and Preventive Dentistry, 7*(1), 77–81.

Foss-Durant, A. M., & McAffee, A. (1997). A comparison of three oral care products commonly used in practice. *Clinical Nursing Research, 6*, 1.

Giger, J., & Davidhizar, R. (2008). *Transcultural nursing: assessment and intervention* (5th ed.). St Louis: Mosby.

Gilbert, G. H., Duncan, R. P., & Shelton, B. J. (2003). Social determinants of tooth loss. *Health Services Research, 38*(6 Pt. 2).

Godard, A., Dufour, T., & Jeanne, S. (2011). Application of self-regulation theory and motivational interview for improving oral hygiene: a randomized controlled trial. *Journal of Clinical Periodontology, 38*(12), 1099–1105.

He, T., et al. (2008). A comparative clinical study of the plaque removal efficacy of an oscillating/rotating power toothbrush and an ultrasonic toothbrush. *The Journal of Clinical Dentistry, 19*(4), 138–142.

Herman, R., & Williams, K. (2009). Elderspeak's influence on resistiveness to care: focus on behavior events. *American Journal of Alzheimer's Disease and Other Dementias, 24*(5), 417–423.

Huebner, C., & Milgrom, P. (2015). Evaluation of a parent-designed programme to support tooth brushing of infants and young children. *International Journal of Dental Hygiene, 13*(1), 65–73. (29 ref).

Jablonski, R., Therrien, B., & Kolanowski, A. (2011). No more fighting and biting during mouth care: applying the theoretical constructs of threat perception to clinical practice. *Research and Theory for Nursing Practice, 25*(3), 163–175.

Iida, H., et al. (2007). Association between infant breastfeeding and early childhood caries in the United States. *Pediatrics, 120*(4), e944–e952.

Ishikawa, A., et al. (2008). Professional oral health care reduces the number of oropharyngeal bacteria. *Journal of Dental Research, 87*(6), 594–598.

Kagihara, L. E., Niederhauser, V. P., & Stark, M. (2009). Assessment, management, and prevention of early childhood caries. *Journal of the American Academy of Nurse Practitioners, 21*(1), 1–10.

Llena, C., & Forner, L. (2008). Dietary habits in a child population in relation to caries experience. *Caries Research, 42*(5), 387–393.

Marinho, V. C., et al. (2003). Fluoride toothpastes for preventing dental caries in children and adolescents. *Cochrane Database of Systematic Reviews*, (1), CD002278.

Meurman, J. H., et al. (1996). Hospital mouth-cleaning aids may cause dental erosion. *Special Care in Dentistry, 16*(6), 247–250.

Panchabhai, T. S., et al. (2009). Oropharyngeal cleansing with 0.2% chlorhexidine for prevention of nosocomial pneumonia in critically ill patients. *Chest, 135*(5), 1150–1156.

Pearson, L. S., & Hutton, J. L. (2002). A controlled trial to compare the ability of foam swabs and toothbrushes to remove dental plaque. *Journal of Advanced Nursing, 39*(5), 480.

Poland, J. M. (1987). Comparing Moi-Stir to lemon-glycerin swabs. *The American Journal of Nursing, 87*(4), 422.

Roberts, A. P., & Mullany, P. (2010). Oral biofilms, a reservoir of transferable bacterial antimicrobial resistance. *Expert Review of Anti-infective Therapy, 8*(12), 1441–1450.

Robinson, P. G. (2011). The safety of oscillating-rotating powered toothbrushes. *Evidence-based Dentistry, 12*(3), 69.

Sambunjak, D., et al. (2011). Flossing for the management of periodontal diseases and dental caries in adults. *Cochrane Database of Systematic Reviews*, (12), CD008829.

Sarin, J., et al. (2008). Reducing the risk of aspiration pneumonia among elderly patients in long-term care facilities through oral health interventions. *Journal of the American Medical Directors Association, 9*(2), 128–135.

Savage, M. F., et al. (2004). Early preventive dental visits: effects on subsequent utilization and costs. *Pediatrics, 114*(4), e418–e423.

Slutzkey, S., & Levin, L. (2008). Gingival recession in young adults: occurrence, severity, and relationship to past orthodontic treatment and oral piercing. *American Journal of Orthodontics and Dentofacial Orthopedics, 134*(5), 652–656.

Tombes, M. B., & Gallucci, B. (1993). The effects of hydrogen peroxide rinses on the normal oral mucosa. *Nursing Research, 42*, 332.

U.S. Department of Health & Human Services Federal Panel on Community Water Fluoridation (2015). *U.S. Public Health Service Recommendation for Fluoride Concentration in Drinking Water for the Prevention of Dental Caries*. Retrieved 2015 from: <http://www.publichealthreports.org/documents/PHS_2015_Fluoride_Guidelines.pdf>.

Van der Sleen, M. I., et al. (2010). Effectiveness of mechanical tongue cleaning on breath odour and tongue coating: a systematic review. *International Journal of Dental Hygiene, 8*(4), 258–268.

Walsh, T., et al. (2010). Fluoride toothpastes of different concentrations for preventing dental caries in children and adolescents. *Cochrane Database of Systematic Reviews*, (1), CD007868.

Watt, R. G. (2010). Motivational interviewing may be effective in dental setting. *Evidence-based Dentistry, 11*(1), 13.

Williams, K., et al. (2008). A study comparing the plaque removal efficacy of an advanced rotation-oscillation power toothbrush to a new sonic toothbrush. *The Journal of Clinical Dentistry, 19*(4), 154–158.

D

Risk for delayed Development

Marsha McKenzie, MA Ed, BSN, RN

NANDA-I

Definition

Vulnerable to delay of 25% or more in one or more of the areas of social or self-regulatory behavior, or in cognitive, language, gross, or fine motor skills, which may compromise health

Risk Factors

Prenatal

Economically disadvantaged; endocrine disorder; functional illiteracy; genetic disorder; infection; inadequate nutrition; insufficient prenatal care; late-term prenatal care; maternal age ≤15 years; maternal age ≥35 years; substance abuse; unplanned pregnancy; unwanted pregnancy

D

Individual

Behavior disorder (e.g., attention deficit, oppositional defiant); brain injury (e.g., abuse, accident hemorrhage, shaken baby syndrome); chronic illness; congenital disorder; failure to thrive; genetic disorder; hearing impairment; history of adoption; inadequate nutrition; involvement with the foster care system; lead poisoning; natural disaster; positive drug screen; prematurity; recurrent otitis media; seizure disorder; substance abuse; technology dependence (e.g., ventilator, augmentative communication); treatment regimen; visual impairment.

Environmental

Economically disadvantaged; exposure to violence

Caregiver

Learning disabilities; mental health issue (e.g., depression, psychosis, personality disorder, substance abuse); presence of abuse (e.g., physical, psychological, sexual)

NOC (Nursing Outcomes Classification)

Suggested NOC Outcomes

Abuse Recovery; Child Development: 1 Month, 2 Months, 4 Months, 6 Months, 12 Months, 2 Years, 3 Years, 4 Years, 5 Years, Middle Childhood, Adolescence; Development: Late Adulthood, Middle Adulthood, Young Adulthood; Knowledge: Parenting, Neglect Recovery

Example NOC Outcome with Indicators

Child Development as evidenced by the following indicators: Appropriate milestones of physical, cognitive, and psychosocial age-appropriate progression. (Rate the outcome and indicators of **Child Development:** 1 = never demonstrated, 2 = rarely demonstrated, 3 = sometimes demonstrated, 4 = often demonstrated, 5 = consistently demonstrated [see Section I].)

Client Outcomes

Client/Parents/Primary Caregiver Will (Specify Time Frame)

- Infant/Child/Adolescent will achieve expected milestones in all areas of development (physical, cognitive, and psychosocial)
- Parent/Caregiver will verbalize understanding of potential impediments to normal development and demonstrate actions or environmental/lifestyle changes necessary to provide appropriate care in a safe, nurturing environment

NIC (Nursing Interventions Classification)

Suggested NIC Interventions

Abuse Protection Support: Child; Caregiver Support; Developmental Enhancement: Child/Adolescent; Home Maintenance Assistance; Immunization/Vaccination Management; Infant Care; Kangaroo Care; Lactation Counseling; Learning Facilitation; Newborn Care; Newborn Monitoring; Nonnutritive Sucking; Normalization Promotion; Nutrition Management; Parent Education: Infant/Adolescent/Childbearing Family; Parenting Promotion; Referral; Risk Identification: Childbearing Family; Teaching: (Infant) Nutrition/Safety/Stimulation; (Toddler) Nutrition/Safety; Temperature Regulation (Infant); Therapeutic Play

Example NIC Activities—Parent Education: Childbearing Family

Instruct parent on normal physiological, emotional, and behavioral characteristics of child

Nursing Interventions and *Rationales*

Preconception/Pregnancy

- Assess for alcohol/drug use during pregnancy. Expectant mothers should be instructed that no amount of alcohol consumption is safe during pregnancy. EB: *Fetal alcohol syndrome (FAS) is thought to be the most preventable cause of mental retardation in the United States (Ethen et al, 2009).*

- Be aware of state legislation requiring mandatory reporting of maternal prenatal drug use. Be aware that mandatory reporting may further hamper prenatal care in that drug addicted mothers may delay or defer care for fear of legal action. EB: *Wu et al (2013) notes that fear of reporting drug use to authorities can create a "flight from care" environment rather than promote improved prenatal care among drug addicted mothers.*
- Advise expectant mothers to stop smoking and assist with methods of smoking cessation. EB: *Smoking during pregnancy increases the risk for miscarriage, impaired fetal growth, low birth weight, and infant mortality (Greener, 2011).*
- Recommend that women of childbearing age take 400 mcg of folic acid daily in order to reduce the risk of neural tube defects. EB: *Taking 400 mcg of folic acid daily, at least 3 months before conception and continuing throughout pregnancy, can prevent as many as 70% of neural tube defects (Greener, 2011).*

D

Neonate/Infant

- Encourage mother/baby interactions when caring for premature infants. EB: *Premature infants have been found to be at risk for developmental delays. Positive mother-infant interactions are important for child development, particularly for premature infants (Nicolaou et al, 2009).*
- Assess infant iron status and encourage iron supplementation for deficient infants. EB: *A study by Angulo-Barroso et al (2011) suggests that fine motor development is delayed for infants with lower iron levels.*

▲ Support early advanced developmental screening tests for male infants who are born prematurely or are medically fragile at birth. EBN: *Male gender can be considered a significant biological risk factor for infants' cognitive and motor development, especially for premature infants (Cho et al, 2010).*

▲ Encourage caution regarding use of glucocorticoids in premature and term infants. EB: *Vázquez et al (2012) note that administration of glucocorticoids in infancy has the potential of causing neurological developmental difficulties, including anxiety and depressive disorders later in life.*

▲ Be aware that socioeconomic factors are predictive of delayed infant development (physical and cognitive) and encourage continued screening along with follow-up care for these infants. Arrange appropriate social services referrals. EBN: *Lower socioeconomic status shows a strong correlation to growth percentile. Hill (2010) found that at 6 months of age, infants on Medicaid are 5.6 times more likely to be in the 10th percentile of weight, 15.2 times more likely to be in the 10th percentile of head circumference, and 9.8 times more likely to be in the 10th percentile of length than other infants.*

▲ Make arrangements for close follow-up monitoring of opioid-exposed infants. EB: *Infants born to mothers who abuse opioids are at a higher risk for developmental delays and physical abuse (Salo et al, 2010).*

Toddler/Preschooler/School-Age

- Provide support and education to parents of toddlers with developmental disabilities (i.e., Down syndrome, cerebral palsy). EB: *Parents should anticipate seeing moderate to significant delays in reaching developmental milestones such as walking and communication (Horovitz & Matson, 2011).*
- Encourage parents of toddlers to obtain age-appropriate developmental screenings to detect early problems. EB: *American Academy of Pediatrics guidelines for developmental screenings should be followed. Screening for autism spectrum disorders should be performed between ages 18 and 24 months (Macias & Lipkin, 2009).*
- Toddlers who are underweight should be offered solid foods first rather than juices. *Excessive juice and milk consumption may interfere with nutritional absorption.*
- Teach parents the importance of avoiding lead-based paints in the home as well as other sources of lead in the environment. EB: *Hou et al (2013) confirmed previous research indicating that when the blood lead level reaches about 50 mcg/L in the body of children, it can impair growth, memory, intelligence, and behavior, even when there is no obvious clinical manifestation.*

▲ Discuss advantages of early speech-language intervention with parents of toddlers having delayed development in communication. EB: *Early intervention makes a significant difference in the developmental course of communication for children with a variety of established conditions (Paul & Roth, 2011).*

- Educate parents on the importance of providing oral care for children with mild/moderate disabilities. Parents may need to assume the responsibility of toothbrushing for the child. EB: *This study showed children with mild/moderate developmental disabilities had nearly three times more decayed teeth on average than children with severe disabilities who received toothbrushing from parents (Liu et al, 2010).*

▲ Encourage mothers with postpartum depression to seek assistance and support as appropriate to ensure normal development of their children. CEB: *In this study the overall incidence of developmental delay at 18 months in children of women displaying depression following pregnancy was 9% (Deave et al, 2008).*

- Teach new mothers the importance of breastfeeding. EB: *Prolonged and exclusive breastfeeding improves children's cognitive development (Kramer et al, 2008).* EB: *Jäger et al (2014) discovered an inverse association between breastfeeding duration and risk of diabetes.*

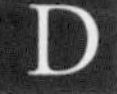

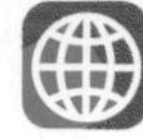

Multicultural

- Recognize cultural risks associated with higher infant mortality. EB: *African American infants are two times more likely to die in the first year of life than Caucasian infants. Low birth weight is a significant determinant of the increased mortality (Dailey, 2009).*

REFERENCES

Angulo-Barroso, R. M., Schapiro, L., Liang, W., et al. (2011). Motor development in 9-month-old infants in relation to cultural differences and iron status. *Developmental Psychobiology, 53*(2), 196–210.

Cho, J., Holditch-Davis, D., & Miles, M. S. (2010). Effects of gender on the health and development of medically at-risk infants. *Journal of Obstetric, Gynecologic, and Neonatal Nursing, 39*(5), 536–549.

Dailey, D. E. (2009). Social stressors and strengths as predictors of infant birth weight in low-income African American women. *Nursing Research, 58*(5), 340–347.

Deave, T., et al. (2008). The impact of maternal depression in pregnancy on early child development. *Obstetrical and Gynecological Survey, 63*(10), 626–628.

Ethen, M. K., et al. (2009). National birth defects prevention study. *Maternal and Child Health Journal, 13*, 274–285.

Greener, M. (2011). The tragedy of congenital abnormalities. *Nurse Prescribing, 9*(3), 117–121.

Hill, A. S. (2010). Predicting the growth percentile of extremely low birthweight infants. *Neonat Pediatr Child Health Nurs, 13*(3), 12–19.

Horovitz, M., & Matson, J. L. (2011). Developmental milestones in toddlers with atypical development. *Research in Developmental Disabilities, 32*, 2278–2282.

Hou, S., Yuan, L., Jin, P., et al. (2013). A clinical study of the effects of lead poisoning on the intelligence and neurobehavioral abilities of children. *Theoretical Biology & Medical Modelling, 10*, 13.

Jäger, S., Jacobs, S., Kröger, J., et al. (2014). Breast-feeding and maternal risk of type 2 diabetes: a prospective study and meta-analysis. *Diabetologia, 57*(7), 1355–1365.

Kramer, M. S., et al. (2008). Breastfeeding and child cognitive development: new evidence from a large randomized trial. *Archives of General Psychiatry, 65*(5), 578–584.

Liu, H., et al. (2010). The impact of dietary and tooth-brushing habits to dental caries of special school children with disability. *Research in Developmental Disabilities, 31*, 1160–1169.

Macias, M. M., & Lipkin, P. H. (2009). Developmental surveillance and screening. *Contemporary Pediatrics, 26*(11), 72–76.

Nicolaou, M., et al. (2009). Mother's experiences of interacting with their premature infants. *Journal of Reproductive and Infant Psychology, 27*(2), 182–194.

Paul, R., & Roth, F. P. (2011). Characterizing and predicting outcomes of communication delays in infants and toddlers: implications for clinical practice. *Language, Speech, and Hearing Services in Schools, 42*, 331–340.

Salo, S., et al. (2010). Early development of opioid-exposed infants born to mothers in buprenorphine-replacement therapy. *Journal of Reproductive and Infant Psychology, 29*(2), 161–179.

Vázquez, D. M., Neal, C. R., Patel, P. D., et al. (2012). Regulation of corticoid and serotonin receptor brain system following early life exposure of glucocorticoids: long term implications for the neurobiology of mood. *Psychoneuroendocrinology, 37*(3), 421–437.

Wu, M., LaGasse, L. L., Wouldes, T. A., et al. (2013). Predictors of inadequate prenatal care in methamphetamine-using mothers in New Zealand and the United States. *Maternal and Child Health Journal, 17*(3), 566–575.

Diarrhea *Mary Beth Flynn Makic, PhD, RN, CNS, CCNS, FAAN, and Betty J. Ackley, MSN, EdS, RN*

NANDA-I

Definition

Passage of loose, unformed stools

Defining Characteristics

Abdominal pain; bowel urgency; cramping; hyperactive bowel sounds; loose liquid stools > 3 in 24 hours

Related Factors

Physiological

Gastrointestinal inflammation; gastrointestinal irritation; infection; malabsorption; parasite

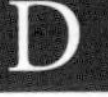

Psychological

Anxiety; increase in stress level

Situational

Enteral feedings; exposure to contaminant; exposure to toxin; laxative abuse; substance abuse; travel; treatment regimen

NOC (Nursing Outcomes Classification)

Suggested NOC Outcomes

Bowel Elimination; Electrolyte and Acid-Base Balance; Fluid Balance; Hydration; Treatment Behavior: Illness or Injury

Example NOC Outcome with Indicators

Bowel Elimination as evidenced by the following indicators: Elimination pattern/Stool soft and formed/Bowel sounds/Liquid stool. (Rate each indicator of **Bowel Elimination:** 1 = severely compromised, 2 = substantially compromised, 3 = moderately compromised, 4 = mildly compromised, 5 = not compromised [see Section I].)

Client Outcomes

Client Will (Specify Time Frame)

- Defecate formed, soft stool every 1 to 3 days
- Maintain the perirectal area free of irritation
- State relief from cramping and less or no diarrhea
- Explain cause of diarrhea and rationale for treatment
- Maintain good skin turgor and weight at usual level
- Have negative stool cultures

NIC (Nursing Interventions Classification)

Suggested NIC Intervention

Diarrhea Management

Example NIC Activities—Diarrhea Management

Evaluate medication profile for gastrointestinal side effects; Suggest trial elimination of foods containing lactose

Nursing Interventions and *Rationales*

- Assess pattern of defecation or have the client keep a diary that includes the following: time of day defecation occurs; usual stimulus for defecation; consistency, amount, and frequency of stool; type of, amount of, and time food consumed; fluid intake; history of bowel habits and laxative use; diet; exercise patterns; obstetrical/gynecological, medical, and surgical histories; medications; alterations in perianal sensations; and present bowel regimen. *Assessment of defecation pattern and factors surrounding diarrhea episode to include changes in diet, medications, exercise, and health history will help direct interventions and treatment Willson et al, 2014).*
- Recommend use of standardized tool to consistently assess, quantify, and then treat diarrhea. CEB/EB: *Stool classification systems include the Hart and Dobb Diarrhea Scale, the Guenther and Sweed Stool Output Assessment Tool, the Bristol Stool Scale, Diarrhea Grading Scale (Hallquist & Fung, 2005; Kyle, 2007; Sabol & Carlson, 2007, Willson et al, 2014).*
- Inspect, auscultate, palpate, and percuss the abdomen, in that order. *Expect increased frequency of bowel sounds with diarrhea (Jarvis, 2012).*

▲ Use an evidence-based bowel management protocol which includes identifying and treating the cause of the diarrhea, obtaining a stool specimen if infectious etiology is suspected, evaluate current medications and osmolality of enteral feedings, assess and treat hydration status of client, review and stop ordered and/or over-the-counter laxatives, provide good skin care and apply barrier creams to prevent skin irritation from diarrhea, and evaluate need for antidiarrheal agents and possible fecal containment device with provider. EB: *The possible cause of the diarrhea needs to be assessed and client hydration and skin protective interventions put into place rapidly to prevent secondary complications associated with the client's diarrhea episodes (Willson et al, 2014; Shahin & Lohrmann, 2015).*

- ▲ Identify cause of diarrhea if possible based on history (e.g., infection; gastrointestinal inflammation; medication effect; malnutrition or malabsorption; laxative abuse; osmotic enteral feedings, anxiety; stress). See Related Factors: *Identification of the underlying cause is important, because the treatment is determined based on the cause of diarrhea.*
- ▲ Testing for diarrhea may consist of laboratory work such as a complete blood count with differential and blood cultures if the client is febrile. Also obtain stool specimens as ordered, to either rule out or diagnose an infectious process (e.g., ova and parasites, *Clostridium difficile* infection, bacterial cultures for food poisoning). *Assessing for signs of systemic infection and inflammatory response as well as evaluation of the stool for infection are important first steps in identifying the cause of diarrhea (Abraham & Sellin, 2012; Dickinson & Surawicz, 2014).*
- ▲ Consider the possibility of *C. difficile* infection if the client has any of the following: watery diarrhea, low-grade fever, abdominal cramps, history of antibiotic therapy, history of gastrointestinal tract surgery, and if the client is taking medications that reduce gastric acid, including proton-pump inhibitors (PPIs). *Any antibiotic can cause* C. difficile *infection but clindamycin, cephalosporins, and fluoroquinolones pose the greatest risk, as do multiple antibiotics and longer duration of antibiotics (Surawicz et al, 2013).* EB: C. difficile *infections have become increasingly common because of the frequent use of broad-spectrum antibiotics, and now there is a hypervirulent form of* C. difficile *causing increased morbidity and mortality. Antibiotics and gastric acid reducing medications can change normal gut flora, increasing the risk for development of* C. difficile *infection, diarrhea, and colitis (Surawicz et al, 2013).*
- • Use standard precautions when caring for clients with diarrhea to prevent spread of infectious diarrhea; use gloves and handwashing. *C. difficile* and viruses causing diarrhea have been shown to be highly contagious. C. difficile *is difficult to eradicate because of spore formation (Surawicz et al, 2013; Martin et al, 2014).* CEB/EB: *A review of client care related to* C. difficile *summarizes care to include contact isolation, soap and water handwashing (alcohol rubs are not effective), use of disposable equipment, and environmental room decontamination (Makic et al, 2011; Centers for Disease Control and Prevention, 2015; Martin et al, 2014).* C. difficile *can survive for at least 24 hours on inanimate surfaces, and spores can survive for months on objects such as toilets, sinks, and bed rails (Makic et al, 2011; CDC, 2015; Martin et al, 2014).*
- ▲ Antibiotic stewardship is an important aspect in prevention of *C. difficile* infections. *Antibiotics should be used judiciously (CDC, 2015; Martin et al, 2014; Surawicz et al, 2013).* If the client has diarrhea associated with antibiotic therapy, consult with the health care provider regarding the use of probiotics, such as yogurt with active cultures, to treat diarrhea, or probiotic dietary supplements; or preferably use probiotics to prevent diarrhea when first beginning antibiotic therapy. EB: *While conclusive evidence on the effectiveness of probiotic in treating and preventing* C. diffcle *and diarrhea is lacking, evidence suggests that probiotics may be helpful for some clients. Probiotics may be used in an attempt to balance intestinal flora and restrict the colonization of* C. difficile *(Williams, 2010; Clauson & Crawford, 2015; Pattani et al, 2013).*
- ▲ If a probiotic is ordered, administer it with food. Recommend that it be taken through the antibiotic course and 10 to 14 days afterward. *Food tends to buffer the stomach acids, allowing more of the probiotic ingredients to pass through the stomach for absorption in the intestines. Beginning this therapy early helps prevent antibiotic-associated diarrhea (Clauson et al, 2015).*
- ▲ Recognize that *C. difficile* can commonly recur and that reculturing of stool is often required before initiating retreatment. EB: *High reinfection rates have been reported within the first 2 months of initial diagnosis. Repeat courses of antibiotics, usually metronidazole or vancomycin, are necessary to treat repeat* C. difficile *infections. New evidence is evolving to support fecal transplant for clients with severe recurrent* C. difficile *infections (Surawicz et al, 2013).*
- • Have the client complete a diet diary for 7 days and monitor the intake of high fructose corn syrup and fructose sweeteners in relation to onset of diarrhea symptoms. If diarrhea is associated with fructose ingestion, intake should be limited or eliminated. EB: *High fructose corn syrup or fructose sweeteners from fruit juices can cause gastrointestinal symptoms of bloating, rumbling, flatulence, and diarrhea at amounts of 25 to 50 g. Malabsorption is demonstrated in clients after 25 g fructose, and most clients develop symptoms with 50 g fructose (Abraham & Sellin, 2012).*

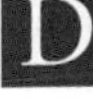

- ▲ If the client has infectious diarrhea, consider avoiding use of medications that slow peristalsis. CEB: *If an infectious process is occurring, such as* C. difficile *infection or food poisoning, medication to slow peristalsis should generally not be given. The increase in gut motility helps eliminate the causative factor, and use of antidiarrheal medication could result in a toxic megacolon (Sunenshine & McDonald, 2006).*
- • Assess for dehydration by observing skin turgor over sternum and inspecting for longitudinal furrows of the tongue. Watch for excessive thirst, fever, dizziness, lightheadedness, palpitations, excessive cramping, bloody stools, hypotension, and symptoms of shock. *Severe diarrhea can cause deficient fluid volume, electrolyte imbalance, extreme weakness, and a possible shock state (El-Sharkawy et al, 2014; Thorson et al, 2008).*
- • Refer to care plans for Deficient **Fluid** volume and Risk for **Electrolyte** imbalance if appropriate.
- ▲ If the client has frequent or chronic diarrhea, consider suggesting use of dietary fiber after consultation with a nutritionist and/or provider. EB: *Use of a fiber supplement decreases the number of incontinent stools and improves stool consistency (Willson et al, 2014).*
- ▲ If diarrhea is chronic and there is evidence of malnutrition, consult with the provider for a dietary consult and possible nutrition supplementation to maintain nutrition while the gastrointestinal system heals (Change & Huang, 2013).
- • Encourage the client to eat small, frequent meals, eating foods that are easy to digest at first (e.g., bananas, crackers, pretzels, rice, potatoes, clear soups, applesauce), but switch to a regular diet as soon as tolerated. Also recommend avoiding milk products, foods high in fiber, and caffeine (dark sodas, tea, coffee, chocolate). *The BRAT diet has been traditionally recommended but may be nutritionally incomplete (Shapiro et al, 2010; International Foundation for Functional Gastrointestinal Disorders, 2014).*
- • Provide a readily available bathroom, commode, or bedpan.
- • Thoroughly cleanse and dry the perianal and perineal skin daily and as needed using a cleanser capable of stool removal. Apply skin moisture barrier cream as needed. Refer to perirectal skin care in the care plan for bowel Incontinence.
- ▲ If the client has enteral tube feedings and diarrhea, consider infusion rate, position of feeding tube, tonicity of formula, possible formula contamination, and excessive intake of hyperosmolar medications, such as sorbitol commonly found in the liquid version of medications (Makic et al, 2011; Chang et al, 2013). Consider changing the formula to a lower osmolarity, lactose-free, or high-fiber feeding. *Determination of the cause of diarrhea should include an abdominal examination, fecal leukocytes, quantification of stool, stool culture for* C. difficile *(and/or toxin assay), serum electrolyte panel, and review of medications (Willson et al, 2014).*
- • Avoid administering bolus enteral feedings into the small bowel. *The stomach has a larger capacity for large fluid volumes, whereas the small bowel can usually only tolerate up to 150 mL/hr (Chang et al, 2013; Sabol & Carlson, 2007).*
- ▲ Dilute liquid medications before administration through the enteral tube and flush the enteral feeding tube with sufficient water before and after medication administration. *Since many liquid medications contain sorbitol or are hyperosmotic, diluting the medication may help decrease occurrence of diarrhea (Chang et al, 2013; Sabol & Carlson, 2007; Thorson et al, 2008).*
- • Teach clients with cancer the types of diarrhea they may encounter, emphasizing not only chemotherapy and radiation induced diarrhea, but also *C. difficile,* along with associated signs and symptoms, and treatments. EB: *Diarrhea in cancer patients is a common complication that causes dehydration, electrolyte imbalances, nutritional deficits, and hospitalization for treatment. Providing the client education focusing on early recognition of diarrhea necessitating early interventions is important in preventing adverse client outcomes (Andreyev et al, 2014).*
- ▲ For chemotherapy induced diarrhea (CID) and radiation induced diarrhea (RID), review rationale for pharmacological interventions, along with soluble fiber and probiotic supplements. Consult a registered dietitian to assist with recommendations to alleviate diarrhea, decrease dehydration, and maintain nutritional status. EBN: *Both CID and RID can occur as often as or more than 50% of the time, dependent on the chemotherapy regimen or combination with radiation (Andreyev et al, 2014; Sun & Yang, 2013).*
- ▲ Acute traveler's diarrhea is the most common illness affecting individuals traveling to, usually, low-income regions of the world. EB: *Improved hygiene and avoidance of foods for which preparation methods are unknown (e.g., street food) can mitigate the severity of gastric distress. Clients should be counseled about precautions they can take while traveling to reduce the severity of diarrhea, and a self-treatment antibiotic series may be prescribed by the health care provider for at risk clients (Steffen et al, 2015).*

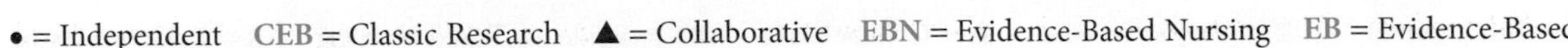

D

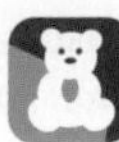

Pediatric

▲ Assess for mild or moderate signs of dehydration with both acute and persistent diarrhea: mild (increased thirst and dry mouth or tongue); moderate (decreased urination; no wet diapers for 3+ hours; feeling of weakness/lightheadedness, irritability, or listlessness; few or no tears when crying) (Pye, 2011). Refer to primary care provider for treatment.

▲ Recommend that parents give the child oral rehydration fluids to drink in the amounts specified by the health care provider especially during the first 4 to 6 hours to replace lost fluid. Once the child is rehydrated, an orally administered maintenance solution should be used along with food. Continue even if child vomits. EB: *Treatment with oral rehydration fluids for children is generally as effective as intravenous fluids (Binder et al, 2014). Oral rehydration therapy (ORT) is an iso-osmolar, glucose-electrolyte solution that has been recognized for more than 40 years to be effective in treating children with dehydration due to acute infectious diarrhea (Binder et al, 2014). Vomiting is not a contraindication to ORT. Adequate ORT is absorbed by most clients during vomiting (Rehydration Project, 2014).*

- Recommend the mother resume breastfeeding as soon as possible.
- Recommend parents avoid giving the child flat soda, fruit juices, gelatin dessert, or instant fruit drink. *These fluids have a high osmolality from carbohydrate contents and can exacerbate diarrhea. In addition they have low sodium concentrations that can aggravate existing hyponatremia (Rehydration Project, 2014; Dekate et al, 2013).*
- Recommend parents give children foods with complex carbohydrates, such as potatoes, rice, bread, cereal, yogurt, fruits, and vegetables. Avoid fatty foods, foods high in simple sugars, and milk products.

▲ Recommend rotavirus vaccine within the child's vaccination schedule. EB: *Two vaccines, Rotarix and Rotateq, have undergone comprehensive studies with findings that they can significantly prevent severe rotavirus diarrhea and death due to dehydration in children (Gray, 2011; Glass et al, 2014).*

Geriatric

▲ Evaluate medications the client is taking. Recognize that many medications can result in diarrhea, including digitalis, propranolol, angiotensin-converting enzyme inhibitors, histamine-receptor antagonists, nonsteroidal anti-inflammatory drugs, anticholinergic agents, oral hypoglycemia agents, and antibiotics, among others. EB: *Numerous medications can cause diarrhea. Evaluate changes in the client's medications as a possible cause of the diarrhea (Willson et al, 2014).*

▲ Monitor the client closely to detect whether an impaction is causing diarrhea; remove impaction as ordered. Clients with fecal impaction commonly experience leakage of mucus or liquid stool from the rectum, rectal irritation, distention, and impaired anal sensation (Meiner, 2010).

▲ Seek medical attention if diarrhea is severe or persists for more than 24 hours, or if the client has history of dehydration or electrolyte disturbances, such as lassitude, weakness, or prostration. *Older adult clients can dehydrate rapidly; especially serious is development of hypokalemia with dysrhythmias.* C. difficile *is a common cause of diarrhea in older clients when they have been subjected to long-term antibiotic therapy (El-Sharkaway et al, 2013; Piacenti & Leuthner, 2013).*

- Provide emotional support for clients who are having trouble controlling unpredictable episodes of diarrhea. Diarrhea can be a great source of embarrassment to older clients and can lead to social isolation and a feeling of powerlessness.

Home Care

Previously mentioned interventions may be adapted for home care use to keep the client well hydrated.

- Assess the home for general sanitation and methods of food preparation. Reinforce principles of sanitation for food handling. *Poor sanitation or mishandling of food may cause bacterial infection or transmission of dangerous organisms from utensils to food.*
- Assess for methods of handling soiled laundry if the client is bed bound or has been incontinent. Instruct or reinforce universal precautions with family and bloodborne pathogen precautions with agency caregivers. *The Bloodborne Pathogen Regulations of the Occupational Safety and Health Administration (OSHA) identify legal guidelines for caregivers.*
- When assessing medication history, include over-the-counter (OTC) drugs, both general and those currently being used to treat the diarrhea. Instruct clients not to mix OTC medications when self-treating. *Mixing OTC medications can further irritate the gastrointestinal system, intensifying the diarrhea or causing nausea and vomiting.*

- Evaluate current medications for indication that specific interventions are warranted. *Blood levels of medications may increase during prolonged episodes of diarrhea, indicating the need for close monitoring of the client or direct intervention.*
- ▲ Evaluate the need for a home health aide or homemaker service referral. Caregiver may need support for maintaining client cleanliness to prevent skin breakdown.
- Evaluate the need for durable medical equipment in the home. The client may need a bedside commode, call bell, or raised toilet seat to facilitate prompt toileting.

Client/Family Teaching and Discharge Planning

- Encourage avoidance of coffee, spices, milk products, and foods that irritate or stimulate the gastrointestinal tract. A list of dietary items that may irritate the gastrointestinal track and trigger diarrhea is available at www.iffgd.org/site/gi-disorders/functional-gi-disorders/diarrhea/nutrition.
- Teach appropriate method of taking ordered antidiarrheal medications; explain side effects.
- Explain how to prevent the spread of infectious diarrhea (e.g., careful handwashing, appropriate handling and storage of food, and thoroughly cleaning the bathroom and kitchen). EB: *Good hand hygiene has repeatedly been found to be the first step in preventing the spread of infectious diarrhea (Dickinson & Surawicz, 2014; Abraham & Sellin, 2012; CDC, 2015).*
- Help the client to determine stressors and set up an appropriate stress reduction plan, if stress is the cause of diarrhea.
- Teach signs and symptoms of dehydration and electrolyte imbalance.
- Teach perirectal skin care.
- ▲ Consider teaching clients about complementary therapies, such as probiotics, after consultation with primary care provider.

REFERENCES

Abraham, B. P., & Sellin, J. H. (2012). Drug-induced, factitious, & idiopathic diarrhea. *Best Practice & Research Clinical Gastroenterology, 26,* 633–648.

Andreyev, J., Ross, P., Donnellan, C., et al. (2014). Guidance on the management of diarrhea during cancer chemotherapy. *The Lancet Oncology, 15,* e447–e460.

Binder, H. J., Brown, I., Ramakrishna, B. S., et al. (2014). Oral rehydration therapy in the second decade of the twenty-first century. *Current Gastroenterology Reports, 16,* 376–383.

Centers for Disease, Control, and Prevention (2015). *Hospital Acquired Infections: Clostridium difficile Infection.* Retrieved April, 13, 2015: <http://www.cdc.gov/HAI/organisms/cdiff/Cdiff_infect.html>.

Chang, S. J., & Huang, H. H. (2013). Diarrhea in enterally fed patients: Blame the diet? *Current Opinion in Clinical Nutrition and Metabolic Care, 2013*(16), 588–594.

Clauson, E. R., & Crawford, P. (2015). What you must know before you recommend a probiotic. *The Journal of Family Practice, 64*(3), 151–155. Retrieved April 13, 2015: <http://www.jfponline.com/fileadmin/qhi/jfp/pdfs/6403/JFP_06403_Article1.pdf>.

Dekate, P., Jayashree, M., & Singhi, S. C. (2013). Management of acute diarrhea in emergency room. *Indian Journal of Pediatrics, 80*(3), 235–246.

Dickinson, B., & Surawicz, C. M. (2014). Infectious diarrhea: An overview. *Current Gastroenterology Reports, 16,* 399.

El-Sharkaway, A. M., Sohota, O., Maughan, R. J., et al. (2013). The pathophysiology of fluid and electrolyte balance in the older adult surgical patient. *Clinical Nutrition, 33,* 6–13.

Glass, R. I., Parashar, U., Patel, M., et al. (2014). Rotavirus vaccines: Successes and challenges. *Journal of Infection, 68,* S9–S18.

Gray, J. (2011). Rotavirus vaccines: safety, efficacy and public health impact. *Journal of Internal Medicine, 270*(3), 206–214.

Hallquist, P., & Fung, A. (2005). Advanced colorectal cancer: Current treatment and nursing management with economic considerations. *Clinical Journal of Oncology Nursing, 9*(5), 541–582.

International Foundation for Functional Gastrointestinal Disorders (March, 2014). *Nutritional strategies for managing diarrhea.* Retrieved April, 13, 2015: <http://www.iffgd.org/site/gi-disorders/functional-gi-disorders/diarrhea/nutrition>.

Jarvis, C. (2012). *Physical examination & health assessment* (6th ed.). St Louis: Saunders/Elsevier.

Kyle, G. (2007). Constipation and palliative care-where are we now? *International Journal of Palliative Nursing, 13*(1), 6–16.

Makic, M. B. F., et al. (2011). Evidence-based practice habits: putting more sacred cows out to pasture. *Critical Care Nurse, 31,* 38–62.

Martin, M., Zingg, W., Knoll, E., et al. (2014). National European guidelines for the prevention of Clostridium difficile infection: a systematic qualitative review. *Journal of Hospital Infection, 87,* 212e219.

Meiner, S. E. (2010). *Gerontologic nursing.* St Louis: Mosby/Elsevier.

Pattani, R., Palda, V. A., Hwang, S. W., et al. (2013). Probiotics for the prevention of antibiotic-associated diarrhea and *Clostridium difficile* infection among hospitalized patients: systematic review and meta-analysis. *Open Medicine, 7*(2), e56. Retrieved April 13, 2015: <http://www.ncbi.nlm.nih.gov/pmc/articles/PMC3863752>.

Piacenti, F. J., & Leuthner, K. D. (2013). Antimicrobial stewardship and Clostridium difficile-Associated diarrhea. *Journal of Pharmacy Practice, 26*(5), 506–513.

Pye, J. (2011). Travel-related health and safety considerations for children. *Nursing Standard, 25*(39), 50–56.

Rehydration Project (2014). Retrieved April 13, 2015: <http://rehydrate.org/ors/ort.htm>.

Sabol, V. K., & Carlson, K. K. (2007). Diarrhea: applying research to bedside practice. *AACN Advanced Critical Care, 18*(1), 32–44.

Shahin, E. S. M., & Lohrmann, C. (2015). Prevalence of fecal and double fecal and urinary incontinence in hospitalized patients. *Journal of Wound, Ostomy, and Continence Nursing, 42*(1), 89–93.

Shapiro, S. D., et al. (2010). Rehydration and refeeding after diarrheal illness. *Advance for NPs & PAs.*

Steffen, R., Hill, D. R., & DuPont, H. L. (2015). Traveler's diarrhea: A clinical review. *JAMA: The Journal of the American Medical Association*, *313*(1), 71–80.

Sun, J. X., & Yang, N. (2013). Role of octreotide in post chemotherapy and/or radiotherapy diarrhea: Prophylaxis or therapy? *Asia-Pacific Journal of Clinical Oncology*, Advance online publication.

Sunenshine, R. H., & McDonald, L. C. (2006). *Clostridium difficile*-associated disease: new challenges from an established pathogen. *Cleveland Clinic Journal of Medicine*, *73*(2), 187–197.

Surawicz, C. M., Brandt, L. B., Binion, D. G., et al. (2013). Guidelines for Diagnosis, Treatment, and Prevention of Clostridium Infections. *The American Journal of Gastroenterology*, *108*, 478–498.

Thorson, M. A., Bliss, D. Z., & Savik, K. (2008). Re-examination of risk factors for non-*Clostridium difficile*-associated diarrhea in hospitalized patients. *Journal of Advanced Nursing*, *62*(3), 354–364.

Williams, N. T. (2010). Probiotics. *American Journal of Health-System Pharmacy*, *67*(6), 449–458. Retrieved April 13, 2015: <http://www.medscape.com/viewarticle/719654_1>.

Willson, M. M., Angyus, M., Beals, D., et al. (2014). Executive summary: A quick reference guide for managing fecal incontinence. *Journal of Wound, Ostomy, and Continence Nursing*, *41*(1), 61–69.

Risk for Disuse syndrome

Betty J. Ackley, MSN, EdS, RN, and Mary Beth Flynn Makic, PhD, RN, CNS, CCNS, FAAN

NANDA-I

Definition

Vulnerable to deterioration of body systems as the result of prescribed or unavoidable musculoskeletal inactivity, which may compromise health

Risk Factors

Alteration in level of consciousness; mechanical immobility; pain; paralysis; prescribed immobility

NOC (Nursing Outcomes Classification)

Suggested NOC Outcomes

Endurance; Immobility Consequences: Physiological; Mobility; Neurological Status: Consciousness; Pain Level

Example NOC Outcome with Indicators

Immobility Consequences: Physiological as evidenced by the following indicators: Pressure sores/Constipation/Compromised nutrition status/Urinary calculi/Compromised muscle strength. (Rate the outcome and indicators of **Immobility Consequences: Physiological:** 1 = severe, 2 = substantial, 3 = moderate, 4 = mild, 5 = none [see Section I].)

Client Outcomes

Client Will (Specify Time Frame)

- Maintain full range of motion in joints
- Maintain intact skin, good peripheral blood flow, and normal pulmonary function
- Maintain normal bowel and bladder function
- Express feelings about imposed immobility
- Explain methods to prevent complications of immobility

NIC (Nursing Interventions Classification)

Suggested NIC Interventions

Energy Management; Exercise Therapy: Joint Mobility; Muscle Control; Positioning

Example NIC Activities—Energy Management

Determine the client's significant other's perception of causes of fatigue; Use valid instruments to measure fatigue, as indicated

Nursing Interventions and *Rationales*

- When client's condition is stable, screen for mobility skills in the following order: (1) bed mobility; (2) supported and unsupported sitting; (3) transition movements such as sit to stand, sitting down, and transfers; (4) standing and walking activities. Use a tool such as the Assessment Criteria and Care Plan for Safe Patient Handling and Movement (Sedlak et al, 2009) or the Banner Mobility Assessment Tool for Nurses (2014). EB: *In healthy adults, muscle strength declines by 1% per day of strict bed rest (De Jonghe et al, 2009).* EBN: *A review of the literature found that mobilizing hospitalized adults assisted with physical, emotional, and social well-being (Kalisch et al, 2013).*

- Assess the level of assistance needed by the client and express in terms of amount of effort expended by the person assisting the client. The range is as follows: total assist, meaning client performs 0% to 25% of task and, if client requires the help of more than one caregiver, it is referred to as a dependent transfer; maximum assist, meaning client gives 25% of effort while caregiver performs majority of the work; moderate assist, meaning client gives 50% of effort; minimal assist, meaning client gives 75% of effort; contact guard assist, meaning no physical assist is given but caregiver is physically touching client for steadying, guiding, or in case of loss of balance; stand by assist, meaning caregiver's hands are up and ready in case needed; supervision, meaning supervision of task is needed even if at a distance; modified independent, meaning client needs assistive device or extra time to accomplish task; independent, meaning client is able to complete task safely without instruction or assistance. CEB: *There are guidelines on how to determine the amount of care the client will need (Granger, 2011; Uniform Data System, 1997).*

▲ Request a referral to a physical therapist as needed so that client's range of motion, muscle strength, balance, coordination, and endurance can be part of the initial evaluation.

- Incorporate bed exercises such as flexing and extending feet and quadriceps or use of Thera-Bands for upper extremities into nursing care to help maintain muscle strength and tone (Koenig et al, 2012).

▲ If not contraindicated by the client's condition, obtain a referral to physical therapy for use of tilt table to help determine the cause of syncope. *Use of the tilt table can help determine if the cause of syncope is autonomic or from another cause (Low & Engstrom, 2012).*

- Perform range of motion exercises for all possible joints at least twice daily; perform passive or active range of motion exercises as appropriate. *If not used, muscles weaken and shorten from fibrosis of the muscle (Wagner et al, 2008; Wood et al, 2014).* EBN: *Range of motion exercises are effective in maintaining joint mobility and muscle integrity (Gillis & MacDonald, 2008; Summers et al, 2009; Kalisch et al, 2013; Wood et al, 2014).*
- Use specialized boots to prevent pressure ulcers on the heels and footdrop; remove boots twice daily to provide foot care. *Boots help keep the foot in normal anatomical alignment to prevent footdrop and prevent pressure ulcer formation on the heel.* EB: *A Cochrane review found that there is not a good evidence base to determine which boots or pressure redistribution system is most effective in preventing heel pressure ulcers (McGinnis & Stubbs, 2011).* CEBN: *A study found that use of a wedge-shaped viscoelastic bed-sized support surface was more effective than use of a pillow to prevent heel ulcers (Heyneman et al, 2009).*
- When positioning a client on the side, tilt client 30 degrees or less while lying on side. *Full (versus tilt) side-lying position places higher pressure on trochanter, predisposing to skin breakdown although more evidence is needed to fully determine the impact of full versus tilted positioning (van Rijswijk, 2009; National Pressure Ulcer Advisory Panel, 2014).*
- Assess skin condition at least daily and more frequently if needed. Use a risk assessment tool such the Braden Scale or the Norton Scale to predict the risk of developing pressure ulcers. EBN: *Use of a risk assessment tool is possibly effective to predict the risk of developing a pressure ulcer (National Pressure Ulcer Advisory Panel, 2014). Refer to care plan for* risk for Impaired **Skin** integrity.
- Discuss with staff and management a "safe handling" policy that may include a "no lift" policy. *Benefits of a safe handling policy include decreased injury to workers, increased safety and comfort for clients, decreased litigation related to injuries, and decreased lost work and wages due to injury, as well as decreased workers' compensation claims (Nelson et al, 2008; Boynton et al, 2014).*
- Turn clients at high risk for pressure/shear/friction frequently. Turn clients at least every 2 to 4 hours on a pressure-reducing mattress/every 2 hours on standard foam mattress. *These are general guidelines for turning, but they do not have a good evidence base. Preferably base the turning schedule on close assessment of the client's condition and predisposing conditions (Krapfl & Gray, 2008; van Rijswijk, 2009; Makic et al, 2014; National Pressure Ulcer Advisory Panel, 2014).*
- Provide the client with a pressure-relieving horizontal support surface. For further interventions on skin care, refer to the care plan for Impaired **Skin** integrity.
- Help the client out of bed as soon as able. *Early mobilization reduces risk of atelectasis, pneumonia, venous thromboembolism (VTE), and pulmonary embolism, and decreases orthostatic hypotension (Makic et al, 2014) as well as reducing risk of skeletal muscle atrophy, joint contractures, insulin resistance, microvascular*

dysfunction, systemic inflammation, and pressure ulcers (Brower, 2009). Bed rest is almost always harmful to clients; early mobilization is better than bed rest for most health conditions (Perme & Chandrashekar, 2009; Kalisch et al, 2013; Hoyer et al, 2014).

- When getting the client up after bed rest, do so slowly and watch for signs of postural (orthostatic) hypotension, tachycardia, nausea, diaphoresis, or syncope. Take the blood pressure with the client lying, sitting, and standing, waiting 2 minutes between each reading. *Consequences of bed rest are increased systemic vascular resistance, muscle atrophy, joint contracture, thromboembolic disease, and insulin resistance as well as microvascular dysfunction (Brower, 2009). Suggest waist-high elastic hosiery such as an elastic "belly binder" and/or bilateral lower extremity ace wraps over TED hose to facilitate venous return if hypotension is an issue (McPhee & Papadakis, 2009).*
- Obtain assistive devices such as braces, crutches, or canes to help the client reach and maintain as much mobility as possible. *Assistive devices can help increase mobility (Yoem et al, 2009; Boynton et al, 2014).*

▲ Apply graduated compression stockings as ordered. Ensure proper fit by measuring accurately. Remove the stockings at least twice a day, in the morning with the bath and in the evening to assess the condition of the extremity, then reapply. Knee length is preferred rather than thigh length. CEBN/EB: *Effectiveness of knee-high compression stockings is equal to thigh-high compression stockings, and knee-high stockings are more comfortable and fit better, adding to client compliance as stockings are most effective when worn continuously during the at-risk period; on during day and off at night (Hilleren-Listerud, 2009; McCaffrey & Blum, 2009). The American College of Chest Physicians (ACCP, 2012) recommends pharmacological or mechanical prophylaxis such as the use of graduated compression stockings to reduce the incidence of VTE in clients who have undergone high-risk orthopedic surgical procedures, clients older than 70 years of age, or clients who are at high risk for VTE for multiple reasons (Kahn et al, 2012). Please refer to the ACCP guidelines for use of mechanical prophylaxis for specific client situations.*

- Observe for signs of VTE, including pain, tenderness, and swelling in the calf and thigh. Also observe for new onset of breathlessness. *Clients commonly complain of a cramp in their lower calf that persists and becomes more painful with time. Symptoms of existing deep vein thrombosis are nonspecific and cannot be used alone to determine the presence of VTE. New onset of breathlessness is commonly associated with development of a pulmonary embolism (Goldhaber, 2012).*
- Have the client cough and deep breathe or use incentive spirometry every 2 hours while awake. *Bed rest compromises breathing because of decreased chest expansion, decreased cilia activity, pooling of mucus, and the effects of organ shift (such as the diaphragm and heart as well as pressure on the esophagus when in the supine position) and leads to partial or complete atelectasis usually of the left lower lobe (Brower, 2009).*
- Monitor respiratory functions, noting breath sounds and respiratory rate. Percuss for new onset of dullness in lungs.
- Note bowel function daily. Provide increased fluids, fiber, and natural laxatives such as prune juice as needed. *Constipation is common in immobilized clients because of decreased activity and fluid and food intake. Refer to care plan for* ***Constipation.***
- Increase fluid intake to 2000 mL/day within the client's cardiac and renal reserve. *Adequate fluids help prevent kidney stones and constipation, both of which are associated with bed rest.*
- Encourage intake of a balanced diet with adequate amounts of fiber and protein. *Consider recommending Practical Interventions to Achieve Therapeutic Lifestyle Changes (TLC), which includes monounsaturated and polyunsaturated fats, oils, margarines, beans, peas, lentils, soy, skinless poultry, lean fish, trimmed cuts of meat, fat-free and low-fat daily foods, omega-3 polyunsaturated fat sources, and whole grains, including soluble fiber sources such as oats, oat bran, and barley (Tucker, 2010).*

Critical Care

▲ Recognize that the client who has been in an intensive care environment may develop a neuromuscular dysfunction acquired in the absence of causative factors other than the underlying critical illness and its treatment, resulting in extreme weakness (Stevens et al, 2009). The client may need a workup to determine the cause before satisfactory ambulation can begin. *Critical care clients can develop disorders such as critical illness myopathy; polyneuropathy due to ischemia, pressure, prolonged recumbency, compartment syndrome, or hematomas; and the third critical care disorder, from prolonged pharmacologic neuromuscular blockade (Stevens et al, 2009).*

▲ Consider use of a continuous lateral rotation therapy bed. EBN: *Implementing kinetic therapy in the intensive care unit resulted in improved oxygenation and decreased length of stay for clients with pulmonary disorders (Swadener-Culpepper et al, 2008; Makic, 2014).*

▲ For the stable client in the intensive care unit, consider mobilizing the client in a four-phase method from dangling at the side of the bed to walking if there is sufficient knowledgeable staff available to protect the client from harm. *Even intensive care unit clients receiving mechanical ventilation can be mobilized safely if a multidisciplinary team is present to support, protect, and monitor the client for intolerance to activity (Perme & Chandrashekar, 2009; Boynton et al, 2014; Kalisch et al, 2013).* CEB: *A study found that whole-body rehabilitation consisting of interruption of sedation and physical and occupational therapy in the early days of critical illness was safe and well tolerated, and resulted in better functional outcomes at discharge (Schweickert et al, 2009).* EBN: *Critical care clients are at high risk for complications related to immobility such as ventilator-associated pneumonia (VAP), atelectasis, and long-lasting functional limitations; therefore, once the client is hemodynamically stable, use progressive mobilization to dangle legs, sit in a chair, stand and bear weight, and walk. Use rotation therapy (kinetic and continuous lateral) to reduce risk of VAP for clients on mechanical ventilation (Rauen et al, 2008; Makic et al, 2014).*

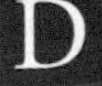

Geriatric

- Get the client out of bed as early possible and ambulate frequently after consultation with the health care provider. *Immobility is a risk factor for VTE; early ambulation can help prevent clot formation (American Association of Chest Physicians, 2012). Functional decline from hospital-associated deconditioning is common in older adults, and acute inpatient rehabilitation can be effective in preventing this condition (Kortebein, 2009; Wood et al, 2014).*
- Use the Exercise Assessment and Screening for You (EASY), which was developed to identify benefits of exercise and to assist older adults to select safe and effective exercises. This tool decreases barriers to exercise. CEBN: *Use of self-efficacy–based interventions resulted in increased exercise (Resnick et al, 2008).*

▲ Refer the client to physical therapy for resistance strength exercise training. CEB: *Disuse, aging, loss of skeletal mass, and malnutrition, referred to as sarcopenia, should be assessed, and strategies to counter sarcopenia such as resistance training should be employed even in very old clients (Bautmans et al, 2009).*

- Monitor for signs of depression: flat affect, poor appetite, insomnia, many somatic complaints. *Depression can commonly accompany decreased mobility and function in older adults and may be misinterpreted as not doing enough to help themselves (Rittenmeyer, 2010; Kalisch et al 2013).*
- Keep careful track of bowel function in older adults; do not allow the client to become constipated. *Older adults can easily develop impactions as a result of immobility. Refer to* **Constipation** *care plan.*

Home Care

- Some of the previous interventions may be adapted for home care use.

▲ Begin discharge planning as soon as possible with case manager or social worker to assess need for home support systems and community or home health services.

▲ Become oriented to all programs of care for the client before discharge from institutional care.

▲ Confirm the immediate availability of all necessary assistive devices for home.

- Perform complete physical assessment and recent history at initial home visit.

▲ Refer to physical and occupational therapies for immediate evaluations of the client's potential for independence and functioning in the home setting and for follow-up care.

- Allow the client to have as much input and control of the plan of care as possible. *Client perception of control increases self-esteem and motivation to follow medical plan of care.*
- Assess knowledge of all care with caregivers. Review as necessary. *Having the necessary knowledge and skills to perform care decreases caregiver role strain and supports safety of the client.*

▲ Support the family of the client in assumption of caregiver activities. Refer for home health aide services for assistance and respite as appropriate. Refer to medical social services as appropriate.

▲ Institute case management of frail elderly to support continued independent living, if possible in the home environment.

Client/Family Teaching and Discharge Planning

- Teach client/family how to perform range-of-motion exercises in bed if not contraindicated; this is referred to as a Home Exercise Program.
- Teach the family how to turn and position the client and provide all care necessary.

NOTE: Nursing diagnoses that are commonly relevant when the client is on bed rest include **Constipation,** risk for Impaired **Skin** integrity, Disturbed **Sleep** pattern, **Frail Elderly** syndrome, and **Powerlessness.**

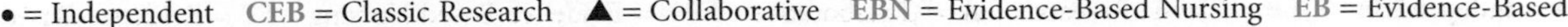

REFERENCES

American Association of Chest Physicians (AACP). *The Antithrombotic Therapy and Prevention of Thrombosis, ed 9: American College of Chest Physicians Evidence-Based Clinical Practice Guidelines.* Retrieved August 24, 2012, from: <http://www.chestnet.org/accp/guidelines/accp-antithrombotic-guidelines-9th-ed-now-available>.

Bautmans, I., Van Puyvelde, K., & Mets, T. (2009). Sarcopenia and functional decline: pathophysiology, prevention and therapy. *Acta Clinica Belgica*, *64*(4), 303–316.

Boynton, T., Kelly, L., Perez, A., et al. (2014). Banner mobility assessment tool for nurses: Instrument validation. *American Journal of Safe Patient Handling & Mobility*, *493*, 86–92.

Brower, R. G. (2009). Consequences of bed rest. *Critical Care Medicine*, *37*(10), S422–S428.

De Jonghe, B., et al. (2009). Intensive care unit-acquired weakness: risk factors and prevention. *Critical Care Medicine*, *37*(10), S309–S315.

Gillis, A. J., & MacDonald, B. C. (2008). Bedrest care guideline. In B. Ackley, et al. (Eds.), *Evidence-based nursing care guidelines: medical-surgical interventions*. Philadelphia: Mosby.

Goldhaber, S. (2012). Deep venous thrombosis and pulmonary thromboembolism. In D. Longo, et al. (Eds.), *Harrison's principles of internal medicine* (18th ed.). New York: McGraw-Hill.

Granger, C. (2011). *Quality and outcome measure for rehabilitation programs*. Medscape Reference Retrieved December 6, 2011, from: <http://emedicine.medscape.com/article/317865-overview#aw2aab6b>.

Heyneman, A., et al. (2009). Effectiveness of two cushions in the prevention of heel pressure ulcers. *Worldviews on Evidence-based Nursing*, *6*(2), 114–120.

Hilleren-Listerud, A. E. (2009). Graduated compression stocking and intermittent pneumatic compression device length selection. *Clinical Nurse Specialist CNS*, *23*(1), 21–24.

Hoyer, E. H., Brotman, D. J., Chan, K., et al. (2014). Barriers to early mobility of hospitalized general medicine patients. *American Journal of Physical Medicine and Rehabilitation*.

Kahn, S., et al. (2012). Prevention of VTE in nonsurgical patients. *Chest, Suppl*, *141*(2), 195S–226S.

Kalisch, B. J., Lee, S., & Dabney, B. W. (2013). Outcomes of inpatient mobilization: A literature review. *Journal of Clinical Nursing*, *23*, 1486–1501.

Koenig, S., Teixeira, J., & Yetzer, E. (2012). Promoting mobility and function. In K. L. Mauk (Ed.), *Rehabilitation nursing, a contemporary approach to practice*. Sudbury, MA: Jones & Bartlett Learning.

Kortebein, P. (2009). Rehabilitation for hospital-associated deconditioning. *American Journal of Physical Medicine and Rehabilitation*, *88*(1), 66–77.

Krapfl, L. A., & Gray, M. (2008). Does regular repositioning prevent pressure ulcers? *Journal of Wound, Ostomy, and Continence Nursing*, *35*(6), 571–577.

Low, P., & Engstrom, J. (2012). Disordered of the autonomic nervous system. In D. Longo, et al. (Eds.), *Harrison's principles of internal medicine* (18th ed.). New York: McGraw-Hill.

Makic, M. B. F., Rauen, C., Watson, R., et al. (2014). Examining the evidence to guide practice: Challenging practice habits. *Critical Care Nurse*, *34*(2), 58–68.

McCaffrey, R., & Blum, C. (2009). Venothrombotic events: evidence-based risk assessment, prophylaxis, diagnosis, and treatment. *Journal for Nurse Practitioners*, *5*(5), 325–333.

McGinnis, E., & Stubbs, N. (2011). Pressure-relieving devices for treating heel pressure ulcers. *Cochrane Database of Systematic Reviews*, (9), CD005485.

McPhee, S. J., & Papadakis, M. A. (2009). *Current medical diagnosis & treatment* (48th ed.). New York: McGraw-Hill.

National Pressure Ulcer Advisory Panel (2014). *Prevention and Treatment of Pressure Ulcers: Quick Reference Guide.* Retrieved June 16, 2015: <http://www.npuap.org/wp-content/uploads/2014/08/Updated-10-16-14-Quick-Reference-Guide-DIGITAL-NPUAP-EPUAP-PPPIA-16Oct2014.pdf>.

Nelson, A., et al. (2008). Myths and facts about safe patient handling in rehabilitations. *Rehabilitation Nursing*, *33*(1), 10–17.

Perme, C., & Chandrashekar, R. (2009). Early mobility and walking program for patients in intensive care units: creating a standard of care. *American Journal of Critical Care*, *18*(3), 212–221.

Rauen, C. A., et al. (2008). Seven evidence-based practice habits: putting some sacred cows out to pasture. *Critical Care Nurse*, *28*(2), 98–113.

Resnick, B., et al. (2008). The exercise assessment and screening for you (EASY) tool: application in the oldest old population. *American Journal of Lifestyle Medicine*, *2*(5), 432–440.

Rittenmeyer, L. (2010). Psychosocial issues in nursing. In K. S. Osborn, C. E. Wraa, & A. B. Watson (Eds.), *Medical-surgical nursing, preparation for practice* (1st ed.). Upper Saddle River, NJ: Pearson.

Schweickert, W. D., et al. (2009). Early physical and occupational therapy in mechanically ventilated, critically ill patients: a randomised controlled trial. *Lancet*, *373*(9678), 1874–1882.

Sedlak, C. A., et al. (2009). Development of the National Association of Orthopaedic Nurses guidance statement on safe patient handling and movement in the orthopaedic setting. *Orthopaedic Nursing*, *28*(Suppl. 2), S2–S8.

Stevens, R. D., et al. (2009). A framework for diagnosing and classifying intensive care unit-acquired weakness. *Critical Care Medicine*, *37*(10), S299–S308.

Summers, D., et al. (2009). Comprehensive overview of nursing and interdisciplinary care of the acute ischemic stroke patient. *Stroke; a Journal of Cerebral Circulation*, *40*, 2911–2944.

Swadener-Culpepper, L., Skaggs, R. L., & Vangilder, C. A. (2008). The impact of continuous lateral rotation therapy in overall clinical and financial outcomes of critically ill patients. *Critical Care Nursing Quarterly*, *31*(3), 270–279.

Tucker, S. (2010). Nutrition. In K. S. Osborn, C. E. Wraa, & A. B. Watson (Eds.), *Medical-surgical nursing, preparation for practice* (1st ed.). Upper Saddle River, NJ: Pearson.

Uniform Data System for Medical Rehabilitation (1997). *Functional independence measure*. Buffalo, NY: University of Buffalo.

Van Rijswijk, L. (2009). Pressure ulcer prevention updates. *The American Journal of Nursing*, *109*(8), 56.

Wagner, L., et al. (2008). Contractures in frail nursing home residents. *Geriatric Nursing (New York, N.Y.)*, *29*(4), 259–265.

Wood, W., Tschannen, D., Trotsky, A., et al. (2014). A mobility program for an inpatient acute care medical unit. *The American Journal of Nursing*, *14*(10), 34–40.

Yoem, H. A., Keller, C., & Fleury, J. (2009). Interventions for promoting mobility in community-dwelling older adults. *Journal of the American Academy of Nurse Practitioners*, *21*, 95–100.

Deficient Diversional activity *Mila W. Grady, MSN, RN*

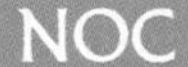

NANDA-I

D

Definition

Decreased stimulation from (or interest or engagement in) recreational or leisure activities

Defining Characteristics

Boredom; current setting does not allow engagement in activity

Related Factors (r/t)

Insufficient diversional activity; extremes of age; prolonged hospitalization; prolonged institutionalization

NOC (Nursing Outcomes Classification)

Suggested NOC Outcomes

Leisure Participation; Play Participation; Social Involvement

Example NOC Outcome with Indicators

Leisure Participation as evidenced by the following indicators: Expresses satisfaction with leisure activities/Feels relaxed from leisure activities/Enjoys leisure activities. (Rate the outcome and indicators of **Leisure Participation:** 1 = never demonstrated, 2 = rarely demonstrated, 3 = sometimes demonstrated, 4 = often demonstrated, 5 = consistently demonstrated [see Section I] (Moorhead et al, 2013).

Client Outcomes

Client Will (Specify Time Frame)

- Engage in personally satisfying diversional activities

NIC (Nursing Interventions Classification)

Suggested NIC Interventions

Recreation Therapy; Self-Responsibility Facilitation

Example NIC Activities—Recreation Therapy

Assist the client to identify meaningful recreational activities; Provide safe recreational equipment

Nursing Interventions and *Rationales*

- Observe for signs of deficient diversional activity: restlessness, unhappy facial expression, and statements of boredom and discontent. EBN: *In a study of residents living in long-term care in Turkey, 67% of the residents were diagnosed with deficient diversional activity (Güler et al, 2012).*
- Observe ability to engage in activities that require good vision and use of hands. *Diversional activities must be tailored to the client's capabilities.*
- Discuss activities with clients that are interesting and feasible in the present environment.
- Encourage the client to share feelings about situation of inactivity. *Work and hobbies provide structure and continuity to life; the client may feel a sense of loss.*
- Encourage the client to participate in any available social or recreational opportunities in the health care environment. EB: *Social engagement is associated with self-reported physical health in older adults (Cherry et al, 2013).*
- Encourage a mix of physical and mental activities if possible (e.g., crafts, crossword puzzles).
- Provide videos and/or DVDs of movies for recreation and distraction.
- Provide magazines and books of interest.

D

- Provide books on CD and CD player, and electronic versions of books for listening or reading as available.
- Set up a puzzle in a community space, or provide individual puzzles as desired.
- Provide access to a portable computer so that the client can access email and the Internet. Give client a list of interesting websites, including games and directions on how to perform Web searches if needed.
- Help client find a support group for the appropriate condition on the Internet if interested. EBN: *A study found that individuals dealing with low survival rate cancers desire online informational support (Buis & Whitten, 2011).*
- ▲ Arrange animal-assisted therapy if desired, with a dog, cat, or bird for the client to care for and interact with. EB: *Animal-assisted therapy has been associated with enhanced socialization, stress reduction, improvement in mood and well-being, a decrease in anxiety and loneliness, and the development of leisure and recreational skills (Muñoz Lasa et al, 2011).*
- Encourage the client to schedule visitors so that they are not all present at once or at inconvenient times. *A schedule prevents the client from becoming exhausted from frequent company.*
- If clients are able to write, help them keep journals or engage them in opportunities for creative writing in a group; if clients are unable to write, have them record thoughts on tape, or on videotape. EB: *A professional writer led creative writing workshop for a small group of older women in a nursing home; these workshops provided enjoyment, promoted the development of personal relationships within the community, and allowed staff to gain deeper insight into the lives of the residents (Wilson et al, 2011).*
- ▲ Request recreational or art therapist to assist with activities. EB: *Art therapy can assist individuals undergoing stroke rehabilitation to reduce anxiety and feelings of isolation (Ali et al, 2014).*
- ▲ Refer to occupational therapy. EB: *Occupational therapists are able to assist persons with compensatory strategies to assist with activities (Arbesman & Lieberman, 2011).*
- Provide a change in scenery; get the client out of the room as possible. *A lack of sensory stimulation has significant adverse effects on clients.*
- Help the client to experience nature through looking at a nature scene from a window, or walking through a garden if possible. EB: *Physical activity in the natural environment can promote emotional well-being (Pasanen et al, 2014).*
- Structure the environment as needed to promote optimal comfort and sensory diversity (e.g., have family bring in posters, banners, or photos; change lighting; change arrangement of furniture). CEBN: *For hospitalized clients needing close observation, consider the use of a S.A.F.E. unit that uses trained "diversional partners" rather than sitters; diversional activities were promoted through the use of TVs and VCRs on rolling carts, radios and CD players with music from various genres, movies, rocking chairs, a storage cabinet stocked with games and art supplies, stuffed animals, soft balls, and towels for folding (Nadler-Moodie et al, 2009).*
- Work with family or music therapist to provide music that is enjoyable to the client. EB: *Hospitalized patients who received an individualized music therapy session and who were provided with a CD for listening demonstrated marginally better quality of life pain scores after hospitalization and were more likely to recommend the hospital to others (Mandel et al, 2014).*
- Structure the client's schedule around personal wishes for time of care, relaxation, and participation in fun activities. *Increased client control fosters increased client self-esteem.*
- Spend time with the client when possible, giving the client full attention and being present in the moment, or arrange for a friendly visitor.

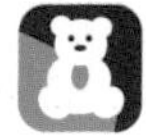

Pediatric

- ▲ Request an order for a child life specialist or, if not available, a play therapist for children. *Child life therapists provide opportunities for self-expression and play for hospitalized children and may help to normalize the environment.*
- Promote a referral to a music therapist. EBN: *Music therapy may lead to a decrease in self-reported pain and anxiety in hospitalized children, and may lead to improved patient and family satisfaction (Colwell et al, 2013).*
- Consider art therapy for children living with chronic illness who have activity restrictions. CEB: *In a study of children with persistent asthma, those who engaged in art therapy demonstrated a reduction in anxiety and an improvement in emotional health (Beebe et al, 2010).*

- Provide opportunities for children to connect with family and friends through technology. EBN: *Children desire to feel connected to the world outside the hospital environment; technology can reduce isolation as well as support educational needs (Lambert et al, 2014).*
- Provide activities such as video projects and use of computer-based support groups for children, such as Starbright World, a computer network where teenagers interact virtually, sharing their experiences and escaping hospital routines (www.starbrightworld.org). CEB: *Starbright World was shown to significantly reduce loneliness and withdrawn behavior in chronically ill children (Battles & Wiener, 2002).*
- Provide animal-assisted therapy for hospitalized children. CEBN: *Animal-assisted therapy produces a number of therapeutic benefits for hospitalized children, including a reduction in pain (Braun et al, 2009).*
- Provide computer games and virtual reality experiences for children, which can be used as distraction techniques during venipuncture, wound care, or other procedures. EBN: *Actively engaging children in serious gaming resulted in lower observed behavioral pain scores and distress for children undergoing wound dressing changes (Nilsson et al, 2013).*

D

Geriatric

- Assess the interests of older adults and the types of activities that they enjoy; encourage creative expression such as storytelling, drama, dance, art, writing, or music. EB: *Art therapy was shown to be effective in reducing anxiety and negative emotions, and improving self-esteem in a group of Korean American older adults (Kim, 2013); participating in music-making with others may improve quality of life, well-being, and physical and mental health in older adults (Creech et al, 2013).*
- If the client is able, arrange for him or her to attend group senior citizen activities. EB: *Social connectedness may assist with older adults' perception that they are aging well (Hodge et al, 2013).*
- Promote activity for older adults through the use of exergames (video games combined with exercise). EB: *A pilot study demonstrated that Wii interactive videogaming is feasible for use with older adults with mild cognitive impairment; participants enjoyed physical, mental, and social stimulation from the intervention (Hughes et al, 2014).*
- Encourage involvement in dance. EB: *Active participation in dance may enhance healthy aging (Noice et al, 2013).*
- Encourage involvement in gardening. EB: *Gardening promotes relief from stress (Van Den Berg & Custers, 2011).*
- Encourage clients to use their ability to help others by volunteering. EB: *Volunteering is associated with better self-reported health, fewer functional limitations, reduced depressive symptoms, and lower mortality (Anderson et al, 2014).*
- Provide an environment that promotes activity (e.g., one that has adequate lighting for crafts, large-print books, and adequate acoustics).
- Balance effortful activities with restful activities. EB: *Older adults had higher happiness scores when they were able to combine effortful activities that were physical, social, or cognitive with activities that were restful (Oerlemans et al, 2011).*
- Provide tai chi as an activity. EB: *In a study of heart failure clients, it was found that participation in tai chi exercises may lead to an improvement in mood, exercise self-efficacy, and quality of life (Yeh et al, 2011).*
- Provide opportunities for storytelling and life review. EBN: *Reflection on one's life assists individuals to discover meaning and purpose; a pilot study demonstrated a significant reduction in depressive symptoms after the creation of life story books (Chan et al, 2014).*

▲ Use reminiscence therapy in conjunction with the expression of emotions. Refer to a reminiscence group if available. EBN: *Participation in a structured reminiscence group led to improved self-esteem and life satisfaction and a decrease in depressive symptoms in a group of institutionalized older veterans (Wu, 2011).*

- Arrange for intergenerational volunteering for individuals with mild to moderate dementia. EB: *In a study of older adults living in an assisted living facility with mild to moderate dementia who visited inner city students, it was found that engagement in singing, reading, writing, and reminiscence led to a decrease in stress and an increase in quality of life (George & Singer, 2011).*
- Use the Eden Alternative for older adults; bring in appropriate plants for the older client to care for and animals such as birds, fish, dogs, and cats as appropriate for the client and children to visit. See rationales for animal-assisted therapy above. *The Eden Alternative offers a more natural human habitat where the quality of life is improved by reducing loneliness, boredom, and helplessness (Baumann, 2008).*

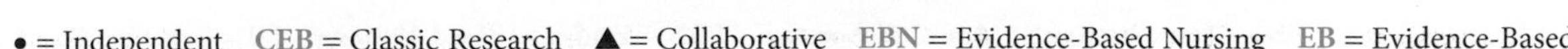

D

- For clients who love gardening but who may have difficulty being outside, bring in seeds, soil, and pots for indoor gardening experiences. Use seeds such as sunflower, pumpkin, and zinnia that grow rapidly. EB: *Gardening may foster socialization, fitness, flexibility, cognitive ability, health, and quality of life (Wang & Macmillan, 2013).*
- For clients with depressive symptoms, facilitate regular music listening. EB: *Listening to pleasant music was found to enhance auditory and verbal memory, focused attention, and mood in patients in the early phase of recovery after stroke (Särkämo & Soto, 2012).*
- For hospitalized clients with cognitive impairment, engage the assistance of volunteers to provide diversional activities. EBN: *A small pilot study demonstrated that patients, caregivers, staff, and volunteers were satisfied with a volunteer program that engaged hospitalized patients in a variety of activities during hospitalization (Shee et al, 2014).*
- For clients in assisted-living facilities, provide leisure educational programs and pleasant dining experiences. EB: *Opportunities for social engagement lead to psychological benefits for older adults in assisted living (Jang et al, 2014).*
- For clients who are interested in reading and writing, promote book or writing groups or journaling, creative or expressive writing. EB: *Participation in reading and writing activities positively influenced quality of life in a group of older adults (Sampaio & Ito, 2013).*
- Prescribe activities to engage passive dementia clients based on their former interests and hobbies. EB: *Residents of long-term care facilities who have dementia spend the majority of their time engaged in no activity at all, and inactivity has been linked to agitated behavior; stimuli such as looking at and sorting pictures, arranging flowers, folding towels, making puzzles, planting seeds, screwing nuts and bolts together, and listening to and singing along with favorite music led to positive affect and a decrease in agitated behavior (van der Ploeg et al, 2013).*
- Initiate opportunities for creative expression such as a TimeSlips storytelling group or Memories in the Making project to foster meaningful activities for clients with dementia. EB: *A creative storytelling program for clients with dementia, TimeSlips, resulted in increased creativity, quality of life, and involvement in meaningful activity and positively altered resident behavior while allowing staff to develop a deeper understanding of residents (George & Houser, 2014).*

Home Care

- Many of the previously listed interventions may be administered in the home setting.
- Explore with the client previous interests; consider related activities that are within the client's capabilities.
- ▲ Assess the client for depression. Refer for mental health services as indicated. EB: *Lack of interest in previously enjoyed activities is part of the syndrome of depression (American Psychiatric Association, 2013).*
- Assess the family's ability to respond to the client's psychosocial needs for stimulation. Assist as able.
- ▲ Refer to occupational therapy. EB: *Clients with low vision who received adequate training in the use of low vision devices tailored to individual goals were able to improve independence at home (Liu et al, 2013).*
- Introduce (or continue) friendly volunteer visitors if the client is willing and able to have the company. If transportation is an issue or if the client does not want visitors in the home, consider alternatives (e.g., telephone contacts, computer messaging).
- For clients who are interested and capable, suggest involvement in a community gardening experience. EB: *Community gardens were identified as a source of individual and community well-being (Okvat & Zautra, 2011).*
- If the client is approaching the end of life, and is interested, assist in making a videotape, audiotape, or memory book for family members with treasured stories, memoirs, pictures, and video clips. CEB: *Leaving a legacy entails passing on the essence of one's self; passing on values and beliefs is important to older adults (Hunter, 2007-2008).*

Client/Family Teaching and Discharge Planning

- Work with the client and family on learning diversional activities in which the client is interested (e.g., knitting, hooking rugs, writing memoirs).
- If the client is in isolation, give the client complete information on why isolation is needed and how it should be accomplished, especially guidelines for visitors; provide diversional activities and encourage visitation. EBN: *Children in isolation feel lonely and bored; access to play, social connections, and education may assist (Austin et al, 2013).*

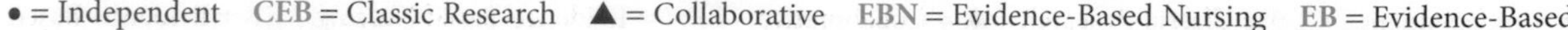

REFERENCES

Ali, K., Gammidge, T., & Waller, D. (2014). Fight like a ferret: A novel approach of using art therapy to reduce anxiety in stroke patients undergoing a hospital rehabilitation. *Medical Humanities, 40*(1), 56–60.

Anderson, N. D., Damianakis, T., Kröger, E., et al. (2014). The benefits associated with volunteering among seniors: A critical review and recommendations for future research. *Psychological Bulletin*, Advanced online publication.

American Psychiatric Association (2013). *Diagnostic and statistical manual of mental disorders* (5th ed.). Washington, DC: American Psychiatric Association.

Arbesman, M., & Lieberman, D. (2011). Methodology for the systematic reviews on occupational therapy for adults with Alzheimer's disease and related dementias. *American Journal of Occupational Therapy, 65*(5), 490–496.

Austin, D., Prieto, J., & Rushforth, H. (2013). The child's experience of single room isolation: A literature review. *Nursing Children and Young People, 25*(3), 18–24.

Battles, H., & Wiener, L. (2002). Starbright world: Effects of an electronic network on the social environment of children with life-threatening illness. *Children's Health Care, 31*(1), 47–68.

Baumann, S. L. (2008). How do you keep the music playing? *Nurs Sci Q, 21*(4), 363–364.

Beebe, A., Gelfand, E. W., & Bender, B. (2010). A randomized trial to test the effectiveness of art therapy for children with asthma. *Journal of Allergy and Clinical Immunology, 126*(2), 263–266.

Braun, C., Stangler, T., Narveson, J., et al. (2009). Animal-assisted therapy as a pain relief intervention for children. *Complementary Therapies in Clinical Practice, 15*(2), 105–109.

Buis, L. R., & Whitten, P. (2011). Comparison of social support content within online communities for high- and low-survival-rate cancers. *Computers, Informatics, Nursing, 29*(8), 461–467.

Chan, M. F., Leong, K. S., Heng, B. L., et al. (2014). Reducing depression among community-dwelling older adults using life-story review: A pilot study. *Geriatric Nursing, 35*(2), 105–110.

Cherry, K. E., Walker, E. J., Brown, J. S., et al. (2013). Social engagement and health in younger, older, and oldest-old adults in the Louisiana healthy aging study. *Journal of Applied Gerontology, 32*(1), 51–75.

Colwell, C. M., Edwards, R., Hernandez, E., et al. (2013). Impact of music therapy interventions (listening, composition, Orff-based) on the physiological and psychosocial behaviors of hospitalized children: A feasibility study. *Journal of Pediatric Nursing, 28*(3), 249–257.

Creech, A., Hallam, S., Varvarigou, M., et al. (2013). Active music-making: A route to enhanced subjective well-being among older people. *Perspectives in Public Health, 133*(1), 36–43.

George, D. R., & Houser, W. S. (2014). "I'm a storyteller!": exploring the benefits of TimeSlips Creative Expression Program at a nursing home. *American Journal of Alzheimer's Disease & Other Dementias.*

George, D. R., & Singer, M. E. (2011). Intergenerational volunteering and quality of life for persons with mild to moderate dementia: Results from a 5-month intervention study in the United States. *American Journal of Geriatric Psychiatry, 19*(4), 392–396.

Güler, E. K., Eser, I., Khorshid, L., et al. (2012). Nursing diagnosis in elderly residents of a nursing home: A case in Turkey. *Nursing Outlook, 60*(1), 21–28.

Hodge, A. M., English, D. R., Giles, G. G., et al. (2013). Social connectedness and predictors of successful ageing. *Maturitas, 75*(4), 361–366.

Hughes, T. F., Flatt, J. D., Fu, B., et al. (2014). Interactive video gaming compared with health education in older adults with mild cognitive impairment: A feasibility study. *International Journal of Geriatric Psychiatry, 29*(9), 890–898.

Hunter, E. G. (2007-2008). Beyond death: Inheriting the past and giving to the future, transmitting the legacy of one's self. *Omega, 56*(4), 313–329.

Jang, Y., Park, N. S., Dominquez, D. D., et al. (2014). Social engagement in older residents of assisted living facilities. *Aging and Mental Health, 18*(5), 642–647.

Kim, S. K. (2013). A randomized, controlled study of the effects of art therapy on older Korean-Americans' healthy aging. *The Arts in Psychotherapy, 40*(1), 158–164.

Lambert, V., Coad, J., Hicks, P., et al. (2014). Social spaces for young children in hospital. *Child: Care, Health & Development, 40*(2), 195–204.

Liu, C. J., Brost, M. A., Horton, V. E., et al. (2013). Occupational therapy interventions to improve performance of daily activities at home for older adults with low vision: A systematic review. *American Journal of Occupational Therapy, 67*(3), 279–287.

Mandel, S., Davis, B. A., & Secic, M. (2014). Effects of music therapy on patient satisfaction and health-related quality of life of hospital inpatients. *Hospital Topics, 92*(2), 28–35.

Moorhead, S., Johnson, M., Maas, M. L., et al. (2013). *Nursing outcomes classification (NOC): Measurement of health outcomes* (5th ed.). St. Louis: Elsevier.

Muñoz Lasa, S., Ferriero, G., Brigatti, E., et al. (2011). Animal-assisted interventions in internal and rehabilitation medicine: A review of the recent literature. *Panminerva Medica, 53*(2), 129–136.

Nadler-Moodie, M., Burnell, L., Fries, J., et al. (2009). A S.A.F.E. alternative to sitters. *Nursing Management, 40*(8), 43–50.

Nilsson, S., Enskär, K., Hallqvist, C., et al. (2013). Active and passive distraction in children undergoing wound dressings. *Journal of Pediatric Nursing, 28*(2), 158–166.

Noice, T., Noice, H., & Kramer, A. F. (2013). Participatory arts for older adults: a review of benefits and challenges. *The Gerontologist, 54*(5), 741–753.

Oerlemans, W. G., Bakker, A. B., & Veenhoven, R. (2011). Finding the key to happy aging: A day reconstruction study of happiness. *Journal of Gerontology Series B, Psychological Science and Social Science, 66*(6), 665–674.

Okvat, H. A., & Zautra, A. J. (2011). Community gardening: A parsimonious path to individual, community, and environmental resilience. *American Journal of Community Psychology, 47*(3–4), 374–387.

Pasanen, T. P., Tyrväinen, L., & Korpela, K. M. (2014). The relationship between perceived health and physical activity indoors, outdoors in built environments, and outdoors in nature. *Applied Psychology: Health and Well Being*, [epub ahead of print].

Sampaio, P. Y., & Ito, E. (2013). Activities with higher influence on quality of life in older adults in Japan. *Occupational Therapy International, 20*(1), 1–10.

Särkämo, T., & Soto, D. (2012). Music listening after stroke: Beneficial effects and potential neural mechanisms. *Annals of the New York Academy of Sciences, 1252*, 266–281.

Shee, A. W., Bev Phillips, K., & Hill, K. D. (2014). Feasibility and acceptability of a volunteer-mediated diversional therapy program for older patients with cognitive impairment. *Geriatric Nursing, 35*(5), 300–305.

Van Den Berg, A. E., & Custers, M. H. (2011). Gardening promotes neuroendocrine and affective restoration from stress. *Journal of Health Psychology, 16*(1), 3–11.

Van Der Ploeg, E., Eppingstall, B., Camp, C. J., et al. (2013). A randomized crossover trial to study the effect of personalized,

D

one-to-one interaction using Montessori-based activities on agitation, affect, and engagement in nursing home residents with dementia. *International Psychogeriatrics*, *25*(4), 565–575.

Wang, D., & Macmillan, T. (2013). The benefits of gardening for older adults: A systematic review of the literature. *Activities, Adaptation & Aging*, *37*(2), 153–181.

Wilson, C. B., Tetley, J., Healey, J., et al. (2011). The best care is like sunshine: Accessing older people's experiences of living in care homes through creative writing. *Activities, Adaptation & Aging*, *35*(1), 1–20.

Wu, L. F. (2011). Group integrative reminiscence therapy on self-esteem, life satisfaction and depressive symptoms in institutionalized older veterans. *Journal of Clinical Nursing*, *20*(15–16), 2195–2203.

Yeh, G. Y., McCarthy, E. P., Wayne, P. M., et al. (2011). Tai chi exercise in patients with chronic heart failure: A randomized clinical trial. *Archives of Internal Medicine*, *171*(8), 750–757.

Risk for Electrolyte imbalance

Susan M. Dirkes, RN, MS, CCRN

NANDA-I

Definition

Vulnerable to changes in serum electrolyte levels, which may compromise health

Risk Factors

Compromised regulatory mechanism; diarrhea; endocrine regulatory dysfunction; fluid imbalance (e.g., glucose intolerance, increase in IGF-1, androgen, DHEA, and cortisol); excessive fluid volume; insufficient fluid volume; renal dysfunction; treatment regimen; vomiting

NOC (Nursing Outcomes Classification)

Suggested NOC Outcomes

Electrolyte and Acid-Base Balance; Fluid Balance; Hydration; Nutritional Status: Biochemical Measures; Nutritional Status: Food and Fluid Intake; Nutritional Status: Nutrient Intake; Kidney Function

Example NOC Outcome with Indicators

Electrolyte and Acid-Base Balance as evidenced by the following indicators: Apical heart rate/Apical heart rhythm/Serum potassium/Serum sodium/Serum calcium, serum magnesium, serum phosphorus. (Rate the outcome and indicators of **Electrolyte and Acid-Base Balance:** 1 = severe deviation from normal range, 2 = substantial deviation from normal range, 3 = moderate deviation from normal range, 4 = mild deviation from normal range, 5 = no deviation from normal range [see Section I].)

Client Outcomes

Client Will (Specify Time Frame)

- Maintain a normal sinus heart rhythm with a regular rate
- Have a decrease in edema
- Maintain an absence of muscle cramping
- Maintain normal serum potassium, sodium, calcium, and phosphorus
- Maintain normal serum pH

NIC (Nursing Interventions Classification)

Suggested NIC Interventions

Electrolyte Monitoring; Electrolyte Management: Hypokalemia, Hyperkalemia, Hypocalcemia, Hypercalcemia, Hyponatremia, Hypernatremia, Hypophosphatemia, and Hyperphosphatemia; Electrolyte Management: Hyponatremia; Fluid/Electrolyte Management; Laboratory Data Interpretation

Example NIC Activities—Electrolyte Monitoring

Identify possible causes of electrolyte imbalances; Monitor the serum level of electrolytes

Nursing Interventions and *Rationales*

- ▲ Monitor vital signs at least three times a day, or more frequently as needed. Notify health care provider of significant deviation from baseline. *Electrolyte imbalance can lead to clinical manifestations such as respiratory failure, arrhythmias, edema, muscle weakness, and altered mental status (Wagner & Hardin-Pierce, 2014).*
- ▲ Monitor cardiac rate and rhythm. Report changes to provider. *Hypokalemia and hyperkalemia can result in electrocardiogram (ECG) changes that can lead to cardiac arrest, and ventricular dysrhythmias. Magnesium and calcium imbalances also can cause cardiac arrhythmias. Low serum magnesium (≤2 mEq/L) is associated with hypokalemia and ECG changes, and high phosphate may indicate kidney injury (Wagner & Hardin-Pierce, 2014).*
- • Monitor intake and output and daily weights using a consistent scale. *Weight gain is a sensitive and consistent sign of fluid volume excess (Wagner & Hardin-Pierce, 2014).*
- • Monitor for abdominal distention and discomfort. *A focused assessment should be done on any patient presenting with hepatic, gastrointestinal or pancreatic dysfunction (Wagner & Hardin-Pierce, 2014).*
- • Monitor the client's respiratory status and muscle strength. *Phosphorus is an essential element in cell structure, metabolism, and maintenance of acid-base processes. Consequences of hypophosphatemia include cardiac and respiratory failure (Wagner & Hardin-Pierce, 2014).*
- • Assess cardiac status and neurological alterations. EB: *Hypophosphatemia can cause myocardial dysfunction, hematological dysfunction, respiratory depression, and neurological changes (Claure-DelGrando & Bouchard, 2012).*
- • *Causes of neurological changes are not well documented. Hyperphosphatemia is associated with hypocalcemia (since it is inversely related to calcium), causing tetany, muscle spasms, and cardiac arrhythmias (Wagner & Hardin-Pierce, 2014).*
- ▲ Review laboratory data as ordered and report deviations to provider. *Laboratory studies may include serum electrolytes: potassium, chloride, sodium, bicarbonate, magnesium, phosphate, calcium; serum pH; comprehensive metabolic panel; and arterial blood gases.*
- • Review the client's medical and surgical history for possible causes of altered electrolytes. *Periods of excess fluid loss can lead to dehydration and resulting loss of electrolytes; fluid can be lost through gastrointestinal illness, renal failure, hyperthermia, blood loss, and perspiration due to strenuous exercise (Wagner & Hardin-Pierce, 2014; Chlibkova et al, 2014). Additional causes of electrolyte imbalances include burns, trauma, sepsis, diabetic ketoacidosis, extensive surgeries, and changes in acid-base balance (Yee, 2010).*
- ▲ Complete pain assessment. Assess and document the onset, intensity, character, location, duration, aggravating factors, and relieving factors. Notify the provider for any increase in pain or discomfort or if comfort measures are not effective. *Symptoms of electrolyte imbalance and dehydration can include muscle cramps, paresthesias, abdominal cramps, skin manifestations, cardiac arrhythmias, and tetany (Wagner & Hardin-Pierce, 2014).*
- ▲ Monitor the effects of ordered medications such as diuretics and heart medications. *Medications can have adverse effects on kidney function and electrolyte balance, particularly contrast agents, chemotherapeutic agents, amphotericin B, aminoglycosides, phosphate ingestion, loop diuretics, and vitamin D (Calazza et al, 2014; Wagner & Hardin-Pierce 2014).*
- ▲ Administer parenteral fluids as ordered and monitor their effects. *Rapid resuscitation with fluids can cause adverse effects such as electrolyte imbalance, increased bleeding, and coagulopathies (Wang et al, 2014). Administration of fluids should be done in order to impact the plasma electrolytes and pH as well as hemodynamic improvement (Vassalos & Rooney, 2013).*

Geriatric

- • Monitor electrolyte levels carefully, including sodium levels and potassium levels, with both increased and decreased levels possible. EB: *Older adults are prone to electrolyte abnormalities because of failure of regulatory mechanisms associated with heart and kidney disease, a decrease in the ability to reabsorb sodium, and a loss of diluting capacity in the kidneys (Bolignano et al, 2014). Many older clients receive selective serotonin reuptake inhibitors for treatment of depression, which can result in hyponatremia (Rudge & Kim, 2014).*

Client/Family Teaching and Discharge Planning

- • Teach client/family the signs of low potassium and the risk factors. *Signs and symptoms of low potassium include muscle weakness, nausea, vomiting, constipation, and irregular pulse (Wagner & Hardin-Pierce, 2014).*

E

- Teach client/family the signs of high potassium and the risk factors. *Signs and symptoms of high potassium include restlessness, muscle weakness, slow heart rate, diarrhea, and cramping (Wagner & Hardin-Pierce, 2014).*
- Teach client/family the signs of low sodium and the risk factors. *Early signs of low sodium include nausea, muscle cramps, disorientation, and mental status changes (Wagner & Hardin-Pierce, 2014).*
- Teach client/family the signs of high sodium and the risk factors. *Signs of high sodium include thirst, dry mucous membranes, rapid heartbeat, low blood pressure, and mental status changes; symptoms can progress to confusion, delirium, and seizures (Wagner & Hardin-Pierce, 2014).*
- Teach client/family the importance of hydration during exercise. Dehydration occurs when the amount of water leaving the body is greater than the amount consumed. *The body can lose large amounts of fluid when it tries to cool itself by sweating (Jequier & Constant, 2010).*
- Teach client/family the warning signs of dehydration. Early signs of dehydration include thirst and decreased urine output. As dehydration increases, symptoms may include dry mouth, muscle cramps, nausea and vomiting, lightheadedness, and orthostatic hypotension. *Severe dehydration can cause confusion, weakness, coma, and organ failure (Wagner & Hardin-Pierce, 2014).*
- Teach client about any medications prescribed. Medication teaching includes the drug name, its purpose, administration instructions such as taking it with or without food, and any side effects to be aware of. EB: *Diuretic use remains a primary cause of low serum potassium levels (Arampatzis et al, 2013).*

▲ Instruct the client to report any adverse medication side effects to his/her health care provider. EB: *Assessing and instructing clients about medications and focusing on important details can help prevent client medication errors (Buckley et al, 2010).*

REFERENCES

Arampatzis, B. D., Funk, G. C., Leichtle, A. B., et al. (2013). Impact of diuretic-therapy electrolyte disorders present on admission to the emergency department: a cross-sectional analysis. *BMC Medicine*, *11*, 83.

Bolignano, D., Mattace-Raso, F., Sijbrands, E. J., et al. (2014). The aging kidney revisited: a systematic review. *Ageing Research Reviews*, 65–80.

Buckley, M. S., LeBlanc, J. M., & Cawley, M. J. (2010). Electrolyte disturbances associated with commonly prescribed medications in the intensive care unit. *Critical Care Medicine*, *38*(6), S253–S264.

Calazza, A., Russo, L., Sabbatini, M., et al. (2014). Hemodynamic and tubular changes induced by contrast media. *BioMed Research International*, *2014*, 578974.

Chlibkova, D., Knechtie, B., Roseman, T., et al. (2014). The prevalence of exercise-associated hyponatremia in 24-hour ultra mountain bikers, 24 hour ultrarunners and multi-stage ultramountain bikers in the Czech Republic. *Journal of the International Society of Sports Nutrition*, *11*(1), 3.

Claure-DelGrando, R., & Bouchard, J. (2012). Acid-based and electrolyte abnormalities during renal support for acute kidney injury: recognition and management. *Blood Purification*, *34*(2), 186–193.

Jequier, E., & Constant, F. (2010). Water as an essential nutrient: the physiological basis of hydration. *European Journal of Clinical Nutrition*, *64*, 115–123.

Rudge, J. E., & Kim, D. (2014). New-onset hyponatraemia after surgery for traumatic hip fracture. *Age and Ageing*.

Wagner, K. D., & Hardin-Pierce, M. G. (2014). *High Acuity Nursing* (6th ed, pp. 359–629). Boston, MA: Prentice Hall, Inc.

Vassalos, A., & Rooney, K. (2013). Surviving sepsis guidelines 2012. *Critical Care Medicine*, *41*(12), 485–486.

Wang, C. H., Hsieh, W. H., Chou, H. C., et al. (2014). Liberal versus restricted fluid resuscitation strategies in trauma patients: a systematic review and meta-analysis of randomized controlled trials and observational studies. *Critical Care Medicine*, *42*(4), 954–961.

Yee, A. H. (2010). Neurologic presentations of acid-base imbalance, electrolyte abnormalities and endocrine emergencies. *Neurologic Clinics*, *28*(1), 1–16.

Labile Emotional Control

Wolter Paans, MSc, PhD, RN

NANDA-I

Definition

Uncontrollable outbursts of exaggerated and involuntary emotional expression

Defining Characteristics

Absence of eye contact; difficulty in use of facial expressions; embarrassment regarding emotional expression; excessive crying without feeling sadness; excessive laughing without feeling happiness; expression of emotion incongruent with triggering factor; involuntary crying; involuntary laughing; tearfulness;

uncontrollable crying; uncontrollable laughing; withdrawal from occupational situation; withdrawal from social situation

Related Factors

Alteration in self-esteem; brain injury; emotional disturbance; fatigue; functional impairment; insufficient knowledge about symptom control; insufficient knowledge of disease; insufficient muscle strength; mood disorder; musculoskeletal impairment; pharmaceutical agent; physical disability; psychiatric disorder; social distress; stressors; substance abuse

E

NOC Outcomes (Nursing Outcomes Classification)

Suggested NOC Outcomes

Coping; Knowledge: Disease Process; Impulse; Self-Control; Self-Esteem; Quality of Life; Personal Well-Being; Stress Level

Example NOC Outcomes with Indicators

Knowledge: Disease Process as evidenced by the following indicator: Specific disease process. (Rate the outcome and indicators of **Knowledge: Disease Process:** 1 = no knowledge, 2 = limited knowledge, 3= moderate knowledge, 4 = substantial knowledge, 5 = extensive knowledge [see Section I].)

Client Outcomes

Client Will (Specify Time Frame)

- Improve coping strategies
- Improved knowledge about disease process, signs and symptoms, triggers, symptom control
- Employ mechanisms to control impulses and ask for help when feeling impulses
- Improve feelings of dignity
- Enhance and improve response to social and environmental stimuli

NIC Interventions (Nursing Interventions Classification)

Suggested NIC Interventions

Coping Enhancement; Teaching: Disease Process; Enhance Self-Esteem; Improved Quality of Life; Improved Well-Being

Example NIC Activities—Labile Emotional Control

Coping Enhancement: Assist the patient to solve problems in a constructive manner; Instruct the patient on the use of relaxation techniques, as needed; Assist the patient to identify positive strategies to deal with limitations and manage needed lifestyle or role changes

Nursing Interventions and *Rationales*

- Provide progressive relaxation exercise techniques. EB: *"Our present study with a randomized controlled group design clearly demonstrates that after two sessions, a single bout of PMR reduces anxiety and psychological stress, and improves subjective well-being" (Georgiev et al, 2012).* EB: *Systematic review demonstrates specific physical therapy interventions, including aerobic and muscle strength exercises, progressive muscle relaxation, and yoga, resulted in beneficial outcomes for psychiatric symptoms, psychosocial distress, anxiety, health-related quality of life, and aerobic and muscular fitness (Vancampfort et al, 2011).*
- Offer instruction regarding alternative coping strategies such as mindfulness and breath awareness. EB: *Increased breath awareness (a fundamental component of mindfulness meditation) has been shown to reduce autonomic and psychological arousal, and this increased capacity to remain calm can help individuals to respond more adaptively to internal and external stressors (Compare et al, 2014).* EB: *Studies have demonstrated the effects of mindfulness and yoga on well-being, somatic effects of stress, immune system, and physical symptoms and chronic conditions (Lazaridou et al, 2013).*

- Use the Pathological Laughter and Crying Scale (PLACS) to identify pathological laughing and crying or related disorders (e.g., IEED, PBA). EB/EBN: *PLACS is an interviewer-administered instrument that has been validated in clients with acute stroke. It has shown excellent interrater and test-retest reliability (Ahmed & Simmons, 2013).*
- Consider using cognitive-behavioral therapy. CEB/EB: *Cognitive-behavioral therapy has been shown to be moderately effective when compared to usual care and to relaxation, counseling, and education/support, although these effects have not been maintained over time (Malouff et al, 2008; Price et al, 2008).*
- Provide, if possible, music therapy. EB: *The use of music therapy can improve mental well-being, social functioning, quality of life, anxiety, pain, mood, relaxation, and comfort in persons with several disorders/diseases such as cancer, schizophrenia, mood disorders, and autism (Kamioka et al, 2014). Music therapy as an addition to standard care helps people with schizophrenia to improve their global state, mental state (including negative symptoms), and social functioning if a sufficient number of music therapy sessions are provided (Mössler et al, 2011).*

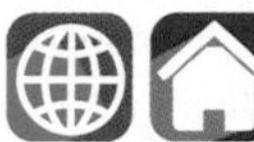

Multicultural, Home Care

- The above interventions may be adapted for multicultural and home care.

Client/Family Teaching and Discharge Planning

- Inform client and family about the emotional lability and talk with them about how to cope with the situation. EBN: *Stroke services should aim to produce easy-to-read literature that explains emotional lability, and offer clients and families reassurance and simple suggestions about how to cope with the condition (Gillespie et al, 2011).*
- Use verbal and nonverbal therapeutic communication approaches including empathy, active listening, and confrontation to encourage the client and family to express emotions such as sadness, guilt, and anger (within appropriate limits); verbalize fears and concerns; and set goals. EB: *Solution focused communication with clients helps focus on goals and helps find solutions (Ruddick, 2011).*
- Provide psychoeducation for stress-related variables to client and family. EB: *Psychoeducation was conducted in seven studies, six of which had positive outcomes on depression, anxiety, or knowledge levels (Bte Iskhandar Shah et al, 2013).* EB: *Learning about stress and extending techniques to cope with stress seems to contribute positively to mental health (Van Daele et al, 2012).*

REFERENCES

Ahmed, A., & Simmons, Z. (2013). Pseudobulbar affect: prevalence and management. *Therapeutics and Clinical Risk Management, 2013*(9), 483–489.

Bte Iskhandar Shah, L., Klainin-Yobas, P., Torres, S., et al. (2013). Efficacy of psychoeducation and relaxation interventions on stress-related variables in people with mental disorders: a literature review. *Archives of Psychiatric Nursing, 28*(2), 94–101.

Compare, A., Zarbo, C., Shonin, E., et al. (2014). Emotional regulation and depression: a potential mediator between heart and mind. *Cardiovascular Psychiatry and Neurology*.

Georgiev, A., Probst, M., Hert, M., et al. (2012). Acute effects of progressive muscle relaxation on state anxiety and subjective well-being in chronic bulgarian patients with schizophrenia. *Psychiatria Danubina, 24*(4), 367–372.

Gillespie, D. C., Joice, S., Lawrence, M., et al. (2011). Interventions for post-stroke disturbances of mood and emotional behavior: recommendations from SIGN 118. *International Journal of Therapy and Rehabilitation, 18*(3), 545–553.

Kamioka, H., Tsutani, K., Yamada, M., et al. (2014). Effectiveness of music therapy: a summary of systematic reviews based on randomized controlled trials of music interventions. *Patient Preference and Adherence, 2014*(8), 727–754.

Lazaridou, A., Philbrook, P., & Tzika, A. (2013). Yoga and mindfulness as therapeutic interventions for stroke rehabilitation: a systematic review. *Evidence-based Complementary and Alternative Medicine*. <http://dx.doi.org/10.1155/2013/357108>.

Malouff, J. M., Thorsteinsson, E. B., Rooke, S. E., et al. (2008). Efficacy of cognitive behavioral therapy for chronic fatigue syndrome: a meta-analysis. *Clinical Psychology Review, 28*(5), 736–745.

Mössler, K., Chen, X., Heldal, T. O., et al. (2011). Music therapy for people with schizophrenia and schizophrenia-like disorders. *The Cochrane Database of Systematic Reviews, 2011*(12), CD004025.

Price, J. R., Mitchell, E., Tidy, E., et al. (2008). Cognitive behavior therapy for chronic fatigue syndrome in adults. *The Cochrane Database of Systematic Reviews, 16*(3), CD001027.

Ruddick, F. (2011). Coping with problems by focusing on solutions. *Mental Health Practice, 14*(8), 28–30.

van Daele, T., Hermans, D., van Audenhove, C., et al. (2012). Stress reduction through psychoeducation: a meta-analytic review. *Health Education Behaviour, 39*(4), 474–485.

Vancampfort, D., Probst, M., Helvik Skjaerven, L., et al. (2011). Systematic review of the benefits of physical therapy within a multidisciplinary care approach for people with schizophrenia. *Physical Therapy, 92*, 11–23.

Risk for dry Eye

Paula D. Hopper, MSN, RN, CNE, and Betty J. Ackley, MSN, EdS, RN

E

NANDA-I

Definition

Vulnerable to eye discomfort or damage to the cornea and conjunctiva due to reduced quantity or quality of tears to moisten the eye, which may compromise health

Risk Factors

Aging; autoimmune diseases (e.g., rheumatoid arthritis, diabetes mellitus, thyroid disease); contact lens wearer; environmental factor (e.g., air conditioning, excessive wind, sunlight exposure, air pollution, low humidity); female gender; history of allergy; hormonal change; lifestyle choice (e.g., smoking, caffeine use, prolonged reading); mechanical ventilation neurological lesions with sensory or motor reflex loss (e.g., lagophthalmos, lack of spontaneous blink reflex); ocular surface damage; treatment regimen; vitamin A deficiency

NOC (Nursing Outcomes Classification)

Suggested NOC Outcomes (Visual)

Dry Eye Severity; Sensory Function: Vision; Vision Compensation Behavior

Example NOC Outcome with Indicators

Dry Eye Severity as evidenced by the following indicators: Decreased tear production/Redness of conjunctiva/burning eye sensation/Itchy eye sensation/Eye pain/Excessive watering/Blurred vision. (Rate each indicator of **Dry Eye Severity:** 1 = severe, 2 = substantial, 3 = moderate, 4 = mild, 5 = none [see Section I].)

Client Outcomes

Client Will (Specify Time Frame)

- State eyes are comfortable with no itching, burning, or dryness
- Have corneal surface that is intact and without injury
- Demonstrate self-administration of eye drops if ordered
- State vision is clear

NIC (Nursing Interventions Classification)

Suggested NIC Interventions

Communication Enhancement: Visual Deficit; Environmental Management

Example NIC Activities—Communication Enhancement: Visual Deficit

Identify yourself when you enter the client's space; Provide adequate room lighting

Nursing Interventions and *Rationales*

▲ Assess for symptoms of dry eyes, such as "irritation, tearing, burning, stinging, dry or foreign body sensation, mild itching, photophobia, blurry vision, contact lens intolerance, redness, mucus discharge, increased frequency of blinking, eye fatigue, diurnal fluctuation, symptoms that worsen later in the day" (American Academy of Ophthalmology [AAO], 2013).

▲ If symptoms are present, refer client to an ophthalmologist for diagnosis and treatment. EB: *Clients with dry eye who are evaluated by non-ophthalmologist health care providers should be referred promptly to the ophthalmologist if moderate or severe pain, lack of response to therapy, corneal infiltration or ulceration, or vision loss occurs (AAO, 2013).*

▲ Administer ordered eye drops. *As the severity of the dry eye increases, aqueous enhancement of the eye using topical agents is appropriate. Emulsions, gels, and ointments can be used (AAO, 2013).*

- Consider use of eyeglass side shields or moisture chambers. EB: *Eyeglass side shields can protect the eyes from drafts. Moisture chambers are a type of eyeglasses that are frequently worn by motorcyclists and mountain climbers and can be purchased at stores or online (AAO, 2013).*
- ▲ Watch for symptoms of blepharitis including crusting and irritation at the base of the lashes and adjacent redness of the eyelid, which may accompany dry eye; refer for treatment as needed. EB: *Contributing ocular factors such as blepharitis should be treated. Particularly effective treatments for evaporative tear deficiency include eyelid therapy for conditions such as blepharitis (AAO, 2013).*
- ▲ Discuss use of caffeine with client's health care provider. EB: *Arita et al (2012) found that use of caffeine capsules increased tear volume.*

Geriatric

- Recognize that symptoms of dry eye are more common in menopausal women and geriatric clients. *Hormonal changes after menopause can disrupt tear production. It is estimated that one in three individuals older than 65 years experiences dry eyes (National Health Service [NHS], 2014).*

Critical Care

- ▲ Provide regular cleaning of the eyes, lubricating eye drops and ointments, and consultation with an ophthalmologist if infection is suspected in clients in the intensive care unit (ICU). *ICU staff may miss ocular complications while caring for life-threatening conditions; ocular complications can seriously impair vision and quality of life.* EB: *"As ICU patients are more susceptible to develop dry eye, keratopathy, and ocular infections, they should be consulted by an ophthalmologist for early diagnosis of ocular surface disorders" (Saritas et al, 2013).*
- Avoid using adhesive tape to keep eyes closed in sedated patients. EBN: *In an audit of eye dryness and corneal abrasions of patients in four ICUs in Iran, patients receiving adhesive tape as an eye care method were twice as likely to develop corneal abrasion (Masoudi et al, 2014).*

Client/Family Teaching and Discharge Planning

- Teach client conditions that can exacerbate dry eye symptoms. *Exacerbating conditions include wind, air travel, decreased humidity, air conditioning or heating, and prolonged activities that reduce blink rate such as reading and computer use (AAO, 2013).*
- Teach client good eye hygiene:
  - Apply warm compresses for 10-minute intervals using a clean cloth and water that has been boiled and cooled (or sterile water).
  - Gently massage around eyelids.
  - Gently clean eyelids to remove excess oil, crusts, and bacteria. Use a few drops of baby shampoo in water that has been boiled and cooled, or in sterile water.
    - *Good hygiene can help improve dry eyes, especially dry eye associated with blepharitis (NHS, 2014).*
- Teach clients methods to decrease problems with dry eye including the following:
  - Avoid drafty (e.g., ceiling fans) and low-humidity environments.
  - Avoid smoking and exposure to second-hand smoke.
- ▲ Discuss avoidance of offending medications with health care provider.
- Drink plenty of water to keep well hydrated. EB: *For patients with a clinical diagnosis of mild dry eye, potentially exacerbating exogenous factors such as antihistamine or diuretic use, cigarette smoking, and exposure to second-hand smoke, and environmental factors such as air drafts and low-humidity environments should be addressed (AAO, 2013). Symptoms of dry eye may be exacerbated by the use of medications such as diuretics, antihistamines, anticholinergics, antidepressants, and systemic retinoids (AAO, 2013). Self-care includes drinking plenty of water to stay hydrated (American Optometric Association, 2014).*
- Teach client to lower the computer screen to below eye level and to blink more frequently. *Measures such as lowering the computer screen to below eye level to decrease lid aperture, scheduling regular breaks, and increasing blink frequency may decrease the discomfort associated with computer and reading activities (AAO, 2013).*
- ▲ Teach client to consult with the health care provider regarding use of omega-3 supplements to decrease dry eye. EB: *Omega-3 fatty acid products without ethyl esters may be beneficial in the treatment of dry eye, although they may increase the risk of prostate cancer (AAO, 2013).*

- Teach client using eye drops how to self-administer eye drops.
- Warn clients with dry eyes that driving at night can be dangerous. *Clients with dry eyes have light sensitivity and decreased refraction.*

REFERENCES

American Academy of Ophthalmology (AAO) (2013). Dry eye syndrome preferred practice patterns—2013. *The Ophthalmic News and Education Network.* Retrieved from <http://one.aao.org/preferred-practice-pattern/dry-eye-syndrome-ppp–2013>.

American Optometric Association (AOA) (2014). *Dry eye.* Retrieved from <http://www.aoa.org/patients-and-public/eye-and-vision-problems/glossary-of-eye-and-vision-conditions/dry-eye?sso=y>.

Arita, R., et al. (2012). Caffeine increases tear volume depending on polymorphisms within the adenosine A2a receptor gene and cytochrome P450 1A2. *Ophthalmology, 119*(5), 972–978.

Masoudi, N., et al. (2014). An audit of eye dryness and corneal abrasion in ICU patients in Iran. *Nursing in Critical Care, 19*(2), 73–77.

National Health Service (NHS) England (2014). *Dry eye syndrome—self-help.* Retrieved from <http://www.nhs.uk/Conditions/Dry-eye-syndrome/Pages/Prevention.aspx>.

Saritas, T. B., et al. (2013). Ocular surface disorders in intensive care unit patients. *Scientific World Journal.* Retrieved from <http://www.ncbi.nlm.nih.gov/pmc/articles/PMC3830763/>.

Risk for Falls

Sherry A. Greenberg, PhD, RN, GNP-BC

NANDA-I

Definition

Vulnerable to increased susceptibility to falling, which may cause physical harm and compromise health

Risk Factors

Adults

Age ≥ 65 years; history of falls; living alone; lower limb prosthesis; use of assistive device (e.g., walker, cane, wheelchair)

Children

Absence of stairway gate; absence of window guard; age ≤ 2 years; inadequate supervision; insufficient automobile restraints; male gender when < 1 year of age

Cognitive

Alteration in cognitive functioning

Environment

Cluttered environment; exposure to unsafe weather-related condition (e.g., wet floors, ice); insufficient lighting; insufficient antislip material in bathroom; unfamiliar setting; use of restraints; use of throw rugs

Pharmaceutical Agents

Alcohol consumption; pharmaceutical agent

Physiological

Acute illness; alteration in blood glucose level; anemia; arthritis; condition affecting the foot; decrease in lower extremity strength; diarrhea; difficulty with gait; faintness when extending neck; faintness when turning neck; hearing impairment; impaired balance; impaired mobility; incontinence; neoplasm; neuropathy; orthostatic hypotension; postoperative recovery period; proprioceptive deficit; sleeplessness; urinary urgency; vascular disease; visual impairment

NOC (Nursing Outcomes Classification)

Suggested NOC Outcomes

Fall Prevention Behavior; Knowledge: Child Physical Safety

Example NOC Outcome with Indicators

Fall Prevention Behavior as evidenced by the following indicators: Uses assistive devices correctly/Eliminates clutter, spills, glare from floors/Uses safe transfer procedures. (Rate each indicator of **Fall Prevention Behavior:** 1 = never demonstrated, 2 = rarely demonstrated, 3 = sometimes demonstrated, 4 = often demonstrated, 5 = consistently demonstrated [see Section I].)

Client Outcomes

Client Will (Specify Time Frame)

- Remain free of falls
- Change environment to minimize the incidence of falls
- Explain methods to prevent injury

F

NIC (Nursing Interventions Classification)

Suggested NIC Interventions

Dementia Management; Fall Prevention; Post-Fall Assessment; Surveillance: Safety

Example NIC Activities—Fall Prevention

Assist unsteady individual with ambulation; Monitor gait, balance, and fatigue level with ambulation

Nursing Interventions and *Rationales*

- Safety Guidelines. Complete a fall-risk assessment for older adults in acute care using a valid and reliable tool such as the Hendrich II Model. Recognize that risk factors for falling include recent history of falls, fear of falling, confusion, depression, altered elimination patterns, cardiovascular/respiratory disease impairing perfusion or oxygenation, postural hypotension, dizziness or vertigo, primary cancer diagnosis, and altered mobility (Gray-Miceli, 2008). *The Hendrich II Fall Risk Model is quick to administer and provides a determination of risk for falling based on gender, mental and emotional status, symptoms of dizziness, and known categories of medications increasing risk (Hendrich, 2006). This tool screens for primary prevention of falls and is integral in a post-fall assessment for the secondary prevention of falls (Gray-Miceli, 2007).*
- Screen all clients for balance and mobility skills (supine to sit, sitting supported and unsupported, sit to stand, standing, walking and turning around, transferring, stooping to floor and recovering, and sitting down). Use tools such as the Balance Scale by Tinetti or the Get Up and Go Scale. *It is helpful to determine the client's functional abilities and then plan for ways to improve problem areas or determine methods to ensure safety (Gray-Miceli, 2008).*
- Recognize that when people attend to another task while walking, such as carrying a cup of water, clothing, or supplies, they are more likely to fall. CEB: *Those who slow down when given a carrying task are at a higher risk for subsequent falls (Lundin-Olsson et al, 1998).*
- Carefully assist a mostly immobile client up. Be sure to lock the bed and wheelchair and have sufficient personnel to protect the client from falls. When rising from a lying position, have the client change positions slowly, dangle legs, and stand next to the bed before walking to prevent orthostatic hypotension. *Encourage client engagement in a monitored exercise program that will strengthen core and lower extremities to reduce fall risk (Grabiner, 2013; Hirase et al, 2014).*
- Use a "high-risk fall" armband/bracelet and fall risk room sign to alert staff for increased vigilance and mobility assistance. *These steps alert the nursing staff of the increased risk of falls (Goodwin et al, 2014; McCarter-Bayer et al, 2005).*

▲ Evaluate the client's medications to determine whether medications increase the risk of falling; consult with health care provider regarding the client's need for medication if appropriate. *Polypharmacy, or taking more than four medications, has been associated with increased falls. Medications such as benzodiazepines, as well as antipsychotic and antidepressant medications given to promote sleep, actually increase the rate of falls (Capezuti et al, 1999; Goodwin et al, 2014).* EB: *Short-to-intermediate-acting benzodiazepine and tricyclic antidepressants may produce ataxia, impaired psychomotor function, syncope, and additional falls (Fick et al, 2003; Molony, 2008).*

- Orient the client to environment. Place the call light within reach and show how to call for assistance; answer call light promptly.
- Use one-fourth to one-half–length side rails only, and maintain bed in a low position. Ensure that wheels are locked on bed and commode. Keep dim light in room at night. *Use of full side rails can result in the client climbing over the rails, leading with the head, and sustaining a head injury. Side rails with widely spaced vertical bars and side rails not situated flush with the mattress have been associated with asphyxiation deaths because of rail and in bed entrapment and should not be used (Capezuti, 2004; Goodwin et al, 2014).*
- Routinely assist the client with toileting on his or her own schedule. Take the client to bathroom on awakening and before bedtime (McCarter-Bayer et al, 2005; Goodwin et al, 2014). Keep the path to the bathroom clear, label the bathroom, and leave the door open.

F

▲ Avoid use of restraints if possible. Obtain health care provider's order if restraints are deemed necessary, and use the least restrictive device. *The use of restraints has been associated with serious injuries including rhabdomyolysis, brachial plexus injury, neuropathy, and dysrhythmias, as well as strangulation, asphyxiation, traumatic brain injuries, and all the consequences of immobility (Evans & Cotter, 2008).* CEB/EB: *A study demonstrated that there was no increase in falls or injuries in a group of clients who were not restrained versus a similar group that was restrained in a nursing home (Capezuti et al, 1999). A study in two acute care hospitals demonstrated that when restraints were not used, there was no increase in client falls, injuries, or therapy disruptions (Mion et al, 2001).*

- In place of restraints, use the following:
  - Well-staffed and educated nursing personnel with frequent client contact with careful consideration during shift changes
  - Nursing units designed to care for clients with cognitive or functional impairments
  - Nonskid footwear, sneakers preferable
  - Adequate lighting, night-light in bathroom
  - Frequent toileting
  - Frequently assess need for invasive devices, tubes, intravenous (IV) access
  - Hide tubes with bandages to prevent pulling of tubes
  - Consider alternative IV placement site to prevent pulling out IV line
  - Alarm systems with ankle, above-the-knee, or wrist sensors
  - Bed or wheelchair alarms
  - Wedge cushions on chairs to prevent slipping
  - Increased observation of the client
  - Locked doors to unit
  - Low or very low height beds
  - Border-defining pillow/mattress to remind the client to stay in bed
- *These alternatives to restraints can be helpful to prevent falls (McCarter-Bayer et al, 2005; Cotter & Evans, 2007; Grabiner 2013).*
- If the client has an acute change in mental status (delirium), recognize that the cause is usually physiological and is a medical emergency. Consider possible causes for delirium. Consult with the health care provider immediately. See interventions for Acute **Confusion.**
- If the client has chronic confusion due to dementia, implement individualized strategies to enhance communication. *Assessment of specific receptive and expressive language abilities is needed in order to understand the client's communication difficulties and facilitate communication.* See interventions for Chronic **Confusion.**
- Ask family to stay with the client to assist with activities of daily living and prevent the client from accidentally falling or pulling out tubes.

▲ If the client is unsteady on his/her feet, have two nursing staff members alongside when walking the client. Use facility approved mobility devices to assist with client ambulation (e.g., gait belts, walkers). Consider referral to physical therapy for gait training and strengthening. *The client can walk independently, but the nurse can rapidly ensure safety if the client becomes weak or unsteady. Interdisciplinary care is most comprehensive and beneficial to the client (Grabiner 2013).*

- Place a fall-prone client in a room that is near the nurses' station. *Such placement allows more frequent observation of the client.*
- Help clients sit in a stable chair with arm rests. Avoid use of wheelchairs except for transportation as needed. CEB: *Clients are likely to fall when left in a wheelchair because they may stand up without locking*

the wheels or removing the footrests. Wheelchairs do not increase mobility; people just sit in them the majority of the time (Simmons et al, 1995).

- Avoid use of wheelchairs as much as possible because they can serve as a restraint device. Most people in wheelchairs do not move. *Wheelchairs unfortunately serve as a restraint device.* CEB: *A study has shown that only 4% of residents in wheelchairs were observed to propel them independently and only 45% could propel them, even with cues and prompts. Another study showed that no residents could unlock wheelchairs without help, the wheelchairs were not fitted to residents, and residents were not trained in propulsion (Simmons et al, 1995).*

▲ Refer to physical therapy or other programs for exercise programs that target strength, balance, flexibility, or endurance. EB: *Programs with at least two of these components have been shown to decrease the rate of falling and number of people falling, (Gillespie et al, 2009).*

Geriatric

- Assess ability to move using the Hendrich II Fall Risk Model, which includes the Get Up and Go test. Ask the client to rise from a sitting position, walk 10 feet, turn, and return to the chair to sit. *Performance on this screening exam demonstrates the client's mobility and ability to leave the house safely. If the client completes the test in less than 20 seconds, he/she usually can live independently. If completing the test takes longer than 30 seconds, the client is more likely to be dependent on others and more likely to sustain a fall (Gray-Miceli, 2007; Goodwin et al, 2014).*
- Complete a fall risk assessment for older adults in acute care using a valid and reliable tool such as the Hendrich II Fall Risk Model. *It is quick to administer and provides a determination of risk for falling based on gender, mental and emotional status, symptoms of dizziness, and known categories of medications increasing risk (Hendrich et al, 2003). This tool screens for primary prevention of falls and is integral in a post-fall assessment for the secondary prevention of falls (Gray-Miceli, 2007; Goodwin et al, 2014).*

▲ If new onset of falling, assess for lab abnormalities, and signs and symptoms of infection and dehydration, and check blood pressure and pulse rate with client in supine, sitting, and standing positions for hypotension and orthostatic hypotension. If the client has borderline high blood pressure, the risk of falling due to administration of antihypertensives may outweigh the benefits of the antihypertensive medication. Discuss with the health care provider on a client-to-client basis. *If orthostatic hypotension is present and there is minimal change in the heart rate, most likely the baroreceptors are not working to maintain blood pressure on arising. This is common in older adults and may be caused by hypovolemia resulting from the excessive use of diuretics, vasodilators, or other types of drugs; dehydration; or prolonged bed rest as well as cardiovascular disease, neurological disease, or the adverse effects of another medication (NINDS, 2011). Insertion of a pacemaker can reduce falls in people with frequent falls associated with carotid sinus hypersensitivity, a condition that may cause changes in heart rate and blood pressure (Gillespie et al, 2009).*

- Complete a fear of falling assessment for older adults. This includes measuring fear of falling, or the level of concern about falling, and falls self-efficacy, the degree of confidence a person has in performing common activities of daily living without falling. Fear of falling may be measured by a single-item question asking about the presence of fear of falling or rating severity of fear of falling on a 1-4 Likert scale as is commonly done in studies. Falls self-efficacy may be measured using a valid and reliable tool such as the Falls Efficacy Scale-International (Yardley et al, 2005; Greenberg, 2011).
- Encourage the client to wear glasses and use walking aids when ambulating.
- If the client experiences dizziness because of orthostatic hypotension when getting up, teach methods to decrease dizziness, such as rising slowly, remaining seated several minutes before standing, flexing feet upward several times while sitting, sitting down immediately if feeling dizzy, and trying to have someone present when standing. CEB/EB: *Always have the client dangle at the bedside before standing to evaluate for postural hypotension. Watch the client closely for dizziness during increased activity. Postural hypotension can be detected in up to 30% of older clients. These methods can help prevent falls as well as maintain adequate fluid intake (Tinetti, 2003; Goodwin et al, 2014).*

▲ If the client is experiencing syncope, determine symptoms that occur before syncope, and note medications that the client is taking. Refer for medical care. The circumstances surrounding syncope often suggest the cause. *Use of many medications, including diuretics, antihypertensives, digoxin, beta-blockers, and calcium channel blockers can cause syncope. Use of the tilt table can be diagnostic in incidences of syncope (Fick & Mion, 2007; Goodwin et al, 2014).*

▲ Observe client for signs of anemia, and refer to health care provider for testing if appropriate.
• Evaluate client for chronic alcohol intake, as well as mental health and neurological function.
▲ Refer to physical therapy for strength training, using free weights or machines, and suggest participation in exercise programs. *Exercise can prevent falls in older people. Greater relative effects are seen in programs that include exercises that challenge balance, use a higher dose of exercise, and do not include a walking program. Service providers can use these findings to design and implement exercise programs for falls prevention (Sherrington et al, 2008; Grabiner, 2013; Hirase et al, 2014).*
▲ If an older woman has symptoms of urge incontinence, refer to a urologist or nurse specialist in incontinence for evaluation and ensure the path to the bathroom is well lit and free of obstructions. CEB: *Urge urinary incontinence was associated with an increased incidence of falls and non-spine, nontraumatic fractures in older women (Brown et al, 2000).*
▲ New evidence-based guidelines for preventing falls in older adults were published by the American Geriatrics Society (AGS) and British Geriatrics Society (BGS) collaboratively and specify recommendations for all clinical settings. The new recommendations include screening and assessment, as well as interventions. Examples of interventions include (1) exercise for balance and for gait and strength training, such as tai chi or physical therapy; (2) environmental adaptation to reduce fall risk factors in the home and in daily activities; (3) cataract surgery when indicated; (4) medication reduction with particular attention to medications that affect the brain such as sleeping medications and antidepressants; (5) assessment and treatment of postural hypotension; (6) identification and appropriate treatment of foot problems; (7) vitamin D supplementation for those with vitamin D (American Geriatrics Society, 2011a,b).

Home Care

• Some of the above interventions may be adapted for home care use.
• Implement evidence-based fall prevention practices in community settings and home health care programs for older adults (Fortinsky et al, 2008).
• If the client was identified as a fall risk in the hospital, recognize that there is a high incidence of falls after discharge, and use all measures possible to reduce the incidence of falls. CEBN: *The rate of falls is substantially increased in the geriatric client who has been recently hospitalized, especially during the first month after discharge (Mahoney et al, 2000).*
▲ If delirium is present, assess for cause of delirium and/or falls with the use of an interprofessional team. Consult with the health care provider immediately. Assess and monitor for acute changes in cognition and behavior. *An acute and fluctuating change in cognition and behavior is the classic presentation of delirium. Delirium is reversible and should be considered a medical emergency. Delirium can become chronic if untreated, and clients may be discharged from hospitals to home care in states of undiagnosed delirium.* EB: *Falls may be a precipitating event or an indication of frailty consistent with acute confusion (Goodwin et al, 2014).*
• Assess home environment for threats to safety including clutter, slippery floors, scatter rugs, and other potential hazards. Additionally, assess external environment (e.g., uneven pavement, unleveled stairs/steps). *Clients suffering from impaired mobility, impaired visual acuity, and neurological dysfunction, including dementia and other cognitive functional deficits, are all at risk for injury from common hazards. These recommendations were shown to be effective to reduce falls (Tinetti, 2003; Goodwin et al, 2014).*
▲ Institute a home-based, nurse-delivered exercise program to reduce falls or refer to physical therapy services for client and family education of safe transfers and ambulation and for strengthening exercises for the client (Grabiner, 2013).
▲ Instruct the client and family or caregivers on how to correct identified hazards for those with visual impairment. Refer to physical and occupational therapy services for assistance if needed. EB: *Interventions to improve home safety were shown to be effective in people at high risk, such as those with severe visual impairment (Gillespie et al, 2009).*
▲ Use a multifactorial assessment along with interventions targeted to the identified risk factors. Key components of the interventions include evaluating need for all medications, balance, gait and strength training, use of strategies to deal with postural hypotension if present, home safety evaluation with needed modifications, and any needed cardiovascular treatment. EB: *As people age, they may fall more often for multiple reasons including problems with balance, poor vision, and dementia. Fear of falling can result in self-restricted activity levels (Gillespie et al, 2009).*

- Encourage the client to eat a balanced diet, with particular inclusion of vitamin D and calcium. *Vitamin D deficiency and hypocalcemia are common in older adults, contributing to falls, musculoskeletal complaints, and functional and mobility deficits. Results show that vitamin D and calcium were superior to calcium supplementation alone in regard to fall prevention, musculoskeletal function, and bone metabolism, especially in recurrent falls and in frail older women with vitamin D deficiency. Older adults with unexplained falls, pain, and gait imbalance may have osteomalacia due to vitamin D deficiency (Dharmarajan, 2005).*
- If the client lives alone or spends a lot of time alone, teach the client what to do if he/she falls and cannot get up, and make sure he/she has a personal emergency response system or a mobile phone that is available from the floor (Tinetti, 2003). If the client is at risk for falls, use a gait belt and additional persons when ambulating. *Gait belts decrease the risk of falls during ambulation.*
- Ensure appropriate nonglare lighting in the home. Ask the client to install indoor strip or "runway" type of lighting to baseboards to help clients balance. Install motion-sensitive lighting that turns on automatically when the client gets out of bed to go to the bathroom.
- Have the client wear supportive, low-heeled shoes with good traction when ambulating. Avoid use of slip-on footwear. Wear appropriate footwear in inclement weather. *Supportive shoes provide the client with better balance and protect the client from instability on uneven surfaces. Antislip shoe devices worn in icy conditions have been shown to reduce falls (Gillespie et al, 2009).*
- Provide a signaling device for clients who wander or are at risk for falls. *Orienting a vulnerable client to a safety net relieves anxiety of the client and caregiver and allows for rapid response to a crisis situation.*
- Provide medical identification bracelet for clients at risk for injury from dementia, diabetes, seizures, or other medical disorders.
- Suggest a tai chi class designed for older adults and selected clients who have sufficient balance to participate. EB: *Participation in once per week tai chi classes for 16 weeks can prevent falls in relatively healthy community-dwelling older people (Voukelatos et al, 2007).*

Client/Family Teaching and Discharge Planning

- Safety Guidelines. Teach the client and the family about the fall reduction measures that are being used to prevent falls (The Joint Commission, 2009).
- Teach the client how to safely ambulate at home, including using safety measures such as hand rails in bathroom and avoiding carrying things or performing other tasks while walking.
- Teach the client the importance of maintaining a regular exercise program. If the client is afraid of falling while walking outside, suggest he/she walk the length of a local mall. *Exercise can prevent falls in older people. Greater relative effects are seen in programs that include exercises that challenge balance and use a higher dose of exercise than just walking programs (Sherrington et al, 2008; Hirase et al, 2014; Grabiner, 2013).*

REFERENCES

The American Geriatrics Society (AGS) 2010 AGS/BGS Clinical Practice Guideline (2011a). *Prevention of falls in older persons. Summary of recommendations.* <http://www.americangeriatrics.org/files/documents/Adv_Resources/2011_PP_Priorities_with_ACA.pdf>.

The American Geriatrics Society (AGS) and British Geriatrics Society (BGS) (2011b). <http://www.americangeriatrics.org/files/documents/health_care_pros/Falls.Summary.Guide.pdf>.

Brown, J. S., Vittinghoff, E., Wyman, J. F., et al. (2000). Urinary incontinence: does it increase risk for falls and fractures? Study of osteoporotic fracture research group. *Journal of the American Geriatrics Society, 48*(7), 721.

Capezuti, E. (2004). Minimizing the use of restrictive devices in dementia patients at risk for falling. *The Nursing Clinics of North America, 39*, 625.

Capezuti, E., Strumph, N., Evans, I., et al. (1999). Outcomes of nighttime physical restrain removal for severely impaired nursing home residents. *American Journal of Alzheimer's Disease and Other Dementias, 14*(3), 157.

Cotter, V. T., & Evans, L. (2007). Try this: best practices in nursing care to older adults. In: *The John A. Hartford Institute for Geriatric Nursing and the Alzheimer's Association: Avoiding restraints in older adults with dementia.* <www.consultgerirn.org/uploads/File/trythis/-dementia.pdf>. Accessed March 15, 2009.

Evans, L. K., & Cotter, V. T. (2008). Avoiding restraints in patients with dementia: understanding, prevention, and management are the keys. *The American Journal of Nursing, 108*(3), 40–49.

Dharmarajan, T. S. (2005). Vitamin D deficiency in community older adults with falls of gait imbalance: an under-recognized problem in the inner city. *Journal of Nutrition for the Elderly, 25*(1), 7–19.

Fick, D., & Mion, L. (2007). Try this: best practices in nursing care to older adults. In: *The John A. Hartford Institute for Geriatric Nursing: Assessing and managing delirium in older adults with dementia*. <www.consultgerirn.org/uploads/File/trythis/AssesMangeDeleriumWDementia.pdf>. Accessed March 15, 2009.

Fick, D. M., Cooper, J. W., Wade, W. E., et al. (2003). Updating the beers criteria for potentially inappropriate medication use in older adults: results of a US consensus panel of experts. *Archives of Internal Medicine, 163*(22), 2716–2724.

Fortinsky, R. H., Baker, D., Gottschalk, M., et al. (2008). Extent of implementation of evidence-based fall prevention practices for older patients in home health care. *Journal of the American Geriatrics Society, 56*(4), 737–743.

Gillespie, L. D., Robertson, M. C., Gillespie, W. J., et al. (2009). Interventions for preventing falls in older people living in the community. *Cochrane Database of Systematic Reviews*, (2), CD007146.

Goodwin, V. A., Abbott, R. A., Whear, R., et al. (2014). Multiple component interventions for preventing falls and fall related injuries among older people: systematic review and meta-analysis. *BMC Geriatrics, 14*, 15–21.

Grabiner, M. D. (2013). Exercise-based fall prevention programmes decrease fall-related injuries. *Evidence-Based Nursing, 17*(4), 125.

Gray-Miceli, D. (2007). Try this: best practices in nursing care to older adults. In: *The John A. Hartford Institute for Geriatric Nursing: Fall risk assessment in older adults: The Hendrich II Model*. <www.consultgerirn.org/uploads/File/trythis/issue08.pdf>. Accessed March 15, 2009.

Gray-Miceli, D. (2008). Delirium: preventing falls in acute care. In E. Capezuti, D. Zwicker, M. Mezey, et al. (Eds.), *Geriatric nursing protocols* (3rd ed.). New York: Springer.

Greenberg, S. A. (2011). Try this: best practices in nursing care to older adults. In: *The John A. Hartford Institute for Geriatric Nursing: Falls Efficacy Scale-International (FES-I)*. <http://consultgerirn.org/uploads/File/trythis/try_this_29.pdf>. Accessed September 9, 2011.

Hendrich, A. (2006). Inpatient falls: lessons from the field. *Patient Safety & Quality Healthcare*, May/June, 26–30.

Hendrich, A. L., Bender, P. S., & Nyhuis, A. (2003). Validation of the hendrich II fall risk model: a large concurrent CASE/control study of hospitalized patients. *Applied Nursing Research, 16*(1), 9–21.

Hirase, T., Inokuchi, S., Matsusaka, N., et al. (2014). A modified fall risk assessment tool that is specific to physical function predicts falls in community-dwelling elderly people. *Journal of Geriatric Physical Therapy (2001), 37*, 159–165.

The Joint Commission on Accreditation of Healthcare Organizations (2009). *Accreditation program: home care. 2010 national patient safety goals. Goal 9. Reduce the risk of patient harm resulting from falls*. <www.jointcommission.org/NR/rdonlyres/E07E8A63–5867–4090–A5AC-210D9565BCDB/0/RevisedChapter_OME_NPSG_20090924.pdf>. Accessed on October 8, 2009.

Lundin-Olsson, L., Nyberg, L., & Gustafson, Y. (1998). Attention, frailty, and falls: the effect of a manual task on basic mobility. *Journal of the American Geriatrics Society, 46*(6), 758–761.

Mahoney, J. E., Palta, M., Johnson, J., et al. (2000). Temporal association between hospitalization and rate of falls after discharge. *Archives of Internal Medicine, 160*(18), 2788.

McCarter-Bayer, A., Bayer, F., & Hall, K. (2005). Preventing falls in acute care: an innovative approach. *Journal of Gerontological Nursing, 31*(3), 25.

Mion, L. C., Fogel, J., Sandhu, S., et al. (2001). Outcomes following physical restraint reduction programs in two acute care hospitals. *The Joint Commission Journal on Quality Improvement, 27*(11), 605–618.

Molony, S. (2008). Try this: best practices in nursing care to older adults. In: *The John A. Hartford Institute for Geriatric Nursing: Beers Criteria for potentially inappropriate medication use in older adults: Part II: 2002 Criteria Considering Diagnoses or Conditions*. <www.consultgerirn.org/uploads/File/trythis/issue16_2.pdf>. Accessed March 15, 2009.

National Institute of Neurological Disorders and Stroke: *NINDS orthostatic hypotension information page*. Last updated 2011. <http://www.ninds.nih.gov/disorders/orthostatic_hypotension/orthostatic_hypotension.htm>. Accessed June 5, 2015.

Sherrington, C., Whitney, J. C., Lord, S. R., et al. (2008). Effective exercise for the prevention of falls: a systematic review and meta-analysis. *Journal of the American Geriatrics Society, 56*(12), 2234–2243.

Simmons, S. F., Schnelle, J. F., MacRae, P. G., et al. (1995). Wheelchairs as mobility restraints: predictors of wheelchair activity in non-ambulatory nursing home residents. *Journal of the American Geriatrics Society, 43*(4), 384–388.

Tinetti, M. E. (2003). Preventing falls in elderly persons. *The New England Journal of Medicine, 348*(1), 42–49.

Voukelatos, A., Cumming, R. G., Lord, S. R., et al. (2007). A randomized controlled trial of tai chi for the prevention of falls: the central sydney tai chi trial. *Journal of the American Geriatrics Society, 55*(8), 1185–1191.

Yardley, L., Beyer, N., Hauer, K., et al. (2005). Development and initial validation of the falls efficacy scale-international (FES-I). *Age and Ageing, 34*(6), 614–619.

F

Dysfunctional Family processes

Gail B. Ladwig, MSN, RN, and Deborah Yvonne Fields, RN, BSN, MA, LICDC, CCMC

NANDA-I

Definition

Psychosocial, spiritual, and physiological functions of the family unit are chronically disorganized, which leads to conflict, denial of problems, resistance to change, ineffective problem solving, and a series of self-perpetuating crises

Defining Characteristics

Behavioral

Agitation; alteration in concentration; blaming; broken promises; chaos; complicated grieving; conflict avoidance; contradictory communication pattern; controlling communication pattern; criticizing; decrease in physical contact; denial of problems; dependency; difficulty having fun; difficulty with intimate relationships; difficulty with life cycle transitions; disturbances in academic performance in children; enabling substance use pattern; escalating conflict; failure to accomplish developmental tasks; harsh self-judgment; immaturity; inability to accept a wide range of feelings; inability to accept help; inability to adapt to change; inability to deal constructively with traumatic experiences; inability to express wide range of feelings; inability to meet the emotional needs of its members; inability to meet the security needs of its members; inability to meet the spiritual needs of its members; inability to receive help appropriately; inappropriate anger expression; ineffective communication skills; insufficient knowledge about substance abuse; insufficient problem solving skills; lying; manipulation; nicotine addiction; orientation favors tension relief rather than goal attainment; paradoxical communication pattern; power struggles; rationalization; refusal to get help; seeking of affirmation; seeking of approval; self-blame; social isolation; special occasions centered on substance use; stress-related physical illnesses; substance abuse; unreliable behavior; verbal abuse of children; verbal abuse of parent; verbal abuse of partner

Feelings

Abandonment; anger; anxiety; confuses love and pity; confusion; depression; dissatisfaction; distress; embarrassment; emotional isolation; failure; fear; feeling different from others; feeling misunderstood; feeling unloved; frustration; guilt; hopelessness; hostility; hurt; insecurity; lack of identity; lingering resentment; loneliness; loss; mistrust; moodiness; powerlessness; rejection; reports feeling misunderstood; repressed emotions; responsibility for substance abuser's behavior; suppressed rage; shame; tension; unhappiness; vulnerability; worthlessness

Roles and Relationships

Change in role function; chronic family problems; closed communication systems; conflict between partners; deterioration in family relationships; diminished ability of family members to relate to each other for mutual growth and maturation; disrupted family rituals; disrupted family roles; disturbance in family dynamics; economically disadvantaged; family denial; inconsistent parenting; ineffective communication with partner; insufficient cohesiveness; insufficient family respect for autonomy of its members; insufficient family respect for individuality of its members; insufficient relationship skills; intimacy dysfunction; neglect of obligation to family member; pattern of rejection; perceived insufficient parental support; triangulating family relationships

Related Factors (r/t)

Addictive personality; biological factors; family history of resistance to treatment; family history of substance abuse; genetic predisposition to substance abuse; ineffective coping skills; insufficient problem-solving skills; substance abuse

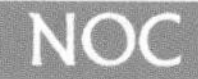

NOC (Nursing Outcomes Classification)

Suggested NOC Outcomes

Family Coping; Family Functioning; Family Health Status; Substance Addiction Consequences

Example NOC Outcome with Indicators

Family Coping as evidenced by the following indicators: Confronts/manages family problems/Involves family members in decision-making. (Rate the outcome and indicators of **Family Coping:** 1 = never demonstrated, 2 = rarely demonstrated, 3 = sometimes demonstrated, 4 = often demonstrated, 5 = consistently demonstrated [see Section I].)

Client Outcomes

Family/Client Will (Specify Time Frame)

- State one way that alcoholism has affected the health of the family
- Identify three healthy coping behaviors that family members can employ to facilitate a shift toward improved family functioning

- Identify one Al-Anon meeting from Al-Anon meeting schedule that family members express a desire to attend
- Attend different types of meetings (lead, big book, discussion, beginner's meeting) to find a good match and commit to attending that group regularly

NIC (Nursing Interventions Classification)

Suggested NIC Interventions

Family Process Maintenance; Substance Use Treatment

F

Example Activities—Family Process Maintenance

Identify effects of role changes on family process; Assist family members to use existing support mechanisms

Nursing Interventions and *Rationales*

- • Refer to care plans for Ineffective **Denial** and Defensive **Coping** for additional interventions.
- ▲ Behavioral screening and intervention (BSI) should be integrated into all health care settings. Different terminology has evolved for screening, intervention, and referral for various behavioral issues. The five As—ask, advise, assess, assist, and arrange—apply to tobacco use. SBIRT (screening, brief intervention, and referral to treatment) pertains to alcohol and drug use. EB: *The U.S. Preventive Services Task Force recommends universal screening and intervention for tobacco use, excessive drinking, and depression. These services improve health outcomes, decrease health care costs, enhance public safety, and generate substantial return on investment (Brown, 2011).*
- • Screen clients for at-risk drinking during routine primary care visits and before surgery using the Alcohol Use Disorders Identification Test (AUDIT). EB: *Complications following total joint arthroplasty were significantly related to alcohol misuse in this group of male patients treated at a VHA facility. The AUDIT-C has three simple questions that can be incorporated into a preoperative evaluation and can alert the treatment team to patients with increased postoperative risk (Harris et al, 2011).*
- • Stress early treatment and brief intervention to resolve the problem. CEBN: *This study demonstrated cost-effectiveness of the early treatment model (project TrEAT; Trial for Early Alcohol Treatment) (Mundt, 2006).*
- • Provide brief education and individual counsel as a routine part of primary care. EB: *Brief interventions may be effective in helping patients engage in nonharmful drinking. The objective of the current study tested the implementation of a telephone-based brief intervention (telephone care management; TCM) with heavy drinkers in primary care. The addition of TCM to primary care provider standard care (screening and brief advice) was compared with standard care alone. Both groups significantly decreased their drinking over time, with 40% of participants no longer engaging in heavy drinking at follow-up, Both groups decreased the number of drinking days and the average number of drinks per day over the follow-up period. Participants reported a decrease in alcohol use frequency and alcohol-related problems (Helstrom et al, 2014).*
- • Refer for family therapy. *Family therapy is generally advisable to restore healthy family dynamics and to provide the appropriate environment and support for full recovery (Psychology Today, 2012).*
- ▲ Refer for possible use of medications to control alcohol dependence. EB: *The Food and Drug Administration has approved three medications for treating alcohol dependence. Naltrexone can help people reduce heavy drinking. Acamprosate makes it easier to maintain abstinence. Disulfiram blocks the breakdown (metabolism) of alcohol by the body, causing unpleasant symptoms such as nausea and flushing of the skin. Those unpleasant effects can help some people avoid drinking while taking disulfiram. It is important to remember that not all people will respond to medications, but for a subset of individuals, they can be an important tool in overcoming alcohol dependence (NIH, 2014).*

Pediatric

- ▲ Encourage early intervention, when parental depression, childhood exposure to conflict and violence and childhood experience with abuse and neglect co-exist with parental substance abuse, their children are more likely to engage in increased teacher-rated unfavorable student behavioral problems. EB: *Early intervention with COSA (children of substance abusers) is necessary to reach children while they are more receptive to treatment (Conners-Burrow et al, 2012).*

- Encourage parent communication about alcohol use with adolescents. EB: *Abar et al (2011) identified parent-adolescent communication as important in delaying the onset and escalation of alcohol use.*
- ▲ Consider the Community Reinforcement Approach (CRA) that encourages clients to become progressively involved in alternative non–substance-related pleasant social activities and to work on enhancing the enjoyment they receive within the "community" of their family and job. EB: *CRA, originally developed for individuals with alcohol use disorders, has been successfully employed to treat a variety of substance use disorders for more than 35 years. Based on operant conditioning, CRA helps adolescents rearrange their lifestyles so that healthy, drug-free living becomes rewarding and thereby competes with alcohol and drug use (Meyers et al, 2010).*
- ▲ Educate family members about available educational and support programs and encourage no/limited alcohol use in the home. EBN: *Both individual and multiperson interventions exert an influential role in family-based therapy for treatment of adolescent drug abuse (Hoque et al, 2006).*
- Encourage adolescents to attend a 12-step program. EB: *Mundt et al (2012) demonstrated that adolescents who attend 12-step groups following alcohol and other drug (AOD) treatment are more likely to remain abstinent and to avoid relapse.*
- Provide a school-based drug-prevention program to junior high students. EB: *Students who received the drug-prevention program during junior high school were less likely to have violations and points on their driving records (Warner et al, 2007).*

Geriatric

- Include assessment of possible alcohol abuse when assessing older family members. EB: *Alcohol abuse and dependence in older people are important problems that frequently remain undetected by health services (Beullens & Aertgeerts, 2004). The majority of older alcoholics are married, have low education levels, and do not belong to high social classes (Shahpesandy et al, 2006).*

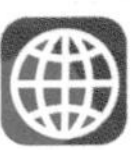

Multicultural

- Acknowledge racial/ethnic differences at the onset of care. EBN: *Acknowledgment of race/ethnicity issues will enhance communication, establish rapport, and promote treatment outcomes (Giger & Davidhizar, 2008).*
- Use a family-centered approach when working with Latino, Asian American, African American, and Native American clients. EBN: *American Indian families may be extended structures that could exert powerful influences over functioning (Kopera-Frye, 2009). Family therapy is important in addressing the needs of Hispanic families with adolescent substance abusers (Kopera-Frye, 2009).*
- Some less-acculturated Latino families may be unwilling to discuss family issues with health care providers until they perceive a close personal relationship with the provider. EBN: *Some Latino families may believe that personal problems should be kept private and may not respond to the health care provider until there is an established personal relationship (Kopera-Frye, 2009).*
- Work with families in a way that incorporates cultural elements. CEB: *Activities such as tundra walks and time with older adults supported in treatment were used successfully for substance abuse treatment with Yup'ik and Cup'ik Eskimos (Mills, 2003).*

Home Care

NOTE: In the community setting, alcoholism as cause of dysfunctional family processes must be considered in two categories: (1) when the client suffers personally from the illness, and (2) when a significant other suffers from the illness, that is, the client is not the active alcoholic but may depend on the alcoholic for caregiving. The following considerations apply to both situations with appropriate adaptation for the circumstances.

- The previous interventions may be adapted for home care use.
- Work with family members to support a sense of valued fit on their part; include them in treatment planning and identify the importance of their roles in the client's care. At the same time, encourage their pursuit of positive outside activities that enhance their sense of belonging. CEBN: *Sense of belonging (valued fit) has been identified as a buffer to depression among both depressed and nondepressed individuals with a family history of alcoholism. A buffering effect was not found for individuals with a family history of drug abuse (Sargent et al, 2002).*

- Educate client and family regarding the interactions of alcohol use with medications and the therapeutic regimen. *Increased awareness of drug interactions decreases the chance of relapse due to over-the-counter and other medications (Weisberg & Hawes, 2005).*
- Alcoholism is a family disease. *If everyone participates in recovery, everyone can be healed (Buddy, 2007).*
- ▲ Refer for psychiatric home health care services for client reassurance and implementation of therapeutic regimen. CEB: *Twelve studies (five randomized controlled trials, one quasi-experimental study, and six uncontrolled cohort studies) found that home and community-based treatment of psychiatric symptoms of socially isolated older adults with mental illness was associated with improved or maintained psychiatric status. All randomized controlled trials reported improved depressive symptoms, and one reported improved overall psychiatric symptoms (Van Citters & Bartells, 2004).*
- ▲ Consider use of a smartphone-based intervention for alcohol use disorders. *Participants in a pilot study indicated the smartphone provided numerous features for addressing ongoing drinking, craving, connection with supportive others, managing life problems, high-risk location alerting, and activity scheduling. These intervention modules were helpful in highlighting alcohol use patterns. Tools related to managing alcohol craving, monitoring consumption, and identifying triggers to drink were rated by participants as particularly helpful. Participants also demonstrated significant reductions in hazardous alcohol use while using the system (Dulin et al, 2014).*

F

Client/Family Teaching and Discharge Planning

- Suggest the client complete a confidential Internet self-screening test for identification of problems and suggestions for treatment if a problem with alcohol is suspected. Many tools are available. *The website* www.AlcoholScreening.org *helps individuals assess their own alcohol consumption patterns to determine if their drinking is likely harming their health or increasing their risk for future harm. Through education and referral, the site urges those whose drinking is harmful or hazardous to take positive action and informs all adults who consume alcohol about guidelines and caveats for lower risk drinking (Boston University School of Public Health, 2005).*
- Provide education for family. EB: *Family education facilitates understanding of the disease and its causes, effects, and treatment (U.S. Department of Health and Human Services, 2005).*
- Facilitate participation in mutual help groups (MHGs). EB: *Mutual help groups appear to mobilize the same change processes such as coping, motivation, and self-efficacy that are mobilized by many different types of professionally led groups (Kelly et al, 2009; Moos, 2008).*

REFERENCES

Abar, C. C., Fernandez, A. C., & Wood, M. D. (2011). Parent-teen communication and pre-college alcohol involvement: a latent class analysis. *Addictive Behaviors*, *36*(12), 1357–1360.

Beullens, J., & Aertgeerts, B. (2004). Screening for alcohol abuse and dependence in older people using DSM criteria: a review. *Aging and Mental Health*, *8*(1), 76–82.

Boston University School of Public Health. *How much is too much?* From: <http://www.alcoholscreening.org>. Retrieved January 18, 2005.

Brown, R. (2011). Configuring health care for systematic behavioral screening and intervention. *Population Health Management*, *14*(6), 299–305.

Buddy, T. Alcoholism is a family disease: why do I need help? He's the alcoholic! *About.com*, updated December 24, 2007. From:<http://alcoholism.about.com/cs/info2/a/aa030597.htm>. Retrieved August 19, 2009.

Conners-Burrow, N., Kyzer, N., Pemberton, J., et al. (2012). Child and family factors associated with teacher-reported behavior problems in young children of substance abusers. *Child and Adolescent Mental Health*, *18*(4), 218–224.

Dulin, P., Gonzalez, V., & Campbell, K. (2014). Results of a pilot test of a self-administered smartphone-based treatment system for alcohol use disorders: usability and early outcomes. *Substance Abuse*, *35*(2), 168–175.

Giger, J., & Davidhizar, R. (2008). *Transcultural nursing: assessment and intervention* (4th ed.). St Louis: Mosby.

Harris, A. H., et al. (2011). Preoperative alcohol screening scores: association with complications in men undergoing total joint arthroplasty. *The Journal of Bone and Joint Surgery*, *93*(4), 321–327.

Helstrom, A., Ingram, E., Wei, W., et al. (2014). Treating heavy drinking in primary care practices: evaluation of a telephone-based intervention program. *Addictive Disorders & Their Treatment*, *13*(3), 101–109.

Hoque, A., et al. (2006). Treatment techniques and outcomes in multidimensional family therapy for adolescent behaviour problems. *Journal of Family Psychology*, *20*(4), 535–543.

Kelly, J. F., Magill, M., & Stout, R. L. (2009). How do people recover from alcohol dependence? A systematic review of the research on mechanisms of behavior change in alcoholics anonymous. *Addiction Research & Theory*, *17*(3), 236–259.

Kopera-Frye, K. (2009). Strengths and challenges within a needs and issues of latino and native american nonparental relative caregivers: strengths and challenges within a cultural context. *Family and Consumer Sciences Research Journal*, *37*, 394.

Meyers, R. J., Roozen, H. G., & Smith, J. E. (2010). The community reinforcement approach: an update of the evidence. *Alcohol Research and Health: The Journal of the National Institute on Alcohol Abuse and Alcoholism*, *33*(4), 380–388.

Mills, P. A. (2003). Incorporating Yup'ik and Cup'ik Eskimo traditions into behavioral health treatment. *Journal of Psychoactive Drugs, 35*(1), 85–88.

Moos, R. H. (2008). Active ingredients of substance use-focused self-help groups. *Addiction (Abingdon, England), 103*(3), 387–396.

Mundt, M. (2006). Analyzing the costs and benefits of brief intervention. *Alcohol Research and Health: The Journal of the National Institute on Alcohol Abuse and Alcoholism, 29*(1), 34–36.

Mundt, M. P., Parthasarathy, S., Chi, F. W., et al. (2012). 12-Step participation reduces medical use costs among adolescents with a history of alcohol and other drug treatment. *Drug & Alcohol Dependence, 126*(1–2), 124–130.

NIH, National Institute on Alcohol Abuse and Alcoholism (2014). *NIH publication No. 14-7974*. Retrieved from: www <http://pubs.niaaa.nih.gov/publications/Treatment/treatment.htm#chapter04>. May 29, 2015.

Psychology Today: Facts about recovery, best in treatment: 16-17, 2012.

Sargent, J., Williams, R. A., Hagerty, B., et al. (2002). Sense of belonging as a buffer against depressive symptoms. *Journal of the American Psychiatric Nurses Association, 8*(4), 120–129.

Shahpesandy, H., et al. (2006). Alcoholism in the elderly: a study of elderly alcoholics compared with healthy elderly and young alcoholics. *Neuro Endocrinology Letters, 27*(5), 651–657.

U.S. Department of Health and Human Services (2005). *What is substance abuse treatment? A booklet for families*. From: <http://www.samhsa.gov>. Retrieved December 10, 2009.

Van Citters, A. D., & Bartels, S. J. (2004). A systematic review of the effectiveness of community-based mental health outreach services for older adults. *Psychiatric Services (Washington, D.C.), 55*(11), 1237–1249.

Warner, L. A., White, H. R., & Johnson, V. (2007). Alcohol initiation experiences and family history of alcoholism as predictors of problem-drinking trajectories. *Journal of Studies on Alcohol, 68*(1), 56–65.

Weisberg, J., & Hawes, G. (2005). *Safe medicine for sober people: how to avoid relapsing on pain, sleep, cold, or any other medication*. New York: St. Martin's Griffin.

F

Interrupted Family processes *Vanessa Flannery, MSN, PHCNS-BC, CNE*

NANDA-I

Definition

Change in family relationships and/or functioning

Defining Characteristics

Alteration in availability for affective responsiveness; alteration in family conflict resolution; alteration in family satisfaction; alteration in intimacy; alteration in participation for problem solving; assigned tasks change; change in communication pattern; change in somatization; change in stress reduction behavior; changes in expressions of conflict with community resources; changes in expressions of isolation from community resources; changes in participation for decision-making; changes in relationship pattern; decrease in available emotional support; decrease in mutual support; ineffective task completion; power alliance change; ritual change

Related Factors (r/t)

Alteration in family finances; change in family social status; changes in interaction with community; developmental crisis; developmental transition; power shift among family members; shift in family roles; shift in health status of a family member; situational crisis; situational transition

NOC (Nursing Outcomes Classification)

Suggested NOC Outcomes

Family Coping; Family Functioning; Family Normalization; Psychosocial Adjustment: Life Change, Role Performance

Example NOC Outcome with Indicators

Family Coping as evidenced by the following indicators: Confronts/manages family problems/Involves family members in decision-making. (Rate the outcome and indicators of **Family Coping:** 1 = never demonstrated, 2 = rarely demonstrated, 3 = sometimes demonstrated, 4 = often demonstrated, 5 = consistently demonstrated [see Section I].)

Client Outcomes

Family/Client Will (Specify Time Frame)

- Express feelings (family)
- Identify ways to cope effectively and use appropriate support systems (family)

- Treat impaired family member as normally as possible to avoid overdependence (family)
- Meet physical, psychosocial, and spiritual needs of members or seek appropriate assistance (family)
- Demonstrate knowledge of illness or injury, treatment modalities, and prognosis (family)
- Participate in the development of the plan of care to the best of ability (significant person)

NIC (Nursing Interventions Classification)

Suggested NIC Interventions

Family Integrity Promotion; Family Process Maintenance; Normalization Promotion

Example NIC Activities—Family Integrity Promotion

Collaborate with family in problem solving and decision-making; Counsel family members on additional effective coping skills for their own use

Nursing Interventions and *Rationales*

- Motivate family members to speak openly about illnesses, keeping in mind the importance of ethnic origin. EBN: *Recognizing ethnic origin to caregivers' open communication can improve the quality of life to allow family members to derive solutions and face challenges (Bachner et al, 2014).*
- Recognize informal roles in medical decision-making by family members. EBN: *Informal roles emerge in critical situations to help fill the gaps in how family members respond to the challenge of end-of-life decision-making (Quinn et al, 2012).*
- Acknowledge the range of emotions and feelings that may be experienced when the health status of a family member changes. EBN: *Nurses can better support caregivers regarding their perception of family support and expressive family functioning (Svavarsdottir & Sigurdardottir, 2013).*
- Encourage family members to list their personal strengths and available resources. EBN: *Families provide the main support network and family strengths are closely associated with the family use of resources (Coym, 2013).*
- Establish relationships among clients, their families, and health care professionals. EBN: *A systems approach to disease management incorporates the family as part of the care team and may improve outcomes for the individual (LaFrance, 2011).*
- Encourage family to visit the client; adjust visiting hours to accommodate family's schedule. EBN: *Incorporating visiting family members in the plan of care is complex and requires balancing the visitor's needs for information and access to a loved one with the nurse's need to safely manage the care of a critically ill individual (Alves, 2013).*
- Allow and encourage family members to assist in the client's treatment. EBN: *Support for family members is an essential part of quality end-of-life care for residents, and health care facilities should embrace the opportunity to demonstrate the value of family participation in care (Oliver et al, 2014).*
- Support family members during emotional and conflict situations in the clinical setting. EBN: *A key element of successful interpersonal relationships is the use of constructive conflict management, such as problem solving, compromise, affection, humor and apology (Baptist et al, 2012).*
- Refer to the care plan Readiness for enhanced **Family** processes for additional interventions.

Pediatric

- Carefully assess potential for reunifying children placed in foster care with their birth parents. EB: *Reunifying children placed in foster care with their birth parents is a primary goal of the child welfare system (Lewis, 2011).*
- Provide parents with both general information and professional support by family-centered early childhood intervention services to their families. EBN: *Providing families with general information (such as making information available in various forms and arranging for a guest speaker) in addition to specialized information about their children is most important to empower parents (Fordham et al, 2012).*
- Encourage and support parents/family to assist in client's care. EBN: *Parents need to be able to negotiate with health staff what this participation will involve and negotiate new roles for themselves in sharing care of their sick child (Kelly & Kelly, 2013).*

▲ Refer parents and other primary caregivers to a mindfulness-based stress reduction (MBSR) program. EBN: *Community-based MBSR programs can be an effective intervention to reduce stress and improve psychological well-being for parents and caregivers of children, especially those with developmental disabilities (Bazzano, 2013).*

Geriatric

- Encourage family members to be involved in the care of relatives who are in residential care settings. EBN: *Family involvement in residential long-term care is important especially when preparing for end-of-life care (Oliver et al, 2014).*
- Support group problem solving among family caregivers and include the older member. EBN: *Health personnel must be aware that family caregiving undergoes a transition, shifting both how and when family members mobilize to meet the needs of the older adult (Wongsawang et al, 2013).*

▲ Refer family for counseling with a psychotherapist who is knowledgeable about gerontology.

- Refer to care plan for readiness for Enhanced **Family** processes for additional interventions.

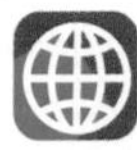

Multicultural

- Refer to the care plan readiness for Enhanced **Family** processes for additional interventions.

Home Care

- The nursing interventions described in the care plan for Compromised family **Coping** should be used in the home environment with adaptations as necessary.
- Encourage family members to find meaning in a serious illness. EBN: *Letting go before the death of a loved one involves a shift in thinking in which there is acknowledgment of impending loss without impeding its natural progression (Molzahn et al, 2012).*

Client/Family Teaching and Discharge Planning

- Refer to Client/Family Teaching and Discharge Planning in Compromised family **Coping** and Readiness for enhanced family **Coping** for suggestions that may be used with minor adaptations.

F

REFERENCES

Alves, M. V. M. F. F., Cordeiro, J. G., Bronzato Luppi, C. H., et al. (2013). Experience of family members as a result of children's hospitalization at the intensive care unit. *Investigacion & Educacion en Enfermeria, 31*(2), 191–200.

Bachner, G., Yosef-Sela, N., & Carmel, S. (2014). Open communication with terminally ill cancer patients about illness and death. *Cancer Nursing, 37*(1), 50–58.

Baptist, J., Thompson, D. E., Norton, A. M., et al. (2012). The effects of the intergenerational transmission of family emotional processes on conflict styles: the moderating role of attachment. *The American Journal of Family Therapy, 40*, 56–73.

Bazzano, A., Wolfe C., Zylowska, L., et al. (2013). Mindfulness based stress reduction (MBSR) for parents and caregivers of individuals with developmental disabilities: a community-based approach. *Journal of Child & Family Studies, 22*(8), 1–11.

Coym, E. (2013). The strengths and resources used by families of young women with breast cancer. *Australian Journal of Cancer Nursing, 14*(2), 10–16.

Fordham, L., Gibson, F., & Bowes, J. (2012). Information and professional support: key factors in the provision of family-centered early childhood intervention services. *Child: Care, Health and Development, 38*(5), 647–653.

Kelly, P., & Kelly, D. (2013). Childhood cancer-parenting work for british bangladeshi families during treatment: an ethnographic study. *International Journal of Nursing Studies, 50*(7), 933–944.

LaFrance, W. C., Jr., Alosco M. L., Davis J. D., et al. (2011). Impact of family functioning on quality of life in patients with psychogenic nonepileptic seizures versus epilepsy. *Epilepsia, 52*(2), 292–300.

Lewis, C. (2011). Providing therapy to children and families in foster care: a systemic-relational approach. *Family Process, 50*(4), 436–452.

Molzahn, A., Sheilds, L., Bruce, A., et al. (2012). People living with serious illness: stories of spirituality. *Journal of Clinical Nursing, 21*(15/16), 2347–2356.

Oliver, D. P., Washington, K., Kruse, R. L., et al. (2014). Hospice family members' perceptions of and experiences with end-of-life care in the nursing home. *Journal of the American Medical Directors Association, 15*(10), 744–750.

Quinn, J. R., Schmitt, M., Baggs, J. G., et al. (2012). Family members' informal roles in end-of-life decision making in adult intensive care units. *American Journal of Critical Care, 21*(1), 43–51.

Svavarsdottir, E. K., & Sigurdardottir, A. O. (2013). Benefits of a brief therapeutic conversation intervention for families of children and adolescents in active cancer treatment. *Oncology Nursing Forum, 40*(5), E346–E357.

Wongsawang, N., Lagampan, S., Lapvongwattana, P., et al. (2013). Family caregiving for dependent older adults in Thai families. *Journal of Nursing Scholarship, 45*(4), 336–343.

Readiness for enhanced Family processes *Kimberly Silvey, MSN, RN*

NANDA-I

Definition

A pattern of family functioning to support the well-being of family members, which can be strengthened

Defining Characteristics

Expresses desire to enhance balance between autonomy and cohesiveness; expresses desire to enhance communication pattern; expresses desire to enhance energy level of family to support activities of daily living; expresses desire to enhance family adaptation to change; expresses desire to enhance family dynamics; expresses desire to enhance family resilience; expresses desire to enhance growth of family members; expresses desire to enhance interdependence with community; expresses desire to enhance maintenance of boundaries between family members; expresses desire to enhance respect for family members; expresses desire to enhance safety of family members.

NOC (Nursing Outcomes Classification)

Suggested NOC Outcomes

Family Coping; Health-Promoting Behavior; Health-Seeking Behavior; Parent-Infant Attachment; Parenting Performance

Example NOC Outcome with Indicators

Family Coping as evidenced by the following indicators: Confronts/manages family problems/Obtains family assistance. (Rate the outcome and indicators of **Family Coping:** 1 = never demonstrated, 2 = rarely demonstrated, 3 = sometimes demonstrated, 4 = often demonstrated, 5 = consistently demonstrated [see Section I].)

Client Outcomes

Family/Client Will (Specify Time Frame)

- Identify ways to cope effectively and use appropriate support systems (family)
- Meet physical, psychosocial, and spiritual needs of members or seek appropriate assistance (family)
- Demonstrate knowledge of potential environmental, lifestyle, and genetic risks to health and use appropriate measures to decrease possibility of risk (family)
- Focus on wellness, disease prevention, and maintenance (family and individual)
- Seek balance among exercise, work, leisure, rest, and nutrition (family and individual)

NIC (Nursing Interventions Classification)

Suggested NIC Interventions

Coping Enhancement; Decision-Making Support; Family Integrity Promotion; Family Involvement Promotion; Family Mobilization; Family Process Maintenance; Parent Education: Adolescent; Childrearing Family; Risk Identification; Role Enhancement

Example NIC Activities—Risk Identification

Determine availability and quality of resources (e.g., psychological, financial, education level, family and other social, and community)

Nursing Interventions and *Rationales*

- Assess the family's stress level and coping abilities during the initial nursing assessment. EB: *Assessing parental stress level will help the nurse to plan interventions to better care for the child and their parents (Burke et al, 2014).*

F

- Consider the use of family-centered theory as the conceptual foundation to help guide interventions. EB: *The concept of family-centered care stresses the importance of the family in children's well-being (Kuo et al, 2012).*
- Use family-centered care and role modeling for holistic care of families. EB: *A holistic approach to care enhances the family's well-being and respects the family's beliefs (Purow et al, 2011).*
- Discuss with family members and identify the perceptions of the health care experience. EBN: *Nurses and parents may perceive the care the child receives differently and it is important to help identify the differences to better care for the child and family (Stuart & Melling, 2014).*
- Support family needs, strengths, and resourcefulness through family interviews. EBN: *Family interviews can give the nurse an understanding of the family's understanding and expectations (Alsem et al, 2014).*
- Spend time with family members; allow them to verbalize their feelings. EB: *Listening to what the family is saying can help the nurse understand how they are feeling (SmithBattle et al, 2013).*
- Encourage family members to find meaning in a serious illness. EBN: *Just because parents have hope for their child does not mean they do not understand their child's prognosis (O'Brien, 2014).*
- Provide family-centered care to explore and use all available resources appropriate for the situation (e.g., counseling, social services, self-help groups, pastoral care). EB: *Family-centered care includes multiple members of the health care team (Hodgetts et al, 2013).*
- Consider focus groups to provide insight to family perceptions of illness and/or disease prevention. EBN: *Focus groups provide insight into the perception of care that is received by the client (Pozzar et al, 2014).*

Pediatric

- Provide a parenting class series based on individual and couple changes in meaning and identity, roles, and relationships and interaction during the transition to parenthood. Address mother and father roles, infant communication abilities, and patterns of the first 3 months of life in a mutually enjoyable, possibility focused manner. EB: *Parenting classes can improve parenting and coping skills to enhance quality of life (Okamoto et al, 2013).*
- Encourage families with adolescents to have family meals. *Eating family meals may enhance the health and well-being of adolescents. Public education on the benefits of family mealtime is recommended (Fruh et al, 2012). Family meals help strengthen a family and provide structure for better development (Utter et al, 2013).*

▲ Consider the use of adventure therapy for adolescents with cancer. EBN: *Adventure therapy is considered a strategy to promote health and in this study cancer survival (Wynn et al, 2012).*

Geriatric

- Carefully listen to residents and family members in the long-term care facility. EBN: *Nurses can improve life and dignity for residents by listening to residents and family members (van der Cingel, 2011).*
- Support caregivers' awareness of the positive effects of their contribution to the well-being of parents. EBN: *Children caring for their elderly parents can have a positive impact on the child and the parent (Lin et al, 2013).*
- Teach family members about the impact of developmental events (e.g., retirement, death, change in health status, and household composition). EBN: *Knowledge helps the family to better cope with health care and the care of the client (Nigolian & Miller, 2011).*
- Encourage social networks; social integration; social engagement and internet social networking with friends, children, and relatives of older adults. EB: *Social networking enables older adults to be more engaged (Cornejo et al, 2013).*

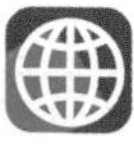

Multicultural

- Assess for the influence of cultural beliefs, norms, and values on the family's perceptions of normal functioning. EBN: *Cultural beliefs will have a considerable impact on a client's functioning (Mutair et al, 2014).*
- Identify and acknowledge the stresses unique to racial/ethnic families. EBN: *Understanding a client's unique racial/ethnic background may help the nurse identify stressors that the client and the family may be experiencing (Balaam et al, 2013).*
- Assess and support spiritual needs of families. EB: *Assessing and supporting the spiritual needs of the client and the family can enhance the understanding of the family's perception of care and the care that was actually received (Chrash et al, 2011; Bernstein et al, 2013).*

- With the client's consent, facilitate a group meeting for family members to discuss how the family is functioning. EBN: *A family meeting opens communication and lets each family member know it is okay to talk about what is happening (Sharma & Dy, 2011).*
- Facilitate modeling and role playing for the client and family regarding healthy ways to start a discussion about the client's prognosis. EBN: *It is helpful to practice communication skills in a safe environment before trying them in a real-life situation (Fisher et al, 2012).*
- Encourage family mealtimes. EB: *Encouraging family mealtimes enhances the communication between the family and health and well-being (Fruh et al, 2012).*

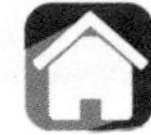

Home Care

- The previous nursing interventions should be used in the home environment with adaptations as necessary.

▲ Encourage virtual support groups to family caregivers. EB: *Use of online support groups gives the caregiver a forum for giving and receiving guidance and support (Diefenbeck et al, 2014). Encourage caregivers of older clients with chronic obstructive pulmonary disease (COPD) receiving long-term oxygen therapy to seek additional services such as social services, respite care, and additional home health visits.* EBN: *Positive support should be given to the caregivers of clients with COPD (Janssen et al, 2012).*

Client/Family Teaching and Discharge Planning

- Refer to Client/Family Teaching and Discharge Planning for readiness for enhanced family **Coping** for suggestions that may be used with minor adaptations.

F

REFERENCES

Alsem, M. W., Siebes, R. C., et al. (2014). Assessment of family needs in children with physical disabilities: development of a family needs inventory. *Child: Care, Health and Development*, *40*(4), 498–506.

Balaam, M.-C., Akerjordet, K., et al. (2013). A qualitative review of migrant women's perceptions of their needs and experiences related to pregnancy and childbirth. *Journal of Advanced Nursing*, *69*(9), 1919–1930.

Bernstein, K., Angelo, L. D., et al. (2013). An exploratory study of HIV+ adolescents' spirituality: will you pray with me? *Journal of Religion & Health*, *52*(4), 1253–1266.

Burke, K., McCarthy, M., et al. (2014). Adapting acceptance and commitment therapy for parents of children with life-threatening illness: pilot study. *Families, Systems and Health: The Journal of Collaborative Family Healthcare*, *32*(1), 122–127.

Chrash, M., Mulich, B., et al. (2011). The APN role in holistic assessment and integration of spiritual assessment for advance care planning. *Journal of the American Academy of Nurse Practitioners*, *23*(10), 530–536.

Cornejo, R., Tentori, M., et al. (2013). Enriching in-person encounters through social media: a study on family connectedness for the elderly. *International Journal of Human-Computer Studies*, *71*(9), 889–899.

Diefenbeck, C. A., Klemm, P. R., et al. (2014). Emergence of Yalom's therapeutic factors in a peer-led, asynchronous, online support group for family caregivers. *Issues in Mental Health Nursing*, *35*(1), 21–32.

Fisher, M. J., Taylor, E. A., & High, P. L. (2012). Parent-nursing student communication practice: role-play and learning outcomes. *The Journal of Nursing Education*, *51*(2), 115–119.

Fruh, S. M., et al. (2012). Benefits of family meals with adolescents: nurse practitioners' perspective. *The Journal for Nurse Practitioners: JNP*, *8*(4), 280–287.

Hodgetts, S., Nicholas, D., et al. (2013). Parents' and professionals' perceptions of family-centered care for children with autism spectrum disorder across service sectors. *Social Science & Medicine*, *96*, 138–146.

Janssen, D. J. A., Spruit, M. A., et al. (2012). Family caregiving in advanced chronic organ failure. *Journal of the American Medical Directors Association*, *13*(4), 394–399.

Kuo, D., Houtrow, A., et al. (2012). Family-centered care: current applications and future directions in pediatric health care. *Maternal & Child Health Journal*, *16*(2), 297–305.

Lin, W., Chen, L., et al. (2013). Adult children's caregiver burden and depression: the moderating roles of parent-child relationship satisfaction and feedback from others. *Journal of Happiness Studies*, *14*(2), 673–687.

Mutair, A. S. A., Plummer, V., et al. (2014). Providing culturally congruent care for Saudi patients and their families. *Contemporary Nurse: A Journal for the Australian Nursing Profession*, *46*(2), 254–258.

Nigolian, C., & Miller, K. L. (2011). Teaching essential skills to family caregivers. *American Journal of Nursing*, *111*(11), 52–58.

O'Brien, R. (2014). Expressions of hope in paediatric intensive care: a reflection on their meaning. *Nursing in Critical Care*, *19*(6), 316–321.

Okamoto, M., Ishigami, H., et al. (2013). Early parenting program as intervention strategy for emotional distress in first-time mothers: a propensity score analysis. *Maternal & Child Health Journal*, *17*(6), 1059–1070.

Pozzar, R. A., Allen, N. A., et al. (2014). Focusing on feedback: how nurse practitioners can use focus group interviews to build a patient-centered practice. *Journal of the American Association of Nurse Practitioners*, *26*(9), 481–487.

Purow, B., Alisanski, S., et al. (2011). Spirituality and pediatric cancer. *Southern Medical Journal*, *104*(4), 299–302.

Sharma, R. K., & Dy, S. M. (2011). Cross-cultural communication and use of the family meeting in palliative care. *The American Journal of Hospice & Palliative Care*, *28*(6), 437–444.

SmithBattle, L., Lorenz, R., et al. (2013). Listening with care: using narrative methods to cultivate nurses' responsive relationships in a home visiting intervention with teen mothers. *Nursing Inquiry*, *20*(3), 188–198.

Stuart, M., & Melling, S. (2014). Understanding nurses' and parents' perceptions of family-centred care. *Nursing Children & Young People*, *26*(7), 16–20.

Utter, J., Denny, S., et al. (2013). Family meals and the well-being of adolescents. *Journal of Paediatrics & Child Health*, *49*(11), 906–911.

van der Cingel, M. (2011). Compassion in care: a qualitative study of older people with a chronic disease and nurses. *Nursing Ethics*, *18*(5), 672–685.

Wynn, B., Frost, A., & Pawson, P. (2012). Adventure therapy proves successful for adolescent survivors of childhood cancers. *Nursing New Zealand*, *18*(1), 28–30.

Fatigue

Victoria K. Marshall, RN, BSN, Paula Riess Sherwood, PhD, RN, CNRN, FAAN, and Barbara A. Given, PhD, RN, FAAN

F

NANDA-I

Definition

An overwhelming, sustained sense of exhaustion and decreased capacity for physical and mental work at the usual level

Defining Characteristics

Alteration in concentration; alteration in libido; disinterest in surroundings; drowsiness; guilt about difficulty maintaining responsibilities; impaired ability to maintain usual physical activity; impaired ability to maintain usual routines; increase in physical symptoms; increase in rest requirement; ineffective role performance; insufficient energy; introspection; lethargy; listlessness; nonrestorative sleep pattern (due to caregiver responsibilities, parenting practices, sleep partner); tiredness

Related Factors (r/t)

Anxiety; depression; environmental barrier (e.g., ambient noise, daylight/darkness exposure, ambient temperature/humidity, unfamiliar setting); increase in physical exertion; malnutrition; negative life event; nonstimulating lifestyle; occupational demands (e.g., shift work, high level of activity, stress); physical deconditioning; physiological condition (e.g., anemia, pregnancy disease); sleep deprivation; stressors

NOC (Nursing Outcomes Classification)

Suggested NOC Outcomes

Concentration; Endurance; Energy Conservation/Restoration; Nutritional Status; Energy; Vitality

Example NOC Outcome with Indicators

Endurance as evidenced by the following indicators: Performance of usual routine/Activity/Energy restored after rest/Blood oxygen level with activity/Muscle endurance. (Rate the outcome and indicators of **Endurance:** 1 = severely compromised, 2 = substantially compromised, 3 = moderately compromised, 4 = mildly compromised, 5 = not compromised [see Section I].)

Client Outcomes

Client Will (Specify Time Frame)

- Identify potential etiology of fatigue
- Identify potential factors that aggravate and relieve fatigue
- Describe ways to assess and track patterns of fatigue over set periods of time (e.g., a few days, a week, a month)
- Describe ways in which fatigue affects the ability to accomplish goals and activities of daily living (ADLs)
- Verbalize increased energy and improved vitality
- Explain energy conservation plan to offset fatigue
- Explain energy restoration plan to offset fatigue

NIC (Nursing Interventions Classification)

Suggested NIC Intervention

Energy management, including both conservation and restoration; conservation interventions are targeted at preserving an individual's energy, whereas restorative interventions are intended to reestablish vitality

Example NIC Activities—Energy Management

Assess client's physiological and psychological status for deficits resulting in fatigue within the context of age, development, and stage of disease or illness; Determine client/significant other's perception of causes of client's fatigue

Nursing Interventions and *Rationales*

- Assess severity of fatigue on a scale of 0 to 10 (average fatigue, worst and best levels); assess frequency of fatigue (number of days per week and time of day), activities and symptoms associated with increased fatigue (e.g., pain), ability to perform ADLs and instrumental ADLs, interference with social and role function, times of increased energy, ability to concentrate, mood, usual pattern of physical activity, and typical sleep cycles. Consider use of an instrument such as the Profile of Mood State Short Form Fatigue Subscale, the Multidimensional Assessment of Fatigue, the Lee Fatigue Scale, the Multidimensional Fatigue Inventory, the HIV-Related Fatigue Scale, or the Brief Fatigue Inventory, Short Form Vitality Subscale, Piper Fatigue Scale, Chalder Fatigue Scale, or Nottingham of Chronic Illness Therapy Fatigue Scale. EBN/CEB: *These assessments have all been shown to have good internal reliability. The Fatigue Severity Scale, Fatigue Impact Scale, and Brief Fatigue Inventory are relatively short with good psychometric properties, making them clinically useful. These measures, along with the Multidimensional Assessment of Fatigue, have shown the ability to detect changes in fatigue over time (Whitehead, 2009). The European Organization for Research and Treatment of Cancer Quality of Life Core Questionnaire (EORTC QLQ-FA 13) (Weis et al, 2013) was proven reliable. Varying populations may respond differently to instruments. The Fatigue Scale for Motor and Cognitive functions and the Unidimensional Fatigue Impact Scale demonstrate good applicability in clients with multiple sclerosis; the Functional Assessment of Chronic Illness Therapy Fatigue subscale and the Fatigue Severity Scale demonstrate good applicability in clients with Parkinson's disease, and the Profile of Mood States Fatigue subscale demonstrates good applicability in clients who have had a stroke (Elbers et al, 2012).*
- Evaluate adequacy of nutrition and sleep hygiene (napping throughout the day, inability to fall asleep or stay asleep). Encourage the client to get adequate rest, limit naps (particularly in the late afternoon or evening), use a routine sleep/wake schedule, plan and prioritize for daily activities as tolerated, allow exposure to sunlight during daytime hours by going outside or opening shades and curtains in the home, use relaxation techniques before bedtime such as meditation, music therapy, or guided imagery (Kwekkeboom et al, 2010), avoid caffeine in the late afternoon or evening, and eat a well-balanced diet that includes fresh fruits, vegetables, and lean meats. Refer to Imbalanced **Nutrition:** less than body requirements or **Insomnia** if appropriate. EBN: *Dysfunction in sleep (too much, too little, or too many interruptions) can aggravate fatigue (Denlinger et al, 2014; Johansson et al, 2010). Inadequate nutrition can also contribute to fatigue, particularly if anemia is present (Bower et al, 2014).*
- Evaluate fluid status and assess for dehydration. Encourage at least eight glasses of water a day. Avoid caffeine, which can cause further dehydration. EB: *Dehydration has been shown to cause fatigue (Ganio et al, 2011; Pross et al, 2013). Some populations such as young children, older adults, and those with other medical conditions are more susceptible to dehydration (Ganio et al, 2011).*

▲ Collaborate with the primary care provider to identify physiological and/or psychological causes of fatigue that could be treated, such as anemia, pain, electrolyte imbalance (e.g., altered potassium levels), thyroid disorders, arthritis, depression, sleep disturbances (insomnia/sleep deprivation), acute or chronic infection, medication use or side effects, alcohol use/abuse, metabolic disorders (diabetes), or a preexisting comorbidity or disease (multiple sclerosis, cancer or cancer treatment, respiratory disease, fibromyalgia, cardiac disease, renal disease or renal replacement therapy, Parkinson's disease) (Berger et al, 2012; Connolly et al, 2013). EB/EBN: *If an etiology for fatigue can be determined, the condition should be treated according to the underlying cause. Anemia is highly correlated with fatigue, particularly in clients with cancer (Kleinman et al, 2012). Fatigue is also related to psychological distress, nausea/vomiting (Oh & Seo, 2011), medication side effects, and nutritional deficit (due to change in taste or cancer affecting swallowing or the digestive tract) in clients with cancer (Berger et al, 2012). Fatigue also negatively impacts a client's quality of life (Connolly et al, 2013; Borneman, 2013).*

▲ Work with the primary care provider to determine if the client has chronic fatigue syndrome, paying attention to risk factors in particular populations. *Chronic fatigue syndrome is unexplained fatigue lasting 6 months or longer that is not associated with a diagnosed physical or psychological condition (White et al, 2011; Stahl et al, 2014).* EB: *Studies also suggest there is a genetic component to chronic fatigue syndrome*

(Pihur et al, 2011). Cognitive behavioral therapy has been shown to be effective in improving symptoms of chronic fatigue syndrome (White et al, 2011; Stahl et al, 2014).

- Encourage the client to express feelings, attribution of cause and behaviors about fatigue, including potential causes of fatigue, and possible interventions to alleviate fatigue. Such interventions could include setting small, easily achieved short-term goals and developing energy management techniques; use active listening techniques to help identify sources of hope. Assess client's level of motivation and willingness to adopt new behaviors that can improve symptoms of fatigue (Connolly et al, 2013). EBN/EB: *Cognitive behavioral therapy has been shown to be effective in reducing fatigue (Berger et al, 2012; Hofmann et al, 2012). Education, counseling, and expressive therapy have also been shown to be effective for managing fatigue (Berger et al, 2012). In addition, cognitive behavioral therapy in combination with hypnosis may improve fatigue in breast cancer clients undergoing radiotherapy (Montgomery et al, 2014).*

F

- Encourage the client to keep a journal of activities that contribute to symptoms of fatigue, patterns of symptoms across days/weeks/months, and feelings, including how fatigue affects the client's normal daily activities and roles. EBN: *Clients who feel as if they have control over their fatigue and its impact on their lives have lower levels of fatigue (Primdahl et al, 2011).*
- Help the client identify sources of support and essential and nonessential tasks to determine which tasks can be delegated to whom. Give the client permission to limit social and role demands if needed (e.g., switch to part-time employment, hire cleaning service). EBN: *Psychoeducational interventions that include fatigue education, self-care (Payne et al, 2012), coping techniques, and activity management have been shown to be effective in reducing cancer-related fatigue (Goedendorp et al, 2009). Emotional support has been linked to decreased level of physical symptoms, including fatigue, for heart failure clients (Heo et al, 2014).*

▲ Collaborate with the primary care provider regarding the appropriateness of referrals to physical therapy for carefully monitored aerobic exercise program and possible physical aids, such as a walker or cane if client has a disability requiring such support. Occupational therapy may also be indicated (Connolly et al, 2013). EBN: *Meta-analyses have shown that exercise, particularly aerobic exercise, can reduce cancer-related fatigue (McMillan & Newhouse, 2011; Berger et al, 2012; Payne et al, 2012).*

- Encourage the client to try complementary and alternative therapy such as guided imagery, massage therapy, mindfulness, and acupressure. EB: *Meta-analyses have suggested that guided imagery may be beneficial, although the studies have not been well developed enough to support analysis (Bernardy et al, 2011; Duijts et al, 2011). Mindfulness-cognitive behavioral therapy has exhibited improved outcomes for those experiencing chronic fatigue (Rimes & Wingrove, 2013). Mindfulness-based stress reduction has also revealed lower fatigue levels for cancer survivors (Johns et al, 2014).*

▲ Refer the client to diagnosis-appropriate support groups such as the National Chronic Fatigue Syndrome Association, Multiple Sclerosis Association, or cancer fatigue websites such as the Oncology Nurses Association (http://www.ons.org) or the National Comprehensive Cancer Network. EB: *Persons with chronic fatigue syndrome have reported needing support to reduce the impact of their disease on their life and regain control (Carvalho Leite et al, 2011).*

▲ For a person with cardiac disease, recognize that fatigue is common after a myocardial infarction, CHF, or chronic cardiac insufficiency. Refer to cardiac rehabilitation for carefully prescribed and monitored exercise program. EBN: *Fatigue is a common finding following cardiovascular insult (Johansson et al, 2010), CHF, and chronic obstructive pulmonary disease (Theander et al, 2014; Sharafkhaneh et al, 2013).*

- If fatigue is associated with cancer or cancer-related treatment, assess for other symptoms that may enhance fatigue (e.g., pain, insomnia, anemia, emotional distress, electrolyte imbalance [nausea, vomiting, diarrhea], or depression). EBN: *Clients with cancer who reported both pain and fatigue reported three times as many other symptoms as clients who reported neither pain nor fatigue; fatigue was linked to the presence of pain, multiple comorbid conditions, and site of cancer (National Comprehensive Cancer Network, 2014). Cancer treatment can increase fatigue and those who have cancer are more likely to experience fatigue than those without cancer (Goedendorp et al, 2013).*
- *Fatigue associated with rheumatoid arthritis can impact a client's quality of life and coping. Group cognitive behavior therapy (CBT) has been shown to be effective in improving fatigue self-management, coping, and fatigue severity. CBT involves using self-management skills such as problem-solving and goal setting to improve self-efficacy while achieving a sense of balance, priority planning, and pacing of activities (Hewlett et al, 2011).*

▲ Collaborate with primary care provider to identify attentional fatigue, which may manifest itself as the inability to direct attention necessary to perform usual activities. Attentional fatigue is associated with sleep disturbances, depressive symptoms, anxiety, psychosocial stressors and can lead to irrational decision-making, inability to plan goals, inability to control emotions or social interactions (Merriman et al, 2013). EBN: *A meta-analysis reported that persons with chronic fatigue syndrome had deficits in the areas of attention, memory, and reaction time (Cockshell & Mathias, 2010).*

▲ Collaborate with primary care providers to identify potential pharmacological treatment for fatigue. EB/EBN: *Pharmacological therapy has been shown to be effective in reducing fatigue, particularly cancer-related fatigue (Minton et al, 2011), although meta-analysis demonstrated small effects in some client populations (Chauffier et al, 2011). Psychostimulants, erythropoiesis-stimulating agents (ESAs) for cancer related fatigue, cytokine blockers, and nutritional supplements have all been shown to improve symptoms of fatigue (Giacalone et al, 2013).*

Geriatric

- Evaluate fatigue in geriatric clients routinely, particularly in clients with limited physical function and lower levels of social support. Chronic conditions related to age can contribute to fatigue in the geriatric client, such as cancer, anemia, multiple medication usage and side effects, depression, insomnia (Naeim et al, 2014), nutritional deficiencies, electrolyte imbalance, and comorbidities involving multiple organ dysfunction (Giacalone et al, 2013). EBN: *Older adults report fatigue that limits functional and social ability and can aggravate comorbid conditions (Yu et al, 2010). Low levels of physical activity have been linked to fatigue in older adults (Avlund, 2013). In persons 80 years old and older, functional capacity, affect, and social support all predicted fatigue (Cho et al, 2012). Fatigue can be as high as 70% in the older cancer population (NCCN, 2014).*
- Review medications to determine possible side effects or interaction effects that could cause fatigue. EB: *The aging process changes the way an individual absorbs, metabolizes, and eliminates medications, leaving the geriatric client susceptible to medication side effects and medication interactions that can cause fatigue, especially when multiple medications are prescribed (Rich & Nienaber, 2014).*
- Review comorbid conditions that may contribute to fatigue, such as congestive heart failure, pulmonary disease, cardiac disease, arthritis, obesity, anemia, depression, insomnia, and cancer. EB: *Fatigue is one of the most common and debilitating symptoms experienced by clients living with chronic conditions and is also commonly experienced in the general U.S. population. (Lai et al, 2014).*
- Identify recent losses; monitor for depression or loneliness as a possible contributing factor to fatigue. EB: *There is a strong correlation between depression and fatigue (Mänty et al, 2014; Oh & Seo, 2011).*
- Review other symptoms the client may be experiencing. Fatigue is often associated with other symptom clusters such as depression and sleep disturbances *(Mänty et al, 2014; NCCN, 2014).*

▲ Review medications for side effects. Certain medications (e.g., diuretics with associated loss of potassium, antihypertensives, antihistamines, pain medications [Rich & Nienaber, 2014], anticonvulsants [Siniscalchi et al, 2013], chemotherapeutic agents [Koornstra et al, 2014], psychiatric medications [Koornstra et al, 2014], and corticosteroids [Koornstra et al, 2014]) may cause fatigue, particularly in older adults.

Home Care

The above interventions may be adapted for home care use.

- Assess the client's history and current patterns of fatigue as they relate to the home environment and environmental and behavioral triggers of increased fatigue. CEB: *Fatigue may be more pronounced in specific settings for physical, environmental (e.g., stairs required to reach bathroom, patterns of movement around home, cleaning activities that require high energy), or psychological (e.g., rooms associated with loss of loved ones) reasons (Wahl et al, 2009) or family responsibilities such as child care (Hazes et al, 2010).*

▲ Encourage planned exercise regimens or physical activities such as walking or light aerobic exercises. This activity can be organized in the home or in a setting such as senior centers or wellness facilities. EB: *Continued physical activity after cancer treatment has been associated with better quality of life, including improved functioning in both physical and social realms (Fong et al, 2012).*

▲ Refer to occupational and/or physical therapy if substantial intervention is needed to assist the client in adapting to home and daily patterns. CEB: *Interventions in older adults led by occupational and physical therapists have been associated with less difficulty in ADLs and instrumental ADLs, which may lead to lower levels of fatigue (Murphy & Niemiec, 2014). Occupational and physical therapy rehabilitation have also been shown to decrease fatigue in cancer survivors (Silver & Gilchrist, 2011). Home-based exercise in stage IV lung and colorectal clients has shown improvement in levels of fatigue (Cheville et al, 2013).*

- For clients receiving chemotherapy, intervene to:
  - ❍ Relieve symptom distress (anxiety, nausea and vomiting, diarrhea, lack of appetite, emotional distress, difficulty sleeping)
  - ❍ Encourage as much physical activity as possible with a specific regimen
  - ❍ Support a positive attitude for the future and reduce uncertainty by being sure clients know expectations and treatment expectations
  - ❍ Support adequate recovery time between treatments

The above factors have been identified as associated with fatigue, particularly during early stages of chemotherapy (NCCN, 2014).

- Teach the client and family the importance of and methods for setting priorities for activities, especially those with high energy demand (e.g., home or family events). Instruct in realistic expectations and behavioral pacing. EBN: *Prioritization of activities can be effective in restoring energy (Goedendorp et al, 2009).*
- Assess effect of fatigue on the client's relatedness; recognize that the client's fatigue affects the whole family. Initiate the following interventions:
  - ❍ Avoid dismissing reports of fatigue; validate the client's experience and foster hope for eventual treatment, if not resolution, of the fatigue.
  - ❍ Identify with the client ways in which he or she continues to be a valued part of his or her social environment.
  - ❍ Identify with the client ways in which he or she continues to participate in equitable exchange with others.
  - ❍ Encourage the client to maintain regular family routines (e.g., meals, sleep patterns) as much as possible.
  - ❍ Initiate cognitive restructuring to refute the client's guilt-producing and negative thought patterns.
  - ❍ Assess and intervene with family's and friends' contributions to guilt-inducing self-talk.
  - ❍ Work with the client to inoculate against the negative thinking of others.
  - ❍ Explore family life and demands to identify accommodations.
  - ❍ Support the client's efforts at limit setting on the demands of others.
  - ❍ Assist the client to move toward a state of parallelism by working to identify and relieve sources of physical or emotional discomfort. Degree of involvement, limited by fatigue, need not be changed.
  - ▲ Refer for family therapy in the event the client's fatigue interferes with normal family functioning. EBN: *The client's fatigue can have a major impact on family members, which is dependent upon the number of familial roles the client holds (Oktay et al, 2011).*

Client/Family Teaching and Discharge Planning

- Help client to reframe cognitively; share information about fatigue and how to live with it, including need for positive self-talk. EBN: *Cognitive behavioral approaches to managing fatigue enhance the client's sense of control over fatigue (White et al, 2011; Hewlett et al, 2011) as well as contributing factors such as depression and insomnia.*
- Teach strategies for energy conservation (e.g., sitting instead of standing during showering, storing items at waist level). EB: *Energy conservation strategies can decrease the amount of energy used (Payne et al, 2012; Goedendorp et al, 2009).*
- Teach the client to carry a pocket calendar, make lists of required activities, and post reminders around the house. EB: *Fatigue is often associated with memory loss and loss of ability to pay attention (Cockshell & Mathias, 2010).* Attentional fatigue is associated with sleep disturbances, depressive symptoms, anxiety, and psychosocial stressors and can lead to irrational decision-making, inability to plan goals, inability to control emotions or social interactions (Merriman et al, 2013).
- Teach the importance of following a healthy lifestyle with adequate nutrition, fluids, and rest; pain relief; insomnia correction; and appropriate exercise to decrease fatigue (i.e., energy restoration).
- See **Hopelessness** care plan if appropriate.

REFERENCES

Avlund, K. (2013). Fatigue in older populations. *Fatigue: Biomedicine, Health & Behavior*, *1*(1–2), 43–63.

Berger, A. M., Gerber, L. H., & Mayer, D. K. (2012). Cancer-related fatigue. *Cancer*, *118*(S8), 2261–2269.

Bernardy, K., Füber, N., Klose, P., et al. (2011). Efficacy of hypnosis/guided imagery in fibromyalgia syndrome—a systematic review and meta-analysis of controlled trials. *BMC Musculoskeletal Disorders*, *12*, 133.

Borneman, T. (2013). Assessment and management of cancer-related fatigue. *Journal of Hospice & Palliative Nursing, 15*(2), 77–86.

Bower, J. E., Bak, K., Berger, A., et al. (2014). Screening, assessment, and management of fatigue in adult survivors of cancer: an american society of clinical oncology clinical practice guideline adaptation. *Journal of Clinical Oncology, 32*(17), 1840–1850.

Carvalho Leite, J. C., de L Drachler, M., Killett, A., et al. (2011). Social support needs for equity in health and social care: a thematic analysis of experiences of people with chronic fatigue syndrome/myalgic encephalomyelitis. *International Journal of Equity in Health, 10*(1), 46.

Chauffier, K., Salliot, C., Berenbaum, F., et al. (2011). Effect of biotherapies on fatigue in rheumatoid arthritis: a systematic review of the literature and meta-analysis. *Rheumatology (Oxford, England), 51*(1), 60–68.

Cheville, A. L., Kollasch, J., Vandenberg, J., et al. (2013). A home-based exercise program to improve function, fatigue, and sleep quality in patients with stage IV lung and colorectal cancer: a randomized controlled trial. *Journal of Pain and Symptom Management, 45*(5), 811–821.

Cho, J., Martin, P., Margrett, J., et al. (2012). Multidimensional predictors of fatigue among octogenarians and centenarians. *Gerontology, 58*(3), 249–257.

Cockshell, S. J., & Mathias, J. L. (2010). Cognitive functioning in chronic fatigue syndrome: a meta-analysis. *Psychological Medicine, 40*(8), 1253–1267.

Connolly, D., O'Toole, L., Redmond, P., et al. (2013). Managing fatigue in patients with chronic conditions in primary care. *Family Practice, 30*(2), 123–124.

Denlinger, C. S., Ligibel, J. A., Are, M., et al. (2014). Survivorship: sleep disorders, version 1.2014. *Journal of the National Comprehensive Cancer Network, 12*(5), 630–642.

Duijts, S. F., Faber, M. M., Oldenburg, H. S., et al. (2011). Effectiveness of behavioral techniques and physical exercise on psychosocial functioning and health-related quality of life in breast cancer patients and survivors-a meta-analysis. *Psycho-Oncology, 20*(2), 115–126.

Elbers, R. G., Rietberg, M. B., van Wegen, E. E., et al. (2012). Self report fatigue questionnaires in multiple sclerosis, Parkinson's disease and stroke: a systematic review of measurement properties. *Quality of Life Research, 21*(6), 925–944.

Fong, D. Y., Ho, J. W., Hui, B. P., et al. (2012). Physical activity for cancer survivors: meta-analysis of randomised controlled trials. *BMJ (Clinical Research Ed.), 344*, e70.

Ganio, M. S., Armstrong, L. E., Casa, D. J., et al. (2011). Mild dehydration impairs cognitive performance and mood of men. *British Journal of Nutrition, 106*(10), 1535–1543.

Giacalone, A., Quitadamo, D., Zanet, E., et al. (2013). Cancer-related fatigue in the elderly. *Supportive Care in Cancer, 21*(10), 2899–2911.

Goedendorp, M. M., Gielissen, M. F., Verhagen, C. A., et al. (2009). Psychosocial interventions for reducing fatigue during cancer treatment in adults. *Cochrane Database of Systematic Reviews*, (1), CD006953.

Goedendorp, M. M., Gielissen, M. F., Verhagen, C. A., et al. (2013). Development of fatigue in cancer survivors: a prospective follow-up study from diagnosis into the year after treatment. *Journal of Pain and Symptom Management, 45*(2), 213–222.

Hazes, J. M., Taylor, P., Strand, V., et al. (2010). Physical function improvements and relief from fatigue and pain are associated with increased productivity at work and at home in rheumatoid arthritis patients treated with certolizumab pegol. *Rheumatology, 49*(10), 1900–1910.

Heo, S., Lennie, T. A., Moser, D. K., et al. (2014). Types of social support and their relationships to physical and depressive symptoms and health-related quality of life in patients with heart failure. *Heart & Lung: The Journal of Acute and Critical Care, 43*(4), 299–305.

Hewlett, S., Ambler, N., Almeida, C., et al. (2011). Self-management of fatigue in rheumatoid arthritis: a randomised controlled trial of group cognitive-behavioural therapy. *Annals of the Rheumatic Diseases, 70*(6), 1060–1067.

Hofmann, S. G., Asnaani, A., Vonk, I. J., et al. (2012). The efficacy of cognitive behavioral therapy: a review of meta-analyses. *Cognitive Therapy and Research, 36*(5), 427–440.

Johansson, I., Karlson, B. W., Grankvist, G., et al. (2010). Disturbed sleep, fatigue, anxiety and depression in myocardial infarction patients. *European Journal of Cardiovascular Nursing, 9*(3), 175–180.

Johns, S. A., Brown, L. F., Beck-Coon, K., et al. (2014). Randomized controlled pilot study of mindfulness-based stress reduction for persistently fatigued cancer survivors. *Psycho-Oncology*, [Epub ahead of print].

Kleinman, L., Benjamin, K., Viswanathan, H., et al. (2012). The anemia impact measure (AIM): development and content validation of a patient-reported outcome measure of anemia symptoms and symptom impacts in cancer patients receiving chemotherapy. *Quality of Life Research, 21*(7), 1255–1266.

Koornstra, R. H., Peters, M., Donofrio, S., et al. (2014). Management of fatigue in patients with cancer–a practical overview. *Cancer Treatment Reviews, 40*(6), 791–799.

Kwekkeboom, K. L., Cherwin, C. H., Lee, J. W., et al. (2010). Mind-body treatments for the pain-fatigue-sleep disturbance symptom cluster in persons with cancer. *Journal of Pain and Symptom Management, 39*(1), 126–138.

Lai, J. S., Cella, D., Yanez, B., et al. (2014). Linking fatigue measures on a common reporting metric. *Journal of Pain & Symptom Management, 48*(4), 639–648.

Mänty, M., Rantanen, T., Era, P., et al. (2014). Fatigue and depressive symptoms in older people. *Journal of Applied Gerontology, 33*(4), 505–514.

McMillan, E. M., & Newhouse, I. J. (2011). Exercise is an effective treatment modality for reducing cancer-related fatigue and improving physical capacity in cancer patients and survivors: a meta-analysis. *Applied Physiology, Nutrition, and Metabolism, 36*(6), 892–903.

Merriman, J. D., Von Ah, D., Miaskowski, C., et al. (2013). Proposed mechanisms for cancer-and treatment-related cognitive changes. *Seminars in Oncology Nursing, 29*(4), 260–269.

Minton, O., Richardson, A., Sharpe, M., et al. (2011). Psychostimulants for the management of cancer-related fatigue: a systematic review and meta-analysis. *Journal of Pain and Symptom Management, 41*(4), 761–767.

Montgomery, G. H., David, D., Kangas, M., et al. (2014). Randomized controlled trial of a cognitive-behavioral therapy plus hypnosis intervention to control fatigue in patients undergoing radiotherapy for breast cancer. *Journal of Clinical Oncology, 32*(6), 557–563.

Murphy, S., & Niemiec, S. S. (2014). Aging, fatigue, and fatigability: implications for occupational and physical therapists. *Current Geriatrics Reports, 3*(3), 135–141.

Naeim, A., Aapro, M., Subbarao, R., et al. (2014). Supportive care considerations for older adults with cancer. *Journal of Clinical Oncology, 32*(24), 2627–2634.

National Comprehensive Cancer Network (2014). *NCCN clinical practice guidelines in oncology cancer-related fatigue version I.2014*. Retrieved from: <http://www.nccn.org/professionals/physician_gls/pdf/fatigue.pdf>.

F

Oh, H. S., & Seo, W. S. (2011). Systematic review and meta-analysis of the correlates of cancer-related fatigue. *Worldviews on Evidence-based Nursing*, *8*(4), 191–201.
Oktay, J. S., Bellin, M. H., Scarvalone, S., et al. (2011). Managing the impact of posttreatment fatigue on the family: breast cancer survivors share their experiences. *Families, Systems and Health: The Journal of Collaborative Family Healthcare*, *29*(2), 127–137.
Payne, C., Wiffen, P. J., & Martin, S. (2012). Interventions for fatigue and weight loss in adults with advanced progressive illness. *Cochrane Database of Systematic Reviews*, *1*.
Pihur, V., Datta, S., & Datta, S. (2011). Meta analysis of chronic fatigue syndrome through integration of clinical, gene expression, SNP and proteomic data. *Bioinformation*, *6*(3), 120–124.
Primdahl, J., Wagner, L., & Horslev-Petersen, K. (2011). Self-efficacy as an outcome measure and its association with physical disease-related variables in persons with rheumatoid arthritis: a literature review. *Musculoskeletal Care*, *9*, 125–140.
Pross, N., Demazieres, A., Girard, N., et al. (2013). Influence of progressive fluid restriction on mood and physiological markers of dehydration in women. *British Journal of Nutrition*, *109*(02), 313–321.
Rich, M. W., & Nienaber, W. J. (2014). Polypharmacy and adverse drug reactions in the aging population with heart failure. In B. I. Jugdutt (Ed.), *Aging and heart failure* (pp. 107–116). New York: Springer.
Rimes, K. A., & Wingrove, J. (2013). Mindfulness-based cognitive therapy for people with chronic fatigue syndrome still experiencing excessive fatigue after cognitive behaviour therapy: a pilot randomized study. *Clinical Psychology & Psychotherapy*, *20*(2), 107–117.
Sharafkhaneh, A., Melendez, J., Akhtar, F., et al. (2013). Fatigue in cardiorespiratory conditions. *Sleep Medicine Clinics*, *8*(2), 221–227.
Silver, J. K., & Gilchrist, L. S. (2011). Cancer rehabilitation with a focus on evidence-based outpatient physical and occupational therapy interventions. *American Journal of Physical Medicine & Rehabilitation*, *90*(5), S5–S15.
Siniscalchi, A., Gallelli, L., Russo, E., et al. (2013). A review on antiepileptic drugs-dependent fatigue: pathophysiological mechanisms and incidence. *European Journal of Pharmacology*, *718*(1), 10–16.
Stahl, D., Rimes, K. A., & Chalder, T. (2014). Mechanisms of change underlying the efficacy of cognitive behaviour therapy for chronic fatigue syndrome in a specialist clinic: a mediation analysis. *Psychological Medicine*, *44*(6), 1331–1344.
Theander, K., Hasselgren, M., Luhr, K., et al. (2014). Symptoms and impact of symptoms on function and health in patients with chronic obstructive pulmonary disease and chronic heart failure in primary health care. *International Journal of Chronic Obstructive Pulmonary Disease*, *9*, 785.
Wahl, H. W., Fänge, A., Oswald, F., et al. (2009). The home environment and disability-related outcomes in aging individuals: What is the empirical evidence? *The Gerontologist*, *49*(3), 355–367.
Weis, J., Arraras, J. I., Conroy, T., et al. (2013). Development of an EORTC quality of life phase III module measuring cancer-related fatigue (EORTC QLQ-FA13). *Psycho-Oncology*, *22*(5), 1002–1007.
White, P. D., Goldsmith, K. A., Johnson, A. L., et al. (2011). Comparison of adaptive pacing therapy, cognitive behaviour therapy, graded exercise therapy, and specialist medical care for chronic fatigue syndrome (PACE): a randomised trial. *The Lancet*, *377*(9768), 823–836.
Whitehead, L. (2009). The measurement of fatigue in chronic illness: a systematic review of unidimensional and multidimensional fatigue measures. *Journal of Pain and Symptom Management*, *37*(1), 107–128.
Yu, D. S., Lee, D. T., & Man, N. W. (2010). Fatigue among older people: a review of the research literature. *International Journal of Nursing Studies*, *47*(2), 216–228.

Fear

Ruth McCaffrey, DNP, ARNP, FNP-BC, GNP-BC, FAAN

NANDA-I

Definition

Response to perceived threat that is consciously recognized as a danger

Defining Characteristics

Apprehensiveness; decrease in self-assurance; excitedness; feeling of dread; feeling of fear; feeling of pain; feeling of terror; feeling of alarm; increase in blood pressure; increase in tension; jitteriness; muscle tension; nausea; pallor; pupil dilation; vomiting

Cognitive

Decrease in learning ability; decrease in problem-solving ability; decrease in productivity; identifies object of fear; stimulus believed to be a threat

Behaviors

Attack behaviors; avoidance behaviors; focus narrowed to the source of fear; impulsiveness; increase in alertness

Physiological

Anorexia; change in physiological response (e.g., blood pressure, heart rate, respiratory rate, oxygen saturation, and end-tidal CO_2); diarrhea; dry mouth; dyspnea; fatigue; increase in perspiration; increase in respiratory rate

Related Factors (r/t)

Innate releasing mechanism to external stimuli (e.g., neurotransmitters); innate response to stimuli (e.g., sudden noise, height); language barrier; learned response; phobic stimulus; sensory deficit (e.g., visual, hearing); separation from support system; unfamiliar setting

F

NOC (Nursing Outcomes Classification)

Suggested NOC Outcome

Fear Self-Control

Example NOC Outcome with Indicators

Fear Self-Control as evidenced by the following indicators: Eliminates precursors of fear/Seeks information to reduce fear/Plans coping strategies for fearful situations. (Rate the outcome and indicators of **Fear Self-Control:** 1 = never demonstrated, 2 = rarely demonstrated, 3 = sometimes demonstrated, 4 = often demonstrated, 5 = consistently demonstrated [see Section I].)

Client Outcomes

Client Will (Specify Time Frame)

- Verbalize known fears
- State accurate information about the situation
- Identify, verbalize, and demonstrate those coping behaviors that reduce own fear
- Report and demonstrate reduced fear

NIC (Nursing Interventions Classification)

Suggested NIC Interventions

Anxiety Reduction; Coping Enhancement; Security Enhancement

Example NIC Activities—Anxiety Reduction

Use a calm, reassuring approach; Stay with the client to promote safety and reduce fear

Nursing Interventions and *Rationales*

- Assess source of fear with the client. EB: *The capacity to experience fear is adaptive, enabling rapid and energetic response to imminent threat or danger (George et al, 2011).* EB: *Fear can cause the inability to manage chronic diseases. The model of chronic pain describes how individuals experiencing acute pain may become trapped into a vicious cycle of chronic disability, suffering, and fear (Crombez et al, 2012). Many clients with chronic diseases such as multiple sclerosis or those with mobility issues have a fear of falling (Topuz et al, 2014).*
- Assess for a history of anxiety. EB: *Participants in a study of older adults who had anxiety were found to have a higher level of fear of pain (Lumley et al, 2011). Fear of pain independently predicts limitations in function and further exacerbation of pain (LeMay et al, 2011).* EB: *Clients experiencing post-traumatic stress disorder often fear uncertainty, which can exacerbate symptoms (Boswell et al, 2013).*
- Have the client draw the object of his or her fear. EBN: *In a study of older adults with a fear of falling, a community-based art program helped them overcome fears and anxiety (Beauvais & Beauvais, 2014).*
- Discuss the situation with the client and help distinguish between real and imagined threats to well-being. EB: *Fear activation occurs before conscious cognitive analysis of the stimulus can occur (George et al, 2011). There is a need to address psychological aspects of fear, catastrophizing, and emotional distress in the management of clients with pain (Westman et al, 2011).*
- Encourage the client to explore underlying feelings that may be contributing to the fear. *Exploring underlying feelings may help the client confront unresolved conflicts and develop coping abilities (Eva et al, 2011).*
- Stay with clients when they express fear; provide verbal and nonverbal (touch and hug with permission and if culturally acceptable) reassurances of safety if safety is within control. EBN: *One study in which nurses stayed with ventilated clients to provide support and reassurance reduced anxiety levels in th*

clients. Clients' ability to interact with the environment served as a basis for identification and management of anxiety or agitation. Health care providers' attributions about anxiety or agitation, and "knowing the patient," contributed to their assessment of client response (Tate et al, 2013).

- Explore coping skills previously used by the client to deal with fear; reinforce these skills and explore other outlets. Provide backrubs and massage for clients to decrease anxiety. EB: *A study of 87 children who received massage prior to a painful treatment had lower levels of fear and anxiety then those who did not receive massage (Celebiogiu et al, 2014). In a group of older adults those who received massage had less pain after hip or knee surgery (Buyukyilmaz & Turkinaz, 2014).*
- ▲ Refer for cognitive behavior therapy. EB: *Therapeutic touch and harp music reduced fear and anxiety in a group of postoperative clients (Lincoln et al, 2014).*
- ▲ *Animal-assisted therapy can be incorporated into the care of clients in hospice situations.*
- Encourage clients to express their fears in narrative form. *Refer to care plans for* ***Anxiety*** *and Death* ***Anxiety****.*

Pediatric

- Explore coping skills previously used by the client to deal with fear. EB: *Children whose mothers were fearful and depressed had increased levels of fearfulness from infancy through the toddler stage (Gartstein et al, 2010).*
- Teach parents to use cognitive behavioral strategies such as positive coping statements ("I am a brave girl [boy]. I can take care of myself in the dark") and rewards of bravery tokens for appropriate behavior.
- EB: *Screen for depression in clients who report social or school fears (Chung et al, 2010).* EB: *Early onset of depression in young people is associated with a poor prognosis. All children with school fears or phobias should be screened for depression early to avoid poor outcomes and lingering depressive symptoms (Chung et al, 2010).*
- Teach relaxation techniques to children to induce calmness. EB: *Using relaxation and distraction techniques will calm children's fears during procedures and in times of stress (Koller & Goldman, 2012).*

Geriatric

- Establish a trusting relationship so that all fears can be identified. Monitor for dementia and use appropriate interventions. EB: *Fear is an early symptom of dementia and may be associated with decreased cognitive and reasoning ability. New onset fear in an older adult should be an indication for cognitive assessment and monitoring (Sigstrom et al, 2011).*
- Provide a protective and safe environment, use consistent caregivers, and maintain the accustomed environmental structure. EBN: *Providing an environment that included safety equipment and balance training reduced the fear of falling among older adults (Gusi et al, 2011).*
- Observe for untoward changes if antianxiety drugs are taken. *Advancing age renders clients more sensitive to both the clinical and toxic effects of many agents (Baldwin et al, 2011).*
- Assess for fear of falls in hospitalized clients with hip fractures to determine risk of poor health outcomes. EBN: *Fear of falling can increase risk of depression and isolation, and further decrease physical performance in older clients (Park et al, 2014).*
- Encourage exercises to improve physical skills and levels of mobility to decrease fear of falling. *Improving physical skills and levels of mobility counteracts excessive fear during activity performance (Perry et al, 2013).*
- Assist the client in identifying and reducing risk factors for falls, including environmental hazards in and out of the home, the importance of good nutrition and activity, proper footwear, and how to stand up after a fall. EB: *Clients receiving education focused on identifying and reducing risk factors for falls were found to have a significant reduction in their fear of falling (Park et al, 2014).*

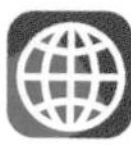

Multicultural

- Assess for the presence of culture-bound anxiety and fear states. EBN: *Allowing clients to define their cultural beliefs, how their cultural beliefs impact their ideas about health and well-being, and how their culture identifies and deals with suffering is a way in which nurses can better understand culture-bound anxiety and fear (Kagawa-Singer, 2011).*
- Assess for the influence of cultural beliefs, norms, and values on the client's perspective of a stressful situation. EBN: *Having insight into clients' illness beliefs about the cause and experience of fear may assist in alleviating pain and create motivation to change detrimental and dysfunctional illness beliefs (Buitenhuis & de Jong 2011).*

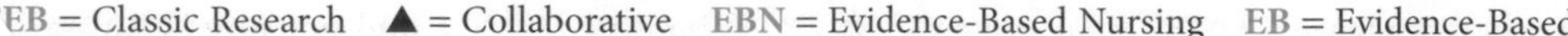

- Identify what triggers fear response. EBN: *Consider all of the aspects of cultural belief including religious or spiritual beliefs when attempting to identify what triggers any fear response (Salman & Zoucha, 2011).* EB: *Culture plays a role in how people perceive themselves in fearful situations Fear, fatalism, and current and historical relationships influence how people perceive themselves (Somayaji & Cloyes, 2014).*
- Identify how the client expresses fear. EBN: *Fear is culturally sensitive; therefore, nurses must attentively and actively listen to all clients to determine what expresses fear to that individual (Salman & Zoucha, 2011).*
- Validate the client's feelings regarding fear. EBN: *The most valid predictor of fear is younger clients with cancer. There is also a strong correlation between level of physical symptoms and fear (Crist & Grunfeld, 2012).*
- Assess for fears of racism in culturally diverse clients.

F

Home Care

- The previous interventions may be adapted for home care use.
- Assess to differentiate the presence of fear versus anxiety. EB: *Study findings suggest that fear and anxiety are largely distinct emotions and that psychological disorders of trait fear and trait anxiety warrant classification in separate higher-order categories (Sylvers et al, 2011). Addressing fear avoidance beliefs, catastrophizing, and emotional distress can reduce fear (Westman et al, 2011).*
- Refer to care plan for **Anxiety.**
- During initial assessment, determine whether current or previous episodes of fear relate to the home environment (e.g., perception of danger in the home or neighborhood or of relationships that have a history in the home). EB: *Fear of falling can negatively affect the ability of older adults to function and complete physical activities in the home (Hornyak et al, 2010).*
- Identify with the client what steps may be taken to make the home a "safe" place to be. EB: *Identifying a given area as a safe place reduces fear and anxiety when the client is in that area. Compared with whites, both blacks and Hispanics were less likely to own a variety of safety devices at baseline, but Hispanics were more likely than blacks to redeem vouchers (Pressley et al, 2010).*

▲ Encourage the client to seek or continue appropriate counseling to reduce fear associated with stress or resolve alterations in irrational thought processes. *Correcting mistaken beliefs reduces anxiety. Creating a fear appeal that helps the client see that the fear is out of proportion to the situation can reduce fear in some clients (Sandkuhler & Lee, 2013).*

▲ Encourage the client to have a trusted companion, family member, or caregiver present in the home for periods when fear is most prominent. Pending other medical diagnoses, a referral to homemaker or home health aide services may meet this need. *Creating periods when fear and anxiety can be reduced allows the client periods of rest and supports positive coping. A healing environment responds to the needs of all the people within a critical care unit—those who receive or give care and those who support clients and staff. Critical care units should be designed to focus on healing the body, the mind, and the senses (Bauzin & Cardon, 2011).*

▲ Offer to sit quietly with a terminally ill client as needed by the client or family, or provide hospice volunteers to do the same. EB: *Skill in communicating and being with dying clients and their families is an important aspect of health care (Curtis et al, 2013).*

Client/Family Teaching and Discharge Planning

- Teach the client the difference between warranted and excessive fear. *Different interventions are indicated for rational and irrational fears. Creating a fear appeal that helps the client see that the fear is out of proportion to the situation can reduce fear in some clients (Sandkuhler & Lee, 2013).*
- Teach clients to use guided imagery when they are fearful; have them use all senses to visualize a place that is "comfortable and safe" for them. *Imagery makes use of subjective symbolism, bypassing the rational mind and making the areas "safe" that the client may otherwise be reluctant to face (Milad et al, 2014).*
- Teach use of appropriate community resources in emergency situations (e.g., hotlines, emergency departments, law enforcement, judicial systems). *Serious emergencies need immediate assistance to ensure the client's safety. Social media has a profound impact on society and affects many aspects of human life. Its applications in combating crises are unanticipated results of social media inventors and many lessons could be learned from its applications in combating real crises (Chen et al, 2014).*
- Encourage use of appropriate community resources in nonemergency situations (e.g., family, friends, neighbors, self-help and support groups, volunteer agencies, churches, recreation clubs and centers,

seniors, youths, others with similar interests). *Social support and coping strategies were able to modify fears and anxiety in young women with eating disorders (Wonderlich-Tierney & Vander Val, 2010).*

- If fear is associated with bioterrorism, provide accurate information and ensure that health care personnel have appropriate training and preparation. *Clear, consistent, accessible, reliable, and redundant information (received from trusted sources) will diminish public uncertainty about the cause of symptoms that might otherwise prompt persons to seek unnecessary treatment. Training for providers is essential.* **EB:** *Using a diverse group of experts and providing a transparent and open line of communication can reduce fear in communities and the nation regarding bioterrorism (Siegrist & Zingg, 2014).*

F

REFERENCES

Baldwin, D., Woods, R., Lawson, R., et al. (2011). Efficacy of drug treatments for generalized anxiety disorder: systematic review and meta-analysis. *British Medical Journal*, *342*, d1199.

Bauzin, D., & Cardon, K. (2011). Creating healing intensive care unit environments: physical and psychological considerations in designing critical care areas. *Critical Care Nursing Quarterly*, *34*(4), 259–267.

Beauvais, A., & Beauvais, J. (2014). Reducing the fear of falling through a community evidence-based intervention. *Home Healthcare Nurse*, *32*(2), 98–105.

Boswell, J., Thompson-Hollands, J., Frachione, T., et al. (2013). Intolerance of uncertainty: a common factor in the treatment of emotional disorders. *Journal of Clinical Psychology*, *69*(6), 630–645.

Buitenhuis, J., & de Jong, P. (2011). Fear avoidance and illness beliefs in post-traumatic neck pain. *Spine*, *36*(Suppl. 25S), S238–S243.

Buyukyilmaz, F., & Turkinaz, A. (2014). *The effect of relaxation techniques and back massage on pain and anxiety in Turkey Total Hip or Knee Pain Management Nursing.*

Celebiogiu, A., Gurol, A., Yildirim, Z. X., et al. (2014). Effects of massage therapy on pain and anxiety arising from interthecal therapy or bone marrow aspiration in children. *International Journal of Nursing Practice*, Published on line on April 1, 2014.

Chen, C., Ractham, P., & Kaewkitipong, L. (2014). *The community-based model of using social media to share knowledge to combat crises. Pacific Asia Conference on Information System.* Accessed on line at: <http://aisel.aisnet.org/pacis2014>.

Chung, M., et al. (2010). A rapid screening test for depression in junior high school children. *Journal of the Chinese Medical Association*, *74*(8), 363–368.

Crist, J., & Grunfeld, E. (2012). Factors reported to influence fear of recurrence in cancer patients: a systematic review. *Psycho-Oncology*, *22*(5), 978–986.

Crombez, G., Eccleston, C., Van Damme, S., et al. (2012). Fear-avoidance model of chronic pain: the next generation. *The Clinical Journal of Pain*, *28*(6), 475–483.

Curtis, R., Back, A., & Ford, D. (2013). Effect of communication skills training for residents and nurse practitioners on quality of communication with patients with serious illness. *Journal of the American Medical Association*, *310*(21), 2271–2281.

Eva, K., Armson, H., Holmboe, E., et al. (2011). Factors influencing responsiveness to feedback on the interplay between fear, confidence and reasoning processes. *Advances in Health Science Education* Available online at: <Springerlink.com>.

Gartstein, M., et al. (2010). A latent growth examination of fear development in infancy: contributions of maternal depression and the risk for toddler anxiety. *Developmental Psychology*, *46*(3), 651–668.

George, S., Calley, D., Valencia, C., et al. (2011). Clinical investigation of pain-related fear and pain catastrophizing for patients with low back pain. *The Clinical Journal of Pain*, *27*(2), 108–115.

Gusi, N., Adsuar, J., Corzo, H., et al. (2011). Balance training reduces fear of falling and improves dynamic balance and isometric strength in institutionalised older people: a randomised trial. *Journal of Physiotherapy*, *58*(2), 97–104.

Hornyak, V., Brach, J., Wert, D., et al. (2010). What is the relation between fear of falling and physical activity in older adults? *Archives of Physical Medicine and Rehabilitation*, *94*(12), 2529–2534.

Kagawa-Singer, M. (2011). Impact of culture on health outcomes. *Journal of Pediatric Hematology*, *33*(2), 590–595.

Koller, D., & Goldman, R. (2012). Distraction techniques for children undergoing procedures: a critical review of pediatric research. *Journal of Pediatric Nursing*, *27*(6), 652–681.

LeMay, K., et al. (2011). Fear of patient with advanced cancer or with chronic non cancer pain. *The Clinical Journal of Pain*, *27*(7), 116–124.

Lincoln, V., Norwak, E., Schommer, B., et al. (2014). Impact of healing touch with healing harp on inpatient acute care pain: a retrospective analysis. *Holistic Nursing Practice*, *28*(3), 164–170.

Lumley, M., Cohen, J., Borszcz, G., et al. (2011). Pain and emotion: a biopsychosocial review of recent research. *Journal of Clinical Psychology*, *67*(9), 942–968.

Milad, M., Rosenblum, B., & Simon, N. (2014). Neuroscience of fear extinction: implications for assessment and treatment of fear-based and anxiety related disorders. *Behavior Research and Therapy*.

Park, J., Cho, H., Shin, J., et al. (2014). Relationship among fear of falling, physical performance, and physical characteristics in rural elderly. *American Journal of Physical Medicine and Rehabilitation*, *93*(5), 379–386.

Perry, S., Finch, T., & Deary, V. (2013). How should we manage fear of falling in older adults living in the community? *British Medical Journal*, *346*, f2933.

Pressley, J., et al. (2010). Race and ethnic differences in home use of safety devices and fears of home safety. *J Trauma Infect Crit Care*, *67*(1), 3–11.

Salman, K., & Zoucha, R. (2011). Considering faith and culture when caring for terminally ill cancer patients. *Hosp Palliat Care*, *12*(3), 156–163.

Sandkuhler, J., & Lee, J. (2013). How to erase memory traces of pain and fear. *Trends in Neuroscience*, *36(6), 343–352.*

Siegrist, M., & Zingg, A. (2014). The role of public trust during pandemics: implications for crisis communication. *European Psychologist*, *19*(1), 23–32.

Sigstrom, R. M., et al. (2011). A population based study on phobic fears in 70 year olds. *Journal of Anxiety Disorders*, *25*(1), 148–153.

Somayaji, D., & Cloyes, K. (2014). Cancer, fear and fatalism. *Cancer Nursing, 2014.*

Sylvers, P., Lilienfield, S., & LaPrarie, J. (2011). Differences between trait fear and trait anxiety. *Clinical Psychology Review*, *31*(1), 122–137.

Tate, J., Dabbs, A. D., Hoffman, L., et al. (2013). Anxiety and agitation in mechanically ventilated patients. *Qualitative Health Research*, *22*(2), 157–173.

Topuz, S., De Schepper, J., Ulger, O., et al. (2014). Do mobility and life setting affect falling and fear of falling in elderly people. *Topics in Geriatric Rehabilitation*, *30*(3), 223–229.
Westman, A., Boersma, K., Leppert, J., et al. (2011). Fear-avoidance beliefs, catastrophizing, and distress: a longitudinal subgroup analysis on patients with musculoskeletal pain. *The Clinical Journal of Pain*, *27*(7), 567–577.
Wonderlich-Tierney, A., & Vander Val, J. (2010). The effects of social support and coping on the relationship between social anxiety and eating disorders. *Eating Behaviors*, *11*(2), 85–91.

Ineffective infant Feeding pattern

Vanessa Flannery, MSN, PHCNS-BC, CNE

F

NANDA-I

Definition

Impaired ability of an infant to suck or coordinate the suck/swallow response, resulting in inadequate oral nutrition for metabolic needs

Defining Characteristics

Inability to coordinate sucking, swallowing, and breathing; inability to initiate an effective suck; inability to sustain an effective suck

Related Factors (r/t)

Neurological delay; neurological impairment (e.g., positive electroencephalogram, head trauma, seizure disorders); oral hypersensitivity; oropharyngeal defect; prematurity; prolonged nil per os (NPO) status

NOC (Nursing Outcomes Classification)

Suggested NOC Outcomes

Breastfeeding Establishment: Infant, Maternal; Breastfeeding: Maintenance; Hydration; Nutritional Status: Food and Fluid Intake

Example NOC Outcome with Indicators

Breastfeeding Establishment: Infant as evidenced by the following indicators: Proper alignment and latch-on/Correct suck and tongue placement/Urinations per day appropriate for age/Weight gain appropriate for age. (Rate the outcome and indicators of **Breastfeeding Establishment: Infant:** 1 = not adequate, 2 = slightly adequate, 3 = moderately adequate, 4 = substantially adequate, 5 = totally adequate [see Section I].)

Client Outcomes

Infant Will (Specify Time Frame)

- Consume adequate calories that will result in appropriate weight gain and optimal growth and development
- Have opportunities for skin-to-skin (kangaroo care) experiences
- Have opportunities for "trophic" (i.e., small volume of breast milk/formula) enteral feedings prior to full oral feedings
- Progress to stable, neurobehavioral organization (i.e., motor, state, self-regulation, attention-interaction)
- Demonstrate presence of mature oral reflexes that are necessary for safe feeding
- Progress to safe, self-regulated oral feedings
- Coordinate the suck-swallow-breathe sequence while nippling
- Display clear behavioral cues related to hunger and satiety
- Display approach/engagement cues, with minimal avoidance/disengagement cues
- Have opportunities to pace own feeding, taking breaks as needed
- Display evidence of being in the "quiet-alert" state while nippling
- Progress to and engage in mutually positive parent/caregiver-infant/child interactions during feedings

Parent/Family Will (Specify Time Frame)

- Recognize necessity of adequate calories for appropriate weight gain and optimal growth and development
- Learn to read and respond contingently to infant's behavioral cues (e.g., hunger, satiety, approach/engagement, stress/avoidance/disengagement)
- Learn strategies that promote organized infant behavior
- Learn appropriate positioning and handling techniques
- Learn effective ways to relieve stress behaviors during nippling
- Learn ways to help infant coordinate suck-swallow-breathe sequence (i.e., external pacing techniques)
- Engage in mutually positive interactions with infant during feeding
- Recognize ways to facilitate effective feedings: feed in quiet-alert state; keep length of feeding appropriate; burp; prepare/structure environment; recognize signs of sensory overload; encourage self-regulation; respect need for breaks and breathing pauses; avoid pulling and twisting nipple during pauses; allow infant to resume sucking when ready; provide oral support (cheek and/or jaw) as needed; use appropriate nipple hole size and flow rate

F

NIC (Nursing Interventions Classification)

Suggested NIC Interventions

Bottle Feeding; Breastfeeding Assistance; Fluid Monitoring; Kangaroo Care; Lactation Counseling; Teaching: Infant Safety

Example NIC Activities—Lactation Counseling

Provide information about psychological and physiological benefits of breastfeeding; Refer to a lactation consultant

Nursing Interventions and *Rationales*

- Refer to care plans for Disorganized **Infant** behavior, Risk for disorganized **Infant** behavior, Ineffective and Interrupted **Breastfeeding,** and Insufficient **Breast Milk** and assess as needed.
- Interventions follow a sequential pattern of implementation that can be adapted as appropriate.
- Assess coordination of infant's suck, swallow, and gag reflex. EBN: *During this first hour when the infant starts seeking the breast, the rooting reflex becomes successively more mature and distinct (Svensson et al, 2013).*
- ▲ Provide developmentally supportive neonatal intensive care for preterm infants. EBN: *To decrease barriers for mothers to optimize breast milk feedings during the infants' first weeks of life (Purdy et al, 2012).*
- Provide opportunities for kangaroo (i.e., skin-to-skin) care. EBN: *Use of kangaroo care increases the interval of breastfeeding and reduces the risk of mortality, infection/sepsis, hypothermia, and length of hospital stay (Gregson & Blacker, 2011).*
- ▲ Before the infant is ready for oral feedings, implement gavage feedings (or other alternative) as ordered, using breast milk whenever possible. EBN: *Gavage feeding is the method used to feed preterm infants or infants with inadequate suck/swallow during feeding (Pineda, 2011).*
- Provide a naturalistic environment for tube feedings (naso-orogastric, gavage, or other) that approximates a pleasurable oral feeding experience: hold infant in semi-upright/flexed position; offer nonnutritive sucking; pace feedings; allow for semi-demand feedings contingent with infant cues; offer rest breaks; burp, as appropriate. EBN: *Nonnutritive sucking during gavage feeding is comforting for the infant and significantly supports breastfeeding ability (Garpiel, 2012).*
- Foster direct breastfeeding as early as possible and enable the first oral feed to be at the breast in the neonatal intensive care unit (NICU). EBN: *Research demonstrates a link between direct breastfeeding behaviors in the NICU and success with provision of milk at discharge (Pineda, 2011).*
- Allow parents to feed the infant when possible. EBN: *Parents who feed effectively early on develop positive feeding relationships with their infants and promote infant feeding self-regulation and normative growth patterns (Horodynski et al, 2011).*
- Position infant in semi-upright position, with head, shoulders, and hips in straight line facing the mother with the infant's nose level with the mother's nipple. EBN: *Good positioning of the baby during breastfeeding is crucial to encourage oxytocin and prolactin release (Hughes, 2011).*

- Feed infant in the quiet-alert state. EBN: *Preterm infants who are in awake states at the beginning of nipple feedings are more successful at ingesting their feeding volumes (McCain et al, 2012).*
- Determine the appropriate shape, size, and hole of nipple to provide flow rate for preterm infants. EBN: *The coordination of rhythmic sucking, swallowing, and breathing patterns during feeding is disorganized in preterm infants with bronchopulmonary dysplasia (McCain et al, 2012).*
- Implement pacing for infants having difficulty coordinating breathing with sucking and swallowing. EBN: *Paced feedings decrease risk of fatigue and oxygen desaturation of the infant (McCain et al, 2012).*
- Provide infants with jaw and/or cheek support, as needed. EBN: *Breastfeeding difficulties can be avoided if good attachment and positioning are achieved at the first and early feeds (Goyal et al, 2011).*
- Allow the stable newborn to breastfeed within the first half hour after birth. EBN: *Mothers of infants who were breastfed within 1 to 2 hours were almost three times more likely to experience breastfeeding problems in the postpartum period than those mothers who breastfed within 30 minutes of birth (Demirtas, 2012).*
- Allow appropriate time for nipple feeding to ensure infant's safety, limiting to 15 to 20 minutes for bottle feeding. EBN: *Bottle feeding mothers need to develop responsive behavior to their infants' hunger and satiety cues (Horodynski et al, 2011).*
- Monitor length of breastfeeding so that it does not exceed 30 minutes. Breast milk transfer may last from as little as 5 to 20 minutes during breastfeeding depending on variations in milk supply during a 24-hour day (Flaherman et al, 2012).
- Encourage transitioning from scheduled to semi-demand feedings, contingent with infant behavior cues. *Flexible feeding schedules allow infants to feed during awake and alert periods in response to infant's readiness and tolerance of nipple feedings (McCain et al, 2012).*

▲ Refer to a multidisciplinary team (e.g., neonatal/pediatric nutritionist, physical or occupational therapist, speech pathologist, lactation specialist) as needed. EB: *Follow-up visits with lactation consultants, nurses, and health care providers are beneficial for breastfeeding mothers (Henry & Britz, 2011).*

Home Care

- The above appropriate interventions may be adapted for home care use.

▲ Infants with risk factors and clinical indicators of feeding problems present before hospital discharge should be referred to appropriate community early-intervention service providers (e.g., community health nurses, early learning programs (individualized per states), occupational therapy, speech pathologists, feeding specialists) to facilitate adequate weight gain for optimal growth and development. EBN: *Late preterm infants are susceptible to multiple complications including feeding and sucking problems (Henry & Britz, 2011).*

Client/Family Teaching and Discharge Planning

- Provide anticipatory guidance for infant's expected feeding course. *Providing written information and education on breastfeeding with culturally sensitive awareness helps guide parents after early discharge (Wiener & Wiener, 2011).*
- Teach various effective feeding methods and strategies to parents. EBN: *Mothers need to be given evidence-based information and support before discharge, giving mothers a sense of security and providing understanding care (Demirtas, 2014).*
- Teach parents how to read, interpret, and respond contingently to infant cues. EBN: *Parents' ability to recognize and react quickly and consistently to their infant's state or cues leads to parental confidence in providing care, promotes parent-child relationship, and strengthens the family unit (Kadivar & Maryam Mozafarinia, 2013).*
- Help parents identify support systems before hospital discharge. *Nurses need to assess the support system of the family and collaborate with other health care team members to meet the mother's needs for successful breastfeeding (Feldman-Winter, 2013).*
- Provide anticipatory guidance for the infant's discharge. *Providing written information and education on breastfeeding with culturally sensitive awareness helps guide parents after early discharge (Wiener & Wiener, 2011).*

REFERENCES

Demirtas, B. (2012). Breastfeeding support received by Turkish first-time mothers. *International Nursing Review*, *59*(3), 338–344.

Demirtas, B. (2014). Multiparous mothers: breastfeeding support provided by nurses. *International Journal of Nursing Practice*.

Feldman-Winter, L. (2013). Evidence-based interventions to support breastfeeding. *Pediatric Clinics of North America*, *60*(1), 169–187.

Flaherman, V. J., Gay, B., Scott, C., et al. (2012). Randomised trial comparing hand expression with breast pumping for mothers of term newborns feeding poorly. *Archives of Disease in Childhood. Fetal and Neonatal Edition*, *97*(1), F18–F23.

Garpiel, S. J. (2012). Premature infant transition to effective breastfeeding: a comparison of four supplemental feeding methods. *JOGNN: Journal of Obstetric, Gynecologic & Neonatal Nursing*, *41*, S143.

Goyal, R. C., Banginwar, A. S., Ziyo, F., et al. (2011). Breastfeeding practices: positioning, attachment (latch-on) and effective suckling—a hospital-based study in Libya. *Journal Of Family & Community Medicine*, *18*(2), 74–79.

Gregson, S., & Blacker, J. (2011). Kangaroo care in pre-term or low birth weight babies in a postnatal ward. *British Journal of Midwifery*, *19*(9), 568–577.

Henry, L., & Britz, S. P. (2011). Breastfeeding the late preterm infant: hospital-based lactation consultants lead the way. *JOGNN: Journal of Obstetric, Gynecologic & Neonatal Nursing*, *40*, S30–S31.

Horodynski, M. A., Olson, B., Baker, S., et al. (2011). Healthy babies through infant-centered feeding protocol: an intervention targeting early childhood obesity in vulnerable populations. *BMC Public Health*, *11*, 868.

Hughes, G. (2011). How to … help with positioning and attachment. *Midwives*, *14*(4), 26.

Kadivar, M., & Maryam Mozafarinia, S. (2013). Supporting fathers in a NICU: effects of the HUG your baby program on fathers' understanding of preterm infant behavior. *Journal of Perinatal Education*, *22*(2), 113–119.

McCain, G. C., Del Moral, T., Duncan, R. C., et al. (2012). Transition from gavage to nipple feeding for preterm infants with bronchopulmonary dysplasia. *Nursing Research*, *61*(6), 380–387.

Pineda, R. (2011). Direct breast-feeding in the neonatal intensive care unit: is it important? *Journal of Perinatology*, *31*(8), 540–545.

Purdy, I. B., Singh, N., Le, C., et al. (2012). Biophysiologic and social stress relationships with breast milk feeding pre- and post-discharge from the neonatal intensive care unit. *JOGNN: Journal of Obstetric, Gynecologic & Neonatal Nursing*, *41*(3), 347–357.

Svensson, K. E., Velandia, M. I., Matthiesen, A.-S. T., et al. (2013). Effects of mother-infant skin-to-skin contact on severe latch-on problems in older infants: a randomized trial. *International Breastfeeding Journal*, *8*(1), 1.

Wiener, R. C., & Wiener, M. A. (2011). Breastfeeding prevalence and distribution in the USA and Appalachia by rural and urban setting. *Rural and Remote Health*, *11*(2), 1–9.

Readiness for enhanced Fluid balance *Susan M. Dirkes, RN, MS, CCRN*

NANDA-I

Definition

A pattern of equilibrium between the fluid volume and chemical composition of body fluids, which can be strengthened

Defining Characteristics

Expresses desire to enhance fluid balance

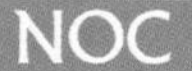

NOC (Nursing Outcomes Classification)

Suggested NOC Outcomes

Fluid Balance; Electrolyte and Acid-Base Balance; Hydration

Example NOC Outcome with Indicators

Maintains **Fluid Balance** as evidenced by the following indicators: BP/Peripheral pulses palpable/Skin turgor/Moist mucous membranes/Serum electrolytes/Hematocrit/Peripheral edema/Neck vein distention/Body weight stable/24-hour intake and output balanced/Urine specific gravity/Adventitious breath sounds. (Rate each indicator of **Fluid Balance:** 1 = severely compromised, 2 = substantially compromised, 3 = moderately compromised, 4 = mildly compromised, 5 = not compromised [see Section I].)

Client Outcomes

Client Will (Specify Time Frame)

- Maintain light yellow urine output of at least 0.5 mL/kg/hr
- Maintain elastic skin turgor, moist tongue, and mucous membranes
- Explain measures that can be taken to improve fluid intake

NIC (Nursing Interventions Classification)

Suggested NIC Interventions

Fluid Management; Fluid Monitoring

Example NIC Activities—Fluid Management

Monitor hydration status as appropriate; Monitor food/fluid ingested and calculate daily caloric intake, as appropriate

Nursing Interventions and *Rationales*

- Discuss normal fluid requirements. *A guideline is 1 to 1.5 mL of fluid per each calorie needed, so an average intake would be between 2000 and 3000 mL/day, or at least 8 cups of fluid. The adequate intake recommendation is 3 L for the 19- to 30-year-old male and 2.2 L for the 19- to 30-year-old female.* EB: *The previous general health recommendation of intake of eight 8-oz glasses of water per day is currently found to have no scientific basis but is used as a recommendation (McCartney, 2011).*
- Recommend the client choose mainly water to meet fluid needs, although fruit juices and milk are also useful for hydration. The intake of beverages containing caffeine or alcohol is no longer thought to cause dehydration. EB: *While caffeinated drinks and alcohol can cause mild diuresis, intake of these beverages is not associated with dehydration (Hobson & Maughan, 2010).*
- Recommend the client choose and prepare foods with less salt, aiming for a maximum of 1500 mg per day, less than a teaspoon. The Centers for Disease Control and Prevention (2012) recommends that all salt-sensitive Americans, including everyone 40 years or older, should decrease daily sodium intake. EB: *A study found that decreased sodium intake helped lower blood pressure, as well as increased flexibility in blood vessels, improving the health of the blood vessels (CDC, 2012).*
- Recommend the client avoid intake of soft drinks with sugar; instead, encourage the client to drink water. EB: *Consumption of sweetened beverages is associated with an increased risk of stroke (Larsson et al, 2014).*
- Recommend the client note the color of urine at intervals when voiding. Normal urine is straw-colored or amber. EB: *Dark-colored urine with an increased specific gravity may reflect increased urine concentration and fluid deficit (Perrier et al, 2013). Observing urine color is an effective and simple method of monitoring for possible dehydration (Jequier & Constant, 2010).*
- Recommend client monitor weight at intervals for alterations. EB: *Decreases in weight may be caused by inadequate fluid intake (Hooper et al, 2014).*

Geriatric

- Encourage older clients to develop a pattern of drinking water regularly. EB: *Thirst sensation diminishes with aging. Some geriatric clients limit fluid intake because of fear of incontinence, inability to drink on their own, due to poor availability and accessibility of fluids, altered sensorium/cognition, or decreased thirst as a part of the aging process. Mild levels of dehydration in older adults can produce disruptions in mood and cognitive functioning (Hooper et al, 2014). Also, older adults experience less hunger (Gregersen et al, 2011).*
- Ensure that when food intake is reduced or limited, it is compensated with an increase in water/fluid intake. EB: *Food contains water, thus any reduction in food intake also involves a reduction in water intake (Popkin et al, 2010).*
- Incorporate regular hydration into daily routines, such as providing an extra glass of fluid with medication or during social activities. EB: *Consider using a beverage cart to routinely offer beverages to clients in extended care facilities (Hooper et al, 2014).*

REFERENCES

Centers for Disease Control and Prevention (CDC) (2012). <http://www.cdc.gov/vitalsigns/Sodium/index.html>. Retrieved June 21, 2014.

Gregersen, N. T., Møller, B. K., Raben, A., et al. (2011). Determinants of appetite ratings: the role of age, gender, BMI, physical activity, smoking habits and diet/ weight concern. *Food & Nutrition Research*, *55*(10).

Hobson, R. M., & Maughan, R. J. (2010). Hydration status and the diuretic action of a small dose of alcohol. *Alcohol (Fayetteville, N.Y.)*, *45*(4), 366–373.

Hooper, L., Bunn, D., Jimoh, F. O., et al. (2014). Water loss dehydration and aging. *Mechanisms of Ageing and Development*, *136–137*, 50–58.

Jequier, E., & Constant, F. (2010). Water as an essential nutrient: the physiological basis of hydration. *European Journal of Clinical Nutrition*, *64*, 115–123.

Larsson, S. C., Akesson, A., & Wolk, A. (2014). Sweetened beverage consumption is associated with increased risk of stroke in women and men. *The Journal of Nutrition*, *144*(6), 856–860.

McCartney, M. (2011). Waterlogged? *British medical journal (Clinical research ed.)*, *343*, <http://dx.doi.org/10.1136/bmj.d4280>.

Perrier, E., Vergne, S., Klein, A., et al. (2013). Hydration biomarkers in free-living.adults with different levels of habitual fluid consumption. *The British Journal of Nutrition*, *109*(9), 1678–1687.

Popkin, B. M., D'Anci, K. E., & Rosenberg, I. H. (2010). Water, hydration and health. *Nutrition Reviews*, *68*(8), 439–458.

Deficient Fluid volume *Susan M. Dirkes, RN, MS, CCRN*

NANDA-I

Definition

Decreased intravascular, interstitial, and/or intracellular fluid. This refers to dehydration, water loss alone without change in sodium level

Defining Characteristics

F

Alteration in mental status; alteration in skin turgor; decrease in blood pressure; decrease in pulse pressure; decrease in pulse volume; decrease in tongue turgor; decrease in urine output; decreased venous filling; dry mucous membranes; dry skin; increase in body temperature; increase in heart rate; increase in hematocrit; increase in urine concentration; sudden weight loss; thirst; weakness

Related Factors

Active fluid volume loss; compromised regulatory mechanisms

NOC (Nursing Outcomes Classification)

Suggested NOC Outcomes

Fluid Balance; Hydration; Nutritional Status: Food and Fluid Intake

Example NOC Outcome with Indicators

Fluid Balance as evidenced by the following indicators: Elastic skin turgor/Moist mucous membranes/Orthostatic hypotension not present/24-hour intake and output balance/Urine specific gravity. (Rate each indicator of **Fluid Balance:** 1 = severely compromised, 2 = substantially compromised, 3 = moderately compromised, 4 = mildly compromised, 5 = not compromised [see Section I].)

Client Outcomes

Client Will (Specify Time Frame)

- Maintain urine output of 0.5 mL/kg/hour or at least more than 1300 mL/day
- Maintain normal blood pressure, heart rate, and body temperature
- Maintain elastic skin turgor; moist tongue and mucous membranes; and orientation to person, place, and time
- Explain measures that can be taken to treat or prevent fluid volume loss
- Describe symptoms that indicate the need to consult with health care provider

NIC (Nursing Interventions Classification)

Suggested NIC Interventions

Fluid Management; Hypovolemia Management; Shock Management: Volume

Example NIC Activities—Fluid Management

Monitor hydration status (e.g., moist mucous membranes, adequacy of pulses, and orthostatic blood pressure) as appropriate; Administer intravenous (IV) therapy, as prescribed

Nursing Interventions and *Rationales*

- Watch for early signs of hypovolemia, including thirst, restlessness, headaches, and inability to concentrate. *Thirst is often the first sign of dehydration (Wagner & Hardin-Pierce, 2014).* CEB: *A study of healthy women showed heart rate was increased by fluid restriction along with increased urine specific gravity, darker urine color, and increased thirst. They also experienced decreased alertness and increased sleepiness, fatigue, and confusion (Pross et al, 2013).*

- Recognize symptoms of cyanosis, cold clammy skin, weak thready pulse, confusion, and oliguria as late signs of hypovolemia. *These symptoms occur after the body has compensated for fluid loss by moving fluid from the interstitial space into the vascular compartment (Wagner & Hardin-Pierce, 2014).*
- Monitor pulse, respiration, and blood pressure of clients with deficient fluid volume every 15 minutes to 1 hour for the unstable client and every 4 hours for the stable client. *Vital sign changes seen with fluid volume deficit include tachycardia, tachypnea, decreased pulse pressure first, then hypotension, decreased pulse volume, and increased or decreased body temperature (Wagner & Hardin-Pierce, 2014).* CEB: *A systematic review demonstrated that hypotension and tachycardia, and occasionally fever, are clinical signs of dehydration (Jequier & Constant, 2010).*
- Check orthostatic blood pressures with the client lying, sitting, and standing. *A decrease in systolic blood pressure of 20 mm Hg or a decrease in diastolic blood pressure of 10 mm Hg within 3 minutes of standing when compared with blood pressure from the sitting position is considered orthostatic hypotension. This can occur with dehydration or cardiovascular disorders (Lanier et al, 2011).*
- Note skin turgor over bony prominences such as the hand or shin.
- Monitor for the existence of factors causing deficient fluid volume (e.g., hypovolemia from vomiting, diarrhea, difficulty maintaining oral intake, fever, uncontrolled type 2 diabetes, diuretic therapy). *Early identification of risk factors and early intervention can decrease the occurrence and severity of complications from deficient fluid volume and acute kidney injury (Ftouh & Lewington, 2014).*
- Observe for dry tongue and mucous membranes, and longitudinal tongue furrows. *These are symptoms of decreased body fluids (Wagner & Hardin-Pierce, 2014).*
- Recognize that checking capillary refill may not be helpful in identifying fluid volume deficit. Capillary refill can be normal in clients with sepsis because increased body temperature dilates peripheral blood vessels and capillary return may be immediate *(Wagner & Hardin-Pierce, 2014).* EBN: *A recent study indicated capillary refill showed good specificity to detect dehydration but had poor sensitivity (Shimizu et al, 2012).*
- Weigh client daily and watch for sudden decreases, especially in the presence of decreasing urine output or active fluid loss. *Body weight changes of 1 kg (2.2 lb) represent a fluid loss of 1 L (Wagner & Hardin-Pierce, 2014).*
- Monitor total fluid intake and output every 4 hours (or every hour for the unstable client or the client who has urine output equal to or less than 0.5 mL/kg/hr). Recognize that urine output is an accurate indicator of fluid balance. EB: *The incidence of kidney injury increased significantly from 24% to 52% when adding the urine output as criteria, as defined by the Acute Kidney Injury Network classification system, to the measurement of serum creatinine-based criteria alone* (Macedo et al, 2011).
- A urine output of less than 0.5 mL/kg/hr is indicative of acute kidney injury (Prowle et al, 2011). *The RIFLE criteria define oliguria as urine output less than 0.5 mL/kg/hr for each of 6 or more consecutive hours, which is thought to confer "risk" of kidney injury; when urine output less than 0.5 mL/kg/hr and persists for 12 or more consecutive hours, the kidneys are considered to be "in injury" (Ratanarat et al, 2013).*
- Note the color of urine, urine osmolality, and specific gravity. *Normal urine is straw-colored or amber. Dark-colored urine with a specific gravity greater than 1.030 and a high urine osmolality reflects fluid volume deficit (Wagner & Hardin-Pierce, 2014; Perrier et al, 2013).*
- Provide fresh water and oral fluids preferred by the client (distribute over 24 hours [e.g., 1200 mL on days, 800 mL on evenings, and 200 mL on nights]); provide prescribed diet; offer snacks (e.g., frequent drinks, fresh fruits, fruit juice); instruct significant other to assist the client with feedings as appropriate. *Distributing the intake over the entire 24-hour period and providing snacks, specifically those with creatine and carnitine, and beverages including caffeine may improve muscular ability, endurance, and alertness (Cherniack, 2012).*

▲ Provide oral replacement therapy as ordered and tolerated with a hypotonic glucose-electrolyte solution when the client has acute diarrhea or nausea/vomiting. Provide small, frequent quantities of slightly chilled solutions. *Maintenance of oral intake stabilizes the ability of the intestines to absorb nutrients and promote gastric emptying (Popkin et al, 2010); glucose-electrolyte solutions increase net fluid absorption while correcting deficient fluid volume. Use diluted carbohydrate-electrolyte solutions such as sports replacement drinks, and ginger ale (Deshpande et al, 2013).* EB: *Many studies have shown that diluted oral replacement fluids resulted in reductions in stool output, decreased vomiting, and less need for IV hydration (Suh et al, 2010).*

▲ Administer antidiarrheals and antiemetics as ordered and appropriate. *The goal is to stop the loss that results from vomiting or diarrhea. Refer to care plan for* ***Diarrhea*** *or* ***Nausea.***

▲ Hydrate the client with ordered isotonic IV solutions if prescribed. *For clients with mild to moderate fluid deficit, crystalloids such as 0.9 saline or lactated Ringer's should be used for fluid volume replacement (Peng & Kellum, 2013).*

• Assist with ambulation if the client has postural hypotension. Hypovolemia causes orthostatic hypotension, which can result in syncope when the client goes from a sitting to standing position (Wagner & Hardin-Pierce, 2014).

Critically Ill

▲ Monitor central venous pressure (CVP), pulmonary artery pressure, or stroke volume for decreasing trends for more accurate fluid volume status. *Hemodynamic pressures such as CVP and pulmonary artery pressures have been demonstrated to be less to predict fluid volume responsiveness, whereas changes in stroke volume measured by a number of noninvasive methods including passive leg lift may more accurately predict fluid volume responsiveness of a client (Marik et al, 2011).*

▲ Monitor serum and urine osmolality blood urea nitrogen (BUN)/creatinine ratio, and hematocrit for elevations. *These are all measures of concentration and will be elevated with decreased intravascular volume (Wagner & Hardin-Pierce, 2014).*

▲ Insert an indwelling urinary catheter if ordered and measure urine output hourly. Notify health care provider if urine output is less than 0.5 mL/kg/hr. *A decrease in urine output is seen with poorly perfused kidneys and a drop in the glomerular filtration rate in the client with normal kidney function, and action, if taken early, can prevent further deterioration (Zheng et al, 2014).*

▲ When ordered, initiate a fluid challenge of crystalloids (e.g., 0.9% normal saline or lactated Ringer's) for replacement of intravascular volume; monitor the client's response to prescribed fluid therapy and fluid challenge, especially noting vital signs, urine output, blood lactate concentrations, and lung sounds. *A fluid challenge can help the client with deficient fluid volume regain intravascular volume quickly, but the client must be carefully observed to ensure that he or she does not go into fluid volume overload in that excess fluid volume can lead to organ edema and increased mortality (Peng & Kellum, 2013; Wang et al, 2014).*

• Position the client flat with legs elevated when hypotensive, if not contraindicated. *This position enhances venous return, thus contributing to the maintenance of cardiac output with an increased blood pressure (Singh et al, 2011).*

▲ Monitor trends in serum lactic acid levels and base deficit obtained from blood gases as ordered. *A trend of increasing lactic acid levels and increasing base deficit can help identify hypoperfusion, which results in decreased survival and increased incidence of organ dysfunction (Richards & Wilcox, 2014).*

▲ Consult provider if signs and symptoms of deficient fluid volume persist or worsen. *Prolonged deficient fluid volume increases the risk for development of complications, including decrease in cognitive function, weakness, tachycardia, hemodynamic instability, and kidney injury (Popkin et al, 2010).*

Pediatric

• Monitor the child for signs of deficient fluid volume, including sunken eyes, decreased tears, dry mucous membranes, poor skin turgor, and decreased urine output (Graves, 2013). **EB:** *These assessment factors are more significant in identifying dehydration, but a combination of physical examination findings is a much better predictor than individual signs (Falszewska et al, 2014).*

▲ Reinforce the health care provider recommendation for the parents to give the child oral rehydration fluids to drink in the amounts specified, especially during the first 4 to 6 hours to replace fluid losses. Consider using diluted oral rehydration fluids. Once the child is rehydrated, an orally administered maintenance solution should be used along with food. **EB:** *A study demonstrated that treatment with oral rehydration fluids for children was generally as effective as IV fluids, and IV fluids did not shorten the duration of gastroenteritis and are more likely to cause adverse effects than oral rehydration therapy (Ciccarelli et al, 2013).* **EB:** *Many studies have shown that diluted oral replacement fluids and some drugs resulted in reductions in stool output, decreased vomiting, and less need for IV hydration (Ciccarelli et al, 2013).*

• Recommend that the mother resume breastfeeding as soon as possible.

• Recommend that parents not give the child decarbonated soda, fruit juices, gelatin dessert, or instant fruit drink mix. Instead give the child oral rehydration fluids ordered and, when tolerated, food. *Antiemetic, antidiarrheal agents, and probiotics have been shown to reduce the duration and severity of infectious diarrhea (Ciccarelli et al, 2013).*

- Once the child has been rehydrated, begin feeding regular food, but avoid milk products *(Guandalini et al, 2014). When a child has diarrhea, dietary modification includes avoiding dairy products, because viral or bacterial infections can cause a transient lactase deficiency (Bolen, 2012).*

Geriatric

- Monitor older clients for deficient fluid volume carefully, noting new onset of headache, weakness, dizziness, and postural hypotension. EB: *Older adults have a decrease in thirst and drink less compared to younger persons (Hooper et al, 2013).*
- *Implement fall precautions for clients experiencing weakness, dizziness, and/or postural hypotension.*
- Evaluate the risk for dehydration using the Dehydration Risk Appraisal Checklist. CEB: *A study demonstrated that the checklist has potential to predict the onset of dehydration in nursing home clients (Mentes & Wang, 2011).*
- Check skin turgor of older clients on the forehead and axilla; check for dry mucous membranes and sunken eyes. *Older people commonly have decreased skin turgor from normal age-related loss of elasticity; therefore checking skin turgor on the arm is not reflective of fluid volume. The presence of longitudinal furrows or dry mucous membrane, tachycardia, and orthostatic hypotension are good indication of dehydration in older adults (Hooper et al, 2013).*
- Encourage fluid intake by offering fluids regularly to cognitively impaired clients. CEB: *A study in women demonstrated that fluid restriction resulted in impaired alertness, increased sleepiness, fatigue, and confusion (Pross et al, 2013).*
- Incorporate regular hydration into daily routines (e.g., extra glass of fluid with medication or social activities) (Hooper et al, 2013).
- Because they have low water reserves, older adults should be encouraged to drink regularly even when not thirsty. Frequent and varied beverage offerings should be made available by hydration assistants to routinely offer increased beverages to clients in extended care. EB: *Strategies to improve fluid intake include making healthy drinks and water easily available and accessible at all times and reminding and encouraging older adults to consume these fluids. Older people should not be encouraged to consume large amounts of fluids at once but rather small amounts throughout the day (Hooper et al, 2013).*
- Flag the food tray of clients with chronic dehydration to indicate if the client is identified as having chronic dehydration and indicate that they should finish 75% to 100% of their food and fluids. Offering beverages in brightly colored cups may improve fluid intake. *Older clients often have a combination of both malnutrition and fluid deficit, and may not have good taste sensation (Hooper et al, 2013).*
- Recognize that lower blood pressures and a higher BUN/creatinine ratio can be significant signs of dehydration in older adults. *Structural changes of the kidney include alterations of renal blood flow of up to 50% from age 20 to 80. As people age, the kidney undergoes age-related changes, which translate in an inexorable and progressive decline in renal function.*
- *In the United States, renal dysfunction has a 15% prevalence in persons older than 70 years (Bolignano et al, 2014).*
- Note the color of urine and compare against a urine color chart to monitor adequate fluid intake. CEB: *A research study on older veterans demonstrated that urine color correlated significantly with urine osmolality, serum sodium, and BUN/creatinine ratio (Jequier & Constant, 2010).*
- Monitor older clients for excess fluid volume during the treatment of deficient fluid volume: auscultate lung sounds, assess for edema, and note vital signs. *The older client has a decreased ability to adapt to rapid increases in intravascular volume and can quickly develop fluid overload.*

Home Care

- Teach family members how to monitor output in the home (e.g., use of commode "hat" in the toilet, urinal, or bedpan, or use of catheter and closed drainage system). Instruct them to monitor both intake and output. Use common terms such as "cups" or "glasses of water a day" when providing education.
- When weighing the client, use same scale each day. Be sure scale is on a flat, not cushioned, surface. Do not weigh the client with scale placed on any type of rug.
- Teach family about complications of deficient fluid volume and when to call the health care provider.
- Teach the family the signs of hypovolemia, especially in older adults, and how to monitor for dizziness or unsteady gait.
- If the client is receiving IV fluids, there must be a responsible caregiver in the home. Teach caregiver about administration of fluids, complications of IV administration (e.g., fluid volume overload, speed of

medication reactions), and when to call for assistance. Assist caregiver with administration for as long as necessary to maintain client safety. *Administration of IV fluids in the home is a high-technology procedure and requires sufficient professional support to ensure safety of the client.*

- Identify an emergency plan, including when to call 911. *Some complications of deficient fluid volume cannot be reversed in the home and are life-threatening. Clients progressing toward hypovolemic shock will need emergency care.*
- Deficient fluid volume may be a symptom of impending death in terminally ill clients. In palliative care situations, treatment of deficient fluid volume should be determined based on client/family goals. Information and support should be provided to assist the client/family in this decision. Support the family/client in a palliative care situation to decide if it is appropriate to intervene for deficient fluid volume or to allow the client to die without fluids. *Deficient fluid volume may be a symptom of impending death in terminally ill clients. There is no defined gold standard for hydrating dying clients, and hydration and nutrition are considered basic acts for care of a dying client (Ong et al, 2012).*

Client/Family Teaching and Discharge Planning

- Instruct the client to avoid rapid position changes, especially from supine to sitting or standing.
- Teach the client and family about appropriate diet and fluid intake.
- Teach the client and family how to measure and record intake and output accurately.
- Teach the client and family about measures instituted to treat hypovolemia and to prevent or treat fluid volume loss.
- Instruct the client and family about signs of deficient fluid volume that indicate they should contact health care provider.

REFERENCES

Bolen, B. B. (2012). *What not to eat with diarrhea.* Retrieved from: <http://ibs.about.com/od/ibsfood/qt/EatforDiarrhea.htm>. Retrieved June 17 2014.

Bolignano, D., Mattace-Raso, F., Sijbrands, E. J., et al. (2014). The aging kidney revisited: a systematic review. *Ageing Research Reviews*, 65–80.

Cherniack, E. P. (2012). Ergogenic dietary aids for the elderly. *Nutrition (Burbank, Los Angeles County, Calif.)*, *28*(3), 225–229.

Ciccarelli, S., Stolfi, I., & Caramia, G. (2013). Management strategies in the treatment of neonatal and pediatric gastroenteritis. *Infection and Drug Resistance*, (6), 133–161.

Deshpande, A., Lever, D. S., & Soffer, E. (2013). *Acute diarrhea.* Cleveland Clinic Continuing Education. Retrieved from <http://www.clevelandclinicmeded.com/medicalpubs/diseasemanagement/gastroenterology/acute-diarrhea/>. Accessed December, 6, 2014.

Falszewska, A., Dziechciarz, P., & Szajewska, H. (2014). The diagnostic accuracy of clinical dehydration scale in identifying children with acute gastroenteritis: a systematic review. *Clinical Pediatrics*, *53*(12), 1181–1188.

Ftouh, S., & Lewington, A. (2014). Prevention, detection and management of acute kidney injury: concise guidelines. *Clinical Medicine (London, England)*, *14*(1), 61–65.

Graves, N. S. (2013). Acute gastroenteritis. *Primary Care*, *40*(3), 727–741.

Guandalini, S., Frye, R. E., Tamer, M. A., et al. (2014). *Diarrhea.* Medscape Reference. From: <http://emedicine.medscape.com/article/928598-overview>. Retrieved December, 6, 2014.

Hooper, L., Bunn, D., Jimoh, F. O., et al. (2013). Water loss dehydration and aging. *Mechanisms of Ageing and Development*, S0047-6374(13)00128-0.

Jequier, E., & Constant, F. (2010). Water as an essential nutrient: the physiological basis of hydration. *European Journal of Clinical Nutrition*, *64*, 115–123.

Lanier, J. B., Mote, M. B., & Clay, E. C. (2011). Evaluation and management of orthostatic hypotension. *American Family Physician*, *84*(5), 527–536.

Marik, P. E., Monnet, X., & Teboul, J.-L. (2011). Hemodynamic parameters to guide fluid therapy. *Annals of Intensive Care*, *1*, 1.

Macedo, E., Malhotra, R., Bouchard, J., et al. (2011). Oliguria is an early predictor of higher mortality in critically ill patients. *Kidney International*, *80*(7), 760–767.

Mentes, J., & Wang, J. (2011). Measuring risk for dehydration in nursing home residents: evaluation of the dehydration risk appraisal checklist. *Research in Gerontological Nursing*, *4(2), 148–156.*

Ong, Y. W., Yee, C. M., & Lee, A. (2012). Ethical dilemmas in the care of cancer patients near the end of life. *Singapore Medical Journal*, *53*(1), 11–16.

Peng, Z. Y., & Kellum, J. A. (2013). Perioperative fluids: a clear road ahead? *Current Opinion in Critical Care*, *19*(4), 353–358.

Perrier, E., Vergne, S., Klein, A., et al. (2013). Hydration biomarkers in free-living adults with different levels of habitual fluid consumption. *The British Journal of Nutrition*, *109*(9), 1678–1687.

Popkin, B. M., D'Anci, K. E., & Rosenberg, I. H. (2010). Water, hydration, and health. *Nutrition Reviews*, *68*(8), 439–458.

Pross, N., Demazieres, A., Girard, N., et al. (2013). Influence of progressive fluid restriction on mood and physiological markers of dehydration in women. *The British Journal of Nutrition*, *109*(2), 313–321.

Prowle, J. R., Liu, Y. L., Licari, E., et al. (2011). Oliguria as a predictive biomarker of acute kidney injury in critically ill patients. *Critical Care (London, England)*, *15*(4), R 172.

Ratanarat, R., Skulratanasak, P., Tangkawattanakul, N., et al. (2013). Clinical accuracy of RIFLE and acute kidney injury network (AKIN) criteria for predicting hospital mortality in critically ill patients with multiorgan dysfunction syndrome. *Journal of the Medical Association of Thailand*, *96*(Suppl. 2), S224–S231.

Richards, J. B., & Wilcox, S. R. (2014). Diagnosis and management of shock in the emergency department. *Emergency Medicine Practice*, *16*(3), 1–22.

Shimizu, M., Kinoshita, K., Hattori, K., et al. (2012). Physical signs of dehydration in the elderly. *Internal Medicine (Tokyo, Japan)*, *51*(10), 1207–1210.

Singh, S., Kuschner, W. G., & Lighthall, G. (2011). Perioperative intravascular fluid assessment and monitoring: a narrative review of established and emerging techniques. *Anesthesiology Research and Practice*, *2011*, 231493.

Suh, J. S., Hahn, W. H., & Cho, B. S. (2010). Recent advances of oral rehydration therapy. *Electrolyte Blood Press*, *8*(2), 82–86.

Wagner, K. D., & Hardin-Pierce, M. G. (2014). *High Acuity Nursing* (6th ed.). Boston, MA: Prentice Hall, Inc.

Wang, C. H., Hsieh, W. H., Chou, H. C., et al. (2014). Liberal versus restricted fluid resuscitation strategies in trauma patients: a systematic review and meta-analysis of randomized controlled trials and observational studies. *Critical Care Medicine*, *42*(4), 954–961.

Zheng, Z., Xu, X., & Deng, H. (2014). Urine output on ICU entry is associated with hospital mortality in unselected critically ill patients. *Journal of Nephrology*, *27*(1), 65–71.

Excess Fluid volume *Susan M. Dirkes, RN, MS, CCRN*

NANDA-I

Definition

Increased isotonic fluid retention

Defining Characteristics

Adventitious breath sounds; alteration in blood pressure; alteration in mental status; alteration in pulmonary artery pressure (PAP); alteration in respiratory pattern; alteration in urine specific gravity; anasarca; anxiety; azotemia; decrease in hematocrit; decrease in hemoglobin; dyspnea; edema; electrolyte imbalance; hepatomegaly; increased central venous pressure (CVP); intake exceeds output; jugular vein distention; oliguria; orthopnea; paroxysmal nocturnal dyspnea; pleural effusion; positive hepatojugular reflex; pulmonary congestion; restlessness; presence of S3 heart sound; weight gain over short period of time

Related Factors

Compromised regulatory mechanism; excessive fluid intake; excessive sodium intake

NOC (Nursing Outcomes Classification)

Suggested NOC Outcomes

Electrolyte and Acid-Base Balance; Fluid Balance; Fluid Overload Severity; Hydration

Example NOC Outcome with Indicators

Fluid Balance as evidenced by the following indicators: Peripheral edema/Neck vein distention/Adventitious breath sounds/Body weight increase. (Rate each indicator of **Fluid Balance:** 1 = severe, 2 = substantial, 3 = moderate, 4 = mild, 5 = none [see Section I].)

Client Outcomes

Client Will (Specify Time Frame)

- Remain free of edema, effusion, anasarca
- Maintain body weight appropriate for the client
- Maintain clear lung sounds; no evidence of dyspnea or orthopnea
- Remain free of jugular vein distention, positive hepatojugular reflex, and S3 heart sound
- Maintain normal CVP, PAP, cardiac output, and vital signs
- Maintain urine output of 0.5 mL/kg/hr or more with normal urine osmolality and specific gravity
- Explain actions that are needed to treat or prevent excess fluid volume including fluid and dietary restrictions, and medications
- Describe symptoms that indicate the need to consult with health care provider

NIC (Nursing Interventions Classification)

Suggested NIC Interventions

Fluid Management; Fluid Monitoring

Example NIC Activities—Fluid Monitoring

Monitor weight; Monitor intake and output

F

Nursing Interventions and *Rationales*

- Monitor location and extent of edema using the 1+ to 4+ scale to quantify edema; also measure the legs using a millimeter tape in the same area at the same time each day. Note differences in measurement between extremities. EBN: *Causes of peripheral edema in clients with heart failure are related to medications, compensatory changes that influence hydrostatic pressure, and fluid retention, among other things (Cooper, 2011).*
- Monitor daily weight for sudden increases; use same scale and type of clothing at same time each day, preferably before breakfast. *Body weight changes reflect changes in body fluid volume.* EB: *Body weight is commonly used to monitor for fluid overload (Wagner & Hardin-Pierce, 2014).*
- Monitor intake and output; note trends reflecting decreasing urine output in relation to fluid intake. EB: *Accurately measuring intake and output is important for the client with fluid volume overload (Macedo et al, 2011). The volume of all fluids should be measured. If the family is measuring, instruct them on common conversions between household measurements and metric.*
- Monitor vital signs; note decreasing blood pressure, tachycardia, and tachypnea. Monitor for S3 heart sounds. If signs of heart failure are present, see the care plan for Decreased **Cardiac** output. *Heart failure results in dyspnea, edema, orthopnea, and elevated CVP. The secondary characteristics are weight gain, hepatomegaly, jugular vein distention, palpitations, crackles, oliguria, coughing, clammy skin, and skin color changes (Wagner & Hardin-Pierce, 2014).*
- Auscultate lung sounds for crackles, monitor respiration effort, and determine the presence and severity of orthopnea. *Acute pulmonary edema may be due either to increased permeability of the alveolar capillary barrier, in the case of acute lung injury, or to increased pulmonary microvascular hydrostatic pressure, in the case of cardiogenic pulmonary edema (Wagner & Hardin-Pierce, 2014).*
- Monitor serum and urine osmolality, serum sodium, blood urea nitrogen (BUN)/creatinine ratio, and hematocrit for abnormalities. EB: *In a client with fluid overload, an increase in urine volume and dilution will usually be observed (Macedo et al, 2011). BUN and creatinine are monitored currently, but they lack sensitivity, and an overall assessment of client fluid status is critical before fluid is administered (Shiffl & Lang, 2012).*
- With head of bed elevated 30 to 45 degrees, monitor jugular veins for distention with the client in the upright position; assess for positive hepatojugular reflex. *Increased intravascular volume results in jugular vein distention, edema, crackles, and S3 heart sound (Peacock & Soto, 2010).*
- Monitor the client's behavior for restlessness, anxiety, or confusion; use safety precautions if symptoms are present. *When excess fluid volume compromises cardiac output, the client may experience cerebral tissue hypoxia and demonstrate restlessness and anxiety. When the excess fluid volume results in hyponatremia, there is a shift of water into the cells, resulting in symptoms ranging from nausea, malaise, and abdominal cramping to confusion, seizure, and coma (Ronco et al, 2012).*

▲ Monitor for the development of conditions that increase the client's risk for excess fluid volume, including heart failure, kidney failure, and liver failure, all of which result in decreased glomerular filtration rate and fluid retention. EB: *Other causes are increased intake of oral or intravenous (IV) fluids in excess of the client's cardiac and renal reserve levels, and increased levels of antidiuretic hormone (Ronco et al, 2012). Many clients with fluid overload have acute kidney injury, and fluid balance is an important indicator of outcomes. Studies show increased morbidity and mortality in clients with fluid overload (Ricci & Ronco, 2013).*

▲ Provide a restricted-sodium diet as appropriate if ordered. *Restricting the sodium in the diet will favor the renal excretion of excess fluid. Take care to avoid hyponatremia, which can cause serious complications including nausea, seizures, coma, and death (Kornusky & Pravikoff, 2011; Rudge & Kimm, 2014).*

- ▲ Monitor serum albumin level and provide protein intake as appropriate. *When plasma proteins, especially albumin, no longer sustain sufficient colloid osmotic pressure to counterbalance hydrostatic pressure, edema develops (Wagner & Hardin-Pierce, 2014).*
- ▲ Administer prescribed diuretics as appropriate; ensure adequate blood pressure before administration. If diuretic is administered intravenously, note and record the blood pressure and urine output following the dose. EB: *Clinical practice guidelines on heart failure state that monitoring input and output is useful for monitoring effects of diuretic therapy (Wagner & Hardin-Pierce, 2014).*
- • Monitor for side effects of diuretic therapy: orthostatic hypotension (especially if the client is also receiving angiotensin-converting enzyme [ACE] inhibitors), hypovolemia, and electrolyte imbalances (hypokalemia and hyponatremia). *Observe for hyperkalemia in clients receiving a potassium-sparing diuretic and in those on beta-blockers and ACE inhibitors (Wagner & Hardin-Pierce, 2014; Rudge & Kimm, 2014).*
- ▲ Implement fluid restriction as ordered, especially when serum sodium is low; include all routes of intake. Schedule limited intake of fluids around the clock, and include the type of fluids preferred by the client. *Fluid restriction may decrease intravascular volume and myocardial workload. Overzealous fluid restriction should not be used because hypovolemia can worsen heart failure. Client involvement in planning will enhance participation in the necessary fluid restriction.*
- • Maintain the rate of all IV infusions, carefully using an IV pump. *This is done to prevent inadvertent exacerbation of excess fluid volume.*
- • Turn clients with dependent edema at least every 2 hours. *Severe edema predisposes clients to skin breakdown and pressure ulcers (Cooper, 2011).*
- ▲ Provide ordered care for edematous extremities including compression, elevation, and muscle exercises. EB: *Treatments for clients with peripheral edema include the use of sequential compression devices, elevation of the extremities above heart level, and exercises that affect the calf muscle pump (i.e., pedal push exercises) and layered compression wraps (Cooper, 2011).*
- • Promote a positive body image and good self-esteem. *Visible edema may alter the client's body image.* Refer to the care plan for Disturbed **Body Image.**
- ▲ Consult with the health care provider if signs and symptoms of excess fluid volume persist or worsen. *Pulmonary edema requires prompt treatment such as preload reducers, afterload reducers, and morphine to relieve anxiety (Mayo Foundation for Medical Education and Research, 2014).*

Critically Ill

- • Insert an indwelling urinary catheter if ordered and measure urine output hourly. Notify health care provider if output is less than 0.5 mL/kg/hr. *Urine output of less than 0.5 mL/kg/hr for 6 or more hours is defined as oliguria (Prowle et al, 2011).*
- ▲ Monitor CVP, mean arterial pressure, PAP, and cardiac output/index; note and report trends of increasing or decreasing pressures over time. *Alterations in these parameters may indicate the client is going into shock. Hemodynamic criteria for cardiogenic shock are sustained hypotension (systolic blood pressure less than 90 mm Hg for at least 30 minutes) and a reduced cardiac index (less than 2.2 L/min/m^2) in the presence of elevated pulmonary capillary occlusion pressure (greater than 15 mm Hg), pulmonary congestion, dyspnea, and hypoxemia (Wagner & Hardin-Pierce, 2014).*
- ▲ Monitor the effects of infusion of diuretic drips. Perform continuous renal replacement therapy (CRRT) as ordered if the client is critically ill and hemodynamically unstable and excessive fluid must be removed. EBN: *CRRT is indicated for hypervolemia, metabolic acidosis, and hyperkalemia (Dirkes, 2014).*

Geriatric

- • Recognize that the presence of fluid volume excess is particularly serious in older adults. EB: *The kidney undergoes age-related changes that include structural and functional changes, which may increase the incidence of acute kidney injury (Bolignano et al, 2014).*
- • Monitor electrolyte levels carefully, including sodium levels and potassium levels, with both increased and decreased levels possible. *Older adults are prone to electrolyte abnormalities due to aging, decreased muscle mass, and decreased total body water (Hooper et al, 2013), plus the large number of medications that are taken that can affect electrolyte levels. Many older clients receive selective serotonin reuptake inhibitors for treatment of depression, which can result in hyponatremia (Mannesse et al, 2013).* Refer to the care plan for risk for **Electrolyte** imbalance.

Home Care

- • Assess client and family knowledge of disease process causing excess fluid volume.
- ▲ Teach about disease process and complications of excess fluid volume, including when to contact the health care provider.
- • Assess client and family knowledge and compliance with medical regimen, including medications, diet, rest, and exercise. Assist family with integrating restrictions into daily living. *Assistance with integration of cultural values, especially those related to foods, with medical regimen promotes compliance and decreased risk of complications.*
- ▲ Teach and reinforce knowledge of medications. Instruct the client not to use over-the-counter (OTC) medications (e.g., diet medications) without first consulting the provider.
- ▲ Instruct the client to make the primary health care provider aware of medications ordered by other health care providers.
- • Identify emergency plan for rapidly developing or critical levels of excess fluid volume when diuresing is not safe at home. *Excess fluid volume can be life threatening.*
- ▲ Teach about signs and symptoms of both excess and deficient fluid volume, such as darker urine and when to call the health care provider. *Urine color may be a simple indicator of hydration (Perrier et al, 2013).*

Client/Family Teaching and Discharge Planning

- • Describe signs and symptoms of excess fluid volume and actions to take if they occur.
- ▲ Teach client on diuretics to weigh self daily in the morning and to notify the health care provider if there is a 2.2 pound (1 kg) or more weight gain (Wagner & Hardin-Pierce, 2014). EB: *Clinical practice guidelines on heart failure suggest that daily weight monitoring leads to early recognition of excess fluid retention, which, when reported, can be offset with additional medication to avoid hospitalization due to heart failure decompensation (Wagner & Hardin-Pierce, 2014).*
- ▲ Teach the importance of fluid and sodium restrictions. Help the client and family devise a schedule for intake of fluids throughout the entire day. Refer to a dietitian concerning implementation of a low-sodium diet.
- • Teach clients how to measure and document intake and output with common household measurements, such as cups.
- ▲ Teach how to take diuretics correctly: take one dose in the morning and second dose (if taken) no later than 4 PM. Adjust potassium intake as appropriate for potassium-losing or potassium-sparing diuretics. Note the appearance of side effects such as weakness, muscle cramps, hypertension, palpitations, or irregular heartbeat (Wagner & Hardin-Pierce, 2014).
- • For the client undergoing hemodialysis, teach client the required restrictions in dietary electrolytes, protein, and fluid. Spend time with the client to detect any factors that may interfere with the client's compliance with the fluid restriction or restrictive diet. EBN: *Recent research has shown an association between albumin level (an important marker of nutritional status and possible inflammation) and psychosocial factors. Also, lower levels of family support were associated with higher risk of nonadherence to medical care (Untas et al, 2011).*

REFERENCES

Bolignano, D., Mattace-Raso, F., Sijbrands, E. J., et al. (2014). The aging kidney revisited: a systematic review. *Ageing Research Reviews*, 65–80.

Cooper, K. L. (2011). Care of lower extremities in patients with acute decompensated heart failure. *Critical Care Nurse*, *31*(4), 21–29.

Dirkes, S. (2014). Continuous renal replacement therapy: dialysis for critically ill patients. *American Nurse Today*, 9(5).

Hooper, L., Bunn, D., Jimoh, F. O., et al. (2013). Water loss dehydration and aging. *Mechanisms of Ageing and Development*, S0047-6374(13)00128-0.

Kornusky, J., & Pravikoff, D. (2011). Hyponatremia. *CINAHL Nursing Guide*.

Macedo, E., Malhotra, R., Claure-Del Granado, R., et al. (2011). Defining urine output criterion for acute kidney injury in critically ill patients. *Nephrology, Dialysis, Transplantation*, *26*(2), 509–515.

Mannesse, C. K., Jansen, P. A., Van Marum, R. J., et al. (2013). Characteristics, prevalence, risk factors, and underlying mechanism of hyponatremia in elderly patients treated with antidepressants: a cross-sectional study. *Maturitas*, *76*(4), 357–363.

Mayo Foundation for Medical Education and Research (MFMER). *Diseases and Conditions: Pulmonary Edema July, 2014*. From: <http://www.mayoclinic.com/health/pulmonary-edema/DS00412/DSECTION=symptoms>. Retrieved December 7, 2014.

Perrier, E., Vergne, S., Klein, A., et al. (2013). Hydration biomarkers in free-living adults with different levels of habitual fluid consumption. *The British Journal of Nutrition*, *109*(9), 1678–1687.

Peacock, W. F., & Soto, K. M. (2010). Current techniques of fluid status assessment. In C. Ronco, et al. (Eds.), *Fluid overload: diagnosis and management. Contribution nephrology*. Basel: Karger.

Prowle, J. R., Liu, Y. L., Licari, E., et al. (2011). Oliguria as predictive biomarker of acute kidney injury in critically ill patients. *Critical Care (London, England), 15*(4), R 172–R 2011.

Ricci, Z., & Ronco, C. (2013). The year in review 2012: critical care-nephrology. *Critical Care (London, England), 17*(6), 246.

Ronco, C., Kaushik, M., Valle, R., et al. (2012). Diagnosis and management of fluid overload in heart failure and cardio-renal syndrome: the 5B approach. *Seminars in Nephrology, 32*(1), 129–141.

Rudge, J. E., & Kim, D. (2014). New-onset hyponatremia after surgery for traumatic hip fracture. *Age and Ageing, 43*(6), 821–826.

Shiffl, H., & Lang, S. M. (2012). Update on biomarkers of acute kidney injury: moving closer to clinical impact? *Molecular Diagnosis and Therapy, 16*(4), 199–207.

Untas, A., Thumma, J., Rascle, N., et al. (2011). The associations of social support and other psychosocial factors with mortality and quality of life in the dialysis outcomes and practice patterns study. *American Society of Nephrology, 6*(1), 142–152.

Wagner, K. D., & Hardin-Pierce, M. G. (2014). *High Acuity Nursing* (6th ed.). Boston, MA: Prentice Hall, Inc.

Risk for Deficient Fluid volume

Betty J. Ackley, MSN, EdS, RN, and Mary Beth Flynn Makic, PhD, RN, CNS, CCNS, FAAN

NANDA-I

Definition

Vulnerable to experiencing decreased intravascular, interstitial, and/or intracellular fluid volumes, which may compromise health

Risk Factors

Active fluid volume loss; barrier to accessing fluid; compromised regulatory mechanism; deviations affecting fluid absorption; deviations affecting fluid intake; excessive fluid loss through normal route; extremes of age; extremes of weight; factors influencing fluid needs; fluid loss through abnormal route; insufficient knowledge about fluid needs; pharmaceutical agent

NIC, NOC, Client Outcomes, Nursing Interventions, Client/Family Teaching, *Rationales*, and References

Refer to care plan for Deficient **Fluid** volume.

Risk for imbalanced Fluid volume

Mary Beth Flynn Makic, PhD, RN, CNS, CCNS, FAAN, and Betty J. Ackley, MSN, EdS, RN

NANDA-I

Definition

Vulnerable to a decrease, increase, or rapid shift from one to the other of intravascular, interstitial, and/or intracellular fluid, which may compromise health; this refers to body fluid loss, gain, or both

Risk Factors

Apheresis; ascites; burns; intestinal obstruction; pancreatitis; sepsis; trauma; treatment regimen

NOC (Nursing Outcomes Classification)

Suggested NOC Outcomes

Fluid Balance; Electrolyte and Acid-Base Balance; Hydration

Example NOC Outcome with Indicators

Maintains **Fluid Balance** as evidenced by the following indicators: BP/Peripheral pulses palpable/Skin turgor/Moist mucous membranes/Serum electrolytes/Hematocrit/Body weight stable/24-hour intake and output balanced/Urine specific gravity. (Rate each indicator of **Fluid Balance:** 1 = severely compromised, 2 = substantially compromised, 3 = moderately compromised, 4 = mildly compromised, 5 = not compromised [see Section I].)

Client Outcomes

- Lung sounds clear, respiratory rate 12 to 20 and free of dyspnea
- Urine output greater than 0.5 mL/kg/hr
- Blood pressure, pulse rate, temperature, and oxygen saturation within expected range
- Laboratory values within expected range, that is, normal serum sodium, hematocrit, and osmolarity
- Extremities and dependent areas free of edema
- Mental orientation appropriate based on previous condition

NIC (Nursing Interventions Classification)

F

Suggested NIC Interventions

Autotransfusion; Bleeding Precautions; Bleeding Reduction: Wound; Electrolyte Management; Fluid Management; Fluid Monitoring; Hemodynamic Regulation; Hypervolemia Management; Hypovolemia Management; Intravenous Therapy; Invasive Hemodynamic Monitoring; Shock Management: Volume; Vital Signs Monitoring

Example NIC Activities—Fluid Management

Maintain accurate intake and output record; Monitor vital signs

Nursing Interventions and *Rationales*

Surgical Clients

- Monitor the fluid balance. If there are symptoms of hypovolemia, refer to the interventions in the care plan for Deficient **Fluid** volume. If there are symptoms of hypervolemia, refer to the interventions in the care plan for Excess **Fluid** volume.

Preoperative

- Collect a thorough history and perform a preoperative assessment to identify clients with increased risk for hemorrhage or hypovolemia, that is, clients with recent traumatic injury, abnormal bleeding or altered clotting times, complicated kidney or liver disease, diabetes, cardiovascular disease, major organ transplant, history of aspirin and/or NSAID use, anticoagulant therapy, or history of hemophilia, von Willebrand's disease, or disseminated intravascular coagulation. Assess the client's use of over-the-counter agents to include herbal products. CEB: *Assessment of the client's use of herbal products is important as some herbs act as anticoagulants and could cause increased blood loss, and some herbs have diuretic or laxative effects (Young et al, 2009; Flanagan, 2001).*
- Recognize that NPO at midnight may or may not be appropriate for each surgical client. Guidelines from the American Society of Anesthesiologists (ASA) in 2011 recommend the following: healthy clients having elective surgery should be allowed to have clear liquids up to 2 hours before surgery. *Research has shown the value of allowing healthy clients to consume clear liquids up to 2 hours before surgery; practice is not consistent (Crenshaw, 2011). Many clients are unnecessarily dehydrated from lack of fluid for an extended period, which can complicate postoperative recovery. It is important to provide clear communication to the client that only clear liquids can be safely consumed up to 2 hours before surgery (Allison & George, 2014).*
- Determine length of time the client has been without normal intake, been NPO, or experienced fluid loss (e.g., vomiting, diarrhea, bleeding). *The length of time and severity of the above factors, along with the presence of a fluid deficit, allow the health care provider to determine a general estimate of preoperative fluid loss, which can affect intraoperative fluid management. However, laboratory testing of hemoglobin, hematocrit, blood urea nitrogen (BUN), and creatinine should be used to corroborate the assessment (Allison & George, 2014).*
- Assess and document the client's mental status. *A baseline assessment is important so that changes in mental status during the postoperative period can be easily identified.*
- Recognize that there is conflicting evidence regarding liberal intraoperative fluid management versus restrictive fluid management. Fluid administration during surgery is more restrictive to prevent pulmonary complications associated with excessive fluid administration (Assaad et al, 2013). CEB: *Using a restrictive approach to intraoperative fluid management resulted in less postoperative pulmonary*

complications, fewer wound healing complications, and decreased length of time for bowel function to resume, than the use of a more liberal fluid regimen (Young et al, 2009). Studies involving clients having bowel resections showed that those clients who had restricted fluids developed hemodynamic instability, and it was concluded that a liberal approach might have improved both cardiopulmonary and renal function in these clients (Bamboat & Bordeianou, 2009). To reduce fluid administration volume, colloids rather than crystalloid fluids may be administered during surgery (Cortes et al, 2015).

- Recognize that an individualized fluid management plan would be developed incorporating client specific assessment parameters (e.g., existing comorbid diseases, age) and type of surgical procedure (Allison & George, 2014). EB: *Perioperative hemodynamic and fluid management that is goal directed improved both short- and long-term outcomes and can easily be achieved (Cannesson, 2011; Cecconi et al, 2015).*
- Recognize the effects of general anesthetics, inhalational agents, and of regional anesthesia on perfusion in the body and decreasing the blood pressure. CEB: *None of these types of anesthesia alone affect circulating blood volume, but anesthetics can cause a drop in blood pressure that is often treated with a fluid bolus, which is especially important in critically ill clients who have poor cardiopulmonary reserves (Bamboat & Bordeianou, 2009).*
- Monitor for signs of intraoperative hypovolemia: dry skin, dry mucous membranes, tachycardia, decreased urinary output, decreased central venous pressure, hypotension, increased pulse, and/or deep rapid respirations.
- Monitor for signs of intraoperative hypervolemia: dyspnea, coarse crackles, increased pulse and respirations, decreased oxygenation, and decreased urinary output, all of which could progress to pulmonary edema.
- In the critically ill surgical client a pulmonary artery catheter or other minimally invasive cardiac output monitoring device may be used to determine fluid balance and guide fluid and vasoactive intravenous (IV) drip administration. EB: *Monitoring devices that directly (pulmonary artery catheter) or indirectly (minimally or noninvasively) assess the client's cardiac output and fluid volume status may be used to "optimize" cardiac function by allowing better fluid regimens. Fluids must be individually titrated based on each client's changes in monitored variables (Cannesson, 2011; Zang et al, 2011; Cecconi et al, 2015).*
- Monitor the client for hyponatremia, that is, headache, anorexia, nausea and vomiting, diarrhea, tachycardia, general malaise, muscle cramps, weakness, lethargy, change in mental status, disorientation, seizures, and death. *Many pathologies can predispose the client to hyponatremia, including adrenal insufficiency, brain tumor, cirrhosis, hypothyroidism, lung cancer, meningitis, renal disease, tuberculosis, use of complementary therapies, and head trauma (Allison & George, 2014).*
- Monitor clients undergoing laparoscopic or hysteroscopic procedures for the development of hyponatremia, hypervolemia, and pulmonary edema when an irrigation fluid is used. CEB: *Use of local or spinal anesthesia for these operations can cause the client to develop symptoms of hyponatremia and hypervolemia sooner than with other anesthetics (Young et al, 2009).*
- Monitor clients undergoing transurethral resection of the prostate (TURP) procedures for development of hyponatremia, and hypervolemia with symptoms of TURP syndrome: headache, visual changes, agitation, lethargy, vomiting, muscle twitching, bradycardia, diminished pupillary reflexes, hypertension, and respiratory distress. *Considerable fluid absorption occurs during TURP procedures and gynecological procedures, which can result in hyponatremia and/or hypervolemia (Young et al, 2009).*
- Measure the irrigation fluid used during urological and gynecological procedures accurately for volume deficit, that is, amount of irrigation used minus amount of irrigation recovered via suction. *Absorption of large amounts of fluid can cause complications for the client (Young et al, 2009).*
- Monitor intraoperative intake and output including blood loss, urine output, and third-space losses, to provide an estimate of fluid volume. EBN: *Weighing used sponges can provide an estimate of blood loss (Blanchard & Burlingam, 2012).* CEB: *Weighing fluid used and returned provides a more accurate measurement of fluid deficit than measuring the fluids (Young et al, 2009).*
- Observe the surgical client for hyperkalemia, that is, dysrhythmias, heart block, asystole, abdominal distention, and weakness. *Hyperkalemia can occur intraoperatively due to massive blood transfusions, tissue breakdown from surgery, shifting of potassium from the cells into the extracellular fluid, decreased potassium excretion due to renal failure or hypovolemia, crush injuries, or burns (Rothrock, 2010).*
- Maintain the client's core temperature at normal levels, using warming devices as needed. *Fluids administration during surgery can increase risk of hypothermia.* CEB: *Research has shown that perioperative hypothermia can adversely affect the cardiopulmonary system (Young et al, 2009).*

Postoperative

- Continue to support restrictive fluid management postoperatively. CEB: *Using restrictive fluid management postoperatively has been found to result in earlier gastric emptying and shorter length of time before passage of flatus and the first postoperative bowel movement than in those receiving standard fluid management (Bamboat & Bordeianou, 2009; Young et al, 2009).*
- Assess the client for development of tissue edema. CEB: *Clients developing tissue edema have been shown to develop poor wound healing, compromised pulmonary function, and delay in return of bowel function (Bamboat & Bordeianou, 2009; Young et al, 2009).*
- Recognize that IV fluid replacement decisions incorporate multiple assessment parameters: hourly urine output, blood pressure, heart rate, respiratory rate, lung sounds, output from drains, and changes in laboratory results (e.g., hemoglobin/hematocrit, serum electrolytes).

F

Geriatric

- Check skin turgor of older client on the forehead, subclavian area, or inner thigh; also look for the presence of longitudinal furrows on the tongue and dry mucous membranes. *Older people commonly have decreased skin turgor from normal age-related loss of elasticity; checking skin turgor on the arm is not reflective of fluid volume (El-Sharkawy et al, 2014).*
- Closely monitor urine output, concentration of urine, and serum BUN/creatinine results. EB: *Reduced renal perfusion and altered renal function as a normal or abnormal change in physiologic aging can compromise the client's fluid volume status (El-Sharkawy et al, 2014).*
- Monitor older clients for excess fluid volume during the treatment of deficient fluid volume: auscultate lung sounds, assess for edema, and trend vital signs.
- Assess the older client's cognitive status. EB: *Cognitive impairment is a risk factor associated with dehydration, especially in the older adult (El-Sharkawy et al, 2014).*

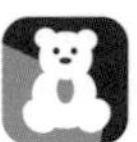

Pediatric

- Assess the pediatric client's weight, length of NPO status, underlying illness, and the surgical procedure to be performed.
- Recognize that newborns require very little fluid replacement when undergoing major surgical procedures during the first few days of life.
- Monitor pediatric surgical clients closely for signs of fluid loss.
- Administer fluids preoperatively until NPO status must be initiated so that fluid deficit is decreased.
- Perform an assessment for signs of fluid responsiveness in the pediatric client. EB: *A systematic review found that respiratory variation was the only assessment parameter to most reliably predict a pediatric client's responsiveness for fluid administration (Gan et al, 2013).* CEB: *Oral rehydration therapy, when possible, is the treatment of choice for children with mild to moderate dehydration (Barclay, 2009).*

REFERENCES

Allison, J., & George, M. (2014). Using preoperative assessment and patient instruction to improve patient safety. *Association of Operating Room Nurses*, *99*(3), 364–375.

American Society of Anesthesiologists. (2011). Practice guidelines for preoperative fasting and the use of pharmacologic agents to reduce the risk of pulmonary aspiration: application to healthy patients undergoing elective procedures: an updated report by the american society of anesthesiologists committee on standards and practice parameters. *Anesthesiology*, *114*(3), 495–511.

Assaad, S., Popescu, W., & Perrino, A. (2013). Fluid management in thoracic surgery. *Current Opinion in Anaesthesiology*, *26*, 31–39.

Blanchard, J., & Burlingam, B. (2012). Perioperative standards and recommended practices. *Association of Operating Room Nurses.*

Bamboat, Z. M., & Bordeianou, L. (2009). Perioperative fluid management. *Clinics in Colon and Rectal Surgery*, *22*, 28–33.

Barclay, L. (2009). *Strategies for diagnosing and treating dehydration in children*. From: <http://www.medscape.com/viewarticle/710684>. Retrieved August 15, 2011.

Cannesson, M. (2011). Guiding fluid management in the surgical setting: part 1 of a 2-part series. *Anesthesiol News.*

Cecconi, M., Garcia, M., Romero, M. G., et al. (2015). The use of pulse pressure variation and stroke volume variation in spontaneously breathing patients to assess dynamic arterial elastance and to predict arterial pressure response to fluid administration. *Anesthesia and Analgesia*, *210*, 76–84.

Crenshaw, J. T. (2011). Preoperative fasting: will the evidence ever be put into practice? *The American Journal of Nursing*, *111*(10), 38–43.

Cortes, D. O., Barros, T. G., Njimi, H., et al. (2015). Crystalloids versus colloids: exploring differences in fluid requirements by systematic review and meta-regression. *Anesthesia and Analgesia*, *120*, 398–401.

El-Sharkawy, A. M., Sahota, O., Maughan, R. J., et al. (2014). The pathophysiology of fluid and electrolyte balance in the older adult surgical patient. *Clinical Nutrition*, *33*, 6–13.

Flanagan, K. (2001). Preoperative assessment: safety considerations for patients taking herbal products. *Journal of Perianesthesia Nursing*, *16*(1), 19–26.

Gan, H., Cannesson, M., Chandler, J. R., et al. (2013). Predicting fluid responsiveness in children: a systematic review. *Anesthesia and Analgesia*, *117*, 1380–1392.

Rothrock, J. (2010). *Alexander's care of the patient in surgery* (14th ed.). St. Louis: Mosby.

Young, E., et al. (2009). Perioperative fluid management. *Association of Operating Room Nurses*, *89*(1), 167–178, quiz 179–182.

Zang, Z., Lu, B., Sheng, X., et al. (2011). Accuracy of stroke volume variation in predicting fluid responsiveness: a systematic review and meta-analysis. *Journal of Anesthesia*, *25*, 904–916.

Frail Elderly syndrome

Noelle L. Fields, PhD, LCSW

F

NANDA-I

Definition

Dynamic state of unstable equilibrium that affects the older individual experiencing deterioration in one or more domain of health (physical, functional, psychological, or social) and leads to increased susceptibility to adverse health effects, particularly disability

Risk Factors

Activity intolerance; bathing self-care deficit; decreased cardiac output; dressing self-care deficit; fatigue; feeding self-care deficit; hopelessness; imbalanced nutrition: less than body requirements; impaired memory; impaired physical mobility; impaired walking; social isolation; toileting self-care deficit

Related Factors

Alteration in cognitive functioning; chronic illness; history of falls; living alone; malnutrition; prolonged hospitalization; psychiatric disorder; sarcopenia; sarcopenic obesity; sedentary lifestyle

NOC Outcomes (Nursing Outcomes Classification)

Suggested NOC Outcomes

Physical Aging; Psychosocial Adjustment: Life Change; Client Satisfaction: Functional Assistance

Example NOC Outcomes with Indicators

Client Satisfaction: Functional Assistance as evidenced by the following indicators: Included in planning for optimal mobility and self-care/Encouraged to be as active as possible/Assistance with physical activity/Allowed to choose food for meals. (Rate the outcome and indicators of **Client Satisfaction: Functional Assistance:** 1 = not at all satisfied, 2 = somewhat satisfied, 3 = moderately satisfied, 4 = very satisfied, 5 = completely satisfied [see Section I].)

Client Outcomes

Client Will (Specify Time Frame)

- Remain living as independently as possible in the home or care setting of his or her choice
- Maintain safety when engaging in activities of daily living and ambulation
- Increase exercise and/or daily physical activity in order to build muscle strength
- Maintain a healthy weight

NIC Interventions (Nursing Interventions Classification)

Suggested NIC Interventions

Physical Exercise; Strength Training; Balance Training

Example NIC Activities—Frail Elderly Syndrome

Promote physical activities that build strength and improve balance and endurance

Nursing Interventions and *Rationales*

- Assess frailty with a tool such as the Edmonton Frail Scale. EB: *The Edmonton Frail Scale is a tool designed to identify frail older adults in clinical settings and requires less than 5 minutes to administer (Clegg & Young, 2011).*

- Recognize that balance and gait impairment are features of frailty and are risk factors for falls. EB: *Cadore et al (2013) did a systematic review of the literature and found that exercise interventions composed of strength, endurance, and balance training improve the rate of falls in frail older adults.*
- Monitor physical frailty indicators such as slow gait speed and low physical activity. EB: *Vermeulen et al (2011) did a systematic review and found that monitoring physical frailty indicators might be useful to identify older adults who could benefit from interventions aimed at preventing disability.*
- Assess falls using a falls risk assessment tool such as the Hendrich II Fall Risk Model. EBN: *Ivziku et al (2011) studied 179 older adult patients in a hospital setting and found that this falls risk assessment tool had predictive properties for patients at risk for fall in acute care settings.*
- Evaluate the client's medications to determine whether medications increase the risk of frailty; if appropriate, consult with the client's health care provider regarding the client's medications. EB: *Polypharmacy, or taking five or more medications, has been associated with frailty in older adults (Gnjidic et al, 2012).*

F

▲ Refer to a dietitian for an individualized therapeutic diet. EB: *Dietary supplements such as protein are needed to promote muscle mass gain during exercise training in frail older adults (Tieland et al, 2012).* EB: *Malafarina et al (2013) did a systematic review of the literature about nutritional supplements in older adults and found that nutritional supplements are effective in the treatment of muscle mass loss, particularly in conjunction with physical exercise.*

- Refer to care plan for Readiness for enhanced **Nutrition** for additional interventions.
- Monitor weight loss. EB: *Weight loss is considered a main component of frailty syndrome (Morley et al, 2013).* CEB: *Milne et al (2009) did a systematic literature review and found that when given to older adults, nutritional supplements containing protein and energy result in weight gain.*
- Encourage clients to engage in active lifestyles. CEB: *Peterson et al (2009) studied 2964 older adults for 5 years and found that sedentary older individuals had a greater likelihood of developing frailty than individuals who were engaged in exercise.*
- Provide an exercise-training program. EB: *Physical exercise training leads to improved cognitive functioning as well as psychological well-being in older adults who are frail (Langlois et al, 2013).* EB: *Theou et al (2011) did a systematic review and found that structured exercise programs performed three times per week for 30 to 35 minutes per session had a positive impact on frail older adults.*
- Promote the benefits of home-based exercise to older clients who are frail. EB: *Clegg et al (2014) conducted a study of 49 frail older adults and found evidence that the deterioration in mobility may be reduced through a 12-week home-based exercise intervention.* EB: *Clegg et al (2012) did a systematic review of the literature and found evidence that home-based exercise interventions may improve disability in older adults with moderate frailty.*
- Use a multidisciplinary and person-centered approach for supporting frail older adults. EBN: *The focus of caring for frail older adults should not only be on medical problems but also on providing supportive services to help individuals maintain their independence and manage their lives despite frailty (Ebrahimi et al, 2014).*
- Develop a trusting and responsive relationship with frail clients. EBN: *Bindels et al (2013) qualitatively interviewed nurses (N = 23) and found that building a trusting relationship, along with competence, responsiveness, and attentiveness were important for providing frail older adults with good care.*

Multicultural, Home Care, Client/Family Teaching

- The above interventions may be adapted for multicultural, home care, and client family teaching.

REFERENCES

Bindels, J., Cox, K., Widdershoven, G., et al. (2013). Care for community-dwelling frail older people: a practice nurse perspective. *Journal of Clinical Nursing*.

Cadore, E. L., Rodríguez-Mañas, L., Sinclair, A., et al. (2013). Effects of different exercise interventions on risk of falls, gait ability, and balance in physically frail older adults: a systematic review. *Rejuvenation Research*, *16*(2), 105–114.

Clegg, A. P., Barber, S. E., Young, J. B., et al. (2012). Do home-based exercise interventions improve outcomes for frail older people? Findings from a systematic review. *Reviews in Clinical Gerontology*, *22*(01), 68–78.

Clegg, A., Barber, S., Young, J., et al. (2014). The home-based older people's exercise (HOPE) trial: a pilot randomised controlled trial of a home-based exercise intervention for older people with frailty. *Age and Ageing*, afu033.

Clegg, A., & Young, J. (2011). The frailty syndrome. *Clinical Medicine, 11*(1), 72–75.
Ebrahimi, Z., Dahlin-Ivanoff, S., Eklund, K., et al. (2014). Self-rated health and health-strengthening factors in community-living frail older people. *Journal of Advanced Nursing*, 825–836.
Gnjidic, D., Hilmer, S. N., Blyth, F. M., et al. (2012). Polypharmacy cutoff and outcomes: five or more medicines were used to identify community-dwelling older men at risk of different adverse outcomes. *Journal of Clinical Epidemiology, 65*(9), 989–995.
Ivziku, D., Matarese, M., & Pedone, C. (2011). Predictive validity of the Hendrich fall risk model II in an acute geriatric unit. *International Journal of Nursing Studies, 48*(4), 468–474.
Langlois, F., Vu, T. T. M., Chassé, K., et al. (2013). Benefits of physical exercise training on cognition and quality of life in frail older adults. *The Journals of Gerontology. Series B, Psychological Sciences and Social Sciences, 68*(3), 400–404.
Malafarina, V., Uriz-Otano, F., Iniesta, R., et al. (2013). Effectiveness of nutritional supplementation on muscle mass in treatment of sarcopenia in old age: a systematic review. *Journal of the American Medical Directors Association, 14*(1), 10–17.
Milne, A. C., Potter, J., Vivanti, A., et al. (2009). Protein and energy supplementation in elderly people at risk from malnutrition. *Cochrane Database of Systematic Reviews, 2*(2).
Morley, J. E., Vellas, B., Abellan van Kan, G., et al. (2013). Frailty consensus: a call to action. *Journal of the American Medical Directors Association, 14*(6), 392–397.
Peterson, M. J., Giuliani, C., Morey, M. C., et al. (2009). Physical activity as a preventative factor for frailty: the health, aging, and body composition study. *The Journals of Gerontology. Series A, Biological Sciences and Medical Sciences, 64*(1), 61–68.
Theou, O., Stathokostas, L., Roland, K. P., et al. (2011). The effectiveness of exercise interventions for the management of frailty: a systematic review. *Journal of Aging Research, 2011*.
Tieland, M., Dirks, M. L., van der Zwaluw, N., et al. (2012). Protein supplementation increases muscle mass gain during prolonged resistance-type exercise training in frail elderly people: a randomized, double-blind, placebo-controlled trial. *Journal of the American Medical Directors Association, 13*(8), 713–719.
Vermeulen, J., Neyens, J. C., van Rossum, E., et al. (2011). Predicting ADL disability in community-dwelling elderly people using physical frailty indicators: a systematic review. *BMC Geriatrics, 11*(1), 33.

F

Risk for Frail Elderly syndrome

Noelle L. Fields, PhD, LCSW

NANDA-I

Definition

Vulnerable to a dynamic state of unstable equilibrium that affects the older individual experiencing deterioration in one or more domains of health (physical, functional, or social) and leads to increased susceptibility to adverse health effects, in particular disability

Defining Characteristics

Activity intolerance; age >70 years; alteration in cognitive functioning; altered clotting process (e.g., factor VII, D-dimers); anorexia; anxiety; average daily physical activity is less than recommended for gender and age; chronic illness; constricted life space; decrease in energy; decrease in muscle strength; decrease in serum 25-hydroxyvitamin D concentration; depression; economically disadvantaged; endocrine regulatory dysfunction (e.g., glucose intolerance, increase in IGF-1, androgen, DHEA, and cortisol); ethnicity other than Caucasian; exhaustion; fear of falling; female gender; history of falls; immobility; impaired balance; impaired mobility; insufficient social support; living alone; low educational level; malnutrition; muscle weakness; obesity; prolonged hospitalization; sadness; sarcopenia; sarcopenic obesity; sedentary lifestyle; sensory deficit (e.g., visual, hearing); social isolation; social vulnerability (e.g., disempowerment, decreased life control); suppressed inflammatory response (e.g., IL-6, CRP); unintentional loss of 25% of body weight over 1 year; unintentional weight loss >10 pounds (>4.5 kg) in 1 year; walking 15 feet requires more than 6 seconds (4 m > 5 seconds)

NIC, NOC, Client Outcomes, Nursing Interventions, *Rationales,* and References

Refer to care plan for **Frail Elderly** syndrome.

Impaired Gas exchange

Debra Siela, PhD, RN, CCNS, ACNS-BC, CCRN-K, CNE, RRT

NANDA-I

Definition

Excess or deficit in oxygenation and/or carbon dioxide elimination at the alveolar-capillary membrane

Defining Characteristics

Abnormal arterial blood gases; abnormal arterial pH; abnormal breathing pattern (e.g., rate, rhythm, depth); abnormal skin color (e.g., pale, dusky, cyanosis); confusion; cyanosis; decrease in carbon dioxide (CO_2) levels; diaphoresis; dyspnea; headache upon awakening; hypercapnia; hypoxemia; hypoxia; irritability; nasal flaring; restlessness, somnolence; tachycardia; visual disturbances

Related Factors (r/t)

Alveolar-capillary membrane changes; ventilation-perfusion imbalance

NOC (Nursing Outcomes Classification)

Suggested NOC Outcomes

Respiratory Status: Gas Exchange, Ventilation

Example NOC Outcome with Indicators

Achieves appropriate **Respiratory Status: Gas Exchange** as evidenced by the following indicators: Cognitive status/Partial pressure of oxygen/Partial pressure of carbon dioxide/Arterial pH/Oxygen saturation. (Rate each indicator of **Respiratory Status:** 1 = severe deviation from normal range, 2 = substantial deviation from normal range, 3 = moderate deviation from normal range, 4 = mild deviation from normal range, 5 = no deviation from normal range [see Section I].)

Client Outcomes

Client Will (Specify Time Frame)

- Demonstrate improved ventilation and adequate oxygenation as evidenced by blood gas levels within normal parameters for that client
- Maintain clear lung fields and remain free of signs of respiratory distress
- Verbalize understanding of oxygen supplementation and other therapeutic interventions

NIC (Nursing Interventions Classification)

Suggested NIC Interventions

Acid-Base Management; Airway Management

Example NIC Activities—Acid-Base Management

Monitor for symptoms of respiratory failure (e.g., low PaO_2 and elevated $PaCO_2$ levels and respiratory muscle fatigue); Monitor determinants of tissue oxygen delivery (e.g., PaO_2, SaO_2, and hemoglobin levels, and cardiac output) if available

Nursing Interventions and *Rationales*

- Monitor respiratory rate, depth, and ease of respiration. Watch for use of accessory muscles and nasal flaring. *Normal respiratory rate is 14 to 16 breaths/minute in the adult (Bickley & Szilagyi, 2012).* EBN: *A study demonstrated that when the respiratory rate exceeds 30 breaths/minute, along with other physiological measures, a significant cardiovascular or respiratory alteration exists (Hagle, 2008).*
- Auscultate breath sounds every 1 to 2 hours. The presence of crackles and wheezes may alert the nurse to airway obstruction, which may lead to or exacerbate existing hypoxia. *In severe exacerbations of chronic obstructive pulmonary disease (COPD), lung sounds may be diminished or distant with air trapping (Bickley & Szilagyi, 2012).*

- Monitor the client's behavior and mental status for the onset of restlessness, agitation, confusion, and (in the late stages) extreme lethargy. *Changes in behavior and mental status can be early signs of impaired gas exchange. In the late stages the client becomes lethargic and somnolent (Burns, 2011).*

▲ Monitor oxygen saturation continuously using pulse oximetry. Note blood gas results as available. *An oxygen saturation of less than 88% (normal: 95% to 100%) or a partial pressure of oxygen of less than 55 mm Hg (normal: 80 to 100 mm Hg) indicates significant oxygenation problems. Pulse oximetry is useful for tracking and/or adjusting supplemental oxygen therapy for clients with COPD (GOLD, 2015).*

- Observe for cyanosis of the skin; especially note color of the tongue and oral mucous membranes. *In central cyanosis both the skin and mucous membranes are affected due to seriously impaired pulmonary function from unventilated or underventilated alveoli. Peripheral cyanosis (skin only) usually indicates vasoconstriction or obstruction to blood flow (Loscalzo, 2013).*
- *Central cyanosis of the tongue and oral mucosa is indicative of serious hypoxia and is a medical emergency. Peripheral cyanosis in the extremities may be due to activation of the central nervous system or exposure to cold and may or may not be serious (Bickley & Szilagyi, 2012).*
- Position the client in a semirecumbent position with the head of the bed at a 30- to 45-degree angle to decrease the aspiration of gastric, oral, and nasal secretions (Grap, 2009; Siela, 2010; Vollman & Sole, 2011). Historically, evidence shows that mechanically ventilated clients have a decreased incidence of aspiration pneumonia if the client is placed in a 30- to 45-degree semirecumbent position as opposed to a supine position.
- If the client has unilateral lung disease, position with head of bed at 30 to 45 degrees with "good lung down" for about 1 hour at a time (Burns, 2011).

▲ If the client is acutely dyspneic, consider having the client lean forward over a bedside table, resting elbows on the table if tolerated. *Leaning forward can help decrease dyspnea, possibly because gastric pressure allows better contraction of the diaphragm (Langer et al, 2009). This is called the tripod position and is used during times of distress, including when walking, leaning forward on the walker.*

- Help the client deep breathe and perform controlled coughing. Have the client inhale deeply, hold the breath for several seconds, and cough two or three times with the mouth open while tightening the upper abdominal muscles as tolerated. *Controlled coughing uses the diaphragmatic muscles, which makes the cough more forceful and effective.* If the client has excessive fluid in the respiratory system, see the interventions for Ineffective **Airway** clearance.

▲ Monitor the effects of sedation and analgesics on the client's respiratory pattern; use judiciously. *Both analgesics and medications that cause sedation can depress respiration at times. However, these medications can be very helpful for decreasing the sympathetic nervous system discharge that accompanies hypoxia (Spruit et al, 2013).*

- Schedule nursing care to provide rest and minimize fatigue. *The hypoxic client has limited reserves; inappropriate activity can increase hypoxia (Spruit et al, 2013).*

▲ Administer humidified oxygen through an appropriate device (e.g., nasal cannula or Venturi mask per the health care provider's order); aim for an oxygen (O_2) saturation level of 90% or above. Watch for onset of hypoventilation as evidenced by increased somnolence. *There is a fine line between ideal and excessive oxygen therapy; increasing somnolence is caused by retention of CO_2 leading to CO_2 narcosis (Wong & Elliott, 2009). Promote oxygen therapy during a COPD exacerbation. Supplemental oxygen should be titrated to improve the client's hypoxemia with a target of 88% to 92% (GOLD, 2015).*

- Once oxygen is started, arterial blood gases should be checked 30 to 60 minutes later to ensure satisfactory oxygenation without carbon dioxide retention or acidosis (GOLD, 2015). EBN: *Use of high-flow nasal cannula oxygen therapy may improve gas exchange and oxygenation in acute respiratory therapy (Roca et al, 2010; Parke et al, 2011; Sztrymf et al, 2012; Lenglet et al, 2012; Rittayamai et al, 2014).*
- Assess nutritional status including serum albumin level and body mass index (BMI). *Weight loss in a client with COPD has a negative effect on the course of the disease; it can result in loss of muscle mass in the respiratory muscles, including the diaphragm, which can lead to respiratory failure (Odencrants et al, 2008; GOLD, 2015).*

▲ Assist the client to eat small meals frequently and use dietary supplements as necessary. Engage dietary in evaluating and creating an optimal nutrition plan. For some clients, drinking 30 mL of a supplement every hour while awake can be helpful.

- If the client is severely debilitated from chronic respiratory disease, consider the use of a wheeled walker to help in ambulation.

▲ Watch for signs of psychological distress including anxiety, agitation, and insomnia.

G

▲ Refer the COPD client to a pulmonary rehabilitation program. *Pulmonary rehabilitation is now considered a standard of care for the client with COPD (Spruit et al, 2013; GOLD, 2015; Nici et al, 2009).*

Critical Care

▲ Assess and monitor oxygen indices such as the PF ratio (FIO_2:pO_2), venous oxygen saturation/oxygen consumption (SVO_2 or $ScVO_2$) (Headley & Guiliano, 2011; Burns, 2011).

▲ Turn the client every 2 hours. Monitor mixed venous oxygen saturation closely after turning. If it drops below 10% or fails to return to baseline promptly, turn the client back into the supine position and evaluate oxygen status. If the client does not tolerate turning, consider use of a kinetic bed that rotates the client from side to side in a turn of at least 40 degrees (Vollman et al, 2011).

▲ If the client has acute respiratory distress syndrome with difficulty maintaining oxygenation, consider positioning the client prone with the upper thorax and pelvis supported. Monitor oxygen saturation and turn the client back to supine position if desaturation occurs. EBN/EB: *Oxygenation levels have been shown to improve in the prone position, probably due to decreased shunting and better perfusion of the lungs (Gattinoni et al, 2013; Vollman & Powers, 2011). Prone ventilation significantly reduced mortality in clients with severe acute hypoxemic respiratory failure, but not in clients with less severe hypoxemia (Sud et al, 2010; Gattinoni et al, 2013).* NOTE: If the client becomes ventilator dependent, see the care plan for Impaired spontaneous **Ventilation.**

▲ High levels of positive end-expiratory pressures likely improve oxygenation and gas exchange (Meade et al, 2008; Suzumura et al, 2014).

Geriatric

▲ Use central nervous system depressants and other sedating agents carefully to avoid decreasing respiration rate.

▲ Maintain low-flow oxygen therapy for clients with impaired gas exchange and hypoxemia (GOLD 2015; Burns, 2011).

Home Care

• Work with the client to determine what strategies are most helpful during times of dyspnea. Educate and empower the client to self-manage the disease associated with impaired gas exchange. EBN/EB: *A study found that use of oxygen, self-use of medication, and getting some fresh air were most helpful in dealing with dyspnea (Thomas, 2009). Evidence-based reviews have found that self-management offers COPD clients effective options for managing the illness, leading to more positive outcomes (Kaptein et al, 2008; Spruit et al, 2013).*

• Collaborate with health care providers regarding long-term oxygen administration for chronic respiratory failure clients with severe resting hypoxemia. Administer long-term oxygen therapy greater than 15 hours daily for pO_2 less than 55 or SaO_2 at or below 88% (GOLD, 2015).

• Assess the home environment for irritants that impair gas exchange. Help the client adjust the home environment as necessary (e.g., install an air filter to decrease the level of dust).

▲ Refer the client to occupational therapy as necessary to assist the client in adapting to the home and environment and in energy conservation (GOLD, 2015).

• Assist the client with identifying and avoiding situations that exacerbate impairment of gas exchange (e.g., stress-related situations, exposure to pollution of any kind, proximity to noxious gas fumes such as chlorine bleach). *Irritants in the environment decrease the client's effectiveness in accessing oxygen during breathing.*

• Refer to GOLD guidelines for management of home care and indications of hospital admission criteria (GOLD, 2015).

• Instruct the client to keep the home temperature above 68° F (20° C) and to avoid cold weather. *Cold air temperatures cause constriction of the blood vessels, which impairs the client's ability to absorb oxygen (Brickley et al, 2012).*

• Instruct the client to limit exposure to persons with respiratory infections. *Viruses, bacteria, and environmental pollutants are the main causes of exacerbations of COPD (Barnett, 2008).*

• Instruct the family in the complications of the disease and the importance of maintaining the medical regimen, including when to call a health care provider.

▲ Refer the client for home health aide services as necessary for assistance with activities of daily living. *Clients with decreased oxygenation have decreased energy to carry out personal and role-related activities.*

- When respiratory procedures are being implemented, explain equipment and procedures to family members, and provide needed emotional support. *Family members assuming responsibility for respiratory monitoring often find this stressful (Langer et al, 2009).*
- When electrically based equipment for respiratory support is being implemented, evaluate home environment for electrical safety, proper grounding, and so on. Ensure that notification is sent to the local utility company, the emergency medical team, and police and fire departments. *Notification is important to provide for priority service.*
- ▲ Assess family role changes and coping ability. Refer the client to medical social services as appropriate for assistance in adjusting to chronic illness. *Inability to maintain the level of social involvement experienced before illness leads to frustration and anger in the client and may create a threat to the family unit (Langer et al, 2009).*
- Support the family of the client with chronic illness. *Severely compromised respiratory functioning causes fear and anxiety in clients and their families. Reassurance from the nurse can be helpful (Rose et al, 2014).*

G

Client/Family Teaching and Discharge Planning

- Teach the client how to perform pursed-lip breathing and inspiratory muscle training, and how to use the tripod position. Have the client watch the pulse oximeter to note improvement in oxygenation with these breathing techniques. CEB: *Studies demonstrated that pursed-lip breathing was effective in decreasing breathlessness and improving respiratory function (Faager et al, 2008). A systematic review found that inspiratory muscle training was effective in increasing endurance of the client and decreasing dyspnea (Langer et al, 2009).*
- Teach the client energy conservation techniques and the importance of alternating rest periods with activity. See nursing interventions for **Fatigue.**
- ▲ Teach the importance of not smoking. Refer to smoking cessation programs, and encourage clients who relapse to keep trying to quit. Ensure that clients receive appropriate medications to support smoking cessation from the primary health care provider. EB: *A systematic review of research demonstrated that the combination of medications and an intensive, prolonged counseling program supporting smoking cessation were effective in promoting long-term abstinence from smoking (Fiore et al, 2008). A Cochrane review found that use of the medication varenicline (Chantix) increased the rate of smoking withdrawal two to three times more than smoking withdrawal without use of medications (Cahill et al, 2008; GOLD, 2015).*
- ▲ Instruct the family regarding home oxygen therapy if ordered (e.g., delivery system, liter flow, safety precautions). *Long-term oxygen therapy can improve survival, exercise ability, sleep, and ability to think in hypoxemic clients. Client education improves compliance with prescribed use of oxygen (GOLD, 2015).*
- ▲ Teach the client the need to receive a yearly influenza vaccine. *Receiving a yearly influenza vaccine is helpful to prevent exacerbations of COPD (Black & McDonald, 2009).*
- Teach the client relaxation techniques to help reduce stress responses and panic attacks resulting from dyspnea. EB: *Relaxation therapy can help reduce dyspnea and anxiety (Langer et al, 2009).*
- Teach the client to use music, along with a rest period, to decrease dyspnea and anxiety (Loscalzo, 2013).

REFERENCES

Barnett, M. (2008). Nursing management of chronic obstructive pulmonary disease. *British Journal of Nursing*, *17*(21), 1314–1318.

Bickley, L. S., & Szilagyi, P. (2012). *Bate's Guide to physical examination* (11th ed.). Philadelphia: Lippincott Williams & Wilkins.

Black, P. N., & McDonald, C. F. (2009). Interventions to reduce the frequency of exacerbations of chronic obstructive pulmonary disease. *Postgraduate Medical Journal*, *85*(1001), 141–147.

Burns, S. M. (2011). Indices of oxygenation. In D. J. Lynn-McHale (Ed.), *AACN Procedure Manual for Critical Care* (6th ed.). Philadelphia: Saunders Elsevier.

Cahill, K., Stead, L. F., & Lancaster, T. (2008). Nicotine receptor partial agonists for smoking cessation. *Cochrane Database of Systematic Reviews*, (3), CD006103.

Faager, G., Ståhle, A., & Larsen, F. F. (2008). Influence of spontaneous pursed lips breathing on walking endurance and oxygen saturation in patients with moderate to severe chronic obstructive pulmonary disease. *Clinical Rehabilitation*, *22*(8), 675–683.

Fiore, M. C., Jaen, C. R., & Baker, T. B. (2008). *Treating tobacco use and dependence clinical practice guideline, 2008 update.* Rockville MD: U.S. Department of Health and Human Services, Public Health Service.

Gattinoni, L., Taccone, P., Carlesso, E., et al. (2013). Prone position in acute respiratory distress syndrome. *American Journal of Respiratory and Critical Care Medicine*, *188*(11), 1286–1293.

GOLD. Global strategy for the diagnosis, management, and prevention of COPD (revised 2015), *Global Initiative for Chronic Obstructive Lung Disease*, <http://www.goldcopd.org/uploads/users/files/GOLD_Report_2015_Apr2.pdf> Retrieved April 23, 2015.

Grap, M. (2009). Not-so-trivial pursuit: mechanical ventilation risk reduction. *American Journal of Critical Care*, *18*(4), 299–309.

Hagle, M. (2008). Vital signs monitoring. An EBP Guideline. In B. Ackley, G. Ladwig, & B. A. Swann (Eds.), *Evidence-based nursing care guidelines: medical-surgical interventions*. Philadelphia: Mosby Elsevier.

Headley, J., & Giuliano, K. (2011). Continuous venous oxygen saturation monitoring. In D. J. Lynn-McHale (Ed.), *AACN Procedure Manual for Critical Care* (6th ed.). Philadelphia: Saunders Elsevier.

Kaptein, A. A., Scharloo, M., Fischer, M. J., et al. (2008). 50 years of psychological research on patients with COPD—road to ruin or highway to heaven? *Respiratory Medicine*, *103*(3), 3–11.

Langer, D., Hendriks, E., Burtin, C., et al. (2009). A clinical practice guideline for physiotherapists treating patients with chronic obstructive pulmonary disease based on a systematic review of available evidence. *Clinical Rehabilitation*, *23*(5), 445–462.

Lenglet, H., Sztrymf, B., Leroy, C., et al. (2012). Humidified high flow nasal oxygen during respiratory failure in the emergency department: feasibility and efficacy. *Respiratory Care*, *57*(11), 1873–1878.

Loscalzo, J. (2013). Hypoxia and cyanosis. In J. Loscalzo (Ed.), *Harrison's pulmonary and critical care medicine* (2nd ed., pp. 21–25). New York: McGraw Hill Education Medical.

Meade, M. O., Cook, D. J., Guyatt, G. H., et al. (2008). Ventilation strategy using low tidal volumes, recruitment maneuvers, and high positive end-expiratory pressure for acute lung injury and acute respiratory distress syndrome: a randomized controlled trial. *Journal of American Medical Association*, *299*(6), 637–645.

Nici, L., Raskin, J., Rochester, C. L., et al. (2009). Pulmonary rehabilitation: what we know and what we need to know. *Journal of Cardiopulmonary Rehabilitation & Prevention*, *29*(3), 141–151.

Odencrants, S., Ehnfors, M., & Ehrenbert, A. (2008). Nutritional status and patient characteristics for hospitalized older patients with chronic obstructive pulmonary disease. *Journal of Clinical Nursing*, *17*(13), 1771–1778.

Parke, R. L., McGuinness, S. P., & Eccleston, M. L. (2011). A preliminary randomized controlled trial to assess effectiveness of nasal high-flow oxygen in intensive care patients. *Respiratory Care*, *56*(3), 265–270.

Rittayamai, N., Tscheikuna, J., & Rujiwit, P. (2014). High-flow nasal versus conventional oxygen therapy after endotracheal extubation: a randomized crossover physiologic study. *Respiratory Care*, *59*(4), 485–490.

Roca, O., Riera, J., Torres, F., et al. (2010). High-flow oxygen therapy in acute respiratory failure. *Respiratory Care*, *55*(4), 408–413.

Rose, L., Dainty, K. N., Jordan, J., et al. (2014). Weaning from mechanical ventilation: a scoping review of qualitative studies. *American Journal of Critical Care*, *23*(5), e54–e71.

Siela, D. (2010). Evaluation standards for management of artificial airways. *Critical Care Nurse*, *30*(4), 76–78.

Spruit, M. A., Singh, S. J., Garvey, C., et al. (2013). An official American Thoracic Society/European Respiratory Society Statement: key concepts and advances in pulmonary rehabilitation. *American Journal of Respiratory and Critical Care Medicine*, *188*(8), e13–e64.

Sud, S., Friedrich, J., Taccone, P., et al. (2010). Prone ventilation reduces mortality in patients with acute respiratory failure and severe hypoxemia: systematic review and meta-analysis. *Intensive Care Medicine*, *36*, 585–599.

Suzumura, E. A., Figueiro, M., Normilio-Silva, K., et al. (2014). Effects of alveolar recruitment maneuvers on clinical outcomes in aptients with acute respiratory distress syndrome: a systematic review and meta-analysis. *Intensive Care Medicine*, *40*, 1227–1240.

Sztrymf, B., Messika, J., Mayot, T., et al. (2012). Impact of high-flow nasal cannula oxygen therapy on intensive care unit patients with acute respiratory failure: a prospective observational study. *Journal of Critical Care*, *27*, 324.e9–324.e13.

Thomas, L. (2009). Effective dyspnea management strategies identified by elders with end-stage chronic obstructive pulmonary disease. *Applied Nursing Research*, *22*(2), 79–85.

Vollman, K., & Powers, J. (2011). Pronation Therapy. In D. J. Lynn-McHale (Ed.), *AACN Procedure Manual for Critical Care* (6th ed.). Philadelphia: Saunders Elsevier.

Vollman, K., & Sole, M. (2011). Endotracheal tube and oral care. In D. J. Lynn-McHale (Ed.), *AACN Procedure Manual for Critical Care* (6th ed.). Philadelphia: Saunders Elsevier.

Wong, M., & Elliott, M. (2009). The use of medical orders in acute care oxygen therapy. *British Journal of Nursing*, *18*(8), 462–464.

Dysfunctional Gastrointestinal motility

Betty J. Ackley, MSN, EdS, RN, and Mary Beth Flynn Makic, PhD, RN, CNS, CCNS, FAAN

NANDA-I

Definition

Increased, decreased, ineffective, or lack of peristaltic activity within the gastrointestinal system

Defining Characteristics

Abdominal cramping; abdominal distention; abdominal pain; absence of flatus; acceleration of gastric emptying; bile-colored gastric residual; change in bowel sounds; diarrhea; difficulty with defecation; hard, formed stool; increase in gastric residual; nausea; regurgitation; vomiting

Related Factors (r/t)

Aging; anxiety; enteral feedings; food intolerance; immobility; ingestion of contaminated material (e.g., radioactive, food, water); malnutrition; prematurity; sedentary lifestyle; treatment regimen

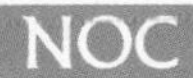

NOC (Nursing Outcomes Classification)

Suggested NOC Outcomes

Gastrointestinal Function; Electrolyte and Acid-Base Balance; Fluid Balance; Hydration; Nausea and Vomiting Control; Treatment Behavior: Illness or Injury

Example NOC Outcome with Indicators

Gastrointestinal Function as evidenced by the following indicators: Bowel sounds/Stool soft and formed/Appetite present without evidence of reflux, nausea, or vomiting/Reported normal abdominal comfort. (Rate the outcome and indicators of **Gastrointestinal Function:** 1 = severely compromised, 2 = substantially compromised, 3 = moderately compromised, 4 = mildly compromised, 5 = not compromised [see Section I].)

Client Outcomes

Client Will (Specify Time Frame)

- Be free of abdominal distention and pain
- Have normal bowel sounds
- Pass flatus rectally at intervals
- Defecate formed, soft stool every day to every third day
- State has an appetite
- Be able to eat food without nausea and vomiting

NIC (Nursing Interventions Classification)

Suggested NIC Intervention

Gastric Motility Management

Example NIC Activities—Gastric Motility Management

Evaluate use of prokinetics for delayed gastric motility; Suggest change in dietary habits to either increase or decrease gastric motility, depending on the presenting complaint

Nursing Interventions and *Rationales*

- • Monitor for abdominal distention, and presence of abdominal pain, weight loss, nausea, vomiting, obstipation, or diarrhea. *The acute onset of abdominal distention in conjunction with symptoms of cramping pain, weight loss, nausea, vomiting, obstipation, or diarrhea warrants further evaluation for disorders that cause intestinal obstruction (Camilleri, 2012).*
- • Inspect, auscultate for bowel sounds noting characteristics and frequency; palpate and percuss the abdomen. *Hypoactive bowel sounds are found with decreased motility as with peritonitis from paralytic ileus or from late bowel obstruction. Hyperactive bowel sounds are associated with increased motility (Jarvis, 2012).*
- • Review history noting any anorexia or nausea/vomiting. Other symptoms may include relation of symptoms to meals, especially if aggravated by food, satiety, postprandial fullness/bloating, and weight loss or weight loss with severe gastroparesis. *These are signs of abnormal gastric motility (Bouras et al, 2013).*
- • Monitor for fluid deficits by checking skin turgor and moisture of tongue, daily weights, input and output, and electrolyte values. Refer to care plan deficient **Fluid** volume if relevant.
- ▲ Monitor for nutritional deficits by keeping close track of food intake. Review laboratory studies that affirm nutritional deficits, such as decreased albumin and serum protein levels, liver profile, glucose, and an electrolyte panel. Refer to care plan for imbalanced **Nutrition:** less than body requirements or Risk for **Electrolyte** imbalance as appropriate.

Slowed Gastric Motility

- • Monitor the client for signs and symptoms of decreased gastric motility, which may include nausea after meals, vomiting, feeling full quickly while eating, abdominal bloating and abdominal pain (Bouras et al, 2013).

- ▲ Monitor daily laboratory studies and point of care testing blood glucose levels ensuring ordered glucose levels are performed and evaluated. *Elevated blood glucose levels can cause delayed gastric emptying; therefore, it is important to normalize blood glucose levels (Powers, 2012).*
- • Obtain a thorough gastrointestinal history if the client has diabetes, because he/she is at high risk for gastroparesis and gastric reflux. *Gastroparesis with delayed emptying of the stomach is a well-known complication of diabetes (Olausson et al, 2014).*
- ▲ If client has nausea and vomiting, provide an antiemetic and intravenous fluids as ordered. Refer to the care plans for **Nausea.**
- ▲ Evaluate medications that the client is taking. Recognize that vasopressors, opioids, or anticholinergic medications can cause gastric slowing (Aderinto-Adike & Quigley, 2014).
- ▲ Review laboratory and other diagnostic tools, including complete blood count, amylase, and thyroid-stimulating hormone level, glucose with other metabolic studies, upper endoscopy, and gastric-emptying scintigraphy. *The diagnosis of diabetic gastroparesis is made when other causes are excluded and postprandial gastric stasis is confirmed by gastric emptying scintigraphy, which is considered the gold standard for diagnosing gastroparesis (Lacy, 2012).*
- ▲ Obtain a nutritional consult, considering a small particle size diet or diets lower or higher in liquids or solids, depending on gastric motility. EB: *A randomized controlled trial found that diets with smaller particle size reduced the symptoms of gastroparesis in diabetic clients (Olausson et al, 2014).*
- ▲ If client is unable to eat or retain food, consult with the registered dietitian and health care provider, considering further nutritional support in the form of enteral or parenteral feedings for the client with gastroparesis. *Some clients require supplementation with either enteral or parenteral nutrition for survival.*
- ▲ If client is receiving gastric enteral nutrition, see the care plan Risk for **Aspiration.**
- ▲ Administer medications that increase gastrointestinal motility as ordered (Chang et al, 2011).

Postoperative Ileus

- • Observe for complications of delayed intestinal motility. Symptoms include vague abdominal pain and distention, nausea, vomiting, anorexia, sometimes bloating, and tympany to percussion. Clients may or may not pass flatus and some stool (Cagir, 2013).
- ▲ Recommend chewing gum for the abdominal surgery client who is experiencing an ileus, is not at risk for aspiration, and has normal dentition. EB: *Gum chewing may decrease postoperative ileus because it acts as a sham feeding, potentially stimulating gastric and bowel motility. A meta-analysis of research found that using chewing gum reduces the time of postoperative ileus (Shan et al, 2013).*
- • Help the client out of bed to walk at least two times per day. Assist client to sit in a rocking chair to rock back and forth. *Exercise may increase gastrointestinal motility.*
- ▲ If postoperative ileus is associated with opioid pain medication, ensure opioids are decreased or ideally discontinued. Use nonsteroidal anti-inflammatory drugs for pain as feasible and if not contraindicated (Cagir, 2013).
- ▲ Note serum electrolyte levels, especially potassium and magnesium. *A low potassium level decreases the function of intestinal smooth muscle and can result in an ileus. A low magnesium level makes the body refractory to potassium replacement (Mount et al, 2012; Cagir, 2013).*

Increased Gastrointestinal Motility

- ▲ Observe for complications of gastric surgeries such as dumping syndrome. *This syndrome is the effect of changes in size and function of the stomach, with rapid dumping of hyperosmolar food into the intestines (Bosnic, 2014).*
- • Watch for nausea, vomiting, bloating, cramping, diarrhea, dizziness, and fatigue. *These are common signs and symptoms of early rapid gastric emptying (Bosnic, 2014).*
- • Monitor for low blood sugar, weakness, sweating, and dizziness 1 to 3 hours after eating as this is when late rapid gastric emptying may occur. Late rapid gastric emptying is associated with low blood sugar (Bosnic, 2014).
- ▲ Order a nutritional consult to discuss diet changes. The diet may vary depending on the kind of surgery causing dumping syndrome. *Encourage small meals that are low in carbohydrates and fats. Space fluids around meal times (Bosnic, 2014).*
- ▲ Give intravenous fluids as ordered for the client complaining of diarrhea with weakness and dizziness. Monitor electrolyte panel. *Severe diarrhea can cause deficient fluid volume with extreme weakness.*

- Offer bathroom, commode, or bedpan assistance, depending on frequency, amount of diarrhea, and condition of client.
- Monitor rectal area for decreased skin integrity, apply barrier creams as needed to protect and treat skin.
- Refer to the care plans for the nursing diagnoses of Deficient **Fluid** volume, **Nausea,** Impaired **Skin** integrity, and **Diarrhea** as relevant.

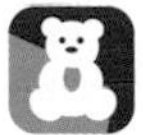

Pediatric

- Assess infants and children with suspected delayed gastric emptying for fullness and vomiting. *Babies and children with delayed gastric emptying take longer to get hungry again and throw up undigested or partially digested food several hours after feeding (Waseem et al, 2012; Ambartsumyan & Rodriguez, 2014).*
- ▲ Observe for nutritional and fluid deficits with assessment of skin turgor, mucous membranes, fontanels, furrows of the tongue, electrolyte panel, fluid status, input and output, and daily weights (Saliakellis & Fotoulaki, 2013).
- ▲ Recommend gentle massage for preterm infants as appropriate. EB: *With massage, there was increased vagal activity. This was then associated with increased gastric motility and greater weight gain (Field et al, 2011).*

G

Geriatric

- Closely monitor diet and medication use/side effects as they affect the gastrointestinal system. Watch for constipation. *Many gastrointestinal functions are slowed in older adults (Grassi et al, 2011).*
- ▲ Watch for symptoms of dysphagia, gastroesophageal reflux disease, dyspepsia, irritable bowel syndrome, maldigestion, and reduced absorption of nutrients. *These are common gastrointestinal disorders in older adults (Grassi et al, 2011).*

Client/Family Teaching and Discharge Planning

- Teach the client and caregivers about medications, reinforcing side effects as they relate to gastrointestinal function.
- Teach client and caregivers to report signs and symptoms that may indicate further complications including increased abdominal girth, projectile vomiting, and unrelieved acute cramping pain (bowel obstruction).
- Review signs and symptoms of dehydration with client and caregivers.

REFERENCES

Aderinto-Adike, A. O., & Quigley, E. M. (2014). Gastrointestinal motility problems in critical care: a clinical perspective. *Chinese Journal of Digestive Diseases*, *15*(7), 335–344.

Ambartsumyan, L., & Rodriguez, L. (2014). Gastrointestinal motility disorders in children. *Gastroenterologia Y Hepatologia*, *10*(1), 16–26.

Bosnic, G. (2014). Nutritional requirements after bariatric surgery. *Critical Care Nursing Clinics of North America*, *26*, 255–262.

Bouras, E. P., Vazquez, M. I., & Aranda-Michel, J. (2013). Gastroparesis: from concepts to management. *Nutrition in Clinical Practice*, *28*(4), 437–447.

Cagir, B. (2013). Ileus: Drugs and diseases. *Medscape*. Retrieved from: <http://emedicine.medscape.com/article/178948-overview>.

Camilleri, M., et al. (2012). Disorders of Gastrointestinal motility. In L. Goldman (Ed.), *Goldman's Cecil medicine* (24th ed.). Philadelphia: Elsevier.

Chang, J., et al. (2011). Diabetic gastroparesis-backwards and forwards. *Journal of Gastroenterology and Hepatology*, *26*, 46–57.

Field, T., Diego, M., & Hernandez-Reif, M. (2011). Potential underlying mechanisms for greater weight gain in massaged preterm infants. *Infant Behavior and Development*, *34*(3), 383–389.

Grassi, M., et al. (2011). Changes, functional disorders, and diseases in the gastrointestinal tract of elderly. *Nutricion Hospitalaria: Organo Oficial de la Sociedad Espanola de Nutricion Parenteral Y Enteral*, *26*(4), 659–668.

Jarvis, C. (2012). *Physical examination and health assessment* (6th ed.). St Louis: Saunders Elsevier.

Lacy, B. E. (2012). Functional dyspepsia and gastroparesis. *The American Journal of Gastroenterology*, *107*(11), 1615–1620.

Mount, D., et al. (2012). Fluid and electrolyte disturbances. In D. Longo (Ed.), *Harrison's textbook of internal medicine* (18th ed.). New York: McGraw-Hill.

Olausson, E. A., et al. (2014). S small particle size diet reduces upper gastrointestinal symptoms in patients with diabetic gastroparesis: a randomized controlled trial. *The American Journal of Gastroenterology*, *109*(3), 375–385. [Epub 2014 Jan 14].

Powers, A. C. (2012). Diabetes Mellitus. In D. L. Longo, et al. (Eds.), *Harrison's Principles of Internal Medicine* (18th ed.). New York: McGraw Hill.

Saliakellis, E., & Fotoulaki, M. (2013). Gastroparesis in children. *Annales de Gastroenterologie et D'hepatologie*, *26*(3), 204–2011.

Shan, L. I., et al. (2013). Chewing gum reduces postoperative ileus following abdominal surgery. *Journal of Gastroenterology and Hepatology*, *28*(7), 1122–1132.

Waseem, S., et al. (2012). Spectrum of gastroparesis in children. *Journal of Pediatric Gastroenterology and Nutrition*, *55*(2), 166–172.

Risk for dysfunctional Gastrointestinal motility

Betty J. Ackley, MSN, EdS, RN, and Mary Beth Flynn Makic, PhD, RN, CNS, CCNS, FAAN

NANDA-I

Definition

Vulnerable to a decrease in normal frequency of defecation accompanied by difficult or incomplete passage of stool, which may compromise health

Risk Factors

Aging, anxiety; change in water source; decrease in gastrointestinal circulation; diabetes mellitus; eating habit change (e.g., foods, eating times); food intolerance; gastroesophageal reflux disease; immobility; infection; pharmaceutical agent; prematurity; sedentary lifestyle; stressors; unsanitary food preparation

NIC, NOC, Client Outcomes, Nursing Interventions, Client/Family Teaching and Discharge Planning, *Rationales,* and References

Refer to care plan for Dysfunctional **Gastrointestinal** motility.

Risk for ineffective Gastrointestinal perfusion

Betty J. Ackley MSN, EdS, RN, and Mary Beth Flynn Makic, PhD, RN, CNS, CCNS, FAAN

NANDA-I

Definition

Vulnerable to decrease in gastrointestinal circulation, which may compromise health

Risk Factors

Abdominal aortic aneurysm; abdominal compartment syndrome; abnormal partial thromboplastin time (PTT); abnormal prothrombin time (PT); acute gastrointestinal hemorrhage; age >60 years; anemia; cerebral vascular accident; coagulopathy (e.g., sickle cell anemia); decrease in left ventricular performance; diabetes mellitus; disseminated intravascular coagulopathy; female gender; gastroesophageal varices; gastrointestinal condition (e.g., ulcer, ischemic colitis, ischemic pancreatitis); myocardial infarction; renal disease (e.g., polycystic kidney, renal artery stenosis, failure); smoking; trauma; treatment regimen; vascular disease

NOC (Nursing Outcomes Classification)

Suggested NOC Outcomes

Tissue Perfusion: Abdominal Organs; Gastrointestinal Function; Tissue Perfusion: Cellular; Circulation Status; Knowledge: Treatment Regimen

Example NOC Outcome with Indicators

Tissue Perfusion: Abdominal Organs as evidenced by the following indicators: Diastolic, systolic, and mean arterial blood pressure within normal limits/Bowel sounds active/Urine output within normal limits for age/Electrolyte and acid-base balance within normal limits. (Rate the outcome and indicators of **Tissue Perfusion: Abdominal Organs:** 1 = severe deviation from normal range, 2 = substantial deviation from normal range, 3 = moderate deviation from normal range, 4 = mild deviation from normal range, 5 = no deviation from normal range [see Section I].)

Client Outcomes

Client Will (Specify Time Frame)

- Maintain blood pressure within normal limits
- Remain free from abdominal distention

- Tolerate feedings without nausea, vomiting, or abdominal discomfort
- Pass stools of normal color, consistency, frequency, and amount
- Describe prescribed diet regimen
- Describe prescribed medication regimen including medication actions and possible side effects
- Verbalize understanding of treatment regimen including monitoring for signs and symptoms that may indicate problems with gastrointestinal tissue perfusion, the importance of diet and exercise to gastrointestinal health

NIC (Nursing Interventions Classification)

Suggested NIC Interventions

Vital Signs Monitoring; Surveillance; Electrolyte Monitoring; Laboratory Data Interpretation

Example NIC Activities—Surveillance

Monitor gastrointestinal function; Monitor vital signs

Nursing Interventions and *Rationales*

Critical Care

▲ Complete a pain assessment. Assess and document the onset, intensity, character, location, duration, aggravating factors, and relieving factors. Determine whether the pain is exacerbated by eating. Notify the provider for any significant increase in pain. *A significant symptom of mesenteric ischemia is pain that is disproportionate to the physical examination findings. It is an emergent condition and positive outcomes are only possible with treatment in the early stages, preferable within 12 hours (Dang & Su, 2014; Hauser, 2011).*

- Perform a physical abdominal examination including inspection, auscultation, percussion, and palpation. Complete the assessment in the described order. *Initially with decreased perfusion there may be increased bowel sounds, and then absence of bowel sounds (Hauser, 2011).*
- Monitor vital signs frequently as needed, watching for hypotension and tachycardia. *Hemodynamic instability with ischemia or infarction of the gastrointestinal blood supply is a serious situation and can result in death of the client, especially older clients (Dang & Su, 2014; Hauser, 2011).*
- Monitor frequency, consistency, color, and amount of stools. *Clients presenting with sudden cramping, left lower abdominal pain, a strong urge to pass stool, and bright red or maroon blood mixed with the stool should be evaluated for colon ischemia. Obvious bleeding from the gastrointestinal tract is an ominous sign and often suggests bowel infarction (Dang & Su, 2014; Hauser, 2011).*
- Assess for abdominal distention. Measure abdominal girth and compare to client's accustomed waist or belt size. *Ischemia of the gastrointestinal system can result in decreased motility and a paralytic ileus with abdominal distention (Dang & Su, 2014).*
- Review the client's medical and surgical history. Certain conditions place clients at higher risk for ineffective tissue perfusion (see risk factors above). In addition to medical or surgical conditions, lifestyle choices such as smoking or cocaine and amphetamine use affect tissue perfusion (Hauser, 2011). *Gastrointestinal complications following cardiac surgery are rare, but substantially increase morbidity and mortality. Risk factors include age, intraoperative hypoperfusion, and need for high-dose vasopressors (Dang & Su, 2014).*
- Recognize that any client who has been in a shock state has decreased gastrointestinal perfusion due to compensatory mechanisms, and watch for symptoms as identified. *In shock, the blood flow is preferentially shunted away from the gut to the brain and heart to preserve life. Ischemia bowel necrosis is part of the multiple organ dysfunction syndrome that follows a shock state, especially septic shock (Munford, 2012).* See care plan for Risk for **Shock.**

▲ Monitor intake and output to evaluate fluid and electrolyte balance, and review laboratory data as ordered.

▲ Prepare client for diagnostic or surgical procedures. Diagnostic studies may include abdominal x-ray study to rapidly rule out intestinal obstruction, computed tomography, angiography, and abdominal ultrasound. Surgical procedures include exploratory laparotomy, thrombectomy, surgical revascularization, and/or stent placement (Dang & Su, 2014).

Pediatric

- Monitor vital signs frequently. Notify health care provider if there is significant deviation from baseline or findings are significantly abnormal. EBN: *Splanchnic hypoperfusion leads to mucosal ischemia and gastrointestinal dysfunction. Temperature instability, bradycardia, and apnea can be early symptoms of necrotizing enterocolitis in the newborn (Gregory et al, 2011).*
- Monitor oxygen saturation and provide oxygen therapy as ordered. Take steps to prevent hypovolemia and hypotensive episodes. *Untreated acute compartment syndrome leading to elevated intraabdominal pressure can result in multiple organ failure and death (Newcombe, 2012).*
- Monitor tolerance of enteral feedings. Measure gastric residual and note color and consistency. *The premature infant's gastrointestinal system is less able to absorb nutrients. The unabsorbed nutrients can lead to proliferation of enteral bacteria, which can produce intestinal gas, which leads to distention, increased pressure in the lumen of the intestine, and decreased circulation (Gregory et al, 2011).*

G

Geriatric

▲ Monitor for gastrointestinal side effects from medications, especially nonsteroidal antiinflammatory drugs (NSAIDs). *NSAIDs cause local tissue hypoxia due to vasoconstriction, resulting in gastric and duodenal ulcers, perforation, and possibly hemorrhage, especially in older adults (Wehling, 2014).*

▲ Recognize that decreased gastrointestinal perfusion, either acute or chronic, is much more common in older adults. *Risk factors for ischemia of the bowel are primarily older age and increased atherosclerosis (Dang & Su, 2014).*

▲ Be aware that gastrointestinal bleeding that is difficult to control in older adults may be associated with decreased gastrointestinal perfusion (Hauser, 2011).

REFERENCES

Dang, C. V., & Su, M. (2014) *Acute Mesenteric Ischemia*. Medscape Diseases. Retrieved from: <http://emedicine.medscape.com/article/189146-overview#aw2aab6b2b6>.

Gregory, K., et al. (2011). Necrotizing enterocolitis in the premature infant: neonatal nursing assessment, disease pathogenesis, and clinical presentation. *Advances in Neonatal Care*, *11*(3), 155–164.

Hauser, S. C. (2011). Vascular diseases of the gastrointestinal tract. In R. L. Cecil, et al. (Eds.), *Goldman's Cecil Medicine* (24th ed.). Philadelphia: Elsevier Saunders.

Munford, R. S. (2012). Severe sepsis and septic shock. In D. L. Longo, et al. (Eds.), *Harrison's Principles of Internal Medicine* (18th ed.). New York: McGraw Hill.

Newcombe, J. (2012). Pediatric critical care nurses' experience with abdominal compartment syndrome. *Annals Intensive Care*, *2*(Suppl. 1), S6. PMCID: PMC3390293.

Wehling, M. (2014). Non-steroidal anti-inflammatory drug use in chronic pain conditions with special emphasis on the elderly and patients with relevant comorbidities: management and mitigation of risks and adverse effects. *European Journal of Clinical Pharmacology*, *70*(10), 1159–1172. [Epub 2014 Aug 28].

Risk for unstable blood Glucose level

Paula D. Hopper, MSN, RN, CNE

NANDA-I

Definition

Vulnerable to variation in blood glucose/sugar levels from the normal range, which may compromise health

Risk Factors

Alteration in mental status; average daily physical activity is less than recommended for gender and age; compromised physical health status; delay in cognitive development; does not accept diagnosis; excessive stress; excessive weight gain; excessive weight loss; inadequate blood glucose monitoring; ineffective medication management; insufficient diabetes management; insufficient dietary intake; insufficient knowledge of disease management; nonadherence to diabetes management plan; pregnancy; rapid growth period

NOC (Nursing Outcomes Classification)

Suggested NOC Outcomes

Compliance Behavior: Prescribed Diet; Compliance Behavior: Prescribed Medication; Coping; Endurance; Knowledge: Diabetes Management; Knowledge: Treatment Regimen; Nutritional Status; Personal Health Status; Self-Management: Diabetes; Weight Maintenance Behavior

Example NOC Outcome with Indicators

Blood Glucose Level as evidenced by the following indicators: Blood glucose/Glycosylated hemoglobin/Fructosamine/Urine glucose/Urine ketones. (Rate the outcome and indicators of **Blood Glucose Level:** 1 = severe deviation from normal range, 2 = substantial deviation from normal range, 3 = moderate deviation from normal range, 4 = mild deviation from normal range, 5 = no deviation from normal range [see Section I].)

G

Client Outcomes

Client Will (Specify Time Frame)

- Maintain A_{1C} less than 7% (normal level 4% to 6%) (American Diabetes Association [ADA], 2014)
- Maintain outpatient preprandial blood glucose in adults between 70 and 130 mg/dL (ADA, 2014a); consult primary care provider for client-specific goals
- Maintain preprandial blood glucose for preschoolers (0 to 6 years) between 100 and 180 mg/dL; school age (6 to 12 years) between 90 and 180 mg/dL; adolescents and young adults (13 to 19 years) between 90 and 130 mg/dL (ADA, 2014a)
- Maintain outpatient peak postprandial (1 to 2 hours after beginning of meal) glucose below 180 mg/dL (ADA, 2014a)
- Maintain preprandial blood glucose for gestational diabetes ≤95 mg/dL, 1-hour pc level at or below 140 mg/dL, and 2-hour pc level at or below 120 mg/dL (ADA, 2014a)
- Maintain premeal, bedtime, and overnight blood glucose for a pregnant mother with preexisting type 1 or 2 diabetes at 60 to 99 mg/dL, peak postprandial glucose at 100 to 129 mg/dL, and A_{1C} <6% (ADA, 2014a)
- Maintain blood glucose in critically ill hospitalized clients between 140 and 180 mg/dL (ADA, 2014a)
- Maintain premeal blood glucose values in non-critically ill hospitalized clients below 140 mg/dL and random blood glucose values below 180 mg/dL (ADA, 2014a)
- *Collaborate with health care provider to individualize goal glucose levels, based on duration of diabetes, age and life expectancy, comorbid conditions, hypoglycemia unawareness, and individual client considerations (ADA, 2014a)*
- Demonstrate how to accurately test blood glucose
- Identify self-care actions to take to maintain target glucose levels
- Identify self-care actions to take if blood glucose level is too low or too high
- Demonstrate correct administration of prescribed medications
- Demonstrate knowledge of appropriate diet and carbohydrate intake

NIC (Nursing Interventions Classification)

Suggested NIC Interventions

Hypoglycemia Management; Hyperglycemia Management

Example NIC Activities—Hypoglycemia Management

Monitor blood glucose levels, as indicated; Provide simple carbohydrate, as indicated

Nursing Interventions and *Rationales*

▲ Obtain blood glucose before meals and snacks. Obtain blood glucose every 4 to 6 hours in the client not receiving nutrition. EB: *Self monitoring of blood glucose (SMBG) is useful in adjusting premeal insulin doses (ADA, 2014a).* EB: *Evidence supports a correlation between SMBG frequency and lower* A_{1C} *(ADA, 2014a).*

▲ Evaluate blood glucose levels in hospitalized clients before administering oral hypoglycemic agents or insulin. Adjust timing of medication appropriately with meal times. *Inappropriately timed insulin can result in hypoglycemia (ADA, 2014a).*

▲ Recognize that SMBG may not be beneficial in clients who have had type 2 diabetes for more than 1 year and who are not taking insulin. EB: *A systematic review of 12 research studies concluded that SMBG in clients with type 2 diabetes for more than 1 year did not significantly affect glycemic control, quality of life, well-being, or client satisfaction (Malanda, 2012).*

▲ Monitor blood glucose every 30 minutes to 2 hours for clients on continuous insulin drips. EB: *More frequent blood glucose testing ranging from every 30 minutes to every 2 hours is required for clients on intravenous insulin infusions (ADA, 2014a).*

• Consider continuous glucose monitoring (CGM) in clients with type 1 diabetes on intensive insulin regimens. EB: *"When used properly, continuous glucose monitoring (CGM) in conjunction with intensive insulin regimens is a useful tool to lower A_{1C} in selected adults (aged ≥25 years) with type 1 diabetes" (ADA, 2014a).* EB: *In a study of children and adults with type 1 diabetes, CGM was associated with reduced time spent in hypoglycemia and a concomitant decrease in A_{1C} (Battelino et al, 2011).*

G

▲ Evaluate A_{1C} level for glucose control over previous 2 to 3 months. EB: *Two primary techniques are available to assess the effectiveness of the management plan on glycemic control: client SMBG or interstitial glucose and A_{1C} (ADA, 2014a).*

• Consider monitoring 1 to 2 hours after meals in individuals who have premeal glucose values within target but have A_{1C} values above target. EB: *"It is clear that postprandial hyperglycemia, like preprandial hyperglycemia, contributes to elevated A_{1C} levels" (ADA, 2014a).*

• Monitor for signs and symptoms of hypoglycemia, such as shakiness, dizziness, sweating, hunger, headache, pallor, behavior changes, confusion, or seizures. EB: *"Mild hypoglycemia may be inconvenient or frightening to patients with diabetes. Severe hypoglycemia can cause acute harm to the person with diabetes or others, especially if it causes falls, motor vehicle accidents, or other injury" (ADA, 2014a).*

▲ Be alert for hypoglycemia in clients receiving 0.6 unit/kg insulin or more daily, and in clients receiving NPH insulin. EB: *"Higher weight-based insulin doses are associated with greater odds of hypoglycemia independent of insulin type … 0.6 unit/kg seems to be a threshold below which the odds of hypoglycemia are relatively low … patients who received NPH trended toward greater odds of hypoglycemia compared with those given other insulins" (Rubin et al, 2011).*

▲ If client is experiencing signs and symptoms of hypoglycemia, test glucose; if result is below 70 mg/dL, administer 15 to 20 g glucose. Pure glucose is the preferred treatment, but any form of carbohydrate that contains glucose will suffice (½ cup fruit juice or regular [not diet] soda, 1 cup milk, 1 small piece of fruit, or 3 to 4 glucose tablets). Avoid treating with foods that contain fat. Repeat test in 15 minutes and repeat treatment if indicated. Once blood glucose returns to normal, the individual should consume a meal or snack to prevent recurrence of hypoglycemia. EB: *Treatment of hypoglycemia (plasma glucose <70 mg/dL) requires ingestion of glucose- or carbohydrate-containing foods. The acute glycemic response correlates better with the glucose content than with the carbohydrate content of the food. Although pure glucose is the preferred treatment, any form of carbohydrate that contains glucose will raise blood glucose. Added fat may retard and then prolong the acute glycemic response" (ADA, 2014a).*

▲ If the client is unable to swallow, parenteral glucagon may be given by a trained family member or by medical personnel. In unresponsive clients, intravenous glucose should be given. EB: *Intravenous dextrose or injected glucagon are alternatives to oral carbohydrate in hypoglycemic clients who cannot take oral glucose (AACE, 2014).*

▲ Clients who do not experience symptoms of hypoglycemia should raise their glucose targets to avoid hypoglycemia for several weeks. EB: *If the client has hypoglycemic unawareness and hypoglycemia-associated autonomic failure, several weeks of hypoglycemia avoidance may reduce the risk or prevent the recurrence of severe hypoglycemia (AACE, 2014).* EB: *Insulin-treated clients with hypoglycemia unawareness or an episode of severe hypoglycemia should be advised to raise their glycemic targets to strictly avoid further hypoglycemia for at least several weeks, to partially reverse hypoglycemia unawareness and reduce risk of future episodes (ADA, 2014a).*

▲ In clients with type 2 diabetes who become hypoglycemic and have been treated with an alpha-glucosidase inhibitor (e.g., acarbose [Precose] or miglitol [Glyset]) in addition to insulin or an insulin release stimulator, oral glucose rather than more complex carbohydrates must be given. EB: *Alpha-glucosidase inhibitors inhibit the breakdown and absorption of complex carbohydrates and disaccharides (AACE, 2014).*

- Monitor for signs and symptoms of hyperglycemia, such as increased thirst or urination, or high blood or urine glucose levels. EB: *"Improved glycemic control is associated with significantly decreased rates of microvascular (retinopathy and nephropathy) and neuropathic complications" (ADA, 2014a).*
- ▲ Ensure an acutely ill client is receiving adequate fluids and nutrition. Adjustment in oral hypoglycemic or insulin therapy may be required. EB: *"The stress of illness, trauma, and/or surgery frequently aggravates glycemic control and may precipitate diabetic ketoacidosis (DKA) or nonketotic hyperosmolar state, life-threatening conditions that require immediate medical care to prevent complications and death" (ADA, 2014a).*
- ▲ Test urine or blood for ketones in ketosis-prone clients during acute illness, trauma, surgery, or stress. *"If accompanied by ketosis, vomiting, or alteration in level of consciousness, marked hyperglycemia requires temporary adjustment of the treatment regimen and immediate interaction with the diabetes care team" (ADA, 2014a).*
- ▲ Prime intravenous (IV) tubing with 20 mL of diluted insulin solution before initiating insulin drip. CEB: *Glucose adsorbs to some IV tubing; priming with 20 mL is enough to minimize this effect (Goldberg et al, 2006; Zahid et al, 2008).*
- ▲ Evaluate client's medication regimen for medications that can alter blood glucose. *Catecholamines, some antipsychotic and antidepressant agents, thiazide diuretics, glucocorticoids, and niacin, among others, can cause hyperglycemia. Alcohol, aspirin, and beta-blockers are among agents that can cause hypoglycemia (National Prescribing Service [NPS], 2011).*
- ▲ Refer client to dietitian for carbohydrate counting instruction. EB: *"Monitoring carbohydrate intake, whether by carbohydrate counting or experience-based estimation, remains a key strategy in achieving glycemic control" (ADA, 2014a).*
- ▲ Refer overweight clients to dietitian for weight loss counseling. EB: *"Modest weight loss may provide clinical benefits (improved glycemia, blood pressure, and/or lipids) in some individuals with diabetes, especially those early in the disease process" (ADA, 2014a).*
- For interventions regarding foot care, refer to the care plan Ineffective peripheral **Tissue Perfusion.**

Geriatric

- Watch for age-related cognitive changes that can impair self-management of diabetes. EBN: *"In older people taking insulin, around one quarter of those aged over 75 years had evidence of cognitive impairment, which significantly reduced their ability to understand the actions required in the event of low blood glucose" (Phillips & Phillips, 2011).*
- Monitor for vision and dexterity impairments that may affect the older client's ability to accurately measure insulin doses. EB: *Medication therapy can present a challenge due to possible visual and dexterity impairments (Pfützner et al, 2011).*
- ▲ Consider relaxing glucose targets for older adults with advanced diabetes complications, life-limiting comorbid illness, or substantial cognitive or functional impairment. EB: *"These patients are less likely to benefit from reducing the risk of microvascular complications and more likely to suffer serious adverse effects from hypoglycemia" (ADA, 2014a).* EB: *"A large cohort study suggested that among older adults with type 2 diabetes, a history of severe hypoglycemia was associated with greater risk of dementia" (ADA, 2014a).*
- Teach older clients the importance of verifying symptoms with a glucometer reading. EB: *A study of older adults found that they were unable to identify whether symptoms indicated high or low blood glucose. Common symptoms included sensations such as tingling or numbness, lightheadedness, dizziness, lack of energy, and blurred vision (Kirk et al, 2011).*

Pediatric

- Be aware that young children (<7 years) may not be aware of symptoms of hypoglycemia. EB: *"For young children (<7 years old), glycemic goals may need to be modified because most children at that age have a form of 'hypoglycemic unawareness,' including immaturity of and a relative inability to recognize and respond to hypoglycemic symptoms. This places them at greater risk for severe hypoglycemia" (ADA, 2014a).*
- Teach children and adolescents (and their parents) with type 1 diabetes or on intensive insulin regimens (MDI or insulin pump therapy) to perform SMBG before meals and snacks, occasionally postprandially, at bedtime, before exercise, when they suspect low blood glucose, after treating low blood glucose until they are normoglycemic, and before critical tasks such as driving. EB: *A database study of almost 27,000*

children and adolescents with type 1 diabetes showed that … increased daily frequency of SMBG was significantly associated with lower A_{1C} (−0.2% per additional test per day, leveling off at five tests per day) and with fewer acute complications (ADA, 2014a). EB: *An "observational study shows a strong association between more frequent SMBG in the range of 0-5 per day and better metabolic control in adolescents above 12 yr of age" (Ziegler et al, 2011).*

- Teach self-efficacy measures to adolescents with type 1 diabetes who are involved in family conflict. CEB: *The effect of family conflict on frequency of SMBG is reduced when adolescents are taught self-efficacy (Sander et al, 2010).*

Home Care

▲ Teach family and others having close contact with the person with diabetes how to use an emergency glucagon kit (if prescribed). *Severe hypoglycemia in which client is unable to take oral glucose should be treated with glucagon (ADA, 2014a).*

G

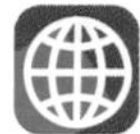

Multicultural

- Provide culturally appropriate diabetes health education. EB: *Ten of 11 studies reviewed showed that structured intervention tailored to ethnic minority groups by integrating elements of culture, language, religion, and health literacy skills produced a positive impact on a range of outcomes (Zeh et al, 2012).*
- Involve Hispanic community workers (promotoras) when working with Hispanic clients with diabetes. CEB: *Improved A_{1C} level was associated with promotora advocacy and participation in promotora-led support groups (Ingram et al, 2007).*
- Provide culturally adapted diabetes self-management education for African American clients with diabetes. EB: *A systematic review of 32 research articles found that culturally appropriate education reduced HbA1c in African American clients by 0.8% (Ricci-Cabello et al, 2013).*
- Encourage involvement of African American client's family and friends in diabetes education activities. CEB: *"Support from family, peers, and health care providers positively influenced adherence behaviors by providing cues to action, direct assistance, reinforcement, and knowledge" (Chlebowy et al, 2010).*

Client/Family Teaching and Discharge Planning

- Provide "survival skills" education or review for hospitalized clients, including information about (1) identification of the health care provider who will provide diabetes care after discharge, (2) diagnosis of diabetes, SMBG, and explanation of home blood glucose goals, (3) information on consistent eating patterns, (4) when and how to take medications including insulin administration, (5) proper use and disposal of needles and syringes if applicable, (6) definition, recognition, treatment, and prevention of hyperglycemia and hypoglycemia, and (7) sick-day management. EB: *"For the hospitalized patient, diabetes 'survival skills' education is generally a feasible approach to provide sufficient information and training to enable safe care at home" (ADA, 2014a).*
- Evaluate clients' monitoring technique initially and at regular intervals. *Accuracy of SMBG is instrument- and user-dependent (ADA, 2014a).*
- Teach client how to match prandial insulin dose to carbohydrate intake, premeal blood glucose, and anticipated activity. EB: *"Results of SMBG can be useful in preventing hypoglycemia and adjusting medications (particularly prandial insulin doses), medical nutrition therapy (MNT), and physical activity" (ADA, 2014a).*

▲ Refer client for Blood Glucose Awareness Training (BGAT) or Web-based training available at http://www.BGAThome.com for instruction in detection, anticipation, avoidance, and treatment of extremes in blood glucose levels. CEB: *BGAT has been shown to significantly reduce both hypoglycemia and hyperglycemia (Cox et al, 2006), and BGAThome resulted in significant clinical improvements (Cox et al, 2008).*

- Teach client to maintain a blood glucose log. A results log can help clients track their response to treatment. Many logs are available online (*ADA, 2014b*).
- Provide group-based training programs for instruction. EB: *"Comprehensive group diabetes education programs including nutrition therapy or individualized education sessions have reported A_{1C} decreases of 0.3% to 1% for type 1 diabetes and 0.5% to 2% for type 2 diabetes" (ADA, 2014a).*
- Teach client the importance of at least 150 minutes/week of moderate-intensity aerobic physical activity (50% to 70% of maximum heart rate), spread over at least 3 days per week. EB: *"Regular exercise has been shown to improve blood glucose control, reduce cardiovascular risk factors, contribute to weight loss, and improve well-being (ADA, 2014a).*

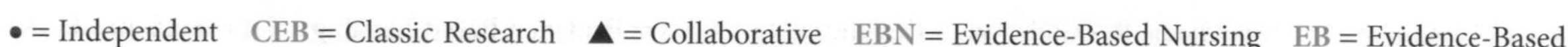

- Discuss recommending resistance training with client's provider. **EB:** *Clinical trials have provided strong evidence for the A_{1C}-lowering value of resistance training in older adults with type 2 diabetes and for an additive benefit of combined aerobic and resistance exercise in adults with type 2 diabetes (ADA, 2014a).*
- Teach client with type 1 diabetes to avoid vigorous activity if ketones are present in urine or blood. Exercise can worsen hyperglycemia and ketosis in people deprived of insulin for 12 to 48 hours *(ADA, 2014a).*
- Teach clients who are treated with insulin or insulin-stimulating oral agents to eat added carbohydrates before exercise if glucose levels are below 100 mg/dL. Physical activity can cause hypoglycemia if medication dose or carbohydrate consumption is not altered (ADA, 2014a).

▲ Teach clients on multiple-dose insulin or insulin pump therapy to perform SMBG before critical tasks such as driving. **EB:** *"Patients should understand ... that hypoglycemia may increase the risk of harm to self or other such as with driving" (ADA, 2014a).*

▲ Teach clients to use alcohol with caution. **EB:** *Alcohol consumption may place people with diabetes at increased risk for delayed hypoglycemia, especially if taking insulin or insulin secretagogues (ADA, 2014a).*

REFERENCES

American Association of Clinical Endocrinologists. (AACE, 2014). Medical guidelines for clinical practice for developing a diabetes mellitus comprehensive care plan. *National Guideline Clearinghouse, Agency for Healthcare Research and Quality,* Retrieved from: <http://www.guideline.gov/content.aspx?id=34038>.

American Diabetes Association. (ADA, 2014a). Clinical practice recommendations. *Diabetes Care, 37*(Suppl. 1).

American Diabetes Association. (ADA, 2014b). *Checking your blood glucose.* Retrieved from: <http://www.diabetes.org/living-with-diabetes/treatment-and-care/blood-glucose-control/checking-your-blood-glucose.html>.

Battelino, T., Phillip, M., Bratina, N., et al. (2011). Effect of continuous glucose monitoring on hypoglycemia in type 1 diabetes. *Diabetes Care, 34*(4), 795–800.

Chlebowy, D. O., Hood, S., & LaJoie, A. S. (2010). Facilitators and barriers to self-management of type 2 diabetes among urban African American adults: focus group findings. *The Diabetes Educator, 36*(6), 897–905.

Cox, D. J., et al. (2006). Blood glucose awareness training: what is it, where is it, and where is it going? *Diabetes Spectrum, 19*(1), 43–49.

Cox, D. J., et al. (2008). Blood glucose awareness training delivered over the Internet. *Diabetes Care, 31*(8), 1527–1528.

Goldberg, P. A., et al. (2006). "Waste not, want not": determining the optimal priming volume for intravenous insulin infusions. *Diabetes Technology and Therapeutics, 8*(5), 598–601.

Ingram, M., et al. (2007). The impact of promotoras on social support and glycemic control among members of a farmworker community on the US-Mexico border. *The Diabetes Educator, 33*(Suppl. 6), 172S–178S.

Kirk, J. K., et al. (2011). Blood glucose symptom recognition: perspectives of older rural adults. *The Diabetes Educator, 37*(3), 363–369.

Malanda, U. L. (2012). Self-monitoring of blood glucose in patients with type 2 diabetes mellitus who are not using insulin. *Cochrane Database of Systematic Reviews,* (1), Art. No.: CD005060, Retrieved from: <http://summaries.cochrane.org/CD005060/self-monitoring-of-blood-glucose-in-patients-with-type-2-diabetes-mellitus-who-are-not-using-insulin#sthash.ML41WJk1.dpuf>.

National Prescribing Service Limited (NPS). (2011). *Medicines that affect blood glucose levels in type 2 diabetes.* Retrieved from: <http://www.nps.org.au/conditions/hormones-metabolism-and-nutritional-problems/diabetes-type-2/for-individuals/medicines-and-treatments/medicines-that-affect-blood-glucose-levels>.

Pfützner, J., et al. (2011). Evaluation of dexterity in insulin-treated patients with type 1 and type 2 diabetes mellitus. *Journal of Diabetes Science and Technology, 5*(1), 158–165.

Phillips, S., & Phillips, A. (2011). Diabetes evidence based management: diabetes and older people: ensuring individualized practice. *Practical Nursing, 22*(4), 196–200.

Ricci-Cabello, I., et al. (2013). Health care interventions to improve the quality of diabetes care in African Americans—a systematic review and meta analysis. *Diabetes Care, 36*(March), 760–768.

Rubin, D., et al. (2011). Weight-based, insulin dose-related hypoglycemia in hospitalized patients with diabetes. *Diabetes Care, 34*(8), 1723–1728.

Sander, E., Odell, S., & Hood, K. (2010). Diabetes-specific family conflict and blood glucose monitoring in adolescents with type 1 diabetes: mediational role of diabetes self efficacy. *Diabetes Spectrum, 23*(2), 89–94.

Zahid, N., et al. (2008). Adsorption of insulin onto infusion sets used in adult intensive care unit and neonatal care settings. *Diabetes Research and Clinical Practice, 80*(3), e11–e13.

Zeh, P., et al. (2012). The impact of culturally competent diabetes care interventions for improving diabetes-related outcomes in ethnic minority groups: a systematic review. *Diabetic Medicine: A Journal of the British Diabetic Association, 29*(10), 1237–1252.

Ziegler, R., et al. (2011). Frequency of SMBG correlates with HbA1c and acute complications in children and adolescents with type 1 diabetes. *Pediatric Diabetes, 12*(1), 11–17.

Grieving

Ruth A. Wittmann-Price, PhD, RN, CNS, CNE, CHSE, ANEF, FAAN

NANDA-I

Definition

A normal complex process that includes emotional, physical, spiritual, social, and intellectual responses and behaviors by which individuals, families, and communities incorporate an actual, anticipated, or perceived loss into their daily lives

Defining Characteristics

Alteration in activity level; alteration in dream pattern; alteration in immune functioning; alteration in neuroendocrine functioning; alteration in sleep pattern; anger; blaming; despair; detachment; disorganization; finding meaning in a loss; guilt about feeling relieved; maintaining a connection to the deceased; pain; panic behavior; personal growth; psychological distress; suffering

Related Factors (r/t)

Anticipatory loss of significant object (e.g., possession, job status); anticipatory loss of significant other; death of significant other; loss of significant object (e.g., possession, job, status, home, body part)

NOC (Nursing Outcomes Classification)

Suggested NOC Outcomes

Grief Resolution; Dignified Life Closure; Hope; Psychosocial Adjustment: Life Change

Example NOC Outcome with Indicators

Grief Resolution as evidenced by the following indicators: Resolves feelings about the loss/Verbalizes reality and acceptance of loss/Maintains living environment/Seeks social support. (Rate the outcome and indicators of **Grief Resolution:** 1 = never demonstrated, 2 = rarely demonstrated, 3 = sometimes demonstrated, 4 = often demonstrated, 5 = consistently demonstrated [see Section I].)

Client/Family Outcomes

Client/Family Will (Specify Time Frame)

- Discuss meaning of the loss to his/her life and the functioning of the family
- Identify ways to support family members and articulate methods of support he/she requires from family and friends
- Accept assistance in meeting the needs of the family from friends/extended family

NIC (Nursing Interventions Classification)

Suggested NIC Interventions

Grief Work Facilitation; Dying Care; Emotional Support: Perinatal Death; Hope Instillation; Support System Enhancement; Family Support; Family Integrity Promotion

Example NIC Activities—Grief Work Facilitation

Identify the loss; Encourage expression of feelings about the loss; Assist to identify personal coping strategies; Identify sources of community support

Nursing Interventions and *Rationales*

Anticipatory Grieving Interventions

- Grieving of a critically ill or dying client and clients' family/relatives for the losses experienced during the deteriorating illness, and the future that will be filled with loss. EB: *Boer et al (2014) validated the use of the Acceptance of Disease and Impairments Questionnaire scale with clients (N = 145) with chronic obstructive pulmonary disease to identify the four stages of grieving that clients go through: denial, resistance, sorrow, and acceptance.*
- Develop a trusting relationship both with the client and with the family by using presence and therapeutic communication techniques. EB: *Hobgood et al (2013) studied emergency medical services personnel's (N = 30) preparation for notifying family about deaths using a program called GRIEVING and found an increase in confidence and competency, but communication was not significantly changed, warranting further research in this population of health care providers.* EBN: *Janze and Henriksson (2014) qualitatively explored family experiences when providing care to a terminally ill partner. Two themes resulted: (1) living in uncertainty and (2) preparing for caregiving in the awareness of death. Both issues can be addressed by therapeutic nursing communication.*
- Keep the family apprised of the client's ongoing condition as much as possible. Consult with the family for decision-making as appropriate. EBN: *McLeod-Sordjan (2014) found that 40% of older clients require decision-making and communication in the final days of life. Part of that communication should be about death preparedness with a health care provider regarding how the client would like their end of life to unfold and developing a plan.*
- Keep the family informed of client's needs for physical care and support in symptom control, and inform them about health care options at the end of life, including palliative care, hospice care, and home care. EB: *In a multicultural qualitative study, Angelo and Wilson (2014) explored participants' (N = 6) experiences in caring for a dying family member. Important themes were food preparation, spirituality, and family gathering.*
- Discuss preferred place of death (PPD) with client. EB: *Kulkarni et al (2014) studied the PPD by questionnaire and found that most people preferred to die at home where they would be more comfortable; therefore, clients should be asked about their PPD.* EBN: *Evans et al (2014) studied whether clients changed their PPD and found that the majority of clients (N = 204) in palliative care were able to identify a PPD and only 15% changed their PPD as the time of death approached.*
- Ask family members if they are receiving sufficient sleep. If a family member desires to be in the room for sleep, provide a reclining chair or portable bed if possible, and bedding to keep the family member comfortable. If needed, find housing for family member from out of town with support of case manager or social worker. EB: *Estevens et al (2014) qualitatively studied primary caregiver's perspective when caring for a terminally ill client and found that caregivers wanted to be in that role and also preferred the death to take place at home.* EBN: *Dosser and Kennedy (2014) completed a participatory action research study to determine family support at the end of life in a hospital setting and identified two things that would assist them: (1) improving nurses' communication skills and (2) improving the environment for family caregivers.*
- Ask family member about having adequate resources to care for themselves and the critically ill family member. EBN: *Cowan (2014) explored the experiences of Sikh (English) clients (N = 6) when caring for a dying client at home and found five themes: (1) being placed in the caring role, (2) emotional effects on the caregiver, (3) impact on family, (4) influence of health care services, and (5) religious influence. Additionally, clients felt a lack of support from health care professionals and did not always know about available services.*
- Listen to the family member's story. EB: *Gillies et al (2014) developed a reliable 30-category codebook with negative and positive themes from analysis of adults (N = 162) who were grieving to help professionals provide support to families who were losing a loved one.*
- Encourage family members to show their caring feelings and talk to the client. EBN: *Devery et al (2014) completed a systematic review of the literature (N = 8) about death bed phenomena (DBP), which is when a dying client recalls a significant dream or sees a dead relative and the experience is deeply meaningful. The research demonstrated that DBP brings comfort, peace, and reassurance; therefore, the significance of DBP should be recognized and health professionals and families should encourage clients to discuss them.*

- Recognize and respect different feelings and wishes from both the family members and the client. EB: *Researchers investigated whether homebound end-of-life clients (N = 77) had anticipatory medications prescribed for comfort and found only 54% had anticipatory medications prescribed and only 15% had prescriptions for recommended anticipatory medications, noting more attention by health professionals needs to be paid to making sure families have the proper medications to care for their loved one (Finucane et al, 2014).*
- If necessary, refer a family member for counseling or to a minister/priest to help him/her cope with the existential questions and current overwhelming reality. EBN: *Ramezani et al (2014) completed a concept analysis of spiritual care (N = 158) and found the attributes include healing presence, therapeutic use of self, intuitive sense, exploration of the spiritual perspective, client-centeredness, and creating a spiritually nurturing environment. Establishing a definition of spiritual care was done to increase nursing knowledge about holistic client care.*
- Recognize that one family member may be in a state of caregiver role strain from a long caregiving situation. EBN: *Yang et al (2014) investigated the role strain of family caregivers (N = 197) of clients with dementia using a cross-sectional correlational survey and found that having resources, predictability, and being prepared moderated the effects of role strain.*
- Promote the family roles as appropriate. EBN: *Al-Gamal (2013) used a cross-sectional descriptive correlational design to understand parents (N = 204) caring for a child with cerebral palsy (CP) and found that parents had high levels of anticipatory grief and lower quality of life compared with other parents who did not have a child with special needs child.*
- Promote mutual goal setting where decisions are made together that affect the family. EBN: *McLeod (2014) studied end-of-life decision-making related to intensive care unit (ICU) clients and families and explored ICU nurses' (N = 6) experiences in withdrawing treatment. The researcher concluded that treatment withdrawal creates significant professional and personal dilemmas that call for open discussion and collaborative decision-making with other health care professionals as well as family members.*

Grieving Interventions When Death of a Loved One Occurs

- Use the following activities when interacting with the bereaved person:
  - Be present and attentive, use active empathetic listening. EBN: *Researchers qualitatively explored the beliefs of recently bereaved clients (N = 46) about death to better understand bereavement care and found three themes: (1) death was described in terms of religious, dualist, eco-spiritualist, materialist, and death-as-transition; (2) life after death such as resurrection, reuniting, and reincarnation; and (3) relationship with the deceased person continuing after death due to a sense of presence (Draper et al, 2014).*
  - Validate the client's feelings of grief and feeling hurt, stressful, anxious, out of control, and further symptoms of grieving. EBN: *Ly Thuy et al (2014) sampled 251 palliative nurses who identified that they need to feel more competent in pain management, psychological and spiritual care, and communication while working with terminally ill oncology clients in order to better handle their clients' feelings and needs.*
  - Provide time and space for the person to tell their story of loss. EBN: *Braband et al (2014) conducted a qualitative study to evaluate the use of the Memory Book intervention for grief and loss recovery and found that it helped children to work through loss and grief when they are assisted in preserving and telling their story. Memory books may be a helpful nursing interaction for older clients also.*
  - Offer condolences: "I am sorry that you lost your husband." EB: *Collins (2014) explored by longitudinal method (18 months) the experiences of older widowed women (N = 26) and found the following themes: (1) family friction, (2) dependence, (3) additional losses, (4) overcommitment, (5) passivity, and (5) feeling different from other women.*
  - Explain that feelings will oscillate as the person does grief work, from coping to accept the loss to coping to build a new life without the loved one. EB: *Funk et al (2013) studied health care workers' (N = 11) grief management related to end-of-life care and reported personnel challenges due to witnessing death and experiencing loss; personnel often felt helplessness and frustration. To overcome negative feelings, participants often used "consoling refrains," such as, "Such is life," "They are better off," "They had a full life," "I did my best," and "I experience rewards."*
  - Intentionally schedule meetings with family members to provide support during grieving. EBN: *Lee and King (2014) found that caregivers of hemodialysis clients experience psychological stress, including death anxiety, unresolved grieving, and burnout, and found in their quantitative study that educational classes decreased participants' level of death anxiety and emotional exhaustion.*

- Refer to mental health providers as needed. EB: *Breen and O'Connor (2013) found inequalities in service delivery for cancer clients and their families (N = 11) living in rural areas. Lack of grief referral availability was categorized as (1) inequity of services, (2) strain being the "Jack of all trades" role, (3) lack of education, and (4) challenges in delivering post-bereavement services.*
- Help the client use a method to give voice to his unique story of loss. Methods include keeping a personal journal to record feelings and insights, retelling of the loss narrative to a caring person, music therapy techniques with a trained therapist or listening to music that has significance to the relationship, use of the "virtual dream," a dreamlike short story written by the grieving person to tell the narrative of the loss.
- Discuss coping methods with the grieving person. Common coping techniques include exercise, telling the story of grief to a caring person, journaling, pets, and developing a legacy for the deceased. EB: *Parikh and Servaty-Seib (2013) studied college students' (N = 23) beliefs about supporting a grieving friend using open-ended questions and found that students listened supportively to a friend in need and found a quiet place to do so.*
- Encourage the family to create a quiet and comfortable healing environment, and follow comforting grief rituals such as prayer, interacting with nature, or lighting votive candles. EB: *A study looked at how parents (N = 155) make meaning out of the loss of a child and found that many clients use spiritual and religious meanings and the cultivation of empathy for the suffering of others (Lichtenthal et al, 2013).*
- Refer the family members for spiritual counseling if desired. EBN: *Hatamipour et al (2015) qualitatively studied spiritual needs of cancer clients (N = 18) in Iran and identified four themes (connection, peace, meaning and purpose, and transcendence) that were integrated with verbalization about social support, normal behavior, inner peace, seeking forgiveness, hope, acceptance of reality, seeking meaning, ending well, change of life meaning, strengthening spiritual belief, communication with God, and prayer.*
- Help the family determine the best way and place to find social support. Encourage family members to continue to use supports as needed for years. EBN: *A qualitative study using a grounded theory method described how nurses (N = 22) engaged with families who had a member in palliative care and found that different families had different expectations, and the best intervention was to provide engaged and consistent care (Namasivavam et al, 2014).*
- Identify available community resources, including bereavement groups at local hospitals and hospice centers. Volunteers who provide bereavement support can also be effective. EBN: *Jennings and Nicholl (2014) investigated the bereavement support of mothers following the death of their child with a qualitative descriptive design study and found that the mothers used a combination of informal and formal bereavement support.*
- Refer to complicated **Grieving** if grieving fails to follow normative (or cultural) expectations and manifests in functional impairment.

Pediatric/Parent

- Treat the child/parents with respect, give him/her opportunity to talk about concerns and answer questions honestly. EB: *Quinn-Lee (2014) studied social workers' experience (N = 22) with grieving children by a qualitative online method and found four main themes: (1) barriers prevent helping grieving students, (2) grief is defined differently by children, (3) social workers are not always prepared to deal with grief, and (4) students may need referrals to outside resources.* EB: *Researchers retrospectively looked at the time between extubation and documented cardiorespiratory in neonates (N = 117) who died in a neonatal intensive care unit in order to provide parents with a realistic time frame to assist with grieving (Saha & Kent, 2014).*
- Listen to the child's expression of grief. EBN: *A qualitative study with parents (N = 8) demonstrated that reactions to young children's grief was a balance between shielding including, informing/frightening, and creating a new life/cherishing the old (Bugge et al, 2014).*
- Help parents recognize that the grieving child does not have to be "fixed"; instead they need support going through an experience of grieving just as adults do. EB: *Researchers performed a mixed-methods investigation to study the impact of maternal death on families and children; findings demonstrated that maternal death has different effects on boy and girl children, and actually increases the risks for girl children to get married and pregnant early and to drop out of school in South Africa. Similar studies are needed in other populations (Yamin et al, 2015).*

G

- Consider the use of art for children in hospice care who are dying or dealing with the death of a parent, sibling, or other family member. EB: *Researchers tested a new intervention (MEND), which includes dialogue and art therapy to address the needs of families (N = 22) with a child with a chronic illnesses. Results demonstrated that the MEND program had positive effects across many psychosocial measures (Distelberg et al, 2014).*
- ▲ Refer grieving children and parents to a program to help facilitate grieving if desired, especially if the death was traumatic. EB: *A qualitative study of Israeli parents (N = 16) whose children were killed in terror attacks revealed, though interviews, four themes: (1) inclusiveness is helpful, (2) the "family of the bereaved' is most important in the healing process, (3) nongovernmental services are preferred, and (4) engaging in the heritage of the Jewish people helped (Possick et al, 2014).*
- Help the adolescent determine sources of support and how to use them effectively. EB: *A study looked at parental death in South African adolescents (N = 381) and its impact on functioning, comparing double, single, and non-orphans and examined bereavement, depression, behavior problems, and violence. Results showed double orphans had increased depression and poorer psychosocial functioning, and were more likely to be abused than single orphans or non-orphans (Sherr et al, 2014).*
- Encourage grieving parents to take good care of their own health. EB: *Aho et al (2013) investigated the experiences of peer supporters (N = 16) of bereavement interventions for grieving parents to analyze the program that included a support package for grieving parents, peer supporters' contact, and health care personnel's contact with parents and found that parents were willing to receive peer support and peer supporters were a good resource to encourage parents to care for themselves during the time of grieving.*
- ▲ Encourage grieving parents to seek mental health services as needed. The death of a child is regarded as among the most traumatic, incomprehensible, and devastating of losses, with the potential to precipitate a crisis of meaning for the bereaved parent. EBN: *Brännström (2014) did literature review (N = 55) about women who experienced a sudden infant death and found three themes: (1) women bear guilt and accountability, (2) social ordering portrays women as principal caregiver, and (3) women are marginalized socially in family policies. The researchers encourage further studies to recognize infant nursing practices, gender equality, and safe parenthood in child health research and nursing practices.*
- Recognize that men and women often grieve differently, and explain this to parents if it becomes an issue. EBN: *Steen (2015) studied multicultural perinatal bereavement interventions (N = 59) by using a cross-sectional method and found differences in interventions by nurses/midwives in different countries regarding knowledge, communication skills, and management of personal feelings, indicating that consistent bereavement information is needed.*
- Recognize that mothers who have a miscarriage/stillbirth grieve and experience sorrow because of loss of the child. EBN: *Tseng et al (2014) completed a qualitative descriptive study about women (N = 21) after stillbirth in which clients described a three-stage emotional journey of recovery: (1) suffering from silent grief, (2) searching for a way out, and (3) achieving peace of mind.*

Geriatric

- Monitor an older adult who has been treated for bereavement-related depression for relapse or recurrence. EB: *Holland et al (2013) studied older clients (N = 169) who lost their spouses to identify what grief experiences predict "intensified grieving" and found that early experiences of nonacceptance significantly predict more intense grief experiences later, suggesting that health professionals working with older clients should pay close attention to nonacceptance.*
- Provide support for the family when the loss is associated with dementia of the family member. EBN: *Graneheim et al (2014) completed a meta-ethnographic study that included 180 descriptions of caregivers' experiences of relinquishing the care of a family member with dementia to a nursing home. The experiences were described as a three-stage grieving process: (1) being responsible for the decision, (2) living with the decision, and (3) adjusting to a role and changed relationship.*
- Determine the social supports of older adults. EBN: *Bellamy et al (2014) interviewed older clients on the telephone about their experiences and sources of bereavement support following the death of a spouse and found that family and friends, as well as community organizations, played a fundamental supporting role for older bereaved adults.*

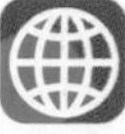

Multicultural

- See interventions and rationales in care plans for complicated **Grieving** and chronic **Sorrow.**

Home Care

- The interventions previously described may be adapted for home care use.
- Assessment of activities of daily living (ADLs) and instrumental ADLs is essential as part of comprehensive care after a home care client has suffered the loss of a loved one. EBN: *Joo and Huber (2014) studied client-centered care provided in the community by conducting an integrative review (N = 6) and found that community-based case management significantly reduced hospital access outcomes, especially readmissions, and increased cost effectiveness, client clinical outcomes, and satisfaction.*
- Actively listen as the client grieves for his or her own death or for real or perceived loss. Normalize the client's expressions of grief for self. Demonstrate a caring and hopeful approach. EB: *Risk (2013) presented a case study of a client suffering from Parkinson's disease and used narrative theory to help the client develop new coping strategies and a new sense of identity as a spiritual, contingent self as the disease eroded the client's physical self and former life.*
- ▲ Refer the client to social services as necessary for losses not related to death. Support is helpful to grief work for all types of losses. Social workers can help the client plan for financial changes as a result of job losses and help with community referrals as appropriate. EB: *Chen et al (2015) conducted a longitudinal study of community-living older residents and used disability, chronic disease, depression, and social service usage data and found changes in levels of disability during the aging process were identified and also found that hypertension and depression were predictors of increased disability among clients and the use of social services such as personal care, homemaker-household, and physical therapy were significantly related to increases in disability.*
- ▲ Refer the bereaved to hospice bereavement programs or an Internet self-help group. Relief of the suffering of clients and families (physical, emotional, and spiritual) is the goal of hospice care. EB: *Hwang et al (2013) compared hospice care and usual care for older clients with terminal hepatocellular carcinoma (N = 729) in a nationwide survey in Taiwan and found that clients in hospice care were treated with better pain control and with less aggressive procedures and medical expenses than clients in hospital care.*

G

REFERENCES

Aho, A. L., Astedt-Kurki, P., & Kaunonen, M. (2013). Peer supporters' experiences of a bereavement follow-up intervention for grieving parents. *Omega: Journal of Death & Dying*, *68*(4), 347–366.

Al-Gamal, E. (2013). Quality of life and anticipatory grieving among parents living with a child with cerebral palsy. *International Journal of Nursing Practice*, *19*(3), 288–294.

Angelo, J., & Wilson, L. (2014). Exploring occupation roles of hospice family caregivers from Māori, Chinese and Tongan ethnic backgrounds living in New Zealand. *Occupational Therapy International*, *21*(2), 81–90.

Bellamy, G., Gott, M., Waterworth, S., et al. (2014). 'But I do believe you've got to accept that that's what life's about': older adults living in New Zealand talk about their experiences of loss and bereavement support. *Health & Social Care in the Community*, *22*(1), 96–103.

Boer, L., Daudey, L., Peters, J., et al. (2014). Assessing the stages of the grieving process in chronic obstructive pulmonary disease (COPD): validation of the acceptance of disease and impairments questionnaire (ADIQ). *International Journal of Behavioral Medicine*, *21*(3), 561–570.

Braband, B. J., Faris, T., & Wilson-Anderson, K. (2014). Evaluation of a memory book intervention with orphaned children in South Africa. *Journal of Pediatric Nursing*, *29*(4), 337–343.

Brännström, I. I. (2014). Speaking discourses and silent lips: women and gender-based portraits in sudden infant death publications. *Journal of Clinical Nursing*, *23*(7/8), 1120–1132.

Breen, L. J., & O'Connor, M. (2013). Rural health professionals' perspectives on providing grief and loss support in cancer care. *European Journal of Cancer Care*, *22*(6), 765–772.

Bugge, K. E., Darebyshire, P., Rokholt, E. G., et al. (2014). Young children's grief: parents' understanding and coping. *Death Studies*, *38*(1), 36–43.

Chen, C., Su, Y., Mullan, J., et al. (2015). Trajectories of disability and their relationship with health status and social service use. *Experimental Aging Research*, *41*(3), 240–258.

Collins, T. (2014). Managing widowhood in later life: the challenges encountered. *International Journal of Therapy & Rehabilitation*, *21*(2), 69–76.

Cowan, M. M. (2014). The lived experiences of the Sikh population of south east England when caring for a dying relative at home. *International Journal of Palliative Nursing*, *20*(4), 179–186.

Devery, K., Rawlings, D., Tieman, J., et al. (2014). Deathbed phenomena reported by patients in palliative care: clinical opportunities and responses. *International Journal of Palliative Nursing*, *21*(3), 117–125.

Distelberg, B., Williams-Reade, J., Tapanes, D., et al. (2014). Evaluation of a family systems intervention for managing pediatric chronic illness: mastering each new direction (MEND). *Family Process*, *53*(2), 194–213.

Dosser, I., & Kennedy, C. (2014). Improving family carers' experiences of support at the end of life by enhancing communication: an action research study. *International Journal of Palliative Nursing*, *20*(12), 608–616.

Draper, P., Holloway, M., & Adamson, S. (2014). A qualitative study of recently bereaved people's beliefs about death: implications for bereavement care. *Journal of Clinical Nursing*, *23*(9/10), 1300–1308.

Estevens Pazes, M. C., Nunes, L., & Barbosa, A. (2014). Factors influencing the experience of the terminal phase and the grieving process: the primary caregiver's perspective. *Revista de Enfermagem Referência*, (3), 95–104.

Evans, R., Finucane, A., Vanhegan, L., et al. (2014). Do place-of-death preferences for patients receiving specialist palliative care change over time? *International Journal of Palliative Nursing, 20*(12), 579–583.

Finucane, A. M., McArthur, D., Stevenson, B., et al. (2014). Anticipatory prescribing at the end of life in Lothian care homes. *British Journal of Community Nursing, 19*(11), 544–547.

Funk, L. M., Waskiewich, S., & Stajduhar, K. I. (2013). Meaning-making and managing difficult feelings: providing front-line end-of-life care. *Omega: Journal of Death & Dying, 68*(1), 23–43.

Gillies, J., Neimeyer, R. A., & Milman, E. (2014). The meaning of loss codebook: construction of a system for analyzing meanings made in bereavement. *Death Studies, 38*(4), 207–216.

Graneheim, U. H., Johansson, A., & Lindgren, B. (2014). Family caregivers' experiences of relinquishing the care of a person with dementia to a nursing home: insights from a meta-ethnographic study. *Scandinavian Journal of Caring Sciences, 28*(2), 215–224.

Hatamipour, K., Rassouli, M., Yaghmaie, F., et al. (2015). Spiritual needs of cancer patients: a qualitative study. *Indian Journal of Palliative Care, 21*(1), 61–67.

Hobgood, C., Mathew, D., Woodyard, D. J., et al. (2013). Death in the field: teaching paramedics to deliver effective death notifications using the educational intervention 'GRIEVING'. *Prehospital Emergency Care, 17*(4), 501–510.

Holland, J. M., Futterman, A., Thompson, L. W., et al. (2013). Difficulties accepting the loss of a spouse: a precursor for intensified grieving among widowed older adults. *Death Studies, 37*(2), 126–144.

Hwang, S., Chang, H., Hwang, I., et al. (2013). Hospice offers more palliative care but costs less than usual care for terminal geriatric hepatocellular carcinoma patients: a nationwide study. *Journal of Palliative Medicine, 16*(7), 780–785.

Janze, A., & Henriksson, A. (2014). Preparing for palliative caregiving as a transition in the awareness of death: family carer experiences. *International Journal of Palliative Nursing, 20*(10), 494–501.

Jennings, V., & Nicholl, H. (2014). Bereavement support used by mothers in Ireland following the death of their child from a life-limiting condition. *International Journal of Palliative Nursing, 20*(4), 173–178.

Joo, J. Y., & Huber, D. L. (2014). An integrative review of nurse-led community-based case management effectiveness. *International Nursing Review, 61*(1), 14–24.

Kulkarni, P., Kulkarni, P., Anavkar, V., et al. (2014). Preference of the place of death among people of Pune. *Indian Journal of Palliative Care, 20*(2), 101–106.

Lee, V. L., & King, A. H. (2014). Exploring death anxiety and burnout among staff members who work in outpatient hemodialysis units. *Nephrology Nursing Journal: Journal of the American Nephrology Nurses' Association, 41*(5), 479–486.

Lichtenthal, W. O., Neimeyer, R. A., Currier, J. M., et al. (2013). Cause of death and the quest for meaning after the loss of a child. *Death Studies, 37*(4), 311–342.

Ly Thuy, N., Yates, P., & Osborne, Y. (2014). Palliative care knowledge, attitudes and perceived self-competence of nurses working in Vietnam. *International Journal of Palliative Nursing, 20*(9), 448–456.

McLeod, A. (2014). Nurses' views of the causes of ethical dilemmas during treatment cessation in the ICU: a qualitative study. *British Journal of Neuroscience Nursing, 10*(3), 131–137.

McLeod-Sordjan, R. (2014). Death preparedness: A concept analysis. *Journal of Advanced Nursing, 70*(5), 1008–1019.

Namasivavam, P., Lee, S., O'Connor, M., et al. (2014). Caring for families of the terminally ill in Malaysia from palliative care nurses' perspectives. *Journal of Clinical Nursing, 23*(1/2), 173–180.

Parikh, S. J., & Servaty-Seib, H. L. (2013). College students' beliefs about supporting a grieving peer. *Death Studies, 37*(7), 653–669.

Possick, C., Shamai, M., & Sadeh, R. (2014). Healing the social self: How parents whose children were killed in terror attacks construct the experience of help. *Community Mental Health Journal, 50*(4), 487–496.

Quinn-Lee, L. (2014). School social work with grieving children. *Children & Schools, 36*(2), 93–103.

Ramezani, M., Ahmadi, F., Mohammadi, E., et al. (2014). Spiritual care in nursing: a concept analysis. *International Nursing Review, 61*(2), 211–219.

Risk, J. L. (2013). Building a new life: A Chaplain's theory based case study of chronic illness. *Journal of Health Care Chaplaincy, 19*(3), 81–98.

Saha, S., & Kent, A. L. (2014). Length of time from extubation to cardiorespiratory death in neonatal intensive care patients and assessment of suitability for organ donation. *Archives of Disease in Childhood. Fetal and Neonatal Edition, 99*(1), F59–F63.

Sherr, L., Croome, N., Clucas, C., et al. (2014). Differential effects of single and double parental death on child emotional functioning and daily life in South Africa. *Child Welfare, 93*(1), 149–172.

Steen, S. E. (2015). Perinatal death: bereavement interventions used by US and Spanish nurses and midwives. *International Journal of Palliative Nursing, 21*(2), 79–86.

Tseng, Y., Chen, C., & Wang, H. (2014). Taiwanese women's process of recovery from stillbirth: a qualitative descriptive study. *Research in Nursing & Health, 37*(3), 219–228.

Yamin, A. E., Bazile, J., Knight, L., et al. (2015). Tracing shadows: How gendered power relations shape the impacts of maternal death on living children in sub Saharan Africa. *Social Science & Medicine, 135*, 143–150.

Yang, C., Liu, H., & Shyu, Y. L. (2014). Dyadic relational resources and role strain in family caregivers of persons living with dementia at home: a cross-sectional survey. *International Journal of Nursing Studies, 51*(4), 593–602.

Complicated Grieving

Ruth A. Wittmann-Price, PhD, RN, CNS, CNE, CHSE, ANEF, FAAN, and Betty J. Ackley, MSN, EdS, RN

NANDA-I

Definition

A disorder that occurs after the death of a significant other in which the experience of distress accompanying bereavement fails to follow normative expectations and manifests in functional impairment

Defining Characteristics

Anger; anxiety; avoidance of grieving; decrease in functioning in life roles; depression; disbelief; distress about the deceased person; excessive stress; experiencing symptoms the deceased experienced; fatigue; feeling dazed; feeling of detachment from others; feeling of shock; feeling stunned; feelings of emptiness; insufficient same of well-being; longing for the deceased person; low levels of intimacy; mistrust; non-acceptance of a death; persistent painful memories; preoccupation with thoughts about a deceased person; rumination; searching for a deceased person; self-blame; separation distress; traumatic distress; yearning for deceased person

Related Factors (r/t)

Death of a significant other; emotional disturbance; insufficient social support (Adapted from the work of NANDA-I)

G

NOC (Nursing Outcomes Classification)

Suggested NOC Outcomes

Anxiety Level; Coping; Depression; Grief Resolution; Mood Equilibrium; Personal Well-Being; Psychosocial Adjustment: Life Change; Sleep

Example NOC Outcome with Indicators

See care plan for **Grieving.**

Client Outcomes

Client Will (Specify Time Frame)

- Express appropriate feelings of guilt, fear, anger, or sadness
- Identify somatic distress associated with grief (e.g., anxiety, changes in appetite, insomnia, nightmares, loss of libido, decreased energy, altered activity levels)
- Seek support in dealing with grief-associated issues
- Identify personal strengths and effective coping strategies
- Function at a normal developmental level and begin to successfully and increasingly perform activities of daily living

NIC (Nursing Interventions Classification)

Suggested NIC Interventions

Grief Work Facilitation; Grief Work Facilitation: Perinatal Death; Guilt Work Facilitation; Hope Installation

Example NIC Activities—Grief Work Facilitation

See care plan for **Grieving.**

Nursing Interventions and *Rationales*

- Assess for signs of complicated grieving that include symptoms that persist at least 6 months after the death and are experienced at least daily or to a disabling degree. Symptoms include feeling emotionally numb, stunned, shocked, and that life is meaningless; dysfunctional thoughts and maladaptive behaviors; experiencing mistrust and estrangement from others; anger and bitterness over the loss; identity confusion; avoidance of the reality of the loss, or excessive proximity seeking to try to feel closer to the deceased, sometimes focused on wishes to die or suicidal statements and behavior; or difficulty moving on with life. *Symptoms must be associated with functional impairment (Maercker et al, 2013; Shear et al, 2013).* EB: *Jordan and Litz (2014) describe the difference between normal bereavement reactions and prolonged grief disorder (PGD), which many times coexists with depression in the clients studied, and they suggest medication should be one treatment considered for PGD.* EB: *McKinnon and Chonody (2014) qualitatively interviewed survivors (N = 14) of loved ones who committed suicide, and their responses ranged from compassionate to coldness; therefore, the researchers concluded that survivors require support for their unique grief, yet they are inconsistently offered care and provided with information regarding available services.*

▲ Determine the client's state of grieving. Use a tool such as the Prolonged Grief Disorder (PGD) scale (Jordan & Litz, 2014), the Grief Support in Health Care Scale (Anderson et al, 2010), the Hogan Grief Reaction Checklist (Hogan et al, 2004), and the Beck Depression Inventory. EBN: *Al-Gamal and Long (2014) modified the MM-CGI Childhood Cancer to evaluate parents' anticipatory grief with children with cerebral palsy (CP) and used a cross-sectional, descriptive, correlational design to validate the subscales accurately measure the dimensions of anticipatory grief with good internal consistency reliability and construct validity.*

G

▲ Determine whether the client is experiencing depression, suicidal tendencies, or other emotional disorders. Refer the client for counseling or therapy as appropriate. EB: *Burke et al (2014) interviewed five families and revealed an association between complicated grief and complicated spiritual grief defined as a spiritual crisis following loss. The researchers found the clients expressed three major themes during the interviews, including (1) resentment for and doubt of God, (2) dissatisfaction with spiritual support, and (3) changes in spiritual beliefs and behaviors.* EB: *Gillies et al (2014) developed a 30-category coding system for positive and negative feelings experienced by clients (N = 162) who suffered the loss of a loved one; statistical analysis supports the coding system as reliable, comprehensive, and useful in studies about grief therapy.*

• Educate the client and his or her support systems that grief resolution is not a sequential process and that the positive outcome of grief resolution is the integration of the deceased into the ongoing life of the griever. EB: *Bentley and O'Connor (2015) interviewed bereaved family members (N = 22) to examine the most appropriate time to interview them about the death of their family member with motor neuron disease (MND) and/or cancer and found that 86% felt comfortable being interviewed within 5 months; of those, 43% reported they could be interviewed within weeks after the death.*

▲ Assess caregivers, particularly younger caregivers, for pessimistic thinking and additional stressful life events. Refer for appropriate support. EB: *Avelin et al (2014) interviewed adolescents (N = 13) who experienced the stillbirth of a half-sibling and found the main theme to be sadness, but the clients expressed feelings of not being totally included in family grief process, implying that half-siblings of the deceased infant need to be fully included in the grieving process.* EBN: *Cinzia et al (2014) performed a literature review (N = 14) to study the experiences and needs of adolescents who lose a parent to a chronic illness and identified four themes: (1) response to the loss, (2) the teenagers' life after the death, (3) coping strategies, and (4) the factors influencing the grieving process. These elements should be addressed by health professionals, parents, teachers, and therapists when counseling adolescents who lose a parent.*

• See the interventions and rationales in the care plans for **Grieving** and Chronic **Sorrow.**

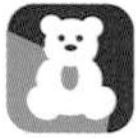

Pediatric/Parent

▲ Refer grieving children and parents to a program to help facilitate grieving if desired, especially if the death was traumatic. EB: *Thienprayoon et al (2015) studied the bereavement services in U.S. pediatric hospitals by an online survey to chaplains (N = 70) and found that 47.8% of respondents felt resources are not adequate and need to include increased staff, financial resources, and consistency in services.* EBN: *Howes (2015) conducted a literature review (N = 8) about the provision of end-of-life care in pediatric intensive care units because the care delivered to a child and family surrounding death can have a lasting effect on the grieving process. Howes identified many challenges facing children, parents, and staff related to family views, staff views, decision-making, medicolegal issues, and resources, indicating the need for further research to inform clinical protocols.*

• Encourage grieving parents to take part in activities that are supportive, such as faith based activities. EB: *A qualitative study of Israeli parents (N = 16) whose children were killed in terror attacks revealed, though interviews, four themes: (1) inclusiveness is helpful, (2) the "family of the bereaved' is most important in the healing process, (3) nongovernmental services are preferred, and (4) engaging in the heritage of the Jewish people helped (Possick et al, 2014). These elements inform the development and delivery of psychosocial services.*

• *Encourage grieving parents to seek mental health services as needed.* EBN: *Steen (2015) surveyed U.S. (N = 44) and Spanish (N = 15) nurses about the interventions used in cases of perinatal death and found that interventions (accompanying, listening, offering keepsakes, baptism discussion, and funeral planning) were significantly different between the two groups, which demonstrates a need to promote an international nursing standard of perinatal bereavement care.* EBN: *A grounded theory study examined black adolescents' (N = 8) experience with perinatal loss, and the results revealed stages that clients went through to ultimately "enduring to gain new perspective." First the clients felt "denying and hesitating" about the pregnancy, then "getting ready for this whole new life," followed by shock of "suffering through the loss," "all that pain for nothing," and "mixed emotions going everywhere." Researchers identified that clients "over time" reached out for support, which has implications for continuing nursing care (Fenstermacher, 2014).*

- Help the adolescent determine sources of support and how to use them effectively. If client is an adolescent exposed to a peer's suicide, watch for symptoms of traumatic grief as well as post-traumatic stress disorder, which include numbness, preoccupation with the deceased, functional impairment, and poor adjustment to the loss. EB: *Quinn-Lee (2014) interviewed 59 school social workers about their experiences with student grieving in an exploratory study using constant comparison and identified four important themes: (1) barriers to helping grieving students, (2) variations on how grief is defined, (3) social workers' preparation for dealing with grief, and (4) referrals of grieving students to outside resources.* EB: *Currier et al (2015) studied bereaved young adults (N = 195) and measured their attachment-related insecurities (anxiety and avoidance), their continuing bond (CB) to the deceased, and their complicated grief (CG) manifestations and found that CBs were less predictive of CG symptoms in clients with high anxiety and low avoidance, and more predictive for clients whose attachment styles were highly avoidant and minimally anxious.*

G

Geriatric

- Assess for deterioration in bereaved older adults' self-care. EBN: *Bellamy et al (2014) conducted telephone interviews with older clients (N = 28) about experiences with bereavement support following the death of a spouse or family member and found that family and friends and community-based organizations play an important supportive role, and they did not see the need for formal bereavement support services because they had life experiences and developed coping mechanisms. This study suggests that community and family supports need to be assessed for older bereaved clients.* EBN: *Gray (2014) studied clients entering the final phase of their lives and noted many older clients have well-established habits and rituals and found that they often struggle to balance addictive behaviors and a disciplined lifestyle in their quest to find a balance between meaningful fulfillment and the need to find pleasure in living the final years.*
- Those who have lived with older adults with dementia and experienced significant feelings of loss before the loved one's death may be at risk for more intense feelings of grief after the death of the client with dementia. EBN: *Lindauer and Harvath (2014) analyzed the concept of pre-death grief in families who were caring for a client with dementia (N = 49) and found it was associated with depression, burden, and caregiver coping.* EBN: *A qualitative study interviewed caregivers (N = 6) of clients with dementia about their counseling experiences and caregivers identified three themes: (1) feeling connected, (2) being understood, and (3) wanting to share information. All participants thought that counseling created "safe space" to disclose and share concerns (Elvish et al, 2014).*
- Monitor the older client for complicated grieving manifesting in physical and mental health problems. EBN: *McLeod-Sordjan (2014) analyzed death preparedness related to communication and end-of-life shared decisions and found that 40% of geriatric clients noted it involved a transition from denial to communication with a health care provider and that the client has to become aware and implement a plan.* EB: *Stahl and Schulz (2013) completed a systematic review (N = 32) to analyze the relationship between late-life spousal bereavement and changes in routine health and found that geriatric clients are at risk for poor nutrition, weight loss, impaired sleep, and increased alcohol consumption, which all have clinical implications for nursing interventions.*

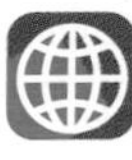

Multicultural

- Assess for the influence of cultural beliefs, norms, and values on the client's grief and mourning practices. EB: *Neimeyer and Young-Eisendrath (2015) developed a bereavement intervention for Buddhist clients (N = 41) to deal with their belief of impermanence, which assists clients to reflect on the natural conditions of impermanence and provides a compassionate environment.* EBN: *Lee et al (2014) studied prolonged grief manifestations among clients (N = 22) who reported near-death experiences (NDEs) using an online survey and found that NDEs are associated with grief, meaning-making, and religion.*
- Encourage discussion of the grief process. EB: *Young et al (2014) conducted interviews about bereavement among people with profound and multiple learning disabilities (PMLDs) and their caregivers and used the information to develop a bereavement learning resource pack specifically for people with PMLD and their caregivers.* EB: *McRitchie et al (2014) qualitatively studied the bereavement experiences of clients (N = 13)*

with intellectual disabilities. Results confirmed that the experiences of such clients follow the patterns of the general population but they feel more disenfranchised, which supports the need for open communication, information, and inclusion.

- Identify whether the client had been notified of the health status of the deceased and was able to be present during illness and death. EB: *Dhiliwal and Muckaden (2015) studied clients (N = 690) using home care services for terminal cancer using the Edmonton Symptom Assessment Scale (ESAS) and found that 50.98% of clients were cared for at home, 28.85% of clients needed hospice referral, and 20.15% of clients needed short-term hospitalizations. Clients receiving home-based palliative care reported improved symptom control, health-related communication, and psychosocial support.* EBN: *Dosser and Kennedy (2014) used participatory action research in an acute care setting and found that improving nurses' communication skills and improving the environment for family caregivers by providing "safe space" away from the bedside of the dying client were nursing interventions that had a positive impact on families' grief experience.*

G

Home Care

- Consider providing support via the Internet. EB: *Varga and Paulus (2014) used discourse analysis to examine 107 initial Internet posts and found that there were three "non-normal" grief reactions: (1) unusual stories of loss, (2) describing uncontrollable emotional and physical states, and (3) engaging in "troubles telling," supporting the use of Internet support groups for complicated grief.* EB: *Jakoby (2014) studied the conversations of bereaved clients in an online survey and identified that clients sought out conversation partners to discuss grieving but they had difficulty in talking openly about grief and were concerned about being a burden to others.*

REFERENCES

Al-Gamal, E., & Long, T. (2014). The MM-CGI Cerebral Palsy: modification and pretesting of an instrument to measure anticipatory grief in parents whose child has cerebral palsy. *Journal of Clinical Nursing, 23*(13/14), 1810–1819.

Anderson, K., Ewen, H., Miles, E., et al. (2010). The grief support in healthcare scale: development and testing. *Nursing Research, 59*(6), 372–379.

Avelin, P., Gyllensward, G., Erlandsson, K., et al. (2014). Adolescents' experiences of having a stillborn half-sibling. *Death Studies, 38*(9), 557–562.

Bellamy, G., Gott, M., Waterworth, S., et al. (2014). 'But I do believe you've got to accept that that's what life's about': older adults living in New Zealand talk about their experiences of loss and bereavement support. *Health & Social Care in the Community, 22*(1), 96–103.

Bentley, B., & O'Connor, M. (2015). Conducting research interviews with bereaved family carers: when do we ask? *Journal of Palliative Medicine, 18*(3), 241–245.

Burke, L. A., Neimeyer, R. A., Young, A. J., et al. (2014). Complicated spiritual grief II: a deductive inquiry following the loss of a loved one. *Death Studies, 38*(4), 268–281.

Cinzia, P. A., Montagna, L., Mastroianni, C., et al. (2014). Losing a parent. *Journal of Hospice & Palliative Nursing, 16*(6), 362–373.

Currier, J. M., Irish, J. E. F., Neimeyer, R. A., et al. (2015). Attachment, continuing bonds, and complicated grief following violent loss: testing a moderated model. *Death Studies, 39*(4), 201–210.

Dhiliwal, S. R., & Muckaden, M. (2015). Impact of specialist home-based palliative care services n a tertiary oncology set up: a prospective non-randomized observational study. *Indian Journal of Palliative Care, 21*(1), 28–34.

Dosser, I., & Kennedy, C. (2014). Improving family carers' experiences of support at the end of life by enhancing communication: an action research study. *International Journal of Palliative Care, 20*(12), 608–616.

Elvish, R., Cawley, R., & Keady, J. (2014). The experiences of therapy from the perspectives of carers of people with dementia: an exploratory study. *Counseling & Psychotherapy Research, 14*(1), 56–63.

Fenstermacher, K. M. (2014). Enduring to gain new perspective: a grounded theory study of the experience of perinatal bereavement in Black adolescents. *Research in Nursing & Health, 37*(2), 135–143.

Gillies, J., Neimeyer, R. A., & Milman, E. (2014). The meaning of loss codebook: construction of a system for analyzing meanings made in bereavement. *Death Studies, 38*(4), 207–216.

Gray, M. T. (2014). Habits, rituals, and addiction: an inquiry into substance abuse in older persons. *Nursing Philosophy: An International Journal for Healthcare Professionals, 15*(2), 138–151.

Hogan, N. S., Worden, J. W., & Schmidt, L. A. (2004). An empirical study of the proposed complicated grief disorder criteria. *Omega, 48*(3), 263–277.

Howes, C. (2015). Caring until the end: A systematic literature review exploring paediatric intensive care unit end-of-life care. *Nursing in Critical Care, 20*(1), 41–51.

Jakoby, N. R. (2014). Talking about grief: conversational partners sought by bereaved people. *Bereavement Care, 33*(1), 13–18.

Jordan, A. H., & Litz, B. T. (2014). Prolonged grief disorder: diagnostic, assessment, and treatment considerations. *Professional Psychology, Research and Practice, 45*(3), 180–187.

Lee, S. A., Feudo, A., & Gibbons, J. A. (2014). Grief among near-death experiencers: pathways through religion and meaning. *Mental Health, Religion, and Culture, 17*(9), 877–885.

Lindauer, A., & Harvath, T. A. (2014). Pre-death grief in the context of dementia caregiving: a concept analysis. *Journal of Advanced Nursing, 70*(10), 2196–2207.

Maercker, A., Brewin, C. R., Bryant, R. A., et al. (2013). Proposals for mental disorders specifically associated with stress in the international classification of diseases-11. *Lancet, 381*, 1683–1685.

McKinnon, J. M., & Chonody, J. (2014). Exploring the formal supports used by people bereaved through suicide: a qualitative study. *Social Work in Mental Health, 12*(3), 231–248.

McLeod-Sordjan, R. (2014). Death preparedness: a concept analysis. *Journal of Advanced Nursing, 70*(5), 1008–1019.

McRitchie, R., McKenzie, K., Quayle, E., et al. (2014). How adults with an intellectual disability experience bereavement and grief: a qualitative exploration. *Death Studies*, *38*(3), 179–185.

Neimeyer, R. A., & Young-Eisendrath, P. (2015). Assessing a Buddhist treatment for bereavement and loss: the mustard seed project. *Death Studies*, *39*(5), 263–273.

Possick, C., Shamai, M., & Sadeh, R. (2014). Healing the social self: how parents whose children were killed in terror attacks construct the experience of help. *Community Mental Health Journal*, *50*(4), 487–496.

Quinn-Lee, L. (2014). School social work with grieving children. *Children & Schools*, *36*(2), 93–103.

Shear, K. M., Ghesquiere, A., & Glickman, K. (2013). Bereavement and complicated grief. *Current Psychiatry Reports*, *15*(11).

Stahl, S., & Schulz, R. (2013). Changes in routine health behaviors following late-life bereavement: a systematic review. *Journal of Behavioral Medicine*, *37*(4), 736–755.

Steen, S. E. (2015). Perinatal death: bereavement interventions used by US and Spanish nurses and midwives. *International Journal of Palliative Care*, *21*(2), 79–86.

Thienprayoon, R., Campell, R., & Winick, N. (2015). Attitudes and practices in the bereavement care offered by children's hospitals: a survey of the pediatric chaplains network. *Omega: Journal of Death & Dying*, *71*(1), 48–59.

Varga, M. A., & Paulus, T. M. (2014). Grieving online: newcomers' constructions of grief in an online support group. *Death Studies*, *38*(7), 443–449.

Young, H., Garrard, B., Lambe, L., et al. (2014). Helping people cope with bereavement. *Learning Disability Practice*, *17*(6), 16–20.

Risk for complicated Grieving *Gail B. Ladwig, MSN, RN, and Jane M. Kendall, RN, BS, CHT*

NANDA-I

Definition

Vulnerable to a disorder that occurs after death of a significant other in which the experience of distress accompanying bereavement fails to follow normative expectations and manifests in functional impairment, which may compromise health

Risk Factors

Death of a significant other; insufficient social support; emotional disturbance

NIC, NOC, Client Outcomes, Nursing Interventions, Client/Family Teaching and Discharge Planning, *Rationales*, and References

Refer to care plan for Complicated **Grieving.**

Risk for disproportionate Growth *Roberta Dobrzanski, MSN, RN*

NANDA-I

Definition

Vulnerable to growth above the 97th percentile or below the 3rd percentile for age, crossing two percentile channels, which may compromise health

Risk Factors

Caregiver

Alteration in cognitive functioning; learning disability; mental health issue (e.g., depression, psychosis, personality disorder, substance abuse); presence of abuse (e.g., physical, psychological, sexual)

Environmental

Deprivation; economically disadvantaged; exposure to teratogen; exposure to violence; lead poisoning; natural disaster

Individual

Anorexia; chronic illness; infection; insatiable appetite; maladaptive feeding behavior by caregiver; maladaptive self-feeding behavior; malnutrition; prematurity; substance abuse

Prenatal

Congenital disorder; exposure to teratogen; genetic disorder; inadequate maternal nutrition; maternal infection; multiple gestation; substance abuse

NOC (Nursing Outcomes Classification)

Suggested NOC Outcomes

Body Image; Child Development: 1 Month, 2 Months, 4 Months, 6 Months, 12 Months, 2 Years, 3 Years, 4 Years, 5 Years, Middle Childhood, Adolescence; Growth; Knowledge: Infant Care; Preconception Maternal Health; Pregnancy; Physical Maturation: Female, Male; Weight: Body Mass

G

Example NOC Outcome with Indicators

Growth as evidenced by the following indicators: Weight percentile for sex/Weight percentile for age/Weight percentile for height/Length/height percentile for age/Length/height percentile for sex. (Rate the outcome and indicators of **Growth:** 1 = severe deviation from normal range, 2 = substantial deviation from normal range, 3 = moderate deviation from normal range, 4 = mild deviation from normal range, 5 = no deviation from normal range [see Section I].)

Client Outcomes

Client/Parents/Primary Caregiver Will (Specify Time Frame)

- State information related to possible teratogenic agents
- Identify components of healthy nutrition that will promote growth
- Maintain or improve weight to be within a healthy range for age and sex

NIC (Nursing Interventions Classification)

Suggested NIC Interventions

Eating Disorders Management; Weight Management; Nutrition Therapy; Nutrition Management; Teaching: Infant Nutrition, Toddler Nutrition

Example NIC Activities—Nutrition Therapy

Determine, in collaboration with dietitian as appropriate, number of calories and type of nutrients needed to meet nutrition requirements; Ensure that diet includes foods high in fiber content to prevent constipation; Refer for diet teaching and planning, as needed

Nursing Interventions and *Rationales*

Preconception/Pregnancy

- Counsel women who smoke to quit smoking prior to conception if possible and to avoid smoking and secondhand smoke while pregnant. EB: *Smoking during pregnancy has been linked to multiple complications for both mother and infant. The findings of this review also revealed that maternal exposure to environmental smoke is correlated with low birth weight in infants as well as numerous other adverse effects (Hawsawi et al, 2015).*
- Assess alcohol consumption of pregnant women and advise those who drink alcohol to discontinue all use of alcohol through the pregnancy. EB: *Current research suggests that alcohol intake of seven or more standard drinks (one standard drink = 13.6 grams of absolute alcohol) per week during pregnancy places the fetus at significant risk for the negative effects of ethanol. Effects of alcohol on the fetus are influenced not only by the amount of alcohol consumed, but also by the pattern of alcohol (binge drinking vs. daily consumption of alcohol) and the exposure threshold amounts of alcohol in the blood, as well as the timing of exposure during gestation (Stade et al, 2009).*
- Assess and limit exposure to all drugs (prescription, "recreational," and over the counter) and give the mother information on known teratogenic agents. EB: *According to the National Research Council, 3% of all birth defects and developmental disabilities are caused by environmental exposures. No drug can be considered safe during pregnancy. It should be emphasized that any drug has the potential to cause a birth defect, so no listing of known teratogens is ever complete (CDC, 2014; Florida Birth Defects Registry, 2015).*

- All women of childbearing age who are capable of becoming pregnant should take 400 mcg of folic acid daily. EB: *Periconceptional use of folic acid reduces the incidence of neural tube defects. Up to 70% of neural tube defects could be prevented if all women who can become pregnant consumed 400 mcg of folic acid from at least 1 month before conception through the first trimester of pregnancy (CDC, 2014; Florida Birth Defects Registry, 2015).*

▲ Promote a team approach toward preconception and pregnancy glucose control for women with diabetes. EB: *Offspring of women with diabetes mellitus type 1 or type 2 have a twofold to fourfold increased risk of birth defects. Available data suggest that excellent preconception and first-trimester glucose control in the mother can greatly reduce, if not eliminate, this risk. Fetal morbidity may still be high in the second and third trimesters if gestational diabetes is not under good control. Programs with a team approach have been the most successful (CDC, 2014; Florida Birth Defects Registry, 2015).*

▲ Advise women with mental health disorders to seek appropriate counseling before pregnancy. EB: *Well-characterized risks are associated with valproate, carbamazepine, lamotrigine, and lithium (Nguyen et al, 2009).*

G

Pediatric

- Consider regular breast milk and protein-fortified breast milk for low-birth-weight infants in the neonatal intensive care unit. CEB: *Observational studies and meta-analyses of trials comparing feeding with formula milk versus donor breast milk suggest that feeding with breast milk has major nonnutrient advantages for preterm or low-birth-weight infants (Henderson et al, 2007). In an earlier study it was concluded that protein-enriched breast milk enables low-birth-weight infants requiring especially intensive care to attain growth at discharge comparable to that of healthier infants not given enriched milk (Funkquist et al, 2006).*
- Provide tube feedings per health care provider's orders when appropriate for clients with neuromuscular impairment. EB: *Malnutrition and gastrointestinal disorders are common in children with cerebral palsy. On the other hand, improved nutritional status seems to have a positive effect on motor function in these children (Bekem et al, 2008).*
- Provide for adequate nutrition and nutritional monitoring in clients with medical disorders requiring long-term medication and those with developmental delay. EB: *One study found a high prevalence of overweight children who had developmental delay. Many factors can contribute to overweight issues in this population, including sedentary lifestyle and medications with weight gain as a side effect (De et al, 2008). Drugs such as SSRIs (selective serotonin reuptake inhibitors), mood stabilizers, psychostimulants, and anti-psychotics can cause weight gain in adolescents. Other medications used to treat chronic conditions, such as stimulants, can cause poor weight gain (Jerrell, 2010).*
- Adequate intake of vitamin D is set at 400 IU/day by the National Academy of Sciences. Because adequate sunlight exposure is difficult to determine, a supplement of 400 IU/day is recommended for the following groups to prevent rickets and vitamin D deficiency in healthy infants and children:
  - All breastfed infants unless they are weaned to at least 500 mL/day of vitamin D–fortified formula or milk
  - All non-breastfed infants who are ingesting less than 500 mL/day of vitamin D–fortified formula or milk
  - Children and adolescents who do not receive regular sunlight exposure, do not ingest at least 500 mL/day of vitamin D–fortified milk, or do not take a daily multivitamin supplement containing at least 400 IU of vitamin D

▲ EB: *It is now recommended that all infants and children, including adolescents, have a minimum daily intake of 400 IU of vitamin D beginning soon after birth. New evidence supports a potential role for vitamin D in maintaining innate immunity and preventing diseases such as diabetes and cancer (Wagner & Greer, 2008).*

- Provide adequate nutrition to clients with active intestinal inflammation. EB: *Nutrition plays a role in inflammatory bowel disease (IBD), primarily in prevention and treatment of malnutrition and growth failure. Furthermore, in Crohn's disease, nutrition can induce remission, maintain remission, and prevent relapse. Malnutrition is common in IBD and the mechanisms involved include decreased food intake, malabsorption, increased nutrient loss, increased energy requirements, and drug-nutrient interactions (Shamir, 2009).*
- Encourage limiting "screen time" (television, video games, Internet, smartphones, and tablets) to less than 2 hours/day for children. EB: *High levels of sedentary behaviors, particularly television viewing, are associated with increased risk of overweight and obesity during youth (Hume et al, 2010). The relationship between*

weight status and time spent in sedentary activities is well documented among older children and adolescents. The formative school years may be an important period when these relationships emerge, providing an opportune time to intervene (Jones et al, 2010).

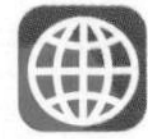

Multicultural

- Assess the influence of cultural beliefs, norms, values, and expectations on parents' perceptions of normal growth and development. EBN: *One binational study found a Mexican cultural norm toward larger ideal body types for children and showed that the vestiges of this cultural norm persist in Mexican immigrant communities in the United States (Jones et al, 2010).*
- Focus nutritional education on promoting good nutrition and physically active lifestyles for healthy child development as opposed to only for prevention or reduction of overweight. EBN: *Programs to address overweight among children of Mexican descent in both the United States and Mexico may be more effective if they focus on alternative benefits of weight control strategies (Jones et al, 2010).*
- Assess for the influence of acculturation. EB: *One study found a marked relationship between acculturation, measured by generational status and language use at home, and failure to meet physical activity recommendations among adolescents aged 10 to 17 (Liu et al, 2009).*
- Assess parents' understanding of appropriate nutrition for infants. CEB: *Some cultures may add semisolid food within the first month of life because of concerns that the infant is not getting enough to eat and the perception that "big is healthy" (Higgins, 2000). Studies have found that the introduction of solids at less than 4 months is a risk factor for increased infant weight gain (Taveras et al, 2010).*
- Assess the influence of family/parents on patterns of nutritional intake. EBN: *In some studies, mothers' pressure on their children to eat has been associated with disinhibited eating and increased child energy intake and body weight (Taveras et al, 2010).*
- *Negotiate with clients regarding which aspects of healthy nutrition can be modified while still honoring cultural beliefs.* CEB: *Give and take with clients will lead to culturally congruent care (Leininger & McFarland, 2002).* EB: *Although black and Hispanic mothers were more likely to initiate breastfeeding, they were less likely to breastfeed their infants exclusively to 6 months of age and were more likely to introduce solid foods before 4 months of age (Taveras et al, 2010).*
- Encourage parental efforts at increasing physical activity and decreasing dietary fat for their children. EB: *Parental role modeling and parental social support are important elements to consider in designing programs to increase physical activity among underserved adolescents (Wright et al, 2010). Fluctuation of resources affects family food purchase and consumption, resulting in unstable eating patterns and unhealthy eating (Kaufman & Karpati, 2007).*

Home Care

- The interventions previously described may be adapted for home care use.
- Assess parental perception of their child's weight. EBN: *If parents do not recognize their child as at risk for overweight, or overweight, they cannot intervene to diminish the risk factors for pediatric obesity and its related complications (Doolen et al, 2009).*
- Assess family meal planning and family participation in mealtime activities such as eating together at a scheduled time. EB: *Lifestyle assessment is an opportunity to identify potential targets for prevention and increase families' self-awareness of current behaviors (Daniels et al, 2009).*

Client/Family Teaching and Discharge Planning

- Educate families and children about providing healthy meals and healthy eating to improve learning ability. EB: *Using standardized tests, results of one study suggest that a nutritional education program can improve academic performance measured by achievement of specific mathematics and English education standards (Shilts et al, 2009).*

REFERENCES

Bekem, O., et al. (2008). Effect of nutritional support in children with spastic quadriplegia. *Pediatric Neurology*, *39*, 330–334.

CDC (Centers for Disease Control and Prevention). *Birth Defects: Research and tracking*. Revised October 10, 2014, Retrieved April 1, 2015, from: <http://www.cdc.gov/ncbddd/birthdefects/research.html>.

Daniels, S. R., et al. (2009). American heart association childhood obesity research summit: executive summary. *Circulation*, *119*(15), 2114–2123.

De, S., Small, J., & Baur, L. A. (2008). Overweight and obesity among children with developmental disabilities. *Journal of Intellectual and Developmental Disability*, *33*(1), 43–47.

Doolen, J., Alpert, P. T., & Miller, S. K. (2009). Parental disconnect between perceived and actual weight status of children: a metasynthesis of the current research. *Journal of the American Academy of Nurse Practitioners*, *21*, 160–166.

Florida Birth Defects Registry. *Prevention strategies index: strategies to prevent birth defects: limit all drug exposures (prescriptions, "recreational," and over-the-counter)*. Retrieved April 1, 2015, from: <http://www.fbdr.org>.

Funkquist, E. L., et al. (2006). Growth and breastfeeding among low birth weight infants fed with or without protein enrichment of human milk. *Upsala Journal of Medical Sciences*, *111*(1), 97–108.

Hawsawi, A., Bryant, L., & Goodfellow, L. (2015). Association between exposure to secondhand smoke during pregnancy and low birthweight: a narrative review. *Respiratory Care*, *60*(1), 135–140. (39 ref).

Henderson, G., Anthony, M. Y., & McGuire, W. (2007). Formula milk versus maternal breast milk for feeding preterm or low birth weight infants. *Cochrane Database of Systematic Reviews*, (4), CD002972.

Higgins, B. (2000). Puerto Rican cultural beliefs: influence on infant feeding practices in western New York. *Journal of Transcultural Nursing*, *11*(1), 19.

Hume, C., et al. (2010). Understanding the correlates of adolescents' TV viewing: social ecological approach. *International Journal of Pediatric Obesity*, *1*(2), 61–168.

Jerrell, J. M. (2010). Neuroendocrine-related adverse events associated with antidepressant treatment in children and adolescents. *CNS Neuroscience & Therapeutics*, *16*(2), 3–90.

Jones, R. A., et al. (2010). Relationships between child, parent and community characteristics and weight status among young children. *International Journal of Pediatric Obesity*, *5*(3), 256–264.

Kaufman, L., & Karpati, A. (2007). Understanding the sociocultural roots of childhood obesity: food practices among Latino families of Bushwick, Brooklyn. *Social Science and Medicine*, *64*(11), 2177–2188.

Leininger, M. M., & McFarland, M. R. (2002). *Transcultural nursing: concepts, theories, research and practices* (3rd ed.). New York: McGraw-Hill.

Liu, J., et al. (2009). Acculturation, physical activity, and obesity among Hispanic adolescents. *Ethnicity and Health*, *14*(5), 509–525.

Nguyen, H. T., Sharma, V., & McIntyre, R. S. (2009). Teratogenesis associated with antibipolar agents. *Advances in Therapy*, *26*(3), 281–294.

Shamir, R. (2009). Nutritional aspects in inflammatory bowel disease. *Journal of Pediatric Gastroenterology and Nutrition*, *48*, S86–S88.

Shilts, M. K., et al. (2009). Pilot study: EatFit impacts sixth graders' academic performance on achievement of mathematics and English education standards. *Journal of Nutrition Education and Behavior*, *41*(2), 127–131.

Stade, B. C., et al. (2009). Psychological and/or educational interventions for reducing prenatal alcohol consumption in pregnant women and women planning pregnancy. *Cochrane Database of Systematic Reviews*, (2), CD004228.

Taveras, E. M., et al. (2010). Racial/ethnic differences in early-life risk factors for childhood obesity. *Pediatrics*, *125*(4), 686–695.

Wagner, C. L., & Greer, F. R. (2008). Prevention of rickets and vitamin D deficiency in infants, children, and adolescents. *Pediatrics*, *122*(5), 1142–1152.

Wright, M. S., et al. (2010). A qualitative study of parental modeling and social support for physical activity in underserved adolescents. *Health Education Research*, *25*(2), 224–232.

Deficient community Health

Gail B. Ladwig, MSN, RN, and Marina Martinez-Kratz, MS, RN, CNE

NANDA-I

Definition

Presence of one or more health problems or factors that deter wellness or increase the risk of health problems experienced by an aggregate

Defining Characteristics

Health problem experienced by aggregates or populations; program unavailable to eliminate health problems of an aggregate or population; program unavailable to enhance wellness of an aggregate or population; program unavailable to prevent health problems of an aggregate or population; program unavailable to reduce health problems of an aggregate or population; risk of hospitalization experienced by aggregates or population; risk of physiological states experienced by aggregates or populations; risk of psychological states experienced by aggregates or population

Related Factors

Inadequate consumer satisfaction with program; inadequate program budget; inadequate program evaluation plan; inadequate program outcome data; inadequate social support for program; insufficient access to healthcare provider; insufficient community experts; insufficient resources (e.g., financial, social, knowledge); program incompletely addresses health problem

NOC (Nursing Outcomes Classification)

Suggested NOC Outcomes

Community Grief Response; Community Health Screening Effectiveness; Community Health Status Community Program Effectiveness; Community Resiliency; Community Risk Control: Obesity; Community Risk Control: Unhealthy Cultural Traditions

Example NOC Outcome with Indicators

Community Health Status as evidenced by the following indicators: Health status of infants/children/adolescents/adults/elders/minority populations/Prevalence of health promotion programs. (Rate the outcome and indicators of **Community Health Status:** 1 = poor, 2 = fair, 3 = good, 4 = very good, 5 = excellent, NA [see Section I].)

H

Client Outcomes

Community/Adolescents/Minority Clients Will (Specify Time Frame)

- Provide programs for healthy behaviors
- Demonstrate goal setting
- Describe and comply with healthy behaviors
- Describe and demonstrate compliance with HBV education and testing

NIC (Nursing Interventions Classification)

Suggested NIC Interventions

Community health development: Identify health concerns, strengths, and priorities with community partners; Assist community members in raising awareness of health problems and concerns

Nursing Interventions and *Rationales*

Refer to care plans: Readiness for Enhanced community **Coping,** Ineffective Community **Coping,** Ineffective **Health** maintenance, Impaired **Home** maintenance, Risk for other-directed **Violence.**

- Assess for the presence of demographic variables that predict community mortality. EB: *The following demographic variables were associated with increased community mortality: age 65 years or older, poverty, and a high concentration of construction and service workers (Chan et al, 2014).*
- Assess for needs related to the community's priority health concerns. EB: *Research results generated from the first study of the National Institutes of Health Sentinel Network identified the top five health concerns of respondents as hypertension, diabetes, cancer, weight, and heart problems (Cottler et al, 2013).*
- Encourage healthy nutrition and exercise among community members using the resources available to the community. EB: *Community-based health communication interventions must address the realities of the community including, literacy levels and existing networks of providers and consumers (Martinez et al, 2012). Community-belonging was strongly related to health behavior change in Canada and may be an important component of population health prevention strategies (Hystad & Carpiano, 2012).*
- Facilitate goal setting in the community for behavior change related to diet and exercise for overweight and obese adults. EB: *In this study goal setting shows promise as a community-based intervention to change behavior specific to diet and exercise (Pearson, 2012).*
- Utilize a community forum approach to increase community knowledge and awareness of community health issues. EBN: *A community forum was effective at disseminating education about domestic violence prevention and increasing awareness of domestic violence prevention programs (Gonzalez-Guarda et al, 2012).*

Pediatric

▲ Consider a community-based program for young people that encourages health-related behavior changes, increasing fruit and vegetable intake, and engaging in activity. EB: *This program for overweight and obese young people helped implement behavior and lifestyle changes that were associated with significant reductions in self-reported weight and body mass index Z-score (standard deviation), without compromising growth in height (Stubbs et al, 2012).*

- ▲ Support religious affiliation and positive school climates for adolescents, particularly for lesbian, gay, and bisexual youths in the community. EB: *Although religious climate was also associated with health behaviors among heterosexual youths, it was more strongly associated with the health behaviors of lesbian, gay, and bisexual youths. Among LGB youths, a supportive religious climate was significantly associated with fewer alcohol abuse symptoms and fewer sexual partners (Hatzenbuehler et al, 2012).*

Geriatric

- ▲ Assess homeless older veterans in the community for post-traumatic stress disorder and/or suicidal behavior and make appropriate referrals. EB: *This study documented the increased prevalence of suicidal behavior in homeless older veterans (Schinka et al, 2012).*
- ▲ Provide community-dwelling older women with psychoeducation about aging skills and behaviors and cognitive function using group discussion. EB: *This new comprehensive educational group intervention reduces negative emotional reactions toward cognitive functioning. It can potentially contribute to the well-being of an important and large group of older adults (Hoogenhout et al, 2012).*

H

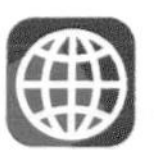

Multicultural

- Provide information and venues for testing about the pervasiveness and deadly consequence of hepatitis B virus (HBV) for Asians in the United States. EB: *Asians in San Francisco are disproportionately affected by chronic HBV infection and its fatal consequences. This information was most likely to drive clients to seek education and testing (Shiau et al, 2012).*
- Provide culturally and linguistically appropriate risk reduction programs to individuals living in rural and border regions of the country. EBN: *Culturally appropriate risk reduction programs will reduce sexual health disparities (Hernandez et al, 2014).*

Home Care and Client/Family Teaching and Discharge Planning

- The above interventions may be adapted for home care and client/family teaching.
- Provide support for establishment of a community garden. EB: *In this study, community garden participants consumed fruits and vegetables 5.7 times per day. Community gardeners met national recommendations to consume fruits and vegetables at least five times per day, compared with 37% of home gardeners and 24% of non-gardeners (Litt et al, 2011).*

REFERENCES

Chan, K. S., Roberts, E., McCleary, R., et al. (2014). Community characteristics and mortality: the relative strength of association of different community characteristics. *American Journal of Public Health, 104*(9), 1751–1758.

Cottler, L. B., McCloskey, D., Aguilar-Gaxiola, S., et al. (2013). Community needs, concerns, and perceptions about health research: findings from the clinical and translational science award sentinel network. *American Journal of Public Health, 103*(9), 1685–1692.

Gonzalez-Guarda, R., Lipman, D., & Cummings, A. M. (2012). A community forum to assess the needs and preferences for domestic violence prevention targeting hispanics. *Hispanic Health Care International, 10*(1), 18–27.

Hatzenbuehler, M., Pachankis, J., & Wolff, J. (2012). Religious climate and health risk behaviors in sexual minority youths: a population-based study. *American Journal of Public Health, 102*(4), 657–663.

Hernandez, K., Mata, H., Provencio Vasquez, E., et al. (2014). Community outreach along the U.S./Mexico border: developing HIV health education strategies to engage rural populations. *Online Journal Of Rural Nursing & Health Care, 14*(1), 3–17.

Hoogenhout, E. M., et al. (2012). Effects of a comprehensive educational group intervention in older women with cognitive complaints: a randomized controlled trial. *Aging and Mental Health, 16*(2), 135–144.

Hystad, P., & Carpiano, R. (2012). Sense of community-belonging and health-behaviour change in Canada. *Journal of Epidemiology and Community Health, 66*(3), 277–283.

Litt, J., et al. (2011). The influence of social involvement, neighborhood aesthetics, and community garden participation on fruit and vegetable consumption. *American Journal of Public Health, 101*(8), 1466–1473.

Martinez, J., et al. (2012). Formative research for a community-based message-framing intervention. *American Journal of Health Behavior, 36*(3), 335–347.

Pearson, E. S. (2012). Goal setting as a health behavior change strategy in overweight and obese adults: a systematic literature review examining intervention components. *Patient Education and Counseling, 87*(1), 32–42.

Schinka, J. A., et al. (2012). Suicidal behavior in a national sample of older homeless veterans. *American Journal of Public Health, 102*(Suppl. 1), S147–S153.

Shiau, R., et al. (2012). Using survey results regarding hepatitis B knowledge, community awareness and testing behavior among Asians to improve the San Francisco Hep B free campaign. *Journal of Community Health, 37*(2), 350–364.

Stubbs, J., et al. (2012). Weight, body mass index and behaviour change in a commercially run lifestyle programme for young people. *Journal of Human Nutrition and Dietetics, 25*, 161–166.

Risk-prone Health behavior

Nicole Jones, MSN, FNP-BC

NANDA-I

Definition

Impaired ability to modify lifestyle/behaviors in a manner that improves health status

Defining Characteristics

Failure to achieve optimal sense of control; failure to take action that prevents health problem; minimizes health status change; nonacceptance of health status change

Related Factors (r/t)

Economically disadvantaged; inadequate comprehension; insufficient social support; low self-efficacy; negative attitude toward health care; smoking; stressors; substance abuse

H

NOC (Nursing Outcomes Classification)

Suggested NOC Outcomes

Participation in Health Care Decisions; Psychosocial Adjustment: Life Change; Risk Detection

Example NOC Outcome with Indicators

Risk Detection as evidenced by the following indicators: Recognizes signs and symptoms that indicate risks/Identifies potential health risks/Participates in screening at recommended intervals/Obtains information about changes in health recommendations. (Rate the outcome and indicators of **Risk Detection:** 1 = never demonstrated, 2 = rarely demonstrated, 3 = sometimes demonstrated, 4 = often demonstrated, 5 = consistently demonstrated [see Section I].)

Client Outcomes

Client Will (Specify Time Frame)

- State acceptance of change in health status
- Request assistance in altering behaviors to adapt to change
- State personal goals for dealing with change in health status and means to prevent further health problems
- State experience of a period of grief that is proportional to the actual or perceived effect of the loss
- Report and/or demonstrate behavior changes mutually agreed upon with nurse as evidence of positive adaptation

NIC (Nursing Interventions Classification)

Suggested NIC Intervention

Self-Efficacy Enhancement

Example NIC Activities—Self-Efficacy Enhancement

Explore individual's perception of his/her capability to perform the desired behavior; Reinforce confidence in making behavior changes and taking action

Nursing Interventions and *Rationales*

- Assess the client's definitions of health and wellness and major barriers to health and wellness. CEB: *Each person has unique, individual perceptions of well-being and illness (Kiefer, 2008).*
- Use motivational interviewing to help the client identify and change unhealthy behaviors. EBN: *In these studies, motivational interviewing helped clients identify and examine their high-risk health behaviors (Wong & Cheng, 2013; Smedslund et al, 2011).*

- • Encourage mindfulness and meditation to help the client cope with changes in health status. EBN: *Mindfulness and meditation can reduce stress, leading to increased quality of life and self-efficacy (Robins et al, 2014).*
- • Allow the client adequate time to express feelings about the change in health status. CEB: *This is an important intervention for the client with a serious illness such as a malignant brain tumor (Khalili, 2007).*
- • Use open-ended questions to allow the client free expression (e.g., "Tell me about your last hospitalization" or "How does this time compare?"). CEB: *Using open-ended questions generates more objective responses with less bias, leading to a more genuine qualitative understanding (Alemi & Harry, 2014).*
- • Help the client work through the stages of grief that occur as part of a psychological adaptation to illness or life change. Assess for signs of nonacceptance to illness or change. CEB: *Clients who exhibit nonacceptance are at higher risk for stronger, delayed grief reactions. Identifying these clients and making appropriate referrals for counseling and support groups may prevent future adverse outcomes (Holland et al, 2013).*
- • Assess the client for depression and refer to for counseling or medical follow-up, as appropriate. CEB: *Depression is often a response to and a comorbid condition of chronic disease. Depression is associated with poorer client outcomes and higher risk behavior (Di Benedetto et al, 2014).*
- • Discuss the client's current goals and assist in modification, if appropriate. Have the client list goals so that they can be referred to and steps can be taken to accomplish them. Support hope that the goals will be accomplished. CEB: *Clarification of the client/family goals and expectations will allow the nurse to clarify what is possible and to identify measures that can facilitate achievement of the goals (Northouse et al, 2002). "Hope theory" may facilitate recovery and clearer and more sustainable goals (Snyder et al, 2006).*
- ▲ Encourage participation in appropriate wellness programs associated with health changes. EBN: *Studies of clients with multiple sclerosis and chronic obstructive pulmonary disease found that wellness programs facilitating positive health choices and self-management demonstrated gains in functional status and decreased anxiety and depression (Hart et al, 2011; Simpson & Jones, 2013).*
- • Provide assistance with activities as needed. CEB: *Clients' feelings of personal control increased when assistance was available to help them do things they could not do by themselves; they felt insecure and experienced emotional discomfort when assistance was lacking (Lauck, 2009).*
- • Give the client positive feedback for accomplishments, no matter how small. Support the client and family and promote their strengths and coping skills. CEB: *Support is necessary to help the client and family throughout the illness. Support leads to hopefulness and is associated with improved outcomes (Soundy et al, 2014).*
- • Manipulate the environment to decrease stress; allow the client to display personal items that have meaning. CEB: *Appraisal uncertainty is a risk factor for a negative adaptation to health change (Dudley-Brown, 2002).*
- • Maintain consistency and continuity in daily schedule. When possible, provide the same caregiver. CEB: *The predictability of interaction with the same nurses as a part of treatment facilitates trust, confidence, and positive adaptation (Richer & Ezer, 2002).*
- ▲ Promote use of positive spiritual influences, as appropriate. EBN: *Faith and spiritual-based resources may promote an atmosphere of forgiveness and stress personal resilience. These resources may also provide a sense of community and belonging and provide an additional support network (Brewer-Smith & Koenig, 2014).*
- ▲ Refer to community resources. Provide general and contact information for ease of use. CEB: *In this study in Canada, community-belonging was strongly related to health behavior change (Hystad & Carpiano, 2012).*

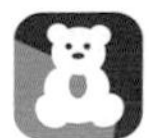

Pediatric

- • Include social history in client assessment to help identify past abuse and traumatic experiences. CEB: *Studies show that clients who have experienced past abuse or trauma are at higher risk to engage in high-risk behaviors (Whetten et al, 2012).*
- • Encourage visitation of children when family members are in intensive care. CEB: *Visitation of children should be supported to facilitate expression of feelings associated with major health changes in family members (Knutsson et al, 2008).*
- • Encourage parents to process and express grief, uncertainty, and discouragement after learning about their child's diagnosis, prognosis, and treatments. Provide parents with resources and tools to help further

their understanding of the illness. CEB: *Providing support has been shown to increase parental sense of empowerment and encourage patient advocacy (Mulligan et al, 2012).*

▲ Refer parents of critically ill children to an intervention program such as COPE, a theory-based intervention program. CEBN: *Research findings indicate that this program reduces short- and long-term stress, anxiety, and post-traumatic stress disorder symptoms often experienced by parents with critically ill children (Peek & Melnyk, 2010).*

- Use visualization and distraction with children undergoing procedures or treatment with unpleasant side effects. EBN: *This study found that visualization and distraction were the most effective coping strategies employed for children with chemotherapy-induced nausea and vomiting (Rodgers et al, 2012).*
- Discuss with parents and children possible adverse or unpleasant side effects associated with a treatment and assist with developing a plan to cope with these effects. EBN: *This study found that predetermined family interventions for developing coping strategies for cancer-related stressors was beneficial (Hildenbrand et al, 2011).*

Geriatric

▲ Assess for signs of depression resulting from illness-associated changes and make appropriate referrals. CEB: *Depression may be a consequence of aging. Assessments of the spouse's perception as well as of the client's factual situation may identify risk factors that are leading to a depressed state (Franzen-Dahlin, 2008).*

- Use open-ended questions in screening for depression in older adults (Magnil et al, 2011).
- Support activities that promote usefulness of older adults. CEB: *Older adults with persistently low perceived usefulness or feelings of uselessness may be a vulnerable group with increased risk for poor health outcomes in later life (Rozanova et al, 2012).*

▲ Encourage social support. EBN: *In this study, social support demonstrated a positive relation with perceived well-being in older adults (Kiefer, 2011).*

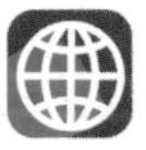

Multicultural

- Assess for the influence of cultural beliefs, norms, and values on the client's ability to modify health behavior. CEB: *What the client considers normal and abnormal health behavior may be based on cultural perceptions (Leininger & McFarland, 2002; Richardson, 2004; Van Bruggen, 2008).*
- Assess the role of fatalism on the client's ability to modify health behavior. CEB: *Fatalistic perspectives, which involve the belief that you cannot control your own fate, may influence health behaviors in some cultures.* CEB: *Fatalism has been identified as a dominant belief among Latinos and is believed to act as a barrier to cancer prevention (Espinosa de los Monteros & Gallo, 2011). Some African American women experience a fatalistic attitude about breast cancer (McQueen et al, 2011).*
- Encourage spirituality as a source of support for coping. CEB: *Many African Americans and Latinos identify spirituality, religiousness, prayer, and church-based approaches as coping resources (Giger et al, 2008).*
- Negotiate with the client regarding the aspects of health behavior that will need to be modified. CEB: *Give-and-take with the client will lead to culturally congruent care (Leininger & McFarland, 2002).*
- Acknowledge client's identified gender and sexual orientation and refer client and family members to support networks that have experience with lesbian, gay, bisexual, or transgender (LGBT) issues, as appropriate. EBN: *Disclosure and support systems are associated with better self-help perception; creating safe and accepting environments for LGBT patients has been shown to improve overall care in this underserved population (Kamen et al, 2015).*

Home Care

- The above interventions may be adapted for home care use.
- Take the client's perspective into consideration and use a holistic approach in assessing and responding to client planning for the future. EBN: *Clients with newly diagnosed diabetes do not want to become their illness (Johansson et al, 2009).*
- Assist the client to adapt to his/her diagnosis and to live with their disease. CEB: *Despite being diagnosed with diabetes, clients still want to continue the same life and be the same persons as before, although they now carry a disease (Johansson et al, 2009).*
- Ensure that evaluations of the client's ability to perform activities of daily living are age appropriate and consider existing, as well as new, diagnoses. CEB: *This study used a geriatric-designed functional*

evaluation that took into account age-related decrease in flexibility and strength, identifying additional areas for potential loss of function (Adamo et al, 2015).

- ▲ Refer the client to a counselor or therapist for follow-up care. Initiate community referrals as needed (e.g., grief counseling, self-help groups). CEB: *Families need assistance and support in coping with health change and caregiving (Honea et al, 2008).*
- • Refer to care plan for **Powerlessness.**

Client/Family Teaching and Discharge Planning

- • Assess family/caregivers for coping and teaching/learning styles. CEB: *The degree of optimism and pessimism influences the coping and health outcomes of caregivers of clients with Parkinson's disease (Lyons et al, 2004).*
- • Foster communication between the client/family and medical staff. CEB: *Family members of individuals undergoing cardiopulmonary resuscitation expressed a need to be involved and present or informed at all times during the process (Wagner, 2004).* CEB: *Psychotherapeutic interventions should not only address the client's problems but also the support-giver's questions, needs, and psychosocial burdens (Frick et al, 2005).*
- • Educate and prepare families regarding the appearance of the client and the environment before initial exposure. CEB: *Families indicated that knowing what to expect was helpful (Clukey, 2008).*
- • Help the client to enjoy a sense of "wellness." Provide support for progress and support enjoyment of the physical, emotional, spiritual, and social aspects of life. EBN: *Nurses provide information and support to facilitate the individual in his/her progress toward achieving a sense of wellness and recognizing that healing will take time (White et al, 2012).*
- • Teach a client and his/her family relaxation techniques (controlled breathing, guided imagery) and help them practice. EBN: *Guided imagery with relaxation may be an easy-to-use self-management intervention to improve the quality of life of older adults with osteoarthritis (Ha & Kim, 2013; Helgadottir & Wilson, 2014).*
- • Allow the client to proceed at own pace in learning; provide time for return demonstrations (e.g., self-injection of insulin). Tailor teaching and learning materials as appropriate for client and caregiver literacy level. EBN: *Use clear and distinct language free of medical jargon and meaningless values. Be sensitive to education levels and cultural environments that may hinder effective communication (Protheroe & Rowlands, 2013).*
- • If long-term deficits are expected, inform the family as soon as possible. CEB: *An honest assessment shared by the nurse of a particular situation is important to the family's sense of what is expected of them in adapting to a health care change (Weiss & Chen, 2002).*
- • Provide clients with information on how to access and evaluate available health information via the Internet. CEB: *Client access to health information and personal health records is becoming increasingly important in today's health care society. MedlinePlus, NIH Senior Health, and* ClinicalTrials.gov *are designed to get medical information directly into the hands of clients (Koonce et al, 2007).*

REFERENCES

Adamo, D., Talley, S., & Goldberg, A. (2015). Age and task differences in functional fitness in older women: comparisons with senior fitness test normative and criterion-referenced data. *Journal of Aging and Physical Activity*, *23*(1), 47–54.

Alemi, F., & Harry, J. (2014). An alternative to satisfaction surveys: let the patients talk. *Quality Management in Healthcare*, *23*(1), 10–19.

Brewer-Smith, K., & Koenig, H. (2014). Could spirituality and religion promote stress resilience in survivors of childhood trauma? *Issues in Mental Health Nursing*, *35*(4), 251–256.

Clukey, L. (2008). Anticipatory mourning: processes of expected loss in palliative care. *International Journal of Palliative Nursing*, *14*(7), 316, 318–325.

Di Benedetto, M., Lindner, H., Aucote, H., et al. (2014). Co-morbid depression and chronic illness related to coping and physical and mental health status. *Psychology, Health & Medicine*, *13*(3), 253–262.

Dudley-Brown, S. (2002). Prevention of psychological distress in persons with inflammatory bowel disease. *Issues Mental Health Nursing*, *23*, 403.

Espinosa de los Monteros, K., & Gallo, L. (2011). The relevance of fatalism in the study of Latinas' cancer screening behavior: a systematic review of the literature. *International Journal of Behavioral Medicine*, *18*(4), 310–318.

Franzen-Dahlin, A. (2008). Predictors of life situation among significant others of depressed or aphasic stroke patients. *Journal of Clinical Nursing*, *17*(12), 1574–1580.

Frick, E., et al. (2005). Social support, affectivity, and the quality of life of patients and their support-givers prior to stem cell transplantation. *Journal of Psychosocial Oncology*, *23*(4), 15–34.

Giger, J., et al. (2008). Church and spirituality in the lives of the African American community. *Journal of Transcultural Nursing*, *19*(4), 375–383.

Ha, Y., & Kim, H. (2013). The effects of audiovisual distraction on children's pain during laceration repair. *International Journal of Nursing Practice*, *19*(Suppl. 3), 20–27.

Hart, D., Memoli, R., Mason, B., et al. (2011). Developing a wellness program for people with multiple sclerosis. *International Journal of MS Care*, *13*(4), 154–162.

Helgadottir, H., & Wilson, M. (2014). A randomized controlled trial of the effectiveness of educating parents about distraction to decrease postoperative pain in children at home after tonsillectomy. *Pain Management Nursing*, *15*(3), 632–640.

Hildenbrand, A., Clawson, K., Alderfer, M., et al. (2011). Coping with pediatric cancer: strategies employed by children and their parents to manage cancer-related stressors during treatment. *Journal of Pediatric Oncology Nursing*, *28*(6), 344–354.

Holland, J., Futterman, A., Thompson, L., et al. (2013). Difficulties accepting the loss of a spouse: a precursor for intensified grieving among widowed older adults. *Death Studies*, *37*(2), 126–144.

Honea, N. J., et al. (2008). Putting evidence into practice: nursing assessment and interventions to reduce family caregiver strain and burden. *Clinical Journal of Oncology Nursing*, *12*(3), 507–516.

Hystad, P., & Carpiano, R. (2012). Sense of community-belonging and health-behaviour change in Canada. *Journal of Epidemiological Community Health*, *66*(3), 277–283.

Johansson, A., Dahlberg, K., & Ekebergh, M. (2009). A lifeworld phenomenological study of the experience of falling ill with diabetes. *International Journal of Nursing Studies*, *46*(2), 197–203.

Kamen, C., Smith-Stoner, M., Heckler, C., et al. (2015). Social support, self-rated health, and lesbian, gay, bisexual, and transgender identity disclosure to cancer care providers. *Oncology Nursing Forum*, *42*(1), 44–51.

Khalili, Y. (2007). Ongoing transitions: the impact of a malignant brain tumour on patient and family. *Axone (Dartmouth, N.S.)*, *28*(3), 5–13.

Kiefer, R. (2008). An integrative review of the concept of well-being. *Holistic Nursing Practice*, *22*(5), 244–252.

Kiefer, R. (2011). The effect of social support on functional recovery and well-being in older adults following joint arthroplasty. *Rehabilitation Nursing*, *36*(3), 120–126.

Knutsson, S., Samuelsson, I., Hellstrom, A., et al. (2008). Children's experiences of visiting a seriously ill/injured relative on an adult intensive care unit. *Journal of Advanced Nursing*, *61*(2), 154–162.

Koonce, T., et al. (2007). Toward a more informed patient: bridging health care information through an interactive communication portal. *Journal of the Medical Library Association*, *95*(1), 77.

Lauck, S. (2009). Patients felt greater personal control and emotional comfort in hospital when they felt secure, informed, and valued. *Evidence-Based Nursing*, *12*(1), 29.

Leininger, M., & McFarland, M. (2002). *Transcultural nursing: concepts, theories, research and practices* (3rd ed.). New York: McGraw-Hill.

Lyons, K. S., et al. (2004). Pessimism and optimism as early warning signs for compromised health for caregivers of patients with Parkinson's disease. *Nursing Research*, *53*(6), 354–362.

Magnil, M., Gunnarsson, R., & Björkelund, C. (2011). Using patient-centred consultation when screening for depression in elderly patients: a comparative pilot study. *Scandinavian Journal of Primary Health Care*, *29*(1), 51–56.

McQueen, A., Kreuter, M., Kalesan, B., et al. (2011). Understanding narrative effects: the impact of breast cancer survivor stories on message processing, attitudes, and beliefs among African American women. *Health Psychology*, *30*(6), 674–682.

Mulligan, J., MacColloch, R., Good, B., et al. (2012). Transparency, hope, and empowerment: a model for partnering with parents of a child with autism spectrum disorder at diagnosis and beyond. *Social Work in Mental Health*, *10*(4), 311–330.

Northouse, L., Walker, J., Schafenacker, A., et al. (2002). A family-based program of care for women with recurrent breast cancer and their family members. *Oncololgy Nursing Forum*, *29*(10), 1411–1419.

Peek, G., & Melnyk, B. M. (2010). Coping interventions for parents of children newly diagnosed with cancer: an evidence review with implications for clinical practice and future research. *Pediatric Nursing*, *36*(6), 306–313.

Protheroe, J., & Rowlands, G. (2013). Matching clinical information with levels of patient health literacy. *Nursing Management*, *20*(3), 20–21.

Richardson, P. (2004). How cultural ideas help shape the conceptualization of mental illness and mental health. *Occupational Therapy*, *9*(1), 5–8.

Richer, M., & Ezer, H. (2002). Living in it, living with it, and moving on: dimensions of meaning during chemotherapy. *Oncology Nursing Forum*, *29*(1), 113–119.

Robins, J., Kiken, L., Holt, M., et al. (2014). Mindfulness: an effective coaching tool for improving physical and mental health. *Journal of the American Association of Nurse Practitioners*, *26*, 511–518.

Rodgers, C., Norville, R., Taylor, O., et al. (2012). Children's coping strategies for chemotherapy-induced nausea and vomiting. *Oncology Nursing Forum*, *39*(2), 202–209.

Rozanova, J., Keating, N., & Eales, J. (2012). Unequal social engagement for older adults: constraints on choice. *Canadian Journal of Aging*, *31*(1), 25–36.

Simpson, E., & Jones, M. (2013). An exploration of self-efficacy and self-management in COPD patients. *British Journal of Nursing*, *22*(19), 1105–1109.

Smedslund, G., et al. (2011). Motivational interviewing for substance abuse. *Cochrane Database of Systematic Reviews*, (5), CD008063.

Snyder, C., Lehman, K., Kluck, B., et al. (2006). Hope for rehabilitation and vice versa. *Rehabilitation Psychology*, *51*(2), 89–112.

Soundy, A., Liles, C., Stubbs, B., et al. (2014). Identifying a framework for hope in order to establish the importance of generalised hopes for individuals who have suffered a stroke. *Advances in Medicine*, Article ID 471874, 8 pages.

Van Bruggen, H. (2008). Mental health as social construct. In J. Creek & L. Lougher (Eds.), *Occupational health and mental health* (4th ed.). London: Churchill Livingstone.

Wagner, J. M. (2004). Lived experience of critically ill patients' family members during cardiopulmonary resuscitation. *American Journal Critical Care*, *13*(5), 416–420.

Weiss, S. J., & Chen, J. L. (2002). Factors influencing maternal mental health and family functioning during the low birthweight infant's first year of life. *Journal Pediatric Nursing*, *17*(2), 114–125.

Whetten, K., Reif, S., Toth, M., et al. (2012). Relationship between trauma and high-risk behavior among HIV-positive men who do not have sex with men (MDSM). *AIDS Care*, *24*(11), 1453–1460.

White, M., et al. (2012). In the shadows of family-centered care: parents of ill adult children. Detail only available. *Hospice Palliative Nursing*, *14*(1), 53–60.

Wong, E., & Cheng, M. (2013). Effects of motivational interviewing to promote weight loss in obese children. *Journal of Clinical Nursing*, *22*, 2519–2530.

Ineffective Health management

Ruth A. Wittmann-Price, PhD, RN, CNS, CNE, CHSE, ANEF, FAAN

NANDA-I

Definition

Pattern of regulating and integrating into daily living a therapeutic regimen for the treatment of illness and its sequelae that is unsatisfactory for meeting specific health goals

Defining Characteristics

Difficulty with prescribed regimen; failure to include treatment regimen in daily living; failure to take action to reduce risk factors; ineffective choices in daily living for meeting health goals

Related Factors (r/t)

Complex treatment regimen; complexity of health care system; decisional conflict; economically disadvantaged; excessive demands; family conflict; family pattern of health care; inadequate number of cues to action; insufficient knowledge of therapeutic regimen; insufficient social support; perceived barrier; perceived benefit; perceived seriousness of condition; perceived susceptibility; powerlessness

H

NOC (Nursing Outcomes Classification)

Suggested NOC Outcomes

Knowledge: Disease Process; Knowledge: Treatment Regimen; Participation in Health Care Decisions

Example NOC Outcome with Indicators

Knowledge: Treatment Regimen as evidenced by the following indicators: Extent of understanding of prescribed medication, activity, exercise, and specific disease process. (Rate the outcome and indicators of **Knowledge: Treatment Regimen:** 1 = no knowledge, 2 = limited knowledge, 3 = moderate knowledge, 4 = substantial knowledge, 5 = extensive knowledge [see Section I].)

Client Outcomes

Client Will (Specify Time Frame)

- Describe daily food and fluid intake that meets therapeutic goals
- Describe activity/exercise patterns that meet therapeutic goals
- Describe scheduling of medications that meets therapeutic goals
- Verbalize ability to manage therapeutic regimens
- Collaborate with health professionals to decide on a therapeutic regimen that is congruent with health goals and lifestyle

NIC (Nursing Interventions Classification)

Suggested NIC Intervention

Health System Guidance; Learning Facilitation; Learning Readiness Enhancement

Example NIC Activities—Learning Facilitation

Present the information in a stimulating manner; Encourage the client's active participation

Nursing Interventions and *Rationales*

Note: This diagnosis does not have the same meaning as the diagnosis **Noncompliance.** This diagnosis is made with the client, so if the client does not agree with the diagnosis, it should not be made. The emphasis is on helping the client direct his or her own life and health, not on the client's compliance with the provider's instructions.

- Establish a collaborative partnership with the client for purposes of meeting health-related goals. EBN: *The concept of "knowing the patient" was studied through an integrative review and found to be a significant factor for clients but the barriers to "knowing the patient" are (1) time, (2) expedited client discharges, and (3) consistency of nursing assignments (Zolnierek, 2014).* CEB: *A study by Musich et al (2014) found that using a health care model based on the health care provider-client relationship decreased health care cost to the client by $86.68/month.*
- Explore the client's perception of their illness experience and identify uncertainties and needs through open-ended questions. EBN: *Nurses understanding the client's meaning of pain as perceived by clients experiencing chronic pain contributed to the client's ability to self-manage and develop coping strategies (Roditi & Robinson, 2011).* EBN: *Having hope even when there is impending death is often misinterpreted by caregivers as denial; therefore, awareness of death, uncertainty, and hope can coexist (Borneman et al, 2014).*

H

- Assist the client to enhance self-efficacy or confidence in his or her own ability to manage the illness. EBN: *A study of women with advanced breast cancer supported self-management's positive relationship to developing self-care skills and feeling empowered (Schulman-Green et al, 2011).* EBN: *Clients who smoke have a higher risk for depression and lower self-efficacy (Mee, 2014).*
- Involve family members in knowledge development, planning for self-management, and shared decision-making. EBN: *Diabetic clients view family participation as support and motivation to care for themselves as supported by three reported themes in a qualitative study: (1) families needed to be recognized, (2) at times clients blamed family for nonadherence, and (3) family involvement made clients feel "cared for" (de Lima Santos & Marcon, 2014).* EBN: *Nurses found that by using an evidence-based structured communication algorithm with families of clients in the intensive care unit, there was increased participation in decision-making with health care providers (Huffines et al, 2013).*
- Review factors of the health belief model (HBM) (individual perceptions of seriousness and susceptibility, demographic and other modifying factors, and perceived benefits and barriers) with the client. EBN: *Studies using the HBM supports the view that individual perceptions along with a variety of modifying factors affect the likelihood of changing health behaviors (Pender et al, 2015).* EBN: *Using the HBM, specifically the concept of acceptance, to assess clients receiving vaccines found that age, perceived susceptibility, and perceived severity of the disease being immunized for, increases the odds of getting vaccines (Adams et al, 2014).*
- Use various formats to provide information about the therapeutic regimen, including group education, brochures, videotapes, written instructions, computer-based programs, and telephone contact. CEB: *Women's knowledge about health care screening for breast cancer in Nigeria was shown to be best disseminated by newspapers, TV/radio programs, libraries, and the Internet, which were accessible to women there (Ugwoke & Ezukwouke, 2014).* EBN: *Telephone calls and text messages supported significantly better control of symptoms and medication adherence for psychiatric clients (Bebe et al, 2014).*
- Help the client identify and modify barriers to effective self-management. CEB: *A qualitative study found that the words used for health promotion during the professional-client interaction affects the client's participation in health care (Moreira et al, 2013).* EBN: *A pre-test, post-test study with overweight African American women (N = 19) demonstrated that client activation and self-efficacy are essential for success in self-management (Onubogu et al, 2014).*
- Help the client self-manage his or her own health through education about strategies for changing habits such as overeating, sedentary lifestyle, and smoking. CEB: *A large-scale Chinese study involving 21 sites found that cessation to quit smoking was directly related to intent to quit and professional status, whereas risk factors for not quitting were related to smoking alone and reported addiction to nicotine (Yang et al, 2014).* CEB: *A study of 114 high school students demonstrated that peer-led interventions were effective at improving students' cigarette smoking knowledge, attitude, and behavior (Raji et al, 2014).*
- Develop a contract with the client to maintain motivation for changes in behavior. CEB: *A study that examined the impact of telephone reinforcement and a tailored maintenance contract on physical activity maintenance in older adults with osteoarthritis found that the contract group changed behavior more often than the telephone group (Desai et al, 2014).* EBN: *A descriptive study explored nurses' learning in the community settings and three major themes emerged: (1) power relationships are different in community settings, (2) clients have more autonomy and self-determination in decision-making, and (3) the development of a self-management plan (Merritt & Boogaerts, 2014).*

- Use focus groups to evaluate the implementation of self-management programs. EBN: *The use of focus groups to foster decision-making in mental health clients contributed to greater self-health management (Mahone et al, 2011).* CEB: *A qualitative study of members of the military with chronic low back pain found developing trusting relationships, establishing a need to be actively engaged in their rehabilitation, and finding workable rehabilitation solutions motivated clients to engage in needed rehabilitation (Harman et al, 2014).*
- Refer to the care plan ineffective Family **Health** management.

Geriatric

- Identify the reasons for behaviors that are not therapeutic and discuss alternatives. EBN: *Researchers found that implementing a programmed learning to encourage staff to help clients reminisce assisted dementia clients to "tell their story" (Cooney et al, 2013).* CEB: *Researchers followed older clients (65 and older) after discharge to home with structured telephone interviews about medication adherence; 69% were nonadherent at 3 months due to (1) the number of medications, (2) changes in medications, and (3) understanding the reason for medication (Pasina et al, 2014).*

H

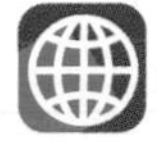

Multicultural

- Assess the influence of cultural beliefs, norms, and values on the individual's perceptions of the therapeutic regimen. EBN: *Identification of factors contributing to adherence of cardiac medication in the Asian population of Canada found clients relied on family members for support to be adherent with their medications (Ens et al, 2014).* CEB: *Infection prevention and control is affected by human behavior, which is influenced by cultural constructs, including (1) power, (2) uncertainty avoidance, and (3) masculinity (Borg, 2014).*
- Discuss all strategies with the client in the context of the client's culture. CEB: *Adherence to antiretroviral therapy in Kenya was studied using cognitive interviewing with pediatric caregivers and HIV-infected adolescents by verbal probing and guided "thinking aloud"; comprehension problems were found as the reason for key missed doses and understanding side effects (Vreeman et al, 2014).* CEB: *Researchers interviewed clients of Arcadian descent on hemodialysis to learn about their intake of the Acadian diet and found that the diet held multiple meanings for different participants, which supports the individualization of care and discourages generalization based on assumptions of homogeneity of all clients within a cultural group (Raed Tarakji et al, 2014).*
- Provide health information that is consistent with the health literacy of clients. EBN: *Chinese clients, when surveyed, indicated that they prefer face to face communication and teaching (You et al, 2014).* EBN: *A study investigated economically and socially disadvantaged clients with type 2 diabetes with low health literacy and found that an educational program designed to be culturally sensitive and meet the needs of individuals with low health literacy improved short-term outcomes (Swaverly et al, 2014).*
- Assess for barriers that may interfere with client follow-up of treatment recommendations. CEB: *Patients discharged from specialty care are more likely to receive follow-up care if referred back to their familiar primary care provider (Tuot et al, 2014).* EBN: *Breastfeeding rates among black infants in the United States are 16% lower than among whites; a data analysis by ZIP code revealed that the largest differences were in hospitals that implemented breastfeeding practices, such as (1) early initiation of breastfeeding, (2) limited use of supplements, and (3) rooming-in, suggesting that there are racial disparities in access to maternity care practices that support breastfeeding (Lind et al, 2014).*
- Use electronic monitoring and dosing to improve management of medications. EBN: *The use of electronic dosing and monitoring devices, in conjunction with other measures of adherence, has contributed to successful client adherence to medication regimens (Cook et al, 2012).* CEB: *Post-discharge home-based, pharmacist-provided medication management services to clients after discharge assisted in resolving medication discrepancies (Pherson et al, 2014).*
- Validate the client's feelings regarding the ability to manage his/her own care and the impact on lifestyle. EBN: *A descriptive correlational study identified self-care ability as being correlated with the concepts of health literacy and self efficacy (McCleary-Jones, 2011).* CEB: *Understanding youth's and parents' changing perceptions of illness during the course of a youth's psychosis was studied and five themes that assisted the child's self-determination and self-management included: 1) symptom recognition, 2) awareness of change, 3) negative appraisals, 4) positive appraisals, and 5) treatment self-management (Gearing et al, 2014).*

Home Care

- Prepare and instruct clients and family members in the use of a medication box. Set up an appropriate schedule for filling of the medication box, and post medication times and doses in an accessible area (e.g., attached by a magnet to the refrigerator). EBN: *Improved self-management of therapeutic regimen is increased through the use of cues and supports that help clients remember to take medications (Cook et al, 2012).* CEB: *Conklin et al (2014) found that post-discharge medication-related problems are largely due to poor health literacy.*
- Monitor self-management of the medical regimen. EBN: *Patient-centered care was analyzed by an extensive multidisciplinary literature review and three themes were identified as being fundamental: (1) client participation and involvement, (2) the relationship between the client and the health care professional, and (3) the context in which care is delivered (Kitson et al, 2013).* CEB: *Mohammed et al (2013) explored decision-making processes used in allocating occupational and physical therapy services for home care clients and found that funding was the primary determinant of home care treatment.*
- Refer to health care professionals for questions and self-care management. CEB: *Prehospital mobile telemedicine communication for stroke victims to receive plasminogen activators by emergency medical personnel was reliable and feasible (Wu et al, 2014).* CEB: *A study examined whether client satisfaction differed when clients were seen by a physician alone or by a physician and medical student and found that clients in rural and community-based outpatient settings were satisfied when a medical student was involved; therefore, medical students are a good interdisciplinary source in promoting client self-management (Law et al, 2014).*

H

Client/Family Teaching and Discharge Planning

- Identify the client and/or family's current knowledge and adjust teaching accordingly. Teach the client and family about all aspects of the therapeutic regimen, providing as much knowledge as the client and family will accept, in a culturally congruent manner. CEB: *The American Association of Diabetes Education found improved self-management when instruction and guidance were based on a collaborative relationship with health care providers that was based on individual monitored outcomes (Stetson et al, 2011).* EBN: *A qualitative study of significant others of dialysis clients found that significant others were involved in the decision-making and had a need to be informed and supported (DeRosenroll et al, 2013).*
- Teach ways to adjust activities of daily living (ADLs) for inclusion in therapeutic regimens. EBN: *Ha and Kim (2014) studied ADLs in clients with dementia and found that five leading factors (urinary and fecal incontinence, regularity of exercise, mental state scores, and stroke history) negatively affected clients when trying to perform ADLs.* CEB: *This study describes patterns of ADL functional disability in primary progressive aphasia (PPA) clients and found that ADL functionality varies between PPA subtypes and therapeutic strategies can be tailored to each client to promote improved ADL functioning (O'Connor et al, 2014).*
- Teach safety in taking medications. CEB: *This database study examines the primary practitioner's role in the prescription of drugs to home-dwelling older adults and found that the client's regular practitioner, not specialists, prescribe the major portion of nonaddictive and addictive medications and is key to coordination of prescriptions (Kann et al, 2014).* EBN: *Explored nurses' perspectives on preventing medication administration errors revealed three themes: (1) nurses' roles and responsibilities in medication safety, (2) nurses' ability to work safely, and (3) nurses' acceptance of safety practices placing nurses in a position to ensure safe medication management (Smeulers et al, 2014).*
- Teach the client to act as a self-advocate with health providers who prescribe therapeutic regimens. EBN: *A review of literature showed that nurses who advocate for clients and become partners in care need clarification to fully incorporate into the multiple roles that nurses already have (Wellard, 2014).* CEB: *A study analyzed data for children (N = 40,242) with special health care needs by a national survey to look at shared decision-making (SDM) in relation to sociodemographic/health characteristics and found that clients in medical homes had six times greater odds of perceived shared decision-making with providers (Smalley et al, 2014).*

REFERENCES

Adams, A., Hall, M., & Fulghum, J. (2014). Utilizing the health belief model to assess vaccine acceptance of patients on hemodialysis. *Nephrology Nursing Journal, 41*(4), 393–407.

Bebe, L., Smith, K. D., & Phillips, C. (2014). A comparison of telephone and texting interventions for persons with schizophrenia spectrum disorders. *Issues in Mental Health Nursing, 35*(5), 323–329.

Borg, M. A. (2014). Cultural determinants of infection control behaviour: understanding drivers and implementing effective change. *Journal of Hospital Infection, 86*(3), 161–168.

Borneman, T., Irish, T., Sidhu, R., et al. (2014). Death awareness, feelings of uncertainty, and hope in advanced lung cancer patients: can they coexist? *International Journal of Palliative Care, 20*(6), 271–277.

Conklin, J. R., Togami, J. C., Burnett, A., et al. (2014). Care transitions service: a pharmacy-driven program for medication reconciliation through the continuum of care. *American Journal of Health-System Pharmacy, 15*, 802–810.

Cook, P., Schmiege, S., McClean, M., et al. (2012). Practical and analytic issues in the electronic assessment of adherence. *Western Journal of Nursing Research, 34*(5), 598–620.

Cooney, A., O'Shea, E., Casey, D., et al. (2013). Developing a structured education reminiscence-based programme for staff in long-stay care facilities in Ireland. *Journal of Clinical Nursing, 22*(13/14), 1977–1987.

de Lima Santos, A., & Marcon, S. S. (2014). How people with diabetes evaluate participation of their family in their health care. *Investigacion & Educacion en Enfermeria, 32*(2), 260–269.

DeRosenroll, A., Smith Higuchi, K., Standish Dutton, K., et al. (2013). Perspectives of significant others in dialysis modality decision-making: a qualitative study. *CANNT Journal, 23*(4), 17–24.

Desai, P. M., Hughes, S. L., Peters, K. E., et al. (2014). Impact of telephone reinforcement and negotiated contracts on behavioral predictors of exercise maintenance in older adults with osteoarthritis. *American Journal of Behavioral Health, 38*(3), 465–477.

Ens, T. A., Seneviratne, C. C., Jones, C., et al. (2014). Factors influencing medication adherence in South Asian people with cardiac disorders: an ethnographic study. *International Journal of Nursing Studies, 51*(11), 1472–1481.

Gearing, R. E., DeVylder, J. E., Chen, F., et al. (2014). Changing perceptions of illness in the early course of psychosis: psychological pathways to self-determination and self-management of treatment. *Psychiatry: Interpersonal & Biological Processes, 77*(4), 344–359.

Ha, E., & Kim, K. (2014). Factors that influence activities of daily living in the elderly with probable dementia. *Journal of Psychiatric & Mental Health Nursing, 21*(5), 447–454.

Harman, K., MacRae, M., Vallis, M., et al. (2014). Working with people to make changes: a behavioural change approach used in chronic low back pain rehabilitation. *Physiotherapy Canada, 66*(1), 82–90.

Huffines, M. J., Johnson, K. L., Naranjo, S. L. L., et al. (2013). Improving family satisfaction and participation in decision making in an intensive care unit. *Critical Care Nurse, 33*(5), 56–69.

Kann, I., Lundqvist, C., & Luras, H. (2014). Prescription of addictive and non-addictive drugs to home-dwelling elderly. *Drugs and Aging, 31*(6), 453–459.

Kitson, A., Marshall, A., Bassett, K., et al. (2013). What are the core elements of patient-centred care? A narrative review and synthesis of the literature from health policy, medicine and nursing. *Journal of Advanced Nursing, 69*(1), 4–15.

Law, M., Hamilton, M., Bridge, E., et al. (2014). The effect of clinical teaching on patient satisfaction in rural and community settings. *Canadian Journal of Rural Medicine, 19*(2), 57–62.

Lind, J. N., Perrine, C. G., Li, R., et al. (2014). Racial disparities in access to maternity care practices that support breastfeeding—United States, 2011. *MMWR: Morbidity & Mortality Weekly Report, 63*(33), 725–728.

Mahone, I. H., Farell, S., Hinton, I., et al. (2011). Shared decision making in mental health treatment: qualitative findings from stakeholder focus groups. *Archives of Psychiatric Nursing, 25*(6), 27–36.

McCleary-Jones, V. (2011). Health literacy and its association with diabetes knowledge, self-efficacy and disease self-management among African Americans with diabetes mellitus. *Association of Black Nursing Faculty Journal, 22*(2), 25–32.

Mee, S. (2014). Self-efficacy: a mediator of smoking behavior and depression among college students. *Pediatric Nursing, 40*(1), 9–37.

Merritt, A., & Boogaerts, M. (2014). Creativity and power: a qualitative, exploratory study of student learning acquired in a community nursing setting that is applied in future settings. *Contemporary Nurse: A Journal for the Australian Nursing Profession, 46*(2), 225–233.

Mohammed, R., Poss, J., Egan, M., et al. (2013). Decision makers' allocation of home-care therapy services: a process map. *Physiotherapy Canada, 65*(2), 125–132.

Moreira, D. R., Lopes, M. R., Freire, D., et al. (2013). Prevention of cervical cancer in pregnant women: a phenomenological study. *Online Brazilian Journal of Nursing, 12*(3), 511–521.

Musich, S., Klemes, A., Kubica, M. A., et al. (2014). Clinical: personalized preventive care reduces healthcare expenditures among medicare advantage beneficiaries. *American Journal of Managed Care, 8*, 613–620.

O'Connor, C. M., Ahmed, S., & Misoshi, E. (2014). Functional disability in primary progressive aphasia. *Aphasiology, 28*(8/9), 1131–1149.

Onubogu, U., Graham, M. E., & Robinson, T. O. (2014). Pilot study of an action plan intervention for self-management in overweight/obese adults in a medically underserved minority population: phase I. *Association of Black Nursing Faculty Journal, 25*(3), 64–71.

Pasina, L., Brucato, A., Falcone, C., et al. (2014). Medication non-adherence among elderly patients newly discharged and receiving polypharmacy. *Drugs and Aging, 31*(4), 283–289.

Pender, N. J., Murdaugh, C. L., & Parsons, M. A. (2015). *Health promotion in nursing practice* (7th ed.). NJ: Upper Saddle River: Prentice Hall.

Pherson, E. C., Shermock, K. M., Efird, L. E., et al. (2014). Development and implementation of a postdischarge home-based medication management service. *American Journal of Health-System Pharmacy, 71*(18), 1576–1583.

Raed Tarakji, A., Surette, M., Frotten, R., et al. (2014). Experiences of people of Acadian descent receiving hemodialysis in southwest Nova Scotia. *Canadian Journal of Dietetic Practice & Research, 75*(2), 342–345.

Raji, M., Abubakar, I., Oche, M., et al. (2014). Using peer led health education intervention to improve in-school adolescents' cigarette smoking related knowledge, attitude and behaviour in a north west Nigeria state. *Health Science Journal, 8*(4), 485–494.

Roditi, D., & Robinson, M. E. (2011). The role of psychological interventions in the management of patients with chronic pain. *Journal of Psychology Research and Behavioral Management*, (4), 41–49.

Schulman-Green, D., Bradley, E., Knobf, M. T., et al. (2011). Self-management and transitions in women with advanced breast cancer. *Journal of Pain Symptom Management, 42*(4), 517–525.

Smalley, L., Kenney, M., Denboba, D., et al. (2014). Family perceptions of shared decision-making with health care providers: results of the national survey of children with special health care needs, 2009-2010. *Maternal & Child Health Journal, 18*(6), 1316–1327.

Smeulers, M., Onderwater, A. T., Zwieten, M. C. B., et al. (2014). Nurses' experiences and perspectives on medication safety

H

practices: an explorative qualitative study. *Journal of Nursing Management*, *22*(3), 276–285.
Stetson, B., Schlundt, D., Peyrot, M., et al. (2011). Monitoring in diabetes self-management: issues and recommendations for improvement. *Population Health Management*, *14*(4), 189–197.
Swaverly, D., Vorderstrasse, A., Maldonado, E., et al. (2014). Implementation and evaluation of a low health literacy and culturally sensitive diabetes education program. *Journal of Healthcare Quality: Promoting Excellence in Healthcare*, *36*(6), 16–23.
Tuot, D. S., Sewell, J. L., Day, L., et al. (2014). Increasing access to specialty care: patient discharges from a gastroenterology clinic. *American Journal of Managed Care*, *20*(10), 812–819.
Ugwoke, B., & Ezukwouke, N. (2014). Information for breast cancer prevention among females in Nigeria: as of patients in two teaching hospitals. *Journal of Hospital Librarianship*, *14*(3), 250–260.
Vreeman, R., Nyandikl, W., Ayaya, S., et al. (2014). Cognitive interviewing for cross-cultural adaptation of pediatric antiretroviral therapy adherence measurement items. *International Journal of Behavioral Medicine*, *21*(1), 186–196.
Wellard, S. J. (2014). Who speaks for whom? Can nurses be patient advocates in renal settings? *Renal Society of Australasia Journal*, *10*(2), 81–83.
Wu, T., Nguyen, C., Ankrom, C., et al. (2014). Prehospital utility of rapid stroke evaluation using in-ambulance telemedicine: a pilot feasibility study. *Stroke; a Journal of Cerebral Circulation*, *45*(8), 2342–2347.
Yang, T., Mao, A., Feng, X., et al. (2014). Smoking cessation in an urban population in China. *American Journal of Behavioral Health*, *38*(6), 933–941.
You, G., Li, X., Xu, Y., et al. (2014). Learning needs of Chinese patients before undergoing elective percutaneous coronary intervention. *Contemporary Nurse: A Journal for the Australian Nursing Profession*, *47*(1/2), 152–158.
Zolnierek, C. D. (2014). An integrative review of knowing the patient. *Journal of Nursing Scholarship*, *46*(1), 3–10.

Ineffective Family Health management

Roberta Dobrzanski, MSN, RN

NANDA-I

Definition

A pattern of regulating and integrating, into family processes, a program for the treatment of illness and its sequelae that is unsatisfactory for meeting specific health goals

Defining Characteristics

Acceleration of illness symptoms of a family member; decrease in attention to illness; difficulty with prescribed regimen; failure to take action to reduce risk factors; inappropriate family activities for meeting health goals

Related Factors (r/t)

Complex treatment regimen; complexity of health care system; decisional conflict; economically disadvantaged; family conflict

NOC (Nursing Outcomes Classification)

Suggested NOC Outcomes

Family Health-Status; Knowledge: Treatment Regimen; Family Participation in Professional Care

Example NOC Outcome with Indicators

Knowledge: Treatment Regimen as evidenced by the following indicator: Understanding conveyed about prescribed medication, activity, exercise, and specific disease process. (Rate the outcome and indicators of **Knowledge: Treatment Regimen:** 1 = no knowledge, 2 = limited knowledge, 3 = moderate knowledge, 4 = substantial knowledge, 5 = extensive knowledge [see Section I].)

Client Outcomes

Client Will (Specify Time Frame)

- Make adjustments in usual activities (e.g., diet, activity, stress management) to incorporate therapeutic regimens of its members

- Reduce illness symptoms of family members
- Desire to manage therapeutic regimens of its members
- Describe a decrease in the difficulties of managing therapeutic regimens
- Describe actions to reduce risk factors

NIC (Nursing Interventions Classification)

Suggested NIC Intervention

Family Involvement Promotion; Family Mobilization; Teaching: Disease Process

Example NIC Activities—Family Involvement Promotion

Identify and respect coping mechanisms used by family members; Provide crucial information to family members about the patient in accordance with client's preference

H

Nursing Interventions and *Rationales*

- Base family interventions on knowledge of the family, family context, family dynamics, family structure, and family function. EBN: *Family research has established that families differ widely from one another, even within cultures (Wright & Leahey, 2013).*
- Use a family approach when helping an individual with a health problem that requires therapeutic management. EBN: *Family relationships can be a source of support for people with diabetes and may influence self-management behavior (Paddison, 2010).*
- Review with family members the congruence and incongruence of family behaviors and health-related goals. EBN: *To attain the motivation needed for changes in health habits, family members should understand the relation of daily habits to health-related goals (Wright & Leahey, 2013).*
- Acknowledge the challenge of integrating therapeutic regimens with family behaviors. EBN: *Therapeutic regimens require modifications of daily activities that have already been established based on family values and beliefs. Acknowledging the difficulty of changing family habits supports families through the process (Wright & Leahey, 2013).*
- Review the symptoms of specific illnesses and work with the family toward development of greater self-efficacy in relation to these symptoms. EBN: *Knowledge of symptoms improves the ability of family members to adjust behaviors to prevent and manage symptoms (Larsen, 2014).*
- Support family decisions to adjust therapeutic regimens as indicated. EBN: *Sometimes families do not have access to health care providers and should make independent decisions because of side effects or adverse effects of therapeutic regimens. Family members need to make informed decisions in their best interests (Wright & Leahey, 2009).*
- Advocate for the family in negotiating therapeutic regimens with health providers. CEB: *Illness regimens generally are neither arbitrary nor absolute; therefore, modifications can be discussed as needed to fit with the family lifestyle (Wright & Leahey, 2009).*
- Help the family mobilize social supports. EBN: *Increased social support helps families meet health-related goals (Pender et al, 2011).*
- Help family members modify perceptions as indicated. EBN: *Individual perceptions of the seriousness of, susceptibility to, and threat of illness may be distorted or inaccurate and may be modified with new information (Pender et al, 2011).*
- Use one or more theories of family dynamics to describe, explain, or predict family behaviors (e.g., theories of Bowen, Satir, and Minuchin). EBN: *Family systems may not be understood by the nurse without adequate knowledge of family theory (Wright & Leahey, 2013).*

▲ Collaborate with expert nurses or other consultants regarding strategies for working with families. EBN: *The family clinical nurse specialist uses components such as time allowance; level of staff's family theory knowledge; level of experience and comfort; institution policy; and interdisciplinary team commitment to positively influence the delivery of family-centered care (Parker, 2011).*

- Coaching methods can be used to help families improve their health. EBN: *Coaching is a beneficial tool for families of many children and teens with attention deficit hyperactivity disorder, executive functioning disorders (Sleeper-Triplett, 2008), and/or behavioral concerns.* CEB: *Coaching processes were shown to improve family outcomes related to improved nutrition and physical activity (Heimendinger et al, 2007).*

Pediatric

- Support kangaroo care for infants at risk at birth. Keep infants in an upright position in skin-to-skin contact until they no longer tolerate it. CEB: *Kangaroo mother care has a positive impact on family and home environment. The results of this study also suggest, first, that both parents should be involved as direct caregivers in the kangaroo mother care procedure, and second, that this intervention should be directed more specifically at infants who are more at risk at birth (Tessier et al, 2009).*

Geriatric

- Recommend that clients use the "Ask Me 3" program when communicating with their pharmacist (What is my main problem? What do I need to do? Why is it important for me to do this?). CEB: *The Ask Me 3 program is a practical tool that created awareness and reinforced principles of clear health communication with pharmacists and community-dwelling well older adults who participated in this study (Miller et al, 2008).*

H

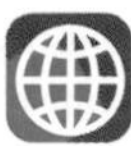

Multicultural

- Acknowledge racial and ethnic differences at the onset of care. CEB: *Acknowledgment of race and ethnicity issues enhances communication, establishes rapport, and promotes treatment outcomes (Giger & Davidhizar, 2008; Leininger & McFarland, 2006).*
- Ensure that all strategies for working with the family are congruent with the culture of the family. CEB: *Many nursing studies among people of a variety of cultures show that cultural variations exist in the management of therapeutic regimens, and these differences should be taken into account when working with families (Hanley, 2008; Leininger & McFarland, 2006).*
- Use a family-centered approach when working with Latino, Asian, African American, and Native American clients. CEB: *Latinos may perceive the family as a source of support, solver of problems, and source of pride. Asian Americans may regard the family as the primary decision-maker and influence on individual family members. Native American families may have extended structures and exert powerful influences over functioning (Hanley, 2008; Leininger & McFarland, 2006). Findings in this study suggest that incorporating family norms is critical when developing interventions to increase formal health service utilization among African Americans (Barksdale & Molock, 2009).*
- Facilitate modeling and role playing for the family regarding healthy ways to communicate and interact. CEB: *It is helpful for families and the client to practice communication skills in a safe environment before trying them in a real-life situation (Degazon, 2006; Wright & Leahey, 2013).*
- Use the nursing intervention of cultural brokerage to help families deal with the health care system. CEB: *In a study based on 24 in-depth interviews, four empirical mechanisms of cultural brokerage were identified: translating between health systems, bridging divergent images of medicine, establishing long-term relationships, and working with patients' relational networks (Lo, 2010).*

Client/Family Teaching and Discharge Planning

- Teach about all aspects of therapeutic regimens. Provide as much knowledge as family members will accept, adjust instruction to account for what the family already knows, and provide information in a culturally congruent manner.
- Teach ways to adjust family behaviors to include therapeutic regimens, such as safety in taking medications and teaching family members to act as self-advocates with health providers who prescribe therapeutic regimens.

REFERENCES

Barksdale, C. L., & Molock, S. D. (2009). Perceived norms and mental health help seeking among African American college students. *The Journal of Behavioral Health Services and Research, 36*(3), 285–299.

Degazon, C. (2006). Cultural influences in nursing in community health. In M. Stanhope & J. Lancaster (Eds.), *Foundations of nursing in the community: community-oriented practice* (2nd ed.). St Louis: Mosby.

Giger, J. N., & Davidhizar, R. (2008). *Transcultural nursing: assessment and intervention* (5th ed.). St Louis: Mosby.
Hanley, K. (2008). Navajos. In J. N. Giger & R. Davidhizar (Eds.), *Transcultural nursing: assessment and intervention* (5th ed.). St Louis: Mosby.
Heimendinger, J., et al. (2007). Coaching process outcomes of a family visit nutrition and physical activity intervention. *Health Education and Behavior, 34*, 71–89.
Larsen, P. D. (2014). *Lubkin's Chronic illness: impact and interventions* (9th ed.). Boston: Jones & Bartlett.
Leininger, M. M., & McFarland, M. R. (2006). *Culture care diversity and universality: a worldwide nursing theory* (2nd ed.). Boston: Jones & Bartlett.
Lo, M. C. M. (2010). Cultural brokerage: creating linkages between voices of lifeworld and medicine in cross-cultural clinical settings. *Health (London, England: 1997), 14*(5), 484–504.
Miller, M. J., et al. (2008). Promoting health communication between the community-dwelling well-elderly and pharmacists: the Ask Me 3 program. *Journal of the American Pharmaceutical Association, 48*(6), 784–792.
Paddison, C. (2010). Family support and conflict among adults with type 2 diabetes: development and testing of a new measure. *Eur Diabetes Nurs, 7*(1), 29–33.
Parker, L. (2011). Enhancing family-centered care in intensive care: the family clinical nurse specialist. *Dynamics (Pembroke, Ont.), 22*(2), 55.
Pender, N. J., Murdaugh, C. L., & Parsons, M. A. (2011). *Health promotion in nursing practice* (6th ed.). Upper Saddle River, NJ: Prentice Hall.
Sleeper-Triplett, J. (2008). Family matters. The effectiveness of coaching for children and teens with AD/HD. *Pediatric Nursing, 34*(5), 433–435.
Tessier, R., et al. (2009). Kangaroo Mother Care, home environment and father involvement in the first year of life: a randomized controlled study. *Acta Paediatrica, 98*(9), 1444–1450.
Wright, L. M., & Leahey, M. (2013). *Nurses and families: a guide to family assessment and intervention* (6th ed.). Philadelphia: FA Davis.

Readiness for Enhanced Health management

Ruth A. Wittmann-Price, PhD, RN, CNS, CNE, CHSE, ANEF, FAAN

NANDA-I

Definition

A pattern of regulating and integrating into daily living a therapeutic regimen for treatment of illness and its sequelae, which can be strengthened

Defining Characteristics

Expresses desire to enhance choices of daily living for meeting goals; expresses desire to enhance management of illness; expresses desire to enhance management of prescribed regimens; expresses desire to enhance management of risk factors; expresses desire to enhance management of symptoms; expresses desire to enhance immunization/vaccination status

NOC (Nursing Outcomes Classification)

Suggested NOC Outcomes

Health-Promoting Behavior; Health-Seeking Behavior; Knowledge: Health Behavior; Health Promotion; Health Resources; Illness Care; Medication; Prescribed Activity; Treatment Regimen

Example NOC Outcome with Indicators

Health-Promoting Behavior as evidenced by the following indicators: Monitors personal behavior for risks/Seeks balance activity and rest/Performs healthy behaviors routinely/Uses financial and social support resources to promote health. (Rate each indicator of **Health-Promoting Behavior:** 1 = never demonstrated, 2 = rarely demonstrated, 3 = sometimes demonstrated, 4 = often demonstrated, 5 = consistently demonstrated [see Section I].)

Client Outcomes

Client Will (Specify Time Frame)

- Describe integration of therapeutic regimen into daily living
- Demonstrate continued commitment to integration of therapeutic regimen into daily living routines

NIC (Nursing Interventions Classification)

Suggested NIC Intervention

Anticipatory Guidance; Mutual Goal Setting; Client Contracting; Self-Modification Assistance; Self-Responsibility Facilitation; Support System Enhancement

Example NIC Activities—Mutual Goal Setting

Assist client and significant others to develop realistic expectations of themselves in performance of their roles; Clarify with the client the roles of the health care provider and the client, respectively

Nursing Interventions and *Rationales*

H

- Acknowledge the expertise that the client and family bring to health management. EBN: *The use of focus groups to acknowledge expertise and foster decision-making in mental health consumers contributed to greater health management (Mahone et al, 2011).* CEB: *This study investigated the influence of factors on the use of speech, the use of sign, spoken language multilingualism, and spoken language of caregivers of children with hearing loss and found that caregivers' decision-making regarding communication mode is influenced by factors that are not equally weighted and that relate to the child, family, community, and advice from others (Crowe et al, 2014).*
- Review factors that contribute to the likelihood of health promotion and health protection. Use Pender's Health Promotion Model and Becker's Health Belief Model to identify contributing factors (Pender et al, 2015). EBN: *Many studies using both the Health Promotion Model and the Health Belief Model (HBM) support the view that individual perceptions and a variety of modifying factors affect the likelihood of improving health behaviors (Pender et al, 2015).* EBN: *When using the HBM to examine weight management barriers in first-year college students, researchers found that students identified resources to assist them with weight management such as curriculum inclusion and methods to promote physical activity and nutrition (Das & Evans, 2014).*
- Further develop and reinforce contributing factors that might change with ongoing management of the therapeutic regimen (e.g., knowledge, self-efficacy, self-esteem, and perceived benefits). EBN: *The purpose of this study was to decrease sun exposure and skin cancer to clients at their workplace through an intervention that significantly improved perceived self-efficacy and increased use of sunscreen protection (Lee et al, 2014).* CEB: *When studying adolescents with food allergy–induced anaphylaxis self-care behaviors, it was identified that adherence was influenced by severity of reaction, barriers to adherence, illness identity, cyclical beliefs, and emotional responses (Jones et al, 2014).*
- Support all efforts to manage therapeutic regimens. EBN: *Ongoing support and assistance from health care providers is needed to identify and enhance factors that contribute to the likelihood of taking action for health promotion and health protection (Pender et al, 2015).* EBN: *The HBM was used to measure and predict the sleep behavior of employed college students (N = 188) and found that it explained 34% of the variance in sleep behavior and the significant elements were perceived severity, perceived barriers, cues to action, and self-efficacy (Knowlden & Sharma, 2014).*
- Review the client's strengths in the management of the therapeutic regimen. CEB: *Researchers studied conversations of hearing-impaired clients to assess knowledge and attitudes about hearing and hearing conversation and use of hearing protection and found a significant relationship between use of hearing protection and the HBM (Saunders et al, 2014).* CEB: *A study examined older clients' reasons for help-seeking for hearing impairment and found the most important factors related to attitudinal beliefs (e.g., perceived benefits of hearing aids) and external cues to action (e.g., support from significant others) (Meyer et al, 2014).*
- Collaborate with the client to identify strategies to maintain strengths and develop additional strengths as indicated. CEB: *A study about chronic pain, identification of strengths regarding pain management, rather than direct elimination of the pain, helped empowered and enabled clients to manage their pain (Roditi & Robinson, 2011).* CEB: *Corcoran and Crowley (2014) studied Latina women's attitudes and perceptions regarding cervical cancer screening and found that the most important factors were culturally appropriate education and improving accessibility to health care.*

- Identify contributing factors that may need to be improved now or in the future. EBN: *Health promotion and protection are complex behaviors that are difficult to implement on a daily basis. Based on the complexity of achieving these behaviors and the perceived barriers to implementation (e.g., time, energy, money), usually one or more contributing factors would benefit from increased focus and attention (Pender et al, 2015).* EBN: *This study identified the health-seeking preferences of older Filipinos in the community, and results indicated that the most important element in terms of health-seeking behavior was the client's experience with the health care provider (de Guzman et al, 2014).*
- Provide knowledge as needed related to the pathophysiology of the disease or illness, prescribed activities, prescribed medications, and nutrition. EBN: *Knowledge is a factor that contributes significantly to the client's taking action for health promotion and protection. Remember, however, that knowledge is necessary but not sufficient to explain why people perform or do not perform actions for health promotion and protection (Pender et al, 2015).* CEB: *Researchers provided veteran clients with a 12-week "Pain Education School" program for chronic pain; quantitative findings suggest that veterans reported (1) learning "new and useful" information, (2) perceived the program as "easy to understand," (3) used the learned information, and (4) recommended the program to others (Watson et al, 2014).*
- Support positive health promotion and health protection behaviors. EBN: *Ongoing support may be needed to maintain these behaviors (Pender et al, 2015).* EBN: *Key predictors of "help-seeking behavior" in adolescents with mental illness were identified and include health beliefs, personality traits, and attitudes, but perceived benefits were a particularly strong indicator (O'Connor et al, 2014).*
- Help the client maintain existing support and seek additional supports as needed. EBN: *In numerous research studies, social support was shown to be a factor contributing to ongoing maintenance of positive health behaviors (Pender et al, 2015).* EBN: *A study used visual imagery depicting super heroes with college students to engage them in a health campaigns about sleep and found that providing health care messaging to college students about sleep health promotion may benefit from visual imaging (Mackert et al, 2014).*

H

Geriatric

- Facilitate the client and family to obtain health insurance and drug payment plans whenever needed and possible. CEB: *Adherence to medications and self-health regimens is facilitated by payers' knowledge and use of value-based insurance designs (Cohen et al, 2012).* CEB: *An investigation probed the continuation of clients' medication from primary care to hospital and back again to primary care and found that clients were using an average of 8.2 drugs before hospital admission. Of those, 0.9 were discontinued while the clients were in the hospital and an average of 1.7 new drugs were started for each client in the hospital and less than half of newly initiated drugs were continued after discharge (Larsen et al, 2014).*

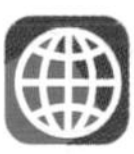

Multicultural

- Assess client's cultural perspectives on health management. EBN: *The effect of an HBM-based nursing intervention was studied on health care outcomes in Chinese clients with chronic obstructive pulmonary disease (COPD). Clients had significantly increased scores of health belief and self-efficacy after receiving HBM-based nursing intervention compared with a control group (Wang et al, 2014).* EBN: *Researchers pilot tested a culturally specific curriculum for African American college students to increase awareness of cardiovascular disease (CVD). The program increased student understanding of family history and strategies to reduce their own risk of CVD (Holland et al, 2014).*
- Assess health literacy in clients of diverse backgrounds. EBN: *The high recurrence rate of chlamydial infection among African American urban women was studied using the HBM. Results of participant interviews suggested knowledge deficits about the seriousness of* Chlamydia *compared to other sexually transmitted infections (Craft-Blacksheare et al, 2014).* EBN: *A study evaluated commonly used printed health materials for readability and found 28% of the teaching material at a 9th grade or higher level and only 23% below a 5th grade level. Researchers then showed providers how to assess readability to improve client outcomes (Ryan et al, 2014).*
- Validate the client's feelings regarding the ability to manage his/her own care and the impact on current lifestyle. CEB: *A descriptive study correlated self-care ability with health literacy and self-efficacy (McCleary-Jones, 2011).* EBN: *There is a high incidence of anxiety and depression in COPD clients. This study educated nurses to screen for depression and anxiety and to offer motivational interviewing for self-management, which increased the clients' capability to manage their condition (Hardy et al, 2014).*

- Facilitate the client and family to obtain financial assistance in the form of health insurance and drug payment plans whenever needed and possible. CEB: *Adherence to medications and health regimens is facilitated by payers' knowledge and use of value-based insurance designs (Cohen et al, 2012).* CEB: *A retrospective analysis of insurance plan drug coverage data for three drug classes (statins, angiotensin II receptor blockers, and protein-tyrosine kinase inhibitors) demonstrated that there was substantially less drug reimbursement with low copays for Medicare plans than for commercial plans, employer plans, or union plans, and with pharmacy benefit management companies (Reignier, 2014).*
- Use electronic monitoring to improve medication adherence. EBN: *The use of electronic dosing and monitoring devices, in conjunction with other measures of adherence, has contributed to adherence to medication regimen (Cook et al, 2012).* EBN: *A study used a Meducation technology health literacy intervention to evaluate medication adherence for clients at risk for CVD for 6 months, at which time medication adherence improved 3.2% and there was a decrease in clients' average systolic blood pressure (0.5 mm Hg), diastolic blood pressure (1.5 mm Hg), and body weight (3.6 pounds) (Zullig et al, 2014).*
- Discuss with clients their beliefs about medication and treatment to enhance medication and treatment adherence. CEB: *A study used the HBM with mixed-race clients from a lower socioeconomic, nonurban environment to look at vaccine efficacy and personal constraints on vaccination behavior and found that vaccine efficacy and personal constraints do not significantly predict vaccination behavior and that convenience was the most important factor (Avery & Lariscy, 2014).* EBN: *This study focused on asthmatic clients and found they are generally nonadherent to medication therapy 30% to 70% of the time and need to engage in appropriate management strategies, which can be assisted by health care professionals who acknowledge and reflect the client's perspectives (Clayton, 2014).*

H

Community Teaching

- Review therapeutic regimens and their optimal integration with daily living routines. EBN: *Improved therapeutic regimen management is increased through the use of cues and supports that help clients remember to take medications (Cook et al, 2012).* EBN: *A case study reveals that a client living with HIV infection requires highly complex HIV care, including antiretroviral adherence therapies, cognitive behavioral therapy to alleviate depression, and motivational interviewing as essential components of complete HIV management (Paparello et al, 2014).*
- Teach disease processes and therapeutic regimens to clients and peer supporters for management of disease processes. CEB: *A study reviewed the role of peer supporters in helping individuals to maximize their medication adherence by promoting self-advocacy and negotiation skills (West, 2011).*

▲ EBN: *A qualitative study explored the lives of hemodialysis clients and their adherence to treatment and quality of life and found that clients' two most important motivators were (1) embracing the disease and dialysis and (2) using management to prevent disease progression (Guerra-Guerrerro et al, 2014).*

REFERENCES

Avery, E. J., & Lariscy, R. W. (2014). Preventable disease practices among a lower SES, multicultural, nonurban, U.S. community: the roles of vaccination efficacy and personal constraints. *Health Communication*, *29*(8), 826–836.

Clayton, S. (2014). Adherence to asthma medication. *Nurse Prescribing*, *12*(2), 68–74.

Cohen, J., Christensen, K., & Feldman, L. (2012). Disease management and medication compliance. *Population Health Management*, *15*(1), 20–28.

Cook, P., Schmiege, S., McClean, M., et al. (2012). Practical and analytic issues in the electronic assessment of adherence. *Western Journal of Nursing Research*, *34*(5), 598–620.

Corcoran, J., & Crowley, M. (2014). Latinas' attitudes about cervical cancer prevention: a meta-synthesis. *Journal of Cultural Diversity*, *21*(1), 15–21.

Craft-Blacksheare, M., Jackson, F., & Graham, T. K. (2014). Urban African American women's explanations of recurrent Chlamydia infections. *JOGNN: Journal of Obstetrical, Gynecological, and Neonatal Nursing*, *43*(5), 589–597.

Crowe, K., McLeod, S., McKinnon, D. H., et al. (2014). Speech, sign, or multilingualism for children with hearing loss: quantitative insights into caregivers' decision making. *Language, Speech & Hearing Services in Schools*, *45*(3), 234–247.

Das, B. M., & Evans, E. M. (2014). Understanding weight management perceptions in first-year college students using the health belief model. *Journal of American College Health*, *62*(7), 488–497.

de Guzman, A. B., Lores, K. V. A., Lorano, M. C. R., et al. (2014). Health-seeking preferences of elderly Filipinos in the community via conjoint analysis. *Educational Gerontology*, *40*(11), 801–815.

Guerra-Guerrerro, V., del Pilar Camargo Plazas, M., Cameron, B. L., et al. (2014). Understanding the life experience of people on hemodialysis: adherence to treatment and quality of life. *Nephrology Nursing Journal*, *41*(3), 289–298.

Hardy, S., Smart, D., Scanlon, M., et al. (2014). Integrating psychological screening into reviews of patients with COPD. *British Journal of Nursing*, *23*(15), 832–836.

Holland, C., Carthron, D. L., Duren-Winfield, V., et al. (2014). An experiential cardiovascular health education program for African

American college students. *Association of Black Nursing Faculty Journal, 25*(2), 52–56.

Jones, C. J., Smith, H. E., Frew, A. J., et al. (2014). Explaining adherence to self-care behaviours amongst adolescents with food allergy: a comparison of the health belief model and the common sense self-regulation model. *British Journal of Health Psychology, 19*(1), 65–82.

Knowlden, A. P., & Sharma, M. (2014). Health belief structural equation model predicting sleep behavior of employed college students. *Family & Community Health, 37*(4), 271–278.

Larsen, M., Rosholm, J., & Halla, J. (2014). The influence of comprehensive geriatric assessment on drug therapy in elderly patients. *European Journal of Clinical Pharmacology, 70*(2), 233–239.

Lee, C., Duffy, S. A., Louzon, S. A., et al. (2014). The Impact of sun solutions educational interventions on select health belief model constructs. *Workplace & Health Safety, 62*(2), 70–79.

Mackert, M., Lazard, A., Guadagno, M., et al. (2014). The role of implied motion in engaging audiences for health promotion: encouraging naps on a college campus. *Journal of American College Health, 62*(8), 542–551.

Mahone, I. H., Farrell, S., Hinton, I., et al. (2011). Shared decision making in mental health treatment: qualitative findings from stakeholder focus groups. *Archives of Psychiatric Nursing, 25*(6), e27–e36.

McCleary-Jones, V. (2011). Health literacy and its association with diabetes knowledge, self-efficacy and disease self-management among African Americans with diabetes mellitus. *Association of Black Nursing Faculty Journal, 22*(2), 25–32.

Meyer, C., Hickson, L., Lovelock, K., et al. (2014). An investigation of factors that influence help-seeking for hearing impairment in older adults. *International Journal of Audiology, 53*, S3–S17.

O'Connor, P. J., Martin, B., Weeks, C. S., et al. (2014). Factors that influence young people's mental health help-seeking behaviour: a study based on the Health Belief Model. *Journal of Advanced Nursing, 70*(11), 2577–2587.

Paparello, J., Zeller, I., & While, A. (2014). Meeting the complex needs of individuals living with HIV: a case study approach. *British Journal of Community Nursing, 19*(11), 526–533.

Pender, N. J., Murdaugh, C. L., & Parsons, M. A. (2015). *Health promotion in nursing practice* (7th ed.). Upper Saddle River, NJ: Prentice Hall.

Reignier, S. A. (2014). How does drug coverage vary by insurance type? Analysis of drug formularies in the United States. *American Journal of Managed Care, 20*(4), 322–331.

Roditi, D., & Robinson, M. E. (2011). The role of psychological interventions in the management of patients with chronic pain. *Psychology Research Behavioral Management, 4*, 41–49.

Ryan, L., Logsdon, M. C., McGill, S., et al. (2014). Evaluation of printed health education materials for use by low-education families. *Journal of Nursing Scholarship, 46*(4), 218–228.

Saunders, G. H., Dann, S. M., Griest, S. E., et al. (2014). Development and evaluation of a questionnaire to assess knowledge, attitudes, and behaviors towards hearing loss prevention. *International Journal of Audiology, 53*(4), 209–218.

Wang, Y., Zang, X., Bai, J., et al. (2014). Effect of a Health Belief Model-based nursing intervention on Chinese patients with moderate to severe chronic obstructive pulmonary disease: a randomised controlled trial. *Journal of Clinical Nursing, 23*(9/10), 1342–1353.

Watson, E. C., Cosio, D., & Lin, E. H. (2014). Mixed-method approach to veteran satisfaction with pain education. *Journal of Rehabilitation Research & Development, 51*(3), 503–514.

West, C. (2011). Powerful choices: peer support and individualized medication self-determination. *Schizophrenia Bulletin, 37*(3), 445–450.

Zullig, L. L., McCant, F., Melnyk, S. D., et al. (2014). A health literacy pilot intervention to improve medication adherence using Meducation((R)) technology. *Patient Education & Counseling, 95*(2), 288–291.

Ineffective Health maintenance

Kathaleen C. Bloom, PhD, CNM, and Barbara J. Olinzock, MSN, EdD, RN

NANDA-I

Definition

Inability to identify, manage, and/or seek out help to maintain health

Defining Characteristics

Absence of adaptive behaviors to environmental changes; absence of interest in improving health behaviors; inability to take responsibility for meeting basic health practices; insufficient knowledge about basic health practices; insufficient social support; pattern of lack of health-seeking behavior

Related Factors (r/t)

Alteration in cognitive functioning; complicated grieving; decrease in fine motor skills; decrease in gross motor skills; impaired decision-making; ineffective communication skills; ineffective coping strategies; insufficient resources (e.g., financial, social knowledge); perceptual impairment; spiritual distress; unachieved developmental tasks.

NOC (Nursing Outcomes Classification)

Suggested NOC Outcomes

Health Beliefs: Perceived Resources; Health-Promoting Behavior; Health-Seeking Behavior

Example NOC Outcome with Indicators

Health-Seeking Behavior as evidenced by the following indicators: Completes health-related tasks/Performs self-screening/Obtains assistance from health professional. (Rate the outcome and indicators of **Health-Seeking Behavior:** 1 = never demonstrated, 2 = rarely demonstrated, 3 = sometimes demonstrated, 4 = often demonstrated, 5 = consistently demonstrated [see Section I].)

Client Outcomes

H

Client Will (Specify Time Frame)

- Discuss fear of or blocks to implementing health regimen
- Follow mutually agreed on health care maintenance plan
- Meet goals for health care maintenance

NIC (Nursing Interventions Classification)

Suggested NIC Intervention

Health Education; Health System Guidance; Support System Enhancement

Example NIC Activities—Health Education

Prioritize identified learner needs based on client preference, skills of nurse, resources available, and likelihood of successful goal attainment; Emphasize immediate or short-term positive health benefits to be received by positive lifestyle behaviors, rather than long-term benefits or negative effects of noncompliance

Nursing Interventions and *Rationales*

- Assess the client's feelings, values, and reasons for not following the prescribed plan of care. See Related Factors. EBN: *A systematic review of 80 studies determined that personal beliefs and values, decisional control preferences, and perception of the decision-making process affect treatment decision-making in older adults diagnosed with cancer (Tariman et al, 2012).*
- Assess for family patterns, economic issues, spiritual, and cultural patterns that influence compliance with a given medical regimen. CEB: *A qualitative study (N = 14) found that critical challenges to increasing physical activity among low-income African American women included financial constraints (Harley et al, 2014).*
- Involve the client in shared decision-making regarding health maintenance. CEB: *A meta-analysis of 32 clinical trials revealed that assessing client preferences and involving them in shared decision-making had higher adherence, higher satisfaction, and better clinical outcomes (Lindhiem et al, 2014).*
- Show genuine interest in client's individual needs. EBN: *A systematic review of 24 qualitative studies concluded that clients' perception of the health care professional's responsiveness, interest in their individual needs, and shared information positively influence self-care for heart failure (Currie et al, 2014).*
- Assist the client in finding methods to reduce stress. EBN: *In a survey of 1257 university students, those who had high levels of perceived stress also engaged in high-risk behaviors such as alcohol consumption, unhealthy diet, physical inactivity, and tobacco and drug use (Deasy et al, 2014).*
- Help the client determine how to manage complex medication schedules (e.g., HIV/AIDS regimens or polypharmacy). EBN: *In a pilot study with 20 older adults taking an average of 13.2 prescription medications, providing an illustrated daily medication schedule improved both self-efficacy and adherence (Martin et al, 2012).*
- Identify complementary healing modalities, such as herbal remedies, acupuncture, healing touch, yoga, or cultural shamans that the client uses in addition to or instead of the prescribed allopathic regimen

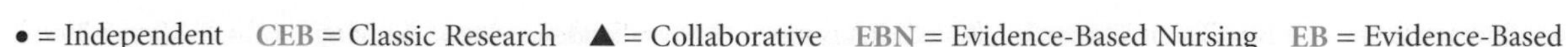

along with the client's perception of the complementary healing modalities. CEB: *Use of complementary healing modalities among clients with chronic disease is relatively high. In an exploratory study with 217 Mexican immigrants, a person's beliefs about complementary and alternative therapies may negatively influence medical adherence (Villagran et al, 2012).*

▲ Refer the client to appropriate medical and social services as needed, providing adequate information on details about the service, including scheduling. EBN: *A metasynthesis of 62 qualitative studies concluded that client participation in services such as cardiac rehabilitation is most strongly associated with perceptions of the nature, suitability, and scheduling, but not the benefits of the rehabilitation program (Clark et al, 2013).*

- Identify support groups related to the disease process. EBN: *Individuals who attend support groups demonstrate improved disease management and enhanced quality of life. A systematic review of 84 studies of group visits for chronic illness found client benefits to include greater satisfaction and improved clinical outcomes (Jones et al, 2014).*
- Use social media such as text messaging to remind clients of scheduled appointments. CEB: *A Cochrane review of eight randomized controlled trials concluded that text messaging reminders increase attendance at health care appointments similar to telephone reminders but better than no reminders or postal reminders (Gurol-Urganci et al, 2013). Additional relevant research: Farmer et al, 2014; McInnes et al, 2014.*
- Use telehealth interventions to facilitate self-care. EBN: *A systematic review of 14 studies supports telehealth as a positive factor in enabling self-care behaviors related to daily weighing, medication management, exercise adherence, fluid and alcohol restriction, salt restriction, and stress reduction in clients with heart failure (Radhakrishnan & Jacelon, 2012).*

H

Geriatric

- Assess the client's perception of health and health maintenance. CEB: *A study of 681 older clients with diabetes or metabolic syndrome found that they often underestimate their cardiovascular risk, with as many as 42% perceiving themselves to be in good or excellent health (Martell-Claros et al, 2013).*
- Assist client to identify both life- and health-related goals. CEB: *A study of 308 women demonstrated beginning evidence that when the health goals of older individuals are congruent with their life goals, they are more likely to participate in health-related activities (Saajanaho et al, 2014).*
- Provide information that supports informed decision-making. CEB: *In a modified grounded theory study (N = 59), participants endorsed the elements of informed decision making, including discussion of the role of the client, the clinical issue, the alternatives, benefits/risks/uncertainties; assessment of client understanding and preference; soliciting input from trusted others, and discussion of the impact on clients' daily lives (Price et al, 2012).*
- Discuss realistic goal setting for changes in health maintenance with the client and support person. EBN: *An integrative review of 13 studies revealed that mutual goal-setting between the client and the health care provider improves overall health behaviors and outcomes for older adults with chronic conditions (Anuruang et al, 2014).*
- Educate the client about the symptoms of life-threatening illness, such as myocardial infarction (MI), and the need for timeliness in seeking care. EBN: *A qualitative study with 42 persons with an MI found that misinformation regarding the symptoms of MI is common; many believe sudden, intense chest pain is the only indication of MI, resulting in delay in seeking treatment (O'Donnell & Moser, 2012).*

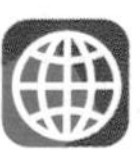

Multicultural

- Assess influence of cultural beliefs, norms, and values on the client's ability to modify health behavior. EBN: *A descriptive qualitative study of 30 Thai Buddhist people revealed that understanding the cultural and religious traditions, influence of family and economics when choosing interventions to help them cope with their illness and empower them to control their disease is essential for effective care (Lundberg & Thrakul, 2012).*
- Assess the effect of fatalism on the client's ability to modify health behavior. CEB: *A population-based study of 2018 adults found that fatalistic beliefs about cancer may hamper screening and delay help-seeking for symptoms (Beeken et al, 2011).*
- Clarify culturally related health beliefs and practices. EBN: *Language, culture, and ethnicity influence the choice of a health care provider and participation in health management strategies. An exploratory*

descriptive study with 23 women found that health/illness beliefs affect both self-care and care seeking (Hjelm et al, 2012).

- Provide culturally appropriate education and health care services. CEB: *In a randomized controlled trial involving 223 Hispanic women, a culturally tailored lifestyle behavior intervention was shown to significantly influence dietary habits, weight, and waist circumference (Koniak-Griffin et al, 2014).* CEB: *In a systematic review of 28 studies of culturally adapted strategies to improve diet and weight outcomes of African American women, strategies that reflected the group's values and beliefs and that drew from the group's experiences were the most successful (Kong et al, 2014).*

Home Care

- The interventions described previously may be adapted for home care use.
- ▲ Provide nurse-led case management. EBN: *A review of relevant research concluded that individualized, systematic, and guideline-based nurse case management promotes cardiovascular risk reduction in home-based, primary care, and community settings (Berra, 2011).*
- Provide a health promotion focus for the client with disabilities, with the goals of reducing secondary conditions (e.g., obesity, hypertension, pressure sores), maintaining functional independence, providing opportunities for leisure and enjoyment, and enhancing overall quality of life. CEB: *A retrospective analysis of data from a national survey comparing health of adults with and without physical or cognitive disabilities found that individuals living with physical disabilities or cognitive impairment receive fewer preventive services and have higher rates of chronic illness (Reichard et al, 2011). A systematic review of 11 studies found that community-based physical activity and educational programs provide fitness and psychosocial benefits for individuals with intellectual disabilities (Heller et al, 2011).*
- Provide support and individual training for caregivers before the client is discharged from the hospital. EBN: *Caregivers are very interested in receiving instruction and hands-on practice of procedures they would need to perform at home.* In a study of hospital-to-home transition of older veterans, caregivers (N = 40) *reported increased confidence in their ability to provide such care and to help their loved ones manage symptoms at home (Hendrix et al, 2011).*
- Assist client to develop confidence in ability to manage the health condition. CEB: *A clinical trial of self-management education targeted at self-efficacy (N = 57) improved physiological outcomes, enhanced coping techniques, and reduced health care use (Labrecque et al, 2011).*

Client/Family Teaching and Discharge Planning

- Provide the family with credible sources where information can be obtained from social media. (Most libraries have Internet access with printing capabilities.) CEB: *In an experimental study (N = 197), researchers concluded that websites containing credible and evidence-based medical information positively affected users' health information seeking. General, non–evidence-based sites were perceived positively by the user, independent of the site's credibility, and often negatively influencing opinions about health practices (Allam et al, 2014).*
- ▲ Develop collaborative multidisciplinary partnerships. CEB: *Multidisciplinary and multifactorial interventions are likely to be more effective in achieving desired outcomes. In a quality improvement study of readmission rates for 463 clients with pneumonia, the clients whose in-hospital and post-discharge diagnosis and care was managed by a multidisciplinary team consisting of health care providers, nurses, and social workers had significantly fewer all-cause readmissions and readmissions for pneumonia (Hussein et al, 2014).*
- Tailor both the information provided and the method of delivery of information to the specific client and/or family. CEB: *A systematic review of 27 studies related to medication adherence and diabetes outcomes was not able to identify a specific intervention, but emphasized the need to tailor interventions to optimize management and improve outcomes (Williams et al, 2014).*
- Explain nonthreatening qualities before introducing more anxiety-producing information regarding possible side effects of the disease or medical regimen. EBN: *In a laboratory study of anxiety and task interference (N = 157), anxiety was found to interfere with concentration and the ability to understand and remember (Lachman & Agrigoroaei, 2012).*

REFERENCES

Allam, A., Schulz, P. J., & Nakamoto, K. (2014). The impact of search engine selection and sorting criteria on vaccination beliefs and attitudes: two experiments manipulating Google output. *Journal of Medical Interest Research, 16*, e100.

Anuruang, S., Hickman, L. D., Jackson, D., et al. (2014). Community-based interventions to promote management for older people: an integrative review. *Journal of Clinical Nursing, 23*, 2110–2120.

Beeken, R. J., Simon, A. E., von Wagner, C., et al. (2011). Cancer fatalism: deterring early presentation and increasing social inequalities? *Cancer Epidemiology, Biomarkers & Prevention, 20*, 2127–2131.

Berra, K. (2011). Does nurse case management improve implementation of guidelines for cardiovascular disease risk reduction? *Journal of Cardiovascular Nursing, 26*, 145–167.

Clark, A. M., King-Shier, K. M., Spaling, M. A., et al. (2013). Factors influencing participation in cardiac rehabilitation programmes after referral and initial attendance: qualitative systematic review and meta-synthesis. *Clinical Rehabilitation, 27*, 948–959.

Currie, K., Strachan, P. H., Spaling, M., et al. (2014). The importance of interactions between patients and healthcare professionals for heart failure self-care: a systematic review of qualitative research into patient perspectives. *European Journal of Cardiovascular Nursing*, pii: 1474515114547648.

Deasy, C., Coughlan, B., Pironom, J., et al. (2014). Psychological distress and lifestyle of students: implications for health promotion. *Health Promotion International*, pii: dau086.

Farmer, T., Brook, G., McSorley, J., et al. (2014). Using short message service text reminders to reduce 'did not attend' rates in sexual health and HIV appointment clinics. *International Journal of STD & AIDS, 25*, 289–293.

Gurol-Urganci, I., de Jongh, T., Vodopivec-Jamsek, V., et al. (2013). Mobile phone messaging reminders for attendance at healthcare appointments. *Cochrane Database of Systematic Reviews*, (12), CD007458.

Harley, A. E., Rice, J., Walker, R., et al. (2014). Physically active, low-income African American women: an exploration of activity maintenance in the context of sociodemographic factors associated with inactivity. *Women and Health, 54*, 354–372.

Heller, T., McCubbin, J. A., Drum, C., et al. (2011). Physical activity and nutrition health promotion interventions: what is working for people with intellectual disabilities? *Intellectual & Developmental Disabilities, 49*, 26–36.

Hendrix, C. C., Hastings, S. N., Van Houtven, C., et al. (2011). Pilot study: individualized training for caregivers of hospitalized older veterans. *Nursing Research, 60*, 436–441.

Hjelm, K., Berntorp, K., & Apelqvist, J. (2012). Beliefs about health and illness in Swedish and African-born women with gestational diabetes living in Sweden. *Journal of Clinical Nursing, 21*, 1374–1386.

Hussein, H., Golden, M., & Hahn, S. (2014). Multidisciplinary intervention to improve readmission rates of patients discharged with a diagnosis of pneumonia. *Chest, 146*, 905A.

Jones, K. R., Kaewluang, N., & Lekhak, N. (2014). Group visits for chronic illness management: implementation challenges and recommendations. *Nursing Economics, 32*, 118–134, 147.

Kong, A., Tussing-Humphreys, L. M., Odoms-Young, A. M., et al. (2014). Systematic review of behavioural interventions with culturally adapted strategies to improve diet and weight outcomes in African American women. *Obesity Reviews, 4*, 62–92.

Koniak-Griffin, D., Brecht, M. L., Takayanagi, S., et al. (2014). A community health worker-led lifestyle behavior intervention for Latina (Hispanic) women: feasibility and outcomes of a randomized controlled trial. *International Journal of Nursing Studies*, pii: S0020-7489(14)00253-3.

Labrecque, M., Rabhi, K., Laurin, C., et al. (2011). Can a self-management education program for patients with chronic obstructive pulmonary disease improve quality of life? *Canadian Respiratory Journal, 18*, e77–e81.

Lachman, M. E., & Agrigoroaei, S. (2012). Low perceived control as a risk factor for episodic memory: the mediational role of anxiety and task interference. *Memory & Cognition, 40*, 287–296.

Lindhiem, O., Bennett, C. B., Trentacosta, C. J., et al. (2014). Client preferences affect treatment satisfaction, completion, and clinical outcome: a meta-analysis. *Clinical Psychology Review, 34*, 506–517.

Lundberg, P. C., & Thrakul, S. (2012). Type w diabetes: how do Thai Buddhist people with diabetes practice self-management? *Journal of Advanced Nursing, 68*, 550–558.

Martell-Claros, N., Aranda, P., González-Albarrán, O., et al. (2013). Perception of health and understanding of cardiovascular risk among patients with recently diagnosed diabetes and/or metabolic syndrome. *European Journal of Preventative Cardiology, 20*, 21–28.

Martin, D., Kripalani, S., & Durapau, V. J. (2012). Improving medication management among at-risk older adults. *Journal of Gerontological Nursing, 38*, 24–34.

McInnes, D. K., Sawh, L., Petrakis, B. A., et al. (2014). The potential for health-related uses of mobile phones and internet with homeless veterans: results from a multisite survey. *Telemedicine Journal and E-Health, 20*, 801–809.

O'Donnell, S., & Moser, D. K. (2012). Slow-onset myocardial infarction and its influence on help-seeking behaviors. *Journal of Cardiovascular Nursing, 27*, 334–344.

Price, E. L., Bereknyei, S., Kuby, A., et al. (2012). New elements for informed decision making: a qualitative study of older adults' views. *Patient Education and Counseling, 86*, 335–341.

Radhakrishnan, K., & Jacelon, C. (2012). Impact of telehealth on patient self-management of heart failure: a review of literature. *Journal of Cardiovascular Nursing, 27*, 33–43.

Reichard, A., Stolzle, H., & Fox, M. H. (2011). Health disparities among adults with physical disabilities or cognitive limitations compared to individuals with no disabilities in the United States. *Disability and Health Journal, 4*, 59–67.

Saajanaho, M., Viljanen, A., Read, S., et al. (2014). Older women's personal goals and exercise activity: an 8-year follow-up. *Journal of Aging and Physical Activity, 22*, 386–392.

Tariman, J. D., Berry, D. L., Cochrane, B., et al. (2012). Physician, patient, and contextual factors affecting treatment decisions in older adults with cancer and models of decision making: a literature review. *Oncology Nursing Forum, 39*, E70–E83.

Villagran, M., Hajek, C., Zhao, X., et al. (2012). Communication and culture: predictors of treatment adherence among Mexican immigrant patients. *Journal of Health Psychology, 17*, 443–452.

Williams, J. L., Walker, R. J., Smalls, B. L., et al. (2014). Effective interventions to improve medication adherence in Type 2 diabetes: a systematic review. *Diabetes Management, 4*, 29–48.

H

Impaired Home maintenance

Kathaleen C. Bloom, PhD, CNM, and Barbara J. Olinzock, MSN, EdD, RN

NANDA-I

Definition

Inability to independently maintain a safe, growth-promoting immediate environment

• = Independent CEB = Classic Research ▲ = Collaborative EBN = Evidence-Based Nursing EB = Evidence-Based

Defining Characteristics

Difficulty maintaining a comfortable environment; excessive family responsibilities; financial crisis (e.g., debt, insufficient finances); insufficient clothing; insufficient cooking equipment; insufficient equipment for maintaining home; insufficient linen; pattern of disease caused by unhygienic conditions; pattern of infection caused by unhygienic conditions; request for assistance with home maintenance; unsanitary environment

Related Factors (r/t)

Alteration in cognitive functioning; condition impacting ability to maintain home (e.g., disease, illness injury); illness impacting ability to maintain home; injury impacting ability to maintain home; insufficient family organization; insufficient family planning; insufficient knowledge of home maintenance; insufficient knowledge of neighborhood resources; insufficient role model; insufficient support system

NOC (Nursing Outcomes Classification)

H

Suggested NOC Outcomes

Safe Home Environment; Self-Care: Activities of Daily Living (ADLs)

Example NOC Outcome with Indicators

Safe Home Environment as evidenced by the following indicators: Elimination of pests/Smoke detector maintenance/Accessibility of assistive devices/Elimination of tobacco smoke. (Rate the outcome and indicators of **Safe Home Environment:** 1 = not adequate, 2 = slightly adequate, 3 = moderately adequate, 4 = substantially adequate, 5 = totally adequate [see Section I].)

Client Outcomes

Client Will (Specify Time Frame)

- Maintain a healthy home environment
- Use community resources to assist with home care needs
- Maintain a safe home environment

NIC (Nursing Interventions Classification)

Suggested NIC Intervention

Home Maintenance Assistance

Example NIC Activities—Home Maintenance Assistance

Involve client/family in deciding home maintenance requirements; Provide information on how to make home environment safe and clean; Help family use social support network

Nursing Interventions and *Rationales*

- Assess the concerns of family members, especially the primary caregiver, about home care for a long time. EBN: *A cross-sectional study of 515 caregiver/client dyads found that caregiver confidence in ability to contribute to their family member's self-care was a significant determinant of how much they were involved in self-care maintenance and management (Vellone et al, 2014).*
- Provide home safety education and, safety equipment when possible. CEB: *A Cochrane review of 98 studies (with meta-analysis of 54 studies) concluded that home safety interventions, especially those delivered in the home, were effective in reducing injury and in increasing uptake of home safety measures, including safe water temperature, functional smoke alarms, a fire escape plan, and storing hazardous items out of reach (Kendrick et al, 2012).*
- ▲ Consider a predischarge home assessment referral to determine the need for accessibility and safety-related environmental changes. CEB: *A randomized controlled trial (RCT) (N = 842 households; 1848 individual occupants) found significantly fewer falls and fall-related injuries in those households*

that had specific low-cost home modifications such as alterations in steps inside and outside the house, grab rails and non-slip bath mats in bathrooms, outside lighting, and alterations in carpeting (Keall et al, 2014).

- Use an assessment tool to identify environmental safety hazards in the home. EBN: *In a study of 130 persons receiving discharge teaching, those who received targeted education and practice using a mock-up of their home regarding home safety modifications had significantly fewer overall and in-home falls 1 year after discharge (Kamei et al, 2014).*
- Establish an individualized plan of care for improved home maintenance with the client and family based on the client's needs and the caregiver's capabilities. EBN: *In a study involving 116 households with 170 children with asthma, an in-home assessment followed by targeted changes in the home environment resulted in a decrease in all measures of asthma severity and health care utilization (Turcotte et al, 2014).*
- Set up a system of relief for the main caregiver in the home and a plan for sharing of household duties and/or outside assistance. EBN: *In a qualitative study, seven mothers providing care to children with complex health care needs verified that respite care provides decreased burden and improved quality of life for the caregiver and the family as a whole (Thomas & Price, 2012).*

H

▲ Provide a multidisciplinary approach to target the home environment and the client's ability to function in the home. EBN: *The Community Aging in Place: Advancing Better Living for Elders (CAPABLE), a program involving teams of nurses, occupational therapists, and handymen, targets the home environment and individual physical function (Pho et al, 2012; Szanton et al, 2014a). There is an ongoing RCT with 300 individuals testing the program's outcomes in terms of functional abilities, mobility, and environmental safety (Szanton et al, 2014b).*

- Assess the quality of relationships among family members. CEB: *In a cross-sectional study of fifth graders (N = 3218), unintentional injuries requiring medical attention were associated with parental marital discord (Schwebel et al, 2012).*

Geriatric

- All of the previously mentioned interventions are applicable for the geriatric population.
- Assess injury prevention knowledge and practices of the client and caregivers and provide information as appropriate. EBN: *A survey of 84 older adults showed that only 36% had a working smoke alarm, 22% had a working carbon monoxide alarm, and 36% had water that was hotter than recommended (Shields et al, 2013).*
- Assess functional ability to manage safely after hospital discharge. CEB: *A validation study of The Assessment of Motor and Process Skills and Cognitive Performance Test were found to reliably predict time to incident of harm post discharge (Douglas et al, 2013).*
- Explore community resources to assist with home maintenance (e.g., senior centers, Department of Aging, hospital case managers, friends and relatives, the Internet, or church parish nurse). CEB: *In a qualitative study with 43 older adults living at home, participants perceived they were both capable and willing to manage many home maintenance tasks. They reported using compensatory means, such as tools and technologies, to do home maintenance and repairs themselves as well as either hiring someone or having friends, neighbors, or family do the task (Kelly et al, 2014).*
- Support "aging in place" by providing assistive technology devices: home modification, daily living aids, mobility aids, seating and positioning devices, and sensory aids. CEB: *Assessment for risk and incorporation of compensatory strategies, home modification for access and safety, and exercises to promote balance and muscle strength in programs such as Advancing Better Living for Elders (ABLE) are cost-effective ways to delay functional decline and mortality in older adults (Jutkowitz et al, 2012).*
- Focus on the interaction between the older client and the technology, assisting the client to be an active participant in choices of and uses for technology. EBN: *A systematic review of 18 studies of communication technologies and assistive strategies concluded that when users of technologies are active in the technological process, assessed in interaction with technology in their everyday practices, the technology can be more efficiently used to meet the needs of the client (Rodeschini, 2011).*
- See the care plans for Risk for **Injury** and Risk for **Falls.**

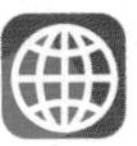

Multicultural

- Acknowledge the stresses unique to racial/ethnic communities. CEB: *A systematic review of 57 studies revealed that cultural factors, including distrust of home visits, language barriers and lifestyle were barriers to home injury prevention interventions (Ingram et al, 2012).*

Home Care

- The previously mentioned interventions incorporate these resources.
- See care plans **Contamination** and Risk for **Contamination.**

Client/Family Teaching and Discharge Planning

- Identify support groups within the community to assist families in the caregiver role. CEB: *Community-based participatory research using focus groups with 39 family caregivers found that caregivers are most in need of effective communication, emotional support, education, and advocacy (Macleod et al, 2012).*
- Provide counseling and support for clients and for caregivers of clients. CEB: *A Cochrane review of 11 RCTs involving 1836 caregiver participants found evidence suggesting that interventions directly supporting the caregiver may help reduce psychological distress (Candy et al, 2011).*
- Focus teaching on environmental hazards identified in the nursing assessment. Areas may include, but are not limited to:
  - **Home Safety.** Identify the need for and use of common safety devices in the home. EB: *An RCT (N = 355) found that an intervention to reduce exposure to injury hazards (including installing smoke detectors, stair gates, and cabinet locks) in homes of young children led to a 70% reduction in injury (Phelan et al, 2011).*
  - **Food Safety.** Instruct client to avoid microbial food-borne illness by storing and cooking food at the proper temperature, regularly washing hands, food contact surfaces, and fruits and vegetables, and monitoring expiration dates. EBN: *A qualitative study of 10 households found that all took risks in terms of not following recommended practices with respect to best practices and that the logic behind food practices was often faulty (Dickinson et al, 2014).*
- Teach clients to assess their homes for potential environmental health hazards in the home, including risks related to structure, moisture/mold, fire, pets, electrical, ventilation, pests, and lifestyle. CEB: *The housing-based hazard index (HHI) is a measure of overall home hazards with good reliability and validity and the ability to discriminate between healthy and nonhealthy homes (N = 643) (Nriagu et al, 2012; Nriagu et al, 2011).*
- See care plans **Contamination,** Risk for **Contamination,** Risk for **Falls,** Risk for **Infection,** and Risk for **Injury.**

REFERENCES

Candy, B., Jones, L., Drake, R., et al. (2011). Interventions for supporting informal caregivers of patients in the terminal phase of a disease. *Cochrane Database of Systematic Reviews*, (6), CD007617.

Dickinson, A., Wills, W., Meah, A., et al. (2014). Food safety and older people: the kitchen life study. *British Journal of Community Nursing, 19*, 226–232.

Douglas, A. M., Letts, L. J., Richardson, J. A., et al. (2013). Validity of predischarge measures for predicting time to harm in older adults. *Canadian Journal of Occupational Therapy, 80*, 19–27.

Ingram, J. C., Deave, T., Towner, E., et al. (2012). Identifying facilitators and barriers for home injury prevention interventions for pre-school children: a systematic review of the quantitative literature. *Health Education Research, 27*, 258–268.

Jutkowitz, E., Gitlin, L. N., Pizzi, L. T., et al. (2012). Cost effectiveness of a home-based intervention that helps functionally vulnerable older adults age in place at home. *Journal of Aging Research, 2012*, Article ID 680265.

Kamei, T., Kajii, F., Yamamoto, Y., et al. (2014). Effectiveness of a home hazard modification program for reducing falls in urban community-dwelling older adults: a randomized controlled trial. *Japan Journal of Nursing Science, 12*(3).

Keall, M. D., Pierse, N., Howden-Chapman, P., et al. (2014). Home modifications to reduce injuries from falls in the Home Injury Prevention Intervention (HIPI) study: a cluster-randomised controlled trial. *Lancet, 385*, 231–238.

Kelly, A. J., Fausset, C. B., Rogers, W., et al. (2014). Responding to home maintenance challenge scenarios: the role of selection, optimization, and compensation in aging-in-place. *Journal of Applied Gerontology, 33*, 1018–1042.

Kendrick, D., Young, B., Mason-Jones, A. J., et al. (2012). Home safety education and provision of safety equipment for injury prevention. *Cochrane Database of Systematic Reviews*, (9), CD005014.

MacLeod, A., Skinner, M. W., & Low, E. (2012). Supporting hospice volunteers and caregivers through community-based participatory research. *Health and Social Care in the Community, 20*, 190–198.

Nriagu, J., Martin, J., Smith, P., et al. (2012). Residential hazards, high asthma prevalence and multimorbidity among children in Saginaw, Michigan. *Science of the Total Environment, 416*, 53–61.

Nriagu, J., Smith, P., & Socier, D. (2011). A rating scale for housing-based health hazards. *Science of the Total Environment, 409*, 5423–5431.

Phelan, K. J., Khoury, J., Xu, Y., et al. (2011). A randomized controlled trial of home injury hazard reduction: the HOME injury study. *Archives of Pediatrics and Adolescent Medicine, 165*, 339–345.

Pho, A. T., Tanner, E. K., Roth, J., et al. (2012). Nursing strategies for promoting and maintaining function among community-living older adults: the CAPABLE intervention. *Geriatric Nursing, 33*, 439–445.

Rodeschini, G. (2011). Gerotechnology: A new kind of care for aging? An analysis of the relationship between older people and technology. *Nursing and Health Sciences, 13*, 521–528.

Schwebel, D. C., Roth, D. L., Elliott, M. N., et al. (2012). Marital conflict and fifth-graders' risk for injury. *Accident, Analysis and Prevention, 47*, 30–35.

Shields, W. C., Perry, E. C., Szanton, S. L., et al. (2013). Knowledge and injury prevention practices in homes of older adults. *Geriatric Nursing, 34*, 19–24.

Szanton, S. L., Roth, J., Nkimbeng, M., et al. (2014a). Improving unsafe environments to support aging independence with limited resources. *Nursing Clinics of North America, 49*, 133–145.

Szanton, S. L., Wolff, J. W., Leff, B., et al. (2014b). CAPABLE trial: a randomized controlled trial of nurse, occupational therapist and handyman to reduce disability among older adults: Rationale and design. *Contemporary Clinical Trials, 38*, 102–112.

Thomas, S., & Price, M. (2012). Respite care in seven families with children with complex care needs. *Nursing Children and Young People, 24*(8), 24–27.

Turcotte, D. A., Alker, H., Chaves, E., et al. (2014). Healthy homes: in-home environmental asthma intervention in a diverse urban community. *American Journal of Public Health, 104*, 665–671.

Vellone, E., D'Agostino, F., Buck, H. G., et al. (2014). The key role of caregiver confidence in the caregiver's contribution to self-care in adults with heart failure. *European Journal of Cardiovascular Nursing*, pii: 1474515114547649.

H

Readiness for enhanced Hope

Gail B. Ladwig, MSN, RN, and Marina Martinez-Kratz, MS, RN, CNE

NANDA-I

Definition

A pattern of expectations and desires for mobilizing energy on one's own behalf, which can be strengthened

Defining Characteristics

Expresses desire to enhance ability to set achievable goals; expresses desire to enhance belief in possibilities; expresses desire to enhance congruency of expectations with goal; expresses desire to enhance connectedness with others; expresses desire to enhance hope; expresses desire to enhance problem solving to meet goal; expresses desire to enhance sense of meaning in life; expresses desire to enhance spirituality

NOC (Nursing Outcomes Classification)

Suggested NOC Outcomes

Hope; Quality of Life

Example NOC Outcome with Indicators

Hope as evidenced by the following indicators: Expresses expectation of a positive future/Expresses faith/Expresses meaning in life/Exhibits a zest for life/Sets goals. (Rate the outcome and indicators of **Hope:** 1 = never demonstrated, 2 = rarely demonstrated, 3 = sometimes demonstrated, 4 = often demonstrated, 5 = consistently demonstrated [see Section I].)

Client Outcomes

Client Will (Specify Time Frame)

- Describe values, expectations, and meanings
- Set achievable goals that are consistent with values
- Design strategies to achieve goals
- Express belief in possibilities

NIC (Nursing Interventions Classification)

Suggested NIC Interventions

Emotional Support; Hope Inspiration; Presence; Support System Enhancement

Example NIC Activities—Hope Inspiration

Assist client and family to identify areas of hope in life; Demonstrate hope by recognizing the client's intrinsic worth; Encourage therapeutic relationships; Help the person expand spiritual self

Nursing Interventions and *Rationales*

- Develop an open and caring and empathetic relationship that enables the client to discuss hope. EBN: *Time nurses spend with clients can inspire hope (Montana & Kautz, 2011). In this study of clients in palliative care, hope was increased when empathy was used (Richardson et al, 2012).*
- Assist clients to identify sources of gratitude in their lives using a future oriented focus. CEB: *Research shows that clients with a regulatory focus of promotion were more likely to express gratitude, which inspired them to strengthen their relationships with helpful and responsive partners (Mathews & Shook, 2013).*
- Assist families to identify sources of gratitude in their lives. CEB: *Research showed that gratitude fostered all facets of post-traumatic growth, such as relationships, personal strengths, and awareness of meaningful possibilities (Ruini & Vescovelli, 2013).*
- Screen the client for hope using a valid and reliable instrument as indicated. CEB: *The HHI is a brief instrument with good psychometric properties that has been developed for clinical use. It has been designed to facilitate the examination of hope at various intervals so that changes in levels of hope can be identified (Van Gestel-Timmermans et al, 2010).*
- Focus on the positive aspects of hope, rather than the prevention of hopelessness. *Hope is essential to life and is therefore a fundamental human need. Without hope, despair and depression take hold with devastating effects (O'Hara, 2010).*
- Assist the client to expect positive outcomes and recognize the pathways to achieve the positive outcomes. CEB: *Research shows that these actions facilitate the development of hope as a strength (Proctor et al, 2011).*
- Assist clients in developing realistic goals for their recovery. EBN: *Realistic goals reflect realistic sense of hope versus false hope (Tutton et al, 2012).*
- Assist clients to set a goal, write down what steps are needed to achieve the goal, and visualize themselves reaching the goal. CEB: *Research found that structured goal setting session was sufficient to foster hope (Feldman & Dreher, 2011).*
- Teach individuals how to become aware of attention that is focused on unwanted aspects of life and how to redirect attention toward things that feel more wanted or desired by using a future directed approach. CEB: *Future directed therapy is effective at decreasing hopelessness and increases positive future expectations (Vilhauer et al, 2013).*
- Engage the client in a therapeutic relationship to enhance social connectedness and social support networks. EBN: *Nursing research found that relationship based interventions improve a client's sense of social connectedness and decrease hopelessness (McCay et al, 2011).*
- Provide emotional support and encourage hope. CEB: *This study illustrates how reestablishment of a hopeful attitude can strengthen a client even with end-stage pulmonary disease and passive suicidal ideation (Anbar & Murthy, 2010).*
- Help the client identify his or her desires and expectations. EBN: *This study indicates that nurses working with clients with serious conditions such as cancer listen carefully to the clients' metaphors and reflect on the implicit meaning of them, helping the clients to see the light on the horizon and helping them to realize that hope and hopelessness are two sides of the same coin (Hammer et al, 2009).*
- Use a family-oriented approach when discussing hope. CEB: *Adaptation is an issue for the whole family and is facilitated by being able to stay close to the client and receive supportive unambiguous information from the staff both during the intensive care unit stay and after discharge (Söderström et al, 2009).*
- Review internal and external resources to enhance hope. EBN: *In a concept analysis of hope, based on a review of 17 research studies of terminally ill clients, the 10 attributes of hope were identified as positive expectation, positive qualities, spirituality, goals, comfort, help/caring, interpersonal relationships, control, legacy, and life review (Johnson, 2007).*
- Identify spiritual beliefs and practices. CEB: *Hope is a spiritual need, as identified in a study of 683 individuals (Flannelly et al, 2006).* CEB: *Spirituality was identified as a factor in increasing hope in clients with mental illness (Schrank et al, 2012).*
- Assist the person to consider possible adaptations to changes. EBN: *A grounded theory study of 41 women looked at refocusing hope after having a diagnosis of fetal abnormality identified by ultrasound. It identified four phases they experienced as "assume normal," "shock," "gaining meaning," and "rebuilding." It showed that they maintained hope by attaching their hopes to reality and adapting to changes as needed (Lalor et al, 2009).*

Home Care

- The above interventions may be adapted for home care use.

Client/Family Teaching and Discharge Planning

- Assess client and family hope before teaching. CEB: *The degree and type of client and family hope may differ from each other, which may interfere with learning and use of knowledge for problem solving (Benzein & Berg, 2005).*
- Incorporate client and family goal setting within teaching content. EBN: *Realistic goal setting fosters and supports hope (Lalor et al, 2009).*
- Teach alternative coping strategies such as physical activity. CEB: *Clients with severe mental illness showed decreased hopelessness after participation in an adjunct exercise program (Sylvia et al, 2013).*
- Provide information to the client and family regarding all aspects of the client's health condition. EBN: *Accurate and complete information sharing empowers, which is more likely to support hope than the perceptions that might occur without accurate and complete information (Forbat et al, 2009; Lalor et al, 2009). The most important need identified in the Critical Care Family Needs Inventory was "hope," followed by the need for adequate and honest information (Linnarsson et al, 2010).*
- Offer emotional support, active listening, and coping assistance to client families. EBN: *Family hopelessness is addressed when nurses offer emotional support (Coco et al, 2013).*

H

REFERENCES

Anbar, R. D., & Murthy, V. V. (2010). Reestablishment of hope as an intervention for a patient with cystic fibrosis awaiting lung transplantation. *Journal of Alternative and Complementary Medicine (New York, N.Y.), 16*(9), 1007–1010.

Benzein, E. G., & Berg, A. C. (2005). The level of and relation between hope, hopelessness and fatigue in patients and family members in palliative care. *Palliative Medicine, 19*, 234–240.

Coco, K., Tossavainen, K., Jääskeläinen, J., et al. (2013). The provision of emotional support to the families of traumatic brain injury patients: perspectives of Finnish nurses. *Journal of Clinical Nursing, 22*(9/10), 1467–1476.

Feldman, D. B., & Dreher, D. E. (2011). Can hope be changed in 90 minutes? Testing the efficacy of a single-session goal-pursuit intervention for college students. *Journal of Happiness Studies, 13*, 745–759.

Flannelly, K. J., Galek, K., & Flannelly, L. T. (2006). A test of the factor structure of the patient spiritual needs assessment scale. *Holistic Nursing Practice, 20*(4), 187–190.

Forbat, L., et al. (2009). The use of technology in cancer care: applying Foucault's ideas to explore the changing dynamics of power in health care. *Journal of Advanced Nursing, 65*(2), 306–315.

Hammer, K., Mogensen, O., & Hall, E. O. C. (2009). The meaning of hope in nursing research: a meta-synthesis. *Scandinavian Journal of Caring Sciences, 23*(3), 549–557.

Johnson, S. (2007). Hope in terminal illness: an evolutionary concept analysis. *International Journal of Palliative Nursing, 13*(9), 451–459.

Lalor, J., Begley, C. M., & Galavan, E. (2009). Recasting hope: a process of adaptation following fetal anomaly diagnosis. *Social Science and Medicine, 68*(3), 362–372.

Linnarsson, J. R., Bubini, J., & Perseius, K. (2010). Review: a meta-synthesis of qualitative research into needs and experiences of significant others to critically ill or injured patients. *Journal of Clinical Nursing, 19*(21/22), 3102–3111.

Mathews, M. A., & Shook, N. J. (2013). Promoting or preventing thanks: regulatory focus and its effect on gratitude and indebtedness. *Journal of Research in Personality, 47*, 191–195.

McCay, E., Quesnel, S., Langley, J., et al. (2011). A relationship-based intervention to improve social connectedness in street-involved youth: a pilot study. *Journal of Child & Adolescent Psychiatric Nursing, 24*(4), 208–215.

Montana, C., & Kautz, D. D. (2011). Turning the nightmare of complex regional pain syndrome into a time of healing, renewal, and hope. *Medsurg Nursing, 20*(3), 139–142.

O'Hara, D. (2010). Hope—the neglected common factor. *Therapy Today, 21*(9), 1748–7846.

Proctor, C., Tsukayama, E., Wood, A. M., et al. (2011). Strengths Gym: the impact of a character strengths based intervention on the life satisfaction and wellbeing of adolescents. *Journal of Positive Psychology, 6*, 377–388.

Richardson, K., MacLeod, R., & Kent, B. (2012). A Steinian approach to an empathic understanding of hope among patients and clinicians in the culture of palliative care. *Journal of Advanced Nursing, 68*(3), 686–694.

Ruini, C., & Vescovelli, F. (2013). The role of gratitude in breast cancer: its relationships with post-traumatic growth, psychological well-being and distress. *Journal of Happiness Studies, 14*, 263–274.

Schrank, B., et al. (2012). Determinants, self-management strategies and interventions for hope in people with mental disorders: systematic search and narrative review. *Social Science and Medicine, 74*(4), 554–564.

Söderström, I. K., et al. (2009). Family adaptation in relation to a family member's stay in ICU. *Intensive and Critical Care Nursing, 25*(5), 250–257.

Sylvia, L., Kopeski, L., Brown, C., et al. (2013). An adjunct exercise program for serious mental illness: who chooses to participate and is it feasible? *Community Mental Health Journal, 49*(2), 213–219.

Tutton, E., Seers, K., Langstaff, D., et al. (2012). Staff and patient views of the concept of hope on a stroke unit: a qualitative study. *Journal of Advanced Nursing, 68*(9), 2061–2069.

Van Gestel-Timmermans, H., et al. (2010). Hope as a determinant of mental health recovery: a psychometric evaluation of the herth hope index—dutch version. *Scandinavian Journal of Caring Sciences, 24*(Suppl.), 67–74.

Vilhauer, J. S., Cortes, J., Moali, N., et al. (2013). Improving quality of life for patients with major depressive disorder by increasing hope and positive expectations with future directed therapy (FDT). *Innovations In Clinical Neuroscience, 10*(3), 12–22.

Hopelessness

Gail B. Ladwig, MSN, RN, and Marina Martinez-Kratz, MS, RN, CNE

NANDA-I

Definition

Subjective state in which an individual sees limited or no alternatives or personal choices available and is unable to mobilize energy on own behalf

Defining Characteristics

Alteration in sleep pattern; decrease in affect; decrease in appetite; decrease in initiative; decrease in response to stimuli; decrease in verbalization; despondent verbal cues (e.g., "I can't," sighing); inadequate involvement in care; passivity; poor eye contact; shrugging in response to speaker; turning away from speaker

H

Related Factors (r/t)

Chronic stress; deterioration in physiological condition; history of abandonment; loss of belief in spiritual power; loss of belief in transcendent values; prolonged activity restriction; social isolation

NOC (Nursing Outcomes Classification)

Suggested NOC Outcomes

Decision-Making; Hope; Mood Equilibrium; Nutritional Status: Food and Fluid Intake; Quality of Life; Sleep

Example NOC Outcome with Indicators

Has a presence of **Hope** as evidenced by the following indicators: Expresses expectation of a positive future/Expresses faith/Expresses will to live. (Rate the outcome and indicators of **Hope:** 1 = never demonstrated, 2 = rarely demonstrated, 3 = sometimes demonstrated, 4 = often demonstrated, 5 = consistently demonstrated [see Section I].)

Client Outcomes

Client Will (Specify Time Frame)

- Verbalize feelings
- Participate in care
- Make positive statements (e.g., "I can" or "I will try")
- Set goals
- Make eye contact, focus on speaker
- Maintain appropriate appetite for age and physical health
- Sleep appropriate length of time for age and physical health
- Express concern for another
- Initiate activity

NIC (Nursing Interventions Classification)

Suggested NIC Intervention

Hope Inspiration

Example NIC Activities—Hope Inspiration

Assist client/family to identify areas of hope in life; Demonstrate hope by recognizing client's intrinsic worth and viewing client's illness as only one facet of the individual; Expand the client's repertoire of coping mechanisms

Nursing Interventions and *Rationales*

▲ Assess for, monitor, and document the potential for suicide. (Refer the client for appropriate treatment if a potential for suicide is identified.) Refer to the care plan risk for **Suicide** for specific interventions. CEB: *In this study of men who had attempted suicide, hopelessness was identified as an important risk factor and thus it is important to be identified by nurses (Hinkkurinen et al, 2011).*

- ▲ Assess and monitor potential for depression. (Refer the client for appropriate treatment if depression is identified.) CEB: *Hopelessness is a potential predictor for depressive and suicidal symptoms (Wang et al, 2013).*
- ▲ Assess for hopelessness with the modified Beck Hopelessness Scale. CEB: *The modified Beck Hopelessness Scale is a valid and reliable tool to measure hopelessness (Fisher & Overholser, 2013).*
- • Engage the client in a therapeutic relationship to enhance social connectedness and social support networks. EBN: *Nursing research found that relationship-based interventions improve a client's sense of social connectedness and decrease hopelessness (McCay et al, 2011).*
- • Assess and monitor family caregivers for symptoms of hopelessness. CEB: *Caregivers of advanced cancer clients are at risk for experiencing hopelessness (Mystakidou et al, 2007a).* EBN: *Adult daughter caregivers experience hopelessness as part of compassion fatigue (Day et al, 2014).*
- • Determine appropriate approaches based on the underlying condition or situation that is contributing to feelings of hopelessness. CEB: *Understanding the source of the hopelessness, such as negative life events, will indicate the approaches that may be most beneficial to the person (Toussaint et al, 2008).* CEBN: *Women with advanced breast cancer and their families and men with prostate cancer and their families benefit from specific strategies of intervention (Northouse et al, 2007).*
- • Assess for pain and respond with appropriate measures for pain relief. CEB: *Pain that interferes with mood and enjoyment in life results in feelings of hopelessness for clients with advanced cancer (Mystakidou et al, 2007b).*
- • Facilitate access to resources to support spiritual well-being. EBN: *Spiritual care that addresses three universal spiritual needs (meaning and purpose, love and relatedness, and forgiveness) is recommended as a valuable intervention to address hopelessness (Taylor, 2012).*
- • Facilitate sources of the client's resilience. CEB: *Higher levels of resilience were associated with lower levels of hopelessness in children of HIV positive parents (Mo et al, 2014).*
- • Assist the client to expect positive outcomes and recognize the pathways to achieve the positive outcomes. CEB: *Research shows that these actions facilitate the development of hope as a strength (Proctor et al, 2011).*
- • Assist the client in looking at alternatives and setting long- and short term goals that are important to him/her. CEBN: *When health professionals work with men with prostate cancer and their family caregivers, they should help them replace avoidant coping strategies with alternate strategies (Northouse et al, 2007). Setting goals is a future oriented action that promotes the development of hope and optimism (Duke et al, 2011).*
- • Encourage clients to discuss hope, because discussion may be helpful in increasing hope. CEBN: *Entering into discussion of hope may be helpful in increasing hope (Cutcliff & Koehn, 2007).* CEBN: *Health-promoting conversations about hope and suffering with couples in palliative care has potential for improving hope (Benzein & Savemant, 2008).*
- • Assist clients in developing realistic goals for their recovery. EBN: *Realistic goals reflect realistic sense of hope versus false hope (Tutton et al, 2012).*
- • Assist clients to set a goal, write down what steps are needed to achieve the goal, and visualize themselves reaching the goal. CEB: *Research found that structured goal setting was sufficient to foster hope (Feldman & Dreher, 2011).*
- • Provide accurate information. CEBN: *Accurate information allows the redefining and transforming of hope (Duggleby & Wright, 2005; Duggleby et al, 2009).*
- • Encourage decision-making and problem solving. EBN: *Hopelessness may be an outgrowth of a perceived loss of control and/or self-efficacy. As changes occur, the nurse interacts with the client to evaluate their impact on life goals and assists in making adaptations that support hopefulness and decrease hopelessness (Kylma, 2005).* CEB: *Problem solving was associated with higher resilience and lower levels of hopelessness (Gooding et al, 2012).*
- • Spend one-on-one time with the client. Use empathy; try to understand what the client is saying and communicate this understanding to the client to create a nonjudgmental trusting environment to develop therapeutic relationships with the client. CEBN: *The therapeutic relationship is an essential component of interventions to address hopelessness (Koehn & Cutcliff, 2007).*
- • Teach alternative coping strategies such as physical activity. CEB: *Clients with severe mental illness showed decreased hopelessness after participation in an adjunct exercise program (Sylvia et al, 2013).*
- • Use a future directed approach that teaches individuals how to become aware of attention that is focused on unwanted aspects of life and how to redirect attention toward things that feel more wanted or desired.

CEB: *Future directed therapy is effective at decreasing hopelessness and increases positive future expectations (Vilhauer et al, 2013).*

- Review the client's strengths and resources in conjunction with the client. CEBN: *Working with the client to identify positive experiences, resources, and personal strengths facilitates the development of hopefulness (Kylma, 2005).*
- Encourage the client to adopt active coping strategies. CEB: *Active coping strategies decreased hopelessness in both curative and palliative cancer patients (van Laarhoven et al, 2011).*
- Involve family and significant others in the plan of care. EBN: *Social support decreased hopelessness and anxiety in parents of children with cancer (Bayat et al, 2008).*
- Offer emotional support, active listening, and coping assistance to client families. EBN: *Family hopelessness is addressed when nurses offer emotional support (Coco et al, 2013).*
- For additional interventions, see the care plans for Readiness for enhanced **Hope, Spiritual** distress, Readiness for enhanced **Spiritual** well-being, and Disturbed **Sleep** pattern.

Geriatric

- Previous interventions may be adapted for geriatric clients.
- ▲ If depression is suspected, confer with the primary health care provider regarding referral for mental health services. CEB: *This study of older adults identified hopelessness as a major risk factor for suicide (Neufeld et al, 2010).*
- Take threats of self-harm or suicide seriously and intervene as needed. CEB: *This study of older adults identified hopelessness as a major risk factor for suicide (Neufeld et al, 2010). Older adults have the highest risk of death by suicide in the United States (Cukrowicz et al, 2011).*
- Use reminiscence and life-review therapies to identify past coping skills. Older people in residential facilities benefit from this therapy (*Wang, 2004*). CEB: *Life review produced a positive outcome when used with individuals with right hemisphere cerebrovascular accidents (Davis, 2004).*
- Encourage visits from children and family members. CEBN: *Social relationships foster hopefulness (Duggleby, 2001).*
- Consider videoconferencing for older adults in nursing homes with relatives as alternatives to "live visits." *Once-a-week videoconferencing effectively improved the nursing home residents' emotional and appraisal social support, depressive status, and loneliness (Tsai et al, 2010).*
- Position the client by a window, take the client outside, or encourage such activities as gardening (if ability allows). *Using nature can help older people expand their perspectives, connect with strength, and expand their coping strategies, while gaining a wider sense of acceptance and completion in life (Berger, 2009).*
- Provide esthetic forms of expression, such as dance, music, literature, and pictures. EBN: *Esthetic experiences are related to feelings of timelessness and spacelessness and serve as sources of gratification (Wikstrom, 2004).*
- Consider "biblio and telephone therapy" (BTT). CEB: *The results of this study of older adults demonstrated that the clients benefited from BTT and that depressive symptoms lessened (Brenes et al, 2010).*

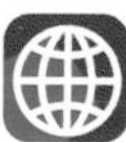

Multicultural

- Assess for the influence of cultural beliefs, norms, and values on the client's feelings of hopelessness. CEB: *In some Latino cultures, talking about depression* (depresión) *may be taboo. Hopelessness* (desanimo) *may be understood differently by clients of various cultural backgrounds and may have a more normative and culturally specific, comfortable sound for clients (Marsiglia et al, 2011).*
- Assess the effect of fatalism on the client's expression of hopelessness. EBN: *Fatalistic perspectives, which involve the belief that one cannot control one's own fate, may influence health behaviors in some Asian, African American, and Latino populations (Marsiglia et al, 2011). This study of African Americans with multiple sclerosis identified fatalism, defined as a surrender of power to external forces in life leading to hopelessness, as being common among some African Americans (Holland et al, 2011).*
- ▲ Assess for depression and refer to appropriate services. CEB: *Hispanic women expressing hopelessness may also be at risk for depression (Marsiglia et al, 2011).*
- Encourage spirituality as a source of support for hopelessness. CEBN: *African Americans and Latinos may identify spirituality, religiousness, prayer, and church-based approaches as coping resources (Samuel-Hodge et al, 2000).* CEBN: *Spiritual beliefs, the role of prayer, and the role of family in caregiving were predominant aspects of the end-of-life experience in Mexican Americans. There is a need to focus on the role*

of religious institutions in Mexican American culture, where spirituality and religion are strong influences in the life experience (Johnston, 2007).

Home Care

- Previously mentioned interventions may be adapted for home care use.
- ▲ Assess for isolation within the family unit. Encourage the client to participate in family activities. If the client cannot participate, encourage him/her to be in the same area and watch family activities. Refer for telephone support. CEBN: *Hope is facilitated by meaningful interpersonal relationships (Koehn & Cutcliff, 2007).* CEB: *Clients show significant improvements in depression and positive affect during the 16 weeks of telephone-administered treatment (Mohr et al, 2005).*
- Reminisce with the client about his/her life. CEBN: *The process of remembering past activities helps find meaning and purpose in life and inspires hope (Duggleby & Wright, 2005).* CEB: *Older people in residential facilities benefit from life review (Chin, 2007).*
- Identify areas in which the client can have control. *Allow the client to set achievable goals in these areas. Assist the client when necessary to negotiate desirable outcomes.* CEBN: *Mobilization of resources to promote self-efficacy promotes hope (Kylma, 2005).*
- If illness precipitated the hopelessness, discuss knowledge of and previous experience with the disease. *Help the client identify past coping strengths.* CEBN: *Knowledge of the disease and previous positive coping experience with the illness provide hope for the future (Duggleby & Wright, 2005).*
- ▲ Provide plant or pet therapy if possible. CEBN: Caring for pets or plants helps to find meaning and purpose and foster hope (*Holtslander & Duggleby, 2009*).

Client/Family Teaching and Discharge Planning

- Provide information regarding the client's condition, treatment plan, and progress. CEBN: *Clear, direct communication of the potential of an intervention to overcome a threat along with honest discussion of negative aspects fosters hope for clients and their families (Duggleby & Wright, 2005; Holtslander et al, 2005).*
- Teach family caregivers skills to provide care in the home. CEBN: *Family caregivers find hope in giving skilled care to their family members (Duggleby et al, 2009).* CEBN: *A psychoeducational program preparing family caregivers for caring for a dying relative at home increased their feeling of caregiving competence and rewards (Hudson et al, 2008).*
- Provide positive reinforcement, praise, and acknowledgment of the challenges of caregiving to family members. EBN: *Positive comments and praise foster hope in family caregivers (Holtslander et al, 2005).*
- ▲ Refer the client to self-help groups, such as "I Can Cope" and "Make Today Count." CEBN: *Self-help and/or professionally led curriculum-based support programs for families are effective in reducing stress and facilitating coping and hope (Northouse et al, 2007).*
- ▲ Consider an Internet-based behavior change intervention when depression is identified by primary care provider in adolescents. CEB: *In this study, a primary care/Internet-based intervention model among adolescents demonstrated reductions in depressed mood over 6 months and may result in fewer depressive episodes (Hoek et al, 2011).*

REFERENCES

Bayat, M., Erdem, E., & Kuzucu, E. G. (2008). Depression, anxiety, hopelessness and social support levels of the parents of children with cancer. *Journal of Pediatric Oncology Nursing, 25*, 247–253.

Benzein, E. V., & Savemant, B. I. (2008). Health-promoting conversation about hope and suffering with couples in palliative care. *International Journal of Palliative Nursing, 14*(9), 409–445.

Berger, R. (2009). Being in nature: an innovative framework for incorporating nature in therapy with older adults. *Journal of Holistic Nursing, 27*(1), 45–50.

Brenes, G., et al. (2010). Feasibility and acceptability of bibliotherapy and telephone sessions for the treatment of late-life anxiety disorders. *Clinical Gerontologist, 33*, 62–68.

Chin, A. (2007). Clinical effects of reminiscence therapy in older adults: a meta-analysis of controlled trials. *Hong Kong Journal of Occupational Therapy, 17*(1), 10–22.

Coco, K., Tossavainen, K., Jääskeläinen, J., et al. (2013). The provision of emotional support to the families of traumatic brain injury patients: perspectives of Finnish nurses. *Journal of Clinical Nursing, 22*(9/10), 1467–1476.

Cukrowicz, K. C., et al. (2011). Perceived burdensomeness and suicide ideation in older adults. *Psychology and Aging, 26*(2), 331–338.

Cutcliff, J. R., & Koehn, C. V. (2007). Hope and interpersonal psychiatric/mental health nursing: a systematic review of the literature—part two. *Journal of Psychiatric and Mental Health Nursing, 14*, 141–147.

Davis, M. C. (2004). Life review therapy as an intervention to manage depression and enhance life satisfaction in individuals with right hemisphere cerebral vascular accidents. *Issues in Mental Health Nursing, 25*(5), 503–515.

Day, J. R., Anderson, R. A., & Davis, L. L. (2014). Compassion fatigue in adult daughter caregivers of a parent with dementia. *Issues in Mental Health Nursing, 35*(10), 796–804.

Duggleby, W. (2001). Hope at the end of life. *J Hosp Palliat Nurs, 3*(2), 51.

Duggleby, W., et al. (2009). Renewing everyday hope: the hope experience of family caregivers of persons with dementia. *Issues in Mental Health Nursing, 30*(8), 514–521.

Duggleby, W., & Wright, K. (2005). Transforming hope: how elderly palliative patients live with hope. *The Canadian Journal of Nursing Research, 37*(2), 70–84.

Duke, N., Borowsky, I., Pettingell, S., et al. (2011). Examining youth hopelessness as an independent risk correlate for adolescent delinquency and violence. *Maternal & Child Health Journal, 15*(1), 87–97.

Feldman, D. B., & Dreher, D. E. (2011). Can hope be changed in 90 minutes? Testing the efficacy of a single-session goal-pursuit intervention for college students. *Journal of Happiness Studies, 13*, 745–759.

Fisher, L. B., & Overholser, J. C. (2013). Refining the assessment of hopelessness: an improved way to look to the future. *Death Studies, 37*(3), 212–227.

Gooding, P., Hurst, A., Johnson, J., et al. (2012). Psychological resilience in young and older adults. *International Journal of Geriatric Psychiatry, 27*(3), 262–270.

Hinkkurinen, J., Isola, A., & Kylmä, J. (2011). Experiences of self-destruction and related hopelessness in men who have attempted suicide [Finnish]. *Hoitotiede, 23*(3), 230–239.

Hoek, W., et al. (2011). Randomized controlled trial of primary care physician motivational interviewing versus brief advice to engage adolescents with an Internet-based depression prevention intervention: 6-month outcomes and predictors of improvement. *Translational Research: The Journal of Laboratory and Clinical Medicine, 158*(6), 315–325.

Holland, B. E., Gray, J., & Pierce, T. G. (2011). The client experience model: synthesis and application to African Americans with multiple sclerosis. *J Theory Constr Test, 15*(2), 36–40.

Holtslander, L., & Duggleby, W. (2009). The hope experience of older bereaved women who cared for a spouse with terminal cancer. *Qualitative Health Research, 19*, 388–400.

Holtslander, L., et al. (2005). The experience of hope for informal caregivers of palliative patients. *Journal of Palliative Care, 21*(4), 285–291.

Hudson, P., et al. (2008). Evaluation of a psycho-educational group program for family caregivers in home-based palliative care. *Palliative Medicine, 22*, 270–280.

Johnston, R. (2007). *Religions in society* (7th ed.). Upper Saddle River, NJ: Pearson Prentice Hall.

Koehn, C. V., & Cutcliff, J. R. (2007). Hope and interpersonal psychiatric/mental health nursing: a systematic review of the literature—part one. *Journal of Psychiatric and Mental Health Nursing, 14*, 134–140.

Kylma, J. (2005). Despair and hopelessness in the context of HIV: a meta-synthesis on qualitative research findings. *Journal of Clinical Nursing, 14*, 813–821.

Marsiglia, F. F., Kulis, S., Perez, H., et al. (2011). Hopelessness, family stress, and depression among mexican-heritage mothers in the southwest. *Health & Social Work, 36*(1), 7–18.

McCay, E., Quesnel, S., Langley, J., et al. (2011). A relationship-based intervention to improve social connectedness in street-involved youth: a pilot study. *Journal of Child & Adolescent Psychiatric Nursing, 24*(4), 208–215.

Mo, P. H., Lau, J. F., Yu, X., et al. (2014). The role of social support on resilience, posttraumatic growth, hopelessness, and depression among children of HIV-infected parents in mainland China. *AIDS Care, 26*(12), 1526–1533.

Mohr, D., Har,t, S., & Julian, L. (2005). Telephone administered psychotherapy for depression. *Archives of General Psychiatry, 62*(9), 1007–1014.

Mystakidou, K., et al. (2007a). Caregivers of advanced cancer patients: feelings of hopelessness and depression. *Cancer Nursing, 30*(5), 412–418.

Mystakidou, K., et al. (2007b). Exploring the relationships between depression, hopelessness, cognitive status, pain and spirituality in patients with advanced cancer. *Archives of Psychiatric Nursing, 21*(3), 150–161.

Neufeld, E., O'Rourke, N., & Donnelly, M. (2010). Enhanced measurement sensitivity of hopeless ideation among older adults at risk of self-harm: reliability and validity of Likert-type responses to the Beck Hopelessness Scale. *Aging and Mental Health, 14*(6), 752–756.

Northouse, L., et al. (2007). Randomized clinical trial of a family intervention for prostate cancer patients and their spouses. *Cancer, 110*, 2809–2811.

Proctor, C., Tsukayama, E., Wood, A. M., et al. (2011). Strengths Gym: the impact of a character strengths based intervention on the life satisfaction and wellbeing of adolescents. *Journal of Positive Psychology, 6*, 377–388.

Samuel-Hodge, C. D., et al. (2000). Influences on day-to-day self-management of type 2 diabetes among African American women: spirituality, the multi-caregiver role, and other social context factors. *Diabetes Care, 23*(7), 928.

Sylvia, L., Kopeski, L., Brown, C., et al. (2013). An adjunct exercise program for serious mental illness: who chooses to participate and is it feasible? *Community Mental Health Journal, 49*(2), 213–219.

Taylor, C. (2012). Rethinking hopelessness and the role of spiritual care when cure is no longer an option. *Journal Of Pain & Symptom Management, 44*(4), 626–630.

Toussaint, L., et al. (2008). Why forgiveness may protect against depression: hopelessness as an explanatory mechanism. *Pers Ment Health, 2*, 89–103.

Tutton, E., Seers, K., Langstaff, D., et al. (2012). Staff and patient views of the concept of hope on a stroke unit: a qualitative study. *Journal of Advanced Nursing, 68*(9), 2061–2069.

Tsai, H. H., et al. (2010). Videoconference program enhances social support, loneliness, and depressive status of elderly nursing home residents. *Aging and Mental Health, 14*(8), 947–954.

van Laarhoven, H., Schilderman, J., Bleijenberg, G., et al. (2011). Coping, quality of life, depression, and hopelessness in cancer patients in a curative and palliative, end-of-life care setting. *Cancer Nursing, 34*(4), 302–314.

Vilhauer, J. S., Cortes, J., Moali, N., et al. (2013). Improving quality of life for patients with major depressive disorder by increasing hope and positive expectations with future directed therapy (FDT). *Innovations In Clinical Neuroscience, 10*(3), 12–22.

Wang, J. (2004). The comparative effectiveness among institutionalized and non-institutionalized elderly people in Taiwan of reminiscence therapy as a psychological measure. *The Journal of Nursing Research, 12*(3), 237–244.

Wang, L., Liu, L., Shi, S., et al. (2013). Cognitive trio: relationship with major depression and clinical predictors in Han Chinese women. *Psychological Medicine, 43*(11), 2265–2275.

Wikstrom, B. (2004). Older adults and the arts: the importance of aesthetic forms of expression in later life. *Journal of Gerontological Nursing, 30*(9), 30–36.

Risk for compromised Human Dignity

Shari D. Froelich, DNP, MSN, MSBA, ANP, BC, ACHPN, PMHNP, BC, and Betty J. Ackley, MSN, EdS, RN

NANDA-I

Definition

Vulnerable for perceived loss of respect and honor, which may compromise health

Risk Factors

Cultural incongruence; dehumanizing treatment; disclosure of confidential information; exposure of the body; humiliation; insufficient comprehension of health information; intrusion by clinician; invasion of privacy; limited decision-making experience; loss of control over body function; stigmatization

NOC (Nursing Outcomes Classification)

Suggested NOC Outcomes

Health Beliefs: Perceived Control; Decision-Making; Spiritual Control; Perceived Social Support

Example NOC Outcome with Indicators

Health Beliefs: Perceived Control as evidenced by the following indicators: Perceived responsibility for health decisions/Requested involvement in health decisions/Efforts at gathering information/Belief that own decisions control health outcomes/Willingness to designate surrogate decision maker. (Rate the outcome and indicators of **Health Beliefs: Perceived Control:** 1 = very weak, 2 = weak, 3 = moderate, 4 = strong, 5 = very strong [see Section I].)

Client-Based Outcome

Client/Caregiver Will (Specify Time Frame)

- Perceive that dignity is maintained throughout hospitalization/encounter
- Consistently call client by name of choice
- Maintain client's privacy

NIC (Nursing Interventions Classification)

Suggested NIC Interventions

Presence; Decision-Making Support; Spiritual Support; Hope Instillation

Example NIC Activities—Presence

Demonstrate accepting attitude; Listen to client's concerns

Nursing Interventions and *Rationales*

- Be authentically present when with the client, try to limit extraneous thoughts of self or others, and concentrate on the well-being of the client. EBN: *Human presence never leaves one unaffected. Expressed as compassion and caring, it is not only the words that are spoken or the eyes that notice, leading to action (Manookian et al, 2014).*
- Enter into and stay within the other's frame of reference. Connect with the inner life world of meaning and spirit of the other. Join in a mutual search for meaning and wholeness of being and becoming to potentiate comfort measures, pain control, a sense of well-being, wholeness, or even spiritual transcendence of suffering. EBN: *Human dignity is a central concept within nursing and the caring professions because it communicates the shared humanity. A shared humanity is evident anywhere where human beings interact, and because nurses are eager to actualize the healing relationship with clients, they have the opportunity to share their humanity (Manookian et al, 2014).*
- Determine the client's perspective about his/her health. Example questions include "Tell me about your health." "What is it like to be in your situation?" "Tell me how you perceive yourself in this situation."

"What meaning are you giving to this situation?" "Tell me about your health priorities." "Tell me about the harmony you wish to reach." CEB: *Such questions usually contribute to helping people find meaning to the crisis in their life (Watson, 2008).* CEB: *Confirm the person's worthiness and sense of self. A genuine respect for the person as a unique human being, with an inherent desire or right to make choices according to his/her subjective needs, was found to be fundamental in advocating autonomy and integrity. Confirming the person's worthiness and sense of self in this way was identified as crucial in dignity preservation. In order to preserve personal dignity and reduce the experienced loss of freedom, autonomy, and integrity, going for frequent walks was given high priority (Tranvag et al, 2013).*

H

- Determine the client's preferences for when and how nursing care is needed and follow the client's guidelines if possible. *The client's autonomy must be recognized as part of dignified nursing care.* CEB: *A summary of older adults' perceptions of the most important nurse caring behaviors is, Knowing what they are doing, Know when it's necessary to call the medical provider, Treat me as an individual, Give my treatments and medications on time, Check my condition very closely, Give my pain medication on time, Know how to handle equipment, Keep my family informed of my progress, Don't give up on me when I am difficult to get along with (Marini, 1999).*
- Include the client in all decision-making; if the client does not choose to be part of the decision or is no longer capable of making a decision, use the named surrogate decision maker. *The Patient Self-Determination Act, effective in 1991, requires that all individuals receiving medical care also receive written information about their right to accept or refuse medical or surgical treatment and their right to initiate advance directives (Dossey & Keegan, 2009).*
- Maintain client's privacy at all times.
- Actively listen to what the client is saying both verbally and nonverbally. CEB: *We must quiet our "inner dialogue" so that we may hear more clearly, allow others to tell the whole story, listen without judgment or advice, and bear witness to the experience. Attentive silence is a communicative act in its own right, an act of compassion. It signifies respect, legitimizes what is said, and creates an atmosphere in which self-discovery can occur (Stanley, 2002).*
- Encourage the client to share thoughts about spirituality as desired. CEB: *The care of the soul remains the most powerful aspect of the art of caring in nursing. The caring occasion becomes "transpersonal" when "it allows for the presence of the spirit of both—then the event of the moment expands the limits of openness and has the ability to expand human capabilities" (Watson, 2008).*
- Use interventions to instill increased hope; see the care plan for Readiness for enhanced **Hope.** CEB: *When hope for a cure is no longer possible, help clients recognize that the relationships change between clients, families, and caregivers but do not end. Hope continues, but has a different focus (Erlen, 2003). Caring does not end but is rather transformed when intensive treatment ends.*
- For further interventions on spirituality, see the care plan for Readiness for enhanced **Spiritual** well-being.

Geriatric

- Always ask the client how he/she would like to be addressed. Avoid calling older clients "sweetie," "honey," "Gramps," or other terms that can be demeaning unless this is acceptable in the client's culture or requested by the client. *Appropriate forms of address must be used with older adults to maintain dignity.* CEB: *A respectful form of address has positive effects, whereas overfamiliarity tends to have a negative impact on self-respect, physical and mental health, and recovery from disease, particularly in older adults and those with dementia (Williams et al, 2008; Woolhead et al, 2006).*
- Treat the older client with the utmost respect, even if delirium or dementia is present with confusion. *Confused clients respond positively to caregivers who approach gently, with positive regard, and treat the confused client with respect and dignity.*

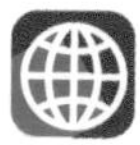

Multicultural

- Assess for the influence of cultural beliefs, norms, and values on the client's way of communicating, and follow the client's lead in communicating in matters of eye contact, amount of personal space, voice tones, and amount of touching. If in doubt, ask the client. *What the client considers normal and appropriate communication that maintains and facilitates dignity is based on cultural perceptions.* CEB: *Client dignity is promoted when staff provide privacy and use interactions that help clients feel comfortable, in control, and valued. Individual staff behavior has a major impact on whether threats to client dignity actually lead to its loss (Baillie, 2009).*

Home Care

- Most of the interventions described previously may be adapted for home care use.
- Recognize that the client with the caregiver has complete autonomy in the home. *The nurse's role is to provide the care needed and desired. The client and caregiver determine if the care offered is acceptable.*

Client/Family Teaching and Discharge Planning

- Teach family and caregivers the need for the dignity of the client to be maintained at all times. How an individual cognitively perceives and emotionally deals with the illness can depend on the person's family and social relationships and ultimately can affect the ability to heal. NOTE: Caring is integral to maintaining dignity. CEB: *According to Jean Watson (2008), a caring occasion is the moment (focal point in space and time) when the nurse and another person come together in such a way that an occasion for human caring is created. Both the one cared for and the one caring can be influenced by the caring moment through the choices and actions decided within the relationship, thereby influencing and becoming part of their own life history.*

H

REFERENCES

Baillie, L. (2009). Patient dignity in an acute care hospital setting: a case study. *International Journal of Nursing Studies, 46*, 23–37.

Dossey, B., & Keegan, L. (2009). *Holistic nursing: a handbook for practice* (5th ed.). Sudbury, MA: Jones & Bartlett.

Erlen, J. (2003). Caring doesn't end. *Orthopaedic Nursing, 22*(5), 446–449.

Manookian, A., Cheraghi, M. A., & Nasrabadi, A. N. (2014). Factors influencing patients' dignity: a qualitative study. *Nursing Ethics, 21*(3), 323–334.

Marini, B. (1999). Institutionalized older adults' perception of nursing caring behaviors: a pilot study. *Journal of Gerontological Nursing, 25*(5), 10–16.

Stanley, K. (2002). The healing power of presence: respite from the fear of abandonment. *Oncology Nursing Forum, 39*(6), 935–940.

Tranvag, O., Petersen, K. A., & Naden, D. (2013). Dignity-preserving dementia care: a metasynthesis. *Nursing Ethics, 20*(8), 861–880.

Watson, J. (2008). *Nursing: the philosophy and science of caring.* Boulder: University Press of Colorado.

Williams, K., et al. (2008). Elderspeak communication: impact on dementia care. *American Journal of Alzheimer's Disease and Other Dementias, 24*(1), 11–20.

Woolhead, G., et al. (2006). "Tu" or "vous"? A European qualitative study of dignity and communication with older people in health and social care settings. *Patient Education and Counseling, 61*(3), 363–371.

Hyperthermia

Mary Beth Flynn Makic, PhD, RN, CNS, CCNS, FAAN

NANDA-I

Definition

Core body temperature above the normal diurnal range due to failure of thermoregulation

Defining Characteristics

Abnormal posturing; apnea; coma; convulsions; flushed skin; hypotension; infant does not maintain suck; irritability; lethargy; seizure; skin warm to touch; stupor; tachycardia; tachypnea; vasodilation

Related Factors (r/t)

Decreased sweat response; dehydration; high environmental temperature; illness; inappropriate clothing; increase in metabolic rate; ischemia; pharmaceutical agent; sepsis; trauma; vigorous activity

NOC (Nursing Outcomes Classification)

Suggested NOC Outcomes

Thermoregulation; Thermoregulation: Newborn

Example NOC Outcome with Indicators

Thermoregulation as evidenced by the following indicators: Increased skin temperature/Decreased skin temperature/Skin color changes/Dehydration/Hyperthermia. (Rate the outcome and indicators of **Thermoregulation:** 1 = severe, 2 = substantial, 3 = moderate, 4 = mild, 5 = none [see Section I].)

Client Outcomes

Client Will (Specify Time Frame)

- Maintain core body temperature within adaptive levels (less than 104° F, 40° C)
- Remain free of complications of malignant hyperthermia
- Remain free of complication of neuroleptic malignant syndrome
- Remain free of dehydration
- Remain free from infection
- Verbalize signs and symptoms of heat stroke and actions to prevent heat stroke
- Verbalize personal risks for malignant hyperthermia and neuroleptic malignant syndrome to be reported during health history reviews to all health care professionals, including pharmacists

H

NIC (Nursing Interventions Classification)

Suggested NIC Interventions

Fever Treatment; Malignant Hyperthermia Precautions; Temperature Regulation

Example NIC Activities—Hyperthermia Treatment

Monitor core body temperature using appropriate device; Monitor for abnormalities in mental status

Nursing Interventions and *Rationales*

Temperature Measurement

- Recognize that hyperthermia is a rise in body temperature above 40° C (104° F) that is not regulated by the hypothalamus, resulting in an uncontrolled increase in body temperature exceeding the body's ability to lose heat, and is a medical emergency (Dinarello & Porat, 2012; Saltzberg, 2013).
- Measure and record a client's temperature every hour and more frequently as clinically indicated. Two modes of temperature monitoring may be indicated. Continuous temperature monitoring using an indwelling method of temperature measurement is usually indicated to monitor effectiveness of interventions in lowering the body temperature. EBN/CEB: *Hyperthermia is a life-threatening crisis that requires accurate temperature measurement. Core temperature is obtained by a pulmonary artery catheter or from the distal esophagus; near core temperature measurements include oral, bladder, rectal, and temporal artery, and peripheral measurements are obtained by skin surface measurements and in the axilla (Davie & Amoore, 2010; Barnason et al, 2012; Hooper et al, 2009). Research is limited on accuracy of temporal artery measurements outside normal ranges; axillary temperature is accurate in neonates but is not well supported in adults; tympanic membrane measurements and chemical dot thermometers are least accurate and should be avoided in caring for the acutely ill adult client (Calonder et al, 2010; Davie & Amoore, 2010; Hooper et al, 2009; Makic et al, 2011; Barnason et al, 2012; Kenney et al, 2014).*
- Use the same site and method (device) for temperature measurement for a given client so that temperature trends are assessed accurately; record site of temperature measurement. EBN/CEB: *There are differences in temperature depending on the site from which temperature measurement is obtained; however, differences between sites should not be greater than 0.3° C to 0.5° C (Bridges & Thomas, 2009; Davie & Amoore, 2010; Dinarello & Porat, 2012; Hooper et al, 2009; Makic et al, 2011; Kenney et al, 2014).*

▲ Work with the health care provider to help determine the cause of the temperature increase, hyperthermia, which will often help direct appropriate treatment. *It is important to treat the underlying cause of the temperature to preserve neurological function of the client as well as implement interventions to rapidly lower the core temperature (Saltzberg, 2013; Dinarello & Porat, 2012; Leon & Helwig, 2010; Bohman & Levine, 2014).*

- Refer to care plan for Ineffective **Thermoregulation** for interventions managing fever (pyrexia).

Heat Stroke

- Recognize that heat stroke may be separated into two categories: classic and exertional. *Classic heat stroke usually involves the very young and older client during environmental heat waves. Exertional heat stroke occurs in young adults performing strenuous exercise in hot climates (Leon & Helwig, 2010; Thomas & Crowhurst, 2013; Kerr et al, 2014).*
- Watch for risk factors for classic heat stroke, which include (Leon & Helwig, 2010):
  - Medications, especially diuretic agents, anticholinergic agents, anti-Parkinson medications
  - Alcoholism
  - Mental illness

▲ EB: *Physiological effects of aging lower onset of sweating and rate of sweating needed to help with dissipation of body heat. Medications can dehydrate the client as well as blunt physiological responses necessary to assist with heat dissipation, increasing the risk of heat stroke in older clients (Brege, 2009; Leon & Helwig, 2010).*

- Risk factors of exertional heat stroke include (Kerr et al, 2014):
  - Preexisting illness
  - Drug use (e.g., alcohol, amphetamines, ecstasy)
  - Wearing protective clothing (uniforms and athletic gear) that limits heat dissipation
- Recognize signs and symptoms of hyperthermia: core body temperature greater than 40°C (104°F), exercise associated muscle cramps, tachycardia, tachypnea, orthostatic dizziness, weakness, vomiting, headache, confusion, delirium, seizures, coma, acute kidney injury (rhabdomyolysis), hot dry skin (classic heat stroke) (Pryor et al, 2013; Brege, 2009; Dinarello & Porat, 2012; Leon & Helwig, 2010).
- Recognize that antipyretic agents are of little use in treatment of hyperthermia. CEB: *Because the cause of the hyperthermia does not involve the hypothalamus, antipyretic agents are ineffective and not indicated in treatment of clients with hyperthermia (Dinarello & Porat, 2012; Hamaya et al, 2015).*

▲ Assess fluid loss and facilitate oral intake or administer intravenous fluids as ordered to accomplish fluid replacement and support the cardiovascular system. *Increased metabolic rate, diuresis, and diaphoresis-associated exertional hyperthermia cause loss of body fluids (Brege, 2009; CDC, 2013).* Refer to the care plan for Deficient **Fluid** volume.

- Use external cooling measures carefully: loosen or remove excessive clothing, give a tepid water bath, provide cool liquids if the client is alert enough to swallow, fan the client's face. EB/EBN: *Hyperthermia must be treated aggressively to lower the body temperature. However, interventions to cool the client should not be so aggressive that the client shivers. Shivering increases heat production, oxygen consumption, and cardiorespiratory effort (Pryor et al, 2013; Brege, 2009; CDC, 2013; Pitoni et al, 2011).*
- Recognize that cooling with ice packs, cooled intravenous solution, or a hypothermia blanket may be required to lower the body temperature quickly (Dinarello & Porat, 2012; Leon & Helwig, 2010). When using a cooling blanket, choose a circulating water cooling device if available and set the temperature regulator to 0.5°C to 1°C (1°F to 2°F) below the client's current temperature to prevent shivering. CEB: *A review examining cooling methods found that skin surface cooling methods using ice and fans provided inconsistent cooling; hydrogel-coated water circulating pads placed on the chest and legs provided better targeted cooling than water circulating cooling blankets that can be placed over or under the client; and intravascular core cooling is an invasive technique that may be used to rapidly cool the body (Polderman & Herold, 2009).*

▲ Continually assess the client's neurological and other organ function, especially kidney function (i.e., signs of rhabdomyolysis), for signs of injury from hyperthermia. EB/EBN: *Hyperthermia can cause permanent neurological injury, acute kidney injury, electrolyte imbalances, and coagulation disorders. Continuous assessment of neurological and other organ function is essential because the client's body temperature is rapidly lowered (CDC, 2013; Hamaya et al, 2015; Pryor et al, 2013; Dinarello & Porat, 2012; Thomas & Crowhurst, 2013).*

Malignant Hyperthermia

▲ If the client has just received general anesthesia, especially sevoflurane, desflurane, enflurane, isoflurane, or succinylcholine, recognize that the hyperthermia may be caused by malignant hyperthermia and requires immediate treatment to prevent death. *Malignant hyperthermia is often a fatal disease and must be treated promptly. Emergent treatment includes rapid administration of the medication dantrolene, increasing oxygenation and assisting ventilation, initiating external cooling measures, and treating*

H

acid-base (e.g., metabolic acidosis) and electrolyte disorders (Seifert et al, 2014; Dinarello & Porat, 2012; Hopkins, 2011).

- Recognize that signs and symptoms of malignant hyperthermia typically occur suddenly after exposure to the anesthetic agent and include rapid rise in core body temperature, hypercarbia (increase in end tidal carbon dioxide), muscle rigidity, arrhythmias, tachycardia, tachypnea, rhabdomyolysis, and acute kidney injury, and elevated serum calcium and potassium, progressing to disseminated intravascular coagulation and cardiac arrest (Seifert et al, 2014; Stewart 2014; Hopkins, 2011).

▲ If the client has malignant hyperthermia, begin treatment as ordered, including cessation of the anesthetic agent and intravenous administration of dantrolene sodium, stat, along with antiarrhythmics, and continued support of the cardiovascular system. *Dantrolene helps decrease the increased muscle activity associated with malignant hyperthermia and can be life-saving (Dinarello & Porat, 2012).*

- Provide client and family education when malignant hyperthermia occurs, as it is an inherited muscle disorder. *Obtaining a thorough health history to include family history of adverse experiences with anesthesia is important in identifying clients at risk for malignant hyperthermia. Genetic testing may also be indicated* (*Malignant Hyperthermia Association of the United States, 2015*).

Neuroleptic Malignant Syndrome

▲ Recognize that neuroleptic malignant syndrome is a rare condition associated with clients who are taking typical and atypical antipsychotic agents (Takanobu K et al, 2015; Paden et al, 2013; Gillman, 2010; Trollor et al, 2009). **EB/EBN:** *The most common agents associated with the condition are dopamine-2 inhibiting agents (e.g., haloperidol, fluphenazine, chlorpromazine, quetiapine, risperidone, and olanzapine). Dopamine antagonist agents have also been found to trigger the syndrome as well (e.g., metoclopramide, promethazine, prochlorperazine) (Takanobu et al, 2015; Paden et al, 2013; Dinarello & Porat, 2012; Gillman, 2010; Trollor et al, 2009).*

- Watch for signs and symptoms that can range from mild to severe and include a sudden change in mental status, rapid rise in body temperature, muscle rigidity, tachycardia, tachypnea, elevated or labile blood pressure, diaphoresis, rhabdomyolysis, and acute kidney injury (Paden et al, 2013).

▲ Begin treatment when diagnosed, including cessation of the neuroleptic or dopamine antagonist agent; order administration of dantrolene and continued support of the cardiovascular, pulmonary, and renal systems (Dinarello & Porat, 2012).

- A client health history that reports extrapyramidal reaction to any medication should be further explored for risk of neuroleptic malignant syndrome, because this syndrome can occur at any time during a client's treatment with typical and atypical antipsychotic agents (*Takanobu et al, 2015; Paden et al, 2013; Trollor et al, 2009).*
- Recognize that clients receiving rapid dose escalation of antipsychotic agents (e.g., haloperidol) intramuscularly for acute treatment of delirium may be at increased risk for neuroleptic malignant syndrome (*Takanobu et al, 2015; Paden et al, 2013*).

Pediatric

- Assess risk factors of malignant hyperthermia as this has an increased prevalence in the pediatric population. *The administration of inhalation anesthesia and succinylcholine is common in this age group. Risk assessment includes a personal or family history of anesthesia-related complications or death (Malignant Hyperthermia Association of the United States, 2015).*

▲ Administer dantrolene, provide oxygen and assist with ventilation, monitor heart rate and rhythm, and treat electrolyte and acid-base disorders (i.e., metabolic acidosis) as ordered if malignant hyperthermia is present. *Dantrolene and airway management/support are necessary during emergent treatment of malignant hyperthermia (Dinarello & Porat, 2012; Seifert et al, 2014).*

Geriatric

- Help the client seek medical attention immediately if elevated core temperature is present. To diagnose the hyperthermia, assess for possible precipitating factors, including changes in medication, environmental changes, and recent medical interventions or infectious exposures. *Older adults are more susceptible to environmentally and medication-induced hyperthermia, due to the greater incidence of underlying chronic medical conditions that impair thermal regulation or prevent removal from a hot environment (Saltzberg, 2013).*
- In hot weather, encourage the client to wear lightweight cotton clothing (Sadler, 2011).

- Provide education on the importance of drinking eight glasses of fluid per day (within their cardiac and renal reserves) regardless of whether they are thirsty. Assess for the need for and presence of fans or air conditioning, and also appropriate clothing. *Older adults are more susceptible to a hot environment than are younger adults because of a decreased sensitivity to heat, decreased sweat gland function, decreased thirst, and decreased mobility (Brege, 2009).*
- ▲ In hot weather, monitor the older client for signs of heat stroke: rising temperature, orthostatic blood pressure drop, weakness, restlessness, mental status changes, faintness, thirst, nausea, and vomiting. If signs are present, move the client to a cool place, have the client lie down, give sips of water, check orthostatic blood pressure, spray with lukewarm water, cool with a fan, and seek medical assistance immediately. *Older adults are predisposed to heat exhaustion and should be watched carefully for occurrence; if present, it should be treated promptly (Sadler, 2011; Brege, 2009).*
- During warm weather, help the client obtain a fan or an air conditioner to increase evaporation, as needed. Help the older client locate a cool environment to which they can go for safety in hot weather.
- Take the temperature of the older client in hot weather. *Older clients may not be able to tell that they are hot because of decreased sensation.*

H

Home Care

- Some of the interventions described previously may be adapted for home care use.
- Determine whether the client or family has a functioning thermometer, and know how to use it. Refer to the interventions above on taking a temperature.
- Help the client and caregivers prevent and monitor for heat stroke/hyperthermia during times of high outdoor temperatures. *Preventive measures include minimizing time spent outdoors, use of air conditioning or fans, increasing fluid intake, and taking frequent rest periods (Sadler, 2011; CDC, 2013).*
- To prevent heat-related injury in athletes, laborers, and military personnel, instruct them to acclimate gradually to the higher temperatures, increase fluid intake, wear vapor-permeable clothing, and take frequent rests (Kerr et al, 2014; CDC, 2013).
- In the event of temperature elevation above the adaptive range, institute measures to decrease temperature (e.g., get the client out of the sun and into a cool place, remove excess clothing, have the client drink fluids, spray the client with lukewarm water, and fan with cool air). Initiate emergency transport. *Hyperthermia is an acute and possibly life-threatening situation (Kerr et al, 2014; CDC, 2013).*

Client/Family Teaching and Discharge Planning

- ▲ Instruct to increase fluids to prevent heat-induced hyperthermia and dehydration in the presence of fever. Liberal fluid intake replaces fluid lost through perspiration and respiration (*Pinto & Walsh, 2011; Sadler, 2011*).
- Teach the client to stay in a cooler environment during periods of excessive outdoor heat or humidity. If the client does go out, instruct him/her to avoid vigorous physical activity; wear lightweight, loose-fitting clothing; and wear a hat to minimize sun exposure. *Such methods reduce exposure to high environmental temperatures, which can cause heat stroke and hyperthermia (Sadler, 2011; Kerr et al, 2014; CDC, 2013).*

REFERENCES

Barnason, S., et al. (2012). Emergency nursing resource: non-invasive temperature measurement in the emergency department. *Journal of Emergency Nursing*, *38*, 523–530.

Bohman, L. E., & Levine, J. M. (2014). Fever and therapeutic normothermia in severe brain injury: an update. *Current Opinion in Critical Care*, *20*, 182–188.

Brege, D. J. (2009). Red flags: recognizing and treating heatstroke. *Nursing Made Incred Easy*, *7*(4), 13–18.

Bridges, E., & Thomas, K. (2009). Noninvasive measurement of body temperature in critically ill patients. *Critical Care Nurse*, *29*(3), 94–97.

Calonder, E. M., et al. (2010). Temperature measurement in patients undergoing colorectal surgery and gynecology surgery: a comparison of esophageal core, temporal artery, and oral methods. *Journal of Perianesthesia Nursing*, *25*(2), 71–78.

Centers for Disease Control and Prevention (CDC) (2013). *Heat stress.* NIOSH workplace safety and health tips. From: <http://www.cdc.gov/niosh/topics/heatstress>. Retrieved June 3, 2015.

Davie, A., & Amoore, J. (2010). Best practice in the measurement of body temperature. *Nursing Standard*, *24*(42), 42–50.

Dinarello, C., & Porat, R. (2012). Fever and hyperthermia. In A. S. Fauci, et al. (Eds.), *Harrison's principles of internal medicine* (18th ed.). New York: McGraw-Hill.

Gillman, P. K. (2010). Neuroleptic malignant syndrome: mechanisms, interactions and causality, a review. *Move Disord*, *25*(12), 1780–1790.

Hamaya, H., Hifumi, T., Kawakita, K., et al. (2015). Successful management of heat stroke associated with multiple-organ dysfunction by active intravascular cooling. *The American Journal of Emergency Medicine*, *33*, 124e5–124e7.

Hooper, V. D., et al. (2009). ASPAN's evidence-based clinical practice guideline for the promotion of perioperative normothermia. *Journal of Perianesthesia Nursing*, *24*(5), 217–287.

Hopkins, P. M. (2011). Malignant hyperthermia: pharmacology of triggering. *British Journal of Anaesthesia*, *107*(1), 48–56.

Kenney, W. L., et al. (2014). Blood pressure regulation III: what happens when one system must serve two masters: Temperature and pressure regulation? *European Journal of Applied Physiology*, *114*, 467–479.

Kerr, Z. Y., Marshall, S. W., Cornstock, D., et al. (2014). Exertional heat stroke management strategies in United States high school football. *The American Journal of Sports Medicine*, *42*(1), 70–81.

Leon, L. R., & Helwig, B. G. (2010). Heat stroke: role of the systemic inflammatory response. *Journal of Applied Physiology*, *109*, 1980–1988.

Makic, M. B. F., et al. (2011). Evidence-based practice habits: putting more sacred cows out to pasture. *Critical Care Nurse*, *31*, 38–62.

Malignant Hyperthermia Association of the United States (2015). *Website*. <http://www.mhaus.org/>. Retrieved June 3, 2015.

Paden, M. S., Franjic, L., & Halcomb, E. (2013). Hyperthermia caused by drug interactions and adverse reaction. *Emergency Medicine Clinics of North America*, *31*, 1035–1044.

Pinto, S., & Walsh, K. (Dec 23, 2011). *Heart stroke. CINAHL Information Systems*. <http://web.ebscohost.com/ehost/pdfviewer/pdfviewer?sid=40ac8537-a3d4-4e3b-b632-5214cbd9402d%40sessionmgr11&vid=12&hid=21>; Accessed August 5, 2012. (2p).

Pitoni, S., Sinclair, H. L., & Andrews, P. J. D. (2011). Aspects of thermoregulation physiology. *Current Opinion in Critical Care*, *17*, 115–121.

Polderman, K. H., & Herold, I. (2009). Therapeutic hypothermia and controlled normothermia in the intensive care unit: practical considerations, side effects, and cooling methods. *Critical Care Medicine*, *37*(3), 1101–1120.

Pryor, R. R., Casa, D. J., Holschen, J. C., et al. (2013). Exertional heat stroke: strategies for prevention and treatment from the sports field to the emergency department. *Clinical Ped Emergency Medicine*, *14*(4), 267–278.

Sadler, C. (2011). When the heat is on. *Nursing Standard*, *25*(40), 18–20.

Saltzberg, J. M. R. (2013). Fever and signs of shock: the essential dangerous fever. *Emergency Medicine Clinics of North America*, *31*, 907–926.

Seifert, P. C., Wahr, J. A., Pace, M., et al. (2014). Crisis management of malignant hyperthermia in the OR. *AORN Journal*, *100*(2), 189–202.

Stewart, M. W. (2014). Anesthetic drugs and malignant hyperthermia. *Journal of Perianesthesia Nursing*, *29*(3), 253–255.

Takanobu, K., Okazaki, D., Ogawa, T., et al. (2015). Hyperosmolar hyperglycemic state secondary to neuroleptic malignant syndrome. *The American Journal of Emergency Medicine*, *33*, 126e1–126e2.

Thomas, J., & Crowhurst, T. (2013). Exertional heat stroke, rhabdomyolysis and susceptibility to malignant hyperthermia. *Internal Medicine Journal*, 1035–1038.

Trollor, J. N., Chen, X., & Sachdev, P. S. (2009). Neuroleptic malignant syndrome associated with atypical antipsychotic drugs. *CNS Drugs*, *23*(6), 477–492.

H

Hypothermia *Mary Beth Flynn Makic, PhD, RN, CNS, CCNS, FAAN*

NANDA-I

Definition

Core body temperature below normal diurnal range due to failure of thermoregulation

Defining Characteristics

Acrocyanosis; bradycardia; cyanotic nail beds; decrease in blood glucose level; decrease in ventilation; hypertension; hypoglycemia; hypoxia; increase in metabolic rate; increase in oxygen consumption; peripheral vasoconstriction; piloerection; shivering; skin cool to touch; slow capillary refill; tachycardia

Accidental Low Body Temperature in Children and Adults

Mild hypothermia, core temperature approaching 32° C to 35° C; moderate hypothermia, core temperature approaching 30° C to 32° C; severe hypothermia, core temperature < 30° C

Injured Adults and Children

Hypothermia, core temperature < 35° C; severe hypothermia, core temperature < 32° C

Neonates

Grade 1 hypothermia, core temperature 36° C to 36.5° C; grade 2 hypothermia, core temperature 35° C to 35.9° C; grade 3 hypothermia, core temperature 34° C to 34.9° C; grade 4 hypothermia, core temperature < 34° C; infant with insufficient energy to maintain sucking; infant with insufficient weight gain (<30 g/d); irritability; jaundice; metabolic acidosis; pallor; respiratory distress

Related Factors (r/t)

Alcohol consumption; damage to hypothalamus; decrease in metabolic rate; economically disadvantaged; extremes of age; extremes of weight; heat transfer (e.g., conduction, convection, evaporation, radiation); inactivity; insufficient caregiver knowledge of hypothermia prevention; insufficient clothing; insufficient supply of subcutaneous fat; low environmental temperature; malnutrition; pharmaceutical agent; radiation; trauma

Neonates

Delay in breastfeeding; early bathing of newborn; high-risk out-of-hospital birth; immature stratum corneum; increased body surface area to weight ratio; increase in oxygen demand; increase in pulmonary vascular resistance; ineffective vascular control; inefficient nonshivering thermogenesis; unplanned out-of-hospital birth

NOC (Nursing Outcomes Classification)

Suggested NOC Outcomes

Thermoregulation; Thermoregulation: Newborn

Example NOC Outcome with Indicators

Thermoregulation as evidenced by the following indicators: Increased skin temperature/Decreased skin temperature/Skin color changes/Dehydration/Hypothermia. (Rate the outcome and indicators of **Thermoregulation:** 1 = severe, 2 = substantial, 3 = moderate, 4 = mild, 5 = none [see Section I].)

Client Outcomes

Client Will (Specify Time Frame)

- Maintain body temperature within normal range
- Identify risk factors of hypothermia
- State measures to prevent hypothermia
- Identify symptoms of hypothermia and actions to take when hypothermia is present
- If hypothermia is medically induced client/family will state goals for hypothermia treatment

NIC (Nursing Interventions Classification)

Suggested NIC Intervention

Hypothermia Treatment; Temperature Regulation; Temperature Regulation: Intraoperative; Vital Signs Monitoring

Example NIC Activities—Temperature Regulation

Institute use of a continuous core temperature-monitoring device, as appropriate; Promote adequate fluid and nutritional intake

Nursing Interventions and *Rationales*

Temperature Measurement

- Recognize hypothermia as a drop in core body temperature below 35° C (95° F) (Danzl et al, 2011; Turk, 2010).
- Measure the client's temperature at least hourly and with changes in client condition (e.g., chills, change in mental status); if more than mild hypothermia is present (temperature lower than 35° C [95° F]), use a continuous temperature-monitoring device. Two modes of temperature monitoring may be indicated. Continuous temperature monitoring using an indwelling method of temperature measurement is usually indicated to monitor effectiveness of treating body alterations in core body temperature. EBN/CEB: *Hypothermia can be a life-threatening crisis that requires accurate temperature measurement. Core temperature is obtained by a pulmonary artery catheter or from the distal esophagus; near core temperature measurements include oral, bladder, rectal, and temporal artery, and peripheral measurements are obtained*

by skin surface measurements and in the axilla (Barnason et al, 2012). Research is limited on accuracy of temporal artery measurements outside normal ranges; axillary temperature is accurate in neonates but is not well supported in adults; tympanic membrane measurements and chemical dot thermometers are least accurate and should be avoided in caring for the acutely ill adult client (Calonder et al, 2010; Hooper et al, 2009; Makic et al, 2011; Barnason et al, 2012).

- Use the same site and method (device) for temperature measurement for a given client so that temperature trends are assessed accurately and record site of temperature measurement. EBN/CEB: *There are differences in temperature depending on the site (esophageal, oral, bladder, rectal, axillary, or temporal artery); however, differences should not be greater than 0.3°C to 0.5°C (Barnason, 2012; Jefferies et al, 2011; Bridges & Thomas, 2009; Davie & Amoore, 2010; Hooper et al, 2009; Makic et al, 2011; Polderman & Herold, 2009).*
- Bladder temperature may be used as an indwelling urinary catheter and is often inserted in the management of hypothermia to monitor diuresis. CEB: *Bladder temperature probes have been shown to be accurate during states of increased diuresis, but measurements may be less accurate when urine volume is low (low rate of diuresis) (Polderman & Herold, 2009; Wollerich et al, 2012). Temperatures obtained by this method may lag, up to 20 minutes during targeted temperature hypothermia interventions (Polderman & Herold, 2009).*
- See the care plan for Ineffective **Thermoregulation** as appropriate.

H

Accidental Hypothermia

- Recognize that there are three types of accidental hypothermia (environmental causes):
  - Acute hypothermia, also called immersion hypothermia, often from sudden exposure to cold through immersion in cold water or snow
  - Exhaustion hypothermia, caused by exposure to cold in association with lack of food and exhaustion
  - Chronic hypothermia that occurs over days or weeks and primarily affects older adults (Guly, 2011; Petrone, 2014)
- Remove the client from the cause of the hypothermic episode (e.g., cold environment, cold or wet clothing) and bring into a warm environment. Cover the client with warm blankets and apply a covering to the head and neck to conserve body heat. *Layering of dry clothing, including wearing a hat, can be effective in warming a client with mild hypothermia; the goal is also to prevent any further heat loss (Petrone, 2014; Danzl et al, 2011).*
- Watch the client for signs of hypothermia: shivering, slurred speech, confusion, clumsy movements, fatigue, and dehydration. As hypothermia progresses, the skin becomes pale, muscles are tense, fatigue and weakness progress, breathing is decreased, and pulmonary congestion is present, compromising oxygenation; pulses are decreased and blood pressure and heart rate decrease, progressing to lethal arrhythmias (e.g., ventricular fibrillation) (*Danzl et al, 2011; Petrone, 2014*).
- ▲ Administer oxygen as ordered. *Oxygenation is hampered by the change in the oxyhemoglobin curve caused by hypothermia (Danzl et al, 2011).*
- Monitor the client's vital signs every hour and as appropriate. Note changes associated with hypothermia, such as initially increased pulse rate, respiratory rate, and blood pressure as well as diuresis with mild hypothermia, and then decreased pulse rate, respiratory rate, and blood pressure as well as oliguria with moderate to severe hypothermia. *With mild hypothermia, there is activation of the sympathetic nervous system, which can increase the values of vital signs. As hypothermia progresses, decreased circulating volume develops, which results in decreased cardiac output and depressed oxygen delivery. Hypoxia, metabolic acidosis, and intrinsic irritability of a cold myocardium result in dysrhythmias (Danzl et al, 2011; Turk, 2010; Petrone, 2014; Soreide, 2014).*
- ▲ Attach electrodes and a cardiac monitor. Watch for dysrhythmias. *With hypothermia, the client is prone to dysrhythmias because of the cold myocardium; dysrhythmias may include atrial fibrillation, ventricular fibrillation, or asystole (Danzl et al, 2011; Petrone, 2014).*
- ▲ Monitor for signs of coagulopathy (e.g., oozing of blood from any open areas or from intravascular catheter sites or mucous membranes). Also note results of clotting studies as available. *Coagulopathy is a common occurrence during hypothermia (Thorsen et al, 2011; Petrone, 2014; Soreide, 2014).*
- For mild hypothermia (core temperature of 32.2°C to 35°C [90°F to 95°F]), rewarm client passively:
  - Set room temperature to 21°C to 24°C (70°F to 75°F)
  - Keep the client dry; remove any damp or wet clothing

- ❍ Layer clothing and blankets and cover the client's head; use insulated metallic blankets
- ❍ Offer warm fluids; avoid alcohol or caffeine

For mild hypothermia, allow the client to rewarm at his/her own pace. Heat is regained through the body's ability to generate heat (Danzl et al, 2011; Petrone, 2014; Kelly et al, 2013). Passive rewarming is not encouraged for clients with temperatures lower than 32.2° C (90° F) because it is a slow process, requires sufficient glycogen stores to be used by the client's body, and may increase oxygen consumption, increasing the risk of adverse cardiac events (Danzl et al, 2011).

▲ For moderate hypothermia (core temperature 28° C to 32.1° C [82.4° F to 90° F]), use active external rewarming methods. The rewarming rate should not exceed 0.5° C to 1° C (1.8° F) per hour. Methods include the following (Danzl et al, 2011; Galvao et al, 2010):

- ❍ Forced-air warming blankets
- ❍ Circulation of water through external heat exchange pads
- ❍ Radiant heat sources

▲ For severe hypothermia (core temperature below 28° C [82.4° F]), use active core rewarming techniques as ordered (Danzl et al, 2011; Petrone, 2014; Soreide, 2014):

- ❍ Recognize that extracorporeal blood rewarming methods, such as coronary artery bypass, are most effective.
- ❍ Use intravascular countercurrent in-line heat exchange to deliver warmed fluid or blood (Danzl et al, 2011).
- ❍ Use heated and humidified oxygen through the ventilator as ordered.
- ❍ Administer heated intravenous (IV) fluids at prescribed temperature.
- ❍ Use heated irrigation of the gastrointestinal tract (nasogastric lavage) or bladder irrigations as ordered.

- • Rewarm clients slowly, generally at a rate of 0.5° C to 1° C every hour. *Slow rewarming helps prevent a phenomenon called "afterdrop," wherein cold, hyperkalemic blood from the periphery returns to the heart, resulting in a biochemical injury, leading to dysrhythmias and severe hypotension (Danzl et al, 2011).*
- • Check blood pressure frequently when rewarming; watch for hypotension. *As the body warms, formerly vasoconstricted vessels dilate, which results in hypotension (Kelly et al, 2013; Petrone, 2014).*
- ▲ Administer IV fluids, using a rapid infuser IV fluid warmer as ordered. *Fluids are often needed to maintain adequate fluid volume. If the client develops untreated fluid depletion, hypotension with decreased cardiac output and acute renal failure can result. A rapid infuser warmer is needed to keep IV fluids warmed sufficiently to be effective in raising the body temperature (Danzl et al, 2011).*
- • Determine the factors leading to the hypothermic episode; see Related Factors. *It is important to assess risk factors and precipitating events to prevent another incident of hypothermia and to direct treatment (Guly, 2011).*
- ▲ Request a social service referral to help the client obtain the heat, shelter, and food needed to maintain body temperature. *A preventive approach that includes adequate food and fluid intake, shelter, heat, and clothing decreases the risk of hypothermia.*
- ▲ Encourage proper nutrition and hydration. *Request a referral to a dietitian to identify appropriate dietary needs. Insufficient calorie and fluid intake predisposes the client to hypothermia, especially in older adults (Danzl et al, 2011).*

Targeted Temperature Hypothermia

- • Recognize that targeted temperature management, also called therapeutic hypothermia, is the active lowering of the client's body temperature, in a controlled manner, to preserve neurological function after an acute myocardial injury or cardiac arrest. CEB: *In the event the client is successfully resuscitated after an acute myocardial injury/arrest, recognize that medically induced targeted temperature management has been shown to provide neurological protection against ischemic neuronal injury after cardiac arrest (Scirica, 2013; Bravo & Kim, 2014; Kim et al, 2015).*
- • Recognize that controlled cooling of clients should be considered for all unconscious survivors of out-of-hospital ventricular tachycardia arrest as well as clients experiencing in-hospital arrests (Neumer et al, 2011; Scirica, 2013; Kim et al, 2015). The optimal targeted temperature for therapy is between 34° and 36° C for up to 48 hours (Azmoon et al, 2011; Neumer et al, 2011; Scirica, 2013; Bravo & Kim, 2014). CEB: *The American Heart Association and the International Liaison Committee on Resuscitation have included therapeutic hypothermia as an intervention to be considered in the management of cardiac arrest patients to optimize neurological outcomes (Neumer et al, 2011; Scirica, 2013).*

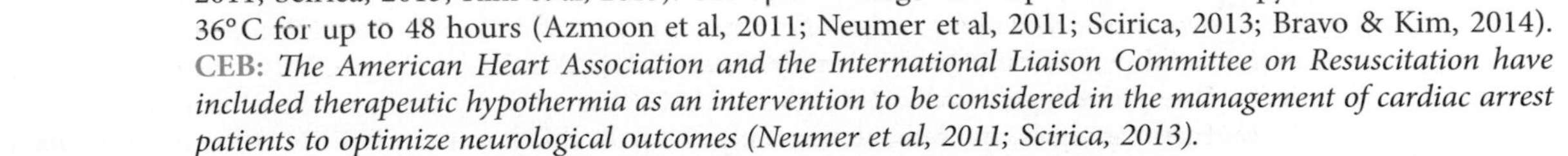

- Monitor core or near core temperatures continuously using two methods of temperature monitoring. CEB: *To ensure that the targeted temperature is achieved and maintained closely within the prescribed temperature range, two methods of core or near core temperature monitoring are recommended (Polderman & Herold, 2009; Barnason et al, 2012).*
- Recognize that cooling may be achieved noninvasively, using fluid-filled cooling devices that are placed next to the client's skin, or invasively, infusing iced solution. EB/EBN: *Invasive cooling provides a more predictable cooling; however, current research has found air- or fluid-filled external devices to provide effective cooling as well. Less optimal methods of cooling include the use of fans, ice packs, or blankets, which do not provide temperature regulation feedback between the machine and client (Galvao et al, 2010; Morita et al, 2011).*
- Obtain vital signs hourly (or via continuous monitoring) to include continuous electrocardiogram monitoring. Observe for signs of hypotension, bradycardia, and arrhythmias. Mechanical ventilation is required to protect the client's airway and breathing during treatment. CEB: *Diuresis is more pronounced during the induction of hypothermia. Hypotension may be more prominent as the client is rewarmed because of vasodilatation, requiring close monitoring and interventions to support blood pressure. Bradycardia associated with hypothermia is often not responsive to atropine. If the client is overcooled (temperature drops below 32° C), the risk of arrhythmias will increase; ventricular fibrillation refractory to defibrillation may occur at temperatures below 30° C (Polderman & Herold, 2009).*

▲ Observe for shivering and administer sedation agents as prescribed. CEB: *Shivering significantly increases the body's metabolic rate and oxygen consumption (Polderman & Herold, 2009).*

▲ Closely inspect the skin before and throughout the cooling intervention to prevent skin breakdown associated with the treatment. Implement frequent turning and other pressure reduction interventions as indicated. *Lowering the body temperature causes vasoconstriction and can compromise perfusion to the skin, increasing the client's risk of skin breakdown (Polderman & Herold, 2009).*

▲ Monitor and treat serum electrolytes (e.g., potassium, magnesium, calcium, and phosphorus) and serum glucose closely during targeted hypothermia and during rewarming of the client. Electrolytes will fluctuate as the client is rewarmed. EB/EBN: *Diuresis, acid-base imbalances, and metabolic responses are responsible for fluctuations of electrolytes and glucose. As the client is rewarmed, electrolyte replacements, especially potassium replacements, should be closely monitored to prevent rebound hyperkalemia that may occur as the body temperature rises (Polderman & Herold, 2009; Turk, 2010; Petrone, 2014).*

▲ Observe for signs and symptoms of coagulopathy during targeted hypothermia treatment. Hemoconcentration may be noticed as fluids shift during treatment. CEB: *For every 1° C decline in temperature, the hematocrit may increase by approximately 2%, requiring monitoring but not treatment. Platelet counts decrease during hypothermic states, but research has not found a significant risk of bleeding during targeted hypothermia treatment (Polderman & Herold, 2009; Thorsen et al, 2011; Turk, 2010; Petrone, 2014).*

- Rewarming should occur in a controlled manner with a rise in body temperature of 0.5° C to 1° C per hour and targeted goal of normothermia, 37° C. CEB: *Aggressive rewarming may cause rebound hyperthermia, cerebral edema, seizures, hypotension, and ventricular fibrillation (Niklasch, 2010; Polderman & Herold, 2009; Bravo & Kim, 2014; Kim et al, 2015).*

▲ Neurological and cognitive function should be assessed during targeted temperature treatment and after rewarming. CEB: *The goal of targeted temperature treatment is neurological protection; close monitoring of neurological function after intervention and serial assessments are indicated (Nunnally et al, 2011; Polderman & Herold, 2009; Scirica, 2013).*

Pediatric

- Recognize that pediatric clients have a decreased ability to adapt to temperature extremes. Take the following actions to maintain body temperature in the infant/child:
  - Keep the head covered.
  - Use blankets to keep the client warm.
  - Keep the client covered during procedures, transport, and diagnostic testing.
  - Keep the room temperature at 22.2° C (72° F).

The combination of a relatively smaller body surface area, smaller body fluid volume, less well-developed temperature control mechanisms, and smaller amount of protective body fat limits the infant's and child's ability to maintain normal temperatures (Pio et al, 2010; Wyckoff, 2014).

▲ For the preterm or low-birth-weight newborn, use specially designed bags, skin-to-skin care, transwarmer mattresses, and radiant warmers to keep the infant warm. EB/EBN: *These methods can help keep the vulnerable newborn warm in the delivery room (McCall et al, 2010). Parents should be taught how to wrap neonates/infants to maintain body temperature (Bissinger & Annibale, 2010), yet there is a need for more studies in this area (McCall et al, 2010).*

▲ Targeted hypothermia may be implemented in the treatment of neonates with hypoxic-ischemic encephalopathy. *Passive cooling may be achieved by withholding external heat sources and requires frequent monitoring of the neonate's temperature to prevent severe hypothermia (Wyckoff, 2014; Sussman & Weiss, 2013).*

Geriatric

- Normal aging often includes changes in touch-related sensations, making it harder to differentiate cool and cold. *Decreased temperature sensitivity increases the risk of hypothermia in the older adult (Dugdale, 2012).*
- Recognize that older adults can develop indoor hypothermia from air conditioning or ice baths. *Clients present with vague complaints of mental and/or other skill deterioration (Heller, 2012).*
- Assess neurological signs frequently, watching for confusion and decreased level of consciousness. CEB: *Mechanisms to control body temperature decrease with age; coupled with a slower counterregulatory response, lower rate of metabolism, and less effective vascular response, this will make hypothermia less obvious. Early signs of hypothermia are subtle (Danzl et al, 2011).*
- Recognize that older adults often wear socks and sweaters to protect themselves from feeling cold, even in warmer weather (Sadler, 2011).

H

Home Care

Hypothermia is not a symptom that appears in the normal course of home care. When it occurs, it is a clinical emergency, and the client/family should access emergency medical services immediately.

- Some of the interventions described earlier may be adapted for home care use.
- Before a medical crisis occurs, confirm that the client or family has a thermometer and can read it. Instruct as needed. Verify that the thermometer registers accurately.
- Instruct the client or family to take the temperature when the client displays cyanosis, pallor, or shivering.

▲ Monitor temperature every hour, as noted previously. If the temperature of the client begins dropping below the normal range, apply layers of clothing or blankets, or adjust environmental heat to the comfort level. Do not overheat. Contact a health care provider. *Passive rewarming is the only method of rewarming that is appropriate for home care under normal circumstances.*

▲ If temperature continues to drop, activate the emergency system and notify a health care provider. *Hypothermia is a clinically acute condition that cannot be managed safely in the home.*

▲ If the client is in hospice care or is terminally ill, follow advance directives, client wishes, and the health care provider's orders. Keep the client free of pain. *The goal of terminal care is to provide dignity and comfort during the dying process.*

Client/Family Teaching and Discharge Planning

- Teach the client and family signs of hypothermia and the method of taking the temperature (age appropriate).
- Teach the client methods to prevent hypothermia: wearing adequate clothing, including a hat and mittens; heating the environment to a minimum of 20° C (68° F); and ingesting adequate food and fluid. *Simple measures such as layering clothes, wearing a hat, and avoiding extremes in temperature prevent significant heat loss (Petrone, 2014).*

▲ Teach the client and family about medications such as sedatives, opioids, and anxiolytics that predispose the client to hypothermia (as appropriate). *If the client has had hypothermia in the past, using alternative medications is an option if there is no contraindication (Danzl et al, 2011).*

REFERENCES

Azmoon, S., et al. (2011). Neurological and cardiac benefits of therapeutic hypothermia. *Cardiology in Review, 19*(3), 108–114.

Barnason, S., et al. (2012). Emergency nursing resource: non-invasive temperature measurement in the emergency department. *Journal of Emergency Nursing, 38*, 523–530.

Bissinger, R. L., & Annibale, D. J. (2010). Thermoregulation in very low birth weight infants during the golden hour. *Advances in Neonatal Care, 10*(5), 230–240.

Bravo, P. E., & Kim, F. (2014). Enhancing approaches to therapeutic hypothermia in patients with sudden circulatory arrest. *Current Atherosclerosis Reports, 16*, 451–456.

Bridges, E., & Thomas, K. (2009). Noninvasive measurement of body temperature in critically ill patients. *Critical Care Nurse, 29*(3), 94–97.
Calonder, E. M., et al. (2010). Temperature measurement in patients undergoing colorectal surgery and gynecology surgery: a comparison of esophageal core, temporal artery, and oral methods. *Journal of Perianesthesia Nursing, 25*(2), 71–78.
Danzl, D. F., et al. (2011). Hypothermia and frostbite. In A. S. Fauci (Ed.), *Harrison's principles of internal medicine* (18th ed.). New York: McGraw-Hill.
Davie, A., & Amoore, J. (2010). Best practice in the measurement of body temperature. *Nursing Standard, 24*(42), 42–50.
Dugdale, D. C. (2012). *Aging changes in the senses. In MedlinePlus medical encyclopedia, U.S. National Library of Medicine.* From: <http://www.nlm.nih.gov/medlineplus/ency/article/004013.htm>. Retrieved June 9, 2015.
Galvao, C. M., Liang, Y., & Clark, A. M. (2010). Effectiveness of cutaneous warming systems on temperature control: meta-analysis. *Journal of Advanced Nursing, 66*(6), 1196–1206.
Guly, H. (2011). History of accidental hypothermia. *Resuscitation, 82*(2), 122–125.
Heller, J. L. *Hypothermia. In MedlinePlus medical encyclopedia, U.S. National Library of Medicine.* From: <http://www.nlm.nih.gov/medlineplus/ency/article/000038.htm>. Retrieved September 4, 2012.
Hooper, V. D., et al. (2009). ASPAN's evidence-based clinical practice guideline for the promotion of perioperative normothermia. *Journal of Perianesthesia Nursing, 24*(5), 217–287.
Jefferies, S., et al. (2011). A systematic review of the accuracy of peripheral thermometry in estimating core temperatures among febrile critically ill patients. *Critical Care and Resuscitation: Journal of the Australasian Academy of Critical Care Medicine, 13*, 194–199.
Kelly, P. A., Cooper, S. K., Krogh, M. L., et al. (2013). Thermal comfort and safety of cotton blankets warmed at 130°F and 200°F. *Journal of Perianesthesia Nursing, 28*(6), 337–346.
Kim, F., Bravo, P. E., & Nichol, G. (2015). What is the use of hypothermia for neuroprotection after out-of-hospital cardiac arrest? *Stroke; a Journal of Cerebral Circulation, 46*, 592–597.
Makic, M. B. F., et al. (2011). Evidence-based practice habits: putting more sacred cows out to pasture. *Critical Care Nurse, 31*, 38–62.
McCall, E. M., et al. (2010). Interventions to prevent hypothermia at birth in preterm and/or low birth weight infants. *Cochrane Database of Systematic Reviews*, (3), CD004210.
Morita, S., et al. (2011). Efficacy of portable and percutaneous cardiopulmonary bypass rewarming versus that of conventional internal rewarming for patients with accidental deep hypothermia. *Critical Care Medicine, 39*(5), 1064–1068.
Neumer, R. W., et al. (2011). Implementation strategies for improving survival after out-of-hospital cardiac arrest in the United States. *Circulation, 123*, 2898–2911.
Niklasch, D. M. (2010). Induced mild hypothermia and the prevention of neurological injury. *Journal of Infusion Nursing, 33*(4), 236–242.
Nunnally, M. E., et al. (2011). Target temperature management in critical care: a report and recommendations from five professional societies. *Critical Care Medicine, 39*(5), 1113–1125.
Petrone, P. (2014). Management of accidental hypothermia and cold injury. *Current Problems in Surgery, 51*(10), 417–431.
Pio, A., Kirkwood, B. R., & Gove, S. (2010). Avoiding hypothermia and intervention to prevent morbidity and mortality from pneumonia in young children. *The Pediatric Infectious Disease Journal, 29*(2), 153–159.
Polderman, K. H., & Herold, I. (2009). Therapeutic hypothermia and controlled normothermia in the intensive care unit: practical considerations, side effects and cooling methods. *Critical Care Medicine, 37*(3), 1101–1120.
Sadler, C. (2011). When the heat is on. *Nursing Standard, 25*(40), 18–20.
Scirica, B. M. (2013). Therapeutic hypothermia after cardiac arrest. *Circulation, 127*, 244–250.
Soreide, K. (2014). Clinical and translational aspects of hypothermia in major trauma patients: from pathophysiology to prevention, prognosis and potential preservation. *Injury, 45*, 647–654.
Sussman, C. B., & Weiss, M. D. (2013). While waiting: early recognition and initial management of neonatal hypoxic ischemic encephalopathy. *Advances in Neonatal Care, 13*(6), 415–423.
Thorsen, K., et al. (2011). Clinical and cellular effects of hypothermia, acidosis and coagulopathy in major injury. *The British Journal of Surgery, 98*, 894–907.
Turk, E. E. (2010). Hypothermia. *Forensic Sci Med Pathol, 6*, 106–115.
Wollerich, H., Ismael, F., Nijsten, M. W., et al. (2012). Comparison of temperature measurements in bladder, rectum and pulmonary artery in patients after cardiac surgery. *Journal of Nursing, 2*, 307–310.
Wyckoff, M. H. (2014). Initial resuscitation and stabilization of the periviable neonate: The golden-hour approach. *Seminars in Perinatology, 38*, 12–16.

Risk for Hypothermia *Mary Beth Flynn Makic, PhD, RN, CNS, CCNS, FAAN*

NANDA-I

Definition

Vulnerable to a failure of thermoregulation that may result in a core body temperature below the normal diurnal range, which may compromise health

Risk Factors

Alcohol consumption; damage to hypothalamus; economically disadvantaged; extremes of age; extremes of weight; heat transfer (e.g., conduction, convection, evaporation, radiation); inactivity; insufficient caregiver knowledge of hypothermia prevention; insufficient clothing; insufficient supply of subcutaneous fat; low environmental temperature; malnutrition; pharmaceutical agent; radiation; trauma

Children and Adults: Accidental

Mild hypothermia, core temperature approaching 35° C; moderate hypothermia, core temperature approaching 32° C; severe hypothermia, core temperature approaching 30° C

Neonates

Decrease in metabolic rate; delay in breastfeeding; early bathing of newborn; grade 1 hypothermia, core temperature approaching 36.5° C; grade 2 hypothermia, core temperature approaching 36° C; grade 3 hypothermia, core temperature approaching 35° C; grade 4 hypothermia, core temperature approaching 34° C; high-risk out-of-hospital birth; immature stratum corneum; increased body surface area to weight ratio; increase in oxygen demand; increase in pulmonary vascular resistance; ineffective vascular control; inefficient nonshivering thermogenesis; unplanned out-of-hospital birth

NIC, NOC, Client Outcomes, Nursing Interventions, Client/Family Teaching and Discharge Planning, *Rationales,* and References

Refer to care plan for **Hypothermia.**

H

Risk for Perioperative Hypothermia

Mary Beth Flynn Makic, PhD, RN, CNS, CCNS, FAAN

NANDA-I

Definition

Vulnerable to an inadvertent drop in core body temperature below 36° C (96.8° F) occurring 1 hour before to 24 hours after surgery, which may compromise health

Risk Factors

American Society of Anesthesiologist (ASA) Physical Status classification score > 1; cardiovascular complications; combined regional and general anesthesia; diabetic neuropathy; heat transfer (e.g., high volume of unwarmed infusion, unwarmed irrigation > 20 L); low body weight; low environmental temperature; low preoperative temperature (<36° C [96.8° F]); surgical procedure

NOC (Nursing Outcomes Classification)

Suggested NOC Outcomes

Thermoregulation

Example NOC Outcome with Indicators

Thermoregulation as evidenced by the following indicators: Increased skin temperature/Decreased skin temperature/Skin color changes/Dehydration/Hypothermia. (Rate the outcome and indicators of **Thermoregulation:** 1 = severe, 2 = substantial, 3 = moderate, 4 = mild, 5 = none [see Section I].)

Client Outcomes

Client Will (Specify Time Frame)

- Maintain body temperature within normal range
- Identify risk factors of hypothermia
- State measures to prevent hypothermia
- Identify symptoms of hypothermia and actions to take when hypothermia is present
- Client will be free of surgical site infection

NIC (Nursing Interventions Classification)

Suggested NIC Interventions

Hypothermia Treatment; Temperature Regulation; Temperature Regulation: Intraoperative; Vital Signs Monitoring

Example NIC Activities—Temperature Regulation

Institute use of a continuous core temperature-monitoring device, as appropriate; Promote adequate fluid and nutritional intake

Nursing Interventions and *Rationales*

Temperature Measurement

- Recognize perioperative hypothermia as a drop in core body temperature below 36° C (96.8° F) (Campbell et al, 2015; CDC, 2015).
- Measure the client's temperature frequently, and with changes in client condition (e.g., chills, change in mental status); if more than mild hypothermia is present (temperature lower than 36° C [96.85° F]), use a continuous temperature-monitoring device. Two modes of temperature monitoring may be indicated. Continuous temperature monitoring using an indwelling method of temperature measurement is usually indicated to monitor effectiveness of treating body alterations in core body temperature. CEB/EBN/CEB: *Hypothermia can be a life-threatening crisis that requires accurate temperature measurement. Core temperature is obtained by a pulmonary artery catheter or from the distal esophagus; near core temperature measurements include oral, bladder, rectal, and temporal artery, and peripheral measurements are obtained by skin surface measurements and in the axilla (Barnason et al, 2012). Research is limited on accuracy of temporal artery measurements outside normal ranges; axillary temperature is accurate in neonates but is not well supported in adults; tympanic membrane measurements and chemical dot thermometers are least accurate and should be avoided in caring for the acutely ill adult client (Winslow et al, 2012; Calonder et al, 2010; Hooper et al, 2009; Makic et al, 2011; Barnason et al, 2012).*
- Use the same site and method (device) for temperature measurement for a given client so that temperature trends are assessed accurately, and record site of temperature measurement. EBN/CEB: *There are differences in temperature depending on the site (esophageal, oral, bladder, rectal, axillary, or temporal artery); however, differences should not be greater than 0.3°C to 0.5°C (Barnason et al, 2012; Jefferies et al, 2011; Bridges & Thomas, 2009; Davie & Amoore, 2010; Hooper et al, 2009; Makic et al, 2011).*
- Bladder temperature may be used as an indwelling urinary catheter and is often inserted in the management of hypothermia to monitor diuresis. CEB: *Bladder temperature probes have been shown to be accurate during states of increased diuresis, but measurements may be less accurate when urine volume is low (low rate of diuresis). Temperatures obtained by this method may lag, up to 20 minutes during targeted temperature hypothermia interventions (Wollerich et al, 2012).*

Unintentional Perioperative Hypothermia

- Keep the client warm throughout the perioperative period (preoperative, intraoperatively, and postoperatively) to prevent unintentional perioperative hypothermia. CEB: *Initiating warming interventions preoperatively has been found to assist with normothermia and client comfort (Burns et al, 2009; Horosz & Malec-Milewska, 2014).*
- *Factors that increase the risk of perioperative hypothermia include anesthetic agents, ambient room air temperature, intravenous (IV) fluid infusion, and cavity solution irrigation, blood product administration, duration and type of surgical procedure, anemia, extremes of ages, neurologic disorders, cachexia; preexisting conditions (e.g., peripheral vascular disease, endocrine disease, pregnancy, burns, open wounds) (Billeter et al, 2014; ASPAN, 2015).*
- Closely monitoring and preventing unintentional perioperative hypothermia is necessary to prevent adverse patient outcomes. CEB: *Adverse outcomes include client discomfort, shivering, cardiac events (e.g., arrhythmias), increased catecholamine release, impaired coagulation, altered drug metabolism, impaired wound healing, and impaired immune function (ASPAN, 2015; Kuchena et al, 2014; Horosz & Malec-Milewska, 2014; Winslow et al, 2012).*
- Several interventions should be implemented to prevent unintentional perioperative hypothermia:
  - Use warming and booties perioperatively
  - Use warming blankets over and under the client perioperatively
  - Use warming blankets under the client on the operating table
  - Adjust environmental room controls to prevent cool ambient room temperature in the perioperative and operative rooms
  - Use warmed forced-air blankets preoperatively, during surgery, and in the postanesthesia care unit

- ❍ Use warmed IV fluids and irrigation solutions
- ❍ Designate responsibility and accountability for thermoregulation

▲ EB: *Maintaining the client's temperature during the surgical procedure has been found to be essential in preventing surgical complications, especially surgical site infections. Maintaining normothermia also enhances client comfort (ASPAN, 2015; IHI, 2012a; CDC, 2015). One study found that clients who experienced unintentional perioperative hypothermia during elective operations experienced a four-fold increase in mortality and stroke (Billeter et al, 2014).*

- Using warmed IV fluids and irrigation solutions during the operative period may assist with reducing the client's risk of unintentional perioperative hypothermia. CEB: *Researchers found that warmed IV fluids and irrigation solutions kept the core temperature of study participants warmer than those in clients receiving room temperature fluids (Campbell et al, 2015).*
- Active warming interventions include the use of warm blankets and forced air warming devices. EBN: *Blankets used for warming client's quickly lose heat. To prevent rapid heat loss from blankets, warming cabinets should be set at 200°F, and reapply blankets frequently (Kelly et al, 2013).* CEB: *Actively warming clients with forced air warming offers a clinically important reduction in time to achieve normothermia in postoperative clients (Warttig et al, 2014).*
- Watch the client for signs of hypothermia: shivering, slurred speech, confusion, clumsy movements, fatigue, dehydration. As hypothermia progresses, the skin becomes pale, muscles are tense, fatigue and weakness progress, breathing is decreased, and pulmonary congestion is present, compromising oxygenation; pulses are decreased and blood pressure and heart rate decrease, progressing to lethal arrhythmias (e.g., ventricular fibrillation) (Danzl, 2012; Petrone, 2014).

▲ Administer oxygen as ordered. *Oxygenation is hampered by the change in the oxyhemoglobin curve caused by hypothermia (Danzl, 2012).*

▲ Attach electrodes and a cardiac monitor. Watch for dysrhythmias. *With hypothermia, the client is prone to dysrhythmias because of the cold myocardium; dysrhythmias may include atrial fibrillation, ventricular fibrillation, or asystole (Danzl, 2012; Petrone, 2014).*

▲ Monitor for signs of coagulopathy (e.g., oozing of blood from any open areas or from intravascular catheter sites or mucous membranes). Also note results of clotting studies as available. *Coagulopathy is a common occurrence during hypothermia (ASPAN, 2015; Petrone, 2014; Soreide, 2014).*

▲ Monitor for signs of surgical site infection (e.g., increased incisional pain, drainage, poor healing, poor incision approximation). *Unintentional perioperative hypothermia has been associated with increased risk of surgical site infections (CDC, 2015; IHI, 2012a; ASPAN, 2015).*

- See care plan for Ineffective **Thermoregulation** and **Hypothermia** as appropriate.

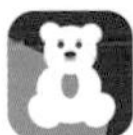

Pediatric

- Interventions implemented in the care of adult clients are similar when providing care to pediatric clients to prevent hypothermia. CEB: *Keep the head covered, use warm blankets or force warm air to keep the client warm; maintain normal ambient room temperature in the perioperative units, and use warmed IV fluids (IHI, 2012b).*

Home Care

▲ Hypothermia is not a symptom that appears in the normal course of postoperative home care. If the client continues to complain of chills or feeling cold after discharge home from a surgical procedure, provide the client with warm blankets and if the client is allowed to drink provide warm fluids by mouth.

▲ Monitor temperature every hour, as noted previously. If the temperature of the client begins dropping below the normal range, apply layers of clothing or blankets, or adjust environmental heat to the comfort level. Do not overheat. Contact a health care provider. *Passive rewarming is the only method of rewarming that is appropriate for home care under normal circumstances.*

▲ If temperature continues to drop, activate the emergency system and notify a health care provider. *Hypothermia is a clinically acute condition that cannot be managed safely in the home.*

Client/Family Teaching and Discharge Planning

- Teach the client/family signs of hypothermia and the method of taking the temperature (age-appropriate).

▲ Teach the client and family about medications such as sedatives, opioids, and anxiolytics that predispose the client to hypothermia (as appropriate). *If the client has had hypothermia in the past, using alternative medications is an option if there is no contraindication (Danzl, 2012).*

REFERENCES

American Society of PeriAnesthesia Nurses (ASPAN) (2015). *Normothermia clinical guideline.* <http://www.aspan.org/Clinical-Practice/Clinical-Guidelines/Normothermia>. Retrieved June 9, 2015.

Barnason, S., et al. (2012). Emergency nursing resource: non-invasive temperature measurement in the emergency department. *Journal of Emergency Nursing, 38,* 523–530.

Billeter, A. T., Hohmann, S. F., Dren, D., et al. (2014). Unintentional perioperative hypothermia is associated with severe complications and high mortality in elective operations. *Surgery, 156,* 1245–1252.

Bridges, E., & Thomas, K. (2009). Noninvasive measurement of body temperature in critically ill patients. *Critical Care Nurse, 29*(3), 94–97.

Burns, S. M., Wojnakowski, M., Pioirowski, K., et al. (2009). Unintentional hypothermia: implications for perianesthesia nurses. *Journal of Perianesthesia Nursing, 24*(5), 167–176.

Calonder, E. M., et al. (2010). Temperature measurement in patients undergoing colorectal surgery and gynecology surgery: a comparison of esophageal core, temporal artery, and oral methods. *Journal of Perianesthesia Nursing, 25*(2), 71–78.

Campbell, G., Alderson, P., Smith, A. F., et al. (2015). Warming of intravenous and irrigation fluids for preventing inadvertent perioperative hypothermia (Review). *The Cochrane Collaboration,* (4), CD009891.

Centers for Disease Control (2015). *Surgical Site Infection Event.* <http://www.cdc.gov/nhsn/PDFs/pscManual/9pscSSIcurrent.pdf>. Retrieved June 9, 2015.

Danzl, D. F. (2012). Hypothermia and frostbite. In A. S. Fauci (Ed.), *Harrison's principles of internal medicine* (18th ed.). New York: McGraw-Hill.

Davie, A., & Amoore, J. (2010). Best practice in the measurement of body temperature. *Nursing Standard, 24*(42), 42–50.

Hooper, V. D., et al. (2009). ASPAN's evidence-based clinical practice guideline for the promotion of perioperative normothermia. *Journal of Perianesthesia Nursing, 24*(5), 217–287.

Horosz, B., & Malec-Milewska, M. M. (2014). Methods to prevent intraoperative hypothermia. *Anaesthesiology Intensive Therapy, 46*(2), 96–100.

Institute for Healthcare Improvement (2012a). *How-to-Guide: Prevent Surgical Site Infections.* Cambridge, MA: Institute for Healthcare Improvement. Available at: <www.ihi.org>. Retrieved June 9, 2015.

Institute for Healthcare Improvement (2012b). *How-to Guide: Prevent Surgical Site Infections, Pediatric Supplement.* Cambridge, MA: Institute for Healthcare Improvement. Available at: <www.ihi.org>. Retrieved June 9, 2015.

Jefferies, S., et al. (2011). A systematic review of the accuracy of peripheral thermometry in estimating core temperatures among febrile critically ill patients. *Critical Care and Resuscitation: Journal of the Australasian Academy of Critical Care Medicine, 13,* 194–199.

Kelly, P. A., Cooper, S. K., Krogh, M. L., et al. (2013). Thermal comfort and safety of cotton blankets warmed at 130^{0}F and 200^{0}F. *Journal of Perianesthesia Nursing, 28*(6), 337–346.

Kuchena, A., Merkel, M. J., & Hutches, M. P. (2014). Postcardiac arrest temperature management: infectious risks. *Current Opinion in Critical Care, 20,* 507–515.

Makic, M. B. F., et al. (2011). Evidence-based practice habits: putting more sacred cows out to pasture. *Critical Care Nurse, 31,* 38–62.

Petrone, P. (2014). Management of accidental hypothermia and cold injury. *Current Problems in Surgery, 51*(10), 417–431.

Soreide, K. (2014). Clinical and translational aspects of hypothermia in major trauma patients: from pathophysiology to prevention, prognosis and potential preservation. *Injury, 45,* 647–654.

Warttig, S., Alderson, P., Campbell, G., et al. (2014). Interventions for treating inadvertent postoperative hypothermia (Review). *The Cochrane Collaboration,* (11), CD009892.

Winslow, E. H., Cooper, S. K., Hawas, D. M., et al. (2012). Unplanned perioperative hypothermia and agreement between oral, temporal artery, and bladder temperatures in adult major surgery patients. *Journal of Perianesthesia Nursing, 27*(3), 165–180.

Wollerich, H., Ismael, F., Nijsten, M. W., et al. (2012). Comparison of temperature measurements in bladder, rectum and pulmonary artery in patients after cardiac surgery. *Journal of Nursing, 2,* 307–310.

Disturbed personal Identity

Gail B. Ladwig, MSN, RN; revised by Ruth A. Wittmann-Price, PhD, RN, CNS, CNE, CHSE, ANEF, FAAN

NANDA-I

Definition

Inability to maintain an integrated and complete perception of self

Defining Characteristics

Alteration in body image; confusion about cultural values; confusion about goals; confusion about ideological values; delusional description of self; feeling of emptiness; feeling of strangeness; fluctuating feelings about self; gender confusion; inability to distinguish between internal and external stimuli; inconsistent behavior; ineffective coping strategies; ineffective relationships; ineffective role performance

Related Factors

Alteration in social role; cult indoctrination; cultural incongruence; developmental transition; discrimination; dissociative identity disorder; dysfunctional family processes; exposure to toxic chemical; low self-esteem; manic states; organic brain disorder; perceived prejudice; pharmaceutical agent; psychiatric disorder; situational crisis; stages of growth

NOC (Nursing Outcomes Classification)

Suggested NOC Outcomes

Anxiety Self-Control; Abuse Recovery (Emotional, physical, sexual); Body Image; Decision-Making; Distorted Thought Self-Control; Identity; Mutilation; Suicide/Self-Restraint

Example NOC Outcome with Indicators

Identity as evidenced by the following indicators: Verbalizes affirmations of personal identity/Exhibits congruent verbal and nonverbal behavior about self/Differentiates self from environment and other human beings. (Rate the outcome and indicators of **Identity:** 1 = never demonstrated, 2 = rarely demonstrated, 3 = sometimes demonstrated, 4 = often demonstrated, 5 = consistently demonstrated [see Section I].)

Client Outcomes

Client Will (Specify Time Frame)

- Demonstrate new purposes for life
- Show interests in surroundings
- Perform self-care and self-control activities appropriate for age
- Acknowledge personal strengths
- Engage in interpersonal relationships

NIC (Nursing Interventions Classification)

Suggested NIC Interventions

Decision-Making Support; Mutual Goal Setting; Self-Awareness Enhancement; Self-Esteem Enhancement; Sexual Counseling; Substance Use Prevention

Example NIC Activities—Self-Esteem Enhancement

Monitor client's statements of self-worth; Encourage client to identify strengths

Nursing Interventions and *Rationales*

- Assess and support family strengths of commitment, appreciation, and affection toward each other, positive communication, time together, a sense of spiritual well-being, and the ability to cope with stress and crisis. EB: *Mayberry et al (2015) studied family behaviors, depression, stress, and adherence for clients (N = 192) with type 2 diabetes and found that obstructive family behaviors were associated with depressive symptoms and nonadherence to treatments.* EBN: *An investigation of the effects of a Family-to-Family Support (FFS) program on the coping strategies and mental health status of caregivers (N = 46) of schizophrenia clients was conducted by Bademli and Duman (2014), who found that the FFS program has a positive impact on caregivers' self-confidence, optimism, and ability to reach out to social supports, thereby increasing their coping strategies.*

▲ Assess for suicidal ideation and make appropriate referral for clients dealing with diversity, mental, or chronic somatic illness. EB: *Finley et al (2015) studied the association of post-traumatic stress disorder, traumatic brain injury, and chronic pain with suicide-related behavior among veteran clients (N = 211,652) and found these conditions significantly increased suicide ideation risk and/or attempts.* EB: *Researchers studied the correlation of adolescent clients' (N = 75,344) gender, sexual orientation, and risk of bullying to suicide ideation and concluded that white and Hispanic gay and bisexual males, white lesbian and bisexual females, and Hispanic bisexual females were at increased risk for being bullied and the sexual minority groups had increased reports of suicide ideation (Mueller et al, 2015).*

- ▲ Assess clients with mood disorders and make appropriate referrals for treatment. EB: *DeLas Cuevas et al (2014) studied clients (N = 160) with depression and their adherence to antidepressant therapy and found that sociodemographic variables did not affect adherence but adherence was related to a positive attitude toward his/her treatment.* EB: *A large, national study found that 50% of clients with eating disorders also suffered from mood or anxiety disorders, but reported to health care professionals fewer symptoms than clients who suffered from mood or anxiety disorders without eating disorders (Meng & D'Arcy, 2015).*
- ▲ Assess and make appropriate referrals for clients with physical or mental disabilities. EB: *Bogart (2014) studied "disability identity" and its relationship to depression and anxiety in clients (N = 106) with multiple sclerosis and found through an Internet survey that "disability identity" predicted lower depression and anxiety.* EB: *An investigation explored self-identity in clients (N = 15) with mental health issues using in-depth interview sessions, which revealed three main themes about employment: (1) they did not like protective work settings, (2) relationships with others in the workplace are important, and (3) they experienced a change in self-identity and were not defined by their mental health problems but as a person who had worth and abilities (Baum & Neuberger, 2014).*
- ▲ Assess clients for substance abuse and make appropriate referral. EB: *Beckwith et al (2015) studied the social identity of addicted clients who were in a therapeutic community (TC) and found that clients who identified with the TC social group and less with the "outside" user group had a more successful recovery.* EB: *A study examined the efficacy of social identity targeting to increase anti-cigarette smoking beliefs among clients (N = 251). Morgan and Sussman (2014) used an online survey to categorize clients' social identity. Using specific anti-smoking ads, they found that social identity targeting increased the effectiveness of smoking cessation.*
- • Use empathetic communication and encourage the client and family to verbalize fears, express emotions, and set goals. EBN: *Buus et al (2014) studied the experiences of two groups of parents of children who had attempted suicide and through thematic analysis the parents communicated that their experience was a double trauma that included the suicide attempts and the psychosocial impact on the family's well-being.* EBN: *Nurse researchers studied psychiatric clients (N = 20) who were in an acute-care facility using qualitative interviews and four themes were prominent: (1) being alone in the world, (2) staff exert power and control, (3) resentment towards staff, and (4) time for meditation (Ezeobele et al, 2014).*
- • Be present for clients physically or by telephone. EBN: *A study used telephone communication by nurses to clients with post-traumatic stress disorder (N = 14) and found qualitative telephone interviews worked well to collect information on sensitive topics and promoted healthy post-traumatic adaptation (Mealer & Jones, 2014).*
- ▲ EB: *Muller et al (2015) studied telephone communication's effect on the development of the therapeutic relationship for clients in self-directed therapy and found that the therapists were able to establish over the phone therapeutic relationships that were client-centered.*
- • Empower the client to set realistic goals and engage in problem solving. EB: *Fisher and Freshwater (2014) studied two types of research methodologies, post-structuralist and narrative, and found that the narrative approach offers greater emancipatory scope to help clients with mental health problems restore their lives and enhance their self-identity.* EB: *Researchers examined the relationships among heart failure (HF) symptoms, social support, social problem solving, depressive symptoms, and self-care behaviors in clients (N = 201) and found that HF symptoms and social support predicted depression and self-care (Graven et al, 2015).*
- • Encourage expression of positive thoughts and emotions. EB: *Researchers surveyed participants (N = 265) about sexual identity compared to activism and collective self-esteem and found a significantly lower collective self-esteem for participants who identified themselves as bisexual, and activism was most likely among those who identified as queer (Gray & Desmarais, 2014).* EB: *A researcher conducted interviews with psychiatric clients (N = 30) about how their diagnosis effected them. The study used and found that metaphors assisted clients to reclaim their identity (Probst, 2015).*
- • Encourage the client to use coping mechanisms. EBN: *da Silva et al (2015) completed a phenomenological study to understand the "musical identity" of palliative care clients (N = 7) and their relatives (N = 5) and found that "musical identity" was related to the client's spirituality and history. Nurses should consider musical identity to empower clients in palliative care.* EB: *Nguyen-Rodriquez et al (2015) investigated the relationship of stress, depressive symptoms, sleep problems, and coping strategies in clients (N = 1676) by survey and discovered a positive relationship between depressive symptoms and sleep problems arising from use of angry coping strategies.*
- • Help clients with serious and chronic conditions to maintain social support networks or assist in building new ones. EB: *Read et al (2015) surveyed clients (N = 28) with cerebral palsy about identity and*

seeking support when needed. Results revealed that the majority of clients did seek support and identified that their personal and their social self was an important part of their total sense of self. EBN: *Rossman et al (2015) studied maternal role development in first-time neonatal intensive care moms (N = 23) and found through interviews that peer support was the most helpful agent in developing their maternal identity.*

▲ Refer women facing diagnostic and curative breast cancer surgery for psychosocial support. EBN: *Budden et al (2014) did a cross-sectional study with women (N = 104) to compare decision satisfaction with breast cancer treatment to psychological distress. Women who were living alone, worked as professionals, and were not involved in decision-making were less satisfied. Additionally, 26% were distressed, 18.3% had anxiety, 19.2% had sleeping problems, and 27.9% experienced depression.* EB: *Researchers evaluated the quality of life (QOL) and social support of clients with breast cancer and their significant others and found that the significant others' QOL was negatively affected. They recommend that significant others need more support that should be tailored to family needs (Salonen et al, 2014).*

• Refer for cognitive behavioral therapy (CBT). EB: *Roscoe et al (2015) evaluated cognitive behavioral therapy for insomnia (CBT-I) in clients with cancer (N = 96) and found that CBT-I resulted in significant improvements in sleep time and quality.* EB: *Researchers developed planned structured sessions of group CBT for detoxification for alcohol dependence and tested it at detoxification centers. Clients perceived that the intervention did indeed prepare them for detoxification (Croxford et al, 2015).*

I

▲ Refer clients with borderline personality disorder (BPD) and dual-diagnosed BPD and substance-dependent female clients for dialectical behavior therapy (DBT) and psychoanalytical-orientated day-hospital therapy. EB: *Feenstra et al (2014) investigated identity integration as a core component of personality disorders in adolescents in both normal (N = 406) and clinical populations (N = 285). Most adolescents receiving inpatient psychotherapy gradually changed toward more healthy levels of identity integration.* EB: *Chen et al (2015) did a pilot study on the use of DBT for adult anorexia nervosa (AN) and addressed over self-control successfully in clients (N = 15). The pilot study indicated that DBT is a positive intervention for AN and should be researched on a larger scale.*

▲ Refer to the care plans for Readiness for enhanced **Communication** and Readiness for enhanced **Spiritual** well-being.

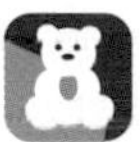

Pediatric

• Encourage adolescents to promote positive self-esteem, to enhance coping, and to prevent behavioral and psychological problems. EB: *Ikizler and Szymanski (2014) studied the development of sexual minority identity in clients (N = 12) from a minority racial/ethnic group and identified themes that needed to be addressed: intersectionality, race/ethnicity, sexual identity development, discrimination, stigma, oppression, and invisibility.* EBN: *Peer support for children/adolescents in families affected by mental illness was studied using an exploratory approach. Clients made connections with others in the program, developed personal strengths, and learned how to contribute to others' well-being (Foster et al, 2014).*

• Evaluate and refer children and adolescents for eating disorder prevention programs to include medical care, nutritional intervention, and mental health treatment and care coordination. EB: *Researchers used a data base to identify 158,679 children aged 12 to 24 years to investigate whether parental mental illnesses are a risk factor for children's eating disorders. They found that it is a significant risk factor for female children in developing eating disorders (Bould et al, 2015).* EB: *Mayes et al (2014) researched 90 children aged 7 to 18 years with bulimia nervosa or AN for suicide ideation and found that it was more prevalent in clients with bulimia nervosa (43%) than clients with AN (20%), indicating a need for specialized nursing interventions for children with different eating disorders.*

• Provide children with low self-esteem with appropriate support. EB: *Kemmery and Compton (2014) researched the self-identities of hearing deficit students (N = 4) and their caregivers/parents (N = 6) to understand the students' self-advocacy development. Interviews demonstrated that identity is affected by interactions with others, setting/context, and life experiences.* EB: *Lingam et al (2014) interviewed children (N = 11) with developmental coordination disorder using an art-based method and found that identity was described by the theme of "We're all different," but subthemes included attitude of the day to day lives and strategies used to overcome difficulties in school and at home.*

• Use computer-mediated support groups to enhance identity formation. EB: *Hou et al (2015) studied how children represent their identity online in a multicultural social environment. Qualitative results showed that children expose their complete identities online to learn about personal, ethnic, and gender identities of others and ignored cultural identity, which led to positive attitudes about others.* EB: *Carey et al (2014) developed a clinical trial to examine stuttering adolescents' (N = 14) responsiveness to the Webcam-delivered Camperdown Program. After 25 sessions, 50% of the clients successfully reduced stuttering.*

Geriatric

- Evaluate the effectiveness of nursing interventions used to promote positive self-identify in older adults. EB: *Bohlmeijer et al (2014) studied processes that affect later life identity by narrative methods and developed a scale that was validated in two studies on middle-aged (N = 319) and older adults (N = 174). The scale was judged reliable to measure effectiveness of interventions aimed at positive identity development, such as life review and narrative therapy.* EB: *Researchers studied older clients' (N = 30) perceptions of age-friendly communities using photographs and found three factors that impact the perceptions of clients: (1) community history and identity, (2) aging in urban, rural, and remote communities, and (3) environmental conditions (Novek & Menac, 2014).*
- Consider the use of telephone/interview/group/computer support for caregivers of family members with dementia. EB: *Lopez et al (2015) interviewed dementia clients' caregivers (N = 108) about optimism, anger, and physical health and found that anger was negatively associated with optimism and vitality, and optimism was positively associated with vitality. The findings suggest that low optimism may be a key in understanding anger and reduced vitality.* EB: *Ho et al (2015) developed a Web-based learning project for dementia family caregivers (N = 279) and evaluated the demographic background and stressfulness of an online dementia educational program. More than 80% of clients showed interest in learning from a computer program, making it a viable teaching tool for caregivers.*
- Encourage clients to discuss "life history." Life history-based interventions and self-esteem and life-satisfaction questionnaires may be used to reinforce personal identity and foster hope. EB: *Gammonley et al (2015) used older clients' oral history interviews to successfully educate staff members in an assisted-living setting about personhood and identity.* EB: *Researchers developed a life story book (LSB) for clients with dementia (N = 23) and found that the development of the LSB provided positive relationships for the clients and their family members (Subramaniam et al, 2014).*

▲ Refer the older client to self-help support groups. EBN: *Baldacchino et al (2014) interviewed older clients (N = 137) about spirituality and discovered that interviews revealed three important themes for the clients: (1) self-empowerment through connectedness with God, self, others, and nature, (2) belongingness to the residence, and (3) the finding of meaning and purpose in life or afterlife, indicating that spiritual coping in self-awareness exercises and support groups is important.*

▲ Refer the client with Alzheimer's disease who is terminally ill to hospice. EBN: *Brooke and Kirk (2014) performed a literature review about end-of-life care needs for dementia clients and their families and found a lack of advance care planning.*

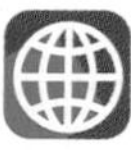

Multicultural

- Assess an individual's sociocultural background in teaching self-management and self-regulation as a means of supporting hope and coping. EB: *Dommelen et al (2015) studied multiple social identities and described an in-group identity as having being included in a group and this predicted participants' attitudes toward out-groups or others.* EB: *Osborne et al (2015) completed a large scale study (N = 6349) whose results supported that income and deprivation were negatively correlated with self-esteem, but group-based relative deprivation was positively correlated with ethnic identity.*
- Decrease discrimination to promote positive ethnic identity. EBN: *Hall et al (2015) assessed minority college students' self-reported stress, ethnic identity, and skin complexion as predictors of racial discrimination and found that skin complexion and ethnic identity had a positive relationship with racial discrimination; therefore, understanding racial discrimination may allow for the development of nondiscriminatory interventions.* EB: *Researchers investigated whether the prevalence of psychotic experiences is higher among ethnic minority youth (N = 1545) by self-report questionnaires and found a significantly increased risk for psychotic experiences in ethnic minority children (Adriaanse et al, 2015).*
- Refer to care plan for Ineffective **Coping.**

Home Care

- The interventions described previously may be adapted for home care use.
- Provide an Internet-based health coach to encourage self-management for clients with chronic conditions such as depression, impaired mobility, and chronic pain. Use computer-mediated support groups to enhance identify formation.

▲ Refer the client to mutual health support groups. Participating in mutual health support groups led to enhanced coping by improving psychological and social functioning. EB: *Gillard et al (2015) developed and researched an open access community support group for clients (N = 38) with personality disorders, and interviews found the model as a useful therapeutic, community-based peer support group and self-referral increased feelings of empowerment and engagement for clients.*

▲ Refer cancer clients and their spouses to family programs that include family-based interventions for communication, hope, coping, uncertainty, and symptom management. EBN: *Sautier et al (2014) studied predictors of participation in client support groups using clients (N = 1281) and assessed support group participation and satisfaction, psychosocial distress (anxiety, fear of cancer recurrence, depression), social support, coping, quality of life, pain, and treatment-related characteristics. The results revealed that unemployment, increased number of treatments, and a high emotion-oriented coping style significantly predicted self-help group participation.* EB: *Researchers compared the effectiveness of conventional Internet and Internet support groups that had a social networking component and found that, in support groups for women (N = 184) with breast cancer that had a social component, clients used more supportive behaviors (emotional, informational, and companionate support), posted more messages that were other-focused and fewer that were self-focused, and expressed less negative emotion (Lepore et al, 2014).*

I

- Refer combat veterans and service members directly involved in combat, as well as those providing support to combatants, including nurses, for mental health services. EB: *Hoglund and Schwartz (2014) investigated the mental health of deployed and nondeployed veterans compared with civilians (N = 41,903) and found that women had more adverse mental health issues than men among civilians, deployed veterans, and nondeployed veterans, and deployed men had more adverse mental health issues than men among civilians and nondeployed veterans.* EB: *This study investigated the relationship of housing, mental health, and service use in a sample of homeless clients with mental illness of veterans (N = 99) and non-veterans (N = 297) and found no significant difference (Bourque et al, 2014).*

Client/Family Teaching and Discharge Planning

- Teach the client about available community resources (e.g., therapists, ministers, counselors, self-help groups, family education groups). EB: *Researchers tracked usage of community-based exercise programs with the proximity of the program to clients' (N= 417) homes and found no differences in awareness or utilization of the community resource (Dondzila et al, 2014).* EBN: *Hanajin et al (2014) found methods to actively support public health and community nurses by providing services to individuals, families, and communities that are based on the best available research evidence.*
- Teach coping skills to family caregivers of cancer clients. EBN: *Gulliford et al (2015) studied a group-based parenting program to teach communication and coping skills to parents (N=14) of preschoolers. The program demonstrated significant changes in the use of productive coping and a reduction in nonproductive coping strategies.* EBN: *Researchers studied personal beliefs and their relationship with learned resourcefulness and adaptive functioning in adults with depression. Results showed that clients (N = 187) with depression when being taught need to have their personal beliefs considered to affect learning resourcefulness and adaptive (Lai et al, 2014).*
- Teach caregivers the COPE intervention (creativity, optimism, planning, expert information) to assist with symptom management. EBN: *Mazurek et al (2014) performed a pre- and post-test pilot study to assess the usability of the COPE (Creating Opportunities for Personal Empowerment) program with adolescents (N = 16) who were depressed or anxious and found that the group COPE intervention was a positive teen experience.*

REFERENCES

Refer to Ineffective **Coping** for additional references.

Adriaanse, M., van Domburgh, L., Hoek, H. W., et al. (2015). Prevalence, impact and cultural context of psychotic experiences among ethnic minority youth. *Psychological Medicine, 45*(3), 637–646.

Bademli, K., & Duman, Z. C. (2014). Effects of a family-to-family support program on the mental health and coping strategies of caregivers of adults with mental illness: a randomized controlled study. *Archives of Psychiatric Nursing, 28*(6), 392–398.

Baldacchino, D. R., Boneilo, L., & Debattista, C. J. (2014). Spiritual coping of older persons in Malta and Australia (part 2). *British Journal of Nursing, 23*(15), 843–846.

Baum, N., & Neuberger, T. (2014). The contributions of persons in the work environment to the self-identity of persons with mental health problems: a study in Israel. *Health & Social Care in the Community, 22*(3), 308–316.

Beckwith, M., Best, D., Dingle, G., et al. (2015). Predictors of flexibility in social identity among people entering a therapeutic community for substance abuse. *Alcoholism Treatment Quarterly, 33*(1), 93–104.

Bogart, K. R. (2014). Disability identity predicts lower anxiety and depression in multiple sclerosis. *Rehabilitation Psychology*, *60*(1), 105–109.

Bohlmeijer, E. T., Westerhof, G. J., & Lamers, S. M. A. (2014). The development and initial validation of the narrative foreclosure scale. *Aging & Mental Health*, *18*(7), 879–888.

Bould, H., Koupil, I., Dalman, C., et al. (2015). Parental mental illness and eating disorders in offspring. *International Journal of Eating Disorders*, *48*(4), 383–391.

Bourque, J., VanTil, L., LeBlanc, S. R., et al. (2014). Correlates of veteran status in a Canadian sample of homeless people with mental illness. *Canadian Journal of Community Mental Health*, *33*(4), 141–159.

Brooke, J., & Kirk, M. (2014). Advance care planning for people living with dementia. *British Journal of Community Nursing*, *19*(10), 490–495.

Budden, L. M., Hayes, B. A., & Buettner, P. G. (2014). Women's decision satisfaction and psychological distress following early breast cancer treatment: a treatment decision support role for nurses. *International Journal of Nursing Practice*, *20*(1), 8–16.

Buus, N., Caspersen, J., Hansen, R., et al. (2014). Experiences of parents whose sons or daughters have (had) attempted suicide. *Journal of Advanced Nursing*, *70*(4), 823–832.

Carey, B., O'Brien, S., Lowe, R., et al. (2014). Webcam delivery of the camperdown program for adolescents who stutter: a phase II trial. *Language, Speech & Hearing Services in Schools*, *45*(4), 314–324.

Chen, E. Y., Segal, K., Weissman, J., et al. (2015). Adapting dialectical behavior therapy for outpatient adult anorexia nervosa—a pilot study. *International Journal of Eating Disorders*, *48*(1), 123–132.

Croxford, A., Notley, C. J., Maskrey, V., et al. (2015). An exploratory qualitative study seeking participant views evaluating group cognitive behavioral therapy preparation for alcohol detoxification. *Journal of Substance Abuse*, *20*(1), 61–68.

da Silva, V. A., Alvim, N. A. T., & Marcon, S. S. (2015). Significances and meanings of the musical identity of patients and relatives receiving oncological palliative care. *Revista Electonica de Enfermagemm*, *16*(1), 132–141.

DeLas Cuevas, C., Penate, W., & Sanz, E. (2014). Risk factors for non-adherence to antidepressant treatment in patients with mood disorders. *European Journal of Clinical Pharmacology*, *70*(1), 89–98.

Dommelen, A., Schmid, K., Hewstone, M., et al. (2015). Construing multiple in-groups: assessing social identity inclusiveness and structure in ethnic and religious minority group members. *European Journal of Social Psychology*, *45*(3), 386–399.

Dondzila, C. J., Swartz, A. M., Keenan, K. G., et al. (2014). Geospatial relationships between awareness and utilization of community exercise resources and physical activity levels in older adults. *Journal of Aging Research*, 1–7.

Ezeobele, I. E., Malecha, A. T., Mock, A., et al. (2014). Patients' lived seclusion experience in acute psychiatric hospital in the United States: a qualitative study. *Journal of Psychiatric & Mental Health Nursing*, *21*(4), 303–312.

Feenstra, D. J., Hutsebaut, J., Verheul, R., et al. (2014). Identity: empirical contribution: changes in the identity integration of adolescents in treatment for personality disorders. *Journal of Personality Disorders*, *28*(1), 101–112.

Finley, E. P., Bollinger, M., Noel, P. H., et al. (2015). A national cohort study of the association between the polytrauma clinical triad and suicide-related behavior among US veterans who served in Iraq and Afghanistan. *American Journal of Public Health*, *105*(2), 380–387.

Fisher, P., & Freshwater, D. (2014). Methodology and mental illness: resistance and restorying. *Journal of Psychiatric & Mental Health Nursing*, *21*(3), 197–205.

Foster, K., Lewis, P., & McCloughen, A. (2014). Experiences of peer support for children and adolescents whose parents and siblings have mental illness. *Journal of Child & Adolescent Psychiatric Nursing*, *27*(2), 61–67.

Gammonley, D., Lester, C. L., Fleishman, D., et al. (2015). Using life history narratives to educate staff members about personhood in assisted living. *Gerontology & Geriatrics Education*, *36*(2), 109–123.

Gillard, S., White, R., Miller, S., et al. (2015). Open access support groups for people experiencing personality disorders: do group members' experiences reflect the theoretical foundations of the SUN project. *Psychology & Psychotherapy: Theory, Research & Practice*, *88*(1), 87–104.

Graven, L. J., Grant, J. S., Vance, D. E., et al. (2015). Predicting depressive symptoms and self-care in patients with heart failure. *American Journal of Health Behavior*, *39*(1), 77–87.

Gray, A., & Desmarais, S. (2014). Not all one and the same: sexual identity, activism, and collective self-esteem. *Canadian Journal of Human Sexuality*, *23*(2), 116–122.

Gulliford, H., Deans, J., Frydenberg, E., et al. (2015). Teaching coping skills in the context of positive parenting within a preschool setting. *Australian Psychologist*, *50*(3), 219–231.

Hall, M. E., Williams, R. D., Penhollow, T. M., et al. (2015). Factors associated with discrimination among minority college students. *American Journal of Health Behavior*, *39*(3), 318–329.

Hanajin, S., Roe, S., O'Dowd, M., et al. (2014). Supporting the use of evidence in community nursing: a national strategic approach. *British Journal of Community Nursing*, *19*(10), 496–501.

Ho, D. W. H., Mak, V., Kwok, T. C. Y., et al. (2015). Development of a web-based training program for dementia caregivers in Hong Kong. *Clinical Gerontologist*, *38*(3), 211–223.

Hoglund, M. W., & Schwartz, R. M. (2014). Mental health in deployed and nondeployed veteran men and women in comparison with their civilian counterparts. *Military Medicine*, *179*(1), 19–25.

Hou, W., Komlodi, A., Lutters, W., et al. (2015). Supporting children's online identity in international communities. *Behaviour & Information Technology*, *34*(4), 375–391.

Ikizler, A. S., & Szymanski, D. M. (2014). A qualitative study of Middle Eastern/Arab American sexual minority identity development. *Journal of LGBT Issues in Counseling*, *8*(2), 206–214.

Kemmery, M. A., & Compton, M. V. (2014). Are you deaf or hard of hearing? Which do you go by: perceptions of identity in families of students with hearing loss. *Volta Review*, *114*(2), 157–192.

Lai, C. Y., Zauszniewski, J. A., Tang, T. C., et al. (2014). Personal beliefs, learned resourcefulness, and adaptive functioning in depressed adults. *Journal of Psychiatric & Mental Health Nursing*, *21*(3), 280–287.

Lepore, S. J., Buzaglo, J. S., Lieberman, M. A., et al. (2014). Comparing standard versus prosocial internet support groups for patients with breast cancer: a randomized controlled trial of the helper therapy principle. *Journal of Clinical Oncology*, *32*(36), 4081–4086.

Lingam, R. P., Novak, C., Emond, A., et al. (2014). The importance of identity and empowerment to teenagers with developmental co-ordination disorder. *Child: Care, Health & Development*, *40*(3), 309–318.

Lopez, J., Romero-Moreno, R., Marquez-Gonzalez, M., et al. (2015). Anger and health in dementia caregivers: exploring the mediation effect of optimism. *Stress & Health: Journal of the International Society for the Investigation of Stress*, *31*(2), 158-165.

Mayberry, L., Egede, L., Wagner, J., et al. (2015). Stress, depression and medication nonadherence in diabetes: test of the exacerbating and buffering effects of family support. *Journal of Behavioral Medicine*, *38*(2), 363–371.

Mayes, S. D., Fernandez-Mendoza, J., Baweja, R., et al. (2014). Correlates of suicide ideation and attempts in children and adolescents with eating disorders. *Eating Disorders*, *22*(4), 352–366.

Mazurek, M. B., Kelly, S., & Lusk, P. (2014). Outcomes and feasibility of a manualized cognitive-behavioral skills building intervention: group COPE for depressed and anxious adolescents in school settings. *Journal of Child & Adolescent Psychiatric Nursing*, *27*(1), 3–13.

Mealer, M., & Jones, J. (2014). Methodological and ethical issues related to qualitative telephone interviews on sensitive topics. *Nurse Researcher, 21*(4), 32–37.

Meng, X., & D'Arcy, C. (2015). Comorbidity between lifetime eating problems and mood and anxiety disorders: results from the Canadian community health survey of mental health and well-being. *European Eating Disorders Review, 23*(2), 156–162.

Morgan, M. B., & Sussman, S. (2014). Translating the link between social identity and health behavior into effective health communication strategies: an experimental application using antismoking advertisements. *Health Communication, 29*(10), 1057–1066.

Mueller, A. S., James, W., Abrutyn, S., et al. (2015). Suicide ideation and bullying among US adolescents: examining the intersections of sexual orientation, gender, and race/ethnicity. *American Journal of Public Health, 105*(5), 980–985.

Muller, I., Kirby, S., & Yardley, L. (2015). The therapeutic relationship in telephone-delivered support for people undertaking rehabilitation: a mixed-methods interaction analysis. *Disability & Rehabilitation, 37*(12), 1060–1065.

Nguyen-Rodriquez, S. T., Lisha, N. E., Spruijt-Metz, D., et al. (2015). Coping mediates the effects of depressive symptoms on sleep problems. *American Journal of Health Behavior, 39*(2), 183–190.

Novek, S., & Menac, V. H. (2014). Older adults' perceptions of age-friendly communities in Canada: a photovoice study. *Ageing & Society, 34*(6), 1052–1072.

Osborne, D., Sibley, C. G., & Sengupta, N. K. (2015). Income and neighbourhood-level inequality predict self-esteem and ethnic identity centrality through individual- and group-based relative deprivation: a multilevel path analysis. *European Journal of Social Psychology, 45*(3), 368–377.

Probst, B. (2015). Queen of the owls: Metaphor and identity in psychiatric diagnosis. *Social Work in Mental Health, 13*(3), 235–251.

Read, S. A., Morton, T. A., & Ryan, M. K. (2015). Negotiating identity: a qualitative analysis of stigma and support seeking for individuals with cerebral palsy. *Disability & Rehabilitation, 37*(13), 1162–1169.

Roscoe, J. A., Garland, S. N., Heckler, C. E., et al. (2015). Randomized placebo-controlled trial of cognitive behavioral therapy and armodafinil for insomnia after cancer treatment. *Journal of Clinical Oncology, 33*(2), 165–171.

Rossman, B., Greene, M. M., & Meier, P. P. (2015). The role of peer support in the development of maternal identity for 'NICU moms'. *JOGNN. Journal of Obstetric, Gynecologic & Neonatal Nursing, 44*(1), 3–16.

Salonen, P., Rantanen, A., Kellokumpu-Lehtinen, P. L., et al. (2014). The quality of life and social support in significant others of patients with breast cancer—a longitudinal study. *European Journal of Cancer Care, 23*(2), 274–283.

Sautier, L., Mehnert, A., Hocker, A., et al. (2014). Participation in patient support groups among cancer survivors: do psychosocial and medical factors have an impact? *European Journal of Cancer Care, 23*(1), 140–148.

Subramaniam, P., Woods, B., & Whitaker, C. (2014). Life review and life story books for people with mild to moderate dementia: a randomised controlled trial. *Ageing & Mental Health, 8*(3), 363–375.

Risk for disturbed personal Identity *Gail B. Ladwig, MSN, RN*

NANDA-I

Definition

Vulnerable to the inability to maintain an integrated and complete perception of self, which may compromise health

Risk Factors

Alteration in social role; cult indoctrination; cultural incongruence; developmental transition; discrimination; dissociative identity disorder; dysfunctional family processes; exposure to toxic chemical; low self-esteem; manic states; organic brain disorder; perceived prejudice; pharmaceutical agent; psychiatric disorder; situational crisis; stages of growth

NOC, NIC, Client Outcomes, Nursing Interventions, Client/Family Teaching and Discharge Planning, *Rationales*, and References

Refer to care plan for Disturbed personal **Identity.**

Ineffective Impulse control *Marina Martinez-Kratz, MS, RN, CNE*

NANDA-I

Definition

A pattern of performing rapid, unplanned reactions to internal or external stimuli without regard for the negative consequences of these reactions to the impulsive individual or to others

Defining Characteristics

Acting without thinking; asking personal questions despite the discomfort of others; gambling addiction; inability to save money or regulate finances; inappropriate sharing of personal details; irritability; overly familiar with strangers; sensation seeking; sexual promiscuity; temper outbursts; violent behavior

Related Factors

Alteration in cognitive functioning; alteration in development; hopelessness; mood disorder; organic brain disorder; personality disorder; smoking; substance abuse

NOC (Nursing Outcomes Classification)

Suggested NOC Outcome

Impulse Self-Control

Example NOC Outcome with Indicators

Impulse Self-Control as evidenced by the following indicators: Identifies harmful impulsive behaviors/Identifies feelings that lead to impulsive actions/Avoids high-risk situations/Controls impulses/Maintains self-control without supervision. (Rate the outcome and indicators of **Impulse Self-Control:** 1 = never demonstrated, 2 = rarely demonstrated, 3 = sometimes demonstrated, 4 = often demonstrated, 5 = continually demonstrated [see Section I].)

I

Client Outcomes

Client Will (Specify Time Frame)

- Be free from harm
- Cooperate with behavioral modification plan
- Verbalize adaptive ways to cope with stress by means other than impulsive behaviors
- Delay gratification and use adaptive coping strategies in response to stress
- Verbalize understanding that behavior is unacceptable
- Accept responsibility for own behavior

NIC (Nursing Interventions Classification)

Suggested NIC Interventions

Impulse Control Training

Example NIC Activities—Impulse Control Training

Use a behavior modification plan, as appropriate, to reinforce the problem-solving strategy that is being taught; Teach client to cue himself/herself to "stop and think" before acting impulsively

Nursing Interventions and *Rationales*

- Refer to mental health treatment for cognitive behavioral therapy (CBT). EB: *CBT has been beneficial in treating substance use disorders and impulse control disorders (Dempsey et al, 2011; Okai et al, 2013).*
- Assess the circumstances that led the client to seek help for their impulse control disorder. EB: *Clients may seek help because they continue to struggle with the desire to engage in the behavior because of the impact of their mounting social, occupational, financial, or legal problems (Grant et al, 2013).*
- Implement motivational interviewing for clients with impulse control disorders. *Motivational interviewing includes treatment components that involve providing feedback to the client concerning current impulsive behaviors and the likely longer term effects associated with such behavior (Farmer & Golden, 2009).*
- Teach client mindfulness meditation techniques. Mindfulness meditation includes observing experiences in the present moment, describing those experiences without judgments or evaluations, and participating fully in one's current context. *Mindfulness meditation is used to assist the individual to develop an attentional focus on the present that is useful in controlling impulsive behavior (Farmer & Golden, 2009).*
- Refer to self-help groups such as Gambler's Anonymous or Overeaters Anonymous as needed. *Methods of psychological and psychosocial management related to specific symptoms are effective strategies for care of impulse control disorders (Dell'Osso et al, 2008; Gallagher, 2010; Greener, 2011).*
- Remove positive reinforcements associated with excessive behavior. *Altering reactivity to immediate environmental cues or circumstances is a contingency management approach effective for impulse control disorders (Farmer & Golden, 2009).*
- Assist the client to recognize patterns and cues of impulsive behavior. *The first step in gaining insight into behaviors is to recognize the causes so long-term therapeutic strategies for stimulus and impulse control can be developed (Dell'Osso et al, 2008).*

- Teach clients to use urge surfing techniques when impulses are triggered. A core skill associated with urge surfing is the ability to observe within oneself the rise and fall of urges and to "surf" or stay with these urges without acting on them. *Urge surfing is a behavioral skill used to facilitate tolerance of urgent action impulses without acting on them (Farmer & Golden, 2009).*
- Implement cue elimination procedures as a stimulus control technique. *Cue elimination is a stimulus control technique in which cues that signal the availability of rewards for problematic behavior are removed (Farmer & Golden, 2009).*
- Implement strategies to engage a high level construal mind-set by asking "why" abstaining from the targeted behavior will benefit the client. EB: *Questions of "why" are effective in priming a high-level construal mind-set, which then is effective at reducing the targeted behavior (Chiou et al, 2013).*

Pediatric

- Assess children who have been exposed to violence in their environment for impulsive behavior. EB: *Research indicates that children exposed to higher levels of violence show an increase in impulsive behavior (Sharkey et al, 2012).*
- Implement in situ training to address impulsive behavior followed by role-play, differential reinforcement, corrective feedback, and rehearsal in young children and adolescents. *In situ training provides children and adolescents with self-management skills that enable them to exhibit on-task and socially appropriate behavior (Farmer & Golden, 2009).*
- Refer to mental health treatment for CBT. *CBT has been beneficial in treating impulse control disorders in pediatric populations (Keeley et al, 2007).*

I

Geriatric

- Assess for impulsive symptoms and maintain increased surveillance of the client whenever use of dopamine agonists has been initiated. *Dopamine agonist therapy is related to the development of impulse control disorders in clients with Parkinson's disease (Greener, 2011; Ambermoon et al, 2011).*
- Implement fall risk screening and precautions for geriatric clients with inattention and impulse control symptoms. *Research demonstrates that older adults with inattention and impulsivity are at highest risk for falls (Harrison et al, 2010).*
- Monitor caregivers for evidence of caregiver burden. *Recent research shows that significantly greater burden was seen in caregivers of Parkinson's disease clients with impulse control disorders (Leroi et al, 2012).*

Client/Family Teaching and Discharge Planning

- Provide families with information about services such as addiction or marriage counseling. *Methods of psychological and psychosocial management related to specific symptoms is an effective strategy for care (Gallagher, 2010).*
- Families should be encouraged to employ practical measures to manage behavior such as limiting access to credit cards and restricting Internet access gambling and casino websites and other addictive social media. *Methods of psychological and psychosocial management related to specific symptoms are an effective strategy for care (Gallagher, 2010).*

REFERENCES

Ambermoon, P., Carter, A., Hall, W. D., et al. (2011). Impulse control disorders in patients with Parkinson's disease receiving dopamine replacement therapy: evidence and implications for the addictions field. *Addiction (Abingdon, England), 106*(2), 283–293.

Chiou, W., Wu, W., & Chang, M. (2013). Think abstractly, smoke less: a brief construal-level intervention can promote self-control, leading to reduced cigarette consumption among current smokers. *Addiction (Abingdon, England), 108*(5), 985–992.

Dell'Osso, B., et al. (2008). Impulsive-compulsive buying disorder: clinical overview. *The Australian and New Zealand Journal of Psychiatry, 42*(4), 259–266.

Dempsey, A., Dyehouse, J., & Schafer, J. (2011). The relationship between executive function, AD/HD, overeating, and obesity. *Western Journal of Nursing Research, 33*(5), 609–629.

Farmer, R., & Golden, J. (2009). The forms and functions of impulsive actions: implications for behavioral assessment and therapy. *International Journal of Behavioral and Consultation Therapy, 5*(1), 12–30.

Gallagher, S. (2010). Treating Parkinson's disease: dopamine dysregulation syndrome and impulse control. *British Journal of Neuroscience Nursing, 6*(1), 24–28.

Grant, J., Schreiber, L., & Odlaug, B. (2013). Phenomenology and treatment of behavioural addictions. *Canadian Journal of Psychiatry, 58*(5), 252–259.

Greener, M. (2011). Managing impulse control disorders. *Nurse Prescrib, 9*(9), 430–434.

Harrison, B. E., et al. (2010). Evaluating the relationship between inattention and impulsivity-related falls in hospitalized older adults. *Geriatric Nursing (New York, N.Y.), 31*(1), 8–16.

Keeley, M., et al. (2007). Pediatric obsessive-compulsive disorder: a guide to assessment and treatment. *Issues in Mental Health Nursing, 28*(6), 555–574.

Leroi, I., et al. (2012). Carer burden in apathy and impulse control disorders in Parkinson's disease. *International Journal of Geriatric Psychiatry*, *27*(2), 160–166.

Okai, D., Askey-Jones, S., Samuel, M., et al. (2013). Trial of CBT for impulse control behaviors affecting Parkinson patients and their caregivers. *Neurology*, *80*(9), 792–799.

Sharkey, P. T., Tirado-Strayer, N., Papachristos, A. V., et al. (2012). The effect of local violence on children's attention and impulse control. *American Journal of Public Health*, *102*(12), 2287–2293.

Bowel Incontinence *Mary Beth Flynn Makic, PhD, RN, CNS, CCNS, FAAN*

NANDA-I

Definition

Change in normal bowel elimination habits characterized by involuntary passage of stool

Defining Characteristics

Bowel urgency; Constant passage of soft stool; Does not recognize urge to defecate; Fecal odor; Fecal staining of bedding; Fecal staining of clothing; Inability to delay defecation; Inability to expel formed stool despite recognition of rectal fullness; Inability to recognize rectal fullness; Inattentive to urge to defecate; Reddened perianal skin

Related Factors

Increase in abdominal pressure; Abnormal increase in intestinal pressure; Alteration in cognitive functioning; Chronic diarrhea; Colorectal lesion; Deficient dietary habits; Difficulty with toileting self-care; Dysfunctional rectal sphincter; Environmental factor (e.g., inaccessible bathroom); Generalized decline in muscle tone; Immobility; Impaction; Impaired reservoir capacity; Incomplete emptying of bowel; Laxative abuse; Lower motor nerve damage; Pharmaceutical agent; Rectal sphincter abnormality; Stressors; Upper motor nerve damage

NOC (Nursing Outcomes Classification)

Suggested NOC Outcomes

Bowel Continence; Bowel Elimination

Example NOC Outcome with Indicators

Bowel Continence as evidenced by the following indicators: Maintains predictable pattern of stool evacuation/Maintains control of stool passage/Evacuates stool at least every 3 days. (Rate the outcome and indicators of **Bowel Continence:** 1 = never demonstrated, 2 = rarely demonstrated, 3 = sometimes demonstrated, 4 = often demonstrated, 5 = consistently demonstrated [see Section I].)

Client Outcomes

Client Will (Specify Time Frame)

- Have regular, complete evacuation of fecal contents from the rectal vault (pattern may vary from every day to every 3 days)
- Have regulation of stool consistency (soft, formed stools)
- Reduce or eliminate frequency of incontinent episodes
- Exhibit intact skin in the perianal/perineal area
- Demonstrate the ability to isolate, contract, and relax pelvic muscles (when incontinence related to sphincter incompetence or high-tone pelvic floor dysfunction)
- Increase pelvic muscle strength (when incontinence related to sphincter incompetence)
- Identify triggers that precipitate change in bowel continence

NIC (Nursing Interventions Classification)

Suggested NIC Interventions

Bowel Incontinence Care; Bowel Incontinence Care: Encopresis; Bowel Training

Example NIC Interventions—Bowel Incontinence Care

Determine physical or psychological cause of fecal incontinence; Instruct client/family to record fecal output, as appropriate

Nursing Interventions and *Rationales*

- • In a private setting, directly question client about the presence of fecal incontinence. If the client reports altered bowel elimination patterns, problems with bowel control, or "uncontrollable diarrhea," complete a focused nursing history including previous and present bowel elimination routines, dietary history, frequency and volume of uncontrolled stool loss, and aggravating and alleviating factors. CEB/EB: *Unless questioned directly, clients are often hesitant to report the presence of fecal incontinence (Fisher et al, 2008). The nursing history determines the patterns of stool elimination, to characterize involuntary stool loss and the likely etiology of the incontinence (Willson et al, 2014).*
- • Recognize that risk factors for fecal incontinence include older individuals, female sex, impaired mobility, cognitive impairment, and structural or functional impairment of bowel function (Aitola et al, 2010; Langemo et al, 2011; Willson et al, 2014). *Although fecal incontinence is more common in women, it is also a problem for men and should not be overlooked when obtaining a health history (Aitola et al, 2010). Physiologic changes of the female pelvis occur with aging, increasing the risk of elimination problems, both constipation and incontinence (Mannella et al, 2013).* CEBN: *Double incontinence, defined as urinary and fecal incontinence, was found in 10.3% of 1869 community-dwelling women aged 45 to 85 years in a large cross-sectional study; thus, if a client is suffering from one form of incontinence, ask the client if he/she suffers from double incontinence as well (Slieker-ten Hove et al, 2010).*
- • Recognize that additional risk factors for bowel incontinence in hospitalized clients include antibiotic therapy, medications, enteral feeding, immobility, inability to communicate elimination needs, acute disease processes and procedures (e.g., cancer, abdominal surgery), sedation, and mechanical ventilation (Hurnauth, 2011; Makic et al, 2011; Chang & Huang, 2013).
- ▲ Conduct a health history assessment that includes a review of current bowel patterns/habits to include constipation and use of laxatives; pelvic floor injury with childbirth; acute trauma to organs, muscles, or nerves involved in defecation; gastrointestinal inflammatory disorders; functional disability; and medications (Nurko & Scott, 2011; Kaiser et al, 2014).
- ▲ Closely inspect the perineal skin and skin folds for evidence of skin breakdown in clients with incontinence. EBN: *An expert consensus statement defined moisture-associated skin damage as inflammation and erosion of the skin caused by prolonged exposure to various sources of moisture (Black et al, 2011). Incontinence-associated dermatitis (IAD) is a form of skin irritation that develops from chronic exposure to urine or liquid stool (Black et al, 2011). A recent meta-analysis found a strong association between IAD and a client developing a pressure ulcer (Beeckman et al, 2014).*
- ▲ Use a validated tool that focuses on bowel elimination patterns to help provide a more clear understanding of the client's individual challenges with fecal incontinence (Gillibrand, 2012; Langemo et al, 2011).
- ▲ Complete a focused physical assessment, including inspection of perineal skin, pelvic muscle strength assessment, digital examination of the rectum for presence of impaction and anal sphincter strength, and evaluation of functional status (mobility, dexterity, visual acuity).
- • Complete an assessment of cognitive function; explore for a history of dementia, delirium, or acute confusion (Bliss et al, 2011; Drennan et al, 2014). EBN: *A study found that critically ill clients who were less cognitively aware were more likely to develop incontinence-associated dermatitis than clients who were more cognitively aware (Bliss et al, 2011).*
- • Document patterns of stool elimination and incontinent episodes through a bowel record, including frequency of bowel movements, stool consistency, frequency and severity of incontinent episodes, precipitating factors, and dietary and fluid intake. *Documented patterns of elimination are used to narrow the likely etiology of stool incontinence and serve as a baseline to evaluate treatment efficacy (Nurko & Scott, 2011; Willson et al, 2014).*
- • Assess stool consistency and its influence on risk for stool loss. *Several classification systems for stool exist and may assist the nurse and client to differentiate among normal soft, formed stool, hardened stools associated with constipation, and liquid stools associated with diarrhea.* CEB: *A study of stool consistency found good reliability when evaluated by nurses and clients. Word-only descriptors yielded equivocal consistency when assessed by subjects, as did tools that combined words with illustrations of various stool consistencies*

(Bliss et al, 2011). Less well-formed (loose or liquid) stool is associated with an increased severity and frequency of fecal incontinence episodes and potential for compromised skin integrity (Bharucha et al, 2008; Black et al, 2011; Langemo et al, 2011; Willson et al, 2014; Beeckman et al, 2014).

- Identify conditions contributing to or causing fecal incontinence. *Fecal incontinence is frequently multifactorial. Accurate assessment of the probable etiology of fecal incontinence is necessary to select a treatment plan likely to control or eliminate the condition (Willson et al, 2014; Unger et al, 2014).*
- Improve access to toileting:
  - ❍ Identify usual toileting patterns and plan opportunities for toileting accordingly.
  - ❍ Provide assistance with toileting for clients with limited access or impaired functional status (mobility, dexterity, access).
  - ❍ Institute a prompted toileting program for persons with impaired cognitive status.
  - ❍ Provide adequate privacy for toileting.
  - ❍ Respond promptly to requests for assistance with toileting.

▲ CEB/EB: *Acute or transient fecal incontinence frequently occurs in the acute care or long-term care facility because of inadequate access to toileting facilities, insufficient assistance with toileting, or inadequate privacy when attempting to toilet (Bliss et al, 2000; Gillibrand, 2012; Park & Kim, 2014).*

I

- Review the client's nutritional history and evaluate methods to normalize stool consistency with dietary adjustments (e.g., avoiding high-fat content foods) and use of fiber (Nurko & Scott, 2011; Willson et al, 2014; International Foundation for Functional Gastrointestinal Disorders [IFFGD], 2014). EB: *Diet modifications have been found to be helpful in the management of fecal incontinence, including restrictions of some foods, adding fiber to the diet, and establishing consistent eating patterns (National Institute for Diabetes and Digestive and Kidney Diseases, 2013; Willson et al, 2014).*
- Encourage the client to keep a nutrition log to track foods that irritate the bowel *(Nurko & Scott, 2011).*
- For hospitalized clients with tube feeding–associated fecal incontinence, involve the nutrition specialist to evaluate the formula composition, osmolality, and fiber content.
- For the client with intermittent episodes of fecal incontinence related to acute changes in stool consistency, begin a bowel reeducation program consisting of:
  - ❍ Cleansing the bowel of impacted stool if indicated
  - ❍ Normalizing stool consistency by adequate intake of fluids (30 mL/kg of body weight/day) and dietary or supplemental fiber
  - ❍ Establishing a regular routine of fecal elimination based on established patterns of bowel elimination (patterns established before onset of incontinence)

Education on bowel patterns and strategies to establish normal defecation patterns and stool consistency to reduce or eliminate the risk of recurring fecal incontinence have been found to be beneficial in controlling fecal incontinence associated with changes in stool consistency (NHS, 2015; IFFGD, 2014).

▲ Implement a scheduled stimulation defecation program for persons with neurological conditions causing fecal incontinence:
  - ❍ Cleanse the bowel of impacted fecal material before beginning the program.
  - ❍ Implement strategies to normalize stool consistency, including adequate intake of fluid and fiber and avoidance of foods associated with diarrhea.
  - ❍ Determine a regular schedule for bowel elimination (typically every day or every other day) based on prior patterns of bowel elimination.
  - ❍ Provide a stimulus before assisting the client to a position on the toilet; digital stimulation, a stimulating suppository, "mini-enema," or pulsed evacuation enema may be used for stimulation.

The scheduled, stimulated program relies on consistency of stool and a mechanical or chemical stimulus to produce a bolus contraction of the rectum with evacuation of fecal material (Penn, 2011).

▲ Begin a reeducation or pelvic floor muscle exercise program for the person with sphincter incompetence or high-tone pelvic floor muscle dysfunction of the pelvic muscles, or refer persons with fecal incontinence related to sphincter dysfunction to a nurse specialist or other therapist with clinical expertise in these techniques of care. EB: *While evidence of overall effectiveness of pelvic floor muscle exercise programs is inconclusive as a treatment strategy for fecal incontinence, the programs are not harmful (Mannella et al, 2013; Unger et al, 2014).*

▲ Consider a sacral nerve stimulation program in clients with urgency to defecate and fecal incontinence related to weakened sphincter muscles or sphincter defect. EB: *Sacral nerve stimulation has been found to significantly reduce incontinence for some clients (Kaiser et al, 2014; Van Koughnett & Wexner, 2013).*

- Institute a structured skin care regimen that incorporates three essential steps: cleanse, moisturize, and protect:
  - Select a cleanser with a pH range comparable to that of normal skin (usually labeled "pH balanced").
  - Moisturize with an emollient to replace lipids removed with cleansing and protect with a skin. Products containing petrolatum, dimethicone, or zinc oxide base or a no-sting skin barrier should be used.
  - Routine incontinence care should include daily perineal skin cleansing and following each episode of incontinence.
  - When feasible, select a product that combines two or all three of these processes into a single step. Ensure that products are available at the bedside when caring for a client with total incontinence in an inpatient facility.
- ▲ Use of absorptive pads or adult containment briefs that are applied next to the client's skin increases the risk of incontinence-associated dermatitis. Absorbent underpads that wick moisture away from skin may be used with immobile clients. EBN: *A structured skin care regimen based on a three-step process (cleanse, moisturize, and protect) is effective for the prevention of incontinence-associated dermatitis (Black et al, 2011; Langemo et al, 2011; Makic et al, 2011; Willson et al, 2014).*
- ▲ Consult the provider if a fungal infection is suspected. An antifungal cream or powder beneath a protective ointment may be indicated (Black et al, 2011; Langemo et al, 2011; Makic et al, 2011; Willson et al, 2014).
- Assist the client to select and apply a containment device for occasional episodes of fecal incontinence. A fecal containment device will prevent soiling of clothing and reduce odors in the client with uncontrolled stool loss. CEBN: *A study of community persons with fecal incontinence who used an absorptive dressing to contain mucus and stool leakage after surgery revealed that the device was preferred over traditional pads in 92% (Bliss et al, 2011).*
- In the client with frequent episodes of fecal incontinence and limited mobility, monitor the sacrum and perineal area for pressure ulcerations. CEB/EBN: *Limited mobility, particularly when combined with fecal incontinence and increased moisture, increases the risk of pressure ulceration. Routine cleansing, pressure reduction techniques, and management of fecal and urinary incontinence reduce this risk (Johanson et al, 1997; Junkin & Selekof, 2007; Schnelle et al, 1997; Willson et al, 2014; Beeckman et al, 2014).*
- With acutely ill clients, anticipate and evaluate the cause of acute diarrhea. Anticipate diarrhea associated with treatment or specific interventions (e.g., medications, initiation of tube feedings). *Interventions to manage acute diarrhea include use of absorbent pads and skin protectant moisturizers or fecal collector/pouch (Makic et al, 2011; Langemo et al, 2011; Willson et al, 2014).*
- ▲ Consult a provider about insertion of a bowel management system in the critically ill client when conservative measures have failed and fecal incontinence is excessive and/or produces perianal skin injury or incontinence-associated dermatitis. *Indwelling bowel management systems (BMSs), also called fecal management systems (FMS), are commercially available and designed to direct, collect, and contain liquid stool in immobile clients. BMS devices are approved by the Food and Drug Administration for up to 29 days for management of liquid stool (Langemo et al, 2011; Makic et al, 2011).* CEB/EBN: *Devices other than BMSs should not be used for indwelling bowel/feces diversion (Beeckman et al, 2009; Wishin et al, 2008; Pittman et al, 2012; Munhall & Jindal, 2013; Willson et al, 2014; Whitely et al, 2014).*

Geriatric

- Evaluate all older clients for established or acute fecal incontinence when the older client enters the acute or long-term care facility and intervene as indicated. EB: *Fecal incontinence often coexists with urinary incontinence, necessitating evidence-based interventions to prevent skin breakdown and/or pressure ulcer development in the older client (Willson et al, 2014; Shahin & Lohrmann, 2015; National Pressure Ulcer Advisory Panel, 2014).*
- Determine the client's cognitive level using a screening tool such as the Mini-Mental State Exam (MMSE), the CAM, or Mini-Cog. CEB/EB: *Use of a standard evaluation tool such as the MMSE can help determine the client's abilities and assist in planning appropriate nursing interventions. Acute or established dementias increase the risk of fecal incontinence among older adults (Borson et al, 2006; Braes et al, 2012).*
  - Teach nursing colleagues, nonprofessional care providers, family, and clients the importance of providing toileting opportunities and adequate privacy for the client in an acute or long-term care facility.

Home Care

- The preceding interventions may be adapted for home care use.
- Assess and teach a bowel management program to support continence. Address timing, diet, fluids, and actions taken independently to deal with bowel incontinence. *Identifying factors that change level of incontinence may guide interventions. If client has been taking over-the-counter medications or home remedies, it is important to consider their influence.*
- Instruct caregiver to provide clothing that is nonrestrictive, can be manipulated easily for toileting, and can be changed with ease. *Avoidance of complicated maneuvers increases the chance of success in toileting programs and decreases the client's risk for embarrassing incontinent episodes.*
- Evaluate self-care strategies of community-dwelling older adults, strengthen adaptive behaviors, and counsel older adults about altering strategies that compromise general health.
- Assist the family in arranging care in a way that allows the client to participate in family or favorite activities without embarrassment. *Careful planning can both help the client retain dignity and maintain integrity of family patterns.*

▲ If the client is limited to bed (or bed and chair), provide a commode or bedpan that can be easily accessed. Involve occupational and physical therapy services as indicated to promote safe transfers.

▲ If the client is frequently incontinent, refer for home health aide services to assist with hygiene and skin care.

▲ Refer the family to support services to assist with in-home management of fecal incontinence as indicated.

NOTE: Refer to nursing diagnoses **Diarrhea** and **Constipation** for detailed management of these related conditions.

REFERENCES

Aitola, P., et al. (2010). Prevalence of fecal incontinence in adults aged 30 years or more in general population. *Colorectal Disease, 12*(7), 687–691.

Beeckman, D., VanLancker, A., VanHecke, A., et al. (2014). A systematic review and meta-analysis of incontinence-associated dermatitis, incontinence, and moisture as risk factors for pressure ulcer development. *Research in Nursing & Health, 37*, 201–218.

Beeckman, D., et al. (2009). Prevention and treatment of incontinence-associated dermatitis: literature review. *Journal of Advanced Nursing, 65*(6), 1141–1154.

Braes, T., Milisen, K., & Foreman, M. D. (2012). *Assessing Cognitive Function*. <http://consultgerirn.org/topics/assessing_cognitive_function/want_to_know_more>. Retrieved April 14, 2014.

Bharucha, A. E., et al. (2008). Relation of bowel habits to fecal incontinence in women. *The American Journal of Gastroenterology, 103*(6), 1470–1475.

Black, J. M., et al. (2011). MASD part 2: incontinence-associated dermatitis and intertriginous dermatitis. *Journal of Wound, Ostomy, and Continence Nursing, 38*(4), 359–370.

Bliss, D. Z., et al. (2000). Fecal incontinence in hospitalized clients who are acutely ill. *Nursing Research, 49*(2), 101–108.

Bliss, D. Z., et al. (2011). Incontinence-associated dermatitis in critically ill adults. *Journal of Wound, Ostomy, and Continence Nursing, 38*(4), 433–445.

Borson, S., et al. (2006). Improving identification of cognitive impairment in primary care. *International Journal of Geriatric Psychiatry, 21*(4), 349–355.

Chang, S. J., & Huang, H. H. (2013). Diarrhea in enterally fed patients: blame the diet? *Current Opinion in Clinical Nutrition and Metabolic Care, 2013*(16), 588–594.

Drennan, V. M., Greenwood, N., & Cole, L. (2014). Continence care for people with dementia at home. *Nursing Times*.

Fisher, K., Bliss, D. Z., & Savik, K. (2008). Comparison of recall and daily self-report of fecal incontinence severity. *Journal of Wound, Ostomy, and Continence Nursing, 35*(5), 515–520.

Gillibrand, W. (2012). Faecal incontinence in the elderly: issues and interventions in the home. *British Journal of Community Nursing, 17*(8), 364–368.

Hurnauth, C. (2011). Management of faecal incontinence in acutely ill patients. *Nursing Standard, 25*(2), 48–56.

International Foundation for Functional Gastrointestinal Disorders (March, 2014). *Nutritional strategies for managing diarrhea*. <http://www.iffgd.org/site/gi-disorders/functional-gi-disorders/diarrhea/nutrition>. Retrieved April 13, 2015.

Johanson, J. F., Irizarry, F., & Doughty, A. (1997). Risk factors for fecal incontinence in a nursing home population. *Journal of Clinical Gastroenterology, 24*, 156.

Junkin, J., & Selekof, J. (2007). Prevalence of incontinence and associated skin injury in an acute care population. *Journal of Wound, Ostomy, and Continence Nursing, 34*(3), 260–269.

Kaiser, A. M., Orangio, G. R., Zutshi, M., et al. (2014). Current status: new technologies for the treatment of patients with fecal incontinence. *Surgical Endoscopy, 28*, 2277–2301.

Langemo, D., et al. (2011). Incontinence and incontinence-associated dermatitis. *Advances in Skin and Wound Care, 24*(3), 126–140.

Makic, M. B. F., et al. (2011). Evidence-based practice habits: putting more sacred cows out to pasture. *Critical Care Nurse, 31*, 38–62.

Mannella, P., Palla, G., Bellini, M., et al. (2013). The female pelvic floor through midlife and aging. *Maturitas, 76*, 230–234.

Munhall, A. M., & Jindal, S. K. (2013). Massive gastrointestinal hemorrhage as a complication of the flexi-seal fecal management system. *American Journal of Critical Care, 22*(6), 537–543.

NHS Choices Information (2015). *Bowel incontinence-treatment*. <http://www.nhs.uk/Conditions/Incontinence-bowel/Pages/Treatment.aspx>. Retrieved April 14, 2015.

National Institute for Diabetes and Digestive and Kidney Diseases (2013). *Fecal Incontinence*. <http://www.niddk.nih.gov/health-information/health-topics/digestive-diseases/fecal-incontinence/Pages/facts.aspx#eating>. Retrieved April 14, 2015.

National Pressure Ulcer Advisory Panel (2014). *Prevention and Treatment of Pressure Ulcers: Quick Reference Guide*. Cambridge Media. <http://www.npuap.org/wp-content/uploads/2014/08/Updated-10-16-14-Quick-Reference-Guide-DIGITAL-NPUAP-EPUAP-PPPIA-16Oct2014.pdf>. Retrieved April 14, 2015.

Nurko, S., & Scott, S. M. (2011). Coexistence of constipation and incontinence in children and adults. *Best Practice and Research. Clinical Gastroenterology*, *25*, 29–41.

Park, K. H., & Kim, K. S. (2014). Effect of a structured skin care regimen on patients with fecal incontinence: a comparison cohort study. *Journal of Wound, Ostomy, and Continence Nursing*, *41*(2), 161–167.

Penn, R. (2011). Not having the right bowel care is demeaning. *Nursing Times*, *107*(12), 16 18.

Pittman, J., Beeson, T., Terry, C., et al. (2012). Methods of bowel management in critical care: a randomized controlled trial. *Journal of Wound, Ostomy, and Continence Nursing*, *39*(6), 633–639.

Schnelle, J. F., et al. (1997). Skin disorders and moisture in incontinent nursing home residents: intervention implications. *Journal of the American Geriatrics Society*, *45*(10), 1182–1188.

Shahin, E. S. M., & Lohrmann, C. (2015). Prevalence of fecal and double fecal and urinary incontinence in hospitalized patients. *Journal of Wound, Ostomy, and Continence Nursing*, *42*(1), 89–93.

Slieker-ten Hove, M. C., et al. (2010). Prevalence of double incontinence, risks and influence on quality of life in a general female population. *Neurourology and Urodynamics*, *29*(4), 454–550.

Unger, C. A., Goldman, H. B., & Jelovesk, J. E. (2014). Fecal incontinence: the role of the urologist. *Current Urology Reports*, *15*, 388–398.

Van Koughnett, J. A., & Wexner, S. D. (2013). Current management of fecal incontinence: choosing amongst treatment options to optimize outcomes. *World Journal of Gastroenterology*, *19*(48), 9216–9230.

Whitely, I., Sinclair, G., Comm, M., et al. (2014). A retrospective review of outcomes using a fecal management system in acute care patients. *Ostomy/Wound Management*, *60*(12), 37–43.

Willson, M. M., Angyus, M., Beals, D., et al. (2014). Executive summary: a quick reference guide for managing fecal incontinence. *Journal of Wound, Ostomy, and Continence Nursing*, *41*(1), 61–69.

Wishin, J., Gallagher, J., & McCann, E. (2008). Emerging options for the management of fecal incontinence in hospitalized patients. *Journal of Wound, Ostomy, and Continence Nursing*, *35*(1), 104–110.

Functional urinary Incontinence

Amanda Andrews, MA, Ed, BSc, DN, RN, HEA Fellow

NANDA-I

Definition

Inability of usually continent person to reach toilet in time to avoid unintentional loss of urine

Defining Characteristics

Completely empties bladder; early morning urinary incontinence; sensation of need to void; time between sensation of urge and ability to reach toilet is too short; voiding prior to reaching toilet

Related Factors (r/t)

Alteration in cognitive functioning; alteration in environmental factor; impaired vision; neuromuscular impairment; psychological disorder; weakened supporting pelvic structure

NOC (Nursing Outcomes Classification)

Suggested NOC Outcomes

Urinary Continence; Urinary Elimination

Example NOC Outcome with Indicators

Urinary Continence as evidenced by the following indicators: Recognizes urge to void/Responds to urge in timely manner/Voids in appropriate receptacle/Underclothing remains dry during day/Underclothing or bedding remains dry during night. (Rate the outcome and indicators of **Urinary Continence:** 1 = never demonstrated, 2 = rarely demonstrated, 3 = sometimes demonstrated, 4 = often demonstrated, 5 = consistently demonstrated [see Section I].)

Client Outcomes

Client Will (Specify Time Frame)

- Eliminate or reduce incontinent episodes
- Eliminate or overcome environmental barriers to toileting

- Use adaptive equipment to reduce or eliminate incontinence related to impaired mobility or dexterity
- Use portable urinary collection devices or urine containment devices when access to the toilet is not feasible

NIC (Nursing Interventions Classification)

Suggested NIC Interventions

Urinary Habit Training; Urinary Incontinence Care

Example NIC Activities—Urinary Habit Training

Keep a continence-specification record for 3 days to establish voiding pattern; Establish interval for toileting of preferably not less than 2 hours

Nursing Interventions and *Rationales*

I

- Introduce yourself to the client and anyone accompanying him or her and inform them of your role. *Introducing yourself to a client helps establish and develop a therapeutic relationship that recognizes the person within the client and forms the bases for building trust on which to base the provision of care (Howatson-Jones et al, 2012).*
- Gain consent to carry out care before proceeding further with the assessment. In clients unable to give consent, liaise with relevant health care professionals and/or family members. *Clients have the right of autonomy both legally and morally and therefore should be fully involved in the decision-making process (Avery, 2013).*
- Wash hands using a recognized technique. *Evidence shows that strict hand hygiene regimens significantly reduce the incidence of methicillin-resistant* Staphylococcus aureus *and* Clostridium difficile *(Health Protection Agency, 2013).*
- Assess usual pattern of bladder management and establish the extent of the problem to include the following: *A detailed and accurate assessment of the client enables the nurse to plan interventions, monitor outcomes, and evaluate care, ensuring no unnecessary treatment is carried out (Matthews, 2011).*
- Bladder Habits:
    - Episodes of incontinence during the day and night
    - Alleviating and aggravating factors
    - Current management strategies to include containing/collection devices, restriction of fluid intake, and avoidance of fluid/food groups that cause bladder irritation
- Lifestyle and Risk Assessment: Toilet facility access and ability to use including:
    - Distance of the toilet from the bed, chair, and living quarters
    - Characteristics of the bed, including presence of side rails and distance of the bed from the floor
    - Characteristics of the pathway to the toilet, including barriers such as stairs, loose rugs on the floor, and inadequate lighting
    - Characteristics of the bathroom, including patterns of use, lighting, height of the toilet from the floor, presence of handrails to assist transfers to the toilet, and breadth of the door and its accessibility for a wheelchair, walker, or other assistive device

For older adults who may have limited mobility, the nurse must assess environmental barriers that may restrict access to the toilet (Dowling-Castronovo & Specht, 2009).

- Physical and Mental Abilities:
    - Ability to rise from chair and bed, transfer to the toilet, and ambulate, and the need for physical assistive devices such as a cane, walker, or wheelchair. *Urinary incontinence can occur as a direct consequence of the inability to reach and use the toilet either independently or with the assistance of aids or caregivers (Ostaszkiewicz et al, 2013).*
    - Ability to manipulate buttons, hooks, snaps, loop and pile closures, and zippers as needed to remove clothing. *Functional continence requires the ability to remove clothing to urinate; individuals with compromised visual acuity, dexterity, and mobility will need specific interventions to assist with these challenges to continence (Abrams et al, 2010).*
    - Functional and cognitive status assessment using a tool such as the Mini Mental Status Examination for the older client with functional incontinence. *Functional continence requires sufficient mental acuity*

to respond to sensory input from a filling urinary bladder by locating the toilet, moving to it, and emptying the bladder. In a cohort of nondisabled older adults, those with severe white matter changes (dementia) were found to have more urinary urge incontinence (Poggesi et al, 2008).
  - Daily fluid intake included amount of types of fluids drank
  - Risk of falls due to dizziness, impaired vision, and hearing
  - Functional ability decline secondary to comorbidities (cerebral vascular incidents, amputation—see Past Medical History)
  - Discuss quality of life issues relating to socialization and family events

A comprehensive assessment enables the problem to be identified, generating a baseline of information from which to accurately diagnose and plan treatment and care (Reid, 2014).

- Past Medical History:
  - Obstetrical/gynecological/urological history and surgeries
  - Relevant comorbidities—cardiac, respiratory, renal, or neurological
  - Recurrent urinary tract infections

Nazarko (2007) identified the importance of considering other conditions that affect an individual's ability to maintain continence.

I

- Teach the client, the client's care providers, or the family to complete a bladder diary; each 24-hour period is subdivided into 1- to 2-hour periods and includes number of urinations occurring in the toilet, actual episodes of incontinence and amount of urine leaked, reasons for episode of incontinence, type and amount of liquid intake, number of bowel movements, and incontinence pads or other products used. EB: *A bladder diary provides a detailed account of patterns and factors related to incontinence and captures bladder activity more accurately than questionnaires (Dowling-Castronovo & Specht, 2009).*
- Consult with the health care provider and carry out a medication review relating to side effects and contraindications. Antimuscarinic medications in clients receiving cholinesterase reuptake inhibitors for Alzheimer's-type dementia may experience adverse drug interactions. EB: *Retrospective clinical evidence suggests that clients receiving both cholinesterase reuptake inhibitors and antimuscarinics experience more rapid functional decline than do clients taking cholinesterase reuptake inhibitors alone (Sink et al, 2008).*
- Provide an appropriate, safe urinary receptacle such as a three-in-one commode, female or male hand-held urinal, no-spill urinal, or containment device when toileting access is limited by immobility or environmental barriers and while other interventions are being put in place. EB: *Toileting aids should be generally considered as a short-term strategy and/or an addition to ongoing treatment. It is recommended that long-term management with such items should only be considered when all other options have been excluded (NICE, 2013).*
- Refer to occupational therapy for help in obtaining assistive devices and adapting the home for optimal toilet accessibility. *An occupational therapist may suggest adaptations to clothing or to the environment to assist with functional incontinence (Keegan & Knight, 2009).*
- Provide advice to clients relating to loose-fitting clothing with stretch waistbands rather than buttoned or zippered waist; minimize buttons, snaps, and multilayered clothing; and substitute a loop-and-pile closure or other easily loosened systems such as Velcro for buttons, hooks, and zippers in existing clothing. *Clients with impaired dexterity or weakness may benefit from clothing that has been modified or is without buttons and zippers (Cohen, 2008).*
- Work with client on retraining the bladder by regular timed toileting regimens (every 2 hours). For the older client in the home or a long-term care facility who has functional incontinence and dementia:
  - Determine the frequency of current urination using an alarm system or check-and-change device.
  - Record urinary elimination and incontinent patterns in a bladder log to use as a baseline for assessment and evaluation of treatment efficacy.
  - Begin a prompted toileting program based on the results of this program; toileting frequency may vary from every 1.5 to 2 hours to every 4 hours.
  - Provide positive reinforcement.

Based on a systematic review of 14 clinical trials, prompted voiding has been shown to improve daytime incontinence and the percentage of appropriate toileting episodes in clients with dementia and functional incontinence (Fink et al, 2008).

- Monitor older clients in a long-term care facility, acute care facility, or home for dehydration. EB: *Dehydration can exacerbate urine loss, and it is essential that it be considered a factor when managing incontinence, particularly in care home settings (Flanagan et al, 2014).*

- Inspect the perineal and perianal skin for evidence of incontinence-associated dermatitis, including inflammation, vesicles in skin exposed to urinary leakage, and especially skin folds or denudation of the skin, particularly when incontinence is managed by absorptive pads or containment briefs. EB: *Skin folds and the perineal skin are at risk for dermatitis and fungal or bacterial infections (Gray, 2010).*
- Begin a preventive skin care regimen for all clients with urinary incontinence and treat clients with incontinence-associated dermatitis or related skin damage. CEB: *Minimizing exposure to urine, gentle cleansing, moisture protection, preferably with an emollient, and application of a skin protectant are the necessary components of a skin protection program (Gray, 2010).*
- Advise the client about the advantages of using disposable or reusable insert pads, pad-pant systems, or replacement briefs specifically designed for urinary incontinence as indicated for short-term/long-term use, including social events. *Using a combination of absorbent products (varied designs for day/night, going out/staying in) may be more effective and less costly than using the same design at all times; gender is a factor in determining the best design for absorbent products (Fader et al, 2008).*
- Consider the use of an indwelling catheter for continuous drainage in the client who is both homebound and bed-bound and is receiving palliative or end-of-life care (requires a health care provider's order). EB: *Indwelling catheters may be used for clients who are at the end of life, when repositioning adds to discomfort or pain (Rogers et al, 2008; Talley et al, 2014).*
- When an indwelling urinary catheter is in place, follow prescribed maintenance protocols for managing the catheter, taping and replacing the catheter, drainage bag, and care of perineal skin and urethral meatus. Teach infection control measures adapted to the home care setting. *Proper care reduces the risk of catheter-associated urinary tract infection (Centers for Disease control and Prevention, 2015).*
- Assist the client in adapting to the catheter. Encourage discussion of the client's response to the catheter. CEB: *Clients living with a catheter are often keenly aware of its presence; adaptation is served by normalizing the experience. Instruction could include the fact that the client will be more aware of some sensations and sounds (e.g., urine sloshing in the bag, the weight of the bag, pressure or pain when urine flow has been altered). Rehearsing emptying of the bag when away from home will support resumption of activities. Discussion of the client's response will assist him/her in dealing with embarrassment or frustration (Wilde, 2002).*
- Provide client with comprehensive written information about bladder care. *Providing clients with well-written, evidence-based information about their condition and treatment can have a beneficial effect on the outcomes of treatment. In addition, clients are more likely to retain important information that will assist them in making informed decisions about their care (Coulter, 2011).*
- Document all care and advice given in a factual and comprehensive manner. *Good record keeping is an integral part of nursing practice and is essential to the provision of safe and effective care (St. Aubyn & Andrews, 2012).*

REFERENCES

Avery, G. (2013). *Law and Ethics in Nursing and Healthcare an Introduction*. London: Sage Publications Inc.

Abrams, P., Andersson, K. E., & Birder, L. (2010). Fourth international consultation on incontinence recommendations of the international scientific committee: evaluations and treatment of urinary incontinence, pelvic organ prolapse, and fecal incontinence. *Neurourol Urodynam*, *29*(1), 213–240.

Centers for Disease Control and Prevention. *Urinary Tract Infection (Catheter-Associated Urinary Tract Infection [CAUTI] and Non-Catheter-Associated Urinary Tract Infection [UTI]) and Other Urinary System Infection [USI]) Events*. <http://www.cdc.gov/nhsn/PDFs/pscManual/7pscCAUTIcurrent.pdf>. Accessed June 9, 2015.

Cohen, D. (2008). Providing an assist. *Rehab Management*, *21*(8), 16–19.

Coulter, A. (2011). *Engaging Patients in Health Care*. Berkshire: McGraw Hill Open University Press.

Dowling-Castronovo, A., & Specht, J. K. (2009). How to try this: assessment of transient urinary incontinence in older adults. *The American Journal of Nursing*, *109*(2), 62–71.

Fader, M., Cottenden, A. M., & Getliffe, K. (2008). Absorbent products for moderate-heavy urinary and/or faecal incontinence in women and men. *Cochrane Database of Systematic Reviews*, (4), CD007408.

Fink, H. A., et al. (2008). Treatment interventions in nursing home residents with urinary incontinence: a systematic review of randomized trials. *Mayo Clinic Proceedings. Mayo Clinic*, *83*(12), 1332–1343.

Flanagan, L., Roe, B., Jack, B., et al. (2014). Factors with the management of incontinence and promotion of continence in older people in care homes. *Journal of Advanced Nursing*, *70*(3), 476–496.

Gray, M. (2010). Optimal management of incontinence-associated dermatitis in the elderly. *American Journal of Clinical Dermatology*, *11*(3), 201–210.

Howatson-Jones, L., Standing, M., & Roberts, S. (Eds.), (2012). *Patient Assessment and Care Planning in Nursing*. London: Sage Publications Inc.

Health Protection Agency (2013). *Ayliffe Hand Washing Technique*. Available at: <www.hpa.org.uk/Topics/InfectiousDiseases/infectionsAZ/Handwashing>. Accessed on 7th June 2015.

Keegan, W., & Knight, J. (2009). Addressing the problem of urinary incontinence. *Pract Nurse, 38*(8), 43–48.

Matthews, E. (2011). *Nursing Care Planning*. London: Lippincott Williams & Wilkins.

Nazarko, L. (2007). Continence problems following stroke. *Nursing Research Care, 9*(4), 152–155.

NICE (2013). *Urinary Incontinence: the management of urinary incontinence in women*. Available at: <www.nice.org.uk/guidance/cg171>. Accessed on 6th June 2015.

Ostaszkiewicz, J., Eustice, S., Roe, B., et al. (2013). *Toileting assistance programmes for the management of urinary incontinence in adults. Cochrane Incontinence Group*. Available at: <http://www.cochrane.org/CD010589/INCONT_toileting-assistance-programmes-for-the-management-of-urinary-incontinence-in-adults>. Accessed on 6th June 2015.

Poggesi, A., et al. (2008). Urinary complaints in non-disabled elderly people with age-related white matter changes: the leukoaraiosis and disability (LADIS) study. *Journal of the American Geriatrics Society, 56*(9), 1638–1643.

Reid, J. (2014). Managing urinary incontinence: guidelines for community nurses. *Journal of Christian Nursing, 28*(6), 20–26.

Rogers, M. A., et al. (2008). Use of urinary collection devices in skilled nursing facilities in five states. *Journal of the American Geriatrics Society, 56*(5), 854–861.

Sink, K. M., et al. (2008). Dual use of bladder anticholinergics and cholinesterase inhibitors: long-term functional and cognitive outcomes. *Journal of the American Geriatrics Society, 56*(5), 847–853.

St. Aubyn, B., & Andrews, A. (2012). Documentation. In M. Aldridge & S. Wanless (Eds.), *Developing Healthcare Skills through Simulation* (p. 2012). London: Sage Publications Inc.

Talley, K. M., Wyam, J. F., Bronas, U. G., et al. (2014). Factors associated with toileting disability in older adults without dementia living in residential care facilities. *Nursing Research, 63*(2), 94–104.

Wilde, M. H. (2002). Urine flowing: a phenomenological study of living with a urinary catheter. *Research in Nursing and Health, 25*, 14–24.

Overflow urinary Incontinence

Jane M. Kendall, RN, BS, CHT

NANDA-I

Definition

Involuntary loss of urine associated with overdistention of the bladder

Defining Characteristics

Bladder distention; high postvoid residual volume, involuntary leakage of small volume of urine, nocturia

Related Factors

Bladder outlet obstruction; detrusor external sphincter dyssynergia; detrusor hypocontractility; fecal impaction; severe pelvic prolapse; treatment regimen; urethral obstruction

NOC, NIC, Client Outcomes, Nursing Interventions, Client/Family Teaching and Discharge Planning, *Rationales*, and References

Refer to care plan for **Urinary Retention.**

Reflex urinary Incontinence

Amanda Andrews, MA, Ed, BSc, DN, RN, HEA Fellow, and Betty J. Ackley, MSN, EdS, RN

NANDA-I

Definition

Involuntary loss of urine at somewhat predictable intervals when a specific bladder volume is reached

Defining Characteristics

Absence of sensation of bladder fullness; absence of urge to void; absence of voiding sensation; inability to voluntarily inhibit voiding; inability to voluntarily initiate voiding; incomplete emptying of bladder with lesion above pontine micturition center; predictable pattern of voiding; sensation of bladder fullness; sensation of urgency to void without voluntary inhibition of bladder contraction

NOTE: Reflex urinary incontinence may be associated with sweating and acute elevation in blood pressure and pulse rate in clients with spinal cord injury. Refer to the care plan for **Autonomic Dysreflexia.**

Related Factors (r/t)

Neurological impairment above level of pontine micturition center; neurological impairment above level of sacral micturition center; tissue damage

NOC (Nursing Outcomes Classification)

Suggested NOC Outcomes

Urinary Continence; Urinary Elimination

Example NOC Outcome with Indicators

Urinary Continence as evidenced by the following indicators: Absence of urinary leakage between catheterizations or containment of micturition by condom catheter and drainage bag/Absence of symptomatic urinary tract infection (absence of leukocytes and absence of bacterial growth or >100,000 colony-forming units per milliliter)/Underclothing dry during day/ Underclothing or bedding dry during night. (Rate the outcome and indicators of **Urinary Continence:** 1 = never demonstrated, 2 = rarely demonstrated, 3 = sometimes demonstrated, 4 = often demonstrated, 5 = consistently demonstrated [see Section I].)

Client Outcomes

Client Will (Specify Time Frame)

- Follow prescribed schedule for bladder emptying
- Have intact perineal skin
- Remain clear of symptomatic urinary tract infection
- Demonstrate how to apply containment device or insert intermittent catheter or be able to provide caregiver with instructions for performing these procedures

NIC (Nursing Interventions Classification)

Suggested NIC Interventions

Urinary Catheterization: Intermittent; Urinary Elimination Management; Urinary Incontinence Care

Example NIC Activities—Urinary Elimination Management

Monitor urinary elimination including frequency, consistency, odor, volume, and color as appropriate; Teach client signs and symptoms of urinary tract infection

Nursing Interventions and *Rationales*

- Introduce yourself to the client and anyone accompanying him/her and inform them of your role. *Introducing yourself to a client helps establish and develop a therapeutic relationship that recognizes the person within the client and forms the bases for building trust on which to base the provision of care (Howatson-Jones, 2012).*
- Gain consent to carry out care before proceeding further with the assessment. *Clients have the right of autonomy both legally and morally and therefore should be fully involved in the decision-making process (Avery, 2013).*
- Wash hands using a recognized technique. EB: *Evidence shows that strict hand hygiene regimens significantly reduce the incidence of methicillin-resistant* Staphylococcus aureus *and* Clostridium difficile *(Health Protection Agency, 2013).*
- Assess usual pattern of bladder management and establish the extent of the problem (refer to Functional urinary **Incontinence** care plan). EB: *A detailed and accurate assessment of the client enables the nurse to plan interventions, monitor outcomes, and evaluate care, ensuring no unnecessary treatment is carried out (Matthews, 2011).*
- Ask the client to complete a bladder diary/log to determine the pattern of urine elimination, any incontinence episodes, and current bladder management program. An electronic voiding diary may be kept whenever feasible. EB: Use *of a bladder diary may reduce client discrepancies in recall and is a valuable tool for assessment of the bladder (Bright et al, 2011).*

- Consult with the health care provider concerning current bladder function and the potential of the bladder to produce hydronephrosis, vesicoureteral reflux, febrile urinary tract infection, or compromised renal function. *Whether the client has urinary retention directs the method of urine management to prevent damage to the renal system from unrelieved obstruction (Dorsher & McIntosh, 2012).*
- Consult with the health care provider and physical therapist concerning the neuromuscular ability to perform bladder management. The type of neurological disorder, as well as the level of neurological impairment and the ability to use the hands effectively, determines the method of urine management in reflex incontinence. EB: *Bladder symptoms and management options need to be in keeping with the client's level of general disability to be effective in managing the problem (Fowler et al, 2009).*
- Inspect the perineal and perigenital skin for signs of incontinence-associated dermatitis and pressure ulcers (Gray et al, 2007). CEB: *Standardizing skin care routines making them an integrated part of essential care for incontinence clients will improve client care in specialized areas, thus helping reduce the incidence of associated dermatitis. A research study on use of products to protect skin found that an evidence-based practice of using a product that cleansed and also protected the skin resulted in improved client care (Foxley & Baadjies, 2009).*
- In consultation with the rehabilitation team, counsel the client and family concerning the merits and potential risks associated with each possible bladder management program, including spontaneous voiding, intermittent self-catheterization, and reflex voiding with condom catheter containment and in some cases, indwelling suprapubic catheterization. *All bladder management programs carry some risk of urinary incontinence or serious urinary system complications (Newman & Willson, 2011).* EB: *Spontaneous voiding and intermittent catheterization carry greater risk of urine loss than condom catheter containment or indwelling catheter. A study demonstrated increased rates of complications and a high rate of infection with indwelling catheter use compared with other modes of management (Singh et al, 2011). Some studies support the use of suprapubic catheters for long-term treatment of reflex incontinence in spinal cord injury clients (Böthig et al, 2012; Colli & Lloyd, 2011).*

I

Intermittent Self-Catheterization (ISC)

- Begin intermittent catheterization as ordered using sterile technique; the client may be taught to use clean technique in the home situation. EB: *Intermittent catheterization is considered the preferred long-term management for a neurogenic bladder. Sterile intermittent catheterization should be used in hospitals, rehabilitation centers, and extended care facilities (Newman & Willson, 2011). There is an associated risk of urinary tract infection with any type of bladder management; however, by performing ISC the risk of urinary tract infections is reduced as the residual volume in the bladder is resolved (Winder, 2012).*
- Schedule the frequency of intermittent catheterization based on the frequency/volume records of previous catheterizations, functional bladder capacity, and the impact of catheterization on the quality of the client's life. *Bladder volumes must be kept lower to prevent development of urinary tract infection from retention of urine, and draining the urine regularly helps prevent movement of bacteria into the bladder long enough to produce symptomatic infection (Dorsher & McIntosh, 2012; Newman & Willson, 2011).*
- Teach the client to recognize signs of symptomatic urinary tract infection and to seek care promptly when these signs occur. The signs of symptomatic infection are the following:
  - Discomfort over the bladder or during urination
  - Acute onset of urinary incontinence
  - Fever
  - Markedly increased spasticity of muscles below the level of the spinal lesion
  - Malaise, lethargy
  - Hematuria
  - Autonomic dysreflexia (hyperreflexia) symptoms

Signs of symptomatic urinary tract infection as indicated above should be treated promptly with antimicrobial therapy, whereas asymptomatic bacteriuria should not generally be treated (Gupta & Trautner, 2011; Newman & Willson, 2011).

- Recognize that intermittent catheterization is typically associated with asymptomatic bacteriuria, and the indwelling catheter is routinely associated with asymptomatic colonization. EB: *Antibiotic treatment of asymptomatic bacteriuria has not proven helpful, but prompt management of symptomatic infection is necessary to prevent urosepsis or related complications (Gupta & Trautner, 2011).*

- Teach intermittent catheterization as the client approaches discharge as per operational guidelines and best practice. Instruct the client and at least one family member in the performance of catheterization. Teach the client with quadriplegia how to instruct others to perform this procedure. EB: *Intermittent catheterization is a safe and effective bladder management strategy for persons with reflex urinary incontinence. Inclusion of a family member is particularly helpful for the client with limited upper extremity dexterity and reflex urinary incontinence (Woodbury et al, 2008).*
- Teach the client managed by intermittent catheterization to self-administer antispasmodic (parasympatholytic) medications as prescribed by consulting health care provider and to recognize and manage potential side effects as needed. *Antimuscarinic medications enhance catheterized volumes and reduce the frequency of incontinence episodes in persons with reflex incontinence owing to spinal cord injury or multiple sclerosis (Fowler, 2011; Verpoorten & Buyse, 2008).*

Condom Catheter/Sheath System

- For a male client with reflex incontinence who does not have urinary retention and cannot manage the condition effectively with spontaneous voiding, does not choose to perform intermittent catheterization, or cannot perform catheterization, teach the client and his family to obtain, select, and apply an external collective device and urinary drainage system. Assist the client and family to choose a product that adheres to the glans penis or penile shaft without allowing seepage of urine onto surrounding skin or clothing, that avoids provoking hypersensitivity reactions on the skin, and that includes a urinary drainage reservoir that is easily concealed under the clothing and does not cause irritation to the skin of the thigh. EB: *Multiple components of the external collection device affect the product's ability to contain urinary leakage, protect underlying skin, and preserve the client's dignity (Kyle, 2011; Wells, 2008). National Institute for Health and Care Excellence (NICE) guidance (2012) advocates that all risks and benefits are discussed relating to the available sheath system options.*
- Teach the client whose incontinence is managed by a condom catheter to routinely inspect the skin with each catheter change for evidence of lesions caused by pressure from the containment device or by exposure to urine, to cleanse the penis thoroughly, and to reapply a new device daily or every other day. CEB: *Skin breakdown is a common complication associated with routine use of the condom catheter (Wells, 2008).*
- Ensure the client is aware of when and how to report any problems and/or complications of reflex incontinence care when at home. *Early detection allows for rapid diagnosis and treatment. Information about this should be individually presented to the clients, specifically tailored to their physical condition and cognitive abilities to encourage self-management (Swain, 2012).*
- Encourage a mindset and program of self-care management. CEB: *Addressing self-care activities through exercise, diet, fluid intake, and protective devices helps the client to exercise control over incontinence and may reduce the substantial burden affecting a significant proportion of spouse, partner, or familial care providers (Post et al, 2005).*
- Assist the family with arranging care in a way that allows the client to participate in family or favorite activities without embarrassment. Elicit discussion of the client's concerns about the social or emotional burden of incontinence. EB: *Urinary incontinence has a substantial negative impact on the quality of life for clients, both socially and financially. Further studies are needed to determine the true extent of the problem and to address it (Tapia et al, 2013).*
- Teach the client to ensure good hydration. Total daily fluid intake should be approximately 2.7 L per day for women and 3.7 L per day for men. *Adequate fluid helps wash out bacteria from the urethra to prevent urinary tract infections, helps prevent kidney stones, and potentially protects the client from development of cancer of the bladder from exposure to carcinogens concentrated in the urine (Newman & Willson, 2011).*
- Teach the client with a spinal injury the signs of autonomic dysreflexia, its relationship to bladder fullness, and management of the condition. Refer to the care plan for **Autonomic Dysreflexia.**
- Provide client with comprehensive written information about bladder care. EB: *Providing clients with well-written, evidence-based information about their condition and treatment can have a beneficial effect on the outcomes of treatment. In addition, clients are more likely to retain important information that will assist them in making informed decisions about their care (Coulter, 2011).*
- Document all care and advice given in a factual and comprehensive manner. *Good record keeping is an integral part of nursing practice and is essential to the provision of safe and effective care (St. Aubyn & Andrews, 2012).*

REFERENCES

Avery, G. (2013). *Law and Ethics in Nursing and Healthcare an Introduction*. London: Sage Publications Inc.

Böthig, R., Hirschfeld, S., & Thietje, R. (2012). Quality of life and urological morbidity in tetraplegics with artificial ventilation managed with suprapubic or intermittent catheterization. *Spinal Cord, 50*(3), 247–251.

Bright, E., Drake, M. J., & Abrams, P. (2011). Urinary diaries: evidence for the development and validation of diary content, format, and duration. *Neurourol Urodynam, 30*(3), 348–352.

Colli, J., & Lloyd, K. (2011). Bladder neck closure and suprapubic catheter placement as definitive management of neurogenic bladder. *The Journal of Spinal Cord Medicine, 34*(3), 273–277.

Coulter, A. (2011). *Engaging Patients in Health Care*. Berkshire: McGraw Hill Open University Press.

Dorsher, P., & McIntosh, P. (2012). Neurogenic bladder. *Advances in Urology*, 816274.

Fowler, C. (2011). Systematic review of therapy for neurogenic detrusor over activity. *Canadian Urological Association Journal, 5*(5 Suppl. 2), S146–S148.

Fowler, C. J., Paniker, J. N., Drake, M., et al. (2009). A UK consensus on the management of the bladder in multiple sclerosis. *Neurology, Neurosurgery and Psychiatry, 80*(5), 470–477.

Foxley, S., & Baadjies, R. (2009). Incontinence-associated dermatitis in patients with spinal cord injury. *British Journal of Nursing (Mark Allen Publishing), 18*(12), 719–723.

Gray, M., et al. (2007). Incontinence-associated dermatitis: a consensus. *Journal of Wound, Ostomy, and Continence Nursing, 24*(1), 45–56.

Gupta, K., & Trautner, B. (2011). Urinary tract infections, pyelonephritis, and prostatitis. In D. L. Longo, et al. (Eds.), *Harrison's principles of internal medicine* (18th ed.). New York: McGraw-Hill.

Health protection Agency. (2013). *Ayliffe Hand Washing Technique*. Available at: <http://www.hpa.org.uk/Topics/InfectiousDiseases/infectionsAZ/Handwashing>. Accessed on June 7, 2015.

Howatson-Jones, L., Standing, M., & Roberts, S. (Eds.), (2012). *Patient Assessment and Care Planning in Nursing*. London: Sage Publications Inc.

Kyle, G. (2011). The use of urinary sheaths in male incontinence. *British Journal of Nursing (Mark Allen Publishing), 20*(6), 338.

Matthews, E. (2011). *Nursing Care Planning*. London: Lippincott Williams & Wilkins.

Newman, D., & Willson, M. (2011). Review of intermittent catheterization and current best practices. *Urologic Nursing, 31*(1), 12–48.

NICE (August 2012). *Urinary Incontinence in neurological disease: Management of lower urinary tract dysfunction in neurological disease. NICE guidance CG128*. Available at: <http://www.nice.org.uk/guidance/CG148/chapter/4-Research-recommendations>. Accessed on 7th June 2015.

Post, M. W., Bloemen, J., & de Witte, L. P. (2005). Burden of support for partners of persons with spinal cord injuries. *Spinal Cord, 43*(5), 311–319.

Singh, R., et al. (2011). Bladder management methods and urological complications in spinal cord injury patients. *Indian Journal of Orthopaedics, 45*(2), 141–147.

St. Aubyn, B., & Andrews, A. (2012). Documentation. In M. Aldridge & S. Wanless (Eds.), *Developing Healthcare Skills through Simulation* (p. 2012). London: Sage Publications Inc.

Swain, S. (2012). *Urinary Incontinence in neurological disease: Management of lower urinary tract dysfunction in neurological disease: summary of NICE guidance*. Available at: <http://www.bmj.com/content/345/bmj.e5074>. Accessed on 7th July 2015.

Tapia, C., Khalaf, K., Berenson, K., et al. (2013). Health-related quality of life and economic impact of urinary incontinence due to detrusor overactivity associated with a neurological condition: a systematic review. *Health & Quality of Life Outcomes*, Available at: <http://www.biomedcentral.com/content/pdf/1477-7525-11-13.pdf>. Accessed on 4th June 2015.

Verpoorten, C., & Buyse, G. M. (2008). The neurogenic bladder: medical treatment. *Pediatric Nephrology (Berlin, Germany), 23*(5), 717–725.

Wells, M. (2008). Managing urinary incontinence with BIODERM external continence device. *British Journal of Nursing (Mark Allen Publishing), 17*(9), 524, 526–529.

Winder, A. (2012). Good Practice in Catheter Care. *Journal of Community Nursing, 26*(6), 15–20.

Woodbury, M. G., Hayes, K. C., & Askes, H. K. (2008). Intermittent catheterization practices following spinal cord injury: a national survey. *The Canadian Journal of Urology, 15*(3), 4065–4071.

I

Risk for Urge Urinary Incontinence

Betty J. Ackley, MSN, EdS, RN

NANDA-I

Definition

Vulnerable to involuntary passage of urine occurring soon after a strong sensation or urgency to void, which may compromise health

Risk Factors

Alcohol consumption; atrophic urethritis; atrophic vaginitis; detrusor hyperactivity with impaired bladder contractility; ineffective toileting habits; involuntary sphincter relaxation; small bladder capacity; treatment regimen

NIC, NOC, Client Outcomes, Nursing Interventions, Client/Family Teaching and Discharge Planning, *Rationales,* and References

Refer to care plan for Urge urinary **Incontinence.**

Stress Urinary Incontinence

Amanda Andrews, MA, Ed, BSc, DN, RN, HEA Fellow

NANDA-I

Definition

Sudden leakage of urine with activities that increase intra-abdominal pressure

Defining Characteristics

Involuntary leakage of small volume of urine (e.g., with coughing, laughing, sneezing, on exertion); involuntary leakage of small volume of urine in the absence of detrusor contraction; involuntary leakage of small volume of urine in the absence of overdistended bladder

Related Factors (r/t)

Degenerative changes in pelvic muscles; increase in intra-abdominal pressure; intrinsic urethral sphincter deficiency; weak pelvic muscles

I

NOC (Nursing Outcomes Classification)

Suggested NOC Outcomes

Urinary Continence; Urinary Elimination

Example NOC Outcome with Indicators

Urinary Continence as evidenced by the following indicators: Experiences no urine leakage with increased abdominal pressure (e.g., sneezing, laughing, lifting)/Voids in appropriate receptacle/Able to move to toilet after strong desire to urinate is perceived/Underclothing remains dry during day/Underclothing or bedding remains dry during night. (Rate the outcome and indicators of **Urinary Continence:** 1 = never demonstrated, 2 = rarely demonstrated, 3 = sometimes demonstrated, 4 = often demonstrated, 5 = consistently demonstrated [see Section I].)

Client Outcomes

Client Will (Specify Time Frame)

- Report fewer stress incontinence episodes and/or a decrease in the severity of urine loss
- Experience reduction in frequency of urinary incontinence episodes as recorded on voiding diary (bladder log)
- Identify containment devices that assist in management of stress incontinence

NIC (Nursing Interventions Classification)

Suggested NIC Interventions

Pelvic Muscle Exercises; Urinary Incontinence Care

Example NIC Activities—Urinary Incontinence Care

Explain etiology of problem and rationale for actions; Modify clothing and environment to provide easy access to toilet

Nursing Interventions and *Rationales*

- Introduce yourself to the client and anyone accompanying him/her and inform them of your role. *Introducing yourself to a client helps establish and develop a therapeutic relationship that recognizes the person within the client and forms the bases for building trust on which to base the provision of care (Howatson-Jones et al, 2012).*
- Gain consent to carry out care before proceeding further with the assessment. In clients unable to give consent, liaise with relevant health care professionals and/or family members. *Clients have the right of autonomy both legally and morally and therefore should be fully involved in the decision-making process (Avery, 2013).*

- Wash hands using a recognized technique. *Evidence shows that strict hand hygiene regimens significantly reduce the incidence of methicillin-resistant* Staphylococcus aureus *and* Clostridium difficile *(Health Protection Agency, 2013).*
- Assess usual pattern of bladder management and establish pattern of bladder management and extent of the problem to include: (refer to Functional urinary **Incontinence** care plan). EB: *A detailed and accurate assessment of the client enables the nurse to plan interventions, monitor outcomes, and evaluate care, ensuring no unnecessary treatment is carried out (Matthews, 2011).*
- Past Medical History (risk factors for stress incontinence): pregnancy, parity, large babies, forceps or breech deliveries, obesity, chronic cough, physical activity, previous urinary tract or gynecological surgery. *Nazarko (2007) identified the importance of considering other conditions that will affect an individual's ability to maintain continence.*
- Medication Review (diuretics, lithium, adrenergic blockers, diabetes, and smoking). EB: *The most common types of urinary incontinence in adult women are stress, urge, or a combination of both (Bradley et al, 2010). Many women are reluctant to initiate a discussion regarding incontinence; identifying women at risk is essential for effective screening (Keyock & Newman, 2011). Stress incontinence is caused by activities that create an increase in intra-abdominal pressure, such as coughing, sneezing, lifting, jumping, stair climbing, or exercise, whereas urge incontinence is caused by detrusor overactivity. Individuals may have mixed incontinence, and it is important to determine which symptom is the most troublesome to the individual in order to treat that first (McKertich, 2008).*
- Bladder Habits
    - Onset and duration of urinary leakage
    - Related lower urinary tract symptoms, including voiding frequency (day/night), urgency, severity (small, moderate, large amounts) of urinary leakage
    - Factors provoking urine loss (diuretics, bladder irritants, alcohol), focusing on the differential diagnosis of stress, urge or mixed stress, and urge urinary symptoms. Consider using a symptom questionnaire that elicits relevant lower urinary tract symptoms and provides differentiation between stress and urge incontinence symptoms.

▲ EB: *Stress urinary incontinence is more common in young and middle-aged women (Strothers & Friedman, 2011), is characterized by incontinence in small amounts (drops, spurts), no nocturia or incontinence at night, and incontinence without sensation of urine loss. With urge incontinence, the client has a strong, uncontrolled urge before losing a moderate to large volume of urine, and experiences frequency and nocturia (Nygaard et al, 2010). Clients with mixed urinary incontinence should be treated first for the predominant problem with conservative management for 8 to 12 weeks (Abrams et al, 2010).*

- Assess for mixed urinary incontinence (a combination of stress and urge incontinence):
    - Can you delay urination for a 2-hour movie or car ride?
    - How often do you arise at night to urinate?
    - When you have the urge to urinate, can you reach the toilet without leaking?

CEB/EB: *Farrell et al (2013) established that by using a questionnaire for urinary tract diagnosis, the client's ability to assess their own incontinence type was enhanced. These three questions have been found to reliably evaluate the presence of urge incontinence (Gray et al, 2001).*

- Lifestyle Assessment: impact on the individual's lifestyle. Inquire about incontinence pad use and change in daily, social, or recreational activities, as well as emotional impact. EB: *Incontinence is distressing and may contribute to decreased quality of life (Lasserre et al, 2009); psychological well-being, social interactions and activities, and sexual and interpersonal relationships may be negatively affected (Bartoli et al, 2010).*
- Inspect the perineal skin for evidence of incontinence-associated dermatitis, including inflammation, vesicles in skin exposed to urinary leakage, and especially skin folds or denudation of the skin, particularly when incontinence is managed by absorptive pads or containment briefs. EB: *Ammonia produced from the breakdown of urea in urine causes an increase in skin pH, which increases the permeability of the skin; excess moisture and damage to the acid mantle further increases permeability and vulnerability to bacterial and fungal infections (Langemo et al, 2011). Skin exposed to urine or stool will become bright red, and the surface may appear shiny due to serous exudate; inflamed areas of individuals with darker skin tones may be a duller red or hypopigmented when compared to adjacent skin. Inspect the skin for a maculopapular red rash typical of candidiasis (Gray, 2010).*
- Refer client for specific testing to further confirm diagnosis. If trained to do so, carry out cough stress test, request 24-hour pad test (if appropriate) and urodynamic studies (to include urine speed and flow, post-void residual measurement, leak point pressure, and pressure flow study). EB: *Markle et al (2011)*

I

established a greater agreement rating between cough stress test and urodynamics than between 24-hour pad test and urodynamics in the assessment of stress incontinence.

- Establish with client his/her current use of containment devices; evaluate the devices for their ability to adequately contain urine loss, protect clothing, and control odor. Assist the client in identifying containment devices specifically designed to contain urinary leakage. CEB: *Recommend the client buy incontinent products specifically designed to contain urine, utilizing hydrogel to contain fluid, and not use sanitary pads. Using a combination of products may be more effective and economical (Fader et al, 2008).* EB: *Recognize that incontinence products may present a significant financial burden to clients, with approximately 70% of expenditures attributed to containment devices, laundry, and dry cleaning expenses, which are often paid out of pocket (Chong et al, 2011).*
- Teach the client to complete a bladder diary by recording voiding frequency, the frequency and degree of urinary incontinence episodes, their association with urgency (a sudden and strong desire to urinate that is difficult to defer), fluid intake, and pad usage over a 3- to 7-day period. An electronic voiding diary may be kept whenever feasible. EB: *Use of a bladder diary may reduce client discrepancies in recall and is a valuable tool for assessment; short (24-hour) duration of the bladder diary may yield inadequate data, and excessive diary duration reduces compliance (Bright et al, 2011).*
- With the client and in close consultation with the health care provider, review treatment options, including behavioral management; drug therapy; use of a pessary, vaginal device, or urethral insert; and surgery. Outline their potential benefits, efficacy, and side effects. CEB: *Behavioral and nonsurgical treatments may improve symptoms in up to 70% of women; referral to a specialist may be indicated if conservative treatment is ineffective (Waetjen, 2008).*

Pelvic Floor Training Program

- *Pelvic floor muscle training is effective in the treatment of stress, urge, and mixed urinary incontinence; participation in a supervised program for at least 3 months may yield improved outcomes (Dumoulin & Hay-Smith, 2010).*
- Teach the client undergoing pelvic floor muscle training to identify, contract, and relax the pelvic floor muscles without contracting distal muscle groups (e.g., abdominal muscles or gluteus muscles) using verbal feedback based on vaginal or anal palpation, biofeedback, or electrical stimulation, utilizing the assistance of an incontinence specialist or health care provider as necessary. EB: *To find the proper muscles, the client may be instructed to think about trying to control the urge to pass gas; women will feel a lifting sensation in the vaginal area and a pulling in of the rectum (Keyock & Newman, 2011).* CEB: *When learning to control pelvic floor muscles, clients may recruit other muscles such as the rectus abdominis or gluteal muscles, which may be counterproductive; these muscles must be relaxed to avoid increasing pressure on the bladder or pelvic floor (Burgio et al, 2009).*
- Incorporate principles of exercise physiology into a pelvic muscle training program using the following strategies:
  - Begin a graded exercise program, usually starting with 5 to 10 repetitions and advancing gradually to no more than 35 to 50 repetitions every day or every other day based on baseline and ongoing evaluation of maximal strength and endurance.
  - Continue exercise sessions over a period of 3 to 6 months.
  - Integrate muscle training into activities of daily living.
  - Assess progress every 2 weeks during the first month and every 4 to 6 weeks thereafter.

Pelvic floor muscle training strengthens urethral sphincter tone (Chong et al, 2011) and is the first-line conservative approach for all types of incontinence and in particular for stress and mixed urinary incontinence; women report an improvement in symptoms and quality of life (Dumoulin & Hay-Smith, 2010).

Bladder Training Program

- Assist the client in completing a bladder diary over a period of a minimum of 3 days or up to 7 days.
  - Review the results with the client, determining typical voiding frequency and establishing goals for voiding frequency.
  - Using baseline voiding frequency, as determined by the diary, teach the client to urinate by the clock when awake, typically every 30 to 120 minutes.
  - Encourage adherence to the program with timing devices, as well as verbal encouragement and support, and address individual reasons for schedule interruption.

- ❍ Gradually increase the time between urinations to the negotiated goal. Time intervals between voiding are typically increased in increments of 15 to 30 minutes for clients with a baseline frequency of less than every 60 minutes and increments of 25 to 30 minutes for clients with a baseline frequency of more than every 60 minutes.

Bladder training reduces the frequency and severity of urinary leakage in women with stress incontinence, urge incontinence, and mixed incontinence. The result of bladder training in ambulatory, community-dwelling women is comparable to that achieved through pelvic floor muscle training (Milne, 2008).

- Teach the client to self-administer duloxetine and imipramine as ordered by consulting health care provider, and to monitor for adverse side effects. CEB/EB: *There are no prescriptive drugs approved for use in stress urinary incontinence in the United States. Nevertheless, several agents are sometimes prescribed to highly selected clients with stress urinary incontinence. They include duloxetine (Schagen van Leeuwen et al, 2008) and imipramine (Andersson, 2000).*
- Teach the client to self-administer topical (vaginal) estrogens as directed, and to monitor for adverse side effects. EB: *Postmenopausal estrogen deprivation may contribute to stress incontinence; topical vaginal medications reverse urogenital atrophic changes and may relieve lower urinary tract dysfunction (Ewies & Alfhaily, 2010).*
- Refer the female client with stress urinary incontinence and pelvic organ prolapse who wishes to employ a pessary to manage stress incontinence to a nurse specialist or gynecologist with expertise in the placement and maintenance of these devices. CEB: *Placement of an appropriately sized dish pessary resolved stress urinary incontinence in 60% of a group of 95 women (Noblett et al, 2008).*
- Discuss potentially reversible or controllable risk factors, such as weight loss, with the client with stress incontinence and assist the client to formulate a strategy to eliminate these conditions. *Although research supports a strong familial predisposition to stress incontinence among women, other risk factors, including obesity, smoking (Mishra et al, 2008), and chronic coughing from smoking, are reversible.* EB: *Being obese may increase pressure on the pelvic floor and doubles the risk for incontinence (Strothers & Friedman, 2011).*
- Provide information about support resources such as the National Association for Continence, The Simon Foundation for Continence, or the Total Control Program.
- Refer the client with persistent stress incontinence to a continence service, health care provider, or nurse who specializes in the management of this condition. *All clients presenting with incontinence should be offered an initial assessment by a suitably trained individual.*
- Teach the client to ensure good hydration. Total daily fluid intake should be approximately 2.7 L per day for women and 3.7 L per day for men. EB: *Adequate fluid helps wash out bacteria from the urethra to prevent urinary tract infections, helps prevent kidney stones, and potentially protects the client from development of cancer of the bladder from exposure to carcinogens concentrated in the urine (Newman & Willson, 2011).*
- Provide client with comprehensive written information about bladder care. EB: *Providing clients with well-written, evidence-based information about their condition and treatment can have a beneficial effect on the outcomes of treatment. In addition, clients are more likely to retain important information that will assist them in making informed decisions about their care (Coulter, 2011).*
- Encourage a mindset and program of self-care management. *Addressing self-care activities through exercise, diet, fluid intake, and protective devices helps the client exercise control over incontinence and may reduce the substantial care provider burden affecting a significant proportion of spouse, partner, or familial care providers (Post et al, 2005).*
- Assist the family with arranging care in a way that allows the client to participate in family or favorite activities without embarrassment. Elicit discussion of the client's concerns about the social or emotional burden of incontinence. EB: *Urinary incontinence has a substantial negative impact on the quality of life for clients, both socially and financially. Further studies are needed to determine the true extent of the problem and to address it (Tapia et al, 2013).*
- Document all care and advice given in a factual and comprehensive manner. *Good record keeping is an integral part of nursing practice and is essential to the provision of safe and effective care (St. Aubyn & Andrews, 2012).*

REFERENCES

Abrams, P., et al. (2010). Fourth international consultation on incontinence recommendations of the international scientific committee: evaluation and treatment of urinary incontinence, pelvic organ prolapse, and fecal incontinence. *Neurourol Urodynam, 29*, 213–240.

Andersson, K. E. (2000). Drug therapy for urinary incontinence. *Baillierė's Best Practice and Research. Clinical Obstetrics and Gynaecology, 14*(2), 291.

Avery, G. (2013). *Law and Ethics in Nursing and Healthcare an Introduction*. London: Sage Publications Inc.

Bartoli, S., Aguzzi, G., & Tarricone, R. (2010). Impact on quality of life of urinary incontinence and overactive bladder: a systematic literature review. *Urology, 75*(3), 491–500.

Bradley, C. S., et al. (2010). The questionnaire for urinary incontinence diagnosis (QUID): validity and responsiveness to change in women undergoing non-surgical therapies for treatment of stress predominant urinary incontinence. *Neurourol Urodynam, 29*(1), 726–733.

Bright, E., Drake, M. J., & Abrams, P. (2011). Urinary diaries: evidence for the development and validation of diary content, format, and duration. *Neurourol Urodynam, 30*(3), 348–352.

Burgio, K. L., et al. (2009). Behavioral treatment of urinary incontinence, voiding dysfunction, and overactive bladder. *Obstetrics and Gynecology Clinics of North America, 36*(3), 475–491.

Chong, E. C., Khan, A. A., & Anger, J. T. (2011). The financial burden of stress urinary incontinence among women in the United States. *Current Urology Reports, 12*(5), 358–362.

Coulter, A. (2011). *Engaging Patients in Health Care*. Berkshire: McGraw Hill Open University Press.

Dumoulin, C., & Hay-Smith, J. (2010). Pelvic floor muscle training versus no treatment, or inactive control treatments, for urinary incontinence in women. *Cochrane Database of Systematic Reviews*, (1), CD005654.

Ewies, A. A., & Alfhaily, F. (2010). Topical vaginal estrogen therapy in managing postmenopausal urinary symptoms: a reality or a gimmick? *Climacteric: The Journal of the International Menopause Society, 13*(5), 405–418.

Fader, M., Cottenden, A. M., & Getliffe, K. (2008). Absorbent products for moderate-heavy urinary and/or faecal incontinence in women and men. *Cochrane Database of Systematic Reviews, 4*, CD007408.

Farrell, S. A., Bent, A., Amir-Khalkhali, B., et al. (2013). Women's ability to assess their own urinary incontinence type using the QUID as an educational tool. *International Urogynaecology Journal, 24*(5), 759–762.

Gray, M. (2010). Optimal management of incontinence-associated dermatitis in the elderly. *American Journal of Clinical Dermatology, 11*(3), 201–210.

Gray, M., et al. (2001). A model for predicting motor urge urinary incontinence. *Nursing Research, 50*(2), 116–122.

Howatson-Jones, L., Standing, M., & Roberts, S. (Eds.), (2012). *Patient Assessment and Care Planning in Nursing*. London: Sage Publications Inc.

Health Protection Agency (2013). *Ayliffe Hand Washing Technique*. Available at: <www.hpa.org.uk/Topics/InfectiousDiseases/infectionsAZ/Handwashing>. Accessed on 7th June 2015.

Keyock, K., & Newman, D. (2011). Understanding stress urinary incontinence. *The Nurse Practitioner, 36*(10), 24–36.

Langemo, D., et al. (2011). Incontinence and incontinence-associated dermatitis. *Advances in Skin and Wound Care, 24*(3), 126–140.

Lasserre, A., et al. (2009). Urinary incontinence in French women: prevalence, risk factors, and impact on quality of life. *European Urology, 56*(1), 177–183.

Markle Price, D., & Noblett, K. (2011). Comparison of the cough stress test and 24hour pad test in the assessment of urinary incontinence. *International Journal of Urogynaecology, 23*(4), 429–433.

Matthews, E. (2011). *Nursing Care Planning*. London: Lippincott Williams & Wilkins.

McKertich, K. (2008). Urinary incontinence assessment in women: stress, urge or both? *Austr Fam Physician, 37*(3), 112–117.

Milne, J. (2008). Bladder training, guideline. In B. Ackley, et al. (Eds.), *Evidence-based nursing care guidelines*. Philadelphia: Mosby.

Mishra, G. D., et al. (2008). Body weight through adult life and risk of urinary incontinence in middle-aged women: results from a British prospective cohort. *International Journal of Obesity (2005), 32*(9), 1415–1422.

Nazarko, L. (2007). Reducing the risk of falls in the care home. *Nursing and Residential Care, 9*, 524–526.

Newman, D., & Willson, M. (2011). Review of intermittent catheterization and current best practices. *Urologic Nursing, 31*(1), 12–48.

Noblett, K. L., McKinney, A., & Lane, F. L. (2008). Effects of the incontinence dish pessary on urethral support and urodynamic parameters. *American Journal of Obstetrics and Gynecology, 198*(5), 592, e1–5.

Nygaard, I., et al. (2010). Clinical practice: idiopathic urgency urinary incontinence. *The New England Journal of Medicine, 363*(10), 1156–1162.

Post, M. W., Bloemen, J., & de Witte, L. P. (2005). Burden of support for partners of persons with spinal cord injuries. *Spinal Cord, 43*(5), 311–319.

Schagen van Leeuwen, J. H., et al. (2008). Efficacy and safety of duloxetine in elderly women with stress urinary incontinence or stress-predominant mixed urinary incontinence. *Maturitas, 60*(2), 138–147.

St. Aubyn, B., & Andrews, A. (2012). Documentation. In M. Aldridge & S. Wanless (Eds.), *Developing Healthcare Skills through Simulation*. London: Sage Publications Inc.

Strothers, L., & Friedman, B. (2011). Risk factors for the development of stress urinary incontinence in women. *Current Urology Reports, 12*, 363–369.

Tapia, C., Khalaf, K., Berenson, K., et al. (2013). Health-related quality of life and economic impact of urinary incontinence due to detrusor overactivity associated with a neurological condition: a systematic review. *Health & Quality of Life Outcomes*, Available at: <http://www.biomedcentral.com/content/pdf/1477-7525-11-13.pdf>. Accessed on 4th June 2015.

Waetjen, L. E. (2008). Management of stress urinary incontinence. *Menopause Manage, May/June*, 14–24.

Urge urinary Incontinence

Amanda Andrews, MA, Ed, BSc, DN, RN, HEA Fellow

NANDA-I

Definition

Involuntary passage of urine occurring soon after a strong sense of urgency to void

Defining Characteristics

Inability to reach toilet in time to avoid urine loss; involuntary loss of urine with bladder contractions; involuntary loss of urine with bladder spasms; urinary urgency

Related Factors (r/t)

Alcohol consumption; atrophic urethritis; atrophic vaginitis; bladder infection; caffeine intake; decrease in bladder capacity; detrusor hyperactivity with impaired bladder contractility; fecal impaction; treatment regimen

I

NOC (Nursing Outcomes Classification)

Suggested NOC Outcomes

Tissue Integrity: Skin and Mucous Membranes; Urinary Continence; Urinary Elimination

Example NOC Outcome with Indicators

Urinary Continence as evidenced by the following indicators: Responds in timely manner to urge/Voids in appropriate receptacle/Has adequate time to reach toilet between urge and evacuation of urine/Underclothing remains dry during day/Underclothing or bedding remains dry during night. (Rate the outcome and indicators of **Urinary Continence:** 1 = never demonstrated, 2 = rarely demonstrated, 3 = sometimes demonstrated, 4 = often demonstrated, 5 = consistently demonstrated [see Section I].)

Client Outcomes

Client Will (Specify Time Frame)

- Report relief from urge urinary incontinence or a decrease in the frequency of incontinent episodes
- Identify containment devices that assist in the management of urge urinary incontinence

NIC (Nursing Interventions Classification)

Suggested NIC Interventions

Urinary Habit Training; Urinary Incontinence Care

Example NIC Activities—Urinary Habit Training

Keep a continence specification record for 3 days to establish voiding pattern; establish interval for toileting of preferably not less than 2 hours

Nursing Interventions and *Rationales*

- Introduce yourself to the client and anyone accompanying him/her and inform them of your role. *Introducing yourself to a client helps establish and develop a therapeutic relationship that recognizes the person within the client and forms the bases for building trust on which to base the provision of care (Howatson-Jones et al, 2012).*
- Gain consent to carry out care before proceeding further with the assessment. *Clients have the right of autonomy both legally and morally and therefore should be fully involved in the decision-making process (Avery, 2013).*

- Wash hands using a recognized technique. *Evidence shows that strict hand hygiene regimens significantly reduce the incidence of methicillin-resistant* Staphylococcus aureus *and* Clostridium difficile *(Health Protection Agency, 2013).*
- Assess usual pattern of bladder management and establish pattern of bladder management and extent of the problem. *A detailed and accurate assessment of the client enables the nurse to plan interventions, monitor outcomes, and evaluate care, ensuring no unnecessary treatment is carried out (Matthews, 2011).* Refer to Functional urinary **Incontinence** care plan.
- Bladder Habits and Quality of Life Issues:
  - Diurnal frequency (voiding more than once every 2 hours while awake)
  - Urgency, daytime frequency and nocturia
  - Involuntary leakage and leakage accompanied by or preceded by urgency
  - Amount of urine loss—moderate or large volume
  - Severity of symptoms
  - Alleviating and aggravating factors
  - Effect on quality of life

▲ EB: *Incontinence is distressing and may contribute to decreased quality of life (Lassere et al, 2009); psychological well-being, social interactions and activities, and sexual and interpersonal relationships may be negatively affected (Bartoli et al, 2010). Urge urinary incontinence occurs when involuntary leakage of urine is accompanied by or immediately preceded by urgency; overactive bladder is characterized by the storage symptoms of urgency with or without incontinence and is usually accompanied by frequency and nocturia (Abrams et al, 2010).*

- Ask specific questions relating to urge presentation:
  - Can you delay urination for a 2-hour movie or car ride?
  - How often do you wake at night to urinate?
  - When you have the urge to urinate, can you reach the toilet without leaking?

▲ EB: *A history of urine loss associated with urgency is the most helpful criterion for diagnosing urge urinary incontinence (Holroyd-Leduc et al, 2011). These three questions have been found to reliably evaluate the presence of urge incontinence (Gray et al, 2001).*

- In close consultation with a health care practitioner or advanced practice nurse, consider administering a symptom questionnaire that elicits relevant lower urinary tract symptoms and differentiates stress and urge incontinence symptoms. CEB: *The Urogenital Distress Inventory, short form (UDI-6) is a reliable and valid tool for identifying types of urinary incontinence (Dowling-Castronovo, 2008).*
- Assess the severity of incontinence as well as the impact on the individual's lifestyle; inquire about incontinence pad use and change in daily, social, or recreational activities, as well as emotional impact. EB: *Incontinence is distressing and may contribute to decreased quality of life, especially for women with mixed incontinence (Lassere et al, 2009).*
- Perform a focused physical assessment, if competent to do so, alternatively in close consultation with a health care practitioner or advanced practice nurse including:
  - Bladder palpation after voiding to check for retention
  - Bladder scanning for post-void residual
  - Inspection of the perineal skin
  - Vaginal examination to determine hypoestrogenic changes in the mucosa (may contribute to urge incontinence)
  - Pelvic examination to determine the presence, location, and severity of vaginal wall prolapse, and reproduction of stress urinary incontinence with the cough test
  - Anal tone and constipation should be assessed. *A thorough abdominal and pelvic examination must be completed to accurately assess incontinence; assess for neurological conditions or heart failure (cause of nocturia) as warranted (McKertich, 2008).*
- Inspect the perineal and perianal skin for evidence of incontinence-associated dermatitis, including inflammation, vesicles in skin exposed to urinary leakage, and especially skin folds or denudation of the skin, particularly when incontinence is managed by absorptive pads or containment briefs. EB: *Ammonia produced from the breakdown of urea in urine causes an increase in skin pH, which increases the permeability of the skin; excess moisture and damage to the acid mantle further increases permeability and vulnerability to bacterial and fungal infections (Langemo et al, 2011). Skin exposed to urine or stool will become bright red, and the surface may appear shiny due to serous exudate; inflamed areas of individuals with darker skin*

tones may be a duller red or hypopigmented when compared to adjacent skin. Inspect the skin for a maculopapular red rash typical of candidiasis (Gray, 2010).

- Teach the client to complete a bladder diary by recording voiding frequency, the frequency and degree of urinary incontinence episodes, their association with urgency (a sudden and strong desire to urinate that is difficult to defer), fluid intake, and pad usage over a 3- to 7-day period. An electronic voiding diary may be kept whenever feasible. In addition to these parameters, the client may be asked to record voided volume and fluid intake. EB: *Use of a bladder diary may reduce client discrepancies in recall and is a valuable tool for assessment; short (24-hour) duration of the bladder diary may yield inadequate data, and excessive diary duration reduces compliance (Bright et al, 2011).*
- Review all medications the client is receiving, paying particular attention to sedatives, opioid analgesics, diuretics, antidepressants, psychotropic drugs, and cholinergics. Consult the health care practitioner or nurse practitioner about altering or eliminating these medications if they are suspected of affecting incontinence. EB: *All medications should be reviewed to determine whether they are contributing to incontinence (Abrams et al, 2010).*
- Assess the client for urinary retention (see the care plan for **Urinary Retention**).
- Assess the client for functional limitations (environmental barriers, limited mobility or dexterity, impaired cognitive function). EBN: *Du Moulin et al (2008) analyzed a group of 2866 clients receiving home care and found that functional impairment (poor mobility) was associated with an increased likelihood of urinary incontinence.* Refer to the care plan for Functional urinary **Incontinence.**
- Consult the health care practitioner concerning diabetic management or pharmacotherapy for urinary tract infection when indicated. In specific cases, urgency and an increased risk of urge incontinence may be related to bacteriuria or urinary tract infection (Rodhe et al, 2008).
- Assess for signs and symptoms of atrophic vaginal changes in the perimenopausal or postmenopausal woman, including vaginal dryness, tenderness to touch, mucosal dryness, friability, and discomfort with gentle palpation. Specifically query the woman with atrophic vaginitis concerning associated lower urinary tract symptoms (usually voiding frequency, urgency, and dysuria). Refer the woman with atrophic vaginal changes and bothersome lower urinary tract symptoms to a gynecologist, urologist, or women's health nurse practitioner for further evaluation and management. *Vaginal topical estrogens may reduce urge incontinence, prevent urogenital atrophy, and prevent recurrent urinary tract infections (Hillard, 2010).*

I

Pelvic Floor Training Program

- *Pelvic floor muscle training is effective in the treatment of stress, urge, and mixed urinary incontinence; participation in a supervised program for at least 3 months may yield improved outcomes (Dumoulin & Hay-Smith, 2010).*
- Teach the client undergoing pelvic floor muscle training to identify, contract, and relax the pelvic floor muscles without contracting distal muscle groups (e.g., abdominal muscles or gluteus muscles) using verbal feedback based on vaginal or anal palpation, biofeedback, or electrical stimulation, utilizing the assistance of an incontinence specialist or health care practitioner as necessary. EB: *To find the proper muscles, the client may be instructed to think about trying to control the urge to pass gas; women will feel a lifting sensation in the vaginal area and a pulling in of the rectum (Keyock & Newman, 2011). When learning to control pelvic floor muscles, clients may recruit other muscles such as the rectus abdominis or gluteal muscles, which may be counterproductive; these muscles must be relaxed to avoid increasing pressure on the bladder or pelvic floor (Burgio, 2009).*
- Incorporate principles of exercise physiology into a pelvic muscle training program using the following strategies:
  - Begin a graded exercise program, usually starting with 5 to 10 repetitions and advancing gradually to no more than 35 to 50 repetitions every day or every other day based on baseline and ongoing evaluation of maximal strength and endurance.
  - Continue exercise sessions over a period of 3 to 6 months.
  - Integrate muscle training into activities of daily living.
  - Assess progress every 2 weeks during the first month and every 4 to 6 weeks thereafter.

Pelvic floor muscle training strengthens urethral sphincter tone (Chong, Khan, & Anger, 2011) and is the first-line conservative approach for all types of incontinence and in particular for stress and mixed urinary incontinence; women report an improvement in symptoms and quality of life (Dumoulin & Hay-Smith, 2010).

Bladder Training Program

- Assist the client in completing a voiding diary over a period of a minimum of 3 days or up to 7 days.
- Review the results with the client, determining typical voiding frequency and establishing goals for voiding frequency based on the longest time interval between voids that is comfortable for the client.
- Using baseline voiding frequency, as determined by the diary, teach the client to void first thing in the morning, every time the predetermined voiding interval passes, and before going to bed at night.
- Encourage adherence to the program with timing devices and verbal encouragement and support, and address individual reasons for schedule interruption.
- Teach distraction and urge suppression techniques (see later discussion) to control urgency while the client postpones urination.
- Gradually increase the time between urinations to the negotiated goal. Time intervals between voiding are typically increased in increments of 15 to 30 minutes for clients with a baseline frequency of less than every 60 minutes and increments of 25 to 30 minutes for clients with a baseline frequency of more than every 60 minutes. The voiding interval should be increased by 15 to 30 minutes each week (based on the client's tolerance) until a voiding interval of 3 to 4 hours is achieved. Utilize a bladder diary to monitor progress. CEB: *Improvement rates using bladder training range from 57% to 87% (Wyman et al, 2009). With bladder training, the goal is to restore normal bladder function through the use of a voiding schedule; the woman voids at predetermined intervals rather than in response to urgency, progressively increasing the intervals between voiding. Distraction and relaxation techniques may be used to postpone voiding (Wyman et al, 2009).*
- Review with the client the types of beverages consumed, focusing on the intake of caffeine, which is associated with a transient effect on lower urinary tract symptoms. Advise all clients to reduce or eliminate intake of caffeinated beverages or over-the-counter medications of dietary aids containing caffeine. Identify and counsel the client to eliminate other bladder irritants that may exacerbate incontinence, such as smoking, carbonated beverages, citrus, sugar substitutes, and tomato products. CEB: *Caffeine is a diuretic, is a bladder irritant, increases detrusor pressure, and is a risk factor for detrusor instability; reducing caffeine may decrease both stress and urge incontinence. Decrease caffeine gradually to avoid caffeine withdrawal. Carbonated beverages, citrus fruits, sugar substitutes, and tomato products may be bladder irritants (Burgio, 2009). Chemicals from smoking are bladder irritants (Wyman et al, 2009).*
- Review with the client the volume of fluids consumed; fluids may be reduced with caution, *particularly in clients who do not drink more than 1500 mL during the day*, to alleviate urinary frequency, especially in the evening after 6 PM or 3 to 4 hours before bedtime to reduce nocturia. EB: *Be aware that adequate fluid intake is essential; six 8-oz glasses per 24 hours, 1500 mL, or 30 mL/kg body weight is recommended. The type and amount of fluid intake is associated with frequency and urge urinary incontinence (Segal et al, 2011). Excessive fluid intake may exacerbate incontinence; fluid restriction may cause an increase in urine concentration, which may cause bladder mucosa irritation that promotes urgency, frequency, and urinary tract infection (Wyman et al, 2009).*
- Teach the client methods to avoid constipation (refer to **Constipation** care plans) such as increasing dietary fiber, moderately increasing fluid intake, exercising, and establishing a routine defecation schedule. CEB: *Women with severe constipation demonstrate changes in pelvic floor neurological function; alleviation of constipation may significantly improve frequency and urgency in older clients (Wyman et al, 2009).*

Urge Suppression

- *Urge suppression skills are essential in helping clients learn a new way of responding to the sense of urgency. Rushing to the toilet increases physical pressure on the bladder, enhances the sensation of fullness, exposes the client to visual cues that can trigger incontinence, and exacerbates urgency (Burgio, 2009).*
- Teach the client the following techniques:
  - When a strong or precipitous urge to urinate is perceived, teach the client to avoid running to the toilet.
  - Pause, sit down, and relax the entire body.
  - Perform repeated, rapid pelvic muscle contractions until the urge is relieved.
  - Use distraction: count backward from 100 by sevens, recite a poem, write a letter, balance a checkbook, do handwork such as knitting, take five deep breaths, focusing on breathing.

   - Relief is followed by micturition within 5 to 15 minutes, using nonhurried movements when locating a toilet and voiding.
   - Use urge suppression strategies on waking during the night. If the urge subsides, the client should be encouraged to go back to sleep. If after a minute or two it does not, clients should be instructed to get up to void to avoid sleep interruption. EB: *Behavioral training for urge incontinence can reduce nocturia (Burgio, 2009).*
- Teach the client to self-administer antimuscarinic (anticholinergic) drugs as directed. Teach dosage side effects and administration of the medication and the importance of combining pharmacotherapy with scheduled voiding, adequate fluid intake, restriction of bladder irritants, and urge suppression techniques. EB: *Antimuscarinic drugs increase bladder capacity, reduce the frequency of incontinence episodes, and diminish voiding frequency. However, they do not cure bladder dysfunction or reduce the time between perception of a strong urge and onset of an overactive detrusor contraction. Approximately two thirds of clients treated with antimuscarinic medication discontinue use within 3 to 4 months; the efficacy of pharmacotherapy for urge incontinence is enhanced when combined with behavioral interventions (Burgio et al, 2010).*
- Assist the client in selecting, obtaining, and applying a containment device for urine loss as indicated. *The use of containment devices can be useful as "stop gap" strategies used alongside long-term management options (Reid, 2014).*
- Provide the client with information about incontinence support groups such as the National Association for Continence and the Simon Foundation for Continence. A helpful website titled Total Control (http://www.totalcontrolprogram.com/Pelvic+Health/Bladder+Health) can be accessed to give support and information to women with incontinence. EB: *Knowledge contributes to effective self-management; women with incontinence often do not seek help from others and prefer to self-manage their incontinence (Holroyd-Leduc et al, 2011).*
- Assess the functional and cognitive status of all clients with urge incontinence; use interventions to improve mobility. EB: *Functional limitations affect the severity and management of urge urinary incontinence; strategies to improve physical function may decrease incontinence (Tamanini et al, 2009).*
- Refer client for occupational therapy for help in obtaining assistive devices and adapting the home for optimal toilet accessibility. *An occupational therapist may suggest adaptations to clothing or to the environment to assist with functional incontinence (Keegan & Knight, 2009).*
- Encourage the client to develop an action plan for self-care management of incontinence. *Making an action plan facilitates behavior change (Lippke et al, 2009).*
- Provide client with comprehensive written information about bladder care. EB: *Providing clients with well-written, evidence-based information about their condition and treatment can have a beneficial effect on the outcomes of treatment. In addition, clients are more likely to retain important information that will assist them in making informed decisions about their care (Coulter, 2011).*
- Document all care and advice given in a factual and comprehensive manner. *Good record keeping is an integral part of nursing practice and is essential to the provision of safe and effective care (St. Aubyn & Andrews, 2012).*

I

REFERENCES

Abrams, P., et al. (2002). The standardization of terminology of lower urinary tract function: report from the standardization sub-committee of the international continence society. *American Journal of Obstetrics and Gynecology, 187*(1), 116–126.

Avery, G. (2013). *Law and Ethics in Nursing and Healthcare an Introduction*. London: Sage Publications Inc.

Bartoli, S., Aguzzi, G., & Tarricone, R. (2010). Impact on quality of life of urinary incontinence and overactive bladder: a systematic literature review. *Urology, 75*(3), 491–500.

Bright, E., Drake, M. J., & Abrams, P. (2011). Urinary diaries: evidence for the development and validation of diary content, format, and duration. *Neurourol Urodynam, 30*(3), 348–352.

Burgio, K. L. (2009). Behavioral treatment of urinary incontinence, voiding dysfunction, and overactive bladder. *Obstetrics and Gynecology Clinics of North America, 36*(3), 475–491.

Burgio, K. L., et al. (2010). The effects of drug and behavior therapy on urgency and voiding frequency. *International Urogynecology Journal, 21*(6), 711–719.

Chong, E. C., Khan, A. A., & Anger, J. T. (2011). The financial burden of stress urinary incontinence among women in the United States. *Current Urology Reports, 12*(5), 358–362.

Coulter, A. (2011). *Engaging Patients in Health Care*. Berkshire: McGraw Hill Open University Press.

Dowling-Castronovo, A. (2008). *Urinary incontinence assessment in older adults: part II-established urinary incontinence.* from Try This: Best Practices in Nursing Care to Older Adults, Hartford Institute for Geriatric Nursing, New York University, College of Nursing. <http://consultgerirn.org/uploads/File/trythis/try_this_11_2.pdf>. Retrieved November 3, 2011.

Dumoulin, C., & Hay-Smith, J. (2010). Pelvic floor muscle training versus no treatment, or inactive control treatments, for urinary incontinence in women. *Cochrane Database of Systematic Reviews*, (1), CD005654.

Du Moulin, M. F., et al. (2008). Prevalence of urinary incontinence among community-dwelling adults receiving home care. *Research in Nursing and Health*, *31*(6), 604–612.

Gray, M. (2010). Optimal management of incontinence-associated dermatitis in the elderly. *American Journal of Clinical Dermatology*, *11*(3), 201–210.

Gray, M., et al. (2001). A model for predicting motor urge urinary incontinence. *Nursing Research*, *50*(2), 116–122.

Hillard, T. (2010). The postmenopausal bladder. *Menopause International*, *16*(2), 74–80.

Holroyd-Leduc, J. M., et al. (2011). Translation of evidence into a self-management tool for use by women with urinary incontinence. *Age and Ageing*, *40*(2), 227–233.

Howatson-Jones, L., Standing, M., & Roberts, S. (Eds.), (2012). *Patient Assessment and Care Planning in Nursing*. London: Sage Publications Inc.

Health Protection Agency (2013). *Ayliffe Hand Washing Technique*. Available at: <www.hpa.org.uk/Topics/InfectiousDiseases/infectionsAZ/Handwashing>. Accessed on 7th June 2015.

Keegan, W., & Knight, J. (2009). Addressing the problem of urinary incontinence. *Pract Nurse*, *38*(8), 43–48.

Keyock, K., & Newman, D. (2011). Understanding stress urinary incontinence. *The Nurse Practitioner*, *36*(10), 24–36.

Langemo, D., et al. (2011). Incontinence and incontinence-associated dermatitis. *Advances in Skin and Wound Care*, *24*(3), 126–140.

Lassere, A., et al. (2009). Urinary incontinence in French women: prevalence, risk factors, and impact on quality of life. *European Urology*, *56*(1), 177–183.

Lippke, S., et al. (2009). Self-efficacy moderates the mediation of intentions into behavior via plans. *American Journal of Health Behavior*, *33*(5), 521–529.

Matthews, E. (2011). *Nursing Care Planning*. London: Lippincott Williams & Wilkins.

McKertich, K. (2008). Urinary incontinence assessment in women: stress, urge or both? *Australian Family Physician*, *37*(3), 112–117.

Reid, J. (2014). Managing urinary incontinence: guidelines for community nurses. *Journal of Christian Nursing*, *28*(6), 20–26.

Rodhe, N., et al. (2008). Bacteriuria is associated with urge urinary incontinence in older women. *Scandinavian Journal of Primary Health Care*, *26*(1), 35–39.

Segal, S., Saks, E. K., & Arya, L. A. (2011). Self-assessment of fluid intake behavior and the relationship to lower urinary tract symptoms in women with urinary incontinence. *Journal of Women's Health*, *20*, 1–5.

St. Aubyn, B., & Andrews, A. (2012). Documentation. In M. Aldridge & S. Wanless (Eds.), *Developing Healthcare Skills through Simulation* (p. 2012). London: Sage Publications Inc.

Tamanini, J. T. N., et al. (2009). Analysis of the prevalence of and factors associated with urinary incontinence among elderly people in the municipality of Sao Paulo, Brazil: SABE study (health, wellbeing and aging). *Cadernos De Saude Publica*, *25*(8), 1756–1762.

Wyman, J. F., Burgio, K. L., & Newman, D. K. (2009). Practical aspects of lifestyle modifications and behavioral interventions in the treatment of overactive bladder and urgency urinary incontinence. *International Journal of Clinical Practice*, *63*(8), 1122–1123.

Disorganized Infant behavior

Mary Alice DeWys, RN, BS, CIMI, and Margaret Elizabeth Padnos, RN, AB, BSN, MA

NANDA-I

Definition

Disintegrated physiological and neurobehavioral responses of infant to the environment

Defining Characteristics

Attention-Interaction System

Impaired response to sensory stimuli (e.g., difficult to soothe, unable to sustain alertness)

Motor System

Alteration in primitive reflexes; exaggerated startle response; finger splaying; fisting; hands to face; hyperextension of extremities; impaired motor tone; jitteriness; tremor; twitching; uncoordinated movement

Physiological

Abnormal skin color (e.g., pale, dusky, cyanosis); arrhythmia; bradycardia; desaturation; feeding intolerance; tachycardia; time-out signals (e.g., gaze, hiccough, sneeze, slack jaw, open mouth, tongue thrust)

Regulatory Problems

Inability to inhibit startle reflex; irritability

State-Organization System

Active-awake (e.g., fussy, worried gaze); diffuse alpha EEG activity with eyes closed; irritable crying; quiet-awake (e.g., staring, gaze aversion); state oscillation

Related Factors

Caregiver

Cue misreading; environmental overstimulation; insufficient knowledge of behavioral cues

Environmental

Inadequate physical environment; insufficient containment within environment; insufficient sensory stimulation; sensory deprivation; sensory overstimulation

Individual

Illness; immature neurological functioning; low postconceptual age; prematurity

Postnatal

Feeding intolerance; impaired motor functioning; invasive procedure; malnutrition; oral impairment; pain

Prenatal

Congenital disorder; exposure to teratogen; genetic disorder

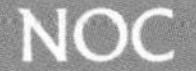

NOC (Nursing Outcomes Classification)

Suggested NOC Outcomes

Child Development; Neurological Status; Preterm Infant Organization; Sleep; Thermoregulation: Newborn; Infant Nutritional Status

Example NOC Outcome with Indicators

Preterm Infant Organization as evidenced by the following indicators: O_2 saturation >85%/Thermoregulation/Sleep-awake state organization/Smooth transition between states/Ability to attend to visual and auditory stimuli/Habituation. (Rate the outcome and indicators of **Preterm Infant Organization:** 1 = severely compromised, 2 = substantially compromised, 3 = moderately compromised, 4 = mildly compromised, 5 = not compromised [see Section I].)

Client Outcomes

Client Will (Specify Time Frame)

Infant/Child

- Display physiological/autonomic stability: cardiopulmonary, digestive functioning
- Display signs of organized motor system (Wyngarden et al, 1999)
- Display signs of organized state system: ability to achieve and maintain a state, and transition smoothly between states (Wyngarden et al, 1999)
- Demonstrate progress toward effective self-regulation (Wyngarden et al, 1999)
- Demonstrate progress toward or ability to maintain calm attention
- Demonstrate progress or ability to engage in positive interactions
- Demonstrate ability to respond to sensory information (visual, auditory, tactile) in an adaptive way

Parent/Significant Other

- Recognize infant/child behaviors as complex communication system that express specific needs and wants (e.g., hunger, pain, stress, desire to engage or disengage)
- Educate parents/caregivers to recognize infant's avenues of neuro-behavioral communication: autonomic/physiological, motor, state, attention/interaction
- Recognize how infants respond to environmental sensory input through stress/avoidance and approach/engagement behaviors
- Recognize and support infant's self-regulatory, coping behaviors used to regain or maintain homeostasis
- Teach parents to "tune in" to their own interactive style and how that affects their infant's behavior
- Teach parents ways to adapt their interactive style in response to infant's style of communication
- Identify appropriate positioning and handling techniques that will enhance normal motor development (Wyngarden et al, 1999)

- Promote infant/child's attention capabilities that support visual and auditory development (Wyngarden et al, 1999)
- Engage in pleasurable parent-infant interactions that encourage bonding and attachment (Wyngarden et al, 1999)
- Structure and modify the environment in response to infant/child's behavior and personal needs (Wyngarden et al, 1999)
- Identify available community resources that provide early intervention services, emotional support, community health nursing, and parenting classes (Wyngarden et al, 1999)

NIC (Nursing Interventions Classification)

Suggested NIC Interventions

Developmental Enhancement; Infant; Positioning; Sleep Enhancement

Example NIC Activities—Developmental Enhancement, Infant

Provide information to parent about child development and child rearing; Promote and facilitate family bonding and attachment with infant

Nursing Interventions and *Rationales*

- Recognize the neurobehavior systems through which infants communicate organization and/or disorganization/stress (i.e., physiological/autonomic, motor, states, attention/interactional, self-regulatory). CEB: *The Assessment of Preterm Infants' Behavior (APIB) is based on theory that each subsystem functions independently and interactively with the other subsystems. Infant's physiological/autonomic subsystem has to be stable/organized, cardiopulmonary system enabling infant to attend and/or interact with animate and inanimate environment (Als et al, 2005).*
- Recognize behavior used to communicate stress/avoidance and approach/engagement. CEB: *The neurobehavior system theory provides a framework for reading, interpreting, and responding to cues that values the infant's importance and ability to affect the environment (Als et al, 2005).*
- Provide high quality individualized developmental care for low-birth-weight preterm infants shown to positively influence neurodevelopmental outcomes. CEB: *Study found positive correlation between neonatal intensive care units (NICUs) providing high-quality individualized developmental care and neurodevelopmental outcomes (Montirosso et al, 2012).*
- Identify and manage pain using appropriate pain management techniques during invasive procedures (e.g., tube insertion, heel sticks, intravenous lines). EB: *Parents shown infant pain cues and comforting techniques were better prepared to take an active role in pain management and felt more positive about their parenting role in the post-discharge period (Franck et al, 2011).* EB: *Pacifier with sucrose is safe and effective for reducing procedural pain from single events (Stevens et al, 2013).* EBN: *Skin-to-skin reduces procedural pain (Johnson et al, 2014).*
- Provide developmentally appropriate positioning to optimize musculoskeletal development and neurological development, and minimize complications; alternate positions over 24-hour period between prone, supine, and lateral side lying to support body alignment, flexion, midline orientation, and hand to mouth and to avoid head and neck hyperextension. CEB: *Positioning using blanket rolls and gel pillows in NICU compensates for preterm infant's immature motor system (Bobish & Stanger, 2007). Developmentally correct positioning can prevent neuromuscular and postural abnormalities (Halverson, 2010).*
- Provide care that supports development of state organization: ability to achieve and maintain quiet sleep and quiet awake states and to transition smoothly between sleep and awake states. EB: *Skin-to-skin holding (kangaroo care) was found to increase quiet sleep (Scher et al, 2009).* EB: *Study found infants experiencing smooth shifts between quiet sleep and awake states had more positive emotions, better cognitive and verbal skills at 5 years of age compared with those having abrupt shifts between states of high arousal, active sleep, and shorter periods of active and quiet sleep (Weisman et al, 2011).* EB: *Swaddled infants had less spontaneous awakening than when unswaddled (Franco et al, 2005).*

- Monitor level of noise in NICU environment; guidelines recommend 49 dB (1 ± 1.4). EB: *Study examined noise level, collected data in three phases, results, reduction of NICU noise level (Wang, 2014).* Recognize and expand infant's ability to focus attention on voices and faces. EBN: *Assist parents to identify and support infant's attention capability (Jean & Stack, 2012).*
- Provide infants with several opportunities for nonnutritive sucking. CEB: *Infants receiving nonnutritive sucking during tube feeding exhibited less defensive behaviors, were less fussy, and fell asleep more easily (Pinelli & Symington, 2010).* CEB: *Study found infants using pacifiers proceeded to oral feedings faster than infants listening only to lullabies (Yildiz & Arikan, 2012).*
- Provide parents opportunities to experience physical closeness through loving touch, massage, cuddling, skin-to-skin (kangaroo care), which enhances parent-infant attachment. EBN: *Match preterm infants' developmental needs with parents' readiness for skin-to-skin care for best results (Lemmen et al, 2013);* EBN: *Kangaroo care positively impacts mother-infant relationship, sleep, and brain maturation (Ludington-Hoe, 2013).*
- Educate parents in ways to support infant's self-regulating behaviors. EB: *"Quality of maternal touch and still-face were associated with infants' self-regulating behaviors and effective component of infants' emotional regulation" (Jean & Stack, 2012).*
- Encourage parents to be active collaborators in their infant's care. EB: *Kangaroo care is an effective way for parents to actively engage by decreasing infant pain during invasive procedures (Akcan et al, 2009).* EBN: *If possible, time intramuscular injections during kangaroo care (Kashaninia et al, 2008).* EBN: *Fathers often hide emotions and need encouragement to express feelings and physically touch their babies (Johnson, 2008).*
- Provide infants with positive sensory experiences (i.e., visual, auditory, tactile, olfactory, vestibular, proprioceptive) to enhance development of sensory pathways. EBN: *Maternal voice along with other sensory events helped develop and maturate infant's overall developmental process and gave mothers more assurance, and infants were discharged earlier from hospital (Cevasco, 2008).* EB: *Classical music by Mozart had positive effect on energy expenditure in growing preterm infants (Lubetzky et al, 2010).* EBN: *Study supported positive results of kangaroo care for parents, and promoting health and development of the preterm infant (Head, 2014).* EB: *Odor of breast milk is an effective method for decreasing transition of preterms from gavage to oral feeding (Yildiz et al, 2011).*

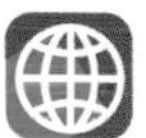

Multicultural

- Identify cultural beliefs, norms, and values of family's perceptions of infant/child behavior. EBN: *The theory of hot and cold espoused by many Mexican Americans has symbolic significance for the nature and process of reproduction and for the relationship between mother and child (Giger & Davidhizer, 2008).*
- Recognize and support positive mother-infant interactive behaviors and be sensitive to cultural differences and ethnic backgrounds. EBN: *Study identified similar and yet different mother-infant interactive behaviors between American Indian and African American mother–infant dyads, an important factor for nurses who work with different ethnic groups to know (Brooks et al, 2013).*

Client/Family Teaching and Discharge Planning

▲ Provide information or refer to community-based follow-up programs for preterm/at-risk infants and their families. EB: *Advance toward seamless communication between NICU staff and community agencies to enhance parents' confidence during the difficult transition from NICU discharge to home (Sherman et al, 2009). Request primary health care provider offer Ages & Stages Questionnaires (ASQ) to parents at regular visits to monitor infant developmental milestones (Bricker & Squires, 1995).*

- Educate parents on safe "Back-to-Sleep" practice before NICU discharge. EB: *Study found that educating parents before NICU discharge on safe to sleep practices, including follow-up phone survey, improved parental compliance of supine positioning from 39% to 83% (Gelfer et al, 2013).*
- Encourage parents during infant awake periods to use a variety of development positions and handling that encourage body movement, hand-to-mouth, eye-hand coordination, and visual scanning; avoid overuse of infant carriers. CEB: *Infants need to experience a variety of different positions during play that encourage movement and play, including pleasurable parent-infant interactions that maximize normal development (Waitzman, 2007).*
- Nurture parents so that they in turn can nurture their infant/child. EBN: *The most difficult and overlooked aspect of care of the high-risk neonate is effective, timely, and compassionate information delivery to parents and family by the medical staff (Sherman et al, 2009).*

Home Care

- The preceding interventions may be adapted for home care use.
- Educate families in ways of preparing the home environment. CEB: *Patterns of sound, light, and caregiving tasks should minimize stress, conserve energy, and protect the developing neonate from inappropriate environmental stimuli (Akers et al, 2007).*
- Prepare families for realistic challenges occurring the first weeks and/or months of transition from NICU to home. EBN: *"Home visits by a nurse were a key component by providing education, support, and nursing care" (Lopez et al, 2012.)* EBN: *NICU discharge is a vulnerable time for parents, and nurses can educate and give opportunities to practice new skills before NICU discharge (Cleveland, 2008).*
- Encourage families to teach extended family and support persons to recognize and respond appropriately to infant's behavioral cues; supportive help may be most appreciated doing physical tasks. CEB: *It is important for families to feel comfortable obtaining support from their regular support systems and supportive persons need to be taught how to support both the family and the infant (Als et al, 2005).* EBN: *Increase knowledge of caring for preterm infants at home from other mothers (Pula-Phillips et al, 2013).*
- Provide families information about community resources, developmental follow-up services, parent-to-parent support programs, and the like; request parents ask primary health care provider to correct age for preterm birth until child is at minimal of 2 years of age, and to monitor developmental milestones to identify adverse neurological development. EB: *Ages and Stages Questionnaire (Bricker & Squires, 1995) is an excellent screening tool to monitor developmental progress.* EB: *Simple cost of ASQ can detect severe developmental delay in preterm children regardless of maternal education; however, children with mild delays may be more limited (Halbwachs et al, 2013).* CEB: *Infants born at 34 to 36 weeks continually can be at risk for neurodevelopmental problems and should have close follow-up (Woythaler et al, 2011).* EB: *Home-based care is effective prevention for preterm infants and can have long-term benefits (Spencer-Smith et al, 2012).*

REFERENCES

Akcan, E., et al. (2009). The effect of kangaroo care on pain in premature infants during invasive procedures. *The Turkish Journal of Pediatrics, 51*(1), 14–18.

Akers, A. L., et al. (2007). In reach: connecting NICU infants and their parents with community early intervention services. *Zero to Three, 27*(3).

Als, H., et al. (2005). The assessment of preterm infants' behavior (APIB): furthering the understanding and measurement of neurodevelopmental competence in preterm and full-term infants. *Mental Retardation and Developmental Disabilities Research Reviews, 11*(1), 94–102.

Bobish, T., & Stanger, M. (2007). Providing services in the clinical setting neonatal intensive care unit and inpatient. In M. Drnach (Ed.), *The clinical practice of pediatric physical therapy*. Baltimore: Lippincott Williams & Wilkins.

Bricker, D., & Squires, J. (1995). *Ages and Stages Questionnaire (ASQ)*. Baltimore, MD: Brooks.

Brooks, J. L., Holditch-Davis, D., & Landerman, L. R. (2013). Interactive behaviors of ethnic minority mothers and their premature infants. *Journal of Obstetric, Gynecologic, & Neonatal Nursing, 42*(3), 357–368.

Cevasco, A. M. (2008). The effects of mothers' singing on full-term and preterm and maternal emotional responses. *Journal of Music Therapy, 45*(3), 273–306.

Cleveland, L. M. (2008). Parenting in the neonatal intensive care unit. *J Obstet Neonatal Nursing, 37*(6), 666–691.

Franck, L. S., et al. (2011). Parent involvement in pain management for NICU infants: a randomized controlled trial. *Pediatrics, 128*(3), 510–518.

Franco, P., et al. (2005). Influence of swaddling on sleep and arousal characteristics of healthy infants. *Pediatrics, 115*(5), 1307–1311.

Gelfer, P., Cameron, R., Masters, K., et al. (2013). Integrating "back to sleep" recommendations into neonatal ICU practice. *Pediatrics, 131*(4), 1264–1270.

Giger, J., & Davidhizar, R. (2008). *Transcultural nursing: assessment and intervention*. St Louis: Mosby.

Halbwachs, M., Muller, J.-B., Nguyen The Tich, S., et al. (2013). Usefulness of parent-completed ASQ for neurodevelopment screening of preterm children at five years of age. *PLoS ONE, 8*(8), e71925.

Halverson, K. (2010). *The Effects of Positiontioning on Premature Infant Development*. <http://commons.pacificu.edu/otcats/>.

Head, L. M. (2014). The effects of kangroo care on neurodevelopmental outcomes in preterm infants. *Journal of Perinatal & Neonatal Nursing, 28*(4), 290–299.

Jean, A. D., & Stack, D. M. (2012). Full-term and very low weight premature infants' self-regulating behaviors during still-face interaction: influences of maternal touch. *Infant Behavior and Development, 35*(4), 779–791.

Johnson, A. (2008). Engaging fathers in NICU: taking down the barriers to the baby. *Journal of Perinatal & Neonatal Nursing, 22*(4), 302–306.

Johnson, C., et al. (2014). Skin-to-skin for pain in neonates. *Cochrane Database of Systematic Reviews*, (1), CD008435.

Kashaninia, Z., et al. (2008). The effect of kangaroo care on behavioral responses to pain of an intramuscular injection in neonates. *Journal for Specialists in Pediatric Nursing, 13*(4), 275–280.

Lemmen, D., Fristedt, P., & Lundqvist, A. (2013). Kangaroo care in a neonatal context: parents' experiences of information and communication of nurse-parents. *The Open Nursing Journal, 7*, 41–48.

Lopez, G. L., et al. (2012). *Neonatal Network, 31*(4), 207–214.

Lubetzky, R., et al. (2010). Effect of music by Mozart on energy expenditure in growing preterm infants. *Pediatrics, 125*(1), 24–28.

Ludington-Hoe, S. M. (2013). Kangaroo care as neonatal therapy. *Newborn and Infant Nursing Reviews, 3*(2).

Montirosso, R., et al. (2012). Level of NICU quality of developmental care and neurobehavioral performance in very preterm infants. *Pediatrics, 129*(5), 1129–1137.

Pula-Phillips, P.L., et al. (2013). Caring for preterm infant at home: a mothers perspective. *Journal of Perinatal and Neonatal Nursing, 27*(4), 335–344.

Pinelli, J., & Symington, A. J. (2010). Non-nutritive sucking calming effect for promoting physiologic stability and nutritive in preterm infants. *Cochrane Database of Systematic Reviews*, (4), CD001071, 2005:updated.

Scher, M. S., et al. (2009). Neurophysiologic assessment of brain maturation after an eight-week trial of skin-to-skin contact with preterm infants. *Clinical Neurophysiology, 120*(10), 1812–1818.

Sherman, M. P., Aylward, G. P., & Shoemaker, C. T. Follow-up of the NICU patient: *updated July 1, 2009*. From: <http://emedicine.medscape.com/article/977318-overview>. Retrieved October 28, 2009.

Sherman, M. P., Aylward, G. P., & Shoemaker, C. T. (2009). *Follow-up of the NICU patient, updated July 1, 2009*. From: <http://emedicine.medscape.com/article/977318overview>. Retrived October 28, 2009.

Spencer-Smith, M. M., et al. (2012). Long-term benefits of home-based preventive care for preterm infants: a randomized trial. *Pediatrics, 130*(6), 1094–1101.

Stevens, B., et al. (2013). Sucrose for analgesia in newborn infants undergoing painful procedures is effective. *Cochrane Database of Systematic Reviews*, (1), CD001069.

Waitzman, K. A. (2007). The importance of positioning the near-term infant for sleep, play, and development. *Newborn & Nursing Reviewers, 7*(2), 76–81.

Wang, D. (2014). Examining the effects of a targeted noise reduction program in a neonatal intensive care unit. *Archives of Disease in Childhood. Fetal and Neonatal Edition, 99*, F203–F208.

Weisman, O., et al. (2011). Sleep-wake transitions in premature neonates predict early development. *Pediatrics, 128*(4), 706–714.

Woythaler, M. S., McCormick, M. C., & Smith, V. C. (2011). Late preterm infants have worse 24 month neurodevelopmental outcomes than term infants. *Pediatrics, 127*(3), 622–629.

Wyngarden, K., DeWys, M., & Padnos, P. (1999). Learnings from the field: the impact of using two new nursing diagnoses, organized infant behavior and disorganized infant behavior [abstract]. *Classification of Nursing Diagnoses: Proceedings of the Thirteenth Conference*. NANDA.

Yildiz, A., & Arikan, D. (2012). The effects of giving pacifiers to premature infants and making them listen to lullabies on their transition period for total oral feeding and sucking success. *Journal of Clinical Nursing, 21*, 644–656.

Yildiz, A., et al. (2011). The effect of the odor of breast milk on the time needed for transition from gavage to oral feeding in preterm infants. *Journal of Nursing Scholarship, 43*(3), 265–273.

I

Readiness for enhanced organized Infant behavior *Gail B. Ladwig, MSN, RN*

NANDA-I

Definition

A pattern of modulation of the physiological and behavioral systems of functioning (i.e., autonomic, motor, state-organization, self-regulatory, and attentional-interactional systems) in an infant, which can be strengthened

Defining Characteristics

Parent expresses desire to enhance cue recognition; parent expresses desire to enhance recognition of infant's self-regulatory behaviors

NOC, NIC, Client Outcomes, Nursing Interventions, Client/Family Teaching and Discharge Planning, *Rationales,* and References

Refer to care plans for Disorganized **Infant** behavior and Risk for disorganized **Infant** behavior.

Risk for disorganized Infant behavior *Gail B. Ladwig, MSN, RN*

NANDA-I

Definition

Vulnerable to alteration in integration and modulation of the physiological and behavioral systems of functioning (i.e., autonomic, motor, state organization, self-regulatory, and attentional-interactional systems), which may compromise health

Risk Factors

Impaired motor functioning; insufficient containment within environment; invasive procedure; oral impairment; pain; parent expresses desire to enhance environmental conditions; prematurity; procedure

NOC, NIC, Client Outcomes, Nursing Interventions, Client/Family Teaching and Discharge Planning, *Rationales,* and References

Refer to Disorganized **Infant** behavior.

Risk for Infection *Ruth M. Curchoe, RN, BSN, MSN, CIC*

NANDA-I

Definition

Vulnerable to invasion and multiplication of pathogenic organisms which may compromise health

Risk Factors

Chronic illness (e.g., diabetes mellitus); inadequate vaccination; insufficient knowledge to avoid exposure to pathogens; invasive procedure; malnutrition; obesity

I

Inadequate Primary Defenses

Alteration in peristalsis; alteration in pH of secretions; alteration in skin integrity; decrease in ciliary action; premature rupture of amniotic membrane; prolonged rupture of amniotic membrane; smoking; stasis of body fluids

Inadequate Secondary Defenses

Decrease in hemoglobin; immunosuppression; leukopenia; suppressed inflammatory response (e.g., IL-6, C-reactive protein [CRP]); inadequate vaccination

Increased Environmental Exposure to Pathogens

Exposure to disease outbreak

NOC (Nursing Outcomes Classification)

Suggested NOC Outcomes

Risk Control: Infectious Process; Immune Status

Example NOC Outcome with Indicators

Risk Control: Infectious Process: Identifies signs and symptoms of infection/Maintains a clean environment/Practices infection control strategies: universal precautions, hand sanitization. (Rate the outcome and indicators of **Risk Control: Infectious Process:** 1 = never demonstrated, 2 = rarely demonstrated, 3 = sometimes demonstrated, 4 = often demonstrated, 5 = consistently demonstrated [see Section I].)

Client Outcomes

Client Will (Specify Time Frame)

- Remain free from symptoms of infection during contact with health care providers
- State symptoms of infection before initiating a health care–related procedure
- Demonstrate appropriate care of infection-prone sites within 48 hours of instruction
- Maintain white blood cell count and differential within normal limits within 48 hours of treatment initiation
- Demonstrate appropriate hygienic measures such as handwashing, oral care, and perineal care within 24 hours of instruction

NIC (Nursing Interventions Classification)

Suggested NIC Interventions

Immunization/Vaccination Management; Infection Control; Infection Protection

Example NIC Activities—Infection Protection and Control

Wash hands before and after each client contact; Ensure aseptic handling of all intravenous lines; Ensure appropriate wound care technique; Teach client and family members how to avoid infections

Nursing Interventions and *Rationales*

- Implement targeted surveillance for methicillin-resistant *Staphylococcus aureus* (MRSA) (screen clients at risk for MRSA on admission) and other multidrug-resistant organisms. EB: *Universal screening for MRSA increased screenings and costs but resulted in few additional cases being detected. Where MRSA is endemic, targeted screening remains the most efficient strategy for early identification of MRSA-positive clients (Creamer et al, 2012).*
- Obtain a travel history from clients presenting to health care site (e.g., emergency department, clinic). EB: *Outbreaks, such as Ebola and avian flu identified in foreign countries, often present with fever and flu-like symptoms (CDC, 2014a).*
- Observe and report signs of infection such as redness, warmth, discharge, and increased body temperature. CEB: *Change in mental status, fever, shaking, chills, and hypotension are indicators of sepsis (Risi, 2009).*
- Assess temperature of neutropenic clients; report a single temperature of greater than 100.5° F. CEB: *Fever is often the first sign of an infection (NCCN, 2006).* CEBN: *The immunocompromised host may present with a very different clinical picture when compared to an immunocompetent host. The progress of the infection may be more rapid, and the infection may quickly become life-threatening; repeat temperature measurement if significant changes occur and report temperature changes from baseline (Risi, 2009).*
- Oral, rectal, tympanic, temporal artery or axillary thermometers may be used to assess temperature in adults and infants. EBN: *The use of axillary in addition to oral, tympanic, and temporal artery temperature measurement is supported (Rubia-Rubia et al, 2011). Rectal and oral temperature measurements are more accurate than other methods of temperature measurement, such as temporal or axillary measurement (Makic et al, 2011).*

▲ Note and report laboratory values (e.g., white blood cell count and differential, serum protein, serum albumin, and cultures). EBN: *While the white blood cell count may be in the normal range, an increased number of immature bands may be present (Versalovic et al, 2011).* CEBN: *A neutropenic client with fever represents an absolute medical emergency (Mahtani, 2010).*

- Assess skin for color, moisture, texture, and turgor (elasticity). Keep accurate, ongoing documentation of changes. EB: *A number of instruments have been developed to assess for risk of pressure ulcers, including the Braden scale, the Norton scale, and the Waterlow scale. All three scales include items related to activity mobility, nutritional status, incontinence, and cognition (Agency for Healthcare Quality and Research, 2011).*
- Carefully wash and pat dry skin, including skinfold areas. Use hydration and moisturization on all at-risk surfaces. EBN: *Moisturizers result in an increase of skin hydration and restoration of the skin barrier function and play a prominent role in the long-term management of atopic dermatitis (Miller et al, 2011).* EB: *Application of moisturizers containing humectants is clearly effective in enhancing skin barrier function (Kottner et al, 2013).*

Refer to care plan for Risk for impaired **Skin** integrity.

▲ Monitor client's vitamin D level. EB: *Vitamin D deficiency has been correlated with increased risk and greater severity of infection, particularly of the respiratory tract. Vitamin D influences the body's immune system by influencing the production of endogenous antimicrobial peptides and regulating the inflammatory cascade (Gunville et al, 2013).*

Refer to care plan Readiness for enhanced **Nutrition** for additional interventions.

- Use strategies to prevent health care–acquired pneumonia (IHI, 2011); assess lung sounds and sputum color and characteristics; provide daily oral care with chlorhexidine; use sterile technique when suctioning; suction secretions above tracheal tube before suctioning; drain accumulated condensation in ventilator tubing into a fluid trap or other collection device before repositioning the client; assess patency and placement of nasogastric tubes; elevate the client's head to 30 degrees or higher to prevent gastric reflux of organisms in the lung (*Peyrani, 2014*). EB: *Hospital mortality of ventilated clients who develop ventilator-associated pneumonia (VAP) is 46% compared to 32% of those ventilated clients without VAP. VAP also adds an estimated cost of $40,000 to a typical hospital admission (IHI, 2011).*

- Encourage fluid intake. EB: *Fluid intake helps thin secretions and replace fluid lost during fever (Guppy et al, 2011).*
- Use appropriate hand hygiene (i.e., handwashing or use of alcohol-based hand rubs). EBN: *Meticulous infection prevention precautions are required to prevent health care–associated infection, with particular attention to hand hygiene and standard precautions (CDC, 2011a).* EB: *Handwashing is currently the recommended strategy for reducing transmission of* Clostridium difficile. *Alcohol gels do not inactivate* C. difficile *spores (Edmonds et al, 2013).*
- When using an alcohol-based hand rub, apply ample amount of product to palm of one hand and rub hands together, covering all surfaces of hands and fingers, until hands are dry. Note that the volume needed to reduce the number of bacteria on hands varies by product. EBN: *Adequate hand antisepsis reduces infection rates. The use of alcohol-based hand rubs is particularly effective; in contrast to handwashing, hand rubs kill susceptible bacteria more rapidly and to a greater extent, and are less time-consuming, and skin health is better preserved when moisturizers are added (Aitken et al, 2011; Hass, 2014).*
- Follow standard precautions and wear gloves during any contact with blood, mucous membranes, nonintact skin, or any body substance except sweat. Use goggles and gowns when appropriate. Standard precautions apply to all clients. You must assume all clients are carrying blood-borne pathogens (CDC, 2007). EBN: *Hands of health care workers are the most common cause of health care–associated infections (Hass, 2014).*

I

- Implement respiratory hygiene/cough etiquette. CEB: *Providing control measures (tissues, masks) and accessibility to hand hygiene materials reduces risks of transmission of respiratory illness (CDC, 2007).*
- Follow transmission-based precautions for airborne-, droplet-, and contact-transmitted microorganisms:
  - **Airborne:** Isolate the client in a room with monitored negative air pressure, with the room door closed and the client remaining in the room. Always wear appropriate respiratory protection when you enter the room. Limit the movement and transport of the client from the room to essential purposes only. Have the client wear a surgical mask during transport.
  - **Droplet:** Keep the client in a private room, if possible. If not possible, maintain a spatial separation of 3 feet from other beds or visitors. The door may remain open. Wear a surgical mask when you must come within 3 feet of the client. Some hospitals may choose to implement a mask requirement for droplet precautions for anyone entering the room. Limit transport to essential purposes and have the client wear a mask, if possible.
  - **Contact:** Place the client in a private room, if possible, or with someone (cohorting) who has an active infection from the same microorganism. Wear clean, nonsterile gloves when entering the room. When providing care, change gloves after contact with any infective material such as wound drainage. Remove the gloves and clean your hands before leaving the room and take care not to touch any potentially infectious items or surfaces on the way out. Wear a gown if you anticipate your clothing may have substantial contact with the client or other potentially infectious items. Remove the gown before leaving the room. Limit transport of the client to essential purposes and take care that the client does not contact other environmental surfaces along the way. Dedicate the use of noncritical client care equipment to a single client. CEB: If use of common equipment is unavoidable, adequately clean and disinfect equipment before use with other clients (CDC, 2007).

▲ Use alternatives to indwelling catheters whenever possible (external catheters, incontinence pads, bladder control techniques). EB: *It is estimated that catheter-associated urinary tract infections increase length of stay by 0.5 to 1 day and increase costs between $1200 and $4700 (2009 dollars) (Umschied et al, 2011; IHI, 2011).*

- If a urinary catheter is necessary, follow catheter management practices: All indwelling catheters should be connected to a sterile, closed drainage system (i.e., not broken), except for good clinical reasons. Cleanse the perineum and meatus twice daily using soap and water. EBN: *A nurse-driven protocol achieved a 32% reduction in the use of catheters (from 0.22 to 0.15 catheters/client-day) and a 45% reduction in catheter-associated urinary tract infection (CAUTI) (from 4.78 to 2.64 infections/1000 catheter-days) (Parry & Srinivasan, 2011).* EB: *Significant rates of inappropriate urinary catheter use underscore the importance of establishing guidelines and implementing policy for appropriate use of urinary catheters (Tiwari et al, 2012).*
- Use evidence-based practices and educate personnel in care of peripheral catheters: use aseptic technique for insertion and care, label insertion sites and all tubing with date and time of insertion, inspect every 8 hours for signs of infection, record, and report. EB: *Use of chlorhexidine gluconate for vascular catheter site care reduces catheter-related bloodstream infections and catheter colonization (CDC, 2011b).*

- Use sterile technique wherever there is a loss of skin integrity. EBN: *Skin and soft tissue infections arise when skin integrity is broken by treatments associated with trauma, surgery, burns, and the like (Apisaranthanara & Mundy, 2014).*
- Ensure the client's appropriate hygienic care with handwashing, bathing, oral care, and hair, nail, and perineal care performed by either the nurse or the client. CEBN: *Daily showers or baths can help to reduce the number of bacteria on the client's skin. The oral cavity is a common site for infection (Coughlan & Healy, 2008; NCCN, 2006).*
- Recommend responsible use of antibiotics; use antibiotics sparingly. EB: *Use and misuse of antibiotics diminishes their therapeutic benefit and facilitates the development of multidrug-resistant organisms (MDROs) and* C. difficile*-associated disease, and increases health care costs. Antibiotic stewardship is essential in reducing current and future resistance in bacteria (Moody et al, 2012).* EB: *The rate of damage to the fallopian tubes increases with subsequent pelvic inflammatory disease episodes, from 34% for the first episode to 54% in women with second and third episodes (Puscheck et al, 2013). Female genital tuberculosis is a symptomless disease inadvertently uncovered during investigation for infertility (Klaus-Dieter et al, 2013).*

Pediatric

I

Note: Many of the preceding interventions are appropriate for the pediatric client.

- Follow meticulous hand hygiene when working with children. EB: *Keep nails short; prohibit false fingernails and limit wearing jewelry as it interferes with effective hand hygiene (AAPeds, 2012). Parents recognize the importance of hand hygiene but in a study only 67% would definitely remind health care workers of its importance (Buser et al, 2012).*
- Cluster nursing procedures to decrease number of contacts with infants, allowing time for appropriate hand hygiene. EBN: *Audit programs to track compliance with hand hygiene identified a drop in the incidence of health care–associated infections in very low-birth-weight infants in the neonatal intensive care unit (Mendicino et al, 2014).*
- Avoid the prophylactic use of topical cream in premature infants. CEB: *Prophylactic application of topical ointment increases the risk of coagulase-negative staphylococcal infection and any health care–acquired infection. A trend toward increased risk of any bacterial infection was noted in infants treated prophylactically (Conner et al, 2004).*
- Encourage early enteral feeding with human milk. *Human milk enhances immune defenses of the infant (Pickering, 2012).*

▲ Monitor recurrent antibiotic use in children.

- Instruct parents on appropriate indicators for medical visits and the risks associated with overuse of antibiotics. EB: *Guidelines addressing treatment of asthma in children state that antibiotics should not be used as part of chronic asthma therapy or for acute exacerbations, with the exception of clients with comorbid bacterial infections such as pneumonia or sinusitis (Paul et al, 2011).*

Geriatric

▲ Suspect pneumonia when the client has symptoms of lethargy or confusion. Assess response to treatment, especially antibiotic therapy. EB: *Leading causes of illness and death among older adults are both community and health care–associated respiratory infections. In long-term care facilities, the risk for pneumonia ranges from 0.3 to 2.5 events per 1000 resident-days (Montoya & Moody, 2011; AOA, 2012).*

- Most clients develop health care-associated pneumonia (HCAP) by either aspirating contaminated substances or inhaling airborne particles. Refer to care plan for Risk for **Aspiration.**

▲ Carefully screen older women with incontinence for urinary tract infections. CEB: *Consider alternatives to chronic indwelling catheters, such as intermittent catheterization. CAUTI has been associated with increased morbidity, mortality, hospital cost, and length of stay (CDC, 2009).*

- Observe and report if the client has a low-grade fever or new onset of confusion. EB: *Those caring for older clients must be alerted to the potential presence of infection when even low-grade temperature elevations appear for short periods (Arinzon et al, 2012).*
- Recommend that the geriatric client receive an annual influenza immunization and one-time pneumococcal vaccine. EB: *Immunization against influenza is an effective intervention that reduces serologically confirmed cases (CDC, 2014b,c).*
- Recognize that chronically ill geriatric clients have an increased susceptibility to *Clostridium difficile* infection; practice meticulous hand hygiene; monitor antibiotic response to antibiotics. EB: *The incidence*

of C. difficile *illness (CDI) is increasing with the greatest impact in persons older than 65 years. More than 90% of deaths from CDI have occurred in this population (CDC, 2012; Kelly & LaMont, 2013).*

Home Care

- Adapt the above interventions for home care as needed.
- Assess and treat wounds in the home. **EBN:** *Promotion of wound healing is a nursing priority. Specific wound care regimens administered depend upon the type, size, and location of the wound and overall treatment goals (Colwell, 2013).*
- Review standards for surveillance of infections in home care. **EB:** *Challenges to surveillance in the home care setting include loss of clients to follow-up, lack of laboratory data, and difficulty in obtaining accurate numerator and denominator data (Yeung, 2014).*
- Maintain infection-prevention policies. **EBN:** *The complexity of client's conditions is frequently high as the incidence of chronic disease and MDROs is increasing (Yeung, 2014).*
- Refer for nutritional evaluation; implement dietary changes to support recovery and maintain health. **EB:** *Medical nutrition therapy (MNT) is important in preventing diabetes, managing existing diabetes, and preventing, or at least slowing, the rate of development of diabetes complications. It is, therefore, important at all levels of diabetes prevention. MNT is also an integral component of diabetes self-management education (or training) (ADA, 2012).*

Client/Family Teaching and Discharge Planning

- Teach the client risk factors contributing to surgical wound infection. **EB:** *The risk of infection is influenced by characteristics of the client such as age, obesity, and nutritional status (Murphy, 2014).*
- Teach the client and family the importance of hand hygiene in preventing postoperative infections. **EB:** *Two thirds of wound infections occur after discharge. Using good hand hygiene practices is effective for preventing these infections (Alexander 2011).*

▲ Encourage high-risk persons, including health care workers, to get vaccinated (CDC, 2011c).

▲ Influenza: Teach symptoms of influenza and importance of vaccination for influenza. **EB:** *Everyone 6 months of age and older should get the flu vaccine. Seasonal flu vaccine is effective and has a very good safety track record (CDC, 2014b,c).* Teach the client and family how to take a temperature. Encourage the family to take the client's temperature between 4 PM and 10 PM at least once daily. **CEBN:** *The lowest body temperature usually occurs between 4 AM and 5 AM, with highest readings being recorded between 4 PM and 8 PM (Peate & Wild, 2012).*

REFERENCES

Administration on aging (AOA) (2012). *A profile of older Americans. AOA website*. Available at: <www.aoa.gov/AoARoot/Aging_Statistics/Profile/2012/3.aspx>.

AAPeds (2012). Infection Control. In L. E. Riley, A. R. Stark, et al. (Eds.), *Guidelines for Perinatal Care* (7th ed., pp. 439–492). Elk Grove Village, IL: American Academy of Pediatrics.

Agency for Healthcare Quality and Research (AHRQ). (2011). Toolkit helps to prevent hospital acquired pressure ulcers: research activities. *AHRQ*, July 2011, No.371.

Aitken, L., et al. (2011). Nursing considerations to complement the surviving sepsis campaign guidelines. *Critical Care Medicine*, *39*(7), 1800–1818.

Alexander, J. W. (2011). Updated recommendations for controlling surgical site infections. *Annals of Surgery*, *253*(96), 1082–1093.

American Diabetes Association. (2012). Nutrition recommendations and interventions for diabetes: a position statement. *Health: A review Home Health Care Management and Practices*, *24*, 298–308.

Apisaranthanara, A., & Mundy, L. (2014). Skin and soft tissue infections. In *APIC test of Infection Control and Epidemiology* (4th ed.). Washington, DC: Association for Professionals in Infection Control and Epidemiology. Last revised 6/6/14, Accessed 8/5/14.

Arinzon, Z., Shabat, S., Peisakh, A., et al. (2012). Clinical presentation of urinary tract infection (UTI) differs with aging women. *Archives of Gerontology and Geriatrics*, *55*(1), 145–147.

Buser, G. L., Fisher, B. T., Shea, J. A., et al. (2012). Parent willingness to remind health care workers to perform hand hygiene. *American Journal of Infection Control*, *41*(6), 492–496.

Centers for Disease Control and Prevention (CDC) (2014a). *Ebola (Ebola Virus Disease), Interim Guidance for Monitoring and Movement of Person with Ebola Virus Disease Exposure*. <http://www.cdc.gov/vhf/ebola/hcp/monitoring-and-movement-of-persons-with-exposure.html>. Retrieved from www Oct 27, 2014.

Centers for Disease Control and Prevention (CDC) (2014b). *Preventing seasonal flu with vaccination*. Available at: <www.CDC.gov/flu/protect/vaccine>. Accessed 8/12/14.

Centers for Disease Control and Prevention (CDC) (2014c). *Vaccine information Statement (VIS) Influenza*. July 2014.

Centers for Disease Control and Prevention (CDC) (2012). Vital signs: preventing *Clostridium difficile* infections. *MMWR. Morbidity and Mortality Weekly Report*, *61*(9), 157–162.

Centers for Disease Control and Prevention (CDC) (2011a). Guideline for hand hygiene in health-care settings. Recommendations of the Healthcare Infection Control Practices Advisory Committee and the HICPAC/SHEA/APIC/IDSA Hand Hygiene Task Force. *MMWR. Recommendations and Reports: Morbidity and Mortality Weekly Report. Recommendations and Reports*, *51*(RR-16), 1–45. From: <http://www.cdc.gov/handhygiene/Guidelines.html>. Retrieved July 21, 2014, Accessed 7/25/14.

Centers for Disease Control and Prevention (CDC) (2011b). *Guideline for the prevention of intravascular catheter related infections.* Retrieved from: <http://www.cdc.gov/hicpac>. Accessed 8/5/14.

Centers for Disease Control and Prevention (CDC) (2011c). Prevention and control of influenza: recommendations of the advisory committee on immunization practices (ACIP). *MMWR. Recommendations and Reports: Morbidity and Mortality Weekly Report. Recommendations and Reports, 60*(33), 1128–1132.

Centers for Disease Control and Prevention (CDC) (2009). *Healthcare Infection Control Practices Advisory Committee: guideline for prevention of catheter-associated urinary tract infections.* From: <http://www.cdc.gov/hicpac/pdf/CAUTI/CAUTIguideline2009final.pdf>. Retrieved August 1, 2014, Accessed 8/8/14.

Centers for Disease Control and Prevention (CDC) (2007). *Healthcare Infection Control Practices Advisory Committee: guideline for isolation precautions: preventing transmission of infectious agents in healthcare settings.* From: <http://www.cdc.gov/ncidad/dh9p/pdf/guidelines/isolation2007.pdf>. Retrieved July 28, 2014, Accessed 7/28/14.

Colwell, J. (2013). Skin integrity and wound care. In *Potter, Perry Fundamentals of Nursing* (8th ed.). St. Louis Missouri: Elsevier.

Conner, J. M., Soll, R. F., & Edwards, W. H. (2004). Topical ointment for preventing infection in preterm infants. *Cochrane Database of Systematic Reviews,* (1), CD001150.

Coughlan, M., & Healy, C. (2008). Nursing care, education and support for patients with neutropenia. *Nursing Standard, 22*(46), 35–41.

Creamer, E., Galvin, S., Dolon, A., et al. (2012). Evaluation of screening risk and nonrisk patients for methicillin-resistant *Staphylococcus aureus* on admission in an acute care hospital. *American Journal of Infection Control, 40*(5), 411–415.

Edmonds, S. L., Zapka, C., Kaspar, D., et al. (2013). Effectiveness of hand hygiene for removal of *Clostridium difficile* spores from hands. *Infection Control and Hospital Epidemiology, 34,* 302–306.

Gunville, C. F., Mourani, P. M., & Ginde, A. A. (2013). The role of vitamin D in prevention and treatment of infection. *Inflammation and Allergy Drug Targets, 12*(4), 239–245.

Guppy, M. P. B., et al. (2011). Advising patients to increase fluid intake for treating acute respiratory infections. *Cochrane Database of Systematic Reviews,* (2), CD0044193.

Hass, J. (2014). Hand Hygiene. In *APIC test of Infection Control and Epidemiology* (4th ed.). Washington, DC: Association for Professionals in Infection Control and Epidemiology. Last revised 6/6/14, Accessed 7/28/14.

Institute for Healthcare Improvement (IHI) (2011). *Implement the IHI ventilator bundle, IHI website.* Available at: <http://www,ihi.org/knowledge/Pages/Changes/ImplementtheVentilatorBundle.aspx>. Accessed 8/1/14.

Institutes for Healthcare Improvement (IHI) (2011). *How to guide: Prevent catheter associated urinary tract infections.* Cambridge, MA: Institute for Healthcare Improvement.

Kelly, C. P., & LaMont, J. T. (2013). Clostridium difficile *in adults treatment. UpToDate Website.* Available at: <http://www.update.com/contents/clostridium-difficile-in-adults-treatment>.

Klaus-Dieter, L., Kim, E. D., Bylund, J. R., et al. (2013). *Tuberculosis of the genitourinary tract Overview of GUTB.* Available at: <www.emedicine.medscape.com>. Updated 6/7/13, Accessed 8/6/14.

Kottner, J., Lichterfelo, A., & Blume-Peytavi, U. (2013). Maintaining skin integrity in the aged. *The British Journalof Dermatology, 169*(3), 528–542.

Mahtani, R. *Neutropenia and infection.* From: <http://www.staging.caring4cancer.com>. Retrieved July 29, 2010.

Makic, M. B., et al. (2011). Evidence-based practice habits: putting more sacred cows out to pasture. *Critical Care Nurse, 31*(2), 38–63.

Mendicino, N., Morrell, G., & Hernandez, S. L. (2014). Neonates. In *APIC test of Infection Control and Epidemiology* (4th ed.). Washington, DC: Association for Professionals in Infection Control and Epidemiology. Last revised 6/6/14, Accessed 8/6/14.

Miller, D. W., Koch, S. B., & Yentzer, B. A. (2011). An over-the-counter moisturizer is as clinically effective as, and more cost-effective than, prescription barrier creams in the treatment of children with mild-to-moderate atopic dermatitis: a randomized, controlled trial. *Journal of Drugs in Dermatology, 10*(6), 531–537.

Montoya, A., & Moody, L. (2011). Common infections in nursing homes: a review of current issues and challenges. *Aging Health, 7*(6), 689–699.

Moody, J., Cosgrove, S. E., Olmstead, R., et al. (2012). Antimicrobial stewardship: a collaborative partnership between infection preventionists and health care epidemiologists. *American Journal of Infection Control, 40*(2), 94–95.

Murphy, R. (2014). Surgical services. In *APIC test of Infection Control and Epidemiology* (4th ed.). Washington, DC: Association for Professionals in Infection Control and Epidemiology. Last revised 6/6/14, Accessed 8/11/14.

National Comprehensive Cancer Network (NCCN) (2006). *Fever and neutropenia treatment guidelines for patients with cancer-version II, March 2006.* From: <http://www.nccn.org/patients/patient_gls/_english/_fever_and_neutropenia/1_introduction.asp>. Retrieved July 30, 2014. Accessed 7/30/14.

Parry, M., & Srinivasan, A. (2011). *Protocol reduces use of urinary catheters, infections [Abstract 357]. Presented April 3, 2011, at the Society for Healthcare Epidemiology of America (SHEA) 20th Annual Scientific Meeting.*

Paul, I., et al. (2011). Antibiotic prescribing during pediatric ambulatory care visits for asthma. *Pediatrics, 127,* 1014–1021.

Peate, I., & Wild, K. (2012). Clinical observations 1/6: assessing body temperature. *British Journal of Healthcare Assistants, 6*(5), 215–219.

Peyrani, P. (2014). Pneumonia. In *APIC test of Infection Control and Epidemiology* (4th ed.). Washington, DC: Association for Professionals in Infection Control and Epidemiology. Last revised 6/6/14, Accessed 8/1/14.

Pickering, L. K. (2012). Report of the committee of infectious diseases, *Redbook* (29th ed.). Elk Grove Village, IL: American Academy of Pediatrics.

Puscheck, E. E., Scott-Lucidi, R., & Woodard, T. L. (2013). *Infertility.* Available at: <www.emedicine.medscape.com>. 013, Accessed 8/6/14.

Rubia Rubia, J., Arias, A., Sierra, A., et al. (2011). Measurement of body temperature in adult patients: comparative study of accuracy, reliability and validity of different devices. *International Journal of Nursing Studies, 48*(7), 872–880.

Risi, G. F. (2009). The immunocompromised host. In *APIC text of infection control and epidemiology* (3rd ed.). Washington, DC: Association for Professionals in Infection Control and Epidemiology.

Tiwari, M. M., Charlton, M. E., Anderson, J. R., et al. (2012). Inappropriate use of urinary catheters: a prospective observational study. *American Journal of Infection Control, 40*(1), 51–54.

Umschied, C. A., Mitchell, M. D., Doshi, J. A., et al. (2011). Estimating the proportion of healthcare associated infections that are reasonably preventable and the related mortality and costs. *Infection Control and Hospital Epidemiology, 32*(2), 101–114.

Versalovic, J., Carroll, K. C., Funke, G., et al. (2011). *Manual of Clinical Microbiology* (10th ed.). VI. Washington, DC: ASM Press.

Yeung, C. (2014). Home Care. In *APIC test of Infection Control and Epidemiology* (4th ed.). Washington, DC: Association for Professionals in Infection Control and Epidemiology. Last revised 6/6/14, Accessed 8/10/14.

Risk for Injury

Julianne E. Doubet, BSN, RN, CEN, NREMT-P

NANDA-I

Definition

Vulnerable to physical damage due to environmental conditions interacting with the individual's adaptive and defensive resources, which may compromise health

Risk Factors

External

Alteration in cognitive functioning; alteration in psychomotor functioning; compromised nutritional source (e.g., vitamins, food types); exposure to pathogen; exposure to toxic chemical; immunization level within community; nosocomial agent; physical barrier (e.g., design, structure, arrangement of community, building, equipment); unsafe mode of transport

I

Internal

Abnormal blood profile; alteration in affective orientation; alteration in sensation (resulting from, e.g., spinal cord injury, diabetes mellitus); autoimmune dysfunction; biochemical dysfunction; effector dysfunction; extremes of age; immune dysfunction; impaired primary defense mechanisms (e.g., broken skin); malnutrition; sensory integration dysfunction; tissue hypoxia

NOC (Nursing Outcomes Classification)

Suggested NOC Outcomes

Personal Safety Behavior; Risk Control; Safe Home Environment; Knowledge: Fall Prevention

Example NOC Outcome with Indicators

Risk Control as evidenced by the following indicators: Monitors environmental risk factors/Develops effective risk control strategies/Follows selected risk control strategies. (Rate the outcome and indicators of **Risk Control:** 1 = never demonstrated, 2 = rarely demonstrated, 3 = sometimes demonstrated, 4 = often demonstrated, 5 = consistently demonstrated [see Section I].)

Client Outcomes

Client Will (Specify Time Frame)

- Remain free of injuries
- Explain methods to prevent injuries
- Demonstrate behaviors that decrease the risk for injury

NOC (Nursing Outcomes Classification)

Suggested NOC Outcomes

Health Education; Environmental Management; Fall Prevention

Example NIC Activities—Health Education

Identify internal or external factors that may enhance or reduce motivation for healthy behavior; Determine current health knowledge and lifestyle behaviors of individual, family, or target group

Nursing Interventions and *Rationales*

Prevent iatrogenic harm to the hospitalized client by following the National Patient Safety goals:

- Accuracy of Client Identification:
  - Use at least two methods (e.g., client's name and medical record number or birth date) to identify the client upon initial entrance to a client's room and before administering medications, blood products, treatments, or procedures.

  - Before beginning any invasive or surgical procedure, have a final verification to confirm the correct client, the correct procedure, and the correct site for the procedure using active communication techniques.
  - Label containers used for blood and other specimens in the presence of the client.
- Effectiveness of Communication Among Care Staff:
  - Verbal or telephone orders should be written and then read back for verification to the individual giving the order. Avoid verbal or telephone orders whenever possible.
  - Standardize use of abbreviations, acronyms, symbols, and dose designations that are used in the institution.
  - Ensure critical test results and values are recorded and reported in a timely manner.
  - Use a standardized approach of "handing off" communications, including opportunities to ask and answer questions.
  - Use only approved abbreviations.
  - Staff should always wear hospital nametags.
- Medication Safety:
  - Standardize and limit the number of drug concentrations used by the institution (e.g., concentrations of medications such as morphine in client-controlled analgesia pumps).
  - Label all medications and medication containers (e.g., syringes, medication cups, or other solutions on or off the surgical field).
  - Identify all of the client's current medications upon admission to a health care facility, and ensure that all health care staff have access to the information.
  - Ensure that accurate medicine information is sent with the client throughout their care.
  - Reconcile all medication at admission and discharge, and provide list to the client.
  - Improve the effectiveness of alarm systems in the clinical area.
  - Standardize a list of medications that look alike or sound alike. This list needs to be updated yearly.
  - Identify and take extra care with clients who are on anticoagulants.
- Infection Control:
  - Reduce the risk of infections by following Centers for Disease Control and Prevention (CDC, 2014) hand hygiene guidelines.
  - Document clearly when clients obtain injuries or die of infectious disease.
  - Use proven guidelines to prevent infections that are difficult to treat.
  - Use proven guidelines to prevent infection of the blood from central lines.
  - Use safe practices to treat the surgical site of the client.
  - Use proven guidelines to prevent catheter-associated urinary tract infections.
- Fall Prevention:
  - Evaluate all clients for fall risk daily and take appropriate actions to prevent falls.
- Client Involvement in Care:
  - Educate the client and family on how to recognize and report concerns about safety issues.
- Identify Clients with Safety Risks:
  - Identify which clients are at risk for harming themselves.
- Identify Clients Who Are Susceptible to Changes in Health Status:
  - Educate staff on how to recognize changes in client condition, how to respond quickly, and how to alert specially trained staff to intervene if needed.
  - Prevent errors in surgery by following established protocols. Update protocols yearly.
  - Standardize steps to educate staff so documents for surgery are ready before surgery.
  - Educate staff to mark the body part scheduled for surgery and engage the client in this process as well.

These actions have been shown to increase client safety and are required actions for accreditation by The Joint Commission (2011).

- See care plan for Risk for **Falls.**
- Avoid use of physical and chemical restraints if at all possible. Restraint-free is now the standard of care for hospitals and long-term care facilities. Obtain a health care provider's order if restraints are necessary. CEB: *The use of restraints has been associated with serious injuries, including rhabdomyolysis, brachial plexus injury, neuropathy, and dysrhythmias, as well as strangulation, traumatic brain injuries, and all the consequences of immobility (Park & Tang, 2007).* EBN: *Besides physical restraints, other nonpharmaceutical*

I

measures that can be used to promote safe mobility in client-centered care are staff education, balance training, sensor mats, exercise, and low-height adjustable beds (Gulpers et al, 2013).

- Consider providing individualized music of the client's choice if a client is agitated. EB: *Livingston et al (2014) maintain that person-centered care with good communication skills, monitored sensory therapy activities, and structured music therapies diminish distress in care-home dementia residents.* EBN: *In reviewing the results of studies that addressed the effects of safe, low-cost, music therapy for agitation in dementia, Blackburn and Bradshaw (2014) found that music therapy is not only promising in the reduction of agitation in older adults with dementia, but also helps lessen anxiety and depression, and seemingly to improve cognitive function.*
- Review drug profile for potential side effects and interactions that may increase risk of injury. EB: *The use of polypharmacy, as prescribed to older adults, is the sole most significant factor in risk injury in those same adults. A mix of medications can cause a reduction in physical function, raise the risk of falls, and cause delirium and other geriatric syndromes, and is a known factor in hospital admissions and death (Scott et al, 2014).* EB: *By using certain structured strategies, such as awareness of life expectancy, comorbidity, goals, and client preferences, there is evidence that health care providers can reduce their client's risk of injury by "de-prescribing" certain medications; any drug that is of little value and/or increases the client's risk of injury should be discontinued, Scott et al (2013) say in their report.*

I

- Provide a safe environment
  - ❍ Use one fourth– to one half–length side rails only, and maintain bed in a low position. Ensure that wheels are locked on bed and commode. Keep dim light in room at night.
  - ❍ Remove all possible hazards in environment such as razors, medications, room clutter, wet floors, and matches.
  - ❍ Place at risk for injury client in a room that is near the nurse's station. EBN: *According to Wang et al (2014), when clients' safety culture is improved, there is a decrease in client adverse events.* EBN: *"A client-centered environment of care is not just the care provided at the client's side. It is seen throughout the facility" (Blackwell, 2014).*
- Assist clients to sit in a stable chair with armrests. Avoid use of wheelchairs and geri-chairs except for transportation. EB: *Unassisted attempts at getting up from a wheelchair are a common cause of falls (Lee et al, 2012).* EB: *In their study of wheelchair-related injuries, Chen et al (2011) found that wheelchair-associated adverse events were closely connected to wheelchair-using behaviors.*
- If the client has a new onset of confusion (delirium), refer to the care plan for Acute **Confusion.** If the client has chronic confusion, see the care plan for Chronic **Confusion.**
- Involve family in helping to provide a culture of safety. EBN: *A client centered approach to care should include the family, in both planning and decision-making (Wrobleski et al, 2014).* EB: *According to a study by Rathert et al (2012), health care policy leaders are promoting the concept that both clients and their families should take a hands-on role in providing client safety.*

▲ Refer the client for physical therapy for strengthening as needed. EB: *Exercise training supervised by a physiotherapist was found to have positive outcomes on physical function and quality of life, and to reduce incidence of falls (Kwok & Tong, 2014).* EB: *According to Beattie (2014), physical therapists, due to their particular place on the health care team, are able to make a major contribution to the promotion of community-based efforts to reduce fall risk and fall injuries in older adults.*

▲ Use nonphysical forms of behavior management for the agitated psychotic client. EB: *Agitated psychotic clients must first have a brief emergency evaluation as to the cause of their distress, which will then direct crisis interventions to calm them (Stowell et al, 2012).* EB: *Okumura et al (2014) state that there is a call for approaches to client agitation that focus on psychosocial interventions, antipsychotic withdrawal, and the need to moderate the overall incidence of antipsychotics use.*

Pediatric

- Teach parents the need for close supervision of young children playing near water. EB: *Semple-Hess and Campwala (2014) state that drowning and submersion injuries are one of the most common, yet avoidable, causes of childhood mortality and morbidity.* EB: *The Centers for Disease Control (2014) maintains that drowning can occur without warning and quickly, wherever there is water (e.g., pools, bathtubs, buckets), even when a lifeguard is present; an adult, who will not be distracted by other activities, should be chosen to oversee children playing in or near water.*
- If the child has an underlying medical problem that puts them at risk for drowning, it is recommended that they be given showers, not tub baths. No unsupervised swimming is ever allowed. EB: *Semple-Hess*

and Campwala (2014) state that those children who have epilepsy, undiagnosed cardiac dysrhythmias, hyperventilate, hypoglycemia, and hypothermia are in greater danger of drowning. EB: *Caregivers should understand the necessity for constant supervision while children are bathing, especially if the child has an underlying condition such as epilepsy (Bamber et al, 2014).*

- Assess the client's socioeconomic status because financial hardship may correlate with increased rates of injury. EB: *According to Anderson et al (2014), there may be a relationship between intentional injury rate and those children in families living below poverty level: these findings may indicate that financial hardship could be an important risk factor for finding these types of injuries.* EB: *Sociodemographic issues were connected to an increased incidence of children's burns, according to Alnababtah et al (2014): factors include low household income, living in deprived areas, living in rented accommodation, young mothers, single-parent families, and being a child of ethnic minorities. Parental education and size of living space could also play some part in the injury.*
- Never leave young children unsupervised around cooking or open flames. EB: *Risks for children's thermal injuries include inattentive attention in a depressed mother, adult alcohol overuse, and socioeconomic level; these risks are modifiable and should be addressed (Jamshidi & Sato, 2013).* EB: *According to Oram et al (2012), the third leading cause of unintentional death in the United States that affects children younger than 14 living at home is fire and burn injuries.*
- Teach parents and children the need to maintain safety for the exercising child, including wearing helmets when biking. EB: *Parents should be educated in the use of bicycle helmets for their children and set a good example by wearing helmets themselves (Baeseman & Corden, 2014).* EB: *It is has been proven that the use of bicycle helmets helps prevent or reduce severe head injuries in bicycle riders (Basch et al, 2014).*
- Encourage parents to insist on safety precautions in all phases of participation sports involving children. EB: *Due to the increased participation in sports by young children, the number of overuse injuries has increased in that age group (Fournier, 2013).*
- ▲ EB: *In their study of children's sports injuries, Stracciolin et al (2013) found that there is insufficient knowledge regarding sports injuries in young children who play physically challenging organized sports for which they lack physical readiness, thus opening themselves to injury.*
- Provide parents of children with traumatic brain injury with written instruction and emergency phone numbers. Ensure that instructions are understood before the child is discharged from a health care setting. Instruct parents to observe for the following symptoms: nausea, mild headache, dizziness, irritability, lethargy, poor concentration, loss of appetite, and insomnia. *Symptoms of concussion may occur up to 2 weeks after injury and need prompt treatment to prevent further injury (Bethel, 2012).*
- ▲ EBN: *Mason (2013) states that even if the child has suffered a mild concussion (traumatic brain injury), it could have lasting effects on health, behavior, and cognitive abilities.*
- Teach both parents and children the need for gun safety; refer to hunting safety courses. EBN: *Barton and Kologi (2014), in their study, found that thousands of children are killed or injured every year in the United States, due to access to loaded firearms not stored safely.* EB: *Health care providers, including pediatricians, can play a significant role in gun safety education, which must teach the necessity for secure storage of any firearms (Mitka, 2014).*
- Educate parents regarding proper car safety seat use. EB: *Child passenger restraint systems have been found to greatly reduce the risk of injury and death among child passengers (Muller et al, 2014).*

Geriatric

- Encourage the client to wear glasses and hearing aids and to use walking aids, including nonslip footwear when ambulating. EB: *It has been observed that gait and balance problems lead to falls and injuries in older people; the use of walking aids are meant to augment gait safety and prevent falls (Hardi et al, 2014).* EB: *Hearing loss is a common chronic health condition in older adults. Hearing aid treatment helps improve the quality of life for older adults with hearing deficits (Cox et al, 2014).*
- Assess for orthostatic hypotension when getting up, teach methods to decrease dizziness, such as rising slowly, remaining seated several minutes before standing, flexing feet upward several times while sitting, sitting down immediately if feeling dizzy, and trying to have someone present when standing. EBN: *Orthostatic hypotension is a fairly common occurrence in the older adult and is most likely due to comorbidities, polypharmacy, and physiological changes that can occur with aging (Lee, 2013).* EB: *Shibao et al (2013) maintain that the management of orthostatic hypotension should be aimed at treatment of symptoms, client's functional status, and decreasing the risk of falls and syncope.*

- Discourage driving at night. EB: *Certain vision tests could be developed to predict night vision problems in the growing number of older drivers, suggest Gruber et al (2013).* EB: *Older adult drivers who drive at night are at heightened risk for injury due to age-related changes in the amount of light reaching the retina, weaker contrast sensitivity, and variations in dark and light adaptation (Boot et al, 2014).*

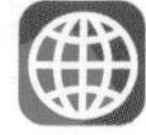

Multicultural

- Acknowledge racial/ethnic differences at the onset of care. EB: *Gagnon et al (2014) assert that minority groups appear to have increased levels of distress in comparison to Caucasians.* EBN: *Alpers and Hanssen (2014) note that experience by itself does not provide nurses with sufficient knowledge for intercultural symptom assessment and culturally competent treatment and care; requirements to produce culturally competent nurses should include formal education, in-service classes, courses, feedback, and access to appropriate information is needed along with their perception of clinical practice.*
- Evaluate the influence of culture on the client's perceptions of risk for injury. EB: *Black (45%) and Hispanic children (46%), in comparison to Caucasian children, are dying in automobile crashes due to not being restrained: effective interventions and education would increase proper restraint use and save a child who is involved in a motor vehicle crash (Sauber-Schatz et al, 2014).* EB: *Spanish speaking children who were hospitalized due to an adverse event, or one that was harmful due to nonstandard practices, were found to be hospitalized longer than their English speaking counterparts: communication barriers should be addressed to help promote client safety, suggest Lion et al (2013).*
- Evaluate whether exposure to community violence is a contributor to a client's risk for injury. EB: *Chang et al (2014) assert in their study that neighborhood environment plays an important part in relation to adolescent health risk behaviors.* EB: *Exposure to violence can result in many negative consequences for youth, including use of tobacco, alcohol, and marijuana, and persisting neighborhood violence (Fagan et al, 2014).*
- Use culturally relevant injury prevention programs when possible. Validate the client's feelings and concerns related to environmental risks. EB: *According to research supported by the findings of Richardson et al (2014), inner-city neighborhoods are linked with school dropouts, substance abuse, crime, violence, homicide, HIV risk related behaviors, and imprisonment for adolescent African American males; therefore, parents of adolescent African American males are tested daily in attempting to keep their children safe in high-risk neighborhoods.* EB: *Wilson-Genderson and Pruchno (2013) found in their research that violent crime in a neighborhood, as well as convictions concerning neighborhood safety, could impact the depressive symptoms felt by community-dwelling older people.*

Home Care and Client/Family Teaching and Discharge Planning

- See Risk for **Trauma** for interventions and rationales.

I

REFERENCES

Alnababtah, K., Kahn, S., & Ashford, R. (2014). Socio-demographic factors and the prevalence of burns in children: an overview of the literature. *Paediatrics and International Child Health, 13*.

Alpers, L. M., & Hansen, I. (2014). Caring for ethnic minority patients: a mixed method study of nurses' self-assessment of cultural competency. *Nursing Education Today, 34*, 999–1004. [Epub 2013 Dec 18].

Anderson, B. L., Pomerantz, W. J., & Gittelman, M. A. (2014). Intentional injuries in young Ohio children: is there an urban/rural variation. *Journal of Trauma and Acute Care Surgery, 77*, 538–540.

Baeseman, Z. J., & Corden, T. E. (2014). A social-ecologic framework for improving bicycle helmet use by children. *Wisconsin Medical Journal, 113*, 49–51.

Bamber, A. R., Pryce, J. W., Ashworth, M. T., et al. (2014). Immersion-related deaths in infants and children: autopsy experience from a specialist center. *Forensic Science Medicine and Pathology, 10*, 363–370.

Barton, B. K., & Kologi, S. M. (2014). Why do you keep them there: a qualitative assessment of firearms storage practices. *Journal of Pediatric Nursing, 10*.

Basch, C., Ethan, D., Rajan, S., et al. (2014). Helmet use among users of the Citi Bike bicycle-sharing program: a pilot study in New York City. *Journal of Community Health, 39*, 503–507.

Beattie, B. L. (2014). Effective fall-prevention demands a community approach. *Journal of Geriatric Physical Therapy, 37*, 31–34.

Bethel, J. (2012). Emergency care of children and adults with head injury. *Nursing Standard, 26*, 49–56.

Blackburn, R., & Bradshaw, T. (2014). Music therapy for service users with dementia: a critical review of the literature. *Journal of Psychiatric and Mental Health Nursing, 10*, 879–888.

Blackwell, L. A. (2014). A successful life safety survey in an ambulatory surgery center (2014). *AORN Journal, 99*, 431–434.

Boot, W. R., Stothart, C., & Charness, N. (2014). Improving the safety of aging road users: a mini-review. *Gerontology, 100*, 90–96.

Centers for Disease Control and Prevention. (2014). Unintentional drowning; get the facts. *Home and Recreational Safety*, From <http://www.cdc.gov/homeandrecreationalsafety/water-safety/waterinjuries-factsheet.html>. Retrieved from October 15, 2014.

Chang, L. Y., Foshee, V. A., Reyes, H. L., et al. (2015). Direct and indirect effects of neighborhood characteristics on the perpetration of dating violence across adolescence. *Journal of Youth and Adolescence, 44*, 727–744.

Chen, W. Y., Jang, Y., Wang, J. D., et al. (2011). Wheelchair related accidents: relationship with wheelchair using behavior in active community wheelchair users. *Archives of Physical Medicine & Rehabilitation, 92*, 892–898.

Cox, R. M., Johnson, J. A., & Xu, J. (2014). Impact of advanced hearing aid technology speech for older listeners with mild to moderate, adult-onset hearing loss. *Gerontology, 60*, 557–608. [Epub 2014 Aug 14].

Fournier, M. (2013). Pediatric lower extremities sports injuries. *Podiatry Management, 32*, 91–98.

Fagan, A. A., Wright, E. M., & Pinchevsky, G. M. (2014). The protective effects of neighborhood collective efficacy on adolescent substance use and violence following exposure to violence. *Journal of Youth and Adolescence, 43*, 1408–1512.

Gagnon, C. M., Matsuura, J. T., Smith, C. C., et al. (2014). Ethnicity and interdisciplinary pain treatment. *Pain Practice, 14*, 532–540.

Gruber, N., Mosiman, U. P., Muri, R. M., et al. (2013). Vision and night driving abilities of elderly drivers. *Traffic Injury Prevention, 14*, 477–485.

Gulpers, M. J., Bleijlevens, M. H., Ambergen, T., et al. (2013). Reduction of belt restraint use: long term effects of EXBELT intervention. *Journal of the American Geriatric Society, 61*, 107–112.

Hardi, I., Bridenbaugh, S. A., Gschwind, Y. J., et al. (2014). The effect of walking aids on spatio-temporal parameters in community dwelling older adults. *Aging Clinical and Experimental Research, 26*, 221–228.

Jamshidi, R., & Sato, T. T. (2013). Initial assessment and management of thermal burn injuries in children. *Pediatrics in Review, 24*, 395–404.

Kwok, T., & Tong, C. Y. (2014). Effects on centre-based training and home-based training on physical function, quality of life an fall incidence in community dwelling older adults. *Physiotherapy Theory and Practice, 30*, 243–248.

Lee, A., Mills, P., & Neilly, J. (2012). Using root cause analysis to reduce falls with injury in community settings. *Joint Commission Journal on Quality and Patient Safety, 38*, 366–374.

Lee, Y. (2013). Orthostatic hypotension in older people. *Journal of the American Association of Nurse Practioners, 25*, 451–458.

Lion, K. C., Rafton, S. A., Shafil, J., et al. (2013). Association between language, serious adverse events, and length of stay among hospitalized children. *Hospital Pediatrics, 3*, 219–225.

Livingston, G., Kelly, L., Lewis-Holmes, E., et al. (2014). A systematic review of the clinical effectiveness and cost effectiveness of sensory psychological and behavioral interventions for managing agitation in older adults with dementia. *Journal of the American Geriatric Society, 18*, 1–226.

Mason, C. N. (2013). Mild traumatic brain injury in children. *Pediatric Nursing, 39*, 267–282.

Mitka, M. (2014). Firearm-related hospitalizations: 20 US teens daily. *JAMA: The Journal of the American Medical Association, 311*, 664.

Muller, V. M., Burke, R. V., Arbogast, H., et al. (2014). Evaluation of a child passenger safety class in increasing parental knowledge. *Accident Analysis & Prevention, 63*, 37–40.

Okumura, Y., Togo, T., & Fujita, J. (2014). Trends in use of psychotropic medications among patients treated with cholinesterase inhibitors in Japan from 2002 to 2010. *International Psychogeriatrics, 12*, 1–9.

Oram, E., Kendrick, D., West, J., et al. (2012). Independent risk factors for injury in pre-school children: three population-based nested case-control studies using routine primary care data. *PLoS ONE, 7*, e3512.

Park, M., & Tang, J. H. (2007). Evidence-based guideline-changing the practice of physical restraint use in acute care. *Journal of Gerontological Nursing, 33*, 9–16.

Rathert, C., Brandt, J., & Williams, E. S. (2012). Putting the patient in patient safety: a qualitative survey of consumers experiences. *Health Expectations, 15*, 327–336.

Richardson, J. B., Jr., Van Brakle, M., & St Vil, C. (2014). Taking boys out of the hood: exile as a parenting strategy for African American male youth. *New Directions for Child and Adolescent Development, 14*, 11–21.

Sauber-Schatz, E. K., West, B. A., & Bergen, G. (2014). Vital signs: restraint use and motor vehicle occupant death rates among children aged 0-12 years—United States, 2002-2011. *Morbidity and Mortality Weekly Report, Centers for Disease Control, 63*, 113–116.

Scott, A., Anderson, K., Freeman, C. R., et al. (2014). First do no harm: a real need to deprescribe in older patients. *Medical Journal of Australia, 201*, 390–392.

Scott, A., Gray, L. B., Martin, J., et al. (2013). Deciding when to stop: evidence-based deprescribing of drugs in older patients. *Evidence-based Medicine, 18*, 121–124. <http://dx.doi.org.ezproxy.jccmi.edu/10.1136/eb-2012-100930>.

Semple-Hess, J., & Campwala, R. (2014). Pediatric submersion injuries and emergency care and resuscitation. *Pediatric Emergency Medicine, 11*, 1–21.

Shibao, C., Lipsitz, L. A., & Biaggioni, I. (2013). Evaluation and treatment of orthostatic hypotension. *Journal of the American Society of Hypertension, 7*, 317–324.

Stowell, K., Florence, P., Herbert, J., et al. (2012). Psychiatric evaluation of the agitated patient consensus statement of the American association for emergency psychiatry project BETA psychiatric evaluation workgroup. *Western Journal of Emergency Medicine, 13*, 11–16.

Stracciolin, A., Casciano, R., Levey-Friedman, H. L., et al. (2013). Pediatric sports injuries: an age comparison of children versus adolescents. *The American Journal of Sports Medicine, 41*, 1932–1939.

The Joint Commission (2011). *National patient safety goals.* From: <http://www.jointcommission.org/PatientSafety/NationalPatientSafetyGoals/07_npsg_facts.htm>. Retrieved December 15, 2011.

Wang, X., Liu, K., You, L. M., et al. (2014). The relationship between patient safety culture and adverse events: a questionnaire survey. *The International Journal of Nursing Studies, 51*, 1114–1122.

Wilson-Genderson, M., & Pruchno, R. (2013). Effects of neighborhood violence and perceptions of neighborhood safety on depressive symptoms of older adults. *Social Science and Medicine, 85*, 43–49.

Wrobleski, D. M. S., Joswiak, M. E., Dunn, D. F., et al. (2014). Discharge planning rounds to the bedside: a patient and family-centered approach. *Medsurg Nursing, 23*, 111–116.

Risk for corneal Injury

Michelle Acorn, DNP, NP PHC-Adult, BA, BScN/PHCNP, MN/ACNP, ENC(C), GNC(C), CAP, CGP

NANDA-I

Definition

Vulnerable to infection or inflammatory lesion in the corneal tissue that can affect superficial or deep layers, which may compromise health

Risk Factors

Blinking less than five times per minute; exposure of the eyeball; Glasgow Coma Scale score < 7; intubation; mechanical ventilation; periorbital edema; pharmaceutical agent; prolonged hospitalization; tracheotomy; use of supplemental oxygen

I

NOC (Nursing Outcomes Classification)

Suggested NOC Outcomes (Visual)

Sensory Function: Vision; Vision Compensation Behavior

Example NOC Outcome with Indicators

Vision Compensation Behavior as evidenced by the following indicators: Wears protective eye wear for prevention/Eye discomfort improves daily with healing. (Rate each indicator of **Vision Compensation Behavior:** 1 = never demonstrated, 2 = rarely demonstrated, 3 = sometimes demonstrated, 4 = often demonstrated, 5 = consistently demonstrated [see Section I].)

Client Outcomes

Client Will (Specify Time Frame)

- Demonstrate relaxed facial expressions
- Remain as independent as possible
- Remain free of physical harm resulting from vision injury risk
- Demonstrate improvement in visual acuity

NIC (Nursing Interventions Classification)

Suggested NIC Interventions

Visual Deficit; Environmental Management

Example NIC Activities—Communication Enhancement: Visual Deficit

Clearly identify yourself when you enter the client's space; Build on client's remaining vision, as appropriate

Nursing Interventions and *Rationales*

Emergency Department Visits or Primary Care Office Visit

▲ Perform a standard ophthalmic exam or examine eye with a slit lamp using fluorescein stain to optimize visualization of the abrasion injury if available.
- Attempt visual acuity measuring using the Snellen Eye chart (corrected with glasses).
- Ensure immunization status is current, namely tetanus-diphtheria-pertussis status (every 10 years).
- Teach the client that fingernail induced corneal abrasions are one of the most common eye injuries and are at risk for complications (Lin et al, 2014). EB: *Treating traumatic corneal abrasions by pressure patching, bandage contact lens, or antibiotic ointment alone was equal in reducing the abrasion area and reducing pain. The epithelium was healed in all clients at day 7. Treatment of choice should be adapted to the needs and preferences of the client (Menghini et al, 2013).* CEB: *Eye patching does not reduce pain in clients with corneal abrasions. Topical nonsteroidal anti-inflammatory agents (e.g., diclofenac) have been found to be effective in reducing pain (Fraser, 2010).*
- Provide analgesia as needed/prescribed. *Clients with all but the most minor abrasions usually require a strong oral narcotic analgesic initially. In addition, topical eye agents may be required to relieve*

pain and photophobia in clients with large abrasions until their healing is nearly complete (Verma & Khan, 2014).

- Injuries that penetrate the cornea are more serious. The outcome depends on the specific injury. *Corneal abrasions usually heal quickly and without vision concerns. Even after the original injury is healed, however, the surface of the cornea is sometimes not as smooth as before. Clients who have had a corneal abrasion may notice that the eye feels irritated for a while after the abrasion heals (Cleveland Clinic, 2015).*

Hospitalization

- Assess for perioperative corneal abrasion risks, including advanced age, general anesthesia, greater blood loss, eye taping during surgery, prone and Trendelenburg positions, and supplemental oxygen use (Segal et al, 2014). EB: *An eye protection method intraoperatively includes eye lubrication with aqueous based gel and application of clear, square occlusive dressings large enough to cover the eyelids and surrounding skin. Standardized documentation of client eye protection should occur (Vetter et al, 2012).*

▲ Corneal abrasion is the most common ophthalmological complication that occurs during general anesthesia for nonocular surgery and can lead to sight-threatening microbial keratitis and permanent scarring. EB: *Taping alone provides protection that is equivalent or superior to other interventions and has fewer side effects. Petroleum gel is flammable and best avoided when electrocautery and open oxygen are used around the face. Preservative-free eye ointment is preferred, in that preservatives can cause corneal epithelial sloughing and conjunctival hyperemia (Grixti et al, 2013).*

- Assess for corneal abrasion and eye dryness, which are common problems in clients in the intensive care unit. Eye dryness is the main risk factor for the development of corneal abrasions. *Clients receiving adhesive tape as an eye care method were twice as likely to develop corneal abrasions (Masoudi et al, 2013).* EB: *Sedated clients or clients in induced comas may experience ineffective eye closure, presenting higher risk for corneal injury (Werli-Alvarenga et al, 2013).* EB: *Consider a humidity chamber with polyethylene fill for best practice (Werli-Alvarenga et al, 2013).* EBN: *Eye care and eye assessment should be essential parts of nursing care for clients in intensive care. To prevent corneal abrasions, use eye lubricants, which is more effective than closing eyes by adhesive tapes (Masoudi et al, 2013).*

Client/Family Teaching and Discharge Planning

▲ First aid principles should be reinforced in the event of an eye injury. Clients should not attempt to remove any object in the eye. Reserve this for the provider. A referral to an ophthalmologist may be required (Jacobs, 2014).

- Teach clients to use caution when using household cleaners. Many household products contain strong acids, alkalis, or other chemicals. Drain and oven cleaners are particularly dangerous. They can lead to blindness if not used correctly (Vorvick, 2014).
- If chemical exposure has occurred, flush the eye immediately with clean water for 10 minutes. Seek prompt health care attention.
- Wear safety goggles at all times when using hand or power tools or chemicals, during high impact sports, or in other situations when eye injury is more likely.
- Wear sunglasses that screen ultraviolet light when outdoors, even in winter.
- Pain is usually improved within 3 days. If pain becomes intolerable, an analgesic may be prescribed short term. Seek medical attention if pain is not resolving.
- Driving should be restricted for safety until client's visual acuity is evaluated.

REFERENCES

Cleveland Clinic (2015). *Corneal Abrasion.* <http://my.clevelandclinic.org/services/cole-eye/diseases-conditions/hic-corneal-abrasion>. Retrieved April 10, 2015.

Fraser, S. (2010). Corneal abrasion. *Clinical Ophthalmology*, *6*, 387–390.

Grixti, A., Sadri, M., & Watts, M. T. (2013). Corneal protection during general anesthesia for nonocular surgery. *The Ocular Surface*, *11*(2), 109–118.

Jacobs, D. S. (2014). *Corneal Abrasions and Injury*. <http://www.uptodate.com/contents/corneal-abrasions-and-corneal-foreign-bodies-management?source=see_link>. Retrieved December 6, 2014.

Lin, Y. B., & Gardiner, M. F. (2014). Fingernail-induced corneal abrasions: case series from an ophthalmology emergency department. I. *Cornea*, *33*(7), 691–695.

Masoudi, A. N., Sharifitabar, Z., Shaeri, M., et al. (2013). An audit of eye dryness and corneal abrasion in ICU patients in Iran. *British Association of Critical Care Nurses*, *19*(2), 73–77.

Menghini, M., Knecht, P. B., Kaufmann, C., et al. (2013). Treatment of traumatic corneal abrasion: a three arm prospective randomized study. *Ophthalmic Research*, *50*(1), 13–18.

Segal, K. L., Fleischut, P. M., Kim, C., et al. (2014). Evaluation and treatment of perioperative corneal abrasions. *Journal of Ophthalmology*, 320–326. <http://dx.doi.org/10.1155/2014/901901>.

Vetter, T. R., Ali, N. M., & Boudreaux, A. M. (2012). A case-control study of an operative corneal abrasion prevention program: holding the gains made with a continuous quality improvement method. *Joint Commission Journal on Quality and Patient Safety*, *38*(11), 490–496.

Werli-Alvarenga, A., Ercole, F. F., Herdman, T. H., et al. (2013). Nursing interventions for adult intensive care patients with risk for corneal injury: a systemic review. *International Journal of Nursing Knowledge*, *24*(1), 25–29.

Verma, A., & Khan, H. R. (2014). *Corneal Abrasion*. <http://emedicine.medscape.com/article/1195402-overview>. Retrieved April 10, 2014.

Vorvick, L. J. (2014). *Corneal Injury*. <http://umm.edu/health/medical/ency/articles/corneal-injury>. Retrieved November 23, 2014.

Risk for urinary tract Injury *Mary Beth Flynn Makic, PhD, RN, CNS, CCNS, FAAN*

NANDA-I

Definition

Vulnerable to damage of the urinary tract structures from use of catheters, which may compromise health

NOTE: This nursing diagnosis overlaps with other diagnoses such as Risk for **Trauma,** Impaired **Urinary** elimination, and Risk for **Infection.** Refer to care plans for these diagnoses if appropriate.

I

Risk Factors

Condition preventing ability to secure catheter (e.g., burn, trauma, amputation); long-term use of urinary catheter; multiple catheterizations; retention balloon inflated to ≥30 mL; use of large-caliber urinary catheter

NOC (Nursing Outcomes Classification)

Suggested NOC Outcomes

Urinary Elimination; Risk Control: Trauma; Infection

Example NOC Outcome with Indicators

Urinary Elimination as evidenced by the following indicators: Urine clarity/Urine odor, fluid intake, pain with urination. (Rate the outcome and indicators of **Urinary Elimination:** 1 = severely compromised 2 = substantially compromised, 3 = moderately compromised, 4 = mildly compromised, 5 = not compromised [see Section I].)

Client Outcomes

Client Will (Specify Time Frame)

- Remain free of urinary tract injury
- State absence of pain with catheter care and during urination
- Experience unobstructed urination after removal of catheter

NIC (Nursing Interventions Classification)

Suggested NIC Intervention

Urinary Elimination Management

Example NIC Activities—Urinary Elimination Management

Monitor urinary elimination, including frequency, consistency, odor, volume, and color, as appropriate; Assess client for pain associated with catheter

Nursing Interventions and *Rationales*

- Monitor urinary elimination, including frequency, consistency, odor, volume, and color, as appropriate; teach client signs and symptoms of urinary tract infection.
- Assess for proper placement of a urinary catheter. Urinary catheters are among the most widely used medical devices. Proper placement is necessary to prevent trauma to the urinary tract structure as well as infections (e.g., catheter-associated urinary tract infection [CAUTI] and urosepsis). EB: *Complications associated with indwelling urinary catheters include delirium, accidental removal, gross hematuria, leakage, urethral injury, restriction of mobility, and infection (Hollingsworth et al, 2013; Burnett et al, 2010).*

- ▲ To prevent injury, educate the client/family as to the reason for the indwelling urinary catheter to prevent harm (Scott et al, 2014). EB: *Accidental or improper removal of catheter can cause urethral injury. Urinary catheters are used in up to 16% of adult hospital inpatients, most frequently in older adults. Older age and older women are more likely to have no clear indication for catheterization (Vincitorio et al, 2014). Studies found that 21% to 54% of all indwelling urinary catheters are inappropriately placed and are not medically indicated (Hooten et al, 2010; Fakih et al, 2010). Understanding the indication for the catheter and encouraging removal of catheters that do not have a clear indication is important to prevent client harm.*
- • Assess clinical indication for urinary catheter daily. EB: *Avoidance of unnecessary indwelling urinary catheters may reduce CAUTI incidence and bloodstream infections (Meddings et al, 2014).*
- • To avoid catheterizations, evaluate alternative strategies for managing urine output for the client. EB: *Developing toileting schedules, providing assistance with toileting, and incorporating toileting activities into frequent, scheduled nursing staff rounding can reduce urgency and incontinence episodes. For clients with limited mobility, use a bedside commode with a toileting schedule (Uberoi et al, 2013), consider condom catheters for male clients (Saint et al, 2013), and use moisture wicking incontinence pads to reduce moisture-associated skin injury (Oman et al, 2012).*
- • If an indwelling urinary catheter is determined to be clinically indicated in the care of a client, proper selection of the right catheter, technique during insertion, and evidence-based care management are needed to reduce infection and injury to the urinary tract structures.
  - ❍ Selecting the smallest catheter size (e.g., smaller than 18 French) reduces irritation and inflammation of the urethra and reduces infection risk (Gray, 2010; Hooten et al, 2010).
  - ❍ Insert the catheter using aseptic technique. Wash hands and use sterile technique when opening the catheterization kit and cleansing the urethral meatus and perineal area with an antiseptic solution. Insert the catheter using a no-touch technique (Gray, 2010; Lo et al, 2014). *Using a no-touch technique may reduce the risk of infection.*
  - ❍ Provide routine hygiene care; once a urinary catheter is placed, optimal management includes care of the urethral meatus according to "routine hygiene" (e.g., daily cleansing of the meatal surface during bathing with soap and water and as needed, e.g., following a bowel movement) (Hooten et al, 2010; Watts et al, 2011). Cleansing with antiseptics, creams, lotions, or ointment has been found to irritate the meatus, possibly increasing the risk of infection (Lo et al, 2014; Watts et al, 2011).
  - ❍ Secure the catheter after placement to reduce friction from movement (Hooten et al, 2010; Watts et al, 2011; Clarke et al, 2013).
  - ❍ Maintain a closed catheter system to reduce the risk of infection (Hooten et al, 2010; Lo et al, 2014; Memorial Sloan Kettering, 2015).
  - ❍ Maintaining the urine collection bag below the level of the bladder minimizes reflux into the catheter itself, preventing retrograde flow of urine and risk for infection (Hooten et al, 2010; Watts et al, 2011; Memorial Sloan Kettering, 2015; Clarke et al, 2013).
  - ❍ Establish workflow protocols to routinely empty the drainage bag frequently and before transport to reduce urine reflux and opportunities for infection.
  - ❍ Use an ultrasound bladder scanner to determine the estimated urine volume in the bladder and the need to insert or reinsert a urinary catheter (Saint et al, 2013).
- ▲ EB: *A quality improvement study found that implementing a nurse-driven protocol based on current best evidence reduced catheter use, risk of infections, and urinary tract harm (Oman et al, 2012).*

Home Care and Client/Family Teaching and Discharge Planning

- • Teach the client/family proper technique for inserting a urinary catheter. Instruct the client/family to never forcefully advance the catheter. Contact a health care provider if resistance is experienced (Herter et al, 2010; Watts et al, 2011).
- • Develop a personalized plan of care to teach the client/family proper catheterization technique. Consider developing a routine bladder draining schedule to avoid bladder distention or other complications (Watts et al, 2011).
- • Cleanse the catheter and surrounding area during a shower (avoid tub baths) using mild soap; dry catheter and skin. Ensure catheter and drainage bag are secured to thigh and lower leg (Memorial Sloan Kettering, 2015).
- • Teach the client/family methods to keep the urinary tract healthy. Refer to Client/Family Teaching in the care plan for Readiness for enhanced **Urinary** elimination.

REFERENCES

Burnett, K. P., Erickson, D., Hunt, A., et al. (2010). Strategies to prevent urinary tract infection from urinary catheter insertion in the emergency department. *Journal of Emergency Nursing*, *36*, 546–550.

Clarke, K., Tong, D., Pan, Y., et al. (2013). Reduction in catheter-associated urinary tract infections by bundling interventions. *International Journal for Quality Health Care*, *25*(1), 43–49.

Fakih, M. G., Shemes, S. P., Pena, M. E., et al. (2010). Urinary catheters in the emergency department: very elderly women are at high risk for unnecessary utilization. *American Journal of Infection Control*, *38*(9), 683–688.

Gray, M. (2010). Reducing catheter-associated urinary tract infection in the critical care unit. *AACN Advanced Critical Care*, *21*(2), 247–257.

Herter, R., & Kazer, M. W. (2010). Best practices in urinary catheter care. *Home Healthcare Nurse*, *2896*, 342–349.

Hollingsworth, J. M., Rogers, M. A., Krein, S. L., et al. (2013). Determining the noninfectious complications of indwelling urethral catheters: a systematic review and meta-analysis. *Annals of Internal Medicine*, *159*(6), 401–410.

Hooten, T. M., Bradley, S. F., Cardenas, D. D., et al. (2010). Diagnosis, prevention, and treatment of catheter-associated urinary tract infection in adults: 2009 international clinical practice guidelines from the infectious diseases society of America. *Clinical Infectious Diseases*, *50*, 625–663.

Lo, E., Nicolle, L. E., Coffin, S. E., et al. (2014). Strategies to prevent catheter-associated urinary tract infections in acute care hospitals: 2014 update. *Infection Control and Hospital Epidemiology*, *35*(Suppl. 2), S32–S47.

Meddings, J., Rogers, M. A. M., Krein, S., et al. (2014). Reducing unnecessary urinary catheter use and other strategies to prevent catheter-associated urinary tract infection: an integrative review. *BMJ Quality and Safety*, *23*(4), 277–289.

Memorial Sloan Kettering Cancer Center (2015). *Caring for your urinary catheter*. <https://www.mskcc.org/cancer-care/patient-education/caring-your-urinary-foley-catheter>. Retrieved June 26, 2015.

Oman, K. S., Makic, M. B. F. M., Fink, R., et al. (2012). Nurse-directed interventions to reduce catheter-associated urinary tract infections. *American Journal of Infection Control*, *40*, 548–553.

Saint, S., Greene, T., Kowalski, C. P., et al. (2013). Preventing catheter-associated urinary tract infection in the United States. *JAMA Internal Medicine*, *173*(10), 874–879.

Scott, R. A., Oman, K. S., Makic, M. B. F., et al. (2014). Reducing indwelling urinary catheter use in the emergency department: a successful quality-improvement initiative. *Journal of Emergency Nursing*, *40*, 237–240.

Uberoi, V., Calixte, N., Coronel, V. R., et al. (2013). Reducing urinary catheter days. *Nursing*, *43*(1), 16–20.

Vincitorio, D., Barbadoro, P., Pennacchietti, L., et al. (2014). Risk factors for catheter-associated urinary tract infection in Italian elderly. *American Journal of Infection Control*, *42*(8), 898–901.

Watts, R., Adams, J., Yearwood, M., et al. (2011). Strategies to promote intermittent self-cauterization in adults with neurogenic bladders. JoAnna Briggs Institute. *Best Practice*, *15*(7), 1–4.

I

Insomnia *Mary Beth Flynn Makic, PhD, RN, CNS, CCNS, FAAN*

NANDA-I

Definition

A disruption in amount and quality of sleep that impairs functioning

Defining Characteristics

Alteration in affect; alteration in concentration; alteration in mood; alteration in sleep pattern; compromised health status; decrease in quality of life; difficulty initiating sleep; difficulty maintaining sleep; dissatisfaction with sleep; early awakening; increase in absenteeism; increase in accidents; insufficient energy; nonrestorative sleep pattern (i.e., due to caregiver responsibilities, parenting practices, sleep partner); sleep disturbance producing next-day consequences

Related Factors (r/t)

Alcohol consumption; anxiety, average daily physical activity is less than recommended for gender and age; depression; environmental barrier (e.g., ambient noise, daylight/darkness exposure, ambient temperature/humidity, unfamiliar setting); fear; frequent naps; grieving; hormonal change; inadequate sleep hygiene; pharmaceutical agent; physical discomfort; stressors

NOC (Nursing Outcomes Classification)

Suggested NOC Outcomes

Comfort Level; Pain Level; Personal Well-Being; Psychosocial Adjustment: Life Change; Quality of Life; Rest; Sleep

Example NOC Outcome with Indicators

Sleep as evidenced by the following indicators: Hours of sleep/Sleep pattern/Sleep quality/Sleep efficiency/Feels rejuvenated after sleep/Sleeps consistently through the night. (Rate the outcome and indicators of **Sleep:** 1 = severely compromised, 2 = substantially compromised, 3 = moderately compromised, 4 = mildly compromised, 5 = not compromised [see Section I].)

Client Outcomes

Client Will (Specify Time Frame)

- Verbalize plan to implement sleep-promoting routines
- Fall asleep with less difficulty a minimum of four nights out of seven
- Wake up less frequently during night a minimum of four nights out of seven
- Sleep a minimum of 6 hours most nights and more if needed to meet next stated outcome
- Awaken refreshed and not be fatigued during day most of the time

NIC (Nursing Interventions Classification)

I

Suggested NIC Intervention

Sleep Enhancement

Example NIC Activities—Sleep Enhancement

Monitor/record client's sleep pattern and number of sleep hours; Encourage client to establish a bedtime routine to facilitate transition from wakefulness to sleep

Nursing Interventions and *Rationales*

- Obtain a sleep history including time needed to initiate sleep, duration of awakenings after the first sleep onset, total nighttime sleep amounts, and satisfaction with sleep amounts. Also explore bedtime routines, use of medications and stimulants, and use of complementary/alternative therapies for stress management (e.g., herbal agents) and relaxation before bedtime. *Assessment of sleep behavior and patterns is an important part of any health status examination (Gooneratne et al, 2014; Salas & Gamaldo, 2011).*
- From the history, assess the degree and chronic nature of insomnia. *Adults can be considered to have insomnia if their daytime tiredness and sleepiness is accompanied by one or more or the following several nights/week: (1) inability to initiate sleep; (2) awakening during the night with inability to reinitiate sleep; and/or (3) short nighttime sleep; insomnia is considered chronic if it continues beyond 4 weeks (Morgan et al, 2011).*
- Avoid negative associations with ability to sleep. EB: *Fear of not sleeping can interfere with sleep initiation and maintenance (Larouche et al, 2014).*
- If feasible, have client arise from bed to participate in calming activities whenever anxious about failure to fall asleep. EB: *Restricting use of bed to sleeping promoted sleep initiation (Matthews, 2011).*
- Avoid a focus on the clock and subsequent worry about sleep time lost to sleeplessness. EB: *Controlling negative stimuli promoted sleep initiation (Matthews, 2011; Larouche et al, 2014).*
- Focus on positive aspects of life. EB: *Subjects' focus on gratitude was related to other positive presleep cognitions, shorter times to fall asleep, longer nighttime sleep, and better daytime function. Using mindfulness cognitive behaviors has been found to reduce insomnia (Larouche et al, 2014). Consider use of full-immersion baths or foot baths in the evening in client settings with close supervision.* CEB: *Small manipulations of core body and skin temperature were found to affect sleep onset in adults, including normal older sleepers and older insomniacs (Raymann & VanSomeren, 2008). Passive body heating via full-immersion or foot baths should be used with caution in older adults because of multiple safety issues including burns, dehydration, and potential for slips/falls in bath area.*

▲ Assist clients with chronic insomnia to limit use of sleeping agents and to select nights for sleeping pill use if complete discontinuance of sleeping pills is not feasible. EB: *Combining learned cognitive behavioral strategies for relaxing the mind and body before sleep and during the night has been found to reduce client's continual need for sleeping pills (Conroy et al, 2014). Melatonin receptor agonist agents are frequently used to treat insomnia, depression, and circadian rhythm sleep-wake disorders (Laudon & Frydman-Marom, 2014).*

▲ For clients with chronic insomnia, refer to a health care provider trained in cognitive behavioral therapies. EB: *Advanced practice nurses trained in cognitive behavioral therapies are effective providers of behavioral sleep medicine (Buysse et al, 2011; Järnefelt et al, 2012).*

▲ Assess pain medication use and, when feasible, recommend pain medications that promote rather than interfere with sleep (see Acute **Pain** and Chronic **Pain** care plans). EB: *Some pain medications also promote sleep, whereas others promote alertness and thus interfere with falling and staying asleep (Laudon & Frydman-Marom, 2014).*

▲ Assess level of anxiety. If chronic insomnia is accompanied by anxiety, use relaxation techniques. (See further Nursing Interventions and *Rationales* for **Anxiety.**) EB: *A recent review of the literature found that mindfulness-based cognitive relaxation techniques were successful in promoting sleep in people with chronic insomnia (Larouche et al, 2014).*

▲ Assess for signs of depression: depressed mood state, statements of hopelessness, poor appetite. Refer for counseling as appropriate. EB: *Many symptoms associated with sleep disruption arise from central nervous system hyperarousal in the depressed client (Melancon et al, 2014).*

▲ Assess for signs of sleep apnea and restless leg syndrome; if present, refer to an accredited sleep clinic for evaluation. If the client is waking frequently during the night, other primary sleep disorders may be the cause (Gooneratne et al, 2014; Matthews, 2011).

▲ Assess for signs of substance overuse/abuse including prescription, over-the-counter, and illicit drugs, as well as alcohol, caffeine, and theophylline use. Suggest lifestyle change and refer for addiction counseling as appropriate. *Stimulants and mood alternators can greatly disrupt the circadian rhythm of sleep and waking (Matthews, 2011; Conroy et al, 2014).*

▲ Evaluate noise and interruptions during the delivery of care of clients. EB: *Noise adversely affects the ability to initiate and sustain sleep. Frequent interruptions can prevent the client from achieving effective sleep (Basner et al, 2015; Kamdar et al, 2013).*

- *Evidence is emerging that blue screens or light emitted from electronic devices in the hours before bedtime or attempting to sleep may delay the client's ability to fall asleep. Research suggests clients exposed to blue light from electronic devices before bedtime may take longer to fall asleep and have less restorative sleep (Chang et al, 2013).*
- Supplement other interventions with teaching about sleep and sleep promotion. (See further Nursing Interventions and *Rationales* for Readiness for enhanced **Sleep.**)

Geriatric

- Assessment of medications used for pain and other symptoms in older adults is important because pain medications may be interfering with the client's ability to initiate and maintain sleep (Matthews, 2011; Gooneratne et al, 2014).
- Clients with heart failure, pulmonary disease, and dementia have a higher risk of sleep apnea, which may be undiagnosed. Consult with a health care provider to evaluate the client for sleep apnea in the older adult (Gooneratne et al, 2014).
- Exercise enhances sleep. Older adults should be encouraged to participate in routine exercise to enhance quality of sleep (Melancon et al, 2014).
- Most interventions discussed previously may be used with geriatric clients. In addition, see the Geriatric section of Nursing Interventions and *Rationales* for Readiness for enhanced **Sleep.**

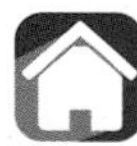

Home Care

- Assessments and interventions discussed previously may be adapted for use in home care.
- In addition, see the Home Care section of Nursing Interventions and *Rationales* for Readiness for enhanced **Sleep.**

Client/Family Teaching

- Teach family about normal sleep and promote adoption of behaviors that enhance it. See Nursing Interventions and *Rationales* for Readiness for enhanced **Sleep.**
- Teach family about sleep deprivation and how to avoid it. See Nursing Interventions and *Rationales* for **Sleep** deprivation.
- Advise family of importance of not disrupting sleep of others unnecessarily. See Nursing Interventions and *Rationales* for Disturbed **Sleep** pattern.

- Advise family of importance of minimizing noise and light, including light from electronic devices in the sleep environment. See Nursing Interventions and *Rationales* for disturbed **Sleep** pattern.
- Help family differentiate insomnia from externally caused sleep disruption and resultant sleep deprivation. Family members may have direct control over interruptions in sleep and thus may help limit sleep deprivation directly. *Insomnia is generally a stress-related, medication-related, or disease-related psychophysiological activation that interferes with the client's ability to calm the mind and body adequately for initiation and maintenance of sleep. Family members can support clients' attempts to manage their health and relax at bedtime, thus having an indirect effect.*

REFERENCES

Basner, M., Brink, M., Brislow, A., et al. (2015). ICBEN review of research on the biological effects of noise 2011-2014. *Noise and Health, 17*, 57–82.

Buysse, D. J., et al. (2011). Efficacy of brief behavioral treatment for chronic *insomnia in older adults. Archives of Internal Medicine, 171*(10), 887–895.

Chang, A. M., Scheer, F. A. J. L., Czeisler, C. A., et al. (2013). Direct effects of light on alertness, vigilance, and the waking electroencephalogram in humans depend on prior light history. *Sleep, 36*(8), 1239–1246.

Conroy, D. A., & Arnedt, J. T. (2014). Sleep and substance order abuse: an update. *Current Psychiatry Reports, 16*, 487–497.

Gooneratne, N. S., & Vitiello, M. V. (2014). *Sleep in older adults: normative changes, sleep disorders, and treatment options.*

Järnefelt, H., et al. (2012). Cognitive behavior therapy for chronic insomnia in occupational health services. *Journal of Occupational Rehabilitation.*

Kamdar, B. B., King, L. M., Collop, N. A., et al. (2013). The effect of a quality improvement intervention on perceived sleep quality and cognition in a medical ICU. *Critical Care Medicine, 41*(3), 800–809.

Larouche, M., Cote, G., Belisle, D., et al. (2014). Kind attention and non-judgement in mindfulness-based cognitive therapy applied to the treatment of insomnia: state of knowledge. *Pathologic Biologie, 62*, 284–291.

Laudon, M., & Frydman-Marom, A. (2014). Therapeutic effects of melatonin receptor agonists on sleep and comorbid disorders. *International Journal of Molecular Sciences, 15*, 15924–15950.

Matthews, E. E. (2011). Sleep disturbances and fatigue in critically ill patients. *AACN Advanced Critical Care, 22*(3), 204–224.

Melancon, M. O., Lorrain, D., & Dionne, I. J. (2014). Exercise and sleep in aging: emphasis on serotonin. *Pathologic Biologie, 62*, 276–283.

Morgan, K., et al. (2011). Insomnia: evidence-based approaches to assessment and management. *Clinical Medicine (London, England), 11*(3), 278–281.

Raymann, R. J., & VanSomeren, E. J. (2008). Diminished capability to recognize the optimal temperature for sleep initiation may contribute to poor sleep in elderly people. *Sleep, 31*(9), 1301–1309.

Salas, R. E., & Gamaldo, C. E. (2011). Diagnostic and therapeutic considerations in sleep disorders: case studies and commentary. *Journal of Clinical Outcomes Management, 18*(3), 129–144.

I

Decreased Intracranial adaptive capacity

Laura Mcilvoy, PhD, RN, CCRN, CNRN

NANDA-I

Definition

Intracranial fluid dynamic mechanisms that normally compensate for increases in intracranial volumes are compromised, resulting in repeated disproportionate increases in intracranial pressure (ICP) in response to a variety of noxious and non-noxious stimuli

Defining Characteristics

Baseline intracranial pressure (ICP) ≥10 mm Hg; disproportionate increases in intracranial pressure (ICP) following stimuli; elevated P2 ICP waveform; repeated increase in intracranial pressure (ICP) ≥10 mm Hg for ≥5 minutes following external stimuli; volume-pressure response test variation (volume: pressure ratio 2, pressure-volume index ≤10); wide-amplitude ICP waveform

Related Factors

Brain injury (e.g., cerebrovascular impairment, neurological illness, trauma, tumor); decreased cerebral perfusion ≥50-60 mm Hg; sustained increase in intracranial pressure (ICP) of 10 to 15 mm Hg; systemic hypotension with intracranial hypertension

NOC (Nursing Outcomes Classification)

Suggested NOC Outcomes

Neurological Status; Neurological Status: Consciousness

Example NOC Outcome with Indicators

Neurological Status as evidenced by the following indicators: Consciousness/Intracranial pressure/Vital signs/Central motor control/Cranial sensory-motor function/Spinal sensory-motor function. (Rate the outcome and indicators of **Neurological Status:** 1 = severely compromised, 2 = substantially compromised, 3 = moderately compromised, 4 = mildly compromised, 5 = not compromised [see Section I].)

Client Outcomes

Client Will (Specify Time Frame)

- Experience fewer than five episodes of disproportionate increases in intracranial pressure (DIICP) in 24 hours
- Have neurological status changes that are not triggered by episodes of DIICP
- Have cerebral perfusion pressure (CPP) remaining greater than 60 to 70 mm Hg in adults

NIC (Nursing Interventions Classification)

I

Suggested NIC Interventions

Cerebral Edema Management; Cerebral Perfusion Promotion; Intracranial Pressure Monitoring; Neurological Monitoring

Example NIC Activities—Cerebral Edema Management

Monitor for confusion, changes in mentation, complaints of dizziness, syncope; Allow ICP to return to baseline between nursing activities

Nursing Interventions and *Rationales*

▲ To assess ICP and CPP effectively:

- ❍ Monitor and display ICP and CPP in clients with severe traumatic brain injury (TBI) and spontaneous intracranial hemorrhage (ICH). EB: *Lack of ICP/CPP monitoring in severe TBI increases mortality (Farahvar et al, 2012; Barmparas et al, 2012).*
- ❍ Maintain ICP less than 20 mm Hg and CPP greater than 60 mm Hg. CEB: *The Guidelines for the Management of Severe Brain Injury established the treatment threshold for ICP as greater than 20 mm Hg and CPP less than 60 mm Hg (Brain Trauma Foundation, 2007).*
- ❍ Monitor neurological status frequently (hourly in acute situations) determining both pupillary size and reaction to light and the Glasgow Coma Scale (GCS) score, noting changes in eye opening, motor response to painful stimuli, and awareness of self, time, and place. EB: *The combination of a GCS score and the pupil size and reactivity are predictive of outcome and aid in discussions of prognosis with family (Hoffmann et al, 2012).*
- ❍ Monitor brain tissue oxygen ($PbtO_2$). EB: *Low brain $PbtO_2$ is predictive of increased mortality in clients with severe TBI (Bohman et al, 2011; Eriksson et al, 2012).*

▲ To prevent harmful increases in ICP:

- ❍ Elevate head of bed 30 to 45 degrees with head in midline position. CEB: *Elevating the head of the bed allows for increased venous drainage that decreases ICP (Fan, 2004; Ledwith et al, 2010).* EB: *If client is suffering acute stroke, CPP may be compromised with head elevation during the first 72 hours after injury (Favilla et al, 2014). See care plan for Risk for ineffective* **Cerebral** *tissue perfusion.*
- ❍ Administer sedation per collaborative protocol. EB: *ICP was maintained <20 mm Hg in a pilot study of acute brain injury using both propofol and dexmedetomidine infusions (James et al, 2012). Sedation was effective in 66% of episodes of decreased $PbtO_2$ (Bohman et al, 2011).*
- ❍ Maintain glycemic control per collaborative protocol. CEB: *Maintain glucose levels between 110 and 180 mg/dL using insulin therapy in critically ill brain-injured clients (Kramer et al, 2012).*
- ❍ Maintain optimal oxygenation and ventilation, applying positive end-expiratory pressure (PEEP) as needed and avoiding hyperventilation. CEB: *PEEP levels of 10 cm H_2O have been found to produce no significant changes in ICP, especially when combined with head of bed elevation of 30 degrees. Hyperventilation has been found to worsen outcomes in TBI clients and should be avoided, especially in the first 24 hours after injury (Brain Trauma Foundation, 2007; Videtta et al, 2002).*

- ❍ Provide hyperbaric oxygen/normobaric hyperoxia if available during the acute phase of severe TBI. EB: *Sixty minutes of hyperbaric oxygen at 1.5 ATA followed by 3 hours of an FiO_2 of 100% every 24 hours during the first 72 hours of severe TBI lowered ICP for the entire 3 day study period in severe TBI clients (Rockswold et al, 2013).*

▲ To prevent and treat harmful decreases in CPP:

- ❍ See care plan for Risk for ineffective **Cerebral** tissue perfusion.

▲ To treat sustained intracranial hypertension (ICP greater than 20 mm Hg):

- ❍ Remove or loosen rigid cervical collars. CEB: *Loosening or removing these collars allows for unrestricted venous drainage that lowers ICP (Mobbs et al, 2002).*
- ❍ Administer hypertonic saline (bolus or continuous infusion) per collaborative protocol. EB: *Hyperosmolar therapy reduces brain water content. A comparison of mannitol and hypertonic saline found that multiple studies, including randomized controlled trials (RCTs), demonstrated superior effectiveness of hypertonic saline in decreasing ICP (Mortazavi et al, 2012).*
- ❍ Drain cerebrospinal fluid (CSF) from an intraventricular catheter system per collaborative protocol. EB: *CSF drainage has been found to be effective in decreasing ICP (Bhargava et al, 2013; Srinivasan et al, 2014).*
- ❍ Induce moderate hypothermia (32° C to 34° C) per collaborative protocol. EB: *A systematic review of 13 RCTs and five observational studies found therapeutic hypothermia effective in controlling ICP in all studies (Sadaka & Veremakis, 2012).*

REFERENCES

Barmparas, G., Singer, M., Ley, E., et al. (2012). Decreased intracranial pressure monitor use at level II trauma centers is associated with increased mortality. *American Surgeon*, *78*(10), 1166–1171.

Bhargava, D., Alalade, A., Ellamushi, H., et al. (2013). Mitigating effects of external ventricular drain usage in the management of severe head injury. *Acta Neurochirurgica*, *155*(11), 2129–2132.

Bohman, L., Heuer, G. G., Macyszyn, L., et al. (2011). Medical management of compromised brain oxygen in patients with severe traumatic brain injury. *Neurocritical Care*, *14*, 361–369.

Brain Trauma Foundation: American Association of Neurological Surgeons, and Congress of Neurological Surgeons, Joint Section on Neurotrauma and Critical Care. (2007). Guidelines for the management of severe traumatic brain injury. *Journal of Neurotrauma*, *24*(Suppl. 1), S1–S106.

Eriksson, E. A., Barletta, J. F., Figueroa, B. E., et al. (2012). The first 72 hours of brain tissue oxygenation predicts patient survival with traumatic brain injury. *Journal of Trauma & Acute Care Surgery*, *72*, 1345–1349.

Fan, J. (2004). Effect of backrest position on intracranial pressure and cerebral perfusion pressure in individuals with brain injury: a systematic review. *Journal of Neuroscience Nursing*, *36*(5), 278–288.

Farahvar, A., Gerber, L. M., Chlu, Y., et al. (2012). Increased mortality in patients with severe traumatic brain injury treated without intracranial pressure monitoring. *Journal of Neurosurgery*, *117*, 729–734.

Favilla, C. G., Mesquita, R. C., Mullen, M., et al. (2014). Optical bedside monitoring of cerebral blood flow in acute ischemic stroke patients during head-of-bed manipulation. *Stroke; a Journal of Cerebral Circulation*, *45*, 1269–1274.

Hoffmann, M., Lefering, R., Rueger, J. M., et al. (2012). Pupil evaluation in addition to glasgow coma scale components in prediction of traumatic brain injury mortality. *British Journal of Surgery*, *99*(Suppl. 1), 122–130.

James, M. L., Olson, D. M., & Graffagnino, C. (2012). A pilot study of cerebral and haemodynamic physiological changes during sedation with dexmedetomidine or propofol in patients with acute brain injury. *Anaesthesia Intensive Care*, *40*, 949–957.

Kramer, A. H., Roberts, D. J., & Zygun, D. A. (2012). Optimal glycemic control in neurocritical care patients: a systematic review and meta-analysis. *Critical Care*, *16*, Retrieved from <http://ccforum.com/content/16/5/R203>.

Ledwith, B., Blood, S., Maloney-Wilensky, E., et al. (2010). Effect of body position on cerebral oxygenation and physiological parameters in patients with acute neurological conditions. *Journal of Neuroscience Nursing*, *42*(5), 280–287.

Mobbs, R., Stoodley, M., & Fuller, J. (2002). Effect of cervical hard collar on intracranial pressure after head injury. *ANZ Journal of Surgery*, *72*(6), 389–391.

Mortazavi, M. M., Romeo, A. K., Deep, A., et al. (2012). Hypertonic saline for treating raised intracranial pressure: literature review with meta-analysis. *Journal of Neurosurgery*, *116*, 210–221.

Rockswold, S. B., Rockswold, G. L., Zaun, D. A., et al. (2013). A prospective, randomized Phase II clinical trial to evaluate the effect of combined hyperbaric and normobaric hyperoxia on cerebral metabolism, intracranial pressure, oxygen toxicity, and clinical outcome in severe traumatic brain injury. *Journal of Neurosurgery*, *118*, 1317–1328.

Sadaka, F., & Veremakis, C. (2012). Therapeutic hypothermia for the management of intracranial hypertension in severe traumatic brain injury: a systematic review. *Brain Injury*, *26*(7–8), 899–908.

Srinivasan, V. M., O'Neill, B. R., Jho, D., et al. (2014). The history of external ventricular drainage. *Journal of Neurosurgery*, *120*, 228–236.

Videtta, W., Villarejo, F., Cohen, M., et al. (2002). Effects of positive end-expiratory pressure on intracranial pressure and cerebral perfusion pressure. *Intracranial Pressure and Brain Biochemical Monitoring Acta Neurochirurgica Supplements*, *81*, 93–97.

Neonatal Jaundice *David Wilson, MS, RNC*

NANDA-I

Definition

The yellow-orange tint of the neonate's skin and mucous membranes that occurs after 24 hours of life as a result of unconjugated bilirubin in the circulation

Defining Characteristics

Abnormal blood profile; bruised skin; yellow mucous membranes; yellow sclera; yellow-orange skin color

Related Factors (r/t)

Age <7 days; deficient feeding pattern; delay in meconium passage; infant experiences difficulty making the transition to extrauterine life; weight loss >10% (Wilson, D, original author)

NOC (Nursing Outcomes Classification)

Suggested NOC Outcomes

Breastfeeding Establishment: Infant; Breastfeeding Maintenance; Bowel Elimination; Parent: Knowledge: Parenting/Infant Care; Risk Detection/Control

Example NOC Outcome with Indicators

Breastfeeding Establishment: Infant as evidenced by the following indicators: Proper alignment and latch-on/Proper areolar grasp/Proper areolar compression/Correct suck and tongue placement/Audible swallow/Minimum eight feedings per day/Urinations per day appropriate for age/Weight gain appropriate for age. (Rate the outcome and indicators of **Breastfeeding Establishment: Infant:** 1 = not adequate, 2 = slightly adequate, 3 = moderately adequate, 4 = substantially adequate, 5 = totally adequate [see Section I].)

Client Outcomes

Client (Infant) Will (Specify Time Frame)

- Establish effective feeding pattern (breast or bottle)
- Receive bilirubin assessment and screening within the first week of life to identify potentially harmful levels of serum bilirubin
- Receive appropriate therapy to enhance indirect bilirubin excretion
- Receive nursing assessments to determine risk for severity of jaundice
- Maintain hydration: moist buccal membranes, 4 to 6 wet diapers in 24-hour period, weight loss no greater than 10% of birth weight
- Evacuate stool within 48 hours of birth, and pass 3 or 4 stools per 24 hours by day 4 of life

Client (Parent[s]) Will (Specify Time Frame)

- Receive information on neonatal jaundice prior to discharge from birth hospital
- Verbalize understanding of physical signs of jaundice prior to discharge
- Verbalize signs requiring immediate health practitioner notification: sleepy infant who does not awaken easily for feedings, fewer than 4 to 6 wet diapers in 24-hour period by day 4, fewer than 3 to 4 stools in 24 hours by day 4, breastfeeds fewer than 8 times per day
- Demonstrate ability to operate home phototherapy unit if prescribed

NIC (Nursing Interventions Classification)

Suggested NIC Interventions

Parent Education: Infant; Phototherapy: Neonate

Example NIC Activities—Phototherapy: Neonate

Review maternal and infant history for risk factors for hyperbilirubinemia (e.g., Rh or ABO incompatibility, polycythemia, sepsis, prematurity, malpresentation); Observe for signs of jaundice

Nursing Interventions and *Rationales*

- Evaluate maternal and delivery history for risk factors for neonatal jaundice (RhD, ABO, G6PD deficiency, direct Coombs). *Assessment of maternal and neonatal risk factors that may cause jaundice is important in the detection of neonatal jaundice (Perry et al, 2014).*
- Perform neonatal gestational age assessment once the newborn has had an initial period of interaction with mother and father. EB: *Gestational age assessment is important to determine potential risk factors in the neonatal population. Infants who are born late preterm (34 to 36 6/7 weeks at birth) and early term (37 and 38 6/7 weeks at birth) are at significantly increased risk for problems related to hyperbilirubinemia, feeding problems, and hospital readmission (Blackburn, 2013; Kuzniewicz et al, 2013).*
- Encourage breastfeeding within the first hour of the neonate's life. EB: *Early feedings increase neonatal intestinal activity, and infant begins establishing intestinal flora; in addition, early breastfeeding promotes enhanced maternal confidence in breastfeeding (Academy of Breastfeeding Medicine Protocol Committee, 2010; Neifert & Bunik, 2013).*
- Encourage skin-to-skin mother-newborn contact shortly after delivery. EB: *Early skin-to-skin mother-baby contact helps promote maternal confidence in nurturing abilities (Academy of Breastfeeding Medicine Protocol Committee, 2010; Neifert & Bunik, 2013).*
- Assess infant's skin color at birth and every 8 hours thereafter until birth hospital discharge for the appearance of jaundice. *Initial and ongoing neonatal skin assessment is important in the detection of jaundice (National Association of Neonatal Nurses, 2010).* CEB: *Jaundice is visible when bilirubin levels reach 5 to 6 mg/dL (Blackburn, 2013) and is reported to first appear on the face and head, then slowly advance to the trunk, arms, and lower extremities (Ambalavanan & Carlo, 2011).* CEB: *Skin color alone is not a reliable assessment for neonatal jaundice; therefore, it is important that such assessments be supported with empirical serum bilirubin measurements or transcutaneous bilirubin measurements when jaundice is suspected (American Academy of Pediatrics, 2004).*
- Encourage and assist mother with frequent breastfeeding (at least 8 to 12 times per day in the first week of life). *Frequent breastfeeding stimulates neonatal gut motility and enhances stooling, thus decreasing intestinal reabsorption of bilirubin; in addition, frequent breastfeeding stimulates breast milk production (Blackburn, 2013). Exclusive breastfeeding is recommended for neonatal feedings yet is associated with the development of hyperbilirubinemia, not directly as a result of the feeding substrate but perhaps due to decreased caloric intake in the first week of life and a substance in breast milk that may interfere with bilirubin excretion (Academy of Breastfeeding Medicine Protocol Committee, 2010; Blackburn, 2013).*
- Assist parents with bottle-feeding neonate. *Adequate caloric intake is essential for the promotion of stooling and the subsequent elimination of bilirubin from the intestine. Parents are assisted in feeding the neonate to ensure adequate growth and development (Blackburn, 2013; Hockenberry & Wilson, 2015).*
- Avoid feeding supplements such as water, dextrose water, or any other milk substitutes in breastfeeding neonate. CEB: *Supplements may act to decrease the effective establishment of breastfeeding (American Academy of Pediatrics, 2004; Blackburn, 2013).*
- Assess neonate's stooling pattern in first 48 hours of life. *Delayed stooling may indicate inadequate breast milk intake and may further increase reabsorption of bilirubin from neonate's intestine (Blackburn, 2013).*

▲ Collect and evaluate laboratory blood specimens as prescribed or per unit protocol. *Because visual assessments of skin color alone are inadequate to determine rising levels of bilirubin, serum bilirubin measurement may be gathered to evaluate risk for pathology (Ambalavanan & Carlo, 2011; National Association of Neonatal Nurses, 2010). The purpose in monitoring, evaluating, and implementing treatment in moderate to severe cases of neonatal hyperbilirubinemia is to prevent acute bilirubin encephalopathy, an early acute central nervous system bilirubin toxicity that is related to the amount of unbound (indirect) bilirubin. Kernicterus describes the yellow staining of brain cells and subsequent necrosis that occurs secondary to exposure to high levels of unconjugated (indirect) bilirubin; kernicterus involves long-term, permanent central nervous system changes (Blackburn, 2013). Bilirubin-induced neurologic dysfunction is a term used to describe the spectrum of symptoms associated with acute bilirubin encephalopathy and kernicterus (Johnson & Bhutani, 2011).*

▲ Monitor transcutaneous bilirubin level in jaundiced neonate per unit protocol or at least once every 8 hours. *Noninvasive bilirubin monitoring is a safe and effective means for monitoring bilirubin levels and determining risk for increasing serum bilirubin levels (National Association of Neonatal Nurses, 2010).*

- Perform hour-specific total serum bilirubin risk assessment before newborn's birth center discharge and document the results. CEB: *The use of an hour-specific nomogram for designation of risk in healthy, late preterm, early term, and term infants, as well as clinical risk factors, may be used to determine the relative risk of rapidly increasing bilirubin levels requiring medical intervention such as phototherapy (American Academy of Pediatrics, 2004; Maisels et al, 2009). The hour-specific nomogram estimates the total serum bilirubin (TSB) in one of four risk zones: low risk, low intermediate risk, high intermediate risk (75th to 94th percentile), and high risk (95th percentile or greater). Infants with TSB values at or above the 75th percentile in addition to risk factors such as preterm birth may require medical intervention such as phototherapy (Maisels et al, 2009). In addition to the hour-specific nomogram, risk factors that have been identified as predicting an increased probability for severe jaundice include lower gestational age, Asian ethnicity, isoimmune or hemolytic disease, significant bruising, and exclusive breastfeeding (Maisels et al, 2009; National Association of Neonatal Nurses, 2010).*

- Monitor newborn for signs of inadequate breast milk or formula intake: dry oral mucous membranes, fewer than 4 to 6 wet diapers per 24 hours, no stool in 24 hours, body weight loss greater than 10%. *Inadequate intake of breast milk in the neonatal period has been identified as a risk factor for the development of hyperbilirubinemia (Academy of Breastfeeding Medicine Protocol Committee, 2010).*
- Assess late preterm infant (born between 34 weeks and 36 6/7 weeks' gestation) for ability to breastfeed successfully and adequate intake of breast milk. *Late preterm infants are at higher risk for breastfeeding and inadequate milk intake due to physiological immaturity. Such infants are also at a much higher risk for severe jaundice than term counterparts (Radtke, 2011; Souto & Hallas, 2011).*
- Assist mother with breastfeeding and assess latch-on. EB: *Successful breastfeeding in the first few weeks of life is associated with decreased levels of serum bilirubin (Blackburn, 2013).*
- Encourage alternate methods for providing expressed breast milk if maternal health status is compromised (use of expressed breast milk) and assist mother with collection of breast milk via use of breast pump or hand expression. EB: *Alternate feeding methods for the ingestion of breast milk may be used to enhance milk intake necessary to promote stooling and enhance bilirubin excretion (Academy of Breastfeeding Medicine Protocol Committee, 2010; Lawrence & Lawrence, 2011).*
- Encourage father's participation in newborn care by changing diapers, helping position newborn for breastfeeding, and holding newborn while mother rests. *Paternal involvement in the care of the newborn helps solidify the father's role as a parent and strengthens the paternal-infant attachment process; paternal participation also helps the mother rest during the recovery from labor and delivery (Hockenberry & Wilson, 2015; Neifert & Bunik, 2013).*
- Weigh newborn daily. EB: *Daily weights assist in the detection of excess weight loss, which is often indicative of inadequate caloric intake (Alex & Gallant, 2008; Lawrence & Lawrence, 2011).*

▲ When phototherapy is ordered, place seminude infant (diaper only) under prescribed amount of phototherapy lights. EB: *Phototherapy is the primary therapy used to treat mild to moderate neonatal indirect (unconjugated) hyperbilirubinemia; phototherapy enhances indirect bilirubin excretion. In order for phototherapy to be effective, the infant must have a large skin surface area exposed to the light source (Blackburn, 2013; Stokowski, 2011).* EB: *Turning the infant periodically has not been shown to reduce circulating bilirubin levels (Stokowski, 2011).*

- Protect infant's eyes from phototherapy light source with eye shields. Remove eye shields periodically when infant is removed from light source for feeding and parent-infant interaction. EB: *Retinal damage may occur from light exposure (Bhutani & American Academy of Pediatrics, 2011; Stokowski, 2011).*
- Monitor infant's hydration status, fluid intake, skin status, and body temperature while undergoing phototherapy. EB: *Transient side effects of phototherapy include increased body temperature, increased insensible water loss, increased gastrointestinal water loss (loose stools), lethargy, irritability, and poor feeding. There is no evidence that removing the infant for parent-infant interaction during feedings and for brief caregiving activities prevents the effectiveness of phototherapy when the infant has mild to moderate hyperbilirubinemia (Blackburn, 2013; Stokowski, 2011).*

▲ Collect and evaluate laboratory blood specimens (total serum bilirubin) while infant is undergoing phototherapy. CEB: *Transcutaneous bilirubin measurements do not provide an adequate estimate of serum bilirubin level and are not effective once phototherapy has been initiated (American Academy of Pediatrics, 2004).*

- Encourage continuation of breastfeeding and brief infant care activities such as changing diapers while infant is being treated with phototherapy; phototherapy may be interrupted for breastfeeding. EB: *In most cases breastfeeding is not interrupted for phototherapy; the benefits of breastfeeding exceed any potential harm (Muchowski, 2014). If the infant's oral intake with breastfeeding is inadequate, supplementation with expressed breast milk or infant formula may be recommended (Lawrence & Lawrence, 2011).*

- Provide emotional support for parents of infants undergoing phototherapy. EB: *Separation of the infant from the mother for phototherapy disrupts parent-infant interaction and may promote parental stress and decrease the effective establishment of breastfeeding (Stokowski, 2011).*

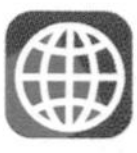

Multicultural

- Assess infants of Asian ethnicity for early rising bilirubin levels, especially when breastfeeding. EB: *Studies have shown Chinese and other Asian newborns to have higher peak serum bilirubin levels than Caucasian and African American newborns (Huang et al, 2009).*
- Encourage early and exclusive breastfeeding among Chinese and other Asian newborns. EB: *Early and exclusive breastfeeding may increase elimination of bilirubin in stool (Blackburn, 2013).*
- Assess Chinese and other Asian newborns suspected of being jaundiced with a serum bilirubin level or transcutaneous monitor. CEB: *Skin color alone is not a reliable assessment for neonatal jaundice; therefore, it is important that such assessments be supported with empirical serum bilirubin measurements or transcutaneous bilirubin measurements when jaundice is suspected (American Academy of Pediatrics, 2004).*

Client/Family Teaching and Discharge Planning

- Teach the breastfeeding mother and support persons about the appearance of jaundice *(yellow or orange color of skin) after birth center discharge, and provide health care resource telephone number for parents to call for concerns related to newborn's care.* EB: *Follow-up for evaluation of jaundice and feeding is recommended within the first 48 hours of discharge (Maisels et al, 2009).*
- Teach parents regarding the signs of inadequate milk intake: fewer than 3 to 4 stools by day 4, fewer than 4 to 6 wet diapers in 24 hours, and dry oral mucous membranes; additional danger signs include a sleepy baby that does not awaken for breastfeeding or appears lethargic (decreased activity level from usual newborn pattern). *Providing information about jaundice and effective breastfeeding may serve to decrease risk factors associated with increasing bilirubin levels (Blackburn, 2013; Seagraves et al, 2014).*
- ▲ Teach parents about the importance of medical follow-up in the first several days of life for the evaluation of jaundice. CEB: *Because of earlier postpartum hospital discharge, follow-up visits in the first 48 hours of discharge are important for the evaluation of breastfeeding, stooling and voiding pattern (hydration), and jaundice (American Academy of Pediatrics, 2004).*
- Teach parents about the use of phototherapy (hospital or home, as prescribed), the proper use of the phototherapy equipment, feedings, and assessment of hydration, body temperature, skin status, and urine and stool output. *Information is provided to the parents of the infant undergoing phototherapy to prevent misinformation about the infant's condition and treatment and to decrease parental anxiety and stress (Hockenberry & Wilson, 2015).*

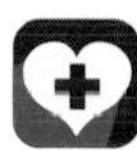

Quality and Safety in Nursing

- **Client safety:** Minimizes risk of harm to client
- Knowledge: Nurses continually assess newborns for risk factors associated with the development of jaundice
- Skills: Nurses use transcutaneous and serum bilirubin measurements to determine the newborn's bilirubin risk according to the hour-specific nomogram
- Attitudes: Nurses appreciate their role as one of promoting safety for the newborn at risk for developing jaundice
- Knowledge: Nurses implement client-focused strategies to promote serum bilirubin reduction; these include but are not limited to placing the newborn to mother's breast in first hours of life and encouraging frequent breastfeeding or no less than 10 to 12 feedings per 24 hours
- Skills: Nurses identify individual clinical risk factors in the neonate that place him/her at risk for jaundice
- Attitudes: Nurses value their role as a health care team member to promote the safe care of the newborn at discharge from the birth center and beyond
- Knowledge: Nurses understand use of phototherapy to reduce levels of indirect bilirubin
- Skills: Nurses use phototherapy lights appropriately
- Skills: Nurses assess infant for untoward effects of phototherapy
- Attitudes: Nurses appreciate the role of phototherapy as a treatment

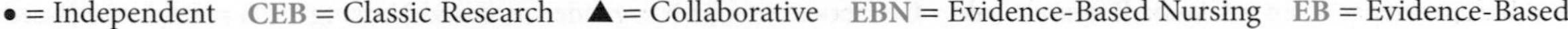

- Attitudes: Nurses value their role in the promotion of safety with the use of phototherapy
- Quality and Safety Education for Nurses: http://www.qsen.org/ksas_graduate.php#safety and http://www.qsen.org/about_qsen.php

REFERENCES

Academy of Breastfeeding Medicine Protocol Committee. (2010). ABM clinical protocol no. 22: guidelines for management of jaundice in the breastfeeding infant equal to or greater than 35 weeks' gestation. *Breastfeeding Medicine*, *5*(2), 87–93.

Alex, M., & Gallant, D. P. (2008). Toward understanding the connections between infant jaundice and infant feeding. *Journal of Pediatric Nursing*, *23*(6), 429–438.

Ambalavanan, N., & Carlo, W. A. (2011). Jaundice and hyperbilirubinemia in the newborn. In R. M. Kliegman, B. F. Stanton, & N. F. Schor (Eds.), *Nelson textbook of pediatrics* (19th ed.). Philadelphia: Saunders/Elsevier.

American Academy of Pediatrics. (2004). Management of hyperbilirubinemia in the newborn infant 35 or more weeks of gestation. *Pediatrics*, *114*(1), 297–316.

Bhutani, V. K., & American Academy of Pediatrics, Committee on Fetus and Newborn. (2011). Phototherapy to prevent severe neonatal hyperbilirubinemia in the newborn infant 35 or more weeks of gestation. *Pediatrics*, *128*(4), e1046–e1052.

Blackburn, S. T. (2013). *Maternal, fetal, & neonatal physiology: a clinical perspective* (4th ed.). St Louis: Elsevier.

Hockenberry, M. J., & Wilson, D. (2015). *Wong's nursing care of infants and children* (10th ed.). St Louis: Elsevier.

Huang, A., et al. (2009). Differential risk for early breastfeeding jaundice in a multi-ethnic Asian cohort. *Annals of the Academy of Medicine, Singapore*, *38*(3), 217–224.

Johnson, L., & Bhutani, V. K. (2011). The clinical syndrome of bilirubin-induced neurologic dysfunction. *Seminars in Perinatology*, *35*(3), 101–113.

Kuzniewicz, M. W., et al. (2013). Hospital readmissions and emergency department visits in moderate preterm, late preterm, and early term infants. *Clinics in Perinatology*, *4*, 753–775.

Lawrence, R. A., & Lawrence, R. M. (2011). *Breastfeeding: a guide for the medical profession* (7th ed.). St Louis: Elsevier/Mosby.

Maisels, M. J., et al. (2009). Hyperbilirubinemia in the newborn infant ≥35 weeks' gestation: an update with clarifications. *Pediatrics*, *124*(4), 1193–1198.

Muchowski, K. E. (2014). Evaluation and treatment of neonatal hyperbilirubinemia. *American Family Physician*, *89*(11), 873–878.

National Association of Neonatal Nurses (March 2010). *Position statement: Prevention of acute bilirubin encephalopathy and kernicterus in newborns*. Glenview, IL: Author.

Neifert, M., & Bunik, M. (2013). Overcoming clinical barriers to exclusive breastfeeding. *Pediatric Clinics of North America*, *60*(1), 115–145.

Perry, S. E., et al. (2014). *Maternal child nursing care* (5th ed.). St Louis: Elsevier/Mosby.

Radtke, J. V. (2011). The paradox of breastfeeding-associated mortality among late preterm infants. *Journal of Obstetric, Gynecologic, and Neonatal Nursing*, *40*(1), 9–24.

Seagraves, K., et al. (2014). Supporting breastfeeding to reduce newborn readmissions for hyperbilirubinemia. *Nursing Women's Health*, *17*(6), 498–507.

Souto, A., & Hallas, D. (2011). Evidence-based care management of the late preterm infant. *Journal of Pediatric Health Care*, *25*(1), 4449.

Stokowski, L. A. (2011). Fundamentals of phototherapy for neonatal jaundice. *Advances in Neonatal Care*, *11*(5S), S10–S21.

Risk for neonatal Jaundice *David Wilson, MS, RN, C*

NANDA-I

Definition

Vulnerable to the yellow orange tint of the neonate's skin and mucous membranes that occur after 24 hours of life as a result of unconjugated bilirubin in the circulation, which may compromise health

Risk Factors

Abnormal weight loss >10%, age <7 days; delay in meconium passage; feeding pattern not well established; infant experiences difficulty making the transition to extrauterine life; prematurity (≤37 weeks) (Wilson D, original author)

NOC (Nursing Outcomes Classification)

See care plan for Neonatal **Jaundice** for suggested NOC outcomes.

Client Outcomes

- Neonatal total serum bilirubin (TSB) will be monitored and there will be no undetected TSB values in the high-risk (95th percentile or greater) or high-intermediate risk (75th to 94th percentile) zones (as determined by the hour-specific nomogram)
- Newborn will receive appropriate therapies to enhance bilirubin excretion
- Newborn will remain free of undetected signs of acute bilirubin neurotoxicity
- Establish effective feeding pattern (breast or bottle)

- Receive bilirubin assessment and screening within the first week of life to detect increasing levels of serum bilirubin
- Receive nursing assessments to determine risk for severity of jaundice prior to discharge from birth hospital
- Maintain hydration: moist buccal membranes, 4 to 6 wet diapers in 24-hour period, weight loss no greater than 10% of birth weight
- Evacuate stool within 48 hours of birth, and pass 3 to 4 stools per 24 hours by day 4 of life

NIC (Nursing Interventions Classification)

See the care plan for Neonatal **Jaundice** for suggested NIC interventions.

Nursing Interventions and *Rationales*

- Identify clinical risk factors that place the infant at greater risk for development of neonatal jaundice: exclusive breastfeeding, isoimmune or hemolytic disease, preterm birth ($38\frac{6}{7}$ weeks' gestation or less), weight loss of 10% or more from birth weight, previous sibling with jaundice, East Asian ethnicity, and significant bruising or cephalhematoma. EB: *Exclusive breastfeeding that is not going well and preterm birth have been identified as being the most predictive of neonatal jaundice (Maisels et al, 2009). The other risk factors listed may also play a significant role in the development of neonatal jaundice and should be considered in the overall assessment.*
- Weigh daily the late preterm infant, early term, and term newborn who is at high risk for inadequate caloric intake for the first week of life. EB: *Daily weights assist in the detection of excess weight loss, which is often indicative of inadequate caloric intake (Alex & Gallant, 2008). Early and late preterm infants are at increased risk for inadequate caloric intake and hyperbilirubinemia; their body weight should be followed closely (Kuzniewicz et al, 2013; Souto et al, 2011).*

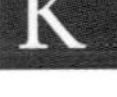

Refer to care plan for Neonatal **Jaundice** for additional interventions for multicultural and discharge planning.

Client/Family Teaching and Discharge Planning

▲ Teach parents about the importance of medical follow-up in the first several days of life for the evaluation of jaundice, especially in the late preterm infant. *Early and late preterm infants are at greater risk for feeding problems and hyperbilirubinemia, and should therefore be followed closely in the first few weeks of life (Souto et al, 2011).*

Refer to care plan for Neonatal **Jaundice** for additional interventions.

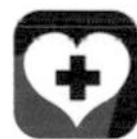

Quality and Safety in Nursing

Refer to care plan for Neonatal **Jaundice** for additional interventions.

REFERENCES

Alex, M., & Gallant, D. P. (2008). Toward understanding the connections between infant jaundice and infant feeding. *Journal of Pediatric Nursing, 23*(6), 429–438.

Kuzniewicz, M. W., et al. (2013). Hospital readmissions and emergency department visits in moderate preterm, late preterm, and early term infants. *Clinics in Perinatology*, (4), 753–775.

Maisels, M. J., et al. (2009). Hyperbilirubinemia in the newborn infant ≥35 weeks' gestation: an update with clarifications. *Pediatrics, 124*(4), 1193–1198.

Souto, A., Pudel, M., & Hallas, D. (2011). Evidence-based care management of the late preterm infant. *Journal of Pediatric Health Care, 25*(1), 44–49.

Deficient Knowledge

Barbara J. Olinzock, MSN, EdD, RN, and Kathaleen C. Bloom, PhD, CNM

NANDA-I

Definition

Absence or deficiency of cognitive information related to a specific topic

Defining Characteristics

Inaccurate follow through of instruction; inaccurate performance on a test; inappropriate behavior (e.g., hysterical, hostile, agitated, apathetic); insufficient knowledge

Related Factors (r/t)

Alteration in cognitive functioning; alteration in memory; insufficient information; insufficient interest in learning; insufficient knowledge of resources; misinformation presented by others

NOC (Nursing Outcomes Classification)

Suggested NOC Outcomes

Knowledge: Disease Process; Energy Conservation; Health Behavior; Health Resources; Healthy Diet; Infection Management; Medication; Personal Safety; Prescribed Activity; Substance Use Control; Treatment Procedure(s); Treatment Regimen

Example NOC Outcome with Indicators

Knowledge: Health Behavior as evidenced by the following indicators: Healthy nutritional practices/Benefits of regular exercise/Safe use of prescribed and nonprescribed medication. (Rate the outcome and indicators of **Knowledge: Health Behavior:** 1 = no knowledge, 2 = limited knowledge, 3 = moderate knowledge, 4 = substantial knowledge, 5 = extensive knowledge [see Section I].)

K

Client Outcomes

Client Will (Specify Time Frame)

- Explain disease state, recognize need for medications, and understand treatments
- Describe the rationale for therapy/treatment options
- Incorporate knowledge of health regimen into lifestyle
- State confidence in one's ability to manage health situation and remain in control of life
- Demonstrate how to perform health-related procedure(s) satisfactorily
- Identify resources that can be used for more information or support after discharge

NIC (Nursing Interventions Classification)

Suggested NIC Interventions

Teaching: Disease Process, Individual, Learning Facilitation

Example NIC Activities—Teaching: Disease Process

Discuss therapy/treatment options; Describe rationale behind management/therapy/treatment recommendations

Nursing Interventions and *Rationales*

- Consider the health literacy and the readiness to learn for all clients and caregivers (e.g., mental acuity, ability to see or hear, existing pain, emotional readiness, motivation, and previous knowledge). EBN: *Findings from a cross-sectional study support the notion that health literacy, as a "sixth vital sign" be addressed in all settings because health literacy can vary depending on the situation and complexities of a chronic condition (Heinrich, 2012).* CEB: *In a descriptive study, Olinzock (2008) found that readiness to learn for persons with spinal cord injury ranged from dependent to self-directed based on situational, physical, and emotional challenges of the client.*
- Focus on the nature of spoken and written communication when teaching clients and caregivers, especially those who may have health literacy needs. EBN: *Lambert and Keogh (2014) provide an overview of tools for effective teaching communication including providing feedback, actively seeking questions, using a teach-back method, and providing age-appropriate client education materials that are in are written in everyday layman language.* EB: *An evaluation study of 97 client education materials in three clinics found more than 90% were beyond the ninth grade reading level, although recommendations are that all educational materials should be on a fifth grade level by all adults regardless of health literacy (Ryan et al, 2014).*

- Consider the context, timing, and order of how information is presented. EB: *A systematic review of 56 studies on educational interventions found that presenting the most important information first and the use of simplifying, "chunking," and grouping information presented in short sessions were effective (Berkman et al, 2011).*
- Use client-centered approaches that engage clients and caregivers as active vs. passive learners. EB: *A systematic review of 38 trials with clients with asthma found that using empathy-building strategies within a framework of person-centered counseling would maximize the effectiveness of self-care interventions for those with poorly controlled asthma (Denford et al, 2014).* EBN: *A synthesis of studies by Cameron (2013) concluded that using multiple or a combination of teaching methods adapted to client learning styles and priority concerns were effective for client outcomes.*
- Reinforce learning through frequent repetition and follow-up sessions. EBN: *A systematic review of six studies found that frequent and regular educational sessions, including "boost" sessions, improved medication and self-care management outcomes for those with a chronic condition, including stroke clients (Chapman & Bogle, 2014).* EB: *In a cohort study of 400 clients at discharge, 59.2% were found to have a misunderstanding of indication, dose, and frequency of their medications, leading investigators to stress the importance of repetition of medication teaching before discharge for all clients regardless of health literacy (Mixon et al, 2014). Additional research: Cameron (2013). Additional source: Forster et al (2012).*
- Use technological and multimedia methods of disbursing information as appropriate. EB: *A Cochrane review of 24 studies with 8112 participants found that the use of multimedia education (video, audio, and self-paced computer programs) as an adjunct with current programs was most effective (Ciciriello et al, 2013).* EB: *In a Cochrane review of 16 trials with 3478 participants, the use of computer programs and the use of mobile phone interventions helped clients with diabetes type 2 improve blood glucose control, although not all clients have access (Pal et al, 2013).*
- Help the client and caregivers locate appropriate post-discharge groups and resources. CEB: *DeWalt et al (2010) offer a detailed health literacy tool kit that includes a guide for how to access nonmedical community and Internet resources for post-discharge and those transitioning home.* EB: *In focus interviews, clients shared that they learned more about themselves and their irritable bowel condition through the experience and input of others, but they were not able to relate in a group setting (Håkanson et al, 2012).*
- Encourage clients and caregivers to maintain and/or expand supportive social networks as self-care learning resources when appropriate. EB: *In a longitudinal study of clients with long-term chronic health conditions (N = 300), those who had sustained or expanded community networks were more likely to sustain self-care management, maintain behavioral change and treatment regimens, and access voluntary caregiving over formal caregiving (Reeves et al, 2014).*

K

Pediatric

- Use family-centered approaches when teaching children and adolescents. EBN: *According to Dunn and Board (2011), relationship building and negotiation of roles among parents and staff is considered essential, especially for families learning to manage complex medical technology and treatment.*
- Guide children and adolescents to credible information about their condition. CEB: *According to Chilman-Blair (2010), children and adolescents need to be connected to credible sources of information that children are familiar with, including visual sources, social media, and social networking groups that are relevant for their condition.*
- Use teaching strategies to enhance learning that are uniquely tailored for the information needs of children and/or adolescents. CEB: *In a study of young children at a diabetes camp, it was found that the children responded well to use of puppets, playthings, and games in teaching sessions because it gives them a sense of control (Pélicand et al, 2006).* EBN: *In a qualitative study of focus groups of adolescents who have undergone kidney transplant, adolescents voiced that they valued on-line discussion boards, mentoring, and sharing of personal experiences, but they were clear that they did not want to relinquish face to face time with health care providers (Korus et al, 2011).*

Geriatric

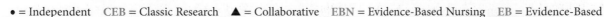

- Educate all older clients on safety issues, including fall prevention and medication management. QSEN: *In a meta-analysis of 19 studies, in client and post-discharge clients receiving targeted fall prevention education face to face or through multimedia had decreased falls than those either receiving no formal education or written education (Lee et al, 2014).* QSEN: *In a study of 162 medical records of older adults with heart failure, 48.1% received incomplete discharge medication instructions, leading investigators to recommend*

that due to complex medication changes, clear and consistent medication information during transition at discharge needs to be improved (Foust et al, 2012).*

- Consider using teaching methods and materials appropriate for older adults, especially those with cognitive challenges. EBN: *Findings in an integrated literature review suggest that the use of simple pictograms (stick figures) vs. written instructions or photographs can be used as a universal language for those with low literacy or language needs in an older adult population (Choi, 2011).* CEB: *The use of Gerogogy or story telling can be used when educating older clients to link new information with familiar concepts from past experiences (Cangelosi & Sorrell, 2008).*
- Assess readiness of older adults for use of technological resources. EBN: *Health care providers need to assess the experience and willingness of older adults to use the Internet as a source of health information and Internet sites need to be assessed for readability, large fonts, and simple structure (Sun Ju & Eun-Ok, 2014).*

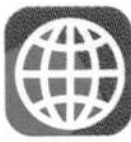

Multicultural

- Use educational interventions that are culturally tailored to the health literacy needs of the client. *A Cochrane review of 33 randomized controlled trials focusing on diabetes type 2 found that culturally appropriate health education improved blood sugar control among participants, compared with those receiving "usual" care, at 3, 6, 12, and 24 months after the intervention (Attridge et al, 2014).* CEB: *Educational programs that focus on the cultural context and not disease symptoms alone are more effective than generic education programs (Bailey et al, 2009).*
- Assess for cultural/ethnic self-care practices. CEB: *Folk and home remedies may interact with medications and treatment (Seeleman et al, 2009).*
- Consider the potential influence of medical interpreters in information sharing and decision-making and of the possible difficulties for clients when using medical interpreters. EBN: *Different categories of interpreters (e.g., trained, untrained, professional) may influence how information is shared and understood (Hadziabdic et al, 2011).*
- Consider involving bilingual members of a community who are considered outside the traditional health care system who may assist in the teaching of community health issues. EB: *Members of an ethnic or cultural group who are well networked may have greater influence when educating peers on needed lifestyle and health-related changes (Henderson et al, 2011).*

Home Care

- All of the previously mentioned interventions are applicable to the home setting.
- Use telehealth and technology-enhanced practices as appropriate. EBN: *Findings from a literature review of 48 papers support previous findings that technology is desired by consumers and can be effective, but the appropriateness for use should take into consideration the abilities of the clients, as well as the credibility of software applications and the accessibility of the type of technology, including computers and mobile devices (Fitzner & Moss, 2013).*

K

REFERENCES

Attridge, M., Creamer, J., Ramsden, M., et al. (2014). Culturally appropriate health education for people in ethnic minority groups with type 2 diabetes mellitus. *Cochrane Database of Systematic Reviews*, (9), 1–591.

Bailey, E. J., Cates, C. J., Kruske, S. G., et al. (2009). Culture-specific programs for children and adults from minority groups who have asthma. *Cochrane Database of Systematic Reviews*, (2), CD006580.

Berkman, N. D., Sheridan, S. L., Donahue, K. E., et al. (2011). *Health literacy interventions and outcomes: An updated systematic review (Evidence Report/Technology Assessment No. 199)* (Prepared by RTI International–University of North Carolina Evidence-based Practice Center under contract No. 290-2007-10056-I. AHRQ Publication Number E006). Rockville, MD.: Agency for Healthcare Research and Quality.

Cameron, V. (2013). Best practices for stroke patient and family education in the acute care setting: a literature review. *Medsurg Nursing*, *22*(1), 51–55.

Cangelosi, P. R., & Sorrell, J. M. (2008). Storytelling as an educational strategy for older adults with chronic illness. *Journal of Psychosocial Nursing & Mental Health Services*, *46*(7), 19–22.

Chapman, B., & Bogle, V. (2014). Adherence to medication and self-management in stroke patients. *British Journal of Nursing*, *23*(3), 158–166.

Chilman-Blair, K. (2010). Communicating with children about illness. *Practice Nursing*, *21*(12), 631–633.

Choi, J. (2011). Literature review: Using pictographs in discharge instructions for older adults with low-literacy skills. *Journal of Clinical Nursing*, *20*(21/22), 2984–2996.

Ciciriello, S., Johnston, R. V., Osborne, R. H., et al. (2013). Multimedia educational interventions for consumers about prescribed and over-the-counter medications. *Cochrane Database of Systematic Reviews*, (4), 1–242.

Denford, S., Taylor, R. S., Campbell, J. L., et al. (2014). Effective behavior change techniques in asthma self-care interventions:

systematic review and meta-regression. *Health Psychology*, *33*(7), 577–587.

DeWalt, D. A., Callahan, L. F., Hawk, V. H., et al. (2010). *Health literacy universal precautions toolkit.* (Prepared by North Carolina Network Consortium, The Cecil G. Sheps Center for Health Services Research, The University of North Carolina at Chapel Hill, under Contract No. HHSA290200710014.) (AHRQ Publication No. 10-0046-EF). Rockville, MD.: Agency for Healthcare Research and Quality.

Dunn, K., & Board, R. (2011). Parents and technology in the inpatient pediatric setting: a beginning model for study. *Pediatric Nursing*, *37*(2), 75–80.

Fitzner, K., & Moss, G. (2013). Telehealth-an effective delivery method for diabetes self management education? *Population Health Management*, *16*(3), 169–177.

Forster, A., Brown, L., Smith, J., et al. (2012). Information provision for stroke patients and their caregivers. *Cochrane Database of Systematic Reviews*, (11), 1–129.

Foust, J. B., Naylor, M. D., Bixby, M. B., et al. (2012). Medication problems occurring at hospital discharge among older adults with heart failure. *Research in Gerontological Nursing*, *5*(1), 25–33.

Hadziabdic, E., Heikkilä, K., Albin, B., et al. (2011). Problems and consequences in the use of professional interpreters: qualitative analysis of incidents from primary healthcare. *Nursing Inquiry*, *18*(3), 253–261.

Håkanson, C., Sahlberg-Blom, E., Ternestedt, B., et al. (2012). Learning about oneself through others: experiences of a group-based patient education programme about irritable bowel syndrome. *Scandinavian Journal of Caring Sciences*, *26*(4), 738–746.

Heinrich, C. (2012). Health literacy: the sixth vital sign. *Journal of the American Academy of Nurse Practitioners*, *24*(4), 218–223.

Henderson, S., Kendall, E., & See, L. (2011). The effectiveness of culturally appropriate interventions to manage or prevent chronic disease in culturally and linguistically diverse communities: a systematic literature review. *Health & Social Care in the Community*, *19*(3), 225–249.

Korus, M., Stinson, J. N., Pool, R., et al. (2011). Exploring the information needs of adolescents and their parents throughout the kidney transplant continuum. *Progress In Transplantation*, *21*(1), 53–60.

Lambert, V., & Keogh, D. (2014). Health literacy and its importance for effective communication. part 2. *Nursing Children & Young People*, *26*(4), 32–36.

Lee, D., Pritchard, E., McDermott, F., et al. (2014). Falls prevention education for older adults during and after hospitalization: a systematic review and meta-analysis. *Health Education Journal*, *73*(5), 530–544.

Mixon, A., Myers, A. P., Cardella, L., et al. (2014). Characteristics associated with postdischarge medication errors. *Mayo Clinic Proceedings*, *89*(8), 1042–1051. Retrieved from <http://www.mayoclinicproceedings.org/article/S0025-6196(14)00387-5/pdf>.

Olinzock, B. J. (2008). Enhancing the learning of patients with SCI: a patient education tool. *SCI Nursing*, *25*(2), 10–20, 2008.

Pal, K., Eastwood, S. V., Michie, S., et al. (2013). Computer-based diabetes self-management interventions for adults with type 2 diabetes mellitus. *Cochrane Database of Systematic Reviews*, (3).

Pélicand, J., Gagnayre, R., Sandrin-Berthon, B., et al. (2006). A therapeutic education programme for diabetic children: recreational, creative methods, and use of puppets. *Patient Education & Counseling*, *60*(2), 152–163.

Reeves, D., Blickem, C., Vassilev, I., et al. (2014). The contribution of social networks to the health and self-management of patients with long term conditions: a longitudinal study. *PLoS ONE*, *9*(6), e98340.

Ryan, L., Logsdon, M. C., McGill, S., et al. (2014). Evaluation of printed health education materials for use by low-education families. *Journal of Nursing Scholarship*, *46*(4), 218–228.

Seeleman, C., Suurmond, J., & Stronks, K. (2009). Cultural competence: a conceptual framework for teaching and learning. *Medical Education*, *43*(3), 229–237.

Sun Ju, C., & Eun-Ok, I. (2014). A path analysis of Internet health information seeking behaviors among older adults. *Geriatric Nursing*, *35*(2), 137–141.

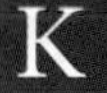

Readiness for enhanced Knowledge

Barbara J. Olinzock, MSN, EdD, RN, and Kathaleen C. Bloom, PhD, CNM

NANDA-I

Definition

A pattern of cognitive information related to a specific topic or its acquisition, which can be strengthened

Defining Characteristics

Expresses desire to enhance learning

NOC (Nursing Outcomes Classification)

Suggested NOC Outcome

Knowledge: Health Promotion

Example NOC Outcome with Indicators

Knowledge: Health Promotion as evidenced by the following indicators: Behaviors that promote health/Reputable health care resources. (Rate the outcome and indicators of **Knowledge: Health Promotion:** 1 = no knowledge, 2 = limited knowledge, 3 = moderate knowledge, 4 = substantial knowledge, 5 = extensive knowledge [see Section I].)

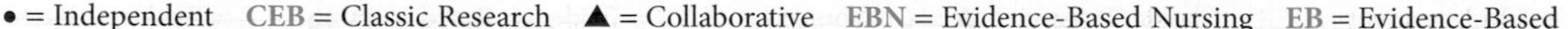

Client Outcomes

Client Will (Specify Time Frame)

- Meet personal health-related goals
- Explain how to incorporate new health regimen into lifestyle
- List sources to obtain information

NIC (Nursing Interventions Classification)

Suggested NIC Interventions

Health Education; Health System Guidance

Example NIC Activities—Health Education
Prioritize identified learner needs based on client preference, skills of nurse, resources available, and likelihood of successful goal attainment

Nursing Interventions and *Rationales*

K

- Assume a facilitator role vs. authority role when engaging clients seeking health-related knowledge. EBN: *According to Tierney et al (2011), advice giving is counterproductive and instead providing information and encouraging clients to "self-generate" solutions to problems can enhance self-control and confidence.* EBN: *A descriptive survey (N = 312) found that nurses may make inaccurate assumptions about the willingness and abilities of clients to become engaged in self-care learning (Wu et al, 2014).*
- Consider "health coaching" and motivational interviewing techniques when focusing on health-related goals, priorities, and preferences. EBN: *According to Howard and Ceci (2013), health coaching and motivational interviewing focus on the client as an autonomous decision-maker.* CEB: *Adult learning theories and models support the use of choice with self-directed autonomous learners (Olinzock, 2008).*
- Seek teachable moments for those with chronic conditions to enhance their knowledge of health promotion. EB: *Findings from a qualitative study suggest that providers often miss opportunities for "teachable moments" on health promotion topics beyond treatment regimens (Cohen et al, 2011).*

▲ Refer clients to lifestyle and health promotion resources delivered in the workplace or community sites outside traditional health care environments. EB: *In a compilation of literature addressing the outcomes of workplace health promotion programs, Goetzel et al (2014) found overwhelming success of programs focusing on areas of wellness, especially in organizations that had a "culture of health."*

- Refer clients to interactive and Web-based technological resources as appropriate. EB: *In a synthesis of literature by Hordern et al (2011), consumer e-health, Internet, and Web-based interventions that are interactive, such as self-care assessment, decision-making, and peer support, are useful in supporting lifestyle changes.*
- Refer to Deficient **Knowledge** care plan.

Pediatric

- Consider the use of mobile text messaging as a resource for delivery of health promotion information. EBN: *A systematic review of eight studies concluded that texting messages is effective for children and adolescents across demographics and can serve as a reminder system as well as augment clinical practice through tailored interactive family-centered care (Militello et al, 2012).*
- Incorporate health promotion education that reflects the unique cultural interests and values of diverse groups. EB: *In a review of 80 papers, Suarez-Balcazar et al (2013) found that adapting physical activities, ethnic dancing, and playing games that are culturally relevant were most effective for promoting health and addressing obesity in African American and Latino youth.*
- Involve children and especially adolescents in designing health promotion programs and teaching methods. EBN: *Young people are more willing to engage in health promotion programs when the program is tailored to their specific needs rather than a standardized program (Tall, 2011).*
- Consider settings outside traditional health care centers and interdisciplinary approaches for engaging children and adolescents in preventive health care. EB: *A systematic review of 55 studies found that schools may be the best place to implement health-related prevention programs to reduce health risk because of the accessibility of youth and the importance of school and peer learning (Hale et al, 2014).*

- Provide a developmentally appropriate environment when addressing health education needs of adolescents. EB: *Sustained involvement in peer educator and service learning programs where adolescents can reflect on health issues. Using guest speakers and Web resources has been shown to be effective and has been linked to reductions in adolescent sexual risk behaviors, violence involvement, and school disconnection (Sieving et al, 2011).*
- Refer to Deficient **Knowledge** care plan.

Geriatric and Multicultural

- Discuss healthy lifestyle changes that promote safety, health promotion, and health maintenance for older clients. EB: *Older people often lack knowledge about safety issues, such as fall prevention and medication management in the home and community (Dickinson et al, 2011).*
- Consider involving bilingual members of a community who are considered outside the traditional health care system who may assist in the teaching of community health issues. EB: *Members of an ethnic or cultural group who are well networked may have greater influence when educating peers on needed lifestyle and health-related changes (Henderson et al, 2011).*
- Refer to Deficient **Knowledge** care plan.

REFERENCES

Cohen, D., Clark, E., Lawson, P., et al. (2011). Identifying teachable moments for health behavior counseling in primary care. *Patient Education & Counseling, 85*(2), e8–e15.

Dickinson, A., Machen, I., Horton, K., et al. (2011). Fall prevention in the community: what older people say they need. *British Journal of Community Nursing, 16*(4), 174–180, 2011.

Goetzel, R. Z., Henke, R. M., Tabrizi, M., et al. (2014). Do workplace health promotion (wellness) programs work? *Journal of Occupational & Environmental Medicine, 56*(9), 927–934.

Hale, D. R., Fitzgerald-Yau, N., & Viner, R. (2014). A systematic review of effective interventions for reducing multiple health risk behaviors in adolescence. *American Journal of Public Health, 104*(5), e19–e41.

Henderson, S., Kendall, E., & See, L. (2011). The effectiveness of culturally appropriate interventions to manage or prevent chronic disease in culturally and linguistically diverse communities: a systematic literature review. *Health and Social Care in the Community, 19*(3), 225–249.

Hordern, A., Georgiou, A., Whetton, S., et al. (2011). Consumer e-health: an overview of research evidence and implications for future policy. *Health Information Management Journal, 40*(2), 6–14.

Howard, L., & Ceci, C. (2013). Problematizing health coaching for chronic illness self-management. *Nursing Inquiry, 20*(3), 223–231.

Militello, L. K., Kelly, S. A., & Melnyk, B. M. (2012). Systematic review of text-messaging interventions to promote healthy behaviors in pediatric and adolescent populations: implications for clinical practice and research. *Worldviews on Evidence based Nursing, 9*(2), 66–77.

Olinzock, B. J. (2008). Enhancing learning for patients with SCI: a patient education tool. *SCI Nursing, 25*(1), 10–19.

Sieving, R. E., Resnick, M. D., Garwick, A. W., et al. (2011). A clinic-based, youth development approach to teen pregnancy prevention. *American Journal of Health Behavior, 35*(3), 346–358.

Suarez-Balcazar, Y., Friesema, J., & Lukyanova, V. (2013). Culturally competent interventions to address obesity among African American and Latino children and youth. *Occupational Therapy In Health Care, 27*(2), 113–128.

Tall, H. (2011). Developing health services designed for young people. *British Journal of School Nursing, 6*(4), 193–198.

Tierney, P., Hughes, C., & Hamilton, S. (2011). Promoting health behaviour change in the cardiac patient. *British Journal of Cardiac Nursing, 6*(3), 126–130.

Wu, S., Tung, H., Liang, S., et al. (2014). Differences in the perceptions of self-care, health education barriers and educational needs between diabetes patients and nurses. *Contemporary Nurse: A Journal for the Australian Nursing Profession, 46*(2), 187–196.

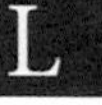

Latex Allergy response *William J. Trees, DNP, FNP-BC, CNP, RN*

NANDA-I

Definition

A hypersensitive reaction to natural latex rubber products

Defining Characteristics

Life-Threatening Reactions Occurring Less Than 1 Hour After Exposure to Latex

Protein

Bronchospasm; cardiac arrest; contact urticaria progressing to generalized symptoms; dyspnea; ede the lips; edema of the throat; edema of the tongue; edema of the uvula; hypotension; respirat syncope; tightness in chest; wheezing

Orofacial Characteristics
Edema of eyelids; edema of sclera; erythema of the eyes; facial erythema; facial itching; itching of the eyes; oral itching; nasal congestion; nasal erythema; nasal itching; rhinorrhea; tearing of the eyes
Gastrointestinal/Characteristics
Abdominal pain; nausea
Generalized Characteristics
Flushing; generalized discomfort; generalized edema; increasing complaint of total body warmth; restlessness

Type IV Reactions Occurring More Than 1 Hour After Exposure to Latex Protein

Discomfort reaction to additives such as thiuram and carbamates; eczema; irritation; redness

Related Factors (r/t)

Hypersensitivity to natural latex rubber protein

NOC (Nursing Outcomes Classification)

Suggested NOC Outcomes

Allergic Response: Localized, Systemic; Immune Hypersensitivity Response; Symptom Severity; Tissue Integrity: Skin and Mucous Membranes

Example NOC Outcome with Indicators

Immune Hypersensitivity Response as evidenced by the following indicators: Respiratory, cardiac, gastrointestinal, renal, and neurological function status IER/Free of allergic reactions. (Rate the outcome indicators of **Immune Hypersensitivity Response:** 1 = severely compromised, 2 = substantially compromised, 3 = moderately compromised, 4 = mildly compromised, 5 = not compromised [see Section I].) *IER,* In expected range.

Client Outcomes

Client Will (Specify Time Frame)

- Identify presence of natural rubber latex (NRL) allergy
- List history of risk factors
- Identify type of reaction
- State reasons not to use or to have anyone use latex products
- Experience a latex-safe environment for all health care procedures
- Avoid areas where there is powder from NRL gloves
- State the importance of wearing a medical alert bracelet and wear one
- State the importance of carrying an emergency kit with a supply of nonlatex gloves, antihistamines, and an autoinjectable epinephrine syringe (EpiPen), and carry one

NIC (Nursing Interventions Classification)

Suggested NIC Interventions

Allergy Management; Latex Precautions

Example NIC Activities—Latex Precautions

Question client or appropriate other about history of systemic reaction or sensitization to NRL (e.g., facial or scleral edema, tearing eyes, urticaria, rhinitis, and wheezing); Place an allergy band on client

Nursing Interventions and *Rationales*

- Identify clients at risk: those persons who are most likely to exhibit sensitivity to NRL that may result in varying degrees of reactivity. Consider the following client groups:
  - Persons with neural tube defects including spina bifida, myelomeningocele/meningocele. CEB: *Clients with spina bifida (myelomeningocele) are at the highest risk of latex allergy because of repeated exposure*

of mucous membranes to latex during surgeries and procedures. The prevalence of latex allergy in these clients ranges from 20% to 67% (Blumchen et al, 2010; Pollart et al, 2009).

- ○ Children with spinal cord injuries. EB: *Sensitization apparently follows multiple procedures involving urinary tract, rectal, and thecal procedures (Schottler et al, 2012).*
- ○ Clients with history of multiple surgeries or other latex-exposing procedures. EB: *Are at an increased risk relative to the general population (Behrman, 2013).*
- ○ Children who have experienced three or more surgeries, particularly as a neonate, and adults who have undergone multiple surgeries. CEB: *A significant correlation between the total number of surgeries, particularly during the first year of life, and degree of sensitization has been established (Venkata & Lerman, 2011).* CEB: *Children who are likely to have multiple surgeries early in life should be treated only with latex-free products. Likewise, adults who have had more than 10 surgeries have a significantly greater risk for developing a latex allergy (Pollart et al, 2009).*
- ○ Atopic individuals (persons with a tendency to have multiple allergic conditions) including allergies to food products. Particular allergies to fruits and vegetables including bananas, avocado, celery, fig, chestnut, papaya, potato, tomato, melon, and passion fruit are significant. CEB: *Atopic individuals generally have a higher prevalence rate, and there are known cross-reactive allergic reactions (Palosuo et al, 2011).*
- ○ Persons who possess a known or suspected NRL allergy by having exhibited an allergic or anaphylactic reaction, positive skin testing, or positive IgE antibodies against latex. CEB: *A formal evaluation for allergy is recommended for clients who have a strong history of an IgE-mediated reaction to latex and a latex-specific IgE value of zero (Siles & Hsieh, 2011).* CEB: *The use of skin prick testing with latex extracts and specific IgE detection for the diagnosis of NRL allergy in suspected clients is directed to identification of risk factors (Venkata & Lerman, 2011).*
- ○ Persons who have had an ongoing occupational exposure to NRL, including health care workers, rubber industry workers, bakers, laboratory personnel, food handlers, hairdressers, janitors, policemen, and firefighters. CEB: *Occupational exposure is different from that among children with spina bifida; it has been suggested that occupational exposure is from NRL glove proteins inhaled through powders rather than particle-bound latex proteins in urinary catheters (Palosuo et al, 2011).* CEB: *Health care workers have a sensitization rate three times higher than the general public, and there is a positive correlation between the risk for latex allergy and the length of employment in the health care industry (Pollart et al, 2009).* EB: Occupational and non-occupational risk pattens are similar in other developed countries. *The focus is on interventions to reduce latex allergy in health care workers such as with use of latex free gloves and instruments and working in latex free environments (Geier et al, 2012; Al-Niaimi, et al, 2013; Turner et al, 2012).* EB: *Exposure to latex in health care workers and clients continues to decrease. Some health care facilities are completely latex-free as the number of latex-free products become available (Chard, 2011).*
- ○ Latex sensitization is also prevalent in older adults but they are often overlooked as a high-risk population. EB: *Latex allergy has not been studied extensively among older adults but a recent study demonstrated that approximately 11.4% of the older adults in the study had latex sensitization (Grieco et al, 2014).*

- • Take a thorough history of the client at risk. CEB: *A clinical history is essential for diagnosing latex allergy (Pollart et al, 2009).* EB: *Prompt diagnosis and management can significantly minimize the risk of serious latex reactions (Kumar, 2012).*
- • Have management protocols in place for treating anaphylaxis. EB: *Prompt initial treatment is essential in anaphylaxis because a few minutes' delay can lead to hypoxic-ischemic brain damage or death (Simons et al, 2013).*
- • Question the client about associated symptoms of itching, swelling, and redness after contact with rubber products such as rubber gloves, balloons, and barrier contraceptives, or swelling of the tongue and lips after dental examinations. CEB: *Latex allergy is an IgE-mediated hypersensitivity to NRL, presenting a wide range of clinical symptoms such as angioedema, swelling, cough, asthma, and anaphylactic reactions (Deval et al, 2008).*
- • Consider the use of a provocation test (cutaneous, sublingual, mucous, conjunctival) for latex allergy diagnosis confirmation. CEB: *Latex allergy diagnosis was confirmed by specific provocation tests (Nucera et al, 2006).* EB: *The nasal provocation test is a more sensitive testing method than the glove use test (Unsel et al, 2009).*

L

- Consider a blood test to measure serum IgE levels. CEB: *Because skin prick testing is not available in the United States, measurement of latex-specific serum IgE levels is the best option (Pollart et al, 2009).* CEB: *In theory, allergy blood testing may be safer, because it does not expose the client to any allergens (Siles & Hsieh, 2011).*
- All latex-sensitive clients are treated as if they have NRL allergy. CEB: *The primary treatment for suspected latex allergy is avoidance of exposure to the latex protein (Gawchik, 2011).* CEB: *Recent studies have demonstrated that adopting latex-free strategies in health care facilities has reduced the prevalence of latex sensitization and allergy in children with spina bifida (26.7% to 4.5%), myelomeningocele (4% to 1.2%), and a history of multiple surgeries (42% to 7%) (Venkata & Lerman, 2011).*
- Clients with spina bifida and others with a positive history of NRL sensitivity or NRL allergy should have all medical/surgical/dental procedures performed in a latex-controlled environment. CEB: *The management strategy recommended by the American Society of Anesthesiology consists of a complete medical history and questionnaire (from the parents), application for a medical alert bracelet, a latex-free card, a list of latex-free devices and alternatives, signage on the client's medical records that highlights his/her latex allergy, and "Latex Allergy" signs in the perioperative area (Venkata & Lerman, 2011).* CEB: *A latex-controlled environment is defined as one in which no latex gloves are used in the room or surgical suite and no latex accessories (catheters, adhesives, tourniquets, and anesthesia equipment) come in contact with the client (Joint Task Force on Practice Parameters, 2010).* CEB: *Clients who are latex allergic should have a surgical procedure performed as the first case in the morning, when the levels of latex aeroallergens in the environment are the lowest (Cleveland Clinic, 2011).*
- In select high-risk atopic individuals, a specific immunotherapy regimen should be discussed with their health care provider. CEB: *Current subcutaneous and sublingual immunotherapy schedules have been tested for treatment of latex allergy with evidence of efficacy, but the risks of adverse events are high (Rolland & O'Hehir, 2008).* CEB: *Sublingual immunotherapy represents an efficient therapeutic tool for the management of latex allergic clients (Nucera et al, 2008).*

L

▲ The most effective approach to preventing NRL anaphylaxis is complete latex avoidance. CEB: *Symptoms of latex allergy resolve quickly with avoidance. However, elevated IgE levels can remain detectable more than 5 years after exposure, suggesting that long-term avoidance of latex should be recommended for clients with known latex allergy (Pollart et al, 2009).* CEB: *The use of no-latex gloves is the best choice from the preventive point of view (Filon & Cerchi, 2008).*

▲ Materials and items that contain NRL must be identified and latex-free alternatives must be found. CEB: *Effective in September 1998, all medical devices were required to be labeled regarding their latex content (Hubbard, 1997).* CEB: *Latex-free synthetic rubber such as neoprene, nitrile, styrene butadiene rubber, butyl, and Viton are polymers that are available as alternatives to natural rubber (Deval et al, 2008).*

▲ In health care settings, general use of latex gloves having negligible allergen content, powder-free latex gloves, and non-latex gloves and medical articles should be considered to minimize exposure to latex allergen. CEB: *The use of low-protein, low-allergenic, powder-free gloves is associated with a significant decrease in the prevalence of type I allergic reactions to NRL among health care workers (Palosuo et al, 2011).*

▲ If latex gloves are chosen for protection from blood or body fluids, a reduced-protein, powder-free glove should be selected. CEB: *Evidence within Europe demonstrates that the many benefits of NRL (gloves) can be retained by purchasing low-allergen, low-protein, and powder-free gloves, thereby reducing the risk for type I and type IV sensitization as well as allergic reactions (Palosuo et al, 2011).*

- CEB: *Clients who are known to be allergic should avoid any product that might contain latex until latex content is determined by contacting the manufacturer. Even products labeled "safe latex" (which indicates lower proportions of natural latex) can cause allergic reactions. There is no safe latex for latex allergy sufferers (Deval et al, 2008).*

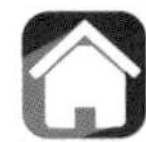

Home Care

- Assess the home environment for presence of NRL products (e.g., balloons, condoms, gloves, and products of related allergies, such as bananas, avocados, and poinsettia plants). CEB: *Strict compliance with latex avoidance instructions is essential both inside and outside the hospital. Greater emphasis should be placed on reducing latex exposure in the home and school environments, because such contact could maintain positive IgE antibody levels (Venkata & Lerman, 2011).*

- At onset of care, assess client history and current status of NRL allergy response. EBN: *A complete and thorough history remains the most reliable screening test to predict the likelihood of an anaphylactic reaction (Sekiya et al, 2011).*
- ▲ Seek medical care as necessary.
- Do not use NRL products in caregiving.
- Assist the client in identifying and obtaining alternatives to NRL products. EBN: *Preventing exposure to latex is the key to managing and preventing this allergy. Providing a safe environment for clients with NRL allergy is the responsibility of all health care professionals (American Association of Nurse Anesthetists, 1998).* CEB: *Avoidance management should be individualized, taking into consideration factors such as age, activity, occupation, hobbies, residential conditions, and the client's level of personal anxiety (Joint Task Force on Practice Parameters, 2010).*

Client/Family Teaching and Discharge Planning

- Provide written information about NRL allergy and sensitivity. CEB: *Client education is the most important preventive strategy. Clients should be carefully instructed about "hidden" latex, cross reactions, particularly with foods, and unforeseen risks during medical procedures (American College of Allergy, Asthma & Immunology, 2010; Joint Task Force on Practice Parameters, 2010).*
- ▲ Instruct the client to inform health care professionals if he or she has an NRL allergy, particularly if the client is scheduled for surgery. CEB: *Although some parents may not realize their children are sensitive to latex, inquiring about their child's responses to touching a toy balloon with their lips or inserting a rubber dam in their mouths during dental surgery, as well as a history of atopy, the number of previous surgeries, and any coexisting medical conditions (including spina bifida and congenital urological abnormalities), should be included in preoperative assessment (Venkata & Lerman, 2011).*
- Teach the client what products contain NRL and to avoid direct contact with all latex products and foods that trigger allergic reactions. EBN: *Once an individual becomes allergic to latex, special precautions are needed to prevent exposures. Teaching is an effective strategy (Society of Gastroenterology Nurses and Associates, 2008).*
- Teach the client to avoid areas where powdered latex gloves are used, as well as where latex balloons are inflated or deflated. CEB: *Powdered gloves have been shown to increase airborne NRL antigens compared with nonpowdered gloves (Palosuo et al, 2011).*
- Instruct the client with NRL allergy to wear a medical identification bracelet and/or carry a medical identification card. CEB: *Clients with a history of severe type I allergy may benefit from wearing a medical alert identification, such as a bracelet, necklace, or keychain (Pollart et al, 2009).*
- Instruct the client to carry an emergency kit with a supply of nonlatex gloves, antihistamines, and an autoinjectable epinephrine syringe (EpiPen). EB: *An autoinjectable epinephrine syringe should be prescribed to sensitized clients who are at risk for an anaphylactic episode with accidental latex exposure (American College of Allergy, Asthma & Immunology, 2010; Joint Task Force on Practice Parameters, 2010).*

L

REFERENCES

Al-Niaimi, F., Chiang, Y. Z., Chiang, Y. N., et al. (2013). Latex allergy: assessment of knowledge, appropriate use of gloves and prevention practices among hospital healthcare workers. *Clinical Experimental Dermatology*, *38*(1), 77–80.

American Association of Nurse Anesthetists. (1998). *AANA latex protocol*. Park Ridge, IL: The Association.

American College of Allergy, Asthma & Immunology. (2010). *Latex allergy*. Retrieved September 16, 2012, from: <http://www.acaai.org/allergist/allergies/Types/latex-allergy/Pages/default.aspx>.

Behrman, A. (2013). *Latex Allergy*. Retrieved September 14, 2014, from: <http://emedicine.medscape.com/article/756632-overview>.

Blumchen, K., et al. (2010). Effects of latex avoidance on latex sensitization, atopy and allergic diseases in patients with spina bifida. *Allergy*, *65*(12), 1585–1593.

Chard, R. (2011). Updating a latex allergy policy and procedure. *AORN*, 501–512.

Cleveland Clinic Foundation. (2011). *How to manage a latex-allergic patient*. Retrieved October 29, from: <http://www.uam.es/departamentos/medicina/anesnet/gtoa/latex/manage.htm>.

Deval, R., et al. (2008). Natural rubber latex allergy. *Indian Journal of Dermatology, Venereology and Leprology*, *74*(4), 304–310.

Filon, F. L., & Cerchi, R. (2008). Epidemiology of latex allergy in healthcare workers. *La Medicina Del Lavoro*, *99*(2), 108–112.

Gawchik, S. (2011). Latex allergy. *The Mount Sinai Journal of Medicine, New York*, *78*(5), 759–772.

Geier, J., Lessmann, H., Mahler, V., et al. (2012). Occupational contact allergy caused by rubber gloves—nothing has changed. *Contact Dermatitis*, *67*(3), 149–156.

Grieco, T., Faina, V., Dies, L., et al. (2014). Latex sensitization in eldery: allergological study and diagnostic protocol. *Immunity and Ageing*, (7), 11.

Hubbard, W. K. (1997). Department of health and human services. Food and drug administration: natural rubber-containing medical devices-user labeling. *Federal register*, *62*, 189.

Joint Task Force on Practice Parameters. (2010). The diagnosis and management of anaphylaxis: a practice parameter, 2010 update. *The Journal of Allergy and Clinical Immunology*, *126*, 477–480.

Kumar, R. P. (2012). Latex allergy in clinical practice. *Indian Journal of Dermatology*, *57*(1), 66–70.

Nucera, E., Schiavino, D., & Pollastrini, E. (2006). Sublingual desensitization in children with congenital malformations and latex allergy. *Pediatric Allergy and Immunology*, *17*(8), 606–612.

Nucera, E., et al. (2008). Sublingual immunotherapy for latex allergy: tolerability and safety profile of rush build-up phase. *Current Medical Research and Opinion*, *24*(4), 1147–1154.

Palosuo, T., et al. (2011). Latex medical gloves: time for a reappraisal. *International Archives of Allergy and Immunology*, *156*(3), 234–246.

Pollart, S., Warniment, C., & Takahiro, M. (2009). Latex allergy. *American Family Physician*, *80*(12), 1413–1418.

Rolland, J. M., & O'Hehir, R. E. (2008). Latex allergy: a model for therapy. *Clinical and Experimental Allergy: Journal of the British Society for Allergy and Clinical Immunology*, *38*(6), 898–912.

Sekiya, K., et al. (2011). Latex anaphylaxis caused by a Swan-Ganz catheter. *Internal Medicine (Tokyo, Japan)*, *50*, 355–357.

Schottler, J., Vogel, L. C., & Sturm, P. (2012). Spinal cord injuries in young children: a review of children injured at 5 years of age and younder. *Developmental Medicine & Child Neurology*, 1138–1143.

Siles, R. I., & Hsieh, F. H. (2011). Allergy blood testing: a practical guide for clinicians. *Cleveland Clinic Journal of Medicine*, *78*(9), 585–592.

Simons, F. E., Ardusso, L. R., Dimov, V., et al. (2013). World allergy organization anaphylaxis guidelines: 2013 update of the evidence base. *International Archives of Allergy and Immunology*, *162*, 193–204.

Society of Gastroenterology Nurses and Associates. (2008). SGNA guidelines for preventing sensitivity and allergic reactions to natural rubber latex in the workplace. *Gastroenterology Nursing*, *31*(3), 239–246.

Turner, S., McNamee, R., Agius, R., et al. (2012). Evaluating interventions aimed at reducing occupational exposure to latex and rubber glove allergens. *Occupational Environmental Medicine*, *69*(12), 925–931.

Unsel, M., et al. (2009). The importance of nasal provocation test in the diagnosis of natural rubber latex allergy. *Allergy*, *64*(6), 862–867.

Venkata, S., & Lerman, J. (2011). Case scenario: perioperative latex allergy in children. *Anesthesiology*, *114*(3), 673–680.

L

Risk for Latex Allergy response

William J. Trees, DNP, FNP-BC, CNP, RN

NANDA-I

Definition

Risk of hypersensitivity to natural latex rubber products

Risk Factors

Allergies to avocados; allergies to bananas; allergies to chestnuts; allergies to kiwis; allergies to poinsettia plants; allergies to tropical fruits; history of allergies; history of asthma; history of reaction to latex; multiple surgical procedures, especially from infancy; professions with daily exposure to latex

NOC (Nursing Outcomes Classification)

Suggested NOC Outcomes

Allergic Response: Systemic; Immune Hypersensitivity Response; Risk Control; Risk Detection; Tissue Integrity: Skin and Mucous Membranes

Example NOC Outcome with Indicators

Immune Hypersensitivity Response as evidenced by the following indicators: Respiratory, cardiac, gastrointestinal, renal and neurological function status IER/Free of allergic reactions. (Rate the outcome and indicators of **Immune Hypersensitivity Response:** 1 = not controlled, 2 = slightly controlled, 3 = moderately controlled, 4 = well controlled, 5 = very well controlled [see Section I].) *IER*, In expected range.

Client Outcomes

Client Will (Specify Time Frame)

- State risk factors for natural rubber latex (NRL) allergy
- Request latex-free environment
- Demonstrate knowledge of plan to treat NRL allergic reaction

NIC Interventions (Nursing Interventions Classification)

Suggested NIC Interventions

Allergy Management; Latex Precautions; Environmental Risk Protection

Example NIC Activities—Latex Precautions

Question client or appropriate other about history of systemic reaction to NRL (e.g., facial or scleral edema, tearing eyes, urticaria, rhinitis, and wheezing); Place an allergy band on client

Nursing Interventions and *Rationales*

- Clients at high risk need to be identified, such as those with frequent bladder catheterizations, occupational exposure to latex, past history of atopy (hay fever, asthma, dermatitis, or food allergy to fruits such as bananas, avocados, papaya, chestnut, or kiwi); those with a history of anaphylaxis of uncertain etiology, especially if associated with surgery; health care workers; and women exposed to barrier contraceptives and routine examinations during gynecological and obstetrical procedures. CEB: *Although the prevalence of latex allergy in the general pediatric population is less than 4%, the prevalence in specific at-risk populations may be as great as 71%. Children at risk for developing latex sensitivity include those with spina bifida; those with congenital urological, gastrointestinal, and tracheoesophageal defects; those who have undergone more than five surgeries; and those with a history of atopy (Venkata & Lerman, 2011).* CEB: *Health care workers have the second highest risk for developing latex allergy, particularly those who work in operating rooms, laboratories, or hemodialysis centers (Pollart et al, 2009).* EB: *Hospital housekeepers who are regularly exposed to latex gloves and other types of rubber demonstrate more frequent glove-related symptoms than other non-clinical health care workers and are considered to be at a higher risk for developing latex allergy. Prevalence of latex allergy is eight times greater in hospital housekeepers than in the general population (Boonchai et al, 2014).* CEB: *A latex-directed history is the primary method of identifying latex sensitivity, although both skin and serum testing are increasingly accurate (Society of Gastroenterology Nurses and Associates, 2008).*
- Clients with spina bifida are a high-risk group for NRL allergy and should remain latex free from the first day of life. CEB: *Latex allergy in spina bifida children is a multifactorial situation related to a disease-associated propensity for latex sensitization, early exposure, and number of surgical procedures. Prophylactic measures to avoid the exposure, not only in the sanitary environment, through the institution of latex-safe routes and every day, prevents potentially serious allergic reactions (Ausili et al, 2007).* CEB: *Children with spina bifida or urogenital abnormalities, or those who are expected to have multiple surgical procedures, should avoid exposure to latex products from birth to prevent development of latex allergy (Pollart et al, 2009).*
- Children who require regular medical treatments at home (e.g., catheterization, home ventilation) should be assessed for NRL allergy. CEB: *The frequency of daily bladder catheterizations with latex catheters has been correlated with latex sensitivity (Venkata & Lerman, 2011).* CEB: *A high level of latex protein was found in medical devices such as elastic bandages, tourniquets, Foley urinary catheters, Penrose drains, and taping (Deval et al, 2008).*
- Assess for NRL allergy in clients who are exposed to "hidden" latex. CEB: *NRL is a ubiquitous allergen as it is a component of more than 40,000 products used in everyday life (Deval et al, 2008).* CEB: *A clinical history is essential because we cannot deny possibility of exposure to latex products in everyday life (Sekiya et al, 2011).*
- See care plan for **Latex Allergy** response.

Home Care

▲ Ensure that the client has a medical plan if a response develops. Prompt treatment decreases potential severity of response.

- See care plan for **Latex Allergy** response. Note client history and environmental assessment.

Client/Family Teaching and Discharge Planning

▲ A client who has had symptoms of NRL allergy or who suspects he or she is allergic to latex needs to give this information to health care providers. EBN: *Health care workers need to implement necessary precautions when a client has known latex allergies. There are specific systems in place to provide "latex-free environments." The systems need to be used (Lankshear et al, 2008).*

- ▲ Provide written information about latex allergy and sensitivity. EB: *Client education is the most important preventive strategy. Clients should be carefully instructed about "hidden" latex; cross reactions, particularly with foods; and unforeseen risks during medical procedures. If clients have a history of anaphylaxis to NRL, it is important for them to carry autoinjectable epinephrine (Joint Task Force on Practice Parameters, 2010).*
- • Health care workers should avoid the use of latex gloves and seek alternatives such as gloves made from nitrile. EB: *Latex-free synthetic rubber such as neoprene, nitrile, styrene butadiene rubber (SBR), butyl, and Viton are polymers that are available as alternatives to natural rubber (Deval et al, 2008).*
- • Health care institutions should develop prevention programs for the use of latex-free gloves and the absence of powdered gloves; they should also establish latex-safe areas in their facilities and emergency management plans for anaphylaxis episodes. CEB: *A facility-wide strategy and commitment is necessary to establish a latex-free health care environment. A multidisciplinary latex-allergy task force should include broad representation from hospital staff and should have policies and protocols for the management of the latex-sensitive client, including educational programs for all health care workers (Venkata & Lerman, 2011).* EB: *This review of scientific evidence reports that main triggers of occupational anaphylaxis are from allergens derived from hymenoptera and natural rubber latex. A written emergency management treatment plan is mandatory for potential anaphylactic episodes with the availability of adrenaline and trained personnel (Moscato et al, 2014).*
- • Institute measures that reduce or completely avoid any latex exposure to clients. EB: *Clients at an early stage of sensitization are less likely to progress to symptomatic disease (Draisci et al, 2011).*

L

REFERENCES

Ausili, E., et al. (2007). *Prevalence of latex allergy in spina bifida: genetic and environmental risk factors. European Review for Medical and Pharmacological Sciences, 11*(3), 149–153.

Boonchai, W., Sirkudta, W., Iamtharachai, P., et al. (2014). Latex glove-related symptoms among health care workers: a self-report questionnaire-based survey. *Dermatitis: Contact, Atopic, Occupational, Drug, 25*(3), 135–139.

Deval, R., et al. (2008). Natural rubber latex allergy. *Indian Journal of Dermatology, Venereology and Leprology, 74*, 304–310.

Draisci, G., Zanfini, B., Nucera, E., et al. (2011). Latex sensitization: a special risk for the obstetric population. *Anesthesiology, 114*(3), 565–569.

Joint Task Force on Practice Parameters. (2010). The diagnosis and management of anaphylaxis: a practice parameter. 2010 update. *The Journal of Allergy and Clinical Immunology, 126*, 477–480.

Lankshear, A., et al. (2008). Making patients safer: nurses' responses to patient safety alerts. *Journal of Advanced Nursing, 63*(6), 567–575.

Moscato, G., Pala, G., Crivellaro, M., et al. (2014). Anaphylaxis as occupational risk. *Current Opinion in Allergy and Clinical Immunology, 14*(4), 328–333.

Pollart, S., Warniment, C., & Takahiro, M. (2009). Latex allergy. *American Family Physician, 80*(12), 1413–1418.

Sekiya, K., et al. (2011). Latex anaphylaxis caused by a Swan-Ganz catheter. *Internal Medicine (Tokyo, Japan), 50*, 355–357.

Society of Gastroenterology Nurses and Associates. (2008). SGNA guidelines for preventing sensitivity and allergic reactions to natural rubber latex in the workplace. *Gastroenterology Nursing, 31*(3), 239–246.

Venkata, S., & Lerman, J. (2011). Case scenario: perioperative latex allergy in children. *Anesthesiology, 114*(3), 673–680.

Risk for impaired Liver function

Betty J. Ackley, MSN, EdS, RN, Mary Beth Flynn Makic, PhD, RN, CNS, CCNS, FAAN, and Janelle M. Tipton, MSN, RN, AOCN

NANDA-I

Definition

Vulnerable to a decrease in liver function, which may compromise health

Risk Factors

HIV co-infection; pharmaceutical agent; substance abuse; viral infection

NOC (Nursing Outcomes Classification)

Suggested NOC Outcome

Knowledge: Health Behavior; Liver Function

Example NOC Outcome with Indicators

Knowledge: Health Behavior as evidenced by the following indicators: Safe use of prescription drugs/Adverse health effects of alcohol misuse/Adverse health effects of recreational drug use/Healthy nutritional practices/Self-screening techniques. (Rate the outcome and indicators of **Knowledge: Health Behavior:** 1 = no knowledge, 2 = limited knowledge, 3 = moderate knowledge, 4 = substantial knowledge, 5 = extensive knowledge [see Section I].)

Client Outcomes

Client Will (Specify Time Frame)

- State the upper limit of the amount of acetaminophen safely taken per day
- Verbalize understanding that over-the-counter (OTC) medications may contain acetaminophen (e.g., OTC cold medicines)
- Have normal liver enzymes, serum and urinary bilirubin levels, white blood cell count, and red blood cell count
- Be free of unexplained weight loss, jaundice, pruritus, bruising, petechiae, gastrointestinal bleeding, and hemorrhage
- Be free of abdominal tenderness/pain, increased abdominal girth, and have normal-colored stool and urine
- Be able to eat frequent small meals per day without nausea and/or vomiting
- If alcohol abuse is factor, state relationship between abuse and worsening gastrointestinal and liver disease

NIC (Nursing Interventions Classification)

L

Suggested NIC Interventions

Teaching: Disease Process; Substance Use Treatment

Example NIC Activities—Teaching Disease Process

Appraise the client's current level of knowledge related to specific disease process; Discuss lifestyle changes that may be required to prevent future complications and/or control the disease process

Nursing Interventions and *Rationales*

- ▲ Watch for signs of liver dysfunction including fatigue, nausea, jaundice of the eyes or skin, pruritus, gastrointestinal bleeding, coagulopathy, infections, increasing abdominal girth, fluid overload, shortness of breath, mental status changes, light-colored stools, dark urine, and increased serum and urinary bilirubin levels. *These are symptoms and laboratory results associated with liver disorders (Ghany et al, 2012).*
- ▲ Evaluate liver function tests. Standard liver panels include the serum enzymes aspartate transaminase (AST), alanine transaminase (ALT), alkaline phosphatase, and γ-glutamyltransferase; total, direct, and indirect serum bilirubin; and serum albumin. EB: *Hepatitis C is often asymptomatic early in the disease state (CDC, 2015b) and may be found during a routine examination when liver function test results are elevated (Ferguson, 2014).*
- ▲ Discuss with the client/family preparations for other diagnostic studies, such as ultrasound, computed tomography, and magnetic resonance imaging exams (Beaumont & Leadbeater, 2011).
- ▲ Evaluate coagulation studies such as international normalized ratio, prothrombin time, and partial thromboplastin time, especially when there is bleeding of the mouth or gums. *Prolonged prothrombin time and decreased production of clotting factors can result in bleeding.*
- • Monitor for signs of hemorrhage, especially in the upper gastrointestinal tract, as it is the most frequent site. *Synthesis of coagulation factors is affected with liver impairment (Lopez & Hendrickson, 2014).*
- • Obtain a list of all medications, including OTC nonsteroidal antiinflammatory drugs, acetaminophen, and herbal remedies. Review risk of drug-induced liver disease. The list includes some antibiotics, anticonvulsants, antidepressants, antiinflammatory drugs, antiplatelets, antihypertensives, calcium channel blockers, cyclosporine, lipid-lowering drugs, chemotherapy drugs, oral hypoglycemics, and tranquilizers, among others (Dienstag, 2012). If client is taking either OTC medications or herbals, discuss signs and symptoms of toxic hepatitis. *Toxic hepatitis is caused by direct toxins, drugs, herbs, and industrial chemicals.*

The risk of toxicity with aspirin, ibuprofen, naproxen sodium, and acetaminophen increases with frequency and in combination with use of alcohol (Lopez & Hendrickson, 2014).

- ▲ In clients receiving drugs associated with liver injury, review risk factors to prevent potentially severe drug reactions. *Drug-induced liver disease accounts for about 50% of hepatitis cases. The most common risk factors are advanced age, alcohol use history, pregnancy, and genetic predisposition (Kim et al, 2010).*
- ▲ Determine the total amount of acetaminophen the client is taking per day. The amount of acetaminophen ingested should not exceed 3.25 g per day, or even lower in the client with chronic alcohol intake (Dienstag, 2012). *It is common for clients to take multiple pain medications, all containing acetaminophen. Toxicity from acetaminophen is increasing because more adolescents are taking acetaminophen in combination with opioids (Bond et al, 2012).*
- ▲ Evaluate the serum acetaminophen-protein adducts in the client with possible liver failure from excessive intake of acetaminophen. CEB: *This diagnostic test was helpful in determining if liver failure is associated with acetaminophen toxicity (Dienstag, 2012).*
- ▲ If the client is on statin medications, ensure that liver enzyme testing is done at intervals. Liver enzymes can become elevated from taking statin medications; it is uncommon, but possible for statins to cause actual liver damage (Zamor & Russo, 2011).
- ▲ If the client is an alcoholic, refer to a cessation program. It is essential the client stop drinking as soon as possible to allow the liver to heal. Alcoholism is associated with malnutrition, which is harmful to the liver (O'Shea et al, 2010). Alcoholism is also associated with formation of proteins called cytokines, which cause inflammation and resultant damage to the liver (Dienstag, 2012). See care plans for Ineffective **Denial** and Dysfunctional **Family** processes.
- ▲ Provide frequent smaller meals for easier digestion. Provide diet with optimal carbohydrates, proteins, and fats. Consult with a registered dietitian to discuss best nutritional support. *Proteins can be increased as tolerated and as serum protein, albumin levels, and bilirubin levels indicate improved liver function. Improved nutrition helps the client with liver dysfunction regain strength and increase activity (Dienstag, 2012).*
- ▲ Recognize that severe malnutrition may result in acute liver failure, which is reversible with improved nutrition.
- ▲ Review medical history with the client, recognizing that obesity and type 2 diabetes, along with hypertriglyceridemia and polycystic ovarian syndrome, are major risk factors in the development of liver disease, specifically nonalcoholic fatty liver disease. *For those clients showing signs of fatty liver involvement, sound nutritional support can reduce the severity as well as mitigate the already existing secondary malnutrition (Kunutsor et al, 2014).*
- • Encourage vaccinations for hepatitis A and B for all ages. *Hepatitis A can affect anyone in the United States. Vaccination can prevent hepatitis A and B, which at times can cause liver failure (CDC, 2015a).*
- • Measure abdominal girth if individual presents with abdominal distention and pain. *Increasing abdominal distention and pain are signs of impending portal hypertension with presence of fluid shifts, resulting in ascites (Ghany et al, 2012).*
- • Assess for tenderness and/or pain level in the right upper quadrant. *Tenderness in this area is a symptom of biliary, liver, and/or pancreatic problems. This pain, along with a palpable mass and weight loss, are a classic triad for malignancies (Kunutsor et al, 2014; Ferguson 2014).*
- • Use standard precautions for handling of blood and body fluids. Review sterile techniques when giving intravenous solution and/or medications. EB: *This is imperative in order to decrease the incidence of infection with hepatitis B and hepatitis C viruses. The viruses have been spread in health care settings when injection equipment and intravenous solutions were mishandled and became contaminated (CDC, 2015a).*
- ▲ Observe for signs and symptoms of mental status changes such as confusion from encephalopathy. Assess ammonia level if mental changes occur (Dienstag, 2012).

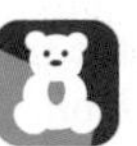

Pediatric/Parents

- ▲ Prescreen pregnant women for hepatitis B surface antigens. If found, recommend nursing case management during pregnancy. EB: *Despite advances in prevention of hepatitis B transmission, approximately half of the infections are caused by mother-to-child transmission. Efforts to prevent transmission are an essential element of perinatal maternal and infant care (Ma et al, 2014).*
- ▲ Recommend implementation of postexposure prophylaxis, including the hepatitis B virus vaccine for an infant born to a hepatitis B surface antigen–positive woman (CDC, 2015b).

- Encourage vaccinations for hepatitis A and B for all ages. *Children should be vaccinated between ages 12 months and 23 months for hepatitis A (CDC, 2015a).*
- ▲ Recognize that children can develop fatty liver disease, which can result in liver failure. Most children are asymptomatic, but others complain of malaise, fatigue, or vague recurrent abdominal pain *(Marzuillo et al, 2014).*
- ▲ During a well-baby visit, assess for signs of potential liver problems. Observe for prolonged jaundice, pale stools, and urine that is anything other than colorless. Consult with health care provider to order a split bilirubin as needed (CDC, 2015b).

Home Care

- Encourage rest, optimal nutrition (high carbohydrates, sufficient protein, essential vitamins and minerals) during initial inflammatory processes of the liver.

Client/Family Teaching and Discharge Planning

- Teach the client and family to examine all medications the client is taking, looking for acetaminophen as an ingredient, and reinforce the 3.25-g upper limit of intake of acetaminophen to protect liver function (Dienstag, 2012).
- For the caregiver or client with hepatitis A, B, or C, teach the need for careful handwashing, use of gloves, and other precautions to prevent spread of any of these diseases.
- Teach avoidance of high-risk behaviors that cause hepatitis and ways to avoid those behaviors.
- Educate clients and their caregivers about treatment options and interventions for hepatitis. Recommend other informational support: risk factors, side effects of the different treatment options, and dietary advice.
- Recommend psychological support if possible during education sessions. EBN: *Hepatitis can result in liver inflammation and chronic liver disease and is a common reason for a liver transplant. The client may feel stigmatized and may have had poor interactions with health care providers, and thus may seek less treatment. Developing a plan and/or services to support and to give client-centered care can provide better support to the client in dealing with liver disease (Grogan & Timmins, 2010).*
- For those clients with mental health problems, collaborate with outreach programs to teach signs/symptoms of hepatitis, risk factors, and factors that increase transmission. EBN: *These clients have higher potential for substance use and injected-drug use, and increased chances of transmission due to homelessness and living conditions in night shelters. Protocols have proven to be successful in developing an effective approach to meeting the needs of clients with or at risk for infection with hepatitis C virus and severe mental health problems (Lewis et al, 2010).*

REFERENCES

Beaumont, T., & Leadbeater, M. (2011). Treatment and care of patients with metastatic breast cancer. *Nursing Standard, 25*(40), 49–56.

Bond, G. R., Ho, M., & Woodward, R. W. (2012). Trends in hepatic injury associated with unintentional overdose of paracetamol (acetaminophen) in products with and without opioid: an analysis using the national poison data system of the American association of poison control centers, 2000–2007. *Drug Safety: An International Journal of Medical Toxicology and Drug Experience, 35*(2), 158.

Centers for Disease Control and Prevention (CDC). (2015a). *Hepatitis A, Q & A for health professionals.* Retrieved June 25, 2015 from: <http://www.cdc.gov/hepatitis/hcv/cfaq.htm>.

Centers for Disease Control and Prevention (CDC). (2015b). *Viral Hepatitis, Perinatal Transmission.* Retrieved June 25, 2015: <http://www.cdc.gov/hepatitis/hbv/perinatalxmtn.htm>.

Dienstag, J. (2012). Toxic and drug-induced hepatitis. In D. L. Longo, et al. (Eds.), *Harrison's principles of internal medicine* (18th ed.). New York: McGraw-Hill.

Ferguson, L. A. (2014). Autoimmune hepatitis: a noninfectious killer. *Journal of the American Association of Nurse Practitioners, 26,* 13–18.

Ghany, M., Hoofnagle, J., et al. (2012). Approach to the patient with liver disease. In D. L. Longo, et al. (Eds.), *Harrison's principles of internal medicine* (18th ed.). New York: McGraw-Hill.

Grogan, A., & Timmins, F. (2010). Patients' perception of information and support received from the nurse specialist during HCV treatment. *Journal of Clinical Nursing, 19,* 2869–2878.

Kim, J., Hattori, A., & Phongsamran, P. (2010). Drug-induced liver disease. *Critical Care Nursing Clinics of North America, 22*(3), 323–334.

Kunutsor, S. K., Apekey, T. A., Seddoh, D., et al. (2014). Liver enzymes and risk of all cause mortality in general populations: a systematic review and meta-analysis. *International Journal of Epidemiology, 43,* 187–201.

Lewis, M., Allen, H., & Warr, J. (2010). The development and implementation of a nurse-led hepatitis C protocol for people with serious mental health problems. *Journal of Psychiatric and Mental Health Nursing, 17*(7), 651–657.

Lopez, A. M., & Hendrickson, R. G. (2014). Toxin induced hepatic injury. *Emergency Medicine Clinics of North America, 32,* 103–125.

L

Ma, L., Alla, N. R., Li, X., et al. (2014). Mother to child transmission of HBV: review of current clinical management and prevention strategies. *Reviews in Medical Virology*, *24*, 396–406.

Marzuillo, P., del Guidice, E. M., & Santoro, N. (2014). Pediatric fatty liver disease: role of ethnicity and genetics. *World Journal of Gastroenterology*, *20*(23), 7347–7355.

O'Shea, R. S., et al. (2010). Alcoholic liver disease. *Hepatology (Baltimore, Md.)*, *51*(1), 307–327.

Zamor, P. J., & Russo, M. W. (2011). Liver function tests and statins. *Current Opinion in Cardiology*, *26*(4), 338–341.

Risk for Loneliness

Julianne E. Doubet, BSN, RN, CEN, NREMT-P

NANDA-I

Definition

Vulnerable to experiencing discomfort associated with a desire or need for more contact with others, which may compromise health

Risk Factors

Affectional deprivation; emotional deprivation; physical isolation; social isolation

NOC (Nursing Outcomes Classification)

Suggested NOC Outcomes

Loneliness Severity; Social Interaction Skills; Social Involvement; Social Support

Example NOC Outcome with Indicators

Loneliness Severity as evidenced by the following indicators: Sense of social isolation/Difficulty in establishing contact with others. (Rate the outcome and indicators of **Loneliness Severity:** 1 = severe, 2 = substantial, 3 = moderate, 4 = mild, 5 = none [see Section I].)

Client Outcomes

Client Will (Specify Time Frame)

- Maintain one or more meaningful relationships (growth-enhancing versus codependent or abusive in nature)
- Sustain relationships that allow self-disclosure and demonstrate a balance between emotional dependence and independence
- Participate in personally meaningful activities and interactions that are ongoing, positive, and relevant socially
- Demonstrate positive use of time alone when socialization is not possible

NIC (Nursing Interventions Classification)

Suggested NIC Interventions

Family Integrity Promotion; Socialization Enhancement; Visitation Facilitation

Example NIC Activities—Socialization Enhancement

Encourage enhanced involvement in already established relationships; Help client increase awareness of strengths and limitations in communicating with others

Nursing Interventions and *Rationales*

- Assess the client's perception of loneliness. (Is the person alone by choice, or are there other factors that contribute to the feelings of loneliness? Is the client in one of the at-risk populations for loneliness?) EB: *According to Schoenmakers et al (2014), there are numerous risk factors that influence loneliness and the caregiver should be alert to the causes and be ready to initiate preventive actions as needed.* EBN: *Loneliness was to be found to be substantially higher for men, those who had never married, primary school graduates, the childless, those who lived alone, and those with a chronic disease and/or in need of continuous medication (Koc, 2012).*

- Refer to care plan for **Social** isolation.
- Use active listening skills. Establish a therapeutic relationship and spend quality time with the client. EB: *Listening is an indispensable part of nurturing care for clients: to tell one's story and be heard is in itself restorative and life supporting (Mowat et al, 2013).* EB: *In their study of clients and families involved in palliative health care, Ciemins et al (2014) found that one expectation of the health care provider included skillful listening abilities.*
- Assess how unmet needs challenge the client. NOTE: See care plan for Disturbed **Body Image** if loneliness is associated with chronic illness and/or afflictions (e.g., multiple sclerosis, skin disturbance, mental illness). EB: *According to Huang et al (2014), job loss is a major factor linked to the increased risk of unmet basic health care needs.* EB: *Unmet needs may exceed what is customary in these clients: minority and low-income community residents; caregivers with lower education; clients with early-stage dementia; those with depression (Black et al, 2013).*

▲ *Assess the bereaved client for risk of suicide and make appropriate referrals as necessary.* EBN: *Sprinks (2014) states in her article that bereavement in older people promotes loneliness, which in turn can lead to depression, therefore increasing the client's risk for suicide.* Refer to care plan for Risk for **Suicide.**

- *Assess the client who is alone for substance abuse and make appropriate referrals.* EBN: *Murdoch's (2014) article emphasizes that all health care professionals are responsible for raising the issue of substance misuse/abuse and referring the client to specialized services if needed.* EB: *The use of heroin is increasing, along with overdose deaths. Current data indicate that the use of nonmedical opioids has intensified and is followed closely by nonmedical users shifting to heroin; interventions should focus on high-risk groups, such as regular nonmedical abusers of opioids (Jones, 2013).*
- Evaluate the client's desire for social interaction. EBN: *In their study, Thomas et al (2013) found that older people need to be involved in leisure pastimes to be socially connected: the authors suggest that new technology and problem-solving techniques assist in keeping clients socially active.*
- Assess the client for feelings of loneliness. EB: *According to Pikhartova et al (2014), the report of loneliness is contingent on sociodemographic factors, such as gender, household income, household living arrangements, and health status.*
- Explore ways to increase the client's support systems. EBN: *Nurses must recognize those who need help in dealing with their loneliness and provide direction and support (Kirkevoid et al, 2013).*
- Show respect for the client's personal attributes. EB: *Grover (2014) characterizes respect as an expression of trust that another person has value.*

L

Adolescents

- Assess the client's social support system. EB: *According to Rowe et al (2014), relationship impediments and a lack of knowledge about where to go for support may hold back an adolescent from seeking help.*
- Evaluate the family stability of adolescent clients. EBN: *In their review of literature, Kao et al (2014) found that family efficacy, characterized as a family's confidence in its ability to manage varied situations and to realize a desired outcome, is associated with the decreased likelihood of adolescents engaging in risky health behaviors.*
- Evaluate peer relationships. EBN: *In comparison to those who describe poor family and peer relationships, it was found that positive familial and peer support are factors in the reduction of adolescents' reports of risky behaviors (Saftner et al, 2011).*
- Encourage social support for clients with disabilities. EB: *In their revisit of a 2006 study involving young adults who suffer from chronic health disorders, Sattoe et al (2014) found that social participation was strongly connected to the client's feelings of independence and self-efficacy.*
- Encourage relationships with peers and involvement with groups and organizations. EBN: *There is a need to provide interventions that will promote connectedness and battle loneliness for at-risk adolescents in the out-of-school time frame (Ruiz-Caseres, 2012).*

Geriatric

- Evaluate the client for any health deviations that may limit or decrease his/her ability to interact with others. EB: *A study by Kvaal et al (2014) makes the point that loneliness is extensive among older people suffering from chronic physical illness.*

- Assess family caregivers of older persons with chronic conditions for depression related to loneliness. EBN: *Caregivers of loved ones many times are subjected to physical, psychological, emotional, social, and financial effects that can be called "caregiver burden": interventions that address caregiver burden may allow the caregivers to postpone placing the client in an extended care facility and enhance the quality of life for both the caregiver and care recipient (Sorrell, 2014).*
- Identify support systems for older adults. EB: *Senior centers are ideal settings for providing evidence-based health programs to the fast growing population of older adults and to help facilitate their continued good health and independence (Felix et al, 2014).*
- When relocation is necessary for older adults, evaluate relocation stress as a contributing factor to loneliness. EB: *This preliminary study by Theurer et al (2014) suggests that mutual support groups have potential to offset loneliness, helplessness, and depression among clients in extended care facilities.*
- Identify risk factors for loneliness in older persons. EBN: *In their study of loneliness in older adults who live at home and in assisted living and extended care facilities, Kirkevoid et al (2013) found loneliness was associated with devastating losses, inactivity, feelings of futility, and social isolation.* EBN: *Practicing clinical nurses should recognize the importance of social, not just family, support for those older persons living in an extended care facility (Drageset et al, 2011).*
- Encourage support for the client when the decision to stop driving must be made. EB: *In the interest of public safety, Reisman (2011) makes a case for a vastly improved policy structure to help get unsafe older drivers off the road.*
- Provide activities that are pleasurable to the client. EB: *In their review of one of the results of the English Longitudinal Study on Aging, Gale et al (2014) found that older people who take pleasure in life tend to live longer, indicating that psychological well-being could be a promising resource for healthier aging.* Refer to the care plan for **Social** isolation for additional interventions.

L

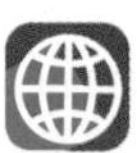

Multicultural

- Refer to the care plan for **Social** isolation.

Home Care

▲ The preceding interventions may be adapted for home care use.

▲ Assess for depression with the lonely older client and make appropriate referrals. EB: *Depression, having no caregiver, and never having been married are all identifiable risks for loneliness in older persons living alone and are indicators of possible poor quality of life and the need for social and medical interventions (Bilotta et al, 2012).* EB: *At risk for intensive loneliness are the divorced, the recently widowed, those who live alone, those who suffer failing health, and those in disadvantaged areas (Ferguson, 2011).*

- If the client has unexplained somatic complaints, evaluate these complaints to ensure that physical needs are being met, and assess for a possible relationship between somatic complaints and loneliness. EBN: *It has been found that treating widespread but underreported pain in older persons, both those confined to an extended care facility and those at home, decreases loneliness and depression (Tse et al, 2012).*
- Evaluate alternatives to being alone. EB: *O'Connor et al (2014) conducted a preliminary study of an online support group for those isolated while caring for clients with dementia; the study establishes the viability of interactive groups in virtual environments to connect members in significant interaction.*
- Refer to the care plan for **Social** isolation.

Client/Family Teaching and Discharge Planning

- Identify the type of loneliness that the client is experiencing: emotional and/or social. EB: *If both emotional and social loneliness are to be reduced in older people, strategies should be directed to widening the ranges of interventions (Dahlberg & McKee, 2014).*
- Encourage family members' involvement, if possible, in helping alleviate client's loneliness. EBN: *Decreased satisfaction with family support was one of the important predictors of depression levels in older people: this is a factor that should be taken into account when planning care (Tanner et al, 2014).*
- Include the family, if possible, in all client-teaching activities, and give them accurate information. EBN: *There is a current call to individualize client and family teaching in discharge planning (Spykopoulos et al, 2011).*

- Provide appropriate education for clients and their support persons about disease transmission and treatment if applicable. EBN: *It is of utmost importance to form an agreeable partnership between the client, his/her family, and/or caregivers who will provide support in the delivery of essential care and the control and prevention of infectious disease (Swanson & Jeanes, 2011).*
- Refer to the care plan for **Social** isolation for additional interventions.

REFERENCES

Bilotta, C., Bowling, A., Nicolini, P., et al. (2012). Quality of life in older outpatients living alone in the community in Italy. *Health and Social Care in the Community*, *20*, 32–41. [Epub 2011 Jul 1].

Black, B. S., Johnston, D., Rabins, P. V., et al. (2013). Unmet needs of community-residing persons with dementia and their informal caregivers: findings from the maximizing independence at home study. *Journal of the American Geriatrics Society*, *61*, 2087–2095.

Ciemins, F. L., Brant, J., Kersten, D., et al. (2014). A qualitative analysis of patient and family perspectives on palliative care. *Journal of Palliative Medicine*, *9*.

Dahlberg, L., & McKee, K. J. (2014). Correlates of social and emotional loneliness in older people: evidence from an English community study. *Aging and Mental Health*, *18*, 504–514. [Epub 2013 Nov 19].

Drageset, J., Kirkveld, M., & Espehaug, B. (2011). Loneliness and social support among nursing home residents without cognitive impairment: a questionnaire survey. *International Journal of Nursing Studies*, *48*, 611–619. [Epub 2010 Oct 13].

Felix, H. C., Adams, B., Cornell, E., et al. (2014). Barriers and facilitators to senior center participating in translational research. *Research on Aging*, *36*, 22–39.

Ferguson, L. (2011). The campaign to end loneliness. *Working With Older People: Community Care Policy & Practice*, *15*, 66–70.

Gale, C. R., Cooper, C., Deary, U., et al. (2014). Psychological well-being and incident frailty in men and women: the English longitudinal study of aging. *Psychological Medicine*, *44*, 697–708. [Epub 2013 Jul 3].

Grover, S. L. (2014). Unraveling respect in organization studies. *Human Relations*, *67*, 27–51.

Huang, J., Birkenmeier, J., & Kim, K. (2014). Job loss and unmet healthcare needs in the economic recession: different associations by family means. *American Journal of Public Health*, *104*, e178–e183.

Jones, C. (2013). Heroin use and heroin use risk behaviors among nonmedical users of prescription opioid pain relievers—United States, 2002–2004 and 2008–2010. *Drug and Alcohol Dependence*, *132*, 95–100. [Epub 2013 Feb 12].

Kao, T. S., Luplya, C. M., & Clemen-Stone, S. (2014). Family efficacy as a protective factor against immigrant adolescent risky behavior: a literature review. *Journal of Holistic Nursing*, *32*, 202–216.

Kirkevoid, M., Moyle, W., Wilkinson, C., et al. (2013). Facing the challenge of adopting a life "alone": the influences of losses. *Journal of Advanced Nursing*, *69*, 394–403. [Epub 2012 Apr 24].

Koc, Z. (2012). Determination of older people's level of loneliness. *Journal of Clinical Nursing*, *21*, 2037–2046.

Kvaal, K., Halding, A. G., & Kvigne, K. (2014). Social provision and loneliness among older people suffering from chronic physical illness. A mixed-methods approach. *Scandanavian Journal of Caring Solutions*, *28*, 104–111. [Epub 2013 Apr 3].

Mowat, H., Bunniss, S., Snowden, A., et al. (2013). Listening as health care. *Scottish Journal of Healthcare Chaplaincy*, *16*, 35–41.

Murdoch, J. (2014). Alcohol misuse: assessment, treatment and aftercare. *Nursing Older People*, *28*, 18–24.

O'Connor, M. F., Arizmendi, B. J., & Kaszniak, A. W. (2014). Virtually supportive: a feasibility pilot study of an on line support group for dementia caregivers in a 3D virtual environment. *Journal of Aging Studies*, *30*, 87–93. [Epub 2014 May 8].

Pikhartova, J., Bowling, A., & Victor, C. (2014). Does owning a pet protect older people against loneliness? *BMC Geriatrics*, *14*, 106.

Reisman, A. (2011). Surrendering the keys: a doctor tries to get an elderly, impaired patient to stop driving. *Health Affairs (Millwood)*, *30*, 358–359.

Rowe, S. L., French, R. S., Henderson, C., et al. (2014). Help-seeking behaviour and adolescent self-harm: a systematic review. *Australian and New Zealand Journal of Psychiatry*, *21*.

Ruiz-Caseres, M. (2012). When it's just me at home, it hits me that I am completely alone: an online survey of adolescents on self care. *Journal of Health Psychology*, *146*, 135–153.

Saftner, M. A., Martyn, K. K., & Lori, J. R. (2011). Sexually active adolescent women: assessing family and peer relationships using event history calendars. *Journal of School Nursing*, *27*, 225–236. [Epub 2011 Jan 28].

Sattoe, J. N. T., Hilberink, S. R., van Staa, A., et al. (2014). Lagging behind or not? Four distinct social participation patterns among young adults with chronic conditions. *Journal of Adolescent Health*, *54*, 397–403.

Schoenmakers, E. C., Van Tilburg, T. G., & Fokkema, T. (2014). Awareness of risk factors for loneliness among third agers. *Ageing and Society*, *34*, 1035–1051.

Sorrell, J. M. (2014). Moving beyond caregiver burden.: identifying helpful interventions for family caregivers. *Journal of Psychosocial Nursing and Mental Health Services*, *52*, 15–18. [Epub 2014 Feb 5].

Spykopoulos, V., Ampleman, S., & Miousse, C. (2011). Cardiac surgery discharge questionnaire: meeting information needs of patients and families. *Canadian Journal of Cardiovascular Nursing*, *21*, 13–19.

Sprinks, J. (2014). Social engagement crucial to tackling loneliness in old age. *Nursing Older People*, *26*, 8–9.

Swanson, J., & Jeanes, A. (2011). Infection control in the community: a pragmatic approach. *British Journal of Community Nursing*, *16*, 282–288.

Tanner, E. F., Martinez, I. L., & Harris, M. (2014). Examining functional and social detriments of depression in community-dwelling older adults: implications for practice. *Geriatric Nursing*, *35*, 236–240.

Theurer, K., Walter, A., Chaudhury, H., et al. (2014). The development and evaluation of mutual support groups in long-term care homes. *Journal of Applied Gerontology*, *33*, 387–415. [Epub 2012 Jun 7].

Thomas, J. E., O'Connell, B., & Gaskin, C. J. (2013). Residents' perceptions and experiences of social interaction and participation in leisure activities in residential aged care. *Contemporary Nurse: A Journal of the Australian Nursing Profession*, *45*, 244–254.

Tse, M., Leung, R., & Ho, S. (2012). Pain and psycho social well-being of older persons living in nursing homes: an exploratory study on planning patient oriented intervention. *Journal of Advanced Nursing*, *68*, 312–321. [Epub 2011 Jun 16].

Risk for disturbed Maternal–Fetal dyad

Dianne Frances Hayward, RN, MSN, WHNP

NANDA-I

Definition

Vulnerable to disruption of the symbiotic maternal–fetal dyad as a result of comorbid or pregnancy-related conditions, which may compromise health

Risk Factors

Alteration in glucose metabolism (e.g., diabetes mellitus, steroid use); compromised fetal oxygen transport (due to anemia, asthma, cardiac disease, hypertension, seizures, premature labor, hemorrhage); inadequate prenatal care; pregnancy complication (e.g., premature rupture of membranes, placenta previa/abruption, multiple gestation); presence of abuse (e.g., physical, psychological, sexual); substance abuse; treatment regimen

NOC (Nursing Outcomes Classification)

Suggested NOC Outcomes

Fetal Status: Antepartum, Intrapartum; Maternal Status: Antepartum, Intrapartum; Depression Level; Diabetes Self-Management; Family Resiliency; Knowledge: Hypertension Management; Substance Use Control; Nausea and Vomiting Severity; Social Support; Spiritual Support

M

Example NOC Outcome with Indicators

Maternal Status: Antepartum as evidenced by the following indicators: Emotional attachment to fetus/Coping with discomforts of pregnancy/Mood lability/Blood pressure/Blood glucose/Hemoglobin. (Rate the outcome and indicators of **Maternal Status: Antepartum:** 1 = severe deviation from normal range, 2 = substantial deviation from normal range, 3 = moderate deviation from normal range, 4 = mild deviation from normal range, 5 = no deviation from normal range [see Section I].)

Client Outcomes

Client Will (Specify Time Frame)

- Cope with discomforts of high-risk pregnancy until delivery of baby
- Adhere to prescribed regimens to maintain homeostasis during pregnancy

NIC (Nursing Interventions Classification)

Suggested NIC Interventions

High-Risk Pregnancy Care; Intrapartal Care: High-Risk Delivery

Example NIC Activities—High-Risk Pregnancy Care

Determine the presence of medical factors that are related to poor pregnancy outcome (e.g., diabetes, hypertension, lupus erythematosus, herpes, hepatitis, HIV, multiple gestation, substance abuse, epilepsy); Provide educational materials that address the risk factors and usual surveillance tests and procedures

Nursing Interventions and *Rationales*

- Standardize internal and external transport forms using SBAR format (situation, background, assessment, recommendation) to provide safe and efficient transport of a high-risk pregnant client. EBN: *The SBAR protocol provides a concise and prioritized structure that supports consistent, comprehensive, and client-centered reports (Cornell et al, 2013).*
- Arrange for psychotherapeutic support when woman expresses intense fear related to high-risk pregnancy and fetal outcomes. Encourage verbalization of feelings, beliefs, and concerns about fetal well-being, maternal health, and family functioning. EB: *A French study emphasizes the importance of delivering*

appropriate psychological support for women with high-risk pregnancies in order to prevent depressive disorders and any potential negative sequelae in the perinatal period (Denis et al, 2012). EB: *When a pregnant woman exhibits symptoms of anxiety, she might need counseling and/or treatment to decrease her anxiety (Rubertsson et al, 2014).*

- Screen all antepartum clients for depression using a tool that evaluates the biopsychosocial-spiritual dimensions in a culturally sensitive way. EBN: *When comprehensive screening is not included during antepartum care, there is less likelihood that significant information will be revealed. Subsequently, undiagnosed clinical depression in pregnancy may lead to serious perinatal complications such as inadequate maternal weight gain, preterm birth, and low infant birth weight (Breedlove & Fryzelka, 2011).*

Additional Relevant Research: Rollans et al, 2013.

- Offer flexible visiting hours, private space for families, and nursing support for management of family stressors; provide distractors such as music, TV, and laptops with Internet access when a woman is hospitalized with a high-risk pregnancy. EBN: *Women on bed rest due to complications of pregnancy face many types of stress, which can lead to emotional distress and the anxiety of being restricted. Interventions that promote a reasonable and safe amount of client control may empower women when many things are beyond their control (Rubarth et al, 2012).*
- Focus on the abilities of a woman with disabilities by encouraging her to identify her support system, resources, and needs for modification of her environment. EBN: *Pregnant women with disabilities, in particular those labeled "high risk," should expect equal ease of access to appropriate maternity care and consultation as that experienced by their "low risk" or "normal" counterparts. Maternity services should encourage independence and autonomy in these vulnerable women as far as practicable and uphold their identity and worth as women and as mothers (Walsh-Gallagher D et al, 2011). Additional Relevant Research: Gajjar et al, 2014.*
- Recognize patterns of physical abuse in all pregnant and postpartum women, regardless of age, race, and socioeconomic status. EB: *Women who were involved in intimate partner violence were more susceptible to negative outcomes such as preterm birth and low birth weight infants (Shneyderman & Kiely, 2013). Women enduring domestic violence are often in denial. Pregnancy and immediately postpartum are highly vulnerable times for mothers and their infants to experience domestic violence. These women also need to be assessed regularly because they may not be ready to seek help at first. This may be the only time a pregnant victim of domestic violence comes in contact with a health care provider who can assess for the abuse and take action to resolve it (Menezes Cooper, 2013).*

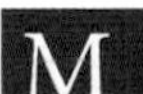

- Perform accurate blood pressure readings at each client's clinic encounter. EB: *Elevated blood pressure during pregnancy, regardless of etiology and even without known risk factors, indicates high risk for preeclampsia and for later cardiovascular disease, chronic kidney disease, and diabetes mellitus. Close clinical monitoring, risk factor assessment, and early intervention could identify and treat women and their babies for hypertension in pregnancy and its sequelae (Mannisto et al, 2013). Additional Relevant Research: Hogan et al, 2012.*
- Provide educational materials and support for personal autonomy about genetic counseling and testing options before pregnancy, that is, preimplantation genetic testing, or during pregnancy, that is, fetal nuchal translucency ultrasound, quadruple screen, cystic fibrosis. EBN: *Ethical principles of autonomy, nonmaleficence, and justice must be considered when discussing genetic counseling and testing with a pregnant woman and her family (Lewis, 2011; McCormick, 2011).* EBN: *Direct to consumer genetic testing has presented several challenges to health care providers in that consumers now have access to tests that they may not fully understand, results of which they may act upon inappropriately (Beery, 2014).*
- Identify adherence barriers and assist with meal selections to maintain optimal nutrition and safe pregnancy weight gain (25 to 35 pounds; 15 to 25 pounds if overweight). Identify cultural beliefs and nutritional patterns. A prenatal vitamin with 400 mcg of folate should also be strongly recommended. EB: *Maternal body weight and diet quality, even before pregnancy, can affect the uterine environment, birth weight, and baby's health into adulthood. A British task force showed that many women are not following nutritional guidelines. Pregnancy provides an opportunity for health care professionals to encourage women to make dietary improvements (e.g., following "myplate.com"), because women tend to be more motivated to change aspects of their diet and lifestyle during this time (Williamson & Wyness, 2013). All women in the reproductive years should consume at least 400 mcg of folic acid per day to reduce the risk for neural tube defects (Littleton-Gibbs & Engebretson, 2013).*
- Teach pregnant women diagnosed with gestational diabetes about management and treatment. EBN: *Gestational diabetes has short- and long-term implications for both the mother and the infant. To reduce*

this morbidity, it is essential to teach the client how to maintain adequate blood glucose levels during pregnancy. When diet and exercise are not enough to control blood glucose levels, drug therapy is the next option. While insulin remains the treatment of choice, insulin therapy requires sufficient education and skills on the part of the woman with gestational diabetes to be properly managed, and may cause hypoglycemia, fear, and anxiety (Mnatsakanyan et al, 2014).

- Use the five A's (tobacco cessation interventions) to treat tobacco use and dependence in pregnant women. CEB: *According to the U.S. Department of Health and Human Services Clinical Practice Guidelines (2008), health care professionals should at every contact (1) ask if a woman is a tobacco user, (2) advise her to quit, (3) assess her willingness to quit, (4) assist with the quit attempt (such as counseling, medication), and (5) arrange for follow-up (telephone support 1-800-QUIT-NOW). The evidence is compelling that even a minimal (less than 3 minute) intervention can make a difference in motivation to quit smoking.*
- When questioning at-risk clients regarding recreational drug use, ask if they have used substances such as marijuana or cocaine within the last month, instead of questioning whether they have used within the last few days. EB: *A study demonstrated that the use of these substances correlates best with the toxicology screens if women are asked if they have used these substances within the month (Yonkers et al, 2011).*
- Refer clients who self-report drug abuse or have positive toxicology screens to a comprehensive addiction program designed for the pregnant woman. Children born to addicted mothers often have poor neonatal outcomes. EBN: *The drug addict is obsessed by the drug of choice because of a change in the pathophysiology of the brain. Treating addiction as a chronic disease instead of a moral weakness is more supportive to women who abuse drugs. It is important to involve a pregnant woman in a treatment program like a methadone clinic to help to stabilize the maternal–fetal dyad. Methadone prevents withdrawal symptoms and eliminates drug craving. Methadone blocks the euphoric effects of illegal self-administered narcotics. It also supports stable maternal opioid levels to protect the fetus from repeated occurrences of withdrawal and decreases the risk for sexually transmitted infections by decreasing drug-seeking behaviors such as prostitution. When a woman makes the decision to enroll in a methadone treatment program, she is taking a significant step toward recovery (Maguire, 2014).*
- Encourage pregnant women to use electronic resources, such as Text4Baby or whattoexpect.com, to track pregnancy progress and provide education and motivation to make healthy lifestyle choices (abstinence from poor nutrition, smoking, alcohol). EBN: *Making education fun, interactive, and personal can encourage women to make behavior modifications for healthier outcomes (Jordan et al, 2011).*

M

REFERENCES

Beery, T. A. (2014). Genetic and genomic testing in clinical practice: what you need to know. *Rehabilitation Nursing*, *39*(2), 70–75.

Breedlove, G., & Fryzelka, D. (2011). Depression screening during pregnancy. *Journal of Midwifery and Women's Health*, *56*(1), 18–25.

Cornell, P., Gervis, M. T., Yates, L., et al. (2013). Improving shift report focus and consistency with the situation, background, assessment, recommendation protocol. *Journal of Nursing Administration*, *43*(7/8), 422–428.

Denis, A., Michaux, P., & Callahan, S. (2012). Factors implicated in moderating the risk for depression and anxiety in high risk pregnancy. *Journal of Reproductive & Infant Psychology*, *30*(2), 124–134.

Gajjar, D. F., Ansar, H., & Singhal, T. (2014). PMM.77Care of pregnant women with physical disabilities. *Archives of Disease in Childhood—Fetal & Neonatal Edition*, 99A147.

Hogan, J., Anglim, B., O'Dwyer, V., et al. (2012). Body mass index and hypertensive disorders of pregnancy. *Pregnancy Hypertens*, *2*(1), 28–31.

Jordan, E. T., Ray, E. M., Johnson, P., et al. (2011). Text4Baby. *Nursing for Women's Health*, *15*, 206–212.

Lewis, J. (2011). Genetics and genomics: impact on perinatal nursing. *The Journal of Perinatal and Neonatal Nursing*, *25*(2), 144–147.

Littleton-Gibbs, L., & Englebretson, J. (2013). *Maternity nursing care.* Clifton Park, NY: Delmar.

Maguire, D. (2014). Drug addiction in pregnancy: disease not moral failure. *Neonatal Network*, *33*(1), 11–18.

Mannisto, T., Mendola, P., Vaarasmaki, M., et al. (2013). Elevated blood pressure in pregnancy and subsequent chronic disease risk. *National Institute of Health: Circulation*, *127*(6), 681–690.

McCormick, M. (2011). Ethical concerns about genetic screening: the Down's dilemma. *Journal of Nurse Practitioners*, *7*(4), 316–320.

Menezes Cooper, T. (2013). Domestic violence and pregnancy: a literature review. *International Journal of Childbirth Education*, *28*(3), 30–33.

Mnatsakanyan, K., Rosario-Sim, M., & Caboral-Stevens, M. (2014). A review of the treatment options for gestational diabetes: the evidence base. *Journal of Diabetes Nursing*, *18*(4), 156–161.

Rollans, M., Schmied, V., Kemp, L., et al. (2013). "We just ask some questions..." the process of antenatal psychosocial assessment by midwives. *Midwifery*, *29*(8), 935–942.

Rubarth, L., Schoening, A., Cosimano, A., et al. (2012). Women's experience of hospitalized bed rest during high-risk pregnancy. *Journal of Obstetric, Gynecologic, and Neonatal Nursing*, *41*, 398–407.

Rubertsson, C., Hellström, J., Cross, M., et al. (2014). Anxiety in early pregnancy: prevalence and contributing factors. *Archives of Women's Mental Health*, *17*(3), 221–228.

Shneyderman, Y., & Kiely, M. (2013). Intimate partner violence during pregnancy: victim or perpetrator? Does it make a difference? *BJOG: An International Journal of Obstetrics & Gynaecology*, *120*(11), 1375–1385.

U.S. Department of Health and Human Services (USDHHS) (2008). *Treating tobacco use and dependence: clinical practice guideline 2008 update. Pregnant smokers.* Retrieved from <http://www.ahrq.gov/clinic/tobacco/treating_tobacco_use08.pdf>.

Walsh-Gallagher, D., Sinclair, M., & Conkey, R. (2011). The ambiguity of disabled women's experiences of pregnancy, childbirth and motherhood: a phenomenological understanding. *Midwifery*, *28*(2), 156–162.

Williamson, C., & Wyness, L. (2013). Nutritional requirements in pregnancy and use of dietary supplements. *Community Practitioner: The Journal of the Community Practitioners' and Health Visitors' Association*, *86*(8), 44–47.

Yonkers, K. A., Howell, H. B., Gotman, N., et al. (2011). Self-report of illicit substance use versus urine toxicology results from at-risk pregnant women. *Journal of Substance Use*, *16*(5), 372–380.

Impaired Memory *Graham J. McDougall, Jr., PhD, RN, FAAN, FGSA*

NANDA-I

Definition

Inability to remember or recall bits of information or behavioral skills

Defining Characteristics

Forgetfulness; forgets to perform a behavior at scheduled time; inability to learn new skill; inability to perform a previously learned skill; inability to recall events; inability to recall factual information; inability to recall if a behavior was performed; inability to retain new information.

Related Factors (r/t)

Alterations in fluid volume; anemia; decrease in cardiac output; distractions in the environment; electrolyte imbalance hypoxia; neurological impairment (e.g., positive EEG, head trauma, seizure disorders)

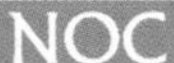

Outcomes (Nursing Outcomes Classification)

Suggested NOC Outcomes

Cognitive Orientation; Memory; Neurological Status: Consciousness

Example NOC Outcome with Indicators

Memory as evidenced by the following indicators: Recalls immediate information accurately/Recalls recent information accurately/Recalls remote information accurately (Rate each indicator of **Memory:** 1 = severely compromised, 2 = substantially compromised, 3 = moderately compromised, 4 = mildly compromised, 5 = not compromised [see Section I].)

Client Outcomes

Client Will (Specify Time Frame)

- Demonstrate use of techniques to help with memory loss
- State he or she has improved memory for everyday concerns

NIC Interventions (Nursing Interventions Classification)

Suggested NIC Intervention

Memory Training; Realistic Appraisal of Memory

Example NIC Activities—Memory Training

Stimulate memory by repeating client's last expressed thought, as appropriate; Provide opportunity to use memory for recent events, such as questioning client about a recent outing; Give examples of external memory strategies, such as using a calendar

Nursing Interventions and *Rationales*

- Assess overall cognitive function and memory. The emphasis of the assessment is everyday memory, the day-to-day operations of memory in real-world ordinary situations. A screening instrument such as the

Mini-Mental State Examination (MMSE) is useful as a first level of evaluation. EB: *The MMSE can help determine whether the client has cognitive impairment and delirium and needs to be referred for further evaluation and treatment (Lacy et al, 2014).*

- Determine whether onset of memory loss is gradual or sudden. If memory loss is sudden, refer the client to a health care provider or neuropsychologist for evaluation. EB: *Acute onset of memory loss may be associated with neurological disease, medication effect, electrolyte disturbances, hypoxia, hypothyroidism, mental illness, post-traumatic stress disorder, drug addiction, or many other physiological factors (Schwabe et al, 2014).*
- Determine amount and pattern of alcohol intake. *Alcohol intake has been associated with blackouts; clients may function but not remember their actions. Higher average weekly quantity and frequency of alcohol consumed in midlife were associated in old age with faster decline in all cognitive domains (Gross et al, 2011; Sabia et al, 2014).*

▲ Note the client's current medications and intake of any mind-altering substances, such as benzodiazepines, ecstasy, marijuana, cocaine, or glucocorticoids. *Benzodiazepines, oxybutynin, amitriptyline, fluoxetine, and diphenhydramine can produce memory loss for events that occur after taking the medication; information is not stored in long-term memory.*

▲ Note the client's current level of anxiety and stress. Ask if there has been a recent traumatic event (Luijten et al, 2014). *Post-traumatic stress and anxiety-inducing general life factors may induce memory problems. Stress or elevated cortisol levels temporarily block memory retrieval (Bauer et al, 2013; Zlomuzica et al, 2014).*

- Encourage the client to develop an aerobic exercise program. EB: *Reviews demonstrated that diet and lifestyle may prevent the onset of age-related problems and can lead to improvements in cognition and memory (Meeusen, 2014; Wang et al, 2014).*
- Determine the client's sleep patterns. If sleep quantity and quality is insufficient, refer to care plan for Disturbed **Sleep** pattern. EB: *A review provided evidence of a range of cognitive deficits identified in untreated obstructive sleep apnea clients. Clients reported difficulty in concentrating, increased forgetfulness, an inability to make decisions, and falling asleep at the wheel of a motor vehicle (Jackson et al, 2011).*

▲ Determine the client's blood sugar levels. If they are elevated, refer to health care provider for treatment and encourage healthy diet and exercise. *Oxidative stress was found to be associated with type 2 diabetes mellitus, but was not a risk factor for the development of Alzheimer's disease (Butterfield et al, 2014). However, the need to rule out diabetes is a relevant concern for a differential diagnosis.*

▲ If signs of depression such as weight loss, insomnia, or sad affect are evident, refer the client for psychotherapy. *Depression may result in deficits in executive functions (Alves et al, 2014; Baune & Renger, 2014).*

▲ Question the client about cholesterol level. If it is high, refer to health care provider or dietitian for help in lowering. Encourage the client to eat a healthy diet, avoiding saturated fats and trans-fat acids. EB: *A systematic review of studies found that statins could not be recommended as a preventive treatment for dementia (Stranahan & Mattso, 2012).*

- Suggest clients use cues, including alarm watches, electronic organizers, calendars, lists, or pocket computers, to trigger certain actions at designated times. *Cues and external cognitive strategies can help remind clients of certain actions, particularly for future intentions known as prospective memory (Yubero et al, 2011).*
- Encourage the client to participate in a multicomponent cognitive rehabilitation program that recommends stress and relaxation training, physical activity, and external memory devices, such as a calendar for appointments and reminder lists. *Using reminders can serve as cues for memory-impaired clients (Nouchi et al, 2012).*
- Help the client set up a medication box that reminds him/her to take medication at prescribed times; assist the client with refilling the box at intervals if necessary. *Medication boxes are effective because clients will know whether medication has been taken when corresponding compartments are empty.*
- If safety is an issue with certain activities (e.g., the client forgets to turn off stove after use or forgets emergency telephone numbers), suggest alternatives such as using a microwave or a whistling teakettle for heating water and programming emergency numbers in the telephone so that they are readily available.

▲ Refer the client to a memory clinic (if available), a neuropsychologist, or an occupational therapist. *Memory clinics can help the client learn ways to improve memory. Clinics may be more effective for minority older adults if work is done in groups because of increased support, reinforcement, and motivation. Of 677*

M

eligible Hispanic clients approached in Los Angeles, 329 (49%) were screened and 77 (23%) met criteria for memory impairment (Harris et al, 2011).

- For clients with memory impairments associated with dementia, see care plan for Chronic **Confusion.**

Geriatric

- Assess for signs of depression. *Depression is an important affective variable for memory loss in older adults. Antidepressant drug therapy has not been associated with reducing the burden of depression in older adults and often causes side effects in older adults, which may limit the effectiveness of treatment for depression (Mulsant et al, 2014).* EB: *In a study, those participants with current depression had significantly higher levels of psychological distress and anxiety, and lower life satisfaction, and performed worse on memory and executive function compared to participants without depression. After controlling for anxiety, the effect on executive function was no longer significant while the effect on memory remained significant. When someone had a history of depression, he/she was likely to have worse executive function, higher levels of psychological distress and anxiety, and lower life satisfaction (Reppermund et al, 2011).*
- Perform a nutritional assessment. If nutritional status is marginal, confer with a dietitian and primary health care practitioner to evaluate whether the client needs supplementation with foods or vitamins. Teach the client the need to eat a healthy diet with adequate intake of whole grains, fruits, and vegetables to decrease cerebrovascular infarcts. *Moderate, long-term deficiencies of nutrients, particularly vitamin B_{12} deficiency in older adults may lead to irreversible neurological damage, anemia, osteoporosis, cerebrovascular cardiovascular diseases, and cognitive deficits. This condition may be preventable or diminished (Chatthanawaree, 2011).* EB: *A large study demonstrated a protective effect against stroke in people who had high daily intake of raw fruits and vegetables (Griep et al, 2011).*
- Evaluate all medications that the client is taking to determine whether they are causing the memory loss. (Evaluate all *herbal and/or nutraceutical products* that the individual might be using to improve memory function, particularly Ginkgo biloba (Diamond & Bailey, 2013).
- Recommend that older clients maintain a positive attitude and active involvement with the world around them and that they maintain good nutrition. CEB: *Of the total of 1672 brain autopsies from the Adult Changes in Thought study, Honolulu-Asia Aging Study, Nun Study, and Oregon Brain Aging Study, 424 met the criteria for cognitively normal (CN). The lesions in each individual and the associated comorbidity varied widely within each study but were similar across studies. There was a convergence of subclinical diseases in the brains of older CN adults that varied widely (Sonnen et al, 2011).*
- Encourage older adults to believe in themselves and to work to improve their memory. Negative attitudes and beliefs may decrease motivation and impair everyday memory function. *Research has shown that there is formation of new neurons in the brain, a process called neurogenesis, throughout the lifespan, and stimulation of the brain is necessary for this formation (McDougall et al, 2010a).* CEB: *Octogenarians were able to improve their memory performance when they challenged their limits, used appropriate strategies, practiced yoga, and invested the energy and time in learning novel memory techniques (McDougall et al, 2015).*
- Refer the client to a memory improvement class that focuses on helping older adults learn memory strategies. CEB/EB: *Research has demonstrated that cognitive training focused on memory strategies and stress reduction may improve memory performance and decrease negative control beliefs (McDougall et al, 2010a). A 195-hour training program used a tablet computer and associated software applications (Chan et al, 2014). Episodic memory and processing speed improved in the older adults in the experimental condition.*

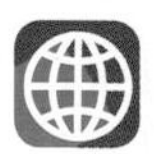

Multicultural

- Assess for the influence of cultural beliefs, norms, and values on the family or caregiver's understanding of impaired memory. *Minority elders have misconceptions in knowledge, awareness, and beliefs about Alzheimer's disease (Darnell et al, 2011).*
- When assessing memory in Mexican Americans, the MMSE has been used with success. EB: *Cultural factors and variables related to preferred language use determined variations in MMSE performance. However, the memory domain of the MMSE is less affected by education and is appropriate to use with other cognitive tests for early detection of cognitive decline in older populations with low education (Matallana et al, 2011).*
- Inform the client's family or caregiver of meaning of and reasons for common behavior observed in the client with impaired memory. CEB: *Memory training in a triethnic sample produced differential benefits.*

Both Hispanics and blacks performed better than whites on visual memory, and blacks performed better over time on instrumental activities of daily living (McDougall et al, 2010b).

- Attempt to validate family members' feelings regarding the impact of the client's behavior on family lifestyle. EBN: *Validation therapy is a communication technique that lets the client with dementia know that the nurse has heard and understands what was said. In this nurse-client relationship, however, there is insufficient evidence to make any conclusion about its efficacy for reducing or reversing symptoms of dementia or cognitive impairment (Zimmerman et al, 2013).*

Home Care

- The above interventions may be adapted for home care use.
- Assess the client's need for outside assistance with recall of treatment, medications, and willingness/ability of family to provide needed support. *During initial phase of home care, increased frequency of visits may be necessary to compensate for the client's inability to recall treatment and medications. Counting of medications may be needed to determine whether the client is following the medication regimen. Telephone calls from family/friends may help remind the client of treatment schedule.*
- Identify a checking-in support system (e.g., Lifeline or significant others). *Checking in ensures the client's safety.*
- Keep furniture placement and household patterns consistent. *Change increases risk of impaired memory and decreased functioning.*

Client/Family Teaching and Discharge Planning

- When teaching the client, determine what the client knows about memory techniques and then build on that knowledge. *New material is organized in terms of what knowledge already exists, and efficient teaching should attempt to take advantage of what is already known in order to graft on new material (McDougall et al, 2014).*
- When teaching a skill to the client, set up a series of practice attempts that will enhance motivation. Begin with simple tasks so the client can be positively reinforced and progress to more difficult concepts. *Distributed practice with correct recall attempts can be a very effective teaching strategy. Widely distribute practice over time if possible (Gross et al, 2014).*
- Teach clients to use memory techniques such as concentrating and attending, repeating information, making mental associations, and placing items in strategic places so that they will not be forgotten. *These methods increase recall of information the client thinks is important. The internal methods of increasing memory can be effective, especially if used along with external methods such as calendars, lists, and other methods (Rebok et al, 2013).*

M

REFERENCES

Alves, M. R., Yamamoto, T., Arias-Carrión, O., et al. (2014). Executive function impairments in patients with depression: a systematic review. *CNS Neurological Disorders Drug Targets*. [Epub ahead of print].

Bauer, M. E., Muller, G. C., Correa, B. L., et al. (2013). Psychoneuroendocrine interventions aimed at attenuating immunosenescence: a review. *Biogerontology*, *14*(1), 9–20.

Baune, B. T., & Renger, L. (2014). Pharmacological and non-pharmacological interventions to improve cognitive dysfunction and functional ability in clinical depression—a systematic review. *Psychiatry Research*, *219*(1), 25–50.

Butterfield, D. A., Di Domenico, F., & Barone, E. (2014). Elevated risk of type 2 diabetes for development of Alzheimer disease: a key role for oxidative stress in brain. *Biochimica et Biophysica Acta*, *1842*(9), 1693–1706.

Chan, M. Y., Haber, S., Drew, L. M., et al. (2014). Training older adults to use tablet computers: does it enhance cognitive function? *The Gerontologist*, pii: gnu057. [Epub ahead of print].

Chatthanawaree, W. (2011). Biomarkers of cobalamin (vitamin B12) deficiency and its application. *Journal of Nutrition Health Aging*, *15*(3), 227–231.

Darnell, K. R., McGuire, C., & Danner, D. D. (2011). African American participation in Alzheimer's disease research that includes brain donation. *American Journal of Alzheimers Disease and Other Dementias*, *26*(6), 469–476.

Diamond, B. J., & Bailey, M. R. (2013). Ginkgo biloba: indications, mechanisms, and safety. *Psychiatric Clinics of North America*, *36*(1), 73–83.

Griep, L. M., Verschuren, W. M., Kromhout, D., et al. (2011). Raw and processed fruit and vegetable consumption and 10-year stroke incidence in a population-based cohort study in the Netherlands. *European Journal Clinical Nutrition*, *65*(7), 791–799.

Gross, A. L., Rebok, G. W., Ford, D. E., et al. (2011). Alcohol consumption and domain-specific cognitive function in older adults: longitudinal data from the johns hopkins precursors study. *Journal Gerontology B Psychological Sciences Social Sciences*, *66*(1), 39–47.

Gross, A. L., Brandt, J., Bandeen-Roche, K., et al. (2014). Do older adults use the method of loci? Results from the ACTIVE study. *Experimental Aging Research*, *40*(2), 140–163.

Harris, D. P., Ortiz, F., Adler, F. M., et al. (2011). Challenges to screening and evaluation of memory impairment among Hispanic elders in a primary care safety net facility. *International Journal Geriatric Psychiatry, 26*(3), 268–276.

Jackson, M. L., Howard, M. E., & Barnes, M. (2011). Cognition and daytime functioning in sleep-related breathing disorders. *Progress Brain Research, 190*, 53–68.

Lacy, M., Kaemmerer, T., & Czipri, S. (2014). Standardized mini-mental state examination scores and verbal memory performance at a memory center: implications for cognitive screening. *American Journal Alzheimers Disease & Other Dementias*, pii: 1533317514539378. [Epub ahead of print].

Luijten, M., Machielsen, M. W., Veltman, D. J., et al. (2014). Systematic review of ERP and fMRI studies investigating inhibitory control and error processing in people with substance dependence and behavioural addictions. *Journal Psychiatry Neuroscience, 39*(3), 149–169.

Matallana, D., de Santacruz, C., Cano, C., et al. (2011). The relationship between education level and mini-mental state examination domains among older Mexican Americans. *Journal Geriatric Psychiatry Neurology, 24*(1), 9–18.

McDougall, G. J., Becker, H., Vaughan, P., et al. (2010a). The SeniorWISE study: improving everyday memory in older adults. *Archives Psychiatric Nursing, 24*(5), 291–306.

McDougall, G. J., Becker, H., Vaughan, P., et al. (2010b). Differential benefits of memory training for minority older adults in the SeniorWISE study. *The Gerontologist, 50*(5), 632–645.

McDougall, G. J., Pituch, K., Stanton, M., et al. (2014). Memory performance and affect: are there gender differences in community-residing older adults? *Issues in Mental Health Nursing, 35*(8), 620–627.

McDougall, G. J., Vance, D., Wayde, E., et al. (2015). Senior WISE memory training plus Yoga for older adults. *Journal of Neuroscience Nursing, 47*(3), 178–188.

Meeusen, R. (2014). Exercise, nutrition and the brain. *Sports Medicine, 44*(Suppl. 1), S47–S56.

Mulsant, B. H., Blumberger, D. M., Ismail, Z., et al. (2014). A systematic approach to pharmacotherapy for geriatric major depression. *Clinical Geriatric Medicine, 30*(3), 517–534.

Nouchi, R., Taki, Y., Takeuchi, H., et al. (2012). Beneficial effects of short-term combination exercise training on diverse cognitive functions in healthy older people: study protocol for a randomized controlled trial. *Trials, 13*, 200.

Rebok, G. W., Langbaum, J. B., Jones, R. N., et al. (2013). Memory training in the ACTIVE study: how much is needed and who benefits? *Journal of Aging and Health, 25*(Suppl. 8), 21S–42S.

Reppermund, S., Brodaty, H., Crawford, J. D., et al. (2011). The relationship of current depressive symptoms and past depression with cognitive impairment and instrumental activities of daily living in an elderly population: the Sydney Memory and Ageing Study. *Journal of Psychiatric Research, 45*(12), 1600–1607.

Sabia, S., Elbaz, A., Britton, A., et al. (2014). Alcohol consumption and cognitive decline in early old age. *Neurology, 82*(4), 332–339.

Schwabe, L., Nader, K., & Pruessner, J. C. (2014). Reconsolidation of human memory: brain mechanisms and clinical relevance. *Biological Psychiatry, 3223*(14), 161–169.

Sonnen, J. A., Sant Cruz, K., Hemmy, L. S., et al. (2011). Ecology of the aging human brain. *Archives Neurology, 68*(8), 1049–1056.

Stranahan, A. M., & Mattson, M. P. (2012). Metabolic reserve as a determinant of cognitive aging. *Journal of Alzheimers Disease, 30*(Suppl. 2), S5–S13.

Wang, C., Yu, J. T., Wang, H. F., et al. (2014). Non-pharmacological interventions for patients with mild cognitive impairment: a meta-analysis of randomized controlled trials of cognition-based and exercise interventions. *Journal of Alzheimers Disease*. [Epub ahead of print].

Yubero, R., Gil, P., Paul, N., et al. (2011). Influence of memory strategies on memory test performance: a study in healthy and pathological aging. *Neuropsychology and Developmental Cognition B Aging Neuropsychological Cognition, 18*(5), 497–515.

Zimmerman, S., Anderson, W. L., Brode, S., et al. (2013). Systematic review: effective characteristics of nursing homes and other residential long-term care settings for people with dementia. *Journal American Geriatrics Society, 61*(8), 1399–1409.

Zlomuzica, A., Dere, D., Machulska, A., et al. (2014). Episodic memories in anxiety disorders: clinical implications. *Frontiers in Behavioral Neuroscience, 8*, 131. eCollection 2014.

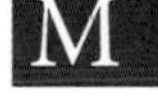

Impaired bed Mobility

Wendie A. Howland, MN, RN-BC, CRRN, CCM, CNLCP, LNCC

NANDA-I

Definition

Limitation of independent movement from one bed position to another

Defining Characteristics

Impaired ability to move between long sitting and supine positions; impaired ability to move between prone and supine positions; impaired ability to move between sitting and supine positions; impaired ability to reposition self in bed; impaired ability to turn from side to side

Related Factors

Alteration in cognitive functioning; environmental barrier (e.g., bed size, bed type, equipment, restraints); insufficient knowledge of mobility strategies; insufficient muscle strength; musculoskeletal impairment; neuromuscular impairment; obesity; pain; pharmaceutical agent; physical deconditioning

NOC Outcomes (Nursing Outcomes Classification)

Suggested NOC Outcomes

Immobility Consequences: Physiological; Mobility; Self-Care: Activities of Daily Living (ADLs)

Example NOC Outcome with Indicators

Immobility Consequences: Physiological as evidenced by the following indicators: Pressure sores/Constipation/Hypoactive bowel/Paralytic ileus/Urinary calculi/Contracted joints/Venous thrombosis/Pneumonia. (Rate the outcome and indicators of **Immobility Consequences: Physiological:** 1 = severely compromised, 2 = substantially compromised, 3 = moderately compromised, 4 = mildly compromised, 5 = not compromised [see Section I].)

Client Outcomes

Client Will (Specify Time Frame)

- Demonstrate optimal independence in positioning, exercising, and performing functional activities in bed
- Demonstrate ability to direct others on how to do bed positioning, exercising, and functional activities

NIC Interventions (Nursing Interventions Classification)

Suggested NIC interventions

Bed Rest Care

M

Example: NIC Activities—Best Rest Care

Position in proper body alignment; Teach bed exercises, as appropriate

Nursing Interventions and *Rationales*

- Choose therapeutic bed positions based on client's history and risk profile; assess to determine if positioning for one condition may negatively affect another; use critical thinking skills for risk-benefit analysis. *Because aspiration is a threat to oxygenation, for some clients this risk is greater and provides a more immediate concern than pressure ulcers risk in critically ill clients (Metheny & Frantz, 2013). Increased acuity of a client should drive turning frequency, which may include small shifts in weight and/or hourly repositioning (Makic et al, 2014).*
- Assess risk for aspiration; if present, elevate head of bed (HOB) to 30 to 45 degrees unless contraindicated and elevate HOB to 90 degrees during oral intake of fluids, solids, and oral medications. EB: *Implementing an aspiration prevention protocol was effective in reducing the occurrence of postoperative pneumonia (Starks & Harbert, 2011).*
- Raise HOB to 30 degrees for clients with acute increased intracranial pressure and brain injury. Refer to care plan for Decreased **Intracranial** adaptive capacity.

▲ Consult health care provider for HOB elevation for acute stroke and monitor response. Refer to care plan for Decreased **Intracranial** adaptive capacity.

- Raise HOB as close to 45 degrees as possible for critically ill ventilated clients to prevent pneumonia (this height may place clients at higher risk for pressure ulcers). Elevating the HOB decreases regurgitation and risk for aspiration of gastric contents. EB: *Researchers reviewed random controlled trials/reviews of prevention of ventilator-associated pneumonia (VAP), and their recommendations included elevating HOB to 30 to 45 degrees unless contraindicated. Implementing an aspiration prevention protocol was effective in reducing the occurrence of postoperative pneumonia (Starks & Harbert, 2011; American Association of Critical-Care Nurses, 2011).*
- Assist client with dysphagia to sit as upright as possible for oral intake, including solids, fluids, and oral medications. Refer to care plan for Impaired **Swallowing.**
- Periodically sit client as upright as tolerated in bed; dangle client, if vital signs and oxygen saturation levels remain stable. *Placing a client who is generally immobilized in a recliner is a good alternative to the bed (Gefen et al, 2013). Being vertical reduces the work of the heart, improves circulation/lung ventilation/strength, and stimulates reflexes and awareness of surroundings.*

- To prevent pressure ulcers, maintain HOB at lowest elevation that is medically possible and raise the foot of the bed to prevent shear-related injury. Assess the client's sacrum, ischial tuberosities, and heels at least every 2 hours. EB: *Shear results when external friction stretches the top layers of the skin as it slides against underlying layers and as internal tissues slide over deeper muscle and bone. These forces increase over the ischial tuberosities and sacrum when the backrest of the bed is elevated and result in tissue damage. Raising the foot of the bed in proportion to the head of the bed to distribute weight brings the body into maximum contact with the supporting surface, helping to eliminate shear. Placing a client who is generally immobilized in a recliner is a good alternative to the bed (Gefen et al, 2013; Berowitz et al, 2014).*
- Try prone positioning for clients with acute respiratory distress syndrome (ARDS), acute lung injury (ALI), and amputation and monitor their tolerance/response. EB: *Evidence varies but suggests that oxygenation, VAP, and mortality may be positively affected by prone positioning. In cases of severe ARDS, early prone positioning sessions significantly decreased 28- and 90-day mortality (Guerin et al, 2013). Prone positioning after both above the knee and below the knee amputations promotes extension, preventing flexor contractions in lower extremity residual joints (Gosselin & Smith, 2014; Wright & Flynn, 2011; Gattinoni et al, 2013).*
- Assess client's risk for falls using a valid fall risk assessment tool, such as the Morse Fall Scale (Morse et al, 1987). CEB: *Establish individualized fall prevention strategies and perform post-fall assessment to further refine fall prevention interventions.* EB: *The fall prevention program should include fall prevention interventions as well as assessment of risk and assessment of a fall (Hill & Fauerbach, 2014).*
- Beds should be kept locked and in the lowest position when occupied. Specialty low beds in which mattresses are approximately 8 to 12 inches from the floor are helpful for clients at risk for falls. Cushioned mats, two to three inches thick, with beveled edges lined with reflective tape and covered by a rubberized material are also helpful. *Mats seemed to provide "a protective effect" for the pelvis during head-first falls and for the thorax during feet-first falls (Hill & Fauerbach, 2014).*

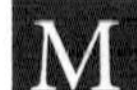

▲ Bed rails and restraints must be prescribed by a health care provider.

▲ While placing all four bed rails up is considered a form of restraint and requires a health care provider's order, two and even three rails up can be a support for bed mobility. *Nursing staff can work with physical and occupational therapists to determine the most effective techniques for bed mobility, including recommendations on the number of bedrails (Hill & Fauerbach, 2014).*

- Place frequently used items within client's reach; demonstrate use of call bell (Hill & Fauerbach, 2014).
- Use a formalized screening tool to identify clients who are at high risk for thromboembolism, or deep venous thrombosis. EB: *Best clinical practice encourages the use of a clinical decision tool that determines deep venous thrombosis risk based on predisposing factors and certain clinical signs and symptoms (Anthony, 2013).*

▲ Implement thromboembolism prophylaxis and treatment as prescribed (e.g., anticoagulants, antiembolic stockings, elastic leg wraps, sequential compression devices, feet/ankle exercises, and hydration). Refer to care plan for Ineffective peripheral **Tissue Perfusion.**

- Use a valid and reliable tool to assess a client's risk for pressure ulcers. EB: *Braden sensory perception and friction/shear subscales and Waterlow mobility and appetite subscales were the most relevant predictors (Serpa et al, 2011).*
- Implement the following interventions to prevent pressure ulcers and complications of immobility:
  - Position sitting clients with special attention to the individual's anatomy, postural alignment, distribution of weight, and foot support.
  - Placing a client who is generally immobilized in a recliner is a good alternative to the bed (Gefen et al, 2013).
  - Turn (logroll) clients at high risk for pressure/shear/friction frequently and regularly. EBN: *Pressure redistribution surfaces cannot replace turning and repositioning. Most pressure ulcers are avoidable; however, clients with hemodynamic instability that is worsened with movement, inability to maintain nutrition and hydration status, and advanced directive prohibiting turning may result in unavoidable pressure ulcers (National Pressure Ulcer Advisory Panel, 2011).*
- Pressure redistribution surfaces cannot replace turning and repositioning.
  - Use static/dynamic bed surfaces and assess for "bottoming out" under susceptible bony areas (body sinks into mattress, thus the recommended 1 inch between mattress/bones is absent). Refer to care plan for Risk for impaired **Skin** integrity.
  - Use heel protection devices that completely float or offload heels (National Pressure Ulcer Advisory Panel, 2011).

- ❍ Implement a 2-hour on/off schedule for heel protector boots or high-top tennis shoes with socks underneath in clients with paralyzed feet, and check condition of heels when removed.
- ❍ Strictly maintain leg abduction in persons with a surgical hip pinning or replacement by placing an abductor splint/pillow between legs as prescribed.
- ❍ Place bariatric beds along a corner wall, which helps keep the bed from moving during repositioning.
- ❍ Identify/modify hospital beds with large gaps between bed rail/mattress that create an entrapment hazard. Ensure that mattresses fit the bed; install gap fillers/rail inserts, then monitor effectiveness.

- • Use devices such as trapeze, friction-reducing slide sheets, mechanical lateral transfer aids, and ceiling-mounted or floor lifts to move (rather than drag) dependent or obese clients in bed to prevent injury to staff.
  - ❍ Use special beds and equipment to move bariatric (very obese) clients, such as mattress overlay, sliding/roller board, trapeze, stirrup, and pulley attached to overhead traction system (holds one leg up during pericare).
  - ❍ Place bariatric clients in free-standing or ceiling-mounted lifts with padded slings while changing bed linen. EB: *The potential for reductions in injury rates in the United States is greatest from improving training and ensuring adequate time for resident care, in that most facilities currently have lifts available (D'Arcy et al, 2012).*
- • Apply elbow pads to comatose and/or restrained clients and to those who use their elbows to prop or scoot up in bed. Apply nocturnal elbow splint as ordered if ulnar nerve palsy exists or if painful elbow with paresthesia in ulnar side of fourth/fifth fingers develops. *The use of pads assists with preventing prolonged compression or flexion pressure on the ulnar nerve, causing neuropathy/nerve damage. Consider using an enclosure bed for agitated clients to alleviate restraints, thus preventing arm abrasions, nerve damage, and pain.*
- • Explain importance of exhaling versus holding one's breath (Valsalva maneuver) and straining during bed activities.
- • Reassess pain level, especially before movement and/or exercising, and accept clients' pain rating and level they think is appropriate for comfort. Administer analgesics based on clients' pain rating. Refer to Acute **Pain** or Chronic **Pain.**

M

Exercise

- • Test strength in bilateral grips, arms at elbow flexion and extension, bilateral arm abduction and adduction, bilateral leg or thigh raise (one at a time in bed or chair), and quadriceps and hamstring strength to extend and flex at knee to assess baseline and interval strength gains.
- • Perform passive range of motion (ROM) of three repetitions, at least twice a day, to immobile joints. *Perform ROM slowly and rhythmically. Do not range beyond point of pain. Range only to point of resistance in those with loss of sensation and mentation. Fast, jerky ROM increases pain and tone. Slow, rhythmical movements relax/lengthen spastic muscles so they can be ranged further. For clients with Parkinson's disease, consult with physical therapy for ROM exercises.*
- • Range or move a hemiplegic arm with the shoulder slightly externally rotated (hand up).
- ▲ Encourage client's practice of exercises taught by therapists (muscle setting, strengthening, contraction against resistance, and weight lifting). *Exercises and weight lifting help maintain muscle tone, strength, and lengthening.*

Bed Positioning

- • Incorporate the following measures to promote normal tone and prevent complications in clients with neurological impairment:
  - ❍ Use a flat head pillow when clients are supine. Use a small pillow behind the head and/or between shoulder blades if neck extension occurs. *Prevents contractures of the cervical spine and abnormal tone of the neck (Potter & Perry, 2013).*
  - ❍ Abduct the shoulders of clients with high paraplegia or quadriplegia horizontally to 90 degrees briefly two to three times a day while client is supine.
  - ❍ Position a hemiplegic shoulder fairly close to the client's body.
- ▲ Elevate a client's paralyzed forearms on a pillow when client is supine and apply Isotoner gloves. Elevate edematous legs on a pillow supporting the knees to prevent hyperextension. Apply elastic wraps and compression garments as prescribed.

- Tilt hemiplegics onto both unaffected and affected sides with the affected shoulder slightly forward (e.g., move/lift the affected shoulder, not the forearm/hand).

▲ Apply resting wrist, hand, and foot/ankle splints or other devices. Range joints before applying splints. Adhere to on/off schedule as prescribed by the physical therapist. *Check underlying tissues for signs of pressure/poor circulation every 2 hours or more often if client resists or manipulates them.*

▲ Recognize that components of normal bed mobility include rolling, bridging, scooting, long sitting, and sitting upright. Activity starts with the client supine, flat in bed, and promotes normal movements that are bilateral, segmental, well timed, and involve set positions such as weight bearing and trunk centering. Refer to a physical therapist (PT) for individualized instructions and mobility strategies.

Geriatric

- Assess caregiver's strength, health history, and cognitive status to predict ability/risk for assisting bed-bound clients at home. *Explore alternatives if risk is too high. Caregivers are often frail older adults with chronic health problems who cannot physically help loved ones.* Refer to care plan for **Caregiver Role Strain.**
- Assess the client's stamina and energy level during bed activities/exercises; if limited, spread out activities and allow rest breaks.

Home Care

▲ Collaborate with nurse case managers, care coordinators, social workers, and physical/occupational therapists to assess home support systems and needs, and to provide for home modifications, durable medical equipment, assistive technology, and home health services.

- Encourage use of the client's bed unless contraindicated. Raise HOB with commercial blocks or grooved-out pieces of wood under legs; set bed against walls in a corner. Emotionally, clients may benefit from sleeping in their own beds with familiar partners.

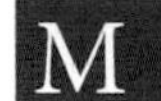

- Stress psychological/physical benefits of clients being as self-sufficient as possible with bed mobility/care even though it may be time-consuming. Allowing independence and autonomy may help prevent disuse syndromes and feelings of helplessness and low self-esteem.
- Offer emotional support and help client identify usual coping responses to help with adjustment and loss issues. The home environment may trigger the reality of lost function and disability.
- Discuss support systems available for caregivers to help them cope. Refer to care plan for **Caregiver Role Strain.**

▲ In the presence of medical disorders, institute case management for frail older adult to support continued independent living.

- Refer to the home care interventions in the care plan for Impaired physical **Mobility.**

Client/Family Teaching and Discharge Planning

- Use various sensory modalities to teach client/caregivers correct range of motion, exercises, positioning, self-care activities, and use of devices. Readiness and learning styles vary but may be enhanced with visual/auditory/tactile/cognitive stimulus as follows:
  - Provide visual information such as demonstrations, sketches, instructional videos, written directions/schedules, notes.
  - Provide auditory information such as verbal instructions, recorded audiotapes, timers, reading aloud written directions, and self-talk during activities.
  - Use tactile stimulation such as motor task practice/repetition, return demonstrations, note taking, manual guidance, or staff's hand-on-client's-hand technique.

▲ Schedule time with family/caregivers for education and practice for nursing, physical therapy, and occupational therapy. Suggest family come prepared with questions and wear comfortable, safe clothing/shoes. Practice provides opportunity for learning; repetition helps memory retention.

▲ Implement safe approaches for caregivers/home care staff and reinforce adequate number of people and handling equipment (e.g., friction pads, slide boards, lifts) during bed mobility, exercise, toileting, and bathing to decrease risk of injury.

▲ Coordinate evaluations for bariatric equipment for home use before discharge, including a weight-rated bed, a wheelchair or mobility device (scooter), and lift device. Doorways may need to be widened, floors reinforced, and ramps added for safety.

REFERENCES

American Association of Critical-Care Nurses (2011). *Practice Alert: Prevention of Aspiration*. Aliso Viejo, CA: American Association of Critical-Care Nurses..

Anthony, M. (2013). Nursing assessment of deep vein thrombosis. *Medsurg Nursing*, *22*(2), 95–98.

Berlowitz, D., Van Deusen-Lukas, C., et al. *AHRQ Quality Indicators Tool Kit. Preventing pressure ulcers in hospitals: a tool kit for improving quality of care*. <www.ahrq.gov/qual/qitoolkit/d4c_pressureulcer_bestpractices.pdf> Retrieved 11/1/2014.

D'Arcy, L. P., Sasai, Y., & Stearns, S. C. (2012). Do assistive devices, training, and workload affect injury incidence? Prevention efforts by nursing homes and back injuries among nursing assistants. *Journal of Advanced Nursing*, *68*(4), 836–845.

Gattinoni, L., Taccone, P., Carlesso, E., et al. (2013). Prone position in acute respiratory distress syndrome: rationale, indications, and limits. *American Journal of Respiratory and Critical Care Medicine*, *188*(11), 1286–1293.

Gefen, A., Farid, K. J., (dnp), & Shaywitz, I. (2013). A review of deep tissue injury development, detection and prevention: shear savvy. *Ostomy/Wound Management*, *59*(2), 26–35.

Gosselin, R. A., & Smith, R. G. (2014). Amputations, Ch. 43. In M. Foltz, R. A. Gosselin, & R. G. Smith (Eds.), *Global Orthopedics*. New York NY: Springer Science + Business Media.

Guerin, C., Reigneir, J., Richard, J.-C., et al. (2013). In cases of severe ARDS, early prone-positioning sessions significantly decreased 28- and 90-day mortality. *The New England Journal of Medicine*, *368*, 2159–2168.

Hill, E., & Fauerbach, L. A. (2014). Falls and fall prevention in older adults. *Journal of Legal Nurse Consulting*, *25*(2), 24–29.

Makic, M. B., Rauen, C., et al. (2014). Examining the evidence to guide practice: challenging practice habits. *Critical Care Nurse*, *34*(2), 28–45.

Metheny, N. A., & Frantz, R. A. (2013). Head-of-bed elevation in critically ill patients: a review. *Critical Care Nurse*, *33*, 53–67.

Morse, J. M., Tylko, S. J., & Dixon, H. A. (1987). Characteristics of the fall-prone patient. *The Gerontologist*, *27*(4), 516–522.

National Pressure Ulcer Advisory Panel. (2011). Pressure ulcers: avoidable or unavoidable? Results of the national pressure ulcer advisory panel consensus conference. *Ostomy/Wound Management*, *57*(2), 24–37.

Serpa, L. F., Santos, V. L., Peres, G. R., et al. (2011). Validity of the Braden and Waterlow subscales in predicting pressure ulcer risk applied nursing research. *Applied Nursing Research*, *24*(4), e23–e28.

Starks, B., & Harbert, C. (2011). Aspiration prevention protocol: decreasing postoperative pneumonia in heart surgery patients. *Critical Care Nurse*, *5*, 38–45.

Wright, A. D., & Flynn, M. (2011). Using the prone position for ventilated patients with respiratory failure: a review. *Nursing in Critical Care*, *16*(1), 19–27.

M

Impaired physical Mobility *Sherry H. Pomeroy, PhD, RN*

NANDA-I

Definition

Limitation in independent, purposeful physical movement of the body or of one or more extremities

Defining Characteristics

Alteration in gait, decrease in fine motor skills; decrease in gross motor skills; decrease in range of motion; decrease in reaction time; difficulty turning; discomfort; engages in substitutions for movement (e.g., attention to other's activity, controlling behavior, focus on pre-illness activity), exertional dyspnea; movement-induced tremor; postural instability; slowed movement; spastic movement; uncoordinated movement

Related Factors (r/t)

Activity intolerance; alteration in bone structure integrity; alteration in cognitive functioning; alteration in metabolism; anxiety; body mass index >75th percentile for age; contractures; cultural belief regarding appropriate activity; decrease in endurance; decrease in muscle control; decrease in muscle mass; decrease in muscle strength; depression; developmental delay; disuse; insufficient environmental support (e.g., physical, social); insufficient knowledge of value of physical activity; joint stiffness; malnutrition; musculoskeletal impairment; neuromuscular impairment; pain; pharmaceutical agent; physical deconditioning; prescribed movement restrictions; reluctance to initiate movement; sedentary lifestyle; sensory-perceptual impairment

NOC (Nursing Outcomes Classification)

Suggested NOC Outcomes

Ambulation; Ambulation: Wheelchair; Mobility; Self-Care: Activities of Daily Living (ADLs); Instrumental Activities of Daily Living (IADLs); Transfer Performance

Example NOC Outcome with Indicators

Ambulation as evidenced by the following indicators: Walks with effective gait/Walks at moderate pace/Walks up and down steps/Walks moderate distance. (Rate the outcome and indicators of **Ambulation:** 1 = severely compromised, 2 = substantially compromised, 3 = moderately compromised, 4 = mildly compromised, 5 = not compromised [see Section I].)

Client Outcomes

Client Will (Specify Time Frame)

- Meet mutually defined goals of increased ambulation and exercise that include individual choice, preference, and enjoyment in the exercise prescription
- Verbalize feeling of increased strength and ability to move
- Verbalize less fear of falling and pain with physical activity
- Demonstrate use of adaptive equipment (e.g., wheelchairs, walkers, gait belts, weighted walking vests) to increase mobility
- Increase exercise to 20 minutes per day for those who were previously sedentary (less than 150 minutes per week). NOTE: Light to moderate intensity exercise may be beneficial in deconditioned persons. In very deconditioned individuals exercise bouts of less than 10 minutes are beneficial.
- Increase pedometer step counts by 1000 steps per day every 2 weeks to reach a daily step count of at least 7000 steps per day, with a daily goal for most healthy adults of 10,000 steps per day (approximately 5 miles)
- Perform resistance exercises that involve all major muscle groups (legs, hips, back, chest, abdomen, shoulders, and arms) performed 2 or 3 days per week
- Perform flexibility exercise (stretching) for each of the major muscle-tendon groups 2 days per week for 10 to 60 seconds to improve joint range of motion; greatest gains occur with daily exercise
- Engage in neuromotor exercise 20 to 30 minutes per day including motor skills (e.g., balance, agility, coordination, and gait), proprioceptive exercise training, and multifaceted activities (e.g., tai chi and yoga) to improve and maintain physical function and reduce falls in those at risk for falling (older persons)
- Engage in purposeful moderate-intensity cardiorespiratory (aerobic) exercise for 30 to 60 minutes per day on at least 5 days per week for a total of 2 hours and 30 minutes (150 minutes) per week

M

NIC (Nursing Interventions Classification)

Suggested NIC Interventions

Exercise Therapy: Ambulation; Joint Mobility; Positioning

Example NIC Activities—Exercise Therapy: Ambulation

Assist the client to use footwear that facilitates walking and prevents injury; Instruct in availability of assistive devices, if appropriate

Nursing Interventions and *Rationales*

- Adults with disabilities should follow the adult guidelines; however, if not possible these persons should be as physically active as their abilities allow and avoid inactivity (U.S. Department of Health & Human Services, 2008). Use "start low and go slow" approach for intensity and duration of physical activity if client highly deconditioned, functionally limited, or has chronic conditions affecting performance of physical tasks. When progressing client's activities, use an individualized and tailored approach based on client's tolerance and preferences (American College of Sports Medicine [ACSM], 2014).
- Screen for mobility skills in the following order: (1) bed mobility; (2) supported and unsupported sitting; (3) transition movements such as sit to stand, sitting down, and transfers; and (4) standing and walking activities. CEB: *Use a tool such as the Assessment Criteria and Care Plan for Safe Patient Handling and Movement (Sedlak et al, 2009).* EBN: *Assess for low mobility, functional difficulties, cognitive impairment and multiple comorbidities that require both client safety and rehabilitation interventions (Kneafsey et al, 2013).*

- Screen for additional measures of physical function to assess strength of muscle groups, including unassisted leg stand, use of a balance platform, elbow flexion and knee extension strength, grip strength, timed chair stands, and the 6-minute walk. CEB: *The nursing assessment should include factors related to mobility problems (e.g., ability to walk and move), with nursing goals and interventions developed to promote maximum mobility (Kneafsey, 2007).* EBN/QSEN: *Client assessment and use of facility or organizational safe client handling algorithms and processes should be used to determine safe client movement (e.g., equipment introduction and safety huddles) and protect nurses from musculoskeletal injuries to reduce preventable disability, nursing turnover, and burnout (Hodgson et al, 2013).*
- Assess the client for cause of impaired mobility. Determine whether cause is physical, psychological, or motivational. *Some clients choose not to move because of psychological factors such as fear of falling or pain, an inability to cope, or depression.* EBN: *Because fear of falling is associated with immobility and functional dependence, it requires effective assessment and measurement (Greenberg, 2012).* Refer to care plans for Risk for **Falls,** Acute **Pain,** Chronic Pain, Ineffective **Coping,** or **Hopelessness.**
- Use Self-Efficacy for Exercise Scale (Resnick & Jenkins, 2000) and the Outcome Expectation for Exercise Scale (Resnick et al, 2001) to determine client's self-efficacy and outcome expectations toward exercise (Resnick & D'Adamo, 2011). CEB: *Use a fear of falling assessment, such as a one-item fear of falling question, Falls Efficacy Scale, or Mobility Efficacy Scale (Messecar, 2008).* EBN: *An integrative review concluded that fear of falling in high-risk community-dwelling older adults is best measured by the Falls Efficacy Scale-International (Greenberg, 2012).*
- Function focused care should be used, such as encouraging self performance of bathing, walking to the bathroom instead of using a bedpan/urinal, and taking the older adult to an exercise class (Resnick & Galik, 2013). EBN: *An integrative review concluded that fear of falling in high-risk community-dwelling older adults is best measured by the Falls Efficacy Scale-International (Greenberg, 2012).*

M

- Monitor and record the client's ability to tolerate activity and use all four extremities; note pulse rate, blood pressure, dyspnea, and skin color before and after activity. Refer to the care plan for **Activity** intolerance. EB: *Use valid and reliable screening procedures and tools to assess the client's preparticipation in exercise health screening and risk stratification for exercise testing (low, moderate, or high risk) (ACSM, 2014).*

▲ Before activity, observe for and, if possible, treat pain with massage, heat pack to affected area, or medication. Ensure that the client is not oversedated. *Pain limits mobility and if exacerbated by specific movements should be temporarily avoided (ACSM, 2014).*

▲ Consult with physical therapist for further evaluation, strength training, gait training, and development of a mobility plan. CEB: *Prescribing a regimen of regular physical activity that includes both aerobic exercise and muscle strengthening activities is beneficial to minimizing impaired mobility; use exercise diary or log to improve adherence to mobility enhancement recommendations. Develop mobility enhancement programs that are specific to gender and ethnicity and are culturally appropriate (Yeom et al, 2009).*

- Before the activity begins, obtain any assistive devices needed for activity, such as gait belt, weighted vest, walker, cane, crutches, or wheelchair, ergonomic shower chairs, ceiling and floor-based lifts, and air-assisted lateral transfer devices. *Assistive devices can help increase mobility (Hodgson et al, 2013).*
- If the client is immobile, perform passive range-of-motion (ROM) exercises at least twice a day unless contraindicated; repeat each maneuver three times. EB: *Physical rehabilitation interventions were found to be safe, reduced disability, and resulted in few adverse events (Foster et al, 2011).*

▲ If the client is immobile, consult with health care provider for a safety evaluation before beginning an exercise program; if program is approved, begin with the following exercises:
  - Active ROM exercises using both upper and lower extremities (e.g., flexing and extending at ankles, knees, hips)
  - Chin-ups and pull-ups using a trapeze in bed (may be contraindicated in clients with cardiac conditions)
  - Strengthening exercises such as gluteal or quadriceps sitting exercises

- If client is immobile, consider use of vertical transfer techniques such as air-assisted lateral transfer devices or gait belt pending weight-bearing status and client cooperation. *Using a transfer chair that can bend into a stretcher position and then upright can help previously immobile clients get out of bed (Gonzalez et al, 2009).* CEB: *Critical care clients are at high risk for complications related to immobility such as ventilator-associated pneumonia (VAP), atelectasis, and long-lasting functional limitations; therefore, once hemodynamically stable, use progressive mobilization to dangle legs, sit in a chair, stand and bear weight, and walk. Use rotation therapy (kinetic and continuous lateral) to reduce risk of VAP for clients on mechanical ventilation (Rauen et al, 2008).*

- • Help the client achieve mobility and start walking as soon as possible if not contraindicated. EBN: *To prevent hospital-acquired disability, organizational values should consider both safety (e.g., fall prevention) and injury protection in concert with a philosophy that enables older adults to be self-directed and independent (Boltz et al, 2013).* CEB: *Early mobilization of orthopedic clients generally prevents medical complications such as deep vein thrombosis, allows clients time to practice using assistive devices or changes in weight-bearing status, and promotes improved function, reduces pain, and facilitates earlier return to independence (Radawiec et al, 2009).*
- • Use a gait-walking belt when ambulating the client. *If the client is able to partially bear weight on one or both lower extremities, use a stand and pivot maneuver with a gait or transfer belt or powered standing assist lift (Gonzalez et al, 2009).*
- ▲ Apply any ordered brace before mobilizing the client. Braces support and stabilize a body part, allowing increased mobility.
- • Initiate a "no lift" policy where appropriate assistive devices are used for manual lifting. EBN: *Relevance of manual client handling policies that may promote overuse of equipment should be openly discussed among nurse managers and direct care providers to avoid hospital-related loss of mobility among clients (Kneafsey et al, 2015).* CEB: *Use the algorithms provided by the National Association of Orthopaedic Nurses for safe client handling and moving during the following high-risk tasks: turning in bed side to side, vertical transfer of postoperative total hip replacement client and extremity cast/splint client, ambulation, and lifting or holding a limb without a cast or splint (Sedlak et al, 2009).*
- • Increase independence in ADLs, encouraging self-efficacy and discouraging helplessness as the client gets stronger. *Providing unnecessary assistance with transfers and bathing activities may promote dependence and a loss of mobility.* EBN: *A function-focused care intervention (designed to optimize physical activity and function in clients with Parkinson's disease) demonstrated a significant effect on increasing outcome expectations for exercise, improving functional performance, and increasing time spent in exercise and physical activity (Pretzer-Abhoff et al, 2011).*
- ▲ If the client has osteoarthritis or rheumatoid arthritis, ask for a referral to a physical therapist to begin an exercise program that includes aerobic exercise, resistance exercise, and flexibility exercise (stretching). EB: *Studies of functional outcomes of exercise in older adults and adults with knee arthritis found only a modest beneficial effect of progressive resistance training and cardiorespiratory programs on pain, strength, and function in both groups (Keysor & Brembs, 2011).* EB: *In a study examining the achievement of physical activity (PA) goals in relation to quality of life and self-reported pain in persons with rheumatoid arthritis (RA), it was found that persons with higher levels of self-efficacy for PA were more likely to achieve personal PA goals. Higher quality of life scores and less perceived arthritis pain were also related to achieving PA goals. Clinicians can therefore support goal achievement by working with clients to foster self-efficacy, set realistic exercise goals with action plans, and provide feedback regarding progress (Knittle, 2011).*
- ▲ If client has had a cerebrovascular accident (CVA) with hemiparesis, consider use of constraint-induced movement therapy, wherein the functional extremity is purposely constrained and the client is forced to use the involved extremity. CEB: *The plasticity of the brain allows the brain to rewire and reroute neural connections to take up the work of the injured area of the brain. Constraint therapy was effective with improved motor function and health-related quality of life (Wu et al, 2007).*
- • If the client has had a CVA, recognize that balance and mobility are likely impaired, and engage client in fall prevention strategies and protect from falling. EBN: *A randomized controlled trial studied the effects of a 6-month treadmill-training program versus a stretching program for stroke survivors. Both groups experienced increased self-efficacy for exercise and a significant increase in outcome expectations for exercise and ADLs on the Stroke Impact Scale (Shaughnessy et al, 2012).*
- • If the client does not feed or groom self, sit side-by-side with the client, put your hand over the client's hand, support the client's elbow with your other hand, and help the client feed self; use the same technique to help the client comb hair. EBN: *Hospitalized older adults who received a family centered intervention to promote functional and cognitive recovery (Family-Centered Function-Focused Care) had improved ADLs and walking ability and less severe and shorter duration of delirium (Boltz et al, 2014).* CEB: *The effectiveness of a restorative care intervention on nursing home resident outcomes included significant improvements in the Tinetti Mobility Score and the subscores for gait and balance, as well as improved walking, bathing, and stair climbing (Resnick et al, 2009).*

M

Geriatric

- Assess ability to move using valid and reliable criterion-referenced standards for fitness testing (e.g., senior fitness test) designed for older adults that can predict the level of capacity associated with maintaining physical independence into later years of life (e.g., get up and go test). *Interventions can subsequently be designed to target weak areas and therefore help reduce the risk of immobility and dependence (Rikli & Jones, 2012).*
- Help the mostly immobile client achieve mobility as soon as possible, depending on physical condition. EB: *A meta-analysis found exercise beneficial in increasing gait speed and improving balance and ADL performance (Chou et al, 2012).*
- For a client who is mostly immobile, minimize cardiovascular deconditioning by positioning the client in the upright position several times daily. *The hazards of bed rest in older adults are multiple, serious, quick to develop, and slow to reverse. Deconditioning of the cardiovascular system occurs within days and involves fluid shifts, fluid loss, decreased cardiac output, decreased peak oxygen uptake, and increased resting heart rate (Longo et al, 2012).* EBN: *A study of function-focused care (FFC) in hospitalized older adults found physical functional declines in both study groups, but less decline was associated with the group receiving FFC. The role of the gerontological rehabilitation nurse is essential throughout the hospital stay and during transitional care (Boltz et al, 2011).*
- ▲ Refer the client to physical therapy for resistance exercise training as able, involving all major muscle groups (e.g., abdominal crunch, leg press, leg extension, leg curl, and calf press) (ACSM, 2014). CEB: *A Cochrane review found that progressive resistance-strength training for physical disability in older clients resulted in increased strength and positive improvements in some limitations (Liu & Latham, 2009).*
- Use the FFC rehabilitative philosophy of care in older adults in residential nursing facilities to prevent avoidable functional decline. The primary goals of FFC are to alter how direct care workers provide care to residents to maintain and improve time spent in physical activity and improve or maintain function. EBN: *Residents in the FFC intervention group had less functional decline and a greater percentage who were not ambulating returned to ambulatory status for short functional distances (Resnick et al, 2011).*
- If client is scheduled for an elective surgery that will result in admission into the intensive care unit and immobility, or recovery from a joint replacement, for example, initiate a prehabilitation program that includes warm-up, aerobic activity, strength, flexibility, neuromotor, and functional task work. EBN: *The risk of declines in functional status when older adults are hospitalized requires using evidence-based strategies to reduce the incidence and impact of decreased mobility, pressure ulcers, pain, dehydration, malnutrition, and sequelae of invasive treatments. Examples of such strategies include completing comprehensive and interdisciplinary geriatric assessment at admission, implementing early mobilization, using assistive devices, ensuring appropriate footwear to encourage mobility and prevent falls, using environmental enhancements such as large clocks and calendars and elevated toilet seats, and evaluating benefits of medications versus side effects (American Academy of Nursing's Expert Panel on Acute and Critical Care, 2012).* CEB: *Aerobic training along with strength and interval training is effective and results in fewer postoperative complications, shorter postoperative stays, and reduced functional disabilities (Carli & Zavorsky, 2005).*
- ▲ Evaluate the client for signs of depression (flat affect, insomnia, anorexia, frequent somatic complaints), anxiety, or cognitive impairment (use Mini-Mental State Exam [MMSE]). Refer for treatment and counseling as needed. CEB: *Interventions to increase physical activity can reduce anxiety in healthy persons. Supervised physical activity (e.g., group or fitness center) as well as individual delivery and moderate to high intensity physical activity seem to be the most effective components in reducing anxiety (Conn, 2010).*
- Watch for orthostatic hypotension when mobilizing older clients. Have the client dangle at the side of the bed with legs hanging over the edge of the bed, flex and extend feet several times after sitting up, then stand up slowly with someone holding the client. If client becomes lightheaded or dizzy, return client to bed immediately. *Postural hypotension is common in older adults (Krecinic et al, 2009).*
- Do not routinely assist with transfers or bathing activities unless necessary. *The nursing staff may contribute to impaired mobility by helping too much. Encourage client independence (Resnick & Galik, 2013).*
- Use gestures and nonverbal cues when helping clients move if they are anxious or have difficulty understanding and following verbal instructions. *Nonverbal gestures are part of a universal language that can be understood when the client is having difficulty with communication.*
- Recognize that wheelchairs are not a good mobility device and often serve as a mobility restraint.
- Ensure that chairs fit clients. Chair seat should be 3 inches above the height of the knee. Provide a raised toilet seat if needed. *Raising the height of a chair can dramatically improve the ability of many older clients*

M

to stand up. Low, deep, soft seats with armrests that are far apart reduce a person's ability to get up and down without help.

- If the client is mainly immobile, provide opportunities for socialization and sensory stimulation (e.g., television and visits). Refer to the care plan for Deficient **Diversional** activity.
- Recognize that immobility and a lack of social support and sensory input may result in confusion or depression in older adults (American Academy of Nursing's Expert Panel on Acute and Critical Care, 2012). Refer to nursing interventions for Acute **Confusion** or **Hopelessness** as appropriate.

Home Care

- The preceding interventions may be adapted for home care use.
- ▲ Begin discharge planning as soon as possible with a personal health navigator (e.g., nurse care coordinator or case manager) to assess need for home support systems, assistive devices, and community or home health services (Paulus et al, 2008).
- ▲ Assess home environment for factors that create barriers to physical mobility. Refer to occupational therapy services if needed to assist the client in restructuring home environment and daily living patterns. EB: *Use the Home Safety Self-Assessment Tool to identify fall risk, prevent falls, and improve mobility and function (Tomita et al, 2014).* EBN: *Assess person-environment fit (P-E Fit) using a reliable and valid instrument such as the Housing Enabler (http://www.enabler.nu) to evaluate the impact of the relationship between the person and his/her environment and subsequently how P-E Fit affects physical activity, mobility, and function (Pomeroy et al, 2011).*
- ▲ Refer to home health aide services to support the client and family through changing levels of mobility. Reinforce need to promote independence in mobility as tolerated. *Providing unnecessary assistance with transfers, bathing, and dressing activities may promote dependence and a loss of mobility rather than optimizing a person's underlying physical capability. Such attentive care may actually prevent older adults from using their remaining abilities (Resnick et al, 2011).*

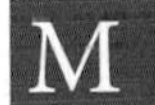

- ▲ Refer to physical therapy for gait training, strengthening, and balance training. Physical therapists can provide direct interventions as well as assess need for assistive devices (e.g., cane, walker). CEB: *An outpatient group exercise intervention (twice per week for 5 weeks) for people with impaired mobility resulted in significantly better balance, sit to stand, and gait; however, strength did not improve (Sherrington et al, 2008).*
- Discuss with client and caregiver the possibility of a service dog to support the more immobile client. CEB: *Service dogs can pull wheelchairs, find keys, open the door, bring the telephone, and more. Use of service dogs was found to increase socialization, increase self-esteem, and give peace of mind to caregivers (Rintala et al, 2005).*
- Assess skin condition at every visit. Establish a skin care program that enhances circulation and maximizes position changes. *Impaired mobility decreases circulation to dependent areas. Decreased circulation and shearing place the client at risk for skin breakdown.*
- Once the client is able to walk independently, suggest the client enter an exercise program, or walk with a friend. *Recommend the client use the Exercise Assessment and Screening for You (EASY) tool to help determine appropriate exercise for the older adult client. This tool is available online at* http://www.easyforyou.info *(Resnick et al, 2008).* EBN: *In a longitudinal data analysis of clients with osteoarthritis, being less sedentary was related to more time spent in physical activity at a moderate to vigorous level and less future functional decline (Semanik et al, 2015).* CEB: *Nurse practitioners providing primary care should prescribe regular physical activity to minimize progressive impaired mobility. Clients should be instructed to use exercise logs or a diary to improve adherence to the mobility enhancement prescription (Yeom et al, 2009).*
- Provide support to the client and family/caregivers during long-term impaired mobility. *Long-term impaired mobility may necessitate role changes within the family and precipitate caregiver stress.* Refer to the care plan for **Caregiver Role Strain.**
- ▲ Institute a personal health navigator (e.g., nurse care coordinator or case manager) and transitional care management of frail older adults to support continued independent living (Paulus et al, 2008).

Client/Family Teaching and Discharge Planning

- Consider using motivational interviewing techniques when working with both children and adult clients to increase their activity. Refer to the care plan for **Sedentary** lifestyle or *rationales* for motivational interviewing.

- Teach the client progressive mobilization (e.g., dangle legs, get out of bed slowly when transferring from the bed to the chair).
- Teach the client relaxation techniques such as deep breathing and stretching to use during activity.
- Teach the client to use assistive devices such as a cane, a walker, gait belt, weighted vest, or crutches or wheelchair to increase mobility (Yeom et al, 2009).
- Teach family members and caregivers to work with clients actively during self-care activities using a restorative care philosophy for eating, bathing, grooming, dressing, and transferring to restore the client to maximum function and independence (Resnick et al, 2009).
- Work with the client using self-efficacy interventions using single or multiple methods. Teach client and family members to assess fear of falling and develop strategies to mitigate its effect on mobility progression. CEB: *Use of self-efficacy-based interventions resulted in increased exercise (Resnick et al, 2009).* EBN: *A study found an association between higher EASY cumulative scores and decreased days limited from usual activity, and decreased unhealthy physical health days (Smith et al, 2011).*
- Work with the client using theory-based interventions (e.g., social cognitive theoretical components such as self-efficacy; transtheoretical model). CEB: *In a study that examined validity of evidence for physical activity stage of change, physical activity stage of change was found to be behaviorally valid evidenced by self-reported exercise, physical activity, pedometers, sedentary behaviors, and physical functioning. Physical fitness and weight indicators were not related to physical activity stage of change (Hellsten et al, 2008).*

REFERENCES

M

American Academy of Nursing's Expert Panel on Acute and Critical Care (2012). *Reducing functional decline in older adults during hospitalization: A best practice approach*, Issue Number 31. From <http://consultgerirn.org/uploads/File/trythis/try_this_31.pdf>.

American College of Sports Medicine (ACSM) (2014). *American College of Sports Medicine's guidelines for exercise testing and prescription* (9th ed.). Philadelphia: Lippincott Williams & Wilkins.

Boltz, M., Capezuti, E., & Shabbat, N. (2011). Nursing staff perceptions of physical function in hospitalized older adults. *Applied Nursing Research, 24*, 215–222.

Boltz, M., Resnick, B., Capezuti, E., et al. (2013). Activity restriction vs. self-direction: hospitalized older adults' responses to fear of falling. *International Journal of Older People Nursing, 9*, 44–53.

Boltz, M., Resnick, B., Chippendale, T., et al. (2014). Testing a family-centered intervention to promote functional and cognitive recovery in hospitalized older adults. *Journal of American Geriatrics Society, 62*, 2398–2407.

Carli, F., & Zavorsky, G. S. (2005). Optimizing functional exercise capacity in the elderly surgical population. *Current Opinion in Clinical Nutrition and Metabolic Care, 8*(1), 23–32.

Chou, C. H., Hwang, C. L., & Wu, Y. T. (2012). Effect of exercise on physical function, daily living activities, and quality of life in the frail older adults: a meta-analysis. *Archives of Physical Medicine and Rehabilitation, 93*(2), 237–244.

Conn, V. S. (2010). Anxiety outcomes after physical activity interventions. *Nursing Research, 59*(3), 224–231.

Foster, A., et al. (2011). Rehabilitation for older people in long-term care. *Cochrane Database of Systematic Reviews*, (1), CD004294.

Gonzalez, C. M., et al. (2009). Recommendations for vertical transfer of a postoperative total hip replacement patient (bed to chair, chair to toilet, chair to chair, or car to chair). *Orthopaedic Nursing, 28*(2S), S13–S17.

Greenberg, S. (2012). Analysis of measurement tools of fear of falling for high-risk, community dwelling older adults. *Clinical Nursing Research, 21*(1), 113–130.

Hellsten, L. A., et al. (2008). Accumulation of behavioral validation evidence for physical activity stage of change. *Health Psychology, 27*(Suppl. 1), 543–553.

Hodgson, M. J., Marz, M. W., & Nelson, A. (2013). Patient handling in the veterans health administration. *American College of Occupational and Environmental Medicine, 55*(10), 1230–1237.

Keysor, J. J. (2011). Brembs A: Exercise: necessary but not sufficient for improving function and preventing disability? *Current Opinion in Rheumatology, 23*(2), 211–218.

Kneafsey, R., Clifford, C., & Greenfield, S. (2015). Perceptions of hospital manual handling policy and impact on nursing team involvement in promoting patients' mobility. *Journal of Clinical Nursing, 24*, 289–299.

Kneafsy, R., Clifford, C., & Greenfield, S. (2013). What is the nursing team involvement in maintaining and promoting the mobility of older adults in hospital? A grounded theory study. *International Journal of Nursing Studies, 50*, 1617–1629.

Kneafsey, R. (2007). A systematic review of nursing contributions to mobility rehabilitation: examining the quality and content of the evidence. *Journal of Clinical Nursing, 16*(11c), 325–340.

Knittle, K. P. (2011). Effect of self-efficacy and physical activity goal achievement on arthritis pain and quality of life in patients with rheumatoid arthritis. *Arthritis Care and Research, 63*(11), 1613–1619.

Krecinic, T., et al. (2009). Orthostatic hypotension in older persons: a diagnostic algorithm. *The Journal of Nutrition, Health and Aging, 13*(6), 572–575.

Liu, C.-J., & Latham, N. (2009). Progressive resistance strength training to improve physical function in older adults. *Cochrane Database of Systematic Reviews*, (3), CD002759.

Longo, D., Fauci, A., Kasper, D., et al. (2012). *Harrison's principles of internal medicine* (18th ed.). New York: McGraw-Hill.

Messecar, D. C. (2008). Review: several interventions reduce fear of falling in older people living in the community. *Evidence-Based Nursing, 11*(1), 21.

Paulus, R. A., Davis, K., & Steele, G. D. (2008). Continuous innovation in health care: implication of the Geisinger experience. *Health Affairs, 27*(5), 1235–1245.

Pomeroy, S. H., et al. (2011). Person-environment fit and functioning among older adults in a long term care setting. *Geriatric Nursing (New York, N.Y.), 32*(5), 368–378.

Pretzer-Aboff, I., Galik, E., & Resnick, G. (2011). Feasibility and impact of a function focused care intervention for Parkinson's disease in the community. *Nursing Research, 60*(4), 276–283.

Radawiec, S. M., et al. (2009). Safe ambulation of an orthopaedic patient. *Orthopaedic Nursing, 28*(2), 24–27.

Rauen, C. A., et al. (2008). Seven evidence-based practice habits: putting some sacred cows out to pasture. *Critical Care Nurse, 28*(2), 98–113.

Resnick, B., & D'Adamo, C. (2011). Factors associated with exercise among older adults in a continuing care retirement community. *Rehabilitation Nursing, 36*(2), 47–53.

Resnick, B., & Galik, E. (2013). Using Function-Focused Care to increase physical activity among older adults. *Annual Review of Nursing Research, 31*, 175–208.

Resnick, B., & Jenkins, L. S. (2000). Testing the reliability and validity of the self-efficacy for exercise scale. *Nursing Research, 49*(3), 154–159.

Resnick, B., Zimmerman, S., & Orwig, D. (2001). Model testing for reliability and validity of the outcome expectations for exercise scale. *Nursing Research, 50*, 5.

Resnick, B., et al. (2008). A proposal for a new screening paradigm and toll called exercise assessment and screening for you (EASY). *Journal of Aging and Physical Activity, 16*(2), 215–233.

Resnick, B., et al. (2009). Nursing home resident outcomes from the res-care intervention. *Journal of the American Geriatrics Society, 57*(7), 1156–1165.

Resnick, B., et al. (2011). Testing the effect of function-focused card in assisted living. *Journal of the American Geriatrics Society, 59*, 2233–2240.

Rikli, R. E., & Jones, J. J. (2012). Development and validation of criterion-referenced clinically relevant fitness standards for maintaining physical independence in later years. *The Gerontologist*. [Epub ahead of print].

Rintala, D. H., et al. (2005). The effects of service dogs on the lives of persons with mobility impairments: a pre-post study design. *SCI Psychosocial Process, 18*(4), 236–249.

Sedlak, C. A., et al. (2009). Development of the national association of orthopaedic nurses guidance statement on safe patient handling and movement in the orthopaedic setting. *Orthopaedic Nursing, 28*(25), 52–58.

Semanik, P. A., Lee, J., Song, J., et al. (2015). Accelerometer-monitored sedentary behavior and observed physical function loss. *American Journal of Public Health, 105*(3), 560–566.

Shaughnessy, M., Michael, K., & Resnick, B. (2012). Impact of treadmill exercise on efficacy expectations, physical activity and stroke recovery. *The Journal of Neuroscience Nursing: Journal of the American Association of Neuroscience Nurses, 44*(1), 27–35.

Sherrington, C., et al. (2008). Group exercise can improve participant's mobility in an outpatient rehabilitation setting: a randomized controlled trial. *Clinical Rehabilitation, 22*(6), 493–502.

Smith, M. L., et al. (2011). Older adults' participation in a community-based falls prevention exercise program: relationships between the EASY tool, program attendance, and health outcomes. *The Gerontologist, 51*(6), 809–821.

Tomita, M., Saharan, S., Rajendran, S., et al. (2014). Psychometrics of the home safety self-assessment tool (HSSAT) to prevent falls in community-dwelling older adults. *The American Journal of Occupational Therapy, 68*, 711–718.

U.S. Department of Health and Human Services (2008). *Physical activity guidelines for Americans, 2008*. Washington, DC: Author.

Wu, C. Y., et al. (2007). A randomized controlled trial of modified constraint-induced movement therapy for elderly stroke survivors: changes in motor impairment, daily functioning, and quality of life. *Archives of Physical Medicine and Rehabilitation, 88*(3), 273–278.

Yeom, H. A., Keller, C., & Fleury, J. (2009). Interventions for promoting mobility in community-dwelling older adults. *Journal of the American Academy of Nurse Practitioners, 21*(2), 95–100.

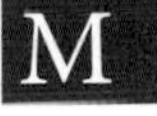

Impaired wheelchair Mobility

Wendie A. Howland, MN, RN-BC, CRRN, CCM, CNLCP, LNCC

NANDA-I

Definition

Limitation of independent operation of wheelchair within environment

Defining Characteristics

Impaired ability to operate power wheelchair on a decline; Impaired ability to operate power wheelchair on an incline; Impaired ability to operate power wheelchair on curbs; Impaired ability to operate power wheelchair on even surface; Impaired ability to operate power wheelchair on uneven surface

Related Factors

Alteration in cognitive functioning; alteration in mood; decrease in endurance; environmental barrier (e.g., stairs, inclines, uneven surfaces, obstacles, distance); impaired vision; insufficient knowledge of wheelchair use; insufficient muscle strength; musculoskeletal impairment; neuromuscular impairment; obesity; pain; physical deconditioning

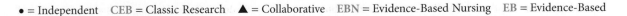

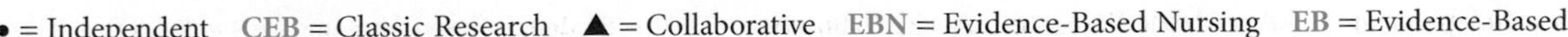

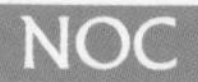 (Nursing Outcomes Classification)

Suggested NOC Outcome

Ambulation: Wheelchair

Example NOC Outcome with Indicators

Ambulation: Wheelchair as evidenced by the following indicators: Propels wheelchair safely/Transfers to and from wheelchair/Maneuvers curbs, doorways, ramps. (Rate the outcome and indicators of **Ambulation: Wheelchair:** 1 = severely compromised, 2 = substantially compromised, 3 = moderately compromised, 4 = mildly compromised, 5 = not compromised [see Section I].)

Client Outcomes

Client Will (Specify Time Frame)

- Demonstrate independence in operating and moving a wheelchair or other device with wheels
- Demonstrate the ability to direct others in operating and moving a wheelchair or other device
- Demonstrate therapeutic positioning, pressure relief, and safety principles while operating and moving a wheelchair or other device equipped with wheels

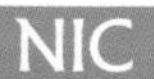 (Nursing Interventions Classification)

Suggested NIC Interventions

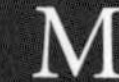

Exercise Therapy: Muscle Control; Positioning: Wheelchair

Example NIC Activities—Positioning: Wheelchair

Select the appropriate wheelchair for the client: standard adult, semi-reclining, fully reclining, amputees; Monitor for client's inability to maintain correct posture in wheelchair

Nursing Interventions and *Rationales*

- Assist client to put on and take off equipment (e.g., braces, orthoses, abdominal binders, compression stockings) in bed. *These provide stabilization and alignment; abdominal binder prevents postural hypotension and increases vital capacity (for hemodynamic stability, binder and stockings must be put on and taken off in bed).*
- Inspect skin where orthoses, braces, and other equipment rested, once they are removed. EB: *Early detection of pressure allows for early pressure relief strategy implementation and a review of outcomes for preventing the development of pressure ulcers and facilitating wound healing (Requejo et al, 2015).*
- ▲ Refer to physical and occupational therapy or wheelchair seating clinic. *Seating for wheelchair-dependent clients should be assessed by health care specialists in conjunction with client/caregiver education on weight shift maneuvers (Sprigle & Sonenbaum, 2011).*
- Recognize that use of support surfaces on chairs and beds redistributes pressure and should be used for at-risk clients as an adjunct to reduce risk of pressure ulcer. However, using support surfaces does not replace the need for repositioning the client on a regular schedule (i.e., weight shifts) (Sprigle & Sonenbaum, 2011; Requejo et al, 2015). *Sitting-acquired pressure ulcers occur primarily over the ischial tuberosities; sacral ulcers primarily result from excessive loading in bed (Gefen et al, 2013; AHRQ, 2014).*
- ▲ EBN/EB: *A randomized clinical trial studied elders at risk for pressure ulcers by pressure mapping and measuring the peak pressure index of subjects placed on standard 3-inch foam cushions compared to two common pressure-reducing cushions. Results demonstrated those with high peak pressure indexes using foam cushions acquired more pressure ulcers than those using pressure-reducing cushions (Akins et al, 2011). There are many pressure-relieving cushions. Several that are commonly used are the ROHO cushion, Varilite Evolution, and Invacare Matrix cushions.*
- Intervene to maintain continence or use absorbent diapers/underpads to help prevent skin breakdown due to excessive moisture and macerated skin. Some wheelchair cushions have moisture-wicking characteristics. *Pressure mapping alone insufficiently describes tissue health (Kim et al, 2012; National Pressure Ulcer Advisory Panel, 2014).*

- Routinely assess client's sitting posture and frequently reposition him/her into alignment. CEB: *A study demonstrated nursing personnel could reliably use the Resident Ergonomic Assessment Profile for Seating to assess posture of persons in their wheelchair (Gavin-Dreschnack et al, 2009).*
- *Assess client satisfaction with function and positioning using a standardized tool if available (Kumar et al, 2013).*
- Sit dysphagic clients as upright as possible in individualized wheelchair versus geri-chair when eating. *Clients with potential risk for aspiration (dysphagic clients) should have aspiration prevention strategies in place.* See care plan for Risk for **Aspiration.**
- Implement use of friction-coated projection hand rims and leather gloves for clients to propel manual wheelchairs. *Friction-coated projection rims are less invasive and slippery than aluminum rims; gloves absorb forces of propulsion and help prevent nerve damage/carpal tunnel.*
- Manually guide or explain to the client to push forward on both wheel rims to move ahead, push the right rim to turn left and vice versa, and pull backward on both wheel rims to back up.
- Recommend that clients back wheelchair into an elevator. If entering face first, instruct them to turn chair around to face the elevator doors. CEB: *Clients can see the control panel, floor monitor display, and doors opening and can exit wheeling forward. Be aware that feet/legs are at risk for injury if door panels close prematurely or if there is insufficient room to accommodate the wheelchair (Pierson & Fairchild, 2008).*

▲ In conjunction with physical therapy for teaching and assessment, reinforce principle of descending a curb backward ("popping a wheelie") if balance, trunk control, strength, and timing are adequate. *Backward descent carries less risk of clients losing control and falling forward out of wheelchair.*

- Ascend curbs in a forward position by popping a wheelie or having someone aid in tilting the chair back, place front wheels over curb, and roll chair up. If surface is muddy or sandy, ascend backward. *Front casters will not roll on soft surfaces; a backward approach requires less energy and prevents getting stuck or falling forward.*

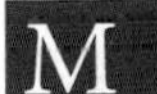

- During assisted wheelies, helper must hold wheelchair until all four wheels are back on the ground and client has control of wheelchair. *Releasing one's grip too soon may alter client's balance and cause injury.*

▲ Follow therapist's recommendations for how clients should propel manual wheelchairs to prevent upper extremity pain and joint degeneration. *Excessive load on the shoulder muscles should be reduced by producing wheelchairs with adjustable chair heights and by using a wheelchair with consideration for an individual's body size (Le et al, 2012).*

- Inform clients that ultra-lightweight, push-rim-activated, power-assisted, or electric wheelchairs may be more therapeutic than manual ones. *Consider push rim-activated power-assist wheelchairs (manual wheel chairs with a motor linked to the pushrim in each rear hub) that reduce energy needed for propulsion and reserve energy for uneven terrain or obstacle negotiation.* EB: *Power-assisted wheelchair propulsion decreased muscle work and forces on the shoulder in all directions (Kloosterman et al, 2012).*
- Help clients transition from a manual to a powered wheelchair/scooter if progressive disability occurs. CEB: *If the client does not have sufficient strength or motor control of the extremities to propel a standard wheelchair, the client may need to be evaluated for a power chair (Pierson & Fairchild, 2008).*

▲ Reduce floor clutter and establish safety rules for drivers of electric/power mobility devices; make referrals to physical or occupational therapy for driver reevaluations if accidents occur or client's health deteriorates. *Safe driving prevents injury to client, pedestrians, and property. Waist belt restraints are attached to the frame of the wheelchair and are designed to prevent the driver from falling out of or sliding forward in the chair (Pierson & Fairchild, 2008).*

- Request and receive client's permission before moving unoccupied wheelchair in room or out to hallway. *Wheelchair-dependent clients may view chair as part of their identity and independence.*
- Reinforce compensatory strategies for unilateral neglect and agnosia (e.g., visual scanning, self-talk, self-questioning as to what could be wrong) as clients propel wheelchair through doorways and around obstacles. *Too often nurses physically move wheelchair or obstacle instead of cueing client to detect and solve problems.* Refer to care plan for **Unilateral Neglect.**
- Offer support to help clients cope with issues related to physical disability. *Depression and anxiety may occur with physical loss.* Refer to care plan for Ineffective **Role** performance.
- Provide information on support group and reliable Internet resource options.
- Provide information about advocacy, accessibility, assistive technology, and issues under the Americans with Disabilities Act.

▲ Make social service or wheelchair clinic referral to educate clients on financial coverage/regulations of third-party payers and Health Care Financing Association for wheelchairs. *It is wise to recognize cost, advantages, and durability of different wheelchair models before purchasing one.*
• Recommend that clients test-drive wheelchairs and try out cushions/postural supports with the advice of a qualified seating professional before purchasing them. *Equipment is expensive, and different models have different advantages and disadvantages.*

Pediatric

▲ EB: *Consult physical or occupational therapist for special considerations for wheelchair fitting and positioning for pediatric client. In children with cerebral palsy, poor trunk control can lead to spinal deformity and pulmonary compromise. Evidence links posture and pulmonary function; special techniques for measuring these may be necessary (Barks & Shaw, 2011).*
▲ Help client/family transition from a manual to a powered wheelchair/scooter if disability is severe. *Compared to a control group using manual wheelchairs, disabled children using power wheelchairs evidenced enhanced development, functional skills, and communication, and decreased caregiver burden (Jones et al, 2012).*

Geriatric

• Avoid using restraints on fidgeting clients who slide down in a wheelchair; rather, assess for deformities, spinal curvatures, abnormal tone, discomfort, and limited joint range.
• Ensure proper seat depth/leg positioning and use custom foot rests (not elevated leg rests) to prevent older adults from sliding down in wheelchairs.
▲ Assess for side effects of medications and potential need for dosage readjustments to increase wheelchair tolerance. Give prescribed hydration and medications to treat orthostatic hypotension. Consider leg wraps. Client should perform warm-up bed exercises (Le, 2012). *Cerebral hypoperfusion is a common cause of orthostatic intolerance and hypotension (Le, 2012). Severe spinal cord injury above T6-8 is a risk factor for orthostatic hypotension due to reduced efferent sympathetic nervous activity and loss of reflex vasoconstriction at arterial baroreceptors below the level of injury (Phillips et al, 2012).*
• Allow client to propel wheelchair independently at his/her own speed. *Older adults may move slowly due to diminished range of motion/strength, stiff/sore joints, and cardiopulmonary compromise.*

M

Home Care

▲ Establish a support system for emergency and contingency care (e.g., remote monitoring, emergency call system, alert local emergency medical system). *Wheelchair dependence may be life-threatening during a crisis (e.g., fall, fire, or other environmental emergency).*
• Recommend the following changes to the home to accommodate the use of a wheelchair:
  ❍ Arrange traffic patterns so they are wide enough to maneuver a wheelchair.
  ❍ Recognize a 5-foot turning space is necessary to maneuver wheelchairs; doorways need to have 32 to 36 inches clear width; and entrance ramps/path slope should be assessed before permanent ramps are installed because standardized slopes may not be appropriate. Temporary ramps are cost-effective and easier to adjust (Sofka, 2011).
  ❍ Replace door hardware with fold-back hinges, remove doorway encasements (if too narrow), remove/replace thresholds (if too high), hang wall-mounted sinks/handrails, grade floors in showers for roll-in chairs, use nonskid/nonslip floor coverings (e.g., nonwaxed wood, linoleum, or Berber carpet).
  ❍ Rearrange room functions, furniture, and storage so that toileting, sleeping, bathing, and preparing/eating meals can safely take place on one level of the home.
  ❍ *Refer to the Easter Seals Summary on Home Accessibility for further details:* http://www.easterseals.com/shared-components/document-library/easy_access_housing.pdf.
▲ Request physical and occupational therapy referrals to evaluate wheelchair fitting, skills, safety, and maintenance. Suggest community resources for servicing and tuning up wheelchairs and/or locating parts so clients can service their own chairs; an annual tune-up is recommended.

Client/Family Teaching and Discharge Planning

▲ Assess pain levels of long-term wheelchair users and make referrals to therapists or wheelchair clinics for modifications as needed.

- Instruct and have client return demonstrate reinflation of pneumatic tires; encourage client to monitor tire pressure every 2 to 3 weeks.
- Instruct family/clients to remove large wheelchair parts (leg rests, arm rests) when lifting wheelchair into car for transport; when reassembling, check that all parts are fastened securely and temperature is tepid. *This reduces weight that needs to be lifted; locked parts and a safe temperature prevent injury/thermal injury.*
- Teach the critical importance of using seatbelts and secure chair tie-downs when riding in motor vehicles in a wheelchair. Never transport a client in an unsecured wheelchair in any kind of vehicle.
- For further information, refer to care plan for Impaired **Transfer** ability.

REFERENCES

AHRQ Quality Indicators Tool Kit, Berlowitz, D., Van Deusen-Lukas, C., et al. *Preventing pressure ulcers in hospitals: a tool kit for improving quality of care.* <www.ahrq.gov/qual/qitoolkit/d4c_pressureulcer_bestpractices.pdf> Retrieved 11/1/2014.

Akins, J. S., Karg, P. E., & Brienza, D. M. (2011). Interface shear and pressure characteristics of wheelchair seat cushions. *Journal of Rehabilitation Research and Development*, *48*(3), 225–234.

Barks, L., & Shaw, P. (2011). Wheelchair positioning and breathing in children with cerebral palsy: study methods and lessons learned. *Rehabilitation Nursing*, *36*, 146–152.

Gavin-Dreschnack, D., Schonfeld, L., Nelson, A., et al. *Development of a screening tool for safe wheelchair seating. In Agency for Healthcare Research and Quality (AHRQ), Department of Defense (DoD)—Health Affairs:* Advances in patient safety: from research to implementation. <www.ncbi.nlm.nih.gov/books/bv.fcgi?rid=aps.section.6773> Accessed December 12, 2011.

Gefen, A., Farid, K. J., (dnp), & Shaywitz, I. (2013). A review of deep tissue injury development, detection and prevention: shear savvy. *Ostomy/Wound Management*, *59*(2), 26–35.

Jones, M. A., McEwen, I. R., et al. (2012). Effect of power wheelchairs on the development and function of young children with severe motor impairments. *Pediatric Physical Therapy*, *24*(2), 131–140.

Kim, J. H., Wang, X., Ho, C. H., et al. (2012). Physiological measurements of tissue health: implications for clinical practice. *International Wound Journal*, *9*, 656–664.

Kloosterman, M. G. M., Eising, H., et al. (2012). Comparison of shoulder load during power-assisted and purely hand-rim wheelchair propulsion. *Clinical Biomechanics*, *27*(5), 428–435. Jour P 51-53.

Kumar, A., Schmeler, M. R., et al. (2013). Test-retest reliability of the functional mobility assessment (FMA): a pilot study. *Disability and Rehabilitation: Assistive Technology*, *8*(3), 213–219.

Le, S.-Y., Kim, S.-C., et al. (2012). Effect of the height of a wheelchair on the shoulder and forearm muscular activation during wheelchair propulsion. *Journal of Physical Therapy Science*, *24*, 51–53.

National Pressure Ulcer Advisory Panel (2014). *Prevention and treatment of pressure ulcers: Quick reference guide* (2nd ed.). NPUAP, Cambridge Media.

Phillips, A. A., Bredin, S. S., Krassioukov, A. V., et al. (2012). Aortic stiffness increased in spinal cord injury when matched for physical activity. *Medicine and Science in Sports and Exercise*, *44*(11), 2065–2070.

Pierson, F. M., & Fairchild, S. L. (2008). Features and activities of wheeled mobility aids. In F. M. Pierson & S. L. Fairchild (Eds.), *Principles & techniques of patient care* (4th ed.). St Louis: Saunders.

Requejo, P. S., Furumasu, J., & Mulroy, S. J. (2015). Evidence-based strategies for preserving mobility for elders and aging manual wheelchair users. *Topics in Geriatric Rehabilitation*, *31*(1), 26–41.

Sofka, K. (2011). *Technology Corner: It's All Downhill-Ramps, Part 1, JNLCP XI.3:438 ff and Part 2, JNLCP XI.4: 476 ff.*

Sprigle, S., & Sonenblum, S. (2011). Assessing evidence supporting redistribution of pressure for pressure ulcer prevention: a review. *Journal of Rehabilitation Research and Development*, *48*(3), 203–214.

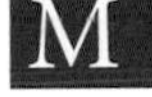

Impaired Mood regulation

Wolter Paans, MSc, PhD, RN

NANDA-I

Definition

A mental state characterized by shifts in mood or affect and which comprises a constellation of affective, cognitive, somatic, and/or physiological manifestations varying from mild to severe

Defining Characteristics

Changes in verbal behavior; disinhibition; dysphoria; excessive guilt; excessive self-awareness; excessive self-blame; flight of thoughts; hopelessness; impaired concentration; influenced self-esteem; irritability; psychomotor agitation; psychomotor retardation; sad affect; withdrawal

Related Factors

Alteration in sleep pattern; anxiety; appetite change; chronic illness; functional impairment; hypervigilance; impaired social functioning; loneliness; pain; psychosis; recurrent thoughts of death; recurrent thoughts of suicide; social isolation; substance misuse; weight change

NOC (Nursing Outcomes Classification)

Suggested NOC Outcomes

Hope: Symptom Control: Mood Equilibrium

Example NOC Outcome with Indicators

Mood Equilibrium as evidenced by the following indicators: Exhibits affect that fits situation/Exhibits impulse control/Shows interest in surroundings. (Rate the outcome and indicators of **Mood Equilibrium:** 1 = never demonstrated, 2 = rarely demonstrated, 3 = sometimes demonstrated, 4 = often demonstrated, 5 = consistently demonstrated [see Section I].)

Client Outcomes

Client Will (Specify Time Frame)

- State feelings related to changes in mood
- Eat appropriate diet for height and weight
- Follow exercise plan
- Have no attempts at self-harm

NIC (Nursing Interventions Classification)

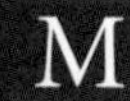

Suggested NIC Interventions

Mood Management; Suicide Prevention; Exercise Promotion; Health Education

Nursing Interventions and *Rationales*

- Provide nutritional intake for a client who is unable to feed self. EB: *This study aimed to define the role of nutritional interventions in the prevention and treatment of malnutrition in head and neck cancer clients undergoing chemo-radiotherapy as well as their impact on CRT-related toxicity and survival. Head and neck cancer clients are frequently malnourished at the time of diagnosis and prior to the beginning of treatment. In addition, chemo-radiotherapy causes or exacerbates symptoms, such as alteration or loss of taste, mucositis, xerostomia, fatigue, and nausea and vomiting, with consequent worsening of malnutrition. Nutritional counseling and oral nutritional supplements should be used to increase dietary intake and prevent therapy-associated weight loss and interruption of radiation therapy (Bossola, 2015). Some of the symptoms (e.g., fatigue, loss of taste) are also present in clients with the diagnostic concept "impaired mood regulation." This study clearly demonstrates that nutritional counseling should be used to increase dietary intake and to prevent weight loss.*
- Encourage regular physical exercise to maintain or advance to a higher level of fitness and health. EB: *Negative affective states such as anxiety, depression, and stress are significant risk factors for cardiovascular disease, particularly in cardiac and postcardiac rehabilitation populations. In this study, yoga is used as physical exercise. Breathing control and meditation can reduce psychosocial symptoms as well as improve cardiovascular and cognitive function (Yeung et al, 2014). This study shows the interest of physical exercise to advance a higher level of health.*
- Reduce the risk of self-inflicted harm for a client in crisis or severe depression with a planned treatment program. CEB/EBN: *This study is about childhood suicidal behavior. This is a complex symptom that requires a carefully planned treatment program that includes multiple modalities of care. Treatment requires a long-term approach that constantly reassesses potential for serious suicidal risk. Psychiatric hospitalization may be required to protect the child from self-inflicted harm and to allow evaluation and appropriate intervention (Pfeffer, 1984). This study is not recent but it confirms that the risk of self-inflicted harm for a client in crisis should be reduced.*
- Facilitate the safe and effective use of prescription and over-the-counter drugs. EB: *This article explains the importance of safe medicine use (Calsbeek, 2007). This article shows clearly that it is important to inform clients about their medicine use.*

Client/Network Interventions

- Provide a treatment involving the cooperation of several aide workers in neighborhood teams and providing customized treatment at the place where the client resides. EB/EBN: *The use of teams is a well-known approach in a variety of settings, including health care, in both developed and developing countries. Team performance comprises teamwork and task work, and ascertaining whether a team is performing as expected to achieve the desired outcome has rarely been done in health care settings in resource-limited countries (Yeboah-Antwi et al, 2013). This article shows that this intervention is still used.*

REFERENCES

Bossola, M. (2015). Nutritional interventions in head and neck cancer patients undergoing chemoradiotherapy: a narrative review. *Nutrients*, 265–276.

Calsbeek, H. (2007). Medicatieveiligheid voor thuiswonende chronisch zieken verdient aandacht. *Huisarts en Wetenschap*, 844–845.

Pfeffer, C. (1984). Modalities of treatment for suicidal children: an overview of the literature on current practice. *American Journal of Psychotherapy*, 364–372.

Yeboah-Antwi, K., Snetro-Plewman, G., Waltensperger, K., et al. (2013). Measuring teamwork and taskwork of community-based “teams” delivering life-saving health interventions in rural Zambia: a qualitative study. *BMC Medical Research Methodology*, 13–84.

Yeung, A., Kiat, H., Denniss, A., et al. (2014). Randomised controlled trial of a 12 week yoga intervention on negative affective states, cardiovascular and cognitive function in post-cardiac rehabilitation patients. *BMC Complementary and Alternative Medicine*, 14–411.

Moral Distress

Ruth A. Wittmann-Price, PhD, RN, CNS, CNE, CHSE, ANEF, FAAN

M

NANDA-I

Definition

Response to the inability to carry out one's chosen ethical/moral decision/action

Defining Characteristics

Anguish about acting on one's moral choice (e.g., powerlessness, anxiety, fear)

Related Factors (r/t)

Conflict among decision makers; conflicting information available for ethical decision-making; conflicting information available for moral decision-making; cultural incongruence; end of life decisions; loss of autonomy; physical distance of decision maker; time constraint for decision-making; treatment decision

NOC (Nursing Outcomes Classification)

Suggested NOC Outcomes

Personal Autonomy; Client Satisfaction: Protection of Rights

Example NOC Outcomes with Indicators

Client Satisfaction: Protection of Rights as evidenced by the following indicators: Requests respected/Included in decisions about care/Care consistent with religious and spiritual needs. (Rate the outcome and indicators of **Client Satisfaction: Protection of Rights**: 1 = not at all satisfied, 2 = somewhat satisfied, 3 = moderately satisfied, 4 = very satisfied, 5 = completely satisfied [see Section I].)

Client Outcomes

Client Will (Specify Time Frame)

- Be able to act in accordance with values, goals, and beliefs
- Regain confidence in the ability to make decisions and/or act in accord with values, goals, and beliefs
- Express satisfaction with the ability to make decisions consistent with values, goals, and beliefs
- Have choices respected

NIC (Nursing Interventions Classification)

Suggested NIC Interventions

Patient Rights Protection; Emotional Support

Example NIC Activities—Patient Rights Protection

Provide environment conducive for private conversations between client, family, and health care professionals

Nursing Interventions and *Rationales*

- Assess if moral distress is present and its relationship to intrinsic or extrinsic factors. EB: *Lester (2014) found in an ethnographic study that women with eating disorders often do not take prescribed medications, purge them, or hoard them because they have a moral imperative that is different from the usually assumed one, which is that everyone strives for health.* EBN: *Hmaideh (2014) studied moral distress among psychiatric nurses and found that it was strongly correlated to case load and burnout.*
- Affirm the distress, commitment "to take care of yourself," and your obligations. Validate feelings and perceptions with others. EBN: *Sirilla (2014) studied moral distress in nurses on different types of nursing units and found high levels of moral distress in oncology nurses who care for clients and families who often make difficult health care decisions.* EBN: *Robinson et al (2014) found that by implementing a course to increase ethical competency among nurses (N = 67) using methods based in adult learning theory, client scenarios, classroom discussion, simulation, and clinical practice, there was a decrease in moral distress and an increase in moral agency, which was defined as the enhanced ability to act to bring about change.*
- Implement strategies to change situations causing moral distress. EBN: *LeBaron et al (2014) used an ethnographic approach to explore moral distress and found that education is the most important aspect when considering moral obligations.* EBN: *Mason et al (2014) studied moral distress in medical intensive care units (ICUs) where there are clients and families faced with sudden life-threatening, life-changing situations and found that as work engagement (helping families, long-time relationships with colleagues, and satisfaction) increased, moral distress decreased.*
- Assess sources and severity of distress. EBN: *A qualitative study identified sources of moral distress as bullying, lateral violence, and retribution. Additionally, inadequate staffing and perceived incompetent coworkers were high items on the moral distress scale (Sauerland et al, 2014a).* EBN: *Strachan et al (2014) conducted a qualitative descriptive study about the experiences of long-term care nurses and residents with heart failure and found that decision-making was negatively influenced by (1) approaching heart failure reactively, (2) not having the skill to identify heart failure signs, (3) poor communication, (4) poor resources, and (5) moral distress.*
- Give voice/recognition to moral distress and express concerns about constraints to supportive individuals. EBN: *Wojtowicz et al (2014) completed a qualitative study about nursing students (N = 13) who reported significant moral distress due to the manner in which nurses and health care providers treated psychiatric clients even when their nursing instructor attempted to change client conditions.* EBN: *Sauerland et al (2014b) did a mixed method study and found that moral distress can be pervasive and the situations in which ethical issues are identified call for open discussion to decrease moral distress.*
- Engage in healthy problem solving. EBN: *Manara et al (2014) used a phenomenological-hermeneutic case analysis and found that moral action requires deliberate reflective thinking about the important things that are happening in a situation.* EB: *Tambuyzer et al (2014) studied mental health care clients' involvement in decision-making as an ethical requirement through a literature search (N = 45) and found a need for a comprehensive model of client involvement for ethical decision-making because three issues were identified: (1) a proliferation of conceptualizations of the topic, (2) vagueness, and (3) a lack of quantitative data.*
- Engage in interdisciplinary problem-solving forums including family meeting and/or interdisciplinary rounds. EB: *Dean et al (2014) did long-term (5-year) review of decision-making to administer sedative drugs during end of life care and found family discussions about sedatives improved by using a decision-making checklist.* EB: *Mah et al (2014) used vignettes in public health policy research to study moral reasoning about food advertising to children and found vignettes can effectively focus on moral conflicts and support moral reasoning for families.*
- Implement multidisciplinary interventions/strategies to address moral distress. EB: *Penny et al (2014) studied moral distress and found that a population that has high moral distress is individuals with chronic*

M

physical disabilities. EB: *Piers et al (2014) used a cross-sectional study of nurses (N = 1,218), junior (N = 180) and senior (N = 227) health care providers in ICUs to assess perceived inappropriate care (PIC) and found by multivariate analysis that nurses have higher PIC rates compared with junior and senior health care providers, but all agreed that excessive care for ICU clients is a major issue and ethical discussions among teams may decrease moral distress.*

- Identify/use a support system. EBN: *Kaplan and Tivnan (2014) used a survey to study college students' (N = 546) moral motivation and emotions and found compassion, distress, anger, and hate among the most reported moral emotions and concluded that increasing emotional awareness positively related to developing better moral decision-making and motivation.* EB: *Schroy et al (2014) used decision aids for colorectal cancer screening in a cross-sectional survey of providers (N = 29). Sixty percent felt that the tool increased client knowledge, helped clients identify a preferred option, improved decision-making, saved time, and increased clients' desire to be screened.*
- Initiate an ethics consult or ethics committee review. EBN: *McLeod (2014) qualitatively studied nurses' (N = 6) ethical principles in relation to treatment withdrawal in ICUs and identified three themes: (1) their personal set of moral beliefs, (2) their experience, and (3) the decision-making process. McLeod concluded that consensus in decision-making is a major factor to reduce moral distress.* EBN: *An investigation of Muslim nurses' (N = 306) attitudes toward do not resuscitate (DNR) orders using a descriptive-comparative research process found that nurses were willing to learn more about DNR orders, but many had negative attitudes toward DNR orders, which may be changed through education (Mogadasian et al, 2014) and use of ethics committees.*

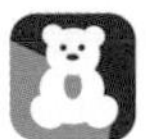

Pediatric

- Consider the developmental age of children when evaluating decisions and conflict. EBN: *Nsar and Rehm (2014) studied the long-term emotional consequences of live liver donations on donors and families by semi-structured interviews (N = 13) and found the experience as transformational with three themes: (1) self-awareness, (2) a clarification of familial relationships, and (3) a change on community perspective.* EBN: *Brandon et al (2014) conducted a before and after cross-sectional study to assess a Pediatric Quality of Life Program's relationship to moral distress of pediatric nurses, health care providers, social workers, therapists, dietitians, chaplains, and administrators and found that a palliative care program reduced moral distress.*

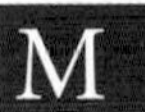

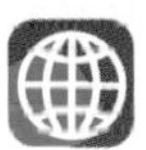

Multicultural

- Acknowledge and understand cultural differences that may influence a client's moral choices. EBN: *Moral et al (2014) used a cross-sectional study of clients' (N = 658) roles in decision-making with health care providers and in 60% of the situations (390 encounters), clients wished they could have been involved in the decision.* EBN: *Karanikola et al (2014) explored moral distress and its relationship to (1) nurse-health care provider collaboration, (2) autonomy, (3) professional satisfaction, (4) intention to resign, and (5) workload among Italian ICU nurses (N = 566) and found that moral distress was correlated with the intention to resign and poor nurse-health care provider interactions.*

Geriatric and Home Care

- Previous interventions may be adapted for geriatric or home care use. EBN: *Boot and Wilson (2014) used advance care planning conversations with terminally ill clients (N = 8) and through interviews found that the top considerations were (1) an assessment of the client's readiness to discuss the topic, (2) the client's physical condition, and (3) the nurse-client (and family) relationship.* EBN: *Lee and King (2014) conducted a quantitative study to assess the effect of educational classes on death anxiety and burnout among outpatient hemodialysis caregivers and found that education decreased the level of death anxiety and emotional exhaustion.*

REFERENCES

Brandon, D., Ryan, D., Shane, R., et al. (2014). Impact of a pediatric quality of life program on providers' moral distress. *The American Journal of Maternal Child Nursing (MCN)*, *39*(3), 189–197.

Boot, M., & Wilson, C. (2014). Clinical nurse specialists' perspectives on advance care planning conversations: a qualitative study. *International Journal of Palliative Nursing*, *20*(1), 9–14.

Dean, A., Miller, B., & Woodwark, C. (2014). Sedation at the end of life: a hospice's decision-making practices in the UK. *International Journal of Palliative Care*, *20*(10), 474–481.

Hmaideh, S. H. (2014). Moral distress and its correlates among mental health nurses in Jordan. *International Journal of Mental Health Nursing*, *23*(1), 33–41.

Kaplan, U., & Tivnan, T. (2014). Multiplicity of emotions in moral judgment and motivation. *Ethics & Behavior*, *24*(6), 421–443.

Karanikola, M. N. K., Albarran, J. W., Drigo, E., et al. (2014). Moral distress, autonomy and nurse-physician collaboration among intensive care unit nurses in Italy. *Journal of Nursing Management*, *22*(4), 472–484.

LeBaron, V., Beck, S. L., Black, F., et al. (2014). Nurse moral distress and cancer pain management. *Cancer Nursing*, *37*(5), 331–344.

Lee, V., & King, A. H. (2014). Exploring death anxiety and burnout among staff members who work in outpatient hemodialysis units. *Nephrology Nursing Journal*, *41*(5), 479–486.

Lester, R. (2014). Health as moral failing: medication restriction among women with eating disorders. *Anthropology & Medicine*, *21*(2), 241–250.

Mah, C. L., Tylor, E., Hoang, S., et al. (2014). Using vignettes to tap into moral reasoning in public health policy: practical advice and design principles from a study on food advertising to children. *American Journal of Public Health*, *104*(10), 1826–1832.

Manara, D. F., Villa, G., & Moranda, D. (2014). In search of salience: phenomenological analysis of moral distress. *Nursing Philosophy*, *15*(3), 171–182.

Mason, V. M., Leslie, G., Clark, K., et al. (2014). Compassion fatigue, moral distress, and work engagement in surgical intensive care unit trauma nurses. *Dimensions of Critical Care Nursing*, *33*(4), 215–225.

McLeod, A. (2014). Nurses' views of the causes of ethical dilemmas during treatment cessation in the ICU: a qualitative study. *British Journal of Neuroscience Nursing*, *10*(3), 131–137.

Mogadasian, S., Abdollahzadeh, F., Rahmani, A., et al. (2014). The attitude of Iranian nurses about do not resuscitate orders. *Indian Journal of Palliative Care*, *20*(1), 21–25.

Moral, R. R., Munguia, L. P., de Torres, L. A. P., et al. (2014). Patient participation in the discussions of options in Spanish primary care consultations. *Health Expectations*, *17*(5), 683–695.

Nsar, A. S., & Rehm, R. S. (2014). Parental live liver donation: a transformational experience. *Progress in Transplantation*, *24*(1), 69–75.

Penny, N. H., Ewing, T. L., Hamid, R. C., et al. (2014). An investigation of moral distress experienced by occupational therapists. *Occupational Therapy in Health Care*, *28*(4), 382–393.

Piers, R. D., Azoulay, E., Ricou, B., et al. (2014). Inappropriate care in European ICUs: confronting views from nurses and junior and senior physicians. *Chest*, *146*(2), 267–275.

Robinson, E. M., Lee, S. M., Zollfrank, A., et al. (2014). Enhancing moral agency: clinical ethics residency for nurses. *Hastings Center Report*, *44*(5), 12–20.

Sauerland, J., Marotta, K., Peinemann, M. A., et al. (2014a). Assessing and addressing moral distress and ethical climate, part 1. *Dimensions of Critical Care*, *33*(4), 234–245.

Sauerland, J., Marotta, K., Peinemann, M. A., et al. (2014b). Assessing and addressing moral distress and ethical climate, part II. *Dimensions of Critical Care*, *34*(1), 33–46.

Schroy, P. C., Mylvaganam, S., & Davidson, P. (2014). Provider perspectives on the utility of a colorectal cancer screening decision aid for facilitating shared decision making. *Health Expectation*, *17*(1), 27–35.

Sirilla, J. (2014). Moral distress in nurses providing direct care on inpatient oncology units. *Clinical Journal of Oncology Nursing*, *18*(5), 536–541.

Strachan, P. H., Kaasalainen, S., Horton, A., et al. (2014). Managing heart failure in the long-term care setting. *Nursing Research*, *63*(5), 357–365.

Tambuyzer, E., Pieters, G., & Van Audenhove, C. (2014). Patient involvement in mental health care: one size does not fit all. *Health Expectations*, *17*(1), 138–150.

Wojtowicz, B., Hagan, B., & Van-Daalen-Smith, C. (2014). No place to turn: nursing students' experiences of moral distress in mental health settings. *International Journal of Mental Health Nursing*, *23*(3), 257–264.

Nausea

Janelle M. Tipton, MSN, RN, AOCN

NANDA-I

Definition

A subjective, phenomenon of an unpleasant feeling in the back of the throat and stomach, which may or may not result in vomiting

Defining Characteristics

Aversion to food; gagging sensation; increase in salivation; increase in swallowing; nausea; sour taste

Related Factors

Biophysical

Biochemical dysfunction (e.g., uremia, diabetic ketoacidosis); esophageal disease; exposure to toxin; gastric distention; gastrointestinal irritation; increase in intracranial pressure; intra-abdominal tumors; labyrinthitis; liver capsule stretch; localized tumors (e.g., acoustic neuroma, brain tumor, bone metastasis); Ménière's disease; meningitis; motion sickness; pancreatic disease; pregnancy; splenetic capsule stretch; treatment regimen

Situational

Anxiety; fear; noxious environmental stimuli; noxious taste; psychological disorder; unpleasant visual stimuli

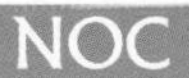

NOC (Nursing Outcomes Classification)

Suggested NOC Outcomes

Comfort Level; Hydration; Nausea and Vomiting Severity; Nutritional Status: Food and Fluid Intake; Nutrient Intake

Example NOC Outcome with Indicators

Nausea and Vomiting Severity as evidenced by the following indicators: Frequency of nausea/Intensity of nausea/ Distress of nausea. (Rate the outcome and indicators of **Nausea and Vomiting Severity:** 1 = severe, 2 = substantial, 3 = moderate, 4 = mild, 5 = none [see Section I].)

Client Outcomes

Client Will (Specify Time Frame)

- State relief of nausea
- Explain methods clients can use to decrease nausea and vomiting (N&V)

NIC (Nursing Interventions Classification)

Suggested NIC Interventions

Distraction; Medication Administration; Progressive Muscle Relaxation; Simple Guided Imagery; Therapeutic Touch

Example NIC Activities—Distraction

Encourage the individual to choose the distraction techniques desired, such as music, engaging in conversation or telling a detailed account of event or story, guided imagery, or humor; Advise client to practice the distraction technique before the time needed, if possible

Nursing Interventions and *Rationales*

- ▲ Determine cause or risk for N&V (e.g., medication effects, infectious causes [viral and bacterial gastroenteritis], disorders of the gut and peritoneum [mechanical obstruction, motility disorders, or other intra-abdominal causes], central nervous system causes [including anxiety], endocrine and metabolic causes [including pregnancy], postoperative-related status). *Because N&V are clinically identifiable symptoms, it is important for the cause to be determined and appropriate plan and interventions to be developed. Reviewing the client's medication record, alcohol history, and electrolytes as appropriate for early identification of cause of nausea (Goel & Wilkinson, 2013).* EB: *Prophylactic interventions given before chemotherapy have proven to be most successful in preventing N&V. Client expectancy of nausea after chemotherapy is predictive of that treatment-related side effect (Tipton, 2014; Kamen et al, 2014).*
- ▲ Evaluate and document the client's history of N&V, with attention to onset, duration, timing, volume of emesis, frequency of pattern, setting, associated factors, aggravating factors, and past medical and social histories. *The onset and duration of N&V may be distinctly associated with specific events and may be treated differently (Grunberg, 2012).*
- • Document each episode of nausea and/or vomiting separately, as well as effectiveness of interventions. Consider an assessment tool for consistency of evaluation. EB: *A systematic approach can provide consistency, accuracy, and measurement needed to direct care. It is important to recognize that nausea is a subjective experience (Wood et al, 2011).*
- • Identify and eliminate contributing causative factors. This may include eliminating unpleasant odors or medications that may be contributing to nausea. *These interventions are theory-based; however, there is no research evidence to support outside of expert opinion.*
- ▲ Implement appropriate dietary measures such as NPO status as appropriate; small, frequent meals; and low-fat meals. It may be helpful to avoid foods that are spicy, fatty, or highly salty. Reverting to previous practices when ill in the past and consuming "comfort foods" may also be helpful at this time. *Expert opinion consensus recommends these interventions, with no research data available (Irwin & Johnson, 2014).*

- ▲ Recognize and implement interventions and monitor complications associated with N&V. This may include administration of intravenous fluids and electrolytes. *Recognition of complications of N&V is critical to prevent and manage complications of dehydration, electrolyte imbalance, and malnourishment. Adequate hydration corrects imbalances and reduces further emesis (Gan et al, 2014)*
- ▲ Administer appropriate antiemetics, according to emetic cause, by most effective route, considering the side effects of the medication, with attention to and coverage for the timeframes that the nausea is anticipated. EB: *Antiemetic medications are effective at different receptor sites and treat different causes of N&V. A combination of agents may be more effective than single agents (Jordan et al, 2014; Rao & Faso, 2012).*
- • Consider nonpharmacological interventions such as acupressure, acupuncture, music therapy, distraction, and slow, deliberate movements. EB: *Nonpharmacological interventions can augment pharmacological interventions because they predominantly affect the higher cortical centers that trigger N&V. Nonpharmacological interventions are often low cost, relatively easy to use, and have few adverse events. The nonpharmacological interventions most likely to be effective include progressive muscle relaxation, hypnosis for anticipatory chemotherapy-induced nausea and vomiting (CINV), and managing client expectations. Effectiveness has not been established for several other nonpharmacological interventions, primarily due to study limitations, lack of effect in small studies, and inconsistent results (Irwin & Johnson, 2014).*
- • Provide oral care after the client vomits. Oral care helps remove the taste and smell of vomitus, thus reducing the stimulus for further vomiting.

Nausea in Pregnancy

- • Early recognition and conservative measures are recommended to successfully manage nausea in pregnancy, and to prevent progression to hyperemesis gravidarum. Dietary and lifestyle modifications should be implemented before pharmacological interventions. Avoidance of any aversive odors or foods is recommended. Eating multiple small meals per day is also recommended to have some food in the stomach at all times, thereby avoiding hypoglycemia and gastric overdistention. Foods with higher protein and carbohydrate and lower fat content are helpful. Drinking smaller volumes of liquids at multiple times throughout the day is recommended. *These are traditional strategies for alleviating nausea during pregnancy and are considered expert opinion (Clark et al, 2014).*
- ▲ Due to the high incidence of coexisting gastroesophageal reflux disease (GERD), it is important to assess and manage these symptoms of heartburn, belching, and indigestion. EB: *Dietary and lifestyle factors are recommended first, with the use of calcium or aluminum-containing antacids. H2 receptor blockers or proton pump inhibitors (PPIs) may be needed if antacids have failed (Clark et al, 2014; Naumann et al, 2012).*
- ▲ It is well-established that *Helicobacter pylori (H. Pylori)* infection is associated with hyperemesis gravidarum. *It may also be recommended to test for* H. pylori *if there are persistent symptoms of nausea with pregnancy, prolonged symptoms of GERD, or a previous history of* H. pylori *infection (Clark et al, 2014).*
- ▲ Coexisting psychosocial factors may also influence the severity of N&V with pregnancy. Symptoms of anxiety and depression can occur in early pregnancy, especially when N&V is severe and can make the treatment of the N&V more challenging and even ineffective. *Timely diagnosis and treatment is recommended (Clark et al, 2014).*
- ▲ The American Congress of Obstetricians & Gynecologists (ACOG) currently recommends a combination of oral pyridoxine hydrochloride (vitamin B6, 25 mg) and doxylamine succinate (antihistamine 12.5 mg) be used as first-line treatment for N&V of pregnancy after failure of pyridoxine alone. This combination agent (Diclegis) is the only U.S. Food and Drug Administration pregnancy Category A approved therapy for N&V of pregnancy. There are, however, several pharmacological treatments outlined by the American College of Obstetrics and Gynecology (ACOG). *A stepwise, cost-effective strategy may be helpful in approaching nausea with pregnancy. Considerable N&V with associated dehydration may require intravenous antiemetics, hydration, and/or parenteral nutrition (Clark et al, 2014).*

Nausea Following Surgery

- ▲ Evaluate for risk factors for postoperative nausea and vomiting (PONV). EB: *Strong evidence suggests that client-related risk factors such as female gender, age group (<50 years), history of PONV, history of motion sickness, nonsmoking behavior, and environmental risk factors such as postoperative opioid use, emetogenic surgery (type and duration), and volatile anesthetics may increase the risk for PONV. It is important to determine this risk in the preoperative period, to better plan strategies to reduce baseline risk (Gan et al, 2014; Kovac, 2013). Childhood risk factors include surgery duration of more than 30 minutes, age older than 3 years, strabismus surgery, and a history of postoperative vomiting or a relative with PONV (Gan, 2014).*

▲ Reduction of risk factors associated with PONV is beneficial for both adults and children. EB: *Avoidance of the use of general anesthesia by the use of regional anesthesia has been associated with a decreased incidence of PONV. The avoidance of both nitrous oxide and volatile anesthetics has also minimized PONV. Decreased and minimal use of intraoperative and postoperative opioids has demonstrated reduction in PONV. Adequate hydration is also an intervention to decrease the risk of PONV (Gan et al, 2014; Skolnik & Gan, 2014).*

▲ Medicate the client prophylactically for nausea as ordered, throughout the period of risk. EB: *Antiemetic medications can reduce the incidence of PONV and use of combination treatment such as 5-HT$_3$ antagonist plus dexamethasone is more effective than monotherapy. This recommendation is for clients at moderate or high risk for PONV. Other antiemetics, such as the neurokinin (NK-1) receptor antagonists, may have a role, particularly in preventing vomiting and severity 24 to 48 hours after surgery (Gan et al, 2014; Kovac, 2013).*

▲ Alleviate postoperative pain using ordered analgesic agents (refer to care plan for Acute **Pain**). *Pain is known to be a factor in the development of PONV.*

• Consider the use of nonpharmacological techniques, such as P6 acupoint stimulation, as an adjunct for controlling PONV, which has been shown to be effective. EB: *Acupuncture and acustimulation have been studied with the most consistent results, similarly effective across methods of stimulation (acupuncture or acupressure or wrist-like electrical stimulation) (Gan et al, 2014).*

• Include client education on the management of PONV for all outpatients and discuss key assessment criteria (Odom-Forren et al, 2014).

Nausea Following Chemotherapy

• Perform risk assessment before chemotherapy administration. Risk factors include female gender, younger age, history of low alcohol consumption, history of morning sickness during pregnancy, anxiety, previous history of chemotherapy, client expectancy of nausea, and emetic potential of the regimen. *It is important to recognize the many risk factors individual clients may have and tailor the antiemetic strategy accordingly. Far too often, the degree of N&V is underestimated by health care providers (Grunberg, 2012; Rao & Faso, 2012).*

N

▲ Initiate antiemetic strategy prophylactically or when N&V occurs in accordance with evidence-based guidelines. *Preventing N&V is important; one failure in antiemetic therapy can result in anticipatory nausea for the remainder of the client's treatments, and interventions are less likely to be effective (Grunberg, 2012; Kamen et al, 2014).*

▲ Drug classes that are recommended for practice include the serotonin receptor antagonists, the neurokinin (NK-1) receptor antagonists, and cannabinoids. *Triple-drug regimens including serotonin receptor antagonists, NK-1 receptor antagonists, and dexamethasone are recommended for adults and children receiving highly emetogenic chemotherapy (Irwin & Johnson, 2014).*

▲ Consider the use of progressive muscle relaxation and guided imagery with antiemetics. EB: *There has been benefit associated with these interventions; however, the evidence has been weak, and further data are warranted (Irwin & Johnson, 2014).*

• Consider managing client expectations about CINV. EBN: *Benefit has been shown, particularly for anticipatory nausea (Irwin & Johnson, 2014).*

Geriatric

• There are no specific guidelines that address the prophylaxis of CINV specifically in older adults. Risk still needs to be assessed, although many older clients are often treated with less emetic chemotherapy. Chemotherapy, however, can cause increased toxicity due to age-related decreases in organ function, comorbidities, and drug-drug interactions secondary to polypharmacy. Additionally, adherence may be an issue, due to cognitive decline, impaired senses, and economic issues. *Increased caution is warranted in this population due to increased safety concerns (Hu et al, 2011).*

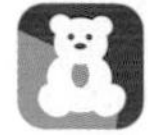

Pediatric

• Interventions for CINV should be implemented before and after chemotherapy. *Despite the extensive use of antiemetics, up to 58% of school-aged and adolescent children receiving highly emetogenic chemotherapy is reported. Delayed CINV occurs most frequently with greater severity and distress (Rodgers et al, 2012).*

• Relatively few studies exist examining the antiemetic medications used for CINV in children. It appears that 5-HT$_3$ antagonists combined with dexamethasone are better than older agents (Basch et al, 2011).

Home Care

- • Previously mentioned interventions may be adapted for home care use.
- ▲ In hospice care clients, assess for causes of nausea, such as constipation, bowel obstruction, adverse effects of medications, and onset of increased intracranial pressure. Refer the client to a primary health care provider if needed. *There can be multiple causes of nausea in clients with advanced cancer (Gordon et al, 2014).* EBN: *Nausea can effectively be controlled if a cause can be identified. An N&V protocol (e.g., Horvitz Center for Palliative Medicine N&V Protocol) can be used to identify and resolve any reversible causes of nausea, such as metabolic abnormalities or medications (Gupta et al, 2013). If none are found and symptoms persist, a flat plate radiograph of the abdomen is done to evaluate for obstruction or constipation. Appropriate medications can then be used to treat central nervous system causes, obstruction, or non-obstructive causes (Gordon et al, 2014).*
- • Assist the client and family with identifying and avoiding irritants in the home that exacerbate nausea (e.g., strong odors from food, plants, perfume, and room deodorizers). All medications except antiemetics should be given after meals to minimize the risk of nausea. EB: *Nausea triggered by odors is related to altered chemoreceptors and pathology (Glare et al, 2011).*

Client/Family Teaching and Discharge Planning

- • Teach the client techniques to use before and after chemotherapy, including antiemetics/medication management schedules and dietary approaches, such as eating smaller meals, avoiding spicy and fatty foods, and avoiding an empty stomach before chemotherapy (Irwin & Johnson, 2014).

REFERENCES

Basch, E., Prestrud, A. A., Hesketh, P. J., et al. (2011). Antiemetics: American Society of Clinical Oncology practice guideline update. *Journal of Clinical Oncology*, Epub ahead of print 9/26/11.

Clark, S. M., Dutta, E., & Hankins, G. D. (2014). The outpatient management and special considerations of nausea and vomiting in pregnancy. *Seminars in Perinatology Epub*, <http://dx.doi.org/10.1053/j.semperi.2014.08.014>.

Gan, T. J., Diemunsch, P., Habib, A. S., et al. (2014). Consensus guidelines for the management of postoperative nausea and vomiting. *Anesthesia & Analgesia*, *118*(1), 85–113.

Glare, P., Miller, J., Nikolova, T., et al. (2011). Treating nausea and vomiting in palliative care: a review. *Clinical Interventions in Aging*, *6*, 243–259.

Goel, R., & Wilkinson, M. (2013). Recommended assessment and treatment of nausea and vomiting. *Prescriber*, *5*, 23–27.

Gordon, P., LeGrand, S. B., & Walsh, D. (2014). Nausea and vomiting in advanced cancer. *European Journal of Pharmacology*, *722*, 187–191.

Grunberg, S. (2012). Patient-Centered management of chemotherapy-induced nausea and vomiting. *Cancer Control: Journal of the Moffitt Cancer Center*, *19*(2), 10–15.

Gupta, M., Davis, M., LeGrand, S., et al. (2013). Nausea and vomiting in advanced cancer: the Cleveland clinic protocol. *The Journal of Supportive Oncology*, *11*(1), 8–13.

Hu, R., Wu, Y., Jiang, X., et al. (2011). Clinical symptoms and chemotherapy completion in elderly patients with newly-diagnosed acute leukemia: a retrospective comparison study with a younger cohort. *BMC Cancer*, *11*(224), 1–8.

Irwin, M., & Johnson, L. A. (2014). Putting evidence into practice: a pocket guide to cancer symptom management. Pittsburgh, PA. *Oncology Nursing Society.*

Jordan, K., Gralla, R., Jahn, F., et al. (2014). International antiemetic guidelines on chemotherapy induced nausea and vomiting (CINV): content and implementation in daily routine practice. *European Journal of Pharmacology*, *722*, 197–202.

Kamen, C., Tejani, M., Chandwani, K., et al. (2014). Anticipatory nausea and vomiting due to chemotherapy. *European Journal of Pharmacology*, *722*, 172–179.

Kovac, A. L. (2013). Update on the management of postoperative nausea and vomiting. *Drugs*, *73*, 1525–1547.

Naumann, C. R., Zelig, C., Napolitano, P. G., et al. (2012). Nausea, vomiting, and heartburn in pregnancy: a prospective look at risk, treatment, and outcome. *The Journal of Maternal-fetal and Neonatal Medicine*, *25*(8), 1488–1493.

Odom-Forren, J., Hooper, V., Moser, D. K., et al. (2014). Postdischarge nausea and vomiting: management strategies and outcomes over 7 days. *Journal of Perianesthesia Nursing*, *29*(4), 275–284.

Rao, K. V., & Faso, A. (2012). Chemotherapy-induced nausea and vomiting: optimizing prevention and management. *American Health & Drug Benefits*, *5*(4), 232–239.

Rodgers, C., et al. (2012). Nausea and vomiting perspectives among children receiving moderate to highly emetogenic chemotherapy treatment. *Cancer Nursing*, *35*(3), 203–210.

Skolnik, A., & Gan, T. J. (2014). Update on the management of postoperative nausea and vomiting. *Current Opinion in Anaesthesiology*, [Epub ahead of print].

Tipton, J. M. (2014). Nausea and vomiting. In C. H. Yarbro, D. Wujcik, & B. H. Gobel (Eds.), *Cancer Symptom Management* (pp. 213–233). Burlington, MA: Jones & Bartlett.

Wood, J. M., Chapman, K., & Eilers, J. (2011). Tools for assessing nausea, vomiting, and retching. *Cancer Nursing*, *34*(1), E14–E24.

Noncompliance

Betty J. Ackley, MSN, EdS, RN, and Gail B. Ladwig, MSN, RN

NANDA-I

Definition

Behavior of person and/or caregiver that fails to coincide with a health-promoting or therapeutic plan agreed on by the person (and/or family and/or community) and health care professional; in the presence of an agreed-on, health-promoting, or therapeutic plan, person's or caregiver's behavior is fully or partially non-adherent and may lead to clinically ineffective or partially ineffective outcomes

Defining Characteristics

Behavior indicative of failure to adhere; evidence of development of complications; evidence of exacerbation of symptoms; failure to keep appointments; failure to progress; objective tests (e.g., physiological measures, detection of physiological markers)

Related Factors (r/t)

Health System

Access to care; communication skills of the provider; convenience of care; credibility of provider; difficulty in client-provider relationship; individual health coverage; provider continuity; provider regular follow-up; provider reimbursement; satisfaction with care; teaching skills of the provider

Health Care Plan

Complexity; cost; duration; financial flexibility of plan; intensity

Individual Factors

Cultural influences; developmental abilities; health beliefs; deficient knowledge relevant to the regimen behavior; individual's value system; motivational forces; personal abilities; significant others; skill relevant to the regimen behavior; spiritual values

N

Network

Involvement of members in health plan; perceived beliefs of significant others; social value regarding plan

NOTE: The nursing diagnosis **Noncompliance** is judgmental and places blame on the client for some things the client has no control over. The authors recommend use of the diagnosis Ineffective **Health** management in place of the diagnosis **Noncompliance.** The diagnosis Ineffective **Health** management has interventions that are developed by both the health care providers and the client. It is a more respectful and efficacious nursing diagnosis.

NIC, NOC, Client Outcomes, Nursing Interventions, Client/Family Teaching Discharge Planning, *Rationales,* and References

Refer to care plans for Ineffective **Health** management.

Readiness for enhanced Nutrition

Betty J. Ackley, MSN, EdS, RN, and Marina Martinez-Kratz, MS, RN, CNE

NANDA-I

Definition

A pattern of nutrient intake that can be strengthened

Defining Characteristics

Expresses desire to enhance nutrition

NOC (Nursing Outcomes Classification)

Suggested NOC Outcomes

Nutritional Status; Nutritional Status: Food and Fluid Intake; Nutrient Intake; Weight Control

Example NOC Outcome with Indicators

Nutritional Status as evidenced by the following indicators: Food and fluid intake/Hydration/Body mass index/Weight-height ratio/Hematocrit. (Rate the outcome and indicators of **Nutritional Status:** 1 = severe deviation from normal range, 2 = substantial deviation from normal range, 3 = moderate deviation from normal range, 4 = mild deviation from normal range, 5 = no deviation from normal range [see Section I].)

Client Outcomes

Client Will (Specify Time Frame)

- Explain how to eat according to the U.S. Dietary Guidelines
- Design dietary modifications to meet individual long-term goal of health, using principles of variety, balance, and moderation
- Maintain weight within normal range for height and age

NIC (Nursing Interventions Classification)

Suggested NIC Interventions

Nutrition Management; Nutritional Counseling; Weight Reduction Assistance

Example NIC Activities—Nutrition Management

Determine the client's motivation for changing eating habits; Develop with the client a method to keep a daily record of intake

Nursing Interventions and *Rationales*

- Assess the meaning and importance of food in the client's life. EB: *Research findings demonstrate that implicit attitudes significantly predict purchases of healthy and unhealthy foods (Prestwich et al, 2011). Research found that youth held some negative associations related to healthy foods and some positive associations linked to unhealthy foods (Harrison & Jackson, 2009).*
- *Assess the client's current nutrition through a 1- to 3-day food diary in which everything ingested orally is recorded. Analyze the following areas:*
  - *Intake of food and beverage calories and fat*
  - *Portion sizes*
  - *Underconsumption or overconsumption of nutrients*
  - *Use of supplements*
  - *Use of meal replacements*
  - *Timing/consistency of meals and snacks*

Use of a food diary is helpful for both the client and the nurse, to examine usual foods eaten and patterns of eating (Shay et al, 2009). EB: *A study found that use of a personal digital assistant for self-monitoring of food intake was more effective than use of a paper record, yet both groups had a similar weight loss (Acharya et al, 2011).*

- Counsel the client to measure regularly consumed foods periodically. Help the client learn usual portion sizes. *Measuring food alerts the client to normal portion sizes. Estimating amounts can be extremely inaccurate.* EB: *A study demonstrated that obese people had significantly larger portion sizes, plus ate later in the day (Berg et al, 2009).*
- Help the client determine his/her body mass index (BMI) and understand the significance of the result. Use a chart or a website such as http://www.cdc.gov/healthyweight/assessing/bmi/index.html (Centers for Disease Control and Prevention [CDC], 2014). *A normal BMI is 20 to 25; 26 to 29 is overweight; and*

a BMI of 30 or greater is obese. Clients with increased muscle mass may be labeled overweight, when in reality they are very physically fit. Also, clients who have lost large amounts of muscle mass may be in the healthy range, when in reality they may be malnourished (Camden, 2009). EB: *An analysis of 57 studies demonstrated that mortality was lowest for people with a BMI of 22.5 to 25. Each 5-unit increase above a BMI of 25 resulted in an increased mortality rate by 30% (Whitlock et al, 2009).*

- Recommend the client follow the U.S. Dietary Guidelines to determine foods to eat, which can be found at http://www.choosemyplate.gov/weight-management-calories/weight-management/better-choices/amount-calories.html. *Dietary guidelines are written by national experts and are based on research in nutrition (U.S. Department of Agriculture, 2014).*
- Recommend the client use Super Tracker (http://www.choosemyplate.gov/food-groups) to determine the number of calories to eat and gain more information on how to eat in a healthy fashion. To lose weight, the client must eat fewer calories (U.S. Department of Agriculture, 2014).
- Recommend the client eat a healthy breakfast every morning. CEB: *A study found that that people who skip breakfast are more likely to overeat in the evening (Masheb & Grillo, 2006). Another study demonstrated that people who skipped breakfast were 450 times more likely to be obese (Ma et al, 2003).*
- Recommend the client avoid eating in fast food restaurants. CEB: *A 15-year study demonstrated that people who frequently eat fast foods gain an average of 10 lb more than those who eat fast food less often and were two times more likely to develop insulin resistance, which can lead to diabetes (Pereira et al, 2005).*
- Demonstrate the use of food labels to make healthful choices. Alert the client/family to focus on serving size, total fat, and simple carbohydrate. *The standardized food label in bold type simplifies the search for information. Fats and sugars contribute the least to a healthful diet and the most to excessive calorie intake.*

Carbohydrates/Sugars

- Encourage the client to decrease intake of sugars, including intake of soft drinks, desserts, and candy. Limit sugar intake to 6.5 teaspoons of added sugars for women and 9.5 teaspoons of added sugar for men daily.
- Share with client the names of sugars include glucose, dextrose, corn syrup, maple syrup, brown sugar, molasses, evaporated cane juice, sucrose, honey, orange juice concentrate, grape juice concentrate, apple juice concentrate, brown rice syrup, high-fructose corn syrup, agave, and fructose (Nutrition Action, 2011). *Sugar predisposes to type 2 diabetes, heart disease, high blood pressure, high triglycerides, gout, and weight gain.* EB: *Studies comparing sugary and diet drinks demonstrated that sugary drinks increase visceral fat, which expands waistlines and drives insulin resistance, predisposing to type 2 diabetes and heart disease (Hu & Malik, 2010; Odegaard et al, 2012).*
- Limit intake of fruit juice to 1 cup per day. EB: *Studies have shown that people who drank more fruit juice had a greater risk of type 2 diabetes or weight gain (Odegaard et al, 2010; Pan et al, 2012).*
- Recommend the client eat whole grains whenever possible, and explain how to find whole grains using the food label. EB: *A review of studies found strong evidence that eating whole grains is associated with a decreased BMI and reduced the risk of being overweight (Williams et al, 2008). Intake of whole grains has been shown to decrease the incidence of heart failure (Nettleton et al, 2008) and, when eaten with other healthier foods, resulted in lower incidence of diabetes in a multiethnic study (Nettleton et al, 2008).*
- Assess the client's usual intake of fiber. Recommended intake is 25 g per day for women and 38 g per day for men. Increase intake of whole grains, beans, fruits, and vegetables to obtain needed fiber. Wheat bran is an excellent source of fiber, but cannot be tolerated by all people; beans are the second-best source of fiber (Nutrition Action, 2011). *In general, high-fiber foods take longer to eat, increase satiety, and contain fewer calories than most other foods (Slavin, 2008).*
- Recommend the client eat five to nine fruits and vegetables per day, with a minimum of two servings of fruit and three servings of vegetables. Encourage client to eat a rainbow of fruits and vegetables because bright colors are associated with increased nutrients. *Both fruits and vegetables are excellent sources of vitamins and also phytochemicals that help protect from disease, strokes, some kinds of cancer, and possibly macular degeneration (Liebman & Hurley, 2009).* EB: *A study done on older men found that ingesting foods high in vitamin C resulted in decreased thickening of the carotid arteries (Ellingsen et al, 2009).*

Fats

- Recommend the client limit intake of saturated fats and avoid trans fatty acids completely; instead increase intake of vegetable oils such as polyunsaturated and monounsaturated oils. EB: *A Cochrane study*

N

showed that decreasing intake of saturated fats, replacing them with unsaturated oils, was effective in decreasing cardiovascular risk (Hooper et al, 2012). Intake of both saturated fat and trans fatty acids raises the low-density lipoprotein (LDL) level, which predisposes to atherosclerosis with cardiovascular disease (Zelman, 2011).

- Recommend client use low-fat choices when selecting and cooking meat, and also when selecting dairy products. EB: *A large population based study found an approximate 50% relative risk reduction of pancreatic cancer, among both men and women who consumed a diet that included low-fat dairy products and lean protein sources (Chan et al, 2013).*
- Recommend that the client eat cold-water fish such as salmon, tuna, or mackerel at least two times per week to ensure adequate intake of omega-3 fatty acids. If client is unwilling to eat fish, suggest sources such as flaxseed, soy, or walnuts. NOTE: Fish oil capsules should be taken cautiously; some brands can be contaminated with mercury or pesticides. Intake of excessive omega-3 fatty acids can result in bleeding. *Ingestion of omega-3 fats results in lower triglycerides and total cholesterol and also decreases the risk of heart disease and stroke (Neville, 2009).* CEB: *The intake of omega-3 fatty acids by eating fish or fish oil capsules results in decreased incidence of sudden cardiac death (von Schacky, 2007).*

Protein

- Recommend the client decrease intake of red meat and processed meats, and instead eat more poultry, fish, soy, and dairy sources of protein. EB: *Red and processed meat intakes were associated with increases in mortality, for cancer, and cardiovascular disease (Sinha et al, 2009).* EB: *A large population-based study found an approximate 50% relative risk reduction of pancreatic cancer among both men and women who consumed a diet that included low-fat dairy products and lean protein sources (Chan et al, 2013).*
- Recommend the client eat meatless meals at intervals and try alternative sources of protein, including nuts, especially almonds (one handful), and nut butters. EB: *Consumption of nuts and peanut butter was shown to decrease the incidence of cardiovascular disease in women with type 2 diabetes (Li et al, 2009). A study found that diabetic people who ate walnuts regularly had improved endothelial function and healthier blood vessels, as well as lower low-density lipoproteins and total cholesterol (Ma et al, 2010).*
- Recommend the client eat beans and soy as an alternative to animal proteins at intervals. Introduce the client to soy products such as flavored soy milk and tofu. NOTE: *Women with diagnosed estrogen-dependent cancer of the breast should generally avoid eating soy foods.* EB: *In a Chinese study, research showed that intake of soy foods as a child may cut the incidence of breast cancer by half and may protect women from breast cancer, but further research is needed (Welland, 2007).*

Fluid and Electrolytes

- Recommend the client choose and prepare foods with less salt, aiming for a maximum of 2300 mg per day (Harvard Health Letter, 2012). *The CDC (2009) recommends that all salt-sensitive Americans, including everyone 40 years or older, should decrease daily sodium intake.* EB: *A study found that decreased sodium intake helped lower blood pressure, as well as increase flexibility in blood vessels, improving the health of the blood vessels (CDC, 2009).*
- If the client drinks alcohol, encourage him or her to drink in moderation—no more than one drink per day for women and two drinks per day for men. EB: *A study found an increased incidence of cancer of the upper gastrointestinal tract, liver cancer, and also renal cancer (Thygesen et al, 2009).*
- Recommend client increase intake of water to at least 2000 mL or 2 quarts per day. A guideline is 1 to 1.5 mL of fluid for each calorie needed, so an average intake would be between 2000 and 3000 mL/day or at least 8 cups of fluid. EB: *The adequate intake recommendation is 3 L for the 19- to 30-year-old male and 2.2 L for the 19- to 30-year-old female. Water balance studies suggest that adult men require 2.5 L per day (Institute of Medicine, 2004).*

Supplements

- Recommend that clients use dietary supplements such as vitamins and minerals only after consulting with their primary health care provider (Mayo Clinic Health Letter, 2012). EB: *A large study performed in women found that those who took more supplements had an increased risk for death, especially with intake of multivitamins, vitamin B_6, folic acid, iron, magnesium, zinc, and copper. Calcium seemed to*

N

decrease the risk of death (Mursu et al, 2011). CEB: *A review of 14 randomized trials demonstrated that intake of antioxidant supplementation did not prevent gastrointestinal cancers, and intake seemed to increase mortality (Bjelakovic et al, 2004).*

Pediatric

- Recommend that families eat together for at least one meal per day. *Mealtime together has been shown to improve children's eating habits: children eat more fruits and vegetables when the family eats together.*
- Recommend involving the family in planning meals and food preparation. Children can learn about nutrition as they help plan and make meals. *Children are more likely to eat foods that they help select or prepare.*
- Suggest that parents work at being good role models of healthy eating. *Setting a good example is key for children; children learn the value of healthy eating early, and it can continue for a lifetime.*
- Recommend that the family try new foods, either a new food or recipe every week. *More variety can increase the intake of fruits and vegetables.*
- Suggest the parents keep healthy snacks on hand. Store the snacks in a purse, the car, a desk drawer. *Suggestions include crackers and peanut butter, small boxes of cereal, fresh fruit, and vegetables (Academy of Nutrition and Dietetics, 2014).*
- Plan ahead before eating out. *Visit restaurant websites to see the nutritional value of foods on the menu; also call ahead to see what is offered for healthy foods. Most mothers want their families to eat healthier, but with busy schedules, this can be difficult.*

Geriatric

- Use a nutritional screening tool designed for older adults, such as the Mini Nutrition Assessment (MNA), the Malnutrition Universal Screening Tool (MUST), or the Nutrition Risk Screening (NRS). *The MNA is helpful for older adults living in the community or in an extended care facility; the NRS is more helpful for clients in the acute care setting (Sieber, 2006).*

- Assess changes in lifestyle and eating patterns. Older clients need to decrease portion size as they age because they do not burn as many calories as when they were younger. *Energy needs decrease an estimated 5% per decade after age 40 years, but often eating patterns remain unchanged from youth (Lutz & Przytulski, 2011).*
- Assess fluid intake. Recommend routine drinks of water regardless of thirst. Monitor older adults for deficient fluid volume carefully, noting new onset of weakness, dizziness, and postural hypotension. *Older adults have a higher osmotic point for thirst sensation and a diminished sensitivity to thirst relative to younger adults (Wotton et al, 2008).*
- Observe for socioeconomic factors that influence food choices (e.g., funds, cooking facilities, food insecurity). *Even those on restricted budgets and with limited facilities can be assisted to choose healthy food sources for a balanced diet.* EB: *Food security is a factor that can indicate a need for nutrition assistance in older adults (Lee et al, 2011).*

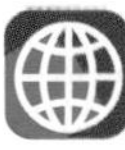

Multicultural

- Assess for the influence of cultural beliefs, norms, and values on the client's nutritional knowledge. *What the client considers normal dietary practices may be based on cultural perceptions (Giger & Davidhizar, 2008).*
- Tailor nutritional interventions to be consistent with cultural beliefs, norms, and values. EBN: *Mexican American women responded positively to nutritional education and physical activity promotion when families were involved (Vincent, 2009).*
- Offer tailored lifestyle counseling via the telephone. EB: *Low socioeconomic status African Americans and Latinos experienced positive nutritional change and weight loss after participating in a community-based translational lifestyle program (Kanaya et al, 2012).*

Client/Family Teaching and Discharge Planning

- The majority of the preceding interventions involve teaching.
- Work with the family members regarding information on how to improve nutritional status.

REFERENCES

Academy of Nutrition and Dietetics: *It's about eating right: nutrition for growing bodies*, 2014. From <http://www.eatright.org/Public/content.aspx?id=6751>. Retrieved September 20, 2014.

Acharya, S. D., Elci, O. U., Sereika, S. M., et al. (2011). Using a personal digital assistant for self-monitoring influences diet quality in comparison to a standard paper record among overweight/obese adults. *Journal of the American Dietetic Association, 111*(4), 583–588.

Berg, C., et al. (2009). Eating patterns and portion size associated with obesity in a Swedish population. *Appetite, 52*(1), 21–26.

Bjelakovic, G., et al. (2004). Antioxidant supplements for prevention of gastrointestinal cancers: a systematic review and meta-analysis. *Lancet, 364*(9441), 1219–1228.

Camden, S. (2009). Obesity: an emerging concern for patients and nurses. *Online Journal of Issues in Nursing, 14*(1), 5–17.

Centers for Disease Control and Prevention (CDC). (2009). Application of lower sodium intake recommendations to adults-United States, 1999-2006. *MMWR. Morbidity and Mortality Weekly Report, 58*(11), 281–283.

Centers for Disease Control and Prevention (CDC): *Healthy weight, it is not a diet, it is a lifestyle. BMI calculator*, 2011. From <http://www.cdc.gov/healthyweight/assessing/bmi/index.html>. Retrieved September 20, 2014.

Centers for Disease Control and Prevention (CDC): *Healthy weight, It's not a diet, it's a lifestyle. BMI calculator*, 2012. From <http://www.cdc.gov/healthyweight/assessing/bmi/index.html>. Retrieved June 13, 2012.

Chan, J. M., Gong, Z., Holly, E. A., et al. (2013). Dietary patterns and risk of pancreatic cancer in a large population-based case-control study in the San Francisco bay area. *Nutrition & Cancer, 65*(1), 157–164.

Ellingsen, I., et al. (2009). Vitamin C consumption is associated with less progression in carotid intima media thickness in elderly men: a 3-year intervention study. *Nutrition, Metabolism, and Cardiovascular Diseases, 19*(1), 8–14.

Giger, J., & Davidhizar, R. (2008). *Transcultural nursing: assessment and intervention* (5th ed.). St Louis: Mosby.

Harrison, M., & Jackson, L. (2009). Meanings that youth associate with healthy and unhealthy food. *Canadian Journal of Dietetic Practice & Research, 70*(1), 6–12.

Harvard Health Letter. (2012). Keep a lookout for sodium. *Harvard Health Letter, 37*(4), 1.

Hooper, L., et al. (2012). Reduced or modified dietary fat for preventing cardiovascular disease. *Cochrane Database of Systematic Reviews, 16*(5), CD002137.

Hu, F. B., & Malik, V. S. (2010). Sugar-sweetened beverages and risk of obesity and type 2 diabetes: epidemiologic evidence. *Physiology and Behavior, 100*(1), 47–54.

Institute of Medicine (2004). *Applications of dietary reference intakes for electrolytes and water*. Washington, DC: National Academies Press.

Kanaya, A. M., Santoyo-Olsson, J., Gregorich, S., et al. (2012). The live well, be well study: a community-based, translational lifestyle program to lower diabetes risk factors in ethnic minority and lower-socioeconomic status adults. *American Journal of Public Health, 102*(8), 1551–1558.

Lee, J. S., Johnson, M. A., & Brown, A. (2011). Older americans act nutrition program improves participants' food security in georgia. *Journal of Nutrition in Gerontology & Geriatrics, 30*(2), 122–139.

Li, T. Y., et al. (2009). Regular consumption of nuts is associated with a lower risk of cardiovascular disease in women with type 2 diabetes. *The Journal of Nutrition, 139*(7), 1333–1338.

Liebman, B., & Hurley, J. (2009). Rating rutabagas: not all vegetables are created equal. *Nutr Action Healthletter, Jan*, 13–15.

Lutz, C. A., & Przytulski, K. R. (2011). *Nutrition and diet therapy* (5th ed.). Philadelphia: FA Davis.

Ma, Y., et al. (2003). Association between eating patterns and obesity in a free-living U.S. adult population. *American Journal of Epidiomology, 158*(1), 85–92.

Ma, Y., et al. (2010). Effects of walnut consumption on endothelial function in type 2 diabetic subjects: a randomized controlled crossover trial. *Diabetes Care, 33*(2), 227–232.

Masheb, R. M., & Grillo, C. M. (2006). Eating patterns and breakfast consumption in obese patients with binge eating disorder. *Behaviour Research and Therapy, 44*(11), 1545–1553.

Mayo Clinic Health Letter: *Risks of vitamin supplements*, March 4, 2012.

Mursu, J., et al. (2011). Dietary supplements and mortality rate in older women: the Iowa women's health study. *Archives of Internal Medicine, 171*(18), 1625–1633.

Nettleton, J. A., et al. (2008). Dietary patterns and risk of incident type 2 diabetes in the multi-ethnic study of atherosclerosis (MESA). *Diabetes Care, 31*(9), 1777–1782.

Neville, K. (2009). Focus on good fats: balancing omega-3s with omega-6s. *Environmental Nutrition, 32*(3), 1–4.

Nutrition Action HealthLetter: *Eat smart: which foods are good for what*, December, 2011.

Odegaard, A. O., et al. (2010). Soft drink and juice consumption and risk of physician-diagnosed incident type 2 diabetes: the Singapore Chinese health study. *American Journal of Epidemiology, 171*(6), 701–708.

Odegaard, A. O., et al. (2012). Sugar-sweetened and diet beverages in relation to visceral adipose tissue. *Obesity (Silver Spring), 20*(3), 689–691.

Pan, A., et al. (2012). Plain-water intake and risk of type 2 diabetes in young and middle-aged women. *The American Journal of Clinical Nutrition, 95*(6), 1454–1460.

Pereira, M. A., et al. (2005). Fast-food habits, weight gain, and insulin resistance (the CARDIA study): 15-year prospective analysis. *Lancet, 365*(9453), 36.

Prestwich, A., Hurling, R., & Baker, S. (2011). Implicit shopping: Attitudinal determinants of the purchasing of healthy and unhealthy foods. *Psychology & Health, 26*(7), 875–885.

Shay, L. E., et al. (2009). Adult weight management: translating research and guidelines into practice. *Journal of the American Academy of Nurse Practitioners, 21*(4), 197–206.

Sieber, C. C. (2006). Nutritional screening tools-how does the MNA compare? Proceedings of the session held in Chicago May 2-3, 2006 (15 Years of Mini Nutritional Assessment). *The Journal of Nutrition, Health and Aging, 10*(6), 488–492.

Sinha, R., et al. (2009). Meat intake and mortality: a prospective study of over half a million people. *Archives of Internal Medicine, 169*(6), 562–571.

Slavin, J. L. (2008). Position of the American Dietetic Association: health implications of dietary fiber. *Journal of the American Dietetic Association, 108*(10), 1716–1731.

Thygesen, L. C., et al. (2009). Cancer incidence among patients with alcohol use disorders—long-term follow-up. *Alcohol and Alcoholism (Oxford, Oxfordshire), 44*(4), 387–391.

U.S. Department of Agriculture (2014) Weight Management, *USDA ChooseMyPlate.gov*. <http://www.choosemyplate.gov/weight-management-calories/weight-management/better-choices/amount-calories.html>. Retrieved June 21, 2015.

N

Vincent, D. (2009). Culturally tailored education to promote lifestyle change in Mexican Americans with type 2 diabetes. *Journal of the American Academy of Nurse Practitioners, 21*(9), 520–527.

von Schacky, C. (2007). Omega-3 fatty acids and cardiovascular disease. *Current Opinion in Clinical Nutrition and Metabolic Care, 10*(2), 129–135.

Welland, D. (2007). Red-flagging food labels: 8 tips to sift fact from fiction. *Environ Nutr, 30*(3), 2.

Whitlock, G., et al. (2009). Body-mass index and cause-specific mortality in 900,000 adults: collaborative analyses of 57 prospective studies. *Lancet, 373*(9669), 1083–1096.

Williams, P. G., Grafenauer, S. J., & O'Shea, J. E. (2008). Cereal grains, legumes, and weight management: a comprehensive review of the scientific evidence. *Nutrition Reviews, 66*(4), 171–182.

Wotton, K., Crannitch, K., & Munt, R. (2008). Prevalence, risk factors and strategies to prevent dehydration in older adults. *Contemporary Nurse: A Journal for the Australian Nursing Profession, 31*(1), 44–56.

Zelman, K. (2011). The great fat debate: a closer look at the controversy—questioning the validity of age-old dietary guidance. *Journal of the American Dietetic Association, 111*(5), 655–658.

Imbalanced Nutrition: less than body requirements

Andrea G. Steiner, MS, RD, LD, CNSC

NANDA-I

Definition

Intake of nutrients insufficient to meet metabolic needs

Defining Characteristics

Abdominal cramping; abdominal pain; alteration in taste sensation; body weight 20% or more below ideal weight range; capillary fragility; diarrhea; excessive loss of hair; food aversion; food intake less than recommended daily allowance; hyperactive bowel sounds; insufficient information; insufficient interest in food; insufficient muscle tone; misinformation; misperception; pale mucous membranes; perceived inability to ingest food; satiety immediately upon ingesting food; sore buccal cavity; weakness of muscles required for mastication; weakness of muscles required for swallowing; weight loss with adequate food intake

N

Related Factors (r/t)

Biological factors; economically disadvantaged; inability to absorb nutrients; inability to digest food; inability to ingest food; insufficient dietary intake; psychological factors

NOC (Nursing Outcomes Classification)

Suggested NOC Outcomes

Nutritional Status; Nutritional Status: Food and Fluid Intake; Nutrient Intake; Weight Control

Example NOC Outcome with Indicators

Nutritional Status as evidenced by the following indicators: Food and fluid intake/Body mass index/Weight-height ratio/Hematocrit. (Rate the outcome and indicators of **Nutritional Status:** 1 = severe deviation from normal range, 2 = substantial deviation from normal range, 3 = moderate deviation from normal range, 4 = mild deviation from normal range, 5 = no deviation from normal range [see Section I].)

Client Outcomes

Client Will (Specify Time Frame)

- Progressively gain weight toward desired goal
- Weigh within normal range for height and age
- Recognize factors contributing to being underweight
- Identify nutritional requirements
- Consume adequate nourishment
- Be free of signs of malnutrition

NIC (Nursing Interventions Classification)

Suggested NIC Interventions

Feeding; Nutrition Management; Nutrition Therapy; Weight Gain Assistance

Example NIC Activities—Nutrition Management

Ascertain the client's food preferences; provide the client with high-protein, high-calorie, nutritious finger foods and drinks that can be readily consumed, as appropriate

Nursing Interventions and *Rationales*

- ▲ Conduct a nutrition screen on all clients within 24 hours of admission and refer to a dietitian as deemed necessary. EB: *A study showed that the presence of early nutrition intervention in severely malnourished clients significantly decreased length of hospital stay (Somanchi et al, 2011).*
- ▲ The screening tool should be based on the client population, and the validity and reliability of the screening tool. The 3-Minute Nutrition Screening (3-MinNS) tool, for example, assesses weight loss, dietary intake, and muscle wasting. EB: *A study found that the best cutoff score to identify all adult clients at risk for malnutrition using the 3-MinNS was 3, and it had a strong correlation with the Subjective Global Assessment, making it a reliable tool for nurses to identify clients at risk for malnutrition (Lim et al, 2012).*
- • Recognize the importance of rescreening and monitoring oral intake in hospitalized individuals to help facilitate the early identification and prevention of nutritional decline.
- • Recognize the characteristics that classify individuals as malnourished and refer to a dietitian for a complex nutritional assessment and intervention. *According to the Academy of Nutrition and Dietetics and the American Society of Parenteral and Enteral Nutrition, two or more of the following characteristics are recommended to support the diagnosis of malnutrition: insufficient energy intake, weight loss, loss of muscle mass, loss of subcutaneous fat, localized or generalized fluid accumulation, and/or decreased functional status (White et al, 2012).*
- • Recognize clients who are likely to experience malnutrition in the context of social or environmental circumstances, characterized by pure chronic starvation and anorexia nervosa without the presence of an inflammatory process (White et al, 2012).
  - ❍ Chronic disease-related malnutrition: those with organ failure, pancreatic cancer, rheumatoid arthritis, sarcopenic obesity
  - ❍ Acute disease or injury-related malnutrition: those with major infection, burns, trauma, closed head injuries accompanied by a marked inflammatory response (White et al, 2012).
- ▲ Note laboratory values cautiously; albumin and prealbumin may be indicators of the inflammatory response that often accompanies acute malnutrition. *Other potential indicators of inflammatory response include C-reactive protein, white blood cell count, and blood glucose values (White et al, 2012).*
- • Weigh the client daily in acute care, weekly to monthly in extended care at the same time (usually before breakfast), with same amount of clothing.
- • Observe for potential barriers to eating such as willingness, ability, and appetite. EB: *Depression, impaired function, and poor oral intake are associated with increased likelihood of weight loss, low BMI, and poor nutrition in nursing home residents (Tamura et al, 2013).*

NOTE: If the client is unable to feed self, refer to Nursing Interventions for Feeding **Self-Care** deficit. If the client has difficulty swallowing, refer to Nursing Interventions for Impaired **Swallowing.** If the client is receiving tube feedings, refer to the Nursing Interventions for Risk for **Aspiration.**

- • Advocate for the implementation of a feeding protocol, if not already in place, to avoid unnecessary and/or prolonged nothing per os (mouth)/clear liquid (NPO/CL) status in hospitalized clients. EB: *A study conducted at a hospital found an NPO order to be appropriate only 58.6% of the time and a CL diet order to be appropriate only 25.6% of the time (Franklin et al, 2011).*
- • For the client with anorexia nervosa, consider offering high-calorie foods and snacks often. EB: *A study found that higher calorie diets led to faster weight gain in hospitalized adolescents with anorexia nervosa compared to lower calorie diets (Garber et al, 2013).*
- • For the client who is able to eat but has a decreased appetite, try the following activities:
  - ❍ Offer oral nutritional supplements (ONS) early after admission and continue to encourage intake of ONS throughout the hospital stay. EB: *A study found that use of ONS in the inpatient population decreased*

length of stay, episode cost, and 30-day readmission risk (Philipson et al, 2013). A meta-analysis found that use of ONS significantly reduced hospital readmissions, particularly in older adults (Stratton et al, 2013). Consumption of ONS was associated with lower risk of underfeeding (Thibault et al, 2011).

- ❍ Avoid interruptions during mealtimes and offer companionship; meals should be eaten in a calm and peaceful environment. EB: *A study found that the implementation of protected mealtimes and use of additional assistant-in-nursing assistance alone and in combination improved nutritional intake of hospitalized clients (Young et al, 2013a).*
- ❍ Allow for access to meals or snacks during "off times" if the client is not available at time of meal delivery, monitor food and ONS intake, and communicate with dietitian/health care provider. EB: *The Alliance Nutrition Care Recommendations include a multidisciplinary approach to address adult hospital malnutrition which includes the rapid implementation of nutrition intervention and continued monitoring (Tappenden et al, 2013).*
- ❍ If the client lacks endurance, schedule rest periods before meals, and open packages and cut up food for the client. *Nursing assistance will conserve the client's energy for eating.*

- • For the client with fracture due to fall, consider the need for vitamin D supplementation. EB: *A study found that 77% of acute rehabilitation clients are 25(OH)D insufficient or deficient at admission, and most inpatients with fracture due to fall were transferred to acute inpatient rehabilitation without supplementation (Pellicane et al, 2011).*
- • For the client who has had a stroke, repeat nutritional screenings weekly and provide timely interventions for those at risk or who may already be malnourished. EB: *According to a recent study, the prevalence of malnutrition and risk of malnutrition in clients with acute stroke increases significantly during the first 10 days of admission (Mosselman et al, 2013). A separate study conducted in stroke clients found a significantly increased risk for malnutrition and continued insufficient oral intake at discharge when compared with the first assessment after hospital admission (Nip et al, 2011).*
- • Recognize the importance of offering high protein foods to most hospitalized individuals (use caution with those with compromised renal/liver function). EB: *A study found that among clients who met their energy and protein requirements less often were those with higher BMI, younger age, cancer, or nausea, or had undergone surgery. This study found that only one in four clients had a protein and energy intake that met their requirements at the fourth day of admission. Protein requirements were met less often than energy requirements (Leistra et al, 2011).*
- • Monitor state of oral cavity (gums, tongue, mucosa, teeth). Provide good oral hygiene before each meal. *Good oral hygiene enhances appetite; the condition of the oral mucosa is critical to the ability to eat. The oral mucosa must be moist, with adequate saliva production to facilitate and aid in the digestion of food.*
- ▲ Administer antiemetics and pain medications as ordered and needed before meals. *The presence of nausea or pain decreases the appetite.*
- • *Anorexia.* If client is nauseated, remove cover of food tray before bringing it into the client's room. *The sudden, concentrated food odors that come when the cover is removed in front of the client can trigger nausea.*
- • Work with the client to develop a plan for increased activity. *Immobility leads to negative nitrogen balance that fosters anorexia.*

N

Critical Care

- • Recognize the need to begin enteral feeding within 24 to 48 hours of admission to the critical care environment, once the client is free of hemodynamic compromise, if the client is unable to eat. CEB: *The guidelines for the provision and assessment of nutrition support therapy in the adult critically ill client call for early enteral feeding (McClave et al, 2009).* EB: *Delay in initiation of enteral feeding has been shown to prolong duration of mechanical ventilation and length of stay in critical care clients (Nguyen et al, 2012).*
- • Recognize that it is important to administer feedings to the client and that frequently checking for gastric residual and fasting clients for procedures can be a limiting factor to adequate nutrition in the tube-fed client. EBN: *A study found that implementing a protocol for managing gastric residual volumes, not fasting clients for procedures, and reducing fasting times when weaning clients for extubation reduced the number of interruptions to enteral feeding (Williams et al, 2013). Refer to care plan* for *Risk for* ***Aspiration.***

Pediatric

- ▲ Use a nutritional screening tool designed for nurses such as the Paediatric Yorkhill Malnutrition Score (PYMS) tool, and if the child has a score of 2 or more, make a referral to a dietitian. EB: *A study found that use of the PYMS was helpful in identifying children with malnutrition and was able to identify children with malnutrition who would not have been referred for treatment (Gerasimidis et al, 2011).*

- Watch for symptoms of malnutrition in the child including short stature, thin arms and legs, poor condition of skin and hair, visible vertebrae and rib cage, wasted buttocks, wasted facial appearance, lethargy, and in extreme cases, edema.
- Weigh and measure the length (height) of the child and use a growth chart to help determine growth pattern, which reflects nutrition. *Age-related growth charts are available from this website:* www.cdc.gov/growthcharts/.

▲ Refer to a health care provider and a dietitian a child who is underweight for any reason. *Good nutrition is extremely important for children to ensure sufficient growth and development of all body systems.*

- Work with the child and parent to develop an appropriate weight gain plan. *The goal for a child is sometimes to maintain existing weight as the body grows taller.*
- Recognize that a large percentage of girls and teenagers are dieting, which can result in nutritional problems.

Geriatric

- Screen for malnutrition in older clients. EB: *A study found that the following screening tools were accurate in identifying malnutrition and can be recommended for use in the older adults who are hospitalized: the Malnutrition Screening Tool (MST), the Mini Nutritional Assessment—Short Form (MNA-SF), the Malnutrition Universal Screening Tool (MUST), the SNAQ (Short Nutritional Assessment Questionnaire), and the Simplified Nutritional Appetite Questionnaire (Young et al, 2013a).*
- Screen for dysphagia in all older clients. EB: *Dysphagia is common in older adults for multiple reasons and is associated with onset of pneumonia (Serra-Prat et al, 2012). See care plan Impaired* ***Swallowing.***
- Recognize that geriatric clients with moderate or severe cognition impairment have a significant risk for developing malnutrition. EBN: *A study demonstrated that older adults with cognitive impairment had a risk for developing malnutrition, regardless of living and housing arrangement (Fagerstrom et al, 2011).*

N

▲ Interpret laboratory findings cautiously. Watch the color of urine for an indication of fluid balance; darker urine demonstrates dehydration. Low axillary moisture could indicate mild to moderate dehydration. CEB/EB: *Because urine color is correlated with urine specific gravity and urine osmolality, observing urine color is a low-cost method of monitoring dehydration (Wakefield et al, 2002). Compromised kidney function makes reliance on blood and urine samples for nutrient analyses less reliable in older adults than in younger persons. Findings of a small pilot study suggest that measuring the axillary moisture of older adults has potential as a simple tool for detecting dehydration at home and in nursing homes (Kinoshita et al, 2013).*

- Consider using dining assistants, trained non-nursing staff, to provide feeding assistance care in extended care facilities to ensure adequate time for feeding clients as needed. EBN: *A study found that dining assistants spent more time assisting residents, and the quality of care was comparable to that of nurse aides (Bertrand et al, 2011).*
- Consider offering healthy snacks such as yogurt, which is a good source of protein, calcium, zinc, B vitamins, and probiotics. EB: *Observational studies suggest that yogurt could play an important role in improving the nutritional health of older adults when combined with a healthy diet (El-Abbadi et al, 2014).*
- Encourage high protein foods for the older client, unless medically contraindicated by organ failure. EB: *A study found protective effects against weight loss in healthy older adults who had protein intakes greater than 1 g/kg/d (Gray-Donald et al, 2014). Anorexia of aging has been found to have an independent association with sarcopenia (Landi et al, 2013). Increased protein is thought to increase muscle protein anabolism and help decrease the development of progressive muscle loss, sarcopenia, with aging. Combining increased protein with resistance exercises is even more effective in maintaining or increasing muscle. Clients taking a high-protein supplement had reduced complications, reduced readmissions to the hospital, improved grip strength, and increased protein intake along with increased energy (Cawood et al, 2012).*
- Encourage physical activity throughout the day as tolerated. EB: *A study found that moderate acute increase in physical activity, such as aerobic exercise, followed by intake of a protein and carbohydrate liquid enhanced skeletal muscle protein synthesis and anabolic responses in healthy older adult. (Timmerman et al, 2012).*
- Recognize the implications of malnutrition on client strength and mobility. EB: *Malnutrition is associated with an increased risk of falling and impaired activity in older long-term care residents; malnourished residents were able to decrease their risk for fall after receiving nutritional intervention (Neyens et al, 2013). A study found that providing oral nutritional supplements and calcium and vitamin D supplementation as*

well as dietitian counseling in malnourished older adults decreased the number of falls and fall incidents (Neelemaat et al, 2012).

- Consider the need for a multivitamin if food intake is low. EB: *According to the Academy of Nutrition and Dietetics: Food and Nutrition for Older Adults: Promoting Health and Wellness, there is strong and imperative evidence to support the recommendation for a multivitamin when food intake is low (Bernstein & Munoz, 2012).*
- Monitor for onset of depression. EB: *A systematic review of the literature found that depression, impaired function, and poor oral intake were factors consistently associated with increased likelihood of weight loss, low BMI, and poor nutrition (Tamura et al, 2013).*
- Consider offering nutritional supplement drinks served in a glass rather than with a straw inserted directly into the container. EBN: *A study found that among people with dementia who are able to feed themselves, they drank statistically significantly more when a nutritional supplement was served in a glass than when consumed directly from the container (Allen et al, 2014).*
- Recommend to families that enteral feedings may or may not be indicated for clients with dementia (Chang & Roberts, 2011). EB: *There is still insufficient evidence regarding the benefits in function, mobility, and quality of life resulting from nutrition support in disabled older adults; the risks associated with the percutaneous endoscopic gastrostomy procedure may exceed potential benefits in such clients as those with dementia (Monod et al, 2011).* For strategies for feeding clients with dementia, please refer to the article by Chang and Roberts (2011).

NOTE: If the client is unable to feed self, refer to Nursing Interventions and *Rationales* for Feeding **Self-Care** deficit. If client has impaired physical function, malnutrition, depression, or cognitive impairment, refer to care plan for **Frail Elderly** syndrome.

- Emphasize importance of good oral care in the older client. EB: *Poor oral health was found to be strongly associated with malnutrition in older hospitalized clients (Poisson et al, 2014).*
- Consult the dietitian if the client has pressure ulcers. EBN: *A study found that an interdisciplinary approach including nutrition intervention improved pressure ulcer wound healing and decreased both hospital length of stay for treatment of pressure ulcer as well as total hospital length of stay in geriatric clients who were admitted with or developed a pressure ulcer from stage 2 to stage 3 during hospitalization (Allen, 2013).*

N

Home Care

- The preceding interventions may be adapted for home care use.
- Screen for malnutrition using the MUST, which is easy and simple. Recognize that the client may also use MUST as a self-screening tool in the home setting. EB: *A study found that most clients were able to complete the self-screen in less than 5 minutes, they found the tool easy to understand and complete, and their results were associated with good agreement with screens conducted by screens conducted by home care providers (Cawood et al, 2012).*
- Monitor food intake. Instruct the client in intake of small frequent meals of foods with increased calories and protein.
- Assess the client's willingness to eat. EB: *Poor intake among older adults has been found to be associated with poor appetite, a diagnosis of infection or cancer, a need for assistance or supervision with feeding, and delirium (Mudge et al, 2011).*
- Consider social factors that may interfere with nutrition (e.g., lack of transportation, inadequate income, lack of social support).
- Continue to encourage intake of ONS to help optimize oral intake. EB: *A meta-analysis of randomized controlled trials suggested that oral nutritional support may be considered for older malnourished medical and surgical clients after discharge from hospital (Beck et al, 2013).*
- ▲ Recognize that the client on home parenteral nutrition requires regularly scheduled lab work for electrolyte monitoring. *Clients should also be educated regarding home parenteral nutrition before discharge from the hospital (Kumpf & Tillman, 2012).*

Client/Family Teaching and Discharge Planning

- Help the client/family identify the area to change that will make the greatest contribution to improved nutrition.
- Build on the strengths in the client/family's food habits. Adapt changes to their current practices.
- Select appropriate teaching aids for the client/family's background.

- • Implement instructional follow-up to answer the client/family's questions.
- • Recommend that clients discuss with their primary health care provider before taking any supplements such as vitamins and minerals. EB: *A large study in women found that those who took more supplements had an increased risk of death, especially with intake of multivitamins, vitamin B6, folic acid, iron, magnesium, zinc, and copper. Calcium seemed to decrease the risk of death (Mursu et al, 2011). A systematic review found no data to support the widespread use of dietary supplements, except possibly vitamin D and omega-3 fatty acids, in industrialized nations; indeed, many of these supplements may be harmful (Marik & Flemmer, 2012).*
- • Suggest community resources, such as Meals on Wheels and community centers as suitable food sources.
- • Teach the client and family how to manage tube feedings or parenteral therapy at home as needed.

REFERENCES

Allen, B. (2013). Effects of a comprehensive nutritional program on pressure ulcer healing, length of hospital stay, and charges to patients. *Clinical Nursing Research*, *22*(2), 186–205.

Allen, V. J., et al. (2014). Impact of serving method on the consumption of nutritional supplement drinks: randomized trial in older adults with cognitive impairment. *Journal of Advanced Nursing*, *70*(6), 1323–1333.

Beck, A. M., et al. (2013). Oral nutritional support for older (65 years+) medical and surgical patients after discharge from hospital: systematic review and meta-analysis of randomized controlled trial. *Clinical Rehabilitation*, *27*(1), 19–27.

Bernstein, M., & Munoz, N. (2012). Position of the academy of nutrition and dietetics: food and nutrition for older adults: promoting health and wellness. *Journal of the Academy of Nutrition and Dietetics*, *112*(8), 1255–1277.

Bertrand, R. M., et al. (2011). The nursing home dining assistant program. *Journal of Gerontological Nursing*, *37*(2), 34–43.

Cawood, A. L., Elia, M., & Stratton, R. J. (2012). Systematic review and meta-analysis of the effects of high protein oral nutritional supplements. *Ageing Research Reviews*, *11*(2), 278–296.

Cawood, A. L., et al. (2012). Malnutrition self-screening by using MUST in hospital outpatients: validity, reliability, and ease of use. *The American Journal of Clinical Nutrition*, *96*(5), 1000–1007.

Chang, C. C., & Roberts, B. (2011). Strategies for feeding patients with dementia. *The American Journal of Nursing*, *11*(4), 36–44.

El-Abbadi, N. H., Dao, M. C., & Meydani, S. N. (2014). Yogurt: role in healthy and active aging. *The American Journal of Clinical Nutrition*, *99*(5), 1263S–1270S.

Fagerstrom, C., et al. (2011). Malnutrition and cognitive impairment among people 60 years of age and above living in regular housing and in special housing in Sweden: a population-based cohort study. *International Journal of Nursing Studies*, *48*(7), 863–871.

Franklin, G. A., et al. (2011). Physician-delivered malnutrition: why do patients receive nothing by mouth or a clear liquid diet in a university hospital setting? *JPEN. Journal of Parenteral and Enteral Nutrition*, *35*(3), 337–342.

Garber, A. K., et al. (2013). Higher calorie diets increase rate of weight gain and shorten hospital stay in hospitalized adolescents with anorexia nervosa. *Journal of Adolescent Health*, *53*(5), 579–584.

Gerasimidis, K., et al. (2011). Performance of the novel paediatric yorkhill malnutrition score (PYMS) in hospital practice. *Clinical Nutrition (Edinburgh, Scotland)*, *30*(4), 430–435.

Gray-Donald, K., et al. (2014). Protein intake protects against weight loss in healthy community-dwelling older adults. *Journal of Nutrition*, *144*(3), 321–326.

Kinoshita, K., et al. (2013). The measurement of axillary moisture for the assessment of dehydration among older patients: a pilot study. *Experimental Gerontology*, *48*(2), 255–258.

Kumpf, V. J., & Tillman, E. M. (2012). Home parenteral nutrition: safe transition from hospital to home. *Nutrition in Clinical Practice*, *27*(6), 749–757.

Landi, F., et al. (2013). Association of anorexia with sarcopenia in a community-dwelling elderly population: results from the ilSIRENTE study. *European Journal of Nutrition*, *52*(3), 1261–1268.

Leistra, E., et al. (2011). Predictors for achieving protein and energy requirements in undernourished hospital patients. *Clinical Nutrition (Edinburgh, Scotland)*, *30*, 484–489.

Lim, S. L., Ong, K. C., Chan, Y. H., et al. (2012). Malnutrition and its impact on cost of hospitalization, length of stay, readmission and 3-year mortality. *Clinical Nutrition (Edinburgh, Scotland)*, *31*(3), 345–350.

Marik, P. E., & Flemmer, M. (2012). Do dietary supplements have beneficial health effects in industrialized nations: what is the evidence? *JPEN. Journal of Parenteral and Enteral Nutrition*, *36*(2), 159–168.

McClave, S. A., et al. (2009). Guidelines for the provision and assessment of nutrition support therapy in the adult critically ill patient: society of critical care medicine (SCCM) and American society for parenteral and enteral nutrition (A.S.P.E.N.). *JPEN. Journal of Parenteral and Enteral Nutrition*, *33*(3), 277–316.

Monod, S., et al. (2011). Ethical issues in nutrition support of severely disabled elderly persons: a guide for health professionals. *JPEN. Journal of Parenteral and Enteral Nutrition*, *5*(3), 295–302.

Mosselman, M. J., et al. (2013). Malnutrition and Risk of Malnutrition in patients with stroke: prevalence during hospital stay. *Journal of Neuroscience Nursing*, *45*(4), 194–204.

Mudge, A. M., et al. (2011). Helping understand nutritional gaps in the elderly (HUNGER): A prospective study of patient factors associated with inadequate nutritional intake in older medical inpatients. *Clinical Nutrition (Edinburgh, Scotland)*, *30*, 320–325.

Mursu, J., et al. (2011). Dietary supplements and mortality rate in older women: the Iowa women's health study. *Archives of Internal Medicine*, *171*(18), 1626–1632.

Neelemaat, F., et al. (2012). Short-term oral nutritional intervention with protein and vitamin D decreases falls in malnourished older adults. *Journal of the American Geriatrics Society*, *60*(4), 691–699.

Neyens, J., et al. (2013). Malnutrition is associated with an increased risk of falls and impaired activity in elderly patients in Dutch residential long-term care (LTC): a cross-sectional study. *Archives of Gerontology and Geriatrics*, *56*(1), 265–269.

Nip, W. F. R., et al. (2011). Dietary intake, nutritional status and rehabilitation outcomes of stroke patients in hospital. *Journal of Human Nutrition and Dietetics*, *24*, 460–469.

Nguyen, N. Q., et al. (2012). Delayed enteral feeding impairs intestinal carbohydrate absorption in critically ill patients. *Critical Care Medicine*, *40*(1), 50–54.

N

Pellicane, A. J., et al. (2011). Prevalence of 25-Hydroxyvitamin D deficiency in the acute inpatient rehabilitation population and its effect on function. *Archives of Physical Rehabilitation, 92*(5), 705–711.

Philipson, T. J., et al. (2013). Impact of oral nutritional supplementation on hospital outcomes. *The American Journal of Managed Care, 19*(2), 121–128.

Poisson, P., Laffond, T., Campos, S., et al. (2014). Relationships between oral health, dysphagia and undernutrition in hospitalised elderly patients. *Gerodontology*, 2014. [Epub ahead of print].

Serra-Prat, M., et al. (2012). Oropharyngeal dysphagia as a risk factor for malnutrition and lower respiratory tract infection in independently living older persons: a population-based prospective study. *Age and Ageing, 41*(3), 376–381.

Somanchi, M., Tao, X., & Mullin, G. E. (2011). The facilitated early enteral and dietary management effectiveness trial in hospitalized patients with malnutrition. *JPEN. Journal of Parenteral and Enteral Nutrition, 35*(2), 209–216.

Stratton, R. J., Hebuterne, X., & Elia, M. (2013). A systematic review and meta-analysis of the impact of oral nutritional supplements on hospital readmissions. *Ageing Research Reviews, 12*(4), 884–897.

Tamura, B. K., et al. (2013). Factors associated with weight loss, low BMI, and malnutrition among nursing home patients: a systematic review of the literature. *Journal of the American Medical Directors Association, 14*(9), 649–655.

Tappenden, K. A., et al. (2013). Critical role of nutrition in improving quality of care: an interdisciplinary call to action to address adult hospital malnutrition. *Journal of the Academy of Nutrition and Dietetics, 113*(9), 1219–1237.

Thibault, R., et al. (2011). Assessment of food intake in hospitalized patients: A 10-year comparative study of a prospective hospital survey. *Clinical Nutrition (Edinburgh, Scotland), 30*(3), 289–296.

Timmerman, K. L., et al. (2012). A moderate acute increase in physical activity enhances nutritive flow and the muscle protein anabolic response to mixed nutrient intake in older adults. *The American Journal of Clinical Nutrition, 95*(6), 1403–1412.

Wakefield, B., et al. (2002). Monitoring hydration status in elderly veterans. *Western Journal of Nursing Research, 24*, 132.

White, J., Guenter, P., & Gordon, J. (2012). Consensus statement of the academy of nutrition and dietetics/American society for parenteral and enteral nutrition: characteristics recommended for the identification and documentation of adult malnutrition. *Journal of the Academy of Nutrition and Dietetics, 112*, 730–738.

Williams, T. A., et al. (2013). Reducing interruptions to continuous enteral nutrition in the intensive care unit: a comparative study. *Journal of Clinical Nursing, 22*(19–20), 2838–2848.

Young, A. M., Kidston, S., Banks, M. D., et al. (2013a). Malnutrition screening tools: comparison against two validated nutrition assessment methods in older medical inpatients. *Nutrition (Burbank, Los Angeles County, Calif.), 29*(1), 101–106.

O

Obesity

Marina Martinez-Kratz, MS, RN, CNE

NANDA-I

Definition

A condition in which an individual accumulates abnormal or excessive fat for age and gender that exceeds overweight

Defining Characteristics

Adult: Body mass index (BMI) >30 kg/m^2; Child <2 years: term not used with children at this age; Child 2 to 18 years: BMI >30 kg/m^2 or >95th percentile for age and gender

Related Factors

Average daily physical activity is less than recommended for gender and age; consumption of sugar sweetened beverages; disordered eating behaviors; disordered eating perceptions; economically disadvantaged; energy expenditure below energy intake based on standard assessment (e.g., WAVE assessment [weight, activity, variety in diet, excess]); excessive alcohol consumption; fear regarding lack of food supply; formula- or mixed-fed infants; frequent snacking; genetic disorder; heritability of interrelated factors (e.g., adipose tissue distribution, energy expenditure, lipoprotein lipase activity, lipid synthesis, lipolysis); high disinhibition and restraint eating behavior score; high frequency of eating restaurant or fried food; low dietary calcium intake in children; maternal diabetes mellitus; maternal smoking; overweight in infancy; parental obesity; portion sizes larger than recommended; premature pubarche; rapid weight gain during childhood; rapid weight gain during infancy, including the first week, first 4 months, and first year; sedentary behavior occurring more than 2 hours per day; shortened sleep time; sleep disorder; solid foods as major food source in infants younger than 5 months of age

NOC (Nursing Outcomes Classification)

Suggested NOC Outcomes

Nutritional Status; Nutritional Status: Food and Fluid Intake; Nutrient Intake; Weight Control

Example NOC Outcome with Indicators

Nutritional Status as evidenced by the following indicators: Food and fluid intake/Hydration/Body mass index/Weight-height ratio/Hematocrit. (Rate the outcome and indicators of **Nutritional Status:** 1 = severe deviation from normal range, 2 = substantial deviation from normal range, 3 = moderate deviation from normal range, 4 = mild deviation from normal range, 5 = no deviation from normal range [see Section I].)

Client Outcomes

Client Will (Specify Time Frame)

- Explain how to eat according to the U.S. Dietary Guidelines
- Design dietary modifications to meet individual long-term goal of health, using principles of variety, balance, and moderation
- Maintain weight within normal range for height and age

NIC (Nursing Interventions Classification)

Suggested NIC Interventions

Nutrition Management; Nutritional Counseling; Weight Reduction Assistance

Example NIC Activities—Nutrition Management

Determine the client's motivation for changing eating habits; Develop with the client a method to keep a daily record of intake

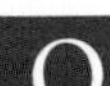

Nursing Interventions and *Rationales*

- Assess the meaning and importance of food in the client's life. EB: *Research findings demonstrate that implicit attitudes significantly predict purchases of healthy and unhealthy foods (Prestwich et al, 2011).*
- Counsel the client to eat breakfast daily. EB: *Research has determined that skipping breakfast is a lifestyle risk significantly associated with a higher BMI (Ghrayeb et al, 2014).*
- Assess the client with a Patient Readiness Scale to determine if the client is ready to discuss weight loss and/or would like weight loss information. EB: *Readiness to change is an important part of treatment for behavior change (Steele et al, 2012).*
- Assess the client's current nutrition through a 1- to 3-day food diary in which everything ingested orally is recorded. Analyze the following areas:
  - Intake of food and beverage calories and fat
  - Portion sizes
  - Underconsumption or overconsumption of nutrients
  - Use of supplements
  - Use of meal replacements
  - Timing/consistency of meals and snacks

Use of a food diary is helpful for both the client and the nurse, to examine usual foods eaten and patterns of eating (Shay et al, 2009). EB: *A study found that use of a personal digital assistant for self-monitoring of food intake was more effective than use of a paper record, yet both groups had a similar weight loss (Acharya et al, 2011).*

- Counsel the client to measure regularly consumed foods periodically. Help the client to learn usual portion sizes. *Measuring food alerts the client to normal portion sizes. Estimating amounts can be extremely inaccurate.* EB: *A study demonstrated that obese people had significantly larger portion sizes, plus ate later in the day (Berg et al, 2009).*
- Assist the client to develop a system of self-management, which may include self-monitoring of weight, BMI, and food intake, interpreting food labels, portion control, recipe modification, restaurant and social

food negotiation, and physical activity. *A key component of successful weight loss and maintenance is regular self-monitoring (Fitch et al, 2013).*

- Document the client's height and weight and teach significance of his/her BMI in relationship to current health. *Use a chart or a website such as http://www.cdc.gov/healthyweight/assessing/bmi/index.html (Centers for Disease Control and Prevention [CDC], 2014).*
- Assist the client to use Super Tracker (http://www.choosemyplate.gov/food-groups) to determine the number of calories to eat and gain more information on how to eat in a healthy fashion. *To lose weight, the client must eat fewer calories (U.S. Department of Agriculture, 2014).*
- Encourage the client to engage in regular physical activity for at least 150 minutes weekly. EB: *Research found that normal weight reproductive-aged women who do not engage in recommended levels of physical activity are at risk for becoming overweight or obese (Hillemeier et al, 2011). Studies determine that increased physical activity in conjunction with improved eating behavior scores resulted in greater weight loss (Jakicic et al, 2011).*
- Recommend the client eat a healthy breakfast every morning. CEB: *A study found that that people who skip breakfast are more likely to overeat in the evening (Masheb & Grillo, 2006).*
- Recommend the client avoid eating in fast food restaurants. CEB: *A 15-year study demonstrated that people who frequently eat fast foods gain an average of 10 lb more than those who eat fast food less often and were two times more likely to develop insulin resistance, which can lead to diabetes (Pereira et al, 2005).*
- Assist the client to reframe slips in weight loss or physical activity behavior as lapses that are a single event and not a full return to previous unhealthy behaviors. *Relapse prevention strategies include managing lapses in healthy behavior, identifying high-risk situations for relapses, enhancing skills for coping, and increasing self-efficacy for avoiding relapse (Fitch et al, 2013).*
- Teach problem-solving strategies to deal with barriers to changing eating and physical activity patterns. *Strategies such as defining the problem, brainstorming solutions, seeking solutions, and evaluating the outcome of the solution are problem-solving strategies that facilitate weight loss (Fitch et al, 2013).*
- Assist clients to engage their social support systems in ways that facilitate weight loss, as well as eating and physical activity behavior change. *Significant others, family, friends, and co-workers can facilitate or hinder weight loss success (Fitch et al, 2013).*
- Assist the client to reframe the goal focus from outcome (weight loss) to process (eating behaviors) for weight loss. EB: *A study of overweight women found that focusing on the process of dieting (the eating behavior) was related to actual weight loss as well as to subjective dieting success (Freund & Hennecke, 2012).*
- Assist the client to develop stimulus control techniques designed to reduce environmental cues associated with eating behaviors. Specifically clients should be taught to limit the presence of high-calorie/high-fat foods in the home; to reduce the visibility of unhealthy food choices in the home; to limit where and when they eat; to avoid distractions like reading, using the computer, or watching television when eating; and to eat more slowly. *Stimulus control strategies are a key to successful weight loss and weight maintenance (Fitch et al, 2013).*
- Use the motivational interviewing technique when working with clients to promote healthy eating and weight loss. EB: *A pilot study with use of motivational interviewing in women found it resulted in a significant weight loss (Low et al, 2012). A review found that use of motivational interviewing was effective in causing weight loss (Armstrong et al, 2011).*
- Refer the client to tailored weight management programs that provide opportunities for ongoing support. CEB: *Tailored weight loss interventions and ongoing support were identified by obese clients as facilitating longer term weight management (Visram et al, 2009).*
- Refer the client to a weight-loss related therapy group. EBN: *A British study showed that addressing psychological factors associated with eating and weight in a group setting offers an important contribution to the treatment of obesity (Yilmaz, 2011).*
- Recommend that clients use dietary supplements such as vitamins and minerals after consulting with their primary health care provider. EB: *Research shows a prevalence of low micronutrient status in obese individuals who can benefit from safeguarding vitamin and mineral adequacy by taking a multinutrient supplement in conjunction with increased intake of nutrient-rich foods (Ruxton, 2011).*
- Behavior methods of losing weight are diverse and effective for weight loss through developing methods to control eating behavior, changing habits, and mindset. EB: *Behavioral-based treatments are safe and effective for weight loss (LeBlanc et al, 2011).* EB: *A study found that behavior treatment that was done*

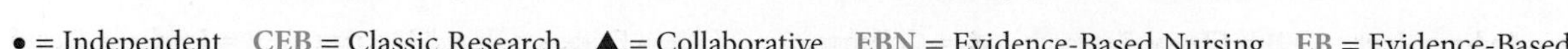

either in person or remotely through computer teaching, email, and the phone resulted in a significant loss of weight in obese clients versus a control group (Appel et al, 2011).

Pediatric

- Offer obese or overweight adolescents healthy methods for weight loss. CEBN: *Research shows that overweight adolescents who demonstrate a desire to lose weight often choose unhealthy methods (Chen et al, 2009).*
- Offer families of obese or overweight children prejudice-free, individually accepting, and supportive interventions to address weight loss. EBN: *Obese children showed signs of stress, stigmatization, and marginalization, while their families reported feeling rejected by health care professionals (Lorentzen et al, 2012).*
- Use motivational interviewing counseling techniques to implement weight loss interventions. EBN: *Obese children treated with motivational interviewing showed significant improvement in their weight-related behavior and obesity-related anthropometric measures (Wong & Cheng, 2013).*
- Recommend that families eat together for at least one meal per day. *Mealtime together has been shown to improve children's eating habits: children eat more fruits and vegetables when the family eats together.*
- Recommend involving the family in planning meals and food preparation. Children can learn about nutrition as they help plan and make meals. *Children are more likely to eat foods that they help select or prepare.*
- Suggest that parents work at being good role models of healthy eating. *Setting a good example is key for children; children learn the value of healthy eating early, and it can continue for a lifetime.*
- Recommend that the family try new foods, either a new food or recipe every week. *More variety can increase the intake of fruits and vegetables.*
- Suggest the parents keep healthy snacks on hand. Store the snacks in a purse, the car, a desk drawer. *Suggestions include crackers and peanut butter, small boxes of cereal, fresh fruit, and vegetables (Academy of Nutrition and Dietetics, 2014).*

Geriatric

- Recognize that it is generally not appropriate to have an older client on a calorie-restrictive diet. *Older clients deserve to eat and not be hungry.* EB: *Strength training and dietary modifications can improve body composition, muscle strength, and physical function in overweight and obese older adults (Straight et al, 2012).*
- Observe for socioeconomic factors that influence food choices (e.g., funds, cooking facilities, food insecurity). *Even those on restricted budgets and with limited facilities can be assisted to choose healthy food sources for a balanced diet.* EB: *Food security is a factor that can indicate a need for nutrition assistance in older adults (Lee et al, 2011).*

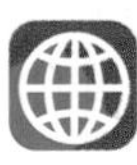

Multicultural

- Tailor nutritional interventions to be consistent with cultural beliefs, norms, and values. CEBN: *Mexican American women responded positively to nutritional education and physical activity promotion when families were involved (Vincent, 2009).*
- Offer tailored lifestyle counseling via the telephone. EB: *Low socioeconomic status African Americans and Latinos experienced positive nutritional change and weight loss after participating in a community-based translational lifestyle program (Kanaya et al, 2012).*
- Integrate weight loss and weight maintenance interventions with church faith based concepts for cultural congruence with African American clients. EB: *Recent research suggests that integrating faith themes into a weight loss maintenance program may increase its long-term impact on participants' health behavior change (Seale et al, 2013).*

Client/Family Teaching and Discharge Planning

- The majority of the preceding interventions involve teaching.
- Work with the family members regarding information on how to support and promote weight loss and healthy intakes.

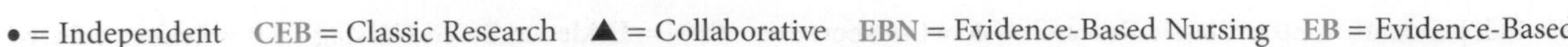

REFERENCES

Academy of Nutrition and Dietetics (2014). *It's about eating right: nutrition for growing bodies.* From: <http://www.eatright.org/Public/content.aspx?id=6751>. Retrieved September 20, 2014.

Acharya, S. D., Elci, O. U., Sereika, S. M., et al. (2011). Using a personal digital assistant for self-monitoring influences diet quality in comparison to a standard paper record among overweight/obese adults. *Journal of the American Dietetic Association, 111*(4), 583–588.

Appel, L. J., Clark, J. M., Yeh, H. C., et al. (2011). Comparative effectiveness of weight-loss interventions in clinical practice. *The New England Journal of Medicine, 365*(21), 1959–1968.

Armstrong, M. J., et al. (2011). Motivational interviewing to improve weight loss in overweight and/or obese patients: a systematic review and meta-analysis of randomized controlled trials. *Obesity Reviews, 12*(9), 709–723.

Berg, C., Lappas, G., Wolk, A., et al. (2009). Eating patterns and portion size associated with obesity in a Swedish population. *Appetite, 52,* 21–26.

Centers for Disease Control and Prevention (2015). *Healthy Weight—it's not a diet, it's a lifestyle!* <http://www.cdc.gov/healthyweight/assessing/bmi/index.html>. Retrieved 6/21/2015.

Chen, M., Fan, J., Jane, S., et al. (2009). Do overweight adolescents perceive the need to reduce weight and take healthy actions? *Journal of Nursing Research (Taiwan Nurses Association), 17*(4), 270–277.

Fitch, A., Everling, L., Fox, C., et al. (2013). *Institute for Clinical Systems Improvement. Prevention and Management of Obesity for Adults.*

Freund, A. M., & Hennecke, M. (2012). Changing eating behaviour vs. losing weight: the role of goal focus for weight loss in overweight women. *Psychology & Health,* 2725–2742.

Ghrayeb, F. A., Mohamed Rusli, A., Al Rifai, A., et al. (2014). PUBLIC HEALTH. Prevalence of lifestyle-related risk factors contributing to non-communicable diseases among adolescents in tarqumia, Palestine. *International Medical Journal, 21*(3), 272–276.

Hillemeier, M. M., Weisman, C. S., Chuang, C., et al. (2011). Transition to overweight or obesity among women of reproductive age. *Journal of Women's Health, 20*(5), 703–710. (15409996).

Jakicic, J. M., Otto, A. D., Lang, W., et al. (2011). The effect of physical activity on 18-month weight change in overweight adults. *Obesity, 19,* 100–109.

Kanaya, A. M., Santoyo-Olsson, J., Gregorich, S., et al. (2012). The live well, be well study: a community-based, translational lifestyle program to lower diabetes risk factors in ethnic minority and lower-socioeconomic status adults. *American Journal of Public Health, 102*(8), 1551–1558.

LeBlanc, E., O'Connor, E., Whitlock, E. P., et al. (2011). *Screening for and management of obesity and overweight in adults. Evidence Report No. 89. AHRQ Publication No. 11-05159-EF-1.* Rockville, MD: Agency for Healthcare Research and Quality.

Lee, J. S., Johnson, M. A., & Brown, A. (2011). Older americans act nutrition program improves participants' food security in Georgia. *Journal of Nutrition in Gerontology & Geriatrics, 30*(2), 122–139.

Lorentzen, V., Dyeremose, V., & Larsen, B. H. (2012). Severely overweight children and dietary changes—a family perspective. *Journal of Advanced Nursing, 68*(4), 878–887.

Low, K. G., et al. (2012). Testing the effectiveness of motivational interviewing as a weight reduction strategy for obese cardiac patients: a pilot study. *International Journal of Behavioral Medicine,* Feb 12, [Epub ahead of print].

Masheb, R., & Grillo, C. (2006). Eating patterns and breakfast consumption in obese patients with binge eating disorder. *Behaviour Research and Therapy, 44*(11), 1545–1553.

Pereira, M., et al. (2005). Fast-food habits, weight gain, and insulin resistance (the CARDIA study): 15-year prospective analysis. *Lancet, 365*(9453), 36.

Prestwich, A., Hurling, R., & Baker, S. (2011). Implicit shopping: Attitudinal determinants of the purchasing of healthy and unhealthy foods. *Psychology & Health, 26*(7), 875–885.

Ruxton, C. S. (2011). Nutritional implications of obesity and dieting. *Nutrition Bulletin, 36*(2), 199–211.

Seale, J. P., Fifield, J., Davis-Smith, Y. M., et al. (2013). Developing culturally congruent weight maintenance programs for African American church members. *Ethnicity & Health, 18*(2), 152–167.

Shay, L., Shobert, J., Seibert, D., et al. (2009). Adult weight management: translating research and guidelines into practice. *Journal of the American Academy of Nurse Practitioners, 21*(4), 197–206.

Steele, M. M., Steele, R. G., & Cushing, C. C. (2012). Weighing the pros and cons in family-based pediatric obesity intervention: parent and child decisional balance as a predictor of child outcomes. *Children's Health Care, 41*(1), 43–55.

Straight, C., et al. (2012). Effects of resistance training and dietary changes on physical function and body composition in overweight and obese older adults. *Journal of Physical Activity and Health, 9*(6), 875–883.

U.S. Department of Agriculture (2014). *Weight Management, USDA ChooseMyPlate.gov.* <http://www.choosemyplate.gov/weight-management-calories/weight-management/better-choices/amount-calories.html>. Retrieved from WWW 6/21/15.

Vincent, D. (2009). Culturally tailored education to promote lifestyle change in Mexican Americans with type 2 diabetes. *Journal of the American Academy of Nurse Practitioners, 21*(9), 520–527.

Visram, S., Crosland, A., & Cording, H. (2009). Triggers for weight gain and loss among participants in a primary care-based intervention. *British Journal of Community Nursing, 14*(11), 495–501.

Wong, E. M., & Cheng, M. M. (2013). Effects of motivational interviewing to promote weight loss in obese children. *Journal of Clinical Nursing, 22*(17/18), 2519–2530.

Yilmaz, J. (2011). Adopting a psychological approach to obesity. *Nursing Standard, 25*(21), 42–46.

O

Impaired Oral Mucous Membrane

Betty J. Ackley, MSN, EdS, RN, and Mary Beth Flynn Makic, PhD, RN, CNS, CCNS, FAAN

NANDA-I

Definition

Injury to the lips, soft tissue, buccal cavity, and/or oropharynx

Defining Characteristics

Bad taste in mouth; bleeding; cheilitis; coated tongue; decrease in taste sensation; desquamation; difficulty eating; difficulty speaking; enlarged tonsils; exposure to pathogen; geographic tongue; gingival hyperplasia; gingival pallor; gingival pocketing deeper than 4 mm; gingival recession; halitosis; hyperemia; fissures; geographic tongue; gingival hyperplasia; gingival pallor; gingival recession; halitosis; hyperemia; impaired ability to swallow; macroplasia; mucosal denudation; oral discomfort; oral edema; oral fissure; oral lesion; oral mucosal pallor; oral nodule; oral pain; oral papule; oral ulcer; oral vesicles; presence of mass (e.g., hemangioma); purulent oral-nasal drainage; purulent oral-nasal exudates; smooth atrophic tongue; spongy patches in mouth; stomatitis; white patches in mouth; white plaque in mouth; white, curd-like oral exudate; xerostomia

Related Factors (r/t)

Alcohol consumption; allergy; alteration in cognitive functioning; autoimmune disease; autosomal disorder; barrier to dental care; barrier to oral self-care; behavior disorder (e.g., attention deficit, oppositional defiant); chemical injury agent (e.g., burn, capsaicin, methylene chloride, mustard agent); cleft lip; cleft palate; decrease in hormone level in women; decrease in platelets; decrease in salivation; dehydration; depression; immunodeficiency; immunosuppression; infection; insufficient knowledge of oral hygiene; insufficient oral hygiene; loss of oral support structure; malnutrition; mechanical factor (e.g., ill-fitting dentures, braces, endotracheal/nasogastric tube, oral surgery); mouth breathing; nil per os (NPO) more than 24 hours; oral trauma; smoking; stressors; syndrome (e.g., Sjögren's); treatment regimen

NOC (Nursing Outcomes Classification)

Suggested NOC Outcomes

Oral Health; Oral Hygiene; Tissue Integrity: Skin and Mucous Membranes

Example NOC Outcome with Indicators

Oral Health as evidenced by the following indicators: Cleanliness of mouth and teeth/Moisture of oral mucosa and tongue/ Color of mucous membranes/Oral mucosa/tongue/gum integrity. (Rate the outcome and indicators of **Oral Health:** 1 = severely compromised, 2 = substantially compromised, 3 = moderately compromised, 4 = mildly compromised, 5 = not compromised [see Section I].)

Client Outcomes

Client Will (Specify Time Frame)

- Maintain intact, moist oral mucous membranes that are free of ulceration, inflammation, infection, and debris
- Demonstrate measures to maintain or regain intact oral mucous membranes

NIC (Nursing Interventions Classification)

Suggested NIC Intervention

Oral Health Restoration

Example NIC Activities—Oral Health Restoration

Monitor condition of client's mouth including character of abnormalities; Instruct client to avoid commercial mouthwashes

Nursing Interventions and *Rationales*

▲ Inspect the oral cavity/teeth at least once daily and note any discoloration, presence of debris, amount of plaque buildup, presence of lesions such as white lesions or patches, edema, or bleeding, and intactness of teeth. Refer to a dentist or periodontist as appropriate. *Systematic inspection can identify impending problems. White lesions are often leukoplakia, which is a precursor to squamous cell carcinoma. If the lesion is cancerous, prompt treatment is needed (Engelke & Pravikoff, 2010; Chen 2014a; Worthington et al, 2011).*

- If the client does not have a bleeding disorder and is able to swallow, encourage the client to brush the teeth with a soft toothbrush using fluoride-containing toothpaste at least twice per day. EB: *Toothbrush is the most effective method for reducing plaque and controlling periodontal disease (Barnes, 2014).*
- Recommend the client use a powered toothbrush if desired for removal of dental plaque and prevent gingivitis. EB: *Two systematic reviews found the powered/oscillating toothbrush to be safe for use on both hard and soft dental tissues and more effective in cleaning teeth (Yaacob et al, 2014; Slade, 2013).*
- Use foam sticks to moisten the oral mucous membranes, clean out debris, and swab out the mouth of the edentulous client. **Do not use foam sticks to clean the teeth** unless the platelet count is very low and the client is prone to bleeding gums. Foam sticks are useful for cleansing the oral cavity of a client who is edentulous. CEB/EB: *Foam sticks are not effective for removing plaque; the toothbrush is much more effective (Pearson & Hutton, 2002; Chen, 2014a).*
- If the client does not have a bleeding disorder, encourage the client to floss once per day or use an inter-dental cleaner. EB: *Floss is useful to remove plaque buildup between the teeth (American Dental Association [ADA], 2015a).*
- Use an antimicrobial mouthwash as ordered or tap water or saline only for a mouth rinse. Do not use commercial mouthwashes containing alcohol or hydrogen peroxide. Also, do not use lemon-glycerin swabs. *Some antimicrobial mouthwashes have demonstrated effective action in decreasing bacterial counts in plaque and decreasing gingivitis (ADA, 2015a).* CEB/EB: *Hydrogen peroxide can cause mucosal damage and is extremely foul-tasting to clients (Tombes & Gallucci, 1993). Use of lemon-glycerin swabs can result in decreased salivary amylase and oral moisture, as well as erosion of tooth enamel (Foss-Durant & McAffee, 1997). Chlorhexidine mouthwash and sodium bicarbonate appropriately diluted may be used during oral care (Chen 2014b).*
- Provide oral hygiene if the client is unable to care for himself/herself. The nursing diagnosis Bathing **Self-Care** deficit is then applicable.
- If the client is unable to brush own teeth, follow this procedure:
  - Position the client sitting upright or on side.
  - Use a soft bristle toothbrush.
  - Use fluoride toothpaste and tap water or saline as a solution.
  - Brush teeth in an up-and-down manner.
  - Suction as needed.

Each client must receive oral care including toothbrushing two times every day to maintain healthy teeth and mouth and to prevent complications associated with periodontitis (the advanced form of gum disease that can cause tooth loss), which is associated with health problems, such as cardiovascular disease, stroke, and bacterial pneumonia (ADA, 2015a).

- Monitor the client's nutritional and fluid status to determine if it is adequate. Refer to the care plan for Deficient **Fluid** volume or Imbalanced **Nutrition:** less than body requirements if applicable. *Dehydration and malnutrition predispose clients to impaired oral mucous membranes.*
- Encourage fluid intake of up to 3000 mL/day if not contraindicated by the client's medical condition. *Fluids help increase moisture in the mouth, which protects the mucous membranes from damage.*
- Determine the client's usual method of oral care and address any concerns regarding oral hygiene.
- ▲ If the client has a dry mouth (xerostomia):
  - Recognize that more than 500 medications may cause xerostomia, and at times the medication can be discontinued to increase the client's comfort (Schub et al, 2010a).
  - Provide saliva substitutes as ordered. *Saliva substitutes are helpful to decrease the discomfort of dry mouth and may help prevent stomatitis (ADA, 2015c).*
  - Suggest the client chew sugarless gum or sugarless sour candy to promote salivary flow. *Both sugarless gum and candy stimulate the formation of saliva (ADA, 2015c; Schub et al, 2010a).*
  - Examine the oral cavity for signs of mucositis ulceration and oral candidiasis. *Untreated xerostomia may result in these conditions (Schub et al, 2010a).*
- Recommend the client decrease or preferably stop intake of soft drinks. Sugar-containing soft drinks can cause cavities, and the low pH of the drink can cause erosion in teeth (*ADA, 2015a*).
- If client has halitosis, review good oral care with the client including brushing teeth, using floss, and brushing the tongue. Halitosis can be a beginning sign of gingivitis and can be eradicated by a good program of dental hygiene (*ADA, 2015b*).

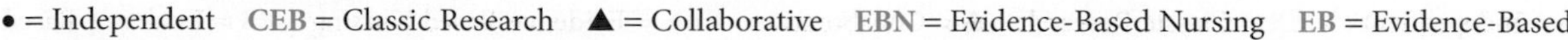

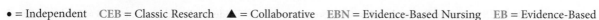

- Instruct the client with halitosis to clean the tongue when performing oral hygiene; brush tongue with tongue scraper or toothbrush and follow with a mouth rinse. CEB: A Cochrane review found that tongue cleaning was effective for short-term control of halitosis (*Van der Sleen et al, 2010; ADA 2015b*).

▲ Assess the client for underlying medical condition that may be causing halitosis. *Causes of halitosis can be subdivided into three categories: oral origin where good mouth care can help prevent, halitosis from the upper respiratory tract including the sinuses and nose, and halitosis from systemic diseases that is blood-borne, volatilized in the lungs, and expelled from the lower respiratory tract. Potential sources of blood-borne halitosis are some systemic diseases, metabolic disorders, medication, and certain foods such as onions and garlic (ADA, 2015b).*

- Keep the lips well lubricated using a lip balm that is water- or aloe-based. *This is a comfort measure (Radvansky et al, 2013).*

Client Receiving Chemotherapy/Radiation

- Ensure that the client receives a comprehensive oral examination before initiation of chemotherapy or radiation, with aggressive preventive dental care given as needed (Radvansky et al, 2013).
- Provide both verbal and written instruction about the need for and method of providing frequent oral care to the client before radiation therapy or chemotherapy. Assess the condition of the oral cavity daily in the client receiving radiation or chemotherapy (Radvansky et al, 2013).
- For measurement of presence or severity of mucositis, use the Oral Mucositis Assessment Scale (OMAS). CEBN: *This is an instrument that has two components: clinician's assessment of presence and severity of mucositis, and client report about pain, difficulty swallowing, and ability to eat (Harris et al, 2008).*
- Use a protocol to prevent/treat mucositis that includes the following:
  - Use a soft toothbrush that is replaced on a regular basis; brush teeth at least two times a day and for at least 90 seconds.
  - Continue to floss teeth daily.
  - Use a bland, alcohol-free rinse to remove debris and moisten the oral cavity. Rinse the mouth often (every 2 hours while awake) if the client has mouth sores.
  - Avoid tobacco, alcohol, and irritating foods (hot, rough, acidic, or spicy).
  - Use a valid and reliable pain assessment tool and treatment of pain as needed.

▲ EB: *Use of an oral care protocol helps to decrease oral mucositis in clients receiving treatment for cancer (Radvansky et al, 2013; Eilers et al, 2014).*

- Help the client use a mouth rinse of normal saline or salt and soda every 1 to 2 hours for prevention and treatment of stomatitis. A typical mixture is 1 teaspoon of salt or sodium bicarbonate per pint of water. Clients are directed to take a tablespoon of the rinse and swish it in the mouth for 30 seconds, then expectorate. *Rinses are helpful to remove debris and hydrate the oral mucous membranes; sodium bicarbonate can discourage yeast colonization (Schub et al, 2010b).*

▲ If the mouth is severely inflamed and it is painful to swallow, contact the health care provider for a topical anesthetic or analgesic order. Modification of oral intake (e.g., soft or liquid diet) may also be necessary to prevent friction trauma. The nursing diagnosis Imbalanced **Nutrition:** less than body requirements may apply.

- If the client's platelet count is lower than 50,000/mm^3 or the client has a bleeding disorder, use a specially made toothbrush designed for sensitive or diseased tissue, or a toothette that is not soaked in glycerin or flavorings; if the client cannot tolerate a toothbrush or a toothette, a piece of gauze wrapped around a finger can be used to remove plaque and debris (Radvansky et al, 2013).

Critical Care—Client on a Ventilator

- Use a soft toothbrush to brush teeth to clean the client's teeth at least every 12 hours; use suction to remove secretions. Provide oral moisturizer to oral mucosa and lips every 4 hours. Recognize that good oral care is paramount in the prevention of ventilator-associated events (VAE) and ventilator-associated pneumonia (VAP). CEB/EBN: *Increased plaque on the teeth is associated with increased contamination of the mouth and incidence of VAP (Munro et al, 2009). An integrative review of the literature found that consistently performing frequent oral care along with other interventions (e.g., head of bed >30°, adequate endotracheal tube cuff pressure to reduce aspiration, daily evaluation of client's readiness for extubation)*

O

and oral moisturizing reduced VAP as well as decreased overall health care expenses (Parsons et al, 2013; Hillier et al, 2013; Chu, 2014; Alhazzani et al, 2013).

▲ Apply chlorhexidine gluconate mouthwash or gel in the oral cavity after performing tooth brushing, which may reduce the risk of the client developing VAE and VAP. EB: *The use of chlorhexidine gluconate has been associated with a 40% reduction in the odds of a client developing VAP (Shi et al, 2013). Routine oral care with chlorhexidine gluconate in the care of the mechanically ventilated cardiac surgery clients reduces the risk of VAP (Klompas et al, 2014; Xue, 2015).*

Geriatric

- Determine the functional ability of the client to provide his/her own oral care. Refer to Bathing **Self-Care** deficit. *Interventions must be directed toward both treatment of the functional loss and care of oral health.*
- Provide appropriate oral care to older adults with a self-care deficit, brushing the teeth after breakfast and in the evening. EBN: *Oral care is often poor for older clients and clients with dementia.* CEB/EB: *Several studies have shown that the rate of pneumonia was decreased by providing oral care (Sarin et al, 2008; Le, 2015).*
- If the client has dementia or delirium and exhibits care-resistant behavior such as fighting, biting, or refusing care, use the following method:
  - Ensure client is in a quiet environment such as own bathroom, sitting or standing at the sink to prime memory for appropriate actions.
  - Approach the client at eye level within his/her range of vision.
  - Approach with a smile and begin conversation with a touch of the hand and gradually move up.
  - Use mirror-mirror technique, standing behind the client, and brush and floss teeth.
  - Use respectful adult speech, not elder speak— sing-song voice, calling "dearie," "honey," and so forth. *Elder speak is a documented trigger for care-resistant behavior (Herman & Williams, 2009).*
  - Promote self-care where client brushes own teeth if possible.
  - Use distractors when needed, such as singing, talking, reminiscing, or use of a teddy bear. EBN: *Use of specific techniques can decrease the fear-evoked response to nursing care and increase the effectiveness of nurses providing oral care to clients (Jablonski et al, 2011).*
- Carefully observe the oral cavity and lips for abnormal lesions such as white or red patches, masses, ulcerations with an indurated margin, or a raised granular lesion. *Malignant lesions are more common in older adults than in younger persons, especially if there is a history of smoking or alcohol use (Engelke & Pravikoff, 2010; Le, 2015).*
- Ensure that dentures are removed and cleaned regularly, preferably after every meal and before bedtime. *Dentures left in the mouth at night may impede circulation to the palate and predispose the client to oral lesions.*

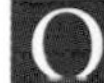

Home Care

- The interventions described previously may be adapted for home care use.

▲ Instruct the client in ways to soothe the oral cavity (e.g., cool beverages, Popsicles, viscous lidocaine).

▲ If necessary, refer for home health aide services to support the family in oral care and observation of the oral cavity.

Client/Family Teaching and Discharge Planning

- Teach the client how to inspect the oral cavity and monitor for signs and symptoms of infection or complications, and when to call the health care provider (Radvansky et al, 2013; Eilers et al, 2014).
- Recommend the client not smoke, use chewing tobacco, or drink excessive amounts of alcohol. *Tobacco use, either smoking or chewing, is a common cause of leukoplakia. Also, alcohol and human papillomavirus have been associated with squamous cell carcinoma in the oral cavity (Engelke & Pravikoff, 2010).*
- Teach the client and family if necessary how to perform appropriate mouth care. Use the motivational interviewing technique. EB: *A study demonstrated improved dental hygiene with decreased amount of plaque when motivational interviewing compared with a usual teaching session on dental care (Godard et al, 2011). A systematic review found motivational interviewing more effective in changing oral health than usual care (Watt, 2010). See Motivational Interviewing in Appendix C.*

REFERENCES

Alhazzani, W., Smith, O., Muscedere, J., et al. (2013). Toothbrushing for critically ill mechanically ventilated patients: a systematic review and meta-analysis of randomized trials evaluating ventilator-associated pneumonia. *Critical Care Medicine*, *41*, 646–655.

American Dental Association (ADA) (2015a). *Oral Health*. From: <http://www.mouthhealthy.org/en/az-topics/o/oral-health>. Retrieved June 24, 2015.

American Dental Association (ADA) (2015b). *Mouth Healthy: Halitosis*. <http://www.mouthhealthy.org/en/az-topics/h/Halitosis>. Retrieved June 24, 2015.

American Dental Association (ADA) (2015c). *Dry mouth*. From: <http://www.mouthhealthy.org/en/az-topics/d/dry-mouth>. Retrieved June 25, 2015.

Barnes, C. M. (2014). Dental hygiene intervention to prevent nosocomial pneumonias. *The Journal of Evidence-Based Dental Practice*, *145*, 103–114.

Chen, Z. (2014a). *Oral care. Joanna Briggs Institute.*

Chen, Z. (2014b). *Mouth wash. Joanna Briggs Institute.*

Chu, V. (2014). *Ventilator-associated pneumonia: Clinician information. Joanna Briggs Institute.*

Eilers, J., Harris, D., Henry, K., et al. (2014). Evidence-based interventions for cancer treatment-related mucositis: putting evidence into practice. *Clinical Journal of Oncology Nursing*, *18*(6), 80–96.

Engelke, A., & Pravikoff, D. (Oct 29, 2010). *Leukoplakia, oral. Nursing Reference Center. CINAHL Nursing Guide.*

Foss-Durant, A. M., & McAffee, A. (1997). A comparison of three oral care products commonly used in practice. *Clinical Nursing Research*, *6*, 1.

Godard, A., Dufour, T., & Jeanne, S. (2011). Application of self-regulation theory and motivational interview for improving oral hygiene: a randomized controlled trial. *Journal of Clinical Periodontology*, *38*(12), 1099–1105.

Harris, D. J., et al. (2008). Putting evidence into practice: evidence-based interventions for the management of oral mucositis. *Clinical Journal of Oncology Nursing*, *12*(1), 141–152.

Herman, R. E., & Williams, K. N. (2009). Elderspeak's influence on resistiveness to care: focus on behavioral events. *American Journal of Alzheimer's Disease and Other Dementias*, *24*(5), 417–423. [Epub Aug 19, 2009].

Hillier, B., Wilson, C., Chamberlain, D., et al. (2013). Preventing ventilator-associated pneumonia through oral care, product selection, and application method: a literature review. *AACN Advanced Critical Care*, *24*(1), 38–58.

Jablonski, R., Therrien, B., & Kolanowski, A. (2011). No more fighting and biting during mouth care: applying the theoretical constructs of threat perception to clinical practice. *Research and Theory for Nursing Practice*, *25*(3), 163–175.

Klompas, M., Speck, K., Howell, M. D., et al. (2014). Reappraisal of routine oral care with chlorhexidine gluconate for patients receiving mechanical ventilation: systematic review and meta-analysis. *JAMA: The Journal of the American Medical Association*, *174*, 751–761.

Le, L. K. D. (2015). *Oral assessment tools: older adults. JoAnna Briggs Institute.*

Munro, C. L., et al. (2009). Chlorhexidine, tooth brushing, and preventing ventilator associated pneumonia in critically ill adults. *American Journal of Critical Care*, *18*(5), 428–437.

Pearson, L. S., & Hutton, J. L. (2002). A controlled trial to compare the ability of foam swabs and toothbrushes to remove dental plaque. *Journal of Advanced Nursing*, *39*, 5.

Parsons, S., Lee, C. A., Strickert, D., et al. (2013). Oral care and ventilator-associated pneumonia: an integrated review of the literature. *Dimensions of Critical Care Nursing*, *3193*, 138–145.

Radvansky, L. J., Pace, M. B., & Siddiqui, A. (2013). Prevention and management of radiation-induced dermatitis, mucositis, and xerostomia. *American Journal of Health-System Pharmacy*, *70*, 1025–1032.

Sarin, J., et al. (2008). Reducing the risk of aspiration pneumonia among elderly patients in long-term care facilities through oral health interventions. *Journal of the American Medical Directors Association*, *9*(2), 128–135.

Schub, T., Grose, S., & Pravikoff, D. (Sept 3, 2010a). *Xerostomia. Nursing Reference Center: CINAHL Nursing Guide.*

Schub, E., Schub, T., & Pravikoff, D. (2010b). *Stomatitis (oral mucositis) therapy. Nursing Reference Center: CINAHL Nursing Guide*. Oct 29.

Shi, Z., Xie, H., Wang, P., et al. (2013). Oral hygiene care for critically ill patients to prevent ventilator-associated pneumonia. *Cochrane Database of Systematic Reviews*, (8), CD008367.

Slade, S. (2013). *Oral health: manual and powered toothbrushing. Joanna Briggs Institute.*

Tombes, M. B., & Gallucci, B. (1993). The effects of hydrogen peroxide rinses on the normal oral mucosa. *Nursing Research*, *42*(6), 332.

Van der Sleen, M. I., et al. (2010). Effectiveness of mechanical tongue cleaning on breath odour and tongue coating: a systematic review. *International Journal of Dental Hygiene*, *8*(4), 258–268.

Watt, R. G. (2010). Motivational interviewing may be effective in dental setting. *Evidence-based Dentistry*, *11*(1), 13.

Worthington, H. V., et al. (2011). Interventions for preventing oral mucositis for patients with cancer receiving treatment. *Cochrane Database of Systematic Reviews*, *2*(4), CD000978.

Xue, Y. (2015). *Ventilator associated pneumonia: oral hygiene care. Joanna Briggs Institute.*

Yaacob, M., Worthington, H. V., Deacon, S. A., et al. (2014). Powered versus manual toothbrushing for oral health. *Cochran Database of Systematic Reviews*, *6*, CD002281.

O

Risk for impaired Oral Mucous Membrane

Mary Beth Flynn Makic, PhD, RN, CNS, CCNS, FAAN

NANDA-I

Definition

Vulnerable to injury to the lips, soft tissues, buccal cavity, and/or oropharynx, which may compromise health

Risk Factors

Alcohol consumption; allergy; alteration in cognitive functioning; autoimmune disease; autosomal disorder; barriers to dental care; barrier to oral self-care; behavior disorder (e.g., attention deficit, oppositional defiant); chemotherapy; decrease in hormone level in women; economically disadvantaged; immunodeficiency; immunosuppression; inadequate nutrition; infection; insufficient knowledge of oral hygiene; insufficient oral hygiene; mechanical factor (e.g., orthodontic appliance, device for ventilation or food, ill-fitting dentures); radiation therapy; smoking; stressors; surgical procedure; syndrome (e.g., Sjögren's); trauma

NIC, Client Outcomes, Nursing Interventions, Client/Family Teaching, *Rationales,* and References

Refer to care plan for Impaired **Oral Mucous Membrane.**

Overweight

Marina Martinez-Kratz, MS, RN, CNE

NANDA-I

Definition

A condition in which an individual accumulates abnormal or excessive fat for age and gender

Defining Characteristics

Children age 2 or younger

Weight-for-length percentiles >95th percentile

Childhood (age 2 to 18 years)

Body mass index (BMI) >85th but <95th percentile or kg/m^2 (whichever is smaller)

Adult

BMI >25 kg/m^2

Related Factors

Average daily physical activity is less than recommended for gender and age; consumption of sugar sweetened beverages; disordered eating behaviors (e.g., binge eating, extreme weight control); disordered eating perceptions; economically disadvantaged; energy expenditure below energy intake based on standard assessment (e.g., weight, activity, variety in diet, excess [WAVE] assessment); excessive alcohol consumption; fear regarding lack of food supply; formula or mixed fed infants; frequent snaking; genetic disorder heritability of interrelated factors (e.g., adipose tissue distribution, energy expenditure, lipoprotein lipase activity, lipid synthesis, lipolysis); high disinhibition and restraint eating behavior score; high frequency of restaurant or fried food; low dietary calcium intake in children; maternal diabetes mellitus; maternal smoking; obesity in childhood; parental obesity; portion sizes larger than recommended; premature pubarche; rapid weight gain during childhood; rapid weight gain during infancy, including the first week, first 4 months, and first year; sedentary behavior occurring for >2 hours/day; shortened sleep time; sleep disorder; solid foods as major food source of <5 months of age

Nursing Interventions and *Rationales*

- Assess the meaning and importance of food in the client's life. EB: *Research findings demonstrate that implicit attitudes significantly predict purchases of healthy and unhealthy foods (Prestwich et al, 2011). Research found that youth held some negative associations related to healthy foods and some positive associations linked to unhealthy foods (Harrison & Jackson, 2009).*
- Counsel the client to eat breakfast daily. EB: *Research has determined that skipping breakfast is a lifestyle risk significantly associated with higher BMI (Ghrayeb et al, 2014).*
- Assess the client with a Patient Readiness Scale to determine if the client is ready to discuss weight loss and/or would like weight loss information. EB: *Readiness to change is an important part of treatment for behavior change (Steele et al, 2012).*

- Assess the client's current nutrition through a 1- to 3-day food diary in which everything ingested orally is recorded. Analyze the following areas:
  - Intake of food and beverage calories and fat
  - Portion sizes
  - Underconsumption or overconsumption of nutrients
  - Use of supplements
  - Use of meal replacements
  - Timing/consistency of meals and snacks
- ▲ EB: *Use of a food diary is helpful for both the client and the nurse, to examine usual foods eaten and patterns of eating (Shay et al, 2009).* EB: *A study found that use of a personal digital assistant for self-monitoring of food intake was more effective than use of a paper record, yet both groups had a similar weight loss (Acharya et al, 2011).*
- Counsel the client to measure regularly consumed foods periodically. Help the client learn usual portion sizes. *Measuring food alerts the client to normal portion sizes. Estimating amounts can be extremely inaccurate.* EB: *A study demonstrated that obese people had significantly larger portion sizes, plus ate later in the day (Berg et al, 2009).*
- Assist the client to develop a system of self-management, which may include self-monitoring of weight, BMI, and food intake, interpreting food labels, portion control, recipe modification, restaurant and social food negotiation, and physical activity. *A key component of successful weight loss and maintenance is regular self-monitoring (Fitch et al, 2013).*
- Document the client's height and weight and teach significance of his/her BMI in relationship to current health. Use a chart or a website such as http://www.cdc.gov/healthyweight/assessing/bmi/index.html (CDC, 2015).
- Assist the client to use Super Tracker (http://www.choosemyplate.gov/food-groups) to determine the number of calories to eat and gain more information on how to eat in a healthy fashion. To lose weight, the client must eat fewer calories (U.S. Department of Agriculture, 2014).
- Encourage the client to engage in regular physical activity for at least 150 minutes weekly. EB: *Research found that normal weight reproductive-aged women who do not engage in recommended levels of physical activity are at risk for becoming overweight or obese (Hillemeier et al, 2011). Studies determined that increased physical activity in conjunction with improved eating behavior scores resulted in greater weight loss (Jakicic et al, 2011).*
- Recommend the client eat a healthy breakfast every morning. CEB: *A study found that that people who skip breakfast are more likely to overeat in the evening (Masheb & Grillo, 2006). Another study demonstrated that people who skipped breakfast were 450 times more likely to be obese (Ma et al, 2003).*
- Recommend the client avoid eating in fast food restaurants. CEB: *A 15-year study demonstrated that people who frequently eat fast foods gain an average of 10 lb more than those who eat fast food less often and were two times more likely to develop insulin resistance, which can lead to diabetes (Peirera et al, 2005).*
- Assist the client to reframe slips in weight loss or physical activity behavior as lapses that are a single event and not a full return to previous unhealthy behaviors. *Relapse prevention strategies include managing lapses in healthy behavior, identifying high-risk situations for relapses, enhancing skills for coping, and increasing self-efficacy for avoiding relapse (Fitch et al, 2013).*
- Teach problem-solving strategies to deal with barriers to changing eating and physical activity patterns. *Strategies such as defining the problem, brainstorming solutions, seeking solutions, and evaluating the outcome of the solution are problem-solving strategies that facilitate weight loss (Fitch et al, 2013).*
- Assist clients to engage their social support systems in ways that facilitate weight loss, as well as eating and physical activity behavior change. *Significant others, family, friends and co-workers can facilitate or hinder weight loss success (Fitch et al, 2013).*
- Assist the client to reframe the goal focus from outcome (weight loss) to process (eating behaviors) for weight loss. EB: *A study of overweight women found that focusing on the process of dieting (the eating behavior) was related to actual weight loss as well as to subjective dieting success (Freund & Hennecke, 2012).*
- Assist the client to develop stimulus control techniques designed to reduce environmental cues associated with eating behaviors. Specifically clients should be taught to limit the presence of high-calorie/high-fat foods in the home; to reduce the visibility of unhealthy food choices in the home; to limit where and when they eat; to avoid distractions like reading, using the computer or watching television when eating;

and to eat more slowly. *Stimulus control strategies are a key to successful weight loss and weight maintenance (Fitch et al, 2013).*

- Use the motivational interviewing technique when working with clients to promote healthy eating and weight loss. EB: *A pilot study with use of motivational interviewing in women found it resulted in a significant weight loss (Low et al, 2012). A review found that use of motivational interviewing was effective in causing weight loss (Armstrong et al, 2011).*
- Refer the client to tailored weight management programs that provide opportunities for ongoing support. CEB: *Tailored weight loss interventions and ongoing support were identified by obese or overweight clients as facilitating longer term weight management (Visram et al, 2009).*
- Refer the client to a weight-loss related therapy group. EBN: *A British study showed that addressing psychological factors associated with eating and weight in a group setting offers an important contribution to the treatment of obesity (Yilmaz, 2011).*
- Recommend that clients use dietary supplements such as vitamins and minerals after consulting with their primary health care provider. EB: *Research shows a prevalence of low micronutrient status in obese individuals who can benefit from safeguarding vitamin and mineral adequacy by taking a multinutrient supplement in conjunction with increased intake of nutrient-rich foods (Ruxton, 2011).*
- Behavior methods of losing weight are diverse and effective for weight loss through developing methods to control eating behavior, changing habits, and mindset. EB: *Behavioral based treatments are safe and effective for weight loss (LeBlanc et al, 2011).* EB: *A study found that behavior treatment that was done either in person or remotely through computer teaching, email, and the phone resulted in a significant loss of weight in obese clients versus a control group (Appel et al, 2011). A Cochrane review found that behavioral therapy used independently as a stand-alone therapy resulted in significant weight loss (Shaw et al, 2009).*

Pediatric

- Offer obese or overweight adolescents healthy methods for weight loss. CEBN: Research shows that overweight adolescents who demonstrate a desire to lose weight often choose unhealthy methods (Chen et al, 2009).
- Offer families of obese or overweight children prejudice-free, individually accepting, and supportive interventions to address weight loss. EBN: *Obese children showed signs of stress, stigmatization, and marginalization, while their families reported feeling rejected by health care professionals (Lorentzen et al, 2012).* EBN: *Obese children treated with motivational interviewing showed significant improvement in their weight-related behavior and obesity-related anthropometric measures (Wong & Cheng, 2013).*
- Recommend that families eat together for at least one meal per day. *Mealtime together has been shown to improve children's eating habits: children eat more fruits and vegetables when the family eats together*
- Recommend involving the family in planning meals and food preparation. Children can learn about nutrition as they help plan and make meals. *Children are more likely to eat foods that they help select or prepare.*
- Suggest that parents work at being good role models of healthy eating. *Setting a good example is key for children; children learn the value of healthy eating early, and it can continue for a lifetime.*
- Recommend that the family try new foods, either a new food or recipe every week. *More variety can increase the intake of fruits and vegetables.*
- Suggest the parents keep healthy snacks on hand. Store the snacks in a purse, the car, and a desk drawer. *Suggestions include crackers and peanut butter, small boxes of cereal, fresh fruit, and vegetables (Academy of Nutrition and Dietetics, 2014).*

Geriatric

- Recognize that it is generally not appropriate to have an older client on a calorie-restrictive diet. *Older clients deserve to eat and not be hungry.* EB: *Strength training and dietary modifications can improve body composition, muscle strength, and physical function in overweight and obese older adults (Straight et al, 2012).*
- Observe for socioeconomic factors that influence food choices (e.g., funds, cooking facilities, food insecurity). *Even those on restricted budgets and with limited facilities can be assisted to choose healthy food sources for a balanced diet.* EB: *Food security is a factor that can indicate a need for nutrition assistance in older adults (Lee et al, 2011).*

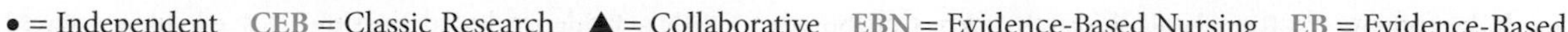

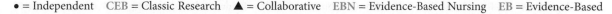

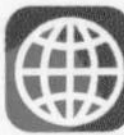

Multicultural

- Tailor nutritional interventions to be consistent with cultural beliefs, norms, and values. CEBN: *Mexican American women responded positively to nutritional education and physical activity promotion when families were involved (Vincent, 2009).*
- Offer tailored lifestyle counseling via the telephone. EB: *Low socioeconomic status African Americans and Latinos experienced positive nutritional change and weight loss after participating in a community-based translational lifestyle program (Kanaya et al, 2012).*
- Integrate weight loss and weight maintenance interventions with church faith based concepts for cultural congruence with African American clients. EB: *Recent research suggests that integrating faith themes into a weight loss maintenance program may increase its long-term impact on participants' health behavior change (Seale et al, 2013).*

Client/Family Teaching and Discharge Planning

- The majority of the preceding interventions involve teaching.
- Work with the family members regarding information on how to support and promote weight loss and healthy intakes.

REFERENCES

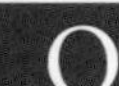

Academy of Nutrition and Dietetics (2014). *It's about eating right: nutrition for growing bodies.* From: <http://www.eatright.org/Public/content.aspx?id=6751>. Retrieved September 20, 2014.

Acharya, S. D., Elci, O. U., Sereika, S. M., et al. (2011). Using a personal digital assistant for self-monitoring influences diet quality in comparison to a standard paper record among overweight/obese adults. *Journal of the American Dietetic Association, 111*(4), 583–588.

Appel, L. J., Clark, J. M., Yeh, H. C., et al. (2011). Comparative effectiveness of weight-loss interventions in clinical practice. *The New England Journal of Medicine, 365*(21), 1959–1968.

Armstrong, M. J., et al. (2011). Motivational interviewing to improve weight loss in overweight and/or obese patients: a systematic review and meta-analysis of randomized controlled trials. *Obesity Reviews, 12*(9), 709–723.

Berg, C., Lappas, G., Wolk, A., et al. (2009). Eating patterns and portion size associated with obesity in a Swedish population. *Appetite, 52*, 21–26.

Centers for Disease Control and Prevention (2015). *Healthy Weight—it's not a diet, it's a lifestyle!* <http://www.cdc.gov/healthyweight/assessing/bmi/index.html>. Retrieved 6/21/2015.

Chen, M., Fan, J., Jane, S., et al. (2009). Do overweight adolescents perceive the need to reduce weight and take healthy actions? *Journal of Nursing Research (Taiwan Nurses Association), 17*(4), 270–277.

Fitch, A., Everling, L., Fox, C., et al. (2013). *Institute for Clinical Systems Improvement. Prevention and Management of Obesity for Adults.*

Freund, A. M., & Hennecke, M. (2012). Changing eating behaviour vs. losing weight: the role of goal focus for weight loss in overweight women. *Psychology & Health*, 2725–2742.

Ghrayeb, F. A., Mohamed Rusli, A., Al Rifai, A., et al. (2014). PUBLIC HEALTH. Prevalence of lifestyle-related risk factors contributing to non-communicable diseases among adolescents in tarqumia, Palestine. *International Medical Journal, 21*(3), 272–276.

Harrison, M., & Jackson, L. (2009). Meanings that youth associate with healthy and unhealthy food. *Canadian Journal of Dietetic Practice & Research, 70*(1), 6–12.

Hillemeier, M. M., Weisman, C. S., Chuang, C., et al. (2011). Transition to overweight or obesity among women of reproductive age. *Journal of Women's Health, 20*(5), 703–710. (15409996).

Jakicic, J. M., Otto, A. D., Lang, W., et al. (2011). The effect of physical activity on 18-month weight change in overweight adults. *Obesity, 19*, 100–109.

Kanaya, A. M., Santoyo-Olsson, J., Gregorich, S., et al. (2012). The live well, be well study: a community-based, translational lifestyle program to lower diabetes risk factors in ethnic minority and lower-socioeconomic status adults. *American Journal of Public Health, 102*(8), 1551–1558.

LeBlanc, E., O'Connor, E., Whitlock, E. P., et al. (2011). *Screening for and management of obesity and overweight in adults. Evidence Report No. 89. AHRQ Publication No. 11-05159-EF-1.* Rockville, MD: Agency for Healthcare Research and Quality.

Lee, J. S., Johnson, M. A., & Brown, A. (2011). Older americans act nutrition program improves participants' food security in Georgia. *Journal of Nutrition In Gerontology & Geriatrics, 30*(2), 122–139.

Low, K. G., et al. (2012). Testing the effectiveness of motivational interviewing as a weight reduction strategy for obese cardiac patients: a pilot study. *International Journal of Behavioral Medicine*, Feb 12, [Epub ahead of print].

Ma, Y., et al. (2003). Association between eating patterns and obesity in a free-living U.S. adult population. *American Journal of Epidemiology, 158*(1), 85–92.

Masheb, R., & Grillo, C. (2006). Eating patterns and breakfast consumption in obese patients with binge eating disorder. *Behaviour Research and Therapy, 44*(11), 1545–1553.

Pereira, M., et al. (2005). Fast-food habits, weight gain, and insulin resistance (the CARDIA study): 15-year prospective analysis. *Lancet, 365*(9453), 36.

Prestwich, A., Hurling, R., & Baker, S. (2011). Implicit shopping: Attitudinal determinants of the purchasing of healthy and unhealthy foods. *Psychology & Health, 26*(7), 875–885.

Ruxton, C. S. (2011). Nutritional implications of obesity and dieting. *Nutrition Bulletin, 36*(2), 199–211.

Seale, J. P., Fifield, J., Davis-Smith, Y. M., et al. (2013). Developing culturally congruent weight maintenance programs for African American church members. *Ethnicity & Health, 18*(2), 152–167.

Shaw, K., O'Rourke, A., & Mar, C. (2009). Psychological interventions for overweight or obesity. *Cochrane Database of Systematic Reviews, (2)*, CD003818.

Shay, L., Shobert, J., Seibert, D., et al. (2009). Adult weight management: translating research and guidelines into practice. *Journal of the American Academy of Nurse Practitioners, 21*(4), 197–206.

Steele, M. M., Steele, R. G., & Cushing, C. C. (2012). Weighing the pros and cons in family-based pediatric obesity intervention: parent and child decisional balance as a predictor of child outcomes. *Children's Health Care, 41*(1), 43–55.

Straight, C., et al. (2012). Effects of resistance training and dietary changes on physical function and body composition in overweight and obese older adults. *Journal of Physical Activity and Health, 9*(6), 875–883.

U.S. Department of Agriculture (2014). *Weight Management, USDA ChooseMyPlate.gov*. <http://www.choosemyplate.gov/weight-management-calories/weight-management/better-choices/amount-calories.html>. Retrieved from WWW 6/21/15.

Vincent, D. (2009). Culturally tailored education to promote lifestyle change in Mexican Americans with type 2 diabetes. *Journal of the American Academy of Nurse Practitioners, 21*(9), 520–527.

Visram, S., Crosland, A., & Cording, H. (2009). Triggers for weight gain and loss among participants in a primary care-based intervention. *British Journal of Community Nursing, 14*(11), 495–501.

Wong, E. M., & Cheng, M. M. (2013). Effects of motivational interviewing to promote weight loss in obese children. *Journal of Clinical Nursing, 22*(17/18), 2519–2530.

Yilmaz, J. (2011). Adopting a psychological approach to obesity. *Nursing Standard, 25*(21), 42–46.

Risk for Overweight*

Marina Martinez-Kratz, MS, RN, CNE

*Previously Risk for imbalanced Nutrition: more than body requirements

NANDA-I

Definition

Vulnerable to abnormal or excessive fat accumulation for age and gender, which may compromise health

Risk Factors

ADULT: Body mass index (BMI) approaching 25 kg/m^2; average daily physical activity is less than recommended for gender and age; CHILD older than 2 years: weight for length approaching 95th percentile; CHILD 2 to 18 years: BMI approaching 85th percentile, or 25 kg/m^2 (whichever is smaller); children who are crossing BMI percentiles upward; children with high BMI percentiles; consumption of sugar-sweetened beverages; disordered eating behaviors (e.g., binge eating, extreme weight control); disordered eating perceptions; eating in response to external cues (e.g., time of day, social situations); eating in response to internal cues other than hunger (e.g., anxiety); economically disadvantaged; energy expenditure below energy intake based on standard assessment (e.g., WAVE [weight, activity, variety in diet, excess]); excessive alcohol consumption; fear regarding lack of food supply; formula- or mixed-fed infants; frequent snacking; genetic disorder; heritability of interrelated factors (e.g., adipose tissue distribution, energy expenditure, lipoprotein lipase activity, lipid synthesis, lipolysis); high disinhibition and restraint eating behavior score; high frequency of eating restaurant or fried food; higher baseline weight at beginning of each pregnancy; low dietary calcium intake in children; maternal diabetes mellitus; maternal smoking; obesity in childhood; parental obesity; portion sizes larger than recommended; premature pubarche; rapid weight gain during childhood; rapid weight gain during infancy, including the first week, first 4 months, and the first year; sedentary behavior occurring for more than 2 hours per day; shortened sleep time; sleep disorder; solid foods as major food sources of less than 5 months of age

Nursing Interventions and *Rationales*

- Assess the meaning and importance of food in the client's life. EB: *Research findings demonstrate that implicit attitudes significantly predict purchases of healthy and unhealthy foods (Prestwich et al, 2011). Research found that youth held some negative associations related to healthy foods and some positive associations linked to unhealthy foods (Harrison & Jackson, 2009).*
- Counsel the client to eat breakfast daily. EB: *Research has determined that skipping breakfast is a lifestyle risk significantly associated with a higher BMI (Ghrayeb et al, 2014).*
- Assess the client with a Patient Readiness Scale to determine if the client is ready to discuss weight loss and/or would like weight loss information. EB: *Readiness to change is an important part of treatment for behavior change (Steele et al, 2012).*
- Assess the client's current nutrition through a 1- to 3-day food diary in which everything ingested orally is recorded. Analyze the following areas:
  - Intake of food and beverage calories and fat
  - Portion sizes

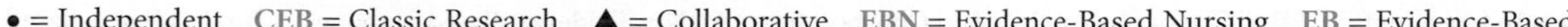

O

- ❍ Underconsumption or overconsumption of nutrients
- ❍ Use of supplements
- ❍ Use of meal replacements
- ❍ Timing/consistency of meals and snacks

▲ EB: *Use of a food diary is helpful for both the client and the nurse, to examine usual foods eaten and patterns of eating (Shay et al, 2009).* EB: *A study found that use of a personal digital assistant for self-monitoring food intake was more effective than use of a paper record, yet both groups had a similar weight loss (Acharya et al, 2011).*

- Counsel the client to measure regularly consumed foods periodically. Help the client learn usual portion sizes. *Measuring food alerts the client to normal portion sizes. Estimating amounts can be extremely inaccurate.* EB: *A study demonstrated that obese people had significantly larger portion sizes, plus ate later in the day (Berg et al, 2009).*
- Assist the client to develop a system of self-management, which may include self-monitoring of weight, BMI and food intake, interpretation of food labels, portion control, recipe modification, restaurant and social food negotiation, and physical activity. *A key component of successful weight loss and maintenance is regular self-monitoring (Fitch et al, 2013).*
- Document the client's height and weight and teach significance of his/her BMI in relationship to current health. *Use a chart or a website such as http://www.cdc.gov/healthyweight/assessing/bmi/index.html (Centers for Disease Control and Prevention, 2015).*
- Assist the client to use Super Tracker (http://www.choosemyplate.gov/food-groups) to determine the number of calories to eat and gain more information on how to eat in a healthy fashion. *To lose weight, the client must eat fewer calories (U.S. Department of Agriculture, 2014).*
- Encourage the client to engage in regular physical activity for at least 150 minutes weekly. EB: *Research found that normal weight reproductive-aged women who do not engage in recommended levels of physical activity are at risk for becoming overweight or obese (Hillemeier et al, 2011). Studies determine that increased physical activity in conjunction with improved eating behavior scores resulted in greater weight loss (Jakicic et al, 2011).*
- Recommend the client eat a healthy breakfast every morning. CEB: *A study found that that people who skip breakfast are more likely to overeat in the evening (Masheb & Grillo, 2006). Another study demonstrated that people who skipped breakfast were 450 times more likely to be obese (Ma et al, 2003).*
- Recommend the client avoid eating in fast food restaurants. CEB: *A 15-year study demonstrated that people who frequently eat fast foods gain an average of 10 lb more than those who eat fast food less often and were two times more likely to develop insulin resistance, which can lead to diabetes (Pereira et al, 2005).*
- Assist the client to reframe slips in weight loss or physical activity behavior as lapses that are a single event and not a full return to previous unhealthy behaviors. *Relapse prevention strategies include managing lapses in healthy behavior, identifying high-risk situations for relapses, enhancing skills for coping, and increasing self-efficacy for avoiding relapse (Fitch et al, 2013).*
- Teach problem-solving strategies to deal with barriers to changing eating and physical activity patterns. *Strategies such as defining the problem, brainstorming solutions, seeking solutions, and evaluating the outcome of the solution are problem-solving strategies that facilitate weight loss (Fitch et al, 2013).*
- Assist clients to engage their social support systems in ways that facilitate weight loss, as well as eating and physical activity behavior change. *Significant others, family, friends, and co-workers can facilitate or hinder weight loss success (Fitch et al, 2013).*
- Assist the client to reframe the goal focus from outcome (weight loss) to process (eating behaviors) for weight loss. EB: *A study of overweight women found that focusing on the process of dieting (the eating behavior) was related to actual weight loss as well as to subjective dieting success (Freund & Hennecke, 2012).*
- Assist the client to develop stimulus control techniques designed to reduce environmental cues associated with eating behaviors. Specifically clients should be taught to limit the presence of high-calorie/high-fat foods in the home; to reduce the visibility of unhealthy food choices in the home; to limit where and when they eat; to avoid distractions like reading, using the computer, or watching television when eating; and to eat more slowly. *Stimulus control strategies are a key to successful weight loss and weight maintenance (Fitch et al, 2013).*

- Use the motivational interviewing technique when working with clients to promote healthy eating and weight loss. EB: *A pilot study with use of motivational interviewing in women found it resulted in a significant weight loss (Low et al, 2012). A review found that use of motivational interviewing was effective in causing weight loss (Armstrong et al, 2011).*
- Refer the client to tailored weight management programs that provide opportunities for ongoing support. CEB: *Tailored weight loss interventions and ongoing support were identified by obese or overweight clients as facilitating longer term weight management (Visram et al, 2009).*
- Refer the client to a weight-loss related therapy group. EBN: *A British study showed that addressing psychological factors associated with eating and weight in a group setting offers an important contribution to the treatment of obesity (Yilmaz, 2011).*
- Recommend that clients use dietary supplements such as vitamins and minerals after consulting with their primary health care provider. EB: *Research shows a prevalence of low micronutrient status in obese individuals who can benefit from safeguarding vitamin and mineral adequacy by taking a multinutrient supplement in conjunction with increased intake of nutrient-rich foods (Ruxton, 2011).*
- Use behavioral methods to control eating behavior, and change habits and mindset. EB: *Behavioral-based treatments are safe and effective for weight loss (LeBlanc et al, 2011).* EB: *A study found that behavior treatment that was done either in person or remotely through computer teaching, email, and the phone resulted in a significant loss of weight for obese clients versus a control group (Appel et al, 2011). A Cochrane review found that behavioral therapy used independently as a stand-alone therapy resulted in significant weight loss (Shaw et al, 2009).*

Pediatric

- Offer obese or overweight adolescents healthy methods for weight loss. EBN: *Research shows that overweight adolescents who demonstrate a desire to lose weight often choose unhealthy methods (Chen et al, 2009).*
- Offer families of obese or overweight children prejudice-free, individually accepting, and supportive interventions to address weight loss. EBN: *Obese children showed signs of stress, stigmatization, and marginalization, while their families reported feeling rejected by health care professionals (Lorentzen et al, 2012).*
- Use motivational interviewing counseling techniques to implement weight loss interventions. EBN: *Obese children treated with motivational interviewing showed significant improvement in their weight-related behavior and obesity-related anthropometric measures (Wong & Cheng, 2013).*
- Recommend that families eat together for at least one meal per day. *Mealtime together has been shown to improve children's eating habits: children eat more fruits and vegetables when the family eats together.*
- Recommend involving the family in planning meals and food preparation. Children can learn about nutrition as they help plan and make meals. *Children are more likely to eat foods that they help select or prepare.*
- Suggest that parents work at being good role models of healthy eating. *Setting a good example is key for children; children learn the value of healthy eating early, and it can continue for a lifetime.*
- Recommend that the family try new foods, either a new food or recipe every week. *More variety can increase the intake of fruits and vegetables.*
- Suggest the parents keep healthy snacks on hand. Store the snacks in a purse, the car, a desk drawer. *Suggestions include crackers and peanut butter, small boxes of cereal, fresh fruit, and vegetables (Academy of Nutrition and Dietetics, 2014).*

Geriatric

- Recognize that it is generally not appropriate to have an older client on a calorie-restrictive diet. *Older clients deserve to eat and not be hungry.* EB: *Strength training and dietary modifications can improve body composition, muscle strength, and physical function in overweight and obese older adults (Straight et al, 2012). Loss of muscle (sarcopenia) occurs with normal aging; when paired with excessive fat, it leads to increased weakness and disability (Jarosz & Bellar, 2009).*
- Observe for socioeconomic factors that influence food choices (e.g., funds, cooking facilities, food insecurity). *Even those on restricted budgets and with limited facilities can be assisted to choose healthy food sources for a balanced diet.* EB: *Food security is a factor that can indicate a need for nutrition assistance in older adults (Lee et al, 2011).*

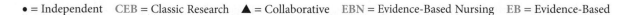

Multicultural

- Tailor nutritional interventions to be consistent with cultural beliefs, norms, and values. CEBN: *Mexican American women responded positively to nutritional education and physical activity promotion when families were involved (Vincent, 2009).*
- Offer tailored lifestyle counseling via the telephone. EB: *Low socioeconomic status African Americans and Latinos experienced positive nutritional change and weight loss after participating in a community-based translational lifestyle program (Kanaya et al, 2012).*
- Integrate weight loss and weight maintenance interventions with church faith based concepts for cultural congruence with African American clients. EB: *Recent research suggests that integrating faith themes into a weight loss maintenance program may increase its long-term impact on participants' health behavior change (Seale et al, 2013).*

Client/Family Teaching and Discharge Planning

- The majority of the preceding interventions involve teaching.
- Work with the family members regarding information on how to support and promote weight loss and healthy intakes.

REFERENCES

Academy of Nutrition and Dietetics (2014). *It's about eating right: nutrition for growing bodies*. From: <http://www.eatright.org/Public/content.aspx?id=6751>. Retrieved September 20, 2014.

Acharya, S. D., Elci, O. U., Sereika, S. M., et al. (2011). Using a personal digital assistant for self-monitoring influences diet quality in comparison to a standard paper record among overweight/obese adults. *Journal of the American Dietetic Association*, *111*(4), 583–588.

Appel, L. J., Clark, J. M., Yeh, H. C., et al. (2011). Comparative effectiveness of weight-loss interventions in clinical practice. *The New England Journal of Medicine*, *365*(21), 1959–1968.

Armstrong, M. J., et al. (2011). Motivational interviewing to improve weight loss in overweight and/or obese patients: a systematic review and meta-analysis of randomized controlled trials. *Obesity Reviews*, *12*(9), 709–723.

Berg, C., Lappas, G., Wolk, A., et al. (2009). Eating patterns and portion size associated with obesity in a Swedish population. *Appetite*, *52*, 21–26.

Centers for Disease Control and Prevention (2015). *Healthy Weight—it's not a diet, it's a lifestyle!* <http://www.cdc.gov/healthyweight/assessing/bmi/index.html>. Retrieved from 6/21/2015.

Chen, M., Fan, J., Jane, S., et al. (2009). Do overweight adolescents perceive the need to reduce weight and take healthy actions? *Journal of Nursing Research (Taiwan Nurses Association)*, *17*(4), 270–277.

Fitch, A., Everling, L., Fox, C., et al. (2013). *Institute for Clinical Systems Improvement. Prevention and Management of Obesity for Adults.*

Freund, A. M., & Hennecke, M. (2012). Changing eating behaviour vs. losing weight: the role of goal focus for weight loss in overweight women. *Psychology & Health*, 2725–2742.

Ghrayeb, F. A., Mohamed Rusli, A., Al Rifai, A., et al. (2014). PUBLIC HEALTH. Prevalence of lifestyle-related risk factors contributing to non-communicable diseases among adolescents in tarqumia, Palestine. *International Medical Journal*, *21*(3), 272–276.

Harrison, M., & Jackson, L. (2009). Meanings that youth associate with healthy and unhealthy food. *Canadian Journal of Dietetic Practice & Research*, *70*(1), 6–12.

Hillemeier, M. M., Weisman, C. S., Chuang, C., et al. (2011). Transition to overweight or obesity among women of reproductive age. *Journal of Women's Health*, *20*(5), 703–710. (15409996).

Jakicic, J. M., Otto, A. D., Lang, W., et al. (2011). The effect of physical activity on 18-month weight change in overweight adults. *Obesity*, *19*, 100–109.

Jarosz, P., & Bellar, A. (2009). Sarcopenic obesity: an emerging cause of frailty in older adults. *Geriatric Nursing*, *30*(1), 64–70.

Kanaya, A. M., Santoyo-Olsson, J., Gregorich, S., et al. (2012). The live well, be well study: a community-based, translational lifestyle program to lower diabetes risk factors in ethnic minority and lower-socioeconomic status adults. *American Journal of Public Health*, *102*(8), 1551–1558.

LeBlanc, E., O'Connor, E., Whitlock, E. P., et al. (2011). *Screening for and management of obesity and overweight in adults. Evidence Report No. 89. AHRQ Publication No. 11-05159-EF-1*. Rockville, MD: Agency for Healthcare Research and Quality.

Lee, J. S., Johnson, M. A., & Brown, A. (2011). Older americans act nutrition program improves participants' food security in Georgia. *Journal of Nutrition in Gerontology & Geriatrics*, *30*(2), 122–139.

Lorentzen, V., Dyeremose, V., & Larsen, B. H. (2012). Severely overweight children and dietary changes—a family perspective. *Journal of Advanced Nursing*, *68*(4), 878–887.

Low, K. G., et al. (2012). Testing the effectiveness of motivational interviewing as a weight reduction strategy for obese cardiac patients: a pilot study. *International Journal of Behavioral Medicine*, Feb 12, [Epub ahead of print].

Ma, Y., et al. (2003). Association between eating patterns and obesity in a free-living U.S. adult population. *American Journal of Epidemiology*, *158*(1), 85–92.

Masheb, R., & Grillo, C. (2006). Eating patterns and breakfast consumption in obese patients with binge eating disorder. *Behaviour Research and Therapy*, *44*(11), 1545–1553.

Pereira, M., et al. (2005). Fast-food habits, weight gain, and insulin resistance (the CARDIA study): 15-year prospective analysis. *Lancet*, *365*(9453), 36.

Prestwich, A., Hurling, R., & Baker, S. (2011). Implicit shopping: Attitudinal determinants of the purchasing of healthy and unhealthy foods. *Psychology & Health*, *26*(7), 875–885.

Ruxton, C. S. (2011). Nutritional implications of obesity and dieting. *Nutrition Bulletin*, *36*(2), 199–211.

Seale, J. P., Fifield, J., Davis-Smith, Y. M., et al. (2013). Developing culturally congruent weight maintenance programs for African American church members. *Ethnicity & Health*, *18*(2), 152–167.

Shaw, K., O'Rourke, A., & Mar, C. (2009). Psychological interventions for overweight or obesity. *Cochrane Database of Systematic Reviews*, (2), CD003818.

Shay, L., Shobert, J., Seibert, D., et al. (2009). Adult weight management: translating research and guidelines into practice. *Journal of the American Academy of Nurse Practitioners, 21*(4), 197–206.

Steele, M. M., Steele, R. G., & Cushing, C. C. (2012). Weighing the pros and cons in family-based pediatric obesity intervention: parent and child decisional balance as a predictor of child outcomes. *Children's Health Care, 41*(1), 43–55.

Straight, C., et al. (2012). Effects of resistance training and dietary changes on physical function and body composition in overweight and obese older adults. *Journal of Physical Activity and Health, 9*(6), 875–883.

U.S. Department of Agriculture (2014). *Weight Management, USDA ChooseMyPlate.gov*. <http://www.choosemyplate.gov/weight-management-calories/weight management/better-choices/amount-calories.html>. Retrieved from WWW 6/21/15.

Vincent, D. (2009). Culturally tailored education to promote lifestyle change in Mexican Americans with type 2 diabetes. *Journal of the American Academy of Nurse Practitioners, 21*(9), 520–527.

Visram, S., Crosland, A., & Cording, H. (2009). Triggers for weight gain and loss among participants in a primary care-based intervention. *British Journal of Community Nursing, 14*(11), 495–501.

Wong, E. M., & Cheng, M. M. (2013). Effects of motivational interviewing to promote weight loss in obese children. *Journal of Clinical Nursing, 22*(17/18), 2519–2530.

Yilmaz, J. (2011). Adopting a psychological approach to obesity. *Nursing Standard, 25*(21), 42–46.

Acute Pain

Maureen F. Cooney, DNP, FNP-BC, Chris Pasero, MS, RN-BC, FAAN, and Denise Sullivan, MSN, ANP-BC

NANDA-I

Definition

An unpleasant sensory and emotional experience associated with actual or potential tissue damage, or described in terms of such damage (International Association for the Study of Pain, 1979); sudden or slow onset of any intensity from mild to severe with an anticipated or predictable end

Defining Characteristics

Appetite change; change in physiological parameter (e.g., blood pressure, heart rate, respiratory rate, oxygen saturation, and end-tidal CO_2); diaphoresis; distraction behavior; evidence of pain using standardized pain behavior checklist for those unable to communicate verbally (e.g., Neonatal Infant Pain Scale, Pain Assessment Checklist for Seniors with Limited Ability to Communicate); expressive behavior (e.g., restlessness, crying, vigilance); facial expression of pain (e.g., eyes lack luster, beaten look, fixed or scattered movement, grimace); guarding behavior; hopelessness; narrowed focus (e.g., time, perception, thought processes, interaction with people and environment); positioning to ease pain; protective behavior; proxy report of pain behavior/activity changes (e.g., family member, caregiver); pupil dilation; self-focused; self-report of intensity using standardized pain scale (e.g., Wong-Baker FACES scale, visual analog scale, numerical rating scale); self-report of pain characteristics using standardized pain instrument (e.g., McGill Pain Questionnaire, Brief Pain Inventory)

Related Factors (r/t)

Biological injury agent (e.g., infection, ischemia, neoplasm); chemical injury agent (e.g., burn, capsaicin, methylene chloride, mustard agent); physical injury agent (e.g., abscess, amputation, burn, cut, heavy lifting, operative procedure, trauma, overtraining)

NOC (Nursing Outcomes Classification)

Suggested NOC Outcomes

Pain Control; Pain Level; Pain: Adverse Psychological Response

Example NOC Outcome

Pain Level as evidenced by severity of observed or reported pain.

NOTE: **Pain Level** is the NOC Outcome label; this text recommends use of the self-report numerical pain rating scale in place of the NOC indicator scales because of the amount of research supporting its use.

P

Client Outcomes

Client Will (Specify Time Frame)

For the client who is able to provide a self-report

- Use a self-report pain tool to identify current pain intensity level and establish a comfort-function goal
- Report that pain management regimen achieves comfort-function goal without side effects
- Describe nonpharmacological methods that can be used to help achieve comfort-function goal
- Perform activities of recovery or activities of daily living (ADLs) easily
- Describe how unrelieved pain will be managed
- State ability to obtain sufficient amounts of rest and sleep
- Notify member of the health care team promptly for pain intensity level that is consistently greater than the comfort-function goal, or occurrence of side effects

For the client who is unable to provide a self-report

- Decrease in pain-related behaviors
- Perform activities of recovery or ADLs easily as determined by client condition
- Demonstrate the absence of side effects of analgesics
- No pain-related behaviors will be evident in the client who is completely unresponsive; a reasonable outcome is to demonstrate the absence of side effects related to the prescribed pain treatment plan

NIC (Nursing Interventions Classification)

Suggested NIC Interventions

Analgesic Administration; Pain Management; Patient-Controlled Analgesia (PCA) Assistance

Example NIC Activities—Pain Management

Ensure client attentive analgesic care; Perform a comprehensive assessment of pain to include location, characteristics, onset/duration, frequency, quality, intensity or severity of pain, and precipitating factors

Nursing Interventions and *Rationales*

P

- During the initial assessment and interview, if the client is experiencing pain, conduct and document a comprehensive pain assessment, using appropriate pain assessment tools. CEB: *Determining location, temporal aspects, pain intensity, characteristics, and the impact of pain on function and quality of life are critical to determine the underlying cause of pain and effectiveness of treatment (McCaffery, 1968; McCaffery et al, 2011). The initial assessment includes all pain information that the client can provide for the development of the individualized pain management plan (McCaffery et al, 2011).* Implement or request orders to implement pain management interventions to achieve a satisfactory level of comfort. Components of this initial assessment include location, quality, onset/duration, temporal profile, intensity, aggravating and alleviating factors, and effects of pain on function and quality of life. **(Please refer to the Hierarchy of Pain Measures presented later for assessment approach in clients who are unable to provide self-report of pain.)**
- Assess if the client is able to provide a self-report of pain intensity, and if so, assess pain intensity level using a valid and reliable self-report pain tool, such as the 0-10 numerical pain rating scale. CEB: *Self-report is considered the single most reliable indicator of pain presence and intensity and single-dimension pain ratings are valid and reliable as measures of pain intensity level (McCaffery et al, 2011).* EB: *Regularly and routinely assess the client for pain presence during activity and rest and with interventions or procedures likely to cause pain.* CEB: *Acute pain should be reliably assessed both at rest (important for comfort) and during movement (important for function and decreased client risk for cardiopulmonary and thromboembolic events) (McCaffery et al, 2011).*
- Ask the client to describe prior experiences with pain, effectiveness of pain management interventions, responses to analgesic medications including occurrence of side effects, and concerns about pain and its treatment (e.g., fear about addiction, worries, or anxiety) and informational needs. EBN: *Obtaining an individualized pain history helps identify potential factors that may influence the client's willingness to report pain, as well as factors that may influence pain intensity, the client's response to pain, anxiety, and pharmacokinetics of analgesics (Pasero 2009a; Pasero & Portenoy, 2011).*
- Using a self-report pain tool, ask the client to identify a comfort-function goal that will allow the client to perform necessary or desired activities easily. EBN: *The comfort-function goal provides the basis for*

individualized pain management plans and assists in determining effectiveness of pain management interventions (McCaffery et al, 2011).

▲ Describe the adverse effects of unrelieved pain. CEB/EBN: *Unrelieved acute pain can have physiological and psychological consequences that facilitate negative client outcomes. Ineffective management of acute pain has the potential for neurohumoral changes, neuronal remodeling, an impact on immune function, and long-lasting physiological, psychological, and emotional distress, and it may lead to persistent pain syndromes (Pasero, 2011; Pasero & Portenoy, 2011).*

• Use the Hierarchy of Pain Measures as a framework for pain assessment (McCaffery et al, 2011): (1) attempt to obtain the client's self-report of pain; (2) consider the client's condition and search for possible causes of pain (e.g., presence of tissue injury, pathological conditions, or exposure to procedures/interventions that are thought to result in pain); (3) observe for behaviors that may indicate pain presence (e.g., facial expressions, crying, restlessness, and changes in activity); (4) evaluate physiological indicators, with the understanding that these are the least sensitive indicators of pain and may be related to conditions other than pain (e.g., shock, hypovolemia, anxiety); and (5) conduct an analgesic trial. EBN: *When a client is unable to use a self-report tool (e.g., cognitively impaired, critically ill, anesthetized or sedated), the presence of pain may be assessed by observing specific client behaviors using a valid and reliable behavioral tool (e.g., Critical Care Observation Tool in critically ill or Checklist of Nonverbal Pain Indicators in cognitively impaired older adults) (Puntillo et al, 2014; McCaffery et al, 2011). In a study involving turning of neurocritically ill clients after elective brain surgery, self-report was obtained when possible, behaviors were found to be valid indicators of pain, and fluctuations in vital signs suggested the presence of pain, but their validity for such use was not supported, suggesting they should only be used in combination with other validated pain assessment tools (Kapoustina et al, 2014).*

• Assume that pain is present if the client is unable to provide a self-report and has tissue injury, a pathological condition, or has undergone a procedure that is thought to produce pain, and conduct an analgesic trial. CEB: *Pain is associated with actual or potential tissue damage such as pathological conditions (e.g., cancer) and procedures (e.g., surgery or trauma, fractures). In the absence of self-report (e.g., anesthetized, critically ill, or cognitively impaired client), the health care provider should use clinical judgment and assume pain is present, then implement pain management interventions accordingly (McCaffery et al, 2011).*

▲ Obtain and review an accurate and complete list of medications the client is taking or has taken. EB: *Accurate medication reconciliation can guide analgesic plan development and prevent errors associated with incorrect medications, dosages, omission of components of the home medication regimen, drug-drug interactions, and toxicity that can occur when incompatible drugs are combined or when allergies are present (Ignatavicius, 2013; Pasero et al, 2011b).*

P

▲ Explain to the client the pain management approach, including pharmacological and nonpharmacological interventions, the assessment and reassessment process, potential side effects, and the importance of prompt reporting of unrelieved pain. EB: *One of the most important steps toward improved control of pain is a better client understanding of the nature of pain, its treatment, and the role the client needs to play in pain control (Ignatavicius, 2013).*

▲ Manage acute pain using a multimodal approach. EB: *A multimodal approach (combining two or more drugs that act by different mechanisms for providing analgesia) enhances pain relief and allows the lowest effective dose of each drug to be administered, resulting in fewer or less severe side effects, such as nausea, sedation, and respiratory depression (Pasero et al, 2011c).*

▲ Select the route for administration of analgesics based upon client condition and pain characteristics. EB: *Routes have different rates of onset and duration. Oral route is preferred because of its convenience and the relatively steady blood levels that can result; the rectal route may be used when the oral route is not feasible; the IV route is preferred for rapid control of severe pain and would therefore not generally be used for chronic pain; intramuscular injections are avoided due to variable absorption and the potential for nerve injury and tissue damage (Pasero et al, 2011c).*

▲ Provide perineural infusions and intraspinal analgesia when appropriate and available. CEBN: *Superior analgesia can be provided through regional analgesic techniques compared with systemic opioids (Nishimori et al, 2012).*

▲ Use diverse analgesic delivery methods such as PCA to increase client's satisfaction with pain management, to lower cost, and to decrease occurrence of adverse reactions. EBN: *Intravenous PCA provides superior analgesia compared to intravenous injection in the first 12 hours after total hysterectomy (Hong & Lee, 2014).*

- ▲ Administer a nonopioid analgesic for mild to moderate pain and add an opioid analgesic if indicated for moderate to severe acute pain. EB: *Nonopioids, such as acetaminophen and nonsteroidal anti-inflammatory drugs, are first-line analgesics for the treatment of mild and some moderate acute pain, while opioids are included for the treatment of moderate to severe acute pain (Pasero et al, 2011a; Young & Buvanendran, 2012).*
- • Administer analgesics around-the-clock for continuous pain (expected to be present approximately 50% of the day, such as postoperative pain) and PRN (as needed) for intermittent or breakthrough pain. CEB: *If pain is present most of the day, the use of PRN medications alone will lead to periods of undermedication and poor pain control and periods of excessive medication and adverse effects (Pasero, 2010).*
- • Prevent pain by administering analgesia before painful procedures whenever possible (e.g., endotracheal suctioning, wound care, heel puncture, venipunctures, and peripherally inserted intravenous catheters). EB: *Adult clients in the intensive care setting experience numerous sources of procedural pain and chest tube removal, wound drain removal, and arterial line insertion are identified as the most painful procedures (Puntillo et al, 2014). The use of topical lidocaine 1% before removal of extremity vacuum-assisted closure wound dressings results in reduced pain and opioid use (Christensen et al, 2013).*
- • Administer supplemental analgesic doses as ordered to keep the client's pain level at or below the comfort-function goal, or desired outcome based on clinical judgment or behaviors if client is unable to provide a self-report. EB: *An order for PRN supplemental analgesic doses between regular doses is essential in providing comprehensive pain management (Pasero et al, 2011c).*
- • Perform nursing care during the peak effect of analgesics to optimize client comfort and participation in care. CEB: *Providing care such as mobilization and bathing should be performed when analgesics have reached peak effect: oral medications peak in 60 minutes, subcutaneous opioids in 30 minutes, and intravenous analgesics in 15 to 30 minutes (McCaffery et al, 2011; Pasero et al, 2011c).*
- ▲ Discuss the client's fears of undertreated pain, side effects, and addiction. EBN: *Cogan et al (2014) report that among 379 clients scheduled for cardiac surgery, 31% stated that it is easy to become addicted to pain medication, 20% report that "good patients" do not talk about their pain, and 35% believe that pain medication should be "saved in case the pain worsens."*
- • The assessment of clients with acute pain on opioids should be done at regular intervals and include frequent assessment of pain level, assessment of respiratory status (including rate, rhythm, noisiness, depth), and systematic assessment of sedation level using a sedation scale (Pasero, 2009b). EB: *Opioid induced respiratory depression occurs with the greatest frequency in postoperative clients during the first 24 hours after surgery, and factors contributing to postoperative respiratory depression include the intervention of multiple prescribers (33%), concurrent administration of nonopioid sedating medications (34%), and inadequate nursing assessments or response (31%) (ASA, 2012; Jarzyna et al, 2011; Lee et al, 2015).*
- ▲ Provide the client with a stool softener and stimulant to prevent/treat opioid related constipation, and ask about other opioid related side effects including nausea, pruritus, lack of appetite, and changes in rest and sleep. EB: *In a study of postoperative orthopedic clients, more than half of the clients experienced one or more opioid related side effects including constipation, nausea, emesis, pruritus, and confusion, and the presence of side effects was associated with increased length of stay (Pizzi et al, 2012).*
- • Review the client's pain flow sheet and medication administration record to evaluate effectiveness of pain relief, previous 24-hour opioid requirements, and occurrence of side effects. EBN: *Systematic tracking of pain is an important factor in improving pain management and making adjustments to the pain management regimen (McCaffery et al, 2011).*
- • Advocate for the use of "as needed" opioid range orders to provide effective and appropriate pain relief. EB: *Correctly prescribed range orders for the delivery of intravenous opioids give nurses the flexibility needed to treat clients' pain in a timely manner while allowing for differences in client response to pain and to analgesia (Pasero et al, 2011c).*
- • Choose analgesic and dose based on orders that reflect the client's report of pain severity and response to the previous dose in terms of pain relief, occurrence of side effects, and ability to perform the activities of recovery or ADLs. EB: *Safe and effective pain management requires opioid dose adjustment based on individualized adequate pain and sedation assessment, opioid administration, and evaluation of the response to treatment (Ignatavicius, 2013).*
- ▲ When converting opioids from parenteral doses to oral doses (the preferred route when the client can tolerate and absorb oral medications), use equianalgesic dosing charts and carefully monitor the client's

P

response to the new medication route and dose. EBN: *Equianalgesic dosing calculations should be used cautiously to guide dose conversion of an opioid from one route to another to avoid the toxicity associated with overdosing and the inadequate pain control due to underdosing (Shaheen et al, 2009).*
- Support the client's use of nonpharmacological methods to supplement pharmacological analgesic approaches to help control pain, such as distraction, imagery, music therapy, simple massage, relaxation, and application of heat and cold. EBN: *Although more evidence is needed to conclude effectiveness, nonpharmacological methods (which are low cost and low risk) can be used to complement pharmacological treatment of pain (Gelinas & Arbour, 2009; Ignatavicius, 2013).*
- Assist client to identify resources for coping with psychological impact of pain. EBN: *Cognitive-behavioral (mind-body) strategies can restore the client's sense of self-control, personal efficacy, and active participation in his or her own care (Bruckenthal, 2010).*
- Teach and implement nonpharmacological interventions when pain is relatively well controlled with pharmacological interventions. EB: *Pain causes cognitive impairment (Moriarty et al, 2011; Pasero et al, 2011a).*

Pediatric

- Assess for the presence of pain using a valid and reliable pain scale based on age, cognitive development, and the child's ability to provide a self-report. EBN: *Scales that depict faces at various levels of pain intensity are commonly used in young children and have been shown to be reliable and valid in children as young as 3 years old (Oakes, 2011).* EB: *Behavioral tools such as the FLACC Scale may be used to assess pain in infants and children who cannot provide a self-report (Crellin et al, 2015).*

▲ Administer prescribed analgesics using a multimodal approach to treat pain in children, infants, and neonates. EB: *PCA may be used by children as young as 4 years of age, and intraspinal and perineural analgesic techniques may be used for major surgical procedures (Oakes, 2011).*

- Prevent procedural pain in neonates, infants, and children by using opioid analgesics and anesthetics, as indicated, in appropriate dosages. EBN: *Czarnecki et al (2011) found that several barriers exist to the treatment of procedural pain in children including insufficient medication orders before procedures, insufficient time to premedicate children before procedures, the perception of low priority given to pain management by medical staff, and parents' reluctance to have their children medicated.*
- Use a topical local anesthetic such as *eutectic* mixture of local anesthetics (EMLA) cream or LMX-4 before performing venipuncture in neonates, infants, and children. EBN: *The use of EMLA with prolonged application time for pediatric venipuncture in the emergency department results in improved venipuncture success and reduced pain (Baxter et al, 2013).*
- For the neonate, use oral sucrose and nonnutritional sucking (NNS) or human milk for pain of short duration such as heel stick or venipuncture. Neonates, especially preterm neonates, are more sensitive to pain than older children. EBN: *In an integrated literature review, Naughton (2013) found that the combination of oral sucrose and NNS is a safe and effective method of relieving pain in neonates and increases the calming effect in infants undergoing painful procedures.*
- Recognize that breastfeeding has been shown to reduce behavioral indicators of pain. EB: *Breastfeeding has not been shown to have a better analgesic effect than sucrose in late preterm infants (Simonse et al, 2012).*

As with adults, use nonpharmacological analgesic interventions to supplement, not replace, pharmacological interventions in pediatric clients. EB: *Heel pain associated with lancet heel sticks in preterm newborns was shown to provide greater reduction in pain scores when pharmacological methods (fentanyl injections) were combined with nonpharmacological techniques (sensory saturation) (Gitto et al, 2012).* CEB: *Complementary therapies such as relaxation, distraction, hypnotics, art therapies, and imagery may play an important role in holistic pain management (Oakes, 2011). Nonpharmacological interventions reduce procedure-related distress (Oakes, 2011).*

Geriatric

- Refer to the Nursing Interventions and *Rationales* in the care plan for Chronic **Pain.**

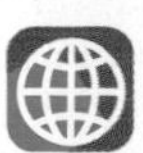

Multicultural

- Refer to the Nursing Interventions and *Rationales* in the care plan for Chronic **Pain.**

P

Home Care

▲ Develop the treatment plan with the client and caregivers. EB: *Client education and motivation play important roles in self-management of clients with pain. Self-management is influenced by client-provider communication (Dorflinger et al, 2013).*

▲ Assess the client's full medication profile, including medications prescribed by all health care providers and all over-the-counter medications for drug interactions, and instruct the client to refrain from mixing medications without health care provider approval. EB: *Pain medications may significantly affect or be affected by other medications and may cause severe side effects; in a study of diabetic pregabalin and duloxetine users, potential duloxetine drug-drug interactions and drug-condition interactions were associated with significant increases in mean health care costs (Johnston et al, 2013).*

▲ Assess the client/family's knowledge of side effects and safety precautions associated with pain medications. EB: *Educational activities related to pain medications are necessary to ensure that clients are knowledgeable about opioid side effects and safety. McCarthy et al (2015) found that clients who were read and given a one page information sheet about hydrocodone-acetaminophen safety had better knowledge of precautions related to acetaminophen dosing, and were less likely to drive a car within 6 hours of taking the medication than those who did not receive this educational intervention.*

- If medication is administered using highly technological methods, assess the home for the necessary resources (e.g., electricity) and ensure that there will be responsible caregivers available to assist the client with administration. EB: *With appropriate assessment of home resources, it is possible to provide home management of clients with complex pain management technologies as demonstrated in a study of children with cleft palate repair who received home infusion of local anesthetic via peripheral nerve block catheter (Visoiu, 2014).*
- Assess the knowledge base of the client and family with regard to highly technological medication administration and provide necessary education, including the procedure to follow if analgesia is unsatisfactory. EB: *With appropriate education and training, outpatient families can successfully manage infusions of local anesthetics through peripheral nerve catheters for analgesia in clients recovering from cleft palate surgery (Visoiu, 2014).*

P

Client/Family Teaching and Discharge Planning

NOTE: To avoid the negative connotations associated with the words "drugs" and "narcotics," use the term "pain medicine" when teaching clients.

- Discuss the various discomforts encompassed by the word "pain" and ask the client to give examples of previously experienced pain. Explain the pain assessment process and the purpose of the pain rating scale. CEB: *It is often difficult for clients to understand the concept of pain and describe their pain experience. Using alternative words and providing a complete description of the assessment process, including the use of scales, ensures that an accurate treatment plan is developed (McCaffery et al, 2011).*
- Teach the client to use the self-report pain tool to rate the intensity of past or current pain. Ask the client to set a comfort-function goal by selecting a pain level on the self-report tool that will allow performance of desired or necessary activities of recovery with relative ease (e.g., turn, cough, deep breathe, ambulate, participate in physical therapy). If the pain level is consistently above the comfort-function goal, the client should take action that decreases pain or notify a member of the health care team so that effective pain management interventions may be implemented promptly. CEB: *The use of comfort-function goals provides the basis for the direction and modification of the treatment plan (McCaffery et al, 2011).*
- Provide written educational materials on various aspects of pain control to improve client understanding of pain and pain-related interventions. EB: *Written materials and other educational tools assist in improving clients' knowledge related to pain management. In knee replacement clients, the use of an educational pamphlet and a compact disc was associated with decreased postoperative pain and increased participation in physical rehabilitation (Chen et al, 2014).*
- Discuss and evaluate the client's understanding about the total plan for pharmacological and nonpharmacological treatment, including the medication plan for around-the-clock administration and supplemental doses, and the use of supplies and equipment. CEB: *Appropriate instruction increases the accuracy and safety of medication administration (Pasero et al, 2011b).*

- Teach basic principles of pain management using a variety of educational strategies, and evaluate learning. EB: *Client educational strategies that have been shown to increase knowledge, decrease anxiety, and increase satisfaction include the use of computer technology, audio and videotapes, written materials, and demonstrations, or combinations of these strategies (Friedman et al, 2011).*
- ▲ Reinforce the importance of taking pain medications to maintain the comfort-function goal. CEB: *Teaching clients to stay on top of their pain and prevent it from getting out of control will improve the ability to accomplish the goals of recovery (McCaffery et al, 2011).*
- ▲ Reinforce that taking opioids for pain relief is not addiction and that addiction is very unlikely to occur. CEB: *The development of addiction when opioids are taken for pain relief is rare (Pasero et al, 2011c).*
- ▲ Demonstrate the use of appropriate nonpharmacological approaches in addition to pharmacological approaches to help control pain, such as application of heat and/or cold, distraction techniques, relaxation breathing, visualization, rocking, stroking, listening to music, and watching television. CEB: *Nonpharmacological interventions are used to complement, not replace, pharmacological interventions (Bruckenthal, 2010).*

REFERENCES

American Society of Anesthesiologists (ASA). (2012). Practice guidelines for acute pain management in the perioperative setting. An updated report by the American society of anesthesiologists task force on acute pain management. *Anesthesiology, 116*, 248–273.

Baxter, A. L., Ewing, P. H., Young, G. B., et al. (2013). EMLA application exceeding two hours improves pediatric emergency department venipuncture success. *Advanced emergency nursing journal, 35*(1), 67–75.

Bruckenthal, P. (2010). Integrating nonpharmacologic and alternative strategies into a comprehensive management approach for older adults with pain. *Pain Management Nursing, 11*(2), S23–S31.

Chen, S. R., Chen, C. S., & Lin, P. C. (2014). The effect of educational intervention on the pain and rehabilitation performance of patients who undergo a total knee replacement. *Journal of Clinical Nursing, 23*(1–2), 279–287.

Christensen, T. J., Thorum, T., & Kubiak, E. (2013). Lidocaine analgesia for removal of wound vacuum-assisted closure dressings: a randomized double-blinded placebo-controlled trial. *Journal of Orthopedic Trauma, 27*(2), 107–112.

Cogan, J., Ouimette, M. F., Vargas-Schaffe, G., et al. (2014). Patient attitudes and beliefs regarding pain medication after cardiac surgery: barriers to adequate pain management. *Pain Management Nursing, 15*(3), 574–579.

Crellin, D. J., Harrison, D., Santamaria, N., et al. (2015). Systematic review of the face, legs, activity, cry, and consolability scale for assessing pain in infants and children: Is it reliable, valid and feasible for use? *Pain, 156*(11), 2132132–2132151.

Czarnecki, M. L., Simon, K., Thompson, J. J., et al. (2011). Barriers to pediatric pain management: a nursing perspective. *Pain Management Nursing, 12*(3), 154–162.

Dorflinger, L., Kerns, R. D., & Auerbach, S. M. (2013). Providers' roles in enhancing patients' adherence to pain self management. *Translational behavioral medicine, 3*(1), 39–46.

Friedman, A. J., Cosby, R., Boyko, S., et al. (2011). Effective teaching strategies and methods of delivery for patient education: a systematic review and practice guideline recommendations. *Journal of Cancer Education, 26*(1), 12–21.

Gelinas, C., & Arbour, C. (2009). Behavioral and physiologic indicators during a nociceptive procedure in conscious and unconscious mechanically ventilated patients: similar or different? *Journal of Critical Care, 24*(4), 7–17.

Gelinas, C., Arbour, C., Michaud, C., et al. (2013). Patients and ICU nurses' perspectives of nonpharmacological interventions for pain management. *Nursing in Critical Care, 18*(6), 307–318.

Gitto, E., Pellegrino, S., Manfrida, M., et al. (2012). Stress response and procedural pain in the preterm newborn: the role of pharmacological and nonpharmacological treatments. *European Journal of Pediatrics, 171*(6), 927–933.

Hong, S.-J., & Lee, E. (2014). Comparing effects of intravenous patient-controlled analgesia and intravenous injection in patients who have undergone total hysterectomy. *Journal of Clinical Nursing, 23*, 967–975.

Ignatavicius, D. (2013). Pain-the 5th vital sign. In D. Ignatavicius & M. L. Workman (Eds.), *Medical-Surgical Nursing: Patient-Centered Collaborative Care* (7th ed., pp. 39–64). St. Louis, MO: W.B. Saunders Company.

International Association for the Study of Pain. (1979). Pain terms: a list with definitions and notes on usage. *Pain, 6*(3), 249–252.

Jarzyna, D., et al. (2011). American society for pain management nursing evidence-based consensus guideline on monitoring of opioid-induced sedation and respiratory depression. *Pain Management Nursing, 12*(3), 118–145.

Johnston, S. S., Udall, M., Cappelleri, J. C., et al. (2013). Cost comparison of drug–drug and drug–condition interactions in patients with painful diabetic peripheral neuropathy treated with pregabalin versus duloxetine. *American Journal of Health-System Pharmacy, 70*(24), 2207–2217

Kapoustina, O., Echegaray-Benites, C., & Gelinas, C. (2014). Fluctuations in vital signs and behavioral responses of brain surgery patients in the intensive care unit: are they valid indicators of pain? *Journal of Advanced Nursing, 70*(11), 2562–2576.

Lee, L. A., Caplan, R. A., Stephens, L. S., et al. (2015). Postoperative opioid-induced respiratory depression: a closed claims analysis. *Anesthesiology, 122*(3), 659–665.

McCaffery, M. (1968). *Nursing practice theories related to cognition, bodily pain, and man-environment interactions.* Los Angeles: University of California at Los Angeles Students' Store.

McCaffery, M., Herr, K., & Pasero, C. (2011). Assessment. In C. Pasero & M. McCaffery (Eds.), *Pain assessment and pharmacologic management* (p. 13176). St Louis: Mosby Elsevier.

McCarthy, D. M., Wolf, M. S., McConnell, R., et al. (2015). Improving patient knowledge and safe use of opioids: a randomized controlled trial. *Academic emergency medicine, 22*(3), 331–339.

Moriarty, O., McGuire, B. E., & Finn, D. P. (2011). The effect of pain on cognitive function: a review of clinical and preclinical research. *Progress in Neurobiology, 93*(3), 385–404.

Naughton, K. A. (2013). The combined use of sucrose and nonnutritive sucking for procedural pain in both term and preterm neonates: an

P

integrative review of the literature. *Advances in Neonatal Care, 13*(1), 9–19.
Nishimori, M., Low, J. H. S., Zheng, H., et al. (2012). Epidural pain relief versus systemic opioid-based pain relief for abdominal aortic surgery. *Cochrane Database of Systematic Reviews*, (7), CD005059.
Oakes, L. (2011). *Compact clinical guide to infant and child pain management*. New York: Springer.
Pasero, C. (2009a). Challenges in pain assessment. *Journal of Perianesthesia Nursing, 24*(1), 50–54.
Pasero, C. (2009b). Assessment of sedation during opioid administration for pain management. *Journal of Perianesthesia Nursing, 24*(3), 186–190.
Pasero, C. (2010). Around-the-clock analgesic dosing. *Journal of Perianesthesia Nursing, 25*(1), 36–39.
Pasero, C. (2011). Persistent post-surgical and post-trauma pain. *Journal of Perianesthesia Nursing, 26*(1), 38–41.
Pasero, C., & Portenoy, R. K. (2011). Neurophysiology of pain and analgesia and the pathophysiology of neuropathic pain. In C. Pasero & M. McCaffery (Eds.), *Pain assessment and pharmacologic management*. St Louis: Mosby/Elsevier.
Pasero, C., Portenoy, R. K., & McCaffery, M. (2011a). Nonopioid analgesics. In C. Pasero & M. McCaffery (Eds.), *Pain assessment and pharmacologic management*. St Louis: Mosby Elsevier.
Pasero, C., et al. (2011b). Adjuvant analgesics. In C. Pasero & M. McCaffery (Eds.), *Pain assessment and pharmacologic management*. St Louis: Mosby Elsevier.
Pasero, C., et al. (2011c). Opioid analgesics. In C. Pasero & M. McCaffery (Eds.), *Pain assessment and pharmacologic management*. St Louis: Mosby Elsevier.
Pizzi, L. T., Toner, R., Foley, K., et al. (2012). Relationship between potential opioid-related adverse effects and hospital length of stay in patients receiving opioids after orthopedic surgery. Pharmacotherapy. *The Journal of Human Pharmacology and Drug Therapy, 32*(6), 502–514.
Puntillo, K. A., Max, A., Timsit, J.-F., et al. (2014). Determinants of procedural pain intensity in the intensive care unit. The European study. *American Journal of Respiratory and Critical Care Medicine, 189*(1), 39–47.
Shaheen, P. E., Walsh, D., Lasheen, W., et al. (2009). Opioid equianalgesic tables: are they all equally dangerous? *Journal of Pain and Symptom Management, 38*(3), 409–417.
Simonse, E., Mulder, P. G., & Van Beek, R. H. (2012). Analgesic effect of breast milk versus sucrose for analgesia during heel lance in late preterm infants. *Pediatrics, 129*(4), 657–663.
Visoiu, M. (2014). Outpatient analgesia via paravertebral peripheral nerve block catheter and On-Q pump—a case series. *Pediatric Anesthesia, 24*(8), 875–878.
Young, A., & Buvanendran, A. (2012). Recent advances in multimodal analgesia. *Anesthesiology Clinics, 30*(1), 91–100.

P

Chronic Pain

Maureen F. Cooney, DNP, FNP-BC, Denise Sullivan, MSN, ANP-BC, and Chris Pasero, MS, RN-BC, FAAN

NANDA-I

Definition

Unpleasant sensory and emotional experience associated with actual or potential tissue damage, or described in terms of such damage (International Association for the Study of Pain, 1979); sudden or slow onset of any intensity from mild to severe, constant or recurring without an anticipated or predictable end and a duration of greater than 3 months

Defining Characteristics

Alteration in ability to continue previous activities; alteration in sleep pattern; anorexia; evidence of pain using standardized pain behavior checklist for those unable to communicate verbally (e.g., Neonatal Infant Pain Scale, Pain Assessment Checklist for Seniors with Limited Ability to Communicate); facial expression of pain (e.g., eyes lack luster, beaten look, fixed or scattered movement, grimace); proxy report of pain behavior/activity changes (e.g., family member, caregiver); self-focused; self-report of intensity using standardized pain scale (e.g., Wong-Baker FACES scale, visual analog scale, numerical rating scale); self-report of pain characteristics using standardized pain instrument (e.g., McGill Pain Questionnaire, Brief Pain Inventory)

Related Factors (r/t)

Age older than 50 years; alteration in sleep pattern; chronic musculoskeletal condition; contusion; crush injury; damage to the nervous system; emotional distress; fatigue; female gender; fracture; genetic disorder; history of abuse (e.g., physical, psychological, sexual); history of genital mutilation; history of indebtedness; history of static work postures; history of substance abuse; history of vigorous exercise; imbalance of neurotransmitters, neuromodulators, and receptors; immune disorder (e.g., HIV-associated neuropathy, varicella-zoster virus); impaired metabolic functioning; increase in body mass index; ineffective sexuality pattern; injury agent (may be present, but not required; pain may be of unknown etiology); ischemic condition; malnutrition; muscle injury; nerve compression; post-trauma related condition (e.g., infection, inflammation); prolonged computer use (>20 hours/week); prolonged increase in cortisol level; repeated handling of heavy loads; social isolation; spinal cord injury; tumor infiltration; whole-body vibration

NOC (Nursing Outcomes Classification)

Suggested NOC Outcomes

Comfort Level; Pain Control; Pain: Disruptive Effects; Pain Level

Example NOC Outcome with Indicators

Pain Level as evidenced by use of a numerical pain rating scale, asking the client to rate the level of pain from 0 to 10. Self-report is considered the single most reliable indicator of pain presence and intensity (American Pain Society [APS], 2008; McCaffery et al, 2011)

NOTE: **Pain Level** is the NOC Outcome label; this text recommends use of the self-report numerical pain rating scale in place of the NOC indicator scales because of the amount of research supporting its use.

Client Outcomes

Client Will (Specify Time Frame)

For the client who is able to provide a self-report

- Provide a description of the pain experience including physical, social, emotional, and spiritual aspects
- Use a self-report pain tool to identify current pain level and establish a comfort-function goal
- Report that the pain management regimen achieves comfort-function goal without the occurrence of side effects
- Describe nonpharmacological methods that can be used to supplement, or enhance, pharmacological interventions and help achieve the comfort-function goal
- Perform necessary or desired activities at a pain level less than or equal to the comfort-function goal
- Demonstrate the ability to pace activity, taking rest breaks before they are needed
- Describe how unrelieved pain will be managed
- State the ability to obtain sufficient amounts of rest and sleep
- Notify a member of the health care team for pain level consistently greater than the comfort-function goal or occurrence of side effect

For the client who is unable to provide a self-report

- Demonstrate decrease or resolved pain-related behaviors
- Perform desired activities as determined by client condition
- Demonstrate the absence of side effects
- No pain-related behaviors will be evident in the client who is completely unresponsive; a reasonable outcome is to demonstrate the absence of side effects related to the prescribed pain treatment plan

NIC (Nursing Interventions Classification)

Suggested NIC Interventions

Analgesic Administration; Pain Management

Example NIC Activities—Pain Management

Ensure that the client receives attentive analgesic care; Perform comprehensive assessment of pain, including location, characteristics, onset and duration, frequency, quality, intensity or severity, and precipitating factors

Nursing Interventions and *Rationales*

- ▲ During the initial assessment and interview, if the client is experiencing pain, conduct and document a comprehensive pain assessment, using appropriate pain assessment tools. EBN: *Determining location, temporal aspects, pain intensity, characteristics, and the impact of pain on function and quality of life are critical to determine the underlying cause of pain and effectiveness of treatment (McCaffery et al, 2011).*
- ▲ Determine the quality of the pain and whether the pain has persisted beyond the usual duration for tissue healing. EB: *Chronic pain is persistent, lasting beyond the expected time or usual time of tissue healing (usually 3 months). Descriptors such as "sharp," "shooting," or "burning" assist in discriminating neuropathic pain from nociceptive pain (Linl et al, 2011; McCaffery et al, 2011).* **Please refer to the acute Pain section for the Hierarchy of Pain Measures for assessment approach in clients who are unable to provide self-report of pain.**
- ▲ Assess pain intensity level in a client using valid and reliable self-report pain tools, such as the 0-10 numerical pain rating scale (NRS), pain relief scale (PRS), or chronic pain grade scale. EB: *Lee et al (2014) report that the NRS together with the PRS increased the objectivity of pain assessment in chronic spinal pain compared to the use of either scale alone.*
- ▲ Ask the client to describe prior experiences with pain, effectiveness of pain management interventions, responses to analgesic medications including occurrence of side effects, and concerns about pain and its treatment (e.g., fear about addiction, worries, or anxiety) and informational needs. EB: *Pain management regimens must be individualized to the client and consider medical, psychological, and physical condition; age; level of fear or anxiety; client goals and preference; and previous response to analgesics (Pasero et al, 2011a).*
- • Using a self-report tool, ask the client to identify a comfort-function goal that will allow the client to perform necessary or desired activities easily. EBN: *The comfort-function goal provides the basis for individualized pain management plans and assists in determining effectiveness of pain management interventions (McCaffery et al, 2011).* Assess the client for the presence of acute pain (see care plan for Acute **Pain**).
- ▲ Assess chronic pain regularly including the impact of chronic pain on activity, sleep, eating habits, social conditions including relationships, finances, and employment. CEB: *Regular assessment of clients with chronic pain is critical because changes in the underlying pain condition, presence of comorbidities, and changes in psychosocial circumstances can affect pain intensity and characteristics and require revision of the pain management plan (Chou et al, 2009).*
- ▲ Assess the client for the presence of psychiatric conditions, including anxiety and depression. EB: *Among chronic pain clients, 30% to 50% have been found to have depression as a comorbidity, and there is a fourfold higher risk of suicide attempt than in the general population (Breivik et al, 2014). Nearly half of chronic pain clients screen positive for anxiety disorders (Kroenke, 2013).*
- ▲ If opioid therapy is considered, assist the provider with aspects of an opioid risk assessment, which includes a comprehensive client interview and examination with a pain focus, mental health screening, use of an opioid risk assessment tool, examination of prescription drug monitoring program results, and urine drug screening. EB: *There is evidence of opioid misuse, abuse, and addiction among chronic noncancer pain clients with varying prevalence rates thus reduce risk and optimize safe opioid use, risk assessment and stratification is recommended (Cheatle & Barker, 2014; Chou et al, 2014).*
- ▲ For the client who is receiving outpatient opioid therapy, at each visit, assess effect of opioids on pain status, function, goal achievement, and presence of side effects including sleep disturbance and sexual dysfunction; assessment for signs of opioid misuse, abuse, and addiction should be included, which may involve the use of random urine drug toxicology screening, pill counts, and review of prescription monitoring database. EB: *Opioid therapy is associated with risk for misuse, abuse, and addiction as well as overdose, while the evidence for the long-term use of opioid therapy in chronic pain is inconclusive. To minimize risk, a number of risk mitigation practices, including careful assessment of the client response to opioid therapy, are recommended (Cheatle & Barker, 2014; Chou et al, 2014).*
- • Ask the client to maintain a diary (if able) of pain ratings, timing, precipitating events, medications, and effectiveness of pain management interventions. EBN: *Systematic tracking of pain has been demonstrated to be an important factor in improving pain management (Hager & Brockopp, 2009; McCaffery et al, 2011). In a study of smartphone-based interventions with diaries among women with chronic widespread pain, it was found that the use of the smartphone intervention with diaries and personalized feedback reduced catastrophizing and prevented increases in functional impairment and symptoms (Kristjansdottir et al, 2013).*

▲ Obtain and review an accurate and complete list of medications the client is taking or has taken. CEB: *Accurate medication reconciliation can guide analgesic plan development and prevent errors associated with incorrect medications, dosages, omission of components of the home medication regimen, drug-drug interactions, and toxicity that can occur when incompatible drugs are combined or when allergies are present (Gleason et al, 2004).*

▲ Explain to the client the pain management approach that has been ordered or revised, including therapies, medication administration, side effects, and complications. EB: *One of the most important steps toward improved control of pain is a better client understanding of the nature of pain, its treatment, and the role the client needs to play in pain control (Pasero & Portenoy, 2011).*

• Discuss the client's fears of undertreated pain, addiction, and overdose. EBN: *Because of the many misconceptions regarding pain and its treatment, education about the ability to control pain effectively and correction of myths about the use of opioids should be included as part of the treatment plan (McCaffery et al, 2011).*

▲ Manage chronic pain using an individualized, multimodal approach. EB: *A multimodal approach (combining two or more drugs that act by different mechanisms for providing analgesia) such as an anticonvulsant, antidepressant, and opioid in chronic pain enhances pain relief and allows the lowest effective dose of each drug to be administered, resulting in fewer or less severe side effects such as nausea, sedation, and respiratory depression (Pasero et al, 2011a; Turk et al, 2011).*

▲ Select the route of administration of analgesics based on client condition and pain characteristics. CEB: *The least invasive route of administration capable of providing adequate pain control is recommended. Oral route is preferred because of its convenience and the relatively steady blood levels that can result (American Geriatric Society [AGS], 2009); the rectal route may be used when the oral route is not feasible; the intravenous route is preferred for rapid control of severe pain and would therefore not generally be used for chronic pain; intramuscular injections are avoided due to variable absorption and the potential for nerve injury and tissue damage (APS, 2008; Pasero et al, 2011a).*

▲ When chronic pain has a neuropathic component, treat with adjuvant analgesics, such as anticonvulsants, antidepressants, and topical local anesthetics. EB: *First-line analgesics for neuropathic pain belong to the adjuvant analgesic group and include anticonvulsants, antidepressants, and some topical local anesthetics. Analgesic efficacy with opioids in chronic neuropathic pain is inconclusive (Gilron et al, 2015; McNicol et al, 2013).*

P

▲ Administer a nonopioid analgesic for mild to moderate chronic pain and as a component of the treatment for all levels of pain for clients with cancer pain. CEB: *Nonopioids, such as acetaminophen and nonsteroidal antiinflammatory drugs (NSAIDs), are first-line analgesics for the treatment of mild and moderate pain conditions (e.g., osteoarthritis pain) and are recommended for cancer pain in all intensities (AGS, 2009; National Comprehensive Cancer Network [NCCN], 2015; Pasero et al, 2011b).*

▲ Recognize that opioid therapy may be indicated for some clients experiencing chronic pain. EB: *Opioids are often used in the management of moderate to severe chronic cancer pain; the evidence to support the long-term use of opioids for chronic, noncancer pain is limited due to a lack of long-term high quality studies, yet with careful client selection, opioids may be considered when nonopioid analgesics are ineffective alone or are contraindicated (AGS, 2009; Chou et al, 2009; Manchikanti et al, 2012; Turk et al, 2011).*

▲ Administer analgesics around-the-clock for continuous pain and PRN (as needed) for intermittent or breakthrough pain as may be experienced by clients with cancer pain. EB: *More than one in two clients with cancer pain also experience breakthrough cancer pain, and if pain is present most of the day, the use of PRN medications alone will lead to periods of undermedication and poor pain control and to periods of excessive medication and adverse effects (Chou, 2009; Deandrea et al, 2014).*

▲ At regular intervals, assess inpatient clients with chronic pain for opioid-related adverse events and include frequent assessment of pain level, assessment of respiratory status (including rate, rhythm, noisiness, depth), and systematic assessment of sedation level using a sedation scale. CEB: *Tolerance to opioid-induced respiratory depression develops within days of regular daily opioid dosing, making this side effect less likely to occur in clients who are taking opioids for underlying chronic pain and are opioid tolerant than in those who are not; however, opioid-tolerant clients are at similar risk for this side effect when they are admitted to the hospital for surgery or experience any other acute pain condition and are given opioid doses in addition to their usual dose (APS, 2008; Pasero et al, 2011a).*

▲ Provide the client with a stool softener and stimulant to prevent/treat opioid-related constipation. Ask about other opioid-related side effects including nausea, pruritus, lack of appetite, and changes in rest and sleep. EB: *While clients may develop tolerance to nausea, pruritus, and other opioid side effects, they do not develop tolerance to opioid-induced constipation. A study of 489 people on long-term opioids revealed varying utilization and responses to laxatives continues to add to the burden of chronic pain (Coyne et al, 2015; Pasero et al, 2011).*

- ▲ Question the client about any disruption in sleep. EB: *Chronic low back pain is associated with reduced sleep duration and quality (Kelly et al, 2011).*
- ▲ In addition to administering analgesics, support the client's use of nonpharmacological methods to help control pain, such as distraction, imagery, relaxation, and application of heat and cold. CEB: *Cognitive behavioral (mind-body) strategies such as cognitive restructuring, relaxation, meditation, goal setting, and pacing can restore the client's sense of self-control, personal efficacy, and active participation in his/her own care. The use of Web-based cognitive behavioral therapy (CBT) has shown that participants improved in self-efficacy for pain management and self-regulation, as well as reduced catastrophizing and fearful avoidance of activity (Bruckenthal, 2010; Carpenter et al, 2012).*
- • Teach and implement nonpharmacological interventions when pain is relatively well controlled with pharmacological interventions. EB: *Pain causes cognitive impairment (Moriarty et al, 2011; Pasero et al, 2011a).*
- ▲ Encourage the client to plan activities around periods of greatest comfort whenever possible. EB: *Some literature supports the use of pacing (a CBT strategy), an active self-management strategy in which individuals learn to balance activity and rest for the purpose of increasing function (Pigeon et al, 2012).*
- ▲ Explore appropriate resources for management of pain on a long-term basis (e.g., hospice, pain care center). EB: *Outpatient pain management resources must be identified to ensure appropriate chronic pain management. A telecare collaborative management study demonstrated that participants with chronic musculoskeletal pain who received telecare management monthly for a year experienced at least 30% improvement in pain scores after 12 months as well as improved secondary pain (Kroenke et al, 2014).*
- ▲ If the client has progressive cancer pain, assist the client and family with handling issues related to death and dying and provide access to palliative care programs and hospice services. EB: *Hui et al (2014) report that in a study of advanced cancer clients, those who were referred to outpatient palliative care had improved end-of-life care compared to those who received inpatient palliative care.*

Pediatric

- • Assess for the presence of pain using a valid and reliable pain scale based on age, cognitive development, and the child's ability to provide a self-report. EBN: *Scales that depict faces at various levels of pain intensity are commonly used in young children and have been shown to be reliable and valid in children as young as 3 years old (Oakes, 2011).* CEB: *Behavioral tools such as the FLACC scale may be used to assess pain in infants and children who cannot provide a self-report (Merkel et al, 2002).*
- ▲ Administer prescribed analgesics using a multimodal approach to treat pain in children, infants, and neonates. EB: *As with adults, pharmacological interventions are first-line approaches to the management of pain in children, infants, and neonates. A multimodal approach using nonopioid and opioid analgesics is recommended (Oakes, 2011).*
- • As with adults, use nonpharmacological analgesic interventions to supplement, not replace, pharmacological interventions in pediatric clients. EBN: *Complementary therapies such as cognitive behavioral strategies, mindfulness-based approaches, and other nonpharmacological approaches may play an important role in chronic pain management in children and adolescents (Song et al, 2014; van der Veek et al, 2013).*

Geriatric

- ▲ An older client's report of pain should be taken seriously and assessed and treated. CEB: *Pain is not an expected part of normal aging and unrecognized, untreated, or undertreated pain may result in adverse effects such as decreased cognition, delirium, mood changes (depression, anxiety), sleep disturbances, and significant physical and social disability (AGS, 2009; McCaffery et al, 2011).*
- • When assessing pain, speak clearly, slowly, and loudly enough for the client to hear, ensure hearing aids and glasses are in place as appropriate; enlarge pain scales and written materials; and repeat information as needed. CEB: *Older clients often have difficulty hearing and seeing, and comprehension is improved when instructions are given slowly and clearly and when clients can see visual aids (Herr & Bjoro, 2008; McCaffery et al, 2011).*
- • Handle the client's body gently and allow the client to move at his or her own speed. CEB: *Older adults are particularly susceptible to injury during care activities. Caregivers must be patient and expect that older*

clients will move more slowly than younger clients; they may also perform better and experience less pain when they are allowed to move themselves (Herr & Titler, 2009).

▲ Use nonopioid analgesics for mild to moderate pain. CEB: *Acetaminophen (maximum dosage 3000 mg/day) is recommended, unless contraindicated, as first-line therapy for older persons with persistent pain; NSAIDs (preferably in topical form due to less system absorption than oral form) should be used short term and with extreme caution due to the higher gastrointestinal, cardiovascular, and renal adverse effects (AGS, 2009; U.S. Food and Drug Administration, 2009).*

▲ Use opioids cautiously in the older client with moderate to severe pain. CEB: *Even though data are lacking in all groups regarding the use of opioids for persistent pain, due to the adverse effects of some nonopioid analgesics in older clients, the initiation of opioids for persistent pain in clients with increased functional impairment or decreased quality of life may be considered, starting with a short-acting low-dose opioid, carefully and slowly titrating to attain therapeutic goal, and converting to a long-acting opioid if needed for persistent around-the-clock pain (AGS, 2009; Pasero et al, 2011a).*

▲ Avoid the use of meperidine (Demerol) in older clients. EB: *Meperidine's metabolite, normeperidine, can produce central nervous system irritability, seizures, and even death; normeperidine is eliminated by the kidneys, which makes meperidine a particularly poor choice for older clients, many of whom have at least some degree of renal insufficiency (Pasero et al, 2011a).*

▲ Use nonpharmacological approaches in addition to analgesics. EB: *Physical and occupational rehabilitation, behavioral approaches, and movement-based interventions tailored to the older person's needs and capabilities have been shown to be effective and should be used to treat chronic pain when possible (Makris et al, 2014; Bruckenthal, 2010).*

▲ Monitor for signs of depression in older clients and refer to specialists with relevant expertise. EB: *Depression is often associated with pain and decreased levels of independence with activities of daily living in the older client. Treatment has been demonstrated to decrease pain and improve functional abilities (Tarakci et al, 2015; AGS, 2009).*

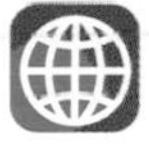

Multicultural

▲ Assess for pain disparities among racial and ethnic minorities. EB: *Individuals of ethnic and racial minorities often receive fewer treatment options and less effective pain treatment than others because of barriers imposed by health care professionals and health care systems (Mossey, 2011; Tait & Chibnall, 2014).*

P

▲ Assess for the influence of cultural beliefs, norms, and values on the client's perception and experience of pain. EBN: *Mexican American women with chronic pain are reluctant to take prescribed analgesics due to perceived negative associations with pain medications (Monsivais, 2012).*

▲ Assess for the effect of fatalism on the client's beliefs regarding the current state of comfort. EBN: *Asian clients' perceived barriers to managing cancer pain were found to be higher than those reported for Western clients, and Asian clients expressed a fatalistic belief that cancer pain is inevitable; these fatalistic beliefs toward pain and pain management may predispose Asian clients to hesitate to report pain and request pain medications (Chen et al, 2012).*

▲ Use a family-centered approach to care. EB: *Involving the family in care through early regular communication and decision-making may reduce anxiety, alleviate uncertainty, and improve coping strategies (Michael et al, 2014).*

• Use culturally relevant pain scales to assess pain in the client. CEB: *Clients from minority cultures may express pain differently than clients from the majority culture. The Faces Pain Scale-Revised was shown to be preferred over other self-report pain rating tools in older minority adults (Ware, 2006) and in Chinese adults (Li et al, 2007). A later study demonstrated that the Iowa Pain Thermometer was the preferred tool in older Chinese adults (Li et al, 2009). The Oucher scale is available in African American and Hispanic versions and is used to assess pain in children (Oakes, 2011). Ensure that directions for medication use are available in the client's language of choice and are understood by the client and caregiver.* CEB: *Use of bilingual instructions for medication administration increased compliance with the pain management plan (Juarez et al, 1998).*

Home Care

• The interventions previously described may be adapted for home care use. Refer to the Nursing Interventions and *Rationales* in the care plan for Acute **Pain.**

Client/Family Teaching and Discharge Planning

NOTE: *To avoid the negative connotations associated with the words "drugs" and "narcotics," use the term "pain medicine" when teaching clients.*

- Discuss the various discomforts encompassed by the word "pain" and ask the client to give examples of previously experienced pain. Explain the pain assessment process and the purpose of the pain rating scale. EB: *It is often difficult for clients to understand the concept of pain and describe their pain experience. Using alternative words and providing a complete description of the assessment process, including the use of scales, ensures that an accurate treatment plan is developed (McCaffery et al, 2011).*
- Teach the client that if the pain level is consistently above the comfort-function goal, the client should take action that decreases pain or should notify a member of the health care team so that effective pain management interventions may be implemented promptly. (See information on teaching clients to use the pain rating scale.) EB: *The use of comfort-function goals provides direction for the treatment plan. Changes are made according to the client's response and achievement of the goals of recovery or rehabilitation (McCaffery et al, 2011).*
- Provide educational materials on various aspects of pain control to improve client understanding of pain and pain-related interventions. EB: *Written materials and other educational tools assist in improving clients' knowledge related to pain management. In knee replacement clients, the use of an educational pamphlet and a compact disc was associated with decreased postoperative pain and increased participation in physical rehabilitation (Chen et al, 2014).*
- Discuss and evaluate the client's understanding about the total plan for pharmacological and nonpharmacological treatment, including the medication plan for around-the-clock administration and supplemental doses, the maintenance of a pain diary, and the use of supplies and equipment. EB: *Appropriate instruction increases the accuracy and safety of medication administration (Pasero et al, 2011a).*
- Reinforce the importance of taking pain medications to maintain the comfort-function goal. EBN: *Teaching clients to stay on top of their pain and prevent it from getting out of control will improve the ability to accomplish the goals of recovery (McCaffery et al, 2011).*

▲ Reinforce that taking opioids for pain relief is not addiction and that addiction is very unlikely to occur. CEB: *The development of addiction when opioids are taken for pain relief is rare (APS, 2008; Pasero et al, 2011a).*

P

- Demonstrate the use of appropriate nonpharmacological approaches in addition to pharmacological approaches for helping control pain, such as application of heat and/or cold, distraction techniques, relaxation breathing, visualization, rocking, stroking, listening to music, and watching television. Teach these methods when pain is relatively well controlled, because pain interferes with cognition. CEB: *Nonpharmacological interventions are used to complement pharmacological interventions (Bruckenthal, 2010; Pasero et al, 2011a).*

▲ Emphasize to the client the importance of participating in a structured, individualized pacing activity and taking rest breaks before they are needed. CEB: *In a study of adults with knee or hip osteoarthritis, it was shown by Murphy et al (2010) that an individualized, tailored activity pacing intervention provides more pain relief and less fatigue than general instructions related to fatigue (Murphy et al, 2010).*

- Teach nonpharmacological methods when pain is relatively well controlled. EB: *Pain interferes with cognition (Moriarty et al, 2011; Pasero et al, 2011a).*

REFERENCES

American Geriatric Society (AGS). (2009). Panel on the pharmacological management of persistent pain in older persons: pharmacological management of persistent pain in older persons. *Journal of the American Geriatrics Society*, *37*(8), 1331–1346.

American Pain Society (APS) (2008). *Principles of analgesic use in acute and chronic pain* (6th ed.). Glenview, IL: American Pain Society.

Breivik, H., Reme, S. E., & Linton, S. J. (2014). High risk of depression and suicide attempt among chronic pain patients: always explore catastrophizing and suicide thoughts when evaluating chronic pain patients. *Scandinavian Journal of Pain*, *5*(1), 1–3.

Bruckenthal, P. (2010). Integrating nonpharmacologic and alternative strategies into a comprehensive management approach for older adults with pain. *Pain Management Nursing*, *11*(2), S23–S31.

Carpenter, K. M., Stoner, S. A., Mundt, J. M., et al. (2012). An online self-help CBT intervention for chronic lower back pain. *The Clinical Journal of Pain*, *28*(1), 14.

Cheatle, M. D., & Barker, C. (2014). Improving opioid prescription practices and reducing patient risk in the primary care setting. *Journal of pain research*, *7*, 301.

Chen, S. R., Chen, C. S., & Lin, P. C. (2014). The effect of educational intervention on the pain and rehabilitation performance of patients who undergo a total knee replacement. *Journal of Clinical Nursing*, *23*(1–2), 279–287.

Chen, C. H., Tang, S. T., & Chen, C. H. (2012). Meta-analysis of cultural differences in western and Asian patient-perceived barriers to managing cancer pain. *Palliative Medicine*, *26*(3), 206–221.

Chou, R., Fanciullo, G. J., Fine, P. G., et al. (2009). Opioids for chronic noncancer pain: prediction and identification of aberrant drug-related behaviors: a review of the evidence for an American pain society and American academy of pain medicine clinical practice guideline. *The Journal of Pain*, *10*(2), 131–146.

Chou, R., et al. (2009). Clinical guidelines for the use of chronic opioid therapy in chronic noncancer pain. *The Journal of Pain*, *10*(2), 113–130.

Coyne, K. S., Margolis, M. K., Yeomans, K., et al. (2015). Opioid-induced constipation among patients with chronic noncancer pain in the United States, Canada, Germany, and the United Kingdom: laxative use, response and symptom burden over time. *Pain Medicine (Malden, Mass.)*.

Deandrea, S., Corli, O., Consonni, D., et al. (2014). Prevalence of breakthrough cancer pain: a systematic review and a pooled analysis of published literature. *Journal of Pain and Symptom Management*, *47*(1), 57–76.

U.S. Food and Drug Administration (FDA): *Joint Meeting of the Drug Safety and Risk Management Advisory Committee with the Anesthetic and Life Support Drugs Advisory Committee and the Nonprescription Drugs Advisory Committee Recommendations*, 2009, From <http://www.fda.gov/downloads/AdvisoryCommittees/CommitteesMeetingMaterials/Drugs/Drug>. Retrieved October 8, 2011.

Gleason, K. M., Grozek, J. M., Sullivan, C., et al. (2004). Reconciliation of discrepancies in medication histories and admission orders of newly hospitalized patients. *American Journal Health-System Pharmacy*, *61*(16), 1689–1695.

Gilron, I., Baron, R., & Jensen, T. (2015). Neuropathic pain: principles of diagnosis and treatment. *Mayo Clinic Proceedings. Mayo Clinic*, *90*(4), 532–545.

Hager, K., & Brockopp, D. (2009). The use of a chronic pain diary in older people. *British Journal of Nursing (Mark Allen Publishing)*, *18*(8), 490–494.

Herr, K., & Bjoro, K. (2008). Assessment of pain in the nonverbal or cognitively impaired older adult. *Clinics in Geriatric Medicine*, *24*(2), 237–262.

Herr, K., & Titler, M. (2009). Acute pain assessment and pharmacological management practices for the older adult with a hip fracture: review of ED trends. *Journal of Emergency Nursing*, *35*(4), 312–320.

Hui, D., Kim, S. H., Roquemore, J., et al. (2014). Impact of timing and setting of palliative care referral on quality of end-of-life care in cancer patients. *Cancer*, *120*(11), 1743–1749.

International Association for the Study of Pain, Subcommittee on Taxonomy. (1979). Classification of chronic pain: descriptions of chronic pain syndromes and definitions of pain terms. *Pain. Supplement*, *3*, S1–S226.

Juarez, G., Ferrell, B. R., & Borneman, T. (1998). Influence of culture on cancer pain management in Hispanic clients. *Cancer Practice*, *6*(5), 262.

Kelly, G. A., Blake, C., Power, C. K., et al. (2011). The association between chronic low back pain and sleep: a systematic review. *Clinical Journal of Pain*, *27*(2), 169–181.

Kristjánsdóttir, Ó. B., Fors, E. A., Eide, E., et al. (2013). A smartphone-based intervention with diaries and therapist-feedback to reduce catastrophizing and increase functioning in women with chronic widespread pain: randomized controlled trial. *Journal of Medical Internet Research*, *15*(1), e5.

Kroenke, K., Krebs, E. E., Wu, J., et al. (2014). Telecare collaborative management of chronic pain in primary care: a randomized clinical trial. *JAMA: The Journal of the American Medical Association*, *312*(3), 240–248.

Kroenke, K., Outcalt, S., Krebs, E., et al. (2013). Association between anxiety, health-related quality of life and functional impairment in primary care patients with chronic pain. *General Hospital Psychiatry*, *35*(4), 359–365.

Lee, J. J., Lee, M. K., Kim, J. E., et al. (2014). Pain relief scale is more highly correlated with numerical rating scale than with visual analogue scale in chronic pain patients. *Pain Physician*, *18*(2), E195–E200.

Li, L., Herr, K., & Chen, P. (2009). Postoperative pain assessment with three intensity scales in Chinese elders. *Journal of Nursing Scholarship*, *41*(3), 241–249.

Li, L., Liu, X., & Herr, K. (2007). Postoperative pain intensity assessment: a comparison of four scales in Chinese adults. *Pain Medicine (Malden, Mass.)*, *8*(3), 223–234.

Linl, C. P., Kupperl, A. E., Gammaitonil, A. R., et al. (2011). Frequency of chronic pain descriptors: implications for assessment of pain quality. *European Journal of Pain*, *15*(6), 628–633.

Makris, U. E., Abrams, R. C., Gurland, B., et al. (2014). Management of persistent pain in the older patient: a clinical review. *JAMA: The Journal of the American Medical Association*, *312*(8), 825–836.

Manchikanti, L., Abdi, S., Atluri, S., et al. (2012). American Society of Interventional Pain Physicians (ASIPP) guidelines for responsible opioid prescribing in chronic non-cancer pain: part I–evidence assessment. *Pain Physician*, *15*(3 Suppl.), S1–S65.

McCaffery, M., Herr, K., & Pasero, C. (2011). Assessment. In C. Pasero & M. McCaffery (Eds.), *Pain assessment and pharmacologic management*. St Louis: Mosby Elsevier.

McNicol, E. D., Midbari, A., & Eisenberg, E. (2013). Opioids for neuropathic pain. *The Cochrane Library.*

Merkel, S., Voepel-Lewis, T., & Malviya, S. (2002). Pain assessment in infants and young children: the FLACC scale: a behavioral tool to measure pain in young children. *American Journal of Nursing*, *102*(10), 55–58.

Michael, N., O'Callaghan, C., Baird, A., et al. (2014). Cancer caregivers advocate a patient- and family-centered approach to advance care planning. *Journal of Pain and Symptom Management*, *47*(6), 1064–1077.

Monsivais, D. B., & Engebretson, J. C. (2012). I'm Just Not That Sick" pain medication and identity in Mexican American women with chronic pain. *Journal of Holistic Nursing*, *30*(3), 188–194.

Moriarty, O., McGuire, B. E., & Finn, D. P. (2011). The effect of pain on cognitive function: a review of clinical and preclinical research. *Progress in Neurobiology*, *93*(3), 385–404.

Mossey, J. M. (2011). (1859–1870). Defining racial and ethnic disparities in pain management. *Clinical Orthopaedics and Related Research*, *469*(7).

Murphy, S. L., et al. (2010). The effect of a tailored activity pacing intervention on pain and fatigue for adults with osteoarthritis. *The American journal of occupational therapy: official publication of the American Occupational Therapy Association*, *64*(6), 869–876. Print.

National Comprehensive Cancer Network. (2015). *NCCN Clinical Practice Guidelines in Oncology.* Adult Cancer Pain. Version 1.2015.

Oakes, L. (2011). *Compact clinical guide to infant and child pain management.* New York: Springer.

Pasero, C., et al. (2011a). Opioid analgesics. In C. Pasero & M. McCaffery (Eds.), *Pain assessment and pharmacologic management* (pp. 277–622). St Louis: Mosby Elsevier.

Pasero, C., Portenoy, R. K., & McCaffery, M. (2011b). Nonopioid analgesics. In C. Pasero & M. McCaffery (Eds.), *Pain assessment and pharmacologic management.* St Louis: Mosby Elsevier.

Pigeon, W. R., Moynihan, J., Matteson-Rusby, S., et al. (2012). Comparative effectiveness of CBT interventions for co-morbid chronic pain & insomnia: a pilot study. *Behaviour Research and Therapy*, *50*(11), 685–689.

Song, Y., Lu, H., Chen, H., et al. (2014). Mindfulness intervention in the management of chronic pain and psychological comorbidity: a meta-analysis. *International Journal of Nursing Sciences, 1*(2), 215–223.

Tait, R. C., & Chibnall, J. T. (2014). Racial/ethnic disparities in the assessment and treatment of pain: psychosocial perspectives. *American Psychologist, 69*(2), 131.

Tarakci, E., Zenginler, Y., & Kaya Mutlu, E. (2015). Chronic pain, depression symptoms and daily living independency level among geriatrics in nursing home. *Journal of the Turkish Society of Algology, 27*(1), 35–41.

Turk, D. C., Wilson, H. D., & Cahana, A. (2011). Treatment of chronic non-cancer pain. *Lancet, 377*, 2226–2235.

van der Veek, S. M., Derkx, B. H., Benninga, M. A., et al. (2013). Cognitive behavior therapy for pediatric functional abdominal pain: a randomized controlled trial. *Pediatrics, 132*(5), e1163–e1172.

Ware, L. J., et al. (2006). Evaluation of the revised faces pain scale, verbal descriptor scale, numeric rating scale, and Iowa pain thermometer in older minority adults. *Pain Management Nursing, 7*(3), 117–125.

Labor Pain *Mary Beth Flynn Makic, PhD, RN, CNS, CCNS, FAAN*

NANDA-I

Definition

Sensory and emotional experience that varies from pleasant to unpleasant, associated with labor and childbirth

Defining Characteristics

Alteration in blood pressure; alteration in heart rate; alteration in muscle tension; alteration in neuroendocrine functioning; alteration in respiratory rate; alteration in sleep pattern; alteration in urinary functioning; decrease in appetite; diaphoresis; distraction behavior; expressive behavior; facial expression of pain (e.g., eyes lack luster, beaten look, fixed or scattered movement, grimace); increase in appetite; narrowed focus; nausea; pain; perineal pressure; positioning to ease pain; protective behavior; pupil dilation; self-focused; uterine contraction; vomiting

P

Related Factors (r/t)

Cervical dilation; fetal expulsion

NIC, NOC, Client Outcomes, Nursing Interventions, Client/Family Teaching and Discharge Planning, *Rationales*, and References

Refer to care plan for Acute **Pain.**

Chronic Pain syndrome *Mary Beth Flynn Makic, PhD, RN, CNS, CCNS, FAAN*

NANDA-I

Definition

Recurrent or persistent pain that has lasted at least 3 months and that significantly affects daily functioning or well-being

Defining Characteristics

Anxiety; constipation; deficient knowledge; disturbed sleep pattern; fatigue; fear; impaired mood regulation; impaired physical mobility; insomnia; obesity; social isolation; stress overload

NIC, NOC, Client Outcomes, Nursing Interventions, Client/Family Teaching and Discharge Planning, *Rationales*, and References

Refer to care plan for Acute **Pain** and Chronic **Pain.**

Impaired Parenting *Kimberly Silvey, MSN, RN*

NANDA-I

Definition

Inability of the primary caretaker to create, maintain, or regain an environment that promotes the optimum growth and development of the child

Defining Characteristics

Infant/Child

Behavioral disorders (e.g., attention deficit, oppositional defiant); delay in cognitive development; diminished separation anxiety; failure to thrive; frequent accidents; frequent illness; history of abuse (e.g., physical, psychological, sexual); history of trauma (e.g., physical, psychological, sexual); impaired social functioning; insufficient attachment behavior; low academic performance; runaway

Parental

Abandonment; decrease in ability to manage child; decrease in cuddling; deficient parent-child interaction; frustration with child; history of childhood abuse (e.g., physical, psychological, sexual); hostility; inadequate child health maintenance; inappropriate caretaking skills; inappropriate childcare arrangements; inappropriate stimulation (e.g., visual tactile auditory); inconsistent behavior management; inconsistent care; inflexibility in meeting needs of child; neglects needs of child; perceived inability to meet child's needs; perceived role inadequacy; punitive; rejection of child; speaks negatively about child; unsafe home environment

Related Factors (r/t)

Infant/Child

Alteration in perceptual abilities; behavior disorder (e.g., attention deficit, oppositional defiant); chronic illness; developmental delay; difficult temperament; disabling condition; gender other than desired; multiple births; parent-child separation; prematurity; temperament conflicts with parental expectations

Knowledge

Alteration in cognitive functioning; ineffective communication skills; insufficient cognitive readiness for parenting; insufficient knowledge about child development; insufficient knowledge about child health maintenance; insufficient knowledge about parenting skills; insufficient response to infant cues; low educational level; preference for physical punishment; unrealistic expectation

Physiological

Physical illness

Psychological

Alteration in sleep pattern; closely spaced pregnancies; depression; difficult birthing process; disability condition; high number of pregnancies; history of mental illness; history of substance abuse; insufficient prenatal care; sleep deprivation; young parental age

Social

Change in family unit; compromised home environment; conflict between partners; economically disadvantaged; father of child not involved; history of abuse (e.g., physical, psychological, sexual); history of being abusive; inability to put child's needs before own; inadequate childcare arrangements; ineffective coping strategies; insufficient family cohesiveness; insufficient parental role model; insufficient problem-solving skills; insufficient resources (e.g., financial social, knowledge); insufficient social support; insufficient transportation; insufficient valuing of parenthood; legal difficulty; low self-esteem; mother of child not involved; relocation; single parent; social isolation; stressors; unemployment; unplanned pregnancy; unwanted pregnancy; work difficulty

NOC (Nursing Outcomes Classification)

Suggested NOC Outcomes

Abuse Cessation; Abuse Protection; Abuse Recovery: Abusive Behavior Self-Restraint; Child Development (all); Coping; Family Functioning; Family Social Climate; Knowledge: Child Physical Safety; Neglect Recovery; Parent-Infant Attachment; Parenting Performance, Psychosocial Safety; Role Performance; Social Support

Example NOC Outcome with Indicators

Parenting Performance: Psychosocial Safety as evidenced by the following indicators: Fosters open communication/Recognizes risks for abuse/Uses strategies to eliminate risks for abuse/Selects appropriate supplemental caregivers/Uses strategies to prevent high-risk social behaviors/Provides required level of supervision/Sets clear rules for behavior/Maintains structure and daily routine in child's life. (Rate the outcome and indicators of **Parenting Performance: Psychosocial Safety:** 1 = never demonstrated, 2 = rarely demonstrated, 3 = sometimes demonstrated, 4 = often demonstrated, 5 = consistently demonstrated [see Section I].)

Client Outcomes

Client Will (Specify Time Frame)

- Initiate appropriate measures to develop a safe, nurturing environment
- Acquire and display attentive, supportive parenting behaviors and child supervision
- Identify appropriate strategies to manage a child's inappropriate behaviors
- Identify strategies to protect child from harm and/or neglect and initiate action when indicated

NIC (Nursing Interventions Classification)

Suggested NIC Interventions

P

Abuse Protection Support: Child; Attachment Promotion; Caregiver Support; Developmental Enhancement: Adolescent, Child; Environmental Management: Family Integrity Promotion; Impulse Control Training; Infant Care; Parent Education: Adolescent, Childrearing Family, Infant; Parenting Promotion; Role Enhancement; Substance Use Prevention, Treatment; Teaching: Infant Stimulation; Toddler Nutrition; Toddler Safety

Example NIC Activities—Family Integrity Promotion

Identify typical family coping mechanisms; Determine typical family relationships for each family; Counsel family members on additional effective coping skills for their own use; Assist family with conflict resolution; Monitor current family relationships; Facilitate a tone of togetherness within and among the family; Encourage family to maintain positive relationships; Refer for family therapy, as indicated

Nursing Interventions and *Rationales*

- Use the Parenting Sense of Competence (PSOC) scale to measure parental self-efficacy. EB: *The PSOC contains three useful factors that reflect satisfaction with the parental role, parenting efficacy, and interest in parenting. Mothers and father will differ in parenting of their children and their sense of competence (Slagt et al, 2012).*
- Examine the characteristics of parenting style and behaviors. Consider dysfunctional child-centered and parent-centered cognitions as potentially critical correlates of abusive behavior. EB: *Dysfunctional parenting can lead to abuse and should be monitored closely (Wolfe & McIsaac, 2011).*
- ▲ Institute abuse/neglect protection measures if evidence exists of an inability to cope with family stressors or crisis, signs of parental substance abuse are observed, or a significant level of social isolation is apparent. EBN: *Helping parents identify stressors will assist parents with coping in a crisis (Mowery, 2011).*
- ▲ For a mother with a toddler, assess maternal depression. Make appropriate referral. EB: *Helping mothers identify systems of depression through self-assessment or home visits is beneficial for both mother and toddler (Bocknek et al, 2012).*

- Appraise the parent's resources and the availability of social support systems. Determine the single mother's particular sources of support, especially the availability of her own mother and partner. Encourage the use of healthy, strong support systems. EB: *Clinicians should help mothers evaluate what resources and support that they have and encourage healthy relationships (Letourneau et al, 2013).* Provide education to at-risk parents on behavioral management techniques such as looking ahead, giving good instructions, providing positive reinforcement, redirecting, planned ignoring, and instituting time-outs. EB: *Parents with mental health issues need education to help them better care for their children (Houlihan et al, 2013).*
- Promotion of better quality relationships between parents and children is an effective strategy that can lead to enhanced learning. Good quality parenting leads to improved cognitive and social skills for children. EB: *Promoting quality relationships promotes optimal health and development (Titze et al, 2014).*
- Support parents' competence in appraising their infant's behavior and responses. EBN: *Encourage and support the presence of the parents with the care of the infant (Felgen, 2011).*
- Aim supportive interventions at minimizing parents' experience of strain. EBN: *Support caregivers to enhance the family relationship (Tomlinson et al, 2012).*
- Model age-appropriate and cognitively appropriate caregiver skills by doing the following: communicating with the child at an appropriate cognitive level of development, giving the child tasks and responsibilities appropriate to age or functional age/level, instituting safety considerations such as the use of assistive equipment, and encouraging the child to perform activities of daily living as appropriate. EBN: *Children learn from the interactions with family, parents, and even medical staff (Rich et al, 2014).*
- Encourage mothers to understand and capitalize on their infant's capacity to interact, particularly in the early months of life. EBN: *Mother-infant bonding is very important during the first months of life (Lee et al, 2013).*

▲ Provide programs for homeless mothers with severe mental illness who have lost physical custody of their children. EB: *Providing education and support to homeless mothers helps empower them (Sleed et al, 2013).*

▲ Provide a recovery program that includes instruction in parenting skills and child development for mothers who are addicted to cocaine. EB: *Women need additional assistance for recovery from substance abuse and need to understand the effect that it will have on their child (Eiden et al, 2011).*

- Refer to Readiness for enhanced **Parenting** for additional interventions.

P

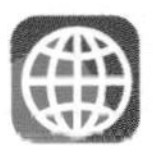

Multicultural

- Acknowledge that value conflicts from acculturation stresses may contribute to increased anxiety and significant conflict with children. EBN: *Help parents develop a plan to address conflicts within the family (Kim, 2011).*
- Approach individuals of color with respect, warmth, and professional courtesy. EBN: *All clients should be cared for in a cultural congruent manner (Wiebe & Young, 2011).*
- Clarify parents' feelings, expectations, perceptions, and availability regarding participation in the care of their sick child. EBN: *Cultural differences in regard to parent participation in the care of ill or hospitalized children should be considered (Mutair et al, 2014).*
- Carefully assess meaning of terms used to describe health status when working with Native Americans. EB: *Health care providers should allow clients to participate in spiritual care according to their beliefs (Hodge & Wolosin, 2014).*
- Provide support for Chinese families caring for children with disabilities. EBN: *The care of the sick in China is based on old world beliefs. It is important to ensure that all aspects of cultural beliefs are included in care (Zhang et al, 2014).*
- Facilitate modeling and role playing to help the family improve parenting skills. EB: *Families need to be able to practice parenting in a safe setting (Franks et al, 2013).*

Home Care

- The interventions previously described may be adapted for home care use.
- Assess parenting stress at each home visit to provide appropriate support and anticipatory guidance to families of children with a chronic disease. EB: *Assessing parental stress in the home assists the health care provider in identifying interventions that can be implemented at home (Gabler et al, 2014).*

▲ Assess the single mother's history regarding childhood and partner abuse and current status regarding depressive symptoms, abusive parenting attitudes (lack of empathy, favorable opinion of corporal punishment, parent-child role reversal, and inappropriate expectations). Refer for mental health services as indicated. EB: *A mother's history can contribute to the stress and the care of her children (Boeckel et al, 2014).*

- Provide a parenting program of Planned Activities Training (PAT). EB: *PAT is a five-session intervention aimed at improving parent-child interactions, increasing child engagement in daily activities, and reducing challenging child behaviors. Parents in this program demonstrated improvements in their parenting behaviors (Bigelow et al, 2008).*
- Provide follow-up support for the PAT via cell phone and text messaging. EB: *Cellular phones afford the opportunity for home visitors to maintain regular communication with parents between intervention visits and thus retain high-risk families in parenting interventions. The use of cell phones may also increase the dosage of intervention provided to families and the fidelity with which parents implement the intervention, thus resulting in improved outcomes for parents and children. Parents have rated text messaging and cell phone call enhancements very positively (Bigelow et al, 2008).*

Client/Family Teaching and Discharge Planning

- Consider individual and/or group-based parenting programs for teenaged mothers. EB: *Offering parenting programs to teenaged parents helps them to better care for their child (Mills et al, 2013).*
- Consider group-based parenting programs for parents of children younger than 3 years with emotional and behavioral problems. EBN: *A study shows that group-based parenting programs assist both the parent and the children (Merry, 2011; Kendall et al, 2013).*
- Consider group-based parenting programs for parents with anxiety, depression, and/or low self-esteem. EB: *Parenting programs assist parent with being able to identify issues they may have (Maher et al, 2011).*
- ▲ Refer adolescent parents for comprehensive psychoeducational parenting classes. EBN: *Adolescent parenting class helps teens to learn the best ways to care for their infant (Allen et al, 2014).*
- Parent training is one of the most effective interventions for behavior problems in young children. EBN: *Parent training programs assist with the improving family functioning and interactions (Arkan et al, 2013). Encourage positive parenting: respect for children, understanding of normal development, and creative and loving approaches to meet parenting challenges rather than using anger, manipulation, punishment, and rewards.* EBN: *Encouraging a male caregiver can reduce challenging behaviors and promote a positive bond with child and caregiver (Salinas et al, 2011).*
- ▲ Initiate referrals to community agencies, parent education programs, stress management training, and social support groups. Consider the use of technology and the media. EB: *Family use of technology to interact with health care providers can broaden the support that the family can receive (Hanlon-Dearman et al, 2014).*
- Provide information regarding available telephone counseling services and Internet support. EBN: *Using the Internet allows parents to communicate with and gain support from others all over the world (Niela-Vilén et al, 2014).* Refer to the care plans for Risk for disproportionate **Growth**, Risk for delayed **Development**, Risk for impaired **Attachment**, and Readiness for enhanced **Parenting** for additional teaching interventions.

P

REFERENCES

Allen, K., El-Beshti, R., et al. (2014). An integrative adlerian approach to creating a teen parenting program. *Journal of Individual Psychology*, *70*(1), 6–20.

Arkan, B., ÜstÜn, B., et al. (2013). An analysis of two evidence-based parent training programmes and determination of the characteristics for a new programme model. *Journal of Psychiatric & Mental Health Nursing*, *20*(2), 176–185.

Bigelow, K. M., Carta, J. J., & Lefever, J. B. (2008). Txt u ltr: using cellular phone technology to enhance a parenting intervention for families at risk for neglect. *Child Maltreatment*, *13*(4), 362–367.

Bocknek, E. L., Brophy-Herb, H. E., et al. (2012). Maternal psychological absence and toddlers' social-emotional development: interpretations from the perspective of boundary ambiguity theory. *Family Process*, *51*(4), 527–541.

Boeckel, M. G., Blasco-Ros, C., et al. (2014). Child abuse in the context of intimate partner violence against women: the impact of women's depressive and posttraumatic stress symptoms on maternal behavior. *Journal of Interpersonal Violence*, *29*(7), 1201–1227.

Eiden, R. D., Schuetze, P., et al. (2011). Maternal cocaine use and mother–infant interactions: Direct and moderated associations. *Neurotoxicology & Teratology*, *33*(1), 120–128.

Felgen, J. (2011). Creating presence. *Creative Nursing*, *17*(1), 3–4.

Franks, S. B., Mata, F. C., et al. (2013). The effects of behavioral parent training on placement outcomes of biological families in a state child welfare system. *Research on Social Work Practice*, *23*(4), 377–382.

Gabler, S., Bovenschen, I., et al. (2014). Foster children's attachment security and behavior problems in the first six months of placement: associations with foster parents' stress and sensitivity. *Attachment & Human Development*, *16*(5), 479–498.

Hanlon-Dearman, A., Edwards, C., et al. (2014). 'Giving voice': evaluation of an integrated telehealth community care model by parents/guardians of children diagnosed with fetal alcohol

spectrum disorder in manitoba. *Telemedicine & e-Health*, *20*(5), 478–484.
Hodge, D. R., & Wolosin, R. J. (2014). American indians and spiritual needs during hospitalization: developing a model of spiritual care. *The Gerontologist*, *54*(4), 683–692.
Houlihan, D., Sharek, D., et al. (2013). Supporting children whose parent has a mental health problem: an assessment of the education, knowledge, confidence and practices of registered psychiatric nurses in Ireland. *Journal of Psychiatric & Mental Health Nursing*, *20*(4), 287–295.
Kendall, S., Bloomfield, L., et al. (2013). Efficacy of a group-based parenting program on stress and self-efficacy among Japanese mothers: a quasi-experimental study. *Nursing & Health Sciences*, *15*(4), 454–460.
Kim, E. (2011). Intergenerational acculturation conflict and korean american parents' depression symptoms. *Issues in Mental Health Nursing*, *32*(11), 687–695.
Lee, G., McCreary, L., et al. (2013). Promoting mother-infant interaction and infant mental health in low-income Korean families: attachment-based cognitive behavioral approach. *Journal for Specialists in Pediatric Nursing*, *18*(4), 265–276.
Letourneau, N., Morris, C. Y., et al. (2013). Social support needs identified by mothers affected by intimate partner violence. *Journal of Interpersonal Violence*, *28*(14), 2873–2893.
Maher, E. J., et al. (2011). Dosage matters: the relationship between participation in the nurturing parenting program for infants, toddlers, and preschoolers and subsequent child maltreatment. *Children and Youth Services Review*, *33*(8), 1426–1434.
Merry, S. N. (2011). 'Timid to Tiger' group parenting training reduces anxiety diagnoses in 3-9-year-olds. *Evidence-Based Mental Health*, *14*(3), 74.
Mills, A., Schmied, V., et al. (2013). Someone to talk to: young mothers' experiences of participating in a young parents support programme. *Scandinavian Journal of Caring Sciences*, *27*(3), 551–559.
Mowery, B. D. (2011). Family matters. Post traumatic stress disorder (PTSD) in parents: is this a significant problem? *Pediatric Nursing*, *37*(2), 89–92.
Mutair, A. S. A., Plummer, V., et al. (2014). Providing culturally congruent care for Saudi patients and their families. *Contemporary Nurse: A Journal for the Australian Nursing Profession*, *46*(2), 254–258.
Niela-Vilén, H., Axelin, A., et al. (2014). Internet-based peer support for parents: a systematic integrative review. *International Journal of Nursing Studies*, *51*(11), 1524–1537.
Rich, C., Goncalves, A., et al. (2014). Teen advisory committee: lessons learned by adolescents, facilitators, and hospital staff. *Pediatric Nursing*, *40*(6), 289–296.
Salinas, A., Smith, J. C., & Armstrong, K. (2011). Engaging fathers in behavioral parent training: listening to fathers' voices. *Journal of Pediatric Nursing*, *26*(4), 304–311.
Slagt, M., Deković, M., et al. (2012). Longitudinal associations between mothers' and fathers' sense of competence and children's externalizing problems: the mediating role of parenting. *Developmental Psychology*, *48*(6), 1554–1562.
Sleed, M., James, J., et al. (2013). A psychotherapeutic baby clinic in a hostel for homeless families: practice and evaluation. *Psychology & Psychotherapy: Theory, Research & Practice*, *86*(1), 1–18.
Titze, K., Schenck, S., et al. (2014). Assessing the quality of the parent-child relationship: validity and reliability of the child-parent relationship test (ChiP-C). *Journal of Child & Family Studies*, *23*(5), 917–933.
Tomlinson, P. S., Peden-McAlpine, C., et al. (2012). A family systems nursing intervention model for paediatric health crisis. *Journal of Advanced Nursing*, *68*(3), 705–714.
Wiebe, A., & Young, B. (2011). Parent perspectives from a neonatal intensive care unit: a missing piece of the culturally congruent care puzzle. *Journal of Transcultural Nursing*, *22*(1), 77–82.
Wolfe, D. A., & McIsaac, C. (2011). Distinguishing between poor/dysfunctional parenting and child emotional maltreatment. *Child Abuse & Neglect*, *35*(10), 802–813.
Zhang, Y., Wei, M., et al. (2014). Chinese family management of chronic childhood conditions: A cluster analysis. *Journal for Specialists in Pediatric Nursing*, *19*(1), 39–53.

Readiness for enhanced Parenting

Kimberly Silvey, MSN, RN

NANDA-I

Definition

A pattern of providing an environment for children or other dependent persons to nurture growth and development, which can be strengthened

Defining Characteristics

Children express desire to enhance home environment; expresses desire to enhance parenting; parent expresses desire to enhance emotional support of children; parent expresses desire to enhance emotional support of other dependent person

NOC (Nursing Outcomes Classification)

Suggested NOC Outcomes

Child Development; Knowledge: Child Physical Safety; Parenting Performance; Parenting: Psychosocial Safety

Example NOC Outcome with Indicators

Parenting Performance as evidenced by the following indicators: Provides preventive and episodic health care/Stimulates cognitive and social development/Stimulates emotional and spiritual growth/Empathizes with child/Expresses satisfaction with parental role/Expresses positive self-esteem. (Rate the outcome and indicators of **Parenting Performance:** 1 = never demonstrated, 2 = rarely demonstrated, 3 = sometimes demonstrated, 4 = often demonstrated, 5 = consistently demonstrated [see Section I].)

Client Outcomes

Client/Family Will (Specify Time Frame)

- Affirm desire to improve parenting skills to further support growth and development of children
- Demonstrate loving relationship with children
- Provide a safe, nurturing environment
- Assess risks in home/environment and take steps to prevent possibility of harm to children
- Meet physical, psychosocial, and spiritual needs or seek appropriate assistance

NIC (Nursing Interventions Classification)

Suggested NIC Interventions

Anticipatory Guidance; Attachment Promotion; Developmental Enhancement: Adolescent; Child; Family Integrity Promotion: Childbearing Family; Infant Care; Newborn Care; Parent Education: Adolescent; Childrearing Family; Infant; Parenting Promotion; Teaching: Infant Stimulation

Example NIC Activities—Parenting Promotion

Assist parents to have realistic expectations appropriate to developmental and ability level of child; Assist parents with role transition and expectations of parenthood

P

Nursing Interventions and *Rationales*

- Use family-centered care and role modeling for holistic care of families. EB: *Incorporating family-centered care helps enhance the parents' role in caring for their child (Kuo et al, 2012).*
- Assess parents' feelings when dealing with a child who has a chronic illness. EB: *Nursing should assist parents (Byczkowski et al, 2014) to identify their feelings about their child to help the parents develop coping mechanisms.*
- Promote low-technology interventions, such as massage and multisensory interventions (maternal voice, eye-to-eye contact, and rocking) and music to reduce maternal and infant stress and improve mother-infant relationship. EBN: *Infant massage and gentle touch may represent a support to the mother-child bonding and to the newborn's development (Leni, 2011).*
- Support kangaroo care for infants at risk at birth; keep infants in an upright position in skin-to-skin contact. EB: *Kangaroo care helps the mother and infant to not only start bonding but also assist in the infant's growth and development (de Leon-Mendoza & Mokhachane, 2011).*
- When the person who is ill is the parent, use family-centered assessment skills to determine the impact of an adult's illness on the child, and then guide the parent through those topics that are most likely to be of concern. EB: *Nurses should be educated on how to communicate and identify the needs of young children when a parent is ill (Sutter & Reid, 2012).*
- Provide practical and psychological assistance for parents of clients with psychiatric diagnoses, such as schizophrenia. EB: *Help parents understand the diagnosis of mental illness and the things they can do to help their child (Kusumi & Ross, 2012).*
- Refer to the care plan for Impaired **Parenting** for additional interventions.

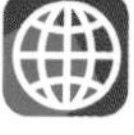

Multicultural

- Assess the influence of cultural beliefs, norms, and values on the client's perception of parenting. EB: *Understanding the cultural beliefs of the family will assist in parental satisfaction with care (Hamilton et al, 2013).*

- Acknowledge racial and ethnic differences at the onset of care and provide appropriate health information and social support. EB: *Acknowledgment of racial and ethnicity issues enhances communication, establishes rapport, and promotes treatment outcomes (Tavallali et al, 2014).*
- Support programs for parents of young children in specific cultural communities. EBN: *Parents and children benefit when a support group is incorporated in the care (Wei et al, 2012).*
- Clarify parents' feelings, expectations, perceptions, and availability regarding participation in the care of their sick child. EBN: *Cultural differences in regard to parent participation in the care of ill or hospitalized children should be considered (Smits et al, 2012).*
- Acknowledge and praise parenting strengths noted. EBN: *Clinicians could explore and support the positive qualities of parenting in a culturally congruent way (Whittaker & Cowley, 2012).*

Home Care

- The nursing interventions previously described should be used in the home environment with adaptations as necessary. EBN: *Clinicians should educate parents on the care the child will need at home and modify to meet the family's needs (Doyle & Buckley, 2012).*
- ▲ Refer to a parenting program to facilitate learning of parenting skills. EBN: *The study shows that parenting programs can increase parental knowledge as well as confidence (Kendall et al, 2013).*

Client/Family Teaching and Discharge Planning

- Refer to Client/Family Teaching and Discharge Planning for Impaired **Parenting** for suggestions that may be used with minor adaptations.
- Teach parents home safety: reduction of hot water temperature, proper poison storage, use of smoke alarms, and installation of safety gates for stairs. EB: *Education may reduce injury and promote children's home safety (Lehna et al, 2014).*
- Teach parents and young teens conflict resolution by using a hypothetical conflict solution with and without a structured conflict resolution guide. Support self-direction of the families with minimal therapist intervention. EB: *Encouraging parent participation in positive-parenting programs can decrease the conflict for parents and teens (Salari et al, 2013).*
- Refer mothers of children with type 1 diabetes for community support in babysitting, child care, or respite. EB: *Mothers raising children with diabetes need to have support and interventions to assist with the care of the child to help reduce their stress (Monaghan et al, 2011).*
- Teach families the importance of monitoring television viewing and limiting exposure to violence. EBN: *Media violence can be hazardous to children's health, and studies overwhelmingly point to a causal connection between media violence and aggressive attitudes, values, and behaviors in some children (McBride, 2011).*
- Promotion of better quality relationships between parents and children is an effective strategy that can lead to enhanced learning. Good quality parenting leads to improved cognitive and social skills for children. EB: *Programs can help parents identify strategies that can develop social skills (Ayoub et al, 2011).*

REFERENCES

See impaired **Parenting** for additional references.

Ayoub, C., Vallotton, C. D., et al. (2011). Developmental pathways to integrated social skills: the roles of parenting and early intervention. *Child Development*, *82*(2), 583–600.

Byczkowski, T. L., Munafo, J. K., et al. (2014). Family perceptions of the usability and value of chronic disease web-based patient portals. *Health Informatics Journal*, *20*(2), 151–162.

de Leon-Mendoza, S., & Mokhachane, M. (2011). "Early" or timely discharge in kangaroo mother care: evidence and experience. *Current Women's Health Reviews*, *7*(3), 270–277.

Doyle, C., & Buckley, S. (2012). An account of nursing a child with complex needs in the home. *Nursing Children & Young People*, *24*(5), 19–22.

Hamilton, L., Lerner, C., et al. (2013). Effects of a medical home program for children with special health care needs on parental perceptions of care in an ethnically diverse patient population. *Maternal & Child Health Journal*, *17*(3), 463–469.

Kendall, S., Bloomfield, L., et al. (2013). Efficacy of a group-based parenting program on stress and self-efficacy among Japanese mothers: a quasi-experimental study. *Nursing & Health Sciences*, *15*(4), 454–460.

Kuo, D., Houtrow, A., et al. (2012). Family-centered care: current applications and future directions in pediatric health care. *Maternal & Child Health Journal*, *16*(2), 297–305.

Kusumi, J., & Ross, R. G. (2012). Prevalence of psychiatric illness in primary caretakers of childhood-onset schizophrenia subjects. *Mental Illness (2036-7457)*, *4*(2), 115–119.

Lehna, C., Janes, E. G., et al. (2014). Community partnership to promote home fire safety in children with special needs. *Burns (03054179)*, *40*(6), 1179–1184.

Leni, E. (2011). Gentle touch and infant massage: means to development and growth, support to child-parents interaction in premature and low birth weight newborns. *Child Nurse Ital J Pediatr Nurs Sci*, *3*(4), 114–117.

P

McBride, D. L. (2011). Commercials on children's television channels. *Journal of Pediatric Nursing, 26*(2), 165–166.

Monaghan, M. M., et al. (2011). Supporting parents of very young children with type 1 diabetes: results from a pilot study. *Patient Education and Counseling, 82*(2), 271–274.

Salari, R., Fabian, H., et al. (2013). The Children and Parents in Focus project: a population-based cluster-randomised controlled trial to prevent behavioural and emotional problems in children. *BMC Public Health, 13*(1), 225–241.

Smits, M., Wagner, C., et al. (2012). The role of patient safety culture in the causation of unintended events in hospitals. *Journal of Clinical Nursing, 21*(23/24), 3392–3401.

Sutter, C., & Reid, T. (2012). How do we talk to the children? Child life consultation to support the children of seriously ill adult inpatients. *Journal of Palliative Medicine, 15*(12), 1362–1368.

Tavallali, A. G., Kabir, Z. N., et al. (2014). Ethnic Swedish Parents' experiences of minority ethnic nurses' cultural competence in Swedish paediatric care. *Scandinavian Journal of Caring Sciences, 28*(2), 255–263.

Wei, Y.-S., Chu, H., et al. (2012). Support groups for caregivers of intellectually disabled family members: effects on physical-psychological health and social support. *Journal of Clinical Nursing, 21*(11/12), 1666–1677.

Whittaker, K. A., & Cowley, S. (2012). A survey of parental self-efficacy experiences: maximising potential through health visiting and universal parenting support. *Journal of Clinical Nursing, 21*(21/22), 3276–3286.

Risk for impaired Parenting *Gail B. Ladwig, MSN, RN*

NANDA-I

Definition

Vulnerable to inability of the primary caretaker to create, maintain, or regain an environment that promotes the optimum growth and development of the child, which may compromise the well-being of the child

Risk Factors

Infant or Child

Altered in perceptual abilities; behavior disorder (e.g., attention deficit, oppositional defiant); developmental delay; difficult temperament; disabling condition; gender other than desired; illness; multiple births; prematurity; prolonged separation from parent; temperament conflicts with parental expectations

Knowledge

Alteration in cognitive functioning; ineffective communication skills; insufficient cognitive readiness for parenting; insufficient knowledge about child development; insufficient knowledge about child health maintenance; insufficient knowledge about parenting skills; insufficient response to infant cues; low educational level preference for physical punishment; unrealistic expectations

Physiological

Physical illness

Psychological

Closely spaced pregnancies; depression; difficult birthing process; disabling condition; high number of pregnancies; history of mental illness; history of substance abuse; nonrestorative sleep pattern (i.e., due to caregiver responsibilities, parenting practices, sleep partner); sleep deprivation; young parental age

Social

Change in family unit; compromised home environment; conflict between partners; economically disadvantaged; father of child not involved; history of abuse (e.g., physical, psychological, sexual); history of being abusive; inadequate child care arrangements; ineffective coping strategies; insufficient access to resources; insufficient family cohesiveness; insufficient parental role model; insufficient prenatal care; insufficient problem-solving skills; insufficient resources (e.g., financial, social, knowledge); insufficient social support; insufficient transportation; insufficient valuing of parenthood; late-term prenatal care; legal difficulty; low self-esteem; mother of child not involved; parent-child separation; relocation; role strain; single parent; social isolation; stressors; unemployment; unplanned pregnancy; unwanted pregnancy; work difficulty

NOC, NIC, Client Outcomes, Nursing Interventions, Client/Family Teaching and Discharge Planning, *Rationales*, and References

Refer to care plans for Readiness for enhanced **Parenting** and Impaired **Parenting.**

Risk for Perioperative Positioning injury

Mary Beth Flynn Makic, PhD, RN, CNS, CCNS, FAAN

NANDA-I

Definition

Vulnerable to inadvertent anatomical and physical changes as a result of posture or equipment used during an invasive/surgical procedure, which may compromise health

Risk Factors

Disorientation; edema; emaciation; immobilization; muscle weakness; obesity; sensory-perceptual disturbance from anesthesia

NOC (Nursing Outcomes Classification)

Suggested NOC Outcomes

Circulation Status; Immobility Consequences: Physiological; Joint Movement; Neurological Status; Respiratory Status; Risk Control; Sensory Function; Skeletal Function; Tissue Integrity: Skin and Mucous Membranes; Tissue Perfusion: Peripheral

Example NOC Outcome with Indicators

Tissue Perfusion: Peripheral as evidenced by the following indicators: Peripheral edema/Localized extremity pain/Skin breakdown/Muscle cramps/Peripheral pulses/Numbness/Tingling/Necrosis. (Rate the outcome and indicators of **Tissue Perfusion: Peripheral:** 1 = severe, 2 = substantial, 3 = moderate, 4 = mild, 5 = none [see Section I].)

Client Outcomes

Client Will (Specify Time Frame)

- Demonstrate unchanged skin condition, with exception of the incision, throughout the perioperative experience
- Demonstrate resolution of redness of the skin at points of pressure within 30 minutes after pressure is eliminated
- Remain injury-free related to surgical positioning, including intact skin and absence of pain and/or numbness associated with surgical positioning
- Demonstrate unchanged or improved physical mobility from preoperative status
- Demonstrate unchanged or improved peripheral sensory integrity from preoperative status

NIC (Nursing Interventions Classification)

Suggested NIC Interventions

Circulatory Precautions; Fall Prevention; Neurological Monitoring; Peripheral Sensation Management; Positioning: Intraoperative; Pressure Ulcer Prevention; Risk Identification; Skin Surveillance; Surgical Precautions

Example NIC Activities—Positioning: Intraoperative

Use an adequate number of personnel to transfer client; Maintain client's proper body alignment

Nursing Interventions and *Rationales*

General Interventions for Any Surgical Client

- Assess the client's skin integrity throughout the perioperative process to avoid skin breakdown during surgical/invasive procedures. EB: *Developing skin breakdown manifested as a skin tear, pressure ulcer, deep tissue injury, or burn is a significant client complication impacted by the duration of surgery and client positioning (Fred et al, 2012; National Pressure Ulcer Advisory Panel and European Pressure Ulcer Advisory Panel [NPUAP/EPUAP], 2014).*

P

Prevention of Pressure Ulcers

- Complete a preoperative assessment to identify physical alterations that may require additional precautions for procedure-specific positioning and to identify specific procedural positioning needs, type of anesthesia, and so on. EBN: *Factors to consider when assessing the surgical client to plan for proper positioning are preexisting conditions, range of motion, presence of prostheses and/or fractures, age, height, and weight (Spruce & Van Wicklin, 2014). Use resources (e.g., positioning aids, padding, transfer devices) to reduce the risk of tissue injury in the care of the older client (AORN, 2015b).*
- Identify risk factors such as length and type of surgery, potential for intraoperative hypotensive episodes, low core temperatures, and decreased mobility on postoperative day 1. EB: *Assess the client for additional risk factors to include the duration of immobilization before and during the surgical procedure, client severity of illness, and preoperative nutritional status (Spruce et al, 2014; NPUAP/EPUAP, 2014). Surgeries lasting more than 4 hours provide a significant risk for pressure ulcer development (Sterner et al, 2011).* EBN: *A recent study showed that vasopressor use is a significant risk factor for pressure ulcer development. The study also showed that the number of surgeries a client has during his/her inpatient stay and the length of surgery (over 1 hour), body mass index, Braden score, mortality risk, and history of diabetes are also risk factors for pressure ulcer development. This study did not show that age was related to pressure ulcer development (Tschannen et al, 2012).*
- Recognize that all surgical clients should be considered at high risk for pressure ulcer development, because pressure ulcers can develop in as little as 20 minutes in the operating room.
- Protect the heels during surgery by elevating the heels completely. EB: *Ensure the heels are free of the surface of the operating table (NPUAP/EPUAP, 2014). Heel pressure ulcers are one of the most common sites for pressure injury during surgery. Traditional devices such as egg crates, booties, and heel pads do not decrease the pressure.*
- Use pressure-reducing devices and pressure-relieving mattresses as necessary to prevent ulcer formation. EB: *Use a high specification reactive or alternating pressure support surface on the operating table for all individuals identified as being at risk for pressure ulcer development (NPUAP/EPUAP, 2014). Additional support surfaces may be indicated to offload pressure points on the face and body when the client is placed in a prone position (Spruce et al, 2014; NPUAP/EPUAP, 2014). Assess for shearing forces that may cause tissue injury when placing the client in Trendelenburg position for selected robotic surgical procedures (Sutton et al, 2013).*
- Avoid using rolled sheets and towels as positioning devices; they tend to produce high and inconsistent pressures. Special positioning devices are available that redistribute pressure. EBN: *Towels and rolled sheets contribute to friction injuries (AORN, 2015).*
- Avoid covering positioning devices or placing extra blankets on top of a pressure-reducing surface. CEB: *Adding material to a pressure reduction surface actually increases the pressure, thus producing a negative result (Aronovitch, 2007; St. Arnaud & Paquin, 2008). Use of rolled sheets and towels beneath overlays decreases the overlay's effectiveness and causes pressure.*
- The nurse should demonstrate knowledge not only of the equipment, but also of anatomy and the application of physiological principles in order to properly position the client. EBN: *Preplanning ensures that the correct positioning devices are available and in good working condition, and that appropriate numbers of personnel are available to position the client safely and appropriately (AORN, 2015a).*
- Monitor pressure being applied to the client intraoperatively by staff, equipment, and/or instruments (AORN, 2015a).
- Pad all bony prominences. EB: *Some positioning devices are solid and can increase pressure over bony prominences (Sutton et al, 2013).*
- Recognize that reddened areas or areas injured by pressure should not be massaged. EB: *Rubbing causes friction that can lead to damage to skin/tissue (NPUAP/EPUAP, 2014).*
- Implement measures to prevent inadvertent hypothermia. *Anesthesia can compromise perfusion by causing hypotension and hypothermia. When coupled with the client being immobile on a noncompliant surface for an extended time period, hypothermia increases vulnerability for pressure ulcer development during surgery (St. Arnaud & Paquin, 2008).*
- Many surgical clients have medical devices placed as a part of the surgical procedure. Avoid positioning the client on the medical device and perform frequent assessments of the skin under and around the device *(Apold et al, 2012; NPUAP/EPUAP, 2014).*

P

Positioning the Perioperative Client

- Ensure that linens on the operating room table are free of wrinkles. *Wrinkles may cause pressure/injury to the skin if the client is unable to move for prolonged periods of time.*
- Lock the operating room table, cart, or bed and stabilize the mattress before transfer/positioning the client. Monitor the client while on the operating room table at all times. EB: *Studies showed that a lack of clear communication about who should be watching the client has contributed to falls (AORN, 2015a).*
- Lift rather than pull or slide the client when positioning to reduce the incidence of skin injury from shearing and/or friction. EB: *Sliding or pulling the client can cause shearing force and/or friction (AORN, 2015a; NPUAP/EPUAP, 2014).*
- Ensure that appropriate numbers of personnel are present to assist in positioning the client. EBN: *A minimum of two people should assist an awake client to transfer from a cart/bed to the operating room table: one person on the stretcher side to assist the client onto the table and a second person on the far side of the table to prevent the client from falling off (AORN, 2015a). A minimum of four persons are necessary when transferring/positioning an anesthetized, unconscious, obese, or weak client (AORN, 2015a).*
- Recognize that, optimally, clients (especially those with limited range of motion/mobility) should be asked to position themselves under the nurse's guidance before induction of anesthesia so that he/she can verify that a position of comfort has been obtained.
- Ensure that nerves are protected by positioning extremities carefully. EB: *Nerves can be injured by stretching and compression, which is caused by a loss of protective muscle tone and pressure between two fixed points. Careful attention to proper body alignment and padding is necessary to prevent peripheral nerve injury (Bouyer-Ferullo, 2013).*
- Use slow and smooth movements during positioning to allow the circulatory system to readjust.
- Reassess the client after positioning and periodically during the procedure to maintain proper alignment and skin integrity. EBN: *Changes in position can expose or injure body parts (e.g., shearing, friction, compression) that were originally protected, and the safety strap can shift and apply increased pressure (AORN, 2012).*
- Frequently assess the eyes and/or monitor intraocular pressure, especially when client is in prone or knee-chest position. CEB/EB: *The cornea can easily be injured during surgery due to a decrease in lacrimation and/or improperly applied face masks, or prolonged prone positioning (Spruce et al, 2014; Ellsworth et al, 2009).*
- Position hips in proper alignment with knees flexed. Unaligned hips can cause pressure to the low back and hip joints.
- Position the arms extended on arm boards so that they do not extend beyond a 90-degree angle. Do not position arms at sides unless surgically necessary. CEB: *Positioning at less than a 90-degree angle, with elbows slightly flexed and hands supine, decreases the risk of a stretching injury to the brachial plexus and possible compression or occlusion injury to the subclavian and axillary arteries (Ellsworth et al, 2009). When positioning arms at sides is necessary, place the arms beneath the sheet and bring the sheet over the top of the arm and then tuck the sheet beneath the mattress, so the arm cannot fall off the mattress and hang over the metal edge of the table, where the surgical team could lean against it (AORN, 2015a).*
- Protect the client's skin surfaces from injury by preventing pooling of preparative solutions, blood, irrigation, urine, and feces. EBN: *Prep solutions may change the pH of the skin and remove protective oils, making the skin more susceptible to pressure and friction. Pooling also increases the risk of maceration (AORN, 2015a).*
- Keep the client appropriately covered during the procedure. *Reducing unnecessary exposure provides privacy and dignity for the client during positioning and helps prevent hypothermia (AORN, 2015a).*
- When positioning the client prone, care should be taken to ensure the head and neck are properly positioned. EB: *Inappropriate positioning of the head and neck in the prone position can lead to vertebral artery obstruction and possible stroke. Standard foam prone pillows should be used because they stabilize the neck in neutral, and the endotracheal tube can be positioned away from the face to decrease excessive pressure (Ellsworth et al, 2009; Spruce et al, 2014).*
- Recognize that clients positioned in lithotomy position should be kept in this position for as short a time as possible. EB: *One research review suggests that the client's legs be removed from lithotomy positioning devices every 2 hours when the procedure is expected to last 4 hours or longer (AORN, 2015a).*

P

- The lowest heel position should be used in the lithotomy position. EBN: *In one study, as the height of the calf support increased, pressure also increased (Lopes & Galvao, 2010).*
- Position the client's legs parallel and uncrossed.
- Maintain normal body alignment. *Misalignment, flexion, extension, and rotation may cause muscle and nerve damage, as well as airway interference; pressure on the carotid sinus can cause arrhythmias; and restricted venous outflow can occur with extreme rotation of the head (St. Arnaud & Paquin, 2008).*
- When applying body supports and restraint straps (safety belt), apply loosely and secure over waist or mid-thigh at least 2 inches above knees, avoiding bony prominences by placing a blanket between the strap and the client. EB: *Belts positioned directly over the knees cause compression of the peroneal nerve against the fibula (St. Arnaud & Paquin, 2008).*
- Assess the client's skin integrity immediately postoperatively. EB: *Assess and document postoperative skin/tissue integrity focusing on areas with constant pressure during the procedure and limb function for nerve damage (St. Arnaud & Paquin, 2008; Sutton et al, 2013; NPUAP/EPUAP, 2014).*
- Ensure that complete, concise, accurate documentation of client assessment and use of positioning devices is in the client's medical record.

REFERENCES

AORN. (2015a). *Clinical Practice Position Statements.* Retrieved June 25, 2015. <http://www.aorn.org/Clinical_Practice/Position_Statements/Position_Statements.aspx>.

AORN. (2015b). *Position statement on the care of the older adult in perioperative settings.* Retrieved June 25, 2015. <http://www.aorn.org/Clinical_Practice/Position_Statements/Position_Statements.aspx>.

Apold, J., & Rydrych, D. (2012). Preventing device-related pressure ulcers: Using data to guide statewide change. *Journal of Nursing Care Quality, 27*(1), 28–34.

Aronovitch, S. A. (2007). Intraoperatively acquired pressure ulcers: are there common risk factors? *Ostomy/Wound Management, 53*(2), 57–69.

Bouyer-Ferullo, S. (2013). Preventing perioperative peripheral nerve injuries. *AORN, 97*(1), 111–121.

Ellsworth, W. A., Basu, C. B., & Iverson, R. E. (2009). Perioperative considerations for patient safety during cosmetic surgery preventing complications. *Can J Plast Surg, 17*(1), 9–16.

Fred, C., Ford, S., Wagner, D., et al. (2012). Intraoperatively acquired pressure ulcers and perioperative normothermia: a look at relationships. *AORN, 96*(3), 251–260.

Lopes, C. M., & Galvao, C. M. (2010). Surgical positioning: evidence for nursing care. *Revista Latino-Americana de Enfermagem, 18*(2), 287–294.

National Pressure Ulcer Advisory Panel (NPUAP) and European Pressure Ulcer Advisory Panel (EPUAP) (2014). E. Haesler (Ed.), *Prevention and Treatment of Pressure Ulcers.* Perth, Australia: Cambridge Media.

Spruce, L., & Van Wicklin, S. A. (2014). Back to basics: positioning the patient. *AORN, 100*(3), 299–302.

St. Arnaud, D., & Paquin, M. J. (2008). Safe positioning for the neurosurgical patient. *AORN Journal, 87*, 1156–1168.

Sterner, E., et al. (2011). Category I pressure ulcers—how reliable is clinical assessment? *Orthopaed Nurs, 30*(3), 194–205.

Sutton, S., Link, T., & Makic, M. B. F. (2013). A quality improvement project for safe and effective patient positioning during robot-assisted surgery. *AORN, 97*(4), 448–456.

Tschannen, D., et al. (2012). Patient-specific and surgical characteristics in the development of pressure ulcers. *American Journal of Critical Care, 21*(2), 116–124.

P

Risk for Peripheral Neurovascular dysfunction

Betty J. Ackley, MSN, EdS, RN, and Mary Beth Flynn Makic, PhD, RN, CNS, CCNS, FAAN

NANDA-I

Definition

Vulnerable to disruption in the circulation, sensation, and motion of an extremity, which may compromise health

Risk Factors

Burns; fractures; immobilization; mechanical compression (e.g., tourniquet, cane, cast, brace, dressing, restraint); orthopedic surgery; trauma; vascular obstruction

NOC (Nursing Outcomes Classification)

Suggested NOC Outcomes

Circulation Status; Neurological Status: Spinal Sensorimotor Function; Tissue Perfusion: Peripheral

Example NOC Outcome with Indicators

Tissue Perfusion: Peripheral as evidenced by the following indicators: Radial or pedal pulse strength/Capillary refill in fingers or toes/Extremity skin temperature/Localized extremity pain/Numbness/Tingling/Skin color/Muscle strength/Skin integrity/Peripheral edema. (Rate the outcome and indicators of **Tissue Perfusion: Peripheral:** 1 = severe deviation from normal range, 2 = substantial deviation from normal range, 3 = moderate deviation from normal range, 4 = mild deviation from normal range, 5 = no deviation from normal range [see Section I].)

Client Outcomes

Client Will (Specify Time Frame)

- Maintain circulation, sensation, and movement of an extremity within client's own normal limits
- Explain signs of neurovascular compromise

NIC (Nursing Interventions Classification)

Suggested NIC Interventions

Exercise Therapy: Joint Mobility; Peripheral Sensation Management

Example NIC Activities—Peripheral Sensation Management

Monitor for paresthesia: numbness, tingling, hyperesthesia, and hypoesthesia; Monitor for thrombophlebitis and deep vein thrombosis

P

Nursing Interventions and *Rationales*

▲ Recognize situations in the Risk Factors that may result in peripheral neurovascular dysfunction. Compartment syndrome may be due to increased volume of the contents of a compartment, or reduced capacity of the compartment sheath. Reduced capacity is associated with tight dressings, bandages, or casts (Mabvuure et al, 2012).

▲ Assess for the early onset of compartment syndrome, and report to health care provider promptly. Perform neurovascular assessment every 15 minutes to every 4 hours as ordered or needed based on client's condition. Use the five Ps of assessment as outlined below. *The goal is to prevent ischemia (cell death). Delay in recognizing compartment syndrome can lead to paralysis, rhabdomyolysis, contracture, and amputation of the limb (Garner et al, 2014). Compartment syndrome is primarily diagnosed by physical examination, and because of the devastating consequences of a missed compartment syndrome, a fasciotomy should be considered. Assess for presence of any of the six Ps.*

- ❍ Pain: Assess severity (on a scale of 1 to 10), quality, radiation, and relief by medications. Pain is usually "out of proportion" to the injury, requiring strong opiates, and is often described as burning, feeling deep in the muscle or structure, and elicited with passive stretching of the compartment (Donaldson et al, 2014).
- ❍ Pulses: Check the pulses distal to the injury. *Palpate pulses in area of concern; for example, for a tibial fracture, assess dorsalis pedis and posterior tibial pulses. Compartment syndrome can occur in the face of an intact pulse. Always assess the uninjured or unaffected side and compare with the area of concern.*
- ❍ Pallor: Check color and temperature changes below the injury site. Check capillary refill. *If pallor is present, record the level of coldness carefully and report to health care provider promptly. A cold, pale, or bluish extremity indicates arterial insufficiency or arterial damage, and a health care provider should be notified.*

- ❍ Paresthesia (change in sensation): Check by lightly touching the skin proximal and distal to the injury. Ask if the client has any unusual sensations such as hypersensitivity, tingling, prickling, decreased feeling, or numbness. Check nerve function (e.g., whether the client can feel a touch to the area of concern, such as the first web space of the foot [deep peroneal nerve] with tibial fracture). *Irreversible damage from compartment syndrome occurs when compression to tissue and nerves is left unchecked (Garner et al, 2014).*
- ❍ Paralysis: Ask the client to perform appropriate range-of-motion exercises in the unaffected and then the affected extremity. *Loss of movement (paralysis) is a late symptom of compartment syndrome. Decreased range of motion and loss of movement can indicate impending muscle, nerve, and cellular death (Donaldson et al, 2014).*
- ❍ Pressure: Check by feeling the extremity; note new onset of firmness or swelling of the extremity, as well as a firm "wooden" feeling upon deep palpation. *Internal pressure or external confinement or restriction can proceed to the point at which cellular exchange is diminished. Swelling and tightness of the involved compartment are indications of increased pressure. Not only are surgical or trauma clients at risk for neurovascular compromise, but also are clients on bed rest because of changes in blood flow through the cardiovascular system (Donaldson et al, 2014).*

▲ All of the Ps may not be present, and they are not specific for compartment syndrome. Have a high index of suspicion for any of the Ps. Noting two or more of the Ps increases the probability of compartment syndrome. Monitor the client for compartment syndrome of the nonoperated leg as well as the operated leg.

- Monitor appropriate application and function of corrective device (e.g., cast, splint, traction) every 1 to 4 hours as needed. *Compartment syndrome can result from improper casting or splinting and is the most serious complication of casting or splinting. The condition results from increased pressure within a closed space that compromises blood flow. After immobilization (casting or splinting), if pain worsens or there is any tingling or numbness, swelling, delayed capillary refill, or change in color of exposed digit, immediate evaluation is needed. Casting or splinting can cause thermal injuries or skin breakdown; therefore, proper padding is essential. Position the extremity in correct alignment with each position change; check every hour to ensure appropriate alignment.*

▲ For prevention of deep vein thrombosis (DVT), nursing care of DVT, and pulmonary embolism, refer to the interventions on DVT prevention and treatment in the care plan for Ineffective peripheral **Tissue Perfusion.**

P

REFERENCES

Donaldson, J., Haddad, B., & Khan, W. S. (2014). The pathophysiology, diagnosis and current management of acute compartment syndrome. *Open Orthop, Suppl 1*(8), 185–193. PMCID: PMC4110398. Published online Jun 27, 2014.

Garner, M. R., et al. (2014). Compartment syndrome: diagnosis, Management, and unique concerns in the twenty-first century. *Hospital for Special Surgery, 10*(2).

Mabvuure, N. T., et al. (2012). Acute compartment syndrome of the limbs: current concepts and management. *Open Ortho J, 6*, 535–543.

Risk for Poisoning

Melodie Cannon, DNP, MSc/FNP, BHScN, RN(EC), NP-PHC, CEN, GNC(C)

NANDA-I

Definition

Vulnerable to accidental exposure to, or ingestion of, drugs or dangerous products in sufficient doses that may compromise health

Risk Factors

External

- Access to dangerous product
- Access to illicit drugs potentially contaminated by poisonous additives
- Access to large supply of pharmaceutical agents in house
- Access to pharmaceutical agent

Internal

- Alteration in cognitive functioning
- Emotional disturbance
- Inadequate precautions against poisoning
- Insufficient knowledge of pharmacological agents
- Insufficient knowledge of poisoning prevention
- Occupational setting without adequate safeguards
- Reduced vision
- Addiction

NOC (Nursing Outcomes Classification)

Suggested NOC Outcomes

Knowledge: Child Physical Safety, Medication, Personal Safety; Parenting Performance; Risk Control; Risk Control: Alcohol Use, Drug Use; Risk Detection; Safe Home Environment

Example NOC Outcome with Indicators

Knowledge: Child Physical Safety as evidenced by the following indicators: Appropriate activities for child's developmental level/Strategies to prevent medication misuse/Strategies to prevent exposure to toxic chemicals or substances. (Rate the outcome and indicators of **Knowledge: Child Physical Safety:** 1 = no knowledge, 2 = limited knowledge, 3 = moderate knowledge, 4 = substantial knowledge, 5 = extensive knowledge [see Section I].)

Client Outcomes

Client Will (Specify Time Frame)

- Prevent inadvertent ingestion of or exposure to toxins or poisonous substances
- Explain and undertake appropriate safety measures to prevent ingestion of or exposure to toxins or poisonous substances
- Verbalize appropriate response to apparent or suspected toxic ingestion or poisoning

P

NIC (Nursing Interventions Classification)

Suggested NIC Interventions

Environmental Management: Safety, First Aid; Health Education; Medication Management; Surveillance; Surveillance: Safety

Example NIC Activities—Environmental Management: Safety

Identify safety hazards in the environment (i.e., physical, biological, and chemical); Remove hazards from the environment, when possible

Nursing Interventions and *Rationales*

- When a client comes to the hospital with possible poisoning, begin care following the ABCs and administer oxygen if needed. EB: *Poisoning is a major cause of morbidity/mortality worldwide. Initial evaluation should include vital signs, mental status, pupil size, oxygenation, finger stick glucose, and cardiac monitoring. Management is geared to supportive care, prevention of poison absorption, antidote use, and elimination techniques (Rhyee, 2013).*

▲ It is important for the triage nurse to call the poison control center. *The poison control hotline is 1-800-222-1222.* Poison centers are a valuable tool for medical consultations. They are staffed by nurses, pharmacists, toxicologists, and other specialists in poisons and toxins who can recommend treatment advice *(American Association of Poison Control Centers, 2014).*

- Obtain a thorough history of what was ingested, how much, and when, and ask to look at the containers. Note the client's age, weight, medications, medical conditions, and any history of vomiting, choking, coughing, or change in mental status. Also take note of any interventions performed before seeking treatment. EB: *The history is important to confirm the diagnosis and is often unreliable when provided by clients with intentional ingestion. Additional information should be obtained from paramedics, police, family, and friends when possible (Rhyee, 2013).*

- Carefully inspect for signs of ingestion of poisons, including an odor on the breath, a trace of the substance on the clothing, burns, or redness around the mouth and lips, as well as signs of confusion, vomiting, or dyspnea. CEB: *It is important to look for signs of ingestion of poison before initiating treatment because up to 40% of children who present with poisoning have not actually been exposed to the suspected toxin (Hwang et al, 2003).*

▲ Note results of toxicology screens, arterial blood gases, blood glucose levels, and any other ordered laboratory tests. *If information about what was ingested is incomplete or inaccurate, laboratory tests may be needed to determine treatment. The poison control center will provide valuable information regarding appropriate labs and investigations specific to the suspected toxin.*

▲ Initiate any ordered treatment for poisoning quickly. The poison control center will specify any treatment or medications that need to be administered. EB: *Client decontamination consisting of water or saline irrigation for topical exposures or the administration of activated charcoal may be required. Early decontamination helps prevent poison absorption (Rhyee, 2013).*

▲ *Ensure recommendations from the poison control center are clearly documented and readily accessible in the client's chart.*

▲ *If the client's condition deteriorates, contact the poison control center again for further direction and notify the most responsible provider.*

Safety Guidelines for Medication Administration

- Prevent iatrogenic harm to the hospitalized client by following these guidelines for administering medications:
  - Use at least two methods to identify the client before administering medications or blood products, such as the client's name and medical record number or birth date. Do not use the client's room number. Use bar code scanning system for client identification if used by your facility.
  - When taking verbal or telephone orders, the orders should be written down and read back for verification to the individual giving the order. The health care provider who gave the orders for the medication then needs to confirm the information that was read back.
- Standardize use of abbreviations, acronyms, symbols, and dose designations and eliminate those that are prone to cause errors. (Refer to The Joint Commission, Critical Access Hospital National Patient Safety Goals for list of abbreviations, acronyms, symbols, and dose designations that should not be used.)
  - Be aware of the medications that look/sound alike and ensure that the correct medication is ordered and administered.
  - Use the eight rights of medication administration to decrease the potential for error:
  - Right client, right medication, right reason, right dose, right frequency, right route, right site, and right time (College of Nurses of Ontario, 2014). Take high-alert medications off the nursing unit, such as potassium chloride. Standardize concentrations of medications such as morphine in patient-controlled analgesia pumps.
  - Follow agency policy/procedures for medications that require two-person check and co-signature.
  - Label all medications and medication containers or other solutions that are on or off a sterile field for a procedure. Label them when they are first taken out of the original packaging to another container. Label with medication name, strength, amount, and expiration date/time. Review the labels whenever there is a change of personnel.
  - Use only intravenous (IV) pumps that prevent free flow of IV solution when the tubing is taken out of the pump.
- Identify all the client's current medications on admission to a health care facility and compare the list with the current ordered medications. Reconcile any differences in medications. Use the expertise of the pharmacy department if there is any uncertainty regarding the accuracy of the client's medications.
- Reconcile the list of medications if the client is transferred from one unit to another, when there is a handoff to the next provider of care, and when the client is discharged.

Adverse drug events occur with disturbing frequency, and communication problems between settings of care are a significant factor in their occurrence (Safer Healthcare Now, 2012).

- Detect possible interactions and cumulative or other adverse effects among prescribed medications, self-administered over-the-counter products, culturally based home treatments, herbal remedies, and foods.

P

Medication reconciliation is an important safety issue due to the number of people taking multiple medications and involves determining what medications the person should be taking, medications they are actually taking, and resolving discrepancies (The Joint Commission, 2014).

Pediatric

- ▲ Evaluate lead exposure risk and consult the health care provider regarding lead screening measures as indicated (public/ambulatory health). *Children can be exposed to lead from multiple sources: house paint, dust, soil, imported toys, imported candy or food, and traditional medications, ceramic housewares, drinking water, and living near lead smelters or battery recycling plants (Barn & Kosatsky, 2011; Ness, 2013).*
- • Provide guidance for parents and caregivers regarding age-related safety measures, including the following:
  - ❍ Store prescription and over-the-counter medications, vitamins, herbs, and alcohol in a locked cabinet far from children's reach.
  - ❍ Do not take medications in front of children (Rodgers et al, 2012).
  - ❍ Store cleaning products including things like dishwashing liquids in a high cabinet, out of children's reach.
  - ❍ Use safety latches on cabinets that contain poisonous substances.
  - ❍ Store potentially harmful substances in the original containers with safety closures intact.
  - ❍ Recognize that no container is completely childproof.
  - ❍ Do not store medications or toxic substances in food containers or near or with food products.
  - ❍ Do not leave alcoholic drinks, cosmetics, or toiletries where children can reach them.
  - ❍ Remove poisonous houseplants from the home. Teach children not to put leaves or berries in their mouths (Oerther, 2011).
  - ❍ Do not suggest that medications are candy.
  - ❍ If interrupted when using a harmful product, take it with you; children can get into it within seconds.
  - ❍ Store poisonous automotive or gardening supplies in a locked area.
  - ❍ Use extreme caution with pesticides and gardening materials close to children's play areas.
  - ❍ When visitors enter the home, place their handbags or backpacks up high where children are unable to reach them, and ask about any potential poisonous substances.
- • Children naturally put things in their mouths and experience new taste sensations as a part of child development. Prevention of this is unrealistic and interventions should target environmental and caregiver behaviors to reduce harm (Rosenberg et al, 2011). EB: *A study found that pediatric poisoning most commonly occurred in 1- to 2-year-olds who ingested prescription or over-the-counter medications (Vilke et al, 2011). Pediatric poisoning deaths most commonly come from ingestion of opioids, other analgesics, cardiovascular medications, antihistamines, and sedatives (Safekids, 2014).*
- • Advise families that syrup of ipecac is no longer recommended to be kept and used in the home. Previous studies have shown unreliable performance with ipecac and the number of poison control centers that have stopped recommending ipecac use for poisonings has increased significantly over the last decades (Gutierrez et al, 2011). Advise families that over-the-counter cough and cold suppressant medications are not recommended and are no longer considered safe for children 2 or younger (U.S. Food and Drug Administration, 2014). *Colds are self-limiting and improve on their own; over-the-counter medications may help relieve symptoms in older children, but will not change the natural course of the illness (U.S. Food and Drug Administration, 2014).* EB: *Since the U.S. Food and Drug Administration advised against the use of cough/cold medicines in children younger than 2 in 2008, there has been a decline in childhood poisonings in this category and a decrease in infant emergency department visits with adverse events due to cough/cold medications (Spiller et al, 2013).*
- • Recognize that some children may have been exposed to methamphetamines or the components used to make methamphetamines. *From year 2000 through the first quarter of 2005, more than 15,000 children were reported as being affected in clandestine laboratory-related incidents (Grant, 2007).*
- • *Advise families to contact state or local government agencies or pharmacies to ask about safe disposal programs for used, excess, or expired medications (U.S. Food and Drug Administration, 2014).*

Geriatric

- • Caution the client and family to avoid storing medications with similar appearances close to one another (e.g., nitroglycerin ointment near toothpaste or denture creams). *Confusion and visual impairment can place the older person at risk of incorrectly identifying the contents. Place medications in a medication organizer that indicates when they are to be taken. Failing eyesight, the use of multiple drugs, and difficulty in remembering whether a medication was taken are among the causes of accidental poisoning in older persons.* EB: *A study demonstrated that older adults who had purposely overdosed had ingested different drugs than younger clients and had poorer outcomes with increased morbidity and mortality (Doak et al, 2009).*

- Remind older clients to store medications out of reach when young children come to visit. Childhood poisonings are common events that involve exposure to both prescription and nonprescription pharmaceuticals in the home, resulting in an increased number of serious outcomes (Spiller et al, 2013). *Medications used by older adults such as heart medication, antihypertensive medication, and antidepressants can be extremely toxic to children; some medications such as calcium channel blockers can cause death with only one pill (Vroman, 2008).*
- Perform medication reconciliation in all older clients entering the health care system as well as upon discharge. *Older clients do not compare drugs that they have at home with new prescriptions and often take multiple drugs with the same indications, leading to toxicity. Encourage older clients to speak with their pharmacist to ensure their medications are reviewed whenever a change occurs. Pharmacists can assist clients with strategies to differentiate medications such as visual, tactile, or audible labeling (Smith & Bailey, 2014). Encourage the consistent use of a pharmacy to promote understanding of medications and any changes. Advise clients who use dosettes or pre-packaged medications that the appropriate changes will need to be made before continuing to use the current administration method.*

Home Care

- The interventions previously described may be adapted for home care use.
- Provide the client and/or family with a poison control poster to be kept on the refrigerator or a bulletin board. Ensure that the telephone number for local poison control information is readily available and/or preprogrammed into household telephones.
- Pre-pour medications for a client who is at risk for ingesting too much of a given medication because of mistakes in preparation. Delegate this task to the family or caregivers if possible. *Older clients who live alone are at greatest risk of poisoning.*
- Identify poisonous substances in the immediate surroundings of the home, such as a garage or barn, including paints and thinners, fertilizers, rodent and bug control substances, animal medications, gasoline, and oil. Label with the name, a poison warning sign, and a poison control center number. Lock out of the reach of children. *Dangerous poisonous substances can be found in areas other than the internal home setting. Curious children are at risk for ingestion when exploring.*
- Identify the risk of toxicity from environmental activities such as spraying trees or roadside shrubs. Contact local departments of agriculture or transportation to obtain material safety data sheets or to prevent the activity in desired areas. *Very young children, women who are of childbearing age or who are pregnant, and older adults are at greatest risk of poisoning.*
- To prevent carbon monoxide poisoning, instruct the client and family in the importance of using a carbon monoxide detector in the home and changing it every 6 months, having the home heating system serviced every year by a qualified technician, and ensuring proper installation and venting of all combustion equipment. Carbon monoxide results from fumes produced by portable generators, stoves, lanterns, gas ranges, running vehicles, or burning charcoal and wood, which can build up in enclosed or partially enclosed spaces and result in harm or death for people and animals exposed (Centers for Disease Control and Prevention, 2014).

P

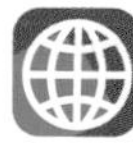

Multicultural

- Assess housing for pathways of lead poisoning. EB: *Refugee children arriving in the United States in recent years have increased rates of lead levels at their time of arrival and are at above average risk for lead poisoning from ongoing exposures after arrival because they often settle into high-risk areas with older housing (Centers for Disease Control and Prevention, 2013).*
- Prompt caregivers to take action to prevent lead poisoning. EB: *A lead poisoning awareness campaign targeted at an urban population of parents of newborns resulted in increased blood lead screening rates and demonstrated that most homes had lead hazards (Campbell et al, 2011).*
- If children live in a high-lead environment, teach the need for handwashing before each meal, annual blood testing for lead levels, and avoidance of high lead areas. EB: *A study of a community-based lead prevention programs was shown to be effective for a rural Native American population who lived near a Superfund site containing contamination from mining waste (Kegler et al, 2010).*

- Work with immigrant Mexican families to implement medication, household cleaners, and carbon monoxide safety interventions in the home to prevent accidental poisoning in children. Use the Hispanic social network. EB: *A study found that urban Mexican immigrant families often lived in unsafe homes, with child-accessible medications and the possibility of carbon monoxide poisoning (Diquiseppi et al, 2012).*

Client/Family Teaching and Discharge Planning

- Teach parents that any substance that is absorbed by the body by a variety of means and can affect health and cause mortality is considered a poison. The increasing use of medications and home cleaning products puts children at risk for poison due to the potential for access in the home environment. EB: *Research has shown that 94% of children who were poisoned accessed the agent in their own home or another home (Nalliah et al, 2014).*

Safety Guidelines

- Counsel the client and family members regarding the following points of medication safety:
  - Avoid sharing prescriptions.
  - Always use good light when preparing medication. Do not dispense medication during the night without a light on.
  - Read the label before you open the bottle, after you remove a dose, and again before you give it.
  - Always use child-resistant caps and lock all medications away from your child or confused older adult.
  - Give the correct dose. *Never* guess.
  - Do not increase or decrease the dose without calling the health care provider.
  - Always follow the weight and age recommendations on the label.
  - Avoid making conversions. If the label calls for 2 tsp and you have a dosing cup labeled only with ounces, do not use it.
  - Be sure the health care provider knows if you are taking more than one medication at a time.
  - Never let young children take medication by themselves.
  - Read and follow labeling instructions on all products; adjust dosage for age.
  - Avoid excessive amounts and/or frequency of doses. ("If a little does some good, a lot should do more.")
- Every day in the United States, about 165 children are treated in emergency departments after getting into medication. Unintentional ingestion of medications is the leading cause of child poisoning among young children and the number of children dying of poisoning has more than doubled since 1999 (Safekids.org, 2014).
- *Each year, thousands of adverse drug-related events occur, including poisoning. Poisoning is a major cause of morbidity and mortality (American Academy of Pediatrics Committee on Injury, Violence, and Poison Prevention, 2003).*
- Advise the family to post first-aid charts and poison control center instructions in an accessible location. Poison control center telephone numbers should be posted close to each telephone and the number programmed into cell phones. *A poison control center should always be called immediately before initiating any first-aid measures. The national toll-free number is (800) 222-1222.*
- Advise family when calling the poison control center to do the following:
  - Give as much information as possible, including your name, location, and telephone number, so that the poison control operator can call back in case you are disconnected or summon help if needed.
  - Give the name of the potential poison ingested and, if possible, the amount and time of ingestion. If the bottle or package is available, give the trade name and ingredients if they are listed.
  - Be prepared to divulge the child's height, weight, age, and medical history.
  - Describe the state of the poisoning victim. Is the victim conscious? Does he or she have any symptoms? What is the person's general appearance, skin color, respiration, breathing difficulties, mental status (alert, sleepy, unusual behavior)? Is the person vomiting? Having convulsions?

Rapid initiation of proper treatment reduces mortality and morbidity rates. Consultation with a poison control center is necessary to assess and treat poisoned clients. EB: *Optimal management of the poisoned client depends on the poison, the severity of the symptoms, and time between exposure and presentation. Poison control centers can provide assistance (Rhyee, 2013).*

- Encourage the client and family to take first-aid and other types of safety-related programs. *These programs raise participants' level of emergency preparation.*
- ▲ Initiate referrals to peer group interventions, peer counseling, and other types of substance abuse prevention/rehabilitation programs when substance abuse is identified as a risk factor.

- Teach parents and other caregivers that cough and cold medication bought over-the-counter are not safe for children younger than 2 unless specifically ordered by a health care provider. Analysis of exposures to cough/cold preparations supports the concept that poisoning exposure occurs in children with substances that they can easily access (Spilller et al, 2013).
- Teach parents about home prevention strategies to prevent accidental poisonings (Gutierrez et al, 2011).
- Teach parents that they can be a source of lead exposure for their children via contaminated work clothing from a lead-related occupation such as transportation workers or automobile repair or if they engage in certain hobbies such as stained glass or ceramic (Schnur & John, 2014). Precautions should be taken to eliminate the risk of exposure.

REFERENCES

American Academy of Pediatrics Committee on Injury, Violence, and Poison Prevention. (2003). Poison treatment in the home, prevention. *Pediatrics*, *112*(5), 1182–1185.

American Association of Poison Control Centers. (2014). *Health Care Providers*. Retrieved from: <http://www.aapcc.org/prevention/health-care-providers/>.

Barn, P., & Kosatsky, T. (2011). Lead in school drinking water: Canada can and should address this important ongoing exposure source. *Canadian Journal of Public Health*, *102*(2), 118–122.

Centers for Disease Control and Prevention. (2014). *Carbon monoxide (CO) poisoning prevention*. Retrieved from: <http://www.cdc.gov/features/copoisoning/>.

Centers for Disease Control and Prevention. (2013). *Immigrant and refugee health: Screening for lead during the domestic medical examination for newly arrived refugees*. Retrieved from: <http://www.cdc.gov/immigrantrefugeehealth/guidelines/lead-guidelines.htl>.

College of Nurses of Ontario. (2014). *Practice standard: Medication*. Retrieved from: <http://www.cno.org/Global/docs/prac/41007_Medication.pdf>.

Campbell, C., Tran, M., Gracely, E., et al. (2011). Primary prevention of lead exposure: the Philadelphia lead safe homes study. *Public Health Reports*, *126*(Suppl.), 76–88.

Doak, M. W., Nixon, A. C., Lupton, D. J., et al. (2009). Self-poisoning in older adults: patterns of drug ingestion and clinical outcomes. *Age and Ageing*, *38*(4), 407–411.

Diquiseppi, C., Goss, C. W., Dao, L., et al. (2012). Safety practices in relation to home ownership among urban Mexican immigrant families. *Journal of Community Health*, *37*(1), 165–175.

Food and Drug Administration. (2014). *Consumer updates, how to dispose of unused medications*. Retrieved from: <http://www.fda.gov/Drugs/ResourcesForYou/Consumers/BuyingUsingMedicineSafely/EEnsuringSafeUseofMedicine/SafeDisposalofMedicine>.

Grant, P. (2007). Evaluation of children removed from a clandestine methamphetamine laboratory. *Journal of Emergency Nursing*, *33*, 31–41.

Gutierrez, J., Negron, J., & Garcia-Fragoso, L. (2011). Parental practices for prevention of home poisoning in children 1-6 years of age. *Journal of Community Health*, *36*, 845–848.

Hwang, C. F., Foot, C. L., & Eddie, G. (2003). The utility of the history and clinical signs of poisoning in childhood: a prospective study. *Therapeutic Drug Monitoring*, *25*(6), 728.

Kegler, M. C., Malcoe, L. H., & Fedirko, M. (2010). Primary prevention of lead poisoning in rural Native American children: behavior outcomes from a community-based intervention in a former mining region. *Family Community Health*, *33*(1), 32–43.

Ness, R. (2013). Practice guidelines for childhood lead screening in primary care. *Journal of Pediatric Health Care*, *27*(5), 395–399.

Nalliah, R. P., Anderson, I. M., Lee, M. K., et al. (2014). Children in the United States make close to 200,000 emergency department visits due to poisoning each year. *Pediatric Emergency Care*, *30*(7), 453–457.

Oerther, S. E. (2011). Plant poisonings: common plants that contain cardiac glycosides. *Journal of Emergency Nursing*, *37*(1), 102–103.

Rhyee, S. H. (2013). General approach to drug poisoning in adults. *UptoDate.*, Retrieved from: <http://www.uptodate.com>.

Rodgers, G. B., Franklin, R. L., & Midgett, J. D. (2012). Unintentional paediatric ingestion poisonings and the role of imitative behavior. *Injury Prevention*, *18*(2), 103–108.

Rosenberg, M., Wood, L., Leeds, M., et al. (2011). But they can't reach that high...": parental perceptions and knowledge relating to childhood poisoning. *Health Promotion Journal of Australia*, *22*(3), 217–222.

Safer Healthcare Now. (2012). *Medication reconciliation*. Retrieved from: <http://www.saferhealthcarenow.ca/EN/Interventions/medrec/Pages/default.aspx>.

Safekids.org. (2014). *Medication safety policy brief, by the numbers*. Retrieved from: <http://www.safekids.org/search?search_api_views_fulltext=poisoning+statistics&=Apply>.

Schnur, J., & John, R. M. (2014). Childhood lead poisoning and the new centers for disease control and prevention guidelines for lead exposure. *Journal of the American Association of Nurse Practitioners*, *26*, 238–247.

Smith, M., & Bailey, T. (2014). Identifying solutions to medication adherence in the visually impaired elderly. *The Consultant Pharmacist*, *29*(2), 131–134.

Spiller, H. A., Beuhler, M. C., Ryan, M. L., et al. (2013). Evaluation of changes in poisoning in young children 2000-2010. *Pediatric Emergency Care*, *29*(5), 635–640.

The Joint Commission. (2014). *National patient safety goals effective January 1, 2014. Hospital accreditation program*. Retrieved from: <http://www.jointcommission.org/assets/1/6HAP_NPSG_Chapter_2014.pdf>.

U.S. Food and Drug Administration. (2014). *Consumer updates > Have a baby or young child with a cold? Most don't need medicines*. Retrieved from: <http://www.fda.gov/ForConsumers/ConsumerUpdates/ucm422465.htm>.

Vilke, G. M., Douglas, D. J., Shipp, H., et al. (2011). Pediatric poisonings in children younger than five years responded to by paramedics. *Journal of Emergency Medicine*, *41*(3), 265–269.

Vroman, R. (2008). Pediatric toxicology: part 2. *EMS Mag*, *37*(5), 88–92.

Post-Trauma syndrome *Mary Jane Roth, RN, BSN, MA*

NANDA-I

Definition

Sustained maladaptive response to a traumatic, overwhelming event

Defining Characteristics

Aggression; alienation; alteration in concentration; alteration in mood; anger; anxiety; avoidance behaviors; compulsive behavior; denial; depression; dissociative amnesia; enuresis; exaggerated startle response; fear; flashbacks; gastrointestinal irritation; grieving; guilt; headache; heart palpitations; history of detachment; hopelessness; horror; hypervigilance; intrusive dreams; intrusive thoughts; irritability; neurosensory irritability; nightmares; panic attacks; rage; reports feeling numb; repression; shame; substance abuse

Related Factors

Destruction of one's home; event outside the range of usual human experience; exposure to disaster (natural or man-made); exposure to epidemic; exposure to event involving multiple deaths; exposure to war; history of abuse (e.g., physical, psychological, sexual); history of being a prisoner of war; history of criminal victimization; history of torture; self-injurious behavior; serious accident (e.g., industrial, motor vehicle); serious injury to loved one; serious threat to loved one; serious threat to self; witnessing mutilation; witnessing violent death

NOC (Nursing Outcomes Classification)

Suggested NOC Outcomes

Abuse Cessation; Abuse Protection; Abuse Recovery: Emotional, Aggression Self-Control, Anxiety Self-Control, Grief Resolution, Impulse Self-Control; Self-Mutilation Restraint; Sleep

Example NOC Outcome with Indicators

Abuse Recovery: Emotional as evidenced by the following indicators: Trauma-induced psychoneurotic behaviors, conduct disorders, and learning difficulties. (Rate outcome and indicators of **Abuse Recovery: Emotional:** 1 = extensive, 2 = substantial, 3 = moderate, 4 = limited, 5 = none [see Section I].)

Client Outcomes

Client Will (Specify Time Frame)

- Return to pretrauma level of functioning as quickly as possible
- Acknowledge traumatic event and begin to work with the trauma by talking about the experience and expressing feelings of fear, anger, anxiety, guilt, and helplessness
- Identify support systems and available resources and be able to connect with them
- Return to and strengthen coping mechanisms used in previous traumatic event
- Acknowledge event and perceive it without distortions
- Assimilate event and move forward to set and pursue life goals

NIC (Nursing Interventions Classification)

Suggested NIC Interventions

Counseling; Support System Enhancement

Example NIC Activities—Counseling

Encourage expression of feelings; Assist client to identify strengths and reinforce them

Nursing Interventions and *Rationales*

- Observe for a reaction to a traumatic event in all clients regardless of age or sex. EB: *Clinicians need to be aware of the differences between injury and PTSD symptoms for women compared with men and assess*

P

for a full range of traumatic combat experiences; injury was more strongly associated with PTSD symptoms for women (Maguen et al, 2012).

- After a traumatic event, assess for intrusive memories, avoidance and numbing, and hyperarousal. EB: *The inability to complete goal-directed behavior by actively maintaining information while inhibiting irrelevant information is specific to symptoms of PTSD (Bornyea et al, 2013).*
- Remain with the client and provide support during periods of overwhelming emotions. EB: *Hansen et al (2014) studied the effects of an intervention for female victims of intimate partner violence on perceived social support and found the overall aim of the stabilization part of this treatment was to provide the woman with a sense of control over her physical safety as well as her psychological and social situation.* CEB: *The importance of trust was found to be a key element in a nurse client relationship (Bell & Duffy, 2009).*
- Help the individual try to comprehend the trauma if possible. CEB: *A stronger sense of coherence as the ability to perceive a stressor as comprehensible, manageable, and meaningful renders the client somewhat resilient to symptoms of PTSD (Engelhan et al, 2003).*
- Use touch with the client's permission (e.g., a hand on the shoulder, holding a hand). *Appropriate physical touching such as holding a person's hand may improve comfort and communication with the client (Baker, 2011).*
- Explore and enhance available support systems. EB: *The efficacy of a self-guided Internet intervention based on techniques from cognitive behavioral therapy (CBT) for prevention of PTSD symptoms was not supported (Mouthaan et al, 2014).*
- Help the client regain previous sleeping and eating habits. EB: *Babson et al (2010) found that post-traumatic stress symptom severity is related to difficulty initiating and maintaining sleep and experiencing nightmares.*

▲ Provide the client pain medication if he/she has physical pain. EB: *A quality of pain care study showed that aggressive medication management by an acute pain services team in a combat support hospital is associated with decreased pain intensity and increased pain relief in combat-injured veterans (Buckenmaier et al, 2012).*

▲ Assess the need for pharmacotherapy. EB: *The two most common interventions for PTSD are pharmacological treatment with SSRIs such as paroxetine and psychological treatment such as trauma-focused cognitive behavioral therapy. This study showed that trauma-focused cognitive behavioral therapy (TF-CBT) was superior to paroxetine in terms of sustainability, effectiveness, and cost effectiveness for the treatment of PTSD (Polak et al, 2012).*

P

▲ Refer for appropriate psychotherapy: cognitive therapy, exposure therapy, eye movement desensitization and reprocessing (EMDR), and CBT. *All of these approaches can help the client gain control of the fear and distress that happen after a traumatic event (Mayo Clinic, 2014).* EB: *Chen et al (2014) confirmed that EMDR significantly reduces the symptoms of PTSD.*

- Help the client use positive cognitive restructuring to reestablish feelings of self-worth. EB: *Anke et al (2013) showed that cognitive therapy was well tolerated and led to a very large improvement in PTSD symptoms, depression, and anxiety; the majority of clients showed reliable improvement that was clinically significant.*
- Provide the means for the client to express feelings through therapeutic drawing. EB: *The creative arts therapies may be particularly effective in the treatment of PTSD because they offer a sensory means for children and adults to express traumatic memories (Green, 2011).*
- Encourage the client to return to the normal routine as quickly as possible. EBN: *For families following an intensive care unit admission, written information about possible psychological sequelae and psychological follow-up was found to be preferable, complemented by telephone support and guidance (Gledhill et al, 2014).*
- Talk to and assess the client's social support after a traumatic event. EB: *Given the high number of physical, mental, and social problems in trauma clients, identifying and strengthening support sources can be effective in the adaption of the effects of an amputation on an individual and improvement of the quality of their life (Valizadeh et al, 2014).*

Pediatric

- Refer to nursing care plan Risk for **Post-Trauma** syndrome.

▲ Carefully assess children exposed to disasters and trauma. Note behavior specific to developmental age. Refer for therapy as needed. EBN: *Zhang et al (2014) found continuous screening is recommended to identify adolescent earthquake survivors with PTSD symptoms, especially survivors who are prone to adapt passive coping strategies and who own external causal attribution.*

Geriatric

- Carefully screen older adults for signs of PTSD, especially after a disaster. CEB: *Clients with PTSD are often not recognized or incorrectly diagnosed. Increased knowledge about vulnerability factors for PTSD can facilitate diagnostic procedures and health management in older adults. Because of age-related changes and associated disease processes, stress reaction in older adults may lead to a deterioration of function and a worsening of existing conditions (Marren & Christianson, 2005).* EB: *The association between PTSD and traumatic stress underscored the importance of screening for traumatic experiences in a geriatric German population (Glaesmer et al, 2011).*
- Consider using the Horwitz Impact of Event Scale, an appropriate instrument to measure the subjective response to stress in the older population. *The Impact of Event Scale—Revised is one of the most widely used self-report measures in the trauma literature (Beck et al, 2008).*
- ▲ Monitor the client for clinical signs of depression and anxiety; refer to a health care provider for medication if appropriate. EB: *Chan et al (2011) found that depressed older adult clients with comorbid PTSD are more functionally impaired and may take longer to respond to depression treatment than those without PTSD, but collaborative care (compared to usual care) produced similar improvements in depression severity in both groups.*
- Instill hope. EBN: *Hope was intentionally used in this study as an intervention in a group setting in a nursing home; it was evident that hope is not static and can change over time (Moore et al, 2014).*

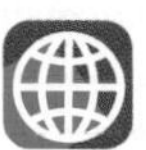

Multicultural

- Assess the influence of cultural beliefs, norms, and values on the client's ability to cope with a traumatic experience. EB: *When receiving treatment, African Americans may feel differently toward a European American clinician due to cultural mistrust. Furthermore, racism and discrimination experienced before or during the traumatic event may compound post-trauma reactions, impacting the severity of symptoms (Williams et al, 2014).*
- Acknowledge racial and ethnic differences at the onset of care. EBN: *Sabri et al (2014) showed that blacks and Asians were less likely than whites to be knowledgeable about workplace violence resources or use resources to address workplace violence.*
- ▲ Carefully assess refugees for PTSD and refer for treatment as appropriate; encourage them to learn the language of their new residence. EB: *Two possible explanations were found for the persistently high prevalence of PTSD among refugees; one is the late onset of PTSD and the other is the low utilization of mental health care (Lamkaddem et al, 2014).*
- Use a family-centered approach when working with Latin, Asian, African American, and Native American clients. CEB: *Latinos may perceive the family as a source of support, solver of problems, and source of pride. Asian Americans may regard the family as the primary decision-maker and influence on individual family members (D'Avanzo & Naegle, 2001).* EB: *Parent and self-reported mental health service use for social anxiety among high school students showed Asian American students endorsed a greater number of social anxiety symptoms than other ethnic groups. There were no differences in parent-reported impairment or service utilization (Brice et al, 2014).*
- When working with Asian American clients, provide opportunities by which the family can save face. CEB: *Asian American families may avoid situations and discussion of issues that they perceive will bring shame on the family unit (D'Avanzo & Naegle, 2001).* EBN: *This study showed that an overwhelming number of abused Chinese women have depression; these women need more attention not only in a health care setting but also in the community, especially if the immigrants are from Mainland China (Wong et al, 2011).*
- Incorporate cultural traditions as appropriate. EBN: *This study identified important culture-specific themes that relate to the treatment of native clients within the setting of trauma medicine; Native American healers were more comfortable with the genre of storytelling as interview rather than with a question-and-answer format (Basset et al, 2012).*

Home Care

- ▲ Assess family support and the response to the client's coping mechanisms. Refer the family for medical social services or other counseling as necessary. EB: *Nicholls et al (2014) studied the role of relationship attachment in psychological adjustment to cancer to improve the ability of those working with cancer clients and their families to better understand and provide for their support needs.*

P

- Assess the impact of the trauma on significant others (e.g., a father may have to take over his partner's parenting responsibility after she has been raped and injured). Provide empathy and caring to significant others. Refer for additional services as necessary. EBN: *Homicide causes negative unintended consequences for family members; a weekend family retreat intervention was studied and found to ameliorate the effects of complicated grief and overwhelming loss (Tuck et al, 2012).*

Client/Family Teaching and Discharge Planning

- Teach positive coping skills and avoidance of negative coping skills. EB: *CBT coupled with an exercise intervention was associated with positive results in an intervention for ovarian cancer client (Moonsammy et al, 2013).*
- Teach stress reduction methods such as deep breathing, visualization, meditation, and physical exercise. Encourage their use especially when intrusive thoughts or flashbacks occur. EB: *Bormann et al (2013) explored the efficacy of private meditation-based mantra intervention for veterans to enhance spiritual well-being in outpatient veterans diagnosed with military-related PTSD.*
- Encourage other healthy living habits of proper diet, adequate sleep, regular exercise, family activities, and spiritual pursuits. EBN: *A cluster randomized study suggested The Health Promotion Model can be used to develop physical activity interventions with spiritual strategies for older African American women in faith communities (Anderson et al, 2012).*
- Refer the client to peer support groups. EB: *Public stereotypes impact help seeking at least early in the course of illness; peer-based outreach and therapy groups may help veterans engage in treatment and resist stigma (Mittal et al, 2013).*
- Consider the use of complementary and alternative therapies. EB: *Stankovic (2011) showed evidence to suggest that PTSD symptoms can be reduced with mindfulness-based stretching exercises.*

REFERENCES

Anderson, K. J., & Pullen, C. H. (2012). Physical activity with spiritual strategies intervention: a cluster randomized trial with older african american women. *Research in Gerontological Nursing*, 12/20/12.

P

Anke, E., Gray, N., Wild, J., et al. (2013). Implementation of cognitive therapy for PTSD in routine clinical care: effectiveness and moderators of outcome in a consecutive sample. *Behaviour Research and Therapy*, *51*(11), 742–752.

Babson, K. A., & Feldner, M. T. (2010). Temporal relations between sleep problems and both traumatic event exposure and PTSD: a critical review of the empirical literature. *Journal of Anxiety Disorders*, *24*(1), 1–15.

Baker, G. (2011). Starting out: students' experiences in the real world of nursing: simply stroking a patient's hand helped relieve his intense pain. *Nursing Standard*, *26*(6), 27.

Basset, D., Tsosie, U., & Nannauck, S. (2012). "Our culture is medicine": perspectives of native healers on posttrauma recovery among American Indian and Alaska native patients. *The Permanente Journal/Winter*, *16*(1).

Beck, J. G., et al. (2008). The impact of event scale—revised: psychometric properties in a sample of motor vehicle accident survivors. *Journal of Anxiety Disorders*, *22*(2), 187–198.

Bell, L., & Duffy, A. (2009). A concept analysis of nurse-patient trust. *British Journal of Nursing (Mark Allen Publishing)*, *8*(1), 46–51.

Bormann, J. E., Thorp, S. R., Wetherell, J. T., et al. (2013). Meditation-Based intervention for veterans with posttraumatic stress disorder: a randomized trial. *Psychological Trauma: Theory, Research, Practice and Policy*, *5*(3), 259–267.

Bornyea, J., Amir, N., & Lang, A. J. (2013). The relationship between cognitive control and posttraumatic stress symptoms. *Journal of Behavioral Therapy and Experimental Psychiatry Psychological Trauma: Theory, Research, Practice and Policy*, *43*(2), 844–848.

Brice, C., Warner, C. M., Okazaki, S., et al. (2014). Social anxiety and mental health service use among asian american high school students. *Child Psychiatry and Human Development*, [epub ahead of print]; PMID: 25300.

Buckenmaier, C. T., Mahoney, P. F., Anton, T., et al. (2012). Impact of an acute pain service on pain outcomes with combat-injured soldiers at camp bastion, afghanistan. *Pain Medicine*, *13*(7), 919–926.

Chan, D., Fan, M. Y., & Unutzer, J. (2011). Long term effectiveness of collaborative depression care in older primary care patients with and without PTSD symptoms. *International Journal of Geriatric Psychiatry*, *26*, 758–764.

Chen, Y. R., Hung, K. W., Tsai, J. C., et al. (2014). Efficacy of eye-movement desensitization and reprocessing for patients with posttraumatic-stress disorder: a meta-analysis of randomized controlled trials. *PLoS ONE*, *9*(8), e103676.

D'Avanzo, C. E., & Naegle, M. A. (2001). Developing culturally informed strategies for substance-related interventions. In M. A. Naegle & C. E. D'Avanzo (Eds.), *Addictions and substance abuse: strategies for advanced practice nursing*. St Louis: Mosby.

Engelhan, I., van den Hout, M., & Vheyen, J. (2003). The sense of coherence in early pregnancy and crisis support and posttraumatic stress after pregnancy loss: a prospective study. *Journal of Behavioral Medicine*, *29*, 80–84.

Glaesmer, H., Brahler, E., Gundel, H., et al. (2011). The association of traumatic experiences and posttraumatic stress disorder with physical morbidity in old age: a German population-based study. *Psychosomatic Medicine*, *73*(5), 401–406.

Gledhill, J., Tareen, A., Cooper, M., et al. (2014). Joint pediatric and psychiatric follow-up for families following paediatric intensive care unit admission: an exploratory study. *Advances in Critical Care*, *2014*, Article ID 897627, 5 pages.

Green, A. (2011). Art and music therapy for trauma survivors. *CATA J*, *24*(2), 14–19.

Hansen, N. B., Ericksen, S. B., & Elklit, A. (2014). Effects of an intervention for female victims of intimate partner violence on psychological symptoms and perceived social support. *European Journal of Psychotraumatology, 5*, 24797.

Lamkaddem, M., Stronks, K., Deville, W. D., et al. (2014). Course of post-traumatic stress disorder and health care utilization among resettled refugees in the Netherlands. *BMC Psychiatry, 14*, 90.

Maguen, S., Luxton, D. D., Skopp, N. A., et al. (2012). Gender differences in traumatic experiences and mental health in active duty soldiers redeployed from Iraq and Afghanistan. *Journal of Psychiatric Research, 46*(2012), 311–316.

Marren, J., & Christianson, S. (2005). Horowitz's impact of event scale: an assessment of post traumatic stress in older adults. *Medsurg Nursing Journal, 14*(5), 329–330.

Mayo Clinic. (2014). *PTSD, treatment and drugs*. From <http://www.mayoclinic.org/diseases-conditions/post-traumatic-stress-disorder/basics/treatment/con-20022540>. Retrieved october 24, 2014.

Mittal, D., Drummond, K. L., Blevins, D., et al. (2013). Stigma associated with PTSD. *Psychiatric Rehabilitation Journal, 36*(2), 89–92.

Moore, S. L., Hall, S. E., & Jackson, J. (2014). Exploring the experience of nursing home residents participation in a hope-focused group. *Nursing Research and Practice, 2014*, Article ID 623082, 9 pages.

Moonsammy, S. H., Guglietti, C. L., Mina, D. S., et al. (2013). A pilot study of an exercise and cognitive behavioral therapy intervention for epithelial ovarian cancer patients. *Journal of Ovarian Research*, <www.ovarianresearch.com/content6/1/21>.

Mouthaan, J., Sijbrandij, M., deVries, G. J., et al. (2014). Internet-based early intervention to prevent posttraumatic stress disorder in injury patients: randomized controlled trial. *Journal of Internal Medical Internet Research, 15*(8), e165, 2013. Plos ONE.

Nicholls, W., Hulbert-Williams, N., & Bramwell, R. (2014). The role of relationship attachment in psychological adjustment to cancer in patients and caregivers: a systematic review of the literature. *Psycho-Oncology*.

Polak, A. R., Wittereen, A. B., Visser, R. S., et al. (2012). Comparison of the effectiveness of trauma-focused cognitive behavioral therapy ad paroxetine treatment in PTSD patients: Design of a randomized controlled study. *BMC Psychiatry, 12*, 166.

Sabri, B., St. Vil, N. M., Campbell, J. C., et al. (2014). Racial and Ethnic Differences in Factors related to Workplace Violence Victimization. *Western Journal of Nursing Research*, <sage.pub.com/journalsPermissions.nav>.

Stankovic, L. (2011). Transforming trauma: a qualititative feasibility study of integrative restoration (iRest) yoga nidra on combat-related post-traumatic stress disorder. *International Journal of Yoga Therapy, 21*, 23–32.

Tuck, I., Baliko, B., Schubert, C. M., et al. (2012). A pilot study of a weekend retreat intervention for family survivors of homicide. *Western Journal of Nursing Research, 34*(6), 766–794.

Valizadeh, S., Dadkhah, B., Mohammadi, E., et al. (2014). The perception of trauma patients from social support in adjustment to lower-limb amputation: a qualitative study. *Indian Journal of Palliative Care, 20*(3), 229–238.

Williams, M. T., Malcoun, E., Sawyer, B. A., et al. (2014). Cultural adaptations of prolonged exposure therapy for treatment and prevention of posttraumatic stress disorder in African Americans. *Behavioral Science, 2014*(4), 102–124.

Wong, J. Y., Tiwari, A., Fong, D. Y., et al. (2011). Depression among women experiencing intimate partner violence in a Chinese community. *Nursing Research, 60*(1), 58–65.

Zhang, W., Lui, H., Jiang, X., et al. (2014). A longitudinal study of posttraumatic stress disorder symptoms and its relationship with coping skill and locus of control in adolescents after an earthquake in china. *PLoS ONE*.

Risk for Post-Trauma syndrome *Mary Jane Roth, RN, BSN, MA*

NANDA-I

Definition

Vulnerable to sustained maladaptive response to a traumatic, overwhelming event, which may compromise health

Risk Factors

Diminished ego strength; displacement from home; duration of traumatic event; environment not conducive to needs; exaggerated sense of responsibility; human service occupations (e.g., police, fire, rescue, corrections, emergency room, mental health); insufficient social support; perceives event as traumatic; survivor role

NOC (Nursing Outcomes Classification)

Refer to the care plan for **Post-Trauma** syndrome for suggested NOC outcomes

Example NOC Outcome with Indicators

Risk Detection as evidenced by the following indicators: Recognizes signs and symptoms that indicate risk/Uses health care services congruent with need. (Rate the outcome and indicators of **Risk Detection:** 1 = never demonstrated, 2 = rarely demonstrated, 3 = sometimes demonstrated, 4 = often demonstrated, 5 = consistently demonstrated [see Section I].)

Client Outcomes

Client Will (Specify Time Frame)

- Identify symptoms associated with PTSD and seek help
- Acknowledge event and perceive it without distortions
- Identify support systems and available resources and be able to connect with them
- State that he/she is not to blame for the event

NIC (Nursing Interventions Classification)

Refer to the care plan for **Post-Trauma** syndrome for suggested NIC interventions

Nursing Interventions and *Rationales*

- Assess for PTSD in a client who has chronic/critical illness, anxiety, or personality disorder; was a witness to serious injury or death; or experienced sexual molestation. EB: *Kross et al (2011) found intensive care unit (ICU) care associated with symptoms of increased PTSD symptoms among family members of clients who die in the ICU.*
- Consider the use of a self-reported screening questionnaire. EB: *Client self-reported screening questionnaires are efficient ways to assess for PTSD (National Center for PTSD, 2014).* EB: *Mouthaan et al (2014) support the use of the SPAN, TSQ, and IES-R for early detection of post-traumatic self-reporting of PTSD symptoms.*
- Assess for ongoing symptoms of dissociation, avoidance behavior, hypervigilance, and reexperiencing. EB: *The symptoms for individuals with PTSD can vary considerably; they generally fall into three categories: reexperience, avoidance, and increased arousal (National Alliance on Mental Illness, 2014).* EB: *Diagnostic criteria for PTSD in the* Diagnostic and Statistical Manual of Mental Disorders, 5th Edition (DSM-5), *includes the above symptoms that continue for more than 1 month after the occurrence of a traumatic event (American Psychiatric Association, 2013).* EB: *He et al (2014) explored the generalizability of the DSM-5 for subpopulations and found differential symptom functioning, such as gender, race, and educational level to be small but recommended that diagnosticians always perform an analysis of subpopulations to ensure validity for research.*

P

- Assess for past experiences with traumatic events. EB: *Multiple lifetime exposures contribute to the development and persistence of PTSD among childhood victims of violence (Kulkarni et al, 2011).*
- Consider screening for PTSD in a client who is a high user of medical care. EB: *Dorrington et al (2014) showed that despite high rates of exposure to trauma, a middle income population had lower rates of PTSD than high-income populations; there are high rates of non-PTSD diagnoses associated with trauma exposure that could be considered in interventions for trauma-exposed populations.*

▲ Provide deployed combat veterans with previous history of low mental or physical health status before deployment with appropriate referral after deployment. EB: *Results of a longitudinal study by Pietrzak et al (2012) indicated that combat exposure, not deployment in general, had an adverse effect on mental health and that health outcomes were affected by both individual characteristics and post-deployment life events that changed over time.*

- Provide peer support to contact co-workers experiencing trauma to remind them that others in the organization are concerned about their welfare. CEB: *Trauma risk management (TRM) is a peer-support system that aims to promote help-seeking in the aftermath of traumatic events. This study showed that using TRM is beneficial and may lead to a valuable culture shift (Greenberg et al, 2010).*
- Provide post-trauma debriefings. Effective post-trauma coping skills are taught, and each participant creates a plan for his/her recovery. During the debriefing, the facilitators assess participants to determine their needs for further services in the form of post-trauma counseling. For maximal effectiveness, the debriefing should occur within 2 to 5 days of the incident (Guess, 2006). EB: *Fakour et al (2014) showed the effectiveness of psychological debriefing in treatment of PTSD after an earthquake; the means of PTSD symptom frequency and severity of avoidance symptoms were reduced during the 3-month period of study.*
- Provide post-trauma counseling. Counseling sessions are extensions of debriefings and include continued discussion of the traumatic event and post-trauma consequences and the further development of coping skills. EB: *Evidence suggests that the response to cognitive behavioral therapy may be enhanced in PTSD clients by preparing them with emotion regulation skills; however, a high attrition of participants during the study limits the conclusions (Bryant et al, 2013).*

- Consider exposure therapy for civilian trauma survivors following a nonsexual assault or motor vehicle crash. EB: *Early intervention with modified prolonged exposure can be successful at reducing symptoms after trauma and is safe and feasible in a civilian emergency department setting (Rothbauma et al, 2012).*

Things to Try: Critical Incident Stress Debriefing

- Instruct the client to use the following critical incident stress management techniques:
  - Within the first 24 to 48 hours, engaging in periods of appropriate physical exercise alternated with relaxation to alleviate some of the physical reactions; structure your time; keep busy; you are normal and are having normal reactions; do not label yourself as "crazy"; talk to people; talk is the most healing medicine; be aware of numbing the pain with overuse of drugs or alcohol; you do not need to complicate the stress with a substance abuse problem; reach out; people do care; maintain as normal a schedule as possible; spend time with others; help your co-workers as much as possible by sharing feelings and checking out how they are doing; give yourself permission to feel rotten and share your feelings with others; keep a journal; write your way through those sleepless hours; do things that feel good to you; realize that those around you are under stress; do not make any big life changes; do make as many daily decisions as possible to give you a feeling of control over your life (e.g., if someone asks you what you want to eat, answer the person even if you are not sure); get plenty of rest; recurring thoughts, dreams, or flashbacks are normal; do not try to fight them because they will decrease over time and become less painful; eat well-balanced and regular meals (even if you do not feel like it). *The critical incident stress debriefing process is specifically designed to prevent or mitigate the development of PTSD among emergency services professions. Critical incident stress debriefing interventions are especially directed toward the mitigation of post-traumatic stress reactions (Agency for Healthcare Research and Quality, 2012).*

▲ Assess for a history of life-threatening illness such as cancer and provide appropriate counseling. *The physical and psychological impact of having a life-threatening disease, undergoing cancer treatment, and living with recurring threats to physical integrity and autonomy constitute traumatic experiences for many cancer clients (National Cancer Institute, 2013).* EB: *Problematic post biopsy symptoms can lead to increased anxiety, distinct from distress related to diagnosis of prostate cancer (Wade et al, 2013).*

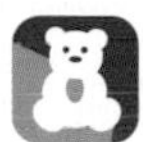

Pediatric

- Children with cancer should continue to be assessed for PTSD into adulthood. EB: *The presence of health outcomes was ascertained using systematic exposure-based medical assessments among adult survivors of childhood cancer; using clinical criteria, the crude prevalence of adverse health outcomes for neurocognitive impairment was 48% (Hudson et al, 2013).*
- Provide protection for a child who has witnessed violence or who has had traumatic injuries. Help the child acknowledge the event and express grief over the event. EB: *Lafta et al (2014) showed that more than half of the total sample in Baghdad had reported multiple experiences of trauma like fear/and or terror and the painful recall of traumatic events pointing to the need for medical educational opportunities.*
- Assess for a medical history of anxiety disorders. EB: *Findings from this study suggest that parents with social anxiety disorder may exhibit a unique pattern of behaviors when interacting with their children that includes high levels of criticism and low levels of warmth; this parenting style has been linked to an increased risk for development of anxiety (Budinger et al, 2013).*

▲ Assess children of deployed parents for PTSD and provide appropriate referrals. EB: *Mansfield et al (2011) reported that, overall, children with parental deployment represented an excess of 6579 mental health diagnoses during the 4-year period of this study compared with children with parents who did not deploy.*

- Consider implementation of a school-based program for children to decrease PTSD after catastrophic events. EB: *Tol et al (2014) used an evidence base from previous studies to draw conclusions about the benefits and risks of school-based intervention in reducing PTSD, anxiety, and depression.*

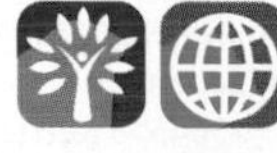

Geriatric and Multicultural

- Refer to the care plan for **Post-Trauma** syndrome.

Home Care

▲ Evaluate the client's response to a traumatic or critical event. If screening warrants, refer to a therapist for counseling/treatment. EBN: *Nurse-Family Partnership is an evidence-based nurse home visitation*

program for disadvantaged first-time mothers. Jack et al (2012) developed an intervention model and modification process to address the needs of women at risk for intimate partner violence or its recurrence.
- Refer to the care plan for **Post-Trauma** syndrome.

Client/Family Teaching and Discharge Planning

- Instruct family and friends to use the following critical incident stress management techniques:
- ▲ Listen carefully; spend time with the traumatized person; offer your assistance and a listening ear, even if the person has not asked for help; help the person with everyday tasks such as cleaning, cooking, caring for the family, and minding children; give the person some private time; do not take the individual's anger or other feelings personally, and do not tell the person that he/she is "lucky it wasn't worse"; such statements do not console traumatized people. Instead, tell the person that you are sorry such an event has occurred and you want to understand and assist him or her (National Interagency Fire Center, CISM Information Sheets, 2014).
- ▲ After exposure to trauma, teach the client and family to recognize symptoms of PTSD and seek treatment for "recurrent and intrusive distressing recollections of the traumatic event," insomnia, irritability, difficulty concentrating, hypervigilance. EB: *Post-traumatic stress symptoms are associated with higher levels of general health symptoms and lower levels of social group functioning over time (Jones et al, 2012).*
- Provide education to explain that acute stress disorder symptoms are normal when preparing combatants for their role in deployment. Instruct clients to seek help if the symptoms persist. EB: *Pre-deployment mental health screening was associated with significant reductions in occupationally impaired mental health problems, medical evacuations from Iraq for mental health reasons, and suicidal ideation (Warner et al, 2011).*

REFERENCES

Agency for Healthcare Research and Quality, Evidence-based Practice Center Systematic Review Protocol, Project Title: *Interventions for the Prevention of Posttraumatic Stress Disorder (PTSD) in Adults After Exposure to Psychological Trauma Amendment Date(s): November 8, 2012; September 26, 2012; July 27, 2012.* From <http://www.ahrq.gov/>. Retrieved October 23, 2014.

American Psychiatric Association (APA) (2013). *Diagnostic and Statistical Manual of Mental Disorders* (5th ed.). DSM-5, Washington: DC, APA.

Bryant, R. A., Mastrodomenico, J., Hopwood, S., et al. (2013). Augmenting cognitive behaviour therapy for post-traumatic stress disorder with emotional tolerance training: a randomized controlled trial. *Focus (San Francisco, Calif.)*, *11*, 379–386.

Budinger, M. C., Drazdowski, T. K., & Ginsburg, G. S. (2013). Anxiety-promoting parenting behaviors: a comparison of anxious parents with and without social anxiety disorder. *Child Psychiatry and Human Development*, *44*, 412–418.

Dorrington, S., Zavoe, H., Ball, H., et al., (2014). *Trauma, post-traumatic stress disorder and psychiatric disorders in a middle-income setting: prevalence and comorbidity.*

Fakour, Y., Mahmoudi Gharaie, J., Mohammadi, M., et al. (2014). The effect of psychosocial supportive interventions on PTSD symptoms after barn severe earthquake. *European Psychiatry*, *29*(Supplement 1).

Greenberg, N., Langston, V., Everitt, B., et al. (2010). A cluster randomized controlled trial to determine the efficacy of trauma risk managemnt (TRiM) in a military population. *Journal of Traumatic Stress*, *23*(4), 430–436.

Guess, K. F. (2006). Posttraumatic stress disorder: early detection is key. *The Nurse Practitioner*, *31*(3), 26–35.

He, Q., Glas, C. A. W., & Veldkamp, B. P. (2014). Assessing impact of differential symptom functioning on post-traumatic Stress disorder (PTSD) diagnosis. *International Journal of Methods in Psychiatric Research Int*, *23*(2), 131–141.

Hudson, M. M., Ness, K. K., Gurney, J. G., et al. (2013). Clinical ascertainment of health outcomes among adults treated for childhood cancer. *JAMA: The Journal of the American Medical Association*, *309*(22), 2371–2381.

Jack, S. H., Ford-Gilboe, M., Wathen, C. N., et al. (2012). Development of a nurse home visitation intervention for intimate partner violence. *BMC Health Services Research*, *12*, 50.

Jones, J. M., Williams, W. H., Jetten, J., et al. (2012). The role of psychological symptoms and social group memberships in the development of post-traumatic stress after traumatic injury. *Br J Health Psych*, *17*(4), 798–811.

Kross, E. K., Engelberh, R. A., & Curtis, J. R. (2011). ICU care associated with symptoms of depression and posttraumatic stress disorder among family members of patients who die in the ICU. *Chest*, *139*(4), 795–801.

Kulkarni, M. R., Graham-Bermann, S., Rauch, S. A., et al. (2011). Witnessing verses experiencing direct violence in childhood as correlates of adult PTSD. *Journal of Interpersonal Violence*, *26*(6), 1264–1281.

Lafta, R. K., Aziz, Z. S., & AlObaidi, A. K. (2014). Post traumatic stress disorder (PTSD) among male adolescents in bagdad. *Psycho Abnorm Child*, *3*, 121.

Mansfield, A. J., Kaufman, J. S., Engle, C. C., et al. (2011). Deployment and mental health diagnoses among children of US army personnel. *Archives of Pediatrics and Adolescent Medicine*, *165*(11), 999–1005.

Mouthaan, J., Sijbrandij, M., Reitsma, J. B., et al. (2014). Comparing screening instruments to predict posttraumatic stress disorder. *PLoS ONE*, *9*(5), e97183.

National Alliance on Mental Illness (NAMI): *What is Post Traumatic Stress Disorder (PTSD)*, 2014, from <http://www.nami.org/Template.cfm?Section=By_Illness&Template=/TaggedPage/TaggedPageDisplay.cfm&TPLID=54&ContentID=23045>. Retrieved October 23, 2014.

National Cancer Institute: *Posttraumatic stress disorder*, 2013, from <http://www.cancer.gov/cancertopics/pdq/supportivecare/post-traumatic-stress/Patient/page4>. Retrieved October 23, 2014.

National Center for PTSD: *Screening for PTSD in primary care settings*, 2014, from <http://www.ptsd.va.gov/professional/assessment/adult-sr/ptsd-checklist.asp & http://www.ptsd.va.gov/professional/assessment/screens/civilian-ptsd-checklist.asp>. Retrieved October 23, 2014.

National Interagency Fire Center: *CISM Information Sheets*, 2014, from <http://gacc.nifc.gov/wgbc/cism/effectsoftrauma.pdf>. Retrieved October 23, 2014.

Pietrzak, E., Pullman, S., Cotea, C., et al. (2012). Effects of deployment on Mental health in modern military forces: a review of longitudinal studies. *Journal of Military and Veterans Health*, *20*(3), 24–36.

Rothbauma, B. O., Kearnsa, M. C., Pricec, M., et al. (2012). Novel therapeutics in psychiatry and addiction. *Biological Psychiatry*, *72*(11), 957–963.

Tol, W. A., Kamproe, I. H., Jordans, M. J. D., et al. (2014). School based mental health intervention for children in war-affected Burundi: a cluster randomized trial. *BMC Medicine*, *12*, 56.

Wade, J., Rosario, D. J., Macefield, R. C., et al. (2013). Psychological Impact of Prostate Biopsy: Physical Symptoms, anxiety, and Depression. *Journal of Clinical Oncology*, 31 @ 2013 by American Society of Clinical Oncology.

Warner, C. H., Appenzeller, G. N., Parker, J. R., et al. (2011). Effectiveness of mental health screening and coordination of in-theater care prior to deployment to Iraq: a cohort study. *The American Journal of Psychiatry*, *168*, 378–385.

Readiness for enhanced Power

Marina Martinez-Kratz, MS, RN, CNE

NANDA-I

Definition

A pattern of participating knowingly in change for well-being, which can be strengthened

Defining Characteristics

Expresses desire to enhance awareness of possible changes; expresses desire to enhance identification of choices that can be made for change; expresses desire to enhance independence with actions for change; expresses desire to enhance involvement in change; expresses desire to enhance knowledge for participation in change; expresses desire to enhance participation in choices for daily living; expresses desire to enhance participation in choices for health; expresses desire to enhance power

NOC (Nursing Outcomes Classification)

Suggested NOC Outcomes

Health Beliefs: Perceived Control; Participation in Health Care Decisions; Personal Autonomy

Example NOC Outcome with Indicators

Health Beliefs: Perceived Control as evidenced by the following indicators: Belief that own actions and decisions control health outcomes/Perceived responsibility for health decisions/Efforts at gathering information. (Rate the outcome and indicators of **Health Beliefs: Perceived Control** as 1 = very weak, 2 = weak, 3 = moderate, 4 = strong, 5 = very strong [see Section I].)

Client Outcomes

Client Will (Specify Time Frame)

- Describe power resources
- Identify realistic perceptions of control
- Develop a plan of action based on power resources
- Seek assistance as needed

NIC (Nursing Interventions Classification)

Suggested NIC Interventions

Mutual Goal Setting; Self-Esteem Enhancement; Self-Responsibility Facilitation

Example NIC Activities—Mutual Goal Setting

Encourage the identification of specific life values; Identify with client the goals of care; Assist client in examining available resources to meet goals

Nursing Interventions and *Rationales*

- Develop partnerships for shared power. EBN: *The client's right to influence their treatment and health care allows the client power (Aasen et al, 2012).*
- Focus on the positive aspects of power, rather than prevention of powerlessness. EBN: *Numerous studies conducted during development of the health promotion model show that promotion differs from prevention and requires a positive rather than negative approach (Fisher & Howell, 2010; Pender et al, 2011).*
- Listen with intent. EBN: *In a study of successful adaptation of women with chronic illness, partnerships with health care providers contributed to positive outcomes. These partnerships were enhanced by careful listening on the part of the health care provider (Cudney et al, 2011).*
- Collaborate with and encourage the person to identify resources to put a plan into action. EBN: *Collaborating with clients provides opportunities for learning and growth and is a client-empowering behavior that improves client health outcomes (Jerofke et al, 2014).*
- Assess the meaning of the event to the person. EBN: *Assessing meaning gives a voice to clients and makes it more likely that solutions reached will have meaning and be useful to the individual (Bevan, 2013).*
- Identify the client's health literacy and provide access to information. EBN: *Providing clients with access to information is a client-empowering behavior that improves client health outcomes (Jerofke et al, 2014).*
- Facilitate trust in self and others. EBN: *Trust in the competence of the health care staff is an empowering to the client (Nygårdh et al, 2012).*
- Help client to mobilize social supports, a power resource. EBN: *Assisting clients with access to resources is a client-empowering behavior that improves client health outcomes (Jerofke et al, 2014).*
- Support beliefs of power and perceptions of behavioral control. CEBN: *A positive correlation was identified between beliefs and motivation toward control of health-promoting behaviors and blood pressure control (Peters & Templin, 2010).*
- Promote the client's optimum level of physical functioning. EBN: *Younger (2011) identifies the relationship between physical health and the ability to heal.*
- Reframe professional image, role, and values to incorporate a vision of clients as the experts in their own care. EBN: *Professional development for nurse practitioners in methods of communication and education was identified as key in promoting effective medication management in people with diabetes (Sibley et al, 2011).*

P

Home Care

- The preceding interventions may be adapted for home care use.

Client/Family Teaching and Discharge Planning

- Assess motivation to learn specific content. CEBN: *Motivation is a basic element of a teaching model and of participation in health care decisions (Pender et al, 2011).*

REFERENCES

Aasen, E. M., Kvangarsnes, M., & Heggen, K. (2012). Perceptions of patient participation amongst elderly patients with end-stage renal disease in a dialysis unit. *Scandinavian Journal of Caring Sciences, 26*(1), 61–69.

Bevan, A. L. (2013). Creating communicative spaces in an action research study. *Nurse Researcher, 21*(2), 14–17.

Cudney, S., Weinert, C., & Kinion, E. (2011). Forging partnerships between rural women with chronic conditions and their health care providers. *Journal of Holistic Nursing, 29*(1), 53–60.

Fisher, M., & Howell, D. (2010). The power of empowerment: an ICF-based model to improve self-efficacy and upper extremity function of survivors of breast cancer. *Rehabil Oncol, 28*(3), 19–25.

Jerofke, T., Weiss, M., & Yakusheva, O. (2014). Patient perceptions of patient-empowering nurse behaviours, patient activation and functional health status in postsurgical patients with life-threatening long-term illnesses. *Journal of Advanced Nursing, 70*(6), 1310–1322.

Nygårdh, A., Malm, D., Wikby, K., et al. (2012). The experience of empowerment in the patient-staff encounter: the patient's perspective. *Journal of Clinical Nursing, 21*(5/6), 897–904.

Pender, N. J., Murdaugh, C. L., & Parsons, M. A. (2011). *Health promotion in nursing practice* (6th ed.). Stamford, CT: Appleton & Lange.

Peters, R., & Templin, T. (2010). Theory of planned behavior, self-care motivation, and blood pressure self-care. *Research and Theory for Nursing Practice*, *24*(3), 172–186.

Sibley, A., et al. (2011). Medication discussion between nurse prescribers and people with diabetes: an analysis of content and participation using MEDICODE. *Journal of Advanced Nursing*, *67*(11), 2323–2336.

Younger, C. (2011). The relationship between physical wellbeing and mental health care. *Ment Health Pract*, *15*(1), 34–36.

Powerlessness *Marina Martinez-Kratz, MS, RN, CNE*

NANDA-I

Definition

The lived experience of lack of control over a situation, including a perception that one's actions do not significantly affect an outcome

Defining Characteristics

Alienation; dependency; depression; doubt about role performance; frustration about inability to perform previous activities; inadequate participation in care; insufficient sense of control; shame

Related Factors

Complex treatment regimen; dysfunctional institutional environment; insufficient interpersonal interactions

NOC (Nursing Outcomes Classification)

Suggested NOC Outcomes

Depression Self-Control; Health Beliefs; Health Beliefs: Perceived Ability to Perform, Perceived Control, Perceived Resources; Participation in Health Care Decisions

Example NOC Outcome with Indicators

Health Beliefs: Perceived Control as evidenced by the following indicators: Perceived responsibility for health decisions/Beliefs that own decisions and actions control health outcomes. (Rate the outcome and indicators of **Health Beliefs: Perceived Control:** 1 = very weak belief, 2 = weak belief, 3 = moderately strong belief, 4 = strong belief, 5 = very strong belief [see Section I].)

Client Outcomes

Client Will (Specify Time Frame)

- State feelings of powerlessness and other feelings related to powerlessness (e.g., anger, sadness, hopelessness)
- Identify factors that are uncontrollable
- Participate in planning and implementing care; make decisions regarding care and treatment when possible
- Ask questions about care and treatment
- Verbalize hope for the future and sense of participation in planning and implementing care

NIC (Nursing Interventions Classification)

Suggested NIC Interventions

Cognitive Restructuring; Complex Relationship Building; Mutual Goal Setting; Self-Esteem Enhancement; Self-Responsibility Facilitation

Example NIC Activities—Self-Responsibility Facilitation

Encourage independence but assist client when unable to perform; Assist client to identify areas in which they could readily assume more responsibility

P

Nursing Interventions and *Rationales*

NOTE: Before implementation of interventions in the face of client powerlessness, nurses should examine their own philosophies of care to ensure that control issues or lack of faith in client capabilities will not bias the ability to intervene sincerely and effectively.

- Observe for factors contributing to powerlessness (e.g., immobility, hospitalization, unfavorable prognosis, lack of support system, misinformation about situation, inflexible routine, chronic illness, addiction, history of trauma, gender). Help clients channel their behaviors in an effective manner. EB: *Many studies identify factors contributing to feelings of powerlessness are related to losses of person, place, health, or social relationships, gender, or the impact of trauma (An & Kim, 2012; Doyle, 2014; Milberg & Strang, 2011; Salomé et al, 2013).*
- Engage with clients using respectful listening and questioning to develop an awareness of clients' most important concerns. EB: *Engaging clients will integrate clinician expertise with client needs and can diminish feelings of powerlessness (Sheridan et al, 2015).*
- Assess the client's locus of control related to his or her health. EBN: *In a quasi-experimental study of hemodialysis clients and the use of interactive media, powerlessness was associated with feelings of loss of control (Wang & Chiou, 2011).*
- Establish a therapeutic relationship with the client by spending one-on-one time with him or her, assigning the same caregiver, keeping commitments (e.g., saying, "I will be back to answer your questions in the next hour"), providing encouragement and social support, and being empathetic. EBN: *In a study of Korean adults with type 2 diabetes, it appears that lower levels of social support are associated with increased measures of powerlessness (An & Kim, 2012).* EBN: *In a study of successful adaptation of women with chronic illness, establishment of a therapeutic relationship contributed to positive outcomes. These relationships were enhanced by careful listening on the part of the health care provider (Cudney et al, 2011).*
- Encourage the client to share his or her beliefs, thoughts, and expectations about his or her illness. CEBN: *The Health Belief Model identifies perceived barriers and perceived susceptibility to disease as powerful predictors of clients' motivation in taking action to prevent disease and participate in self-care management (Pender et al, 2010).*
- Help the client assist in planning care and specify the health goals he or she would like to achieve, prioritizing those goals with regard to immediate concerns and identifying actions that will achieve the goals. Goals may need to be small to be attainable (e.g., dangle legs at bedside for 2 days, then sit in chair 10 minutes for 2 days, then walk to window). CEBN: *People need goals that have value for them; the discrepancy between these goals and reality motivates action to reduce the discrepancy. Goals must be realistic and achievable; otherwise, the inability to perceive progress will increase hopelessness and powerlessness (Pender et al, 2010).*
- Encourage the client in goal-directed activities that promote a sense of accomplishment, especially regular exercise. EB: *People with arthritis were asked to set goals for themselves in terms of exercise. Self-efficacy was found to be a mediator between accomplishment of goals and quality of life. Goal direction enhances self-efficacy (Knittle et al, 2011).*
- Empower clients by providing access to health education in conjunction with counseling and opportunities for discussion. EBN: *A study reported that clients had a reduction in health risk behaviors and an increase in knowledge, self-efficacy, and health-related quality of life with a targeted empowerment program (Ok Ham & Jeong, 2011).*
- Encourage the client to take control of as many activities of daily living (ADLs) as possible; keep the client informed of all care that will be given. Keep items the client uses and needs within reach (e.g., a urinal, tissues, telephone, and television controls). CEBN: *Choice in ADLs such as eating, sleeping, and grooming contributes to a sense of control. Clients are more amenable to therapy if they know what to expect and can perform some tasks independently. Dependence can be alleviated by fostering an expectation of control over activities, which leads to the development of a sense of mastery (Pender et al, 2010).*
- Give realistic and sincere praise for accomplishments. CEBN: *Frequent positive reinforcement helps clients feel successful and competent, especially when it is immediate and is used to balance feedback about errors (Pender et al, 2010).*
- Use a Rehabilitative Behavioral Learning Model that assists clients to understand how the mechanisms of habit and ritual work to reinforce powerlessness in their lives. *For clients with addiction, understanding the learning processes and mechanisms of powerlessness is an important part of recovery (Butler et al, 2015).*

P

- Consider using one of the measures of powerlessness that are available for general and specific client groups:
  - Measure of Powerlessness for Adult Patients (De Almeida & Braga, 2006)
  - Personal Progress Scale—Revised, tested with women (Johnson et al, 2005)
  - Life Situation Questionnaire—Powerlessness subscale, tested with stroke caregivers (Larson et al, 2005)
  - Making Decisions Scale, tested in clients with mental illness (Hansson & Bjorkman, 2005)
- Refer to the care plans for **Hopelessness** and **Spiritual** distress.

Pediatric

- Assess for power differentials in the dating relationships of female adolescent clients and provide teaching that addresses relationship power and dating violence. EBN: *Research indicates that romantic relationships are an important part of adolescent development. Adolescent clients that report relationship control and power imbalances will benefit from learning about relationship equity, effective communication, and negotiation skills to positively influence relationship power and improve health outcomes (Volpe et al, 2012).*
- Provide nursing care that shifts the focus from the illness to the child. EBN: *Research indicates that children with a new diagnosis of cancer feel powerless and can benefit from being viewed as a competent individual who requires information and is able to participate in their care (Darcy et al, 2014).* Recognize that a sense of powerlessness can prevent children and adolescents from reporting peer victimization. Be supportive, encourage disclosure without pressure, and help the child or adolescent problem-solve options to deal with stressors. EBN: *School nurses are poised to provide a supportive and safe haven for children who are being bullied (Carter, 2011).*

Geriatric

- In addition to the preceding interventions as appropriate:
  - Assist older adults to retain a sense of power and control as they are making the transition to residential care. EB: *Older adults report greater satisfaction during transition to residential care when they have the feeling of power and control over the process and are able to perceive their residence as their new home (Riedl, 2011).*
  - Initiate focused assessment questioning and education of client and caregivers regarding syndromes common in the older adults, including dementia. EB: *A disease management model used by a multidisciplinary team in a nursing home was found to improve quality of life in older clients (Boorsma et al, 2011).*
  - Assess for the presence of elder abuse. Initiate referral to Adult Protective Services and help client regain a sense of safety and control. EB: *Elder abuse can be seen in the form of emotional, financial, physical, and sexual abuse. In addition, neglect and self-neglect can be viewed as forms of abuse (Mosqueda & Dong, 2011).*

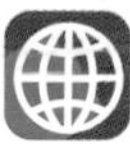

Multicultural

- In addition to the preceding interventions as appropriate:
  - Assess for the influence of communication patterns, cultural differences in medical consultations, and client perceptions of inequalities in care quality as contributors to client feelings of powerlessness. EB: *Understanding and addressing client perceptions of power disparities may decrease clients' feelings of powerlessness (Akhavan & Karlsen, 2013).*

Home Care

- In addition to the preceding interventions as appropriate:
  - Develop a therapeutic relationship in the home setting that respects the client's domain. EB: *Respect for the client's living quarters supports development of a therapeutic relationship that fosters trust (Harkness & DeMarco, 2011).*
  - Empower the client by encouraging the client to guide specifics of care such as wound care procedures and dressing and grooming details. Confirm the client's knowledge and document in the chart that the client is able to guide procedures. Document in the home and in the chart the preferred approach to procedures. Orient the family and caregivers to the client's role. EBN: *The use of focus groups to acknowledge expertise and foster decision-making in mental health consumers contributed to greater self-health management (Mahone et al, 2011).*

P

- ○ Assess the affective climate within the family and family support system, including other caregivers. Instruct the family in appropriate expectations of the client and in the specifics of the client's illness. Assist the family and caregivers to assert personal needs and develop closer proximity to health care providers. EB: *Caregivers and family members often experience a sense of isolation and powerlessness that goes unrecognized by health care providers. Assessment will identify support needs that go beyond the physical and emotional care of the dying client (Clark et al, 2011).*
- ○ Evaluate the powerlessness of caregivers to ensure they continue their ability to care for the client. Provide assistance using interventions from this care plan. EB: *Powerlessness of caregivers of terminally ill clients was studied during care and 3 to 9 months after the client's death. Some aspects that protected the family members from powerlessness were access to information regarding palliative care, believing they were doing good for the client, and social support (Milberg & Strang, 2011).*
- ○ Assist family caregivers, especially fathers, to take an active role in the client's care. EBN: *A study determined that cooperation between the adult client with chronic mental illness, parental caregivers, and health care providers could increase the parent caregiver's ability to support the client, understand the illness, and manage the symptoms. This in turn would decrease feelings of caregiver powerlessness (Johansson et al, 2012).*
- ○ Assess for denial in clients with cancer and provide support for caregivers. EB: *While denial may be a protective mechanism for the client with cancer, it can create additional burdens for caregivers who may experience powerlessness and an inability to meet their own needs (Kogan et al, 2013).*
- ○ Be aware of and assist clients with potential needs for help in negotiating the health care system. EBN: *The use of electronic dosing and monitoring devices, in conjunction with other measures of adherence, has contributed to adherence to medication regimen (Cook et al, 2012).* EB: *Adherence to medications and self-health regimens is facilitated by payers' knowledge and use of value-based insurance designs (Cohen et al, 2012).*
- ○ Teach stress reduction, relaxation, and imagery. Many audio recordings are available on relaxation and meditation. CEBN: *In this study of clients with breast cancer, participants reported the importance of engaging passive and active imagery. Imagery practice improved mood state (Freeman et al, 2008).*
- ○ Teach cognitive-behavioral activities, such as active problem solving, reframing (reappraising the situation from a different perspective), or thought stopping (in response to a negative thought, such as picturing a large stop sign and replacing the image with a prearranged positive alternative). Teach the client to confront his or her own negative thought patterns (cognitive distortions). CEBN: *Through cognitive-behavioral interventions, clients become more aware of their cognitive choices in adopting and maintaining their belief systems, thereby exercising greater control over their own reactions (Hagerty & Patusky, 2008).*
- ○ Identify the strengths of the caregiver and efforts to gain control of unpredictable situations. Help the caregiver stay connected with a client who may be behaving differently than usual to make life as routine as possible, help the client set goals and sustain hope, and allow the client space to experience progress. EBN: *A positive correlation was identified between beliefs and motivation toward control of health-promoting behaviors and blood pressure control (Peters & Templin, 2010).*

P

Client/Family Teaching and Discharge Planning

- The preceding interventions may be adapted for home care use.

REFERENCES

Akhavan, S., & Karlsen, S. (2013). Practitioner and client explanations for disparities in health care use between migrant and non-migrant groups in Sweden: a qualitative study. *Journal of Immigrant & Minority Health*, *15*(1), 188–197.

An, G., & Kim, M. (2012). Powerlessness, social support, and glycemic control in Korean adults with type 2 diabetes. *Contemporary Nurse: A Journal for the Australian Nursing Profession*, *42*(2), 272–279.

Boorsma, M., et al. (2011). Effects of multidisciplinary integrated care on quality of care in residential care facilities for elderly people: a cluster randomized trial. *CMAJ*, *183*(11), E724–E732.

Butler, M. H., Meloy, K. C., & Call, M. L. (2015). Dismantling powerlessness in addiction: empowering recovery through rehabilitating behavioral learning. *Sexual Addiction & Compulsivity*, *22*(1), 26–58.

Carter, S. (2011). Bullies and power: a look at the research. *Issues in Comprehensive Pediatric Nursing*, *34*(2), 97–102.

Clark, P. G., Brethwaite, D. S., & Gnesdiloff, S. (2011). Providing support at time of death from cancer: results of a 5-year post-bereavement group study. *Journal of Social Work In End-of-Life & Palliative Care*, *7*(2/3), 195–215.

Cohen, J., Christensen, K., & Feldman, L. (2012). Disease management and medication compliance. *Popul Health Manage*, *15*(1), 20–28.

Cook, P., et al. (2012). Practical and analytic issues in the electronic assessment of adherence. *Western Journal of Nursing Research*, *34*(5), 598–620.

Cudney, S., Weinert, C., & Kinion, E. (2011). Forging partnerships between rural women with chronic conditions and their health care providers. *Journal of Holistic Nursing*, *29*(1), 53–60.
Darcy, L., Knutsson, S., Huus, K., et al. (2014). The everyday life of the young child shortly after receiving a cancer diagnosis, from both children's and parent's perspectives. *Cancer Nursing*, *37*(6), 445–456.
De Almeida, L. M., & Braga, C. G. (2006). Construction and validation of an instrument to assess powerlessness. *International Journal of Nursing Terminologies and Classifications*, *17*, 67.
Doyle, S. (2014). The impact of power differentials on the care experiences of older people. *Journal of Elder Abuse & Neglect*, *26*(3), 319–332.
Freeman, L., et al. (2008). The experience of imagery as a post-treatment intervention in patients with breast cancer: program, process, and patient recommendations. *Oncology Nursing Forum*, *35*(6), E116–E121.
Hagerty, B., & Patusky, K. (2008). Mood disorders: depression and mania. In K. M. Fortinash & P. A. Holoday-Worret (Eds.), *Psychiatric mental health nursing* (4th ed.). St Louis: Mosby.
Hansson, L., & Bjorkman, T. (2005). Empowerment in people with a mental illness: reliability and validity of the Swedish version of an empowerment scale. *Scandinavian Journal of Caring Sciences*, *19*, 32.
Harkness, G. A., & DeMarco, R. (2011). *Community and public health nursing: evidence for practice*. New York: Lippincott Williams & Wilkins.
Johansson, A., Anderzen-Carlsson, A., Åhlin, A., et al. (2012). Fathers' everyday experiences of having an adult child who suffers from long-term mental illness. *Issues in Mental Health Nursing*, *33*(2), 109–117.
Johnson, D. M., Worell, J., & Chandler, R. K. (2005). Assessing psychological health and empowerment in women: the personal progress scale revised. *Women and Health*, *41*(1), 109.
Knittle, K. P., et al. (2011). Effect of self-efficacy and physical activity goal achievement on arthritis pain and quality of life in patients with rheumatoid arthritis. *Arthritis Care and Research*, *63*(11), 1613–1619.
Kogan, N. R., Dumas, M., & Cohen, S. R. (2013). The extra burdens patients in denial impose on their family caregivers. *Palliative & Supportive Care*, *11*(2), 91–99.
Larson, J., et al. (2005). Spouse's life situation after partner's stroke: psychometric testing of a questionnaire. *Journal of Advanced Nursing*, *52*, 300.
Mahone, I. H., et al. (2011). Shared decision making in mental health treatment: qualitative findings from stakeholder focus groups. *Archives of Psychiatric Nursing*, *25*(6), 27–36.
Milberg, A., & Strang, P. (2011). Protection against perceptions of powerlessness and helplessness during palliative care: the family members' perspective. *Palliative and Supportive Care*, *9*(3), 251–262.
Mosqueda, L., Dong, X. (2011). Elder abuse and self-neglect: "I don't care anything about going to the doctor, to be honest. *JAMA: The Journal of the American Medical Association*, *306*(5), 532–540.
Ok Ham, K., & Jeong Kim, B. (2011). Evaluation of a cardiovascular health promotion programme offered to low-income women in Korea. *Journal of Clinical Nursing*, *20*(9/10), 1245–1254.
Pender, N. J., & Murdaugh, C. L. (2010). *Parsons MA: Health promotion in nursing practice* (6th ed.). Upper Saddle River, NJ: Prentice-Hall.
Peters, R., & Templin, T. (2010). Theory of planned behavior, self-care motivation, and blood pressure self-care. *Research and Theory for Nursing Practice*, *24*(3), 172–186.
Riedl, M. (2011). Psychophysical and social changes in elderly people after the entry into a residential home—a systematic literature research [German]. *Pflegewissenschaft*, *13*(5), 299–311. (50 ref).
Salomé, G. M., Openheimer, D. G., de Almeida, S. A., et al. (2013). Feelings of powerlessness in patients with venous leg ulcers. *Journal of Wound Care*, *22*(11), 628, 630, 632–4.
Sheridan, N. F., Kenealy, T. W., Kidd, J. D., et al. (2015). Patients' engagement in primary care: powerlessness and compounding jeopardy. A qualitative study. *Health Expectations*, *18*(1), 32–43.
Volpe, E. M., Hardie, T. L., & Cerulli, C. (2012). Associations among depressive symptoms, dating violence, and relationship power in urban, adolescent girls. JOGNN. *Journal Of Obstetric, Gynecologic & Neonatal Nursing*, *41*(4), 506–518.
Wang, L. M., & Chiou, C. P. (2011). Effectiveness of interactive multimedia CD on self-care and powerlessness in hemodialysis patients. *The Journal of Nursing Research*, *19*(2), 102–111.

P

Risk for Powerlessness *Gail B. Ladwig, MSN, RN*

NANDA-I

Definition

Vulnerable to the lived experience of lack of control over a situation, including a perception that one's actions do not significantly affect the outcome, which may compromise health

Risk Factors

Anxiety; caregiver role; economically disadvantaged; illness; ineffective coping strategies; insufficient knowledge to manage a situation; insufficient social support; low self-esteem; pain; progressive illness; social marginalization; stigmatization; unpredictability of illness trajectory

NOC, NIC, Client Outcomes, Nursing Interventions, Client/Family Teaching and Discharge Planning, *Rationales*, and References

See the care plan for **Powerlessness**.

Risk for Pressure ulcer

Karen Zulkowski, DNS, RN, and Mary Beth Flynn Makic, PhD, RN, CNS, CCNS, FAAN

NANDA-I

Definition

Vulnerable to localized injury to the skin and/or underlying tissue usually over a bony prominence as a result of pressure, or pressure in combination with shear (NPUAP, 2007)

Risk Factors

Adult

Braden scale score <18; alteration in cognitive functioning; alteration in sensation; American Society of Anesthesiologist (ASA) Physical Status classification score ≥2; anemia; cardiovascular disease

Child

Braden Q scale ≤16; decrease in mobility; decrease in serum albumin level; decrease in tissue oxygenation; decrease in tissue perfusion; dehydration; dry skin; edema; elevated skin temperature by 1° C to 2° C; extended period of immobility on hard surface (e.g., surgical procedure ≥2 hours); extremes of age; extremes of weight; female gender; hip fracture; history of cerebral vascular accident; history of pressure ulcer; history of trauma; hyperthermia; impaired circulation; inadequate nutrition; incontinence; insufficient caregiver knowledge of pressure ulcer prevention; low score on Risk Assessment Pressure Sore (RAPS) scale; lymphopenia; New York Heart Association (NYHA) functional classification ≥2; nonblanchable erythema; pharmaceutical agents (e.g., general anesthesia, vasopressors, antidepressant, norepinephrine); physical immobilization; pressure over bony prominence; reduced triceps skin fold thickness; scaly skin; self-care deficit; shearing forces; skin moisture; smoking; surface friction; use of linens with insufficient moisture wicking property

NOC Outcomes (Nursing Outcomes Classification)

P

Suggested NOC Outcomes

Tissue Integrity: Skin and Mucous Membranes

Example NOC Outcome with Indicators

Intact Tissue Integrity: Skin and Mucous Membranes as evidenced by the following indicators: Skin intactness/Skin lesions absent/Tissue perfusion/Skin temperature. (Rate the outcome and indicators of **Tissue Integrity: Skin and Mucous Membranes:** 1 = severely compromised, 2 = substantially compromised, 3 = moderately compromised, 4 = mildly compromised, 5 = not compromised [see Section I].)

Client Outcomes

Client Will (Specify Time Frame)

- Report any altered sensation or pain at site of tissue impairment
- Skin, without redness over bony prominences and capillary refill of less than 6 seconds over areas of redness
- Be repositioned off of bony prominences frequently if risk for pressure ulcers is high (e.g., Braden scale score <18)
- Demonstrate understanding of plan to reduce pressure ulcer risk
- Describe measures to protect the skin

NIC Interventions (Nursing Interventions Classification)

Suggested NIC Interventions

Pain Management; Pressure Ulcer Care; Pressure Ulcer Prevention; Risk Identification; Skin Care: Topical Treatments; Skin Surveillance

Example NIC Activities—Pressure Ulcer Care

Monitor color of skin, temperature, edema, erythema, moisture, and appearance of surrounding skin; Note characteristics of skin over bony prominences or medical devices

Nursing Interventions and *Rationales*

- *Skin breakdown in the form of pressure ulcers is defined as localized injury to the skin and/or underlying tissue usually over a bony prominence as a result of pressure, or pressure in combination with shearing forces (National Pressure Ulcer Advisory Panel/European Pressure Ulcer Advisory Panel [NPUAP/EPUAP], 2014).*
- Routinely assess clients for risk of pressure ulcers using a valid and reliable risk assessment tool (NPUAP/EPUAP, 2014). A validated risk assessment tool such as the Norton or Braden scale should be used to identify clients at risk for pressure related skin breakdown (NPUAP/EPUAP, 2014). EB: *Targeting variables (e.g., Braden Scale Risk Subscale Categories, age, severity of illness) can focus assessment on particular risk factors (e.g., pressure, immobility, perfusion) and help guide the plan of prevention and care (NPUAP/EPUAP, 2014; McCulloch & Kloth, 2010; Sussman & Bates-Jensen, 2012).*
- Pressure ulcer risk assessment should be completed on admission, daily, and after procedures or changes in the client's condition (Kelleher et al, 2012; NPUAP/EPUAP, 2014).
- Inspect the skin daily, especially bony prominences and dependent areas for pallor, redness, and breakdown In addition to assessing pressure ulcer risk client specific interventions should be implemented to prevent tissue injury. Implement interventions to prevent tissue breakdown:
  - ❍ Assist client to turn at least every 2 hours unless contraindicated
  - ❍ Position client properly; use pressure-reducing or pressure-relieving devices (e.g., pillows, gel or foam cushions, alternating pressure mattress, air-fluidized bed, kinetic bed) if indicated
  - ❍ Lift and move client carefully using a turn sheet and adequate assistance; keep bed linens dry and wrinkle-free
  - ❍ Perform actions to keep client from sliding down in bed (e.g., bend knees slightly when head of bed is elevated 30 degrees or higher) in order to reduce the risk of skin surface abrasion and shearing
  - ❍ Instruct or assist client to shift weight at least every 30 minutes
  - ❍ Keep client's skin clean; thoroughly dry skin after bathing and as often as needed, paying special attention to skin folds and opposing skin surfaces (e.g., axillae, perineum, beneath breasts); pat skin dry rather than rub; use a mild soap for bathing and apply moisturizing lotion at least once a day
  - ❍ Protect the skin from contact with urine and feces (e.g., keep perineal area clean and dry, apply a protective ointment or cream to perineal area)
  - ❍ Encourage a fluid intake of 2500 mL/day unless contraindicated
  - ❍ Apply a protective covering such as a hydrocolloid or transparent membrane dressing to areas of the skin susceptible to breakdown (e.g., coccyx, heels, elbows)
  - ❍ Consult with nutrition/dietary specialist to evaluate client's nutritional status
  - ❍ Increase activity as allowed

▲ EB: *Pressure ulcers result in additional pain and treatment for the client as well as additional health care services and costs. A comprehensive assessment of the client's risk for pressure ulcers and proactive interventions are necessary to reduce the risk for tissue injury (NPUAP/EPUAP, 2014).*

- A medical device–related pressure ulcer (MDRPU) is a localized injury to the skin or underlying tissue as a result of sustained pressure from a medical device. The tissue injury will often have the same configuration as the device (NPUAP 2014; Baharestani, 2013; Black, 2010).
  - ❍ The head/face/neck, heel/ankle/foot, coccyx/buttocks, abdomen, and extremities are common body regions for MDRPU.
  - ❍ Common devices associated with pressure-related tissue injury include oxygen delivery and monitoring devices (e.g., face mask, nasal cannula, pulse oximetry, BiPAP mask); feeding tubes (e.g., nasogastric, gastric, jejunal tubes); endotracheal devices (oral and/or nasal endotracheal tubes, tracheostomy tubes); urinary and bowel elimination (indwelling urinary catheter, fecal containment catheter); musculoskeletal (cervical collar, splints, braces).
  - ❍ Assess and evaluate the purpose and function of the medical device

P

- ❍ Assess proper fit of the medical device and securement to prevent rubbing, torque, or pulling on the device and skin
- ❍ Protect the skin below and around the device to reduce pressure

▲ EB: *Incorporate daily and frequent skin inspection around and under the medical device. See the National Pressure Ulcer Advisory Panel Best Practice flyer to help provide education about MDRPU (http://www.npuap.org/wp-content/uploads/2013/04/BestPractices-CriticalCare1.pdf).*

- Critically ill clients are at increased risk for pressure ulcers, often requiring frequent skin risk assessment and preventive interventions. EB: *Support surfaces are often needed to reduce pressure risk in the critically ill client (Behrendt et al, 2014). Frequently reposition the client often more frequently than every 2 hours (Makic et al, 2014; NPUAP/EPUAP, 2014). Frequently assess skin for shear injury as well as pressure areas when the client is in prone positioning or lateral rotation therapy is used (NPUAP/EPUAP, 2014).*
- *Interprofessional pressure ulcer prevention programs in acute and long-term care facilities are needed to reduce client's risk for developing pressure ulcers and associated complications (Padula et al, 2014; Niederhauser et al, 2012).*
- If tissue breakdown occurs, notify a health care provider or wound care specialist. See care plan for Impaired **Skin** integrity for additional interventions if a pressure ulcer occurs.

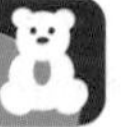

Pediatric

- Perform an age-appropriate pressure ulcer risk assessment using a valid and reliable tool. CEB/EB: *The Braden Q and Glamorgan Scale are valid and reliable scales to assess pediatric client risks for compromised skin integrity related to pressure (Anthony et al, 2010; Galvin et al, 2012; Tume et al, 2013). The Neonatal Skin Risk Assessment Scale was developed to assess unique skin breakdown risk in neonates (Huffines et al, 1997; Dolack et al, 2013).*
- Implement a comprehensive plan to reduce the client's risk of skin breakdown from pressure. Assessment should include the following:
  - ❍ Client independent activity and mobility levels
  - ❍ Body mass index and/or birth weight; lower weight may increase client risk of pressure associated skin breakdown
  - ❍ Skin maturity
  - ❍ Adequate nutritional and hydration status
  - ❍ Perfusion and oxygenation
  - ❍ Presence of external devices
  - ❍ Duration of hospital stay

▲ EB: *Pediatric clients with medical devices are at higher risk for pressure ulcers. Inspect the skin under and around the device at least twice a day. Frequent (e.g., daily and after procedures) and ongoing assessment of the client's risk for pressure ulcer is an important prevention intervention. Carefully assess the skin on the client's occiput as part of the assessment (NPUAP/EPUAP, 2014).*

- Select an age-appropriate support surface for premature neonates and pediatric clients at high risk for pressure ulcers. EBN: *A longitudinal study found that the use of continuous and reactive low-pressure mattresses reduced the observed incidence of pressure ulcers (Garcia-Molina et al, 2012). Select a support surface to prevent occipital pressure ulcers for at-risk clients (NPUAP/EPUAP, 2014).*
- *Engage the client/family/legal guardian in the development of a client specific plan of care to reduce pressure-related risk for skin breakdown (NPUAP/EPUAP, 2014).*
- Document risk assessment and interventions implemented to reduce the client's risk for pressure ulcer development.

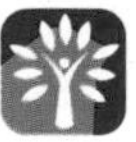

Geriatric

- Consider the older client's cognitive status when assessing the skin and in developing a comprehensive plan of care to prevent pressure ulcers (NPUAP/EPUAP, 2014).
- Aging skin, medications (e.g., steroids), and moisture place the older client at increased risk for pressure-associated skin breakdown. EB: *Assess the client for pressure ulcer risk as well as skin tear and moisture associated skin breakdown. It is important to differentiate the cause of the older client's skin breakdown to effectively implement prevention and treatment strategies. Frequently interventions complement each other in the overall goal to prevent a compromise in the client's skin integrity (NPUAP/EPUAP, 2014; Holmes et al, 2013).*

- *Use atraumatic wound dressings to prevent and treat pressure ulcers to reduce further injury to frail older client's skin (NPUAP/EPUAP, 2014).*
- For older clients with continence concerns, develop and implement an individualized continence management program (NPUAP/EPUAP, 2014). EB: *Use skin barrier products and moisture wicking pads to reduce moisture-associated skin irritation that increases the risk for pressure ulcer development; avoid the use of diapers except when the client is ambulating (NPUAP/EPUAP, 2014; Willson et al, 2014; Makic et al, 2011).*
- *Regularly reposition the older client who is unable to reposition independently. Consider pressure redistribution support surface for client's assessed to be at high risk for pressure ulcers (NPUAP/EPUAP, 2014; Makic et al, 2014).*

Home Care

- The interventions described previously may be adapted for home care use.
- Instruct and assist the client and caregivers in how to assess the skin for excessive pressure. Provide written instructions for actions they can implement to reduce the risk of pressure ulcer development.
- Educate client and caregivers on proper nutrition and when to call the agency and/or healthcare provider with concerns.

▲ It may be beneficial to initiate a consultation in a case assignment with a wound, ostomy, continence nurse (or wounds specialist) to establish a comprehensive plan for pressure ulcer risk reduction for clients at high risk for skin breakdown.

REFERENCES

Anthony, D., Willock, J., & Baharestani. (2010). A comparison of Braden Q, Garvin, and Glamorgan risk assessment scales in paediatrics. *J of Tissue Viability, 19*, 98–105.

Baharestani, M. (2013). *Medical device related pressure ulcers: The hidden epidemic across the life span. Presentation on Behalf of the National Pressure Ulcer Advisory Panel.*

Behrendt, R., Ghaznavi, A., Mahan, M., et al. (2014). Continuous bedside pressure mapping and rates of hospital-associated pressure ulcers in a medical intensive care unit. *American Journal of Critical Care, 23*(2), 127–133.

Black, J. M., Cuddigan, J. E., Walko, M. A., et al. (2010). Medical device related pressure ulcers in hospitalized patients. *International Wound J., 7*(5), 358–365.

Dolack, M., Huffines, B., Stikes, R., et al. (2013). Updated neonatal skin risk assessment scale. *Ky Nurs., 61*(4), 6.

Galvin, P. A., & Curley, M. A. Q. (2012). The braden Q+P: a pediatric perioperative pressure ulcer risk assessment and intervention tool. *AORN, 96*(3), 261–270.

Garcia-Molina, P., Balaguer-Lopez, E., Torra, I., et al. (2012). A prospective, longitudinal study to assess use of continuous and reactive low-pressure mattresses to reduce pressure ulcer incidence in a pediatric intensive care unit. *Ostomy Wound Manag, 58*(7), 32–39.

Holmes, R., Davidson, M., Thompson, B., et al. (2013). Skin tears: care and management of the older adult at home. *Home Healthcare Nurse, 31*(2), 90–101.

Huffines, B., & Logsdon, M. C. (1997). The neonatal skin risk assessment scale for predicting skin breakdown in neonates. *Issues in Comprehensive Pediatric Nursing, 20*(2), 103–114.

Kelleher, A. D., Moorer, A., & Makic, M. B. F. (2012). Peer to peer nursing rounds and hospital-acquired pressure ulcer prevalence in a surgical intensive care unit: a quality improvement project. *JWOCN, 3992*, 152–157.

Makic, M. B. F., VonRueden, K. T., Rauen, C. A., et al. (2011). Evidence-based practice habits: putting more sacred cows out to pasture. *Critical Care Nurse, 31*, 38–62.

Makic, M. B. F., Rauen, C., Watson, R., et al. (2014). Examining the evidence to guide practice: challenging practice habits. *Critical Care Nurse, 34*, 28–46.

McCulloch, J. A., & Kloth, L. C. (2010). *Wound healing evidenced-based management* (4th ed.). Philadelphia: FA Davis.

National Pressure Ulcer Advisory Panel (NPUAP) (2007). *Updated Pressure Ulcer Stages*. Available at: <http://www.npuap.org/resources/educational-and-clinical-resources/pressure-ulcer-categorystaging-illustrations>.

National Pressure Ulcer Advisory Panel (NPUAP) and European Pressure Ulcer Advisory Panel (EPUAP) (2014). E. Haesler (Ed.), *Prevention and Treatment of Pressure Ulcers*. Perth, Australia: Cambridge Media.

Niederhauser, A., Lukas, C., Parker, V., et al. (2012). Comprehensive programs for preventing pressure ulcers: a review of the literature. *Advances in Skin & Wound Care, 25*(4), 168–190.

Padula, W. V., Makic, M. B., Wald, H., et al. (2015). Hospital-acquired pressure ulcers at academic medical centers in the United States, 2008-2012: tracking changes since the CMS nonpayment policy. *Joint Commission J on Quality and Patient Safety, 41*(6), 257–263.

Sussman, C., & Bates-Jensen, B. M. (2012). *Wound care: a collaborative practice manual for healthcare professionals* (4th ed.). Ambler, PA: Lippincott Williams & Wilkins.

Tume, L. N., Siner, S., Scott, E., et al. (2013). The prognostic ability of early Braden Q scores in critically ill children. *Nursing in Crit Care, 19*(2), 98–103.

Willson, M. M., Angyus, M., Beals, D., et al. (2014). Executive summary: a quick reference guide for managing fecal incontinence. *Journal of Wound, Ostomy, and Continence Nursing, 41*(1), 61–69.

P

Ineffective Protection

Ruth M. Curchoe, RN, BSN, MSN, CIC

NANDA-I

Definition

Decrease in the ability to guard self from internal or external threats such as illness or injury

Defining Characteristics

Altered in clotting; alteration in perspiration; anorexia; chilling; coughing; deficient immunity; disorientation; dyspnea; fatigue; immobility; insomnia; itching, maladaptive stress response; neurosensory impairment; pressure ulcer; restlessness; weakness

Related Factors (r/t)

Abnormal blood profiles; cancer; extremes of age; immune disorder (e.g., HIV-associated neuropathy varicella zoster virus); inadequate nutrition; pharmaceutical agent; substance abuse; treatment regimen)

NOC (Nursing Outcomes Classification)

Suggested NOC Outcomes

Health-Promoting Behavior; Blood Coagulation; Endurance; Immune Status

Example NOC Outcome with Indicators

Immune Status as evidenced by the following indicators: Recurrent infections/Tumors/Weight loss. (Rate the outcome and indicators of **Immune Status:** 1 = severe, 2 = substantial, 3 = moderate, 4 = mild, 5 = none [see Section I].)

Client Outcomes

Client Will (Specify Time Frame)

P

- Remain free of infection while in contact during contact with health care
- Remain free of any evidence of new bleeding as evident by stable vital signs
- Explain precautions to take to prevent infection including hand hygiene
- Explain precautions to take to prevent bleeding including fall prevention

NIC (Nursing Interventions Classification)

Suggested NIC Interventions

Bleeding Precautions; Infection Prevention; Infection Protection

Example NIC Activities—Infection Protection

Monitor for systemic and localized signs and symptoms of infection; Inspect skin and mucous membranes for redness, extreme warmth, or drainage

Nursing Interventions and *Rationales*

- Take temperature, pulse, and blood pressure (e.g., every 1 to 4 hours). EBN: *Changes in vital signs can indicate the onset of bleeding or infection. Rectal and oral temperature measurements are more accurate than other methods of temperature measurement such as temporal or axillary measurement (Makic et al, 2011).*
- ▲ Observe nutritional status (e.g., weight, serum protein and albumin levels, muscle mass, and usual food intake). Work with the dietitian to improve nutritional status if needed. EB: *Clients diagnosed with asthma or repeated respiratory infections should have a nutritional assessment.* EB: *Vitamin D influences the body's immune system by influencing the production of endogenous antimicrobial peptides and regulating the inflammatory cascade (Gunville et al, 2013).*
- Observe the client's sleep pattern; if altered, see Nursing Interventions and *Rationales* for Disturbed **Sleep** pattern.

- Identify stressors in the client's life. If stress is uncontrollable, see Nursing Interventions and *Rationales* for Ineffective **Coping.** EB: *Nearly 30% of older clients experience delirium during hospitalization; the incidence is higher in intensive care units. Among older clients who have had surgery, the risk for delirium varies from 10% to more than 50% (Francis & Young, 2012).*

Prevention of Infection

▲ Monitor for and report any signs of infection (e.g., fever, chills, flushed skin, drainage, edema, redness, abnormal laboratory values, and pain) and notify the health care provider promptly. EBN: *While the white blood cell count may be in the normal range, an increased number of immature bands may be present (Versalovic, 2011).* CEBN: *A neutropenic client with fever represents an absolute medical emergency (Mahtani, 2010).* If the client's immune system is depressed, notify the health care provider of elevated temperature, even in the absence of other symptoms of infection. EB: *Clients with depressed immune function are unable to mount the usual immune responses to the onset of infection; fever may be the only sign of infection. A neutropenic client with fever represents an absolute medical emergency.* CEBN: *A neutropenic client with fever represents an absolute medical emergency (Mahtani, 2010).*

- If white blood cell count is severely decreased (i.e., absolute neutrophil count of less than 1000/mm^3), initiate the following precautions:
  - ❍ Take vital signs every 2 to 4 hours
  - ❍ Complete a head-to-toe assessment twice daily, including inspection of oral mucosa, invasive sites, wounds, urine, and stool; monitor for onset of new reports of pain

▲ Avoid any invasive procedures, including catheterization, injections, or rectal or vaginal procedures unless absolutely necessary. EBN: *Classic organisms such as influenza cause infections in the immunocompromised host; often their presentation is different and more serious (Flood, 2014).*

- ❍ Consider warming the client before elective surgery. *Normothermia is associated with low postoperative infection rates (Alexander, 2011).*

▲ Administer granulocyte growth factor as ordered. EB: *Clients most likely to benefit from therapy would be those with profound neutropenia or neutropenia with infections not responding to antimicrobial therapy (Flood, 2014).* EB: *Granulocyte macrophage colony-stimulating factor is mostly well tolerated, although some cancer and kidney disease clients have demonstrated significant complications such as leukopenia (Tovey et al, 2011).*

- ❍ Take meticulous care of all invasive sites; use chlorhexidine gluconate for cleansing. EB: *Use of chlorhexidine gluconate for vascular catheter site care reduces catheter-related bloodstream infections and catheter colonization (Centers for Disease Control and Prevention [CDC], 2011).*
- ❍ Provide frequent oral care. EBN: *The effects of chemotherapy or radiation can cause changes in taste and smell resulting in pain and nutritional deficiencies (Poirier, 2013).*
- ❍ Follow Standard Precautions, especially performing hand hygiene to prevent health care–associated infections. EBN: *Hands of health care workers are the most common cause of health care–associated infections (CDC, 2011; Haas, 2014).*

▲ Refer for appropriate prophylactic antifungal treatment and avoid pathogen exposure (through air filtration, regular hand hygiene, and avoidance of plants and flowers). *Practical measures can be taken to avoid exposing the client to fungi (Flood, 2014).* EB: *Highly active imidazoles have had a major impact on human fungal infections (Ferrara et al, 2011).*

- ❍ Have the client wear a mask when leaving the room. EB: *To prevent health care–acquired pulmonary aspergillosis during hospital construction, neutropenic clients may be at lesser risk if masked when leaving their room (Thom, 2013). Limit and screen visitors to minimize exposure to contagion.*
- ❍ Help the client bathe daily.
- ❍ Practice food safety; a neutropenic diet may not be necessary. EBN: *No clear evidence exists that the neutropenic diet makes a difference in overall rates of infection (Thom, 2013).*
- ❍ Ensure that the client is well nourished. Provide food with protein, and consider vitamin supplements. If appetite is suppressed, institute a dietary referral. Keep track of serum albumin levels, as well as transferrin and prealbumin levels. CEB: *Levels of the visceral proteins (albumin, transferrin, and prealbumin) are an indirect measure of nutritional status (Geismar, 2014).*
- ❍ Help the client cough and practice deep breathing regularly. Maintain an appropriate activity level.
- ❍ Obtain a private room for the client. Use high-energy particulate air filters if available and appropriate. Protective isolation is not recommended. Recognize that cotton cover gowns may not be effective in decreasing infection. EBN: *Complete an infection control risk assessment (ICRA) considering such issues*

as the type of transplant performed, the environment, and prior infection rates. Use the ICRA to decide the types of infections, processes, practices, and risk to be monitored (Harris, 2014).

▲ Watch for signs of sepsis, including change in mental status, fever, shaking, chills, and hypotension. If present, notify the health care provider promptly. *Change in mental status, fever, shaking, chills, and hypotension are indicators of sepsis (Curchoe, 2013).*
- Refer to care plan for Risk for **Infection.**
- Refer to care plan for Readiness for enhanced **Nutrition** for additional interventions.

Pediatric

- Suggest kangaroo care, frequent and exclusive or nearly exclusive breastfeeding, and early discharge from hospital for low-birth-weight infants. EBN: *Kangaroo mother care, frequent and exclusive or nearly exclusive breastfeeding, and early discharge from hospital was associated with a decreased risk of mortality) and severe infection/sepsis for low-birth-weight infants (Conde-Agudelo et al, 2011).*
- Assess postoperative fever in pediatric oncology clients promptly. EB: *Fever is a physiological mechanism that has beneficial effects in fighting infection. There is no evidence that fever itself worsens the course of an illness or that it causes long-term neurological complications (Sullivan & Farrer, 2011).*
- For hand hygiene with low-birth-weight infants, use alcohol hand rub and gloves. EBN: *Audit programs to track compliance with hand hygiene identified a drop in the incidence of health care–associated infections in very low-birth-weight infants in the neonatal intensive care unit (Academy of Pediatrics, 2012).*

Geriatric

- If not contraindicated, promote exercise to promote improved quality of life in older adults. EB: *A study of 95 healthy adults 65 years and older suggests that the effects of resistance-type exercise training can counteract the loss of muscle mass and strength with aging (Leenders et al, 2013).* Give older clients with imbalanced nutrition a vitamin D supplement to reduce risk of fracture. EB: *Lack of vitamin D may exacerbate osteoporosis in older or postmenopausal women (Rizzoli et al, 2013).*
- Refer to the care plan for Risk for **Infection** for more interventions related to the prevention of infection.

P

Prevention of Bleeding

▲ Monitor the client's risk for bleeding; evaluate results of clotting studies and platelet counts. *Laboratory studies give a good indication of the seriousness of the bleeding disorder.*
- Watch for hematuria, melena, hematemesis, hemoptysis, epistaxis, bleeding from mucosa, petechiae, and ecchymoses. EBN: *A study of 200 clients with idiopathic thrombocytopenic purpura revealed that 57% had ecchymoses, 42% petechiae, 23% bleeding from the gums, and 31.5% epistaxis; 8% had two or more signs and symptoms and 73% were asymptomatic when the diagnosis was established (Garcia-Stivalet et al, 2014).*

▲ Give medications orally or intravenously only; avoid giving intramuscularly, subcutaneously, or rectally (Shuey, 1996).
- Apply pressure for a longer time than usual to invasive sites, such as venipuncture or injection sites. *Additional pressure is needed to stop bleeding of invasive sites in clients with bleeding disorders.*
- Take vital signs often; watch for changes associated with fluid volume loss. Excessive bleeding causes decreased blood pressure and increased pulse and respiratory rates.
- Monitor menstrual flow if relevant; have the client use pads instead of tampons. EB: *Menstruation can be excessive in clients with bleeding disorders. Adolescents presenting with heavy menstrual bleeding at or near menarche assessment should include bleeding disorders (Singh, 2013).*
- Have the client use a moistened toothette or a very soft child's toothbrush instead of an adult toothbrush. Follow the dentist's recommendation for flossing and appropriate rinses to use. Control gum bleeding by applying pressure to gums with gauze pad soaked in ice water. *These actions help prevent trauma to the oral mucosa, which could result in bleeding (Medline Plus, 2011).*
- Ask the client either to not shave or to use only an electric razor. *This helps prevent any unnecessary trauma that could result in bleeding (Shuey, 1996).*

▲ To decrease risk of bleeding, avoid administering salicylates or nonsteroidal antiinflammatory drugs (NSAIDs) if possible. CEB: *Gastrointestinal bleeding due to NSAIDs, acetylsalicylic acid, or warfarin was the most common adverse drug reaction that resulted in hospital admission and represented 40% of all ADRs (12 of 30), according to WHO causality criteria (Brvar et al, 2009).*

Home Care

- • Some of the interventions previously described may be adapted for home care use.
- ▲ Consider using a nurse-led client-centered medical home (PCMH) for monitoring anticoagulant therapy. EBN: *Establishment of nurse-led medical homes to monitor anticoagulation therapy management clinics leads to improvements in quality of care in terms of improved control of international normalized ratio and reduced complications. Data support a conclusion that PCMHs do improve quality, access, and cost (Scudder, 2011).*
- • For terminally ill clients, teach and institute all of the aforementioned noninvasive precautions that maintain quality of life. Discuss with the client, family, and health care provider the consequences of contracting infection. Determine which precautions do not maintain quality of life and should not be used (e.g., physical assessment twice daily or multiple vital sign assessments). CEB: *Multiple assessments and other invasive procedures are recovery-based and cure-focused activities. The client and provider must agree on an approach to care for the clients during their remaining life (Periyakoil et al, 2013).*

Client/Family Teaching and Discharge Planning

Depressed Immune Function

- • Teach the client and family how to take a temperature. Encourage the family to take the client's temperature between 3 PM and 7 PM at least once daily. EBN: *For most people, the difference between high and low values throughout the day is approximately 2° F (1.1° C) (97° to 99° F [36.1° to 37.2° C]), with the lowest value typically occurring in the early morning hours (2* am *to 5* am*) and the highest values commonly occurring in the evening (Fetzer, 2013).*
- • Teach precautions to use to decrease the chance of infection (e.g., avoiding uncooked fruits and vegetables, using appropriate self-care including good hand hygiene, and ensuring a safe environment). Teach the client to avoid crowds and contact with persons who have infections. Teach the need for good nutrition, avoidance of stress, and adequate rest to maintain immune system function. CEBN: *Approaches to avoiding infection at home for the client with neutropenia include good hand hygiene and careful management of food, drink, and the client's environment (Hawkins, 2009).*

Bleeding Disorder

- • Teach the client to wear a medical alert bracelet and notify all health care personnel of the bleeding disorder. CEB: *Emergency identification schemes such as medical alert bracelets use emblems that alert health care professionals to potential problems and can ensure appropriate and prompt treatment (National Comprehensive Cancer Network, 2006).* Teach the client and family the signs of bleeding, precautions to take to prevent bleeding, and action to take if bleeding begins. Caution the client to avoid taking over-the-counter medications without the permission of the health care provider. *Medications containing salicylates can increase bleeding.*
- • Teach the client to wear loose-fitting clothes and avoid physical activity that might cause trauma.

P

REFERENCES

Alexander, J. W. (2011). Updated recommendations for controlling surgical site infections. *Annals of Surgery, 253*(96), 1082–1093.

American Academy of Pediatrics and American College of Obstetricians and Gynecologists. (2012). Infection Control. In L. E. Riley, A. R. Stark, et al. (Eds.), *Guidelines for Perinatal Care* (7th ed., pp. 439–492). Elk Grove Village, IL.: American Academy of Pediatrics.

Brvar, M., et al. (2009). The frequency of adverse drug reaction related admissions according to method of detection, admission urgency and medical department specialty. *BMC Clinical Pharmacology, 4*(9), 8.

Centers for Disease Control and Prevention (CDC). (2011). Guideline for hand hygiene in health-care settings. Recommendations of the healthcare infection control practices advisory committee and the HICPAC/SHEA/APIC/IDSA hand hygiene task force. *MMWR. Recommendations and Reports: Morbidity and Mortality Weekly Report. Recommendations and Reports, 51*(RR–16), 1–45. Accessed 7/25/14, from <http://www.cdc.gov/handhygiene/Guidelines.html>; May 19, Retrieved July 21, 2014.

Centers for Disease Control and Prevention (CDC). (2011). *Hospital Infection Control Advisory Committee, Guideline for the prevention of intravascular catheter related infections*, from <http://www.cdc.gov/hicpac>. Retrieved Aug 28, 2011.

Conde-Agudelo, A., Belizán, J. M., & Diaz-Rossello, J. (2011). Kangaroo mother care to reduce morbidity and mortality in low birthweight infants. *Cochrane Database of Sys Rev*, (3), CD002771.

Curchoe, R. M. (2013). Infection Prevention and Control. In *Potter, Perry Fundamentals of Nursing* (8th ed.). St. Louis Missouri: Elsevier.

Ferrara, J., MacDougall, C., & Gallagher, J. (2011). Empiric antifungal therapy in patients with febrile neutropenia. *Pharmocol Ther, 31*(4), 369–385.

Fetzer, S. J. (2013). Vital signs. In *Potter, Perry Fundamentals of Nursing* (8th ed.). St. Louis Missouri: Elsevier.

Flood, A. (2014). The Immunocompromised Host. In *APIC text of infection control and epidemiology* (4th ed.). Washington, DC: Association for Professionals in Infection Control and Epidemiology, Inc (APIC).

Francis, J., & Young, G. B. (2012). *Patient information: Delirium (Beyond the basics)*. Available at <www.uptodate.com/contents/delirium-beyond-the-basics> Accessed 8/20/14.

Garcia-Stivalet, L. A., Munoz-Flores, A., Montiel-Jarquin, A. J., et al. (2014). Clinical analysis of 200 cases of idiopathic thrombocytopenia purpura. *Revista medica del Instituto Mexicano del Seguro Social*, *52*(3), 322–325.

Geismar, K. (2014). Nutrition and Immune Function. In *APIC text of Infection Control and Epidemiology* (4th ed.). Washington, DC: Association for Professionals in Infection Control and Epidemiology, (APIC). [Accessed 8/22/2014] last revised 6/6/14.

Gunville, C. F., Mourani, P. M., & Ginde, A. A. (2013). The role of vitamin D in prevention and treatment of infection. *Inflammation and Allergy Drug Targets*, *12*(4), 239–245.

Haas, J. (2014). Hand Hygiene. In *APIC text of Infection Control and Epidemiology* (4th ed.). DC: Association for Professionals in Infection Control and Epidemiology, (APIC). [Accessed 7/28/14] last revised 6/6/14.

Harris, P. L. (2014). Solid Organ Transplantation. In *APIC text of Infection Control and Epidemiology* (4th ed.). Washington, DC: Association for Professionals in Infection Control and Epidemiology, (APIC). [Accessed 8/23/2014] last revised 6/6/14.

Hawkins, J. (2009). Supportive care: managing febrile neutropenia. *Paediatric Nursing*, *21*(4), 33–37.

Leenders, M., Verdjik, L. B., van der Hoeven, L., et al. (2013). Elderly men and women benefit equally from prolonged resistance-type exercise training. *The Journal of Gerontology Series*, *68*(7), 769–779.

Mahtani, R. (2010). *Neutropenia and infection*, From <http://www.caring4cancer>. Retrieved July 29, 2011.

Makic, M. B., et al. (2011). Evidence-based practice habits: putting more sacred cows out to pasture. *Am Assoc Crit Care Nurses*, *31*(2), 38–63.

Medline Plus (2011) *Bleeding gums*, from <http://www.nlm.nih.gov/medlineplus/ency/article/003062.htm>. Retrieved August 1.

National Comprehensive Cancer Network (NCCN). (2006). *Fever and neutropenia: treatment guidelines for patients with cancer-version II, March 2006*, From <http://www.nccn.org/patients/patient_gls/english/feverandneutropenia/1introduction.asp>. Retrieved July 30, 2014. Accessed 8/27/14.

Periyakoil, V. S., Stevens, M., & Kraemer, H. (2013). Multicultural long-term care nurses' perceptions of factors influencing patient dignity at the end-of-life. *Journal of American Geriatrics Society*, *61*(3), 440–446.

Poirier, P. (2013). Nursing-led management of side effects of radiation: evidence-based recommendations for practice. *Nursing Research and Reviews*, *3*, 47–57.

Rizzoli, R., Boonen, S., Brandi, M.-L., et al. (2013). Vitamin D supplementation in elderly or postmenopausal women: a 2013 update of the 2008 recommendations from the European society for clinical and economic aspects of osteoporosis and osteoarthritis (ESCEO). *Current Medical Research & Opinion*, *29*(4), 305–313.

Scudder, L. (2011). Nurse-led medical homes: current status and future plans. *Medscape nurses*, April 20.

Shuey, K. M. (1996). Platelet-associated bleeding disorders. *Seminars in Oncology Nursing*, *12*(1), 15–27.

Singh, S., Best, C., Dunn, S., et al. (2013). Abnormal uterine bleeding in pre-menopausal women. *Journal of Obstetrics and Gynaecology Canada*, *35*(5), 473–475.

Sullivan, J., & Farrer, H. (2011). Fever and antipyretic use in children. *Pediatrics*, *127*(3), 580–587.

Thom, K. A., Kleinberg, M., & Roghmann, M. C. (2013). Infection prevention in the cancer center. *Clinical Infectious Diseases*, Available at: <www.cid.oxford.org/content/early/2013/06/06/cid.cit290>. Accessed 8/22/2014.

Tovey, M. G., Legrand, J., & Lallemand, C. (2011). Overcoming immunogenicity associated with the use of biopharmaceuticals. *Expert Rev Clin Pharmacol*, *4*(5), 623–631.

Versalovic, J., Carroll, K. C., Funke, G., et al. (2011). *Manual of Clinical Microbiology* (10th ed.). VI, Washington, DC: ASM Press.

Rape-Trauma syndrome

Julianne E. Doubet, BSN, RN, CEN, NREMT-P

NANDA-I

Definition

Sustained adaptive response to a forced, violent sexual penetration against the victim's will and consent

Defining Characteristics

Aggression; agitation; anger; anxiety; change in relationships; confusion; denial; dependence; depression; disorganization; dissociative disorders; embarrassment; fear; guilt; helplessness; humiliation; hyperalertness; impaired decision-making; loss of self-esteem; mood swings; muscle spasms; muscle tension; nightmares; paranoia; phobias; physical trauma; powerlessness; revenge; self-blame; sexual dysfunction; shame; shock; sleep disturbances; substance abuse; suicide attempts; vulnerability

Related Factors (r/t)

Rape

NOC (Nursing Outcomes Classification)

Suggested NOC Outcomes

Abuse Cessation; Abuse Protection; Abuse Recovery: Emotional, Sexual, Coping; Impulse Self-Control; Self-Mutilation Restraint

Example NOC Outcome with Indicators

Abuse Recovery: Sexual as evidenced by the following indicators: Acknowledgment of right to disclose abusive situation/ Expression of right to have been protected from abuse. (Rate the outcome and indicators of **Abuse Recovery: Sexual:** 1 = none, 2 = limited, 3 = moderate, 4 = substantial, 5 = extensive [see Section I].)

Client Outcomes

Client Will (Specify Time Frame)

- Share feelings, concerns, and fears
- Recognize that the rape or attempt was not client's own fault
- State that, no matter what the situation, no one has the right to assault another
- Describe medical/legal treatment procedures and reasons for treatment
- Report absence of physical complications or pain
- Identify support resources and attend psychotherapy/group assistance in coping with the trauma and effects of the traumatic experience
- Function at same level as before crisis, including sexual functioning
- Recognize that it is normal for full recovery to take a minimum of 1 year

NIC (Nursing Interventions Classification)

Suggested NIC Interventions

Counseling; Rape-Trauma Treatment

Example NIC Activities—Rape-Trauma Treatment

Explain rape protocol and obtain consent to proceed through protocol; Implement crisis intervention counseling

R

Nursing Interventions and *Rationales*

- Escort the client to a treatment room immediately upon arrival to the emergency department. Stay with (or have a trusted person stay with) the client. EBN: *Victims of sexual assault require special attention from caregivers, so as not to feel victimized a second time in the medical facility; the presence of the nurse at every step of the care process supports the victim (Durieux, 2014).* EB: *Cybulski (2013) states that the immediate needs of sexual assault victims begin with privacy and safety.*
- Assure the client of confidentiality. EB: *It is suggested that not all criminal justice and medical professionals understand the statutory provision of privilege to communications between rape victim advocates and victims (Cole, 2011).* EB: *Burns et al (2014) noted in their research that U.S. servicewomen did not report sexual assaults due to humiliation and anxiety concerning confidentiality.*

▲ Provide a sexual assault response team (SART), if available, that includes a sexual assault nurse examiner (SANE), rape counseling advocate, and representative of law enforcement for best possible outcomes. EB: *According to a study by Patterson (2014), a team of forensic nurses and victim advocates partner together to provide treatment not only for the necessary physical and medical requirements of sexual assault survivors, but also for dealing with the complex legal and mental health needs that necessitate follow-up.* EBN: *A study of the available literature demonstrates that SANE/SART programs provide emotional and mental support that allows a victim of sexual assault to take control over her/his options and choices, and assists the client in navigating the criminal justice system and accessing health services (Henry & Force, 2011).*

- Observe for signs of physical injury. EBN: *Assessment and documentation of injuries and physical findings are all-important, both in furnishing a baseline for determining intervention priorities and for any possible legal action (Carter-Snell, 2011).* EB: *Some locations to assess for obvious genital injuries would include tears or abrasions of the posterior fourchette labia, abrasion or bruising of the labia minora and fossa navicularis, and ecchymosis or tears of the hymen; document these injuries as evidence for any future legal proceedings (Linden, 2011).*

- Document the client's chief complaint and request an event history of the sexual assault in her/his own words. EB: *Taking time to listen to the victim's story is essential in directing the forensic examination and subsequent samples that are collected (Rey-Salmon, 2012).* EB: *It is agreed that awareness of the client's sexual victimization history is invaluable in personalizing cases and determining treatment interventions (Probst et al, 2011).*
- Encourage the client to verbalize her/his feelings. EB: *There is widely accepted documentation that early intervention in cases of trauma significantly lessens the risk of anxiety, depression, self-harm, addiction issues, eating disorders, and suicide (Marshall, 2012).*
- Make sure that the victim understands everything you are doing. EBN: *The preservation of client dignity must be maintained, not only for the victim's protection, but also to show respect and caring; respecting dignity is one of the essential behaviors that nurtures caring (Gustafsson et al, 2013).* EBN: *Clarify the medical aspects of the forensic examination for the victim and obtain consent, but ensure that the client is aware that, although she/he has given consent for the exam, she/he can stop it at any point (Learner, 2012).*
- Explain to the client that all or some of the client's clothing may be kept for evidential purposes and photographs may be taken (with consent) to document the client's injuries. EBN: *For victims of sexual assault, the forensic examination is the inaugural step in the advancement of justice. Assessment and treatment of victims, as well as the precise collection and documentation of evidence, are critical for a solid case (Fitzpatrick et al, 2012).*

▲ If a law enforcement interview is permitted, provide support by staying with the client at her/his request. EB: *A study authorized by the Bureau of Justice (Kruttschnitt et al, 2014) surmises that we must take into consideration the frequency and environment under which rape and sexual assault are committed, because this is vital information in targeting resources for law enforcement and support for victims.* EBN: *By keeping the victim of sexual assault calm and comfortable, the nurse's actions at the bedside may benefit the legal investigation and leave the victim less traumatized and better able to give a complete report of the assault (Campbell et al, 2011).*

- Use the sexual assault evidence collection kits that have been reviewed by the SART members and provided by your state to collect adequate and accurate evidence for analysis by a forensic laboratory. EB: *The health care provider who examines victims of sexual assault must be responsible to act in accordance with state and local statutory or policy requirements for the use of evidence-gathering kits (ACOG, 2014).* EB: *Standardized evidence-collection kits usually contain forms for documentation to assist examiners. Evidence collection requires the victim's permission during each of the necessary steps, and the client should be given the opportunity to set the tempo of the exam and to be aware that she/he may decline any part of the examination (Linden, 2011).*

R

▲ Discuss the possibility of pregnancy and sexually transmitted infections (STIs) and the treatments available. EB: *Victims of sexual assault should be advised that they are at risk for pregnancy, sexually transmitted infections, and post-traumatic stress disorder; as a victim of sexual assault, she/he should be monitored and offered emergency contraception and STI prophylaxis (Committee on Health Care for Underserved Women, 2014).* EB: *Treatment of injuries and prevention of unwanted pregnancy and sexually transmitted infections, including HIVs, should be offered to any victim of sexual assault (Cybulski, 2013).*

▲ Encourage the client to report the sexual assault to law enforcement agency. EB: *Rape survivors' decisions to assist in legal actions are influenced by three social groups: family/friends, service providers, and police (Anders & Christopher, 2011).* EBN: *In her study, Marchetti (2012) concludes that sexual assault (SA) and the underreporting of SA are highly prevalent in the United States and that regret may play a considerable part in the unwillingness to report the rape.*

▲ For those interested in a spiritual connection, make the appropriate recommendation. EBN: *According to Hellman (2014), research should be introduced to develop theory using religious and spiritual beliefs to aid in the recovery process of sexual assault victims.*

▲ Stress the necessity of follow-up care with a mental health professional to recognize and intervene with problems associated with the effects of rape-trauma/sexual assault. EB: *In the aftermath of rape, victims often experience evidence of depression, anxiety, post-traumatic stress disorder (PTSD), self-harm, and increased risk of suicide (Marshall, 2012).* EB: *Price et al (2014) state that although sexual assault increases the risk for psychiatric disorders and while there is treatment available, few victims choose mental health care after their attack.*

- Stress the importance of awareness throughout the community of the scope and severity of the effects of sexual abuse as a means of additional healing empowerment. EB: *Ullman and Peter-Hagene (2014) suggest in their study of community reactions to a victim's divulgence of sexual assault that negative community reactions were associated with greater PTSD symptoms due to the victim's inability to cope and a sense of loss of control.* EB: *Recovery from sexual assault/rape is frequently hindered by the public's failure to believe the victim and the need to obtain justice (Chapleau & Oswald, 2014).*

Geriatric

- Build a trusting relationship with the client. EBN: *Trust begins by acting with integrity and caring, which then conveys investment in another's welfare (Laskowski-Jones, 2011).*
- All examinations should be done in older adults as they would be done on any adult client after sexual assault, with modifications for comfort if necessary. EB: *In a study by Nobrega et al (2014) of the forensic assessment of older victims of sexual assault, the forensic evaluation was found to be essential in positive judicial outcomes and invaluable in identifying physical and biological confirmation of sexual assault.* EBN: *Elder abuse can be difficult to identify (Kleba & Falk, 2014), in that accidental injuries are more common in older adults and mental disorders, such as dementia, can impede the victim's capacity to recall the occurrences of abuse.*
- Assess for mobility limitations and cognitive impairment. EB: *As the aging population swells, a rise in morbidity can be validated, and with it, not only an increase in chronic illnesses, but also the recognition of significant cognitive changes and physical disabilities (Kizie et al, 2014).*
- Explain and encourage the client to report sexual abuse. EB: *In this study, it was found that the case worker and the older victims might hold contradictory views regarding the perpetrators' motivations for abuse and what would be the likely outcomes of reporting it; this was most likely to occur when the perpetrator was a family member. Adjusting these differences can raise the likelihood of effective interventions (Jackson & Hafemeister, 2011).* EBN: *According to Marchetti (2012), new approaches are called for in the development of a basis for medical professionals to assist victims of sexual assault in making decisions concerning their health care.*
- Observe for psychosocial distress. EBN: *Changes in behavior, such as becoming more withdrawn, depressed, confused, fearful, or agitated, may be the consequences of sexual abuse in older adults (Nazarko, 2011).* EB: *According to Barton et al (2014), older adults with anxiety disorders have difficulty dealing with their everyday lives and are therefore at risk for comorbidities such as depression, falls, physical and functional disability, and loneliness.*

▲ Consider arrangements for safe housing. EB: *Practical implications—collaboration and an integrated community response are vital to enhancing the safety and quality of life of the older victim of abuse (Brandl & Dawson, 2011).* EB: *In Dakin's (2014) study involving a diverse group of older women who were given scenarios, in which the scenario subjects, due to circumstances, had the option of choosing autonomy or protection; when asked which alternative the subject should pick, the majority of women chose protection, suggesting that autonomy may be limited and would only delay needed security and health care at a later time.*

R

Male Rape

▲ EB: *Male rape is markedly under-reported and, consequently, the victim rarely receives essential sexual assault aftercare (McClean, 2013).* EB: *Hiquet and Gromb-Monnoyeaur (2013) maintain that the cause of the underreporting of male sexual assault is due to the stigma attached to the victim's disclosure of rape.*

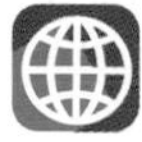

Multicultural

- Assess for the influence of cultural beliefs, norms, and values on the client's ability to cope with the trauma of the rape experience. EBN: *It is suggested that divergences among minority women in the frequency of rape, reports of rape, and use of available resources will vary based on ethnicity, race, cultural standards, help-seeking behaviors, and availability of accessible services (Lawson, 2011).* EB: *A paper by Huong (2012) highlights the fact that rape disclosure in a collective society is often contiguous with the concepts of family honor, kinship, gender, society, and responsibility.*
- Assess to determine if physically abused women are also victims of sexual assault. EB: *Care for those victims of sexual assault and domestic violence should include crisis services: legal advocacy, medical advocacy, counseling, support group, and shelter (Macy et al, 2011).*

Home Care

- Some of the interventions described previously may be adapted for home care use.
- Corroborate the client's feelings of self-worth. This study proposes that the feeling of self-worth moderates the effects of violence—especially violent loss—on PTSD and depression (Mancini et al, 2011). EB: *It is theorized by Ban Hong et al (2012) that there is a connection between the signs of insecure attachment, which appear in victims of interpersonal trauma and is linked to post-traumatic stress and a diminished feeling of self-worth.*
- Assist the client with realistically assessing the home setting for safety and/or selecting a safe environment in which to live. EBN: *The protection or safeguarding of vulnerable adults must be an integral part of everyday nursing practice (Straughair, 2011).*

▲ Ensure that the client has systems in place for long-term support. EB: *Survivors of abuse noted that a cooperative model of health care, particularly between mental health and physical health professionals, was an asset to their recovery (Dunleavy & Slowik, 2012).* EB: *According to Brandl and Dawson (2011), it is imperative that community and private resources join together to promote safety and the quality of life for the older adult victims of trauma.*

▲ Design a practical discharge plan to include a safe shelter if needed, follow-up care for physical injury, and follow-up referral for psychological support. EB: *Safety, medical, and psychological plans for discharge are critical to the victim of sexual assault (Linden, 2011).* EBN: *It is vital to abused older adults to be sheltered in a safe, protected, violence free, and medically suitable environment (Heck & Gillespie, 2013).*

▲ Assess for other client vulnerabilities such as mental health issues or addiction and refer the client to social agencies for implementation of a therapeutic regimen. EB: *Client support should be in response to the whole person; the assault should be addressed in both its social and cultural elements, with sensitivity to the client's distinct needs and by sharing information with other social services, if so allowed by the client (Marshall, 2012).*

Client/Family Teaching and Discharge Planning

- Emphasize the client's needs for safety and to decrease the opportunities for repeat attacks. EBN: *The client should be made aware that the results of continued abuse may include more abuse, chronic pain, physical and emotional illness, and even death (Symes, 2011).*
- *Recognize the vulnerability of the client.* EB: *Conceptualizations of present control over the recovery process were related to lower levels of psychological distress (Walsh & Bruce, 2011).* EBN: *In a qualitative study by Arend et al (2013) involving survivors of sexual assault in South Africa, it was found that nurses have numerous opportunities to improve the quality of post–sexual assault care, which in turn advances the clients' emotional and psychosocial outcomes.*
- NOTE: PTSD has a high probability of being a psychological sequela to rape. Research demonstrated two effective treatments for improvement of PTSD in rape victims: prolonged exposure and stress inoculation training. Prolonged exposure involves reliving the rape experience; by imagining it as vividly as possible, describing it aloud in the present tense, taping this description, and listening to the tape at least once daily. Stress inoculation training uses breathing exercises to diminish anxiety and instruction in coping skills, thought stopping, cognitive restructuring, self-dialogue, and role playing. Research suggests that a combination of both treatments may provide the optimal effect. Furthermore, for those who reported the assault to police, lower levels of legal system success and satisfaction were linked to higher levels of perceived control over present recovery.

R

REFERENCES

American College of Obstetrics and Gynecology. (2014). Committee on health care for underserved women. *Obstetrics and Gynecology, 123*, 726–730.

Anders, M., & Christopher, P. A. (2011). A socioecological model of rape survivors' decisions to aid in case prosecutions. *Psychology of Women Quarterly, 35*, 92–108.

Arend, E., Maw, A., deSwardt, C., et al. (2013). South African sexual assault survivors' experiences of post-exposure prophylaxis and individualized nursing care: a qualitative study. *Journal of the Association of Nurses in AIDS Care, 24*, 154–165. [Epub 2012 Jul 25].

Ban Hong, L., Adams, L. A., & Lilly, M. M. (2012). Self-worth as a mediator between attachment and posttraumatic stress in interpersonal trauma. *The Journal of Interpersonal Violence, 27*, 2030–2061. [Epub 2012 Feb10].

Barton, S., Kamer, C., Salih, F., et al. (2014). Clinical effectiveness of interventions for treatment resistant anxiety in older people. *Health Technology Assessment, 18*, 1–60.

Brandl, B., & Dawson, L. (2011). Responding to victims of abuse in later life in the United States. *The Journal of Adult Protection, 13*, 315–322.

Burns, B., Grindlay, K., Holt, K., et al. (2014). Military sexual trauma among US servicewomen during deployment: a qualitative study. *The American Journal of Public Health, 104*, 345–349. [Epub 2013 Dec 12].

Campbell, R., Greeson, M., & Patterson, D. (2011). Defining the boundaries: how sexual assault nurse examiners (SANE) balance patient care and law enforcement collaboration. *Journal of Forensic Nursing, 7*, 17–26.

Carter-Snell, C. (2011). Injury documentation: Using the BALD STEP mnemonic and the RCMP sexual assault kit. *Outlook, 34*, 15–20.

Chapleau, K. M., & Oswald, D. L. (2014). A system justification view of sexual violence: legitimizing gender inequality and reduced moral outrage are connected to greater rape myth acceptance. *Journal of Trauma and Dissociation, 15*, 204–218.

Cole, J. (2011). Victim confidentiality on sexual assault response teams (SART). *The Journal of Interpersonal Violence, 26*, 360–376. [Epub 2010 May 4].

Cybulski, B. (2013). Immediate medical care after sexual assault. *Best Practice & Research: Clinical Obstetrics and Gynaecology, 27*, 141–149. [Epub 2012 Nov 29].

Dakin, E. (2014). Protection as care: moral reasoning and moral orientation among ethnically and socioeconomically diverse older women. *The Journal of Aging Studies, 28*, 44–56. [Epub 2013 Dec 22].

Dunleavy, K., & Slowik, A. (2012). Emergence of delayed posttraumatic stress disorder symptoms related to sexual trauma: patient-centered and trauma-cognizant management by physical therapists. *Physical Therapy, 95*, 339–351. <http://dx.doi.org.ezproxy.jccmi.edu/10.2522/ptj.2012.92.6.873>.

Durieux, J. (2014). Nursing care of victims of sexual violence. *Revue de L'infirmiere, 201*, 39–41.

Fitzpatrick, M., Ta, A., Lenchus, J., et al. (2012). Sexual assault forensic examiners' training and assessment using simulation technology. *Journal of Emergency Nursing, 38*, 85–90. [Epub 2011 Jan 6].

Gustafsson, L. K., Wingerblad, A., & Lindwall, L. (2013). Respecting dignity in forensic cases: the challenge faced by nurses of maintaining patient's dignity in clinical caring situations. *Journal of Psychiatric and Mental Health Nursing, 20*, 1–8. [Epub 2012 Mar 14].

Heck, L., & Gillespie, G. (2013). Interprofessional program to provide emergency shelter to abused elders. *Advanced Emergency Nursing Journal, 35*, 170–181. <http://dx.doi.org.ezproxy.jccmi.edu/10.1097/TME0b013e31828ecc06>.

Hellman, A. (2014). Examining sexual assault survival of adult women: responses, mediators and current theories. *Journal of Forensic Nursing, 10*, 175–184.

Henry, D., & Force, L. (2011). From our readers. Strategies for implementing an effective sexual assault nurse examiners program (SANE). *American Nurse Today, 6*, 3.

Hiquet, J., & Gromb-Monnoyeaur, S. (2013). Men victim of sexual assault of concern into the first emergency medical unit for victims of assaults in France. *Journal of Forensic and Legal Medicine, 20*, 836–841. <http://dx.doi.org.ezproxy.jccmi.edu/10.1016/j.jflm.2013.06.024>.

Huong, N. T. (2012). Rape disclosure: the interplay of gender, culture and kinship in contemporary Viet Nam. *Culture, Health & Sexuality, 27*, 39–46. [Epub 2012 May 16].

Jackson, S., & Hafemeister, T. (2011). Lessons learned from APS caseworkers and elderly victims they serve. *Victimization of the Elderly and Disabled, 14*, 1–15.

Kizie, C. C., daSilva Talmelli, L. F., Diniz, M. A., et al. (2014). Assessment of cognitive status and frailty of older elderly living at home. *Cienc Cuid Saude, 13*, 120–127.

Kleba, P. A., & Falk, N. L. (2014). The elder justice act: what nurses need to know. *American Journal of Nursing, 114*, 65–68.

Kruttschnitt, C. J., Kalsbeek, W. D., & House, C. C. (2014). *Estimating the incidence of rape and sexual assaults.* Committee on National Statistics; Division on Behavioral and Social Sciences and Education; National Research Council. Washington (DC): National Academies Press (US).

Laskowski-Jones, L. (2011). Building a foundation of trust. *Nursing, 41*, 6. <http://dx.doi.org.ezproxy.jccmi.edu/10.1097/01.NURSE.0000403276.91298.da>.

Lawson, S. (2011). Sexual assault: disparities within health care and the criminal justice system for minority women. *Hispanic Health Care International, 9*, 58–60. <http://dx.doi.org.ezproxy.jccmi.edu/10.1891/1540-4153.9.2.58>.

Learner, S. (2012). Compassion in time of crisis. *Nursing Standard, 27*, 22–30.

Linden, J. (2011). Care of the adult patient after sexual assault. *New England Journal of Medicine, 365*, 834–841.

Macy, R. J., Johns, M., Rizo, C. F., et al. (2011). Domestic violence and sexual assault service goal priorities. *Journal of Interpersonal Violence, 26*, 3361–3382. [Epub 2011 Jan 30].

Mancini, A., Prati, G., & Black, S. (2011). Self worth mediates the effects of violent loss on PTSD symptoms. *Journal of Trauma Stress, 24*, 116–120. [Epub 2011 Jan 6].

Marchetti, C. (2012). Regret and police reporting among individuals who have experienced sexual assault. *Journal of American Psychiatric Nursing, 18*, 32–39. [Epub 2012 Jan 18].

Marshall, D. (2012). Twenty-four-hour sexual assault care-incorporating courtesy, dignity, privacy and respect. *Healthcare Counsel Psychotherapy Journal, 21*, 5–20.

McClean, I. A. (2013). The male victim of sexual assault. Best practice and research: clinical. *Obstetrics Gynaecology, 27*, 39–46. [Epub 2012 Aug 28].

Nazarko, L. (2011). Safeguarding and protection in health and social care. *Nursing and Residential Care, 13*, 264–268.

Nobrega, P. A., Rodrigues, F., Dinis-Oliveria, R. C., et al. (2014). Sexual offenses against elderly people: forensic evaluation and judicial outcome. *Journal of Elder Abuse and Neglect, 26*, 189–204.

Patterson, D. (2014). Interdisciplinary team communication among forensic nurses and rape victim advocates. *Social Work Healthcare Journal, 53*, 382–397.

Price, M., Davidson, T. M., Ruggiero, K. J., et al. (2014). Predictors of using mental health services after sexual assault. *Journal of Trauma Stress, 27*, 331–337. [Epub 2014 May 22].

Probst, D., Turchek, J., & Zimak, E. (2011). Assessment of sexual assault in clinical practice: available screening tools for use with different adult populations. *Journal of Aggression Maltreatment and Trauma, 20*, 199–226. <http://dx.doi.org.ezproxy.jccmi.edu/10.1080/10926771.2011.546754>.

Rey-Salmon, C. (2012). Examination and care of sexual assault victims. *La Revue Du Praticien, 62*, 803–805, 807–808.

Straughair, C. (2011). Safeguarding vulnerable adults: the role of the registered nurse. *Nursing Standard, 25*, 49–56.

Symes, L. (2011). Abuse across the lifespan: prevalence, risk, and protective factors. *Nursing Clinics of North America, 46*, 391–411. [Epub 2011 Oct 6].

Ullman, S. E., & Peter-Hagene, L. (2014). Social reactions to sexual assault disclosure, coping, perceived control and PTSD symptoms in sexual assault victims. *Journal of Community Psychology, 42*, 495–508.

Walsh, R. M., & Bruce, S. E. (2011). The relationships between perceived levels of control, psychological distress, and legal system variables in a sample of sexual assault survivors. *Violence Against Women, 22*, 603–618. <http://dx.doi.org.ezproxy.jccmi.edu/10.1177/1077801211407427>.

R

Ineffective Relationship *Gail B. Ladwig, MSN, RN*

NANDA-I

Definition

A pattern of mutual partnership that is insufficient to provide for each other's needs

Defining Characteristics

Delay in meeting of developmental goals appropriate for family life-cycle stage; dissatisfaction with complementary relationship between partners; dissatisfaction with emotional need fulfillment between partners; dissatisfaction with idea sharing between partners; dissatisfaction with information sharing between partners; dissatisfaction with physical need fulfillment between partners; inadequate understanding of partner's compromised functioning (e.g., physical, psychological social); insufficient balance in autonomy between partners; insufficient balance in collaboration between partners; insufficient mutual respect between partners; insufficient mutual support in daily activities between partners; partner not identified as support person; unsatisfying communication with partner

Related Factors

Alteration in cognitive functioning in one partner; developmental crisis; history of domestic violence; incarceration of one partner; ineffective communication skills; stressors; substance abuse; unrealistic expectations

NOC, NIC, Client Outcomes, Nursing Interventions, Client/Family Teaching and Discharge Planning, *Rationales,* and References

Refer to care plan Readiness for enhanced **Relationship.**

Readiness for enhanced Relationship

Gail B. Ladwig, MSN, RN, and Marina Martinez-Kratz, MS, RN, CNE

NANDA-I

R

Definition

A pattern of mutual partnership to provide for each other's needs, which can be strengthened

Defining Characteristics

Expresses desire to enhance autonomy between partners; expresses desire to enhance collaboration between partners; expresses desire to enhance communication between partners; expresses desire to enhance emotional need fulfillment for each partner; expresses desire to enhance mutual respect between partners; expresses desire to enhance satisfaction with complementary relationship between partners; expresses desire to enhance satisfaction with emotional need fulfillment for each partner; expresses desire to enhance satisfaction with idea sharing between partners; expresses desire to enhance satisfaction with information sharing between partners; expresses desire to enhance satisfaction with physical need fulfillment for each partner; expresses desire to enhance understanding of partner's functional deficit (e.g., physical, psychological social)

NOC (Nursing Outcomes Classification)

Suggested NOC Outcomes

Coping; Family Functioning/Integrity; Role Performance; Social Support

Example NOC Outcome with Indicators

Family Integrity as evidenced by the following indicators: Members share thoughts, feelings, interests, concerns/Members communicate openly and honestly with one another/Members encourage individual autonomy and independence/Members assist one another in performing roles and daily tasks. (Rate the outcome and indicators of **Family Integrity:** 1 = never demonstrated, 2 = rarely demonstrated, 3 = sometimes demonstrated, 4 = often demonstrated, 5 = consistently demonstrated [see Section I].)

Client Outcomes

Family/Client Will (Specify Time Frame)

- Share thoughts and feelings with each other
- Communicate openly with each other
- Assist in performing family roles and tasks
- Provide support for each other
- Obtain appropriate assistance

NIC (Nursing Interventions Classification)

Suggested NIC Interventions

Coping Enhancement; Family Integrity Promotion; Role Enhancement

Example NIC Activities—Family Integrity Promotion

Facilitate a tone of togetherness within/among the family; Encourage family to maintain positive relationships; Facilitate open communication among family members

Nursing Interventions and *Rationales*

- ▲ Assess for signs of depression in the family when one partner is depressed, and make appropriate referrals. EB: *Depressive symptoms affect functioning of the whole family (Hinton et al, 2009).*
- ▲ Assist couples to identify sources of their own perceived *dyadic* empathy in the relationship. EB: *Higher perceived empathy toward the relationship partner is associated with relationship satisfaction (Kimmes et al, 2014).*
- Assist families to identify sources of gratitude in their lives. EB: *Research showed that gratitude fostered all facets of post-traumatic growth, such as relationships, personal strengths, and awareness of meaningful possibilities (Ruini & Vescovelli, 2013).*
- Assist clients to identify sources of gratitude in their lives using a future oriented focus. EB: *Research shows that clients with a regulatory focus of promotion were more likely to express gratitude, which inspired them to strengthen their relationships with helpful and responsive partners (Mathews & Shook, 2013).*
- Support "relationship talk" between couples (talking with a partner about the relationship, what one needs from one's partner, and/or the relationship implications of a shared stressor). Such discussions in couples with lung cancer have been shown to help partners better define their relationships and repair relationships that are functioning poorly (Badr et al, 2008). EB: *These discussions may help alleviate the negative impact that sexual problems have on prostate cancer clients' and their partners' marital adjustment (Badr & Taylor, 2009).*
- Encourage couples to participate and share in exciting and satisfying leisure activities and to share stories. EB: *This study demonstrated that couples feel connected with their partners and more satisfied with their relationships when they engage in these types of activities (Graham, 2008). When stories are used as a way to understand the lives of couples, they have the potential for enhancing individual and relational growth (Skerrett, 2010).*
- Assist couples in establishing boundaries between work and home. *This study demonstrates that for both men and women, job demands foster their own work-family conflict (WFC), which in turn contributes to their partner's home demands, family-work conflict (FWC), and exhaustion. In addition, social undermining mediates the relationship between an individual's WFC and his/her partner's home demands (Bakker et al, 2008).*
- Assist couples in regulating negative emotions. EB: *The results of this study of newlyweds support theories suggesting that the ability to regulate negative emotions may help intimates avoid perpetrating intimate partner violence (IPV), particularly when faced with a partner's IPV perpetration (McNulty & Hellmuth, 2008).*
- Assist couples in dealing with anger and communication when the diagnosis is cancer. EB: *The anger-expression styles of both clients and their partners seem to modify the family atmosphere, and together, they are important determinants of the long-term quality of life of the cancer clients. Interventions for couples facing cancer should include a focus on ways of dealing with anger and thereby support dyadic coping with*

cancer (Julkunen et al, 2009). Couples who are survivors of prostate cancer are faced with interruptions in their intimate relationships, communication, and overall quality of life. They need recommendations for appropriate resources (Galbraith et al, 2011).

- Refer to care plans Readiness for enhanced **Family** processes and Readiness for enhanced family **Coping.**

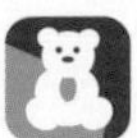

Pediatric

- Provide guidance and information on communication techniques for teenagers, especially those involved in intimate relationships. EBN: *The findings of this study suggest that many female adolescents desired the love of a male partner and were willing to concede to his request of practicing unprotected sex. Findings support the urgent need for interventions that will promote skill-building techniques to negotiate safer sex behaviors among youth who are most likely to be exposed to STIs through risky behaviors (Bralock & Koniak-Griffin, 2009).*
- Encourage supportive relationships among parents and teenagers. EB: *This study suggests that parenting may be associated with multiple benefits to teenagers' sexual relationships including delayed intercourse and greater condom use (Parkes et al, 2011).*

Geriatric

▲ Assess for spousal depression when one partner has cardiovascular disease, and make appropriate referrals. EB: *Exposure to spousal suffering is an independent and unique source of distress in married couples that contributes to psychiatric and physical morbidity (Schulz et al, 2009).*

▲ Assess for depression and anxiety, and make appropriate referrals for "prewidows" caring for spouses with chronic life-limiting conditions. EB: *In this study, health deficits associated with spousal bereavement may be evident earlier in the marital transition than previously thought, warranting attention to the health of older adults whose spouses have chronic/life-limiting conditions (Williams et al, 2008).*

- Support older couples' positive collaborative communication. EB: *In this study of older couples, the couples displayed a unique blend of warmth and control during collaborative communication, suggesting that a greater focus on emotional and social concerns during problem solving is important (Smith et al, 2009).*
- Encourage collaborative coping (i.e., spouses pooling resources and problem solving jointly) among older adults. EB: *This study of older adults whose husbands had prostate cancer suggested that collaborative coping may be associated with better daily mood and greater marital satisfaction because of heightened perceptions of efficacy in coping with stressful events and problems surrounding illness (Berg et al, 2008).*

R

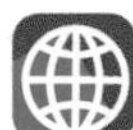

Multicultural

- Provide culturally tailored community-level interventions to raise awareness about HIV and bisexuality, and decrease HIV and sexual orientation stigma. EB: *Culturally tailored interventions may increase comfort of African American and Latino MSMWs (men who have sex with men and women) in communicating with their female partners about sexuality, HIV, and condoms (Mutchler et al, 2008). Sociocultural factors and HIV-related misinformation contribute to the increasing number of Chilean women living with HIV. Future HIV prevention should stress partner communication, empowerment, and improving the education of women vulnerable to HIV (Cianelli et al, 2008).*

Home Care

- Provide home-based psychoeducation to assist new parent couples with parenting and their couple relationship. EB: *The best outcomes for psychoeducational interventions for effective parenting of infants and sustaining a mutually satisfying couple relationship seem to be achieved when programs are accessible by couples at home, when skill training is provided, and possibly when programs target couples at high risk for maladjustment to parenthood (Petch & Halford, 2008).*

Client/Family Teaching and Discharge Planning

- Encourage clients and spouses to participate together in interventions to lower low-density lipoprotein cholesterol (LDL-C). Teach spouses how to provide emotional and instrumental support, allow clients to decide which component of the intervention they would like to receive, and have clients determine their own goals and action plans. Provide telephone calls to clients and spouses separately. During each client telephone call, client progress is reviewed, and clients create goals and action plans for the upcoming month. During spouse telephone calls, which occur within 1 week of client calls, spouses are informed of clients' goals and action plans and devise strategies to increase emotional and instrumental support.

EB: *The behaviors required to lower LDL-C levels may be difficult to adhere to if they are inconsistent with spouses' health practices, and, alternatively, may be enhanced by enlisting support from the spouse. Interventions that teach spouses to provide instrumental and emotional support may help clients initiate and adhere to behaviors that lower their LDL-C levels. Moreover, allowing clients to retain autonomy by deciding which behaviors they would like to change, and how, may improve adherence and clinical outcomes (Voils et al, 2009). Interventions to reduce cardiovascular risk factors should be addressed jointly to both members of a marital couple (Di Castelnuovo et al, 2009).*

REFERENCES

Badr, H., Acitelli, L. K., & Taylor, C. L. (2008). Does talking about their relationship affect couples' marital and psychological adjustment to lung cancer? *Journal of Cancer Survivorship*, *2*(1), 53–64.

Badr, H., & Taylor, C. L. (2009). Sexual dysfunction and spousal communication in couples coping with prostate cancer. *Psycho-Oncology*, *18*(7), 735–746.

Bakker, A. B., Demerouti, E., & Dollard, M. F. (2008). How job demands affect partners' experience of exhaustion: integrating work-family conflict and crossover theory. *The Journal of Applied Psychology*, *93*(4), 901–911.

Berg, C. A., et al. (2008). Collaborative coping and daily mood in couples dealing with prostate cancer. *Psychology and Aging*, *23*(3), 505–516.

Bralock, A., & Koniak-Griffin, D. (2009). What do sexually active adolescent females say about relationship issues? *Journal of Pediatric Nursing*, *24*(2), 131–140.

Cianelli, R., Ferrer, L., & McElmurry, B. J. (2008). HIV prevention and low-income Chilean women: machismo, marianismo and HIV misconceptions. *Culture, Health and Sexuality*, *10*(3), 297–306.

Di Castelnuovo, A., et al. (2009). Spousal concordance for major coronary risk factors: a systematic review and meta-analysis. *American Journal of Epidemiology*, *169*(1), 1–8.

Galbraith, M. E., Fink, R., & Wilkins, G. G. (2011). Couples surviving prostate cancer: challenges in their lives and relationships. *Seminars in Oncology Nursing*, *27*(4), 300–308.

Graham, J. M. (2008). Self-expansion and flow in couples' momentary experiences: an experience sampling study. *Journal of Personality and Social Psychology*, *95*(3), 679–694.

Hinton, L., et al. (2009). Longitudinal influences of partner depression on cognitive functioning in Latino spousal pairs. *Dementia and Geriatric Cognitive Disorders*, *27*(6), 491–500.

Julkunen, J., Gustavsson-Lilius, M., & Hietanen, P. (2009). Anger expression, partner support, and quality of life in cancer patients. *Journal of Psychosomatic Research*, *66*(3), 235–244.

Kimmes, J. G., Edwards, A. B., Wetchler, J. L., et al. (2014). Self and other ratings of dyadic empathy as predictors of relationship satisfaction. *American Journal of Family Therapy*, *42*(5), 426–437.

Mathews, M. A., & Shook, N. J. (2013). Promoting or preventing thanks: regulatory focus and its effect on gratitude and indebtedness. *Journal of Research in Personality*, *47*, 191–195.

McNulty, J. K., & Hellmuth, J. C. (2008). Emotion regulation and intimate partner violence in newlyweds. *Journal of Family Psychology*, *22*(5), 794–797.

Mutchler, M. G., et al. (2008). Psychosocial correlates of unprotected sex without disclosure of HIV-positivity among African-American, Latino, and white men who have sex with men and women. *Archives of Sexual Behavior*, *37*(5), 736–747.

Parkes, A., et al. (2011). Is parenting associated with teenagers' early sexual risk-taking, autonomy and relationship with sexual partners? *Perspect Sexual Reproduct Health*, *43*(1), 30–40.

Petch, J., & Halford, W. K. (2008). Psycho-education to enhance couples' transition to parenthood. *Clinical Psychology Review*, *28*(7), 1125–1137.

Ruini, C., & Vescovelli, F. (2013). The role of gratitude in breast cancer: its relationships with post-traumatic growth, psychological well-being and distress. *Journal of Happiness Studies*, *14*, 263–274.

Schulz, R., et al. (2009). Spousal suffering and partner's depression and cardiovascular disease: the cardiovascular health study. *The American Journal of Geriatric Psychiatry*, *17*(3), 246–254.

Skerrett, K. (2010). "Good Enough Stories": Helping couples invest in one another's growth. *Family Process*, *49*(4), 503–516.

Smith, T. W., et al. (2009). Conflict and collaboration in middle-aged and older couples: I. Age differences in agency and communion during marital interaction. *Psychology and Aging*, *24*(2), 259–273.

Voils, C. I., et al. (2009). Study protocol: couples partnering for lipid enhancing strategies (CouPLES)—a randomized, controlled trial. *Trials*, *6*(10), 10.

Williams, B. R., et al. (2008). Marital status and health: exploring pre-widowhood. *Journal of Palliative Medicine*, *11*(6), 848–856.

R

Risk for ineffective Relationship *Gail B. Ladwig, MSN, RN*

NANDA-I

Definition

Vulnerable to developing a pattern that is insufficient for providing a mutual partnership to provide for each other's needs

Risk Factors

Alteration in cognitive functioning in one partner; developmental crisis; history of domestic violence; incarceration of one partner ineffective communication skills; stressors; substance abuse; unrealistic expectations

NOC, NIC, Client Outcomes, Nursing Interventions, *Rationales*, and References

Refer to care plan for Ineffective **Relationship.**

Impaired Religiosity

Lisa Burkhart, PhD, RN, ANEF, and Barbara Baele Vincensi, PhD, RN, FNP

NANDA-I

Definition

Impaired ability to exercise reliance on beliefs and/or participate in rituals of a particular faith tradition

Defining Characteristics

Desire to reconnect with previous belief pattern; desire to reconnect with previous customs; difficulty adhering to prescribed religious beliefs; difficulty adhering to prescribed religious beliefs; difficulty adhering to prescribed religious rituals (e.g., ceremonies, regulations, clothing, prayer, services, holiday observances); distress about separation from faith community; questioning of religious belief patterns; questioning of religious customs

Related Factors (r/t)

Developmental and Situational

Aging; end-stage life crises; life transitions

Physical

Illness; pain

Psychological

Anxiety; fear of death; history of religious manipulation; ineffective coping strategies; insufficient social support; personal crisis

Sociocultural

Cultural barriers to practicing religion; environmental barriers to practicing religion; insufficient social integration; insufficient sociocultural interaction

Spiritual

Spiritual crises; suffering

NOC (Nursing Outcomes Classification)

Suggested NOC Outcomes

Client Satisfaction: Cultural Needs Fulfillment

Example NOC Outcome with Indicators

Client Satisfaction: Cultural Needs Fulfillment as evidenced by the following indicators: Respect for religious beliefs/Respect for cultural health behaviors/Incorporation of cultural beliefs in health teaching/Respect for personal values. (Rate each indicator of **Client Satisfaction: Cultural Needs Fulfillment:** 1 = not at all satisfied, 2 = somewhat satisfied, 3 = moderately satisfied, 4 = very satisfied, 5 = completely satisfied [see Section I].)

Client Outcomes

Client Will (Specify Time Frame)

- Express satisfaction with the ability to express religious practices
- Express satisfaction with access to religious materials and rituals
- Demonstrate balance between religious practices and healthy lifestyles
- Avoid high-risk, controlling religious relationships that inflict physical, sexual, or emotional harm and/or exploitation

R

NIC (Nursing Interventions Classification)

Suggested NIC Interventions

Religious Ritual Enhancement; Culture Brokerage; Religious Addiction Prevention

Example NIC Activities—Religious Ritual Enhancement

Encourage the use of and participation in usual religious rituals that are not detrimental to health

Nursing Interventions and *Rationales*

- Recognize when clients integrate religious practices in their life. EBN: *Eighty percent of clients with emphysema who participated in the randomized 2-year longitudinal study of the National Emphysema Treatment Trial increased their use of religiosity and spirituality as coping strategies to improve their quality of life (Green et al, 2011).* EB: *In clients with traumatic brain injury, religious well-being (personal connection to a higher power) predicted life satisfaction, whereas public religious practice did not (Waldron-Perrine et al, 2011).*
- Encourage and/or coordinate the use of and participation in usual religious rituals or practices that support coping. EB: *In a cross-sectional correlational descriptive study of 292 people living with HIV/AIDS, a relationship was found between decreased use of religious coping strategies and higher rates of depressive symptoms, which affected HIV medication adherence, immune function, and health-related quality of life (HRQOL) (Dalmida et al, 2013).*
- Encourage the use of prayer or meditation as appropriate. CEB: *A controlled study of 84 college students revealed that those who participated in a religious spiritual meditation exercise experienced significantly ess anxiety and more positive mood, spiritual health, and spiritual experiences and higher pain tolerance (Wachholtz & Pargament, 2005).*
- Promote family coping using religious practices to help cope with loss, as appropriate. EB: *A descriptive correlational study found one's religious beliefs and values moderated perinatal grief and despair in women who had experienced traumatic late pregnancy loss due to fetal death or serious fetal anomalies (Cowchock et al, 2011).*
- ▲ Refer to religious leader, professional counseling, or support group as needed. EBN: *In a grounded theory study, it was found that chaplains promoted spirituality, which was validated in a psychometric study (Burkhart et al, 2011).*

Geriatric

- Promote established religious practices in older adults. EBN: *Increasing physical limitations and worsening chronic disease (emphysema) promoted a higher level of use of religious coping practices in older adults in a randomized longitudinal study (Green et al, 2011).*

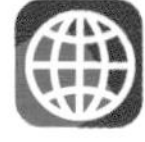

Multicultural

- Promote religious practices that are culturally appropriate:
  - **African American.** EBN/EB: *Higher levels of praying for one's health and use of spiritual and religious practices were found among African Americans in a cross-sectional study of 9105 cancer survivors by Canada et al (2013).* EBN: *In a descriptive-correlational study, 17 African American women with breast cancer were found to use more positive religious coping to decrease distress and improve spiritual well-being (Gaston-Johansson et al, 2013).*
  - **Korean.** EB: *In a cross-sectional study by Lee and Woo (2013), 147 Korean-born immigrants identified religious and cultural practices as increasing general well-being and coping with health concerns.*
  - **African.** EBN: *In a qualitative study on help-seeking behaviors in childbearing women in Ghana, the majority used their religious or spiritual healers or leaders for spiritual protection during pregnancy, a time considered a vulnerable period in a woman's life (Farnes et al, 2011).*
  - **Jordanian.** EBN: *In a qualitative study by Nabolsi and Carson (2011), 19 Jordanian Muslim men with coronary artery disease found direction from their religious beliefs and values to pursue health seeking behaviors.*

R

REFERENCES

Burkhart, L., Schmidt, L., & Hogan, N. (2011). Development and psychometric testing of the spiritual care inventory instrument. *Journal of Advanced Nursing*, *67*(11), 2463–2472.

Canada, A., Fitchett, G., Murphy, P., et al. (2013). Racial/ethnic differences in spiritual well-being among cancer survivors. *Journal of Behavioral Medicine*, *36*, 441–453.

Cowchock, F., Ellestad, S., Meador, K., et al. (2011). Religiosity is an important part of coping with grief in pregnancy after traumatic second trimester loss. *Journal of Religion and Health*, *50*, 901–910.

Dalmida, S., Koenig, H., Holstad, M., et al. (2013). The psychological well-being of people living with HIV/AIDS and the role of religious coping and social support. *International Journal of Psychiatry in Medicine*, *46*(1), 57–83.

Farnes, C., Beckstrand, R., & Callister, L. (2011). Help-seeking behaviors in childbearing women in Ghana, West Africa. *International Nursing Review*, *58*, 491–497.

Gaston-Johansson, F., Haisfield-Wolfe, M., Reddick, B., et al. (2013). The relationship among coping strategies, religious coping, and spirituality in African American women with breast cancer receiving chemotherapy. *Oncology Nursing Forum*, *40*(2), 120–131.

Green, M., Emery, C., Kozora, E., et al. (2011). Religious and spiritual coping and quality of life among patients with emphysema in the national emphysema treatment trial. *Respiratory Care*, *56*(10), 1514–1521.

Lee, K., & Woo, H. (2013). Stressors, social support, religious practice and general well-being among Korean adult immigrants. *Journal of Evidenced Based Social Work*, *10*(5), 421–434.

Nabolsi, M., & Carson, A. (2011). Spirituality, illness and personal responsibility: the experience of Jordanian Muslim men with coronary artery disease. *Scandinavian Journal of Caring Sciences*, *25*, 716–724.

Wachholtz, A., & Pargament, K. (2005). Is spirituality a critical ingredient of meditation? Comparing the effects of spiritual meditation, secular meditation, and relaxation on spiritual, psychological, cardiac, and pain outcomes. *Journal of Behavioral Medicine*, *28*(4), 367–384.

Waldron-Perrine, B., Rapport, L., Hanks, R., et al. (2011). Religion and spirituality in rehabilitation outcomes among individuals with traumatic brain injury. *Rehabilitation Psychology*, *56*(2), 107–116.

Readiness for enhanced Religiosity

Lisa Burkhart, PhD, RN, ANEF, and Barbara Baele Vincensi, PhD, RN, FNP

NANDA-I

Definition

A pattern of reliance on religious beliefs and/or participation in rituals of a particular faith tradition, which can be strengthened

Defining Characteristics

R

Expresses desire to enhance belief patterns used in past; expresses desire to enhance connection with a religious leader; expresses desire to enhance forgiveness; expresses desire to enhance participation in religious experiences; expresses desire to enhance participation in religious practices (e.g., ceremonies, regulations, clothing, prayer, services, holiday observances); expresses desire to enhance religious customs used in the past; expresses desire to enhance religious options; expresses desire to enhance use of religious material

NIC, NOC, Client Outcomes, Nursing Interventions, Client/Family and Discharge Planning, *Rationales*, and References

See care plan for Impaired **Religiosity.**

Pediatric

- Provide spiritual care for children based on developmental level. CEB: *When nurses are comfortable providing spiritual care, they can implement numerous spiritual care activities and interventions to meet the spiritual needs of the child and family. After determining the child's spiritual beliefs and spiritual needs, a plan of care is developed based on the child's developmental age (Burkhart, 2011; Elkins & Cavendish, 2004; Fowler, 1981, 1987).*
    - **Infants:** Have the same nurse care for the child on a daily basis. Encourage holding, cuddling, rocking, playing with, and singing to the infant. CEB: *Continuity of care will promote the establishment of trust because nurses provide much of the needed ongoing support. The infant who is ill or dying still needs to be sung to, talked to, played with, held, cuddled, and rocked (Elkins & Cavendish, 2004).*
    - **Toddlers:** Provide consistency in care and familiar toys, music, stories, clothing blankets, pillows, and any other individual object of contentment. Schedule home religious routines into the plan of care, and support home routines regarding good and bad behavior. CEB: *The importance of consistency in care and routine with this age group cannot be overemphasized. The nurse should support parents' home routines during hospitalization as much as possible and encourage them to continue to have the same*

expectations regarding good and bad behavior. If particular religious routines are carried out at certain times of the day, the nurse should schedule them in the care plan (Elkins & Cavendish, 2004). EB: *In a qualitative exploratory study, McCarthy (2013) explored interrelated themes regarding age and culturally appropriate nonverbal, visuals, sound, touch, and storytelling as different ways the arts can be used to help toddlers cope with illness and the world around them within a spiritual caregiving framework.*

- ❍ **School-age children and adolescents:** Encourage both groups to express their feelings regarding spirituality. Ask them, "Do you wish to pray, and what do you want to pray about?" Offer age-appropriate complementary therapies such as music, art, videos, and connectedness with peers through cards, letters, and visits. EBN: *Three hundred and ten African American (AA) female teens who frequently participated in spiritual health activities, such as attending church services and praying, had significantly higher self-rated health scores and were more likely to participate in healthy lifestyle choices (Powell-Young, 2012).* EB: *In a systematic literature review, religiosity and spirituality were identified as protective factors, providing children and adolescents with a sense of meaning, self-esteem, coherence, and purpose in life, while promoting positive coping strategies and reducing stress (Bryant-Davis et al, 2012).*

REFERENCES

Burkhart, L. (2011). Religious/spiritual influences on health in the family. In M. Craft-Rosenberg & S. Pehler (Eds.), *Encyclopedia of family health*. Washington, DC: Sage.

Bryant-Davis, T., Ellis, M., Burke-Maynard, E., et al. (2012). Religiosity, spirituality and trauma recovery in the lives of children and adolescents. *Professional Psychology, Research and Practice*, *43*(4), 306–314.

Elkins, M., & Cavendish, R. (2004). Developing a plan for pediatric spiritual care. *Holistic Nursing Practice*, *18*(4), 179–184.

Fowler, J. (1981). *Stages of faith: the psychology of human development and quest for meaning*. San Francisco: Harper & Row.

Fowler, J. (1987). *Faith development and pastoral care*. Philadelphia: Fortress Press.

McCarthy, M. (2013). Children's spirituality and music learning: Exploring deeper resonances with arts based research. *International Journal of Education and the Arts*, *14*(4), 1–14.

Powell-Young, Y. (2012). Household income and spiritual well-being but not body mass index as determinants of poor self-rated health among African American adolescents. *Research in Nursing & Health*, *35*, 219–230.

Risk for impaired Religiosity

Gail B. Ladwig, MSN, RN

NANDA-I

Definition

Vulnerable to an impaired ability to exercise reliance on religious beliefs and/or participate in rituals of a particular faith tradition, which may compromise health

R

Risk Factors

Developmental

Life transitions

Environmental

Barriers to practicing religion; lack of transportation

Physical

Hospitalization; illness; pain

Psychological

Depression; ineffective caregiving; ineffective coping strategies; insecurity; insufficient social support

Sociocultural

Cultural barrier to practicing religion; insufficient social interaction

Spiritual

Suffering

NOC, NIC, Client Outcomes, Nursing Interventions, *Rationales*, and References

Refer to care plan for Impaired **Religiosity.**

Relocation stress syndrome

Rebecca Johnson, PhD, RN, FAAN, FNAP, and Jessica Bibbo, MA

NANDA-I

Definition

Physiological and/or psychosocial disturbance following transfer from one environment to another

Defining Characteristics

Alienation; aloneness; alteration in sleep pattern; anger; anxiety; concern about relocation; dependency; depression; fear; frustration; increase in illness; increase in physical symptoms; increase in verbalization of needs; insecurity; loneliness; loss of identity; loss of self-worth; low self-esteem; pessimism; unwillingness to move; withdrawal; worried

Related Factors (r/t)

Compromised health status; history of loss; impaired psychosocial functioning; ineffective coping strategies; insufficient predeparture counseling; insufficient support system; language barrier; move from one environment to another; powerlessness; social isolation; unpredictability of experience

NOC (Nursing Outcomes Classification)

Suggested NOC Outcomes

Relocation Adaptation; Anxiety Self-Control; Child Adaptation to Hospitalization; Coping; Depression Level; Depression Self-Control; Loneliness Severity; Psychosocial Adjustment: Life Change, Quality of Life; Stress Level

Example NOC Outcome with Indicators

Relocation Adaptation as evidenced by the following indicators: Recognizes reason for change in living environment/ Participates in decision-making in new environment/Expresses satisfaction with daily routine/Expresses satisfaction with level of independence/Compares care needs with available resources/Expresses satisfaction with social relationships/Expresses satisfaction with variety of food/Expresses satisfaction with food preparation/Expresses satisfaction with retained personal belongings/Expresses satisfaction with living arrangements/Exhibits positive mood/Appears content/Respects others' rights/Maintains positive relationships with family/Maintains positive relationships with friends/Maintains positive relationships with others in new environment/ Participates in social activities/Seeks information to reduce anxiety/Plans coping strategies for stressful situations/Uses effective coping strategies/Uses relaxation techniques to reduce anxiety/Maintains social relationships/Maintains adequate sleep/Controls anxiety response. (Rate the outcome and indicators of **Relocation Adaptation:** 1 = never demonstrated, 2 = rarely demonstrated, 3 = sometimes demonstrated, 4 = often demonstrated, 5 = consistently demonstrated [see Section I].)

Client Outcomes

Client Will (Specify Time Frame)

- Recognize and know the name of at least one staff member or new neighbor within 1 week of relocating
- Express concern about move when encouraged to do so during individual contacts within 24 hours of awareness of impending relocation
- Carry out activities of daily living (ADLs) in usual manner
- Maintain previous mental and physical health status (e.g., nutrition, elimination, sleep, social interaction, physical activity) within 2 months of relocating

NIC (Nursing Interventions Classification)

Suggested NIC Interventions

Anxiety Reduction; Coping Enhancement; Discharge Planning; Hope Instillation; Self-Responsibility Facilitation; Animal-Assisted Therapy; Art Therapy; Music Therapy; Massage; Mood Management; Active Listening

Example NIC Activities—Anxiety Reduction

Stay with client to promote safety and reduce fear; Provide objects that symbolize safeness to the client

Nursing Interventions and *Rationales*

- Be aware that relocation to supportive housing may be a positive change. CEB: *Relocation stress syndrome is not a universally occurring phenomenon. Relocation was found to be no more stressful than other life changes (Walker et al, 2007).*
- Begin relocation planning as early in the decision process as possible. CEB/EBN: *Having a well-organized plan for the move with support and advocacy through the process may reduce anxiety (Davis, 2005; Johnson, 2008; Kao et al, 2004; Sörensen et al, 2011).*
- Obtain a history, including the reason for the move, the client's usual coping mechanisms, history of losses, and family support for the client. EBN: *A history helps the nurse determine the amount of support needed and appropriate interventions to decrease relocation stress (Brownie et al, 2014).*
- Identify to what extent the client can participate in the relocation decisions and advocate for this participation. EBN: *Engaging older adults in the decision making process is likely to increase the level of adjustment following the relocation (Bekhet & Zauszniewski, 2013) and promote psychological well-being (Ewen & Chahal, 2013; Street & Burge, 2012).* CEB: *Older adults with poor mental functioning may be less able to be involved in the decisions and more vulnerable to disempowerment by others (Johnson et al, 2010).*
- Assess client's readiness to relocate and relocation self-efficacy. CEB: *A validated relocation readiness instrument was used successfully with older adults (Rossen, 2007; Rossen & Gruber, 2007).*
- Consult an evidence-based practice guide for relocation. EBN: *Researchers compiled latest findings to develop a protocol to assist in relocating older adults (Hertz et al, 2007).*
- Assess family members' perceptions of client's ability to participate in relocation decisions. Particularly in cases of dementia, be alert to care workers' involvement in making the decision to relocate. They may need support and encouragement through the process. EB: *Care workers were found to be highly stressed during the relocation decision-making process and "walking a tightrope" between the older adult's needs and those of the person's family members (Hortana et al, 2010).*
- Consider the client's and family's cultural and ethnic values as much as possible when choosing roommates, foods, and other aspects of care. CEB/EBN: *Nurses need to be aware of the differences in values and practices of different cultures and ensure that they give culturally appropriate care that is respectful of older adults and family caregivers' beliefs about elder care (Caron & Bowers, 2003; Johnson, 2008; Johnson & Tripp-Reimer, 2001a, 2001b; Bekhet & Zauszniewski, 2013).*
- Promote clear communication between all participants in the relocation process. CEB: *Case studies revealed the importance of using an integrated approach to planning with clear communication among practitioners (LeClerc & Wells, 2001).*
- Observe the following procedures if the client is being transferred to an extended care facility or assisted living facility:
    - Facilitate the client's participation in decisions and choice of placement, and arrange a preadmission visit if possible. CEB/EBN: *Clients who are more involved in the decision-making process appear to have fewer problems adjusting to the new environment (Newson, 2008b). Research has shown a link between the loss of independence with transfer to a nursing home and depression (Johnson, 2008; Loeher et al, 2004). Decreased relocation control was significantly related to poorer adjustment (Bekhet et al, 2008).*
    - If the client cannot visit the new facility, arrange for a visit or telephone call by a member of the staff to welcome the client and show a videotape or at least provide pictures of the new care facility.
    - Have a familiar person accompany the client to the new facility. *This lessens client and family anxiety, confusion, and dissatisfaction.*
    - Recommend that the caregiver write a journal of thoughts and feelings regarding the relocation of his/her loved one. CEB: *Writing has been found to improve physical and emotional health among caregivers of older adults (Dellasega & Haagen, 2004).*
    - Continue to assess caregiver psychological distress during a 6-month period following relocation. *Caregivers experience distress because of the responsibility of moving their loved one.* EB: *Caregivers may begin to resolve conflicted feelings during this time and need support (Smit et al, 2011).*
- Identify previous routines for ADLs. Try to maintain as much continuity with the previous schedule as possible. CEB: *Continuity of routines has been shown to be a crucial factor in positively influencing adjustment to a new environment (Kao et al, 2004).*
- Bring in familiar items from home (e.g., pictures, clocks, afghans). Familiarity eases transition and symbolizes safeness.

R

- Establish the way the client would like to be addressed (Mr., Mrs., Miss, first name, nickname). *Calling clients by their desired name shows respect.*
- Thoroughly orient the client and the family to the new environment and routines; repeat directions as needed. CEB: *The stress of the move may interfere with the client's ability to remember directions. A progressive introduction and orientation for both the client and the family should be done (Kao et al, 2004).*
- Spend one-to-one time with the client. Allow the client to express feelings and convey acceptance of them; emphasize that the client's feelings are real and individual and that it is acceptable to be sad or angry about moving. CEB: *Expressing feelings can help the client deal with the change and facilitate grief work that accompanies loss of independence (Tracy & DeYoung, 2004).*
- Allocate a caring staff member to help the client adjust to the move. Assign the same staff members to the client for care if compatible with client; maintain consistency in the personnel with whom the client interacts. CEB/EB: *Consistency hastens adjustment and increases quality of care (Iwasiw et al, 2003). A caring practitioner can support the client through the journey of adapting to a new environment (Newson, 2008b).*
- Ask the client to state one positive aspect of the new living situation each day. Helping the client focus on the positive aspects of the move can help change attitude and reframe the situation in a positive fashion. EBN: *Learned resourcefulness through positive thinking significantly affected relocation adjustment (Bekhet et al, 2008).*
- Ask the client to state one positive aspect of the new living situation each day. *Helping the client focus on the positive aspects of the move can help change attitude and reframe the situation in a positive fashion.* CEB: *Learned resourcefulness through positive thinking significantly affected relocation adjustment (Bekhet et al, 2008).*
- Monitor the client's health status and provide appropriate interventions for problems with social interaction, nutrition, sleep, new onset of infection, or elimination problems. CEB/EBN: *Health problems may appear first as declines in ADLs (e.g., bathing, eating, and dressing) (Chen & Wilmoth, 2004). Older adults who moved in the previous year reported increased comorbidity, disability, functional limitation, and worse self-rated health (Hong & Chen, 2009).*
- If the client is being transferred within a facility, have staff members from the new unit visit the client before transfer.
- Work with the caregivers and family members helping them deal with stages of "making the best of it," "making the move," and "making it better." EBN: *A study demonstrated that relatives of clients entering a nursing home can work in partnership with health care staff to ease the transition for their loved one more effectively (Newson, 2008b).*
- If a client is being transferred from the intensive care unit (ICU), have previous staff make occasional visits until the client is comfortable in the new surroundings. Ensure that the family is told relevant information. CEB: *Leaving the ICU staff may be the most negative component of transfer (McKinney & Deeny, 2002). A review of the literature in this area demonstrated that information needs were most important to families of clients transferred out of ICU (Mitchell et al, 2003).*
- Watch for coping problems (e.g., withdrawal, regression, angry behavior, impaired sleeping, refusal to eat, flat affect, anxiety) and intervene immediately. EB: *Research has shown a link between the loss of independence with transfer to a nursing home and depression (Johnson, 2008).*
- Encourage the client to express grief for the loss of the old situation; explain that it is normal to feel sadness over change and loss. CEB/EB: *Older adults in long-term care grieve loss of home, possessions, and independence (Newson, 2008a; Pilkington, 2005).*
- Pay special attention to assessing and giving psychosocial care. EB: *Although physical care may predicate the relocation, meeting psychosocial care needs must be individualized via careful assessment (Salarvand et al, 2008).*
- Encourage the client to participate in care as much as possible and make own decisions when possible (e.g., placement of the bed, choice of roommate, bathing routines). *Having choices helps prevent feelings of powerlessness that may lead to depression.* CEB: *Research showed that residents who viewed the nursing home move negatively after 3 months felt powerless, vulnerable, and isolated (Iwasiw et al, 2003).*

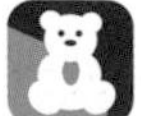

Pediatric

- Assess family history and contact information from children relocated to rescue shelters. EB: *No unified system exists in the United States to reunite children with their families after natural disaster or terrorist attack, so nursing has a major role to play in locating children's families and facilitating reunification (Chung & Shannon, 2007).*

- Be aware that community relocation may be beneficial for children, and assess community resources of new location. EB: *African American children who relocated from an inner city to a suburb benefitted especially from available institutional resources (Keels, 2008).*
- Provide support for a child and family who must relocate to be near a transplant center. CEB: *Recognizing the unique needs of parents who must relocate for a child's transplantation procedure supports the delivery of individualized nursing care and the effective allocation of program resources (Stubblefield & Murray, 2002).*
- In divorce situations, recommend alternative dispute resolution versus traditional litigated settlement. EBN: *This nonadversarial approach may mitigate some of the trauma of divorce experienced by children (Stein & Oler, 2010).*
- Encourage child to verbalize concerns in divorce situations when they and/or a parent relocate. CEB: *Relocation of a parent in divorce has been linked with children's financial concerns, hostility toward parents, views of parents as not socially supportive, and poorer self-perceived health (Braver et al, 2003).*
- Assess presence of allergies before and after relocation. EB: *Six-year-old children who relocated were found to have significant allergy sensitization over those who did not relocate (Herberth et al, 2007).*
- If the client is an adolescent, try to avoid a move in the middle of the school year, find a newcomers' club for the adolescent to join, and refer for counseling if needed. CEB/EB: *Most adolescents who relocate suffer a brief period of loss of companionship and intimacy with close friends (Vernberg et al, 2006; McBride, 2015).*
- Assess adolescents' perceptions of their acceptance by peers. CEB: *Poor perceptions of peer acceptance have been related to less initiation of social interactions in new settings (Aikins et al, 2005; McBride 2015).*
- Help parents recognize that relocation stress syndrome may persist for prolonged periods (e.g., 2 years) in adolescents. EB: *Adolescents were found to commonly express their ideology of the relocation (Nuttman-Shwartz et al, 2010).*
- Be aware that young people may cope with the transition by exerting control in particular domains. EBN: *Adolescents may be at risk of developing eating disorders following a major transition (Berge et al, 2012).*
- The effects of frequent relocation may not manifest immediately and may have long-term impacts on physical and mental health. EBN: *Longitudinal analysis found that frequent relocation in adolescence were associate with higher rates of stress and physical exhaustion in adulthood (Lin et al, 2012).*

Geriatric

- Monitor the need for transfer and transfer only when necessary. CEB: *Older adults often experience loss of function after relocation (Chen & Wilmoth, 2004).* EBN: *Relocation has been associated with death (Laughlin et al, 2007).*
- Implement discharge planning early so that it is not rushed. CEB: *Early discharge planning enhanced information levels for older adults and decreased their concerns (Kleinpell, 2004).*
- Protect the client from injuries such as falls. CEB: *Older adults who fell were more likely to be admitted to a nursing home (Seematter-Bagnoud et al, 2006). Having one fall increases the likelihood of additional falls (Quadri et al, 2005).*
- Utilize technologies such as sensing devices to measure average in-home gait speed (AIGS) as a predictor of fall risk. EBN: *AIGS was found to be a more reliable and valid predictor of fall risk than traditional physical performance assessments (Stone et al, 2015).*
- Implement a registered nurse (RN) care coordination model to restore older adults' health, maintain their independence, and reduce care costs. EBN: *RN care coordination was found to significantly and positively impact older adult outcome variables and to result in lesser costs of care (Rantz et al, 2014).*
- After the transfer, determine the client's mental status. *Document and observe for any new onset of confusion. Confusion can follow relocation because of the overwhelming stress and sensory overload.*
- Facilitate visits from companion animals. CEB: *A randomized trial of 6 weeks of animal-assisted therapy (dog visits) decreased loneliness among nursing home residents (Banks & Banks, 2002).*
- Encourage reminiscence of happy times. EB: *Nine weeks of group reminiscence therapy enhanced self-esteem among 24 nursing home residents in a two-group, nonrandomized study (Chao et al, 2006).*

Client/Family Teaching and Discharge Planning

- Teach family members and remind direct care staff about relocation stress syndrome. Encourage them to monitor for signs of the syndrome. CEB: *Relocation stress syndrome begins to ease at approximately 4 weeks after the move (Hodgson et al, 2004).*
- Help significant others learn how to support the client in the move by setting up a schedule of visits, arranging for holidays, bringing familiar items from home, and establishing a system for contact when

R

the client needs support. **EBN:** *Social support of family and friends was significantly related to relocation adjustment (Bekhet et al, 2008).*

- Assist family members and the relocating older adult to use webcam technology for interaction to supplement in-person visits. **EB:** *When older adults in a care facility have less than one visitor per week, interaction can be supplemented with technological "visits" (Meyer et al, 2011).*

REFERENCES

Aikins, J. W., Bierman, K. L., & Parker, J. G. (2005). Navigating the transition to junior high school: the influence of pre-transition friendship and self-system characteristics. *Social Development (Oxford, England)*, *14*, 42–60.

Banks, M., & Banks, W. (2002). The effects of animal-assisted therapy on loneliness in an elderly population in long-term care facilities. *The Journals of Gerontology. Series A, Biological Sciences and Medical Sciences*, *57A*(7), M428–M432.

Bekhet, A. K., Zauszniewski, J. A., & Wykle, M. L. (2008). Milieu change and relocation adjustment in elders. *Western Journal of Nursing Research*, *30*, 113–129.

Bekhet, A. K., & Zauszniewski, J. A. (2013). Resourcefulness, positive cognitions, relocation controllability and relocation adjustment among older people: a cross-sectional study of cultural differences. *International Journal of Older People Nursing*, *8*(3), 244–252.

Berge, J. M., Loth, K., Hanson, C., et al. (2012). Family life cycle transitions and the onset of eating disorders: a retrospective grounded theory approach. *Journal of Clinical Nursing*, *21*, 1355–1363.

Braver, S. L., Ellman, I. M., & Fabricius, W. V. (2003). Relocation of children after divorce and children's best interests: new evidence and legal considerations. *Journal of Family Psychology*, *17*(2), 206–219.

Bronskill, S. E., et al. (2004). Neuroleptic drug therapy in older adults newly admitted to nursing homes: incidence, dose, and specialist contact. *Journal of the American Geriatrics Society*, *52*(5), 749–755.

Brownie, S., Horstmanshof, L., & Garbutt, R. (2014). Factors that impact residents' transition and psychological adjustment to long-term aged care: a systematic literature review. *International Journal of Nursing Studies.*

Caron, C. D., & Bowers, B. J. (2003). Deciding whether to continue, share, or relinquish caregiving: caregiver views. *Qualitative Health Research*, *13*(9), 1252–1271.

Chao, S., et al. (2006). Effects of group reminiscence therapy on depression, self-esteem and life satisfaction of elderly nursing home residents. *The Journal of Nursing Research*, *14*(1), 36–45.

Chen, P. C., & Wilmoth, J. (2004). The effects of residential mobility on ADL and IADL limitations among the very old living in the community. *J Gerontol B Soc Sci*, *59B*(3), S164–S172.

Chung, S., & Shannon, M. (2007). Reuniting children with their families during disasters: a proposed plan for greater success. *American Journal of Disaster Medicine*, *2*(3), 113–117.

Davis, S. (2005). Meleis' theory of nursing transitions and relatives' experiences of nursing home entry. *Journal of Advanced Nursing*, *52*, 658–671.

Dellasega, C., & Haagen, B. (2004). A different kind of caregiving support group. *Journal of Psychosocial Nursing and Mental Health Services*, *42*(8), 46–55.

Ewen, H. H., & Chahal, J. (2013). Influence of late life stressors on the decisions of older women to relocate into congregate senior housing. *Journal of Housing for the Elderly*, *27*(4), 392–408.

Herberth, G., et al. (2007). The stress of relocation and neuropeptides: an epidemiological study in children. *Journal of Psychosomatic Research*, *63*, 451–452.

Hertz, J. E., et al. (2007). Management of relocation in cognitively intact older adults. *Journal of Gerontological Nursing*, *33*(11), 12–18.

Hodgson, N., et al. (2004). Biobehavioral correlates of relocation in the frail elderly: salivary cortisol, affect, and cognitive function. *Journal of the American Geriatrics Society*, *52*(11), 1856–1862.

Hong, S. I., & Chen, L. M. (2009). Contribution of residential relocation and lifestyle to the structure of health trajectories. *Journal of Aging and Health*, *21*, 244–265.

Hortana, B., Fahlstrom, G., & Ahlstrom, G. (2010). Experiences of relocation in dementia care workers. *International Journal of Older People Nursing*, *6*(2), 93–101.

Iwasiw, C., et al. (2003). Resident and family perspectives: the first year in a long-term care facility. *Journal of Gerontological Nursing*, *29*(1), 45.

Johnson, R. A. (2008). Relocation stress syndrome guideline. In B. Ackley, et al. (Eds.), *Evidence-based nursing care guidelines: medical-surgical interventions*. Philadelphia: Mosby.

Johnson, R. A., Radina, M., & Popejoy, L. (2010). Older adults' participation in nursing home placement decisions. *Clinical Nursing Research*, *19*(4), 358–375.

Johnson, R. A., & Tripp-Reimer, T. (2001a). Aging, ethnicity and social support: a review-part 1. *Journal of Gerontological Nursing*, *27*(6), 15–21.

Johnson, R. A., & Tripp-Reimer, T. (2001b). Relocation among ethnic elders: a review-part 2. *Journal of Gerontological Nursing*, *27*(6), 22–27.

Kao, H. F., Travis, S. S., & Acton, G. J. (2004). Relocation to a long-term care facility: working with patients and families before, during, and after. *Journal of Psychosocial Nursing Mental Health Services*, *42*(3), 10.

Keels, M. (2008). Neighborhood effects examined through the lens of residential mobility programs. *American Journal of Community Psychology*, *42*(3–4), 235–250.

Kleinpell, R. (2004). Randomized trial of an intensive care-based early discharge planning intervention for critically ill elderly patients. *American Journal of Critical Care*, *13*, 335–345.

Kydd, P. (2001). Using music therapy to help a client with Alzheimer's disease adapt to long-term care. *American Journal of Alzheimer's Disease and Other Dementias*, *16*(2), 103.

Laughlin, A., et al. (2007). Predictors of mortality following involuntary interinstitutional relocation. *Journal of Gerontological Nursing*, *33*(9), 20–26.

LeClerc, M., & Wells, D. L. (2001). Process evaluation of an integrated model of discharge planning. *Canadian Journal of Nursing Leadership*, *14*(2), 19–26.

Lin, K. C., Twisk, J. W. R., & Huang, H. C. (2012). Longitudinal impact of frequent geographic relocation from adolescence to adulthood on psychological stress and vital exhaustion at ages 32 and 42 years: the Amsterdam growth and health longitudinal study. *Journal of Epidemiology*, *22*(5), 469–476.

Loeher, K. E., et al. (2004). Nursing home transition and depressive symptoms in older medical rehabilitation patients. *Clinical Gerontologist*, *27*(1–2), 59–70.

McBride, M. E. (2015). Beyond butterflies: generalized anxiety disorder in adolescents. *The Nurse Practitioner*, *40*(3), 29–36.

McKinney, A. A., & Deeny, P. (2002). Leaving the intensive care unit: a phenomenological study of the patients' experience. *Intensive and Critical Care Nursing*, *18*(6), 320.

R

Meyer, D., Marx, T., & Ball-Seiter, V. (2011). Social isolation and telecommunication in the nursing home: a pilot study. *Gerontechnology, 10*(1), 51–58.
Mitchell, M. L., Courtney, M., & Coyer, F. (2003). Understanding uncertainty and minimizing families' anxiety at the time of transfer from intensive care. *Nursing and Health Sciences, 5*(3), 207.
Newson, P. (2008a). Relocation to a care home, part one: exploring reactions. *Nursing and Resident Care, 10*(7), 321–324.
Newson, P. (2008b). Relocation to a care home, part two: exploring helping strategies. *Nursing and Resident Care, 10*(8), 373–377.
Nuttman-Shwartz, O., Huss, E., & Altman, A. (2010). The experience of forced relocation as expressed in children's drawings. *Clinical Social Work Journal, 38*, 397–407.
Pilkington, F. B. (2005). Grieving a loss: the lived experience for elders residing in an institution. *Nursing Science Quarterly, 18*(3), 233–242.
Quadri, P., et al. (2005). Lower limb function as predictor of falls and loss of mobility with social repercussions one year after discharge among elderly inpatients. *Aging Clinical and Experimental Research, 17*(2), 82–89.
Rantz, M., et al. (2014). The continued success of registered nurse care coordination in a state evaluation of aging in place in senior housing. *Nursing Outlook, 62*(4), 237–246.
Rossen, E. J. (2007). Assessing older persons' readiness to move to independent congregate living. *Clinical Nurse Specialist, 21*, 292–296.
Rossen, E. J., & Gruber, K. J. (2007). Development and psychometric testing of the relocation self-efficacy scale. *Nursing Research, 56*, 244–251.
Salarvand, S., et al. (2008). The emotional experiences of elderly people living in nursing homes. *Annimals of General Psychiatry, 7*(Suppl. 1), 1.
Seematter-Bagnoud, L., et al. (2006). Healthcare utilization of elderly persons hospitalized after a noninjurious fall in a Swiss academic medical center. *Journal of the American Geriatrics Society, 54*(6), 891–897.
Smit, D., et al. (2011). The long-term effect of group living homes versus regular nursing homes for people with dementia on psychological distress of informal caregivers. *Ageing and Mental Health, 15*(5), 557–561.
Sörensen, S., Mak, W., & Pinquart, M. (2011). Planning and decision making for care transitions. *Annual Review of Gerontology and Geriatrics, 31*(1), 142–173.
Stein, S., & Oler, C. (2010). Emotional and legal considerations in divorce and relocation: a call for alternative dispute resolution. *Journal of Individual Psychology, 66*(3), 290–301.
Stone, E., Skubic, M., Rantz, M., et al. (2015). Average in-home gait speed: investigation of a new metric for mobility and fall risk assessment of elders. *Gait and Posture, 41*(1), 57–62.
Street, D., & Burge, S. W. (2012). Residential context, social relationships, and subjective well-being in assisted living. *Research on Aging, 34*(3), 1–30.
Stubblefield, C., & Murray, R. L. (2002). Waiting for lung transplantation: family experiences of relocation. *Pediatric Nursing, 28*(5), 501.
Tracy, J. P., & DeYoung, S. (2004). Moving to an assisted living facility: exploring the transitional experience of elderly individuals. *Journal of Gerontological Nursing, 30*(10), 26.
Vernberg, E., Greenhoot, A., & Biggs, B. (2006). Intercommunity relocation and adolescent friendships: who struggles and why? *Journal of Consulting and Clinical Psychology, 74*(3), 511–523.
Walker, C. A., Curry, L. C., & Hogstel, M.O. (2007). Relocation stress syndrome in older adults transitioning from home to a long-term care facility: myth or reality? *Journal of Psychosocial Nursing, 45*, 35–45.

R

Risk for Relocation stress syndrome

Betty J. Ackley, EdS, MSN, RN, and Mary Beth Flynn Makic, PhD, RN, CNS, CCNS, FAAN

NANDA-I

Definition

Vulnerable to physiological and/or psychosocial disturbance following transfer from one environment to another that may compromise health

Risk Factors

Compromised health status; deficient mental competence; history of loss; ineffective coping strategies; insufficient predeparture counseling; insufficient support system; move from one environment to another; powerlessness; significant environmental change; unpredictability of experience

NIC, NOC, Client Outcomes, Nursing Interventions, Client/Family Teaching and Discharge Planning, *Rationales,* and References

Refer to care plan for **Relocation** stress syndrome.

Risk for ineffective Renal perfusion

Pauline McKinney Green, PhD, RN, CNE

NANDA-I

Definition

Vulnerable to a decrease in blood circulation to the kidney that may compromise health

Risk Factors

Abdominal compartment syndrome; alteration in metabolism; bilateral cortical necrosis; burns; cardiac surgery; cardiopulmonary bypass; diabetes mellitus; exposure to nephrotoxin; extremes of age; female gender; glomerulonephritis; hypertension; hypovolemia; hypoxemia; hypoxia; infection; interstitial nephritis; malignancy; malignant hypertension; polynephritis; renal disease (e.g., polycystic kidney, renal artery stenosis, failure); smoking; substance abuse; systemic inflammatory response syndrome; trauma; treatment regimen; vascular embolism; vasculitis

NOC (Nursing Outcomes Classification)

Suggested NOC Outcomes

Tissue Perfusion: Renal; Kidney Function

Example NOC Outcome with Indicators

Kidney Function as evidenced by the following indicators: 24-hour intake and output balance/Blood urea nitrogen/Serum creatinine/Urine color/Serum electrolytes. (Rate the outcome and indicators of **Kidney Function:** 1 = severely compromised, 2 = substantially compromised, 3 = moderately compromised, 4 = mildly compromised, 5 = not compromised [see Section I].)

Client Outcomes

Client Will (Specify Time Frame)

- Maintain normal blood urea nitrogen and serum creatinine levels
- Maintain urine output of 0.5 mL/kg/hr
- Maintain urine output that is yellow and clear
- Maintain serum electrolytes (K^+, PO_4, Na^+) within normal limits
- Maintain glomerular filtration rate of 60 to 89 mL/min/1.73 m^2
- Maintain normal fluid balance

NIC (Nursing Interventions Classification)

Suggested NIC Interventions

R

Medication Management; Acid-Base Monitoring; Fluid/Electrolyte Management; Laboratory Data Interpretation; Electrolyte Management

Example NIC Activities—Fluid/Electrolyte Management

Monitor for serum electrolyte levels, as available; Weigh daily and monitor trends; Monitor vital signs, as appropriate

Nursing Interventions and *Rationales*

▲ Be aware of major risk factors that increase the risk for decreased renal perfusion. EB: *The KDIGO (Kidney Disease Improving Global Outcomes) guidelines indicate shock, nephrotoxic exposure, intravenous contrast media with iodine, cisplatin, amphotericin B, autoimmune disease, infection, sepsis, hypoxemia, and multisystem failure are major risk factors for ineffective pre renal and intrarenal perfusion and the development of acute kidney injury (Kellum & Lameire, 2013; Chao et al, 2014).*

▲ Be aware of the RIFLE classification system used to indicate progression in severity of acute kidney injury in adults. CEB/EB: *The RIFLE system classifies kidney injury based on serum creatinine and urine output determinants, and includes the following categories:* ***R****isk,* ***I****njury,* ***F****ailure,* ***L****oss of kidney function, and* ***E****nd stage kidney disease (Akcan-Arikan et al, 2007). A retrospective observational study of post discharge information on 49,518 admissions showed effective discrimination with both the RIFLE criteria and the KDIGO criteria for kidney damage and hospital mortality (Fujii et al, 2014).*

- Review client's medical and social history for evidence of chronic conditions such as hypertension and diabetes, exposure to tropical disease, and exposure to nephrotoxins at work, home, or recreation. EB: *Certain conditions and exposures adversely affect renal perfusion (Kellum & Lameire, 2013).*
- Assess clients for fluid imbalance by examining 24-hour fluid intake and output measurements. *Initiating intake and output measurement is standard practice for clients with diseases or conditions that place them at risk for fluid overload or deficit.*

- Assess vital signs, carefully noting new onset of hypertension, hypotension, or dysrhythmia; communicate findings promptly to health care provider. EB: *Normal systolic pressure is less than 120 mm Hg and normal diastolic pressure is less than 80 mm Hg. Mean arterial pressure (MAP) of 72 to 82 mm Hg is necessary to avoid acute kidney insufficiency in clients with septic shock (Badin et al, 2011).*
- Assess for early signs of fluid deficit (skin turgor, tongue turgor, thirst, decreased urinary output). *Dehydration from high output renal damage can lead to hypovolemia and decreased renal perfusion.*
- *Weigh the client daily. Fluid retention related to decreased renal perfusion will cause weight to increase.*
- Assess for early signs of fluid overload. *Fluid overload secondary to decreased renal perfusion will be reflected in bounding pulse, lung sounds (rales), distended neck veins, polyuria, dependent edema, and weight gain over a short period of time.*
- Assess for early changes in mental status (irritability, drowsiness, headache, muscle weakness, difficulty concentrating, disorientation, confusion). *Changes in mental status may result from fluid/electrolyte disturbances from impaired renal function.* Refer to care plan for Acute **Confusion.**

▲ Monitor at-risk clients for increasing levels of serum creatinine and decreasing glomerular filtration rate and urine output. EB: *Clinical practice guidelines recommend evaluation of kidney function using the following indicators: increase in serum creatinine of 0.3 mg/dL within 48 hours despite fluid resuscitation; increase in serum creatinine to 1.5 times baseline or within the last 7 days; urine output <0.5 mL/kg/hr for 6 consecutive hours (KDIGO Work Group, 2012).*

▲ Use isotonic crystalloids rather than colloids (albumin or starches) to provide expansion of intravascular volume in hypovolemic clients who are at risk for or have acute kidney injury. EB: *A Cochrane review concluded that there is no evidence that the use of colloids, instead of crystalloids, reduces the risk for death in clients with trauma or burns, or following surgery (Kellum & Lameire, 2013.)*

▲ Maintain normal to somewhat increased levels of glucose in critically ill clients with insulin therapy. EB: *Maintaining plasma glucose at a target level of 110 to 149 mg/dL prevents complications from hyperglycemia and hypoglycemia that can adversely affect perfusion to the renal macrovasculature and microvasculature (Kellum & Lameire, 2013).*

▲ *Advocate for at risk clients by notifying health care providers when clients have concurrent use of nephrotoxic drugs. Administration of multiple nephrotoxic drugs increases risk for renal toxicity.*

▲ Communicate to radiology departments when clients scheduled for testing with contrast media had contrast media testing within the last 24 hours or recently received cisplatin or high-dose methotrexate. EBN: *Intravenous contrast media with iodine or gadolinium increases risk for contrast-induced nephropathy (Matich, 2014).*

▲ Monitor that peak and trough serum levels of aminoglycosides are within acceptable ranges when multiple daily dosing is administered for more than 24 hours. EB: *Risk for acute kidney injury with aminoglycoside use is high; KDIGO guidelines recommend not using aminoglycosides for infections unless no suitable, less nephrotoxic therapeutic alternative exists (Kellum & Lameire, 2013).*

- Ensure that at-risk clients having diagnostic testing with contrast media are well hydrated with intravenous isotonic sodium chloride or sodium bicarbonate solutions as ordered before and after the procedure. CEB: *Hydration with crystalloids has been shown to prevent acute kidney injury (KDIGO, 2012).* Refer to care plan for Risk for adverse reaction to iodinated **Contrast Media.**
- Collect a 24-hour urine specimen for examination as ordered. *A 24-hour urine specimen to measure urinary excretion of electrolytes is used to assess kidney function; in addition, a glomerular filtration rate can be determined if a blood creatinine is also obtained (Dugdale, 2013).*

▲ Note the results of diagnostic studies such as renal ultrasound, radionuclide scanning, abdominal/pelvic computed tomography (CT), magnetic resonance angiography, magnetic resonance imaging (MRI), and arteriography. *These tests are commonly done for diagnosing acute kidney injury and renal failure (American College of Radiology, 2013).*

- Monitor results of serum and urine tests of kidney function as ordered or per protocol and promptly notify health care provider of abnormal results. EB: *Results of laboratory tests of kidney function are used to distinguish prerenal from intrarenal causes of acute kidney injury (White et al, 2011).*

Geriatric

- Be aware that advanced age is a risk factor that increases the probability of ineffective renal perfusion. CEB: *Older clients have less renal reserve because of reduced glomerular filtration rates due to the aging process and comorbid conditions (Yilmaz & Erdem, 2009).*

- Assess for signs of dehydration in older adults who have less thirst and consume less fluid than young adults when experiencing fluid deprivation. Refer to care plan for Deficient **Fluid** volume.
- Ensure older clients receive sufficient fluids to prevent dehydration and hypovolemia (Pinto & Schub, 2013).

Pediatric

- Be aware that renal development in infants and neonates may be adversely affected by nephrotoxic drugs. EB: *Nephrotoxic medication during fetal and postnatal life may interfere with nephron generation and further increase risk for renal failure (Misurac, et al, 2013).*

▲ Be aware of the Pediatric RIFLE classification system used to indicate progression in severity of acute kidney injury in children. CEB: *The Pediatric RIFLE system supports recognition and classification of kidney injury in children (Akcan-Arikan et al, 2007).*

Client/Family Teaching and Discharge Planning

- Instruct at-risk clients and families to inform health care professionals about their kidney status if scheduled for a CT scan, MRI scan, or angiogram (National Kidney Foundation, 2013a).
- Instruct at-risk clients to avoid overuse of analgesics such as acetaminophen and nonsteroidal antiinflammatory drugs (NSAIDs). EB: *Studies in both adults and children demonstrated a significant increase in acute kidney injury in clients who ingested NSAIDs (Leonard et al, 2012; Misurac et al, 2013).*
- Instruct clients about risk factors for renal insufficiency or acute renal failure including signs and symptoms of acute renal failure and lifestyle changes that can improve renal function. *Client education is a vital part of nursing care for the client with possible renal disease (National Kidney Foundation, 2013a).*

▲ Instruct at-risk clients to alert health care providers about renal status before obtaining new medication prescriptions. *Promote client safety for at-risk clients by encouraging communication with health care providers regarding issues with renal status.*

▲ Encourage smoking cessation. Effects of nicotine include increased pulse and blood pressure and constriction of blood vessels; vasoconstriction and atherosclerosis exacerbate existing problems with kidney perfusion (National Kidney Foundation, 2013b).

REFERENCES

R

Akcan-Arikan, A., Zappiteli, M., & Loftus, L. L. (2007). Modified RIFLE criteria in critically ill children with acute kidney injury. *Kidney International*, *71*(10), 1028–1035.

American College of Radiology. (2013). *ACR appropriateness criteria*. Retrieved from <http://www.acr.org/Quality-Safety/Appropriateness-Criteria>.

Badin, J., Boulain, T., & Ehrmann, S. (2011). Relation between mean arterial pressure and renal function in the early phase of shock: a prospective, explorative cohort study. *Critical Care*, *15*(3), R135. [Epub 2011 Jun 6].

Chao, C.-T., Tsai, H.-B., & Lin, Y.-F. (2014). Acute kidney injury in the elderly: only the tip of the iceberg. *Journal of Clinical Gerontology and Geriatrics*, *5*, 7e12.

Dugdale, D. C. (2013). Glomerular Filtration Rate. *MedlinePlus*. U.S. National Library of Medicine/National Institute of Health. Retrieved from <http://www.nlm.nih.gov/medlineplus/ency/article/007305.htm>.

Fujii, T., Uchino, S., Takinami, M., et al. (2014). Validation of the kidney disease improving global outcomes criteria for AKI and comparison of three criteria in hospitalized patients. *Clinical Journal of American Society Nephrology*, *9*(5), 848–854. [Epub 2014 Feb 27].

Kellum, J. A., & Lameire, N. (2013). Diagnosis, evaluation, and management of acute kidney injury: a KDIGO summary (Part 1). *Critical Care*, *17*, 2004.

Kidney Disease Improving Global Outcomes Work Group (KDIGO). (2012). KDIGO clinical practice guidelines for acute kidney injury. *Kidney International*, Suppl, *2*, 1–138.

Leonard, C. E., et al. (2012). Proton pump inhibitors and traditional nonsteroidal anti-inflammatory drugs and the risk of acute interstitial nephritis and acute kidney injury. *Pharmacoepidemiology and Drug Safety*, *21*(11), 1155–1172. [Epub 2012 Aug 9].

Matich, S. M. (2014). Just pediatrics: kids, contrast media, contrast-induced nephropathy, and nephrogenic systemic fibrosis. *Journal of Radiology Nursing*, *33*(2), 88–89.

Misurac, J. M., et al. (2013). Nonsteroidal anti-inflammatory drugs are an important cause of acute kidney injury in children. *The Journal of Pediatrics*, *62*(6), 1153–1159.e1.

National Kidney Foundation. (2013a). *Contrast dyes and the kidney*. Retrieved from <http://www.kidney.org/atoz/content/Contrast-Dye-and-Kidneys.cfm>.

National Kidney Foundation. (2013b). *Smoking and your kidneys*. Retrieved from <http://www.kidney.org/news/ekidney/May12/Smoking.cfm>.

Pinto, S., Schub, T., & Pravikoff, D. (2013). Hydration: maintaining oral hydration in older adults. *Cinahl Information Systems*, Oct 11, 2p, Evidence-based care sheet.

White, M. T., Diebel, L. N., & Lawrence, N. (2011). The significance of a serum creatinine in defining renal function in seriously injured and septic patients. *Journal of Trauma-Injury Infection & Critical Care*, *70*(2), 421–427.

Yilmaz, R., & Erdem, Y. (2009). Acute kidney injury in the elderly population. *International Urology and Nephrology*.

Impaired Resilience

Shelly Eisbach, PhD, RN, PMHNP-BC

NANDA-I

Definition

Decreased ability to sustain a pattern of positive responses to an adverse situation or crisis

Defining Characteristics

Decreased interest in academic activities; decreased interest in vocational activities; depression; guilt; impaired health status; ineffective coping strategies; low self-esteem; renewed elevation of distress; shame; social isolation

Related Factors (r/t)

Community violence; demographics that increase chance of maladjustment; economically disadvantaged; ethnic minority status; exposure to violence; female gender; inconsistent parenting; insufficient impulse control; large family size; low intellectual ability; low maternal educational level; parental mental illness; perceived vulnerability; psychological disorder; substance abuse

NOC (Nursing Outcomes Classification)

Suggested NOC Outcomes

Personal Resiliency; Decision-Making; Self-Esteem

Example NOC Outcome with Indicators

Personal Resiliency as evidenced by the following indicators: Adapts to adversities as challenges. (Rate the outcome and indicators of **Personal Resiliency:** 1 = never demonstrated, 2 = rarely demonstrated, 3 = sometimes demonstrated, 4 = often demonstrated, 5 = consistently demonstrated [see Section I].)

Client Outcomes

Client Will (Specify Time Frame)

- Demonstrate reduced or cessation of drug and alcohol usage
- State effective life events on feelings about self
- Seek help when necessary
- Verbalize or demonstrate cessation of abuse
- Adapt to unexpected crises or challenges
- Verbalize positive outlook on illness, family, situation, and life
- Use available resources to meet coping needs
- Identify role models
- Identify available assets and resources
- Be able to verbalize meaning of one's life

NIC (Nursing Interventions Classification)

Suggested NIC Interventions

Resiliency Promotion; Self-Esteem Enhancement

Example NIC Activities—Resiliency Promotion

Encourage positive health-seeking behaviors; Facilitate family communication

Nursing Interventions and *Rationales*

- Encourage positive, health-seeking behaviors. EBN: *Promoting health will provide a foundation for enhancing the abilities of individuals to cope, find resources, use resources, and evaluate resources for appropriate decision-making (Landau, 2010).*

R

- Ensure access to biological, psychological, and spiritual resources. EBN: *Identifying and linking persons to available resources will foster engagement in resources that enhance protective factors and resilience (Landau, 2010; Tuck & Anderson, 2014).*
- Foster communication skills through basic communication skill training. EBN: *Individuals who are skilled communicators have fewer problems with family relationships and are able to articulate their own viewpoint (Szanton & Gill, 2010).*
- Foster cognitive skills in decision-making. EB: *Assist in the identification of problems and situational factors that contribute to problems, offering options for resolution (Burton et al, 2010).*
- Assist client in cognitive restructuring of negative thought processes. EBN: *Positive thinking has been associated with increased feelings of coherence and resourcefulness when dealing with adversity (Everly et al, 2014).*
- Facilitate supportive family environments and communication. EBN: *Individuals found to be resilient if raised in families with greater levels of parental supervision and consistent expectations, rules, and consequences for problem behaviors, and effective systems for monitoring children and adolescents (Schofield et al, 2014).*
- Promote engagement in positive social activities. EB: *Facilitating involvement with positive peers decreases the potential for involvement in risky behavior (Veselska et al, 2009).*
- Assist client to identify strengths, and reinforce these. EBN: *Positive self-esteem can be seen as an essential feature of mental health, as well as a facilitator of social engagement (Veselska et al, 2009).*
- Help the client identify positive emotions in the midst of adverse situations. EBN: *Recovering from negative emotions in the midst of adverse situations and focusing on positive emotions helps buffer against life adversity (Szanton & Gill, 2010).*
- Build on supportive counseling and therapy. EB: *Facilitating and mobilizing supportive systems external to individuals and families promote social connectedness, problem solving, resource accessing, and cognitive restructuring (Burton et al, 2010).*
- Identify protective factors such as assets and resources to enhance coping. EB: *According to the protective factor model of resilience, a protective factor that interacts with a stressor reduces the likelihood of negative outcomes (Vahia et al, 2011).*
- Provide positive reinforcement and emotional support during the learning process. EBN: *Positive outcomes and adherence to interventions are attained when clients are supported and reinforced for positive behavior or steps in the learning process (Tetlie et al, 2009).* EB: *Clients with positive, supportive educational environments show self-efficacy in attaining goals in the midst of adverse situations (Masten, 2014).*
- Encourage mindfulness, a conscious attention and awareness of self. EB: *This will help the client identify strengths, as well as promote relaxation and stress reduction (Coholic, 2011).*
- Educate and encourage the use of stress reduction techniques such as guided imagery in which the client focuses on positive images and emotions. EB: *Negative thoughts influence both emotions and behaviors. Positive imagery has been shown to reduce subjective feelings of stress (Park et al, 2013).*
- Enhance knowledge and use of self-care strategies. EB: *Promoting stress reduction and enhancing self-care has been shown to positively impact quality of life (Bryant & Nickerson, 2014).*
- Assist the client to have an optimistic world view. EBN: *Promoting positive thinking and empowering individuals to address adverse situations in a positive frame has been associated with reduced mortality and improved psychological well-being (Szanton & Gill, 2010).*

Pediatric

- The preceding interventions may be adapted for the pediatric client.
- Promote nurturing, supportive relationships with family. CEB: *Secure attachment and early life experience affect the development of the brain, which provides integral foundation for learning and health (National Scientific Council on the Developing Child, 2004).*
- Support the seeking of opportunities to improve cognitive abilities, such as tutoring and other resources; the development of positive and supportive relations, such as family, community members, or mentors; and the improvement of general health. EBN: *These activities help encourage the promotion of protective factors of adolescent resilience such as positive coping and positive self-esteem (Lau & van Niekerk, 2011).*
- Promote the development of positive mentor relationships. EB: *Avoidance of risk-taking behavior is linked to attachment with caring adults (Yadav et al, 2010).* EB: *Children exposed early to caring adults experienced support, encouragement, guidance, and admonishment (Anthony et al, 2009).*

R

▲ Consider referral to appropriate community resources, such as faith-based communities for children who have had adverse childhood experiences. *There is a critical need to identify cost-effective community resources that optimize stress resilience. Faith-based communities may promote forgiveness rather than retaliation, opportunities for cathartic emotional release, and social support, all of which have been related to neurobiology, behavior, and health outcomes. While spirituality and religion can be related to guilt, neurotic, and psychotic disorders, they also can be powerful sources of hope, meaning, peace, comfort, and forgiveness for the self and others (Brewer-Smyth & Koenig, 2014).*

REFERENCES

Anthony, E. K., Alter, C. F., & Jenson, J. M. (2009). Development of a risk and resilience-based out-of-school time program for children and youths. *Social Work*, *54*(1), 45–55.

Brewer-Smyth, K., & Koenig, H. G. (2014). Could spirituality and religion promote stress resilience in survivors of childhood trauma? *Issues in Mental Health Nursing*, *35*(4), 251–256.

Bryant, R. A., & Nickerson, A. (2014). Acute Intervention. In L. A. Zollner & N. C. Feeny (Eds.), *Facilitating Resilience and Recovery Following Trauma*. New York: Guilford Press.

Burton, N. W., Pakenham, K. I., & Brown, W. J. (2010). Feasibility and effectiveness of psychosocial resilience training: a pilot study of the READY program … REsilience and Activity for every DaY. *Psychology Health Medicine*, *15*(3), 266–277.

Coholic, D. (2011). Exploring the feasibility and benefits of arts-based mindfulness-based practices with young people in need: aiming to improve aspects of self-awareness and resilience. *Child and Youth Care Forum*, *40*(4), 303–317.

Everly, G. S., McCabe, L., Sermon, N., et al. (2014). The development of a model of psychological first aid for non-mental health trained public health personnel: the Johns Hopkins RAPID-PFA. *Journal of Public Health Management and Practice*, *20*(5), S24–S29.

Landau, J. (2010). Communities that care for families: the LINC model for enhancing individual, family, and community resilience. *American Journal of Orthopsychiatry*, *80*(4), 516–524.

Lau, U., & van Niekerk, A. (2011). Restoring the self: an exploration of young burn survivors' narratives of resilience. *Qualitative Health Research*, *21*(9), 1165–1181.

Masten, A. (2014). *Ordinary Magic: Resilience in Development*. New York: Guilford Press.

National Scientific Council on the Developing Child. (2004). *Young Children Develop in an Environment of Relationships: Working Paper No. 1*. Retrieved from <www.developingchild.harvard.edu>.

Park, E. R., Traeger, L., Vranceanu, A., et al. (2013). The Development of a Patient-Centered Program Based on the Relaxation Response: The Relaxation Response Resiliency Program *(3RP)*. *Psychosomatics*, *54*(2), 165–174.

Schofield, T. J., Conger, R. D., & Neppl, T. K. (2014). Positive Parenting, Beliefs About Parental Efficacy, and Active Coping: Three Sources of Intergenerational Resilience. *Journal of Family Psychology*, Advance online publication. <http://dx.doi.org/10.1037/fam000002>.

Szanton, S. L., & Gill, J. M. (2010). Facilitating resilience using a society-to-cells framework: a theory of nursing essentials applied to research and practice. *Advances in Nursing Science*, *33*(4), 329–343.

Tuck, I., & Anderson, L. (2014). Forgiveness, flourishing, and resilience: the influences of expressions of spirituality on mental health recovery. *Issues in Mental Health Nursing*, *35*(4), 277–282.

Tetlie, T., Heimsnes, M. C., & Almvik, R. (2009). Using exercise to treat patients with severe mental illness: how and why? *Journal of Psychosocial Nursing and Mental Health Services*, *47*(2), 32–40.

Vahia, I. V., Chattillion, E., Kavirajan, H., et al. (2011). Psychological protective factors across the lifespan: implications for psychiatry. *Psychiatric Clinics of North America*, *34*(1), 231–248. [Epub 2010 Dec 18].

Veselska, Z., et al. (2009). Self-esteem and resilience: the connection with risky behavior among adolescents. *Addictive Behaviors*, *34*, 287–291.

Yadav, V., O'Reilly, M., & Karim, K. (2010). Secondary school transition: does mentoring help "at-risk" children? *Community Practitioner: The Journal of the Community Practitioners' and Health Visitors' Association*, *83*(4), 24–28.

R

Readiness for enhanced Resilience

Shelly Eisbach, PhD, RN, PMHNP-BC

NANDA-I

Definition

A pattern of positive responses to an adverse situation or crisis, which can be strengthened

Defining Characteristics

Demonstrates positive outlook; exposure to crisis; expresses desire to enhance available resources; expresses desire to enhance communication skills; expresses desire to enhance environmental safety; expresses desire to enhance goal setting; expresses desire to enhance involvement in activities; expresses desire to enhance own responsibility for action; expresses desire to enhance progress toward goal; expresses desire to enhance relationships with others; expresses desire to enhance resilience; expresses desire to enhance self-esteem; expresses desire to enhance sense of control; expresses desire to enhance support system; expresses desire to enhance use of conflict management strategies; expresses desire to enhance use of coping skills; expresses desire to enhance use of resource

NOC (Nursing Outcomes Classification)

Suggested NOC Outcomes

Personal Resiliency; Family Resiliency; Quality of Life

Example NOC Outcome with Indicators

Personal Resiliency as evidenced by the following indicator: Adapts to adversities and challenges. (Rate the outcome and indicators of **Personal Resiliency:** 1 = never demonstrated, 2 = rarely demonstrated, 3 = sometimes demonstrated, 4 = often demonstrated, 5 = consistently demonstrated [see Section I].)

Client Outcomes

Client Will (Specify Time Frame)

- Adapt to adversities and challenges
- Communicate clearly and appropriately for age
- Take responsibility for own actions
- Make progress towards goals
- Use effective coping strategies
- Express emotions

NIC (Nursing Interventions Classification)

Suggested NIC Interventions

Resiliency Promotion; Self-Efficacy Enhancement; Counseling; Emotional Support

Example NIC Activities—Self-Efficacy Enhancement

Explore individual's perception of his or her capability to perform the desired behavior

R

Nursing Interventions and *Rationales*

- Listen to and encourage expressions of feelings and beliefs. EBN: *Communication assists individuals and families resolve conflicts and facilitate potential for growth, identify inherent strengths, and problem solve effectively (Doherty & Thompson, 2014).*
- Establish a therapeutic relationship based on trust and respect. EBN: *Therapeutic relationships between therapists, nurses, and clients are essential to help individuals establish goals, communicate concerns, and empower the client (Halldórsdóttir & Svavarsdóttir, 2012).*
- Assist client in rating current level of resilience: www.resiliencescale.com. EBN: *Provides a baseline assessment of current status so that the nurse can identify the effectiveness of interventions (Wagnild, 2009).*
- Facilitate supportive family environments and communication. EBN: *Individuals were found to be resilient if raised in families with greater levels of parental supervision and consistent expectations, rules, and consequences for problem behaviors, and effective systems for monitoring children and adolescents (Schofield et al, 2014).*
- Assist client to identify and reinforce strengths. EB: *Fostering the use of protective factors promotes the ability of an individual to overcome adverse situations (Poteat et al, 2014).*
- Enhance skills associated with social and executive functioning. EB: *Research has shown that social and self-regulation skills enhance one's ability to respond sensitively and are associated with better school adjustment, increased competence, and life success (Masten, 2014).*
- Provide positive reinforcement and emotional support during implementation of care. EB: *Providing positive reinforcement and emotional support will enhance a client's self-esteem, which is a key component of physical and mental health; individuals with higher self-esteem are more likely to be resilient than peers with less self-esteem (Veselska et al, 2008; Masten, 2014).*

- ▲ Facilitate the development of mentorship and volunteer opportunities. EB: *Mentoring programs have been shown to prevent negative outcomes and foster a sense of social and community engagement for clients across the lifespan (Yadav et al, 2010; Klinedinst & Resnick, 2014).*
- • Determine how family behavior affects the client. EB: *Resilience models are based on the presupposition that individuals and families are connected to each other and their community and have collective strengths, which help them compensate for their adversity (Swanson et al, 2011; Masten, 2014).*
- • Promote use of mindfulness and other stress reduction techniques. EB: *Mindfulness-based approaches have been shown to assist in coping with stress and provide a sense of relaxation and awareness of self, others, and the environment (Davis & Kurzban, 2012).* Establish individual/family/community goals. EBN: *Individuals, families, and communities that set goals will focus on attaining or achieving positive outcomes despite adversity (Masten, 2014).*

Pediatric

- The preceding interventions may be adapted for the pediatric client.
- Encourage the promotion of protective factors by fostering the seeking of opportunities to improve cognitive abilities, such as tutoring and other resources; the development of positive and supportive relations such as family, community members, or mentors; and the improvement of general health. EBN: *These factors are associated with adolescent resilience and promote positive coping and positive self-esteem (Ahern et al, 2008).*

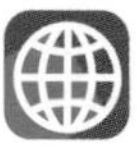

Multicultural

- Use teaching strategies that are culturally and age appropriate. EB: *Nurses who use currently existing family and community resources will promote a context that allows solutions to emerge in a culturally appropriate and sustainable way (Ungar, 2010).*

REFERENCES

Ahern, N. R., Ark, P., & Byers, J. (*2008*). Resilience and coping strategies *in adolescents. Paediatric Nursing, 20*(10), *32–36*.

Davis, L., & Kurzban, S. (2012). Mindfulness-based treatment for people with severe mental illness: a literature review. *American Journal of Psychiatric Rehabilitation*, *15*, 202–232.

Doherty, M., & Thompson, H. (2014). Enhancing person-centered care through the development of the therapeutic relationship. *British Journal of Community Nursing*, *19*(10), 502–507.

Halldórsdóttir, B. S., & Svavarsdóttir, E. K. (2012). Purposeful therapeutic conversations: are they effective for families of individuals with COPD: a quasi-experimental study. *Nordic Journal of Nursing Research & Clinical Studies*, *32*(1), 48–51.

Klinedinst, N. J., & Resnick, B. (2014). Resilience and volunteering: a critical step to maintaining function among older adults with depressive symptoms and mild cognitive impairment. *Topics in Geriatric Rehabilitation*, *30*(3), 181–187.

Masten, A. (2014). *Ordinary Magic: Resilience in Development*. New York: Guilford Press.

Poteat, V. P., Scheer, J. R., & Mereish, E.H. (2014). Factors affecting academic achievement among sexual minority and gender-variant youth. *Advances in Child Development and Behavior*, *47*, 261–300.

Schofield, T. J., Conger, R. D., & Neppl, T. K. (2014). Positive Parenting, Beliefs About Parental Efficacy, and Active Coping: Three Sources of Intergenerational Resilience. *Journal of Family Psychology*, Advance online publication. <http://dx.doi.org/10.1037/fam000002>.

Swanson, J., et al. (2011). Predicting early adolescents' academic achievement, social competence, and physical health from parenting, ego resilience, and engagement coping. *The Journal of Early Adolescence*, *31*(4), 548–576.

Ungar, M. (2010). Families as navigators and negotiators: facilitating culturally and contextually specific expressions of resilience. *Family Process*, *49*(3), 421–435.

Veselska, Z., et al. (2008). Self-esteem and resilience: the connection with risky behaviors among adolescents. *Addictive Behaviors*, *34*, 287–291.

Wagnild, G. M. (2009). Assessing resilience. *Journal of Psychosocial Nursing and Mental Health Services*, *47*, 28–33.

Yadav, V., O'Reilly, M., & Karim, K. (2010). Secondary school transition: does mentoring help "at-risk" children? *Community Practitioner: The Journal of the Community Practitioners' and Health Visitors' Association*, *83*(4), 24–28.

Risk for impaired Resilience

Shelly Eisbach, PhD, RN, PMHNP-BC

NANDA-I

Definition

Vulnerable to decreased ability to sustain a pattern of positive response to an adverse situation or crisis, which may compromise health

R

Risk Factors

Chronicity of existing crisis; multiple coexisting adverse situations: new crisis (e.g., unplanned pregnancy, loss of housing, death of family member)

NOC (Nursing Outcomes Classification)

Suggested NOC Outcomes

Personal Resiliency; Family Resiliency; Knowledge: Health Resources

Example NOC Outcome with Indicators

Personal Resiliency as evidenced by the following indicator: Takes responsibility for own actions. (Rate the outcome and indicators of **Personal Resiliency:** 1 = never demonstrated, 2 = rarely demonstrated, 3 = sometimes demonstrated, 4 = often demonstrated, 5 = consistently demonstrated [see Section I].)

Client Outcomes

Client Will (Specify Time Frame)

- Identify available community resources
- Propose practical, constructive solutions for disputes
- Identify and access community resources for assistance
- Accept assistance with activities of daily living from family and friends
- Verbalize an enhanced sense of control
- Verbalize meaningfulness of one's life

NIC (Nursing Interventions Classification)

Suggested NIC Interventions

Resiliency Promotion; Assertiveness Training; Values Clarification; Parenting Promotion

R

Example NIC Activities—Resiliency Promotion

Encourage family involvement with child's schoolwork and activities; Assist family in providing atmosphere conducive to learning

Nursing Interventions and *Rationales*

- Determine how family behavior affects client. EBN: *The model of resilience is based on the presupposition that individuals and families are connected to each other and their community and have collective strengths, which will help them compensate for their adversity (West et al, 2011; Deist & Greeff, 2015).*
- Help identify personal rights, responsibilities, and conflicting norms. EB: *Maintaining a sense of control and positive perspective about one's environment helps individuals positively cope with adversity (Kia-Keating et al, 2011).*
- Encourage consideration of values underlying choices and consequences of the choice. EB: *Improving social skills, enhancing self-efficacy, and considering values behind choices will promote character building and life satisfaction (Kia-Keating et al, 2011).*
- Help client practice conversational and social skills. EB: *Social competence and social support have been shown to improve academic achievement for minority low-income school children; cognitive skills are protective factors to assist individuals with resilience (Elias & Haynes, 2008).*
- Assist client to prioritize values. EB: *Nurses can help individuals prioritize positive values in order to resist engagement in risky behaviors such as smoking, drinking, or violence (Veselska et al, 2009).*
- Create an accepting, nonjudgmental atmosphere. EB: *Assisting families and individuals to create stable and positive communication skills helps minimize unreasonable expectations and concentrate on positive outcomes (Anthony et al, 2009).*
- Help identify self-defeating thoughts. EBN: *Cognitive reframing is a tool that assists individuals in reflecting and shifting negative thinking toward positive perspectives (Resnick, 2014).*

- ▲ Refer to community resources/social services as appropriate. EB: *Attending community resources, such as support groups, helps disseminate and develop health promotion activities that improve well-being and quality of life (Landau, 2010).*
- ▲ Help clarify problem areas in interpersonal relationships. EBN: *Individuals who were socially connected to their environment, family, and sense of self are able to maintain a supportive mindset and experience a good quality of life despite compromising health conditions, serious diagnosis, and poor prognosis (Stuckey et al, 2014).*
- ▲ Promote a sense of an individual's autonomy and control over choices to be made in one's environment. EBN: *Autonomy promotes a sense of self-efficacy and has been linked to increased quality of life and positive health outcomes for clients (Resnick, 2014).* Identify and enroll high-risk families in follow-up programs. EBN: *Families with adequate resources and positive relationships have a better chance of managing stress and restoring balance in the presence of adversity and limited resources (West et al, 2011; Lester et al, 2013).*

REFERENCES

Anthony, E. K., Alter, C. F., & Jenson, J. M. (2009). Development of a risk and resilience-based out-of-school time program for children and youths. *Social Work, 54*(1), 45–55.

Deist, M., & Greeff, A. P. (2015). Resilience in family members caring for a family member diagnosed with dementia. *Educational Gerontology, 41*(2), 93–105.

Elias, J., & Haynes, N. M. (2008). Social competence, social support, and academic achievement, in minority low income urban elementary school children. *School Psychol Q, 32*(4), 474–495.

Kia-Keating, M., et al. (2011). Protecting and promoting: an integrative conceptual model for healthy development of adolescents. *The Journal of Adolescent Health, 48*(3), 220–228.

Landau, J. (2010). Communities that care for families: the LINC model for enhancing individual, family, and community resilience. *The American Journal of Orthopsychiatry, 80*(4), 516–524.

Lester, P., Stein, J. A., Saltzman, W., et al. (2013). Psychological health of military children: longitudinal evaluation of a family-centered prevention program to enhance family resilience. *Military Medicine, 178*(8), 838–845.

Resnick, B. (2014). Resilience in older adults. *Topics in Geriatric Rehabilitation, 30*(3), 155–163.

Stuckey, H. L., Mullan-Jensen, C. B., Reach, G., et al. (2014). Personal accounts of the negative and adaptive psychosocial experiences of people with diabetes in the second diabetes attitudes, wishes and needs (DAWN2) study. *Diabetes Care, 37*(9), 2466–2474.

Veselska, Z., et al. (2009). Self-esteem and resilience: the connection with risky behavior among adolescents. *Addictive Behaviors, 34*, 287–291.

West, C., Usher, K., & Foster, K. (2011). Family resilience: towards a new model of chronic pain management. *Collegian (Royal College of Nursing, Australia), 18*(1), 3–10.

R

Parental Role conflict *Kimberly Silvey, MSN, RN*

NANDA-I

Definition

Parent's experience of role confusion and conflict in response to crisis

Defining Characteristics

Anxiety; concern about family (e.g., functioning, communication, health); disruption in caregiver routines; fear; frustration; guilt; perceived inadequacy to provide for child's needs (e.g., physical, emotional); perceived loss of control over decisions relating to child; reluctance to participate in usual caregiver activities

Related Factors (r/t)

Change in marital status; home care of a child with special needs; interruptions in family life due to home care regimen (e.g., treatments, caregivers, lack of respite); intimidated by invasive modalities (e.g., intubation); intimidation by restrictive modalities (e.g., isolation); living in nontraditional setting (e.g., foster, group or institutional care); parent-child separation

NOC (Nursing Outcomes Classification)

Suggested NOC Outcomes

Caregiver Lifestyle Disruption; Coping; Parenting Performance; Family Coping

Example NOC Outcome with Indicators

Family Coping as evidenced by the following indicators: Establishes role flexibility/Manages family problems/Uses family-centered stress reduction activities. (Rate the outcome and indicators of **Family Coping:** 1 = never demonstrated, 2 = rarely demonstrated, 3 = sometimes demonstrated, 4 = often demonstrated, 5 = consistently demonstrated [see Section I].)

Client Outcomes

Client Will (Specify Time Frame)

- Express feelings and perceptions regarding impacts of illness, disability, and/or hospitalization on parental role
- Participate in hospital and home care as much as able given the availability of resources and support systems
- Exhibit assertiveness and responsibility in active family decision-making regarding care of the child
- Describe and select available resources to support parental management of the child's and family's needs

NIC (Nursing Interventions Classification)

Suggested NIC Interventions

Caregiver Support; Counseling; Decision-Making Support; Family Process Maintenance; Family Therapy; Role Enhancement

Example NIC Activities—Role Enhancement

Teach new behaviors needed by client/parent to fulfill a role; Serve as role model for learning new behaviors as appropriate

Nursing Interventions and *Rationales*

- Assess and support parent's previous coping behaviors. EBN: *Understanding what experience a parent has with coping will enable the nurse to support the parents in the current situation (Dashiff et al, 2011).*
- Determine parent/family sources of stress, usual methods of coping, and perceptions of illness/condition. Maximize the identified strengths. EB: *Helping to identify stressors in a family's life can help parents better cope with theirs child's illness (Pritchard & Montgomery-Hönger, 2014).*
- Evaluate the family's perceived strength of its social support system, including religious beliefs. Encourage the family to use social support. EB: *Parents use their support from their family to help reduce anxiety (Nabors et al, 2013).*
- Determine the older childbearing woman's support systems and expectations for motherhood. EBN: *Supporting mothers will help mothers better care for their infants (Rossiter et al, 2012).*
- Consider the use of family-centered theory as the conceptual foundation to help guide interventions. EB: *When planning care for a child, family is always the constant in their lives and should be included in all decision-making (Kuo et al, 2012).*
- Be available to accept and support parents by listening and discussing concerns. EBN: *The nurse's ability to observe and listen to parents helps parents gain confidence in caring for their child (Panicker, 2013).*

▲ Maintain parental involvement in shared decision-making with regard to care by using the following steps: incorporate parents' information concerning the child's typical routines, behaviors, fears, likes, and dislikes; provide clear and direct firsthand information concerning the child's condition and progress; normalize the home/hospital environment as much as possible; collaborate in care by providing choices when possible. EB: *Understanding the ways decision are made by the parents will help the nurse better care for the child (Schmidt, 2014).*

- Seek and support parental participation in care. EBN: *Nurses should support the parents in whatever way they choose to participate in care and involve them in as much as the parents feel comfortable (Romaniuk et al, 2014).*
- Provide support for each parent's primary coping strategies and needs. EBN: *Parent support at home can enhance parents' confidence in caring for their child (Callery et al, 2013).*

▲ Inform parents of financial resources, respite care, and home support to assist them in maintaining sufficient energy and personal resources to continue caregiving responsibilities. EB: *There can be a financial*

R

burden on parents of children with chronic illness and a need to help the family identify their resources (George et al, 2011).

- Encourage the parent to meet his/her own needs for rest, nutrition, and hygiene. Provide bed space so that the parent may stay with the sick child. EB: *Children with an illness can have an impact on parent sleep, which in turn can cause parental fatigue and lead to other health problems (Mörelius & Hemmingsson, 2014).*
- Provide family-centered care: allow parents to touch and talk to the child, and assist in the handling of medical equipment; offer a comfortable chair, preferably a rocking chair. Provide opportunities and offer praise for successful caregiving. EBN: *Allowing the parents to participate in care as they feel comfortable enhances family-centered care (Romaniuk et al, 2014).*
- Refer parents to available telephone and/or Internet support groups. EB: *Many parents find that Internet support groups help in coping with their child's illness (Clifford & Minnes, 2013).*
- Involve new mother's partner or parents in clinical encounters and invite family members to discuss their expectations and parenting experiences. EB: *Health care providers realize the importance of involving partners and family members in the care of the infant to help the mother caring for the infant (Gremigni et al, 2011).*

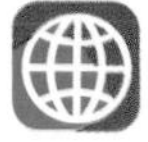

Multicultural

- Acknowledge racial/ethnic differences at the onset of care. EB: *Providing culturally competent care is important to health care equality (Bagchi et al, 2012).*
- Assess for the influence of cultural beliefs, norms, and values on the client's perceptions of the parental role. EB: *Understanding the cultures and beliefs of parents can enhance the interactions between nurse and family (Grant & Luxford, 2011).*
- Acknowledge that value conflicts arising from acculturation stresses may contribute to increased anxiety and significant conflict with the parental role. EBN: *Nurses should assess for any care that may interfere with a family's cultural beliefs and practices (Majdalani et al, 2014).*
- Promote the female parenting role by providing a treatment environment that is culturally based and woman-centered. EBN: *Mothers should be the main focus for shorter hospital stays and better infant bonding (Miah, 2013).*
- Support the client's parenting role in her usual setting via social exchange, including online support. EBN: *Online messaging boards can be very helpful and support the client's parenting role (Porter & Ispa, 2013).*

Home Care

- The interventions described previously may be adapted for home care use.
- Assess family adjustment prenatally and postpartum; assist new parents to renegotiate parenting roles and responsibilities with co-parenting. Encourage the father to take an active role in infant care with the mother's support. EBN: *Home visits can have a positive impact on both the mother and father (Ferguson & Vanderpool, 2013).*

Client/Family Teaching and Discharge Planning

- Offer family-led education interventions to improve participants' knowledge about their condition and its treatment and decreasing their information needs. EBN: *Education of client and family on the condition can improve self-care at home (Swerczek et al, 2013).*
- For children and their parents involved in bereavement support groups, identify the family's positive way of coping. EB: *Support groups and bereaving programs can help parents better cope with the death of a child (Ayers et al, 2013).*

▲ Refer parents of children with behavioral problems to parenting programs. EB: *Parenting programs can help parents identify and reduce problem behaviors in children (Salari et al, 2013).*

- Involve parents in formal and/or informal social support situations, such as Internet support groups. EBN: *Online support groups can allow families to receive support from their peers from around the world and share the knowledge and problems of their child (Mo & Coulson, 2014).*
- Teach the client about available community resources (e.g., therapists, ministers, counselors, self-help groups). EBN: *Community-based resources can support caregivers and ensure that they can identify needed services (Borrow et al, 2011).*
- Encourage parents with chronic illnesses to implement custody plans for their children. EBN: *Support chronically ill parents to plan for the future care of their children (Janotha, 2011).*

R

REFERENCES

Ayers, T. S., Wolchik, S. A., et al. (2013). The family bereavement program: description of a theory-based prevention program for parentally-bereaved children and adolescents. *Omega: Journal of Death & Dying*, *68*(4), 293–314.

Bagchi, A., af Ursin, R., et al. (2012). Assessing cultural perspectives on healthcare quality. *Journal of Immigrant & Minority Health*, *14*(1), 175–182.

Borrow, S., Munns, A., et al. (2011). Community-based child health nurses: an exploration of current practice. *Contemporary Nurse: A Journal for the Australian Nursing Profession*, *40*(1), 71–86.

Callery, P., Kyle, R. G., et al. (2013). Enhancing parents' confidence to care in acute childhood illness: triangulation of findings from a mixed methods study of community children's nursing. *Journal of Advanced Nursing*, *69*(11), 2538–2548.

Clifford, T., & Minnes, P. (2013). Logging on: evaluating an online support group for parents of children with autism spectrum disorders. *Journal of Autism & Developmental Disorders*, *43*(7), 1662–1675.

Dashiff, C., et al. (2011). Parents' experiences supporting self-management of middle adolescents with type 1 diabetes mellitus. *Pediatric Nursing*, *37*(6), 304–310.

Ferguson, J., & Vanderpool, R. (2013). Impact of a kentucky maternal, infant, and early childhood home-visitation program on parental risk factors. *Journal of Child & Family Studies*, *22*(4), 551–558.

George, A., Vickers, M., et al. (2011). Financial implications for parents working full time andcaring for a child with chronic illness. *Australasian Journal of Early Childhood*, *36*(3), 131–140.

Grant, J., & Luxford, Y. (2011). Culture it's a big term isn't it'? An analysis of child and family health nurses' understandings of culture and intercultural communication. *Health Sociology Review*, *20*(1), 16–27.

Gremigni, P., Mariani, L., et al. (2011). Partner support and postpartum depressive symptoms. *Journal of Psychosomatic Obstetrics & Gynecology*, *32*(3), 135–140.

Janotha, B. L. (2011). Supporting parents with chronic illnesses. *Nursing*, *41*(1), 59–62.

Kuo, D., Houtrow, A., et al. (2012). Family-centered care: current applications and future directions in pediatric health care. *Maternal & Child Health Journal*, *16*(2), 297–305.

Majdalani, M. N., Doumit, M. A. A., et al. (2014). The lived experience of parents of children admitted to the pediatric intensive care unit in Lebanon. *International Journal of Nursing Studies*, *51*(2), 217–225.

Miah, R. (2013). Does transitional care improve neonatal and maternal health outcomes? A systematic review. *British Journal of Midwifery*, *21*(9), 634–646.

Mo, P. K. H., & Coulson, N. S. (2014). Are online support groups always beneficial? A qualitative exploration of the empowering and disempowering processes of participation within HIV/AIDS-related online support groups. *International Journal of Nursing Studies*, *51*(7), 983–993.

Mörelius, E., & Hemmingsson, H. (2014). Parents of children with physical disabilities-perceived health in parents related to the child's sleep problems and need for attention at night. *Child: Care, Health & Development*, *40*(3), 412–418.

Nabors, L. A., Kichler, J. C., et al. (2013). Factors related to caregiver state anxiety and coping with a child's chronic illness. *Families, Systems & Health: The Journal of Collaborative Family HealthCare*, *31*(2), 171–180.

Panicker, L. (2013). Nurses' perceptions of parent empowerment in chronic illness. *Contemporary Nurse: A Journal for the Australian Nursing Profession*, *45*(2), 210–219.

Porter, N., & Ispa, J. M. (2013). Mothers' online message board questions about parenting infants and toddlers. *Journal of Advanced Nursing*, *69*(3), 559–568.

Pritchard, V. E., & Montgomery-Hönger, A. (2014). A comparison of parent and staff perceptions of setting-specific and everyday stressors encountered by parents with very preterm infants experiencing neonatal intensive care. *Early Human Development*, *90*(10), 549–555.

Romaniuk, D., O'Mara, L., et al. (2014). Are parents doing what they want to do? Congruency between parents' actual and desired participation in the care of their hospitalized child. *Issues in Comprehensive Pediatric Nursing*, *37*(2), 103–121.

Rossiter, C., Fowler, C., et al. (2012). Supporting depressed mothers at home: Their views on an innovative relationship-based intervention. *Contemporary Nurse: A Journal for the Australian Nursing Profession*, *41*(1), 90–100.

Salari, R., Fabian, H., et al. (2013). The children and parents in focus project: a population-based cluster-randomised controlled trial to prevent behavioural and emotional problems in children. *BMC Public Health*, *13*(1), 225–241.

Schmidt, J. (2014). Primary care decision making among first-time parents in Aotearoa/New Zealand. *Women's Studies Journal*, *28*(1), 18–35.

Swerczek, L. M., Banister, C., et al. (2013). A telephone coaching intervention to improve asthma self-management behaviors. *Pediatric Nursing*, *39*(3), 125–145.

R

Ineffective Role performance

Gail B. Ladwig, MSN, RN, and Marina Martinez-Kratz, MS, RN, CNE

NANDA-I

Definition

Patterns of behavior and self-expression that do not match the environmental context norms and expectations

Defining Characteristics

Alteration in role perceptions; anxiety; change in capacity to resume role; change in other's perception of role; change in self-perception of role; change in usual patterns of responsibility; depression; discrimination; domestic violence; harassment; inappropriate developmental expectations; ineffective adaptation to change;

ineffective coping strategies; ineffective role performance; insufficient confidence; insufficient external support for role enactment; insufficient knowledge of role requirements; insufficient motivation; insufficient opportunity for role enactment; insufficient self management; insufficient skills; pessimism; powerlessness; role ambivalence; role conflict; role confusion; role denial; role dissatisfaction; role strain; system conflict; uncertainty

Related Factors (r/t)

Knowledge

Insufficient role model; insufficient role preparation (e.g., role transition, skill rehearsal, validation); low education level; unrealistic role expectations

Physiological

Alteration in body image; depression; fatigue; low self-esteem; mental health issue (e.g., depression, psychosis, personality disorder, substance abuse); neurological defect; pain; physical illness; substance abuse

Social

Conflict; developmental level inappropriate for role expectation; domestic violence; economically disadvantaged; inappropriate linkage with the healthcare system; insufficient resources (e.g., financial, social, knowledge); insufficient rewards; insufficient role socialization; insufficient support system; stressors; young age

NOC (Nursing Outcomes Classification)

Suggested NOC Outcomes

Coping; Psychosocial Adjustment: Life Change; Role Performance

Example NOC Outcome with Indicators

Role Performance as evidenced by the following indicators: Knowledge of role transition periods/Reported comfort with role changes. (Rate the outcome and indicators of **Role Performance:** 1 = not adequate, 2 = slightly adequate, 3 = moderately adequate, 4 = substantially adequate, 5 = totally adequate [see Section I].)

Client Outcomes

Client Will (Specify Time Frame)

- Identify realistic perception of role
- State personal strengths
- Acknowledge problems contributing to inability to carry out usual role
- Accept physical limitations regarding role responsibility and consider ways to change lifestyle to accomplish goals associated with role performance
- Demonstrate knowledge of appropriate behaviors associated with new or changed role
- State knowledge of change in responsibility and new behaviors associated with new responsibility
- Verbalize acceptance of new responsibility

R

NIC (Nursing Interventions Classification)

Suggested NIC Intervention

Role Enhancement

Example NIC Activities—Role Enhancement

Assist client to identify behaviors needed for role development; Assist client to identify positive strategies for managing role changes

Nursing Interventions and *Rationales*

Social

- Assess the client's level of resilience and implement nursing actions that increase client resilience. EBN: *High resilience is associated with higher role functioning (Melvin et al, 2012).*

- Assess the impact of uncertainty on the client's role. EB: *Role uncertainty may interfere with the individual's ability to articulate his/her role expectations (Stewart et al, 2012).*
- Ask the client direct questions regarding new roles and how the health care system can help him or her continue in roles. EBN: *All participants in this study of clients who had had a stroke described the loss of valued roles that they had previously enjoyed. Health care professionals need to recognize and provide psychological support for clients and significant others who are adjusting to these changes (Thompson, 2008).*
- ▲ Allow the client to express feelings regarding the role change; refer for support as needed. EBN: *For women with cancer and with children living at home, the demands of being a good mother while undergoing treatments and recovering from illness have been described as a difficult life process. All of the women included in this study expressed the need for professional support to help them endure treatment procedures as well as sustain their moral responsibility as good mothers (Elmberger et al, 2008).*
- ▲ Assist the client to identify rewards associated with his or her roles. EB: *Research indicates that role rewards buffers the negative impact of stress on social functioning and depression (Lanza di Scalea et al, 2012).*
- ▲ Refer for support as needed for home caregivers of military families during the deployment of spouses. EBN: *Caregivers affiliated with the National Guard and those with more months of deployment reported significantly poorer emotional well-being and more household and relationship hassles. Given the important effect that maternal well-being has on child and family functioning, it is critical to understand how the stress of deployment is affecting mothers in their daily routines, especially during potentially high-stress periods (Lara-Cinisomo et al, 2012).*
- ▲ Refer the client to Acceptance and Commitment Therapy (ACT). EB: *ACT is a therapy that focuses on the development of psychological flexibility through acceptance of what is out of personal control and a commitment to action that improves and enriches one's life (Hayes et al, 2011).*
- Reinforce the client's strengths and internalized values. CEB: *Participants in this study whose intentions were more aligned with their moral norm were more likely to perform healthy behaviors (driving within speed limit, applying universal precautions, exercising, not smoking) (Godin et al, 2005).*
- Support the client's religious practices. EBN: *Clients dealing with role change associated with health crisis may be at risk for spiritual crisis and need an interdisciplinary approach to assist them through this time (Agrimson & Taft, 2009).*

Physiological

R

- Identify ways to compensate for physical disabilities (e.g., have a ramp built to provide access to house, put household objects within the client's reach from wheelchair) and provide technological assistance when available. CEB: *Among people with disability, use of assistive technology was associated with use of fewer hours of personal assistance (Hoenig et al, 2003).*
- Refer to the care plans for Readiness for enhanced family **Coping,** Readiness for enhanced **Decision-Making,** Impaired **Home** maintenance, Impaired **Parenting,** Risk for **Loneliness,** Readiness for enhanced community **Coping,** Readiness for enhanced **Self-Care,** and Ineffective **Sexuality** pattern.

Pediatric

- Assist new parents to adjust to changes in workload associated with childbirth. Mothers may need additional support. EB: *In most cases, mothers are the primary caregivers and are, therefore, responsible for the majority of the work related to infant care tasks (Barkin et al, 2010).*
- Assess mothers who present with depressive symptoms in the postpartum period for evidence of role performance distress. EBN: *Nursing research indicates that role performance disturbances are correlated with depressive symptoms in the postpartum period (Cavalcanti et al, 2014).*
- ▲ Refer teen parents and families to a community-based, multifamily group intervention strategy (e.g., Families and Schools Together babies). EB: *This program showed statistically significant increases in parental self-efficacy for the teenage mothers, improved parent-child bonds, reduced stress and family conflict, and increased social support (McDonald et al, 2009).*
- ▲ Refer to home health agency for home visits when there is an infant who has excessive crying. EBN: *Mother-infant relationships can be improved through early home visiting interventions by trained nursing staff (Geçkil et al, 2009). The crying baby is the most common presentation in every clinician's office in the first 16 weeks of life (Kvitvær et al, 2012).*
- Provide parents with coping skills when the role change is associated with a critically and chronically ill child. CEB: *Results from mothers who received the Creating Opportunities for Parent Empowerment (COPE)*

program indicate the need to educate parents regarding their children's responses as they recover from critical illness and how they can assist their children in coping with the stressful experience (Melnyk et al, 2006). Involving parents of chronically ill children in ongoing discussions about their positions in management may help promote their active and informed participation (Swallow, 2008).

- ▲ Assist families how to manage day-to-day needs of a child with cerebral palsy (CP). Teach family members to value the small things children do, connect with other families, locate community resources, and understand the short- and long-term needs of the child. CEB: *In families of children with CP, strategies for optimizing caregiver physical and psychological health include supports for behavioral management and daily functional activities as well as stress management and self-efficacy techniques. These data support clinical pathways that require biopsychosocial frameworks that are family centered (Raina et al, 2005).*
- • Consider the use of media-based behavioral treatments for children with behavioral disorders. EBN: *Behavior problems in children are common. For straightforward cases, media-based interventions may be enough to make clinically significant changes in a child's behavior. Media-based therapies appear to have both clinical and economic implications for the treatment of children with behavioral problems (Montgomery, 2005).* EB: *This paper discussed using media-based strategies for delivery of parenting interventions (Barlow & Calam, 2011).*

Geriatric

- • Assess older adults' choices regarding their care and enable them to live as they wish and receive the help they want by carefully listening to their stories. EB: *In this study, "appreciative inquiry" was used to enable older adults, some with dementia, to tell their stories and describe their choices for care (Seebohm et al, 2010). This study showed an association of perceived control and successful aging (Infurna et al, 2010).*
- • Provide support and practice for older adults to use assistive devices. EB: *This study indicates that frail older people need specifically developed support in the process of becoming assistive device users (Skymne et al, 2012).*
- • Support the client's religious beliefs and activities and provide appropriate spiritual support persons. EB: *For individuals like most participants in this study (Christians), incorporating spirituality/religion into counseling for anxiety and depression was desirable (Stanley et al, 2011).*
- • Explore community needs after assessing the client's strengths. Encourage older adults to participate in volunteer programs. EB: *Engagement in social and generative activities has benefits for the well-being of older adults; programs such as Experience Corps Baltimore provide a social model for health promotion for older adult volunteers in public schools (Martinez et al, 2006).*
- • Provide educational materials for older clients who are recovering from hip surgery or fractures to promote early mobility. EBN: *The results of this study of older adults suggest that the provision of basic information is essential for successful recovery (early mobility) from hip surgery. Hip fracture clients should be provided with an educational booklet containing basic information on mobility to promote optimal recovery (Murphy et al, 2011).*
- ▲ Refer to appropriate support groups for mental stress related to role changes. EB: *Within this sample, caregivers of clients with Parkinson's disease reported far greater burden from "mental stress" (e.g., worrying about individual's safety) than from "physical stress" (e.g., lifting individual into bed) (Roland et al, 2010).*
- ▲ Refer clients to therapeutic recreation programs that use humor. EB: *Older adults' life satisfaction showed significant improvement when participating in "the happiness and humor group" (Mathieu, 2008).*
- • Provide music of choice for clients with Alzheimer's disease. EB: *The findings in this study suggest that music enhances autobiographical recall for clients with Alzheimer's disease by promoting positive emotional memories (El Haj et al, 2012).*
- • Provide support for grandparents raising grandchildren. EBN: *Grandparent caregivers are at risk for multiple physical, mental, and emotional problems due to the stresses and strains of care provision (Lo & Liu, 2009).*

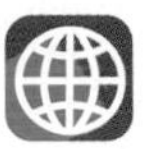

Multicultural

- • Assess for the influence of cultural beliefs, norms, values, and expectations on the individual's role. CEB: *The individual's role may be based on cultural perceptions (Leininger & McFarland, 2002).* EBN: *It is important to gain an understanding of cultural beliefs and traditional practices relating to the postpartum care of women and their babies (Geçkil et al, 2009).*
- • Assess for conflicts between the caregiver's cultural role, obligations, and competing factors, such as employment or school. CEB: *Mexican immigrant children provide essential help to their families, including*

R

translating, interpreting, and caring for siblings (Orellana, 2003). A recent study found that African American caregivers experienced a wide range of caregiver role strain (Wallace Williams et al, 2003).

- Negotiate with the client regarding the aspects of their role that can be modified and still honor cultural beliefs. CEB: *Give-and-take with the client will lead to culturally congruent care (Leininger & McFarland, 2002).*
- Encourage family to use support groups or other service programs to assist with role changes. EB: *Black clients have a history of not participating in support groups (Seebohm et al, 2010).*
- Refer new moms to a new mothers' Internet-based social support network. EBN: *Many single, low-income African-American mothers lack social support, experience psychological distress, and encounter difficulties caring for their infants during the transition to parenthood. The New Mothers Network may be an effective social support nursing intervention for improving single, low-income African American mothers' psychological health outcome, parenting outcome, and health care utilization outcomes (Hudson et al, 2008).*

Home Care

- The preceding interventions may be adapted for home care use.
- ▲ Offer a referral to medical social services to assist with assessing the short- and long-term impacts of role change. EB: *The discharge planner's role, especially for older adults, is important (Preyde et al, 2009).*

Client/Family Teaching and Discharge Planning

- Provide educational materials to family members on client behavior management plus caregiver stress-coping management. EB: *The capacity for caregivers to rate mild cognitive change in Parkinson disease (PD) may be useful to assist in early screening and intervention approaches (Naismith et al, 2011).*
- Help the client identify resources for assistance in caring for a disabled or aging parent (e.g., adult day care, nursing home placement). EBN: *There is a need for support when a family member is placed in a nursing home (Wilkes et al, 2008). In this study, day care was effective in reducing behavioral and psychological symptoms of clients with dementia and in alleviating caregivers' burden (Mossello et al, 2008).*
- Consider pet therapy for college students in a new role, their first semester away from home. EBN: *In this study, students away from home for the first time felt that a pet therapy program could temporarily fill the absence of previous support systems and be a catalyst for establishing new social relationships (Adamle et al, 2009).*

REFERENCES

Adamle, K. N., Riley, T. A., & Carlson, T. (2009). Evaluating college student interest in pet therapy. *Journal of American College Health: J of ACH*, *57*(5), 545–548.

Agrimson, L. B., & Taft, L. B. (2009). Spiritual crisis: a concept analysis. *Journal of Advanced Nursing*, *65*(2), 454–461.

Barkin, J. L., et al. (2010). Development of the barkin index of maternal functioning. *Journal of Women's Health (2002)*, *19*(12), 2239–2246.

Barlow, J., & Calam, R. (2011). A public health approach to safeguarding in the 21st century. *Child Abuse Review*, *20*(4), 238–255.

Cavalcanti, B., Marques, D., Guimarães, F., et al. (2014). Ineffective role performance" nursing diagnosis in postpartum women: a descriptive study. *Online Brazilian Journal Of Nursing*, *13*(2), 246–254.

El Haj, M., Postal, V., & Allain, P. (2012). Music enhances autobiographical memory in mild Alzheimer's disease. *Educational Gerontology*, *38*(1), 30–41.

Elmberger, E., et al. (2008). Being a mother with cancer: achieving a sense of balance in the transition process. *Cancer Nursing*, *31*(1), 58–66.

Geçkil, E., Sahin, T., & Ege, E. (2009). Traditional postpartum practices of women and infants and the factors influencing such practices in South Eastern Turkey. *Midwifery*, *25*(1), 62–71.

Godin, G., Conner, M., & Sheeran, P. (2005). Bridging the intention-behavior "gap": the role of moral norm. *The British Journal of Social Psychology*, *44*(Pt. 4), 497–512.

Hayes, S., Strosahl, K., & Wilson, K. (2011). *Acceptance and Commitment Therapy, Second Edition: The Process and Practice of Mindful Change* (2nd ed.). New York: Guilford.

Hoenig, H., Taylor, D. H., Jr., & Sloan, F. A. (2003). Does assistive technology substitute for personal assistance among the disabled elderly? *American Journal of Public Health*, *93*(2), 330–337.

Hudson, D. B., et al. (2008). New Mothers Network: the development of an Internet-based social support intervention for African American mothers. *Issues in Comprehensive Pediatric Nursing*, *31*(1), 23–35.

Infurna, F. J., et al. (2010). The nature and cross-domain correlates of subjective age in the oldest old: evidence from the OCTO Study. *Psychology and Aging*, *25*(2), 470–476.

Kvitvær, B. G., Miller, J., & Newell, D. (2012). Improving our understanding of the colicky infant: a prospective observational study. *Journal of Clinical Nursing*, *21*(1–2), 63–69.

Lanza di Scalea, T., Matthews, K. A., Avis, N. E., et al. (2012). Role stress, role reward, and mental health in a multiethnic sample of midlife women: results from the study of women's health across the nation (SWAN). *Journal of Women's Health (15409996)*, *21*(5), 481–489.

Lara-Cinisomo, S., et al. (2012). A mixed-method approach to understanding the experiences of non-deployed military caregivers. *Maternal and Child Health Journal*, *16*(2), 374–384.

Leininger, M. M., & McFarland, M. R. (2002). *Transcultural nursing: concepts, theories, research and practices* (3rd ed.). New York: McGraw-Hill.

Lo, M., & Liu, Y. H. (2009). Quality of life among older grandparent caregivers: a pilot study. *Journal of Advanced Nursing, 65*(7), 1475–1484.

Martinez, I. L., et al. (2006). Engaging older adults in high impact volunteering that enhances health: recruitment and retention in the experience corps baltimore. *Journal of Urban Health: Bulletin of the New York Academy of Medicine, 83*(5), 941–953.

Mathieu, S. I. (2008). Happiness and humor group promotes life satisfaction for the senior center participants. *Activities, Adaptation and Aging, 32*(2), 134–148.

McDonald, L., et al. (2009). An evaluation of a groupwork intervention for teenage mothers and their families. *Child and Family Social Work, 14*(1), 45–57.

Melnyk, B. M., Feinstein, N., & Fairbanks, E. (2006). Two decades of evidence to support implementation of the COPE program as standard practice with parents of young unexpectedly hospitalized/critically ill children and premature infants. *Pediatric Nursing, 32*(5), 475–481.

Melvin, K. C., Gross, D., Hayat, M. J., et al. (2012). Couple functioning and post-traumatic stress symptoms in US army couples: The role of resilience. *Research In Nursing & Health, 35*(2), 164–177.

Montgomery, M. (2005). Media-based behavioral treatments for behavioral disorders in children. *Cochrane Database of Systematic Reviews*, (1), CD002206.

Mossello, E., et al. (2008). Day care for older dementia patients: favorable effects on behavioral and psychological symptoms and caregiver stress. *International Journal of Geriatric Psychiatry, 23*(10), 1066–1072.

Murphy, S., et al. (2011). An intervention study exploring the effects of providing older adult hip fracture patients with an information booklet in the early postoperative period. *Journal of Clinical Nursing, 20*(23–24), 3404–3413.

Naismith, S. L., et al. (2011). How well do caregivers detect mild cognitive change in Parkinson's disease? *Movement Disorders, 26*(1), 161–164.

Orellana, M. F. (2003). Responsibilities of children in Latino immigrant homes. *New Directions for Youth Development, 100*, 25–39.

Preyde, M., Macaulay, C., & Dingwall, T. (2009). Discharge planning from hospital to home for elderly patients: a meta-analysis. *Journal of Evidence-Based Social Work, 6*(2), 198–216.

Raina, P., et al. (2005). The health and well-being of caregivers of children with cerebral palsy. *Pediatrics, 115*(6), e626–e636.

Roland, K. P., Jenkins, M. E., & Johnson, A. M. (2010). An exploration of the burden experienced by spousal caregivers of individuals with Parkinson's disease. *Movement Disorders, 25*(2), 189–193.

Seebohm, P., et al. (2010). Using appreciative inquiry to promote choice for older people and their carers. *Mental Health Social Inclusion, 14*(4), 13–21.

Seebohm, P., Munn-Giddings, C., & Brewer, P. (2010). What's in a name? A discussion paper on the labels and location of self-organising community groups, with particular reference to mental health and Black groups. *Ment Health Soc Inclusion, 14*(3), 23–29.

Skymne, C., et al. (2012). Getting used to assistive devices: ambivalent experiences by frail elderly persons. *Scand K Occup Ther, 19*(2), 194–203.

Stanley, M. A., et al. (2011). Older adults' preferences for religion/spirituality in treatment for anxiety and depression. *Aging and Mental Health, 15*(3), 334–343.

Stewart, A., Polak, E., Young, R., et al. (2012). Injured workers' construction of expectations of return to work with sub-acute back pain: the role of perceived uncertainty. *Journal of Occupational Rehabilitation, 22*(1), 1–14.

Swallow, V. (2008). An exploration of mothers' and fathers' views of their identities in chronic-kidney-disease management: parents as students? *Journal of Clinical Nursing, 23*, 3177–3186.

Thompson, H. S. (2008). A review of the psychosocial consequences of stroke and their impact on spousal relationships. *British Journal of Neurosciences Nursing, 4*(4), 177–184.

Wallace Williams, S., Dilworth-Anderson, P., & Goodwin, P. Y. (2003). Caregiver role strain: the contribution of multiple roles and available resources in African American women. *Aging and Mental Health, 7*(2), 103–112.

Wilkes, L., Jackson, D., & Vallido, T. (2008). Placing a relative into a nursing home: family members' experiences after the move. A review of the literature. *Geriaction, 26*(1), 24–29.

Sedentary lifestyle *Sherry H. Pomeroy, PhD, RN*

NANDA-I

Definition

Reports a habit of life that is characterized by a low physical activity level

Defining Characteristics

Average daily physical activity is less than recommended for gender and age; physical deconditioning; preference for activity low in physical activity

Related Factors (r/t)

Insufficient interest in physical activity; insufficient knowledge of health benefits associated with physical exercise; insufficient motivation for physical activity; insufficient resources for physical activity; insufficient training for physical exercise

NOC (Nursing Outcomes Classification)

Suggested NOC Outcomes

Ambulation; Activity Tolerance; Endurance; Exercise Participation; Health Promoting Behavior; Lifestyle Balance; Personal Health Status; Physical Fitness; Exercise Promotion

Example NOC Outcome with Indicators

Ambulation as evidenced by the following indicators: Walks with effective gait/Walks at moderate pace/Walks up and down steps/Walks moderate distance. (Rate the outcome and indicators of **Ambulation:** 1 = severely compromised, 2 = substantially compromised, 3 = moderately compromised, 4 = mildly compromised, 5 = not compromised [see Section I].)

Client Outcomes

Client Will (Specify Time Frame)

- Engage in purposeful moderate-intensity cardiorespiratory (aerobic) exercise for 30 to 60 minutes per day on 5 or more days per week for a total of 2 hours and 30 minutes (150 minutes) per week
- Increase exercise to 20 minutes per day (less than 150 minutes per week); light to moderate intensity exercise may be beneficial in deconditioned persons
- Increase pedometer step counts by 1000 steps per day every 2 weeks to reach a daily step count of at least 7000 steps per day, with a daily goal for most healthy adults of 10,000 steps per day
- Perform resistance exercises that involve all major muscle groups (legs, hips, back, chest, abdomen, shoulders, and arms) performed on 2 to 3 days per week
- Perform flexibility exercise (stretching) for each of the major muscle-tendon groups 2 days per week for 10 to 60 seconds to improve joint range of motion; greatest gains occur with daily exercise
- Engage in neuromotor exercise 20 to 30 minutes per day including motor skills (e.g., balance, agility, coordination, and gait), proprioceptive exercise training, and multifaceted activities (e.g., tai chi and yoga) to improve and maintain physical function and reduce falls in those at risk for falling (older persons)
- Meet mutually defined goals of exercise that include individual choice, preference, and enjoyment in the exercise prescription (American College of Sports Medicine [ACSM], 2011b)

NIC (Nursing Interventions Classification)

Suggested NIC Interventions

Exercise Therapy: Ambulation; Joint Mobility; Positioning; Exercise Promotion; Activity Therapy; Energy Management

Example NIC Activities—Exercise Therapy: Ambulation

Assist the client to use footwear that facilitates walking and prevents injury; Instruct in availability of assistive devices, if appropriate

S

Nursing Interventions and *Rationales*

- Observe the client for cause of sedentary lifestyle. Determine whether cause is physical, psychological, social, or ecological. *Some clients choose not to move because of physical pain, social or psychological factors such as an inability to cope, fear, loneliness, or depression, or environmental factors that can influence physical activity (Resnick et al, 2010).* See care plans for Ineffective **Coping** or **Hopelessness.**

▲ Assess for reasons why the client would be unable to participate in an exercise program; refer for evaluation by a primary health care provider as needed. *Reducing barriers may increase activity level.*

- Use the Self-Efficacy for Exercise Scale (Resnick & Jenkins, 2000) and the Outcome Expectation for Exercise Scale (Resnick et al, 2001) to determine client's self-efficacy and outcome expectations toward exercise (Resnick & D'Adamo, 2011). CEB: *In a meta-analysis of interventions to promote physical activity among chronically ill adults, interventions increased physical activity by an equivalent of 945 steps per day, or 48 minutes of physical activity per week per participant, although the effects on physical activity were variable (Conn et al, 2008; Ruppar & Conn, 2010). Interventions most effective in promoting physical activity were those that focused only on the targeted behavior of physical activity and those that used behavioral strategies (e.g., rewards, contracts, goal setting, feedback and cueing) and self-monitoring (e.g., tracking physical activity using logs or websites). Supervised exercise, tailoring, contracting, exercise prescription, intensity recommendations, behavioral cueing, and fitness testing were also effective, although only modestly supported (Ruppar & Conn, 2010).*

- Recommend the client enter an exercise program with a person who supports exercise behavior (e.g., friend or exercise buddy). EBN: *Recommend using fitness smartphone applications for customizing, cueing, tracking, and analyzing an exercise program (Altena, 2012).*
- Recommend the client begin a walking program using the following criteria:
  - Obtain a pedometer by purchase or from community/public health resources.
  - Determine common times when brisk walking for at least 10-minute intervals can be incorporated into lifestyle and daily activities.
  - Set incremental walking goal and increase it by 1000 steps per day every 2 weeks for a minimum of 7,000 steps per day with a daily goal for most healthy adults of 10,000 steps per day (approximately 5 miles) (ACSM, 2011a).
  - Toward the end of day, if client has not met walking goal, look for opportunities to increase activity level (e.g., park farther from destination; use stairs) or go for a walk indoors or outdoors until designated goal of 7000 to 10,000 steps per day is reached (ACSM, 2011a).

▲ EB: *Use of a pedometer with health care provider counseling and referral to a community action site resulted in a significant increase in physical activity after 6 weeks with inactive participants (Trinh et al, 2011).* EBN: *A nurse-monitored 7-week group exercise training program (ETP) with obese women improved adherence to some type of physical activity program 1 year after the intervention period and the likelihood of adherence increased with the number of ETP sessions attended (del Rey-Moya et al, 2013). Recommend client begin performing resistance exercises for additional health benefits of increased bone strength and muscular fitness.*

- Encourage prescriptive resistance exercise of each major muscle group (hips, thighs, legs, back, chest, shoulders, and abdomen) using a variety of exercise equipment such as free weights, bands, stair climbing, or machines 2 to 3 days per week. Involve the major muscle groups for 8 to 12 repetitions to improve strength and power in most adults; 10 to 15 repetitions to improve strength in middle-aged and older persons starting exercise; 15 to 20 repetitions to improve muscular endurance. Intensity should be between moderate (5 to 6) and hard (7 to 8) on a scale of 0 to 10 (ACSM, 2014, 2011b).
- Encourage gradual progression of greater resistance, more repetitions per set, and/or increasing frequency using concentric, eccentric, and isometric muscle actions. Perform bilateral and unilateral single and multiple joint exercises. Optimize exercise intensity by working large before small muscle groups, multiple joint exercises before single-joint exercises, and higher intensity before lower intensity exercises (ACSM, 2011b). CEB: *After 8 weeks of high-resistance muscle strength exercise and low-resistance exercise for persons with osteoarthritis, there was significant improvement in both groups for pain, function, walking time, and muscle torque (Jan et al, 2008).*

Pediatric

- Children and adolescents should participate in 60 minutes (1 hour) or more of physical activity daily.
- Aerobic: Sixty or more minutes a day should be either moderate- or vigorous-intensity aerobic physical activity, and should include vigorous-intensity physical activity at least 3 days a week.
- Muscle-strengthening: As part of daily physical activity, children and adolescents should include muscle-strengthening physical activity on at least 3 days of the week.
- Bone-strengthening: As part of daily physical activity, children and adolescents should include bone-strengthening physical activity on at least 3 days of the week.
- Providing activities that are age appropriate, enjoyable, and offer a variety will encourage young people to participate in physical activities (U.S. Department of Health and Human Services, 2012).
- Encourage child to increase the amount of walking done per day; if child is willing, ask him/her to wear a pedometer to measure number of steps. EB: *A study demonstrated that the recommended number of steps per day to have a healthy body composition for the 6- to 12-year-old is 10,000 to 13,000 steps for a girl and 12,000 to 16,000 steps for a boy. Evidence shows that adolescents steadily decrease steps/day until approximately 8000 to 9000 steps/day are observed in 18-year-olds (Tudor-Locke et al, 2011).*
- Recommend the child decrease television viewing, watching movies, and playing video games. Ask parents to limit television to 1 to 2 hours per day maximum. CEB: *A study demonstrated that watching television was not connected to an increased body mass index (BMI), but watching television advertising, including food advertisements, was associated with obesity in children (Zimmerman & Bell, 2010).*

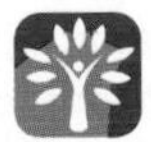

Geriatric

- Use valid and reliable criterion-referenced standards for fitness testing (e.g., Senior Fitness Test) designed for older adults that can predict the level of capacity associated with maintaining physical independence

S

into later years of life (e.g., get up and go test). *Interventions can subsequently be designed to target weak areas and therefore help reduce the risk of immobility and dependence (Rikli & Jones, 2012).*

- Recommend the client begin a regular exercise program, even if generally active. EB: *A meta-analysis of the association between time in sedentary behavior and hospitalizations, mortality, cardiovascular disease, cancer, and diabetes found prolonged sedentary time associated as an independent risk factor for poor health outcomes despite engagement in physical activity (Biswas et al, 2015).* CEB: *Walking is an effective exercise in older adults (Resnick, 2009).* EB: *A meta-analysis to determine the effect sizes of exercise on physical function, activities of daily living (ADLs), and quality of life of frail older adults found exercise beneficial in increasing gait speed and improving balance and ADL performance (Chou et al, 2012).*

▲ Refer the client to physical therapy for resistance exercise training, as able, involving all major muscle groups. CEB: *A Cochrane review found that progressive resistance-strength training for physical disability in older clients resulted in increased strength and positive improvements in some limitations (Liu & Latham, 2009).*

- Use the Function-Focused Care (FFC) rehabilitative philosophy of care with older adults in residential nursing facilities to prevent avoidable functional decline. EBN: *The primary goals of FFC are to alter how direct care workers provide care to residents to maintain and improve time spent in physical activity and improve or maintain function. Residents receiving FFC had less functional decline, and a greater percentage who were not ambulating returned to ambulatory status for short functional distances, while residents with dementia also had a significant decrease in falls (28% vs. 50% in the control group) (Resnick et al, 2011; Galik et al, 2013).*
- Recommend the client practice tai chi. CEB: *Tai chi resulted in increased function and quality of life for clients with osteoarthritis of the knee (Lee et al, 2009). Another study demonstrated that clients performing tai chi had better balance (Wong et al, 2009).*
- If client is scheduled for an elective surgery that will result in admission into the intensive care unit and immobility, or recovery from a joint replacement, for example, initiate a prehabilitation program that includes a warm-up followed by aerobic, strength, flexibility, neuromotor, and functional task work. EBN: *A study of FFC with hospitalized older adults found physical functional declines in both study groups, but less decline was associated with the group receiving FFC. The role of the gerontological rehabilitation nurse is essential throughout the hospital stay and during transitional care (Boltz et al, 2011).*

Home Care

- The preceding interventions may be adapted for home care use.

▲ Assess home environment for factors that create barriers to mobility. Refer to physical and occupational therapy services if needed to assist the client in restructuring home environment and daily living patterns. Use home safety assessment tool to prevent falls and improve mobility and function such as the tool found at http://agingresearch.buffalo.edu/hssat/index.htm. EBN: *Assess person-environment fit (P-E fit) using a reliable and valid instrument such as the Housing Enabler (*http://www.enabler.nu/*) to evaluate the impact of the relationship between the person and his/her environment and subsequently how P-E fit affects physical activity and function (Pomeroy et al, 2011).*

S

Client/Family Teaching and Discharge Planning

- Work with the client using theory-based interventions (e.g., social, cognitive, theoretical components such as self-efficacy; transtheoretical model). EBN: *Residents living in senior housing who attended a 12-week intervention including education, motivational modalities, and exercise classes reported stronger outcome expectations for exercise, less pain, and decreased intake of fat and salt (Resnick et al, 2014).* CEB: *In a behavioral validity study that examined the evidence for physical activity stage of change across nine studies, physical activity stage of change was found to be behaviorally valid, evidenced by self-reported exercise, physical activity, pedometers, sedentary behaviors, and physical functioning. Physical fitness and weight indicators were not related to physical activity stage of change (Hellsten et al, 2008).*
- Recommend the client use the Exercise Assessment and Screening for You (EASY) tool to help determine appropriate exercise for the older adult client. This tool is available online at http://www.easyforyou.info (Resnick, 2009). EBN: *A study found an association between higher EASY cumulative scores with decreased days limited from usual activity and decreased unhealthy physical health outcomes (Smith et al, 2011).*
- Consider using motivational interviewing techniques when working with both children and adult clients to increase their activity. EBN: *A study found that use of motivational interviewing along with evidence-based nutritional guidelines and exercise prescriptions was effective in decreasing the BMI and size of*

waistline in children (Tripp et al, 2011). EB: *Another study found that clients with low back pain who received motivational interviewing were more compliant with performing ordered exercises and had improved physical function (Vong et al, 2011).* CEB: *A study that evaluated compliance of diabetic clients with prescribed exercise found that use of motivational interviewing resulted in increased oxygenation and improved muscle strength and lipid profile (Lohmann et al, 2010).*

REFERENCES

Altena, T. (2012). *DIY: How a smartphone can benefit your health.* From: <http://www.acsm.org/docs/other-documents/2012winterfspn_diyexercise.pdf> Retrieved Oct 1, 2012.

American College of Sports Medicine (ACSM) (2011a). *Selecting and effectively using a walking program.* From: <http://www.acsm.org/docs/brochures/> Retrieved Sept 20, 2012.

American College of Sports Medicine (ACSM). (2011b). Quantity and quality of exercise for developing and maintaining cardiorespiratory, musculoskeletal, and neuromotor fitness in apparently healthy adults: guidance for prescribing exercise. *Medicine and Science in Sports and Exercise, 43*(7), 1334–1359.

American College of Sports Medicine (ACSM) (2014). *American College of Sports Medicine's guidelines for exercise testing and prescription* (9th ed.). Philadelphia: Lippincott Williams & Wilkins.

Biswas, A., Oh, P., Faulkner, G., et al. (2015). Sedentary time and its association with risk for disease incidence, mortality, and hospitalization in adults. *Annals of Internal Medicine, 162,* 123–132.

Boltz, M., et al. (2011). Function-focused care and changes in physical function in Chinese American and non-Chinese American hospitalized older adults. *Rehabilitation Nursing, 36*(6), 233–240.

Chou, C. H., Hwang, C. L., & Wu, Y. T. (2012). Effect of exercise on physical function, daily living activities, and quality of life in the frail older adults: a meta-analysis. *Archives of Physical Medicine and Rehabilitation, 93*(2), 237–244.

Conn, V. S., et al. (2008). Meta-analysis of patient education interventions to increase physical activity among chronically ill adults. *Patient Education and Counseling, 70,* 157–172.

Galik, E., Resnick, B., Hammersla, M., et al. (2013). Optimizing function and physical activity among nursing home residents with dementia: testing the impact of function-focused care. *The Gerontologist, 54*(6), 930–943.

Del Rey-Moya, L., Alvarez, C., Pichiule-Castaneda, M., et al. (2013). Effect of a group intervention in the primary healthcare setting on continuing adherence to physical exercise routines in obese women. *Journal of Clinical Nursing, 22,* 2114–2121.

Hellsten, L. A., et al. (2008). Accumulation of behavioral validation evidence for physical activity stage of change. *Health Psychology, 27*(Suppl. 1), S543–S553.

Jan, M. H., et al. (2008). Investigation of clinical effects of high and low resistance training for patients with knee osteoarthritis: a randomized controlled trial. *Physical Therapy, 88*(4), 427–436.

Lee, H. J., et al. (2009). Tai Chi Qigong for the quality of life of patients with knee osteoarthritis: a pilot, randomized, waiting list controlled trial. *Clinical Rehabilitation, 23*(6), 504–511.

Liu, C. J., & Latham, N. K. (2009). Progressive resistance strength training for improving physical function in older adults. *Cochrane Database of Systematic Reviews,* (3), CD002759.

Lohmann, H., Siersma, V., & Olivarius, N. F. (2010). Fitness consultations in routine care of patients with type 2 diabetes in general practice: an 18-month non-randomised intervention study. *BMC Family Practice, 11,* 83.

Pomeroy, S. H., et al. (2011). Person-environment fit and functioning among older adults in a long term care setting. *Geriatric Nursing (New York, N.Y.), 32*(5), 368–378.

Resnick, B. (2009). Promoting exercise for older adults. *Journal of the American Academy of Nurse Practitioners, 21*(2), 77–78.

Resnick, B., & D'Adamo, C. (2011). Factors associated with exercise among older adults in a continuing care retirement community. *Rehabilitation Nursing, 36*(2), 47–53, 82.

Resnick, B., Hammersla, M., Michael, K., et al. (2014). Changing behavior in senior housing residents: testing of phase I of the PRAISEDD-2 Intervention. *Applied Nursing Research, 27*(3), 162–169.

Resnick, B., & Jenkins, L. S. (2000). Testing the reliability and validity of the self-efficacy for exercise scale. *Nursing Reviews, 49*(3), 154–159.

Resnick, B., Zimmerman, S., & Orwig, D. (2001). Model testing for reliability and validity of the outcome expectations for exercise scale. *Nursing Research, 50*(5), 293.

Resnick, B., et al. (2010). Perceptions and performance of function and physical activity in assisted living communities. *Journal of the American Medical Directors Association, 11*(6), 406–414.

Resnick, B., et al. (2011). Testing the effect of function-focused care in assisted living. *Journal of the American Geriatrics Society, 59,* 2233–2240.

Rikli, R. E., & Jones, C. J. (2012). Development and validation of criterion-referenced clinically relevant fitness standards for maintaining physical independence in later years. *The Gerontologist,* [Epub ahead of print].

Ruppar, T. M., & Conn, V. S. (2010). Interventions to promote physical activity in chronically ill adults. *The American Journal of Nursing, 110*(7), 30–37.

Smith, M. L., et al. (2011). Older adults' participation in a community-based falls prevention exercise program: relationships between the EASY tool, program attendance, and health outcomes. *The Gerontologist, 51*(6), 809–821.

Trinh, L., et al. (2011). Physicians promoting physical activity using pedometers and community partnerships: a real world trial. *British Journal of Sports Medicine, 46*(4), 284–290.

Tripp, S., et al. (2011). Providers as weight coaches: using practice guides and motivational interview to treat obesity in the pediatric office. *Journal of Pediatric Nursing, 26*(5), 474–479.

Tudor-Locke, C., et al. (2011). How many steps/day are enough for children and adolescents. *The International Journal of Behavioral Nutrition and Physical Activity, 8,* 78.

U.S. Department of Health and Human Services (2012). *Physical Activity Guidelines for Americans Midcourse Report Subcommittee of the President's Council on Fitness, Sports & Nutrition. Strategies to Increase Physical Activity Among Youth.* Washington, DC: U.S. Department of Health and Human Services.

Vong, S. K., et al. (2011). Motivational enhancement therapy in addition to physical therapy improves motivational factors and

S

treatment outcomes in people with low back pain: a randomized controlled trial. *Archives of Physical Medicine and Rehabilitation, 92*(2), 176–183.

Wong, A. M., et al. (2009). Is Tai Chi Chuan effective in improving lower limb response time to prevent backward falls in the elderly? *Age, 31*(2), 163–170.

Zimmerman, F. J., & Bell, J. F. (2010). Associations of television content type and obesity in children. *American Journal of Public Health, 100*(2), 334–340.

Readiness for enhanced Self-Care

Ruth A. Wittmann-Price, PhD, RN, CNS, CNE, CHSE, ANEF, FAAN

NANDA-I

Definition

A pattern of performing activities for oneself to meet health-related goals, which can be strengthened

Defining Characteristics

Expresses desire to enhance independence with health; expresses desire to enhance independence with life; expresses desire to enhance independence with personal development; expresses desire to enhance independence with well-being; expresses desire to enhance knowledge of self-care strategies; expresses desire to enhance self-care

NOC (Nursing Outcomes Classification)

Suggested NOC Outcomes

Adherence Behavior; Health-Seeking Behavior; Self-Care Status

Example NOC Outcome with Indicators

Health-Seeking Behavior as evidenced by the following indicators: Completes health-related tasks/Performs self-screening/Obtains assistance from health professionals. (Rate the outcome and indicators of **Health-Seeking Behavior:** 1 = never demonstrated, 2 = rarely demonstrated, 3 = sometimes demonstrated, 4 = often demonstrated, 5 = consistently demonstrated [see Section I].)

S

Client Outcomes

Client Will (Specify Time Frame)

- Evaluate current levels of self-care as optimum for abilities
- Express the need or desire to continue to enhance levels of self-care
- Seek health-related information as needed
- Identify strategies to enhance self-care
- Perform appropriate interventions as needed
- Monitor level of self-care
- Evaluate the effectiveness of self-care interventions at regular intervals

NIC (Nursing Interventions Classification)

Suggested NIC Interventions

Coping Enhancement; Energy Management; Learning Facilitation; Multidisciplinary Care Conference; Mutual Goal Setting; Self-Care Assistance

Example NIC Activity—Self-Care Assistance

Encourage person to perform normal activities of daily living to level of ability

Nursing Interventions and *Rationales*

- For assessment of self-care, use a valid and reliable screening tool if available for specific characteristics of the person, such as arthritis, diabetes, stroke, heart failure, or dementia. **EBN:** *Graven et al (2015) used a cross-sectional study to examine the relationships among heart failure (HF) clients' (N = 201) physical symptoms, social support, problem solving, depressive symptoms, and self-care behaviors and found that the most reliable predictors of self-care behavior were social support and physical symptoms.* **EBN:** *Asplin et al (2014) developed a new scale to measure basic mobility and self-care, the interdisciplinary Traffic Light System-BasicADL. Testing of the new assessment, which measured the function of older clients in acute care settings, demonstrated high interrater and fair intrarater reliability, making it useful for other self-care studies.*
- Conduct mutual goal setting with the person. **EBN:** *Miertova et al (2014) analyzed two case studies of self-care changes in clients with Parkinson's disease (PD) using semistructured interviews, observation, and analysis of health care records and found that self-care needs to be addressed in the initial stages of PD to promote self-sufficiency in activities of daily living (ADLs).* **EBN:** *Basak et al (2014) studied the effects of the multiple sclerosis (MS), ADLs, and self-care in clients (N = 67) who have had MS for 10 years and found that self-care levels are mainly dependent on the duration of the disease and nursing care should be planned with the client accordingly.*
- Support the person's awareness that enhanced self-care is an achievable, desirable, and positive life goal. **EBN:** *A study was completed to determine the items needed in a prostate cancer survivor's toolkit by asking men (N = 22) who underwent a radical prostatectomy. The preferred items were those that aided in managing urinary symptoms for early postoperative clients, and managing erectile dysfunction aids were preferred by men who were postoperative over 100 days (Weber & Roberts, 2015).* **EBN:** *Using a secondary data analysis, researchers evaluated clients (N = 803) with lower extremity primary lymphedema report of self-care, symptom burden, and reported infections and found a significant relationship among self-care, symptom burden, and reported infections that prompted almost half of them to conduct positive self-care activities, such as using compression garments and participating in skin care (Deng et al, 2015).*
- Show respect for the person, regardless of characteristics and/or background. **EBN:** *This study examined foot care among diabetic Jordanian clients (N = 1085) by questionnaire and found a discrepancy between knowledge and practice, prompting efforts to improve foot self-care education that is appropriate to the client's education and culture (Abu-Qamar, 2014).* **EBN:** *Bagnasco et al (2014) performed a systematic review to find the factors that influence self-management of type 2 diabetes by clients searching specifically for interventions, comparators, outcomes, and study design, which were found to be variables for self-care motivation and empowerment.*
- Promote trust and enhanced communication between the person and health care providers. **EBN:** *Akohoue et al (2015) conducted focus groups to improve type 2 diabetes self-management among low-income minority clients (N = 17), caregivers (N = 5), and health care providers (N = 15) and found the most important self-management issues to be providers' accessibility and compassion, and flexible clinic hours.* **EBN:** *Researchers descriptively studied the relationship between quality of life (QOL) and self-care agency in hemodialysis clients (N = 112) and found a relationship between dialysis adequacy, the emotional role, and physical functioning; therefore, communication about dialysis adequacy is important for the client's self-care agency (Kalender & Tosum, 2014).*
- Promote opportunities for spiritual care and growth. **EBN:** *Hatamipour et al (2015) qualitatively studied the spiritual needs of clients diagnosed with cancer (N = 18) and identified fours themes (connection, peace, meaning and purpose, and transcendence) that should be recognized to assist cancer clients with self-care.* **EB:** *Researchers studied the uncertainty experienced by clients (N = 200) with multiple sclerosis (MS) and their spiritual well-being and found that health care professionals should afford clients opportunities to reflect on their spirituality, experiences, feelings, actions, and reactions as a method to constructive self-care learning (Iranmanesh et al, 2014).*
- Promote social support through facilitation of family involvement. **EB:** *Researchers examined clients (N = 100) with type 2 diabetes and the relationship of coping skills and social support with self-care activities and glycated hemoglobin and found a significant relationships between self-care activities producing glycated hemoglobin control, coping styles, and social support (Shaveghian et al, 2015).* **EBN:** *Leikkola et al (2014) assessed aspects of nursing staff support provided to postoperative herniation or spinal stenosis clients (N = 92) and family members (N = 55) and found the most important factor for family and clients in promoting self-care was client education.*

S

- Provide opportunities for ongoing group support through establishment of self-help groups on the Internet. EB: *Koenig et al (2014) studied the relationship between biopsychosocial functioning and pain and pain self-efficacy in clients (N = 99) with low back pain and found that lower biological and social functioning predicted higher pain severity; lower social functioning was found to significantly predict lower pain self-efficacy.* EB: *Hartmann-Boyce et al (2015) reviewed 23 weight loss studies and found that interactive interventions were most effective in the first 6 months.*
- Help the person identify and reduce the barriers to self-care. EBN: *Researchers descriptively studied the relationship between fatigue, self-care, and loneliness in hemodialysis clients (N = 325) and found that as the levels of loneliness and fatigue increased, self-care ability decreased (Akin et al, 2014).* EB: *Shreck et al (2014) studied the relationship between risk perceptions and diabetic self-care (diet and exercise) in a year-long randomized trial in clients (N = 526) who were taking at least one oral diabetes medication; they found no relationships between risk perceptions and glycemic control, but did find a difference in dietary and exercise adherence.*
- Provide literacy-appropriate education for self-care activities. EBN: *Clients with heart failure (HF) may have mild cognitive impairment (MCI). A descriptive correlation study assessed levels of self-care and knowledge and found that clients had the knowledge but were unable to maintain self-care scores, indicating that different methods are needed to educate HF clients with MCI on self-care (Davis et al, 2015).* EB: *Watson et al (2014) studied veterans (N = 219) with chronic pain by providing them with a 12-week educational program and found the program useful and easy to use, and could be integrated into their self-care. Additionally, veterans would recommend the program to others.*
- Facilitate self-efficacy by ensuring the adequacy of self-care education. EBN: *Wu et al (2014) examined perceptions of clients with type 2 diabetes (N = 312) and nurses (N = 202) about self-care activities in Taiwan and found that clients perceived themselves to be more successful at completing self-care tasks than nurses, indicating additional self-care education may be needed.* EBN: *A quasi-experimental single group pre-test, post-test investigation was conducted to evaluate an intervention for self-management in overweight African American clients (N = 19). The results demonstrated that patient activation and self-efficacy were strongly related to self-management (Onubogu et al, 2014).*
- Provide alternative mind-body therapies such as reiki, guided imagery, yoga, and self-hypnosis. EBN: *Sackett et al (2014) conducted an integrative review (N = 25) of older clients' use of folk medicine and other nontraditional therapies and found that there is significant use by older adults for self-care purposes.* EBN: *Fouladbakhsh et al (2014) studied yoga intervention for clients with non–small cell lung cancer and its relationship to sleep mood, salivary cortisol levels, and QOL and found that it did not compromise breathing and had a positive mind-body effect on managing stress, improving mood and sleep, and potentially enhancing QOL.*
- Promote the person's hope to maintain self-care. EBN: *Self-care needs of clients with HF were studied by systematic review of the literature (N = 47); researchers concluded that clients with HF often had difficulty translating self-care into ADLs, thereby indicating that individual self-care approaches would best assist clients with HF (Harkness et al, 2015).* EBN: *Warnock and Tod (2014) used a qualitative interview technique to explore the experiences, concerns, and priorities of clients (N = 10) with advanced malignant spinal cord compression Maintaining hope emerged as an important theme in maintaining a positive outlook.*

S

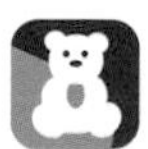

Pediatric

- Assess and evaluate a child's level of self-care and adjust strategies as needed. EBN: *Quaranta et al (2014) conducted focus groups with rural-dwelling adolescents (N = 7) to explore self-management of asthma and its relationship to influences from health care providers, school nurses, teachers, family, and friends. The researchers found that the clients did not perceive that others expected them to change their lifestyle to control their asthma and that they were just expected to use medication.* EB: *Chien et al (2014) studied children's hand skills to assess self-care in children with disabilities (N = 114) compared to typically developed children (N = 139) and found through regression analysis that children's hand skill was the strongest variance for children's self-care function. Assessment of hand skill in real-life contexts is needed.*
- Assist families to engage in and maintain social support networks. EB: *Interviews of adolescents (N = 28) about their first episode of psychosis identified five themes that assisted clients with self-management; (1) symptom recognition, (2) awareness of change, (3) negative appraisals, (4) positive appraisals, and (5) treatment self-management (Gearing et al, 2014).* EB: *Meaux et al (2014) qualitatively studied adolescent clients' (N = 4) and parents' (N = 6) transition to self-management after heart transplantation using online focus*

groups and found that medication management was the most important issue identified for both parents and adolescents.

- Encourage activities that support or enhance spiritual care. EBN: *Riet et al (2014) reported about a healing environment called a "Fairy Garden" created for sick children to enhance holistic care and found that the Fairy Garden supported psychosocial and physical benefits. These benefits improve hospital stay and provide potential for improved clinical self-care outcomes.* EB: *Researchers used a qualitative methodology in children (N = 9) and themes that were important to children in their relationships with adults were identified, including making sense of spirituality and keeping spirituality confidential (Karlsen et al, 2014).*

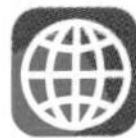

Multicultural

- Identify cultural beliefs, values, lifestyle practices, and problem-solving strategies when assessing the client's level of self-care. EBN: *Yang et al (2014) used a secondary data analysis to identify variables related to self-care behaviors among hypertensive, older, low-income Korean women (N = 234) and found that significant self-care factors included (1) self-efficacy about hypertension control, (2) social support, and (3) age.* EB: *Rajagopal et al (2014) studied the standards of palliative care from 57% of Indian palliative care organizations that participated in the study to establish a "standards tool" that can be applied to assist clients to maintain self-care while on palliative care protocols.*
- Enhance cultural knowledge by seeking out information regarding different cultural or ethnic groups. EBN: *Kleier and Welch Dittman (2014) studied African American clients (N = 100) with diabetes mellitus and variables believed to be important in self-care. The researchers found understanding of diabetes, its treatment, and engagement in self-care activities did not correlate with body mass index and A1c values.* EB: *Researchers qualitatively examined the policies for aging in place for older Czech citizens and study results revealed that allowing clients to remain at home despite their worsening capacity to manage ADLs increased the need for practical support in order for older clients to maintain self-care (Kubalcikova & Havlikova, 2015).*
- Recognize the impact of culture on self-care behaviors. EB: *Paxton et al (2014) consented African American clients (N = 291) with breast cancer to test the validity and reliability of a modified Sedentary Behavior Strategy Self-Management Scale and found that the tool was reliable and valid and considered weight, education, and years since diagnosis of breast cancer but did not consider age. Therefore, further tests are needed to use the tool with older breast cancer survivors.* EBN: *PeAarrieta-de Cardova et al (2014) studied the validation the Self-care in Chronic Conditions Partners in Health Scale to use as a screening tool to assess the self-care skills and abilities of Mexican clients with a chronic illness. Study results demonstrated high reliability and validity of the instrument with three themes identified: knowledge, adherence, and dealing with and managing side effects.*
- Provide culturally competent care. EBN: *Researchers performed a systematic review to develop a self-management program for clients with chronic kidney disease in China and used evidence from studies (N = 22) to develop clinical guidelines. The researchers sent the program to a panel of experts and the content validity score was 0.98; now it is ready to use and be tested in client populations (Yu-Chin et al, 2014).* EB: *Iten et al (2014) investigated the relationship between Mexican clients' experience of health care, diabetes self-management, and clinical outcomes and found no significant differences in measures of diabetes management between undocumented and documented immigrants, including clinical outcomes in glycemic, systolic blood pressure, and lipid control.*
- Support independent self-care activities. EBN: *Omisakin (2014) examined the health care support of clients (N = 88) living with HIV/AIDS and found five different needs including (1) medical support for medication and emergency services, (2) physical support of supplies for the home and nutritional supplement, (3) psychosocial help for emotional and spiritual issues, (4) socioeconomic help with jobs and engagement in community life, and (5) information about HIV/AIDS.* EB: *Sav et al (2015) conducted qualitative interviews about how rural residents (N = 32) living with chronic conditions self-managed their chronic conditions in locations with limited resources and found that self-managing required creativity in order for clients to take care of their health care needs.*

Home Care

- The nursing interventions described previously may also be used in home care settings. EB: *Lawn et al (2014) examined interprofessional health care provider-client interactions during care planning for the home setting (N = 19) and found that health care providers need to be more aware of their power and their communication style in order for clients with chronic condition to improve their self-care management at home.* **EBN:** *This study examined outpatient oncology treatments using a client report checklist that looked at 12 symptoms: hair loss, feeling sluggish, nausea, taste change, loss of appetite, depression, difficulty sleeping, weight loss, difficulty concentrating, constipation, skin changes, and numb fingers and toes. Helpful self-care strategies reported included diet and nutrition changes, lifestyle changes, mind-body control, and spiritual activities (Williams et al, 2014).*

- Support the new sense of self that may occur with complex health problems. **EBN:** *Peng et al (2014) examined goal-setting practices of physical therapists in the community who worked with clients (N = 296) with chronic conditions and found no significant relationship between sex, age, or number of chronic conditions and self-management goals, thereby acknowledging that it is possible to set goals regardless of the client's sex, age, or number of chronic conditions.* **EB:** *A study examined whether older clients (N = 200) would decrease sarcopenia and impaired self-sufficiency during acute illnesses with nutritional therapy and intensive rehabilitation and the interventions prevented the muscle loss, thereby improving function when compared to a control group (Hegerova et al, 2015).*
- Assist individuals and families to prevent exacerbations of chronic illness symptoms so rehospitalization is not necessary. **EBN:** *Bratzke et al (2015) completed a literature review about self-management related to priority setting and decision-making among clients with multiple morbidities and found most studies (N = 13) addressed processes, facilitators, and self-management barriers, and health care providers need to be cognizant that individuals with multiple morbidities engage in day-to-day priority setting and decision-making as self-care activities for multiple chronic illnesses and treatments.*
- In complex chronic illnesses such as heart failure, help individuals and families to accept continued functional disabilities and work toward maintenance of optimum functional status, considering the reality of illness status. **EB:** *Evangelista et al (2015) used remote monitoring systems to determine its effect on activation, self-care, and QOL in older clients (N = 21) with HF and found greater improvements in activation, self-care, and QOL.* **EBN:** *Tao et al (2014) qualitatively studied families/clients' (N = 7) self-care behavior when caring for their colostomy and identified that "taking good care of myself" involved (1) "taking care of my colostomy with a proper degree of independence," (2) "taking care of my life by dealing with limitations," and (3) "taking care of my mood in a positive way."*
- Use educational guidelines for stroke survivors. **EB:** *Hale et al (2014) examined the UK Bridges stroke self-management program through case study analysis with a focus group (N = 60) and neurorehabilitation therapists (N = 17) and found the program to be acceptable and beneficial for developing skills to self-manage recovery following stroke.* **EBN:** *Researchers studied self-management interventions in clients who experienced a stroke to specifically look at medication adherence. A literature review (N = 6) demonstrated that interventions to assist with self-care improved medication adherence in this population (Chapman & Bogle, 2014).*
- Ensure appropriate interdisciplinary communication to support client safety. **EBN:** *Cramm et al (2014) investigated whether communication and coordination is greater between primary care health care professionals and community health nurses than among other professionals and found that it was and assisted with the self-care of older adults in the community setting.* **EB:** *Maneze et al (2014) explored multidisciplinary care of clients with type 2 diabetes (N = 13) and qualitatively demonstrated that clients found it a barrier to be referred to multiple professionals and that communication among the health care team members was poor.*
- Enhance individual and family coping with chronic illnesses. **EBN:** *Shaw and Oneal (2014) studied asthma-related emergency department using a grounded-theory approach (N = 20) and identified the theoretical basis of "living with asthma" included categories of balancing, losing control, seeking control, and transforming, all of which can assist the health care provider in understanding clients' asthma self-care.* **EBN:** *Arestedt et al (2014) studied the lived experience of living as a family in the midst of chronic illness and narrative interviews (N = 7) revealed a phenomenon that is ongoing and moves the family toward well-being. Analysis identified two themes: co-creating a context for living with illness and co-creating alternative ways for everyday life, demonstrating ways that family members manage situations together.*
- Implement a community care management program. **EBN:** *The development of a self-care program for clients aged 65 years and older demonstrated an increased QOL and coherence among older adults who were living at home (Tan et al, 2014).* **EB:** *Cassani (2014) states that studies demonstrate that intermittent self-catheterization is a better option than long-term catheters for clients in the community because they decrease morbidity, increase QOL, and decrease health care visits.*

Client/Family Teaching and Discharge Planning

- Teach clients how to regularly assess their level of self-care.
- Instruct clients that a variety of interventions may be needed to enhance self-care.
- Help clients to understand that enhanced self-care is an achievable goal.
- Empower clients.
- Teach clients about the decision-making process and self-care activities needed to manage their illness state and promote well-being.
- Continuously stress that all self-care activities must be regularly evaluated to ensure that enhanced levels of self-care can be maintained.

REFERENCES

Abu-Qamar, M. Z. (2014). Knowledge and practice of foot self-care among Jordanians with diabetes: an interview-based survey study. *Journal of Wound Care*, *23*(5), 247–254.

Akin, S., Mendi, B., Ozturk, B., et al. (2014). Assessment of relationship between self-care and fatigue and loneliness in haemodialysis patients. *Journal of Clinical Nursing*, *23*(5/6), 856–864.

Akohoue, S. A., Patel, K., Adkerson, L. L., et al. (2015). *Patients', caregivers', and providers' perceived strategies for diabetes care.*

Arestedt, L., Persson, C., & Benzein, E. (2014). Living as a family in the midst of chronic illness. *Scandinavian Journal of Caring Sciences*, *28*(1), 29–37.

Asplin, G., Kjellby-Wendt, G., & Fagevik Olsen, M. (2014). TLS-BasicADL: development and reliability of a new assessment scale to measure basic mobility and self-care. *International Journal of Therapy & Rehabilitation*, *21*(9), 421–426.

Bagnasco, A., Di Giacomo, P., Da Rin Della Mora, R., et al. (2014). Factors influencing self-management in patients with type 2 diabetes: a quantitative systematic review protocol. *Journal of Advanced Nursing*, *70*(1), 187–200.

Basak, T., Unver, V., & Demirkaya, S. (2014). Activities of daily living and self-care agency in patients with multiple sclerosis for the first 10 years. *Rehabilitation Nursing*, *40*(1), 60–65.

Bratzke, L. C., Muehrer, R. J., Kehl, K. A., et al. (2015). Self-management priority setting and decision-making in adults with multimorbidity: a narrative review of literature. *International Journal of Nursing Studies*, *52*(3), 744–755.

Cassani, R. (2014). Promoting intermittent self-catheterisation to encourage self-care in district nursing patients. *British Journal of Community Nursing*, *19*(4), 177–181.

Chapman, B., & Bogle, V. (2014). Adherence to medication and self-management in stroke patients. *British Journal of Neuroscience Nursing*, *Apr-May*(Suppl.), 32–38.

Chien, C. W., Brown, T., McDonald, R., et al. (2014). The contributing role of real-life hand skill performance in self-care function of children with and without disabilities. *Child: Care, Health & Development*, *40*(1), 134–144.

Cramm, J. M., Hoeijmakers, M., & Nieboer, A. P. (2014). Relational coordination between community health nurses and other professionals in delivering care to community-dwelling frail people. *Journal of Nursing Management*, *22*(2), 170–176.

Davis, K. K., Dennison, H., Cheryl, R., et al. (2015). Predictors of heart failure self-care in patients who screened positive for mild cognitive impairment. *Journal of Cardiovascular Nursing*, *30*(2), 152–160.

Deng, J., Radina, E. L., Fuy, M. R., et al. (2015). Self-care status, symptom burden, and reported infections in individuals with lower-extremity primary lymphedema. *Journal of Nursing Scholarship*, *47*(2), 126–134.

Evangelista, L. S., Jung-Ah, L., Moore, A. A., et al. (2015). Examining the effects of remote monitoring systems on activation, self-care, and quality of life in older patients with chronic heart failure. *Journal of Cardiovascular Nursing*, *30*(1), 51–57.

Fouladbakhsh, J. M., Davis, J. E., & Yarandi, H. N. (2014). A pilot study of the feasibility and outcomes of yoga for lung cancer survivors. *Oncology Nursing Forum*, *41*(2), 162–174.

Gearing, R. E., DeVylder, J. E., Chen, F., et al. (2014). Changing perceptions of illness in the early course of psychosis: psychological pathways to self-determination and self-management of treatment. *Psychiatry: Interpersonal & Biological Processes*, *77*(4), 344–359.

Graven, L. J., Grant, J. S., Vance, D. E., et al. (2015). Predicting depressive symptoms and self-care in patients with heart failure. *American Journal of Health Behavior*, *39*(1), 77–87.

Harkness, K., Spaling, M. A., Currie, K., et al. (2015). A systematic review of patient heart failure self-care strategies. *Journal of Cardiovascular Nursing*, *30*(2), 121–135.

Hale, L., Jones, F., Mulligna, H., et al. (2014). Developing the Bridges self-management programme for New Zealand stroke survivors: a case study. *International Journal of Therapy & Rehabilitation*, *21*(8), 381–388.

Hartmann-Boyce, J., Jebb, S. A., Fletcher, B. R., et al. (2015). Self-help for weight loss in overweight and obese adults: systematic review and meta-analysis. *American Journal of Public Health*, *105*(3), e43–e57.

Hatamipour, K., Rassouli, M., Yaghmaie, F., et al. (2015). Spiritual needs of cancer patients: a qualitative study. *Indian Journal of Palliative Care*, *21*(1), 61–67.

Hegerova, P., Dedkova, Z., & Sobotka, L. (2015). Early nutritional support and physiotherapy improved long-term self-sufficiency in acutely ill older patients. *Nutrition (Burbank, Los Angeles County, Calif.)*, *31*(1), 166–170.

Iranmanesh, S., Tirgari, B., Tofighi, M., et al. (2014). Spiritual wellbeing and perceived uncertainty in patients with multiple sclerosis in south-east Iran. *International Journal of Palliative Nursing*, *20*(10), 483–492.

Iten, A., Jacobs, E., Lahiff, M., et al. (2014). Undocumented immigration status and diabetes care among mexican immigrants in two immigration 'sanctuary' areas. *Journal of Immigrant & Minority Health*, *16*(2), 229–238.

Kalender, N., & Tosum, N. (2014). Determination of the relationship between adequacy of dialysis and quality of life and self-care agency. *Journal of Clinical Nursing*, *23*(5/6), 820–828.

Karlsen, M. L., Coyle, A., & Williams, E. (2014). "They never listen": towards a grounded theory of the role played by trusted adults in

S

the spiritual lives of children. *Mental Health, Religion & Culture, 17*(3), 297–312.

Kleier, J. A., & Welch Dittman, P. (2014). Attitude and empowerment as predictors of self-reported self-care and A1C values among African Americans with diabetes mellitus. *Nephrology Nursing Journal, 41*(5), 487–494.

Koenig, A. L., Kupper, A. E., Skidmore, J. R., et al. (2014). Biopsychosocial functioning and pain self-efficacy in chronic low back pain patients. *Journal of Rehabilitation Research & Development, 51*(8), 1277–1286.

Kubalcikova, K., & Havlikova, J. (2015). The potential of domiciliary care service in the Czech Republic to promote ageing in place. *European Journal of Social Work, 18*(1), 65–80.

Lawn, S., Delany, T., Sweet, L., et al. (2014). Control in chronic condition self-care management: how it occurs in the health worker-client relationship and implications for client empowerment. *Journal of Advanced Nursing, 70*(2), 383–394.

Leikkola, P., Helminen, M., Paavilainen, E., et al. (2014). Staff support for back surgical patients and family members: does it improve coping at home? *Orthopaedic Nursing, 33*(6), 352–358.

Maneze, D., Dennis, S., Huei-Yang, C., et al. (2014). Multidisciplinary care: experience of patients with complex needs. *Australian Journal of Primary Care, 20*(1), 20–26.

Meaux, J. B., Green, A., Nelson, M. K., et al. (2014). Transition to self-management after pediatric heart transplant. *Progress in Transplantation, 24*(3), 226–233.

Miertova, M., Tomagova, M., Jarosova, M., et al. (2014). Self-care in patients with Parkinson's disease. *Central European Journal of Nursing & Midwifery, 5*(2), 54–62.

Omisakin, F. (2014). Qualitative study of self-management needs of people living with HIV/AIDS in a semi-rural area in Kwazulu-natal South Africa. *West African Journal of Nursing, 25*(1), 84–95.

Onubogu, U., Graham, M. E., & Roinson, T. O. (2014). Pilot study of an action plan intervention for self-management in overweight/obese adults in a medically underserved minority population: phase I. *Association of Black Nursing Faculty Journal (ABNF J), 25*(3), 64–71.

Paxton, R. J., Yong, G., Hermann, S. D., et al. (2014). Measurement properties of the sedentary behavior strategy self-management instrument in African-American breast cancer survivors. *American Journal of Health Behavior, 39*(2), 175–182.

PeAarrieta-de Cardova, I., Flores Barrios, F., Gutierrez-Gomes, T., et al. (2014). Self-management in chronic conditions: partners in health scale instrument validation. *Nursing Management—UK, 20*(10), 32–37.

Peng, K., Bourret, D., Khan, U., et al. (2014). Self-management goal setting: Identifying the practice patterns of community-based physical therapists. *Physiotherapy Canada, 66*(2), 160–168.

Quaranta, J., Wool, M., Logvis, K., et al. (2014). Interpersonal influences on the asthma self-management skills of the rural adolescent. *Online Journal of Rural Nursing & Health Care, 14*(2), 97–122.

Rajagopal, M. R., Joad, A. K., Muckaden, M., et al. (2014). Creation of minimum standard tool for palliative care in India and self-evaluation of palliative care programs using it. *Indian Journal of Palliative Care, 20*(3), 201–207.

Riet, P., Jitsacorn, C., Junlapeeva, P., et al. (2014). Nurses' stories of a 'Fairy Garden' healing haven for sick children. *Journal of Clinical Nursing, 23*(23/24), 3544–3554.

Sackett, K., Carter, M., & Stanton, M. (2014). Elders' use of folk medicine and complementary and alternative therapies. *Professional Case Management, 19*(3), 113–125.

Sav, A., King, M. A., Kelly, F., et al. (2015). Self-management of chronic conditions in a rural and remote context. *Australian Journal of Primary Health, 21*(1), 90–95.

Shaveghian, Z., Aguilar-Vafaie, M. E., Besharat, M. A., et al. (2015). Self-care activities and glycated haemoglobin in Iranian patients with type 2 diabetes: can coping styles and social support have a buffering role? *Psychology & Health, 30*(2), 153–164.

Shaw, M. R., & Oneal, G. (2014). Living on the edge of asthma: a grounded theory exploration. *Journal for Specialists in Pediatric Nursing, 19*(4), 296–307.

Shreck, E., Gonzalez, J., Cohen, H., et al. (2014). Risk perception and self-management in urban, diverse adults with type 2 diabetes: the improving diabetes outcomes study. *International Journal of Behavioral Medicine, 21*(1), 88–98.

Tan, K., Chan, S. W., & Vehvilainen-Julkunen, K. (2014). Self-care program for older community-dwellers: protocol for a randomized controlled trial. *Central European Journal of Nursing and Midwifery, 5*(4), 145–155.

Tao, H., Songwathana, P., Isaramalai, S., et al. (2014). Taking good care of myself: a qualitative study on self-care behavior among Chinese persons with a permanent colostomy. *Nursing & Health Sciences, 16*(4), 483–489.

Yang, S., Jeong, G. H., Kim, S., et al. (2014). Correlates of self-care behaviors among low-income elderly women with hypertension in South Korea. *JOGNN. Journal of Obstetric, Gynecologic & Neonatal Nursing, 43*(1), 97–106.

Yu-Chin, L., Shu-Fang, V. W., Mei-Chen, L., et al. (2014). The use of systematic review to develop a self-management program for CKD. *Journal of Nursing, 61*(6), 66–77.

Warnock, C., & Tod, A. (2014). A descriptive exploration of the experiences of patients with significant functional impairment following a recent diagnosis of metastatic spinal cord compression. *Journal of Advanced Nursing, 70*(3), 564–574.

Watson, E. C., Cosio, D., & Lin, E. H. (2014). Mixed-method approach to veteran satisfaction with pain education. *Journal of Rehabilitation Research & Development, 51*(3), 503–514.

Weber, B. A., & Roberts, B. L. (2015). Refining a prostate cancer survivor's toolkit. *Urologic Nursing, 35*(1), 22–29.

Williams, P. D., Lantican, L. S., Bader, J. O., et al. (2014). Symptom monitoring, alleviation, and self-care among Mexican Americans during cancer treatment. *Clinical Journal of Oncology Nursing, 18*(5), 547–554.

Wu, S. V., Tung, H., Liang, S., et al. (2014). Differences in the perceptions of self-care, health education barriers and educational needs between diabetes patients and nurses. *Contemporary Nurse: A Journal for the Australian Nursing Profession, 46*(2), 187–196.

Bathing Self-Care deficit

Linda S. Williams, RN, MSN

NANDA-I

Definition

Impaired ability to perform or complete bathing activities for self

Defining Characteristics

Impaired ability to dry body; impaired ability to access bathroom; impaired ability to access water; impaired ability to gather bathing supplies; impaired ability to regulate bath water; impaired ability to wash body

Related Factors (r/t)

Alteration in cognitive functioning; anxiety; decrease in motivation; environmental barrier; impaired ability to perceive body part; impaired ability to perceive spatial relationships; musculoskeletal impairment; neuromuscular impairment; pain; perceptual impairment; weakness

NOC (Nursing Outcomes Classification)

Suggested NOC Outcomes

Self-Care: Activities of Daily Living (ADLs); Self-Care: Bathing; Self-Care: Hygiene

Example NOC Outcome with Indicators

Self-Care: Activities of Daily Living (ADLs) as evidenced by the following indicators: Bathing/Hygiene. (Rate outcome and indicators of **Self-Care: Activities of Daily Living (ADLs):** 1 = severely compromised, 2 = substantially compromised, 3 = moderately compromised, 4 = mildly compromised, 5 = not compromised [see Section I].)

Client Outcomes

Client Will (Specify Time Frame)

- Remain free of body odor and maintain intact skin
- State satisfaction with ability to use adaptive devices to bathe
- Use methods to bathe safely and effectively with minimal difficulty
- Bathe with assistance of caregiver as needed and report satisfaction, and dignity maintained during bathing experience
- Bathe with assistance of caregiver as needed without exhibiting defensive (aggressive) behaviors

NIC (Nursing Interventions Classification)

Suggested NIC Intervention

Self-Care Assistance: Bathing/Hygiene

Example NIC Activities—Self-Care Assistance: Bathing/Hygiene

Determine amount and type of assistance needed; Consider the culture of the client when promoting self-care activities; Provide assistance until client is fully able to assume self-care

Nursing Interventions and *Rationales*

- **QSEN** (Patient-Centered): Ask patients their bathing preferences, which can increase patient privacy and satisfaction. EBN: *Perceptions of patients (N = 71) after an acute myocardial infarction who received bed baths were not as positive as those of patients who took showers (Lopes et al, 2013).*
- **QSEN** (Safety): Warm bathing area above 25.1° C (77.18° F) while bathing, especially on cold days. EB: *Bathing and ambient temperature decreasing from 25.1° C can be a trigger for increasing occurrence of out-of-hospital cardiac arrest (Nishiyama et al, 2011).*

- **QSEN** (Safety): Use chlorhexidine-impregnated cloths rather than soap and water for daily patient bathing. EB: *Chlorhexidine reduces hospital-acquired infection risk from the potentially harmful pathogens methicillin-resistant* Staphylococcus aureus *(MRSA) and vancomycin-resistant* Enterococcus *(VRE) (Kassakian et al, 2011).*
- **QSEN** (Safety): Consider using a prepackaged bath, especially for patients at high risk for infection (older adult, immunocompromised, invasive procedures, wounds, catheters, drains), to avoid patient exposure to multidrug-resistant pathogens from contaminated bath basins. EB: *In a 44-month study by Marchaim et al (2012), hospital bath basins (N = 1103) were found 62.2% of the time to be contaminated with hospital-acquired pathogens.*
- **QSEN** (Safety): Use chlorhexidine gluconate for bath basin bathing. EBN: *Powers et al (2012) found in a study (N = 90) that when patients are bathed with chlorhexidine gluconate and a bath basin that the bacterial growth in the bath basin is significantly reduced.*
- **QSEN** (Patient-Centered): Use patient-centered bathing interventions: plan for patient's comfort and bathing preferences, show respect in communications, critically think to solve issues that arise, and use a gentle approach. CEB: *Focusing on the patient rather than the task of bathing results in greater comfort and fewer aggressive behaviors, which are likely defensive behaviors that result from feeling threatened or anxious, and increase with shower (especially) and tub bathing (Hoeffer et al, 2006).*

▲ Provide pain relief measures, such as ice packs, heat, and analgesics for sore joints 45 minutes before bathing; move extremities slowly and carefully; and inform the client before movements associated with pain occur (walking; transferring to a new location; moving joints; and washing genitals, face, and between toes and under arms). Have the client wash painful areas; recognize indicators of pain and apologize for any pain caused. CEB: *Pain relief and client participation reduce discomfort, preserve dignity, and give a sense of control (Rader et al, 2006).*

- Use a comfortable padded shower chair with foot support, or adapt a chair: pad it with towels/washcloths, cover the cold back with dry towels, and cover the arms with foam pipe insulation. CEB: *Unpadded shower chairs with large openings and no foot support contribute to pain by allowing clients to sink into the opening with their feet unsupported (Rader et al, 2006).*
- Ensure that bathing assistance preserves client dignity through use of privacy with a traffic-free bathing area and posted privacy signs, timeliness of personal care, and conveyance of honor and recognition of the deservedness of respect and esteem of all persons. CEBN: *Older adults report that dignity is promoted via respect, independence, exerting control, timeliness, privacy for the body, cleanliness, independence and sufficient time from staff, attitudes to older people, and communication (Webster & Bryan, 2009).*
- For cognitively impaired clients, avoid upsetting factors associated with bathing: instead of using the terms *bath, shower,* or *wash,* use comforting words, such as *warm, relaxing,* or *massage.* Start at the client's feet and bathe upward; bathe the face last after washing hands and using a clean cloth. Use a beautician/barber or wash hair at another time to avoid water dripping in the face. CEB: *Some words are associated with unpleasant bathing experiences, whereas others convey a pleasant bathing experience. Starting with the face or hair is distressing, because water drips on the face and the head becomes cold and wet (Rader et al, 2006).*
- Use towel bathing to bathe client in bed, a bath blanket, and warm towels to keep the client covered the entire time. Warm and moisten towels/washcloths and place in plastic bags to keep them warm. Use the towels to massage large areas (front, back) and one washcloth for facial areas and another one for genital areas. No rinsing or drying is needed as is commonly thought for bathing. CEB: *Towel bathing is a gentle experience with less discomfort that significantly reduces aggression as well as bathing time and soap residue over showering without accumulation of pathogenic bacteria (Hoeffer et al, 2006).*
- **QSEN** (Patient-Centered): For shower bathing: use patient-centered techniques, keep patient covered with towels and cleanse under the towels, use no-rinse products, use favorite bathing items, and use a handheld shower with adjustable spray. CEB: *Covering the patient is an easy means to maintain dignity, reduce embarrassment, and keep the patient warm and unexposed without increasing bathing time (Rader et al, 2006).*

▲ **QSEN** (Teamwork and Collaboration): Request referral of patient who has had a stroke to rehabilitation services. EB: *In a systematic review of 19 studies, Mehrholz et al (2012) found that electromechanical and robot-assisted arm training devices used in rehabilitation may assist in improving arm function after stroke, which is important for activities of daily living such as bathing.*

▲ **QSEN** (Patient-Centered): Use a wrapped warm footbath for relaxation in patients with cancer. EBN: *Yamamoto and Nagata (2011) found in a randomized controlled trial that the wrapped warm footbath in patients with cancer can increase relaxation and provide pain relief.*

S

Geriatric

- **QSEN** (Patient-Centered, Safety): Advocate for the use of the Bathing Without a Battle educational program for patients with dementia. EB: *In a randomized crossover diffusion study, the Bathing Without a Battle educational program that trains caregivers in methods for improving the bathing experience of patients with dementia in nursing homes was found to be effective in reducing the rate of aggressive and agitated behaviors (Gozalo et al, 2014).*
- **QSEN** (Patient-Centered): Provide night time bathing options for nursing home residents. EBN: *Hashimoto (2014) in an interview survey of administrators of nursing homes (N = 3) found that night time bathing options provided more flexibility for bathing needs, improved sleep and quality of life for the residents, and for caregivers improved care quality and ability to provide patient-centered care.*
- Design the bathing environment for comfort: **Visual.** Reduce clutter and use partitions to hide equipment storage. Laminate and put artwork or decorative objects in bather's view, or place cue cards to bathing process (wall, ceiling, shower). Stand or sit in bather's position to experience what he/she sees. Decrease glare from tiles, white walls, and artificial lights. Use contrasting colors and soft but adequate lighting on a dimming switch for adjustment. *Bathing rooms are sterile, institutional, and frightening spaces filled with unfamiliar equipment—tubs with sides that open up and look like they might swallow you, or gurneys with arms that look like construction cranes. Overhead lights can be bright and shine into the bather's eyes. Glare can cause visual discomfort, especially in clients with visual changes or cataracts (Calkins, 2005).*
- Arrange the bathing environment to promote sensory comfort: **Auditory.** Reduce noise of voices and water. Do not allow traffic into bathing room. Add fabric to absorb sound (three to four times the width of the opening for sound-absorbing folds). Play soft music. CEB: *Noise discomfort can result from high-echo tiled walls, loud voices, and running water. Traffic can compromise privacy. Absorb negative sounds, and add positive sounds through music (Calkins, 2005).* EBN: *In an observational study (N = 53) by Joosse (2012), sound was a predictor of agitation for those with dementia.*
- Design the bathing environment for comfort: **Tactile.** Use heat lamps or radiant heat panels to keep the room warm. Use powder-coated grab bars in decorative colors with nonslip grip. Provide a soft rug to stand on. Ensure that flooring is not slippery (a high coefficient of friction, ideally above 80, is desired and obtained through flooring coatings). CEB: *If the caregiver is warm to the point of sweating, room temperature is about right for an older person being bathed. Appealing, stable grab bars are needed for balance. Preventing the floor from becoming slippery from water is essential (Calkins, 2005).*
- Use music during shower for clients with dementia. *Music may reduce agitation and improve moods to increase job satisfaction (Ray & Fitzsimmons, 2014).*
- Train caregivers bathing clients with dementia to avoid behaviors that can trigger assault: confrontational communication, invalidation of the resident's feelings, failure to prepare a resident for a task, initiating shower spray or touch during bathing without verbal prompts beforehand, washing the hair/face, speaking disrespectfully to the client, and hurrying the pace of the bath. CEB: *During bathing, assaults (defensive behavior) by nursing home residents with dementia are frequently triggered by caregiver actions that startle, frighten, hurt, or upset the resident. This might happen when caregivers spray water on a resident without warning or when they touch a resident's feet, axilla, or perineum, possibly due to the startle reflex (Somboontanont et al, 2004).*
- Develop awareness of the ethics of presence during bathing to better meet clients' needs. Raholm (2012) found in a phenomenological study of nurses in elder care (N = 7) who discussed bathing that one must go beyond being physically present and enter into a caring relationship in which there is no indifference to the client's unique needs.
- Focus on the abilities of the client with dementia to obtain client's participation in bathing. EBN: *The use of an abilities-focused approach increases the ability of people with dementia to participate in their care (Sidani et al, 2012).*
- **QSEN** (Patient-Centered): Use a Chinese herb formula in bath water to reduce paraplegia spasm. EB: *In a randomized controlled trial by Liu et al (2014), Chinese herbs placed in bath water (N = 160) reduced paraplegia spasticity.*

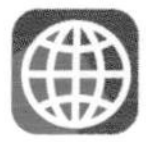

Multicultural

- **QSEN** (Patient-Centered): Ask the patient for input on bathing habits and cultural bathing preferences. CEB: *Bathing is a personal experience with variability in attitudes, preferences, and adaptations to disability to be considered when developing interventions for bathing (Ahluwalia et al, 2010).*

S

Home Care

- If in a typical bathing setting for the client, assess the client's ability to bathe self via direct observation using physical performance tests for ADLs. *Observation of bathing performed in an atypical bathing setting may result in false data.*
- **QSEN** (Safety): Turn down temperature of water heater and recommend use of a water temperature-sensing shower valve to prevent scalding. *Older or disabled people have slower reflexes to respond to hot water and may be unable to regulate water temperature, yet they may be left unattended. Water at 130° F produces a first-degree burn in 20 seconds; at 135° F to 140° F, exposure for 5 to 6 seconds causes third-degree burns (Fathers, 2004).*

Client/Family Teaching and Discharge Planning

- Inform clients with extremity casts or bandages of inexpensive options to protect these devices during showering such as with plastic newspaper bags or bread bags. In a case study, Naram et al (2011) report on the use of inexpensive or free cast and bandage protector bags.

REFERENCES

Ahluwalia, S. C., et al. (2010). Perspectives of older persons on bathing and bathing disability: a qualitative study. *Journal of American GeriatricSociety, 58*, 450–456.

Calkins, M. (2005). Designing bathing rooms that comfort. *Nursing Homes, 54*(1), 54–55.

Fathers, B. (2004). Bathing safety for the elderly and disabled. *Nursing Homes, 53*(9), 50–52.

Gozalo, P., Prakash, S., Qato, D. M., et al. (2014). Effect of the bathing without a battle training intervention on bathing-associated physical and verbal outcomes in nursing home residents with dementia: a randomized crossover diffusion study. *Journal of the American Geriatrics Society, 62*(5), 797–804.

Hashimoto, T. (2014). Investigation into the actual conditions of night bathing for the elderly in nursing homes [Japanese]. *Journal of the Japanese Society of Balneology, Climatology & Physical Medicine, 77*(4), 314–323.

Hoeffer, B., et al. (2006). Assisting cognitively impaired nursing home residents with bathing: effects of two bathing interventions on caregiving. *The Gerontologist, 46*(4), 524–532.

Joosse, L. L. (2012). Do sound levels and space contribute to agitation in nursing home residents with dementia? *Research in Gerontological Nursing, 5*(3), 174–184.

Kassakian, S. Z., et al. (2011). Impact of chlorhexidine bathing on hospital-acquired infections among general medical patients. *Infection Control and Hospital Epidemiology, 32*(3), 238–243.

Liu, X., Meng, Q., Yu, D., et al. (2014). Novel medical bathing with traditional Chinese herb formula alleviates paraplegia spasticity. *International Journal of Nursing Practice, 20*(3), 227–232.

Lopes, J., Nogueira-Martins, L. A., & Barros, A. L. (2013). Bed and shower baths: comparing the perceptions of patients with acute myocardial infarction. *Journal of Clinical Nursing, 22*(5/6), 733–740.

Marchaim, D., Taylor, A. R., Hayakawa, K., et al. (2012). Hospital bath basins are frequently contaminated with multidrug-resistant human pathogens. *American Journal of Infection Control, 40*(6), 562–564.

Mehrholz, J., Hädrich, A., Platz, T., et al. (2012). Electromechanical and robot-assisted arm training for improving generic activities of daily living, arm function, and arm muscle strength after stroke. *Cochrane Database of Systematic Reviews*, (6).

Naram, A., Makhijani, S. N., & Chao, J. D. (2011). Inexpensive alternatives for extremity cast and bandage protection. *Orthopaedic Nursing, 30*(2), 117–118.

Nishiyama, C., Iwami, T., Nichol, G., et al. (2011). Association of out-of-hospital cardiac arrest with prior activity and ambient temperature. *Resuscitation, 82*(8), 1008–1012.

Powers, J., Peed, J., Burns, L., et al. (2012). Chlorhexidine bathing and microbial contamination in patients' bath basins. *American Journal of Critical Care, 21*(5), 338–343.

Rader, J., et al. (2006). The bathing of older adults with dementia: easing the unnecessarily unpleasant aspects of assisted bathing. *American Journal of Nursing, 106*(4), 4–49.

Raholm, M.-B. (2012). The ethics of presence when bathing patients in a nursing home. *International Journal For Human Caring, 16*(4), 30–35.

Ray, K. D., & Fitzsimmons, S. (2014). Music-assisted bathing: making shower time easier for people with dementia. *Journal of Gerontological Nursing, 40*(2), 9–13.

Sidani, S., Streiner, D., & LeClerc, C. (2012). Evaluating the effectiveness of the abilities-focused approach to morning care of people with dementia. *International Journal of Older People Nursing.*

Somboontanont, W., et al. (2004). Assaultive behavior in Alzheimer's disease: identifying immediate antecedents during bathing. *Journal of Gerontological Nursing, 30*(9), 22–29.

Webster, C., & Bryan, K. (2009). Older people's views of dignity and how it can be promoted in a hospital environment. *Journal of Clinical Nursing, 18*(12), 1784–1792.

Yamamoto, K., & Nagata, S. (2011). Physiological and psychological evaluation of the wrapped warm footbath as a complementary nursing therapy to induce relaxation in hospitalized patients with incurable cancer: a pilot study. *Cancer Nursing, 34*(3), 185–192.

Dressing Self-Care deficit *Linda S. Williams, RN, MSN*

NANDA-I

Definition

Impaired ability to perform or complete dressing activities for self

Defining Characteristics

Decrease in motivation; discomfort; environmental barrier; fatigue; impaired ability to choose clothing; impaired ability to fasten clothing; impaired ability to gather clothing; impaired ability to maintain appearance; impaired ability to pick up clothing; impaired ability to put clothing on lower body; impaired ability to put clothing on upper body; impaired ability to put on various items of clothing (e.g., shirt, socks, shoes); impaired ability to remove clothing item (e.g., shirt, socks, shoes); impaired ability to use assistive device; impaired ability to use zipper; musculoskeletal impairment; neuromuscular impairment; pain

Related Factors (r/t)

Alteration in cognitive functioning; anxiety; perceptual impairment; weakness

NOC (Nursing Outcomes Classification)

Suggested NOC Outcomes

Self-Care: Activities of Daily Living (ADLs), Dressing, Hygiene

Example NOC Outcome with Indicators

Self-Care: Dressing as evidenced by the following indicators: Gets clothing from drawer and closet/Puts clothing on upper body and lower body. (Rate outcome and indicators of **Self-Care: Dressing:** 1 = severely compromised, 2 = substantially compromised, 3 = moderately compromised, 4 = mildly compromised, 5 = not compromised [see Section I].)

Client Outcomes

Client Will (Specify Time Frame)

- Dress and groom self to optimal potential
- Use assistive technology to dress and groom
- Explain and use methods to enhance strengths during dressing and grooming
- Dress and groom with assistance of caregiver as needed

NIC (Nursing Interventions Classification)

Suggested NIC Intervention

Self-Care Assistance: Dressing/Grooming

Example NIC Activities—Self-Care Assistance: Dressing/Grooming

Be available for assistance in dressing, as necessary; Reinforce efforts to dress self; Maintain privacy while the client is dressing

Nursing Interventions and *Rationales*

- ▲ QSEN (Teamwork and Collaboration): Assess functional impairment and report functional changes to health care provider to aid in earlier cancer diagnosis. EB: *Functional impairments were found to be symptoms during the diagnostic phase that occurred in clusters based on cancer site: head/neck—impairments in dressing, eating/feeding, bathing, toileting, and walking (Fodeh et al, 2013).*
- QSEN (Patient-Centered): Assess a patient's range of movement, upper limb strength, balance, coordination, functional grip, dexterity, sensation, and ability to detect limb position. *Dressing requires complex functions, and any impairment in these areas causes problems with dressing (Swann, 2011a).*

- ▲ **QSEN** (Patient-Centered): Assess independence in dressing and bathing skills after rehabilitation to determine the need for follow-up care. EB: *It was found that dressing and bathing independence at rehabilitation discharge were predictors of independence at 5 years after stroke (De Wit et al, 2014).*
- ▲ **QSEN** (Teamwork and Collaboration): Refer patients with hand deformities due to rheumatoid arthritis to occupational therapy for self-care rehabilitation. EB: *Patients with rheumatoid arthritis who had hand deformities were found to have difficulty with dressing and grooming (Köybaş et al, 2011).*
- • **QSEN** (Patient-Centered): Recognize that dressing is a private task; encourage patient to participate as much as possible regardless of length of time needed. *Patients may be embarrassed when needing assistance to dress, so discreet help should be provided (Swann, 2011a).*
- • **QSEN** (Safety): Encourage patient to sit while dressing to reduce exertion and provide safety for poor balance or postural hypotension. *Dressing and undressing is a complex and tiring event that can be carried out from a seated position (Swann, 2011a).*
- • **QSEN** (Patient-Centered: Dress the affected side first, then the unaffected side; reverse the process for undressing. *Dressing the affected side first allows for easier manipulation of clothing (Swann, 2011a).*
- • **QSEN** (Patient-Centered): Use adaptive dressing and grooming equipment as needed (e.g., long-handled brushes, long grasping devices, button hooks, elastic shoelaces, Velcro shoes, soap-on-a-rope, suction holders). *Adaptive devices increase self-care ability and can decrease exertion (Swann, 2011b).*

Geriatric

- • **QSEN** (Patient-Centered): Offer residents choices in what to wear and ensure staff is trained to do so. *A controlled study by Schnelle et al (2013) provided training of nursing aides on how to offer long-term care residents (N = 169) morning care choices that resulted in increased frequency of choice being offered in timing for getting out of bed, clothing selection, and incontinence care.*
- • **QSEN** (Patient-Centered): Allow post-stroke patients who are cognitively impaired, especially if unimanual, to practice dressing. EB: *Fletcher-Smith et al (2012) found that bimanual cognitively impaired stroke survivors did better with dressing skills than those who are unimanual although with practice those with arm paresis improved significantly.*
- • **QSEN** (Patient-Centered): Maintain resident's individualized style in clothing as select adaptive clothing: loose clothing; elastic waistbands and cuffs; square, large arm holes; seamless or reversible clothing without a specific front or back; dresses that open down the back and short coats (for wheelchair users); Velcro fasteners; larger or magnetic buttons; zipper pulls for grasping; and absorbent scarves for drooling that can be easily changed. *Adapting clothing can make dressing easier for those with impaired mobility or fine motor skills and help prevent pressure sores (Swann, 2011b).*
- • **QSEN** (Patient-Centered): Lay clothing upon a contrasting color surface for patient selection. *Ensure patients can see clothing for selection by placing it on a contrasting surface (Swann, 2011a).*
- • **QSEN** (Patient-Centered): Inform patient that a winter coat with a funnel sleeve design can be easier to put on. EB: *Green et al (2011) found that older adults (N = 8) required less shoulder range of motion in putting on a winter coat with a funnel sleeve design, which could reduce social isolation in winter.*
- • Use clocks and explanations for the client with dementia to convey that it is morning and time to get ready for the day's activities by dressing. *Clients with memory issues can be assisted to establish a routine for dressing by (Swann, 2011a).*
- • Lay clothing out (with label in back facing up) in the order that it will be put on by the client, either one item at a time or in piles with first item on top of pile. *Clients with dementia may have difficulty recognizing what a clothing item is and in what order and how to put it on (Swann, 2011a).*

S

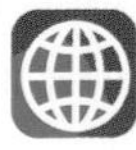

Multicultural

- • Consider use of assistive technology versus personal care assistance for Native Americans. CEB: *Older American Indians use more assistive technology for assistance with ADLs than the general same-age population (Goins et al, 2010).*

Home Care

- • **QSEN** (Patient-Centered): Teach assisted living staff the philosophy and methods to increase resident participation in dressing. EBN: *Staff awareness and knowledge increased significantly after a training program to encourage residents to participate more in dressing themselves (Walker et al, 2013).*
- • **QSEN** (Patient-Centered): Refer and encourage patients to participate in occupational therapy home rehabilitation programs. EB: *A case study revealed that rehabilitation in the home setting showed significant*

functional improvement over inpatient rehabilitation, with the client reporting more empowerment in the home setting (Lackie & Bisset, 2012).

Client/Family Teaching and Discharge Planning

- **QSEN** (Patient-Centered): Assess previously independent patients upon hospital admission for risk factors for new-onset disability that will require assistance with ADLs to plan preventive disability care and/or discharge care. EB: *Mehta et al (2011) found that a clinical index can identify previously independent hospitalized older adults for new onset disability: age older than 80 years, dependence in three or more IADLs 2 weeks before admission, mobility 2 weeks before admission, dependent for 2 or more ADLs, metastatic cancer or stroke, severe cognitive impairment, albumin less than 3 g/dL.*
- ▲ **QSEN** (Patient-Centered): Request referral for occupational therapy for clients who have had a stroke for dressing rehabilitation. EB: *A descriptive study of energy expenditure of upper and lower body dressing in clients after stroke (N = 23) found that more energy was used to dress the upper body and length of time to dress was four times longer than in the control group (Singh et al, 2011).*

REFERENCES

De Wit, L., Putman, K., Devos, H., et al. (2014). Long-term prediction of functional outcome after stroke using single items of the Barthel Index at discharge from rehabilitation centre. *Disability & Rehabilitation*, *36*(5), 353–358.

Fletcher-Smith, J., Walker, M. F., & Drummond, A. (2012). The influence of hand use on dressing outcome in cognitively impaired stroke survivors. *British Journal of Occupational Therapy*, *75*(1), 2–9.

Fodeh, S. J., Lazenby, M., Bai, M., et al. (2013). Functional impairments as symptoms in the symptom cluster analysis of patients newly diagnosed with advanced cancer. *Journal of Pain & Symptom Management*, *46*(4), 500–510.

Green, S., Boger, J., & Mihailidis, A. (2011). Toward enabling winter occupations: testing a winter coat designed for older adults. *Canadian Journal of Occupational Therapy*, *78*(1), 57–64.

Goins, R. T., et al. (2010). Assistive technology use of older American Indians in a southeastern tribe: the native elder care study. *Journal of the American Geriatrics Society*, *58*(11), 2185–2190.

Köybaşi, M., Ayhan, F., Borman, P., et al. (2011). Problems of self-care activities encountered in rheumatoid arthritis and their relationship with disease activity and hand deformity. *Turkish Journal of Rheumatology (Turkish League Against Rheumatism/Turkiye Romatizma Arastirma Ve Savas Dernegi)*, *26*(2), 89–93.

Lackie, R., & Bisset, L. (2012). The power of home rehabilitation: a single case study. *International Journal of Therapy & Rehabilitation [serial online]*, *19*(12), 697–703.

Mehta, K. M., Pierluissi, E., Boscardin, W. J., et al. (2011). A clinical index to stratify hospitalized older adults according to risk for new-onset disability. *Journal of the American Geriatrics Society*, *59*(7), 1206–1216.

Schnelle, J. F., Rahman, A., Durkin, D. W., et al. (2013). A controlled trial of an intervention to increase resident choice in long term care. *Journal of the American Medical Directors Association*, *14*(5), 345–351.

Singh, A., Stewart, A., Franzsen, D., et al. (2011). Energy expenditure of dressing in patients with stroke. *International Journal of Therapy & Rehabilitation*, *18*(12), 683–693.

Swann, J. I. (2011a). Managing dressing after having a stroke. *Nursing & Residential Care*, *13*(5), 219–221.

Swann, J. (2011b). Helping residents who struggle to dress. *Nursing & Residential Care*, *13*(12), 598–601.

Walker, B. L., Harrington, S. S., & Cole, C. S. (2013). Teaching philosophy and methods of restorative care to assisted living owners and staff. *Educational Gerontology*, *39*(1), 28–36.

Feeding Self-Care deficit *Linda S. Williams, RN, MSN*

NANDA-I

Definition

Impaired ability to perform or complete self-feeding activities

Defining Characteristics

Impaired ability to bring food to the mouth; impaired ability to chew food; impaired ability to get food onto utensils; impaired ability to handle utensils; impaired ability to manipulate food in mouth; impaired ability to open containers; impaired ability to pick up cup; impaired ability to prepare food; impaired ability to self-feed a complete meal; impaired ability to self-feed in an acceptable manner; impaired ability to swallow food; impaired ability to swallow sufficient amount of food; impaired ability to use assistive device

Related Factors (r/t)

Alteration in cognitive functioning; anxiety; decrease in motivation; discomfort; environmental barrier; fatigue; musculoskeletal impairment; neuromuscular impairment; pain; perceptual impairment weakness

NOTE: Specify level of independence using a standardized functional scale.

NOC (Nursing Outcomes Classification)

Suggested NOC Outcomes

Self-Care: Activities of Daily Living (ADLs), Eating

Example NOC Outcome with Indicators

Self-Care: Eating as evidenced by the following indicators: Opens containers/Uses utensils/Completes a meal. (Rate the outcome and indicators of **Self-Care: Eating:** 1 = severely compromised, 2 = substantially compromised, 3 = moderately compromised, 4 = mildly compromised, 5 = not compromised [see Section I].)

Client Outcomes

Client Will (Specify Time Frame)

- Feed self safely and effectively
- State satisfaction with ability to use adaptive devices for feeding
- Use assistance with feeding when necessary (caregiver)

NIC (Nursing Interventions Classification)

Suggested NIC Intervention

Self-Care Assistance: Feeding

Example NIC Activities—Self-Care Assistance: Feeding

Provide adaptive devices to facilitate the client's feeding self (e.g., long handles, handle with large circumference, or small strap-on utensils), as needed; Provide frequent cueing and close supervision as appropriate

S

Nursing Interventions and *Rationales*

- **QSEN** (Safety): Consider assessment of patients in the intensive care unit (ICU) and stepdown patients or of patients with acute stroke for readiness of an oral diet with a 3-oz water swallow challenge by a trained provider. EB: *If a 3-oz water swallow challenge, administered by a trained provider to a patient in ICU or to a stepdown patient, is passed, then an individualized diet plan can be made safely (Leder et al, 2011).* EB: *Leder et al (2012) studied (N = 75) patients with acute stroke who were given a 90-mL water swallow challenge and found that specific oral diets could be successfully recommended after passing the 90-mL water swallow challenge.*
- **QSEN** (Patient-Centered): Conduct repeat structured observations of patients at mealtime after a stroke to detect patients with eating difficulties to prevent possible social and functional consequences. EBN: *In a longitudinal and comparative study (N = 36), Medin et al (2012) found eating difficulties continued among clients 3 months after stroke despite improvement in other physical functions, indicating that factors such as psychological well-being should be assessed.*

▲ **QSEN** (Patient-Centered): Develop an overriding guideline for assisted feeding so it is less dependent on a caregiver's own beliefs, time pressures, and organizational characteristics. EBN: *Martinsen and Norlyk (2012a) conducted a qualitative study interviewing caregivers (N = 12) on their experience with assisted feeding and found a focus on nutrition blended with their own beliefs and societal norms about eating.*

▲ **QSEN** (Patient-Centered): Prioritize assisted feeding as important in a caregiver's assignment to allow adequate dedicated time to the activity. EBN: *The experience of assisted feeding for clients with language impairment (N = 42) depends on the caregiver's availability and goal for efficiency rather than the relational and affective aspects of meals, which institutions could address with flexible feeding assistance times that are free from other responsibilities (Martinsen & Norlyk, 2012b).*

▲ **QSEN** (Teamwork and Collaboration): Give priority to continuity in the cooperation between the parties involved in assisted feeding for those who are completely dependent. CEBN: *The continuity in the cooperation between the parties involved in assisted feeding is significant in creating a new eating pattern (Martinsen et al, 2008).*

• **QSEN** (Patient-Centered): Consult patient on the benefit or desire to use assistive devices for feeding. CEBN: *The value of a particular assistive device can only be determined by the patient, who may feel that it is insulting (Martinsen et al 2008).*

• **QSEN** (Safety): Presentation of feeding: provide 1 teaspoon of solid food or 10 to 15 mL of liquid at a time; wait until patient has swallowed the prior food/liquid. CEB: *Feeding large volumes and feeding quickly occurred commonly because caregivers lacked knowledge that this could exacerbate dysphagia and increase the risk of health problems (Pelletier, 2004).* EBN: *For a water swallow to accurately identify dysphagia, it is critical to administer 10 teaspoons (Martino et al, 2014).*

• **QSEN** (Safety): Ensure oral care is provided to all patients regardless of type of feeding. EBN: *Patients receiving tube feedings had inferior oral hygiene in comparison to those receiving oral feeding, creating a higher risk for aspiration pneumonia for patients receiving tube feedings (Maeda et al, 2011).*

Geriatric

• **QSEN** (Safety): Assess for tooth loss in older patients prior to feeding. EB: *Tooth loss contributes to swallowing difficulties that can increase risk of aspiration in the older patient (Okamoto et al, 2012).*

• **QSEN** (Patient-Centered): Assess the ability of patients with dementia to self-feed, and supervise the feeding of those with moderate dependency by providing verbal or physical assistance. CEBN: *Although low-dependency patients can self-feed, and those with severe dependency are fed, food intake among residents with moderate dependence is often ignored (Lin et al, 2010).*

• **QSEN** (Patient-Centered): Implement Montessori interventions for patients with dementia who have eating problems, such as playing music to signal learning session start for hand-eye coordination, scooping, pouring, and squeezing activities. EBN: *In an experimental crossover design, Lin et al (2011) confirmed that use of a Montessori intervention method for those with dementia helps maintain self-feeding ability and can reduce caregiver feeding frequency.*

▲ **QSEN** (Patient-Centered): Reduce interruptions during mealtimes and provide additional feeding assistance for older patients, especially those with cognitive impairment. EB: *Additional assistance with feeding and protected mealtimes while hospitalized can improve nutritional intake in older clients (Young et al, 2013).*

• **QSEN** (Patient-Centered): Use high-calorie oral supplements for patients with advanced dementia. EB: *Desirable weight gain has been shown with the use of high-calorie oral supplements in patients with dementia who have feeding problems (Hanson et al, 2011).*

S

• **QSEN** (Patient-Centered): Provide nutritional supplement drinks in a glass to older adults with cognitive impairment. EBN: *Allen et al (2014) conducted a non-blind randomized control trial that identified that the best method to provide nutritional supplement drinks to older adults with cognitive impairment is in a glass/beaker rather than using a straw in the container.*

• **QSEN** (Patient-Centered): Allow a resident an average of 42 minutes of staff time per meal and 13 minutes per between-meal snack to improve oral intake. CEB: *When these time frames are provided for staff to assist with meals and snacks, improved oral intake and weight gain in residents at risk for weight loss results (Simmons et al, 2008).*

• **QSEN** (Patient-Centered): Discuss meaningful life topics, as identified by family members, with residents with dementia during mealtimes. EB: *Cleary et al (2012) found that conversations during meals that generated reminiscence may improve food intake during the reminiscence state for residents with dementia.*

• **QSEN** (Patient-Centered): Encourage family visits at mealtimes for patients with dementia. EB: *Family participation at mealtimes increased feeding assistance and helped promote satisfactory adaptation to the nursing home environment, Durkin et al (2014) found in a study of 74 residents and their visitors during mealtimes.*

• **QSEN** (Patient-Centered): Play familiar music during meals for clients with dementia. EB: *Agitation often increases at mealtimes in patients with dementia, which music seems to reduce (Whear et al, 2014).*

• Use aromatherapy with the smell of baking bread for those with dementia. CEB: *The smell of baking bread increased intake of food and self-feeding in those with dementia (Cleary et al, 2008).*

▲ **QSEN** (Teamwork and Collaboration): Provide feeding training and education programs for nursing home staff. EBN: *Wen et al (2014) did a systematic review of the literature about interventions for mealtime* *difficulties in older adults with dementia and found that training and education programs for professionals demonstrated moderate evidence to increase eating time and decrease feeding difficulty.*

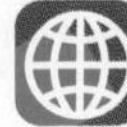

Multicultural

- **QSEN** (Patient-Centered): For those with impaired hand function who use chopsticks, suggest adapted chopsticks. CEB: *In a pilot equipment study, adapted chopsticks, which can be inexpensive and easily constructed, for those with lower cervical spinal cord injury and residual gross grasp were found to convert gross grasp into 2-point pinch (Chang et al, 2006).*
- **QSEN** (Patient-Centered): Use the simplified Chinese Edinburgh Feeding Evaluation in Dementia scale to measure feeding problems in people with dementia from Mainland China and other Chinese cultural groups. EBN: *Identifying patient behaviors during feeding allows development of effective interventions for feeding (Liu et al, 2014).*

Home Care

- **QSEN** (Teamwork and Collaboration): Request referral for physical therapy and occupational therapy to assess client's ability to position and self-feed and provide client and caregiver support with feeding. EB: *Ingestive skill difficulties are frequent among acutely-hospitalized frail elderly patients (Hansen et al, 2012).*

Client/Family Teaching and Discharge Planning

- **QSEN** (Teamwork and Collaboration): Discuss with family caregivers, who are involved in the feeding of a family member with advanced dementia, the feeding experience to provide support to ensure that the mealtime purpose is preserved. EBN: *Lopez et al (2011) in a phenomenological study interviewed family caregivers (N = 16) of those with advanced dementia who indicated that the feeding assistance experience was like living in a time warp with an uncertain future.*

▲ **QSEN** (Patient-Centered): Educate family members that neither insertion of a feeding tube nor timing of its insertion affects client survival for those with advanced dementia who have eating problems. EB: *Teno et al (2012) studied all nursing home residents with advanced dementia who had eating problems from 1999 to 2007 (N = 36,492) and found that survival was not affected by insertion of or timing of insertion of a percutaneous endoscopic gastrostomy feeding tube.*

REFERENCES

Allen, V. J., Methven, L., & Gosney, M. (2014). Impact of serving method on the consumption of nutritional supplement drinks: randomized trial in older adults with cognitive impairment. *Journal of Advanced Nursing, 70*(6), 1323–1333.

Chang, B., Huang, B., Chou, C., et al. (2006). A new type of chopsticks for patients with impaired hand function. *Archives of Physical Medicine & Rehabilitation, 87*(7), 1013–1015.

Cleary, S., Hopper, T., & Van Soest, D. (2012). Reminiscence therapy, mealtimes and improving intake in residents with dementia. *Canadian Nursing Home, 23*(2), 8–13.

Cleary, S., Van Soest, D., Milke, D., et al. (2008). Using the smell of baking bread to facilitate eating in residents with dementia. *Canadian Nursing Home, 19*(1), 6.

Durkin, D. W., Shotwell, M. S., & Simmons, S. F. (2014). The impact of family visitation on feeding assistance quality in nursing homes. *Journal of Applied Gerontology, 33*(5), 586–602.

Hanson, L. C., Ersek, M., Gilliam, R., et al. (2011). Oral feeding options for people with dementia: a systematic review. *Journal of the American Geriatrics Society, 59*(3), 463–472.

Hansen, T., Lambert, H. C., & Faber, J. (2012). Ingestive skill difficulties are frequent among acutely-hospitalized frail elderly patients, and predict hospital outcomes. *Physical & Occupational Therapy in Geriatrics, 30*(4), 271–287.

Leder, S. B., Suiter, D. M., Warner, H. L., et al. (2012). Success of recommending oral diets in acute stroke patients based on passing a 90-cc water swallow challenge protocol. *Topics in Stroke Rehabilitation, 19*(1), 40–44.

Leder, S., Suiter, D., Warner, H., et al. (2011). Initiating safe oral feeding in critically ill intensive care and step-down unit patients based on passing a 3-ounce (90 milliliters) water swallow challenge. *Journal of Trauma, 70*(5), 1203–1207.

Lin, L., Huang, Y., Watson, R., et al. (2011). Using a Montessori method to increase eating ability for institutionalised residents with dementia: a crossover design. *Journal of Clinical Nursing, 20*(21/22), 3092–3101.

Lin, L., Watson, R., & Wu, S. (2010). What is associated with low food intake in older people with dementia? *Journal of Clinical Nursing, 19*(1–2), 53–59.

Liu, W., Watson, R., & Lou, F. (2014). The Edinburgh feeding evaluation in dementia scale (EdFED): cross-cultural validation of the simplified Chinese version in mainland China. *Journal of Clinical Nursing, 23*(1/2), 45–53.

Lopez, R. P., & Amella, E. J. (2011). Time travel: the lived experience of providing feeding assistance to a family member with dementia. *Research in Gerontological Nursing, 4*(2), 127–134.

Maeda, E., Nakamoto, S., Ikeda, T., et al. (2011). Oral microorganisms in the homebound elderly: a comparison between oral feeding and tube feeding. *Journal of Japan Academy of Nursing Science, 31*(2), 34–41.

Martino, R., Maki, E., & Diamant, N. (2014). Identification of dysphagia using the toronto bedside swallowing screening test: are 10 teaspoons of water necessary? *International Journal of Speech-Language Pathology, 16*(3), 193–198.

Martinsen, B., Harder, I., & Biering-Sorensen, F. (2008). The meaning of assisted feeding for people living with spinal cord injury: a phenomenological study. *Journal of Advanced Nursing*, *62*(5), 533–540.
Martinsen, B., & Norlyk, A. (2012a). Caregivers' lived experience of assisted feeding. *Journal of Clinical Nursing*, *21*(19/20), 2966–2974.
Martinsen, B., & Norlyk, A. (2012b). Observations of assisted feeding among people with language impairment. *Journal of Clinical Nursing*, *21*(19/20), 2949–2957.
Medin, J., Windahl, J., von Arbin, M., et al. (2012). Eating difficulties among patients 3 months after stroke in relation to the acute phase. *Journal of Advanced Nursing*, *68*(3), 580–589.
Okamoto, N., Tomioka, K., Saeki, K., et al. (2012). Relationship between swallowing problems and tooth loss in community-dwelling independent elderly adults: the Fujiwara-Kyo study. *Journal of the American Geriatrics Society*, *60*(5), 849–853.
Pelletier, C. (2004). What do certified nurse assistants actually know about dysphagia and feeding nursing home residents? *American Journal of Speech-language Pathology*, *13*(2), 99–113.
Simmons, S. F., Keeler, E., Zhuo, X., et al. (2008). Prevention of unintentional weight loss in nursing home residents: a controlled trial of feeding assistance. *Journal of American Geriatric Society*, *56*(8), 1466–1473.
Teno, J. M., Gozalo, P. L., Mitchell, S. L., et al. (2012). Does feeding tube insertion and its timing improve survival? *Journal of the American Geriatrics Society*, *60*(10), 1918–1921.
Wen, L., Jooyoung, C., & Thomas, S. A. (2014). Interventions on mealtime difficulties in older adults with dementia: a systematic review. *International Journal of Nursing Studies*, *51*(1), 14–27.
Whear, R., Abbott, R., Thompson-Coon, J., et al. (2014). Effectiveness of mealtime interventions on behavior symptoms of people with dementia living in care homes: a systematic review. *Journal of the American Medical Directors Association*, *15*(3), 185–193.
Young, A. M., Mudge, A. M., Banks, M. D., et al. (2013). Encouraging, assisting and time to EAT: improved nutritional intake for older medical patients receiving protected mealtimes and/or additional nursing feeding assistances. *Clinical Nutrition*, *32*(4), 543–549.

Toileting Self-Care deficit

Linda S. Williams, RN, MSN

NANDA-I

Definition

Impaired ability to perform or complete self-toileting activities

Defining Characteristics

Impaired ability to complete toilet hygiene; impaired ability to flush toilet; impaired ability to manipulate clothing for toileting; impaired ability to reach toilet; impaired ability to rise from toilet; impaired ability to sit on toilet

Related Factors (r/t)

Alteration in cognitive functioning; anxiety; decrease in motivation; environmental barrier; fatigue; impaired ability to transfer; impaired mobility; musculoskeletal impairment; neuromuscular impairment; pain; perceptual impairment; weakness

S

NOC (Nursing Outcomes Classification)

Suggested NOC Outcomes

Self-Care: Activities of Daily Living (ADLs), Toileting

Example NOC Outcome with Indicators

Self-Care: Toileting as evidenced by the following indicators: Responds to full bladder and urge to have a bowel movement in a timely manner/Gets to toilet between urge and passage of urine/between urge and evacuation of stool. (Rate the outcome and indicators of **Self-Care: Toileting:** 1 = severely compromised, 2 = substantially compromised, 3 = moderately compromised, 4 = mildly compromised, 5 = not compromised [see Section I].)

Client Outcomes

Client Will (Specify Time Frame)

- Remain free of incontinence and impaction with no urine or stool on skin
- State satisfaction with ability to use adaptive devices for toileting
- Explain and demonstrate use of methods to be safe and independent in toileting

NIC (Nursing Interventions Classification)

Suggested NIC Interventions

Environmental Management; Self-Care Assistance: Toileting

Example NIC Activities—Self-Care Assistance: Toileting

Assist client to toilet/commode/bedpan/fracture pan/urinal at specified intervals; Institute a toileting schedule, as appropriate

Nursing Interventions and *Rationales*

- **QSEN** (Safety): Assess patients for fall risk using established and valid fall risk assessment tools (Morse, Heindrich) and implement fall prevention interventions for those at risk for falling or in physical restraints. EBN: *In a retrospective study of 3 years of acute care fall incident reports (N = 547), Huey-Ming and Chang-Yi (2012) found 45.2% of falls were related to toileting and that predictors of toileting-related falls were having a previous fall, being physically restrained, and being a fall risk.*
- **QSEN** (Patient-Centered): Assess patient's prior use of incontinence briefs and avoid use for hospitalized continent but limited mobility patient. EBN: *Use of adult incontinence briefs for low-mobility continent clients versus self-toileting occurs more frequently for females and can be associated with adverse outcomes (Zisberg, 2011).*
- **QSEN** (Patient-Centered): Assess patients who have had sphincter-saving surgery for self-care strategies to manage bowel symptoms in order to help support these strategies. EBN: *In a quantitative descriptive study of self-care strategies used by patients who had sphincter-saving surgery and bowel symptoms (N = 143), the strategy of proximity and knowing the location of a toilet at all times was used most by those with more bowel symptoms (Landers et al, 2014).*
- **QSEN** (Safety): Make assistance call button readily available to the client and answer call light promptly. CEBN: *Falls often occur related to toileting, and individualized planning for safe transfer to toilet is essential to safety (Tzeng, 2010).*
- **QSEN** (Safety): Provide folding commode chairs in client bathrooms/at bedside. EBN: *Availability of a folding commode chair as part of a fall prevention program can increase accessibility and efficiency in patient care (Tzeng, 2011).*
- **QSEN** (Patient-Centered): Before use of a bedpan, discuss its use with clients. CEBN: *When nurses facilitate discussion about bedpan use with orthopedic patients, they may be less anxious about its use (Cohen, 2009).*
- **QSEN** (Patient-Centered): Use necessary assistive toileting equipment. EB: *Amyotrophic lateral sclerosis clients reported satisfaction and usefulness of all bathroom assistive technology such as elevated toilet seat and arm rails by the toilet (Gruis et al, 2011).*
- **QSEN** (Safety): Close toilet lid before flushing toilet and teach patient to do so. EB: *A literature review of studies of toilet plume aerosols found that potential infectious aerosols during toilet flushing are produced, which can continue to expose toilet users later when some of the aerosols become droplet nuclei in air currents (Johnson et al, 2013).* EB: *A study revealed viral contamination of aerosol and surfaces through toilet use (Verani et al, 2014).*

Geriatric

- Assess residents without dementia for risk factors associated with toileting disability: rating health as fair or poor, living in a residence with four or less residents or that is for-profit, incontinence, physical, visual or hearing impairment, and need for ADL or transferring assistance, to guide prevention interventions. EBN: *In a cross-sectional analysis of adults 65 years or older without dementia in residential care facilities (N = 2395), 15% were found to have toileting disability that was associated with rating health as fair or poor, living in a residence with four or fewer residents or that is for-profit, incontinence, physical, visual, or hearing impairment, and need for ADL or transferring assistance (Talley et al, 2014).*
- **QSEN** (Patient-Centered): Consider use of urine alarms systems for patients with dementias. EB: *Caregivers preferred use of urine alarms over time toileting to reduce urinary accidents (Lancioni et al, 2011).*
- **QSEN** (Patient-Centered): Assess the patient's functional ability to manipulate clothing for toileting, and if necessary modify clothing with Velcro fasteners, elastic waists, drop-front underwear, or slacks. *For*

S

clients with impaired dexterity or weakness, wearing dresses, athletic bottoms, or skirts with a stretch waistband makes it easier to use the toilet than wearing clothing with buttons and zippers (Cohen, 2008).

- **QSEN** (Patient-Centered): Provide patients with dementia access to regular exercise. EBN: *ADL performance improved with a regular exercise program of stretching, walking, and leg weight bearing (Chang et al, 2011).*

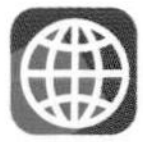

Multicultural

- **QSEN** (Patient-Centered): Remove barriers to toileting, support patient's cultural beliefs, and preserve dignity. CEB: *The physical and sociocultural environments in long-term care require older patients to overcome greater physical and cognitive challenges to maintain their participation, autonomy, and dignity in toileting than if they were at home (Sacco-Peterson & Borell, 2004).*

Home Care

- **QSEN** (Patient-Centered): To design a bathroom for an older adult, consider adaptable bath fixtures/furniture and safety needs. EB: *Poor bathroom design requires use of assistive adaptive devices, reduces quality of life, and contributes to safety concerns such as falls (Burton et al, 2011).*

Client/Family Teaching and Discharge Planning

- Teach men who perform routine clean intermittent catheterization that a 40-cm intermittent catheter was found to provide ease of use, instill confidence in bladder emptying, and draining of urine into a receptacle. EB: *Costa et al (2013) found in a randomized controlled study of self-catheterizing wheelchair-using men (N = 81) that a 40-cm intermittent catheter was preferred over one that was 30 cm.*
- Have the family install a toilet seat of a contrasting color. CEB: *Visualization of the toilet is aided by installing a toilet seat of a contrasting color (Gerdner et al, 2002).*
- Explain to family and caregivers of clients with dementia that toilet self-care activities decrease when self-awareness is lost. *An observational study of toileting self-care in older adults with dementia revealed that toilet activities are affected and decline when self-awareness is lost (composed of theory of mind, self-evaluation, and self-consciousness) (Uchimoto et al, 2013).*

REFERENCES

Burton, M., Reed, H., & Chamberlain, P. (2011). Age-related disability and bathroom use. *International Journal of Integrated Care, 19*(1), 37–43.

Chang, S. H., Chen, C. Y., Shen, S. H., et al. (2011). The effectiveness of an exercise programme for elders with dementia in a Taiwanese day-care centre. *International Journal of Nursing Practice, 17*(3), 213–220.

Cohen, D. (2008). Providing an assist. *Rehabilitation Management, 21*(8), 16–19.

Cohen, S. (2009). Orthopaedic patient's perceptions of using a bed pan. *Journal of Orthopedic Nursing, 13*(2), 78–84.

Costa, J. A., Menier, M., Doran, T. J., et al. (2013). Catheter length preference in wheelchair-using men who perform routine clean intermittent catheterization. *Spinal Cord, 51*(10), 772–775.

Gerdner, L. A., Buckwalter, K. C., & Reed, D. (2002). Impact of a psychoeducational intervention on caregiver response to behavioral problems. *Nursing Research, 51*(6), 363.

Gruis, K., Wren, P., & Huggins, J. (2011). Amyotrophic lateral sclerosis patients' self-reported satisfaction with assistive technology. *Muscle and Nerve, 43*(5), 643–647.

Huey-Ming, T., & Chang-Yi, Y. (2012). Toileting-related inpatient falls in adult acute care settings. *Medsurg Nursing, 21*(6), 372–377.

Johnson, D. L., Mead, K. R., Lynch, R. A., et al. (2013). Lifting the lid on toilet plume aerosol: a literature review with suggestions for future research. *American Journal of Infection Control, 41*(3), 254–258.

Lancioni, G., Singh, N., O'Reilly, M., et al. (2011). Persons with mild or moderate Alzheimer's disease learn to use urine alarms and prompts to avoid large urinary accidents. *Research in Developmental Disabilities, 32*(5), 1998–2004.

Landers, M., McCarthy, G., Livingstone, V., et al. (2014). Patients' bowel symptom experiences and self-care strategies following sphincter-saving surgery for rectal cancer. *Journal of Clinical Nursing, 23*(15/16), 2343–2354.

Sacco-Peterson, M., & Borell, L. (2004). Struggles for autonomy in self-care: the impact of the physical and socio-cultural environment in a long-term care setting. *Scandinavian Journal of Caring Science, 18*(4), 376–386.

Talley, K. C., Wyman, J. F., Bronas, U. G., et al. (2014). Factors associated with toileting disability in older adults without dementia living in residential care facilities. *Nursing Research, 63*(2), 94–104.

Tzeng, H. (2010). Understanding the prevalence of inpatient falls associated with toileting in adult acute care settings. *Journal of Nursing Care Quality, 25*(1), 22–30.

Tzeng, H. (2011). A feasibility study of providing folding commode chairs in patient bathrooms to reduce toilet-related falls in an adult acute medical-surgical unit. *Journal of Nursing Care Quality, 26*(1), 61–68.

Uchimoto, K., Yokoi, T., Yamashita, T., et al. (2013). Investigation of toilet activities in elderly patients with dementia from the viewpoint of motivation and self-awareness. *American Journal of Alzheimer's Disease & Other Dementias, 28*(5), 459–468.

Verani, M., Bigazzi, R., & Carducci, A. (2014). Viral contamination of aerosol and surfaces through toilet use in health care and other settings. *American Journal of Infection Control, 42*(7), 758–762.

Zisberg, A. (2011). Incontinence brief use in acute hospitalized patients with no prior incontinence. *Journal of Wound Ostomy Continence Nursing, 38*(5), 559–564.

Readiness for enhanced Self-Concept

Gail B. Ladwig, MSN, RN, and Marina Martinez-Kratz, RN, MS, CNE

NANDA-I

Definition

A pattern of perceptions or ideas about the self, which can be strengthened

Defining Characteristics

Acceptance of limitations; acceptance of strengths; actions are congruent with verbal expression; confidence in abilities; expresses desire to enhance role performance; expresses desire to enhance self-concept; satisfaction with body image; satisfaction with personal identity; satisfaction with sense of worth; satisfaction with thoughts about self

NOC (Nursing Outcomes Classification)

Suggested NOC Outcomes

Self-Esteem; Personal Well-Being; Psychosocial Adjustment Life Change

Example NOC Outcome with Indicators

Self-Esteem as evidenced by the following indicators: Verbalizations of self-acceptance/Open communication/Confidence level/ Description of pride in self. (Rate the outcome and indicators of **Self-Esteem:** 1 = never positive, 2 = rarely positive, 3 = sometimes positive, 4 = often positive, 5 = consistently positive [see Section I].)

Client Outcomes

Client Will (Specify Time Frame)

- State willingness to enhance self-concept
- State satisfaction with thoughts about self, sense of worthiness, role performance, body image, and personal identity
- Demonstrate actions that are congruent with expressed feelings and thoughts
- State confidence in abilities
- Accept strengths and limitations

S

NIC (Nursing Interventions Classification)

Suggested NIC Intervention

Self-Esteem Enhancement

Example NIC Activities—Self-Esteem Enhancement

Encourage client to identify strengths; Assist client in setting realistic goals to achieve higher self-esteem

Nursing Interventions and *Rationales*

- Assess and support activities that promote developmental self-concept. EB: *Early identification of developmental coordination disorder and associated negative outcomes, also based on child's self-reports, should receive special attention in intervention programs in order to enhance children's self-confidence, feelings of belonging, optimal development, and participation in daily activities (Engel-Yeger & Hanna Kasis, 2010).*
- Engage client in relaxation training. EB: *Results indicate that relaxation training is a useful clinical intervention for clients who have breast cancer and who are experiencing low self-esteem (Kovačič & Kovačič, 2011).*

- Refer to nutritional and exercise programs to support weight loss. CEB: *Changes in weight using a community wellness center with exercise and nutrition information resulted in body satisfaction and an increase in the physical self-concept scale (Annesi, 2007).*
- Refer clients to massage therapy as an adjunct treatment. CEB: *Clients with advanced cancer who received six 30-minute massages over 2 weeks reported less pain and improved mood after each session (Kutner et al, 2008).*
- Refer homeless clients to work skills training programs. EB: *Research found that homeless clients that completed a work skills training program had improvements in self-esteem and self-efficacy, which also predicted stable housing situations at follow-up (Nelson et al, 2012).*
- Refer clients receiving government assistance to Welfare to Work programs. EBN: *Participants who participated in a Work Wellness program credited the program with decreasing negative thoughts and improving self-esteem (Martin et al, 2012).*
- Support establishing church-based community health promotion programs with the following key elements: partnerships, positive health values, availability of services, access to church facilities, community-focused interventions, health behavior change, and supportive social relationships. EB: *This study supported that "spiritual dwelling" (students at Protestant University) is associated with well-being (Jankowski & Sandage, 2012).*

▲ For clients who have had breast surgery and need a prosthesis, provide the appropriate prosthesis before the client leaves the health care facility. EBN: *A good-quality external breast prosthesis and prosthesis-fitting service is an integral part of the recovery process after mastectomy (Gallagher et al, 2010).*

- Offer client choices in clothing while client is hospitalized. CEBN: *Client clothes were experienced as being comfortable and practical, but also as being stigmatizing symbols of illness, confinement, and depersonalization (Edvardsson, 2009).*

▲ Refer clients with history of childhood sexual abuse for intensive therapy that uses narrative life stories to promote positive sense of self. *The participants in this study of women with a history of childhood sexual abuse experienced a more positive sense of self after being in the program (Saha et al, 2011).*

Pediatric

- Consider the development of a Healthy Kids Mentoring Program that has four components: (1) relationship building, (2) self-esteem enhancement, (3) goal setting, and (4) academic assistance (tutoring). Mentors met with students twice each week for 1 hour each session on school grounds. During each meeting, mentors devoted time to each program component. CEB: *The Healthy Kids Mentoring Program results indicated that students' overall self-esteem, school connectedness, peer connectedness, and family connectedness were significantly higher at posttest than at pretest (Kelly et al, 2011).*
- Provide activities to bolster physical self-concept. EB: *Research indicates that physical self-concept acts a moderator for negative events in a child's life (Nguyen & Scott, 2013).*

▲ Consider wheelchair dancing for disabled adolescents. EB: *A wheelchair dancing intervention was associated with an improvement in self-esteem among disabled adolescents (de Villiers et al, 2013).*

▲ Provide overweight adolescents to access to group-based weight control interventions. EB: *Findings demonstrate benefits of group-based weight-control treatment for enhancing adolescent self-perceived social functioning across multiple domains including self-concept (Jelalian et al, 2011).*

▲ Assess and provide referrals to mental health professionals for clients with unresolved worries associated with terrorism. EBN: *The National Association of Pediatric Nurse Practitioners initiated a national campaign titled Keep Your Children/Yourself Safe and Secure. Interventions are urgently needed to assist children and teens in coping with the multitude of stressors related to growing up in today's society (Melnyk et al, 2002).*

- Provide an alternative school-based program for pregnant and parenting teenagers. CEB: *The girls who attended this program developed close relationships with their peers and teachers. Many of them experienced academic success for the first time and reported that pregnancy and impending motherhood motivated them to do better in school (Spear, 2002).*

Geriatric

- Encourage clients to consider a web-based support program when they are in a caregiving situation. EBN: *Technology, such as telephone networks and the Internet, helps in supporting isolated and lonely older people. It helps to alleviate anxiety and increase self-confidence (Cattan et al, 2011).*

- Encourage activity and a strength, mobility, balance, and endurance training program. EB: *Participants in this physical activity program demonstrated increased self-worth (Huberty et al, 2008).*
- Provide opportunities for clients to engage in life skills (themed collections of everyday items based upon general activities that residents may have previously carried out). *Life skill centers offer residents a means of purposeful occupation in tasks that they have undertaken for decades using skills that are inherent and not forgotten (Swann, 2009).*
- Provide information on advance directives. EBN: *In this study elders stated that the optimal time for advance care planning was during periods of wellness. They are ready and eager to discuss advance planning (Malcomson & Bisbee, 2009).*
- Use an approach that reduces the emphasis put on "old age" self-concept attributions when working with older clients. EB: *Research found that older adult clients who attribute the onset of chronic illness (e.g., heart disease, cancer, diabetes) to old age predicted the experience of more perceived health symptoms (Stewart et al, 2012).*

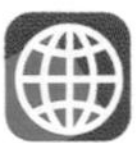

Multicultural

- Carefully assess each client and allow families to participate in providing care that is acceptable based on the client's cultural beliefs. EBN: *An understanding of client suffering that is shaped by traditional cultural values helps nurses communicate empathy in a culturally sensitive manner to facilitate the therapeutic relationship and clinical outcomes (Hsiao et al, 2006). Spiritual well-being, the perception of health and wholeness, can boost self-confidence and self-esteem. These behaviors were demonstrated by older Amish in this study. This information will assist nurses in serving this population (Sharpnack et al, 2011).*
- Provide education and support for health-promoting behaviors and self-concept for clients from diverse cultures. EB: *This study of older adults in Korea demonstrated significant changes in self-esteem, depression, and social network after completing the Older Paraprofessional Training Program (Lee & Choi, 2012).*
- Refer to the care plans Disturbed **Body Image,** Readiness for enhanced **Coping,** Chronic low **Self-Esteem,** and Readiness for enhanced **Spiritual** well-being.

Home Care

- Previously discussed interventions may be used in the home care setting.

REFERENCES

S

Annesi, J. J. (2007). Relations of changes in exercise self-efficacy, physical self-concept, and body satisfaction with weight changes in obese white and African American women initiating a physical activity program. *Ethnicity and Disease*, *17*(1), 19–22.

Cattan, M., Kime, N., & Bagnall, A. (2011). The use of telephone befriending in low level support for socially isolated older people-an evaluation. *Health and Social Care in the Community*, *19*(2), 198–206.

de Villiers, D., van Rooyen, F. C., Beck, V. V., et al. (2013). Wheelchair dancing and self-esteem in adolescents with physical disabilities. *South African Journal of Occupational Therapy*, *43*(2), 23–27.

Edvardsson, D. (2009). Balancing between being a person and being a patient—a qualitative study of wearing patient clothing. *International Journal of Nursing Studies*, *46*(1), 4–11.

Engel-Yeger, B., & Hanna Kasis, A. (2010). The relationship between developmental co-ordination disorders, child's perceived self-efficacy and preference to participate in daily activities. *Child: Care, Health and Development*, *36*(5), 670–677.

Gallagher, P., et al. (2010). External breast prostheses in post-mastectomy care: women's qualitative accounts. *European Journal of Cancer Care*, *19*(1), 61–71.

Hsiao, F. H., et al. (2006). Cultural attribution of mental health suffering in Chinese societies: the views of Chinese patients with mental illness and their caregivers. *Journal of Clinical Nursing*, *15*(8), 998–1006.

Huberty, J. L., et al. (2008). Women bound to be active: a pilot study to explore the feasibility of an intervention to increase physical activity and self-worth in women. *Women's Health (Hillsdale, N.J.)*, *48*(1), 83–101.

Jankowski, P., & Sandage, S. (2012). Spiritual dwelling and well-being: the mediating role of differentiation of self in a sample of distressed adults. *Mental Health Religion & Culture*, *15*(4), 417–434.

Jelalian, E., Sato, A., & Hart, C. N. (2011). The effect of group-based weight-control intervention on adolescent psychosocial outcomes: perceived peer rejection, social anxiety, and self-concept. *Children's Health Care*, *40*(3), 197–211.

Kelly, S., et al. (2011). Correlates among healthy lifestyle cognitive beliefs, healthy lifestyle choices, social support, and healthy behaviors in adolescents: implications for behavioral change strategies and future research. *Journal of Pediatric Health Care*, *25*(4), 216–223.

Kovačič, T., & Kovačič, M. (2011). Impact of relaxation training according to Yoga in daily life system on self-esteem after breast cancer surgery. *Journal of Alternative & Complementary Medicine*, *17*(12), 1157–1164.

Kutner, J. S., et al. (2008). Massage therapy versus simple touch to improve pain and mood in patients with advanced cancer: a randomized trial. *Annals of Internal Medicine*, *149*(6), 369–379.

Lee, M., & Choi, J. S. (2012). Positive side effects of a job-related training program for older adults in South Korea. *Educational Gerontology*, *38*(1), 1–9.

Malcomson, H., & Bisbee, S. (2009). Perspectives of healthy elders on advance care planning. *Journal of the American Academy of Nurse Practitioners*, *21*(1), 18–23.

Martin, C., Keswick, J. L., Crayton, D., et al. (2012). Perceptions of self-esteem in a welfare-to-wellness-to-work program. *Public Health Nursing, 29*(1), 19–26.

Melnyk, B. M., et al. (2002). Mental health worries, communication, and needs in the year of the U.S. terrorist attack: national KySS survey findings. *Journal of Pediatric Health Care, 16*(5), 222.

Nelson, S., Gray, H., Maurice, I., et al. (2012). Moving ahead: evaluation of a work-skills training program for homeless adults. *Community Mental Health Journal, 48*(6), 711–722.

Nguyen, H. T., & Scott, A. N. (2013). Self-concept and depression among children who experienced the death of a family member. *Death Studies, 37*(3), 197–211.

Saha, S., Chung, M. C., & Thorne, L. (2011). A narrative exploration of the sense of self of women recovering from childhood sexual abuse. *Counselling Psychology Quarterly, 24*(2), 101–113.

Sharpnack, P., et al. (2011). Self-transcendence and spiritual well-being in the Amish. *Journal of Holistic Nursing, 29*(2), 91–97.

Spear, H. J. (2002). Reading, writing, and having babies: a nurturing alternative school program. *The Journal of School Nursing, 18*(5), 293.

Stewart, T. L., Chipperfield, J. G., Perry, R. P., et al. (2012). Attributing illness to 'old age:' Consequences of a self-directed stereotype for health and mortality. *Psychology & Health, 27*(8), 881–897.

Swann, J. (2009). Life-skill stations: tools for reminiscence and activity. *Nursing & Residential Care, 11*(2), 96–98.

Chronic low Self-Esteem

Gail B. Ladwig, MSN, RN; revised by Marina Martinez-Kratz, MS, RN, CNE

NANDA-I

Definition

Longstanding negative self-evaluating/feelings about self or self-capabilities

Defining Characteristics

Dependent on others' opinions; exaggerates negative feedback about self; excessive seeking of reassurance; guilt; hesitant to try new experiences; indecisive behavior; nonassertive behavior; overly conforming; passivity; poor eye contact; rejection of positive feedback; repeatedly unsuccessful in life events; shame; underestimates ability to deal with situation

Related Factors (r/t)

Cultural incongruence; exposure to traumatic situation; inadequate belonging; inadequate respect from others; ineffective coping with loss; insufficient group membership; psychiatric disorder; receiving insufficient affection; receiving insufficient approval from others; repeated failures; repeated negative reinforcement; spiritual incongruence

S

NOC (Nursing Outcomes Classification)

Suggested NOC Outcome

Self-Esteem

Example NOC Outcome with Indicators

Demonstrates improved **Self-Esteem** as evidenced by the following indicators: Verbalizations of acceptance of self and limitations/Open communication. (Rate the outcome and indicators of **Self-Esteem:** 1 = never positive, 2 = rarely positive, 3 = sometimes positive, 4 = often positive, 5 = consistently positive [see Section I].)

Client Outcomes

Client Will (Specify Time Frame)

- Demonstrate improved ability to interact with others (e.g., maintains eye contact, engages in conversation, expresses thoughts/feelings)
- Verbalize increased self-acceptance through positive self-statements about self
- Identify personal strengths, accomplishments, and values
- Identify and work on small, achievable goals
- Improve independent decision-making and problem-solving skills

NIC (Nursing Interventions Classification)

Suggested NIC Intervention

Self-Esteem Enhancement

Example NIC Activities—Self-Esteem Enhancement

Encourage patient to identify strengths; Assist in setting realistic goals to achieve higher self-esteem

Nursing Interventions and *Rationales*

- Actively listen to and respect the client. EBN: *Listening and nurturing are important aspects of care (Parrish et al, 2008).* EB: *This study described active listening as essential in uncovering patients' emotions (Del Piccolo et al, 2014).*
- Assess the client's environmental and everyday stressors, including physical health concerns and the potential for abusive relationships. EBN: *It is difficult to determine whether a woman's depressive symptoms are related to physical abuse or to other risk factors (Al-Modallal et al, 2008).* EB: *Findings in this study suggest that early adverse conditions have lasting implications for physical health and that continued exposure to increased levels of both social and nonsocial stress in adolescence, as well as the presence of depression, might be important mechanisms by which early adversity impacts later physical health (Raposa et al, 2014).*
- Assess existing strengths and coping abilities, and provide opportunities for their expression and recognition. CEB: *Supporting a client's beliefs and self-reflection and helping him/her cope can affect self-esteem (Räty & Gustaffson, 2006). Persons with psychiatric illness need help to stop their "negative self-image" and become more conscious of affirmative self-evaluation (Kunikata, 2010).*
- Assess the client's self-esteem using valid and established tools like the Rosenberg Self-Esteem Scale. EBN: *The use of valid and established measures of self-esteem will facilitate the identification of appropriate nursing interventions that strengthen self-esteem (McMullen & Resnick, 2013).*
- Reinforce the personal strengths and positive self-perceptions that a client identifies. EB: *In this study of clients with spinal cord injury, clients attributed their success in rehabilitation to positive self-esteem (Belciug, 2012).*
- Identify client's negative self-assessments. EBN: *Body-esteem and self-esteem are significantly related to one another (Jones et al, 2008).*
- Encourage realistic and achievable goal setting and resources and identify impediments to achievement. CEB: *This promotes self-acceptance, which is associated with psychological well-being (Macinnes, 2006).*
- Demonstrate and promote effective communication techniques; spend time with the client. EBN: *Presence and caring during communication are important (Mantha et al, 2008).*
- Encourage independent decision-making by reviewing options and their possible consequences with client. EBN: *Decision-making capacity is vital to a sense of autonomy (Burke et al, 2008).*
- Assist client to challenge negative perceptions of self and performance. CEBN: *Reduction in negative thinking will increase self-esteem (Day & Deutsch, 2004).*
- Use failure as an opportunity to provide valuable feedback. CEB: *This allows clients to change expectations of what would happen given the reality of what did happen (Pierce & Hicks, 2001).*
- Promote maintaining a level of functioning in the community. EB: *Driving cessation is one factor associated with increased depressive symptoms and decreased social integration among older adults (Mezuk & Rebok, 2008).*
- Assist client with evaluating the effect of family and peer group on feelings of self-worth. EBN: *Nurses are encouraged to actively assess the condition of social contacts among older adults in their care and to assist in strengthening relationships with family members and others (Yao et al, 2008).*
- Support socialization and communication skills. EBN: *Social support increases the client's ability to cope with problems (Johnson, 2008).*
- Encourage journal/diary writing as a safe way of expressing emotions. EB: *Daily diary writing has been shown to decrease symptoms of depression (Hopko & Mullane, 2008).*
- Encourage clients to develop their artistic abilities. EB: *Using an art kit and DVD increased self-confidence and self-esteem and socialization in this study of clients in hospitals and hospices in the United Kingdon (Hull & Stickley, 2010).*

S

Pediatric

- Assess children/adolescents with chronic illness for evidence of reduced self-esteem and make needed referrals. EB: *Children and adolescents with chronic illness have lower levels of self-esteem when compared with their healthy peers; experiences of success and positive peer relations are important sources of self-esteem (Pinquart, 2013).*
- Encourage mothers of premature infants to use kangaroo care for at least 30 minutes per day. EBN: *Research shows that mothers of premature infants who used 30 minutes of kangaroo care showed improved measures of self-esteem (Lee & Bang, 2011).*
- Implement interventions that promote and maintain positive peer relations for adolescent patients. EB: *Peer relationships had the greatest impact on self-esteem for adolescent patients (Farineau et al, 2013).*
- ▲ Assess children/adolescents with low self-esteem for evidence of cyber bullying either as a victim or an offender. EB: *Students who experienced cyber bullying, either as a victim or an offender had significantly lower self-esteem than those who had little or no experience with cyber bullying (Patchin & Hinduja, 2010).*
- ▲ Provide bully prevention programs and include information on cyber bullying. EBN: *This study supported those students who were victims or offenders of bullying and demonstrated low self-esteem. Technology, computers, and cell phones are means for bullying so prevention programs need to address these issues (Patchin & Hinduja, 2010).*

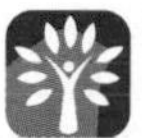

Geriatric

- Support client in identifying and adapting to functional changes. EBN: *The ability to adjust goals was shown to be critical as a way of preventing the development of depressive symptoms following negative life events in older adults (Bailly et al, 2012).*
- Use reminiscence therapy and productive activities. EB: *This study suggests that productive activities with reminiscence therapy may alleviate depressive symptoms and improve task performance of older people with dementia (Nakamae et al, 2014).*
- Encourage older adult clients to participate in flexibility, toning, and balance exercise. EB: *Older adults showed improvements in attractiveness esteem after participation in physical activity that emphasized toning, flexibility, and balance (Gothe et al, 2011).*
- Encourage participation in peer group activities. CEB: *Withdrawal and social isolation are detrimental to feelings of self-worth (Stuart-Shor et al, 2003).*
- Encourage activities in which a client can support/help others. EB: *The findings of this study reveal that late-life productive engagement is widespread, with the majority of older individuals involved in multiple forms of activity concurrently. Non–market-based activities such as caregiving, informal assistance, and volunteering are most prevalent (Hinterlong, 2008).*

S

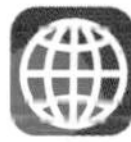

Multicultural

- Assess for the influence of cultural beliefs, norms, and values on the client's sense of self-esteem. CEB: *How the client values self may be based on cultural perceptions (Giger & Davidhizar, 2008). Asian American youths demonstrate lower levels of self-esteem than their non-Asian peers (Rhee et al, 2003).*
- Assess socioeconomic issues. EB: *Racial minorities and those who are economically disadvantaged are up to three times more likely to experience disability than are whites and those who are not economically disadvantaged, respectively (Louie & Ward, 2011).*
- Assess for drug and alcohol use in individuals with low self-esteem. CEB: *Among Mexican American female adolescents, poor self-confidence predicts higher levels of alcohol use (Swaim & Wayman, 2004).*
- Validate the client's feelings regarding ethnic or racial identity. CEB: *Individuals with strong ethnic affiliation have higher levels of self-esteem than others (Greig, 2003).*

Home Care

- Assess a client's immediate support system/family for relationship patterns and content of communication. CEBN: *Family strength assessments help the nurse to incorporate family strengths into nursing care, especially in times of crisis (Sittner et al, 2007).*
- Encourage the client's family to provide support and feedback regarding client value or worth. CEBN: *There are significant relationships between adolescents' practice of healthy behaviors, self-efficacy of those behaviors, self-care abilities, and their support systems, among other factors (Callaghan, 2006).*

▲ Refer to medical social services to assist the family in pattern changes that could benefit the client. EB: *The best nursing plan may be to access specialty services for the client and family (Holmberg et al, 2012).*

▲ If a client is involved in counseling or self-help groups, monitor and encourage attendance. Help the client identify the value of group participation after each group encounter. *Discussion about group participation clarifies and reinforces group feedback and support.*

▲ If a client is taking prescribed psychotropic medications, assess for knowledge of medication side effects and reasons for taking medication. Teach as necessary. EBN: *Education that helps clients understand their illness, particular symptoms, and how medications help them may be beneficial in promoting adherence (Wu et al, 2008).*

▲ Assess medications for effectiveness and side effects and monitor client for compliance. EBN: *A positive working relationship with the health care provider may result in improved adherence to taking medications to assist with problems (Wu et al, 2008).*

Client/Family Teaching and Discharge Planning

▲ Refer to community agencies for psychotherapeutic counseling. EB: *Family-led programs are an effective resource for families with mental illness (Pickett-Schenk et al, 2008). Cognitive behavioral therapy has a unique role in realizing and overcoming negative core beliefs and feelings of low self-worth (Johnson, 2012).*

▲ Refer to psychoeducational groups on stress reduction and coping skills. EB: *Research findings indicated that participants reported improved self-esteem and knowledge of healthy relationship dynamics after enrollment in psychoeducation groups (Marrs Fuchsel, 2014).*

▲ Refer to self-help support groups specific to needs. EB: *Research shows that client participation in support groups increases self-esteem (Seebohm et al, 2013).*

REFERENCES

Al-Modallal, H., Peden, A., & Anderson, D. (2008). Impact of physical abuse on adult depressive symptoms among women. *Issues in Mental Health Nursing, 29*, 299–314.

Bailly, N., et al. (2012). Coping with negative life events in old age: the role of tenacious goal pursuit and flexible goal adjustment. *Aging and Mental Health, 16*(4), 431–437.

Belciug, M. (2012). Patients' perceptions of the causes of their success and lack of success in achieving their potential in spinal cord rehabilitation. *International Journal of Rehabilitation Research. Internationale Zeitschrift fur Rehabilitationsforschung. Revue Internationale de Recherches de Readaptation, 35*(1), 48–53.

Burke, L., et al. (2008). A descriptive study of past experiences with weight-loss treatment. *Journal of the American Dietetic Association, 108*, 640–647.

Callaghan, D. (2006). Basic conditioning factors' influences on adolescents' health, self efficacy, and self-care. *Issues in Comprehensive Pediatric Nursing, 29*(4), 191–204.

Day, P., & Deutsch, S. (2004). Using mindfulness-based therapeutic interventions in psychiatric nursing practice-part 1: description and empirical support for mindfulness-based interventions and part 2: mindfulness-based approaches for all phases of psychotherapy-clinical case study. *Archives of Psychiatric Nursing, 18*(5), 164–177.

Del Piccolo, L., Danzi, O., Fattori, N., et al. (2014). How psychiatrist's communication skills and patient's diagnosis affect emotions disclosure during first diagnostic consultations. *Patient Education & Counseling, 96*(2), 151–158.

Farineau, H. M., Stevenson Wojciak, A., & McWey, L. M. (2013). You matter to me: important relationships and self-esteem of adolescents in foster care. *Child & Family Social Work, 18*(2), 129–138.

Giger, J., & Davidhizar, R. (2008). *Transcultural nursing: assessment and intervention* (4th ed.). St Louis: Mosby.

Gothe, N., Mullen, S., Wójcicki, T., et al. (2011). Trajectories of change in self-esteem in older adults: exercise intervention effects. *Journal of Behavioral Medicine, 34*(4), 298–306.

Greig, R. (2003). Ethnic identity development: implications for mental health in African-American and Hispanic adolescents. *Issues in Mental Health Nursing, 24*(3), 317–331.

Hinterlong, J. E. (2008). Productive engagement among older Americans: prevalence, patterns, and implications for public policy. *Journal of Aging and Social Policy, 20*(2), 141–164.

Holmberg, M., Valmari, G., & Lundgren, S. M. (2012). Patients' experiences of homecare nursing: balancing the duality between obtaining care and to maintain dignity and self-determination. *Scandinavian Journal of Caring Sciences, 26*(4), 705–712.

Hopko, D., & Mullane, C. (2008). Exploring the relation of depression and overt behavior with daily diaries. *Behaviour Research and Therapy, 46*, 1085–1089.

Hull, A., & Stickley, T. (2010). Artistic activities can improve patients' self-esteem. *Mental Health Practice, 14*(4), 30–32.

Johnson, J. (2008). Informal social support networks and the maintenance of voluntary driving cessation by older rural women. *Journal of Community Health Nursing, 25*(2), 65–72.

Johnson, P. (2012). The prevalence of low self-esteem in an intellectually disabled forensic population. *Journal of Intellectual Disability Research, 56*(3), 317–325.

Jones, J. E., et al. (2008). Impact of exudate and odour from chronic venous leg ulceration. *Nursing Standard, 22*(45), 53–61.

Kunikata, H. (2010). Psychiatric illness persons' structure of mind, body and behavior when they felt low self-esteem [Japanese]. *Journal of Japan Academy of Nursing Science, 30*(4), 36–45.

Lee, J., & Bang, K. (2011). The effects of kangaroo care on maternal self-esteem and premature infants' physiological stability. *Korean Journal of Women Health Nursing, 17*(5), 454–462.

Louie, G., & Ward, M. (2011). Socioeconomic and ethnic differences in disease burden and disparities in physical function in older adults. *American Journal of Public Health, 101*(7), 1322–1329.

Macinnes, D. L. (2006). Self-esteem and self-acceptance: an examination into their relationship and their effect on psychological health. *Journal of Psychiatric and Mental Health Nursing, 13*(5), 483.

Mantha, S., et al. (2008). Providing responsive nursing care. *MCN. the American Journal of Maternal Child Nursing*, *33*(5), 307–314.

Marrs Fuchsel, C. L. (2014). Exploratory evaluation of Sí, Yo Puedo: a culturally competent empowerment program for immigrant Latina women in group settings. *Social Work With Groups*, *37*(4), 279–296.

McMullen, T., & Resnick, B. (2013). Self-esteem among nursing assistants: reliability and validity of the Rosenberg self-esteem scale. *Journal of Nursing Measurement*, *21*(2), 335–344.

Mezuk, B., & Rebok, G. (2008). Social integration and social support among older adults following driving cessation. *The Journals of Gerontology. Series B, Psychological Sciences and Social Sciences*, *63*(5), 298–303.

Nakamae, T., Yotsumoto, K., Tatsumi, E., et al. (2014). Effects of productive activities with reminiscence in occupational therapy for people with dementia: a pilot randomized controlled study. *Hong Kong Journal of Occupational Therapy*, *24*(1), 13–19.

Parrish, E., Penden, A., & Staten, R. (2008). Strategies used by advanced practice psychiatric nurses in treating adults with depression. *Perspectives in Psychiatric Care*, *44*(6), 232–240.

Patchin, J., & Hinduja, S. (2010). Cyberbullying and self-esteem. *Journal of School Health*, *80*(12), 614–621.

Pickett-Schenk, S., et al. (2008). improving knowledge about mental illness through family-led education: the journey of hope. *Psychiatric Services (Washington, D.C.)*, *59*, 49–56.

Pierce, P., & Hicks, F. (2001). Patient decision-making behavior: an emerging paradigm for nursing science. *Nursing Research*, *50*(5), 267.

Pinquart, M. M. (2013). Self-esteem of children and adolescents with chronic illness: a meta-analysis. *Child: Care, Health & Development*, *39*(2), 153–161.

Raposa, E., Hammen, C., O'Callaghan, F., et al. (2014). Early adversity and health outcomes in young adulthood: the role of ongoing stress. *Health Psychology*, *33*(5), 410–418.

Räty, L., & Gustaffson, B. (2006). Emotions in relation to healthcare encounters affecting self-esteem. *The Journal of Neuroscience Nursing: Journal of the American Association of Neuroscience Nurses*, *38*(1), 42.

Rhee, S., Chang, J., & Rhee, J. (2003). Acculturation, communication patterns, and self-esteem among Asian and Caucasian American adolescents. *Adolescence*, *38*(152), 749–768.

Seebohm, P., Chaudhary, S., Boyce, M., et al. (2013). The contribution of self-help/mutual aid groups to mental well-being. *Health & Social Care in the Community*, *21*(4), 391–401.

Sittner, B., Hudson, D. B., & DeFrain, J. (2007). Using the concept of family strengths to enhance nursing care. *MCN. the American Journal of Maternal Child Nursing*, *32*(6), 353–357.

Stuart-Shor, E. M., et al. (2003). Are psychosocial factors associated with the pathogenesis and consequences of cardiovascular disease in the elderly? *The Journal of Cardiovascular Nursing*, *18*(3), 169.

Swaim, R. C., & Wayman, J. C. (2004). Multidimensional self-esteem and alcohol use among Mexican American and white non-Latino adolescents: concurrent and prospective effects. *The American Journal of Orthopsychiatry*, *74*(4), 559–570.

Wu, J., et al. (2008). Factors influencing medication adherence in patients with heart failure. *Heart and Lung: The Journal of Critical Care*, *37*(1), 8–16.

Yao, K., Yu, S., & Chen, I. (2008). Relationships between personal, depression and social network factors and sleep quality in community-dwelling older adults. *The Journal of Nursing Research*, *16*(2), 131–139.

Risk for chronic low Self-Esteem

Gail B. Ladwig, MSN, RN

NANDA-I

Definition

Vulnerable to longstanding negative self-evaluating/feelings about self or self-capabilities, which may compromise health

Risk Factors

Cultural incongruence; exposure to traumatic situation; inadequate affection received; inadequate group membership; inadequate respect from others; ineffective coping with loss; insufficient feeling of belonging; psychiatric disorder; repeated failures; repeated negative reinforcement; spiritual incongruence

NOC, NIC, Client Outcomes, Nursing Interventions, *Rationales*, and References

Refer to care plan for Chronic low **Self-Esteem.**

Risk for situational low Self-Esteem

Gail B. Ladwig, MSN, RN, and Marina Martinez-Kratz, MS, RN, CNE

NANDA-I

Definition

Vulnerable to developing a negative perception of self-worth in response to a current situation, which may compromise health

S

Risk Factors

Alteration in body image; alteration in social role; behavior inconsistent with values; decrease in control over environment; developmental transition; functional impairment; history of abandonment; history of abuse (e.g., physical, psychological, sexual); history of loss; history of neglect history of rejection; inadequate recognition; pattern of failure; pattern of helplessness; physical illness; unrealistic self-expectations

NOC (Nursing Outcomes Classification)

See chronic low **Self-Esteem** for suggested NOC outcomes.

Client Outcomes

Client Will (Specify Time Frame)

- State accurate self-appraisal
- Demonstrate the ability to self-validate
- Demonstrate the ability to make decisions independent of primary peer group
- Express effects of media on self-appraisal
- Express influence of substances on self-esteem
- Identify strengths and healthy coping skills
- State life events and change as influencing self-esteem

NIC (Nursing Interventions Classification)

See chronic low **Self-Esteem** for suggested NIC interventions.

Nursing Interventions and *Rationales*

S

- Assess the client's previous experiences with health care and coping with illness to determine the level of education and support needed. EBN: *Accessing illness self-concept in developing a treatment plan may prove useful (Morea et al, 2008).*
- Assess for low and negative affect (expression of feelings). EB: *In this study, both an increase in anxiety and a decrease in self-esteem were associated with emotional responses such as paranoia, depression, or anger/irritability (Thewissen et al, 2011).*
- Assess the client's self-esteem using valid and established tools like the Rosenberg Self-Esteem Scale. EBN: *The use of valid and established measures of self-esteem will facilitate the identification of appropriate nursing interventions that strengthen self-esteem (McMullen & Resnick, 2013).*
- Encourage client to maintain highest level of community functioning. EB: *In this study, clients with serious mental illness were matched with community volunteers for weekly social activities. Clients experienced increased self-esteem, self-worth, and self-confidence (McCorkle et al, 2009).*
- Treat the client with respect and as an equal to maintain positive self-esteem. CEB: *Clients with higher self-esteem need to be confirmed as being equal with care providers (Räty & Gustaffson, 2006).*
- Help the client identify and encourage use of available resources and social support networks. Make referrals as needed. EBN: *Transitions might be significantly enhanced by the presence of intimate ties, positive perceptions of one's health limitations, and residence in a healthy, safe, and resource-rich physical environment that provides the social support needed (Low et al, 2008).*
- Encourage the client to find a self-help or therapy group that focuses on self-esteem enhancement. Encourage utilization of above. CEBN: *Cognitive behavioral group therapy decreases depression levels and increases self-esteem in depressed clients (Chen et al, 2006).*
- Encourage the client to create a sense of competence through short-term goal setting and goal achievement. EBN: *Sense of competence is related to global self-esteem when goals are set and met (Lauder et al, 2008).*
- ▲ Assess the client for symptoms of depression and anxiety. Refer to specialist as needed. Prompt and effective treatment can prevent exacerbation of symptoms or safety risks. EB: *Well-documented suicide risk assessments are a core measure of quality of care (Simon, 2009).*
- See care plans for Disturbed personal **Identity,** Situational low **Self-Esteem,** and Chronic low **Self-Esteem.**

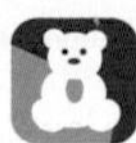

Pediatric

- Assess children/adolescents with chronic illness for evidence of reduced self-esteem and make needed referrals. EB: *Children and adolescents with chronic illness have lower levels of self-esteem when compared with their healthy peers; experiences of success and positive peer relations are important sources of self-esteem (Pinquart, 2013).*
- Identify environmental and/or developmental factors that increase risk for low self-esteem, especially in children/adolescents, to make needed referrals. CEB: *Self-esteem enhancement programs can improve self-esteem in school-age children (Dalgas-Pelish, 2006).*
- Assess children/adolescents who are either a victim or an offender of cyber bullying for low self-esteem. EB: *Students who experienced cyber bullying, either as a victim or an offender, had significantly lower self-esteem than those who had little or no experience with cyber bullying (Patchin & Hinduja, 2010).*
- ▲ Provide support for children who do not have supportive families, and provide a haven outside of the home. EB: *This study demonstrates that children from dysfunctional families are at risk for low self-esteem (Okada et al, 2012).*
- ▲ Encourage a combination of extracurricular activity for adolescents in a safe, supportive, and empowering environment. EB: *Research shows that participation in a variety of extracurricular activities has a positive effect on self-esteem, develops personal identity, and validates a sense of self (Kort-Butler, 2012).*

Geriatric

- Support humor as a coping mechanism. EB: *This study identified a sense of humor as a mechanism for managing the inevitable stresses of aging (Marziali et al, 2008).*
- Assist the client in life review and identifying positive accomplishments. *Life review is a developmental task that increases a person's sense of peace and serenity.*
- Help client establish a peer group and structured daily activities. *Social isolation and lack of structure increase a client's sense of feeling lost and worthless.*
- See care plans for Situational low **Self-Esteem** and Chronic low **Self-Esteem.**

Home Care

- Assess current environmental stresses and identify community resources. *Accessing resources to help decrease environmental stress will increase the client's ability to cope.* CEB: *Nurses who identify older women with low self-esteem, high depressive symptoms, and low quality of life before relocation can make interventions to ease the transition process (Rossen & Knafl, 2007).*
- Encourage family members to acknowledge and validate the client's strengths. *Validation allows the client to increase self-reliance and to trust personal decisions.*
- Assess the need for establishing an emergency plan. *Openly assessing safety risks increases the client's sense of limits, boundaries, and safety.*
- See care plans for Situational low **Self-Esteem** and Chronic low **Self-Esteem.**

Client/Family Teaching and Discharge Planning

- ▲ Refer the client/family to community-based self-help and support groups. EB: *Research shows that clients who participate in support groups show increased self-esteem (Seebohm et al, 2013).*
- ▲ Refer the client to educational classes on stress management, relaxation training, and so on. CEB: Cognitive behavioral therapy, psychoeducation for anxiety disorders appears to be helpful for a number of clients and largely acceptable for most clients who attend *(Houghton & Saxon, 2007).*
- ▲ Refer the client to community agencies that offer support and environmental resources. Make referrals as needed.
- See care plans for Situational low **Self-Esteem** and Chronic low **Self-Esteem.**

REFERENCES

Chen, T., et al. (2006). The evaluation of cognitive-behavioral group therapy on patient depression and self-esteem. *Archives of Psychiatric Nursing, 20*(1), 3–11.

Dalgas-Pelish, P. (2006). Effects of a self-esteem intervention program on school-aged children. *Pediatric Nursing, 32*(4), 241.

Houghton, S., & Saxon, D. (2007). An evaluation of large group CBT psycho-education for anxiety disorders delivered in routine practice. *Patient Education and Counseling, 68*, 107–110.

Kort-Butler, L. A. (2012). Extracurricular activity involvement and adolescent self-esteem. *Prevention Researcher, 19*(2), 13–16.

Lauder, W., et al. (2008). Measuring competence, self-reported competence and self-efficacy in pre-registration students. *Nursing Standard*, *22*(20), 35–43.

Low, G., Molzahn, A., & Kalfoss, M. (2008). Quality of life in older adults in Canada and Norway: examining the Iowa model. *Western Journal of Nursing Research*, *30*(4), 458–476.

Marziali, E., McDonald, L., & Donahue, P. (2008). The role of coping humor in the physical and mental health of older adults. *Aging and Mental Health*, *12*(6), 713–718.

McCorkle, B. H., et al. (2009). Compeer friends: a qualitative study of a volunteer friendship programme for people with serious mental illness. *The International Journal of Social Psychiatry*, *55*(4), 291–305.

McMullen, T., & Resnick, B. (2013). Self-esteem among nursing assistants: reliability and validity of the Rosenberg self-esteem scale. *Journal of Nursing Measurement*, *21*(2), 335–344.

Morea, J., Friend, R., & Bennett, R. (2008). Conceptualizing and measuring illness self concept: a comparison with self-esteem and optimism in predicting fibromyalgia adjustment. *Research in Nursing and Health*, *31*, 563–575.

Okada, A., et al. (2012). Importance and usefulness of evaluating self-esteem in children. *BioPsychoSocial Medicine*, *6*, 9.

Patchin, J., & Hinduja, S. (2010). Cyberbullying and self-esteem. *Journal Of School Health*, *80*(12), 614–621.

Pinquart, M. M. (2013). Self-esteem of children and adolescents with chronic illness: a meta-analysis. *Child: Care, Health & Development*, *39*(2), 153–161.

Räty, L., & Gustaffson, B. (2006). Emotions in relation to healthcare encounters affecting self-esteem. *The Journal of Neuroscience Nursing: Journal of the American Association of Neuroscience Nurses*, *38*(1), 42.

Rossen, E., & Knafl, K. (2007). Women's well-being after relocation to independent living communities. *Western Journal of Nursing Research*, *29*(2), 183–199.

Seebohm, P., Chaudhary, S., Boyce, M., et al. (2013). The contribution of self-help/mutual aid groups to mental well-being. *Health & Social Care in the Community*, *21*(4), 391–401.

Simon, R. (2009). Enhancing suicide risk assessment through evidenced-based psychiatry. *Psychiatr Times*.

Thewissen, V., et al. (2011). Emotions, self-esteem, and paranoid episodes: an experience sampling study. *The British Journal of Clinical Psychology*, *50*(2), 178–195.

Situational low Self-Esteem

Gail B. Ladwig, MSN, RN, and Marina Martinez-Kratz, MS, RN, CNE

NANDA-I

Definition

Development of a negative perception of self-worth in response to a current situation

Defining Characteristics

Helplessness; indecisive behavior; nonassertive behavior; purposelessness; self-negating verbalizations; situational challenge to self-worth; underestimates ability to deal with situation

Related Factors (r/t)

S

Alteration in body image; alteration in social role; behavior inconsistent with values; developmental transition; functional impairment; history of loss; history of rejection; inadequate recognition; pattern of failure

NOC (Nursing Outcomes Classification)

Refer to Chronic low **Self-Esteem** for suggested NOC outcomes.

Client Outcomes

Client Will (Specify Time Frame)

- State effect of life events on feelings about self
- State personal strengths
- Acknowledge presence of guilt and not blame self if an action was related to another person's appraisal
- Seek help when necessary
- Demonstrate self-perceptions are accurate given physical capabilities
- Demonstrate separation of self-perceptions from societal stigmas

NIC (Nursing Interventions Classification)

Refer to Chronic low **Self-Esteem** for suggested NIC interventions.

Nursing Interventions and *Rationales*

▲ Assess the client for signs and symptoms of depression and potential for suicide and/or violence. If present, immediately notify the appropriate personnel of symptoms. See care plans for Risk for other directed **Violence** and Risk for **Suicide.** EB: *Well-documented suicide risk assessments are a core measure of quality of care (Simon, 2009).*

- Assess the client's environmental and everyday stressors, including evidence of abusive relationships. EBN: *High everyday stressors and a history of abuse in relationships are associated with low self-esteem and depression (Al-Modallal et al, 2008).*
- ▲ Assess the client's self-esteem using valid and established tools like the Rosenberg Self-Esteem Scale. EBN: *The use of valid and established measures of self-esteem will facilitate the identification of appropriate nursing interventions that strengthen self-esteem (McMullen & Resnick, 2013).* Assess for unhealthy coping mechanisms, such as substance abuse, and make appropriate referrals. EB: *Numerous factors influence the onset and continuation of alcohol use, including the complex ways that genes interact with one another and with the environment (Faye et al, 2015). A health risk assessment that helps refer clients to medical management programs helped increase overall wellness in this health care plan (Case Management Advisor, 2012).*
- Assist in the identification of problems and situational factors that contribute to problems, offering options for resolution. EBN: *Recognize that the client's own personal resources strengthen client's self-determination (Meijers & Gustafsson, 2008).*
- Mutually identify strengths, resources, and previously effective coping strategies. EBN: *A common action for supporting self-determination is supplying the client with information and engaging the client in making a plan (Meijers & Gustafsson, 2008).* EB: *Helping the client identify positive traits may contribute to living a "happier life" (Bernard et al, 2010).*
- Have client list strengths. EBN: *In this study of women with addiction, it was identified that helping the client identify strengths empowered her in the recovery process (Payne, 2010).*
- Accept client's own pace in working through grief or crisis situations. EBN: *Recommended therapeutic communication skills such as eye contact, use of therapeutic touch, and active listening can be enhanced by an understanding of the grief process (Wright & Hogan, 2008).*
- Accept the client's own defenses in dealing with the crisis. EBN: *The SAUC modes (Sympathy-Acceptance-Understanding-Competence) help strengthen and preserve the individual's positive self-relation (Meijers & Gustafsson, 2008).*
- Provide information about support groups of people who have common experiences or interests. EBN: *Research shows that client participation in support groups increases self-esteem (Seebohm et al, 2013).*
- Teach the client mindfulness techniques to cope more effectively with strong emotional responses. EB: *Mindfulness training has direct positive effects on self-esteem (Pepping et al, 2013).*
- Support client's decisions in health care treatment. EBN: *Self-esteem is enhanced when clients are able to make their own decisions regarding cancer treatment (Kitamura, 2010).*
- Encourage objective appraisal of self and life events and challenge negative or perfectionist expectations of self. CEB: *Positive life events improve self-esteem and positive affect (Drew & Mabry, 2004).*
- Provide psychoeducation to client and family. EB: *Research findings indicated that participants reported improved self-esteem and knowledge of healthy relationship dynamics after enrollment in psychoeducation groups (Marrs Fuchsel, 2014).*
- Validate confusion when feeling ill but looking well. CEB: *Validation of emotions is related to a client's experience of caring (Räty & Gustafsson, 2006).*
- Acknowledge the presence of societal stigma. Teach management tools. EBN: *Stigma toward mental illness is poorly understood, often unrecognized by nurses, and affects both treatment-seeking behavior and treatment adherence (Pinto-Foltz & Logsdon, 2008).*
- Validate the effect of negative past experiences on self-esteem and work on corrective measures. CEB: *People with low self-esteem have a need to be affirmed regarding their value (Räty & Gustaffson, 2006).*
- See care plan for Chronic low **Self-Esteem.**

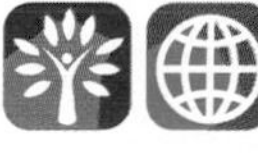

Geriatric and Multicultural

- See care plan for Chronic low **Self-Esteem.**

Home Care

- Establish an emergency plan and contract with the client for its use. *Having an emergency plan is reassuring to the client. Establishing a contract validates the worth of the client and provides a caring link between the client and society.*
- Access supplies that support a client's success at independent living.
- See care plan for Chronic low **Self-Esteem.**

S

Client/Family Teaching and Discharge Planning

- Assess the person's support system (family, friends, and community) and involve them if desired. CEB: *Family strength assessments help the nurse incorporate family strengths into nursing care, especially in times of crisis (Sittner et al, 2007).*
- Educate client and family regarding the grief process. *Understanding this process normalizes responses of sadness, anger, guilt, and helplessness. Recommended therapeutic communication skills such as eye contact, use of therapeutic touch, and active listening can be enhanced by an understanding of the grief process (Wright & Hogan, 2008).*
- Teach client and family that the crisis is temporary. *Knowing that the crisis is temporary provides a sense of hope for the future.*
- ▲ Refer to appropriate community resources or crisis intervention centers.
- ▲ Refer to resources for handicap and/or disability services.
- Refer to illness-specific consumer support groups. *Mutual help support groups aid the client with chronic illness to cope with their illness (Chen et al, 2008).*
- See care plan for Chronic low **Self-Esteem.**

REFERENCES

Al-Modallal, H., Peden, A., & Anderson, D. (2008). Impact of physical abuse on adult depressive symptoms among women. *Issues in Mental Health Nursing, 29*, 299–314.

Bernard, M. E., et al. (2010). Albert Ellis: unsung hero of positive psychology. *The Journal of Positive Psychology, 5*(4), 302–310.

Case Management Advisor. (2012). Health plan reduces high-risk conditions. *Case Management Advisor, 23*(4), 42–43.

Chen, Y., Pai, J., & Li, C. (2008). Haemodialysis: the effects of using the empowerment concept during the development of a mutual support group in Taiwan. *Journal of Clinical Nursing, 17*(5), 133–142.

Drew, L., & Mabry, J. (2004). Predictors of positive life events: self-esteem and positive effect. *The Gerontologist, 44*(1), 230.

Faye, C., et al. *NIAAA's strategic plan to address health disparities.* From: <http://www.niaaa.nih.gov/-publications/HealthDisparities/Strategic.html> Retrieved January 2, 2015.

Kitamura, Y. (2010). Decision-making process of patients with gynecological cancer regarding their cancer treatment choices using the analytic hierarchy process. *Japan Journal of Nursing Science, 7*, 148–157.

Marrs Fuchsel, C. L. (2014). Exploratory evaluation of Sí, Yo Puedo: a culturally competent empowerment program for immigrant Latina women in group settings. *Social Work With Groups, 37*(4), 279–296.

McMullen, T., & Resnick, B. (2013). Self-esteem among nursing assistants: reliability and validity of the Rosenberg Self-Esteem Scale. *Journal of Nursing Measurement, 21*(2), 335–344.

Meijers, K. E., & Gustafsson, B. (2008). Patient's self-determination in intensive care: from an action- and confirmation theoretical perspective. *Intensive and Critical Care Nursing, 24*(4), 222–232.

Payne, L. (2010). Self-acceptance and its role in women's recovery from addiction. *Journal of Addictions Nursing, 21*(4), 207–214.

Pepping, C. A., O'Donovan, A., & Davis, P. J. (2013). The positive effects of mindfulness on self-esteem. *Journal Of Positive Psychology, 8*(5), 376–386.

Pinto-Foltz, M., & Logsdon, M. (2008). Stigma towards mental illness: a concept analysis using postpartum depression as an exemplar. *Issues in Mental Health Nursing, 29*, 21–36.

Räty, L., & Gustafsson, B. (2006). Emotions in relation to healthcare encounters affecting self-esteem. *The Journal of Neuroscience Nursing: Journal of the American Association of Neuroscience Nurses, 38*(1), 42.

Seebohm, P., Chaudhary, S., Boyce, M., et al. (2013). The contribution of self-help/mutual aid groups to mental well-being. *Health & Social Care In The Community, 21*(4), 391–401.

Simon, R. (2009). Enhancing suicide risk assessment through evidence-based psychiatry. *Psychiatr Times.*

Sittner, B. J., Hudson, D. B., & DeFrain, J. (2007). Using the concept of family strengths to enhance nursing care. *MCN. The American Journal of Maternal Child Nursing, 32*(6), 353–357.

Wright, P., & Hogan, S. (2008). Grief theories and models applications to hospice nursing practice. *Journal of Hospice & Palliative Nursing, 10*(6), 350–356.

Self-Mutilation

Kathleen L. Patusky, MA, PhD, RN, CNS

NANDA-I

Definition

Deliberate self-injurious behavior causing tissue damage with the intent of causing nonfatal injury to attain relief of tension

Defining Characteristics

Abrading; biting; constricting a body part; cuts on body; hitting; ingestion of harmful substances; inhalation of harmful substances; insertion of object into body orifice; picking at wounds; scratches on body; self-inflicted burn; severing of a body part

Related Factors (r/t)

Absence of family confidant; adolescence; alteration in body image; autism; borderline personality disorder; character disorder; childhood illness; childhood surgery; depersonalization; developmental delay; dissociation; disturbance in interpersonal relationships; eating disorders; emotional disorder; family divorce; family history of self destructive behaviors; family substance abuse; feeling threatened with loss of significant relationship; history of childhood abuse (e.g., physical, psychological, sexual); history of self-directed violence; impaired self-esteem; impulsiveness; inability to express tension verbally; incarceration; ineffective communication between parent and adolescent; ineffective coping strategies; irresistible urge for self-directed violence; irresistible urge to cut self; isolation from peers; labile behavior; living in nontraditional setting (e.g., foster, group or institutional care); low self-esteem; mounting tension that is intolerable; negative feeling (e.g., depression, rejection, self-hatred, separation anxiety, guilt, depersonalization); pattern of inability to plan solutions; pattern of inability to see long-term consequences; peers who self-mutilate; perfectionism; psychotic disorder; requires rapid stress reduction; sexual identity crisis; substance abuse; use of manipulation to obtain nurturing relationship with others; violence between parental figures

NOC (Nursing Outcomes Classification)

Suggested NOC Outcomes

Self-Control; Distorted Thought Self-Control; Impulse Self-Control; Mood Equilibrium; Risk Detection; Self-Mutilation Restraint

Example NOC Outcome with Indicators

Self-Mutilation Restraint as evidenced by the following indicators: Refrains from gathering means for self-injury/Obtains assistance as needed/Upholds contract not to harm self/Maintains self-control without supervision/Refrains from injuring self. (Rate the outcome and indicators of **Self-Mutilation Restraint:** 1 = never demonstrated, 2 = rarely demonstrated, 3 = sometimes demonstrated, 4 = often demonstrated, 5 = consistently demonstrated [see Section I].)

Consider using a measure of self-harm risk that is available for clients: Self-Injury Questionnaire addresses intention for self-harm (Santa Mina et al, 2006).

Client Outcomes

Client Will (Specify Time Frame)

- Have injuries treated
- Refrain from further self-injury
- State appropriate ways to cope with increased psychological or physiological tension
- Express feelings
- Seek help when having urges to self-mutilate
- Maintain self-control without supervision
- Use appropriate community agencies when caregivers are unable to attend to emotional needs

NIC (Nursing Interventions Classification)

Suggested NIC Interventions

Active Listening; Anger Control Assistance; Behavior Management: Self-Harm; Calming Technique; Environmental Management: Safety; Limit Setting; Mood Management; Mutual Goal Setting; Risk Identification; Self-Responsibility Facilitation

Example NIC Activities—Behavior Management: Self-Harm

Anticipate trigger situations that may prompt self-harm and intervene to prevent it; Teach client and reinforce effective coping behaviors and appropriate expression of feelings

Nursing Interventions and *Rationales*

NOTE: Before implementing interventions in the face of self-mutilation, nurses should examine their own knowledge base and emotional responses to incidents of self-harm to ensure that interventions will not be based on countertransference reactions. EBN/EB: *Lack of educational background on self-harm can influence response to self-harm clients. Nurses' tendency to focus on physical care, especially when working under stressful conditions, can hinder awareness of and response to psychosocial issues (Cleaver, 2014; Muehlenkamp et al, 2013).*

- ▲ Provide medical treatment for injuries. Use aseptic technique when caring for wounds. Care for the wounds in a matter-of-fact manner. EBN: *A significant impediment to wound healing is infection. A matter-of-fact approach avoids positive reinforcement and may decrease repetition of behavior (Catledge et al, 2012).*
- • Assess for risk of suicide or other self-damaging behaviors. EBN: *Although self-mutilation should not be viewed simply as failed suicide, it is a significant indicator of suicide risk. Clients may also engage in other self-damaging behaviors, including substance abuse or eating disorders (Cleaver, 2014; Moller et al, 2013).* Refer to the care plan for Risk for **Suicide.**
- • Assess for signs of psychiatric disorders, including depression, anxiety, borderline personality disorder, dissociative disorders, eating disorders, and impulsivity. EB: *Self-mutilation has been associated with multiple psychiatric disorders (Moller et al, 2013).*
- • Assess for presence of hallucinations. Ask specific questions such as, "Do you hear voices that other people do not hear? Are they telling you to hurt yourself?" CEB: *Command hallucinations occurring with schizophrenia or brief psychotic episodes may direct the client to hurt himself or herself or others (Barrowcliff & Haddock, 2010).*
- ▲ Assure the client that he or she will be safe during hallucinations, and engage supportively. Provide referrals for medication. EBN: *Hallucinations can be very frightening; therefore, clients need reassurance that they will be kept safe, while avoiding a sense of intrusion that overstimulates clients (Ray et al, 2011).*
- ▲ Assess for the presence of medical disorders, mental retardation, medication effects, or disorders such as autism that may include self-mutilation. Initiate referral for evaluation and treatment as appropriate. CEB: *Self-mutilation has been reported as a presenting or ongoing symptom with medical disorders, such as the genetic Lesch-Nyhan syndrome (Robey et al, 2003). (Additional relevant research: Singh et al, 2006.)*
- ▲ Case finding and referral by school nurses for psychological or psychiatric treatment is critical. CEB: *Treatment includes starting therapy and medications, increasing coping skills, facilitating decision making, encouraging positive relationships, and fostering self-esteem (McDonald, 2006).*
- • Monitor the client's behavior closely, using engagement and support as elements of safety checks while avoiding intrusive overstimulation. *When lack of control exists, client safety is an important issue, and close observation is essential.* EBN: *Clients were found to feel overstimulated by intrusive close observation, resulting in agitation (Ray et al, 2011).*
- • Establish trust, listen to client, convey safety, and assist in developing positive goals for the future. EBN: *Clients reported that nurses were helpful when they took charge of unsafe situations, performed bodily interventions (e.g., holding hand), conveyed safety, and respected the autonomy of the client (Schoppmann et al, 2007). Promoting trust and enhancing privacy are considered important (Catledge et al, 2012).*
- • Recognize that self-mutilation may serve a variety of functions for the client. EBN: *Self-mutilation is identified by clients as a way to help with the regulation of dysphoric affect and cope with dissociative states (Catledge et al, 2012).*
- ▲ Refer to family or group psychotherapy as appropriate. EBN: *A systematic review of treatment modalities suggests that systemic family therapy or developmental group psychotherapy (using a combination of cognitive behavior therapy, dialectic behavior therapy, and psychodynamic therapy) can be effective (Pryjmachuk & Trainor, 2010).*
- ▲ Use a collaborative approach for care. A collaborative approach to care is more helpful to the client.
- • Refer to the care plan for Risk for **Self-Mutilation** for additional information.

Home Care and Client/Family Teaching and Discharge Planning

- • See the care plan for Risk for **Self-Mutilation.**

REFERENCES

Barrowcliff, A. L., & Haddock, G. (2010). Factors affecting compliance and resistance to auditory command hallucinations: perceptions of a clinical population. *Journal of Mental Health*, *19*, 542.

Catledge, C. B., Scharer, K., & Fuller, S. (2012). Assessment and identification of deliberate self-harm in adolescents and young adults. *JNP The Journal for Nurse Practitioners*, *8*(4), 299–305.

Cleaver, K. (2014). Attitudes of emergency care staff towards young people who self-harm: a scoping review. *International Emergency Nursing*, *22*, 52–61.

McDonald, C. (2006). Self-mutilation in adolescents. *The Journal of School Nursing, 22*, 193.

Moller, C. I., Tait, R. J., & Byrne, D. G. (2013). Deliberate self-harm, substance use, and negative affect in nonclinical samples: a systematic review. *Substance Abuse, 34*(2), 188–207.

Muehlenkamp, J. J., Claes, L., Quigley, K., et al. (2013). Association of training on attitudes towards self-injuring clients across health professionals. *Archives of Suicide Research, 17*(4), 462–468.

Pryjmachuk, S., & Trainor, G. (2010). Helping young people who self-harm: perspectives from England. *Journal of Child and Adolescent Psychiatric Nursing, 23*(2), 52–60.

Ray, R., Perkins, E., & Meijer, B. (2011). The evolution of practice changes in the use of special observations. *Archives of Psychiatric Nursing, 25*, 90.

Robey, K. L., et al. (2003). Modes and patterns of self-mutilation in persons with Lesch-Nyhan disease. *Developmental Medicine and Child Neurology, 45*, 167.

Santa Mina, E. E., et al. (2006). The Self-Injury Questionnaire: evaluation of the psychometric properties in a clinical population. *Journal of Psychiatric and Mental Health Nursing, 13*, 221.

Schoppmann, S., et al. (2007). "Then I just showed her my arms…." Bodily sensations in moments of alienation related to self-injurious behaviour. A hermeneutic phenomenological study. *Journal of Psychiatric and Mental Health Nursing, 14*, 587.

Singh, N. N., et al. (2006). Mindful parenting decreases aggression, noncompliance, and self-injury in children with autism. *Journal of Emotional and Behavioral Disorders, 14*, 169.

Risk for Self-Mutilation

Kathleen L. Patusky, MA, PhD, RN, CNS

NANDA-I

Definition

Vulnerable to deliberate self-injurious behavior causing tissue damage with the intent of causing nonfatal injury to attain relief of tension

Risk Factors

Adolescence; alteration in body image; battered child; borderline personality disorders; character disorders; childhood illness; childhood surgery; depersonalization; developmental delay; dissociation; disturbed interpersonal relationships; eating disorders; emotional disorder; family divorce; family history of self-destructive behavior; family substance abuse; feeling threatened with loss of significant relationship; history of childhood abuse (e.g., physical, psychological, sexual); history of self-directed violence; impaired self-esteem; impulsiveness; inability to express tension verbally; incarceration; ineffective coping strategies; irresistible urge for self-directed violence; isolation from peers; living in nontraditional setting (e.g., foster, group, or institutional care); loss of control over problem-solving situation; loss of significant relationship (s); low self-esteem; mounting tension that is intolerable; negative feelings (e.g., depression, rejection, self-hatred, separation anxiety, guilt, depersonalization); pattern of inability to plan solutions; pattern of inability to see long term consequences; peers who self-mutilate; perfectionism; psychotic disorder; requires rapid stress reduction, sexual identity crisis; substance abuse; use of manipulation to obtain nurturing relationship with others; violence between parental figures

S

NOC (Nursing Outcomes Classification)

See care plan for **Self-Mutilation** for suggested NOC outcomes.

Client Outcomes

Client Will (Specify Time Frame)

- Refrain from self-injury
- Identify triggers to self-mutilation
- State appropriate ways to cope with increased psychological or physiological tension
- Express feelings
- Seek help when having urges to self-mutilate
- Maintain self-control without supervision
- Use appropriate community agencies when caregivers are unable to attend to emotional needs

NIC (Nursing Interventions Classification)

See care plan for **Self-Mutilation** for suggested NIC interventions.

Nursing Interventions and *Rationales*

Note: Before implementing interventions in the face of self-injury, nurses should examine their own knowledge base and emotional responses to incidents of self-injury to ensure that interventions will not be based on countertransference reactions. EBN: *Lack of educational background on self-harm can influence response to self-harm clients. Nurses' tendency to focus on physical care, especially when working under stressful conditions, can hinder awareness of and response to psychosocial issues (Cleaver, 2014; Muehlenkamp et al, 2013a).*

- Assess client's ability to regulate his/her own emotional states, which may be influenced by the client's perception of his or her body. EB: *Clients who self-injure are more likely to be lower in emotional self-regulation than persons who do not self-injure. They may use self-harm to increase or decrease feelings. Self-injury has been associated with low body regard (Muehlenkamp, et al, 2013b).*
- Assess client's degree of self-criticism and use of effective coping skills. Self-harm serves as a coping mechanism for clients. CEB: *Persecutory self-criticism and limited coping skills are linked with self-harm (Gilbert et al, 2010; Hall & Place, 2010).*
- Assess client's perception of powerlessness. Refer to the care plan for **Powerlessness.** CEB: *Testing of the Cry of Pain model of suicidality and repeat self-harm, which identifies defeat, no escape potential, and no rescue as contributory, supports use of this model to understand self-harm (Rasmussen et al, 2010).*
- Assessment data from the client and family members may have to be gathered at different times; allowing a family member or trusted friend with whom the client is comfortable to be present during the assessment may be helpful. EBN: *Self-mutilation sometimes occurs if clients have been victims of abuse or other types of adverse family experiences (Catledge et al, 2012). Clients or family members may be more willing to disclose the presence of abuse if greater privacy is afforded them, or if presence of a trusted family member or friend helps clients to respond more comfortably to the interview situation.*
- Assess for risk factors of self-mutilation described above. CEB: *Self-mutilation has been associated with multiple psychiatric disorders and psychosocial difficulties (Barnes et al, 2010; Holm & Severinsson, 2010; Joyce et al, 2010; Peebles et al, 2011).*
- Perform a thorough skin assessment at least annually and check for behavioral cues of self-harm. EBN: *Skin assessment must cover body areas normally clothed. Signs of self-harm include scratches, burns, lacerations, objects embedded under the skin (e.g., razor blades), multiple scars, or carved words. Scars may vary in age and depth. Behavioral cues include wearing long sleeves and pants, wristbands or bulky bracelets, and avoiding situations that would result in exposed skin (e.g., physical education class) (Catledge et al, 2012).*
- Assess for co-occurring disorders that require response, specifically childhood abuse, substance abuse, and suicide attempts. Implement reporting or referral as indicated. EB: *Self-mutilation has been associated with multiple psychiatric disorders (Moller et al, 2013).*
- Assess family dynamics and the need for family therapy and community support. EBN: *Self-harm is associated with childhood abuse and family dysfunction (Catledge et al, 2012).*
- Assess for the presence of medical disorders, mental retardation, medication effects, or disorders such as autism that may include self-mutilation. Initiate referral for evaluation and treatment as appropriate. CEB: *Lesch-Nyhan syndrome is a rare genetic disorder, which is characterized by compulsive self-mutilation (Zilli & Hasselmo, 2008).*
- Be alert to other risk factors of self-mutilation in clients with psychosis, including acute intoxication, dramatic changes in body appearance, preoccupation with religion and sexuality, and anticipated or perceived object loss. *Many psychiatric disorders have shown a connection with self-mutilation.* CEB: *Command hallucinations occurring in schizophrenia or brief psychotic episodes may direct the client to hurt himself or herself or others (Barrowcliff & Haddock, 2010).*
- Monitor the client's behavior closely, using engagement and support as elements of safety checks while avoiding intrusive overstimulation. Offer activities that will serve as a distraction. *When lack of control exists, client safety is an important issue and close observation is essential.* EBN: *Clients were found to feel overstimulated by intrusive close observation, resulting in agitation (Ray et al, 2011).*
- Establish trust, listen to client, convey safety, and assist in developing positive goals for the future. EBN/EB: *Clients reported that nurses were helpful when they took charge of unsafe situations, performed bodily interventions (e.g., holding hand), conveyed safety, and respected the autonomy of the client (Schoppmann et al, 2007). Promoting trust and enhancing privacy are considered important (Catledge et al, 2012).*
  Refer to mental health counseling. Multiple therapeutic modalities are available for treatment. EBN: *A systematic review of treatment modalities suggests that systemic family therapy or developmental group*

psychotherapy (using a combination of cognitive behavior therapy, dialectic behavior therapy, and psychodynamic therapy) can be effective (Pryjmachuk & Trainor, 2010). Inform the client of expectations for appropriate behavior and consequences within the unit. Emphasize that the client must comply with the rules. Give positive reinforcement for compliance and minimize attention paid to disruptive behavior while setting limits. *Clients benefit from clear guidance regarding behavioral expectations and consequences, providing much-needed structure. It is important to reinforce appropriate behavior to encourage repetition.* CEB: *Treatment should involve assisting the client to learn healthier affective regulation skills (Gilbert et al, 2010; Hall & Place, 2010).*

- Clients need to learn to recognize distress as it occurs and express it verbally rather than as a physical action against the self. CEB: *Treatment should involve assisting the client to learn healthier affective regulation skills (Gilbert et al, 2010; Hall & Place, 2010).*
- Assist the client to identify the motives/reasons for self-mutilation that have been perceived as positive. Self-harm serves as a defense mechanism. CEB: *Persecutory self-criticism and limited coping skills are linked with self-harm (Gilbert et al, 2010; Hall & Place, 2010).*
- Help the client identify cues that precede impulsive behavior. CEBN: *The dialectical behavior therapy (DBT) technique of behavioral chain analysis was found to reduce self-harm behaviors by processing events that precipitate self-mutilation (Alper & Peterson, 2001).*
- Assist clients to identify ways to soothe themselves and generate hopefulness when faced with painful emotions. CEB: *Women with a history of childhood abuse may not have developed the internal ability to comfort themselves, or self-soothe, resulting in neurobiological disruptions that lead to self-harm as a means of relieving pain (Gallop, 2002). Generating hopefulness is an important self-comforting intervention (Weber, 2002).*
- Reinforce alternative ways of dealing with depression and anxiety, such as exercise, engaging in unit activities, or talking about feelings. *Goal direction enhances self-efficacy, an important antecedent of empowerment (Self-injury.net, 2012).*
- Keep the environment safe; remove all harmful objects from the area. Use of unbreakable glass is recommended for the client at risk for self-injury. *Client safety is a nursing priority. Unbreakable glass would eliminate this type of injury.*
- Anticipate trigger situations and intervene to assist the client in applying alternatives to self-mutilation. CEB: *When triggers occur, client stress level may obstruct ability to apply recent learning. Cognitive strategies can be useful to correct irrational beliefs that are part of the trigger (Claes & Vandereycken, 2007).*
- If self-mutilation does occur, use a calm, nonpunitive approach. Whenever possible, assist the client to assume responsibility for consequences (e.g., dress self-inflicted wound). Refer to the care plan for **Self-Mutilation.** *This approach does not promote inappropriate attention-getting behavior, may decrease repetition of behavior, and reinforces self-responsibility and self-care management.*
- If the client is unable to control self-mutilation behavior, provide interactive supervision, not isolation. *Isolation and deprivation take away the individual's coping abilities and place him or her at risk for self harm. Implementing seclusion for clients who have injured themselves in the past may actually facilitate self-injury. Clients are extraordinarily resourceful at identifying environmental objects with which to self-mutilate.*
- Involve the client in planning his/her care and problem solving, and emphasize that the client can make choices. CEB: *Clients reported negative responses to having no input into their treatment plan (Fish & Duperouzel, 2008; Rasmussen et al, 2010).*

▲ Refer to protective services if evidence of abuse exists. *It is the nurse's legal responsibility to report abuse.*

- Refer to the care plan for **Self-Mutilation.**

Pediatric

- The same dynamics described previously apply to adolescents. EBN: *Self-harm is a major public health issue arising in persons aged 12 to 24 years, most often in females (Catledge et al, 2012).*
- Maintaining a therapeutic relationship with teens requires explicit assurances of confidentiality, consistency of clinical routines, and a nonjudgmental communication style. CEB: *Even adolescents younger than age 18 years need assurances that confidentiality will be maintained unless there is a serious risk of harm to themselves or others. However, teens of all ages should be advised that parental notification will be made to ensure the teen's safety and to implement a treatment plan (Derouin & Bravender, 2004).*
- Encourage expression of painful experiences and provide supportive counseling. EBN: *Among female adolescents, themes from a qualitative study included living with childhood trauma, feeling abandoned, being*

S

an outsider, loathing self, silently screaming, releasing the pressure, feeling alive, being ashamed, and being hopeful (Lesniak, 2010; Rissanen et al, 2011).

- Multiple treatment modalities may be used in addressing the themes of young people who self-harm. EBN: *A systematic review identified individual, family, group, and psychopharmacological therapies as being used for treatment; however, limited research exists to determine which are most effective (Pryjmachuk & Trainor, 2010).*
- Teach coping skills as an important intervention for adolescents. EB: *Studies suggest that negative emotional coping skills such as rumination, self-blame, and helplessness contribute to self-harm. Social and active coping was significantly associated with noncutting behavior (Hall & Place, 2010).*
- Assess for the presence of an eating disorder or substance abuse. Attend to the themes that preoccupy teens with eating disorders who self-mutilate. CEB: *Self-harmers with a history of childhood sexual abuse reported more eating disorders (Murray et al, 2008; Wright et al, 2009).*
- Evaluate for suicidal ideation/suicide risk. Refer to the care plan for Risk for **Suicide** for additional information. CEB: *Adolescents who attempted suicide by overdose admitted to some method of self-mutilation. The self-mutilators were significantly more likely than non-self-mutilators to be diagnosed with oppositional defiant disorder, major depression, and dysthymia and had higher scores on measures of hopelessness, loneliness, anger, risk-taking, and alcohol use (Guertin et al, 2001).*
- Be aware that there is not complete overlap between self-mutilation and suicidal behavior. The motivation may be different (coping with difficult feelings rather than ending life), and the method is usually different. CEB: *In one study, about half of the participants reported both attempted suicide and self-mutilation; the other half reported no overlap in types of acts (Bolognini et al, 2003).*
- Use treatment approaches detailed in nursing interventions, with modifications as appropriate for this age group.

Geriatric

- Provide hand or back rubs and calming music when older clients experience anxiety. *Calming music or hand massage can soothe agitation for up to 1 hour. No additional benefit was found from combining the two interventions.*
- Provide soft objects for older clients to hold and manipulate when self-mutilation occurs as a function of delirium or dementia. Apply mitts, splints, helmets, or restraints as appropriate. *Delirious or demented clients may scratch or pick at themselves. Soft objects may provide a substitute object to pick at; mitts or restraints may be necessary if the client is unable to exercise self-restraint. They should only be used for a limited amount of time as they may contribute to delirium.*
- Be aware that older adults may demonstrate self-neglect. Older adults who show self-destructive behaviors should be evaluated for dementia. EB: *In a qualitative study of unsupervised assisted living residents, more than half of participants showed self-neglect behaviors (Caspi, 2014).*

Home Care

- Communicate degree of risk to family/caregivers; assess the family and caregiving situation for ability to protect the client and to understand the client's self-mutilative behavior. Provide family and caregivers with guidelines on how to manage self-harm behaviors in the home environment. *Client safety between home visits is a nursing priority. Appropriate family/caregiver support is important to the client. Appropriate support will only be forthcoming if all parties understand the basis of the behavior and how to respond to it.*
- Establish an emergency plan, including when to use hotlines and 911. Develop a contract with the client and family for use of the emergency plan. Role-play access to the emergency resources with the client and caregivers. *Having an emergency plan reassures the client and caregivers and promotes client safety. Contracting gives guided control to the client and enhances self-esteem.*
- Assess the home environment for harmful objects. Have family remove or lock objects as able. *Client safety is a nursing priority.*

▲ If client behaviors intensify, institute an emergency plan for mental health intervention. The degree of disturbance and the ability to manage care safely at home determine the level of services needed to protect the client.

▲ Refer for homemaker or psychiatric home health care services for respite, client reassurance, and implementation of therapeutic regimen. *Responsibility for a person at high risk for self-mutilation provides high caregiver stress. Respite decreases caregiver stress. The presence of caring individuals is reassuring to both the client and caregivers, especially during periods of client anxiety. A client with self-mutilative behavior, especially if accompanied by depression, can benefit from the interventions described previously, modified for the home setting.*

▲ If the client is on psychotropic medications, assess client and family knowledge of medication administration and side effects. *Teach as necessary. Knowledge of the medical regimen promotes compliance and promotes safe use of medications.*

▲ Evaluate the effectiveness and side effects of medications. Accurate clinical feedback improves health care provider's ability to prescribe an effective medical regimen specific to client needs.

Client/Family Teaching and Discharge Planning

- Explain all relevant symptoms, procedures, treatments, and expected outcomes for self-mutilation that is illness based (e.g., borderline personality disorder, autism). CEB: *Clients prefer to participate in their treatment planning to gain a sense of control (Fish & Duperouzel, 2008; Rasmussen et al, 2010).*
- Assist family members to understand the complex issues of self-mutilation. Provide instruction on relevant developmental issues and on actions that parents can take to avoid media that glorify self-harm behaviors. CEB: *Family members need to understand the behaviors they are dealing with, receive positive reinforcement that will promote their patience and perseverance, and know that they can take positive action to remove media triggers for self-mutilation (Rasmussen et al, 2010; Rissanen et al, 2009).*
- Provide written instructions for treatments and procedures for which the client will be responsible. *A written record provides a concrete reference so that the client and family can clarify any verbal information that was given.*
- Instruct the client in coping strategies (assertiveness training, impulse control training, deep breathing, progressive muscle relaxation). *Clients who self-mutilate have difficulty dealing with stress and painful emotions, which serve as triggers to self-harm. Once clients are able to identify these triggers, they need to learn how to respond to them more effectively through assertiveness, impulse control, or relaxation, as appropriate.*
- Role play responses to stressful situations (e.g., say, "Tell me how you will respond if someone ignores you"). *Role playing is the most commonly used technique in assertiveness training. It deconditions the anxiety that arises from interpersonal encounters by allowing the client to practice how he or she might respond in a given situation. Anxiety levels tend to be higher in situations that are unfamiliar.*
- Teach cognitive-behavioral activities, such as active problem solving, reframing (reappraising the situation from a different perspective), or thought-stopping (in response to a negative thought, picture a large stop sign and replace the image with a prearranged positive alternative). Teach the client to confront his or her own negative thought patterns (or cognitive distortions), such as catastrophizing (expecting the very worst), dichotomous thinking (perceiving events in only one of two opposite categories), or magnification (placing distorted emphasis on a single event). *Cognitive-behavioral activities address clients' assumptions, beliefs, and attitudes about their situations, fostering modification of these elements to be as realistic and optimistic as possible. Through cognitive-behavioral interventions, clients become more aware of their cognitive choices in adopting and maintaining their belief systems, thereby exercising greater control over their own reactions (Hagerty & Patusky, 2011).*

▲ Provide the client and family with phone numbers of appropriate community agencies for therapy and counseling. Continuous follow-up care should be implemented; therefore, the method to access this care must be given to the client.

▲ Give the client positive things on which to focus by referring to appropriate agencies for job-training skills or education. CEB: *Clients expressed the desire for goals they could aim for as a means of regaining a positive view of the future (Fish & Duperouzel, 2008).*

S

REFERENCES

Alper, G., & Peterson, S. J. (2001). Dialectical behavior therapy for patients with borderline personality disorder. *Journal of Psychosocial Nursing and Mental Health Services*, *39*(10), 38, 52.

Barnes, A. J., Eisenberg, M. E., & Resnick, M. D. (2010). Suicide and self-injury among children and youth with chronic health conditions. *Pediatrics*, *125*, 889.

Barrowcliff, A. L., & Haddock, G. (2010). Factors affecting compliance and resistance to auditory command hallucinations: perceptions of a clinical population. *Journal of Mental Health*, *19*, 542.

Bolognini, M., et al. (2003). Adolescents' self-mutilation: relationship with dependent behaviour. *Swiss Journal of Psychology*, *62*(4), 241.

Caspi, E. (2014). Does self-neglect occur among older adults with dementia when unsupervised in assisted living? An exploratory, observational study. *Journal of Elder Abuse & Neglect.*, *26*(2), 123–149.

Catledge, C. B., Scharer, K., & Fuller, S. (2012). Assessment and identification of deliberate self-harm in adolescents and young adults. *JNP The Journal for Nurse Practitioners*, *8*(4), 299–305. *Journal for Nurse Practitioners*, *8*(4), 299–305.

Claes, L., & Vandereycken, W. (2007). Is there a link between traumatic experiences and self-injurious behaviors in eating-disordered patients? *Eating Disord*, *15*, 305.

Cleaver, K. (2014). Attitudes of emergency care staff towards young people who self-harm: a scoping review. *International Emergency Nursing*, *22*, 52–61.

Derouin, A., & Bravender, T. (2004). Living on the edge: the current phenomenon of self-mutilation in adolescents. *MCN. the American Journal of Maternal Child Nursing*, *29*(1), 12.

Fish, R., & Duperouzel, H. (2008). "Just another day dealing with wounds": self-injury and staff-client relationships. *Learning Disability Practice*, *11*, 12.

Gallop, R. (2002). Failure of the capacity for self-soothing in women who have a history of abuse and self-harm. *Journal of the American Psychiatric Nurses Association*, *8*, 20.

Gilbert, P., et al. (2010). Self-harm in a mixed clinical population: the roles of self-criticism, shame, and social rank. *The British Journal of Clinical Psychology*, *49*, 563.

Guertin, T., et al. (2001). Self-mutilative behavior in adolescents who attempt suicide by overdose. *Journal of the American Academy of Child and Adolescent Psychiatry*, *40*(9), 1062.

Hagerty, B., & Patusky, K. (2011). Mood disorders: depression and mania. In K. M. Fortinash & P. A. Holoday-Worret (Eds.), *Psychiatric mental health nursing* (5th ed.). St Louis: Mosby.

Hall, B., & Place, M. (2010). Cutting to cope-a modern adolescent phenomenon. *Child: Care, Health and Development*, *36*, 623.

Holm, A. L., & Severinsson, E. (2010). Desire to survive emotional pain related to self-harm: a Norwegian hermeneutic study. *Nursing and Health Sciences*, *12*(1), 52.

Joyce, P. R., et al. (2010). Self-mutilation and suicide attempts: relationships to bipolar disorder, borderline personality disorder, temperament and character. *The Australian and New Zealand Journal of Psychiatry*, *44*, 250.

Lesniak, R. G. (2010). The lived experience of adolescent females who self-injure by cutting. *Advanced Emergency Nursing Journal*, *32*(2), 137.

Moller, C. I., Tait, R. J., & Byrne, D. G. (2013). Deliberate Self-Harm, Substance Use, and Negative Affect in Nonclinical Samples: a Systematic Review. *Substance Abuse*, *34*(2), 188–207.

Muehlenkamp, J. J., Claes, L., Quigley, K., et al. (2013a). Association of training on attitudes towards self-injuring clients across health professionals. *Archives of Suicide Research*, *17*(4), 462–468.

Muehlenkamp, J. J., Bagge, C. L., Tull, M. T., et al. (2013b). Body regard as a moderator of the relation between emotion dysregulation and nonsuicidal self-injury. *Suicide & Life-Threatening Behavior*, *43*(5), 479–493.

Murray, C. D., MacDonald, S., & Fox, J. (2008). Body satisfaction, eating disorders and suicide ideation in an Internet sample of self-harmers reporting and not reporting childhood sexual abuse. *Psychology, Health and Medicine*, *13*, 29.

Peebles, R., Wilson, J. L., & Lock, J. D. (2011). Self-injury in adolescents with eating disorders: correlates and provider bias. *The Journal of Adolescent Health*, *48*, 310.

Pryjmachuk, S., & Trainor, G. (2010). Helping young people who self-harm: perspectives from England. *Journal of Child and Adolescent Psychiatric Nursing*, *23*(2), 52.

Rasmussen, S. A., et al. (2010). Elaborating the Cry of Pain model of suicidality: testing a psychological model in a sample of first-time and repeat self-harm patients. *The British Journal of Clinical Psychology*, *49*(Part1), 15.

Ray, R., Perkins, E., & Meijer, B. (2011). The evolution of practice changes in the use of special observations. *Archives of Psychiatric Nursing*, *25*, 90.

Rissanen, M., Kylma, J., & Laukkanen, E. (2009). Helping adolescents who self-mutilate: parental descriptions. *Journal of Clinical Nursing*, *18*, 1711.

Rissanen, M., Kylma, J., & Laukkanen, E. (2011). A systematic literature review: self-mutilation among adolescents as a phenomenon and help for it-what kind of knowledge is lacking? *Issues in Mental Health Nursing*, *32*, 575.

Schoppmann, S., et al. (2007). "Then I just showed her my arms…." Bodily sensations in moments of alienation related to self-injurious behaviour. A hermeneutic phenomenological study. *Journal of Psychiatric and Mental Health Nursing*, *14*, 587.

Self-injury.net *Distractions*. From: <http://self-injury.net/information-recovery/recovery/distractions> Retrieved February 22, 2012.

Weber, M. T. (2002). Triggers for self-abuse: a qualitative study. *Archives of Psychiatric Nursing*, *16*, 118.

Wright, F., et al. (2009). Co-occurrence of self-reported disordered eating and self-harm in UK university students. *The British Journal of Clinical Psychology*, *48*(Pt. 4), 397.

Zilli, E. A., & Hasselmo, M. E. (2008). A model of behavioral treatments for self-mutilation behavior in Lesch-Nyhan syndrome. *Neuroreport*, *19*(4), 459–462.

S

Self-Neglect *Susanne W. Gibbons, PhD, C-ANP/GNP*

NANDA-I

Definition

A constellation of culturally framed behaviors involving one or more self-care activities in which there is a failure to maintain a socially accepted standard of health and well-being (Gibbons et al, 2006)

Defining Characteristics

Insufficient environmental hygiene; insufficient personal hygiene; nonadherence to health activities

Related Factors (r/t)

Alteration in cognitive functioning; Capgras syndrome; deficient executive function; fear of institutionalization; frontal lobe dysfunction; functional impairment; inability to maintain control; learning disability; lifestyle choice; malingering; psychiatric disorder; psychotic disorder; stressors; substance abuse

NOC (Nursing Outcomes Classification)

Suggested NOC Outcomes

Self Neglect; Self-Care Status; Self-Care: Activities of Daily Living (ADLs); Risk Detection; Nutritional Status; Social Support

Examples of NOC Outcome with Indicator

Self-Care Status as evidenced by the following indicators: Maintains personal cleanliness, recognizes safety needs in the home. (Rate outcome and indicators of **Self-Care Status:** 1 = severely compromised, 2 = substantially compromised, 3 = moderately compromised, 4 = mildly compromised, 5 = not compromised [see Section I].)

Client Outcomes

Client Will (Specify Time Frame)

- Show improvement in mental health problems
- Show improvement in chronic medical problems
- Reveal improvement in cognition (e.g., if reversible and treatable)
- Demonstrate improvement in functional status (e.g., basic and instrumental activities of daily living)
- Demonstrate adherence to health activities (e.g., medications and medical appointments)
- Exhibit improved personal hygiene
- Exhibit improved environmental hygiene
- Have fewer hospitalizations and emergency room visits
- Increase safety of client
- Increase safety of community in which client lives
- Agree to necessary personal and environmental changes that eliminate risk/endangerment to self or others (e.g., neighbors)

NOTE: Because self-neglect is a culturally framed and socially defined phenomenon, change in a client's status must occur in such a way that it respects individual rights while ensuring individual health and well-being. This is accomplished through client-nurse partnership as well as interdisciplinary collaboration and team work, and in some instances, assistance of next of kin and/or adult protective services (APS) may be needed (e.g., a state agency or local social services program).

NIC (Nursing Interventions Classification)

S

Suggested NIC Interventions

Self Neglect; Self-Care Assistance: Activities of Daily Living; Support System Enhancement

Example NIC Activities—Self-Care Assistance: Activities of Daily Living

Determine individual's need for assistance with ADLs (e.g., shopping, cooking, housekeeping, laundry, use of transportation, managing money, managing medications, use of communication, and use of time)

Nursing Interventions and *Rationales*

- Monitor individuals with acute or chronic mental and complex physical illness for defining characteristics for self-neglect. EBN/EB: *Medical and psychiatric conditions probably underlie most cases of self-neglect, as demonstrated in studies of impaired older adults (Dong et al, 2012; Gibbons et al, 2006; Pavlou & Lachs, 2008).*
- Assist individuals with complex mental and physical health issues to adopt positive health behaviors so that they may maintain their health status in the community. EBN/EB/CEB: *A variety of mental illnesses have been correlated with self-neglect in younger adults. However, in the older adult population, depression has been particularly associated with self-neglecting behavior, with inadequately treated medical disease identified more often in self-neglecters who are also depressed (Burnett et al, 2006; Gibbons et al, 2006).*
- Assess persons with complex health issues for adequate coping abilities, and assist those with coping problems to maintain their health and well-being in the community. EBN: *Personal control and protecting*

self are coping strategies seen in community-dwelling self-neglecters and in those identified by APS. Individuals use these strategies to compensate, which sometimes causes them to appear uncooperative or resistant to care and change (Gibbons, 2009; Lauder & Roxburgh, 2012).

- Assist individuals with reconnecting with family, friends, and other social networks available to them. CEB/EBN: *Social isolation is a risk for self-neglect: as seen in a case control study, 91 confirmed self-neglecting older adults were more likely to live alone, even if married, had less frequent visits from family, friends, and neighbors, and were less likely to participate in religious activities (Burnett et al, 2006; Gibbons, 2009).*
- Assist individuals whose self-care is failing with managing their medication regimen. EBN/EB: *Individuals who exhibit self-neglect may have difficulty managing medication, as seen in a community study of 100 APS-confirmed older adults with self-neglect, in which researchers found the average rate of medication adherence to be 59% (Turner et al, 2014).*
- Assess individuals with failing self-care for noncompliance (e.g., diagnostic testing, medication regimen, therapeutic regimen, and safety precautions). EBN: *Individuals who exhibit self-neglect may demonstrate noncompliance with other therapeutic regimens as well (Gibbons et al, 2006; Naik et al, 2008).*
- Assist persons with self-care deficits due to ADL or IADL impairments. EBN/EB/CEB: *Individuals with self-care deficits may have difficulty with ADLs. Greater self-neglect severity has been associated with lower levels of physical function among older adults (Ernst & Smith, 2011; Dong et al, 2009).*
- Assess persons with failing self-care for changes in cognitive function (e.g., dementia or delirium). EBN: *Individuals with failing self-care may have changes in cognition. Decline in executive function has been associated with risk of reported and confirmed elder self-neglect, and decline in global cognitive function has been associated with risk of greater self-neglect severity (Naik et al, 2008).*

▲ Refer persons with failing self-care to appropriate specialists (e.g., psychologist, psychiatrist, social work) and therapists (e.g., physical therapy, occupational therapy). EBN/EB: *Individuals with self-care deficits may need assistance from other health professionals (Burnett et al, 2014; Lauder & Roxburgh, 2012).*

- Use behavioral modification as appropriate to bring about client changes that lead to improvement in personal hygiene, environmental hygiene, and adherence to medical regimen. EBN/EB/CEB: *Behavioral modification approaches have been effective in reversing self-neglect in older adults who had triggers or events that brought about the behavior (Fraser, 2006; Gibbons, 2009; Thibault, 2008).*
- Monitor persons with substance abuse problems (i.e., drugs, alcohol, smoking) for adequate safety. EBN/EB: *Because mental health and substance use disorders can go unrecognized and untreated in this population, identified self-neglecting clients should be screened as appropriate by nurses and other health professionals (Gibbons, 2009; Paveza et al, 2008). Self-neglecters demonstrate a unique pattern of controlled prescription drug use as seen in a matched control community study of pain, insomnia, and anxiety, where self-neglecting subjects were less likely to take non-opioid pain medications (e.g., Tylenol) and were four times as likely to use benzodiazepines (Culberson et al, 2011).*

S

▲ Refer persons with failing self-care who are significantly impaired cognitively or functionally and who are suspected victims of abuse to APS. EB/CEB: *Self-neglect has been associated with mistreatment in older adults, especially those who live alone (Dyer et al, 2007; Pavlou & Lachs, 2008).*

- Monitor clients with changes in cognitive function for adequate safety. EB: *Dementia is one of the leading causes for self-neglect (Dong et al, 2010; Dong et al, 2012; Dyer et al, 2007).*
- Monitor clients with functional impairments for adequate safety. EBN/CEB: *Functional impairment, often associated with depression in the older adult, is correlated with self-neglect (Lachs et al, 2002).*
- Assist individuals with complex mental and physical health needs with maintaining their health and well-being in the community. EB: *Those self-neglecters institutionalized in nursing homes have a higher mortality rate than those never identified, and for this reason, maintaining a client's health and well-being in the community setting is essential to a more positive outcome (Gibbons, 2009; Lauder & Roxburgh, 2012).*

Geriatric

▲ Assess client's socioeconomic status and refer for appropriate support. EB: *Findings from several studies associate elder self-neglect/neglect with frail older adults' and their families' lack of resources to pay for essential goods and services, leading to inadequate health care and lack of other formal support programs for these older adults and their caregivers (Choi et al, 2009; Dong et al, 2009).*

▲ Refer persons demonstrating a significant decline in self-care abilities (e.g., posing a threat to themselves or to their community) for evaluation of capacity and executive function. EB: *Current evidence indicates that executive dyscontrol contributes to self-neglect in the older adult population, where it might be considered a geriatric syndrome (Dyer et al, 2007; Pavlou & Lachs, 2006).*

▲ Obtain the assistance of APS in the case of refusal of professional health care services when there is a clear indication of self-endangerment. EB: *Evidence from a systematic review of the medical literature and a roundtable discussion with an interdisciplinary group of experts in the field of gerontology and elder mistreatment led to this important distinction for intervention (Pavlou & Lachs, 2008).*

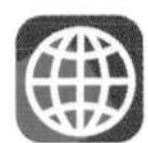

Multicultural

- Deliver health care that is sensitive to the culture and philosophy of individuals whose self-care appears inadequate. EBN: *Nurses must be careful not to prematurely judge clients' health choices or living arrangements, because personal choice or lifestyle does not necessarily indicate self-neglect until client behavior poses a risk to self and/or others. For this reason, it is imperative that nurses assess values and beliefs of persons with inadequate self-care to better identify their individual health needs (Gibbons et al, 2006).*
- Awareness that racial differences for self-neglect may exist, putting some older adults more at risk than others. EB/CEB: *When assessing psychological health and social factors of self-neglecters identified in a biracial community, it was found that there was a significant association between self-neglect severity and health and social factors. Older black adults had more days away from usual activities and less social engagement and suffered greater mortality related to self-neglect than their white counterparts (Dong et al, 2010a; Dong et al, 2011).*

REFERENCES

Burnett, J., Coverdale, J. H., Pickens, S., et al. (2006). What is the association between self-neglect, depressive symptoms and untreated medical conditions? *Journal of Elder Abuse and Neglect, 18*, 25–34.

Burnett, J., Dyer, C. B., Halphen, J. M., et al. (2014). Four subtypes of self-neglect in older adults: results of a latent class analysis. *Journal of the American Geriatrics Society, 62*, 1127–1132.

Choi, N. G., Kim, J., & Asseff, J. (2009). Self-neglect and neglect of vulnerable older adults: reexamination of etiology. *Journal of Gerontological Social Work, 52*, 171–187.

Culberson, J. W., Ticker, R. L., Burnett, J., et al. (2011). Prescription medication use among self-neglecting elderly. *Journal of Addictions Nursing, 22*, 63–68.

Dong, X. Q., Mendes de Leon, C. F., & Evans, D. A. (2009). Is greater self-neglect severity associated with lower levels of physical functioning? *Gerontologic Care, 21*(4), 596–610.

Dong, X. Q., Simon, M., Beck, T., et al. (2010a). A cross-sectional population-based study of elder self-neglect and psychological, health, and social factors in a biracial community. *Ageing and Mental Health, 14*(1), 74–84.

Dong, X. Q., Simon, M. A., Wilson, R. S., et al. (2010b). Decline in cognitive function and risk of elder self-neglect. *Journal of the American Geriatrics Society, 58*(12), 2292–2299.

Dong, X. Q., Wilson, R. S., Mendes De Leon, C. F., et al. (2010c). Self-neglect and cognitive function among community-dwelling older persons. *International Journal of Geriatric Psychiatry, 25*, 798–806.

Dong, X. Q., Simon, M. A., Fulmer, T., et al. (2011). A prospective population-based study of differences in elder self-neglect and mortality between black and white older adults. *The Journals of Gerontology. Series A, Biological Sciences and Medical Sciences, 66*, 695–704.

Dong, X. Q., Simon, M. A., Mosqueda, L., et al. (2012). The prevalence of elder self-neglect in a community-dwelling population: hoarding, hygiene, and environmental hazards. *Journal of Aging and Health, 24*(3), 507–524.

Dyer, C. B., Goodwin, J. S., Pickens, S., et al. (2007). Self-neglect among the elderly: a model based on more than 500 patients seen by a geriatric medicine team. *American Journal of Public Health, 97*(9), 1671–1676.

Ernst, J. S., & Smith, C. A. (2011). Adult protective services clients confirmed for self-neglect: characteristics and service use. *Journal of Elder Abuse & Neglect, 23*, 289–303.

Fraser, A. (2006). Psychological therapies in the treatment of abused adults. *Journal of Adult Protection, 8*(2), 31–38.

Gibbons, S. (2009). Theory synthesis for self-neglect: a health and social phenomenon. *Nursing Research, 58*(3), 194–200.

Gibbons, S., Lauder, W., & Ludwick, R. (2006). Self-neglect: a proposed new NANDA diagnosis. *International Journal of Nursing Terminologies and Classifications, 17*(1), 10–18.

Lachs, M. S., Williams, C. S., O'Brien, S., et al. (2002). Adult protective service use and nursing home placement. *The Gerontologist, 42*, 734–739.

Lauder, W., & Roxburgh, M. (2012). Self-neglect consultation rates and co-morbidities in primary care. *International Journal of Nursing Practice, 18*, 454–461.

Naik, A., Lai, J. M., Kunik, M. E., et al. (2008). Assessing capacity in suspected cases of self-neglect. *Geriatrics, 63*(2), 24–31.

Paveza, G., Vande Weerd, C., & Laumann, E. (2008). Elder self-neglect: a discussion of typology. *Journal of the American Geriatrics Society, 56*(Suppl. 2), S271–S275.

Pavlou, M. P., & Lachs, M. S. (2006). Could self-neglect in older persons be a geriatric syndrome? *Journal of the American Geriatrics Society, 54*, 831–842.

Pavlou, M. P., & Lachs, M. S. (2008). Self-neglect in older adults: a primer for physicians. *Journal of General Internal Medicine, 23*(11), 1841–1846.

Thibault, J. M. (2008). Analysis and treatment of self-neglectful behaviors in three elderly female patients. *Journal of Elder Abuse & Neglect, 19*(3/4), 151–166.

Turner, A., Hochschild, A., Burneett, J., et al. (2014). High Prevalence of medication non-adherence in a sample of community-dwelling older adults with adult protective services-validated self-neglect. *Drugs and Aging, 29*, 741–749.

S

Sexual dysfunction

Elaine E. Steinke, PhD, APRN, CNS-BC, FAHA, FAAN

NANDA-I

Definition

A state in which an individual experiences a change in sexual function during the sexual response phases of desire, excitation, and/or orgasm, which is viewed as unsatisfying, unrewarding, or inadequate

Defining Characteristics

Alteration in sexual activity; alteration in sexual excitation; alteration in sexual satisfaction; change in interest toward others; change in self-interest; change in sexual role; decrease in sexual desire; perceived/actual sexual limitation; seeks confirmation of desirability; undesired change in sexual function

Related Factors (r/t)

Absent of privacy; absence of significant other; alteration in body function (due to anomaly, age disease, medication, pregnancy, radiation, surgery, trauma); alteration in body structure (due to anomaly, disease, pregnancy, radiation, surgery, trauma); inadequate role model; insufficient knowledge about sexual function; misinformation about sexual function; presence of abuse (e.g., physical, psychological, sexual); psychosocial abuse (e.g., controlling, manipulation, verbal abuse); value conflict; vulnerability

NOC (Nursing Outcomes Classification)

Suggested NOC Outcomes

Abuse Recovery: Sexual; Knowledge: Sexual Function, Physical Aging; Psychosocial Adjustment: Life Change; Risk Control: Sexually Transmitted Diseases (STDs); Sexual Functioning; Sexual Identity

Example NOC Outcome with Indicators

Sexual Functioning as evidenced by the following indicators: Expresses comfort with sexual expression/Expresses comfort with body/Expresses sexual interest. (Rate the outcome and indicators of **Sexual Functioning:** 1 = never demonstrated, 2 = rarely demonstrated, 3 = sometimes demonstrated, 4 = often demonstrated, 5 = consistently demonstrated [see Section I].)

S

Client Outcomes

Client Will (Specify Time Frame)

- Identify individual cause of sexual dysfunction
- Identify stressors that contribute to dysfunction
- Discuss alternative, satisfying, and acceptable sexual practices for self and partner
- Identify the degree of sexual interest by the client and partner
- Adapt sexual technique as needed to cope with sexual problems
- Discuss with partner concerns about body image and sex role

NIC (Nursing Interventions Classification)

Suggested NIC Interventions

Sexual Counseling; Teaching: Sexuality

Example NIC Activities—Sexual Counseling

Provide privacy and ensure confidentiality; Discuss necessary modifications in sexual activity, as appropriate; Provide referral/consultation with other members of the health care team, as appropriate

Nursing Interventions and *Rationales*

- Gather the client's sexual history, noting normal patterns of functioning and the client's vocabulary, and encouraging clients to ask questions or discuss sexual problems experienced. EBN: *Women should be evaluated for female sexual dysfunction (FSD), with attention to problems with desire, arousal, orgasm, and pain, as part of a complete history and physical exam (Albaugh, 2014).* EB: *In a cross-sectional study of 388 men evaluated in the cardiology office setting, 56% had erectile dysfunction (ED), and of these 46% expressed interest in discussing ways to improve sexual function with the cardiologist, and 55% wanted a consultation with a specialized nurse (Nicolai et al, 2014b).*

▲ Assess duration and risk factors for sexual dysfunction and explore potential causes such as medications, medical problems, aging process or psychosocial issues. EB: *Erectile dysfunction shares many of the same risk factors of cardiovascular disease (CVD), and a systematic review suggests that erectile dysfunction may be an early marker of CVD in men, preceding CVD by an average of 3 years (Gandaglia et al, 2014).* EB: *Novel approaches may be needed for effective ED care; e-medicine has been shown to improved uniform questioning, history taking, physical exam, screening, and client education, with outcomes greater than that with more traditional care and with improved client-provider communication (Smith et al, 2013).*

• Assess for history of sexual abuse. EB: *Risk factors for adult sexual victimization included being a woman, living alone, economically disadvantaged, and a history of childhood abuse/neglect or parental psychopathology; adult sexual victimization was linked with post-traumatic stress disorder and drug abuse (Xu et al, 2013).*

• Determine the client and partner's current knowledge and understanding, and validate that it is normal to have sexual concerns. EBN: *A qualitative study of women's understanding of sexual problems illustrated that while diagnostic criteria typically do not take into account the partner, women expressed that partner and relationship factors are fundamental factors within the context of the sexual relationship, and inclusive of physical and psychological perspectives (Bellamy et al, 2013).* EBN: *Only 41% of 115 clients with MI and 31% of partners reported a discussion of sex and relationships with health care professionals, and in comparing sexual knowledge from 1 month post-MI to 1 year, knowledge increased for clients and not for partners, illustrating the need to include partners in discussions; the Sex After MI Knowledge Test could be used to facilitate discussion and evaluate knowledge (Brännström et al, 2014).*

▲ Assess and provide treatment for sexual dysfunction, involving the person's partner in the process, and evaluating pharmacological and nonpharmacological interventions. EB: *The use of phosphodiesterase type 5 (PDE5) inhibitors is generally safe in men with cardiovascular disease, although they should be avoided for those receiving nitrate therapy (Levine et al, 2012).* EB: *A review of trials related to sexual satisfaction and PDE5 inhibitors showed a positive relationship between erectile function and both individual sexual satisfaction and satisfaction with erections, as well as satisfaction between the couple and the sexual relationship (Mulhall et al, 2011).*

• Assess risk factors for sexual dysfunction, especially with varying sexual partners. EB: *Men having sex with men had sexual dysfunction with progressive HIV infection (Shindel et al, 2011).* EB: *In Chinese men who had sex with men, sexual dysfunction was prevalent in more than half of study participants, although contributing factors to sexual dysfunction is not well understood in China or other countries (Tsui et al, 2014).*

• Observe for stress and anxiety as possible causes of dysfunction. EBN: *A survey of cardiac rehabilitation clients revealed that ED and lack of interest in sex were commonly reported, with deterioration in sexual function after a cardiac event, and higher anxiety and being male predictive of sexual problems (Byrne et al, 2013).* EB: *Sexual problems and concerns were prevalent among women post-MI, including fears about causing another MI and the risks and safety in resuming sexual activity (Abramsohn et al, 2013).*

▲ Assess for depression as a possible cause of sexual dysfunction, and institute appropriate treatment, as depression is commonly observed in clients with chronic disease and chronic pain. EB: *Adolescents in a trial using a group delivered HIV prevention intervention, and either a general health or sexual health intervention, reported significantly fewer depressive symptoms for both groups, and even more so for those in the sexual health intervention group (Brown et al, 2014).* EBN: *Sexually active cardiac clients reported less sexual depression than those not sexually active; measures to promote sexual function and treatment of sexual dysfunction are important for sexual quality of life (Steinke et al, 2013b). (Additional relevant research: Mosack et al, 2011.)*

• Observe for grief related to loss (e.g., amputation, mastectomy, ostomy), as a change in body image often precedes sexual dysfunction. See care plan for Disturbed **Body Image.** EB: *Changes in body image occur in over half of cancer survivors and 41% experience a decrease in sexual function (Averyt & Nishimoto, 2014).* EB: *A study using a psychoeducational group intervention to examine quality of life in breast cancer survivors had improved relationship adjustment and increased satisfaction with sex (Rowland et al, 2011).*

- ▲ Explore physical causes of sexual dysfunction such as diabetes, cardiovascular disease, arthritis, or benign prostatic hypertrophy (BPH). EB: *In men and women with heart failure, approximately 60% experienced sexual problems related to performance, overall sexual function, and decreased sexual pleasure and satisfaction. Contributing factors included lack of energy, decreased exercise capacity, and depressed mood (Jaarsma et al, 2014).* EB: *Women with diabetes who were insulin dependent were more likely to report problems with vaginal lubrication and orgasm than nondiabetic women, and in all diabetic women, factors associated with decreased sexual function were heart disease, stroke, renal dysfunction, and peripheral neuropathy (Copeland et al, 2012).*
- • Certain chronic diseases such as cancer often have significant effects on sexual function. Both the disease process and treatment can contribute to sexual dysfunction. EBN: *Side effects from cancer treatments such as surgery, chemotherapy, radiation, and other medications contribute to FSD in women with cancer, making treatment such as medications, devices, counseling, and support important interventions (Anderson, 2013).* EB: *In male and female colorectal cancer survivors (N = 261), older age and destructive surgery were associated with poorer erectile function in men, and for women, older age and decreased overall quality of life were associated with lower sexual function scores (Milbury et al, 2013).*
- • Consider that neurological diseases such as multiple sclerosis (MS) affect sexual function directly, but with secondary effects due to disability related to the illness, social, and emotional effects. EBN: *Approximately one half to three fourths of men and women with MS experience sexual problems, which may include erectile dysfunction, delayed ejaculation, and decreased sensation in men, while women may experience decreased libido, impaired genital sensation, problems with orgasm, and vaginal dryness (Ward-Abel & Hall, 2012).*
- • Explore behavioral or other causes of sexual dysfunction, such as smoking, dietary factors, or obesity. EB: *In a small case controlled study of Iranian women, higher body mass index (BMI) was significantly associated with sexual dysfunction, particularly for sexual arousal and pain (Raisi et al, 2013).* EB: *Dyslipidemia contributed to impaired sexual function in men and women with coronary artery disease, in addition to any sexual dysfunction such as ED (Assari et al, 2014).*
- ▲ Consider medications as a cause of sexual dysfunction. EB: *A systematic review of the effects of cardiovascular drugs on sexual function revealed overall negative effects of beta blockers, cardiac glycosides, and diuretics; neutral effects with alpha blockers, angiotensin converting enzyme inhibitors, and calcium channel blockers; and positive effects from angiotensin receptor blockers and statins on sexual function, although there are mixed results for some of these drug classes (Nicolai et al, 2014a).* EB: *A meta-analysis from 63 studies of second generation antidepressants in clients with major depressive disorder showed that bupropion conferred a significantly lower risk of sexual dysfunction, and citalopram and paroxetine were significantly associated with higher risk of sexual dysfunction, when compared with other second generation drugs (Reichenpfader et al, 2014).*
- • Provide privacy when discussing sexual problems and be verbally and nonverbally nonjudgmental. EB: *It is important for health care professionals to balance the sensitivity of discussing sexual issues with the support and educational needs of clients and partners (Steinke et al, 2013b).* EB: *The use of open-ended questions can facilitate sexual discussions (Steinke & Jaarsma, 2014).*
- • Explain the need for the client to share concerns with partner. EB: *Among cardiac clients, partner concerns are prevalent, including fear of causing another cardiac event with sexual activity (Steinke et al, 2013a).*
- ▲ Refer to appropriate medical providers for consideration of medication for premature ejaculation, erectile dysfunction, or orgasmic problems. EB: *Phosphodiesterase type 5 (PDE5) inhibitors are often first line of treatment for ED, with first time response rates of 60% to 70%, overall treatment success rates of 89%, and similar efficacy among the currently available drugs (Smith et al, 2013).* EB: *In a Japanese study, self-confidence and sexual spontaneity in men taking vardenafil and tadalafil were significantly higher than those taking sildenafil, but with clients' time concerns, a preference was shown for taking sildenafil versus tadalafil, which seemed to be related to feeling pressured by having to keep track of time related to drug action and sexual activity (Tsujimura et al, 2014).*
- • Refer women for possible pharmacological intervention for sexual dysfunction. EBN: *Therapies for female sexual dysfunction include testosterone replacement therapy, DHEA, and topical preparations for arousal disorders, atrophy (e.g., topical estrogen), or pain (e.g., lidocaine) (Albaugh, 2014).*

Geriatric

- ▲ Carefully assess the sexuality needs and sexual dysfunction of older adults and refer for counseling if needed. EB: *In older men and women with heart failure, sexual problems occurred in 59%, compared with*

56% in community controls, and sexual problems occurred more frequently in men and those partnered; discussion of sexual problems and implementing appropriate management is an integral part of heart failure care (Hoekstra et al, 2012).

- Teach about normal changes that occur with aging that may be perceived as sexual dysfunction, such as reduction in vaginal lubrication and reduction in duration and resolution of orgasm for women; and for men, increased time required for erection and for subsequent erections, erection without ejaculation, less firm erection, and decreased volume of seminal fluid. EB: *A significant barrier among older adults included the perception that sexual problems were a normal part of aging, and older adults were more likely to seek help if a proactive approach by health care providers was used to assess sexual health (Hinchliff & Gott, 2011).*
- Explore various sexual gratification alternatives (e.g., caressing, sharing feelings) with the client and partner. EBN: *Many satisfying alternatives are available for expressing sexual feelings and, if sexual intercourse is not possible, exploring other types of sexual activities such as hugging, kissing, and sexual touching (Steinke, 2013).*
- Discuss the difference between sexual function, sexuality, and sexual dysfunction, including that all individuals possess sexuality from birth to death, regardless of changes occurring over the life span. EBN: *Sexual problems can be caused by psychological, interpersonal, or social problems and can significantly affect both physical and psychological well-being (Garrett, 2014).* EB: *Successful aging includes positive sexual satisfaction, although sexual problems related to arousal, desire, and ability to climax are associated with increased age (Thompson et al, 2011).*
- If prescribed, instruct clients with chronic pain to take pain medication before sexual activity. EBN: *Nitroglycerin can be used for anginal pain; pain inhibits satisfying sexual activity (Steinke et al, 2013a).* EBN: *Treatment of chronic pain can improve libido and sexual function (Richards et al, 2011).*
- See care plan for Ineffective **Sexuality** pattern.

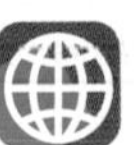

Multicultural

- Evaluate culturally influenced risk factors for sexual dysfunction. EBN: *Women may be reluctant to discuss sexual dysfunction because the topic may be viewed as taboo, and sociocultural factors such as arranged marriages or non-satisfying relationships (Erten et al, 2013).* EB: *Nationally targeted communication campaigns related to HIV often overlook black heterosexual men in prevention efforts, although these men report wanting more information on HIV prevention to better protect themselves and their partners, as well as to educate and protect their children (Bowleg et al, 2013).*
- Validate client feelings and emotions regarding the changes in sexual behavior, letting the client know that the nurse heard and understands what was said, and promoting the nurse-client relationship. EB: *Assessment of sexual dysfunction throughout cancer treatment is important to facilitate discussion and to evaluate the needs and concerns of clients (Averyt & Nishimoto, 2014).* EBN: *A holistic approach that considers cultural, relationship, psychosocial, and health-related concerns is important to avoid "medicalizing" the sexual problems of women (Bellamy et al, 2013).*

Home Care

- Previously discussed interventions may be adapted for home care use.

▲ Identify specific sources of concern about sexual dysfunction and provide reassurance and instruction on appropriate expectations as indicated. EB: *Clients with schizophrenia and sexual dysfunction had significantly worse subjective quality of life, and aspects of physical arousal such as vaginal lubrication and penile erection were commonly affected; it is important to address causes of sexual dysfunction and implement management strategies tailored to the client (Bushong et al, 2013).*

▲ Confirm that physical reasons for dysfunction have been addressed, and refer for therapy and/or support groups if appropriate. EB: *For all cancers, cancer treatments affected intimacy and sexual functioning related to fatigue, treatment-related hair loss, weight gain, scarring, or organ loss, along with other disease-specific changes such as gastrointestinal problems with colorectal cancer, dyspnea with lung cancer, and incontinence with prostate cancer (Flynn et al, 2011).* EB: *In clients with post-traumatic pelvic fracture, urinary tract injury and open surgical treatment were independently associated with sexual dysfunction, and significant predictors of decreased quality of life were male gender, severity of the fracture, pain, and sexual dysfunction (Harvey-Kelly et al, 2014).*

- Reinforce or teach the client about sexual functioning, alternative sexual practices, and necessary sexual precautions, and update teaching as client status changes. EB: *Attendance at a rural nurse led clinic for* women resulted in significant increases in sexual desire, satisfaction, and quality of orgasm at both 1 and 6 months after the last clinic visit (Hakanson et al, 2014).*

- See care plan for Ineffective **Sexuality** pattern.

Client/Family Teaching and Discharge Planning

- Provide accurate information for clients concerning sexual activity after a cardiac event; consider using cognitive and behavioral strategies. EB: *Interventions that have been successfully used for sexual counseling include cognitive behavioral therapy, social and psychological support, specific and deliberate sexual counseling, a team approach, sexual counseling over several sessions, and the inclusion of both the client and their partner (Steinke et al, 2013a).*
- Include the partner/family in discharge instructions, because partner concerns are often overlooked in regard to sexual issues. EBN: *Psychoeducational interventions and counseling have been shown to improve urinary and/or fecal incontinence, and erectile function in men after radical prostatectomy, and may assist both the client and the client's partner in recovery (Lassen et al, 2013).* EB: *Partners may have even greater sexual concerns than clients themselves, thus it is important to include partners in sexual counseling (Steinke et al, 2013a).*
- Teach the client and partner about condom use, for those at risk. EB: *A meta-analysis evaluated sexual communication and condom use among adolescents, finding that those who engaged in sexual communication with their partners were more likely to use condoms, illustrating that encouraging sexual communication between the adolescent and sexual partner is critical (Widman et al, 2014).*
- ▲ Teach the client with cardiovascular disease that sexual activity can be resumed within a few weeks for those with minimal symptoms with moderate physical activity, although clients at higher risk or with exercise intolerance may need further evaluation. EB: *Clients can usually resume sexual activity after 1 week for an uncomplicated MI, or in 3 to 4 weeks for most clients; some clients may need to undergo exercise testing to determine tolerance for sexual activity before sexual activity can be resumed (Levine et al, 2012; Steinke et al, 2013a).*
- For cardiac clients, discuss being well rested, reporting any cardiac warning signs, using foreplay to determine tolerance for sexual activity, not using alcohol or eating heavy meals before sex, and having sex with a familiar partner and in the usual setting to decrease any stress the couple might feel. EB: *Sexual activity can be discussed in the context of exercise, comparing the energy expenditure to that required for sexual activity; clients who are able to walk one mile on a flat surface in 20 minutes, briskly climb 2 flights of stairs in 10 seconds, or walk 4 minutes on a treadmill using the Bruce protocol without symptoms, can generally safely resume sexual activity (Nehra et al, 2012).*
- Provide written educational materials that address sexual issues for clients and families of clients with implantable cardiac defibrillators (ICDs). EBN: *Addressing the fears and concerns related to sexual function of ICD clients and partners is essential to rehabilitation and recovery, and the areas of greatest concern for clients were lack of sexual interest, ED, and an overprotective partner, and fewer clients were sexually active after ICD implantation than before (Berg et al, 2013).*
- Discuss sexual problems and adaptations needed for sexual activity with spinal cord injury. EB: *Women with spinal cord injury reported that intimacy was negatively affected by urinary incontinence, they had excessive concern about autonomic dysreflexia, and body image was negatively affected, often delaying sexual activity or ceasing activity altogether (Cramp et al, 2014).*
- ▲ Refer to appropriate community resources, such as a clinical specialist, family counselor, or cardiac rehabilitation, including the partner if appropriate; for complex issues, a referral to a sex counselor, urologist, gynecologist, or other specialist may be needed. EB: *Sexuality was rated as an important issue by clients after stroke (71%), although sexual dysfunction was common (47%); clients expressed the need for counseling by health care providers, within cardiac rehabilitation, and within 1 year of their stroke (Stein et al, 2013).* EB: *A pilot study of a telephone-based sexual counseling intervention for couples that emphasized establishing rapport, couple communications, and enhancing intimacy, provided participants with successful skills to cope with the effects of cancer treatment and to maintain their sexuality (Reese et al, 2012).*
- Teach the importance of diabetic control and its effect on sexuality to clients with diabetes. EB: *Predictors of ED in men with diabetes mellitus type 2 were HbA1c, fasting plasma glucose, and systolic blood pressure; age and taking calcium channel blockers were independent predictors of ED (Sharifi et al, 2012).* EB: *The role of HbA1c was studied in clients with type 2 diabetes mellitus who had a penile prosthesis implanted, finding that HbA1c was reduced, along with improved sexual functioning (Talib et al, 2014).*

S

- ▲ Refer for medical advice when ED lasts longer than 2 months or is recurring. EB: *ED can be treated, and underlying causes need to be investigated through a thorough medical and sexual history (Glina et al, 2014).* EB: *There are four commonly used PDE5 inhibitors available in the U.S. that have shown effectiveness in treating ED; these drugs include sildenafil, vardenafil, tadalafil, and avanafil (Huang & Lie, 2013).*
- • Teach the following interventions to decrease the likelihood of ED: limit or avoid the use of alcohol, stop smoking, exercise regularly, reduce stress, get enough sleep, deal with anxiety or depression, and see a health care provider for regular checkups and medical screening tests. EB: *Worse scores for erectile function were associated with older age, smoking status, BMI, and resting heart rate (P <.001) in men without a history of CVD or MI; long-term cigarette smoking interfered with sympathovagal balance and negatively affected erectile tumescence (Harte, 2014).*
- • See care plan for Ineffective **Sexuality** pattern.

REFERENCES

Abramsohn, E. M., Decker, C., Garavalia, B., et al. (2013). "I'm not just heart, I'm a whole person here": a qualitative study to improve sexual outcomes in women with myocardial infarction. *Journal of the American Heart Association, 2*, e000199.

Albaugh, J. L. (2014). Female sexual dysfunction. *International Journal of Urologic Nursing, 8*(1), 38–43.

Anderson, J. L. (2013). Acknowledging female sexual dysfunction in women with cancer. *Clinical Journal of Oncology Nursing, 17*, 233–235.

Assari, S., Ahmadi, K., & Saleh, D. K. (2014). Gender differences in the association between lipid profile and sexual function among patients with coronary artery disease. *International Cardiovascular Research Journal, 8*(1), 9–14.

Averyt, J. C., & Nishimoto, P. W. (2014). Addressing sexual dysfunction in colorectal cancer survivorship care. *Journal of Gastrointestinal Oncology, 5*, 388–394.

Bellamy, G., Gott, M., & Hinchliff, S. (2013). Women's understandings of sexual problems; Finding from an in-depth interview study. *Journal of Clinical Nursing, 22*, 3240–3248.

Berg, S. K., Elleman-Jensen, L., Zwisler, A.-D., et al. (2013). Sexual concerns and practices after ICD implantation: findings from the COPE-ICD rehabilitation trial. *European Journal of Cardiovascular Nursing, 12*(5), 468–474.

Bowleg, L., Mingo, M., & Massie, J. S. (2013). "The skill is using your big head over your little head": black heterosexual men say they know, want, and need HIV prevention. *American Journal of Men's Health, 7*(Suppl. 4), 31S–42S.

Brännström, M., Kristofferzon, M.-L., Ivarsson, B., et al. (2014). Sexual knowledge in patients with myocardial infarction and their partners. *Journal of Cardiovascular Nursing, 29*, 332–339.

Brown, J. L., Sales, J. M., Swartzendruber, A. L., et al. (2014). Added benefits: reduced depressive symptom levels among African-American female adolescents participating in and HIV prevention intervention. *Journal of Behavioral Medicine, 37*, 912–920.

Bushong, M. E., Nakonezny, P. A., & Byerly, M. J. (2013). Subjective quality of life and sexual dysfunction in outpatients with schizophrenia or schizoaffective disorder. *Journal of Sex & Marital Therapy, 39*, 336–346.

Byrne, M., Doherty, S., Murphy, A. W., et al. (2013). The CHARMS study: cardiac patients' experiences of sexual problems following cardiac rehabilitation. *European Journal of Cardiovascular Nursing, 12*, 558–566.

Copeland, K. L., Brown, J. S., Creasman, J. M., et al. (2012). Diabetes mellitus and sexual function in middle-aged and older women. *Obstetrics & Gynecology, 120*, 331–340.

Cramp, J., Courtois, F., Connolly, M., et al. (2014). The impact of urinary incontinence on sexual function and sexual satisfaction in women with spinal cord injury. *Sex & Disability, 32*, 397–412.

Erten, Z. K., Zincir, H., Özkan, F., et al. (2013). Sexual lives of women with diabetes mellitus (type 2) and impact of culture on solution for problems related to sexual life. *Journal of Clinical Nursing, 23*, 995–1004.

Flynn, K. E., Jeffery, D. D., Keefe, F. J., et al. (2011). Sexual functioning along the cancer continuum: focus group results from the patient-reported outcomes measurement information system (PROMIS). *Psycho-Oncology, 20*, 378–386.

Gandaglia, G., Briganti, A., Jackson, G., et al. (2014). A systematic review of the association between erectile dysfunction and cardiovascular disease. *European Urology, 65*, 968–978.

Garrett, D. (2014). Psychosocial barriers to sexual intimacy for older people. *British Journal of Nursing, 23*, 327–331.

Glina, S., Cohen, D. J., & Vieira, M. (2014). Diagnosis of erectile dysfunction. *Current Opinion in Psychiatry, 27*, 394–399.

Hakanson, C., Douglas, C., Robertson, J., et al. (2014). Evaluation of a rural nurse-led clinic for female sexual dysfunction. *The Australian Journal of Rural Health, 22*, 33–39.

Harte, C. B. (2014). Concurrent relations among cigarette smoking status, resting heart rate variability, and erectile response. *Journal of Sexual Medicine, 11*, 1230–1239.

Harvey-Kelly, K. F., Kanakaris, N. K., Obakponovwe, O., et al. (2014). Quality of life and sexual function after traumatic pelvic fracture. *Journal of Orthopaedic Trauma, 28*(1), 28–35.

Hinchliff, S., & Gott, M. (2011). Seeking medical help for sexual concerns in mid- and later life: a review of the literature. *Journal of Sex Research, 48*(2–3), 106–117.

Hoekstra, T., Lesman-Leegte, I., Luttik, M. L., et al. (2012). Sexual problems in elderly male and female patients with heart failure. *Heart (British Cardiac Society), 98*, 1647–1652.

Huang, S. A., & Lie, J. D. (2013). Phosphodiesterase-5 (PDE_5) inhibitors in the management of erectile dysfunction. *Pharmacy & Therapeutics, 38*, 407, 414–419.

Jaarsma, T., Fridlund, B., & Mårtensson, J. (2014). Sexual dysfunction in heart failure patients. *Current Heart Failure Reports, 11*, 330–336.

Lassen, B., Gattinger, H., & Saxer, S. (2013). A systematic review of physical impairments following radical prostatectomy: effect of psychoeducational interventions. *Journal of Advanced Nursing, 69*, 2602–2612.

Levine, G. N., Steinke, E. E., Bakaeen, F. G., et al. (2012). Sexual activity and cardiovascular disease: a scientific statement from the American heart association. *Circulation, 125*, 1058–1072.

Milbury, K., Cohen, L., Jenkins, R., et al. (2013). The association between psychosocial and medical factors with long-term sexual dysfunction after treatment for colorectal cancer. *Supportive Care in Cancer, 21*, 793–802.

S

Mosack, V., Steinke, E. E., Wright, D. W., et al. (2011). Effects of depression on sexual activity and sexual satisfaction in heart failure. *Dimensions of Critical Care Nursing*, *30*, 218–225.

Mulhall, J. P., Kaminetsky, J. C., Althof, S. E., et al. (2011). Correlations of satisfaction measures in men treated with phosphodiesterase inhibitors for erectile dysfunction. *American Journal of Men's Health*, *5*, 261–271.

Nehra, A., Jackson, G., Miner, M., et al. (2012). The princeton III consensus recommendations for the management of erectile dysfunction and cardiovascular disease. *Mayo Clinic Proceedings*, *87*, 766–778.

Nicolai, M. P. J., Liem, S. S., Both, S., et al. (2014a). A review of the positive and negative effects of cardiovascular drugs on sexual function: a proposed table for use in clinical practice. *Netherland Heart Journal*, *22*, 11–19.

Nicolai, M. P., van Bavel, J., Somsen, G. A., et al. (2014b). Erectile dysfunction in the cardiology practice—a patients' perspective. *American Heart Journal*, *167*, 178–185.

Raisi, M., Tehran, H. A., Jafarbegloo, E., et al. (2013). Association of body mass index with sexual dysfunction in women referred to health centers of Qom City, 2010, Iran. *Qom University of Medical Sciences Journal*, *7*(5). Available at <http://journal.muq.ac.ir/en/index.php/jmuqen/article/view/353>.

Reese, J. B., Porter, L. S., Somers, T. J., et al. (2012). Pilot feasibility study of a telephone-based couples intervention for physical intimacy and sexual concerns in colorectal cancer. *Journal of Sex & Marital Therapy*, *38*, 402–412.

Reichenpfader, U., Gartlehner, G., Morgan, L. C., et al. (2014). Sexual dysfunction associated with second-generation antidepressants in patients with major depressive disorder: results from a systematic review with network meta-analysis. *Drug Safety*, *37*, 19–31.

Richards, T. A., Bertolotti, P. A., Doss, D., et al. (2011). Sexual dysfunction in multiple myeloma: survivorship care plan of the international myeloma foundation nurse leadership board. *Clinical Journal of Oncology Nursing*, *15*(4), 53–65.

Rowland, J. H., Meyerowitz, B. E., Crespi, C. M., et al. (2011). Addressing intimacy and partner communication after breast cancer: a randomized controlled group intervention. *Breast Cancer Research and Treatment*, *118*(1), 99–111.

Sharifi, F., Asghari, M., Jaberi, Y., et al. (2012). Independent predictors of erectile dysfunction in type 2 diabetes mellitus: is it true what they say about risk factors? *ISRN Endocrinology*, 1–5; Article ID 502353.

Shindel, A. W., Horberg, M. A., Smith, J. F., et al. (2011). Sexual dysfunction, HIV, and AIDS in men who have sex with men. *AIDS Patient Care and Stds*, *25*, 341–349.

Smith, W. B., II, McCaslin, I. R., Gokce, A., et al. (2013). PDE5 inhibitors: considerations for preference and long-term adherence. *The International Journal of Clinical Practice*, *67*, 768–780.

Stein, J., Hillinger, M., Clancy, C., et al. (2013). Sexuality after stroke: patient counseling preferences. *Disability & Rehabilitation*, *35*, 1842–1847.

Steinke, E. E. (2013). Sexuality and chronic illness. *Journal of Gerontological Nursing*, *39*(11), 18–27.

Steinke, E. E., & Jaarsma, T. (2014). Sexual counseling and cardiovascular disease: practical approaches. *Asian Journal of Andrology*, *16*, 1–8.

Steinke, E. E., Jaarsma, T., Barnason, S., et al. (2013a). Sexual counseling for individuals with cardiovascular disease and their partners: a consensus document from the American heart association and the ESC council on cardiovascular nursing and allied health professionals (CCNAP). *Circulation*, *128*(18), 2075–2076.

Steinke, E. E., Mosack, V., & Hill, T. J. (2013b). Sexual self-perception and adjustment of cardiac patients: a psychometric analysis. *Journal of Research in Nursing*, *18*, 191–201.

Talib, R. A., Canguiven, O., & Ansari, A. (2014). Impact of sexual activity on glycated hemoglobin levels in patients with type 2 diabetes mellitus after penile prosthesis implantation. *Urology Journal*, *11*, 1813–1818.

Thompson, W. K., Charoh, L., Vahia, I. V., et al. (2011). Association between higher levels of sexual function, activity, and satisfaction and self-rated successful aging in older postmenopausal women. *Journal of the American Geriatric Society*, *59*, 1503–1508.

Tsui, H. Y., Lau, J. T., Feng, T., et al. (2014). Sexual dysfunction and unprotected anal intercourse among men who have sex with men in two Chinese cities. *Journal of Sex & Marital Therapy*, *40*, 139–148.

Tsujimura, A., Kiuchi, H., Soda, T., et al. (2014). Sexual life of Japanese patients with erectile dysfunction taking phosphodiesterase type 5 inhibitors: an internet survey using the psychological and interpersonal relationship scales-short form questionnaire. *International Journal of Urology*, *21*, 821–825.

Ward-Abel, N., & Hall, J. (2012). Sexual dysfunction in multiple sclerosis: part 1. *British Journal of Neuroscience Nursing*, *8*(1), 32–38.

Widman, L., Noar, S. M., Choukas-Bradley, S., et al. (2014). Adolescent sexual health communication and condom use: a meta-analysis. *Health Psychology*, *33*, 1113–1124.

Xu, Y., Olfson, M., Villegas, L., et al. (2013). A characterization of adult victims of sexual violence: results from the national epidemiological survey for alcohol and related conditions. *Psychiatry*, *76*, 223–240.

S

Ineffective Sexuality pattern

Elaine E. Steinke, PhD, APRN, CNS-BC, FAHA, FAAN

NANDA-I

Definition

Expressions of concern regarding own sexuality

Defining Characteristics

Alterations in relationship with significant other; alteration in sexual activity; alteration in sexual behavior; change in sexual role; difficulty with sexual activity; difficulty with sexual behavior; value conflict

Related Factors (r/t)

Absence of privacy; absence of significant other; conflict about sexual orientation; conflict about variant preference; fear of pregnancy; fear of sexually transmitted infection; impaired relationship with a significant other; inadequate role model; insufficient knowledge about alternatives related to sexuality; skill deficit about alternatives related to sexuality

NOC (Nursing Outcomes Classification)

Suggested NOC Outcomes

Abuse Recovery: Sexual, Body Image; Child Development: Middle Childhood/Adolescence; Client Satisfaction: Teaching; Knowledge: Sexual Function; Psychosocial Adjustment: Life Change; Risk Control: Sexually Transmitted Diseases (STDs); Risk Control: Unintended Pregnancy; Role Performance; Self-Esteem; Sexual Functioning; Sexual Identity

Example NOC Outcome with Indicators

Risk Control: Sexually Transmitted Diseases (STDs) as evidenced by the following indicators: Acknowledges personal risk factors for STD/Uses strategies to prevent STD transmission. (Rate the outcome and indicators of **Risk Control: Sexually Transmitted Diseases (STDs):** 1 = never demonstrated, 2 = rarely demonstrated, 3 = sometimes demonstrated, 4 = often demonstrated, 5 = consistently demonstrated [see Section I].)

Client Outcomes

Client Will (Specify Time Frame)

- State knowledge of difficulties, limitations, or changes in sexual behaviors or activities
- State knowledge of sexual anatomy and functioning
- State acceptance of altered body structure or functioning
- Describe acceptable alternative sexual practices
- Identify importance of discussing sexual issues with significant other
- Describe practice of safe sex with regard to pregnancy and avoidance of STIs

NIC (Nursing Interventions Classification)

Suggested NIC Interventions

Sexual Counseling; Teaching: Sexuality

Example NIC Activities—Sexual Counseling

Provide privacy and ensure confidentiality; Provide information about sexual functioning, as appropriate

Nursing Interventions and *Rationales*

- After establishing rapport or therapeutic relationship, give the client permission to discuss issues dealing with sexuality, for example: "Have you been or are you concerned about functioning sexually because of your health status?" EBN/EB: *Use the PLISSIT model to uncover additional concerns (Permission, Limited Information, Specific Suggestions, referral to Intensive Therapy), and begin with more general questions and then those more personal; for example, discuss exercise recommendations and then sex as another form of exercise (McLeod & Hamilton, 2013; Steinke et al, 2013a).*
- Use assessment questions and standardized instruments to assess sexual problems, where possible. EBN/EB: *Use specific assessment questions to obtain information on current level of sexual activity, changes in sexual satisfaction, the nature of any problems experienced, underlying causes, and beliefs and misconceptions (Steinke, 2013; Steinke & Jaarsma, 2014).*

▲ Assess any risks associated with sexual activity, particularly coronary risks. EB: *Cardiac patients without angina or with mild angina who can exercise at a rate of at least 3 to 5 METS (amount of energy expenditure), and without experiencing angina, ischemic ST segment changes, or excess dyspnea are generally at low risk for cardiac events with sexual activity; those at high risk or if risk classification has not been deter-*

S

mined, exercise stress testing is recommended (Lange & Levine, 2014; Levine et al, 2012). **EBN:** *If a cardiac patient is able to engage in physical activity at the rate of 3 to 5 METS or 3 to 4 miles per hour on a treadmill, or climb two flights of stairs briskly, sexual activity can generally be resumed (Steinke & Jaarsma, 2014).*

- Include the client's partner in discussing sexual concerns and in providing sexual counseling. **EBN:** *Information provided to partners is often inadequate, and discussing sexual issues increases partner understanding and may minimize overprotectiveness by the partner; in post-MI patients and partners, patient knowledge about sex after MI improved at 1 year, while partners' knowledge did not change (Brännström et al, 2014).* **EBN:** *Partners' ratings of their intimate relationships were high both before and after the patient's MI, with women providing somewhat lower ratings before MI and improved ratings at 1 year, while men's ratings declined somewhat, illustrating the need to discuss sexual concerns with patients and their partners, and to encourage open communication by the couple (Fransson et al, 2013; Dalteg et al, 2011).*
- Encourage the client to discuss concerns with his or her partner. **EBN:** *Not communicating sexual concerns as a couple can lead to stress and deterioration in the relationship, while open and honest discussions with one's partner can promote sexual intimacy; an ideal time for such discussions might be during a daily walk together (Steinke et al, 2013a; Steinke, 2013).*
- Explore attitudes about sexual intimacy and changes in sexuality patterns. **EBN:** *Patients with chronic heart failure and their partners reported considerable changes in sexual activity (65%), sexual interest, pleasure and sexual satisfaction, and decline in sexual performance, illustrating the importance of nurses discussing changes in sexual function, considering both psychological and physical perspectives (van Driel et al, 2014).* **EB:** *Adults burned as children felt sexually attractive and confident about sexual activity, showing that sexual attitudes and behaviors may not be negatively affected by prior burn injury (Meyer et al, 2011).*
- Assess psychosocial function such as anxiety, fear, depression, and low self-esteem. **EBN:** *Cardiac patients who were sexually active had less sexual anxiety and depression, and higher sexual self-efficacy and satisfaction, when compared to those not sexually active, who reported negative effects on sexual function for these variables (Steinke et al, 2013b).* **EB:** *Women experiencing sexual distress was significantly associated with decreased pleasure, sexual frequency, and negative partner emotions, and greater distress was experienced by older women and those in unsatisfying relationships (Stephenson & Meston, 2012). (Additional relevant research: Mosack et al, 2011.)*
- Discuss alternative sexual expressions for altered body functioning or structure, including closeness and sexual and nonsexual touching as other forms of expression. **EBN:** *The meaning of sex and sexuality is individually defined, with some engaging in sexual intercourse, whereas others may prefer touching, holding one another, or kissing (Steinke, 2013).* **EB:** *Most sexually active older women reported sexual satisfaction, and sexual satisfaction increased with age, although being sexually active was not contingent on sexual activity (Trompeter et al, 2012).*
- Some clients choose masturbation for sexual release, an acceptable form of sexual expression, and for some with chronic illnesses, it may be an alternative to sexual intercourse when exercise tolerance is low. **EBN:** *Discuss sexual activities in the context of exercise tolerance and suggest acceptable alternatives to the client when sexual intercourse is not possible (Steinke, 2013; Steinke et al, 2013a).* **CEB:** *For some clients with severe heart failure, activities such as mutual masturbation, oral sex, or sexual intercourse may not be possible if exercise capacity is compromised, making other expressions of intimacy of greater importance (Medina et al, 2009).*
- Assess the client's sexual orientation and usual pattern of sexual activities, and discuss prevention of illnesses for which the client may be at increased risk (e.g., anorectal cancer), asking specific questions about sexual orientation, for example, "Do you have sexual relationships with men, women, or both?" Assess use of safer sex practices (e.g., condom use); the frequency of anal intercourse; number of sexual partners in the last year; last HIV screening/results; and use of medications, alcohol, and illicit drugs. **EB:** *Among young men who identified themselves as gay, bisexual, or other men who had sex with men, risk behaviors were highest among those with lower socioeconomic status and foreign-born individuals living in the United States, illustrating that assessment beyond race and ethnicity is important to reach those at risk (Halkitis & Figueroa, 2013).* **EB:** *A sexual genogram is a useful tool to assess issues related to sex and sexuality and to frame intervention, as well as to explore overt and covert messages about sexual behaviors, communication patterns about intimacy, sexual secrets, missing information, and partner communication and perceptions (Belous et al, 2012).*

S

- Specific guidelines for sexual activity for clients who have had total hip arthroplasty include the following: sexual activity can be generally resumed 1 to 2 months after surgery, and a supine position ("missionary") at maximum abduction in extension to prevent hip dislocation, avoiding the lateral decubitus positions, which carry a higher risk of adduction and internal rotation of the hip. EBN: *Although literature supports the use of the supine position and a passive role for the patient, others suggestions include the man and woman standing, with the woman's legs slightly bent and the man approaching the woman from behind (McFadden, 2013).* EB: *In degenerative osteoarthritis patients undergoing total hip or knee replacement, improvements occurred for sexual self-image (55%), improved libido (42%), and increased intercourse duration (36%) and frequency (41%), although fear of damaging the replaced joint (10%) affected sexual function in some patients (Rathod et al, 2013). (Other relevant research: Wall et al, 2011.)*
- Specific guidelines for those who have had a myocardial infarction (MI) include the following: sexual activity can generally be resumed within a few weeks after MI unless complications are experienced, such as arrhythmias or cardiac arrest; engaging in sexual activity in familiar surroundings with the usual partner; a comfortable room temperature, when well rested to minimize cardiac stress; avoiding heavy meals or alcohol for 2 to 3 hours before sexual activity, and choosing a position of comfort to minimize stress of the cardiac client. EB: *Guidelines from the American Heart Association and the European Society of Cardiology suggest that resumption of sexual activity after MI is safe for most patients, and occurrence of MI with sexual activity is estimated to be less than 1% (Levine et al, 2012; Steinke et al, 2013a).* EB: *Studies of cardiac nurses reveal that increased attention is needed for sexual counseling by cardiac nurses, including cardiac rehabilitation nurses (Barnason et al, 2011; Steinke et al, 2011).*
- Specific guidelines for those who had complete coronary revascularization, in addition to those mentioned with MI, include those with successful percutaneous cardiovascular revascularization without complication can resume sex within a few days; those who have had coronary artery bypass grafting (CABG) or noncoronary open heart surgery may resume sex in 6 to 8 weeks; incisional pain with sexual activity can be managed by premedicating with a mild pain reliever; and reassurance should be provided to the partner that sexual activity will not harm the sternum as long as direct pressure is avoided. EB: *Women, particularly those with large breasts, may report more issues related to pain in the breast, chest numbness, and difficulty healing; therefore, encourage the woman to choose a position of comfort, support with pillows, and take a pain reliever such as acetaminophen before sexual activity (Steinke & Jaarsma, 2014).*
- Specific guidelines for those with an implantable cardioverter defibrillator (ICD) include assuring the client and partner that fears about being shocked during sexual activity are normal, and sex can be resumed after the ICD is placed as long as strain on the implant site is avoided; if the ICD discharges with sexual activity, the client should stop, rest, and later notify the health care provider that the device fired so that a determination can be made if this was an appropriate shock or not. The client should be instructed to report any dyspnea, chest pain, or dizziness with sexual activity. EBN: *In a randomized controlled trial of 196 patients who received exercise training and psychoeducational follow-up, the greatest reported concerns were lack of interest in sex, erectile dysfunction, and an overprotective partner; sexual activity had declined from pre- to post-ICD implantation; and sexual concerns and sexual activity did not differ between the intervention and usual care groups (Berg et al, 2013).* EB: *A high level of shock-related anxiety in patients with congenital heart disease with an ICD was associated with poor sexual function scores in both men and women and with depressive symptoms (Cook et al, 2013).*
- Specific guidelines for those with chronic lung disease include planning for sexual activity when energy level is highest; use of controlled breathing techniques; avoiding physical exertion prior to sexual activity; using positions that minimize shortness of breath, such as a semi-reclining position; engaging in sexual activity when medications are at peak effectiveness; and use of an oxygen cannula, if prescribed, to provide oxygen before, during, or after sex (Steinke, 2013). CEB/EBN: *In patients with COPD and post-lung transplantation, sexual desire was improved, but continued problems with breathing capacity and fears were a barrier to sexual activity. Openly discussing sexual fears, assessing fitness for sexual activity, and discussing different positions and other strategies to minimize breathing problems is helpful (Thomsen & Jensen, 2009; Steinke, 2013).* EB: *In women living with lung cancer, those who had regular sexual activity had closer couple relationships; satisfaction with information provided by health professionals and psychological support played a role for both men and women (Préau et al, 2011).*
- Specific guidelines for those with multiple sclerosis include treatment of symptoms with prescribed medications, assessing changes in body image, and supportive therapies to assist with a more satisfying sexual experience, including treatment of neuropathic pain, sexual positions that are most supportive,

S

discussing changes in sensation and stimulation with the partner, use of stretching exercise for tight muscles prior to sexual activity, and avoiding a distended bowel or bladder that may cause discomfort. EB: *Clients experiencing pain from MS had reduced sexual function and body image dissatisfaction; therefore, nonpharmacological and pharmacological management of pain may be helpful to enhance sexual function (Knafo et al, 2011; Ward-Abel & Hall, 2012).* EB: *Both positive and negative partner support yielded significant improvements in sexual satisfaction over time in women with systemic sclerosis (Blackmore et al, 2011).*

- Refer to the care plan **Sexual** dysfunction for additional interventions.

Pediatric

- Provide age-appropriate information for adolescents regarding HIV/AIDS and sexual behavior, and discuss sexually transmitted infections, particularly human papillomavirus, including the risks of perinatal transmission and methods to reduce risks among HIV-infected adolescents. EBN: *Knowledge of sexually transmitted diseases and HIV and discussion of gender roles were identified as important elements of prevention program for Latino adolescents, as well as privacy and confidentiality (Lee et al, 2013).* EB: *African American female adolescents who participated in an HIV prevention intervention with specific sexual health telephone counseling contacts had greater improvement in depressive symptoms than the comparison group; more than 40% had moderate to severe depression at baseline, illustrating the importance of addressing depression in intervention programs (Brown et al, 2014).*
- Encourage client and partner communication in HIV prevention strategies. EB: *In African American adolescent females, partner communication frequency was an important mediator for consistent use and condom protected sex; therefore, strategies to empower adolescent communication with their sexual partner about safe-sex practices are needed (Sales et al, 2012).* EB: *Teenagers and young adults who are identified as "straight" may also engage in homosexual activity, making addressing preventive strategies widely to all youth of importance (McCabe et al, 2011).*
- Provide age-appropriate information regarding potential for sexual abuse. EBN: *Women and adolescents after sexual assault experienced poorer physical health (e.g., STIs, genitourinary complaints) and mental health (e.g., depression, post-traumatic stress disorder), and engaged in greater unhealthy behaviors such as alcohol and drug abuse, illustrating the importance of discussing and screening for potential sexual abuse with adolescents (Wadsworth & Records, 2013).*

Geriatric

S

- Carefully assess the sexuality needs of the older client and refer for counseling if needed; the ability to form satisfying social relationships and to be intimate with others, including building strong emotional intimate connections, contributes to adaptation and successful aging (Steinke, 2013). EB: *Older adults continue to have sexual feelings, and while sexual functioning may be affected by age, the sexual response cycle is the same as in other adults, and many continue to be sexually active (Hartmans et al, 2013).* EB: *The emphasis in older adults' sexuality should be focused on sharing pleasure as a couple, with more emphasis on sexual desire and satisfaction, and less on orgasm and intercourse; engaging in sexual play provides a more realistic focus with less emphasis on performance (McCarthy et al, 2013).*

▲ Explore possible changes in sexuality related to health status, menopause, medications, and sexual risk, and make appropriate referrals. EB: *In community dwelling older adults, the absence of cognitive impairment is an important consideration for maintaining sexual interest, and conversely continuing to be sexually active may be associated with better overall cognitive functioning (Hartmans et al, 2013).* EB: *The number of older adults who are HIV-positive continues to grow due to advances in medical treatment; however, older adults have increased risk related to multiple comorbidities, social isolation, and multiple effects from long-term retroviral therapy. It is important for health care providers to be well educated in managing the long-term health of this population (Cahill & Valadéz, 2013).*

- Allow the client to verbalize feelings regarding loss of sexual partner, and acknowledge problems such as disapproving children, lack of available partner for women, and environmental variables that make forming new relationships difficult. EBN: *Lack of an available partner, negative media portrayals, few studies with sufficient representation of older adults, and fears about entering new relationships are a few of the factors influencing sexuality in older ages (Garrett, 2014).*

▲ Provide a milieu that allows for discussion of sexual issues and a higher level of sexual satisfaction, including allowing couples to room together and the provision of privacy. EB: *Negative attitudes by long-term care facility staff in regard to older adults' sexuality may result in sexual needs being overlooked or sexual*

expression actively discouraged. Although keeping residents safe is important, their right to decision-making regarding intimacy must be considered (Tarzia et al, 2012).
- See care plan for **Sexual** dysfunction.

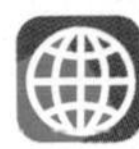

Multicultural

- Assess for the influence of cultural beliefs, norms, and values on client's perceptions of normal sexual behavior. EB: *Mexican migrant women in Mexico and the U.S. reported access to reproductive health care and lack of control over their sexual health as barriers to self-care, as well as sociocultural expectations of when seeking health care is appropriate, and perceived trust and confidentiality concerns (Espinoza et al, 2014).* EBN: *Interviews with Mexican American and African American young men revealed that they struggled to maintain physical and psychological closeness to their partners, and they distanced themselves because of their own unmet psychological needs (Collins & Champion, 2011).*

Home Care

- Previously discussed interventions may be adapted for home care use. Also see care plan for **Sexual** dysfunction.
- Help the client and significant other identify a place and time in the home and daily living for privacy in sharing sexual or relationship activity, and if necessary, help the client communicate the need for privacy to family members. EBN: *Staff in care homes often influence resident perceptions about the appropriateness of sexual expression and may view normal sexual expression as problem behavior; education of staff is important to ensure that acceptance of sexual rights and the dignity of the individual is maintained, while at the same time being of aware of resident safety and sexual abuse (Doll, 2013).*
- Confirm that physical reasons for dysfunction have been addressed, and provide support for coping behaviors, including participation in support groups or therapy if appropriate. EBN: *A 1-day retreat for men with prostate cancer and their partners increased level of knowledge about strategies for sexual recovery, and peer support was rated as an important component of the intervention, although it did not yield better communication among couples or increase sexual activity as hypothesized (Wittmann et al, 2013).* EB: *A pilot study of a Web-based support group for women with gynecologic cancer was well received, with women reporting satisfaction with the intervention and lowered sexual distress (Classen et al, 2013).*
- Reinforce or teach about sexual functioning, alternative sexual practices, and necessary sexual precautions, and update teaching as client status changes. EB: *A couple-focused HIV prevention intervention in young Latino parents reduced the proportion of unprotected sex episodes and increased the intent to use condoms at 6 months, but the results were not sustained at 12 months, although knowledge about AIDS was increased at 6 months and maintained at 12 months (Koniak-Griffin et al, 2011).*

Client/Family Teaching and Discharge Planning

▲ Refer to appropriate community agencies (e.g., certified sex counselor, Reach to Recovery, Ostomy Association, American Association of Sex Educators, Counselors, and Therapists). EBN: *Sexuality concerns should be addressed with all clients for whom sexual function might be affected due to an acute or chronic condition (Steinke, 2013).*

- Sexuality education is important to all populations, whether hearing or deaf, sighted or blind, disabled or not disabled. Discuss contraceptive choices as appropriate, and refer to a health professional (e.g., gynecologist, urologist, nurse practitioner). EB: *Sexuality education of older adults is often overlooked, and they may have less knowledge regarding sexual health risks, such as HIV transmission or use of condoms (Cahill & Valdéz, 2013).*

▲ Teach safe sex to all clients including older adults, including using latex condoms, washing with soap immediately after sexual contact, not ingesting semen, avoiding oral-genital contact, not exchanging saliva, avoiding multiple partners, abstaining from sexual activity when ill, and avoiding recreational drugs and alcohol when engaging in sexual activity. EB: *Suspicion of self-infection during penile-vaginal intercourse among a clinic sample resulted in 63% reporting condom use; nurses helping clients to realistically assess risk may result in greater protective behaviors (Crosby et al, 2014).*

REFERENCES

Barnason, S., Steinke, E., Mosack, V., et al. (2011). Comparison of cardiac rehabilitation and acute care nurses' perceptions of providing sexual counseling for cardiac patients. *Journal of Cardiopulmonary Rehabilitation*, *31*, 157–163.

Belous, C. K., Timm, T. M., Chee, G., et al. (2012). Revisiting the sexual genogram. *The American Journal of Family Therapy*, *40*, 281–296.

Berg, S. K., Elleman-Jensen, L., Zwisler, A.-D., et al. (2013). Sexual concerns and practices after ICD implantation: findings from the COPE-ICD rehabilitation trial. *European Journal of Cardiovascular Nursing*, *12*, 468–474.

Blackmore, D. E., Hart, S. L., Albiani, J. J., et al. (2011). Improvements in partner support predict sexual satisfaction among individuals with multiple sclerosis. *Rehabilitation Psychology*, *56*(2), 117–122.

Brännström, M., Kristofferzon, M.-L., Ivarsson, B., et al. (2014). Sexual knowledge in patients with myocardial infarction and their partners. *Journal of Cardiovascular Nursing*, *29*(4), 332–339.

Brown, J. L., Sales, J. M., Swartzendruber, A. L., et al. (2014). Added benefits: reduced depressive symptom levels among African-American female adolescents participating in and HIV prevention intervention. *Journal of Behavioral Medicine*, *37*, 912–920.

Cahill, S., & Valadéz, R. (2013). Growing older with HIV/AIDS: new public health challenges. *American Journal of Public Health*, *103*, e7–e15.

Classen, C. C., Chivers, M. L., Urowitz, S., et al. (2013). Psychosexual distress in women with gynecologic cancer: a feasibility study of an online support group. *Psycho-Oncology*, *22*, 930–935.

Collins, J. L., & Champion, J. D. (2011). An exploration of young ethnic minority males' beliefs about romantic relationships. *Issues in Mental Health Nursing*, *32*(3), 146–157.

Cook, S. C., Valente, A. M., Maul, T. M., et al. (2013). Shock-related anxiety and sexual function in adults with congenital heart disease and implantable cardioverter-defibrillators. *Heart Rhythm*, *10*, 805–810.

Crosby, R. A., Milhausen, R. R., Graham, C. A., et al. (2014). Likelihood of condom use when sexually transmitted diseases are suspected. *Health Education & Behavior*, *41*, 449–454.

Dalteg, T., Benzein, E., Fridlund, B., et al. (2011). Cardiac disease and its consequences in the partner relationship: a systematic review. *European Journal of Cardiovascular Nursing*, *10*, 140–149.

Doll, G. M. (2013). Sexuality in nursing homes, practice and policy. *Journal of Gerontological Nursing*, *39*(7), 30–37.

Espinoza, R., Martinez, I., Levin, M., et al. (2014). Cultural perceptions and negotiations surrounding sexual and reproductive health among migrant and non-migrant indigenous Mexican women from Yucatan, Mexico. *Journal of Immigrant and Minority Health*, *16*, 356–364.

Fransson, E. I., Arenhall, E., Steinke, E. E., et al. (2013). Perceptions of intimate relationships in partners before and after a patient's myocardial infarction. *Journal of Clinical Nursing*, *23*, 2196–2204.

Garrett, D. (2014). Psychosocial barriers to sexual intimacy for older people. *British Journal of Nursing*, *23*, 327–331.

Halkitis, P. N., & Figueroa, R. P. (2013). Sociodemographic characteristics explain differences in unprotected sexual behavior among young HIV-negative gay, bisexual, and other YMSM in New York City. *AIDS Patient Care and Stds*, *27*(3), 181–190.

Hartmans, C., Comijs, H., & Jonker, C. (2013). Cognitive functioning and its influence on sexual behavior in normal aging and dementia. *International Journal of Geriatric Psychiatry*, *29*, 441–446.

Knafo, R., Haythornthwaite, J. A., Heinberg, L., et al. (2011). The association of body image dissatisfaction and pain with reduced sexual function in women with systemic sclerosis. *Rheumatology*, *50*, 1125–1130.

Koniak-Griffin, D., Lesser, J., Takayanagi, S., et al. (2011). Couple-focused human immunodeficiency virus prevention for young Latino parents: randomized clinical trial of efficacy and sustainability. *Archives of Pediatrics & Adolescent Medicine*, *165*, 306–312.

Lange, R. A., & Levine, G. N. (2014). Sexual activity and ischemic heart disease. *Current Cardiology Reports*, *16*, 445.

Lee, Y.-M., Dancy, B., Florez, E., et al. (2013). Factors related to sexual practices and successful sexually transmitted infection/HIV intervention programs for Latino adolescents. *Public Health Nursing*, *30*, 390–401.

Levine, G. N., Steinke, E. E., Bakaeen, F. G., et al. (2012). Sexual activity and cardiovascular disease: a scientific statement from the American Heart Association. *Circulation*, *125*, 1058–1072.

McCabe, J., Brewster, K. L., & Tillman, K. H. (2011). Patterns of correlates of same-sex sexual activity among U.S. teenagers and young adults. *Perspectives on Sexual and Reproductive Health*, *43*, 142–150.

McCarthy, B., Farr, E., & McDonald, D. (2013). Couple sexuality after 60. *Journal of Family Psychotherapy*, *24*, 38–47.

McFadden, B. (2013). Is there a safe coital position after a total hip arthroplasty? *Orthopaedic Nursing*, *32*, 223–226.

McLeod, D. L., & Hamilton, J. (2013). Sex talk an cancer: who is asking? *Canadian Oncology Nursing Journal*, *23*, 197–201.

Medina, M., Walker, C., Steinke, E. E., et al. (2009). Sexual concerns and sexual counseling in heart failure. *Progress in Cardiovascular Nursing*, *24*, 141–148.

Meyer, W. J., Russell, W., Thomas, C. R., et al. (2011). Sexual attitudes and behavior of young adults who were burned as children. *Burns: Journal of the International Society for Burn Injuries*, *37*, 215–221.

Mosack, V., Steinke, E. E., Wright, D. W., et al. (2011). Effects of depression on sexual activity and sexual satisfaction in heart failure. *Dimensions of Critical Care Nursing*, *30*(4), 218–225.

Préau, M., Bouhnik, A. D., Rey, D., et al. (2011). Two years after cancer diagnosis, which couples become closer? *European Journal of Cancer Care*, *20*, 380–388.

Rathod, P. A., Deshmukh, A. J., Ranawat, A. S., et al. (2013). *Sexual function improves significantly after primary total hip and knee arthroplasty: A prospective study.* Paper presented at the 2013 Annual Meeting of the American Academy of Orthopeadic Surgeons, Chicago, IL. Abstract retrieved from <http://www.abstractsonline.com/Plan/ViewAbstract.aspx?sKey=2ce37c65-d7aa-4d3e-860e-04a0ef9e9f7d&cKey=36be0540-651d-4f68-b7aa-dcab018eac7d&mKey={342D5FB6-3E41-46BB-82B4-861286ECFB41}>.

Sales, J. M., Lang, D. L., DiClemente, R. J., et al. (2012). The mediating role of partner communication frequency on condom use among African American adolescent females participating in an HIV prevention intervention. *Health Psychology*, *31*(1), 63–69.

Steinke, E. E. (2013). Sexuality and chronic illness. *Journal of Gerontological Nursing*, *39*(11), 18–27.

Steinke, E. E., Jaarsma, T., Barnason, S. A., et al. (2013a). Sexual counseling for individuals with cardiovascular disease and their partners: a consensus document from the American heart association and the ESC council on cardiovascular nursing and allied health professionals (CCNAP). *Circulation*, *128*, 2075–2076.

Steinke, E. E., & Jaarsma, T. (2014). Sexual counseling and cardiovascular disease: practical approaches. *Asian Journal of Andrology*, *16*, 1–8.

Steinke, E. E., Mosack, V., Barnason, S., et al. (2011). Progress in sexual counseling by cardiac nurses, 1994 to 2009. *Heart and Lung: The Journal of Critical Care*, *40*(3), e15–e24.

Steinke, E. E., Mosack, V. M., & Hill, T. J. (2013b). Sexual self-perception and adjustment in cardiac patients: a psychometric analysis. *Journal of Research in Nursing*, *18*(3), 191–201.

Stephenson, K. R., & Meston, C. M. (2012). Consequences of impaired female functioning: individual differences and associations with sexual distress. *Sexual and Relationship Therapy*, *27*, 344–357.

Tarzia, L., Fetherstonhaugh, D., & Bauer, M. (2012). Dementia, sexuality and consent in residential aged care facilities. *Journal of Medical Ethics, 38*, 609–613.

Thomsen, D., & Jensen, B. O. (2009). Patients' experiences of everyday life after lung transplantation. *Journal of Clinical Nursing, 18*, 3472–3479.

Trompeter, S. E., Bettencourt, R., & Barrett-Connor, E. (2012). Sexual activity and satisfaction in healthy community-dwelling women. *The American Journal of Medicine, 125*, 37–43.

van Driel, A. G., de Hosson, M. J., & Gamel, C. (2014). Sexuality of patients with chronic heart failure and their spouses and the need for information regarding sexuality. *European Journal of Cardiovascular Nursing, 13*, 227–234.

Wadsworth, P., & Records, K. (2013). A review of the health effects of sexual assault on African American women and adolescents. *Journal of Obstetric, Gynecologic, and Neonatal Nursing, 42*, 249–273.

Wall, P. D. H., Hossain, M., Ganapathi, M., et al. (2011). Sexual activity and total hip arthroplasty: a survey of patients' and surgeons' perspectives. *Hip International, 22*, 199–205.

Ward-Abel, N., & Hall, J. (2012). Sexual dysfunction in multiple sclerosis: part 1. *British Journal of Neuroscience Nursing, 8*(1), 32–38.

Wittmann, D., He, C., Mitchell, S., et al. (2013). A one-day couple group intervention to enhance sexual recovery for surgically treated men with prostate cancer and their partners: a pilot study. *Urologic Nursing, 33*(3), 140–147.

Risk for Shock *June M. Como, EdD, RN, CNS*

NANDA-I

Definition

Vulnerable to an inadequate blood flow to the body's tissues that may lead to life-threatening cellular dysfunction, which may compromise health

Risk Factors

Hypotension; hypovolemia; hypoxemia; hypoxia; infection; sepsis; systemic inflammatory response syndrome (SIRS)

NOC (Nursing Outcomes Classification)

Suggested NOC Outcomes

Cardiac Pump Effectiveness; Fluid Balance; Infection Severity; Respiratory Status: Gas Exchange; Neurological Status: Autonomic; Tissue Perfusion: Cellular

Example NOC Outcome with Indicators

Neurological Status: Autonomic as evidenced by the following indicators: Apical heart rate/Systolic blood pressure/Urinary elimination pattern/Thermoregulation. (Rate the outcome and indicators of **Neurological Status: Autonomic:** 1 = severely compromised, 2 = substantially compromised, 3 = moderately compromised, 4 = mildly compromised, 5 = not compromised [see Section I].)

Client Outcomes

Client Will (Specify Time Frame)

- Discuss precautions to prevent complications of disease
- Maintain adherence to agreed upon medication regimens
- Maintain adequate hydration
- Monitor for infection signs and symptoms
- Maintain a mean arterial pressure above 65 mm Hg
- Maintain a heart rate between 60 and 100 with a normal rhythm
- Maintain urine output greater than 0.5 mL/kg/hr
- Maintain warm, dry skin

NIC (Nursing intervention Classification)

Suggested NIC Interventions

Admission Care; Allergy Management; Cardiac Care; Cerebral Perfusion Promotion; Electrolyte Monitoring; Fever Treatment; Fluid Management; Hemodynamic Regulation; Infection Precaution; Medication

Management; Oxygen Therapy; Postanesthesia Care; Risk Identification; Shock Prevention; Teaching: Disease Process; Temperature Regulation; Vital Signs Monitoring

Example NIC Activities—Shock Prevention

Monitor circulatory status; Monitor for signs of inadequate tissue oxygenation; Administer oxygen and/or mechanical ventilation, as appropriate; Instruct client and/or family on precipitating factors of shock

Nursing Interventions and *Rationales*

- Review data pertaining to client risk status including age, primary diseases, immunosuppression, antibiotic use, and presence of hemodynamic alterations. EB: *Administration of calcium-channel blockers and macrolide antibiotics such as erythromycin and clarithromycin may potentially cause significant hypotension and shock (Henneman & Thornby, 2012). Many clients who develop shock have underlying circumstances that predispose them to shock states as evidenced by hypotension and inadequate organ perfusion (Aitken et al, 2011; Kalil, 2014).*
- Review client's medical and surgical history, noting conditions that place the client at higher risk for shock, including trauma, myocardial infarction, pulmonary embolism, head injury, dehydration, infection, and complicated pregnancy. EB: *Certain clinical conditions place clients at higher risk for shock, which requires prompt identification and treatment to improve morbidity and mortality outcomes (Delgado et al, 2013; American Heart Association [AHA], 2011).*
- Complete a full nursing physical examination. *A full nursing physical examination is crucial in identifying all factors that might place that client at risk for the development of shock, such as hypoperfusion of internal organs (manifesting as decreases in bowel sounds and urinary output, and shortness of breath); tissue hypoperfusion (manifesting as cool, clammy, mottled skin, diminished pulses).* EBN/QSEN: *Educational strategies aimed at improving nurse's role in recognizing and responding to patient deterioration include use of clinical decision-making models, use of competency development in management of clinical deterioration and inclusion of such content in nursing education (Liaw et al, 2011). A systematic review published by Johanna Briggs International indicates that the use of extremity skin temperatures cannot be validated or supported due to a lack of consensus in the studies reviewed (Woo & Childs, 2012).* CEBN: *A systematic review found that capillary refill may not be helpful in the assessment of hypoperfusion states; use of vital signs, pulse oximetry, Doppler ultrasound, grading of peripheral pulses, color, and warmth of skin are more sensitive measures (Dufalt et al, 2008).*
- Monitor circulatory status (e.g., blood pressure [BP], mean arterial pressure [MAP], skin color, skin temperature, heart sounds, heart rate and rhythm, presence and quality of peripheral pulses, Doppler ultrasound, and pulse oximetry). EB: *The initial phase of shock is characterized by decreased cardiac output and tissue perfusion, which results in immediate compensatory changes evidenced by changes in blood pressure, increased heart rate, and shunting of blood away from the periphery, resulting in pale, cooler, damp skin, with reduced peripheral pulses (Kalil, 2014).*
- Maintain intravenous (IV) access and provide isotonic IV fluids such as 0.9% normal saline or Ringer's lactate as ordered; these fluids are commonly used in the prevention and treatment of shock. EB: *Restrictive fluid resuscitation and permissive hypotension (achievement of systolic pressure around 90 mm Hg) may have an advantage over standard higher volume fluid resuscitation in regards to overall and early intraoperative survival benefit (Duke et al, 2012; Sweeney, 2013). In a retrospective review of 778 clients the highest mortality rates were seen in those clients with positive fluid balances and with central venous pressures greater than 12 mm Hg (Boyd et al, 2011).* EB: *A Cochrane review found no difference in risk of dying in the use of colloids compared to crystalloids in trauma, burns, or surgery (Perel & Roberts, 2011).*
- Monitor for inadequate tissue oxygenation (e.g., apprehension, increased anxiety, changes in mental status, agitation, oliguria, cool/mottled periphery) and determinants of tissue oxygen delivery (e.g., PaO_2, SpO_2, $ScvO_2/SvO_2$, MAP, hemoglobin levels, lactate levels, cardiac output [CO]). *Assessment of tissue oxygen delivery and oxygenation patterns provides data to assess trends in client's status and evaluates treatment responses (Kalil, 2014).* EBN: *Tissue oxygenation endpoints, including central venous oxygen saturation ($ScvO_2$), tissue oxygenation (StO_2), and lactate levels, provide data on microcirculation, a key factor in the management of hemodynamic alterations in shock, especially in sepsis (Aitken et al, 2011).* EB: *Lactate or base deficit levels were found to not be correlated with triage vital signs in a study of 75 clients; however, the odds of surgical intervention were found to be four times greater in clients with higher lactate levels (Caputo et al, 2013).*

S

- ▲ Maintain vital signs (BP, pulse, respirations, and temperature), and pulse oximetry within normal parameters. EB: *Unrecognized shock based on the typical presentation of vital signs that are interpreted as being within acceptable boundaries may result in inappropriate triage of clients resulting in delays in treatment (Yeh & Velmahos, 2012).* EB: *Increased heart rate (above 90 beats/min), hypotension (BP below 90 mm Hg systolic), tachypnea (greater than 20 breaths/min), hypoxia (SpO_2 below 90%), and lactate levels (above 2 mmol/L) are indicators of shock (Dellinger et al, 2013, Kalil, 2014). Temperature greater than 38°C or less than 36°C with white blood cell count greater than 12,000/mm^3 or less than 4000/mm^3 plus symptoms listed earlier are indicators of SIRS (Dellinger et al, 2013).*
- ▲ Administer oxygen immediately to maintain SpO_2 greater than 90% and antibiotics and other medications as prescribed to any client presenting with symptoms of early shock. EBN: *The experienced nurse has an important role in the implementation of the Surviving Sepsis Campaign (SSC), which includes specific early goal-directed therapies that enhance client survival (Turi & Von Ah, 2013; Kleinpell et al, 2013).* EB: *Administration of high-flow oxygen, hydration, antibiotics, insulin, and vasoactive medications provides early correction of risks for shock and improves survival of shock. Antibiotics as prescribed administered within 1 hour of diagnosis of a sepsis state facilitates a better rate of survival. For each hour in delayed antibiotic administration, survival decreases by 7.6% (Aitken et al, 2011; Havel et al, 2011).* EB: *A prospective study on compliance with the hemodynamic components of the sepsis resuscitation bundle found that there was a lower mortality rate in clients who were placed on the protocol sooner (Coba et al, 2011).* EB: *Emergency medical services personnel may serve as an important resource for the early diagnosis and treatment of sepsis in the field before hospitalization (Wang et al, 2010).*
- ▲ Monitor trends in noninvasive hemodynamic parameters (e.g., MAP) as appropriate. EB: *Identification of alterations in hemodynamic parameters provides data necessary for early and immediate implementation of prescribed therapies for prompt stabilization, preventing progression of and treating early onset of shock (Werdan et al, 2012).* EB: *Restoring MAP to desired levels (above 65 mm Hg) facilitates adequate perfusion to organs; however, initial impaired tissue oxygenation has been associated with impaired organ function over 24 hours in 33 intensive care unit clients (Dellinger et al, 2013; Mesquida et al, 2012).* CEB: *An overarching goal of cardiovascular support is optimization of blood flow to tissues; however, there is no single optimum MAP that can be applied to all (Jones et al, 2010). Monitor hydration status including skin turgor, daily weights, postural blood pressure changes, serum electrolytes (sodium, potassium, chloride, and blood urea nitrogen), and intake and output. Consider insertion of an indwelling urinary catheter as ordered to measure hourly output.* EB: *Daily weights are an important indicator of fluid status; however, the feasibility of obtaining accurate daily weights and correlating them to fluid balance in the critically ill is challenging (Schneider et al, 2012).* EBN: *Skin turgor is a measure of hydration, as are intake and output. Serum electrolyte levels help monitor fluid status (Schneider et al, 2012).*
- ▲ Monitor serum lactate levels, interpreting them within the context of each client. EB: *Elevations in serum lactate (above 2 mmol/L) may indicate circulatory failure and resultant tissue hypoxia from anaerobic metabolism that results in toxin accumulation, cellular inflammation, and cellular death. Progression to shock may result as characterized by the onset of systemic inflammatory response syndrome (SIRS). Two or more of the following indicators suggest SIRS: altered temperatures, heart rates above 90 beats/min, tachypnea or hypocarbia, and/or leukocytosis/leukopenia, which may or may not be related to infection as other causative factors exists (Kaplan & Pinsky, 2014).* EBN: *The degree of serum lactate elevation correlates with morbidity and mortality in sepsis; early detection facilitates early treatment and is a more accurate triage tool than vital signs (Aitken et al, 2011). Monitor blood glucose levels frequently and administer insulin as prescribed to maintain normal blood sugar levels (blood glucose levels of 70 to 110 mg/dL [3.9 to 6.1 mmol/L]).* EB: *Research suggests that tight glycemic control decreases mortality and morbidity in surgical clients; the Surviving Sepsis Campaign and clinical practice guidelines for cardiogenic shock suggests maintaining blood glucose below 150 mg/dL (8.3 mmol/L) (Dellinger et al, 2013; Werdan et al, 2012).*

Critical Care

- ▲ Prepare the client for the placement of an additional IV line, central line, and/or a pulmonary artery catheter as prescribed. *Adequate IV and central line access may be required for fluid resuscitation and medication delivery. Maintaining more than one IV access ensures rapid IV medication and fluid delivery in a crisis situation. Large amounts of fluid can be delivered more efficiently through centrally placed vascular access sites. Most vasoactive agents, especially vasopressors, should be delivered only through central lines because of risk of tissue sloughing.* EB: *A Cochrane systematic review of 13 studies on 5686 clients found no difference in mortality rates or days spent in an ICU between those clients with a pulmonary artery catheter and those without (Rajaram et al, 2013).* EBN: *Stroke volume assessment offers more precise evaluation of fluid and inotrope therapies in shock management (Aitken et al, 2011).* CEB: *Monitoring of hemodynamic parameters such as CVP, CO, cardiac index (CI), systemic vascular resistance (SVR), stroke volume (SV), and pulmonary artery pressure (PAP) through a pulmonary artery line can facilitate rapid assessment of physiological changes associated with the onset of shock (Wilmont, 2010).*

▲ Monitor trends in hemodynamic parameters (e.g., CVP, CO, CI, SVR, PAP, and MAP) as appropriate. *Hemodynamic indices will be altered depending on the underlying form of shock (hypovolemic, distributive, or cardiogenic). Dehydration will result in reduced CVP, CO, PAP, and ultimately MAP due to hypovolemia. Vasodilation as seen in distributive shock patterns (forms of third spacing as in neurogenic, anaphylactic, and septic shock states) will decrease CVP (a surrogate for intravascular volume) and other hemodynamic indices. Cardiogenic shock will result in low CO and MAP with higher PAP and CVP indices due to heart failure and subsequent congestion of the cardiopulmonary systems. Compensatory mechanisms to address reductions in CO and MAP include tachycardia and reduced urinary output (less than 0.5 mL/kg/hr). Both CO and SVR may temporarily increase with the onset of shock because of compensatory mechanisms; however, as shock progresses, both CO and SVR decline (Dellinger et al, 2013; Kalil, 2014; Werdan et al, 2012).*

▲ Monitor electrocardiography. Tachycardia may be present as a result of decreased fluid volume, which will be seen before a decrease in blood pressure as a compensatory mechanism. EB: *As oxygen demands increase, cardiac dysrhythmias may be evident, such as premature ventricular contractions (Dellinger et al, 2013).*

▲ Monitor arterial blood gases, coagulation, chemistries, point-of-care blood glucose, cardiac enzymes, blood cultures, and hematology. EB: *Abnormalities can identify the cause of the perfusion deficits and identify complications related to the decreased perfusion or shock state. Cardiogenic shock may be identified by elevations in cardiac enzymes as a result of myocardial infarction in association with low MAP. Elevation/reductions in white blood cell counts may be indicative of septic shock when associated with alterations in MAP (Aitken et al, 2011; Kalil, 2014).*

▲ Administer vasopressor agents as prescribed. EB: *A Cochrane collaborative review found that there is not sufficient evidence to prove that any one vasopressor is superior to others in the assessed doses. Choice of specific vasopressor is to be individualized based on the prescriber's discretion (Havel et al, 2011).*

▲ If the client is in shock, refer to the following care plans: Risk for ineffective **Renal** perfusion, Risk for ineffective **Gastrointestinal** perfusion, Impaired **Gas** exchange, and Decreased **Cardiac** output.

Client/Family Teaching and Discharge Planning

▲ *Teach client and family or significant others about any medications prescribed. Instruct the client to report any adverse side effects to his/her health care provider. Medication teaching includes the drug name, purpose, administration instructions (e.g., with or without food), and any side effects to be aware of. Provision of such information using clear communication principles and with an understanding of what the health literacy level of the client/family/significant others may be can facilitate appropriate adherence to the therapeutic regimen (Balentine, 2014; Nielsen-Bohlman et al, 2004; National Institutes of Health, 2011).*

- Instruct the client and family on disease process and rationale for care. EB: *Tailored interventions targeted to the level of the learner enhance client activation (Hibbard & Greene, 2013). Knowledge empowers clients and family members, allowing them to be active participants in their care (Finchman, 2013).* CEB: *When clients and their family members have sufficient understanding of their disease process, they can participate more fully in care and healthy behaviors (Finchman, 2013; Nielsen-Bohlman et al, 2004).*
- Instruct clients and their family members on the signs and symptoms of low blood pressure to report to their health care provider (dizziness, lightheadedness, fainting, dehydration and unusual thirst, lack of concentration, blurred vision, nausea, cold, clammy, pale skin, rapid and shallow breathing, fatigue, depression). EBN: *Teach back methods were found to be significantly associated with self-care activities and fewer hospitalizations in a sample of 276 clients with heart failure (White et al, 2013).* EB: *Use of the teach back method enhances an individual's knowledge and adherence behaviors (Negarandeh et al, 2013). Early recognition and treatment of these symptoms may avoid more serious sequelae (AHA, 2011).*
- Implement educational initiatives to reduce health care–associated infections (HAIs). EB: *Implementation of evidence-based educational interventions may considerably reduce HAIs (Aitken et al, 2011).*
- Promote a culture of client safety and individual accountability. EBN: *Health promotion related nursing interventions are considered by nurses to be an important component of their practice but may be hindered*

by organizational obstacles (Kemppainen et al, 2012). EB: *Include health literacy strategies into all aspects of client-centered care and weave into organizational values (Koh et al, 2013). Everyone involved in the health care of clients should adopt an attitude of accountability and promulgate zero tolerance in relation to HAIs (Aitken et al, 2011).*

REFERENCES

Aitken, L., et al. (2011). Nursing considerations to complement the Surviving Sepsis Campaign guidelines. *Critical Care Medicine, 39*, 1800–1818.

American Heart Association (AHA). (2011). *When is blood pressure too low?* Retrieved <http://www.heart.org?HEARTORG/HealthcareResearch>.

Balentine, J. (2014). *Sepsis (blood infection).* <http://www.emedicinehealth.com/sepsis_blood_infection/article_em.htm> Retrieved October 11, 2012.

Boyd, J. H., Forbes, J., Nakada, T. A., et al. (2011). Fluid resuscitation in septic shock: a positive fluid balance and elevated central venous pressure are associated with increased mortality. *Critical Care Medicine, 39*, 259–265.

Caputo, N., Fraser, R., Paliga, A., et al. (2013). Triage vital signs do not correlate with serum lactate or base deficit, and are less predictive of operative intervention in penetrating trauma patients: a prospective cohort study. *Emergency Medicine Journal, 30*, 546–550.

Coba, V., et al. (2011). Resuscitation bundle compliance in severe sepsis and septic shock: improves survival, is better late than never. *Journal of International Critical Care Medicine, 26*, 304–313.

Delgado, M. K., Liu, V., Pines, J. M., et al. (2013). Risk factors for unplanned transfer to intensive care within 24 hours of admission from the emergency department in an integrated healthcare system. *Journal of Hospital Medicine, 8*, 13–19.

Dellinger, R. P., Levy, M. M., Rhodes, A., et al. (2013). Surviving Sepsis Campaign: international guidelines for management of severe sepsis and septic shock, 2012. *Intensive Care Medicine, 39*, 165–228.

Dufalt, M., et al. (2008). Translating best practices in assessing capillary refill. *Worldviews on Evidence Based Nursing, 5*, 36–44.

Duke, M. D., Guidry, C., Guice, J., et al. (2012). Restrictive fluid resuscitation in combination with damage control resuscitation: time for adaptation. *Journal of Trauma & Acute Care Surgery, 73*, 674–678.

Finchman, J. (2013). The public health importance of improving health literacy. *American Journal of Pharmaceutical Education, 77*, 41.

Havel, C., et al. (2011). Vasopressor for hypotensive shock. *Cochrane Database of Systematic Reviews*, CD003709.

Henneman, A., & Thornby, K.-A. (2012). Risk of hypotension with concomitant use of calcium-channel blockers and macrolide antibiotics. *American Journal of Health-System Pharmacy, 69*, 1038–1043.

Hibbard, J. H., & Greene, J. (2013). What the evidence shows about patient activation: better health outcomes and care experiences; fewer data on costs. *Health Affairs, 32*, 207–214.

Jones, A., Treciak, S., & Dellinger, R. (2010). Arterial pressure optimization in the treatment of septic shock: a complex puzzle. *Critical Care, 14*, 102–103.

Kalil, A. (2014). *Septic shock, 2014. Medscape Reference: Drugs, Disease, & Procedures.* From <http://emedicine.medscape.com/article/168402-overview> Retrieved October 31, 2014.

Kaplan, L., & Pinsky, M. (2014). *Systemic inflammatory response syndrome.* From <http://emedicine.medscape.com/article/1168943-overview> Retrieved October 30, 2014.

Kemppainen, V., Tossavainen, K., & Turunen, H. (2012). Nurses' roles in health promotion practice: an integrative review. *Health Promotion International.*

Kleinpell, R., Aitken, L., & Schorr, C. A. (2013). Implications of the new international sepsis guidelines for nursing care. *American Journal of Critical Care, 22*, 212–222.

Koh, H. K., Brach, C., Harris, L. M., et al. (2013). A proposed 'health literate care model' would constitute a systems approach to improving patients' engagement in care. *Health Affairs, 32*, 357–367.

Liaw, S. Y., Scherpbier, A., Klainin-Yobas, P., et al. (2011). A review of educational strategies to improve nurses' roles in recognizing and responding to deteriorating patients. *International Nursing Review, 58*, 296–303.

Mesquida, J., Espinal, C., Gruartmoner, G., et al. (2012). Prognostic implications of tissue oxygen saturation in human septic shock. *Intensive Care Medicine, 38*, 592–597.

National Institutes of Health (NIH). (2011). *Clear communication: an NIH health literacy initiative.* <http://www.nih.goc/clearcommunication> Retrieved July 29, 2011.

Negarandeh, R., Mahmoodi, H., Noktehdan, H., et al. (2013). Teach back and pictorial image educational strategies on knowledge about diabetes and medication/dietary adherence among low health literate patients with type 2 diabetes. *Primary Care Diabetes, 7*, 111–118.

Nielsen-Bohlman, L., Panzer, A., & Kindig, D. (Eds.), (2004). *Health literacy: a prescription to end confusion.* Washington, D. C.: The National Academies Press.

Perel, P., & Roberts, I. (2011). Colloids versus crystalloids for fluid resuscitation in critically ill patients. *Cochrane Database of Systematic Reviews*, CD000567.

Rajaram, S., Desai, N., Kalra, A., et al. (2013). Pulmonary artery catheter for adults in intensive care. *Cochrane Database of Systematic Reviews.*

Schneider, A. G., Baldwin, I., Freitag, E., et al. (2012). Estimation of fluid status changes in critically ill patients: fluid balance chart or electronic bed weight? *Journal of Critical Care, 27*, 745.e7–e12.

Sweeney, J. (2013). Mass transfusion to combat trauma's lethal triad. *Journal of Emergency Nursing, 39*, 37–39.

Turi, S. K., & Von Ah, D. (2013). Implementation of early goal-directed therapy for septic patients in the emergency department: a review of the literature. *Journal of Emergency Nursing, 39*, 13–19.

Wang, H., et al. (2010). Opportunities for emergency medical services care of sepsis. *Resuscitation, 18*, 193–197.

Werdan, K., Ruß, M., Buerke, M., et al. (2012). Cardiogenic shock due to myocardial infarction: diagnosis, monitoring and treatment. *Deutsches Aerzteblatt International, 109*, 343–351.

White, M., Garbez, R., Carroll, M., et al. (2013). Is "teach-back" associated with knowledge retention and hospital readmission in hospitalized heart failure patients? *Journal of Cardiovascular Nursing, 28*, 137–146.

Woo, F., & Childs, C. (2012). A systematic review on the role of extremity skin temperature as a non-invasive marker for hypoperfusion in critically ill adults in the intensive care setting. *JBI Library of Systematic Reviews, 10*, 1504–1548.

Yeh, D. D., & Velmahos, G. C. (2012). Vital signs are unreliable. *ANZ Journal of Surgery, 82*, 574–576.

S

Impaired Sitting

Ruth A. Wittmann-Price, PhD, RN, CNS, CNE, CHSE, ANEF, FAAN

NANDA-I

Definition

Limitation of ability to independently and purposefully attain and/or maintain a rest position that is supported by the buttocks and thighs, in which the torso is upright

Defining Characteristics

Impaired ability to adjust position of one or both lower limbs on uneven surface; impaired ability to attain a balanced position of the torso; impaired ability to flex or move both hips; impaired ability to flex or move both knees; impaired ability to maintain the torso in balanced position; impaired ability to stress torso with body weight; insufficient muscle strength

Related Factors

Alteration in cognitive functioning; impaired metabolic functioning; insufficient endurance; insufficient energy; malnutrition; neurological disorder; orthopedic surgery; pain; prescribed posture; psychological disorder; sarcopenia; self-imposed relief posture

NOC Outcomes (Nursing Outcomes Classification)

Suggested NOC Outcomes

Endurance

Participate in desired activities; Meet own self-care need; Achieve measurable increased activity tolerance evidenced by ability to properly sit longer without fatigue and maintain vital signs within acceptable limits

Activity Tolerance

Demonstrate measurable increased ability to sit properly with vital signs within normal limits and skin warm, pink, and dry; Report absence of musculoskeletal pain while sitting

Pain Control

Demonstrate and initiate behavioral modifications of lifestyle and appropriate sitting posture; Report chronic lower back pain decreased in frequency, duration, and severity; Demonstrate relief of pain as evidenced by stable vital signs and absence of muscle tension and restlessness

Self-Management

Verbalize understanding of condition; Identify individual risk factors; Initiate lifestyle changes

Tissue Perfusion: Peripheral

Maintain skin integrity while sitting; Demonstrate sitting behaviors and techniques to prevent skin breakdown

Example NOC Outcome with Indicators

Increased sitting endurance as evidenced by the following indicators: participating in necessary and desired activities while sitting; reporting measurable increase in activity tolerance; and demonstrating a decrease in physiological signs of intolerance of sitting. (Rate ability to sit for 1 = 15 minutes; 2 = 30 minutes; 3 = 45 minutes; or 4 = one hour or more without difficulty.)

Client Outcomes

Client Will (Specify Time Frame)

- Verbalize importance of being able to sit as a method to engage in activities of daily living
- Understand somatic physiology of posture control

- Choose health care options that enhance ability to sit
- Engage in physical conditioning exercises to enhance sitting ability
- Understand relationship of posture and emotions
- Control pain to increase ability to sit

NIC Interventions (Nursing Interventions Classification)

Suggested NIC Interventions

Fall Prevention; Energy Management Including both Conservation and Restoration; Physical Exercise, Strength Training, Balance Training

Example NIC Activities—Exercise Therapy: Sitting

Assist client to use chair that facilitates sitting and prevents injury; Transfer safely from bed to chair; Encourage to sit in chair, as tolerated; Provide activities that can be completed while sitting

Nursing Interventions and *Rationales*

- Acknowledge the importance of being able to sit as a method to engage in activities of daily living. EB: *Niekerk et al (2014) studied adolescents' (N = 12) sitting postural changes while on the computer and found that dynamic (purposeful) movement prevented musculoskeletal pain.* EBN: *Harris and Shahid (2014) studied getting clients (N = 21) out of bed early who were in the intensive care unit using an interdisciplinary plan, which included nurses, and found it a safe and cost-effective strategy to improve client outcomes.*
- Understands the somatic physiology of posture control. EB: *Gorman et al (2014) studied clients' (N = 125) scores on the Function In Sitting Test (FIST) between inpatient rehabilitation admission and discharge and compared them to balance and function indicators. The researchers found that the FIST correlated balance and function indicators and both tests demonstrated client improvement in sitting wellness.* EB: *Curran et al (2014) studied how clients (N = 12) sit and sitting's relationship to low back pain and overall body discomforts and found that forward-leaning chairs resulted in greater low back and overall body discomfort than sitting on a flat seat.*
- Choose the musculoskeletal options that enhance ability to sit properly. EBN: *Kiraly and Gondos (2014) analyzed the relationship between clients' (N = 109) total hip replacement (THR) and quality of life and found that THR improves the feeling of well-being and increases mobility of clients 5 years after the operation.* EB: *Masahiro et al (2014) investigated two different trunk muscle activities during sitting focusing on low back pain and found that sitting in a stable seat produced muscle imbalance, while in an unstable seat muscles were not imbalanced, demonstrating muscle control is needed for proper sitting.*
- Engage in physical conditioning exercises to enhance proper sitting ability. EBN: *Huang et al (2014) studied pediatric/surgical intensive care clients' (N = 21) pressure ulcers and developed a successful project to decrease the incidence of pressure ulcers, which included developing a series of pictures to illustrate proper sitting, lying, and changing positions.* EB: *Sung-Jin et al (2014) compared whole body vibration on the sitting balance of stroke clients (N = 30) with clients in a control group and found that the experimental participants had a significant improvement in the Modified Functional Reach Test while sitting.*
- Understands the relationship of posture and somatic functioning. EB: *Thorp et al (2014) studied alternating sitting and standing every 30 minutes in overweight office workers to determine if it reduced postprandial glucose, insulin, and triglyceride responses and found that it had a positive effect on postprandial glucose responses but not on insulin and triglyceride serum levels.* EB: *Pedersen et al (2014) studied desk-based employees (N = 17) with the intent of increasing workday energy by interrupting prolonged occupational sitting time with short bursts of physical activity and found a significant increase in calories expenditure when compared to a control group that did not participate in interspaced physical activity.*
- Understands the relationship of posture and emotions. EB: *Michalak et al (2014) studied the relationship of sitting posture of clients (N = 30) and depression and found that clients in a slumped (depressed) posture demonstrated more of a bias toward negative words than clients an upright (nondepressed) posture when shown words on a computer screen.* EB: *Jussila et al (2014) studied the relationship between psychosocial lifestyle and musculoskeletal pain in adolescence (N = 1773) and found an association between emotional and behavioral problems in both genders with musculoskeletal pain.*

- Maintain pain levels below 3 to 4 on a 0- to 10-scale to increase ability to sit. EBN: *Backaberg et al (2014) studied the high prevalence of musculoskeletal discomfort among nursing students (N = 348) and the most commonly reported everyday activities was prolonged sitting.* EB: *Wells et al (2014) studied using Pilates exercise for people with chronic low back pain (CLBP) by surveying physical therapists (N = 30) and it was recommended that people with CLBP should use Pilates twice a week because it involves body awareness, breathing, movement control, posture, and education.*

Pediatric

- Increase cognitive and physical functioning by promoting proper sitting ability. EB: *Surkar et al (2015) investigated children (N = 19) affected by cerebral palsy to determine if their focused attention changed as sitting postural control improved and found that sitting postural control was correlated with focused attention.* EB: *Harbourne et al (2014) investigated the relationship of developing sitting postural control using infants with motor delays (N = 16) and a control group (N = 28) and found infants with delayed sitting have a greater difficulty in looking at and focusing on objects.*

Geriatric

- Increase cognitive and physical functioning by promoting prober sitting ability. EBN: *Wallace et al (2014) measured the effectiveness of a 12-week exercise program to reduce the health risks in people older than age 60 years and found the intervention produced significant difference between intervention and comparison groups' fitness at 6 months (P >.01) and 12 months (P >.001).* EBN: *Strupeit et al (2014) did a longitudinal study of geriatric clients' mobility and their quality of life (QOL) and found that mobility and QOL increased for 6 months after rehabilitation discharge but then decreased at 12 months. Additionally, over time, men were found to have better function than women.*

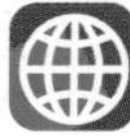

Multicultural

- Understand the importance of unimpaired sitting to different populations. EB: *Wang et al (2014) studied extended computer use in Taiwan and developed a program to remind people to take a break and stretch their bodies and the program increased participants awareness of the dangers of prolonged sitting.* EB: *Watanabe et al (2014) did a study on Japanese men (N = 9) to determine the effects of slumped sitting on muscle health and found that slumped sitting decreases abdominal muscle contraction and thickness.*

Home Care

- Encourage proper sitting posture in the home environment to promote health. EB: *Ivengar et al (2014) studied post-stroke clients (N = 45) and postural control and found that head position while sitting correlated directly with sitting postural control and both were related to upper extremity stroke recovery.* EB: *Bassett et al (2014) used two monitors on adults (N = 15) that recorded sitting/lying down, standing, and stepping to determine accuracy of monitoring clients activity and found that the current method allowed researchers to obtain detailed information about posture.*

REFERENCES

Backaberg, S., Rask, M., Brunt, D., et al. (2014). Impact of musculoskeletal symptoms on general physical activity during nursing education. *Nurse Education in Practice*, *14*(4), 385–390.

Bassett, D. R., John, D., Conger, S., et al. (2014). Detection of lying down, sitting, standing, and stepping using two ActivPAL monitors. *Medicine & Science in Sports & Exercise*, *46*(10), 2025–2059.

Curran, M., Dankaerts, W., O'Sullivan, P., et al. (2014). The effect of a backrest and seatpan inclination on sitting discomfort and trunk muscle activation in subjects with extension-related low back pain. *Ergonomics*, *57*(5), 733–743.

Gorman, S. L., Harro, C. C., Platko, C., et al. (2014). Examining the function in sitting test for validity, responsiveness, and minimal clinically important difference in inpatient rehabilitation. *Archives of Physical Medicine and Rehabilitation*, *95*(12), 2304–2311.

Harbourne, R. T., Ryalls, B., & Stergiou, N. (2014). Sitting and looking: a Comparison of stability and visual exploration in infants with typical development and infants with motor delay. *Physical & Occupational Therapy in Pediatrics*, *34*(2), 197–212.

Harris, C. L., & Shahid, S. (2014). Physical therapy-driven quality improvement to promote early mobility in the intensive care unit. *Baylor University Medical Center Proceedings*, *27*(3), 203–207.

Huang, W., Chang, S., & Tang, C. (2014). Reducing patient pressure sore incidence density in the pediatric surgical intensive care unit. *Journal of Nursing*, S60–S67.

Ivengar, Y. R., Vijavakumar, K., Abraham, J. M., et al. (2014). Relationship between postural alignment in sitting by photogrammetry and seated postural control in post-stroke subjects. *Neurorehabilitation*, *35*(2), 181–190.

Jussila, L., Paananen, M., Nayha, S., et al. (2014). Psychosocial and lifestyle correlates of musculoskeletal pain patterns in adolescence: a 2-year follow-up study. *European Journal of Pain*, *18*(1), 139–146.

Kiraly, E., & Gondos, T. (2014). The effect of functional movement ability on the quality of life after total hip replacement. *Journal of Clinical Nursing, 23*(1/2), 124–131.
Masahiro, W., Koji, K., Yusuke, W., et al. (2014). Trunk muscle activity with different sitting postures and pelvic inclination. *Journal of Back & Musculoskeletal Rehabilitation, 27*(4), 531–536.
Michalak, J., Mischnat, J., & Teismann, T. (2014). Sitting posture makes a difference-embodiment effects on depressive memory bias. *Clinical Psychology & Psychotherapy, 21*(6), 519–524.
Niekerk, S., Louw, Q. A., & Grimmer-Sommers, K. (2014). Frequency of postural changes during sitting whilst using a desktop computer—exploring an analytical methodology. *Ergonomics, 57*(4), 545–554.
Pedersen, S. J., Cooley, P. D., & Mainsbidge, C. (2014). An e-health intervention designed to increase workday energy expenditure by reducing prolonged occupational sitting habits. *Work (Reading, Mass.), 49*(2), 289–295.
Strupeit, S., Wolf-Ostermann, K., Buss, A., et al. (2014). Mobility and quality of life after discharge from a clinical geriatric setting focused on gender and age. *Rehabilitation Nursing, 39*(4), 198–206.
Sung-Jin, C., Won-Seob, S., Bok-Kyun, O., et al. (2014). Effect of training with whole body vibration on the sitting balance of stroke patients. *Journal of Physical Therapy Sciences, 26*(9), 1411–1414.
Surkar, S. M., Edelbrock, C., Stergiou, N., et al. (2015). Sitting postural control affects the development of focused attention in children with cerebral palsy ... including commentary by S Saavedra and D Bellows. *Pediatric Physical Therapy, 27*(1), 16–23.
Thorp, A. A., Kingwell, B. A., Sethi, P., et al. (2014). Alternating bouts of sitting and standing attenuate postprandial glucose responses. *Medicine & Science in Sports & Exercise, 46*(11), 2053–2061.
Wallace, R., Lees, C., Massoumeh, M., et al. (2014). Effects of a 12-week community exercise programme on older people. *Nursing Older People, 26*(1), 20–26.
Wang, S., Jiang, C., & Chen, J. (2014). Promoting healthy computer use: timing-informed computer health animations for prolonged sitting computer users. *Behaviour & Information Technology, 33*(3), 294–300.
Watanabe, S., Kobar, K., Yoshimura, Y., et al. (2014). Influence of trunk muscle co-contraction on spinal curvature during sitting. *Journal of Back & Musculoskeletal Rehabilitation, 27*(1), 55–61.
Wells, C., Kolt, G. S., Marshall, P., et al. (2014). The definition and application of Pilates exercise to treat people with chronic low back pain: a Delphi survey of Australian physical therapists. *Physical Therapy, 94*(6), 792–805.

Impaired Skin integrity

Karen Zulkowski, DNS, RN

NANDA-I

Definition

Altered epidermis and/or dermis

Defining Characteristics

Alteration in skin integrity; foreign matter piercing skin

S

Related Factors

External

Chemical injury agent (e.g., burn, capsaicin, methylene chloride, mustard agent); extremes of age; humidity; hyperthermia; hypothermia; mechanical factors (e.g., shearing forces, pressure, physical immobility); moisture; pharmaceutical agent; radiation therapy

Internal

Alteration in fluid volume; alteration in metabolism; alteration in pigmentation; alteration in sensation (e.g., resulting from spinal cord injury, diabetes mellitus); alteration in skin turgor; hormonal change; immunodeficiency; impaired circulation; impaired nutrition; pressure over bony prominence

NOC (Nursing Outcomes Classification)

Suggested NOC Outcomes

Tissue Integrity: Skin and Mucous Membranes; Wound Healing: Primary Intention, Secondary Intention

Example NOC Outcome with Indicators

Tissue Integrity: Skin and Mucous Membranes will be intact as evidenced by the following indicators: Skin integrity/Skin lesions not present/Tissue perfusion/Skin temperature/Skin thickness. (Rate the outcome and indicators of **Tissue Integrity: Skin and Mucous Membranes:** 1 = severely compromised, 2 = substantially compromised, 3 = moderately compromised, 4 = mildly compromised, 5 = not compromised [see Section I].)

Client Outcomes

Client Will (Specify Time Frame)

- Regain integrity of skin surface
- Report any altered sensation or pain at site of skin impairment
- Demonstrate understanding of plan to heal skin and prevent reinjury
- Describe measures to protect and heal the skin and to care for any skin lesion

NIC (Nursing Interventions Classification)

Suggested NIC Interventions

Incision Site Care; Pain Management; Pressure Ulcer Care; Pressure Ulcer Prevention; Risk Identification; Skin Care: Topical Treatments; Skin Surveillance; Wound Care; Wound Irrigation

Example NIC Activities—Pressure Ulcer Care

Monitor color of wound bed, temperature, edema, erythema, moisture, and appearance of surrounding skin; Note characteristics of any drainage

Nursing Interventions and *Rationales*

- Assess site of skin impairment and determine cause or type of wound (e.g., acute or chronic wound, burn, dermatological lesion, pressure ulcer, skin tear). EB: *The cause of the wound must be determined before appropriate interventions can be implemented. This will provide the basis for additional testing and evaluation to start the assessment process (Baranoski & Ayello, 2012; McCulloch & Kloth, 2010).*
- Use a risk assessment tool to systematically assess client risk factors for skin breakdown due to pressure. EB: *A validated risk assessment tool such as the Norton or Braden scale should be used to identify clients at risk for immobility-related skin breakdown (National Pressure Ulcer Advisory Panel [NPUAP] and European Pressure Ulcer Advisory Panel [EPUAP], 2014). Targeting variables (e.g., age and Braden Scale Risk Category) can focus assessment on particular risk factors (e.g., pressure) and help guide the plan of prevention and care (McCulloch & Kloth, 2010; NPUAP/EPUAP, 2014; Sussman & Bates-Jensen, 2012).*
- Determine the extent of the skin impairment (e.g., partial-thickness wound, stage I or stage II pressure ulcer). The following classification system and definition is for pressure ulcers: Pressure ulcer: localized injury to the skin and/or underlying tissue usually over a bony prominence, as a result of pressure, or pressure in combination with shear (NOTE: Friction is not included in the definition) (NPUAP/EPUAP, 2014).
  - **Category/Stage I:** Intact skin with nonblanchable erythema of a localized area, usually over a bony prominence. Darkly pigmented skin may not have visible blanching. The area may be painful, firm, soft, warmer, or cooler than adjacent tissue. *Category/Stage I may be difficult to detect in individuals with dark skin tones and may indicate "at risk" persons.*
  - **Category/Stage II:** Partial-thickness skin loss of dermis presenting as a shallow open ulcer with a red pink wound bed, without slough, that may also present as intact or open/ruptured and serum-filled. Presents as a shiny or dry shallow ulcer without slough or bruising. *This category/stage should not be used to describe skin tears, tape burns, incontinence-associated dermatitis, maceration, or excoriation.*
  - Bruising may indicate suspected deep tissue injury; for wounds deeper into subcutaneous tissue, muscle, or bone (category/stage III or stage IV pressure ulcers), see the care plan for Impaired **Tissue** integrity (NPUAP/EPUAP, 2014).
- Inspect and monitor site of skin impairment at least once a day for color changes, redness, swelling, warmth, pain, or other signs of infection. Determine whether the client is experiencing changes in sensation or pain. Closely assess high-risk areas such as bony prominences, skinfolds, the sacrum, and heels. *Systematic inspection can identify impending problems early (Baranoski & Ayello, 2012; NPUAP/EPUAP, 2014).*
- Monitor the client's skin care practices, noting type of soap or other cleansing agents used, temperature of water, and frequency of skin cleansing. *Cleansing should not compromise the skin (Baranoski & Ayello, 2012).*

S

- Consider using normal saline to clean the pressure ulcer or as ordered by the health care provider, but if necessary tap water suitable for drinking may be used to clean the wound. EB: *A Cochrane review found no evidence that using tap water to cleanse acute wounds in adults or children increases or reduces infection (Fernandez et al, 2012).*
- Individualize plan according to the client's skin condition, needs, and preferences. EBN: *Avoid harsh cleansing agents, hot water, extreme friction or force, or cleansing too frequently (Wound, Ostomy, and Continence Nurses Society [WOCN], 2010).*
- Monitor the client's continence status, and minimize exposure of skin impairment to other areas of moisture from perspiration or wound drainage. EBN: *Moisture from incontinence may contribute to pressure ulcer development by macerating the skin (Borchert et al, 2010; WOCN, 2010).*
- If the client is incontinent, implement an incontinence management plan to prevent exposure to chemicals in urine and stool that can damage the skin. Use a skin protectant cream to protect the skin after each incontinence episode. Refer to a continence care specialist, urologist, or gastroenterologist for incontinence assessment (Borchert et al, 2010). EB: *Implementing an incontinence prevention plan with the use of a skin protectant or a cleanser protectant can significantly decrease skin breakdown and pressure ulcer formation (Borchert et al, 2010; Scemons 2013).*
- For clients with limited mobility and activity, use a risk assessment tool to systematically assess immobility and activity-related risk factors. EB: *A validated risk assessment tool such as the Norton or Braden scale should be used to identify clients at risk for immobility-related skin breakdown (NPUAP/EPUAP, 2014).* EBN: *A study found that the most commonly reported interventions to reduce skin breakdown in acutely ill patients were protocol development, staff education, new use of a risk assessment tool, performance monitoring, development of a team approach, use of new beds/support surfaces, implementation of guidelines, providing feedback to staff, and linking staff with resources (Stotts et al, 2013).*
- Do not position the client on site of skin impairment. If consistent with overall client management goals, reposition the client as determined by individualized tissue tolerance and overall condition. Reposition and transfer the client with care to protect against the adverse effects of external mechanical forces such as pressure, friction, and shear. EB: *Do not position an individual directly on a pressure ulcer. Continue to turn/reposition the individual regardless of the support surface in use. Establish turning frequency based on the characteristics of the support surface and the individual's response (NPUAP/EPUAP, 2014). If the goal of care is to keep the client (e.g., a terminally ill client) comfortable, turning and repositioning may not be appropriate (NPUAP/EPUAP, 2014).*
- Evaluate for use of support surfaces (specialty mattresses, beds), chair cushions, or devices as appropriate. Maintain the head of the bed at the lowest possible degree of elevation to reduce shear and friction, and use lift devices, pillows, foam wedges, and pressure-reducing devices in the bed (NPUAP/EPUAP, 2014; WOCN, 2010).
- Implement a written treatment plan for topical treatment of the site of skin impairment. *A written plan ensures consistency in care and documentation (Baranoski & Ayello, 2012).*
- Select a topical treatment that will maintain a moist wound-healing environment (stage II) and that is balanced with the need to absorb exudate. Stage I pressure ulcers may be managed by keeping the client off of the area and using a protective dressing (Baranoski & Ayello, 2012). EBN: *Choose dressings that provide a moist environment, keep periwound skin dry, and control exudate and eliminate dead space (NPUAP/EPUAP, 2014; WOCN, 2010).*
- Avoid massaging around the site of skin impairment and over bony prominences. EB: *Research suggests that massage may lead to deep tissue trauma (NPUAP/EPUAP, 2014).*
- Assess the client's nutritional status. Refer for a nutritional consult and/or institute dietary supplements as necessary. EB: *Optimizing nutritional intake, including calories, fatty acids, protein, and vitamins, is needed to promote wound healing. Both the EPUAP and NPUAP (2014) endorse the application of reasonable nutritional assessment and treatment for clients at risk for and with pressure ulcers.*
- Identify the client's phase of wound healing (inflammation, proliferation, maturation) and stage of injury. EBN: *The selection of the dressing is based on the tissue in the ulcer bed (wound bed), the condition of the skin around the ulcer bed, and the goals of the person with the ulcer. Generally, maintaining a moist ulcer bed is the ideal when the ulcer bed is clean and granulating to promote healing and closure (NPUAP/EPUAP, 2014). No single wound dressing is appropriate for all phases of wound healing.*

S

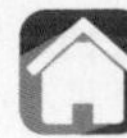

Home Care

- The interventions described previously may be adapted for home care use.
- Instruct and assist the client and caregivers in how to change dressings and maintain a clean environment. Provide written instructions and observe the client completing the dressing change before hospital discharge and in the home setting.
- Educate client and caregivers on proper nutrition, signs and symptoms of infection, and when to call the agency and/or health care provider with concerns.
- It may be beneficial to initiate a consultation in a case assignment with a wound, ostomy, continence nurse (or wounds specialist) to establish a comprehensive plan for complex wounds.

Client/Family Teaching and Discharge Planning

- Teach skin and wound assessment and ways to monitor for signs and symptoms of infection, complications, and healing. Early assessment and intervention help prevent serious problems from developing. EB: *A home visit by a wound care specialist can provide essential in-home education, client specific plan of care, and reduce health care costs (Vrtis, 2013).*
- Teach the client why a topical treatment has been selected. EBN: *The type of dressing needed may change over time as the wound heals and/or deteriorates (NPUAP/EPUAP, 2014; WOCN, 2010).*
- If consistent with overall client management goals, teach how to reposition as client condition warrants. EB: *If the goal of care is to keep a client (e.g., terminally ill client) comfortable, turning and repositioning may not be appropriate (NPUAP/EPUAP, 2014).*
- Teach the client to use pillows, foam wedges, chair cushions, and pressure-redistribution devices to prevent pressure injury. EB: *The use of effective pressure-reducing seat cushions for older wheelchair users significantly prevented sitting-acquired pressure ulcers (Brienza et al, 2012).*

REFERENCES

Baranoski, S., & Ayello, E. A. (Eds.), (2012). *Wound care essentials: practice principles* (3rd ed.). Ambler, PA: Lippincott Williams & Wilkins.

Borchert, K., et al. (2010). The incontinence-associated dermatitis and its severity instrument. *Journal of Wound, Ostomy, and Continence Nursing, 37*(5), 527–535.

Brienza, D. M., et al. (2012). Pressure redistribution: seating, positioning, and support surfaces. In S. Baranoski & E. A. Ayello (Eds.), *Wound care essentials: practice principles* (3rd ed.). Ambler, PA: Lippincott Williams & Wilkins.

Fernandez, R., & Griffiths, R. (2012). Water for wound cleansing. *Cochrane Database of Systematic Reviews*, (2), Art. No.: CD003861.

McCulloch, J. A., & Kloth, L. C. (2010). *Wound healing evidenced-based management* (4th ed.). Philadelphia: EA Davis.

National Pressure Ulcer Advisory Panel (NPUAP) and European Pressure Ulcer Advisory Panel (EPUAP) (2014). *Prevention and treatment of pressure ulcers.* Emily Haesler (ed). Perth, Australia: Cambridge Media.

Scemons, D. (2013). Urinary incontinence in adults. *Nursing, 43*(11), 52–60.

Stotts, N. A., Brown, D. S., Donaldson, N. E., et al. (2013). Eliminating hospital-acquired pressure ulcers: within our reach. *Advances in Skin & Wound Care, 26*(1), 13–18.

Sussman, C., & Bates-Jensen, B. M. (2012). *Wound care: a collaborative practice manual for healthcare professionals* (4th ed.). Ambler, PA: Lippincott Williams & Wilkins.

Vrtis, M. C. (2013). The economic impact of complex wound care on home health agencies. *Journal of Wound, Ostomy and Continence Nursing, 40*(4), 360–363.

Wound, Ostomy, and Continence Nurses Society (WOCN) (2010). *Guideline for prevention and management of pressure ulcers. WOCN clinical practice guideline series no 2.* Mount Laurel, NJ.

S

Risk for impaired Skin integrity

Karen Zulkowski, DNS, RN

NANDA-I

Definition

Vulnerable to alteration in epidermis and/or dermis, which may compromise health

Risk Factors

External

Chemical injury agent (e.g., burn, capsaicin, methylene chloride, mustard agent); excretions; extremes of age; humidity; hyperthermia; hypothermia; mechanical factors (e.g., shearing forces, pressure, physical immobility); moisture; radiation therapy; secretions

Internal

Alteration in metabolism; alteration in pigmentation; alteration in sensation (e.g., resulting from spinal cord injury, diabetes mellitus); alteration in skin turgor; hormonal change; immunodeficiency; impaired circulation; inadequate nutrition; pharmaceutical agent; pressure over bony prominence; psychogenetic factor

NOTE: Risk should be determined by the use of a risk assessment tool (e.g., Norton scale, Braden scale).

NOC (Nursing Outcomes Classification)

Suggested NOC Outcomes

Immobility Consequences: Physiological; Tissue Integrity: Skin and Mucous Membranes

Example NOC Outcome with Indicators

Tissue Integrity: Skin and Mucous Membranes will be intact as evidenced by the following indicators: Skin intactness/Skin lesions not present/Tissue perfusion/Skin temperature. (Rate the outcome and indicators of **Tissue Integrity: Skin and Mucous Membranes:** 1 = severely compromised, 2 = substantially compromised, 3 = moderately compromised, 4 = mildly compromised, 5 = not compromised [see Section I].)

Client Outcomes

Client Will (Specify Time Frame)

- Report altered sensation or pain at risk areas as soon as noted
- Demonstrate understanding of personal risk factors for impaired skin integrity
- Verbalize a personal plan for preventing impaired skin integrity

NIC (Nursing Interventions Classification)

Suggested NIC Interventions

Positioning: Pressure Management; Pressure Ulcer Care; Pressure Ulcer Prevention, Skin Surveillance

Example NIC Activities—Pressure Ulcer Care

Monitor color of wound bed, temperature, edema, erythema, moisture, and appearance of surrounding skin; Note characteristics of any drainage

Nursing Interventions and *Rationales*

- Identify clients at risk for impaired skin integrity as a result of immobility, chronological age, malnutrition, incontinence, compromised perfusion, immunocompromised status, or chronic medical condition, such as diabetes mellitus, spinal cord injury, or renal failure. EB: *These client populations are known to be at high risk for impaired skin integrity (Baranoski & Ayello, 2012). Targeting variables (e.g., age and Braden Scale Risk Category) can focus assessment on particular risk factors (e.g., pressure) and help guide the plan of prevention and care (NPUAP/EPUAP, 2014).*
- Inspect and monitor skin condition at least once a day for color or texture changes, redness, localized heat, edema or induration, pressure damage, dermatological conditions, or lesions and any incontinence-associated dermatitis. Determine whether the client is experiencing loss of sensation or pain. *Systematic inspection can identify impending problems early (NPUAP/EPUAP, 2014; Baranoski & Ayello, 2012).*
- Monitor the client's skin care practices, noting type of soap or other cleansing agents used, temperature of water, and frequency of skin cleansing. *Individualize plan according to the client's skin condition, needs, and preferences (Baranoski & Ayello, 2012).*
- Cleanse the skin gently with pH-balanced cleansers. Avoid harsh cleansing agents, hot water, extreme friction or force, or too-frequent cleansing (WOCN, 2010).

▲ Monitor the client's continence status and minimize exposure of the site of skin impairment (incontinence-associated dermatitis) and other areas to moisture from incontinence, perspiration, or wound drainage. If the client is incontinent, implement an incontinence management plan to prevent exposure to chemicals in urine and stool that can strip or erode the skin. Use a skin barrier product and/or moisture wicking pads to reduce risk of exposure. Refer to a health care provider (e.g., continence care specialist, urologist, gastroenterologist) for an incontinence assessment (WOCN, 2010). EB: *Implementing an incontinence prevention plan with the use of a skin protectant or a cleanser protectant can significantly decrease skin breakdown and pressure ulcer formation (NPAUP/EPUAP 2014; WOCN, 2010; Baranoski & Ayello, 2012; Borchert et al, 2010).*

- For clients with limited mobility, inspect and monitor condition of skin covering bony prominences. *Pressure ulcers usually occur over bony prominences, such as the sacrum, coccyx, trochanter, and heels, as a result of unrelieved pressure between the prominence and support surface, or with shearing and friction (NPUAP/EPUAP, 2014; WOCN, 2010; Baranoski & Ayello, 2012).*
- Implement and communicate a client specific prevention plan. EB: *A plan of care clearly documented in the client's electronic health record will assist in ensuring consistency in care and documentation (Baranoski & Ayello, 2012).*
- At risk clients should be frequently repositioning. Frequency of repositioning will be influenced by variables concerning the individual's independent mobility and the support surface in use. Frequency of repositioning should be determined by the individual's tissue tolerance and medical condition (NPUAP/EPUAP, 2014). Reposition the client with care to protect against the adverse effects of external mechanical forces (e.g., pressure, friction, shear) (WOCN, 2010).
- Evaluate for use of specialty mattresses, beds, or devices as appropriate (Brienza et al, 2012; Lippoldt et al, 2014). *Maintain the head of the bed at the lowest possible degree of elevation to reduce shear and use lift devices, pillows, foam wedges, and pressure-reducing devices in the bed (WOCN,2010; Lippoldt et al, 2014). If the goal of care is to keep the client (e.g., a terminally ill client) comfortable, turning and repositioning may not be appropriate; reposition the client for position of comfort and provide pain relief measures (Horn et al, 2014).*
- Avoid massaging over bony prominences. *Massage may lead to deep tissue trauma (WOCN, 2010; NPUAP/EPUAP, 2014).*

▲ Assess the client's nutritional status; refer for a nutritional consult, and/or institute dietary supplements. EB: *Meeting nutritional needs of the client is important to prevention of skin breakdown as well as preventing complications of illness. Adequate nutrition is important for maintaining overall homeostasis and health (O'Hanlon et al, 2015).*

Geriatric

- Limit number of complete baths to two or three per week, and alternate them with partial baths. Use a tepid water temperature (between 90° F and 105° F) for bathing or use a no rinse alternative product. EB: *Excessive bathing, especially in hot water, depletes aging skin of moisture and increases dryness. The ability to retain moisture is decreased in aging skin due to diminished amounts of dermal proteins. One of the most common age-related changes to the skin is damage to the stratum corneum (Baranoski & Ayello, 2012).*
- Use lotions and moisturizers to prevent skin from drying out, especially in the winter. EB: *Avoid skin care products that contain allergens such as lanolin, latex, and dyes (Baranoski & Ayello 2012).*
- Increase fluid intake within cardiac and renal limits to a minimum of 1500 mL per day. *Dry skin is caused by loss of fluid; increasing fluid intake hydrates the skin (Baranoski & Ayello, 2012).*
- Increase humidity in the environment, especially during the winter, by using a humidifier or placing a container of water on a warm object. *Increasing the moisture in the air helps keep moisture in the skin.*

Home Care

- Assess client and caregiver ability to recognize potential risk for skin breakdown. Provide resources for client/caregiver to contact health care provider with questions/concerns related to skin and incontinence care as needed (Vrtis, 2013).

▲ Initiate a consultation in a case assignment with a wound care specialist or wound, ostomy, and continence nurse to establish a comprehensive plan as soon as possible (Vrtis, 2013).

- See the care plan for Impaired **Skin** integrity.

Client/Family Teaching and Discharge Planning

- Teach the client skin assessment and ways to monitor for impending skin breakdown. *Early assessment and intervention help prevent the development of serious problems.* EB: *Basic elements of a skin assessment are assessment of temperature, color, moisture, turgor, and intact skin (Baranoski & Ayello, 2012).*
- If consistent with overall client management goals, teach how to turn and reposition the client. EB: *Do not position an individual directly on a pressure ulcer. Continue to turn/reposition the individual even if a*

S

low-airloss support surface is in use. Establish turning frequency based on the characteristics of the support surface and the individual's response (NPUAP/EPUAP, 2014). If the goal of care is to keep the client (e.g., a terminally ill client) comfortable, turning and repositioning may not be appropriate (NPUAP/EPUAP, 2014; Horn et al, 2014).

- Teach the client and or caregivers to use pillows, foam wedges, and pressure-reducing devices to prevent pressure injury (WOCN, 2010; NPUAP/EPUAP, 2014). CEB: *The use of effective pressure-reducing seat cushions for older wheelchair users may significantly prevent sitting-acquired pressure ulcers (Brienza et al, 2012).*

REFERENCES

Baranoski, S., & Ayello, E. A. (2012). Skin an essential organ. In S. Baranoski & E. A. Ayello (Eds.), *Wound care essentials: practice principles* (3rd ed.). Ambler, PA: Lippincott, Williams & Wilkins.

Borchert, K., et al. (2010). The incontinence-associated dermatitis and its severity instrument. *Journal of Wound, Ostomy and Continence Nursing, 37*(5), 527–535.

Brienza, D. M., Geyer, M. J., Springle, S., et al. (2012). Pressure redistribution: seating, positioning, and support surfaces. In S. Baranoski & E. A. Ayello (Eds.), *Wound care essentials: practice principles* (3rd ed.). Ambler, PA: Lippincott, Williams & Wilkins.

Horn, J., & Iroin, G. L. (2014). The integument: current concepts in care at end of life. *Journal of Acute Care Physical Therapy, 5*(1), 11–16.

Lippoldt, J., & Staudinger, T. (2014). Interface pressure at different degrees of backrest elevation with various types of pressure redistribution surfaces. *American Journal of Critical Care, 23*(2), 119–126.

National Pressure Ulcer Advisory Panel (NPUAP) and European Pressure Ulcer Advisory Panel (EPUAP) (2014). *Prevention and treatment of pressure ulcers.* Emily Haesler (ed). Perth, Australia: Cambridge Media.

O'Hanlon, C., Dowsett, J., & Smyth, N. (2015). Nutrition assessment of the intensive care unit patient. *Topics in Clinical Nutrition, 30*(1), 47–70.

Vrtis, M. C. (2013). The economic impact of complex wound care on home health agencies. *Journal of Wound, Ostomy and Continence Nursing, 40*(4), 360–363.

Wound, Ostomy, and Continence Nurses Society (WOCN) (2010). *Guideline for prevention and management of pressure ulcers. WOCN clinical practice guideline series no 2.* Mount Laurel, NJ.

Readiness for enhanced Sleep

Mary Beth Flynn Makic, RN, PhD, CNS, CCNS, FAAN

NANDA-I

Definition

A pattern of natural, periodic suspension of relative consciousness to provide rest and sustain a desired lifestyle, which can be strengthened

Defining Characteristics

Expresses desire to enhance sleep

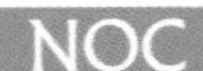

NOC (Nursing Outcomes Classification)

Suggested NOC Outcomes

Personal Well-Being; Rest; Sleep

Example NOC Outcome with Indicators

Sleep as evidenced by the following indicators: Hours of sleep/Sleep pattern/Sleep quality/Sleep efficiency/Feels rejuvenated after sleep/Napping appropriate for age. (Rate each indicator of **Sleep:** 1 = severely compromised, 2 = substantially compromised, 3 = moderately compromised, 4 = mildly compromised, 5 = not compromised [see Section I].)

Client Outcomes

Client Will (Specify Time Frame)

- Verbalize an interest in what constitutes normal sleep
- Verbalize an interest in nonpharmacological approaches to sleep promotion
- Establish an environment conducive to sleep initiation and maintenance throughout the night

NIC (Nursing Interventions Classification)

Suggested NIC Intervention

Sleep Enhancement

Example NIC Activities—Sleep Enhancement
Assess client's sleep/activity pattern; Assist/encourage client to create an environment that facilitates sleep; Assist/encourage client to adopt personal practices that enhance sleep

Nursing Interventions and *Rationales*

- Obtain a sleep history including bedtime routines, sleep patterns, use of medications and stimulants, and use of complementary and alternative medical practices for stress management and relaxation before bedtime. *Assessment of sleep behavior and patterns is an important part of any health status examination (Gooneratne et al, 2014; Salas & Gamaldo, 2011).*
  - From the history, assess the client's ability to initiate and maintain sleep, obtain adequate amounts of sleep, and manage daytime responsibilities free from fatigue and sleepiness. CEB: *A systematic review found that most adults who average 8 hours of sleep per night (range of 7 to 9 hours) were at decreased risk for all-cause mortality (Gallicchio & Kalesan, 2009).* CEBN: *Gender and cultural beliefs influenced sleep patterns and sleep preferences (Sok, 2008). Difficulty sleeping is a side effect of psychoactive substances contained in foodstuffs, as well as prescription and over-the-counter medications (Kloss et al, 2011; Woodward, 2012).*
- Based on assessment, teach one or more of the listed sleep promotion practices as appropriate. EB: *In adult acute care settings, improved sleep quality and less use of sleeping medication was reported when multicomponent sleep promotion protocols were tested (Gooneratne et al, 2014).*
  - Establish a regular schedule for sleep, exercise, napping, and mealtimes. *Regular schedules are believed to promote sleep initiation and sleep maintenance by maintaining a circadian rhythm of alertness/drowsiness (Kloss et al, 2011; Woodward, 2012).*
  - Avoid long periods of daytime sleep. EB: *Whereas regular, short napping in the morning or early afternoon improved mood and performance in older adults, long periods of sleep during the day may interfere with quality nighttime sleep (Sterniczuk et al, 2014).*
  - Arise at the same time each day even if sleep was poor during the previous night. *Although many factors can interfere with falling and staying asleep, forcing a regular arise time helps establish a circadian rhythm and ensures better sleep the following night (Kloss et al, 2011; Woodward, 2012).*
  - Limit caffeine. *Caffeine, colas, teas, and chocolate contain the stimulant caffeine and can adversely affect the client's ability to fall asleep. Nicotine is also a stimulant that may result in smokers sleeping poorly (National Institutes of Health [NIH], 2012).*
  - Avoid large meals before bed. *A large meal can cause indigestion, interfering with comfort and ability to fall asleep (NIH, 2012).*
  - Limit alcohol use. EBN: *Limited alcohol use (one to two drinks) shortened time needed to fall asleep and increased depth of sleep the first 2 hours, but also suppressed REM sleep, which sometimes led to REM-rebound, that is, lighter, more fragmented sleep later in the night (Dean et al, 2010).*
  - Avoid long-term use of sleeping pills. *Long-term use of sleeping pills can be habit forming, and typically dependence and withdrawal symptoms occur while the therapeutic effect diminishes over time (Woelk et al, 2010; Woodward, 2012).*
  - Engage in relaxing activities before bed. EBN: *Several systematic reviews show that all forms of relaxation improve quantity and quality of sleep to some extent (Hellstrom et al, 2011).*
  - Provide backrub or other forms of massage. EBN: *Use of a back massage has been shown effective for promoting relaxation (Hellstrom et al, 2011).*
  - Teach relaxation techniques. *Engaging in relaxation and mindfulness techniques have been found to shorten time to fall asleep and enhance quality of sleep (NIH, 2012; Larouche et al, 2014).*
  - Teach complementary and alternative interventions as culturally congruent. *Using complementary and alternative medicine such as tai chi, acupuncture, acupressure, yoga, and meditation have improved sleep in clinical populations (Gooneratne et al, 2014).*

S

- ❍ Lower lighting in sleep area. EB: *Light affects hormonal secretions related to circadian rhythms of sleepiness (NIH, 2012).*
- ❍ Mask noise in sleep area when it cannot be eliminated. EBN: *"White noise" (i.e., sounds covering the entire range of human hearing, e.g., ocean sounds) and music decrease time needed to fall asleep and nighttime awakenings (Hellstrom et al, 2011).*
- ❍ For anxious clients, consider use of a lavender oil preparation in the health care setting. EB: *A multisite clinical trial found scent of lavender lowered anxiety and improved self-reported sleep (Woelk et al, 2010).*

Geriatric

- Interventions discussed previously may be adapted for use with geriatric clients.
- Counsel the older adult regarding normal age-related changes in sleep: EB: *As people age, increased time is needed to fall asleep; frequency and duration of waking after sleep onset increases; and, nighttime sleep amount tends to decrease (Woodward, 2012).*
- Elicit the older adult's expectations for sleep and correct misconceptions. *The older person may be unduly concerned with normal age-related changes in sleep patterns; lighter sleep and occasional awakenings may be misconstrued as sleep disorders (Morin, 2011).*
- Assess and refer as appropriate if coexisting conditions may be disrupting sleep. EBN: *Depression, sleep apnea, and restless leg syndrome are commonly missed coexisting conditions in older adults (Woodward, 2012).*
- Discuss appropriate and inappropriate self-help measures for improving sleep. EB: *Older adults have been found to choose sleep interventions that can worsen rather than improve sleep (Gooneratne et al, 2011).*
- Encourage walking and other exercise outdoors unless contraindicated. *Exercise and exposure to natural light reinforce circadian rhythms that control sleep (Melancon et al, 2014; NIH, 2012).*
- Help older adults engage with others who enjoy similar events. *Social interactions reinforce circadian rhythms that control sleep (Gooneratne et al, 2014).*

Home Care

- Interventions discussed previously may be adapted for home care use.
- Some complementary and alternative medicine interventions may be more easily tried at home than in health care facilities. EB: *A multisite clinical trial found scent of lavender lowered anxiety and improved self-reported sleep (Woelk et al, 2010).*
- Assess the conduciveness of the home environment for both caregivers and clients' sleep. *Many factors in the home environment can promote or interfere with the sleep readiness of clients/family members (Kloss et al, 2011; Woodward, 2012).* EBN: *A multicomponent sleep promotion program improved sleep quality in family caregivers of persons with dementia (Simpson & Carter, 2010).*

S

REFERENCES

Dean, G. E., et al. (2010). Sleep in lung cancer: the role of anxiety, alcohol and tobacco. *Journal of Addictions Nursing, 21*, 130–137.

Gallicchio, L., & Kalesan, B. (2009). Sleep duration and mortality: a systematic review and meta-analysis. *Journal of Sleep Research, 18*, 148–158.

Gooneratne, N. S., et al. (2011). Perceived effectiveness of diverse sleep treatments in older adults. *Journal of the American Geriatrics Society, 59*, 297–303.

Gooneratne, N. S., & Vitiello, M. V. (2014). Sleep in older adults: normative changes, sleep disorders, and treatment options. *Clinics in Geriatric Medicine, 30*, 591–627.

Hellstrom, A., et al. (2011). Promoting sleep by nursing interventions in health care settings: a systematic review. *Worldviews on Evidence-Based Nursing (3rd quarter)*, 128–142.

Kloss, J. D., et al. (2011). The delivery of behavioral sleep medicine to college students. *The Journal of Adolescent Health, 48*, 553–561.

Larouche, M., Cote, G., Belisle, D., et al. (2014). Kind attention and non-judgement in mindfulness-based cognitive therapy applied to the treatment of insomnia: state of knowledge. *Pathologic Biologie, 62*, 284–291.

Melancon, M. O., Lorrain, D., & Dionne, I. J. (2014). Exercise and sleep in aging: emphasis on serotonin. *Pathologic Biologie, 62*, 276–283.

Morin, C. M. (2011). Psychological and behavioral treatments for insomnia 1: approaches and efficacy. In M. H. Kryger, T. Roth, & W. C. Dement (Eds.), *Principles and practice of sleep medicine* (5th ed.). St Louis: Saunders.

National Institutes of Health (NIH), MedlinePlus. (2012). *Tips for getting a goodnight sleep. 7*(2), 20. <http://www.nlm.nih.gov/medlineplus/magazine/issues/summer12/articles/summer12pg20.html> Retrieved June 22, 2015.

Simpson, C., & Carter, P. A. (2010). Pilot study of a brief behavioral sleep intervention for caregivers of individuals with dementia. *Research in Gerontological Nursing, 3*(1), 19–29.

Sok, S. R. (2008). Sleep patterns and insomnia management in Korean-American older adult immigrants. *Journal of Clinical Nursing, 17*(1), 135–143.

Sterniczuk, R., Rusak, B., & Rockwood, K. (2014). Sleep disturbance in older ICU patients. *Clinical Interventions in Aging*, *9*, 969–977.

Woelk, H., et al. (2010). A multi-center, double-blind, randomised study of the lavender oil preparation Silexan in comparison to lorazepam for generalized anxiety disorder. *Phytomedicine: International Journal of Phytotherapy and Phytopharmacology*, *17*(2), 94–99.

Woodward, M. (2012). Sleep in older people. *Reviews in Clinical Gerontology*, *22*(2), 130–149.

Sleep deprivation

Mary Beth Flynn Makic, PhD, RN, CNS, CCNS, FAAN

NANDA-I

Definition

Prolonged periods of time without sleep (sustained natural, periodic suspension of relative consciousness)

Defining Characteristics

Agitation, alteration in concentration, anxiety, apathy, combativeness, confusion, decrease in functional ability, decrease in reaction time, drowsiness, fatigue, fleeting nystagmus, hallucinations, hand tremors, heightened sensitivity to pain, irritability, lethargy, listlessness, malaise, perceptual disorders, restlessness, transient paranoia

Related Factors (r/t)

Age-related sleep stage shifts, average daily physical activity less than recommended for gender and age, conditions with periodic limb movement (e.g., restless leg syndrome, nocturnal myoclonus), dementia, environmental barrier, familial sleep paralysis, idiopathic central nervous system hypersomnolence, narcolepsy, nightmares, nonrestorative sleep pattern (e.g., due to caregiver responsibilities, parenting practices, sleep partner), overstimulating environment, prolonged discomfort (e.g., physical, psychological), sleep apnea, sleep terror, sleep walking, sleep-related enuresis, sleep-related painful erections, Sundowner syndrome, sustained circadian asynchrony, sustained inadequate sleep hygiene, treatment regimen

NOC (Nursing Outcomes Classification)

Suggested NOC Outcomes

Rest; Sleep; Symptom Severity

Example NOC Outcome with Indicators

Sleep as evidenced by the following indicators: Hours of sleep/Sleep pattern/Sleep quality/Sleep efficiency/Feels rejuvenated after sleep/Sleeps through the night consistently. (Rate the outcome and indicators of **Sleep:** 1 = severely compromised, 2 = substantially compromised, 3 = moderately compromised, 4 = mildly compromised, 5 = not compromised [see Section I].)

Client Outcomes

Client Will (Specify Time Frame)

- Verbalize plan that provides adequate time for sleep
- Identify actions that can be taken to ensure adequate sleep time
- Awaken refreshed once adequate time is spent sleeping
- Be less sleepy during the day once adequate time is spent sleeping

NIC (Nursing Interventions Classification)

Suggested NIC Intervention

Sleep Enhancement

Example NIC Activities—Sleep Enhancement

Monitor/record client's sleep pattern and number of sleep hours; Encourage client to establish a schedule that allows age-appropriate hours of sleep with minimal environmental and personal disruptions

Nursing Interventions and *Rationales*

- Obtain a sleep history to identify the specific personal and environmental factors that may be depriving clients of the amount of sleep needed for optimal functioning. EB: *Two detailed case studies by Salas and Gamaldo (2011) showed uniquely complex combinations of personal and environmental factors contribute to sleep deprivation.* EBN: *A systematic review of 17 studies of heart surgery patients showed factors that led to insufficient sleep during hospitalization were personal factors including pain, dyspnea, nocturia, anxiety, and depression and environmental factors including noise, light, and provision of care (Liao et al, 2011).*
  - Minimize environmental factors that disturb the client's sleep. See Nursing Interventions and *Rationales* for Disturbed **Sleep** pattern.
  - Minimize personal factors that disturb the client's sleep. See Nursing Interventions and *Rationales* for **Insomnia.**
- Assess the amount of sleep obtained each night compared with the amount of sleep needed. EB: *A national survey of 10,896 adults found that more than one third (37.1%) sleep less than 7 hours per night, an amount at which physiological and neurobehavioral deficits manifest and become progressively worse under chronic conditions (Centers for Disease Control and Prevention, 2011).*
- Assess for hypersensitivity to pain. EB: *In a repeated-measures sleep laboratory experiment with 18 adults, sleep deficiency led to increased sensitivity to pain (Roehrs et al, 2012).* EB: *In a laboratory study of 34 subjects, those with shortened sleep due to chronic insomnia were twice as likely as healthy controls with no sleep loss to report experiencing spontaneous pain; they also had lower pain thresholds for discomfort due to heat and pressure (Haack et al, 2012).*
- When daytime drowsiness occurs despite long, undisturbed periods of sleep, consider sleep apnea as a possible cause. EB: *In a household survey of more than 7000 adults, unexplained excessive daytime sleepiness was identified as a predictor of undiagnosed sleep apnea (Dosman et al, 2014).*
- Encourage a regular schedule of napping as a way to compensate for sleep deficiency whenever severely restricted sleep amounts cannot be avoided. CEB: *In a study of 92 adults, naps of no more than 45 minutes were found to supplement rather than replace nighttime sleep (Floyd, 1995).* EB: *In a pre-test/post-test study of 22 older adults, a consistent regimen of daily napping for 45 minutes enhanced waking function without negatively affecting nighttime sleep (Campbell et al, 2011).*
- Monitor caffeine intake in clients who may use caffeinated drinks to overcome sleep deficiency. EB: *In a double-blind, crossover study of 63 adults, even a single cup of caffeinated coffee consumed before bedtime in real-life conditions caused a deterioration in the quality of sleep in caffeine-sensitive subjects (Lloret-Linares et al, 2012).* CEB: *In an analysis of results from randomized controlled trials representing 156 subjects, caffeine abstinence for the whole day resulted in improved sleep quality at night (Sin et al, 2008).*
- If evidence-based interventions are inadequate, consider and carefully evaluate unstudied but commonly used countermeasures for fighting drowsiness. EB: *A descriptive study of 77 middle-aged adults identified the following unstudied strategies as possibly effective interrupters of drowsiness: (1) change physical position; (2) change in ventilation (e.g., get fresh air, turn on fan, open window); (3) reduce air temperature (e.g., turn on air conditioning; turn on fan); (4) increase auditory stimulation (e.g., play music, sing, engage in conversation, listen to debate); (5) engage in interesting visual activity (e.g., board games, watching TV sports events, watching serial TV dramas) (Davidsson, 2012).*

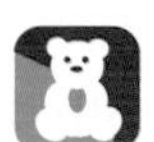

Pediatric

- Assess the amount of sleep obtained each night compared with the amount of sleep needed. EB: *An integrative review of 16 studies suggested that amount of sleep obtained in children was reduced from 9 hours in late childhood to 6 to 7 hours during adolescence, but that amount of sleep needed did not decline from childhood to young adulthood; thus, adolescents are often very sleep deprived (Carskadon, 2011).*

S

- Encourage daily schedules that allow for late awakening times for adolescents. EB: *In an integrative review of 16 studies, biological rhythms were found to shift during puberty, leading to delayed sleep initiation times and subsequent sleep deprivation if early arise times were required (Carskadon, 2011).*
- See the Pediatric section of Nursing Interventions and *Rationales* for: Readiness for enhanced **Sleep,** Disturbed **Sleep** pattern, and **Insomnia.**

Geriatric

- Assess the amount of sleep obtained each night compared with the amount of sleep needed. EB: *An integrative review of research published since 2000 suggested that sleep need in adults does not change across the lifespan, but obtaining adequate sleep becomes more difficult for older adults due to gradual changes in circadian functioning and sleep structure (Rybarczyk et al, 2013).*
- See the Geriatric section of Nursing Interventions and *Rationales* for disturbed **Sleep** pattern and **Insomnia.**

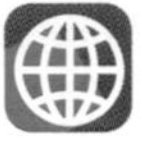

Multicultural

- Be aware of racial and ethnic disparities in sleep deprivation. EB: *A national survey of 10,896 adults found that sleep deficiency is more common among non-Hispanic blacks (53.0%) than among non-Hispanic whites (34.5%), Mexican Americans (35.2%), and persons of other races/ethnicities (41.7%) (Centers for Disease Control and Prevention, 2011).*

Home Care

- Teach family members about the short-term and long-term consequences of inadequate amounts of sleep for both clients and family caregivers. CEB: *In an integrative review of 10 studies, insufficient sleep was associated with poor attention, decreased performance, increased mortality and morbidity, and cardiovascular risk factors, including hypertension, insulin resistance, hormonal deregulation, and inflammation (Mullington et al, 2009).*
- Teach client/family caregivers about the need for those with chronic conditions to avoid schedules and commitments that interfere with obtaining adequate amounts of sleep. EBN: *In a study of 21 subjects with left-ventricular assist devices, clients obtained inadequate sleep persisting up to 6 months after surgery (Casida et al, 2011).*
- Promote adoption of behaviors that ensure adequate amounts of sleep for all family members. See Nursing Interventions and *Rationales* for Readiness for enhanced **Sleep.**
- Teach family members ways to avoid chronic sleep loss. See Nursing Interventions and *Rationales* for Disturbed **Sleep** pattern.
- Advise against the sleep deprived client's chronic use of caffeinated drinks to overcome daytime fatigue and or drowsiness; focus on elimination of factors that lead to chronic sleep loss. CEB: *In an integrative review of 26 controlled laboratory studies, caffeine was found helpful in the temporary management of sleepiness, but overuse and late-day use contributed to subsequent sleep disruption and caffeine habituation (Roehrs & Roth, 2008).*

S

REFERENCES

Campbell, S. S., Stanchina, M. D., Schlang, J. R., et al. (2011). Effects of a month-long napping regimen in older individuals. *Journal of the American Geriatric Society*, *59*(2), 224–232.

Carskadon, M. A. (2011). Sleep in adolescents: the perfect storm. *Pediatric Clinics of North America*, *58*(3), 637–647.

Casida, J. M., Davis, J. E., Brewer, R. J., et al. (2011). Sleep and daytime sleepiness of patients with left ventricular assist devices: a longitudinal pilot study. *Progress in Transplantation*, *21*(2), 131–136.

Centers for Disease Control and Prevention (CDC). (2011). Effect of short sleep duration on daily activities: United States, 2005–2008. *Morbidity and Mortality Weekly Report*, *60*, 239–252.

Davidsson, S. (2012). Countermeasure drowsiness by design: using common behaviour. *Work (Reading, Mass.)*, *41*, 5062–5067.

Dosman, J., Gjevre, J., Karunanayake, C., et al. (2014). Predicting sleep apnea in the clinic. *Chest*, *145*(3), Suppl, 595A.

Floyd, J. A. (1995). Another look at napping in the older adult. *Geriatric Nursing*, *16*, 136–138.

Haack, M., Scott-Sutherland, J., Santangelo, G., et al. (2012). Pain sensitivity and modulation in primary insomnia. *European Journal of Pain*, *16*(4), 522–533.

Liao, W. C., Huang, C. Y., Huang, T. Y., et al. (2011). A systematic review of sleep patterns and factors that disturb sleep after heart surgery. *Journal of Nursing Research*, *19*(4), 275–288.

Lloret-Linares, C., Lafuente-Lafuente, C., Chassany, O., et al. (2012). Does a single cup of coffee at dinner alter the sleep? A controlled cross-over randomised trial in real-life conditions. *Nutrition & Dietetics*, *69*, 250–255.

Mullington, J. M., Haack, M., Toth, M., et al. (2009). Cardiovascular, inflammatory, and metabolic consequences of sleep deprivation. *Progress in Cardiovascular Diseases*, *51*(4), 294–302.

Roehrs, T. A., Harris, E., Randall, S., et al. (2012). Pain sensitivity and recovery from mild chronic sleep loss. *Sleep, 35*(12), 1667–1672.

Roehrs, T., & Roth, T. (2008). Caffeine: sleep and daytime sleepiness. *Sleep Medicine Review, 12*(2), 153–162.

Rybarczyk, B., Lund, H. G., Garroway, A. M., et al. (2013). Cognitive behavioral therapy for insomnia in older adults: background, evidence, and overview of treatment protocol. *Clinical Gerontologist, 36*, 70–93.

Salas, R. E., & Gamaldo, C. E. (2011). Diagnostic and therapeutic considerations in sleep disorders: case studies and commentary. *Journal of Clinical Outcomes Management, 18*(3), 129–144.

Sin, C. W. M., Ho, J. S. C., & Chung, J. W. Y. (2008). Systematic review on the effectiveness of caffeine abstinence on the quality of sleep. *Journal of Clinical Nursing, 18*, 13–21.

Disturbed Sleep pattern

Mary Beth Flynn Makic, PhD, RN, CNS, CCNS, FAAN

NANDA-I

Definition

Time limited interruptions of sleep amount and quality due to external factors

Defining Characteristics

Alteration in sleep pattern; difficulty in daily functioning; difficulty initiating sleep; dissatisfaction with sleep; feeling unrested; unintentional awakening

Related Factors

Disruption caused by sleep partner; environmental barrier (e.g., ambient noise, daylight/darkness exposure, ambient temperature, humidity, unfamiliar settings); immobilization; insufficient privacy; nonrestorative sleep pattern (e.g., due to caregiver responsibilities, parenting practices, sleep partner)

NOC (Nursing Outcomes Classification)

Suggested NOC Outcomes

Personal Well-Being; Rest; Sleep

Example NOC Outcome with Indicators

Sleep as evidenced by the following indicators: Hours of sleep/Sleep pattern/Sleep quality/Sleep efficiency/Feels rejuvenated after sleep. (Rate the outcome and indicators of **Sleep:** 1 = severely compromised, 2 = substantially compromised, 3 = moderately compromised, 4 = mildly compromised, 5 = not compromised [see Section I].)

Client Outcomes

Client Will (Specify Time Frame)

- Verbalize plan to implement sleep promotion routines
- Maintain a regular schedule of sleep and waking
- Fall asleep without difficulty
- Remain asleep throughout the night
- Awaken naturally, feeling refreshed and is not fatigued during day

NIC (Nursing Interventions Classification)

Suggested NIC Intervention

Sleep Enhancement

Example NIC Activities—Sleep Enhancement

Determine external factors leading to sleep fragmentation; Reduce environmental disrupters of sleep

S

Nursing Interventions and *Rationales*

- Obtain a sleep history to identify (1) noise and light levels in the sleep environment, (2) activities occurring in the sleep environment during hours of sleep, (3) number of times awakened during the sleep period, and (4) when during the sleep period, time is available for undisturbed sleep. EBN: *A systematic review of 17 studies of heart surgery clients showed environmental disturbances during hospitalization were caused by noise, light, and provision of care (Liao et al, 2011).* EB: *Two case studies by Salas and Gamaldo (2011) illustrated how causes of sleep disruptions vary by setting.*
- Keep environment quiet during sleep periods. EB: *Recorded intensive care unit (ICU) noise led to more fragmented sleep, less slow-wave (deep) sleep, more arousals, and more time awake when played during sleep (N = 17) (Waye et al, 2013).* CEB: *A descriptive study of 48 hospitalized older adults found a median sound level of almost 50 dB(A) with peaks over 90 dB(A), which exceeds World Health Organization recommendations of 35 dB(A) or less (Missildine et al, 2010b).*
- Consider masking hospital noise that cannot be eliminated. EBN: *A systematic review of nine experimental studies found recorded natural sounds, music, and music videos effective for masking noise in health care settings (Hellstrom et al, 2011).*
- Offer earplugs when feasible. EB: *Results of a randomized controlled trial (RCT) (N = 136) showed perception of sleep in critical care improved with initial earplug use (Van Rompaey et al, 2012).* EBN: *Using a sequential pre-test/post-test research design, 22% of hospitalized clients who were offered earplugs (N = 50) reported that earplugs were helpful for improving sleep (Jones & Dawson, 2012).*
- Dim the lights during client sleep periods. EB: *A sequential pre/post study (N = 171) found the number of awakenings decreased when monitored lighting levels were part of a multicomponent program to decrease sleep disruption in intensive care (Patel et al, 2014).*
- Offer eye covers when lighting cannot be dimmed. CEB: *A descriptive study of 48 hospitalized adults found nighttime light levels were elevated an average of 5.25 hours per night (Missildine et al, 2010b).* EBN: *In a clinical evaluation study, 28% of hospitalized clients who were offered eye covers (N = 50) reported that eye covers were helpful for improving sleep (Jones & Dawson, 2012).*
- Be aware that use of eye covers in intubated clients may lead to sensory deprivation and anxiety. EB: *An experimental study of eye cover use in ICU clients (N = 18) reported less sleep fragmentation, but 72% of intubated clients refused eye covers or removed them prematurely due to restlessness (30%), discomfort (20%), or anxiety (11%) (Simons et al, 2012).*
- Consolidate essential care to provide opportunity for uninterrupted sleep the first 3 to 4 hours of the sleep period. Follow with periods of 90 to 110 minutes between interruptions. CEB: *A meta-analysis using data from 159 studies found the deepest stages of sleep occurred during the first 3 to 4 hours of the sleep period followed by several 90- to 110-minute sleep cycles that consisted of increasingly lighter percentages of sleep (Floyd, 2002).*
- If client must be disturbed the first 3 to 4 hours of the sleep period, attempt to protect 90- to 110-minute blocks of time between awakenings. CEB: *In three studies of hospitalized clients, researchers found that the high frequency of nocturnal care interactions left clients with no 90-minute blocks of uninterrupted time for sleep (Missildine, 2008; Missildine et al, 2010a, 2010b).* EB: *In an experimental study that included protocols for consolidating care, the number of client nights that contained a 3-hour window of interrupted sleep was increased (Patel et al, 2014).*
- Assess for medications and other stimulants that fragment sleep. Use caution when administering sleep medications. See Nursing Interventions and *Rationales* for **Insomnia.**
- Schedule newly ordered medications to avoid the need to wake the client the first few hours of the night. EBN: *A survey of sleep promotion protocols used by nurses in hospitals in The Netherlands (N = 68) identified the need for providers to plan ahead when initiating new medication regimens to help ensure uninterrupted sleep periods (Hofhuis et al, 2012).*
- Combine as many of the above interventions as feasible to create a sleep-promotion care bundle. EB: *A sequential pre/post study (N = 171) found efforts to limit noise and bright lighting along with efforts to consolidate care could successfully be combined into a care bundle effective for limiting sleep fragmentation (Patel et al, 2014).*

Pediatric

- Adapt interventions for pediatric clients with caution due to lack of empirical evidence regarding the effects of their use. EB: *A survey of 341 pediatric critical care providers worldwide found use of earplugs, eye masks, noise reduction, and lighting optimization for sleep promotion was uncommon (Kudchadkar et al, 2014).*

Geriatric

- Use of earplugs and eye covers with ataxic clients and clients with dementia may contribute to disorientation. EB: *A case report and integrative review of the literature suggested sensory deficits in clients with dementia, which can be augmented by use of earplugs and eye covers, decrease their quality of life, increase their risk for delirium and falls, and pose a higher risk for poor outcomes (Haque et al, 2012).*

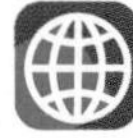

Multicultural

- Be aware that cultural sleep practices may alter the kinds of environmental sleep disruptors that require management. EB: *An integrative review of the literature on family sleep practices demonstrated that bed sharing and other aspects of the sleep environment were influenced most by ethnic factors (Jain et al, 2011).*

Home Care

- Consider the unique characteristics of each home sleep environment when addressing sleep disruption. EBN: *A longitudinal study of postpartum women (N = 142) found new mothers' sleep was disturbed 56% of the time by their infant's cries, but other environmental disrupters included (1) family, friends, and pets in the home, (2) sleeping with the television on, (3) traffic sounds, and (4) other outside noise from neighbors and traffic (Doering, 2013).* EBN: *In two RCTs, modification of homes to promote parental sleep found that interventions were more effective for low socioeconomic status (SES) parents (N = 118) than more advantaged parents (N = 122) (Lee & Gay, 2011).*
- In addition, see the Home Care section of Nursing Interventions and *Rationales* for Readiness for enhanced **Sleep.**

REFERENCES

Doering, J. J. (2013). The physical and social environment of sleep in socioeconomically disadvantaged postpartum women. *Journal of Obstetric, Gynecologic, & Neonatal Nursing, 42*, E33–E43.

Floyd, J. A. (2002). Sleep and aging. *Nursing Clinics of North America, 37*(4), 719–731.

Haque, R., Abdelrehman, N., & Alavi, Z. (2012). "There's a monster under my bed": hearing aids and dementia in long-term care settings. *The Annals of Long-term Care, 20*(8), 28.

Hellstrom, A., Fagerstrom, C., & Willman, A. (2011). Promoting sleep by nursing interventions in health care settings: a systematic review. *Worldviews on Evidence-based Nursing, 8*(3), 128–142.

Hofhuis, J. G. M., Langevoort, G., Rommes, J. H., et al. (2012). Sleep disturbances and sedation practices in the intensive care unit: a postal survey in the Netherlands. *Intensive Care Critical Care Nursing, 28*, 141–149.

Jain, S., Romack, B. S., & Jain, R. (2011). Bed sharing in school-age children—clinical and social implications. *Journal of Child and Adolescent Psychiatric Nursing, 24*, 185–189.

Jones, C., & Dawson, D. (2012). Eye masks and earplugs improve patient's perception of sleep. *Nursing in Critical Care, 17*(5), 247–254.

Kudchadkar, S. R., Yaster, M., & Punjabi, N. M. (2014). Sedation, sleep promotion, and delirium screening practices in the care of mechanically ventilated children: a wake-up call for the pediatric critical care community. *Critical Care Medicine, 42*(7), 1592–1600.

Lee, K. A., & Gay, C. L. (2011). Can modifications to the bedroom environment improve the sleep of new parents? Two randomized controlled trials. *Research in Nursing & Health, 34*, 7–19.

Liao, W. C., Huang, C. Y., Huang, T. Y., et al. (2011). A systematic review of sleep patterns and factors that disturb sleep after heart surgery. *Journal of Nursing Research, 19*(4), 275–288.

Missildine, K. (2008). Sleep and the sleep environment of older adults in acute care settings. *Journal of Gerontological Nursing, 34*(6), 15–21.

Missildine, K., Bergstrom, N., Meininger, J., et al. (2010a). Case studies: is the sleep of hospitalized elders related to delirium? *Medsurg Nursing, 19*(1), 39–46.

Missildine, K., Bergstrom, N., Meininger, J., et al. (2010b). Sleep in hospitalized elders: a pilot study. *Geriatric Nursing, 31*(4), 263–272.

Patel, J., Baldwin, J., Bunting, P., et al. (2014). The effect of a multicomponent multidisciplinary bundle of interventions on sleep and delirium in medical and surgical intensive care patients. *Anaesthesia, 69*, 540–549.

Salas, R. E., & Gamaldo, C. E. (2011). Diagnostic and therapeutic considerations in sleep disorders: case studies and commentary. *Journal of Clinical Outcomes Management, 18*(3), 129–144.

Simons, K. S., Van den Boogaard, M., & De Jager, C. P. C. (2012). Reducing sensory input in critically ill patients: are eyemasks a blind spot? *Critical Care, 16*, 439.

Van Rompaey, B., Elseviers, M. M., Van Drom, W., et al. (2012). The effect of earplugs during the night on the onset of delirium and sleep perception: a randomized controlled trial in intensive care patients. *Critical Care, 16*, R73.

Waye, P. K., Elmenhorst, E. M., Croy, I., et al. (2013). Improvement of intensive care using sound environment and analysis of consequences on sleep: an experimental study. *Sleep Medicine, 14*, 1334–1340.

Impaired Social interaction

Gail B. Ladwig, MSN, RN, and Marina Martinez-Kratz, MS, RN, CNE

NANDA-I

Definition

Insufficient or excessive quantity or ineffective quality of social exchange

Defining Characteristics

Discomfort in social situations; dissatisfaction with social engagement (e.g., belonging, caring, interest, shared history); dysfunctional interaction with others; family reports change in interaction (e.g., style, pattern); impaired social functioning

Related Factors (r/t)

Absence of significant others; communication barriers; disturbance in self-concept; disturbance in thought processes; environmental barrier; impaired mobility; insufficient knowledge about how to enhance mutuality; insufficient skills to enhance mutuality; sociocultural dissonance; therapeutic isolation

NOC (Nursing Outcomes Classification)

Suggested NOC Outcomes

Child Development: Middle Childhood, Adolescence; Play Participation; Role Performance; Social Interaction Skills; Social Involvement

Example NOC Outcome with Indicators

Social Involvement as evidenced by the following indicator: Interacts with close friends, neighbors, family members, and members of work groups. (Rate the outcome and indicators of **Social Involvement:** 1 = never demonstrated, 2 = rarely demonstrated, 3 = sometimes demonstrated, 4 = often demonstrated, 5 = consistently demonstrated [see Section I].)

S

Client Outcomes

Client Will (Specify Time Frame)

- Identify barriers that cause impaired social interactions
- Discuss feelings that accompany impaired and successful social interactions
- Use available opportunities to practice interactions
- Use successful social interaction behaviors
- Report increased comfort in social situations
- Communicate, state feelings of belonging, demonstrate caring and interest in others
- Report effective interactions with others

NIC (Nursing Interventions Classification)

Suggested NIC Intervention

Socialization Enhancement

Example NIC Activities—Socialization Enhancement

Encourage patience in developing relationships; Help client increase awareness of strengths and limitations in communicating with others

Nursing Interventions and *Rationales*

- Monitor the client's use of defense mechanisms and support healthy defenses (e.g., the client focuses on the present and avoids placing blame on others for personal behavior). CEBN: *Solution-focused techniques have been demonstrated to be beneficial. Therapy focuses on the client's present and future, capitalizing on the strengths and resources of the client and significant others around them (Wand, 2010).*
- Spend time with the client. EBN: *In this study of spirituality at end of life, presence was identified as important in itself. By his/her caring presence, the nurse identifies with the client in his/her suffering and conveys dignity, respect, and compassion (Milligan, 2011).*
- Encourage physical activity, such as aerobics or stretching and toning. EB: *A Cochrane Systematic Review indicated that physical activity was beneficial to the social functioning of cancer survivors (Mishra et al, 2012).*
- Have group members support each other in a group setting. EB: *Assertive community treatment is beneficial in reestablishing or maintaining bonds between family, friends, and acquaintances (Tempier et al, 2012).*
- Model appropriate social interactions and use focused imitation interventions. Give positive verbal and nonverbal feedback for appropriate behavior (e.g., make statements such as, "I'm proud that you made it to work on time and did all the tasks assigned to you"; make eye contact). If not contraindicated, touch the client's arm or hand when speaking. CEBN: *Shared feelings increased communication with stroke and aphasia clients without words (Sundin et al, 2000). Use of focused imitation interventions improved social functioning in children with autism spectrum disorders (Ingersoll, 2012).*
- Consider use of social cognition and interaction training (SCIT) combined with social mentoring to improve social functioning. EB: *A randomized controlled trial using SCIT and social mentoring demonstrated improved social cognition and social functioning in individuals with severe mental illness living in the community (Hasson-Ohayon et al, 2014).*
- Use client-centered humor as appropriate. EB: *Humor may be helpful in working with clients with depression (Bokarius et al, 2011).*
- Consider use of animal therapy; arrange for visitation. EB: *Equine-facilitated therapy (working with horses) is described as a parallel experience to working in groups, "social interaction" (Akaltun & Banning, 2012).*
- Consider use of videophone or other visual communication devices to promote social interaction in clients with visual impairments. EB: *The use of videophone technology increased accessibility to social interaction including cultivation and maintenance of friendships with peers (Emerson & Bishop, 2012).*

▲ Refer client for social cognition training to increase social skills. EB: *Social cognition training using targeted programs are most effective at improving social functioning in clients with a diagnosis of psychosis or schizophrenia (Henderson, 2013).*

▲ Refer rehabilitation clients for assistive technologies to increase therapeutic engagement and promote social engagement. EB: *Rehabilitation clients' desire to use mainstream technologies (cell phones, tablets, computers) underscores the need for accessible options that will provide opportunities to engage in therapeutically meaningful activities and promote social interaction (Fager & Burnfield, 2014).*

- Refer to care plans for Risk for **Loneliness** and **Social** isolation for additional interventions.

Pediatric

- Encourage social support and counseling for clients with visual and hearing impairments. EB: *Social support is needed for mothers of children with hearing impairment, because it is a "hidden" disability (Dehkordi et al, 2011). Emotional support and counseling were both effective in improving social functioning in clients with visual impairment.*
- Provide supervised interaction opportunities for children of chronically ill parents. EBN: *Research has identified that social isolation is a challenge for children with parents who experience chronic disabling pain (Umberger et al, 2015).*
- Provide computers and Internet access to children with chronic disabilities that limit socialization. EB: *Children with autism showed more active other-awareness using a technology with a supportive interface and when collaborating with a peer (Holt & Yuill, 2014).*

▲ Refer overweight adolescents to group based weight loss programs. EB: *Overweight adolescents who participated in group based weight loss programs showed improvements in social functioning that were related to increases in self-concept dimensions (Jelalian et al, 2011).*

S

▲ Refer children with autism for family-centered music therapy (FCMT). EB: *Research demonstrated that family participation in FCMT improved social interactions in the home and community as well as the parent-child relationship (Thompson et al, 2014).*

- Consider the use of animal-assisted activities for children on the autistic spectrum. EB: *Research demonstrated significant improvements in social functioning and decreases in social withdrawal behaviors after 8 weeks of animal exposure in a school classroom in addition to sixteen 20-minute animal-interaction sessions (O'Haire et al, 2014).*
- Consider the use of a theater skills training to facilitate social skills. EB: *Brain injured youth showed improvements in social skills and participation with the use of an arts based intervention (Agnihotri et al, 2012).*

Geriatric

- Encourage socialization through education, support groups, and programs for older adults in the community. EB: *Neighborhood social cohesion may be protective against stroke mortality (Clark et al, 2011).*
- Assess for depression in clients with impaired social functioning. EB: *Research shows higher depressive symptoms were associated with smaller numbers of close, inner circle relationships (Shouse et al, 2013).*
- Assess cognitive functioning in clients who present with decreased social interaction. EB: *Researchers identified a link between decreased social interaction and a decline in cognitive abilities (Dickinson et al, 2011).*
- Assess the communication patterns of clients with verbal domain problems for enactment strategies, paralinguistic features, and nonvocal communication. EBN: *Research has demonstrated that clients with semantic dementia spontaneously use enactment (acting out scenes), paralinguistic features (pitch and volume of tone), and nonvocal communication (e.g., body posture, pointing, and facial expression) to compensate for loss of verbal abilities (Kindell et al, 2013).*
- Consider having clients participate in playing Wii. EB: *This study of older adults who played with the Wii experienced well-being, particularly social connection and enjoyment (Kahlbaugh et al, 2011).*

▲ Refer depressed clients to services for cognitive behavioral therapy (CBT). EB: *A systematic review indicated that CBT was likely to be efficacious for depression and accompanying symptoms such as impaired social functioning in older people (Jayasekara et al, 2015).*

- Refer to care plans for **Frail Elderly** syndrome, Risk for **Loneliness,** and **Social** isolation for additional interventions.

S

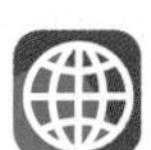

Multicultural

- Assess for the effect of racism on the client's perceptions of social interactions. EB: *In this study of clients in group drug treatment plans, women, but not men, of different races acted differently in mixed-race, mixed-gender cocaine treatment groups, with African American women exhibiting fewer of several behaviors (Johnson et al, 2011).*
- Approach individuals of color with respect, warmth, and professional courtesy. EBN: *To provide client- and family-centered care, nurses must acknowledge their cultural differences, be willing to incorporate their beliefs within the health care treatment plan, and respect their values and lifeways of differing cultures (Hart & Mareno, 2015).*
- Use interpreters as needed. EB: *Primary care nurses act as gatekeepers to interpreting services (McCarthy et al, 2013).*
- Refer to care plan for **Social** isolation for additional interventions.

Home Care

- Previously discussed interventions may be adapted for home care use.

▲ Refer clients to or support involvement in supportive groups and counseling. EBN: *Clients who received direct support and resources had better outcomes with improvement of psychiatric symptoms, social functioning, and self-efficacy (Sono et al, 2012).*

Client/Family Teaching and Discharge Planning

▲ Refer to appropriate social agencies for assistance (e.g., family therapy, self-help groups, creative activities, crisis intervention), especially individuals who are seriously ill. EB: *Clients who received direct support and resources had better outcomes with improvement of psychiatric symptoms, social functioning, and self-efficacy (Sono et al, 2012). Music therapy as an addition to standard care helps people with schizophrenia improve their global state, mental state (including negative symptoms), and social functioning, if a sufficient number of music therapy sessions are provided by qualified music therapists (Mössler et al, 2011).*

REFERENCES

Agnihotri, S., Gray, J., Colantonio, A., et al. (2012). Two case study evaluations of an arts-based social skills intervention for adolescents with childhood brain disorder. *Developmental Neurorehabilitation, 15*(4), 284–297.

Akaltun, E., & Banning, N. (2012). When the therapist is a horse. *Ther Today, 23*(2).

Bokarius, A., et al. (2011). Attitude toward humor in patients experiencing depressive symptoms. *Innovations in Clinical Neuroscience, 8*(9), 20–23.

Clark, C. J., et al. (2011). Neighborhood cohesion is associated with reduced risk of stroke mortality. *Stroke; a Journal of Cerebral Circulation, 42*(5), 1212–1217.

Dehkordi, M., et al. (2011). Stress in mothers of hearing impaired children compared to mothers of normal and other disabled children. *Audiology, 20*(1), 128.

Dickinson, W., Potter, G., Hybels, C., et al. (2011). Change in stress and social support as predictors of cognitive decline in older adults with and without depression. *International Journal of Geriatric Psychiatry, 26*(12), 1267–1274.

Emerson, J., & Bishop, J. (2012). Videophone technology and students with deaf-blindness: a method for increasing access and communication. *Journal of Visual Impairment & Blindness, 106*(10), 622–633.

Fager, S. K., & Burnfield, J. M. (2014). Patients' experiences with technology during inpatient rehabilitation: opportunities to support independence and therapeutic engagement. *Disability & Rehabilitation: Assistive Technology, 9*(2), 121–127.

Hart, P. L., & Mareno, N. (2015). Cultural challenges and barriers through the voices of nurses. *Journal of Clinical Nursing, 23*(15/16), 2223–2233. *CINAHL Plus with Full Text*, EBSCO*host* (accessed June 27, 2015).

Hasson-Ohayon, I., Mashiach-Eizenberg, M., Avidan, M., et al. (2014). Social cognition and interaction training: preliminary results of an RCT in a community setting in Israel. *Psychiatric Services, 65*(4), 555–558.

Henderson, A. R. (2013). The impact of social cognition training on recovery from psychosis. *Current Opinion in Psychiatry, 26*(5), 429–432.

Holt, S. 1., & Yuill, N. (2014). Facilitating other-awareness in low-functioning children with autism and typically-developing preschoolers using dual-control technology. *Journal of Autism and Developmental Disorders, 44*(1), 236–248.

Ingersoll, B. (2012). Brief report: effect of a focused imitation intervention on social functioning in children with autism. *Journal of Autism & Developmental Disorders, 42*(8), 1768–1773.

Jayasekara, R., Procter, N., Harrison, J., et al. (2015). Cognitive behavioural therapy for older adults with depression: a review. *Journal of Mental Health, 24*(3), 168–171.

Jelalian, E., Sato, A., & Hart, C. N. (2011). The effect of group-based weight-control intervention on adolescent psychosocial outcomes: perceived peer rejection, social anxiety, and self-concept. *Children's Health Care, 40*(3), 197–211.

Johnson, J. E., et al. (2011). Gender, race, and group behavior in group drug treatment. *Drug and Alcohol Dependence, 119*(3), e39–e45.

Kahlbaugh, P., et al. (2011). Effects of playing Wii on well-being in the elderly: physical activity, loneliness, and mood. *Activities, Adaptation and Aging, 35*(4), 331–344.

Kindell, J., Sage, K., Keady, J., et al. (2013). Adapting to conversation with semantic dementia: using enactment as a compensatory strategy in everyday social interaction. *International Journal of Language & Communication Disorders, 48*(5), 497–507.

McCarthy, J., Cassidy, I., Graham, M. M., et al. (2013). Conversations through barriers of language and interpretation. *British Journal of Nursing, 22*(6), 335–339.

Milligan, S. (2011). Addressing the spiritual care needs of people near the end of life. *Nursing Standard, 26*(4), 47–56.

Mishra, S., Scherer, R., Geigle, P., et al. (2012). Exercise interventions on health-related quality of life for cancer survivors. *Cochrane Database of Systematic Reviews*, (8), N.PAG.

Mössler, K., et al. (2011). Music therapy for people with schizophrenia and schizophrenia-like disorders. *Cochrane Database of Systematic Reviews*, (12), CD004025.

O'Haire, M. E., McKenzie, S. J., McCune, S., et al. (2014). Effects of classroom animal-assisted activities on social functioning in children with autism spectrum disorder. *Journal of Alternative & Complementary Medicine, 20*(3), 162–168.

Shouse, J. N., Rowe, S. V., & Mast, B. T. (2013). Depression and cognitive functioning as predictors of social network size. *Clinical Gerontologist, 36*(2), 147–161.

Sono, T., Oshima, I., Ito, J., et al. (2012). Family support in assertive community treatment: an analysis of client outcomes. *Community Mental Health Journal, 48*(4), 463–470.

Sundin, K., et al. (2000). Communicating with people with stroke and aphasia: understanding through sensation without words. *Journal of Clinical Nursing, 9*(4), 481.

Tempier, R., et al. (2012). Does assertive community outreach improve social support? Results from the Lambeth study of early-episode psychosis. *Psychiatric Services (Washington, D.C.), 63*(3), 216–222.

Thompson, G. A., McFerran, K. S., & Gold, C. (2014). Family-centred music therapy to promote social engagement in young children with severe autism spectrum disorder: a randomized controlled study. *Child: Care, Health and Development, 40*(6), 840–852. [Epub 2013 Nov 22].

Umberger, W. A., Risko, J., & Covington, E. (2015). The forgotten ones: challenges and needs of children living with disabling parental chronic pain. *Journal of Pediatric Nursing, 30*(3), 498–507.

Wand, T. (2010). Mental health nursing from a solution focused perspective. *International Journal of Mental Health Nursing, 19*(3), 210–219.

S

Social Isolation *Julianne E. Doubet, BSN, RN, CEN, NREMT-P*

NANDA-I

Definition

Aloneness experienced by the individual and perceived as imposed by others and as a negative or threatening state

Defining Characteristics

Absence of support system; aloneness imposed by others; cultural incongruence; desire to be alone; development delay; developmentally inappropriate interests; disabling condition; feeling different from others; flat affect; history of rejection; hostility; illness; inability to meet expectations of others; insecurity in public; meaningless actions; member of a subculture; poor eye contact; preoccupation with own thoughts; purposelessness; repetitive actions; sad affect; values incongruent with cultural norms; withdrawn

Related Factors (r/t)

Alterations in mental status; alterations in physical appearance; altered state of wellness; developmentally inappropriate interests; factors impacting satisfying personal relationships (e.g., developmental delay); inability to engage in satisfying personal relationships; insufficient personal resources (e.g., poor achievement, poor insight, affect unavailable and poorly controlled); social behavior incongruent with norms; values incongruent with cultural norms; may be present but is not required; pain may be of unknown etiology

NOC (Nursing Outcomes Classification)

Suggested NOC Outcomes

Loneliness Severity; Mood Equilibrium; Personal Well-Being; Play Participation; Social Anxiety Level; Social Interaction Skills; Social Involvement; Social Support

Example NOC Outcome with Indicators

Social Involvement as evidenced by the following indicator: Interacts with close friends, neighbors, family members, and members of work groups. (Rate the outcome and indicators of **Social Involvement:** 1 = never demonstrated, 2 = rarely demonstrated, 3 = sometimes demonstrated, 4 = often demonstrated, 5 = consistently demonstrated [see Section I].)

S

Client Outcomes

Client Will (Specify Time Frame)

- Identify feelings of isolation
- Practice social and communication skills needed to interact with others
- Initiate interactions with others; set and meet goals
- Participate in activities and programs at level of ability and desire
- Describe feelings of self-worth

NIC (Nursing Interventions Classification)

Suggested NIC Intervention

Socialization Enhancement

Example NIC Activities—Socialization Enhancement

Encourage patience in developing relationships; Help patient increase awareness of strengths and limitations in communicating with others

Nursing Interventions and *Rationales*

- Establish a therapeutic relationship with the client. EBN: *In her study, Skingley (2013) suggests that many of the circumstances that contribute to social isolation are amendable and that the community nurse is in the position to affect changes by using one-to-one interventions, by involving the client in group activities, and by community engagement.* EBN: *Nurses are one of the fundamental client advocate groups that promote the prevention of social isolation (Wilson et al, 2011).*

- Observe for barriers to social interaction. EBN: *This study by Drury (2014) states that social isolation can be measured by objective indicators, such as the client's social network, and his/her participation in community activities, and by subjective indicators, including a client's self-rating of loneliness and perception of support.* EB: *Ohayon and Roberts (2014) maintain that stress and social isolation were important influences for depression among young adults.*
- Discuss/assess causes of perceived or actual isolation. EBN: *Some variables that were recognized by Nicholson et al (2014) as precursors to diminished social interaction included severe health problems, symptoms of depression, smoking, and decreased religious participation.* EB: *Social isolation is a known risk factor for morbidity and mortality in human beings, according to Cacioppo et al (2014).*
- Allow the client opportunities to describe his/her daily life and to introduce any issues that may be of concern. EBN: *McDonald (2014) surmises that the biggest problem in health care today is lack of communication skills, which can then be related to poor client outcomes; she maintains that the nurse of today must be proficient in effective communication.* EBN: *Therapeutic communication consists of certain techniques that promote a relationship involving mutual trust and respect between nurse and client (Thomas et al, 2013).*
- Promote social interactions. EB: *Positive social interactions may act as a basis for the client to establish new social group relationships (Cruwys et al, 2014).* EB: *In recent studies, it was found that the quality of social interactions, whether positive or negative, impact physical health and the feeling of well-being (Cyranowski et al, 2013).*
- Assist the client in identifying specific health and social problems; involve him/her in their resolution. EBN: *Pearce (2013) maintains that interventions customized to fit a client's disorganized lifestyle reduce their social isolation.* EBN: *Intervention programs that are meant to prevent or reduce loneliness in older adults may be valuable in safeguarding the client from future mental health problems (Bekhet & Zauszniewski, 2012).*
- Assist the client in identifying activities that encourage socialization. EB: *According to this study, the sooner the older client is supported in mobility and social participation, the sooner he/she is able to experience a sense of well-being and lessening of the feelings of social isolation (Elbasan et al, 2013).* EB: *Studies have shown that people with regular social connections present with significantly less cognitive decline when compared to those who are lonely and/or isolated (Ristau, 2011).*
- Identify available support systems and involve those individuals in the client's care. EBN: *According to Mattila et al (2014), nurse support of clients and their families is effective in establishing a positive outlook, mental well-being, and thoughts of getting well.* EB: *"Clinicians should be aware of social isolation and loneliness in late life and discuss nonpharmacologic treatment options with their aging patients" (Canham, 2014).*

S

▲ Refer clients and caregivers to support groups as necessary. EB: *Webster et al (2013) maintain that the family is no longer as strong a force in the struggle to reduce social isolation and that interventions should be based in the community.* EB: *Caring for a family member who is physically and/or mentally challenged can be a drain on caregivers, causing a negative effect both on the client and the caregiver: effective outside assistance might be a factor in modifying the challenges confronted by these families (Thompson et al, 2014).*

- Encourage interactions with others with similar interests. EBN: *Culley et al (2013) believe that their study is the forerunner to understanding the potential for improving connectiveness and alleviating isolation by the use of technology.* EBN: *According to this research study, a community integrative therapy program will allow those involved to form new relationships, gather emotional support, reinforce ties, and reduce social isolation (da Roche et al, 2013).*
- See the care plan for Risk for **Loneliness.**

Pediatric

▲ Refer obese adolescents for diet, exercise and psychosocial support. EB: *Nesbit et al (2014) suggest that to combat adolescent obesity, interventions should target sedentary behavior and promote the increase of physical activity, but also should address parental concerns about neighborhood safety and access to safe areas for physical activity development.* EBN: *This study found that family meals two to three times per week during adolescence is an important factor in preventing obesity in young adulthood (Berge et al, 2015).*

▲ Assess socially isolated adolescents. Refer to appropriate rehabilitation programs as needed. EB: *A study by Plaiser and Konijn (2013) implies that both peers and media have a firm influence on adolescents and that peer rejection may be cause for the adolescent to turn to antisocial media content.* EB: *This study suggests that there are racial/ethnic, gender, and socioeconomic differences in substance abuse types of treatment (Lo & Ching, 2013).*

Geriatric

▲ Assess physical and mental status to establish an early baseline for referring at-risk individuals to community resources. EBN: *In this study, Nicholson (2012) states that health professionals have the opportunity to take measures that will allow early detection of social isolation in at-risk, older clients and match them to suitable community resources; this may serve to prevent negative health outcomes.* EB: *Older individuals should be routinely screened for depression, as it may be an important factor in giving rise to later social isolation (Pritchard et al, 2014).*

- Assess for hearing. EB: *It is well-documented that hearing loss is common in older adults: it is also considered a known factor in the cause of social isolation, depression, and dementia (Genther et al, 2014).* EB: *Because hearing loss is more prevalent with aging, it is important that the nurse be aware of options open to older adults with hearing impairment; early detection is essential (Jupiter, 2012).*
- Involve client in planning activities. EBN: *Assessment of an older person's goals, as identified by the individual in need of home care, allows the health care provider to personalize the client's activities, which then leads to betterment of the client's quality of life (Parsons et al, 2012).* EB: *"Regular and structured physical activity is known to be effective in preventing and/or reducing the physical and mental decline associated with aging," according to Marini et al (2014).*
- Involve nonprofessionals in activities and projects with the client. EBN: *Group music therapy relieved agitated activity in older adults who suffer from dementia and promoted emotional relaxation, encouraged interpersonal interactions, and appeared to reduce further agitated episodes (Lin et al, 2011).* EB: *Pettigrew et al (2014) write that both group activities and a focused approach to those clients who are at risk for social isolation may be the way to manage the problem.*
- Suggest varied social activities that would decrease isolation and encourage participation. EB: *Leisure activities can play a significant part in an older person's social life and improve their quality of life; these could include volunteer work, cultural activities, sports, reading books, hobbies, and shopping (Toepoel, 2013).* EB: *According to Morrow-Howell et al (2014), there are community volunteer programs that have been shown to open new social, civic, and work-related paths for older adults.*

▲ Consider the use of simulated presence therapy (see the care plan for **Hopelessness**). EB: *A video of the simulated presence of a family member appeared to reduce unwillingness of the adult with dementia to involve himself in basic, everyday self-care tasks (O'Connor et al, 2011).* EB: *Obdrzalek et al (2013) promote an automated exercise coaching system for older adults living in assisted homes: this technique is designed to allow remote interaction with a coach and to strengthen the social aspects of exercise.*

- Consider using computers and the Internet to alleviate or reduce loneliness and social isolation. EB: *The use of technology that is tailored to older people may aid in better self-management of health conditions and thus, may produce an increased improvement in social connectedness (Morris et al, 2014).* EB: *According to Gitlow (2014), many older adults are socializing through technological devices (phones, email, surfing the net), but there are still numerous barriers that keep them from fully using technology to its fullest; these include lack of knowledge, negativity, and age-related changes in vision and hearing.*

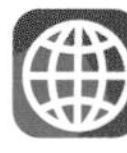

Multicultural

- Acknowledge racial/ethnic differences at the onset of care. EBN: *It is necessary for nurses to be aware of cultural differences, be responsive to clients' needs, and include them in the plan of care (Kwok & White, 2011).* EB: *Every client has a unique culture that has many aspects, is vibrant, and cannot be labeled by race or language group (Hawes & Viera, 2014).*
- Assess for the influence of cultural beliefs, norms, values, and the client's personal cultural needs. EB: *Cultural standpoints concerning medical decision-making and the client's expectations of his/her children, may cause the medical surrogate (who in many cultures is the firstborn) to experience stress, family conflict, and difficulty coping; health care professionals should support the surrogate in communication with the client and with his/her extended family (Su et al, 2014).* EBN: *Culturally responsive caregiver involvement is necessary to make certain that people of culturally and linguistically dissimilar backgrounds have the proper skills to self-manage their multifaceted medical conditions (Williams et al, 2014).*

- Use a culturally competent, professional approach when working with clients of various ethnic groups. EBN: *Today's professional nurse must be aware of the role of cultural competency and cultural safety in his or her practice (Rowan et al, 2013).* EBN: *Miller et al (2013) found that interventions to reduce depression in an immigrant couple required, not only the lessening of immigration-related problems, but also concentration on gender diversity and promoting family and social support.*
- Promote a sense of ethnic attachment. EBN: *Provide care in a way that respects and considers the client's cultural and religious needs (Black, 2011).* EB: *According to Enguidanos et al (2014), there is a need for client-centered intervention and prevention standards that incorporate the client's cultural background, health care requirements, and individual preferences.*
- Assess the client's feelings regarding social isolation. EBN: *In this study of African American women with breast cancer, it is suggested that personal stress can be measured by the level of the client's isolation and proposed that nurses should generate interventions to decrease that isolation and assist clients in developing supportive bonds with other clients and community members (Heiney et al, 2011).* EB: *Cooley and Garcia (2012) suggest that the client's past history and diverse relationship experiences will determine their approach to interactions with others.*
- Assist those ethnic minorities who are underserved to access essential health care. EBN: *Jeffreys and Dogan (2013) maintain that a comprehensive nursing assessment is the first step necessary in providing culturally specialized care, recognition of high risk groups, and reduction of health care inequality.* EBN: *According to Waite et al (2014), it is vital that clinicians recognize the necessity of cultural competence in their practice to both improve and maintain health care for their clients.*

Home Care

- The interventions described previously may be adapted for home care use.
- Confirm that the home setting has health-safety systems in place. EB: *Those older persons who are socially isolated and have no support are especially vulnerable in an emergency, and their preparation to react to a disaster is questionable (Staley et al, 2011).* EB: *The medical and safety goals for older adults should be taken into account when redesigning an approach for home care delivery (Depuccio & Hoff, 2014).*
- Consider the use of the computer and Internet to decrease isolation. EB: *Older adults who use the Internet may derive benefits, such as a reduction in loneliness and an improvement in social interaction (Cotton et al, 2013).* EBN: *A study by Culley et al (2013) illustrated the ability of technology to develop connectedness and diminish the feeling of isolation in community-dwelling older adults.*
- *Assess options for living that allow the client privacy, but not isolation.* EB: *The medical community must respect the client's values of autonomy, safety, privacy and health and consider their unique sociocultural and historical dynamics (Weber et al, 2012).* EBN: *Rulliere (2014) explains that a person's dignity and privacy must be preserved, regardless of his/her cognitive ability, not only when receiving nursing care but also in all phases of life.*
- Assist clients to interact with neighbors in the community when they move to supported housing. EB: *The participants in this study, residents of supported housing, reported that it was important to them to feel a part of the community when interacting with their neighbors, especially in regard to neighbor relations, community safety, neighborhood satisfaction, and tolerance of mental illness (Townley & Kloos, 2011).* EB: *Results of a study by Cho et al (2012) found that housing professionals should consider a supportive neighborhood and social opportunities when promoting community housing for older adults.*

S

Client/Family Teaching and Discharge Planning

- Assist the client in initiating contacts with self-help groups, counselors, and therapists. EBN: *Appropriate interventions are needed to educate the client concerning the problems caused by loneliness; the proper management of chronic disease; referrals, not only to monitor physical status, but also to enhance social networking; and referrals to social services to address personal needs (Jarve & Dool, 2011).* EBN: *Seebohm et al (2013) advise as a result of their study that policy-makers might partner with the local population to provide support for diverse types of residents to facilitate their own self-help/mutual aid groups.*
- Provide information to the client about senior citizen services and community resources. EB: *Those who are Spanish-speaking and those older adults who are living independently are the populations most in need for increased senior center outreach programs, according to Schneider et al (2014).* EB: *Senior centers are excellent locations to deliver evidence-based health support programs that will bolster this rapidly growing age group in remaining healthy and independent (Felix et al, 2014).*

- Refer socially isolated caregivers to appropriate support groups. **EBN:** *Nurses demonstrate a keen knowledge of the needs of relatives and reported efficacious interventions in supporting those needs (Buckley & Andrews, 2011).* **EBN:** *Eriksson et al (2013) maintain that woman who are 24/7 caregivers need choices that can be recommended by health care professionals who will not disregard their ethical concerns.*
- See the care plan for **Caregiver Role Strain.**

REFERENCES

Bekhet, A. K., & Zauszniewski, A. (2012). Mental health of elders in retirement communities: is loneliness a key factor? *Archives of Psychiatric Nursing*, *26*, 214–224. [Epub 2011 Dec 10].

Berge, J. M., Wall, M., Hsueh, T. F., et al. (2015). The protective role of family meals for youth obesity: 10 years longitudinal associations. *Journal of Pediatrics*, *166*(2), 296–301.

Black, P. (2011). Understanding religious beliefs of patients needing a stoma. *Gastrointestinal Nursing*, *9*, 17–22.

Buckley, P., & Andrews, T. (2011). Intensive care nurses' knowledge of critical care family needs. *Intensive and Critical Care Nursing*, *27*, 263–272.

Cacioppo, S., Capitanio, J. P., & Cacioppo, J. T. (2014). Toward a neurology of loneliness. *Psychology Bulletin*, 15.

Canham, S. L. (2014). What's loneliness got to do with it? Older woman who use benzodiazepines. *Australian Journal of Aging*, 26. [Epub ahead of print].

Cho, J., Cook, C., & Bruin, M. J. (2012). Functional ability, neighborhood resources and housing satisfaction among older adults in the U.S. *Journal of Housing for the Elderly*, *26*, 395–412.

Cooley, E. L., & Garcia, A. L. (2012). Attachment style differences and depression in African American and European American college women: normative adaption? *Journal of Multicultural Counseling and Development*, *40*, 216–225.

Cotton, S. R., Anderson, W. A., & McCullough, B. M. (2013). Impact of internet use on loneliness and contact with others among older adults: cross sectional analysis. *Journal of Medical Internet Research*, *15*, e39.

Cruwys, T., Dingle, G. A., Hornsby, M. J., et al. (2014). Social isolation schema responds to positive social experiences: longitudinal evidence from vulnerable populations. *British Journal of Clinical Psychology*, *53*, 265–280. [Epub 2014 Jan 13].

Culley, J. M., Herman, J., Smith, D., et al. (2013). Effects of technology and connectedness in community dwelling older adults. *Online Journal of Nursing Informatics*, *17*, 1–6. <http://ojni.org/issues/?p=2864>.

Cyranowski, J. M., Bode, R., Butt, Z., et al. (2013). Assessing social support, companionship, and distress: national institute of health (NIH) toolbox adult social relationship scales. *Health Psychology*, *32*, 293–301.

da Roche, I. A., al Sa, A. N., Braga, L. A., et al. (2013). Community integrative therapy: situations of emotional suffering and patients' coping Strategies. *Rev Gaucha Enferm (The Nursing Journal of Rio Grande do Sol)*, *34*, 135–162.

Depuccio, M. J., & Hoff, T. J. (2014). Medical home interventions and quality outcomes for older adults: a systematic review. *Quality Management in Health Care*, *23*, 226–239.

Drury, R. (2014). Social Isolation and loneliness in the elderly: an exploration of some of the issues. *British Journal of Community Nursing*, *19*, 125–128.

Elbasan, B., Yilmaz, G. D., Cirak, Y., et al. (2013). Cultural adaption of the friendship scale and health-related quality of life and functional mobility parameters in the elderly living at home and in the nursing home. *Topics in Geriatric Rehabilitation*, *29*, 265–280.

Enguidanos, S. M., Deliema, M., Aguilar, I., et al. (2014). Multicultural voices: attitudes of older adults in the United States about elder mistreatment. *Ageing and Society*, *34*, 877–903.

Eriksson, H., Sandberg, J., & Hellstrom, I. (2013). Experience of long-term home care as an informa; care giver to a spouse: gendered meanings in everyday life for female caregivers. *International Journal of Older People Nursing*, *8*, 159–165.

Felix, H. C., Adams, B., Cornell, C., et al. (2014). Barriers and facilitators to senior center participating in translational research. *Research on Aging*, *36*, 22–39.

Genther, D. J., Betz, J., Pratt, S., et al. (2014). Association of hearing impairment and morbidity in older adults. *The Journals of Gerontology*, *14*.

Gitlow, L. (2014). Technology use by older adults and barriers to using technology. *Physical and Occupational Therapy in Geriatrics*, *32*, 271–280.

Hawes, E. M., & Viera, A. J. (2014). Immigrant and refugee health: cross cultural communication. *FP Essentials*, *423*, 30–39.

Heiney, S. P., Hazlett, L. J., Weinrich, S. P., et al. (2011). Antecedents and mediators of community connection in African American women with breast cancer. *Research and Theory in Nursing Practice*, *25*, 252–270.

Jarve, R., & Dool, D. (2011). Simple tools to increase patient satisfaction with the referral process. *Family Practice Management*, *18*, 9–14.

Jeffreys, M., & Dogan, E. (2013). Evaluating cultural competence in the clinical practicum. *Nursing Education Perspectives*, *34*, 88–94.

Jupiter, T. (2012). Cognition screening for hearing loss in nursing home residents. *Journal of the American Medical Directors Association*, *13*, 744–747. [Epub 2012 Aug 11].

Kwok, C., & White, K. (2011). Cultural and linguistic isolation: the breast cancer experience of Chinese-Australian women—a qualitative study. *Contemporary Nurse*, *30*, 85–94.

Lin, Y., Chu, H., Yang, C. Y., et al. (2011). Effectiveness of group music intervention against agitated behavior in elderly persons with dementia. *International Journal of Geriatric Psychiatry*, *26*, 670–678. [Epub 2010 Jul 29].

Lo, C. C., & Chung, T. C. (2013). American youths' access to substance abuse treatment: does type of treatment facility matter? *Journal of Child and Adolescent Substance Abuse.*, *22*, 191–213.

Marini, M., Monaci, M., Manetti, M., et al. (2014). Can practice of DanceSport as physical activity be associated with the concept of "successful aging"? *The Journal of Sports and Physical Fitness*, 8.

Mattila, E., Kaunonen, M., Aalto, P., et al. (2014). The method of nursing support in hospital and patients' and family members' experiences of the effectiveness of the support. *Scandinavian Journal of Caring Sciences*, *28*, 305–314.

McDonald, A. M. (2014). *Simulation education of communication skills and the effects on nurse empowerment* (p. 201). Teachers College, Columbia University Ed.D.

Miller, A. M., Sorokin, O., & Fogg, L. (2013). Individual family, social and cultural predictions of depressed mood in former Soviet immigrant couples. *Research in Nursing and Health*, *36*, 271–283. [Epub 2013 Feb 13].

Morris, M. E., Adair, B., Ozanne, E., et al. (2014). Smart technologies to enhance social connectiveness in older people who live at home. *Australasian Journal of Ageing, 33*, 142–152. [Epub 2014 Apr 15].

Morrow-Howell, N., Lee, Y. S., McCrary, S., et al. (2014). Volunteering as a pathway to productive social engagement among older adults. *Health Education and Behavior, 41*, 84S–90S.

Nesbit, K. C., Kolobe, T. H., Sisson, S. B., et al. (2014). A model of environment correlates of adolescent obesity in the United States. *Journal of Adolescent Health, 55*, 394–401. <http://dx.doi.org.ezproxy.jccmi.edu/10.1016/j.jadohealth.2014.02.022>.

Nicholson, N. R. (2012). A review of social isolation: an important but underassessed condition in older adults. *Journal of Primary Prevention., 33*, 137–152.

Nicholson, R., Dixon, J. K., & McCorkle, A. U. (2014). Predictions of dementia levels of social integration in older adults. *Research in Gerontological Nursing, 7*, 33–43. [Epub 2013 Sep 25].

Obdrzalek, S., Kurillo, G., Seto, E., et al. (2013). Architecture of an automated coaching system for elderly populations. *Studies in Health Technologies and informatics, 184*, 309–311.

O'Connor, C. M., Smith, R., Nott, M. T., et al. (2011). Using video simulated presence to reduce resistance to care and increase participation of adults with dementia. *American Journal of Alzheimers Disease and Other Dementias, 26*, 317–325. [Epub 2011 May 29].

Ohayon, M., & Roberts, L. W. (2014). Links between occupational activities and depressive mood in young adult population. *Journal of Psychiatric Research, 49*, 10–17. [Epub 2013 Oct 11].

Parsons, J., Rouse, P., & Robinson, M. (2012). Goal setting as a feature of homecare services for older people: does it make a difference? *Age and Ageing, 40*, 24–29. [Epub 2011 Sep 6].

Pearce, L. (2013). Self care success. *Nursing Standard, 27*, 19.

Pettigrew, S., Donavon, R., Boldy, D., et al. (2014). Older people's perceived causes of and strategies for dealing with social isolation. *Aging and Mental Health, 18*, 914–920. [Epub 2014 Mar 31].

Plaiser, X. S., & Konijn, A. (2013). Rejected by peers-attracted to antisocial media content: rejection-based anger impairs moral judgment among adolescents. *Developmental Psychology, 49*, 1105–1173. [Epub 2012 Jul 16].

Pritchard, E., Barker, A., Day, L., et al. (2014). Factors impacting the recreation participation of older adults living in the community. *Disability and Rehabilitation*, 24.

Ristau, S. (2011). People do need people: social interaction boosts brain health in older age. *Generations (San Francisco, Calif.), 35*, 70–76.

Rowan, M. S., Ruckholm, E., Bourque-Bearskin, L., et al. (2013). Cultural competence and cultural safety in Canadian schools of nursing: a mixed methods study. *International Journal of Nursing Education Scholarship, 10*, 1–10.

Rulliere, N. (2014). Privacy and dignity in nursing homes. *Revue de l'Infirmiere, 200*, 37–38.

Schneider, A. E., Ralph, N., Olson, C., et al. (2014). Predictions of senior center use in older adults in New York City public housing. *Journal of Urban Health*, 14.

Seebohm, P., Chaudnary, S., Boyce, M., et al. (2013). The contribution of self help/mutual aid groups to mental well-being. *Health and Social Care in the Community, 21*, 391–401.

Skingley, A. (2013). Older people, isolation and loneliness: implications for community nursing. *British Journal of Community Nursing, 18*, 84–90.

Staley, J., Alemagno, S., & Straffer-King, P. (2011). Senior adult emergency preparedness: what does it really mean? *Journal of Emergency Management, 9*, 47–55.

Su, C. T., McMahan, R. D., Williams, B. A., et al. (2014). Family matters: effects of birth order, culture and family dynamics on surrogate decision-making. *Journal of the American Geriatric Society, 62*, 175–182. [Epub 2014 Jan 2].

Thomas, J. E., O'Connell, B., & Gasken, C. J. (2013). Residents' perceptions and experiences of social interaction and participation in leisure activities in residential aged care. *Contemporary Nurse, 45*, 244–254.

Thompson, R., Kerr, M., Glynn, M., et al. (2014). Caring for a family with intellectual disability and epilepsy: practical, social and emotional perspectives. *Seizure-The European Journal of Epilepsy*, 19. [Epub ahead of print].

Toepoel, V. (2013). Ageing, leisure, and social connectedness: how could leisure help reduce social isolation of older people? *Social Indicators Research, 113*, 355–372.

Townley, G., & Kloos, B. (2011). Examining the psychological sense of community for individuals with serious mental illness residing in supported housing environments. *Community Mental Health Journal, 47*, 436–446.

Waite, R., Nardi, D., & Killian, P. (2014). Examination of cultural knowledge and provider sensitivity in nurse managed health centers. *Journal of Cultural Diversity, 21*, 74–79.

Weber, K., Bittner, U., Manzeschke, A., et al. (2012). Taking patient privacy and autonomy more seriously: why an Orwellian account is not sufficient. *American Journal of Bioethics, 12*, 51–53.

Webster, N. J., Ajrouch, K. J., & Antonucci, T. C. (2013). Living healthier, living stronger: the benefits of residing in community. *Generations-Journal of the American Society on Aging, 37*, 28–32.

Williams, A., Manias, E., Cross, W., et al. (2014). Motivational interviewing to explore culturally and linguistically diverse people's medication self-efficacy. *The Journal of Clinical Nursing*, 30. [Epub ahead of print].

Wilson, D., Harris, A., Hollis, V., et al. (2011). Upstream thinking and health promotion planning for older adults at risk of social isolation. *International Journal of Older People Nursing*, 6, 282–288. [Epub 2010 Dec 30].

S

Chronic Sorrow

Betty Ackley, MSN, EdS, RN, and Tracy P. George, DNP, APRN-BC, CNE

NANDA-I

Definition

Cyclical, recurring, and potentially progressive pattern of pervasive sadness experienced (by parent, caregiver, individual with chronic illness or disability) in response to continual loss throughout the trajectory of an illness or disability

Defining Characteristics

Reports feelings of sadness (e.g., periodic, recurrent); reports feelings that interfere with ability to reach highest level of personal well-being; reports feelings that interfere with ability to reach highest level of social well-being; reports negative feelings (e.g., anger, being misunderstood, confusion, depression, disappointment, emptiness, fear, frustration, guilt, helplessness, hopelessness, low self-esteem, being overwhelmed, recurring loss, self-blame)

Related Factors (r/t)

Crisis in management of the disability; crises in management of the illness; crises related to developmental stages; death of a loved one; experiences chronic disability (e.g., physical or mental); experiences chronic illness (e.g., physical or mental); missed opportunities; missed milestones; unending caregiving

NOC (Nursing Outcomes Classification)

Suggested NOC Outcomes

Acceptance: Health Status; Depression Level; Depression Self-Control; Grief Resolution; Hope; Mood Equilibrium

Example NOC Outcome with Indicators

Grief Resolution with plans for a positive future as evidenced by the following indicators: Describes meaning of loss or death/Reports decreased preoccupation with loss/Reports adequate nutritional intake/Reports adequate sleep/Expresses positive expectations about the future. (Rate the outcome and indicators of **Grief Resolution:** 1 = never demonstrated, 2 = rarely demonstrated, 3 = sometimes demonstrated, 4 = often demonstrated, 5 = consistently demonstrated [see Section I].)

Client Outcomes

Client Will (Specify Time Frame)

- Express appropriate feelings of guilt, fear, anger, or sadness
- Identify problems associated with sorrow (e.g., changes in appetite, insomnia, nightmares, loss of libido, decreased energy, alteration in activity levels)
- Seek help in dealing with grief-associated problems
- Plan for the future one day at a time
- Function at normal developmental level

S

NIC (Nursing Interventions Classification)

Suggested NIC Interventions

Grief Work Facilitation; Grief Work Facilitation: Perinatal Death

Example NIC Activities—Grief Work Facilitation

Encourage client to verbalize memories of loss, both past and current; Assist client in identifying personal coping strategies

Nursing Interventions and *Rationales*

- Determine the client's degree of sorrow. EBN: Use the Adapted Burke Questionnaire for the individual or caregiver as appropriate. *The Adapted Burke Questionnaire is designed to measure chronic sorrow, and it assesses eight mood states including grief, shock, anger, disbelief, sadness, hopelessness, fear, and guilt on a four-point scale (Whittingham et al, 2013).*
- Assess for the four discrete stages of grieving in chronic obstructive pulmonary disease (COPD) clients. EB: *The four stages of grief for clients with COPD can be assessed by the Acceptance of Disease and Impairments Questionnaire (Boer et al, 2014).*
- Provide coping strategies for caregivers who may experience chronic sorrow. EBN: *Coping strategies for the caregivers of clients with schizophrenia may include discussing their feelings about the situation with*

others, reading, praying, being physically active; emotional strategies like crying; and cognitive strategies like thinking positively about the situation (Olwit et al, 2015). See care plan for **Caregiver Role Strain.**

- Assess clients for chronic sorrow and provide them with coping strategies. EBN: *Clients who come to the emergency department frequently may be at an increased risk for chronic sorrow (Joseph, 2012).*
- Develop a trusting relationship with the client by using empathetic therapeutic communication techniques. CEB: *An empathetic person who takes the time to listen, offers support and reassurance, recognizes and focuses on feelings, and appreciates the uniqueness of each individual and family is helpful to clients experiencing chronic sorrow (Isaksson & Ahlstrom, 2008).*
- Help the client understand that sorrow may be ongoing. CEB: *Studies have demonstrated that feelings of sadness, guilt, anger, frustration, and fear occur periodically throughout the lives of people experiencing chronic loss, resulting in chronic sorrow (Isaksson & Ahlstrom, 2008).*
- Help the client recognize that, although sadness will occur at intervals for the rest of his/her life, it will become bearable. CEB: *In time the client may develop a relationship with grief that is lifelong but livable, and as much filled with comfort as it is with sorrow (Moules et al, 2007).*
- Urge the client to use positive coping techniques:
  - EBN: *Encourage the client to participate in a support group, talk with others, or communicate via an online support group (Vitale & Falco, 2014).* CEB: *Social support has been shown to help bereaved individuals as they put their lives back together and find new meaning in life (Isaksson & Ahlstrom, 2008).* EBN: *Encourage the client to participate in a support group, talk with others, or communicate via an online support group (Vitale & Falco, 2014).* CEB: *Social support has been shown to help bereaved individuals as they put their lives back together and find new meaning in life (Isaksson & Ahlstrom, 2008).*
  - EBN: *Encourage the client to engage in a hobby or physical activity (Vitale & Falso, 2014).*
  - EBN: *Encourage the client to think positively about the situation (Vitale & Falco, 2014).*
  - EBN: *Encourage the client to discuss his/her situation with a health care practitioner, such as a nurse, physician, or social worker (Vitale & Falco, 2014).*
  - EBN: *Discuss the need for the client to anticipate triggers that may increase chronic sorrow (Vitale & Falco, 2014).* EB: *Triggers for parents of children with cerebral palsy may include times in which there is awareness of the actual versus expected achievements of the child or during times of medical intervention (Whittingham et al, 2013).*
  - CEB: *Refer for professional counseling or spiritual or pastoral support if needed (Gordon, 2009).*
- ▲ CEB: *Consider the need for medications for anxiety and depression if needed (Gordon, 2009).*
  - CEB: *Refer clients for financial assistance with equipment and supplies if needed (Gordon, 2009).*

Pediatric

S

- Encourage the parents of children with uncommon diseases to use online resources to manage their chronic sorrow. EBN: *In a study of 16 mothers of children with a rare disease, online communication was used effectively to manage chronic sorrow (Glenn, 2015).*
- Educate parents that an increase in chronic sorrow can occur after stressful events. EB: *An increase in chronic sorrow was noted in parents with children who have cerebral palsy after triggering events, indicating that recurring grieving can occur after the diagnosis is made. Triggers can include when the child would have met a developmental milestone or started school (Whittingham et al, 2013).*
- Nurses should assess for chronic sorrow and discuss coping strategies for parents of children who have been in the neonatal intensive care unit (NICU). EBN: *Chronic sorrow is a useful framework for families impacted by an NICU stay (Vitale & Falco, 2014).*
- *Allow children the opportunity to talk about the impending death of a parent or loved one.* EB: *In a qualitative study of seven children whose parent was dying, children often were not encouraged to discuss their feelings, developed anxiety, and developed ways to deal with the stress (Buchwald et al, 2012).*
- Encourage parents to listen to their child's expression of grief. EB: *It is important for parents whose child is grieving to listen to their child's concerns and create a balance between making new memories while holding onto the old memories (Bugge et al, 2014).*
- Consider the use of art for children in hospice care who are dying or dealing with the death of a parent, sibling, or other family member. CEB: *Art can be used in both children and adults to communicate feelings, especially when clients are unable to verbally discuss their feelings (Devlin, 2006).*
- ▲ Refer grieving children and parents to a program to help facilitate grieving. EB: *Parents and families who have lost a child should be referred to peer-led support groups and grief counseling if desired (Wender, 2012).*

- Encourage children experiencing grief to participate in bereavement activities and camps. EB: *In children who participated in a ropes course as activities based counseling during bereavement camp, five themes were noted: grief as a process, expression of feelings, support, coping, and empowerment and hope (Swank, 2013).*
- Help the adolescent with chronic sorrow determine sources of support and refer for counseling if needed. EB: *Cognitive behavioral therapy along with parental counseling has been useful in adolescents who experience prolonged grief (Spuij et al, 2015).*
- Provide family-centered care to parents of children with disabilities, and encourage parents to attend support groups. EB: *Caring for a child with cerebral palsy impacts the quality of life for families and is related to anticipatory grieving among parents (Al-Gamal, 2013).*
- Encourage parents with chronic sorrow to participate in a support group and learn coping strategies. EB: *Bereavement support groups for parents who have lost children can be helpful for managing grief (Grinyer, 2012).*
- Recognize that mothers who have a miscarriage grieve and experience sorrow because of loss of the child. *Understanding, listening, providing respect, and being supportive are important interventions for women who have experienced the loss of a pregnancy (Ancker et al, 2012).*

Geriatric

- Identify previous losses and assess the client for depression. EB: *Bereavement may result in major depression in some older adults, and participation support groups can be helpful in depression management (Ghesquiere et al, 2013).*
- Evaluate the social support system of the older client and refer for bereavement counseling if needed. EB: *In a study of 28 geriatric clients who had recently experienced a death, older adults often used family and friends as a support network following death, but community-based organizations also play an important role in bereavement support (Bellamy et al, 2014).*

Home Care

- In-home bereavement follow-up by nurses should be considered if available. EBN: *In Australia, home health nurses provide bereavement visits in which they provide comfort, counseling, client education, and encouragement and also evaluate the client who has recently experienced a loss (Brownhill et al, 2013).*
- Assess the client for depression. EB: *Clients experiencing bereavement are at risk for depression, so assessment for depression is necessary (Ghesquiere et al, 2013).*
- Refer for mental health services and counseling as indicated. CEB: *It is important to refer clients for mental health services and counseling when needed (Gordon, 2009).*
- Encourage the client to participate in activities that are diversionary and uplifting as tolerated (e.g., outdoor activities, hobby groups, church-related activities, pet care). EBN: *Diversionary activities decrease the time spent in sorrow, can give meaning to life, and provide a sense of well-being (Vitale & Falso, 2014).*
- Encourage the client to participate in support groups appropriate to the area of loss or illness. EBN: *Support groups can increase an individual's sense of belonging (Vitale & Falco, 2014).*
- Provide empathetic communication for family/caregivers. CEB: *Family/caregivers who feel supported are often able to provide greater and more consistent support to the affected person (Isaksson & Ahlstrom, 2008).*
- The interventions described previously may be adapted for home care use.
- See the care plans for Chronic low **Self-Esteem**, Risk for **Loneliness,** and **Hopelessness.**

S

REFERENCES

Al-Gamal, E. (2013). Quality of life and anticipatory grieving among parents living with a child with cerebral palsy. *International Journal of Nursing Practice*, *19*(3), 288–294.

Ancker, T., Gebhardt, A., Andreassen, S., et al. (2012). Early bereavement: women's experiences of miscarriage. *Nordic Journal Of Nursing Research & Clinical Studies/Vård I Norden*, *32*(1), 32–36.

Bellamy, G., Gott, M., Waterworth, S., et al. (2014). But I do believe you've got to accept that that's what life's about': older adults living in New Zealand talk about their experiences of loss and bereavement support. *Health & Social Care in the Community*, *22*(1), 96–103.

Boer, L., Daudey, L., Peters, J., et al. (2014). Assessing the stages of the grieving process in chronic obstructive pulmonary disease (COPD): validation of the acceptance of disease and impairments questionnaire (ADIQ). *International Journal of Behavioral Medicine*, *21*(3), 561–570.

Brownhill, S., Chang, E., Bidewell, J., et al. (2013). A decision model for community nurses providing bereavement care. *British Journal of Community Nursing*, *18*(3), 133–139.

Buchwald, D., Delmar, C., & Schantz-Laursen, B. (2012). How children handle life when their mother or father is seriously ill and dying. *Scandinavian Journal of Caring Sciences*, *26*(2), 228–235.

Bugge, K. E., Darbyshire, P., Røkholt, E. G., et al. (2014). Young children's grief: parents' understanding and coping. *Death Studies*, *38*(1), 36–43.

Devlin, B. (2006). Art therapy. The art of healing and knowing in cancer and palliative care. *International Journal of Palliative Nursing, 12*(1), 16–19.

Ghesquiere, A., Shear, M. K., & Duan, N. (2013). Outcomes of bereavement care among widowed older adults with complicated grief and depression. *Journal of Primary Care & Community Health, 4*(4), 256–264.

Glenn, A. D. (2015). Using online health communication to manage chronic sorrow: mothers of children with rare diseases speak. *Journal of Pediatric Nursing, 30*(1), 17–24.

Gordon, J. (2009). An evidence-based approach for supporting parents experiencing chronic sorrow. *Pediatric Nursing, 35*(2), 115–119.

Grinyer, A. (2012). A bereavement group for parents whose son or daughter died from cancer: how shared experience can lessen isolation. *Mortality, 17*(4), 338–354.

Isaksson, A., & Ahlström, G. (2008). Managing chronic sorrow: experiences of patients with multiple sclerosis. *Journal of Neuroscience Nursing, 40*(3), 180–191.

Joseph, H. A. (2012). Recognizing chronic sorrow in the habitual ED patient. *JEN: Journal of Emergency Nursing, 38*(6), 539–540.

Moules, N., Simonson, K., Fleiszer, A., et al. (2007). The soul of sorrow work: grief and therapeutic interventions with families. *Journal of Family Nursing, 13*(1), 117–141.

Olwit, C., Musisi, S., Leshabari, S., et al. (2015). Chronic sorrow: lived experiences of caregivers of patients diagnosed with schizophrenia in Butabika Mental Hospital, Kampala, Uganda. *Archives of Psychiatric Nursing, 29*(1), 43–48.

Spuij, M., Dekovic, M., & Boelen, P. A. (2015). An open trial of 'grief-help': a cognitive-behavioural treatment for prolonged grief in children and adolescents. *Clinical Psychology & Psychotherapy, 22*(2), 185–192.

Swank, J. M. (2013). Obstacles of grief: the experiences of children processing grief on the ropes course. *Journal of Creativity In Mental Health, 8*(3), 235–248.

Vitale, S. A., & Falco, C. (2014). Children born prematurely: risk of parental chronic sorrow. *Journal of Pediatric Nursing, 29*(3), 248–251.

Wender, E. (2012). Supporting the family after the death of a child. *Pediatrics, 130*(6), 1164–1169.

Whittingham, K., Wee, D., Sanders, M. R., et al. (2013). Sorrow, coping and resiliency: parents of children with cerebral palsy share their experiences. *Disability & Rehabilitation, 35*(17), 1447–1452.

Spiritual distress

Lisa Burkhart, PhD, RN, ANEF, and Barbara Baele Vincensi, PhD, RN, FNP

NANDA-I

Definition

A state of suffering related to the impaired ability to experience meaning in life through connectedness with self, others, world, or a superior being

Defining Characteristics

Anxiety; crying; fatigue; fear; insomnia; questioning identity; questioning meaning of life; questioning meaning of suffering.

Connections to Self

Anger; decrease in serenity; feeling of being unloved; guilt; inadequate acceptance; ineffective coping strategies; insufficient courage; perceived insufficient meaning in life

Connections with Others

Alienation; refuses to interact with spiritual leader; refuses to interact with significant other; separation from support system

Connections with Art, Music, Literature, and Nature

Decrease in expression of previous pattern of creativity; disinterest in nature; disinterest in reading spiritual literature

Connections with Power Greater Than Self

Anger toward power greater than self; feeling abandoned; hopelessness; inability for introspection; inability to experience the transcendent; inability to participate in religious activities; inability to pray; perceived suffering; request for a spiritual leader; sudden change in spiritual practice

Related Factors

Actively dying; aging; birth of a child; death of significant other; exposure to death; illness; imminent death; increasing dependence on another; life transition; loneliness; loss of a body part; loss of function of a body part; pain; perception of having unfinished business; receiving bad news; self-alienation; social alienation; sociocultural deprivation; treatment regimen; unexpected life event

S

NOC (Nursing Outcomes Classification)

Suggested NOC Outcomes

Coping; Dignified Life Closure; Grief Resolution; Hope; Spiritual Health; Stress Level

Example NOC Outcome with Indicators

Spiritual Health as evidenced by the following indicators: Quality of faith, hope, meaning, and purpose in life/ Connectedness with inner-self and with others to share thoughts, feelings, and beliefs. (Rate each indicator of **Spiritual Health:** 1 = severely compromised, 2 = substantially compromised, 3 = moderately compromised, 4 = mildly compromised, 5 = not compromised [see Section I].)

Client Outcomes

Client Will (Specify Time Frame)

- Express meaning and purpose in life
- Express sense of hope in the future
- Express sense of connectedness with self
- Express sense of connectedness with family/friends
- Express ability to forgive
- Express acceptance of health status
- Find meaning in relationships with others
- Find meaning in relationship with higher power
- Find meaning in personal and health care treatment choices

NIC (Nursing Interventions Classification)

Suggested NIC Interventions

Active Listening; Forgiveness Facilitation; Grief Work Facilitation; Hope Inspiration; Humor; Music Therapy; Presence; Referral; Reminiscence Therapy; Self-Awareness Enhancement; Simple Guided Imagery; Simple Massage; Simple Relaxation Therapy; Spiritual Support; Therapeutic Touch; Touch

Example NIC Activities—Spiritual Support

Encourage use of spiritual resources if desired; Be available to listen to client's feelings

S

Nursing Interventions and *Rationales*

- Observe clients for cues indicating difficulties in finding meaning, purpose, or hope in life. CEB: *In a grounded theory study, spiritual care begins by recognizing a client cue for needing spiritual care (Burkhart & Hogan, 2008).* EBN: *In this cross-sectional study involving 202 cognitively intact nursing home residents, Haugan (2014) found a significant relationship between the nurse-patient interaction on patients' development of hope, meaning in life, and self-transcendence, which were found to be important resources for health and global well-being.*
- Observe clients with chronic illness, poor prognosis, or life-changing conditions for loss of meaning, purpose, and hope in life. EB: *In a retrospective study, meaninglessness, helplessness, brokenness, and despair were reported, indicating spiritual distress in younger adult patients with advanced cancer admitted to an acute palliative care unit (Hui et al, 2011).* EBN: *In a metasynthesis, Lin et al (2011) discovered that quality of life often reflected spiritual well-being in those living with rheumatoid arthritis.*
- Offer spiritual care in disaster relief. EB: *In a case study of Hurricane Katrina survivors, spirituality and religion were found to be important sources of resilience and coping in disaster relief, particularly for the African American community (Alawiyah et al, 2011).*
- Promote a sense of love, caring, and compassion in nursing encounters. EBN: *In a cross-sectional, descriptive study of 202 cognitively intact nursing home residents, the nurse-patient interaction had a significant impact on the development of meaning in life, hope, and self-transcendence, potentially promoting health and well-being in this population (Haugan, 2014).*

- Be physically present and actively listen to the client. CEB: *In a grounded theory study, spiritual care included promoting client connectedness with self (Burkhart & Hogan, 2008).* EBN: *In a cross-sectional correlational study by Haugan et al (2014), nurses were found to facilitate both interpersonal and intrapersonal transcendence for long-term nursing home residents by their presence and by encouraging connections with oneself and others in meaningful ways.*
- Help the client find a reason for living, be available for support and promote hope. EBN: *A cross-sectional descriptive study in 44 different nursing homes found nurse-resident interaction was a resource for hope, meaning in life, and self-transcendence for residents (Haugan, 2014).*
- Listen to the client's feelings about suffering and/or death. Be nonjudgmental and allow time for grieving. EBN: *In a cross-sectional descriptive study of 120 patients with chronic renal insufficiency, 25.7% were able to self-identify as having spiritual distress while another 25.8% were identified by expert nurses as such; however, patients were reluctant to discuss their spiritual needs because of fear of judgment by the nurses or disinterest of the health care team (Chaves et al, 2011).*
- Respect the client's beliefs; avoid imposing your own spiritual beliefs on the client. Be aware of your own belief systems and accept the client's spirituality. EB: *In a systematic literature review, assuring an adequate religious, spiritual, and cultural assessment has been made of children, adolescents, and their families regarding their need for spiritual and religious care before referral decreased potential for stereotyping by the nurse and assured specific needs, rituals, and desires of the patient and family were met (Wiener et al, 2013).* CEB: *Taylor and Mamier (2005) reported that most cancer clients and caregivers welcomed interventions that were less intimate, commonly used, and not overtly religious.*
- Monitor and promote supportive social contacts. EB: *In a correlational descriptive study by Dalmida et al (2013), the three variables found to play an important role in mitigating depression in people living with HIV/AIDS were social support and religious and spiritual coping interventions.*
- Integrate family into spiritual practices as appropriate. CEB: *In a phenomenological study, lung cancer clients identified maintaining contact with family and friends for support and prayer as helpful self-care strategies (John, 2010).* EB: *In a cross-sectional, descriptive study, high levels of participation in religious practices and use of social supports were found to improve the general well-being of Korean adult immigrants in the United States (Lee & Woo, 2013).*
- Assist family in searching for meaning in client's health care situation. CEB: *A qualitative study of young adult daughters with parents experiencing cancer identified exploring meaning as a theme (Puterman & Cadell, 2008).* EB: *In a cross-sectional descriptive study of the spirituality of 129 parents whose children had a life-limiting illness, Knapp et al (2011) found higher scores for spirituality and meaning/peace in non-Caucasian parents, parents who were married, and children who had higher hearing and vision scores; recommendations included incorporating the family's spirituality and search for meaning in illness into the palliative care team's routine care. Offer spiritual support to caregivers.* EBN: *In a descriptive study, individual spiritual well-being predicted higher levels of better mental health in cancer survivor/caregiver dyad couples (Kim et al, 2011).*

▲ Refer the client to a support group or counseling. EB: *In a cross sectional randomized study by Lyon et al (2011), a relationship was found between providing family support within a support group, on the spirituality of adolescents living with HIV and adherence to highly active antiretroviral therapy.*

- Support meditation, guided imagery, journaling, relaxation, and involvement in art, music, or poetry. Support outdoor activities. EB: *In a randomized clinical study comparing differences between groups of participants with metastatic carcinoma who used either spiritual or secular meditation techniques, Cole et al (2012) found those who used spiritual meditation had significantly reduced depression and increased physical and psychological well-being than those who used the secular method.* CEB: *In a qualitative study of stroke caregivers, being one with nature emerged as a theme (Pierce et al, 2008).*

▲ Offer or suggest visits with spiritual and/or religious advisors. CEB: *In a grounded theory study, spiritual care included promoting connectedness with others, including chaplains (Burkhart & Hogan, 2008).* EBN: *In a descriptive clinical study to improve quality of care for oncology patients, Blanchard et al (2012) found adequate assessment of patients' spiritual care needs by nurses allowed for appropriate referrals to chaplains or religious/spiritual leaders, improving patients' perception of their overall care and meeting the patients' religious/spiritual needs while hospitalized.*

- Provide privacy or a "sacred space." CEB: *In a qualitative survey of chronically ill individuals, participants wanted access to a garden and a quiet space available in the hospital to think through decisions (Dale & Hunt, 2008).* EBN: *In educating college students on cultural awareness, Walton (2011) used mixed methods research of qualitative and quantitative (descriptive) design to identify five themes that had significant*

S

differences in findings before and after an education program; a primary theme was the development of sacred space on the dialysis unit to encourage participation in dialysis by Native Americans.

- Allow time and a place for prayer. EBN: *In a grounded theory study, spiritual care included promoting religious rituals and prayer and was validated in a psychometric study (Burkhart et al, 2011).* CEB: *In a quantitative study of 156 clients with cancer and 68 caregivers, Taylor (2006) found that one of the most prevalent spiritual needs was understanding or relating to God.*
- Coordinate or encourage attending spiritual retreats, courses, or programming. CEB: *In a study of 128 male clients who expressed interest in attending an informational intervention, topics included spirituality (Manii & Ammerman, 2008).* EBN: *In a qualitative study, Baldacchino (2011) identified that the nurse's awareness of patients' spiritual needs, and the ability of the nurse to meet patients' spiritual needs, increased after attending a specific learning module on Spiritual Coping During Illness.*

Geriatric

- Identify the client's past spiritual practices that have been helpful. Help the client explore his/her life and identify those experiences that are noteworthy. EBN: *In a systematic literature review, past spiritual rituals helped patients with dementia connect to deeply rooted memories and provided a centering experience that promoted a sense of control and connection for the patient (Enis & Kazer, 2013).* EBN: *A cross-sectional study of 202 cognitively intact nursing home residents revealed a significant relationship between promotion of intrapersonal and interpersonal self-transcendence and meaning in life for the resident and the type of nurse-resident interaction (Haugan, 2014).*
- Offer opportunities to practice one's religion. EB: *Eighty percent of patients involved in the National Emphysema Treatment Trial, a randomized longitudinal study, used religious practices or spiritual interventions to cope with their disease (Green et al, 2011).* CEB: *In a descriptive cross-sectional study, the geriatric population uses religious services in naturally occurring retirement communities (Lun, 2010).*

Pediatric

- Offer adolescents opportunities for reflection and storytelling to express their spirituality. EB: *In a systematic literature review, Bryant-Davis et al (2012) found incorporating stories, songs, or passages from sacred script allowed children and adolescents to use their spirituality and religion as a means of coping with distress.*

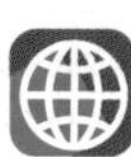

Multicultural

S

- Recognize the importance of spirituality and provide culturally competent spiritual care to specific populations:
  - Arab Muslims. EBN: *In a phenomenological qualitative study of Jordanian Muslim men with coronary artery disease (CAD), participants believed that their illness was fate or God's will, their faith directed them to make sound health decisions, and their spirituality provided the support to accept their illness and suffering (Nabolsi & Carson, 2011).*
  - Chinese elders. EBN: *Using a life review program with Chinese elders with advanced cancer improved psychosocial well-being and enabled elders to make preparations for death, reconcile past conflicts, and make peace within themselves and with others (Xiao et al, 2011).*
  - Korean immigrants: EB: *In a cross-sectional exploratory study, high social support, and religious and spiritual practices were significantly associated with high general well-being in 147 adult Korean immigrants in the United States (Lee & Woo, 2013).*
  - Latinos. EB: *Faith based approaches to coping with cancer were found to be an important part of identity for Latinos in a cross-sectional descriptive study by Canada et al (2013).*
  - African Americans. EB: *In a descriptive study by Canada et al (2013), African Americans were found to use spirituality to cope with advanced cancer more than Hispanics or Caucasians.* EB: *A descriptive study with 100 African Americans with cancer identified positive affect and emotional functioning were influenced by religious and spiritual well-being, with religious beliefs and behaviors significant predictors of finding meaning in life, a positive affect, and use of religious coping interventions (Holt et al, 2011).*
  - Thai. EBN: *In a randomized controlled study of 79 Buddhist Thai elders in Thailand, those participants in the groups who practiced Vipassana meditation or only chanting had significantly improved spiritual well-being and sleep quality compared to the control group who practiced neither (Wiriyasombat et al, 2011).*

- ❍ African women. EBN: *In an ethnographic study in Ghana, the belief that pregnancy makes women's souls vulnerable to spiritual illnesses is the reason many seek spiritual protection through their spiritual or religious leaders during pregnancy (Farnes et al, 2011).* CEB: *In Uganda, 85% of African women with HIV/AIDS use spirituality as a coping mechanism, including support from other believers, prayer, and trusting in God (Hodge & Roby, 2010).*

Veterans of Armed Services

- Recognize the unique spiritual needs of veterans and provide spiritual support or appropriate referrals. EB: *In a grounded theory developed by Chang et al (2012), feelings of guilt and seeking forgiveness as well as finding peace within themselves and with others were spiritual needs of veterans that were discovered.*

Home Care

- All of the nursing interventions described previously apply in the home setting.

REFERENCES

Alawiyah, T., Bell, H., Pyles, L., et al. (2011). Spirituality and faith-based interventions: pathways to disaster resilience for African American hurricane Katrina survivors. *Journal of Religion and Spirituality in Social Work: Social Thought, 30*, 294–319.

Baldacchino, D. (2011). Teaching on spiritual care: the perceived impact on qualified nurses. *Nurse Education in Practice, 11*, 47–53.

Blanchard, J., Dunlap, D., & Fitchett, G. (2012). Screening for spiritual distress in the oncology inpatient: a quality improvement pilot project between nurses and chaplains. *Journal of Nursing Management, 20*, 1076–1084.

Burkhart, L., & Hogan, N. (2008). An experiential theory of spiritual care in nursing practice. *Qualitative Health Reseach, 18*(7), 928–938.

Burkhart, L., Schmidt, L., & Hogan, N. (2011). Development and psychometric testing of the spiritual care inventory instrument. *Journal of Advanced Nursing, 67*(11), 2463–2472.

Bryant-Davis, T., Ellis, M., Burke-Maynard, E., et al. (2012). Religiosity, spirituality and trauma recovery in the lives of children and adolescents. *Professional Psychology, Research and Practice, 43*(4), 306–314.

Canada, A., Fitchett, G., Mutphy, P., et al. (2013). Racial/ethnic differences in spiritual well-being among cancer survivors. *Journal of Behavioral Medicine, 36*, 441–453.

Chang, B.-H., Stein, N., Trevino, K., et al. (2012). End-of-life spiritual care3 at a VA medical center: chaplains perspectives. *Palliative and Supportive Care, 10*, 273–278.

Chaves, E., de Carvalho, E., Beijo, L., et al. (2011). Efficacy of different instruments for the identification of the nursing diagnosis spiritual distress. *Latin-American Journal of Nursing, 19*(4), 902–910.

Cole, B., Hopkins, C., Spiegel, J., et al. (2012). A randomized clinical trial of the effects of spiritually focused meditation for people with metastic melanoma. *Mental Health, Religion & Culture, 15*(2), 161–174.

Dale, H., & Hunt, J. (2008). Perceived need for spiritual and religious treatment options in chronically ill individuals. *Journal of Health Psychology, 13*, 712–718.

Dalmida, S., Koenig, H., Holstad, M., et al. (2013). The psychological well-being of people living with HIV/AIDS and the role of religious coping and social support. *International Journal of Psychiatry in Medicine, 46*(1), 57–83.

Enis, E., & Kazer, M. (2013). The role of spiritual nursing interventions on improved outcomes in older adults with dementia. *Holistic Nursing Practice, 27*(2), 106–113.

Farnes, C., Beckstrand, R., & Callister, L. (2011). Help-seeking behaviors in childbearing women in Ghana, West Africa. *International Nursing Review, 58*, 491–497.

Green, M., Emery, C., Kozora, E., et al. (2011). Religious and spiritual coping and quality of life among patients with emphysema in the national emphysema treatment trial. *Respiratory Care, 56*(10), 1514–1521.

Haugan, G. (2014). Nurse-patient interaction is a resource for hope, meaning in life and self-transcendence in nursing home patients. *Scandinavian Journal of Caring Sciences, 28*, 74–88.

Haugan, G., Rannestad, T., Hammervold, R., et al. (2014). The relationships between self-transcendence and spiritual well-being in cognitively intact nursing home patients. *International Journal of Older People Nursing, 9*, 65–78.

Hodge, D., & Roby, J. (2010). Sub-Sahara African women living with HIV/AIDS: an exploration of general and spiritual coping strategies. *Social Work, 55*(1), 27–37.

Holt, C., Wang, M., Caplan, L., et al. (2011). Role of religious involvement and spirituality in functioning among Afriacn Americans with cancer: testing a mediational model. *Journal of Behavioral Medicine, 34*, 437–448.

Hui, D., de la Cruz, M., Thorney, S., et al. (2011). The frequency and correlates of spiritual distress among patients with advanced cancer admitted to an acute palliative care unit. *American Journal of Hospice and Palliative Medicine, 28*(4), 264–270.

John, L. (2010). Self-care strategies used by patients with lung cancer to promote quality of life. *Oncology Nursing Forum, 37*(3), 339–347.

Kim, Y., Carver, C., Spillers, R., et al. (2011). Individual and dyadic relations between spiritual well-being and quality of life among cancer survivors and their spousal caregivers. *Psycho-Oncology, 20*(7), 762–770.

Knapp, C., Madden, V., Wang, H., et al. (2011). Spirituality of parents of children in palliative care. *Journal of Palliative Medicine, 14*(4), 437–443.

Lee, K., & Woo, H. (2013). Stressors, social support, religious practice, and general well-being among Korean adult immigrants. *Journal of Evidence-Based Social Work, 10*(5), 421–434.

Lin, W.-C., Gau, M.-L., Lin, H.-C., et al. (2011). Spiritual well-being in patients with rheumatoid arthritis. *Journal of Nursing Research, 19*(1), 1–12.

Lun, M. (2010). The correlate of religion involvement and formal service use among community-dwelling elders: an explorative case of naturally occurring retirement community. *Journal of Religion and Spirituality in Social Work: Social Thought, 29*, 207–217.

S

Lyon, M., Garvie, P., Kao, E., et al. (2011). Spirituality in HIV-infected adolescents and their families: FAmily CEntered (FACE) advance care planning and medication adherence. *Journal of Adolescent Health, 48*(6), 633–636.
Manii, D., & Ammerman, D. (2008). Men and cancer: a study of the needs of male cancer patients in treatment. *Journal of Psychosocial Oncology, 26*(2), 87–102.
Nabolsi, M., & Carson, A. (2011). Spirituality, illness and personal responsibility: the experience of Jordanian Muslim men with coronary artery disease. *Scandinavian Journal of Caring Sciences, 21*, 716–724.
Pierce, L., Steiner, V., Havens, H., et al. (2008). Spirituality expressed bycaregivers of stroke survivors. *Western Journal of Nursing Research, 30*(5), 606–619.
Puterman, J., & Cadell, S. (2008). Timing is everything: the experience of parental cancer for young adult daughters—a pilot study. *Journal of Psychosocial Oncology, 26*(2), 103–121.
Taylor, E. (2006). Prevalence and associated factors of spiritual needs among patients with cancer and family caregivers. *Oncology Nursing Forum, 33*(4), 729–735.
Taylor, E., & Mamier, I. (2005). Spiritual care nursing: what cancer patients and family caregivers want. *Journal of Advanced Nursing, 49*(3), 260–267.
Walton, J. (2011). Can a one- hour presentation make an impact on cultural awareness? *Nephrology Nursing Journal, 38*(1), 21–31.
Wiener, L., McConnell, D., Latella, L., et al. (2013). Cultural and religious considerations in pediatric palliative care. *Palliative and Supportive Care, 11*, 47–67.
Wiriyasombat, R., Pothiban, L., Panuthai, S., et al. (2011). Effectiveness of Buddhist doctrine practice-based programs in enhancing spiritual well-being, coping and sleep quality of Thai elders. *Pacific Rim International Journal of Nursing Research, 15*(3), 203–218.
Xiao, H., Kwong, E., Pang, S., et al. (2011). Perceptions of a life review programme among Chinese patients with advanced cancer. *Journal of Clinical Nursing, 21*, 564–572.

Risk for Spiritual distress

Gail B. Ladwig, MSN, RN

NANDA-I

Definition

Vulnerable to an impaired ability to experience and integrate meaning and purpose in life through connectedness within self, literature, nature, and/or a power greater than oneself, which may compromise health

Risk Factors

Developmental

Life transition

Environmental

Environmental change; natural disaster

S

Physical

Chronic illness; physical illness; substance abuse

Psychosocial

Anxiety; barrier to experiencing love; change in religious ritual; change in spiritual practice; cultural conflict; depression; inability to forgive; ineffective relationships; loss; low self-esteem; racial conflict; separation from support system; stressors

NIC, NOC, Client Outcomes, Nursing Interventions, *Rationales,* and References

Refer to care plan for **Spiritual Distress.**

Readiness for enhanced Spiritual well-being

Lisa Burkhart, PhD, RN, ANEF, and Barbara Baele Vincensi, PhD, RN, FNP

NANDA-I

Definition

A pattern of experiencing and integrating meaning and purpose in life through connectedness with self, others, art, music, literature, nature, and/or a power greater than oneself, which can be strengthened

Defining Characteristics

Connections to Self

Expresses desire to enhance acceptance; expresses desire to enhance coping; expresses desire to enhance courage; expresses desire to enhance hope; expresses desire to enhance joy; expresses desire to enhance love; expresses desire to enhance meaning in life; expresses desire to enhance meditative practice; expresses desire to enhance purpose in life; expresses desire to enhance satisfaction with philosophy of life; expresses desire to enhance self-forgiveness; expresses desire to enhance serenity (e.g., peace); expresses desire to enhance surrender; meditation

Connections with Others

Expresses desire to enhance forgiveness from other; expresses desire to enhance interaction with significant other; expresses desire to enhance interaction with spiritual leaders; expresses desire to enhance service to others

Connections with Art, Music, Literature, and Nature

Expresses desire to enhance creative energy (e.g., writing, poetry, music); expresses desire to enhance spiritual reading; expresses desire to enhance time outdoors

Connections with Power Greater Than Self

Expresses desire to enhance mystical experiences; expresses desire to enhance participation in religious activity; expresses desire to enhance prayerfulness; expresses desire to enhance reverence

NOC (Nursing Outcomes Classification)

Suggested NOC Outcomes

Personal Health Status; Coping; Dignified Life Closure; Grief Resolution; Hope; Personal Health Status; Psychosocial Adjustment: Life Change; Quality of Life; Social Involvement; Spiritual Health

Example NOC Outcome with Indicators

Hope as evidenced by the following indicators: Expresses expectation of a positive future/Faith/Optimism/Belief in self/Sense of meaning in life/Belief in others/Inner peace. (Rate each indicator of **Hope:** 1 = never demonstrated, 2 = rarely demonstrated, 3 = sometimes demonstrated, 4 = often demonstrated, 5 = constantly demonstrated [see Section I].)

S

Client Outcomes

Client Will (Specify Time Frame)

- Express hope
- Express sense of meaning and purpose in life
- Express peace and serenity
- Express love
- Express acceptance
- Express surrender
- Express forgiveness of self and others
- Express satisfaction with philosophy of life
- Express joy
- Express courage
- Describe being able to cope
- Describe use of spiritual practices
- Describe providing service to others
- Describe interaction with spiritual leaders, friends, and family
- Describe appreciation for art, music, literature, and nature

NIC (Nursing Interventions Classification)

Suggested NIC Interventions

Active Listening; Coping Enhancement; Counseling; Crisis Intervention; Decision-Making Support; Grief Work Facilitation; Hope Instillation; Meditation Facilitation; Mutual Goal Setting; Presence; Religious Ritual Enhancement; Imagery; Simple Relaxation Therapy; Socialization Enhancement; Spiritual Growth Facilitation; Spiritual Support; Support System Enhancement; Touch; Values Clarification

Example NIC Activities—Spiritual Support

Encourage use of spiritual resources if desired; Be available to listen to client's expression of feelings

Nursing Interventions and *Rationales*

- Perform a spiritual assessment that includes the client's relationship with God, meaning and purpose in life, religious affiliation, and any other significant beliefs. EBN: *A descriptive cross-sectional study examining the relationship between spiritual well-being, perceived stress, coping, and smoking in 125 African American women (smokers, ex-smokers, non-smokers) found increased spiritual well-being and a supportive faith community offered a protective quality against stress and smoking (Franklin, 2011).*
- Be present and actively listen to the client. EBN: *In a grounded theory study, spiritual care included promoting client connectedness with self, and was validated in a psychometric study (Burkhart et al, 2011).*
- Encourage the client to pray or engage in other spiritual meditative practices. EB: *In a descriptive, correlational study, spiritual and religious practices were a coping mechanism utilized by those with chronic disease (Green et al, 2011).* CEB: *Meraviglia (2006) found that prayer was associated with higher psychological well-being.*
- Coordinate or encourage attending spiritual retreats or courses. EBN: *In a qualitative study, Baldacchino (2011) identified nurses' awareness of patients' spiritual needs, and their ability to meet these needs increased after attending a specific learning module on Spiritual Coping During Illness.*
- Promote hope. EBN: *Using a cross-sectional descriptive design, Haugan (2014) found important factors for health in cognitively intact nursing home patients were nurse-patient interactions, which promoted hope and self-transcendence.*
- Encourage clients to reflect on what is meaningful to them in life. EBN: *In a descriptive, cross-sectional design of 202 cognitively intact nursing home patients, the ability to use reflection to discover meaning in life was enhanced by patients' interactions with the nurse (Haugan, 2014).*
- Encourage increased quality of life through social support and family relationships. EB: *Providing family support was one way to enhance the spirituality of adolescents in a quasi-experimental study by Lyon et al (2011).*
- Assist the client in identifying religious or spiritual beliefs that encourage integration of meaning and purpose in the client's life. EBN: *Religion and religious support were identified in a hermeneutic study of 17 participants as part of one's spirituality and caring (Rykkje et al, 2013).* EBN: *Haugan (2014) discovered in a cross-sectional descriptive study that nurses' interactions with the patient positively affect hope, meaning in life, and intrapersonal self-transcendence of the patient.*
- Support meditation, guided imagery, journaling, relaxation, and involvement in art, music, or poetry. Support outdoor activities. EB: *In a systematic literature review, Guerin et al (2011) identified music and other arts promote the spiritual connections to self, others, and community.* CEB: *In a randomized controlled trial, a spiritual meditation intervention was associated with fewer migraine headaches, less anxiety and a greater pain tolerance, headache-related self-efficacy, daily spiritual experiences, and existential well-being (Wachholtz & Pargament, 2008).*
- Encourage outdoor activities. CEB: *In a qualitative study of stroke caregivers, being one with nature emerged as a theme (Pierce et al, 2008).*
- Encourage expressions of spirituality. EB: *Kristeller et al (2011) used a cross-sectional exploratory design in their study of 114 individuals receiving cancer care and found higher levels of religious and spiritual engagement contributed to more positive adjustment to a cancer diagnosis.*

- Encourage integration of spirituality in healthy lifestyle choices. EB: *In a cross-sectional study of 100 adults, higher levels of spiritual well-being were found to be cardioprotective with a significant relationship to lowered blood pressure, C-reactive protein, triglycerides, fasting blood sugars, body mass index, stress, and depression (Holt-Lunstad et al, 2011).*

Geriatric

- Identify the client's past spiritual practices that have been growth-filled. Help the client explore his or her life and identify those experiences that are noteworthy. EB: *In a descriptive correlational study in which participants fell into two of four groups, those with higher levels of spirituality with or without high levels of religion, had higher levels of self-actualization and higher levels of growth initiative; both groups also had higher scores on meaning in life measures (Ivtzan et al, 2013).*
- Offer opportunities to practice one's religion. EB: *Freeze and DiTommaso (2014) identified in their descriptive study and development of a structural equation model (SEM) that a secure connection to God through religious behaviors and prayers lessened emotional distress and increased a sense of purpose in life.* EBN: *In a systematic literature review on improving outcomes in older adults with dementia through spiritual nursing care, spiritual and religious rituals such as praying, attending church, and paying tribute to God were found to be deeply embedded memories and helped to enhance reality orientation and emotional calming while decreasing agitation in this population (Enis & Kazer, 2013).*

Pediatric

- Offer adolescents opportunities for reflection and storytelling to express their spirituality. EBN: *In a cross-sectional correlational study of 310 African American adolescents, there was a relationship between frequency of participation in activities to promote spiritual well-being and positive self-reported health status (Powell-Young, 2012).*

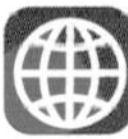

Multicultural

- Recognize the importance of spirituality and provide culturally competent spiritual care to specific populations:
  - Arab/Jordanian Muslims. EB: *Jordanian Muslim men living with coronary artery disease (CAD) shared a belief in this phenomenological study that their disease was God's will but their faith directed them to make sound health decisions while their spirituality enabled them to accept their illness and suffering (Nabolsi & Carson, 2011).*
  - Thai. EBN: *In a randomized controlled study of 79 Buddhist Thai elders in Thailand, those in the groups who practiced Vipassana meditation or chanting had significantly improved spiritual well-being and sleep quality compared to the control group who practiced neither (Wiriyasombat et al, 2011).*
  - Latinos. EB: *In a cross-sectional study examining racial/ethnic differences in spiritual well-being among cancer survivors, 80% of Latinos used their spirituality or faith to help them cope with their cancer experiences (Canada et al, 2013).* CEB: *Latinos may identify spirituality, religiousness, prayer, and church-based approaches as coping resources (Simoni et al, 2006).*
  - African Americans. EBN: *Spirituality was used as a coping mechanism to decrease perceptions of stress and the urge to smoke in a cross-sectional study of 125 AA women who were smokers, ex-smokers, and non-smokers (Franklin, 2011).* Integrate spiritual practices in health-promoting programs, particularly within the African American community. EB: *A cross-sectional study revealed that African Americans use spirituality and religion more than Hispanics and Caucasians to cope as a cancer survivor (Canada et al, 2013).* EB: *A study of African American breast cancer survivors indicated that spirituality may facilitate cancer adjustment (Lewis et al, 2012).*
  - Sheltered homeless. EBN: *In a cross-sectional correlational study examining the relationship between spirituality and health-promoting behaviors in 90 sheltered homeless women, a significant relationship was found between higher levels of spirituality and health-promoting behaviors (physical activity, nutrition, spiritual growth, interpersonal relations, and stress management) (Hurlbut et al, 2011).*
  - Chinese. EBN: *In a descriptive qualitative study, Chinese patients with advanced cancer were found to have improved psycho-spiritual well-being after participating in a life-review program (Xiao et al, 2011).*

Home Care

- All of the nursing interventions described previously apply in the home setting.

S

REFERENCES

Baldacchino, D. (2011). Teaching on spiritual care: the perceived impact on qualified nurses. *Nurse Education in Practice*, *11*, 47–53.

Burkhart, L., Schmidt, L., & Hogan, N. (2011). Development and psychometric testing of the spiritual care inventory instrument. *Journal of Advanced Nursing*, *67*(11), 2463–2472.

Canada, A., Fitchett, G., Mutphy, P., et al. (2013). Racial/ethnic differences in spiritual well-being among cancer survivors. *Journal of Behavioral Medicine*, *36*, 441–453.

Enis, E., & Kazer, M. (2013). The role of spiritual nursing interventions on improved outcomes in older adults with dementia. *Holistic Nursing Practice*, *27*(2), 106–113.

Franklin, W. (2011). African American women and smoking: spiritual well-being makes a difference. *Journal of Christian Nursing*, *28*(3), 162–167.

Freeze, T., & DiTommaso, E. (2014). An examination of attachment, religiousness, spirituality and well-being in a Baptist faith sample. *Mental Health, Religion and Culture*, *17*(7), 690–702.

Green, M., Emery, C., Kozora, E., et al. (2011). Religious and spiritual coping and quality of life among patients with emphysema in the national emphysema treatment trial. *Respiratory Care*, *56*(10), 1514–1521.

Guerin, P., Guerin, B., Tedmanson, D., et al. (2011). How can country, spirituality, music and arts contribute to indigenous mental health and wellbeing? *Australasian Psychiatry*, *19*(S38), S38–S41.

Haugan, G. (2014). Nurse-patient interaction is a resource for hope, meaning in life and self-transcendence in nursing home patients. *Scandinavian Journal of Caring Sciences*, *28*, 74–88.

Holt-Lunstad, J., Steffen, P., Sandberg, J., et al. (2011). Understanding the connections between spiritual well-being and physical health: an examination of ambulatory blood pressure, inflammation, blood lipids and fasting glucose. *Journal of Behavioral Medicine*, *24*, 477–488.

Hurlbut, J., Bobbins, L., & Hoke, M. (2011). Correlations between spirituality and health-promoting behaviors among sheltered homeless women. *Journal of Community Health Nursing*, *28*(2), 81–91.

Ivtzan, I., Chan, C., Gardner, H., et al. (2013). Linking religion and spirituality with psychological well-being: examining self-actualisation, meaning in life, and personal growth initiative. *Journal of Religion and Health*, *52*, 915–929.

Kristeller, J., Sheets, V., Johnson, T., et al. (2011). Understanding religious and spiritual influences on adjustment to cancer: individual patterns and differences. *Journal of Behavioral Medicine*, *34*, 550–561.

Lewis, P., et al. (2012). Psychosocial concerns of young African American breast cancer survivors. *Journal of Psychosocial Oncology*, *2*, 168–184.

Lyon, M., Garvie, P., Kao, E., et al. (2011). Spirituality in HIV-infected adolescents and their families: FAmily CEntered (FACE) advance care planning and medication adherence. *Journal of Adolescent Health*, *48*(6), 633–636.

Meraviglia, M. (2006). Effects of spirituality in breast cancer survivors. *Oncology Nursing Forum*, *33*(1), E1–E7.

Nabolsi, M., & Carson, A. (2011). Spirituality, illness and personal responsibility: the experience of Jordanian Muslim men with coronary artery disease. *Scandinavian Journal of Caring Sciences*, *21*, 716–724.

Pierce, L., Steiner, V., Havens, H., et al. (2008). Spirituality expressed by caregivers of stroke survivors. *Western Journal of Nursing Research*, *30*(5), 606–619.

Powell-Young, Y. (2012). Household income and spiritual well-being but not body mass index as determinants of poor self-rated health among African American adolescents. *Research in Nursing & Health*, *35*, 219–230.

Rykkje, L., Eriksson, K., & Maj-Britt, R. (2013). Spirituality and caring in old age and the significance of religion—a hermeneutical study from Norway. *Scandinavian Journal of Caring Sciences*, *27*, 275–284.

Simoni, J., Frick, P., & Huang, B. (2006). Longitudinal evaluation of a social support model of medication adherence among HIV-positive men and women on antiretroviral therapy. *Health Psychology*, *25*(1), 74–81.

Wachholtz, A., & Pargament, K. (2008). Migraines and meditation: does spirituality matter? *Journal of Behavioral Medicine*, *31*(4), 351–366.

Wiriyasombat, R., Pothiban, L., Panuthai, S., et al. (2011). Effectiveness of Buddhist doctrine practice-based programs in enhancing spiritual well-being, coping and sleep quality of Thai elders. *Pacific Rim International Journal of Nursing Research*, *15*(3), 203–218.

Xiao, H., Kwong, E., Pang, S., et al. (2011). Perceptions of a life review programme among Chinese patients with advanced cancer. *Journal of Clinical Nursing*, *21*, 564–572.

S

Impaired Standing *Tracy P. George, DNP, APRN-BC, CNE*

NANDA-I

Definition

Limitation of ability to independently and purposefully attain and/or maintain the body in an upright position from feet to head

Defining Characteristics

Impaired ability to adjust position of one or both lower limbs on uneven surface; impaired ability to attain a balanced position of the torso; impaired ability to extend one or both hips; impaired ability to extend one or both knees; impaired ability to flex one or both hips; impaired ability to flex one or both knees; impaired ability to maintain the torso in balanced position; impaired ability to stress torso with body weight; insufficient muscle strength

Related Factors

Circulatory perfusion disorder; emotional disturbance; impaired metabolic functioning; injury to lower extremity; insufficient endurance; insufficient energy; malnutrition; neurological disorder; obesity; pain; prescribed posture; sarcopenia; self-imposed relief posture; surgical procedure

NOC Outcomes (Nursing Outcomes Classification)

Suggested NOC Outcomes

Body mechanics performance

Uses correct standing posture

Body Positioning: Self-Initiated

Moves from sitting to standing

Comfort Status: Physical

Comfortable position

Risk Control Hypotension

Monitors for orthostatic hypotension when changing position

Example NOC Outcome with Indicators

Client will use personal actions to maintain proper body alignment and to prevent musculoskeletal strain by using correct standing posture 1 = never demonstrated, 2 = rarely demonstrated, 3 = sometimes demonstrated, 4 = often demonstrated, 5 = consistently demonstrated (see Section I).

Client Outcomes

Client Will (Specify Time Frame)

- Demonstrate optimal independence and safety when standing
- Demonstrate the proper use of assistive devices
- State benefits of standing

NIC Interventions (Nursing Interventions Classification)

Suggested NIC Interventions

Body mechanics promotion

Example NIC Activities

Instruct client on structure and functioned spine and optimal posture for moving and using the body

Nursing Interventions and *Rationales*

- Encourage clients to stand at intervals throughout the day. EB: *In a randomized control trial of overweight or obese Australian office workers, participants who completed work while alternating between sitting and standing at 30-minute intervals throughout the day demonstrated a 11.1% decrease in glucose levels after meals (Thorp et al, 2014).*
- Advise patients of the physical and psychological benefits of being upright and active. EB: *In patients 1 to 3 years after suffering a stroke, depression, left hemisphere infarction, visual neglect, and difficulty with mobility and balance were associated with being less active (Kunkel et al, 2015).*

Geriatric

- Advise older clients who have difficulty standing to use assistive devices. EB: *In a Swedish study using the Psychosocial Impact of Assistive Devices Scale, Nordström et al (2014) found that the frequent use of standing assistive devices was associated with higher psychosocial scores in older adults.*

- Encourage trunk exercises after clients have had strokes. EB: *In a meta-analysis of six randomized controlled studies, trunk exercises were associated with improvements in standing and walking for clients following strokes (Sorinola et al, 2014).*
- Encourage clients post-stroke to participate in rehabilitation interventions that promote standing. EB: *In a meta-analysis using 11 studies, interventions used following strokes to improve standing were associated with faster sitting to standing position times and improved lateral symmetry during sitting to standing position changes (Pollock et al, 2014).* EB: *A study of seven participants found that a home-based intervention, Rehab@home, can be used effectively to improve the rehabilitation of balance and the movement from the sitting to standing position in patients with neurological deficits, without the presence of a physical therapist (Faria et al, 2015).*
- Raise the height of the bed and encourage the use of the client's hands when an older adult is rising from a sitting to standing position. EB: *In a study of 24 older clients, Lindemann et al (2014) found that raising the bed height and using the hands while transferring from a sitting to standing position resulted in less effort.*
- Educate older adults who have fallen about the need for balance and muscle training of the ankle joint. EB: *In a randomized controlled trial of 26 older clients who were at risk of falling and had fallen previously, Jung-Hyun and Nyeon-Jun (2015) found that balance and ankle muscle training resulted in improvements in the gait of older adults.*
- Educate adults older than age 80 years on the need for vitamin D. EB: *Low serum 25-hydroxyvitamin D (25OHD) levels were associated with orthostatic hypotension in a study involving community-dwelling clients 80 years of age and older (N = 329) (Annweiler et al, 2014).*

Client/Family Teaching and Discharge Planning

- Educate clients that standing can be beneficial for their health. EB: *In a Canadian prospective cohort study in which participants were followed for a mean duration of 12 years, Katzmarzyk (2014) found that increased daily standing times was associated with decreased cardiovascular and all-cause mortality rates.* EB: *In a study of participants with chronic pain (N = 18) and participants without chronic pain (N = 19), Raijmakers et al (2015) found that patients with chronic pain spent more time lying and less time sitting and standing over a 1-week period.*
- Teach clients about the need to take frequent breaks when standing for long periods. EB: *With 45 minutes of standing to 15 minutes of sitting (3:1 ratio), 55% of participants experienced low back pain while standing, so this ratio may be not be adequate and alternate rest activities may be needed (Gallagher et al, 2014).*
- Instruct clients about the use of yoga for individuals who have difficulty with standing balance. EB: *In a randomized control of obese adults with poor standing balance, participation in yoga classes three times per week was associated with improved static and dynamic standing balance (Chaiyong et al, 2015).*

REFERENCES

Annweiler, C., Schott, A., Rolland, Y., et al. (2014). Vitamin D deficiency is associated with orthostatic hypotension in oldest-old women. *Journal of Internal Medicine, 276*(3), 285–295.

Chaiyong, J., Jutaluk, K., Chiraprapa, P., et al. (2015). Effect of yoga training on one leg standing and functional reach tests in obese individuals with poor postural control. *Journal of Physical Therapy Science, 27*(1), 59–62.

Faria, C., Silva, J., & Campilho, A. (2015). Rehab@home: a tool for home-based motor function rehabilitation. *Disability & Rehabilitation: Assistive Technology, 10*(1), 67–74.

Gallagher, K. M., Campbell, T., & Callaghan, J. P. (2014). The influence of a seated break on prolonged standing induced low back pain development. *Ergonomics, 57*(4), 555–562. [Epub 2014 Mar 19].

Jung-Hyun, C., & Nyeon-Jun, K. (2015). The effects of balance training and ankle training on the gait of elderly people who have fallen. *Journal of Physical Therapy Science, 27*(1), 139–142.

Katzmarzyk, P. T. (2014). Standing and mortality in a prospective cohort of Canadian adults. *Medicine & Science in Sports & Exercise, 46*(5), 940–946.

Kunkel, D., Fitton, C., Burnett, M., et al. (2015). Physical inactivity post-stroke: a 3-year longitudinal study. *Disability & Rehabilitation, 37*(4), 304–310.

Lindemann, U., van Oosten, L., Evers, J., et al. (2014). Effect of bed height and use of hands on trunk angular velocity during the sit-to-stand transfer. *Ergonomics, 57*(10), 1536–1540.

Nordström, B., Nyberg, L., Ekenberg, L., et al. (2014). The psychosocial impact on standing devices. *Disability & Rehabilitation: Assistive Technology, 9*(4), 299–306.

Pollock, A., Gray, C., Culham, E., et al. (2014). Interventions for improving sit-to-stand ability following stroke. *Cochrane Database of Systematic Reviews, 5*.

Raijmakers, B. G., Nieuwenhuizen, M. G., Beckerman, H., et al. (2015). Differences in the course of daily activity level between persons with and without chronic pain. *American Journal of Physical Medicine & Rehabilitation, 94*(2), 101–167.

Sorinola, I., Powis, I., & White, C. (2014). Does additional exercise improve trunk function recovery in stroke patients? A meta-analysis. *Neurorehabilitation, 35*(2), 205–213.

Thorp, A. A., Kingwell, B. A., Sethi, P., et al. (2014). Alternating bouts of sitting and standing attenuate postprandial glucose responses. *Medicine & Science In Sports & Exercise, 46*(11), 2053–2061.

Stress overload *June M. Como, EdD, RN, CNS*

NANDA-I

Definition

Excessive amounts and types of demands that require action

Defining Characteristics

Excessive stress; feeling of pressure; impaired decision-making; impaired functioning; increase in anger; increase in anger behavior; increase in impatience; negative impact from stress (e.g., physical symptoms, psychological distress, feeling sick); tension

Related Factors (r/t)

Excessive stress; insufficient resources (e.g., financial, social, knowledge); repeated stressors; stressors

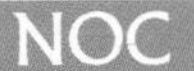

NOC (Nursing Outcomes Classification)

Suggested NOC Outcomes

Anxiety Level; Caregiver Stressors; Stress Level; Health-Promoting Behavior; Knowledge: Stress Management

Example NOC Outcome with Indicators

Stress Level as evidenced by the following indicators: Increased blood pressure, restlessness, emotional outbursts, anxiety, diminished attention to detail. (Rate the outcome and indicators of **Stress Level:** 1 = severe, 2 = substantial, 3 = moderate, 4 = mild, 5 = none [see Section I].)

Client Outcomes

Client Will (Specify Time Frame)

- Review the amounts and types of stressors in daily living
- Identify stressors that can be modified or eliminated
- Mobilize social supports to facilitate lower stress levels
- Reduce stress levels through use of health promoting behaviors and other strategies

NIC (Nursing Interventions Classification)

Suggested NIC Interventions

Active Listening; Anger Control Assistance; Anxiety Reduction; Aroma Therapy; Counseling; Crisis Intervention; Emotional Support; Family Integrity Promotion; Presence; Support System Enhancement

Example NIC Activities—Support System Enhancement

Identify psychological response to situation and availability of support system; Determine adequacy of social networks; Explain to concerned others how they can help; Refer to a self-help group or Internet-based resource as appropriate; Provide services in a caring and supportive manner

Nursing Interventions and *Rationales*

- Assist client in identification of stress overload during vulnerable life events. EBN: *Research suggests that role overload, associated with high stress levels, among nurses and volunteer caregivers may negatively impact health, well-being, and job performance (Kath et al, 2013; Akintola et al, 2013).* EB: *In a systematic review of 40 studies it was found that at least 33% of surrogates experience stressful emotional burden on making treatment decisions for others (Wendler & Rid, 2011).* CEB: *Women with breast cancer who were involved in group therapy focusing on stress reduction and muscle relaxation were 56% less likely to succumb to the disease and 45% less likely to experience a recurrence (Andersen et al, 2008). Men with high stress have higher all-cause mortality, the effects being more pronounced among middle-aged men (Nielsen et al, 2008).*

- Listen actively to descriptions of stressors and the stress response. **EBN:** *In a recent longitudinal study of clients with heart failure, researchers found that clients with high anxiety experienced shorter periods of event-free (hospitalization, mortality) survival than those with lower anxiety (P = .03) (Dejong et al, 2011).* **EB:** *Adolescents exposed to daily stress demonstrate increased risky decision-making compared to those with low stress (Galván, 2012).*
- In younger adult women, assess interpersonal stressors. **EB:** *In a sample of 127 spouse caregivers of clients with Alzheimer's disease who were predominantly female (71%), greater stress was associated with more depressive symptoms and these symptoms were significantly associated with decreased personal mastery (P = .006), self-efficacy (P <.001), increased avoidance coping (P <.001), and activity restriction (P = .040) (Mausbach et al, 2012).* **CEB:** *A systematic review and meta-analysis of 30 studies found that maternal exposure to the stress of domestic violence results in significantly increased risk of low birth weight and preterm birth (Shah & Shah, 2010).*
- Categorize stressors as modifiable or nonmodifiable. **EB:** *Strategizing on nonavoidance coping and increased socialization along with enhanced personal mastery and self-efficacy in use of problem-solving coping may minimize depression symptoms in Alzheimer's disease caregivers (Mausbach et al, 2012).* **CEBN:** *Removing or minimizing some stressors, changing responses to stressors, and modifying the long-term effects of stress are all actions that can assist those with chronic illnesses and stress (Upton & Solowiej, 2010).*
- Help clients modify or mitigate stressors identified as modifiable. **EBN:** *In a sample of 480 nurse managers from 36 hospitals in Southwestern United States, role overload was found to be the most significant predictor of work-related stress followed by organizational constraints and role conflict (all P <.01 [two-tailed]); all three are areas that organizational leaders need to be aware of to mitigate stress overload in managerial staff (Kath et al, 2013).* **CEB:** *There are numerous possible strategies to modify stressors, including time management, improved organizational skills, problem solving, changing perceptions of stress, breathing, relaxation techniques, visual imagery, and soothing rituals (Lloyd et al, 2005).*
- Help clients distinguish among short-term, chronic, and secondary stressors. **EB:** *Cellular aging, identified by leukocyte telomere length (TL), was found to be different in a sample of 36 ethnically diverse, older adults between four pain/stress groups (P = .01) where those with chronic pain/higher stress had the shortest TL indicative of cellular aging (Sibille, 2012).* **CEBN:** *Social support is a critical dimension of health and health promotion and serves as a buffer in the stress response (Pender et al, 2010).*
- Provide information as needed to reduce stress responses to acute and chronic illnesses. **EBN:** *Nursing interventions including strategies to deal with child behavior, a focus on physical health, and planning to meet resource needs may enhance the well-being of African American grandmothers raising grandchildren (Kelley, 2013). Pro-active nursing interventions including assessment of caregiver needs for support and preparedness including early psycho-educational interventions can enhance caregiver ability to navigate the challenges associated with caring for a relative with Alzheimer's disease (Ducharme, 2011).*

▲ Explore possible therapeutic approaches such as cognitive-behavioral therapy, biofeedback, neurofeedback, acupuncture, pharmacological agents, and complementary and alternative therapies. **EBN:** *Non-pharmacological nursing interventions through the use of nature-based sounds played through headsets was found to effectively decrease the stress response in mechanically-ventilated clients in a sample of 60 Iranian clients aged 18-65 (Saadatmand, 2013).* **EB:** *In a sample of 111 healthy adults, those who exercised regularly were more resistant to acute stress (Childs, 2014). Mindfulness techniques have been suggested as an effective means of reducing stress in adolescents (Broderick, 2012), nursing personnel (Zeller, 2013), and older adults (Gallegos, 2013).*

- Help the client to reframe his or her perceptions of some of the stressors. **EBN:** *A study on 335 Thai nursing students found that coping mediated the effects of stress on physical and psychological health (Klainin-Yobas, 2014). Researchers found that nursing students with higher anxiety states were 62% less optimistic, findings supporting that individuals with pessimistic outlooks perceive situations as more threatening (Warning, 2011).*
- Assist the client to mobilize social supports for dealing with recent stressors. **CEBN:** *Emotional support in Taiwanese caregivers is suggested as a moderator of stressors experienced by caregivers of clients with Alzheimer's disease or stroke, particularly in caregivers with lower household incomes (Huang et al, 2009).* **EB:** *In a sample of 79 German adults a predicted association between needed and received emotional support and well-being was found in younger adults (aged 23-34) (Wolff, 2013).*

Pediatric

- With children, nurses should work with parents to help them to reduce children's stressors. EB: *A longitudinal study on 115 children aged 7 to 12 suggests that early life stress and trauma may result in increased limbic activity, a biomarker that may have implications as a risk for later psychiatric diagnoses (Suzuki, 2014). A study on 181 18- to 20-year-olds suggests that more positive parenting behaviors are statistically significantly (P <0.01) associated with more adaptive cognitions in the emerging adult which may impact stress/health outcomes (Donnelly, 2013).*
- Help children to manage their feelings related to self-concept. CEB: *Perceived isolation as experienced in high school associated with victimization results in higher stress and longer-lasting negative psychological outcomes (Newman, Holden, & Delville, 2005).*
- Help children to deal with bullies and other sources of violence in schools and neighborhoods. EB: *In a sample of 1,420 children and adolescents the number of times that the individual was bullied predicted higher levels of C-reactive protein (CRP) (a risk factor for negative health consequences later in life) where those who bullied had lower levels of CRP (Copeland, 2014). Violence in schools and neighborhoods has significant effects on children's stress. In a recent study of college-aged respondents (N = 1339), researchers found that a history of being bullied (victimized) was associated with both increased stress and use of avoidant behaviors (Newman, Holden, & Delville, 2011).*
- Help children to manage the complexities of chronic illnesses. EB: *Individuals who grow up with a chronic illness have lower odds of graduating college, being employed, having a good income, and a higher need for public assistance although do succeed socially as evident by similar odds of marriage, having children, and living with their parents when compared to those without chronic illness (Maslow, 2011).* CEB: *Teenagers who had recently been diagnosed with diabetes described high levels of stress that often related to the complexities of managing the illness (Davidson et al, 2004).*

Geriatric

- Assess for chronic stress with older adults and provide a variety of stress relief techniques. EB: *In a sample of over 9,000 U.S. adults over the age of 60 lifetime post-traumatic stress disorder (PTSD) was found to be associated with greater odds of being diagnosed with hypertension, angina pectoris, tachycardia, other heart disease, stomach ulcer, gastritis, and arthritis (Pietrzak, 2012).*

▲ Encourage older adults to seek appropriate counseling. EB: *Treatment modalities for PTSD in older adults may vary dependent on whether the PTSD was experienced early or late in life; however, trauma confrontation and cognitive restructuring combined with age-specific life review in cognitive behavioral therapy may hold the most promise (Böttche, 2012).* CEB: *Bereavement-related major depression differs from major depression seen in other stressful life events only in relation to older age at onset, individuals are more likely to be female, lower levels of treatment-seeking, higher levels of guilt, fatigue, and loss of interest and therefore should not be excluded from a diagnosis of major depression (Kendler, Myers, & Zisook, 2008).*

S

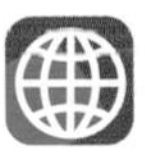

Multicultural

- Review cultural beliefs and acculturation level in relation to perceived stressors. EBN: *A study done to assess how the type of premigration trauma, postmigration stressors and resources predicted PTSD and major depressive disorder (MDD) symptoms it was found that postmigration-related stressors greatly increased the odds (nearly 16-fold) of being in a comorbid group (PTSD or MDD) (Norris, 2011).* EB: *A review of qualitative studies found that organizational constraints, work overload, and interpersonal conflict were universally experienced stressors in studies that assessed occupational stress on an international perspective (Mazzola et al, 2011).* Assess families for whether they experience high stress or low stress. EB: *In a sample of 97 native Norwegian adolescents and 59 immigrant adolescents from an urban Norwegian secondary school, global victimization was found to be higher in the immigrant group compared to the native group although there was no difference in the report of depressive symptoms (Fandrem et al, 2012).* CEB: *Stress related to racial microaggressions experienced by African Americans may have a negative cumulative effect on health outcomes (Sue et al, 2007).*

Home Care

- The preceding interventions may be adapted for home care use.
- Develop community-based programs for stress management as needed for groups with increased risk of stress overload (e.g., firefighters, policemen, military personnel, and nurses). CEB: *Some situations have*

higher risks of stress overload. Stress management interventions may prevent or modify the experience of stress overload (McNulty, 2005).

- Support and encourage neighborhood stability. CEB: *A "significant proportion of health differentials across neighborhoods is due to disparate stress levels across [Detroit] neighborhoods" and neighborhood stability was a buffer to reduce the negative effects of high stress (Boardman, 2004).*

Client/Family Teaching and Discharge Planning

- Diagnose the possibility of stress overload before teaching.
- Establish readiness for learning.
- Provide manageable amounts of information at the appropriate educational level.
- Evaluate the need for additional teaching and learning experiences.

REFERENCES

Akintola, O., Hlengwa, W., & Dageid, W. (2013). Perceived stress and burnout among volunteer caregivers working in AIDS care in South Africa. *Journal of Advanced Nursing*, *69*, 2738–2749.

Andersen, B., et al. (2008). Psychologic intervention improves survival for breast cancer. *Cancer*, *113*(12), 3450–3458.

Boardman, J. (2004). Stress and physical health: the role of neighborhoods as mediating and moderating mechanisms. *Social Science Medicine*, *58*(12), 2473–2483.

Böttche, M., Kuwert, P., & Knaevelsrud, C. (2012). Posttraumatic stress disorder in older adults: an overview of characteristics and treatment approaches. *International Journal of Geriatric Psychiatry*, *27*, 230–239.

Broderick, P. C., & Jennings, P. A. (2012). Mindfulness for adolescents: a promising approach to supporting emotion regulation and preventing risky behavior. *New Directions for Youth Development*, *2012*, 111.

Childs, E., & de Wit, H. (2014). Regular exercise is associated with emotional resilience to acute stress in healthy adults. *Frontiers In Physiology*, *5*, 161.

Copeland, W. E., Wolke, D., Lereya, S. T., et al. (2014). Childhood bullying involvement predicts low-grade systemic inflammation into adulthood. *Proceedings of the National Academy of Sciences of the United States of America*, *111*, 7570–7575.

Davidson, M., et al. (2004). Stressors and self-care challenges faced by adolescents living with type 1 diabetes. *Applied Nursing Research*, *2*, 72–80.

Dejong, M., et al. (2011). Linkages between anxiety and outcomes in heart failure. *Heart and Lung: The Journal of Critical Care*, *40*, 393–404.

Donnelly, R., Renk, K., & McKinney, C. (2013). Emerging adults' stress and health: the role of parent behaviors and cognitions. *Child Psychiatry and Human Development*, *44*, 19–38.

Ducharme, F., Lévesque, L., Lachance, L., et al. (2011). Challenges associated with transition to caregiver role following diagnostic disclosure of Alzheimer disease: a descriptive study. *International Journal of Nursing Studies*, *48*, 1109–1119.

Fandrem, H., Strohmeier, D., & Jonsdottir, K. A. (2012). Peer groups and victimisation among native and immigrant adolescents in Norway. *Emotional & Behavioural Difficulties*, *17*, 273–285.

Gallegos, A. M., Hoerger, M., Talbot, N. L., et al. (2013). Emotional benefits of mindfulness-based stress reduction in older adults: the moderating roles of age and depressive symptom severity. *Aging & Mental Health*, *17*, 823–829.

Galván, A., & McGlennen, K. M. (2012). Daily stress increases risky decision-making in adolescents: a preliminary study. *Developmental Psychobiology*, *54*, 433–440.

Huang, C., et al. (2009). Stressors, social support, depressive symptoms and general health status of Taiwanese caregivers of persons with stroke or Alzheimer's disease. *Journal of the Clinics in Nursing*, *18*(4), 502–511.

Kath, L. M., Stichler, J. F., Ehrhart, M. G., et al. (2013). Predictors of nurse manager stress: a dominance analysis of potential work environment stressors. *International Journal of Nursing Studies*, *50*, 1474–1480.

Kelley, S. J., Whitley, D. M., & Campos, P. E. (2013). Psychological distress in African American grandmothers raising grandchildren: the contribution of child behavior problems, physical health, and family resources. *Research In Nursing & Health*, *36*, 373–385.

Kendler, K., Myers, J., & Zisook, M. (2008). Does bereavement-related major depression differ from major depression associated with other stressful life events? *American Journal of Psychiatry*, *165*(11), 1449–1455.

Klainin-Yobas, P., Keawkerd, O., Pumpuang, W., et al. (2014). The mediating effects of coping on the stress and health relationships among nursing students: a structural equation modelling approach. *Journal of Advanced Nursing*, *70*, 1287–1298.

Lloyd, C., Smith, J., & Weinger, K. (2005). Stress and diabetes: a review of the links. *Diabetes Spectrum*, *18*(2), 121–127.

Maslow, G. R., Haydon, A., McRee, A.-L., et al. (2011). Growing up with a chronic illness: social success, educational/vocational distress. *Journal of Adolescent Health*, *49*, 206–212.

Mausbach, B. T., Roepke, S. K., Chattillion, E. A., et al. (2012). Multiple mediators of the relations between caregiving stress and depressive symptoms. *Aging & Mental Health*, *16*, 27–38.

Mazzola, J., Schonfeld, I., & Spector, P. (2011). What qualitative research has taught us about occupational stress. *Stress Health*, *27*, 93–110.

McNulty, P. (2005). Reported stressors and health care needs of active duty Navy personnel during three phases of deployment in support of the war in Iraq. *Military Medicine*, *170*, 530–535.

Newman, M., Holden, G., & Delville, Y. (2005). Isolation and the stress of being bullied. *Journal of Adolescence*, *28*, 343–357.

Newman, M., Holden, G., & Delville, Y. (2011). Coping with the stress of being bullied: consequences of coping strategies among college students. *Social Psychological Perspectives in Science*, *2*, 205–211.

Nielsen, N., et al. (2008). Perceived stress and cause-specific mortality among men and women: results from a prospective cohort study. *American Journal of Epidemiology*, *168*(5), 481–491.

Norris, A. E., Aroian, K. J., & Nickerson, D. M. (2011). Premigration persecution, postmigration stressors and resources, and postmigration mental health: a study of severely traumatized U.S. Arab immigrant women. *Journal of the American Psychiatric Nurses Association*, *17*, 283–293.

S

Pender, N., Murtaugh, C., & Parsons, M. (2010). *Health promotion in nursing practice* (6th ed.). Upper Saddle River NJ: Prentice Hall.
Pietrzak, R. H., Goldstein, R. B., Southwick, S. M., et al. (2012). Physical health conditions associated with posttraumatic stress disorder in U.S. older adults: results from wave 2 of the national epidemiologic survey on alcohol and related conditions. *Journal of the American Geriatrics Society*, *60*, 296–303.
Saadatmand, V., Rejeh, N., Heravi-Karimooi, M., et al. (2013). Effect of nature-based sounds' intervention on agitation, anxiety, and stress in patients under mechanical ventilator support: a randomised controlled trial. *International Journal of Nursing Studies*, *50*, 895–904.
Shah, P., & Shah, J. (2010). Maternal exposure to domestic violence and pregnancy and birth outcomes: a systematic review and meta-analysis. *Journal of Womens Health*, *19*, 2017–2031.
Sibille, K. T., Langaee, T., Burkley, B., et al. (2012). Chronic pain, perceived stress, and cellular aging: an exploratory study. *Molecular Pain*, *8*, 12.
Sue, D., et al. (2007). Racial microaggressions in everyday life. *American Psychologist*, *62*(4), 271–286.
Suzuki, H., Luby, J. L., Botteron, K. N., et al. (2014). Early life stress and trauma and enhanced limbic activation to emotionally valenced faces in depressed and healthy children. *Journal of the American Academy of Child and Adolescent Psychiatry*, *53*, 800–813, e810.
Upton, D., & Solowiej, K. (2010). Pain and stress as contributors to delayed wound healing. *Wound Practice & Research*, *18*, 114–122.
Warning, L. (2011). Are you positive? The influence of life orientation on the anxiety levels of nursing students. *Holistic Nursing Practice*, *25*, 254–257.
Wendler, D., & Rid, A. (2011). Systematic review: the effect on surrogates of making treatment decisions for others. *Annals of Internal Medicine*, *154*, 336–346.
Wolff, J. K., Schmiedek, F., Brose, A., et al. (2013). Physical and emotional well-being and the balance of needed and received emotional support: age differences in a daily diary study. *Social Science & Medicine (1982)*, *91*, 67–75.
Zeller, J. M., & Levin, P. F. (2013). Mindfulness interventions to reduce stress among nursing personnel: an occupational health perspective. *Workplace Health & Safety*, *61*, 85–89.

Risk for Sudden Infant Death syndrome

Betty Ackley, MSN, EdS, RN

NANDA-I

Definition

Vulnerable to unpredicted death of an infant

Risk Factors

Modifiable

Delay in prenatal care; infant overheating; infant overwrapping; infant placed to sleep in the prone position; infants placed to sleep in the side-lying position; bed sharing; lack of prenatal care; smoke exposure; soft underlayment (loose items in the sleep environment)

Potentially Modifiable

Low birth weight, prematurity, young parental age

Nonmodifiable

Ethnicity (e.g., African American or Native American), male gender, season of the year (i.e., winter and fall), infant age of 2 to 4 months

S

NOC (Nursing Outcomes Classification)

Suggested NOC Outcomes

Knowledge: Infant Care; Parenting Performance; Safe Home Environment; Safe Sleep Environment

Example NOC Outcome with Indicators

Knowledge: Infant Care as evidenced by the following indicators: Proper infant positioning/Age-appropriate cardiopulmonary resuscitation techniques. (Rate the outcome and indicators of **Knowledge: Infant Care:** 1 = no knowledge, 2 = limited knowledge 3 = moderate knowledge, 4 = substantial knowledge, 5 = extensive knowledge [see Section I].)

Client Outcomes

Client Will (Specify Time Frame)

- Explain appropriate measures to prevent sudden infant death syndrome (SIDS)
- Demonstrate correct techniques for positioning and blanketing the infant, protecting the infant from harm

NIC (Nursing Interventions Classification)

Suggested NIC Interventions

Infant Care; Teaching: Infant Safety 0 to 3 Months

Example NIC Activities—Teaching: Infant Safety

Instruct parent/caregiver to place infant on back to sleep and keep loose bedding, pillows, and toys out of crib; Instruct parent/caregiver to avoid holding infant while smoking or holding hot liquids

Nursing Interventions and *Rationales*

- Position the infant supine to sleep during naps and night; do not position in the prone position or side-lying position (American Academy of Pediatrics [AAP], 2014a). CEB/EB: *In a retrospective review of hundreds of SIDS cases, more than 70% of the incidences happened when the infant was in a prone or side-lying position (Ostfeld et al, 2010). In two case studies, infants who were lying on their side during breast-feeding in the maternity ward apparently suffocated (Feldman & Whyte, 2013).*
- Avoid use of bedding, such as blankets and loose sheets for sleeping. Also keep quilts, pillows, bumpers, sheepskins and soft toys out of the infant's bed. Dress the child in one-piece sleepers or wearable blankets (AAP, 2014b). *Infants can suffocate from close proximity to these soft items.*
- Avoid overbundling, overheating, and swaddling the infant. The infant should not feel hot to touch. *Overheating the infant has been associated with increased risk of SIDS. The head is often covered preceding death (AAP, 2014a).* EB: *Swaddling has been associated with infant death, especially when the infant has shown the ability to roll over (McDonnell & Moon, 2014).*
- Provide the infant a certain amount of time in prone position while the infant is awake and observed. Change the direction that the baby lies in the crib from one week to the next; avoid too much time in car seats and carriers. *Prolonged time in the supine position can result in a flat head shape and decreased strength of the neck and shoulder muscles (AAP, 2014a).*
- Consider offering the infant a pacifier during sleep times. EB: *Use of a pacifier was associated with a decreased incidence of SIDS (Moon et al, 2012). Another study found that many infant caregivers were not aware that use of pacifiers was associated with decreased incidence of SIDS (Walsh et al, 2014).*

▲ Use electronic respiratory or cardiac monitors to detect cardiorespiratory arrest only if ordered by the health care provider. *There is no evidence that use of such home monitors decreases the incidence of SIDS (AAP, 2014a).*

Home Care

- Most of the interventions and client teaching information are relevant to home care.
- Evaluate home for potential safety hazards, such as inappropriate cribs, cradles, or strollers.
- Determine where and how the child sleeps, and provide instructions on safe sleeping positions and environments as needed.

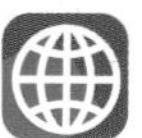

Multicultural

- Encourage pregnant American Indian mothers and native Alaskan Indian mothers to avoid drinking alcohol and to avoid wrapping infants in excessive blankets or clothing. EB: *A study of death rate of infants of Indian mothers found an increased rate of SIDS, as compared with the white population, which was thought to be associated with alcohol ingestion and excessive clothing and blankets used by the mothers (Wong et al, 2014).*
- Encourage Hispanic and black mothers to find alternatives to bed sharing or placing infants for sleep on adult beds, sofas, or cots, and to avoid placing pillows, soft toys, and soft bedding in the sleep

S

environment. EB: *A study found that both Hispanic and black mothers were more likely to share a bed with an infant, and as a result there is an increasing rate of SIDS in their infants (Colson et al, 2013).*

Client/Family Teaching and Discharge Planning

- Teach the safety guidelines for infant care in the previous interventions.
- Recommend breastfeeding. EB: *A meta-analysis demonstrated that breastfeeding was protective against SIDS, especially with exclusive breastfeeding (Hauck et al, 2011).*
- Teach parents the need to obtain a crib that conforms to the safety standards of the Consumer Product Safety Commission (CPSC). *Drop-side rail cribs are now prohibited; cribs need stronger slats and mattress supports, and better quality hardware (CPSC, 2013).*
- Teach the need to stop smoking during pregnancy and to not smoke around the infant. Do not allow the infant to be exposed to any secondhand smoke EB: *Both prenatal and postnatal smoking was shown to have a significant association with SIDS in a large retrospective meta-analysis (Zhang & Wang, 2013; Behm et al, 2012).*
- Teach parents, especially mothers, not to use alcohol, medications, or illicit drugs while caring for or bed sharing with an infant. EB: *Research has shown that mothers who were previously diagnosed with alcoholism had infants with a significant risk for SIDS (O'Leary et al, 2013; Phillips et al, 2011).*
- Teach parents not to sleep in the same bed with the infant, regardless of alcohol, medications, smoking, or illicit drug use. EB/CEB: *A study of more than 1000 SIDS cases found that bed sharing with an infant resulted in an increased incidence of SIDS even without illicit drugs, alcohol, or smoking (Carpenter et al, 2013). Another study of mothers of infants found that 39 of almost 300 mothers reported incidences when they had rolled partially or fully over the infant in the bed (Ateah & Hamelin, 2008).*
- Teach parents not to place the infant on a cushion to sleep, or a sofa chair or other soft surface. Infants should sleep in a crib *(AAP, 2014a).*
- Recommend an alternative to sleeping with an infant of placing the infant's crib near their bed to allow for more convenient breastfeeding and parent contact. *Parents should be advised to place the baby in his/her own crib next to the parent's bed (AAP, 2014a).*
- Recommend that parents with infants in child care make it very clear to the employees that the infant must always be placed in the supine position to sleep, not prone or in a side-lying position (AAP, 2014a).

REFERENCES

American Academy of Pediatrics (AAP) (2014a) *Preventing SIDS.* Retrieved from: <http://www.healthychildren.org/English/ages-stages/baby/sleep/Pages/Preventing-SIDS.aspx.>

American Academy of Pediatrics (AAP) (2014b) *Winter safety tips,* Retrieved from: <http://www.aap.org/en us/about-the-aap/aap-press-room/news-features-and-safety-tips/Pages/Winter-Safety-Tips.aspx.>

Ateah, C. A., & Hamelin, K. J. (2008). Maternal bedsharing practices, experiences, and awareness of risks. *Journal of Obstetric, Gynecologic, and Neonatal Nursing, 37*(3), 274–281.

Behm, I., et al. (2012). Increasing prevalence of smoke-free homes and decreasing rates of sudden infant death syndrome in the United States: an ecological association study. *Tobacco Control, 21*(1), 6–11.

Carpenter, R., et al. (2013). Bed sharing when parents do not smoke: is there a risk of SIDS? An individual level analysis of five major case-control studies. *BMJH Open, 3*(5), pii, e002299.

Colson, R. R., et al. (2013). Trends and factors associated with infant bed sharing, 1993-2010; the national infant sleep position study. *JAMA Pediatr, 167*(11).

Consumer Product Safety Commission (CPSC) (2013) *The new crib standard: questions and answers.* Retrieved from: <http://www.cpsc.gov/onsafety/2011/06/the-new-crib-standard-questions-and-answers/.>

Feldman, K., & Whyte, R. K. (2013). Two cases of apparent suffocation of newborns during side-lying breastfeeding. *Nurs Womens Health., 17*(4), 337–341.

Hauck, F. R., et al. (2011). Breastfeeding and reduced risk of sudden infant death syndrome: a meta-analysis. *Pediatrics, 128*(1), 103–110.

McDonnell, E., & Moon, R. Y. (2014). Infant deaths and injuries associated with wearable blankets, swaddle wraps, and swaddling. *The Journal of Pediatrics, 164*(5), 1152–1156. [Epub 2014 Feb 7].

Moon, R. Y., et al. (2012). Pacifier use and SIDS: evidence for a consistently reduced risk. *Maternal and Child Health Journal, 16*(3), 609–614, 2012.

O'Leary, C. M., et al. (2013). Maternal alcohol use and sudden infant death syndrome and infant mortality excluding SIDS. *Pediatrics, 131*(3), e770–e778. [Epub2013 Feb 25].

Phillips, D. P., Brewer, K. M., & Wadenweiler, P. (2011). Alcohol as a risk factor for sudden infant death syndrome (SIDS). *Addiction (Abingdon, England), 106*(3), 516–525.

Walsh, P., et al. (2014). Using a pacifier to decrease sudden infant death syndrome: an emergency department educational intervention. *Peer, 13*(2), e309. [eCollection 2014].

Wong, C. A., et al. (2014). American Indian and Alaska native infant and pediatric mortality, United States, 1999–2009. *American Journal of Public Health, S3*(Suppl. 3), S320–S328.

Zhang, K., & Wang, X. (2013). Maternal smoking and increased risk of sudden infant death syndrome: a meta analysis. *Legal Medicine, 15*(3), 115–121.

Risk for Suffocation

Melodie Cannon, DNP, MSc/FNP, BHScN, RN(EC), NP-PHC, CEN, GNC(C), and Betty Ackley, MSN, EdS, RN

NANDA-I

Definition

Vulnerable to inadequate air availability for inhalation, which may compromise health

Risk Factors

External

Access to empty refrigerator/freezer; eating large mouthfuls of food; gas leak; low-strung clothesline; pacifier around infant's neck; playing with plastic bag; propped bottle placed in infant's crib; small object in airway; smoking in bed; soft underlayment (e.g., loose items placed near infant); unattended in water; unvented fuel-burning heater; vehicle running in closed garage

Internal

Alteration in cognitive functioning; alteration in olfactory function; emotional disturbance; face/neck disease; face/neck injury; impaired motor functioning; insufficient knowledge of safety precautions

NOC (Nursing Outcomes Classification)

Suggested NOC Outcomes

Knowledge: Infant Care; Personal Safety; Parenting: Adolescent Physical Safety, Early/Middle Childhood Physical Safety; Infant/Toddler Physical Safety; Risk Control; Risk Detection; Safe Home Environment; Substance Addiction Consequences

Example NOC Outcome with Indicators

Knowledge: Infant Care as evidenced by the following indicators: Strategies to prevent choking/Appropriate activities for child's developmental level/First aid techniques. (Rate the outcome and indicators of **Knowledge: Infant Care:** 1 = no knowledge, 2 = limited knowledge, 3 = moderate knowledge, 4 = substantial knowledge, 5 = extensive knowledge [see Section I].)

S

Client Outcomes

Client Will (Specify Time Frame)

- Undertake appropriate measures to prevent suffocation
- Demonstrate correct techniques for emergency rescue maneuvers (e.g., Heimlich maneuver, rescue breathing, cardiopulmonary resuscitation [CPR]) and describe situations that require them

NIC (Nursing Interventions Classification)

Suggested NIC Interventions

Aspiration Precautions; Environmental Management: Safety; Infant Care; Positioning; Security Enhancement; Surveillance; Surveillance: Safety; Teaching: Infant Safety

Example NIC Activities—Environmental Management: Safety

Identify safety hazards in the environment (i.e., physical, biological, and chemical); Remove hazards from the environment, when possible

Nursing Interventions and *Rationales*

- Identify hospitalized clients at particular risk for suffocation, including the following:
  - Clients with altered levels of consciousness
  - Infants or young children
  - Clients with developmental delays
  - Clients with mental illness, especially schizophrenia
  - Clients who have been physically or chemically restrained

Restraint use has been associated with chest compression and death by strangulation. If use of restraints is unavoidable, proper application and close client monitoring is essential (Berzlanovich et al, 2012).

Institute safety measures such as proper positioning and feeding precautions. See the care plans for Risk for ***Aspiration*** *and Impaired* ***Swallowing*** *for additional interventions. Vigilance and special protective measures are necessary for clients at greater risk for suffocation.* CEB: *Mental health clients have an increased incidence of choking and suffocation incidents (Corcoran & Walsh, 2003).*

Pediatric

- Counsel families on the following for care of an infant:
  - Position infants on their back to sleep; do not position them on their side or prone *(Registered Nurses' Association of Ontario, 2014).*
  - Obtain a new crib that conforms to the safety standards of the Federal Safety Commission. *Drop-side rail cribs are now prohibited; cribs need stronger slats and mattress supports, and better quality hardware (American Academy of Pediatrics [AAP], 2011).*
  - Place the infant in the crib with a properly fitted mattress, only to sleep, not on an adult bed, sofa, chair, baby seats, swings, or playpen. *Babies can suffocate when their faces become wedged against or buried in a mattress, pillow, bumper pads, infant cushion, or other soft bedding or when someone in the same bed rolls over onto them (Parachute Preventing Injuries Saving Lives, 2012).* EB: *A study demonstrated that bed sharing was a risk factor for sudden infant death syndrome, especially for very young infants, or a parent who smoked (Vennemann et al, 2012).*
  - Avoid use of loose bedding such as blankets and sheets for sleeping. If blankets are used, they should be tucked in around the crib mattress so the infant's face is less likely to become covered by bedding. The blanket should end at the level of the infant's chest. EB: *Evidence exists that that a firm sleep surface and the absence of soft items and loose bedding has a net benefit in reducing the risk of sudden unexpected infant death (AAP, 2011). See care plan Risk for* ***Sudden Infant Death*** *syndrome for further interventions.*
- Assess for signs and symptoms of abuse such as Munchausen syndrome by proxy (MSBP). CEB: *Suffocation in MSBP is one important differential diagnosis in suspected cases of SIDS (Vennemann et al, 2005)*
- Conduct risk factor identification, noting special circumstances in which preventive or protective measures are indicated. Note the presence of environmental hazards, including the following: plastic bags; cribs with slats wider than 2 inches; ill-fitting crib mattresses that can allow the infant to become wedged between the mattress and crib; pillows/loose bedding in cribs; placement of crib near windows with blinds or cords; co-sleeping; abandoned large appliances such as refrigerators, dishwashers, or freezers; clothing with cords or hoods that can become entangled; bibs; pacifiers on a string; necklaces in infants and children; drapery cords; pull-toy strings. *Suffocation by airway obstruction is a leading cause of death in children younger than 6 years of age. Families need to be taught child protection.* EB: *Home visits, safety education, and injury prevention kits have proven effective in reducing home hazards and injuries, including choking and suffocation (Cyr, 2012).*
- Counsel families to evaluate household furniture for safety, including large dressers, televisions, book shelves, and appliances that may need to be anchored to the wall, to prevent the child from climbing on the furniture, and it falling forward and suffocating the child. EB: *A review of nine deaths of children demonstrated that they could have been prevented by attaching large pieces of furniture to the wall or by better supervision of the child (Wolf & Harding, 2011).*
- Counsel families to not serve these foods to the child younger than 4 years of age: nuts, seeds, hot dogs, popcorn, pretzels, chips, chunks of meat, hard pieces of fruit or vegetables, raisins, whole grapes, hard candies gum, chewable vitamins, fish with bones, snacks on toothpicks, and marshmallows. EB: *A meta-analysis found that nuts, magnets, and small toys are the most common items associated with fatal choking*

S

incidences in children (Foltran et al, 2012). EB: *Most foods implicated are small and round and conform to the contours of a child's airway (Cyr, 2012).*

- Counsel families to keep the following items away from the sight and reach of infants and toddlers:
  - Buttons, beads, jewelry, pins, nails, marbles, coins, stones, magnets, balloons. Choose age appropriate toys and games for children and check for any small parts that may be a choking hazard because children have the need to put everyday objects in their mouths (safekids.org. 2013). *A project that collects data on child safety found that pearls, balls, marbles, and coins were observed most commonly as a cause of aspiration and suffocation (Susy Safe Working Group, 2012).*
- Stress water and pool safety precautions, including vigilant, uninterrupted parental supervision. EB: *Recognize that small portable pools can also be a source of danger for drowning in children younger than 5 years of age (Shields et al, 2011).* EB: *The majority of pediatric immersion-related deaths could be prevented with supervision (Bamber et al, 2014). An intense drive for exploration combined with a lack of awareness of danger makes drowning a threat to small children. A child's high center of gravity and poor coordination make buckets and toilets a threat because a child looking inside can fall over and become lodged (Shields et al, 2011). Pools should be surrounded completely by fencing that is difficult to climb and regularly assessed for structural defects, and has self-closing latches.*
- Underscore the necessity of not allowing children to play with or near electric garage doors and of keeping garage door openers out of the reach of young children. *Children close to the ground may not be large enough to trigger reversal mechanisms on the door and may become trapped.*
- For adolescents, watch for signs of depression that could result in suicide by suffocation. EB: *A study in Canada found that suffocation was a common method for female children and adolescents to commit suicide (Skinner & McFaull, 2012).*

Geriatric

- Assess the status of the swallow reflex. Offer appropriate foods and beverages accordingly. *Older adults, especially those receiving antipsychotic medications, have an increased incidence of choking. Refer to Impaired* ***Swallowing.*** EB: *Dysphagia is a common problem in adults with mental health illness and has a significant mortality risk due to choking asphyxiation (Aldridge & Taylor, 2012).*
- Use care in pillow placement when positioning frail older clients who are on bed rest. *Frail older clients are at risk for suffocation if the head becomes lodged against pillows and the client cannot reposition himself or herself because of weakness. Older adults who are cognitively impaired require assessment of the safety of their sleep environment for potential hazards similar to sleeping risks for the very young (Byard & Gilbert, 2011).*
- Recognize that older adults in depression may use hanging, strangulation, and suffocation as a means of suicide (Shah & Buckley, 2011).

S

Home Care

- Assess the home for potential safety hazards in systems that are not likely to be fixed (e.g., faulty pilot lights or gas leaks in gas stoves, carbon monoxide release from heating systems, kerosene fumes from portable heaters).
- Assist the family in having these areas assessed and making appropriate safety arrangements (e.g., installing detectors, making repairs, home safety inspections). *Assessment and correction of system problems prevent accidental suffocation.*

Client/Family Teaching and Discharge Planning

- Recommend that families who are seeking day care or in-home care for children, geriatric family members, or at-risk family members with developmental or functional disabilities inspect the environment for hazards and examine the first aid preparation and vigilance of providers. *Many working families must trust others to care for family members.*
- Ensure family members learn and practice rescue techniques, including treatment of choking and lack of breathing, as well as CPR. *Family members need preparation to deal with emergency situations and should take part in the American Heart Association Basic Lifesaving Course or the American Red Cross Infant/Child CPR Course.*
- *Use client/family encounters to provide age appropriate anticipatory guidance for safety precautions for infants and children, and education regarding risk reduction for suffocation for vulnerable older adults or clients with physical or mental disabilities.*

REFERENCES

Aldridge, K. J., & Taylor, N. F. (2012). Dysphagia is a common and serious problem for adults with mental illness: a systematic review. *Dysphagia, 27*, 124–137.

American Academy of Pediatrics, (2011). *New crib standards: what parents need to know*. Retrieved from: <http://www.healthychildren.org/English/safety-prevention/at-home/Pages/New-Crib-Standards-What-Parents-Need-to-Know.aspx.>

American Academy of Pediatrics (2011). *SIDS and other sleep-related infant deaths: expansion of recommendations for a safe infant sleeping environment. Task Force on Sudden Infant Death Syndrome.* Retrieved from: <http://pediatrics.aappublications.org/content/early/2011/10/12/peds.2011-2284.>

American Academy of Pediatrics (2011). *SIDS and other sleep-related infant deaths: expansion of recommendations for a safe infant sleeping environment. Task Force on Sudden Infant Death Syndrome.* Retrieved from: <http://pediatrics.aappublications.org/content/early/2011/10/12/peds.2011-2284.>

Bamber, A. R., Pryce, J. W., Ashworth, M. T., et al. (2014). Immersion-related deaths in infants and children: autopsy experience from a specialist center. *Forensic Science Medicine Pathology, 10*, 363–370.

Berzlanovich, A. M., Schöpfer, J., & Keil, W. (2012). Deaths due to physical restraint. *Deutsches Arzteblatt International, 109*(3), 27–32.

Byard, R. W., & Gilbert, J. D. (2011). Sleeping accidents in the elderly. *Journal of Forensic Sciences, 56*(6), 1645–1647.

Corcoran, E., & Walsh, D. (2003). Obstructive asphyxia: a cause of excess mortality in psychiatric patients. *Irish Journal of Psychological Medicine, 20*(3), 88–90.

Cyr, C. (2012). Canadian paediatric society. Injury prevention committee. Preventing choking and suffocation in children. *Abridged version: Paediatric Child Health, 17*(2), 91–92.

Foltran, F., Ballali, S., Passali, F. M., et al. (2012). Foreign bodies in the airways: a meta-analysis of published papers. *International Journal of Pediatric Otorhinolaryngology, 76*(Suppl. 1), S12–S19.

Parachute Preventing Injuries Saving Lives (2012). Retrieved from: <http://www.parachutecanada.org/safekidsCanada.>

Registered Nurses' Association of Ontario (2014). *Working with families to promote safe sleep for infants 0-12 months of age.* Toronto, ON: Registered Nurses' Association of Ontario. Retrieved from: <http://www rnao.ca/bpg/guidelines>.

Safekids.org. (2013). *Choking and Strangulation Prevention Tips.* Retrieved from: <http://www.safekids.org/sites/default/files/documents/choking_and_strangulation_prevention_tips.pdf.>

Shah, A., & Buckley, L. (2011). The current status of methods used by the elderly for suicides in England and Wales. *Journal of Injury and Violence Research, 3*(2), 68–73.

Shields, B. J., Pollack-Nelson, C., & Smith, G. A. (2011). Pediatric submersion events in portable above-ground pools in the United States, 2001-2009. *Pediatrics, 128*(1), 45–52.

Skinner, R., & McFaull, S. (2012). Suicide among children and adolescents in Canada: trends and sex differences, 1980-2008. *Canadian Medical Association Journal, 184*(9), 1029–1034.

Susy Safe Working Group. (2012). The Susy Safe project overview after the first four years of activity. *International Journal of Pediatric Otorhinolaryngology, 76*(Suppl. 1), S3–S11.

Vennemann, B., Bajanowski, T., Karger, B., et al. (2005). Suffocation and poisoning-the hard hitting side of Munchausen syndrome by proxy. *International Journal of Legal Medicine, 119*, 98–102.

Vennemann, M., Hense, H. W., Bajanowski, T., et al. (2012). Bed sharing and the risk of sudden infant death syndrome: can we resolve the debate? *Journal of Pediatrics, 160*(1), 44–48, e2.

Wolf, B. C., & Harding, B. E. (2011). Household furniture tip-over deaths of young children. *Journal of Forensic Science, 56*(4), 918–921.

Risk for Suicide

Kathleen L. Patusky, MA, PhD, RN, CNS

NANDA-I

Definition

Vulnerable to self-inflicted, life threatening injury

Related Factors (r/t)

Behavioral

Changing a will; giving away possessions; history of suicide attempt; impulsiveness; making a will; marked change in attitude; marked change in behavior; marked change in school performance; purchase of a gun; stockpiling medication; sudden euphoric recovery from major depression

Demographic

Age (e.g., older people, young adult males, adolescents); divorced status; ethnicity (e.g., white, Native American); male gender; widowed

Physical

Chronic pain; physical illness; terminal illness

Psychological

Family history of suicide; guilt; history of childhood abuse (e.g., physical, psychological, sexual); homosexual youth; psychiatric disorder; substance abuse

Situational

Access to weapon; adolescents living in nontraditional settings (e.g., juvenile detention center, prison, halfway house, group home); economically disadvantaged; institutionalization; living alone; loss of autonomy; loss of independence; relocation; retired

Social

Cluster suicides; disciplinary problems; disrupted family life; grieving; helplessness; hopelessness; insufficient social support; legal difficulty; loneliness; loss of important relationship; social isolation

Verbal

Reports desire to die; threats of killing self

NOC (Nursing Outcomes Classification)

Suggested NOC Outcomes

Depression Level; Impulse Self-Control; Loneliness Severity; Mood Equilibrium; Risk Detection; Suicide Self-Restraint

Example NOC Outcome with Indicators

Suicide Self-Restraint as evidenced by the following indicators: Expresses feelings/Refrains from attempting suicide/Verbalizes suicidal ideas/Controls impulses. (Rate the outcome and indicators of **Suicide Self-Restraint:** 1 = never demonstrated, 2 = rarely demonstrated, 3 = sometimes demonstrated, 4 = often demonstrated, 5 = consistently demonstrated [see Section I].)

Consider using one of the measures of suicide risk that are available for clients: Nurses' Global Assessment of Suicide Risk (Cutcliffe & Barker, 2004); Center for Epidemiological Studies Depression Scale measures depressed mood level (Chiu et al, 2010); Beck Suicide Intent Scale identifies a strong intent to die (Astruc et al, 2004); Suicide Assessment Checklist (Rogers et al, 2002).

Client Outcomes

Client Will (Specify Time Frame)

- Not harm self
- Maintain connectedness in relationships
- Disclose and discuss suicidal ideas if present; seek help
- Express decreased anxiety and control of impulses
- Talk about feelings; express anger appropriately
- Refrain from using mood-altering substances
- Obtain no access to harmful objects
- Yield access to harmful objects
- Maintain self-control without supervision

S

NIC (Nursing Interventions Classification)

Suggested NIC Interventions

Anxiety Reduction; Coping Enhancement; Crisis Intervention; Delusion Management; Mood Management; Substance Use Prevention; Suicide Prevention; Support System Enhancement; Surveillance

Example NIC Activities—Suicide Prevention

Determine presence and degree of suicidal risk; Encourage patient to seek out care providers to talk as urge to harm self occurs

Nursing Interventions and *Rationales*

The American Psychiatric Nurses Association (APNA, 2015) has adapted a set of essential competencies for psychiatric nurses, all of which can be useful for generalist nurses. These competencies have been incorporated below.

- Before implementing interventions in the face of suicidal behavior, nurses should examine their own emotional responses to incidents of suicide to ensure that interventions will not be based on countertransference reactions. EBN: *Understanding of nurses' responses to suicidal clients can facilitate suicide prevention and recovery (Talseth & Gilje, 2011; APNA, 2015).*
- Pursue an understanding of suicide as a phenomenon at all levels of nursing practice. Elements to be considered include the terminology used with suicidality and self-harm phenomena, the epidemiology of suicide, the risk and protective influences on suicide, and the evidence-based best practices in preventing and responding to suicidality (APNA, 2015).
- Assess for suicidal ideation when the history reveals the following: depression, substance abuse; bipolar disorder, schizophrenia, anxiety disorders, post-traumatic stress disorder, dissociative disorder, eating disorders, substance use disorders, antisocial or other personality disorders; attempted suicide, current or past; recent stressful life events (divorce and/or separation, relocation, problems with children); recent unemployment; recent bereavement; adult or childhood physical or sexual abuse; gay, lesbian, or bisexual gender orientation; family history of suicide, history of chronic trauma. *Clinicians should be alert for suicide when the aforementioned factors are present in asymptomatic persons (APA, 2015; Li et al, 2011).* EB: *In a 10-year longitudinal study, 83% of persons who committed suicide received health care within the previous year; only 24% had been diagnosed with a mental disorder in the 4 weeks prior to death. Medical specialty and primary care accounted for the most common visits (Ahmedani et al, 2014).* Assess all medical clients and clients with chronic illnesses, traumatic injuries, or pain for their perception of health status and suicidal ideation. *Medical clients who perceived their health to be poor or who were in chronic pain were significantly more likely to report current suicidal ideation.* EB: *Research, including systematic review, support the association of both type 1 and type 2 diabetes with an increase in suicidal ideation (Ceretta et al, 2012; Pompili et al, 2014). Myocardial infarction has been connected with higher suicide rates, especially during the first month after discharge, and with impaired prognosis (Larsen, 2013). Persons living with HIV/AIDS who had depressive symptoms and low life satisfaction were at significantly higher risk of suicide (Davis et al, 2011).*
- Assess the client's ability to enter into a no-suicide contract. Contract (verbally or in writing) with the client for no self-harm if the client is appropriate for a contract; recontract at appropriate intervals. *Discussing feelings of self-harm with a trusted person provides relief for the client. A contract gets the subject out in the open and places some of the responsibility for safety with the client.* CEB: *Some clients are not appropriate for a contract: those under the influence of drugs or alcohol or unwilling to abstain from substance use, and those who are isolated or alone without assistance to keep the environment safe (Hauenstein, 2002). If the client will not contract, the risk of suicide should be considered higher.* CEBN: *Note: Although contracting is a common practice in psychiatric care settings, research has suggested that self-harm is not prevented by contracts. Thorough, ongoing assessment of suicide risk is necessary, whether or not the client has entered into a no-self-harm contract. Contracts may not be appropriate in community settings (McMyler & Pryjmachuk, 2008).*
- Be alert for warning signs of suicide: making statements such as, "I can't go on," "Nothing matters anymore," "I wish I were dead"; becoming depressed or withdrawn; behaving recklessly; getting affairs in order and giving away valued possessions; showing a marked change in behavior, attitudes, or appearance; abusing drugs or alcohol; suffering a major loss or life change. *Suicide is rarely a spontaneous decision. In the days and hours before people kill themselves, clues and warning signs usually appear.*
- Take suicide notes seriously and ask if a note was left in any previous suicide attempts. Consider themes of notes in determining appropriate interventions. *Clients who leave a suicide note may be at higher risk of future completed suicide in the future. A note should be viewed as indication of a failed but serious attempt.*
- Question family members regarding the preparatory actions mentioned. *Clinicians should be alert for suicide when these factors are present in asymptomatic persons (APA, 2015).*
- Determine the presence and degree of suicidal risk. A number of questions will elicit the necessary information: Have you been thinking about hurting or killing yourself? How often do you have these thoughts and how long do they last? Do you have a plan? What is it? Do you have access to the means to carry out that plan? How likely is it that you could carry out the plan? Are there people or things that could prevent you from hurting yourself? What do you see in your future a year from now? Five years from now? What do you expect would happen if you died? What has kept you alive up to now? CEB: *Using the acronym SAL, the nurse can evaluate the client's suicide plan for its specificity (how detailed and clear is the plan?), availability (does the client have immediate access to the planned means?), and lethality*

S

(could the plan be fatal, or does the client believe it would be fatal?). Assessment of reasons for living is another important part of evaluating suicidal clients (Malone et al, 2000).

- Observe, record, and report any changes in mood or behavior that may signify increasing suicide risk and document results of regular surveillance checks. EB: *Suicidal ideation often is not continuous; it may decrease, then increase in response to negative thinking or exposure to stressors (e.g., family visits). Documentation of surveillance will alert all members of the health care team to changes in the clients' potential risk for suicide so they may be prepared to respond in the event of suicidal behavior (APNA, 2015).*
- Develop a positive therapeutic relationship with the clients; do not make promises that may not be kept. *Be aware that some clients may offer to self-disclose if the nurse will promise not to tell anyone what they have said. Clarify with the clients that anything they share will be communicated only to other staff but that secrets cannot be kept.* EBN: *Nurses reconnect suicidal clients with humanity by guiding the client, helping them learn how to live, and helping them connect appropriately with others. Positive support can buffer against suicide, whereas conflictual interactions can increase suicide risk (Hirsch & Barton, 2011; APNA, 2015).*
- Express desire to help client. Provide education about suicide and the effectiveness of intervention. Validate the client's experience of psychological pain while maintaining a safe environment for the client. *The nurse must reconcile their goal of preventing suicide with a recognition of the client's goal to alleviate their psychological pain (APNA, 2015).*
- ▲ Refer for mental health counseling and possible hospitalization if evidence of suicidal intent exists, which may include evidence of preparatory actions (e.g., obtaining a weapon, making a plan, putting affairs in order, giving away prized possessions, preparing a suicide note). EB: *Clients vary in the preparation for suicide attempts, and professional assessment is required to determine the need for hospitalization (APA, 2015). The following interventions may be instituted.*
- Perform risk assessment for possible suicidality on admission to the hospital and thereafter during hospitalization. Alert treatment team to level of risk. *Risk assessment includes evaluating each client's risk factors, ameliorating factors, stated suicidal intent, mental status, history of physical or psychological trauma, triggers that prompt distress, tendency to minimize or exaggerate symptoms, sources of assistance, warning signs of acute risk, and history of previous suicidal or self-harm behavior (APNA, 2015).*
- Determine client's need for supervision and assign a hospitalized client to a room located near the nursing station. *Close assignment increases ease of observation and availability for a rapid response in the event of a suicide attempt (APNA, 2015).*
- Search the newly hospitalized client and the client's personal belongings for weapons or potential weapons and hoarded medications during the inpatient admission procedure, as appropriate. Remove dangerous items. *Clients who are intent on suicide may bring the means with them. Action is necessary to maintain a hazard-free environment and client safety (APNA, 2015).*
- Limit access to windows and exits unless locked and shatterproof, as appropriate. *Suicidal behavior may include attempts to jump out of windows or to escape the unit to find other means of suicide (e.g., gaining roof access for a jump). Hospitals should ensure that exits are secure.*
- Monitor the client during the use of potential weapons (e.g., razor, scissors). *Clients with suicidal intent may take advantage of any opportunity to harm themselves (APNA, 2015).*
- Increase surveillance of a hospitalized client at times when staffing is predictably low (e.g., staff meetings, change of shift report, periods of unit disruption). *Clients who remain intent on suicide will be watchful of periods when staff surveillance lessens to permit completion of a suicide plan.*
- Ensure that all oncoming staff members have adequate information to assist the client, using the acronym SBARR: situation (current status, observations), background (relevant client history), assessment (including nurse's current risk assessment and relevant lab findings), recommendations (what the nurse beliefs is necessary going forward), and response feedback (verification of oncoming staff member's understanding) (APNA, 2015).
- ▲ If imminent suicide is suspected or an attempt has occurred, call for assistance and do not leave the client alone. Client and staff safety will be served by assistance in the response. The client may attempt additional self-harm if left alone.
- Place the client in the least restrictive, safe, and monitored environment that allows for the necessary level of observation. Assess suicidal risk at least daily and more frequently as warranted. *Close observation of the client is necessary for safety as long as intent remains high. Suicide risk should be assessed at frequent intervals to adjust suicide precautions and limitations on the client's freedom of movement and to ensure*

S

that restrictions continue to be appropriate. **EB:** *Inpatient root cause analyses of suicide attempts and environmental safety checklists for units can be helpful in maintaining safety (Mills et al, 2008; APNA, 2015).*

- Consider strategies to decrease isolation and opportunity to act on harmful thoughts (e.g., use of a sitter). **CEB:** *Clients have reported feeling safe and having their hope restored in response to close observation (Bowers & Park, 2001).*
- Explain suicide precautions and relevant safety issues to the client and family (e.g., purpose, duration, behavioral expectations, and behavioral consequences). **CEB:** *Suicide precautions may be viewed as restrictive. Clients have reported the loss of privacy as distressing (Bowers & Park, 2001).*

▲ Refer for treatment and participate in the management of any psychiatric illness or symptoms that may be contributing to the client's suicidal ideation or behavior. *Psychiatric disorders have been associated with suicidal behavior. Symptoms of the disorder may require treatment with antidepressant, antipsychotic, or antianxiety medications.* **EB:** *A systematic review has shown a highly significant effect for cognitive behavior therapy in reducing suicidal behavior (Tarrier et al, 2008).*

▲ Verify that the client has taken medications as ordered (e.g., conduct mouth checks after medication administration). *The client may attempt to hoard medications for a later suicide attempt.*

▲ Maintain increased surveillance of the client whenever use of an antidepressant has been initiated or the dose increased. Antidepressant medications take anywhere from 2 to 6 weeks to achieve full efficacy. *During that period the client's energy level may increase, although the depression has not yet lifted, which increases the potential for suicide.*

- Involve the client in treatment planning and self-care management of psychiatric disorders. *Self-care management promotes feelings of self-efficacy, particularly for clients with depression. Suicidal ideation may occur in response to a sense of hopelessness, a sense that the client has no control over life circumstances. The more clients participate in their own care, the less powerless and hopeless they feel.* Refer to the care plan for **Powerlessness.**
- Explore with the client all circumstances and motivations related to the suicidality. Listen to the client's own views on his or her problems. **EB:** *Primary reasons for suicide attempts were found to be feelings of loneliness or hopelessness, and mental illness/psychological problems (APA, 2015).*
- Explore with the client all perceived consequences that could act as a barrier to suicide (e.g., effect on family, religious beliefs). **CEB:** *The most common barrier to suicide is consequences to family members (Bell, 2000).*
- Keep discussion oriented to the present and future. *Clients under stress have difficulty focusing their thoughts, which leads to a sense of being overwhelmed by problems. Focusing on the present and future helps the client to address problem solving with regard to current stressors.*
- Discuss plans for dealing with suicidal ideation in the future (e.g., how to identify precipitating factors, whom to contact, where to go for help, how to respond to desire for self-harm). *Clients are supported in self-care management when they are helped to identify actions they can take if suicidal ideation recurs.*

- Assist the client in identifying a network of supportive persons and resources (e.g., clergy, family, care providers). **EB:** *Social support and positive events were found to have a protective support against suicidal ideation (Kleiman et al, 2014).*

▲ Refer family members and friends to local mental health agencies and crisis intervention centers if the client has suicidal ideation or a suspicion of suicidal thoughts exists. *Clients at risk should receive evaluation and help (APA, 2015).*

▲ Document client behavior in detail to support outpatient commitment or an overnight psychiatric observation program for an actively suicidal client. *Involuntary outpatient commitment can improve treatment, reduce the likelihood of hospital readmission, and reduce episodes of violent behavior in persons with severe psychiatric illnesses. Overnight psychiatric observation followed by outpatient referral also can be an effective alternative to traditional hospitalization without leading to an increase in suicide gestures or attempts.*

- Utilize cognitive-behavioral techniques that help the client to modify thinking styles that promote depression, hopelessness, and a belief that suicide is a valid means of escaping the current situation. *Suicide has been shown to be associated with constriction in cognitive style, leading to decreased problem solving and information processing.* **EB:** *Cognitive behavioral therapy has been shown to be effective in decreasing suicide attempts with improvement in problem-solving skills (Ghahramanlou-Holloway et al, 2012).*
- Engage the client in group interventions that can be useful to address recurrent suicide attempts. *Group therapy was shown to decrease suicidality.*
- With the client's consent, facilitate family-oriented crisis intervention. Family-oriented crisis intervention can clarify stresses and allow assessment of family dynamics. **EBN:** *An educational intervention addressing*

ability to care, stress levels, and attitudes toward the suicidal family member was effective in promoting attitudes toward and ability to care for a suicidal family member (Sun et al, 2014).

- Involve the family in discharge planning (e.g., illness/medication teaching, recognition of increasing suicidal risk, client's plan for dealing with recurring suicidal thoughts, community resources). *Suicidal clients often are ambivalent about hurting themselves; they may not want to die so much as to escape an intolerable situation. Consequently they often leave clues about their state of mind.* EBN: *Family members must learn before clients leave the hospital how to respond to clues early, support the treatment regimen, and encourage the client to initiate the emergency plan. Nurses help in guiding families through the process (Sun et al, 2014).*
- ▲ Before discharge from the hospital, ensure that the client has a supply of ordered medications, has a plan for outpatient follow-up, understands the plan or has a caregiver able and willing to follow the plan, and has the ability to access outpatient treatment. *Clients may be discharged before they have recovered substantial functional ability and may have difficulty concentrating on the plan for follow-up. They may need the assistance of others to ensure that prescriptions are filled, that they attend appointments, or that they have transportation to the outpatient care setting.*
- ▲ In the event of successful suicide, refer the family to a therapy group for survivors of suicide. Recommended clinical interventions include addressing psychological distress, normalizing denial as an effective coping strategy, working with concerns about family disintegration, and helping families deal with stigmatization. EB: *Psychoeducational support group participants found relief in sharing a personal narrative of their suicide bereavement with others (Feigelman & Feigelman, 2011a, 2011b).*
- See the care plans for Risk for self-directed **Violence, Hopelessness,** and Risk for **Self-Mutilation.** *Clients with suicidal ideation often are reacting to a feeling of hopelessness.*

Pediatric

- The preceding interventions may be appropriate for pediatric clients.
- Use brief self-report measures to improve clinical management of at-risk cases. CEBN: *The Home, Education, Activities, Drug use and abuse, Sexual behavior, and Suicidality and depression (HEADSS) instrument has been found useful in suicide risk assessment of adolescents (Biddle et al, 2010).*
- Recognize that the developmental issues of childhood and adolescence may heighten suicide risks and involve different issues from those with adults. Assess specific stressors for the pediatric client, including bullying. EBN: *The experience of being bullied can contribute to suicidality (Cooper et al, 2012).* CEBN: *A model accounting for 41.9% of adolescents' suicide risk showed that negative life events and rumination contributed to suicidal risk behaviors, whereas resilience and social support could decrease the risk (Thanoi et al, 2010).*
- Assess for exposure to suicide of a significant other. CEB: *Among risk factors of previous psychiatric history, poor psychosocial function, dysphoric mood, and psychomotor restlessness, suicide of a significant other was shown to create risk for adolescents diagnosed with adjustment disorder (Pelkonen et al, 2005).*
- Be alert to the presence of school victimization around lesbian, gay, bisexual, and transgender issues and be prepared to advocate for the client. EBN/EB: *Male adolescents experience greater levels of depression and suicidal ideation in response to high rates of LGBT school victimization (Hatzenbuehler, 2011; Russell et al, 2011; Lea et al, 2014).*
- Evaluate for the presence of self-mutilation and related risk factors. Refer to care plan for Risk for **Self-Mutilation** for additional information. *Self-mutilation and suicidality may co-occur.*
- Be aware that complete overlap does not exist between suicidal behavior and self-mutilation. The motivation may be different (ending life rather than coping with difficult feelings), and the method is usually different. CEB: *In one study, about half of the participants reported both attempted suicide and self-mutilation; in the other half there was no overlap in types of acts (Bolognini et al, 2003).*
- Involve the adolescent in multimodal treatment programs. CEBN: *A systematic review identified individual, family, group, and psychopharmacological therapies as being used for treatment; however, limited research exists to determine which are most effective (Pryjmachuk & Trainor, 2010). Cognitive behavior therapy was cited as showing promise in one study included in a systematic review, but further study was recommended (Robinson et al, 2011).*
- Before discharge from the hospital, ensure that the client's parent has a supply of ordered medications, has a plan for outpatient follow-up, has a caregiver who understands the plan or is able and willing to follow the plan, and has the ability to access outpatient treatment. CEB: *A compliance enhancement intervention (including contracting interviews with parent and adolescent and telephone contacts) improved*

S

attendance at follow-up appointments only when barriers to service were controlled (e.g., delays in getting appointments, placement on a waiting list, inability to switch therapists, problems with insurance coverage) (Spirito et al, 2002).

- Parental education groups can influence suicide risk factors. CEB: *A program of parent education groups focused on improved communication skills and relationships with adolescents. Students in the intervention group reported increased maternal care, decreased conflict with parents, decreased substance abuse, and decreased delinquency (Toumbourou & Gregg, 2002).*
- Support the implementation of school-based suicide prevention programs. *School nurses can be key to early intervention.* EB: *School-based suicide prevention programs have been shown in systematic review to improve knowledge, attitude, and help-seeking behavior, with some reports of decreased suicidal ideation (Cusimano & Sameem, 2011). A randomized controlled trial including more than 11,000 students in the European Union were divided into three groups: a question and refer group, a mental health awareness group, and a professional screening group. No differences between the groups showed up at 3 months. At 12 months the mental health awareness group showed significant reduction in suicide attempts and severe suicidal ideation (Wasserman et al, 2015).*

Geriatric

- Evaluate the older client's mental and physical health status and financial stressors. EB: *Depression in particular is more prevalent in persons with chronic medical conditions, including cardiac disease, diabetes mellitus, cancer, and more. Psychological distress, daily hassles, and marital status, along with chronic illnesses and substance abuse, have been associated with suicidal ideation (Bosse et al, 2011; Shelef et al, 2014).*
- Explore with client any concerns or pressures (physical and financial) regarding ability to secure support of medical care, especially perceived pressures about being a burden on family. EB: *"Perceived burdensomeness" has been found to be a risk factor of older adults' suicidality, whether clinical depression is present or not, accounting for 68.3% of variance of suicidal ideation (Jahn et al, 2011). The presence of stressful life events in the previous year and the presence of untreated major depression were also found to increase suicidal behavior (Pompili et al, 2014).*
- Conduct a thorough assessment of clients' medications. EB: *The use of psychotropic medications, especially long-term use and high doses of benzodiazepines, has been significantly associated with suicidal ideation or death thoughts (Bosse et al, 2011).*
- When assessing suicide risk factors, incorporate a higher degree of risk for older men and for some older adults who have lost a loved one in the previous year. CEB: *Although mortality for oldest old adults (80+) has increased, the suicide mortality has not decreased. In one study, oldest old men had the highest increase in suicide risk after death of a partner (more so than oldest old women) and took a longer time to recover from the death of a spouse (Erlangsen et al, 2004). Suicide rate may be rising among men older than age 65, and marriage may no longer be the protective factor it was once considered to be (Lamprecht et al, 2005).*
- Explore triggers of and barriers to suicidal behavior, with particular attention to real and perceived losses (e.g., professional role, health). EB: *A qualitative study found that older adults' reflections preceding their suicide attempt included loss of a significant other, loneliness, loss of control, and unwillingness to live under these conditions (Bonnewyn et al, 2014). "Perceived burdensomeness" has been found to be a risk factor of older adults' suicidality, whether clinical depression is present or not, accounting for 68.3% of variance of suicidal ideation (Jahn et al, 2011).*
- An older adult who shows self-destructive behaviors should be evaluated for dementia. EB: *Reviews of older adult psychiatric care for both the medical and psychiatric communities emphasize the possible overlap of depression, dementia, and suicidality (DeMers et al, 2013).*
- ▲ Advocate for the older client with other professionals in securing treatment for suicidal states. Primary care providers have been noted to underrecognize and undertreat older adult clients with depression. EB: *In a 10-year longitudinal study, 83% of persons who committed suicide received health care within the previous year; only 24% had been diagnosed with a mental disorder in the 4 weeks prior to death. Medical specialty and primary care accounted for the most common visits (Ahmedani et al, 2014).*
- Encourage physical activity in older adults. EB: *Suicide and sleep disturbances have been linked. Exercise has been associated with improved sleep and lower suicide risk (Davidson et al, 2013).*
- ▲ Refer older adults in primary care settings for care management. EBN: *The Depression Care for Patients at Home (Depression CAREPATH) program provided assistance for medical and surgical homebound clients as a routine part of clinical practice (Bruce et al, 2011).*

- Consider telephone contacts as an effective intervention for suicidal older adults. EB: *One study predicted that, over a 10-year period, telephone and chat services could avoid about 36% of suicides and attempts in a high-risk population with a modest effect on quality-adjusted-life-years (Pil et al, 2013).*

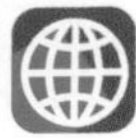

Multicultural

- Assess for the influence of cultural beliefs, norms, and values on the client's perceptions of suicide, as well as on the nurse's perception and approach to suicide. EBN: *A qualitative study of suicidal ideation in Korean college students found that the facilitators of suicidal ideation included physical, psychological, and societal factors. Inhibitors were religious and cultural factors. Buddhism and Confucianism influenced reason not to attempt suicide (Jo et al, 2011).* EB: *A systematic review of psychological autopsies across multiple countries concluded that cultural influences in the diagnosis of a mental disorder might account for the variance in cases without a psychiatric diagnosis (Milner et al, 2013).*
- Identify and acknowledge the stresses unique to culturally diverse individuals. *Financial difficulties and maintaining cultural values are two of the most common family stressors in women of color.* EB: *Acculturative stress and perceived discrimination, moderated by hopelessness, can increase vulnerability to suicide. A strong ethnic identity can serve as a buffer (Polanco-Roman & Miranda, 2013).*
- Identify and acknowledge unique cultural responses to stressors in determining sensitive interventions to prevent suicide. CEB: *In a randomized controlled trial, the Mexican American Problem Solving (MAPS) program addressed depression symptoms of immigrant Mexican women and their fourth- and fifth-grade children using home visits and after-school programs. Family problem-solving communication improved, and children's depression symptoms decreased (Cowell et al, 2009).* Encourage family members to demonstrate and offer caring and support to each other. EB: *Connectedness had been identified as a culture-based protective factor against suicide among young Alaska natives (Mohatt et al, 2011).*
- Validate the individual's feelings regarding concerns about the current crisis and family functioning. *Validation lets the client know that the nurse has heard and understood what was said, and it promotes the nurse-client relationship (APNA, 2015).*

Home Care

- Communicate the degree of risk to family and caregivers; assess the family and caregiving situation for ability to protect the client and to understand the client's suicidal behavior. Provide the family and caregivers with guidelines on how to manage self-harm behaviors in the home environment. *Client safety between home visits is a nursing priority. Family and caregivers may become frightened by the client's suicidal ideation, may be angry at the client's perceived lack of self-control, or may feel as if they are walking on eggshells awaiting another suicide attempt.*
- Assess risk factors in the home. *The presence of a gun must be determined. Safe gun ownership should address the five Ls: locked, loaded, little children, feeling low, learned owner (Pinholt et al, 2014).*
- If the client's suicidal ideation intensifies, or if a suicide plan with access to means becomes evident, institute an emergency plan for mental health intervention. CEB: *More than a quarter (29%) of clients who had previously self-harmed died within 3 months of discharge from psychiatric care and 36% had missed their last service appointment. Measures that may prevent suicide pacts in the mentally ill include the effective treatment of depression and closer supervision in both inpatient and community settings (Hunt et al, 2009).*
- Identify the client's concerns and implement interventions to address the consequences of disability in a client with medical illness. EB: *Depression, perceived social support, and disability have been found to be predictors of suicidal ideation. Lower levels of family support have been implicated in higher levels of suicidal ideation (Park et al, 2014).* Refer to the care plans for **Hopelessness** and **Powerlessness.**

▲ Refer for homemaker or psychiatric home health care services for respite, client reassurance, and implementation of a therapeutic regimen. *Respite decreases the high degree of caregiver stress that goes with the responsibility of caring for a person at risk for suicide.* EBN: *The Depression Care for Patients at Home (Depression CAREPATH) program provided assistance for medical and surgical homebound clients as a routine part of clinical practice (Bruce et al, 2011).*

▲ If the client is on psychotropic medications, assess the client's and family's knowledge of medication administration and side effects. Teach as necessary. *Knowledge of the medical regimen promotes compliance and promotes safe use of medications.*

▲ Evaluate the effectiveness and side effects of medications and adherence to the medication regimen. Review with the client and family all medications kept in the home; encourage discarding of old

S

prescriptions. Monitor the amount of medications ordered/provided by the health care provider; limiting the amount of medications to which the client has access may be necessary. *Accurate clinical feedback improves the health care provider's ability to prescribe an effective medical regimen specific to the client's needs. At home, clients may have greater access to medications, including old prescriptions that may be used to overdose.*

Client/Family Teaching and Discharge Planning

- Establish a supportive relationship with family members. EBN: *Family members experience a great deal of stress around suicidal ideation and benefit from nurses' support (Sun et al, 2014).*
- Explain all relevant symptoms, procedures, treatments, and expected outcomes for suicidal ideation that is illness based (e.g., depression, bipolar disorder). CEBN: *The Health Belief Model identifies perceived barriers and perceived susceptibility to disease as powerful predictors of clients' motivation in taking action to prevent disease and participate in self-care management (Pender et al, 2010).*
- Teach the family how to recognize that the client is at increased risk for suicide (changes in behavior and verbal and nonverbal communication, withdrawal, depression, or sudden lifting of depression). EBN: *A client may be at peace because a suicide plan has been made and the client has the energy to carry it out. Therefore, when depression lifts, increased vigilance is necessary (Sun et al, 2014).*
- Provide written instructions for treatments and procedures for which the client will be responsible. EBN: *A written record provides a concrete reference so that the client and family can clarify any verbal information that was given (Sun et al, 2014).*
- Instruct the client in coping strategies (assertiveness training, impulse control training, deep breathing, progressive muscle relaxation). CEBN: *Suicidal ideation may be triggered by stress and painful emotions. Once clients are able to identify these triggers, they need to learn how to respond to them more effectively through assertiveness, impulse control, or relaxation techniques, as appropriate (Lakeman & FitzGerald, 2008).*
- Teach cognitive-behavioral activities, such as active problem solving, reframing (reappraising the situation from a different perspective), or thought stopping (in response to a negative thought, picturing a large stop sign and replacing the image with a prearranged positive alternative). Teach the client to confront his or her own negative thought patterns (or cognitive distortions), such as catastrophizing (expecting the very worst), dichotomous thinking (perceiving events in only one of two opposite categories), or magnification (placing distorted emphasis on a single event). *Cognitive-behavioral activities address clients' assumptions, beliefs, and attitudes about their situations and foster modification of these elements to be as realistic and optimistic as possible. Through cognitive-behavioral interventions, clients become more aware of their cognitive choices in adopting and maintaining their belief systems and thereby exercise greater control over their own reactions (Hagerty & Patusky, 2011).*
- Provide the client and family with phone numbers of appropriate community agencies for therapy and counseling. The National Alliance on Mental Illness (NAMI) is an excellent resource for client and family support. *Continuous follow-up care should be implemented; therefore, the method to access this care must be given to the client (NAMI, 2012).*

REFERENCES

Ahmedani, B. K., Simon, G. E., Stewart, C., et al. (2014). Health care contacts in the year before suicide death. *Journal of General Internal Medicine*, *29*(6), 870–877. [Epub 2014 Feb 25].

American Psychiatric Association (APA), (2015). *Practice guidelines for the treatment of psychiatric disorders: Compendium*, <http://psychiatryonline.org/guidelines.>

American Psychiatric Nurses Association. (2015). *Psychiatric-mental health nurse essential competencies for assessment and management of individuals at risk for suicide.* Retrieved from <http://www.apna.org/i4a/pages/index.cfm?pageid=5684.>

Astruc, B., et al. (2004). A history of major depressive disorder influences intent to die in violent suicide attempters. *J Clin Psychiatr*, *65*, 690.

Bell, M. A. (2000). *Losing connections: a process of decision-making in late-life suicidality* [doctoral dissertation]. Tucson: University of Arizona.

Biddle, V. S., et al. (2010). Identification of suicide risk among rural youth: implications for the use of HEADSS. *Journal of Pediatric Health Care*, *24*(3), 152.

Bolognini, M., et al. (2003). Adolescents' self-mutilation: relationship with dependent behaviour. *Swiss J Psychol*, *62*(4), 241.

Bonnewyn, C. A., Shah, C. A., Bruffaerts, R., et al. (2014). Reflections of older adults on the process preceding their suicide attempt: a qualitative approach. *Death Studies*, *38*(6–10), 612–618.

Bosse, C., et al. (2011). Suicidal ideation, death thoughts, and use of benzodiazepines in the elderly population. *Can J Community Ment Health*, *30*, 1.

Bowers, L., & Park, A. (2001). Special observation in the care of psychiatric inpatients: a literature review. *Issues in Mental Health Nursing*, *22*, 769.

Bruce, M. L., et al. (2011). Depression care for patients at home (Depression CAREPATH): intervention development and implementation, Part 1. *Home Healthc Nurs*, *29*, 416.

Ceretta, L. B., Reus, G. Z., Abelaira, H. M., et al. (2012). Increased prevalence of mood disorders and suicidal ideation in type 2 diabetic patients. *Acta Diabetologica*, *49*(Suppl. 1), S227–S234.

Chiu, S., et al. (2010). Validation of the center for epidemiologic studies depression scale in screening for major depressive disorder among retired firefighters exposed to the world trade center disaster. *Journal of Affective Disorders*, *121*(3), 212–219.

Cooper, G. D., Clements, P. T., & Holt, K. E. (2012). Examining childhood bullying and adolescent suicide: implications for school nurses. *Journal of School Nursing*, *28*(4), 275–283.

Cowell, J. M., et al. (2009). Clinical trial outcomes of the Mexican American Problem Solving Program (MAPS). *Hispanic Health Care Int*, *7*, 178.

Cusimano, M. D., & Sameem, M. (2011). The effectiveness of middle and high school-based suicide prevention programmes for adolescents: a systematic review. *Injury Prevention*, *17*, 43–49.

Cutcliffe, J. R., & Barker, P. (2004). The nurses' global assessment of suicide risk (NGASR): developing a tool for clinical practice. *Journal of Psychiatric and Mental Health Nursing*, *11*(4), 393.

Davidson, C. L., Babson, K. A., Bonn-Miller, M. O., et al. (2013). The impact of exercise on suicide risk: examining pathways through depression, PTSD, and sleep in an inpatient sample of veterans. *Suicide & Life-Threatening Behavior*, *43*(3), 279–289.

Davis, S. J., et al. (2011). Recognizing suicide risk in consumers with HIV/AIDS. *Journal of Rehabilitation*, *77*, 14.

DeMers, S., Dinsio, K., & Carlson, W. (2014). Psychiatric care of the older adults: an overview for primary care. *Medical Clinics of North America*, *98*(5), 1145–1168.

Erlangsen, A., et al. (2004). Loss of partner and suicide risks among oldest old: a population-based register study. *Age and Ageing*, *33*(4), 378–383.

Feigelman, B., & Feigelman, W. (2011a). Suicide survivor groups: comings and goings, Part I. *Illn Crisis Loss*, *19*, 57.

Feigelman, B., & Feigelman, W. (2011b). Suicide survivor groups: comings and goings, Part II. *Illn Crisis Loss*, *19*, 165.

Ghahramanlou-Holloway, M., Bhar, S. S., Brown, G. K., et al. (2012). Changes in problem-solving appraisal after cognive therapy for the prevention of suicide. *Psychological Medicine*, *42*(6), 1185–1193.

Hagerty, B., & Patusky, K. (2011). Mood disorders: depression and mania. In K. M. Fortinash & P. A. Holoday-Worret (Eds.), *Psychiatric mental health nursing* (5th ed.). St Louis: Mosby.

Hatzenbuehler, M. L. (2011). The social environment and suicide attempts in lesbian, gay, and bisexual youth. *Pediatrics*, *127*, 896.

Hauenstein, E. J. (2002). Case finding and care in suicide: children, adolescents, and adults. In M. A. Boyd (Ed.), *Psychiatric nursing: contemporary practice* (2nd ed.). Philadelphia: Lippincott Williams & Wilkins.

Hirsch, J., & Barton, A. (2011). Positive social support, negative social exchanges, and suicidal behavior in college students. *Journal of American College Health: J of ACH*, *59*(5), 393–398.

Hunt, I. M., While, D., Windfuhr, K., et al. (2009). Suicide pacts in the mentally ill: a national clinical survey. *Psychiatry Research*, *167*(1–2), 131–138.

Jahn, D. R., et al. (2011). The mediating effect of perceived burdensomeness on the relation between depressive symptoms and suicide ideation in a community sample of older adults. *Aging and Mental Health*, *15*, 214.

Jo, K., An, G. J., & Sohn, K. (2011). Qualitative content analysis of suicidal ideation in Korean college students. *Collegian (Royal College of Nursing, Australia)*, *18*, 87.

Kleiman, E. M., Riskind, J. H., & Schaefer, K. E. (2014). Social support and positive events as suicide resiliency factors: examination of synergistic buffering effects. *Archives of Suicide Research*, *18*(2), 144–155.

Lakeman, R., & FitzGerald, M. (2008). How people live with or get over being suicidal: a review of qualitative studies. *Journal of Advanced Nursing*, *64*, 114.

Lamprecht, H. C., et al. (2005). Deliberate self-harm in older people revisited. *International Journal of Geriatric Psychiatry*, *20*, 1090.

Larsen, K. K. (2013). Depression following myocardial infarction—an overseen complication with prognostic importance. *Danish Medical Journal*, *60*(8), B4689.

Lea, T., deWit, J., & Reynolds, R. (2014). Minority stress in lesbian, gay, and bisexual young adults in Australia: associations with psychological distress, suicidality, and substance use. *Archives of Sexual Behavior*, *43*(8), 1571–1578.

Li, Z., et al. (2011). Attributable risk of psychiatric and socio-economic factors for suicide from individual-level, population-based studies: a systematic review. *Social Science and Medicine*, *72*, 608.

Malone, K. M., et al. (2000). Protective factors against suicidal acts in major depression: reasons for living. *The American Journal of Psychiatry*, *157*, 1084.

McMyler, C., & Pryjmachuk, S. (2008). Do "no-suicide" contracts work? *Journal of Psychiatric and Mental Health Nursing*, *15*, 512.

Mills, P. D., et al. (2008). National patient safety goals. Inpatient suicide and suicide attempts in Veterans Affairs hospitals. *Joint Comm J Qual Patient Saf*, *34*, 482.

Milner, A., Sveticic, J., & DeLeo, D. (2013). Suicide in the absence of mental disorder? A review of psychological autopsy studies across countries. *International Journal of Social Psychiatry*, *59*(6), 545–554.

Mohatt, N. V., Fok, C. C., Burket, R., et al. (2011). Assessment of awareness of connectedness as a culturally-based protective factor for Alaska native youth. *Cultural Diversity and Ethnic Minority Psychology*, *17*(4), 444–455.

NAMI: *National Alliance on Mental Illness*. Retrieved Oct 11, 2012, from <http://www.nami.org/.>

Park, J., Han, M., Kim, M., et al. (2014). Predictors of suicidal ideation in older individuals receiving home-care services. *International Journal of Geriatric Psychiatry*, *29*(4), 367–376.

Pelkonen, M., et al. (2005). Suicidality in adjustment disorder: clinical characteristics of adolescent outpatients. *European Child and Adolescent Psychiatry*, *14*, 174.

Pender, N. J., Murdaugh, C. L., & Parsons, M. A. (2010). *Health promotion in nursing practice* (6th ed.). Upper Saddle River, NJ: Prentice-Hall.

Pil, L., Pauwels, K., Muijzers, E., et al. (2013). Cost effectiveness of a helpline for suicide prevention. *Journal of Telemedicine & Telecare*, *19*(5), 273–281.

Pinholt, E. M., Mitchell, J. D., Butler, J. H., et al. (2014). "Is There a Gun in the Home?" Assessing the risks of gun ownership in older adults. *Journal of the American Geriatrics Society*, *62*(6), 1142–1146.

Polanco-Roman, L., & Miranda, R. (2013). Culturally related stress, hopelessness, and vulnerability to depressive symptoms and suicidal ideation in emerging adulthood. *Behavior Therapy*, *44*, 74–87.

Pompili, M., Forte, A., Lester, D., et al. (2014). Suicide risk in type 1 diabetes mellitus: a systematic review. *Journal of Psychosomatic Research*, *76*(5), 352–360.

Pompili, M., Innamorati, M., DiVottorio, C., et al. (2014). Sociodemographic and clinical differences between suicide ideators and attempters: a study of mood disordered patients 50 years and older. *Suicide & Life Threatening Behavior*, *44*, 34–45.

Pryjmachuk, S., & Trainor, G. (2010). Helping young people who self-harm: perspectives from England. *Journal of Child and Adolescent Psychiatric Nursing*, *23*(2), 52.

Robinson, J., Hetrick, S. E., & Martin, C. (2011). Preventing suicide in young people: systematic review. *Australian and New Zealand Journal of Psychiatry*, *45*, 3–26.
Rogers, J. R., Lewis, M. M., & Subich, L. M. (2002). Validity of the suicide assessment checklist in an emergency crisis center. *Journal of Counseling and Development*, *80*, 493.
Russell, S. T., et al. (2011). Lesbian, gay, bisexual, and transgender adolescent school victimization: implications for young adult health and adjustment. *The Journal of School Health*, *81*(5), 223.
Shelef, A., Hiss, J., Cherkashin, G., et al. (2014). Psychosocial and medical aspects of older adult suicide completers in Israel: a 10-year survey. *International Journal of Geriatric Psychiatry*, *29*(8), 846–851.
Spirito, A., et al. (2002). An intervention trial to improve adherence to community treatment by adolescents after a suicide attempt. *Journal of the American Academy of Child and Adolescent Psychiatry*, *41*(4), 435.
Sun, F., Chiang, C., Lin, Y., et al. (2014). Short-term effects of a suicide education intervention for family caregivers of people who are suicidal. *Journal of Clinical Nursing*, *23*(102), 91–102.
Talseth, A., & Gilje, F. L. (2011). Nurses' responses to suicide and suicidal patients: a critical interpretive synthesis. *Journal of Clinical Nursing*, *20*, 1651.
Tarrier, N., Taylor, K., & Gooding, P. (2008). Cognitive-behavioral interventions to reduce suicidal behavior. *Behavior Modification*, *32*, 77.
Thanoi, W., et al. (2010). The adolescent suicide risk behaviors: a model of negative life events, rumination, emotional distress, resilience, and social support. *Pac Rim Int J Nurs Res*, *14*, 187.
Toumbourou, J. W., & Gregg, M. E. (2002). Impact of an empowerment-based parent education program on the reduction of youth suicide risk factors. *The Journal of Adolescent Health*, *31*, 277.
Wasserman, D., Hoven, C. W., Wasserman, C., et al. (2015). School-based suicide prevention programmes: the SEYLE cluster-randomized, controlled trial. *The Lancet*, <http://www.mdlinx.com/internal-medicine/print-preview.cfm/5874195>; January 15 online.

Delayed Surgical recovery

Nicole Jones, MSN, FNP-BC

NANDA-I

Definition

Extension of the number of postoperative days required to initiate and perform activities that maintain life, health, and well-being

Defining Characteristics

Discomfort; evidence of interrupted healing of surgical area; excessive time required for recuperation; impaired mobility; inability to resume employment; loss of appetite; postpones resumption of work; requires assistance for self-care

Related Factors (r/t)

American Society of Anesthesiologists Physical Status classification score ≥3; diabetes mellitus; edema at surgical site; extensive surgical procedure; extremes of age; history of delayed wound healing; impaired mobility; malnutrition; obesity; pain; perioperative surgical site infection; persistent nausea; persistent vomiting; pharmaceutical agent; postoperative emotional response; prolonged surgical procedure; psychological disorder in postoperative period; surgical site contamination; trauma at surgical site

NOC (Nursing Outcomes Classification)

Suggested NOC Outcomes

Endurance; Infection Severity; Mobility; Pain Control; Self-Care: Activities of Daily Living (ADLs); Wound Healing: Primary Intention; Surgical Recovery: Convalescence/Immediate Postoperative

Example NOC Outcome with Indicators

Surgical Recovery/Convalescence as evidenced by the following indicators: Extent of physiological, psychological, and role function following discharge from postanesthesia care to the final postoperative clinic visit/Vital signs/Performance of normal activities, self-care activities. (Rate the outcome and indicators of **Surgical Recovery:** 1 = severe deviation from normal range, 2 = substantial deviation from normal range, 3 = moderate deviation from normal range, 4 = mild deviation from normal range, 5 = no deviation from normal range [see Section I].)

S

Client Outcomes

Client Will (Specify Time Frame)

- Have surgical area that shows evidence of healing: no redness, induration, draining, or immobility
- State that appetite is regained
- State that no nausea is present
- Demonstrate ability to move about
- Demonstrate ability to complete self-care activities
- State that no fatigue is present
- State that pain is controlled or relieved after nursing interventions
- Resume employment activities/activities of daily living (ADLs)
- State no depression or anxiety related to surgical procedure

NIC (Nursing Interventions Classification)

Suggested NIC Interventions

Incision Site Care; Nutrition Management; Pain Management; Self-Care Assistance; Surgical Assistance

Example NIC Activities—Incision Site Care

Teach the client and/or the family how to care for the incision, including signs and symptoms of infection; Inspect the incision site for redness, swelling, or signs of dehiscence or evisceration

Nursing Interventions and *Rationales*

- Encourage smoking cessation prior to surgery. EB: *Smoking cessation improves tissue oxygenation and improves pulmonary function. A meta-analysis shows that smoking cessation leads to improved surgical recovery and fewer complications (Mills et al, 2011).*
- Preoperatively, perform a thorough assessment of the client, including risk factors. Allow time to be with the client, and actively listen to client's concerns and questions about care, functional status, and recovery. CEB: *Assessment of clients preoperatively by nursing and medical staff is an important part of the surgical experience to ensure that appropriate interventions are used and recovery from surgery is as quick as possible (Layzell, 2008).* EB: *Clients with higher presurgery levels of emotional distress appear to be at greater risk for experiencing higher levels of postsurgery side effects (Sadati et al, 2013).* Assess for the presence of medical conditions and treat appropriately before surgery. If the client is diabetic, maintain normal blood glucose levels before surgery. CEB: *High blood glucose levels slow healing and increase risk of infection. The American Diabetes Association (ADA) recommends that blood glucose should be less than 180 mg/dL for people in the hospital or having surgery. For some, the goal is less than 110 mg/dL (ADA, 2014).* EB: *In some cases, complications and poor client satisfaction and joint function can be directly attributable to obesity (Choong & Dowsey, 2011).*
- Carefully assess client's use of dietary supplements such as feverfew, fish oil, ginkgo biloba, garlic, ginseng, ginger, valerian, kava, St. John's wort, ephedra (Ma huang or metabolite), and echinacea. It is recommended that all clients be advised to stop all dietary supplements at least 1 week before major surgical or diagnostic procedures. EB: *Due to increasingly complicated medication regimens and polypharmacy, it is important to assess client's use of herbal and dietary supplements, because they can cause medication reactions or have unintended medical side effects (Nieva et al, 2012).* EB: *Herbal remedies are common in clients presenting for anesthesia. Because of the potential interactions between anesthetic drugs or techniques and such medication, it is important for anesthetists to be aware of their use (Bajwa & Panda, 2012; Kaye, 2014).* Assess and treat for depression and anxiety in a client before surgery and postoperatively. EB: *Clients with depression or anxiety are less likely to regain former level of functioning or following surgery (Barry et al, 2011).* CEB: *Clients with higher levels of preoperative anxiety and depression report increased postoperative pain, nausea, and fatigue (Montgomery et al, 2010).* EB: *Early identification of clients with high preoperative anxiety allows the nurse to prepare postoperative interventions and support systems that may lessen or alleviate client suffering (Yilmaz et al, 2012).*
- Play music of the client's choice preoperatively, intraoperatively, and postoperatively. EBN: *Listening to self-selected music during the preoperative period can effectively reduce anxiety levels and should be a useful*

tool for preoperative nursing (Ni et al, 2012). EBN: *Results of this research provide evidence to support the use of music and/or a quiet rest period to decrease pain and anxiety. The interventions pose no risks and have the benefits of improved pain reports and decreased anxiety (Pittman & Kridli, 2011).*

- Consider using healing touch and other mind-body-spirit interventions such as stress control, therapeutic massage, and imagery in the perianesthesia setting. EBN: *Research shows that use of holistic therapies in the perioperative setting can decrease pain, surgical trauma, and anesthesia complications, leading to increased client satisfaction with health care (Selimen & Andsoy, 2011).* EB: *Therapeutic touch may help restore client's integrity by providing consolation and a sense of safety (Airosa et al, 2013).* Use warmed cotton blankets to reduce heat loss during surgery. EB: *Monitoring of body temperature and avoidance of unintended perioperative hypothermia through active and passive warming measures are the keys to preventing its complications (Hart et al, 2011).*
- Postoperatively, discuss with surgeon vital sign parameters, signs, and symptoms that could indicate early postoperative infection. EB: *Surgical site infections are a leading cause of prolonged hospitalization, which increase cost of care and are associated with poorer outcomes (Tanner et al, 2013).*
- Use careful aseptic technique when caring for wounds. EBN: *Handwashing continues to be the most important factor in reducing health care–associated infection, but the use of an aseptic technique will further cut the risk of infection (Harrington, 2014).* EBN: *Dressings should be changed by nurses who are trained in antiseptic, non-touch technique.*
- Clients should be allowed to shower after surgery to maintain cleanliness if not contraindicated because of the presence of pacemaker wires. EB: *In an analysis of existing studies, it was determined that there was no statistically significant increase in wound infection related to early bathing. Avoiding washing may have an adverse effect on the wound due to accumulation of sweat or dirt at the site. The decision to bathe the client immediately postoperatively should be specific to surgical type and site (Toon et al, 2013).* Promote early ambulation and deep breathing. CEB: *When looking across all of the intervention types, the most frequently reported positive outcomes were associated with measures of ambulatory ability (Chudyk et al, 2009). Deep breathing clears the lungs and prevents pneumonia.*
- The client should be provided with a complete, balanced therapeutic diet after the immediately postoperative period (24 to 48 hours). EBN: *Optimal wound healing requires adequate nutrition. Nutrition deficiencies impede the normal processes that allow progression through stages of wound healing. Malnutrition has also been related to decreased wound tensile strength and increased infection rates (Collins & Sloan, 2013).*
- Encourage the client to use prayer as a form of spiritual coping if this is comfortable for the client. EB: *Prayer has been shown to reduce pain intensity and provide a stabilizing effect on cardiovascular measurements (Jegindø et al, 2013).*
- Carefully assess functional status of client postoperatively using a fall-risk stratification tool such as the Morse Fall Scale to identify clients at high risk for fall. EBN: *The Morse Fall Scale has been validated in numerous studies, and helps to identify clients at high risk for falls. All clients identified as high risk should have increased monitoring and nursing and be placed under increased safety precautions until discharge, regardless of functional improvement (Baek et al, 2014).*
- See the care plans for **Anxiety,** Acute **Pain, Fatigue,** Risk for deficient **Fluid** volume, Risk for **Perioperative Positioning** injury, Impaired physical **Mobility,** and **Nausea.**

S

Pediatric

- Encourage children to ask questions about their procedures and postoperative expectations regarding pain, function, and long-term social and emotional care needs. EBN: *Children often report having little input or understanding of their medical conditions and requirements for surgical and functional interventions. Parents and children report higher levels of satisfaction, decreased preoperative anxiety, and better experiences if they are given the opportunity preoperatively to discuss all aspects of the surgery, including realistic postoperative expectations (Bray et al, 2012; Alanazi, 2014).*
- Teach imagery and encourage distraction for children for postsurgical pain relief. EBN: *Distraction decreases pain in children undergoing painful procedures (Helgadottir & Wilson, 2014; Ha & Kim, 2013).*

Geriatric

- Perform a thorough preoperative assessment, including a cardiac, social support, and skin assessment. EB: *The condition of the client's skin should be noted before and after the procedure and should be fully documented using an objective evaluation tool such as the Braden scale to allow early identification of older clients at higher risk for developing surgical site infections or other skin breakdown (Cohen et al, 2012).* CEB: *Older clients, those with preoperative comorbidities, and those without a caregiver at home experience delays in functional recovery and discharge. These findings support the addition of functional recovery and social support risk items to the preoperative cardiac surgery risk assessment (Anderson et al, 2006).*

- Routinely assess pain in postoperative clients using a pain scale that is appropriate for clients with impaired cognition or inability to verbalize. EB: *The Pain Assessment in Advanced Dementia (PAINAD) and Pain Assessment Checklist for Seniors with Limited Ability to Communicate (PACSLAC) have been validated for reliability (Herr, 2011).*
- Serially evaluate the client's vital signs, including temperature. Know what is normal and abnormal for each client. Check baseline vital signs and monitor trends. EB: *Physiologic changes of aging often result in lower baseline body temperatures and decreased heart rates, and prevent the older client from developing fever. Medications, such as blood pressure agents, may prevent client from having an increased heart rate (Gonik et al, 2011).*
- Provide tools such as clocks, calendars, and other orientation tools to help prevent delirium in the postoperative or extended-stay client. Ensure that hearing aids and glasses are also available as needed. EB: *Older adults are at higher risk for developing delirium following anesthesia or prolonged hospitalization. Delirious clients are at higher risk for falls or other adverse events, have longer inpatient stays, and have higher mortality rates (Mouchoux et al, 2011).*
- Offer spiritual support. EB: *Religiousness is related to significantly fewer depressive symptoms, better quality of life, less cognitive impairment, and less perceived pain. Clinicians should consider taking a spiritual history and ensuring that spiritual needs are addressed among older clients in rehabilitation settings (Lucchetti et al, 2011).*

Home Care

- The preceding interventions may be adapted for the home setting.
- Provide supportive telephone calls from nurse to client as a means of decreasing anxiety and providing the psychosocial support necessary for recovery from surgery. CEB: *A study of clients who underwent surgery for breast cancer showed that a telephone intervention 1 week after surgery was helpful and the timing was appropriate. The intervention group showed significantly better body image, worried less about the future, and had fewer postoperative side effects than the control group (Salonen et al, 2009).*

Client/Family Teaching and Discharge Planning

- Provide discharge planning and teaching in language that is appropriate to the client and caregiver's education and literacy level. EBN: *Do not use technical or medical jargon, and be aware that clients and caregivers may to be reluctant to ask for explanation or clarification due to embarrassment and may verbalize dishonestly understanding. Allow the client to repeat their understanding of the discharge plan (Ross, 2013).*
- Meet with client and caregivers to create a discharge plan that includes measurable goals for functional activities of daily living and pain levels, discuss expectations for recovery, and address signs and symptoms of postoperative complications. EBN: *In a study on successful discharge planning, it was found that plans that were detailed and precise, and addressed client and caregiver feedback, situations, preferences, and agreement with the care plan had greater satisfaction and plan adherence (Tomura et al, 2011).*
- Provide individualized teaching plans for the client with an ostomy. Assess client's ability to manage basic needs: (1) maintenance of a pouching seal for a consistent, predictable wear time; (2) maintenance of peristomal skin integrity; and (3) social and professional support of the client. Referrals for home wound care or nursing visits may be necessary to help client maintain hygiene and prevent readmission for complications. EBN: *Careful assessment of client's ability to manage colostomy will help the nurse anticipate possible problems with routine care requiring close follow-up and referrals for skilled care following discharge (Walker & Lachman, 2013).*

REFERENCES

Airosa, F., Falkenberg, T., Ohlen, G., et al. (2013). Tactile massage or healing touch: caring touch for patients in emergency care—a qualitative study. *European Journal of Integrative Medicine*, *5*(4), 374–381.

Alanazi, A. (2014). Reducing anxiety in preoperative patients: a systematic review. *British Journal of Nursing*, *23*(7), 387–393.

Anderson, J., Petersen, N., Kistner, C., et al. (2006). Determining predictors of delayed recovery and the need for transitional cardiac

S

rehabilitation after cardiac surgery. *Journal of American Academy of Nurse Pracitioners, 18*(8), 386–392.

ADA: American Diabetes Association. (2014). Standards of medical care in diabetes—2014. *Diabetes Care, 37*(s.1).

Baek, S., Piao, J., Jinshi, J., et al. (2014). Validity of the morse fall scale implemented in an electronic medical record system. *Journal of Clinical Nursing, 23*(17/18), 2434–2441.

Bajwa, S. J., & Panda, A. (2012). Alternative medicine and anesthesia: implications and considerations in daily practice. *Ayu [Ayu], 33*(4), 475–480.

Barry, L., Murphy, T., & Gill, T. (2011). Depression and functional recovery after a disabling hospitalization in older persons. *Journal of the American Geriatrics Society, 59*(7), 1320–1325.

Bray, L., Callery, P., & Kirk, S. (2012). A qualitative study of the pre-operative preparation of children, young people and their parents' for planned continence surgery: experiences and expectations. *Journal of Clinical Nursing, 21*(13/14), 1964–1973.

Choong, P., & Dowsey, M. (2011). Update in surgery for osteoarthritis of the knee. *International Journal of Rheumatological Disease, 14*(2), 167–174.

Chudyk, A. M., Jutai, J., Petrella, R., et al. (2009). Systematic eview of hip fracture rehabilitation practices in the elderly. *Archives of Physical Medicine and Rehabilitation, 90*(2), 246–262.

Cohen, R., Lagoo-Deenadayalan, S. A., Heflin, M. T., et al. (2012). Exploring predictors of complication in older surgical patients: a deficit accumulation index and the Braden Scale. *Journal of the American Geriatrics Society, 60*(9), 1609–1615.

Collins, N., & Sloan, C. (2013). Back to basics: nutrition as part of the overall wound treatment plan. *Ostomy/Wound Management, 59*(4), 16–19.

Gonik Chester, J., & Rudolph, J. L. (2011). Vital signs in older patients: age-related changes. *Journal of the American Medical Directors Association, 12*(5), 337–343.

Ha, Y., & Kim, H. (2013). The effects of audiovisual distraction on children's pain during laceration repair. *International Journal of Nursing Practice, 19*(Suppl. 3), 20–27.

Harrington, P. (2014). Prevention of surgical site infection. *Nursing Standard, 28*(48), 50–58.

Hart, S., Bordes, B., Hart, J., et al. (2011). Unintended perioperative hypothermia. *The Oschner Journal, 11*(3), 259–270.

Helgadottir, H., & Wilson, M. (2014). A randomized controlled trial of the effectiveness of educating parents about distraction to decrease postoperative pain in children at home after tonsillectomy. *Pain Management Nursing, 15*(3), 632–640.

Herr, K. (2011). Pain Assessment Strategies in Older Patients. *The Journal of Pain, 15*(11), 1069–1202.

Jegindø, E., Vase, L., Skewes, J., et al. (2013). Expectations contribute to reduced pain levels during prayer in highly religious participants. *Journal of Behavioral Medicine, 36*(4), 413–426.

Kaye, A. (2014). Critical care medicine and the emerging challenges of dietary supplements, including herbal products. *Critical Care Medicine, 42*(4), 1014–1016.

Layzell, M. (2008). Current interventions and approaches to postoperative pain management. *British Journal of Nursing (Mark Allen Publishing), 17*(7), 414–419.

Lucchetti, G., Lucchetti, A., Granero, L., et al. (2011). Religiousness affects mental health, pain and quality of life in older people in an outpatient rehabilitation setting. *Journal of Rehabilitation Medicine, 43*(4), 316–322.

Mills, E., Eyawo, O., Lockhart, I., et al. (2011). Smoking cessation reduces postoperative complications: a systematic review and meta-analysis. *American Journal of Medicine, 124*(2), 144–154.

Montgomery, G., Schnur, J., Erblich, J., et al. (2010). Presurgery psychological factors predict pain, nausea, and fatigue one week after breast cancer surgery. *Journal of Pain and Symptom Management, 39*(6), 1043–1052.

Mouchoux, C., Rippert, P., Duclos, A., et al. (2011). Impact of a multifaceted program to prevent postoperative delirium in the elderly: the CONFUCIUS stepped wedge protocol. *BMC Geriatrics, 11*(25).

Ni, C., Tsai, W., Lee, L., et al. (2012). Minimising preoperative anxiety with music for day surgery patients—a randomised clinical trial. *Journal of Clinical Nursing, 21*(5), 620–625.

Nieva, R., Safavynia, S., Lee Bishop, K., et al. (2012). Herbal, vitamin, and mineral supplement use in patients enrolled in a cardiac rehabilitation program. *Journal of Cardiopulmonary Rehabilitation & Prevention, 32*(5), 270–277.

Pittman, S., & Kridli, S. (2011). Music intervention and preoperative anxiety: an integrative review. *International Nursing Review, 58*(2), 157–163.

Ross, J. (2013). Preoperative assessment and teaching of postoperative discharge instructions: the importance of understanding health literacy. *Journal of PeriAnestheisa Nursing, 38*(5), 318–320.

Sadati, L., Pazouki, A., Mehdizadeh, A., et al. (2013). Effect of preoperative nursing visit on preoperative anxiety and postoperative complications in candidates for laparoscopic cholecystectomy: a randomized clinical trial. *Scandinavian Journal of Caring Sciences, 27*(4), 994–998.

Salonen, P., Tarkka, M., Kellokumpu-Lehtinen, P., et al. (2009). Telephone intervention and quality of life in patients with breast cancer. *Cancer Nursing, 32*(3), 177–190.

Selimen, D., & Andsoy, I. (2011). The importance of a holistic approach during the perioperative period. *AORN Journal, 93*(4), 482–490.

Tanner, J., Padley, W., Kiernan, M., et al. (2013). A benchmark too far: findings from a national survey of surgical site infection surveillance. *Journal of Hospital Infection, 83*(2), 87–91.

Tomura, H., Yamamoto-Mitani, N., Nagata, S., et al. (2011). Creating an agreed discharge: discharge planning for clients with high care needs. *Journal of Clinical Nursing, 20*(3/4), 444–453.

Toon, C. D., Sinha, S., Davidson, B. R., et al. (2013). Early versus delayed post-operative bathing or showering to prevent wound complications. *The Cochrane Library*, Retrieved from: <http://onlinelibrary.wiley.com/doi/10.1002/14651858.CD010075.pub2/pdf/standard>; published online 12 OCT.

Walker, C., & Lachman, V. (2013). Gaps in the discharge process for patients with an ostomy: an ethical perspective. *Medsurg Nursing, 22*(1), 61–64.

Yilmaz, M., Sezer, H., Gurler, H., et al. (2012). Predictors of preoperative anxiety in surgical inpatients. *Journal of Clinical Nursing, 21*(7), 956–964.

S

Risk for delayed Surgical recovery

Nicole Jones, MSN, FNP-BC

NANDA-I

Definition

Vulnerable to an extension of the number of postoperative days required to initiate and perform activities that maintain life, health, and well-being, which may compromise health

Risk Factors

American Society of Anesthesiologists Physical Status classification score ≥3; diabetes mellitus; edema at surgical site; extensive surgical procedure; extremes of age; history of delayed wound healing; impaired mobility; malnutrition; obesity; pain; perioperative surgical site infection; persistent nausea; persistent vomiting; pharmaceutical agent; postoperative emotional response; prolonged surgical procedure; psychological disorder in postoperative period; surgical site contamination; trauma at surgical site

NIC, NOC, Client Outcomes, Nursing Interventions, Client/Family Teaching and Discharge Planning, *Rationales,* and References

See the care plan for Delayed **Surgical** recovery.

Impaired Swallowing

Dennis C. Tanner, PhD, Stephanie C. Christensen, PhD, CCC-SLP, and Betty J. Ackley, MSN, EdS, RN

NANDA-I

Definition

Abnormal functioning of the swallowing mechanism associated with deficits in oral, pharyngeal, or esophageal structure or function

Defining Characteristics

S

First Stage: Oral

Abnormal oral phase of swallow study; choking prior to swallowing; coughing prior to swallowing; drooling; food falls from mouth; food pushed out of mouth; gagging prior to swallowing; inability to clear oral cavity; incomplete lip closure; inefficient nippling; inefficient suck; insufficient chewing; nasal reflux; piecemeal deglutition; pooling of bolus in lateral sulci; premature entry of bolus; prolonged bolus formation; prolonged mealtime with inefficient consumption; tongue action ineffective in forming bolus

Second Stage: Pharyngeal

Abnormal pharyngeal phase of swallow study; alteration in head position; choking; coughing; delayed swallowing; fevers of unknown etiology; food refusal; gagging sensation; gurgling voice quality; inadequate laryngeal elevation; nasal reflux; recurrent pulmonary infection; repetitive swallowing

Third Stage: Esophageal

Abnormal esophageal phase of swallow study; acidic-smelling breath; bruxism; difficulty swallowing; epigastric pain; food refusal; heartburn; hematemesis; hyperextension of head; nighttime awakening; nighttime coughing; odynophagia; regurgitation; repetitive swallowing; reports "something stuck;" unexplained irritability surrounding mealtimes; volume limiting; vomiting; vomitus on pillow

Related Factors

Congenital Defects

Behavioral feeding problem; conditions with significant hypotonia; congenital heart disease; failure to thrive; history of enteral feeding; mechanical obstruction; neuromuscular impairment; protein-energy malnutrition; respiratory condition; self-injurious behavior; upper airway abnormality

Neurological Problems

Achalasia; acquired anatomic defects; brain injury (e.g., cerebrovascular impairment, neurological illness, trauma, tumor); cerebral palsy; cranial nerve involvement; developmental delay; esophageal reflux disease; laryngeal abnormality; laryngeal defect; nasal defect; nasopharyngeal cavity defect; neurological problems; oropharynx abnormality; prematurity; tracheal defect; trauma; upper airway anomaly

NOC (Nursing Outcomes Classification)

Suggested NOC Outcomes

Swallowing Status: Esophageal Phase, Oral Phase, Pharyngeal Phase

Example NOC Outcome with Indicators

Swallowing Status as evidenced by the following indicators: Delivery of bolus to hypopharynx is timed with swallow reflex/Ability to clear oral cavity/Number of swallows appropriate for bolus size and texture/Voice quality/Choking, coughing, gagging/Normal swallow effort. (Rate the outcome and indicators of **Swallowing Status:** 1 = severely compromised, 2 = substantially compromised, 3 = moderately compromised, 4 = mildly compromised, 5 = not compromised [see Section I].)

Client Outcomes

Client Will (Specify Time Frame)

- Demonstrate effective swallowing without signs of aspiration (see defining characteristics above)
- Remain free from aspiration (e.g., lungs clear, temperature within normal range)

NIC (Nursing Interventions Classification)

Suggested NIC Interventions

Aspiration Precautions; Swallowing Therapy

Example NIC Activities—Swallowing Therapy

Assist client to sit in erect position (as close to 90 degrees as possible) for feeding/exercise; Instruct client not to talk during eating, if appropriate

S

Nursing Interventions and *Rationales*

▲ Do not feed clients with impaired swallowing orally until an appropriate diagnostic workup is completed. *Feeding a client who cannot adequately swallow can result in aspiration and possibly death (Forster et al, 2011).*

▲ Ensure proper nutrition by consulting with a health care provider regarding alternative nutrition and hydration when oral nutrition is not safe/adequate. EB: *Nasogastric tube feedings (NGT) and percutaneous endoscopic gastrostomy (PEG) tubes after stroke may reduce death rates (Geeganage et al, 2012). PEG feedings are preferable to NGT when longer term feeding is required (Geeganage et al, 2012).*

▲ Refer to a speech-language pathologist for evaluation and diagnostic evaluation of swallowing to determine swallowing problems and solutions as soon as oral and/or pharyngeal dysphagia is suspected. *Safe nursing care includes a consultation with a speech-language pathologist whenever doubts arise regarding a client's ability to tolerate oral-supported nutrition in any form (Tanner, 2013).*

▲ *To manage impaired swallowing, use a multidisciplinary dysphagia team composed of a speech pathologist, dietitian, nursing, health care provider, and medical staff. A comprehensive assessment from a multidisciplinary dysphagia team can lead to personalized therapeutic interventions that can help the client learn to swallow safely and maintain a good nutritional status (Forster et al, 2011).*

▲ *Observe the following feeding guidelines:*

- ❍ Before giving oral feedings, determine the client's readiness to eat (e.g., alert, able to hold head erect, follow instructions, move tongue in mouth, and manage oral secretions). *If one of these elements is missing, it may be advisable to withhold oral feeding and use enteral feeding for nourishment.*
- ❍ Monitor client during oral feedings and provide cueing as needed to ensure client follows swallowing guidelines/aspiration precautions recommended by speech language pathologist or dysphagia

specialist. NOTE: General aspiration precautions include the following: sit at 90 degrees for all oral feedings; take small bites/sips, slow rate, no straws. However, client specific strategies will be determined via bedside and/or instrumental swallowing evaluation performed by dysphagia specialist. *Postural changes, sensory enhancements, swallow maneuvers, or voluntary controls exerted over the swallow can improve swallow but the use and effectiveness of these treatments will vary systematically with the client's medical diagnosis (Logemann & Larsen, 2012).*

❍ If the client is older or has gastroesophageal reflux disease, ensure the client is kept in an upright posture for an hour after eating. CEB: *An upright posture after eating has been associated with a decreased incidence of pneumonia in older adults (Coleman, 2004).*

- During meals and all oral intake, observe for signs associated with swallowing problems such as coughing, choking, spitting of food, drooling, difficulty handling oral secretions, double swallowing or delay in swallowing, watering eyes, nasal discharge, wet or gurgling voice, decreased ability to move the tongue and lips, decreased mastication of food, decreased ability to move food to the back of the pharynx, slow or scanning speech. CEB: *Perceptual judgments of a clear post-swallow voice quality provided reasonable evidence that aspiration and dysphagia were absent as measured by videofluoroscopy (Waito et al, 2011).*

▲ Watch for uncoordinated chewing or swallowing; coughing immediately after eating or delayed coughing; pocketing of food; wet-sounding voice; sneezing when eating; delay of more than 1 second in swallowing; or a change in respiratory patterns. If any of these signs of dysphagia and/or aspiration is present, remove all food from the oral cavity, stop feedings, and consult with speech and language pathologist and dysphagia team. *Placing a client with suspected dysphagia on NPO (nothing by mouth) status is the strongest measure that can be taken to prevent choking and aspiration (Tanner & Culbertson, 2014).*

▲ If signs of aspiration or pneumonia are present, auscultate lung sounds after feeding. Note new onset of crackles or wheezing, or elevated temperature. CEB: *Bronchial auscultation of lung sounds was shown to be specific in identifying clients at risk for aspiration (Shaw et al, 2004).*

▲ Watch for signs of malnutrition and dehydration and keep a record of food intake. *Clients with dysphagia are at serious risk for malnutrition and dehydration, which can lead to aspiration pneumonia resulting from depressed immune function and weakness, lethargy, and decreased cough.*

▲ Evaluate nutritional status daily. Weigh the client weekly to help evaluate nutritional status. If the client is not adequately nourished, work with the dysphagia team to determine whether the client needs therapeutic feeding only or needs enteral feedings until the client can swallow adequately. CEB: *PEG feedings are preferable to NGT when longer term feeding is required (Geenganage et al, 2010).*

▲ *Assist client in following dysphagia specialist's recommendations and provide open, accurate, and effective communication with dysphagia team regarding client's diet tolerance. Understanding and following dysphagia specialist's recommendations is a pivotal role that nurses play in helping ensure positive dysphagia management outcomes (Tanner & Culbertson, 2014).*

S

▲ Document and notify the health care provider and dysphagia team of changes in medical, nutritional, or swallowing status. *Many negative dysphagia management outcomes can be avoided by ensuring dysphagia communication is accurate, complete, and disseminated among and between health care professionals; nurses are pivotal in this process (Tanner & Culbertson, 2014).*

▲ Work with the client on swallowing exercises prescribed by the dysphagia team. EB: *Exercise programs can improve airway closure, the range of oral or pharyngeal structure movement during swallow, cricopharyngeal opening, and tongue strength (Logemann & Larsen, 2012).*

▲ If needed, provide meals in a quiet environment away from excessive stimuli, such as a community dining room, for some clients who are easily distracted. *A noisy environment can be an aversive stimulus and can decrease effective chewing and swallowing.*

▲ For many adult clients, avoid the use of straws if recommended by the speech pathologist. *Use of straws can increase the risk of aspiration, because straws can result in spilling of a bolus of fluid rapidly in the posterior pharynx.*

▲ Recognize that the client can aspirate oral feedings, even if there are no symptoms of coughing or distress. *This phenomenon is called silent aspiration and is common.* EB: *It is estimated that up to 60% of stroke clients with dysphagia have silent aspiration (Ickenstein et al, 2012).*

▲ Ensure oral hygiene is maintained. EB: *Oral health care including tooth brushing after each meal, cleaning dentures once a day, and consistent professional oral health care reduces the incidence of aspiration pneumonia (van der Maarel-Wierink et al, 2013).*

▲ Check the oral cavity for proper emptying after the client swallows and after the client finishes the meal. Provide oral care at the end of the meal. It may be necessary to manually remove food from the client's mouth. If this is the case, use gloves and keep the client's teeth apart with a padded tongue blade. *Food may become pocketed on the affected side and cause stomatitis, tooth decay, and possible later aspiration.*

▲ Praise the client for successfully following directions and swallowing appropriately. *Praise reinforces behavior and sets up a positive atmosphere in which learning takes place.*

▲ Keep the client in an upright position for 45 minutes to an hour after a meal. CEB: *Matsui and colleagues (2002) found the number of older clients who developed a fever was significantly reduced when clients were kept sitting upright after eating.*

▲ Recognize that impaired swallowing may be caused by the medications the client is taking. Side effects of medications include xerostomia (antidepressants, anticholinergics, antihistamines, bronchodilators, antineoplastic, anti-Parkinson), central nervous system depression (anticonvulsants, benzodiazepines, antispasmodics, antidepressants, antipsychotics), myopathy (corticosteroids, lipid-lowering agents, colchicines), and decreased esophageal sphincter tone (antihistamines, diuretics, opiates, antipsychotics, antihypertensives, anticholinergics). *Medications can cause impaired swallowing in multiple ways.*

▲ For clients receiving mechanical ventilation with a tracheostomy tube, request a referral to speech language pathologist or dysphagia specialist for a instrumental swallowing evaluation before beginning oral diet. *Dysphagia occurs in approximately 50% of clients with a tracheostomy receiving mechanical ventilation; objective swallowing studies are the best way to determine safest oral intake and rule out silent aspiration in these clients (Seckel & Schulenburg, 2011).*

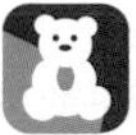

Pediatric

▲ Refer a child who has difficulty swallowing and symptoms such as difficulty manipulating food, delayed swallow response, and pocketing of a bolus of food to speech-language pathologist (or dysphagia specialist) and a dietitian. *Adequate nutrition is extremely important for children to ensure sufficient growth and development of all body systems.*

▲ Consult with speech-language pathologist or dysphagia specialist regarding modifications to nipple; appropriate positioning and feeding strategies; and other therapeutic activities deemed most appropriate based on bedside and instrumental swallowing evaluation. *Speech-language pathologists are trained to evaluate and treat pediatric dysphagia. Consultation with a speech-language pathologist or feeding therapist with pediatric expertise improves the diagnostic utility of a feeding assessment and can result in better outcomes.*

▲ The following are general feeding guidelines. Specific strategies to eliminate aspiration and maximize intake should be individualized and determined by swallowing specialist through bedside and instrumental swallowing evaluation.

• Attempt feedings when infant is in an optimal behavioral feeding state (e.g., awake, alert, and not agitated) and halt feedings if infant is not able to maintain or regain a proper feeding state. *Infants' feeding state can fluctuate rapidly and caregiver's attention to this state can influence feedings (Lau, 2014).*

• In preterm infant, provide opportunities for patterned nonnutritive sucking (NNS). EB: *Although adequate NNS is not sufficient to predict adequacy of oral feeding (Lau, 2014), providing skilled training in patterned NNS has been demonstrated to accelerate the transition from NNS to oral feeding (Lau et al, 2012).*

• In preterm infant, alter nipple flow rate to one that is easily managed by infant to facilitate intake while achieving physiologic stability. CEB: *Increased flow rate should only be considered when doing so assists the infant in obtaining adequate intake while maintaining physiologic stability. Aspiration risk is increased with faster flow rates.*

• Watch for indicators of aspiration and physiologic instability during feeding: coughing, a change in vocal quality or wet vocal quality, perspiration and color changes, sneezing, apnea, and/or increased heart rate and breathing. Infants and children with silent aspiration may only have indicators of increased respiratory mucous, congestion and chronic wheeze or rhonchi, recurrent bronchitis, or recurrent pneumonia (Tutor & Gosa, 2012).

• Watch for warning signs of reflux: sour-smelling breath after eating, sneezing, lack of interest in feeding, crying and fussing extraordinarily when feeding, pained expressions when feeding, and excessive chewing and swallowing after eating. *Many premature and medically fragile children experience growth deficits and respiratory problems from an underlying dysphagia. Some infants may need to work harder to breathe than others and as a result develop a decreased tolerance for food intake. They also demonstrate inconsistent arousal and poor/uncoordinated suck-swallow-breath synchrony. Many of these infants require supplemental tube feedings and the use of special nipples or bottles to boost oral intake.*

- Observe infant's behavior and cues and adjust feeding to promote a safe pleasurable feeding experience while eliminating aspiration and maximizing intake. *Individualize interventions based on infant's cues related to swallowing, breathing, physiologic stability, postural control, and state regulation to help infant maintain or regain stability. Some approaches include reducing noise/light levels, adjusting feeding position, letting infant regulate milk flow, and varying number and/or duration of feedings to reduce adverse events (Lau, 2014).*

Geriatric

▲ Recognize that age-related changes can impact swallowing and these changes have a more pronounced effect when superimposed on disease such as neurological and other chronic medical problems. *Subtle motor changes and age-related decrements in oral moisture, taste, and smell can contribute to less efficient and effective swallowing in older adults (Sura et al, 2012).*

▲ Evaluate medications the client is presently taking and consult with the pharmacist for assistance in monitoring for incorrect doses and drug interactions that could result in dysphagia. *Most older clients take numerous medications, which when taken individually can slow motor function, cause anxiety and depression, and reduce salivary flow. When taken together, these medications can interact, resulting in impaired swallowing function.*

▲ Ensure all nursing home residents are screened for swallowing problems. *It is estimated that up to 40% to 60% of nursing home residents have swallowing problems (Tanner, 2013).*

▲ Encourage and provide good oral hygiene when indicated. EB: *Good oral health care reduces the incidence of aspiration pneumonia (van der Maarel-Wierink et al, 2013).*

▲ Consult with occupational therapist for adaptive equipment when appropriate. *The use of adaptive equipment such as cups without rims and angled utensils can improve outcomes for older clients with dysphagia (Sura et al, 2012).*

▲ Recognize that the older client with dementia may need a longer time to eat and is often easily distracted. Help optimize hydration and nutrition using the following techniques:

- ❍ Encourage six small meals and hydration breaks per day.
- ❍ Offer foods that are sweet, spicy, or sour to increase sensory input.
- ❍ Allow clients to touch food and self-feed, if necessary (Tanner, 2013).
- ❍ Eliminate from the tray or table nonfoods such as salt and pepper, or anything that can be distracting. *Dementia clients are often impulsive and easily distracted.*
- ❍ Keep desserts out of sight until the end of the meal.
- ❍ Offer finger foods to the client who has trouble holding still to eat.
- ❍ Allow clients to eat immediately when they come for the meal.
- ❍ Recognize that the client with advanced dementia, who is unable to swallow, may or may not benefit from enteral tube feedings. *Some dementia clients enter into a catabolic state with negative protein balance, and it may be irreversible. In addition, there is often an increased risk for aspiration pneumonia in the tube fed client.*

S

Home Care

▲ Refer to speech therapy. Speech-language pathologists can work with clients to enhance swallowing ability and teach compensatory strategies.

Client/Family Teaching and Discharge Planning

▲ Teach the client and family exercises prescribed by the dysphagia team.

▲ Teach the client a systematic method of swallowing effectively as prescribed by the dysphagia team.

- Educate the client, family, and all caregivers about rationales for food consistency and choices. *It is common for family members to disregard necessary dietary restrictions and give the client inappropriate foods that predispose to aspiration.*
- Teach the family how to monitor the client to prevent and detect aspiration during eating.

REFERENCES

Coleman, P. R. (2004). Pneumonia in the long-term care setting: etiology, management, and prevention. *Journal of Gerontological Nursing*, *30*(4), 14.

Forster, A., Samaras, N., Gold, G., et al. (2011). Oropharyngeal dysphagia in older adults: a review. *European Geriatric Medicine*, *2*(6), 356–362.

Geeganage, C., Beavan, J., Elender, S., et al. (2012). Interventions for dysphagia and nutritional support in acute and subacute stroke. *Cochrane Database of Systematic Reviews, 10*.

Ickenstein, G. W., Hohlig, C., Proseigel, M., et al. (2012). Prediction of outcome in neurogenic oropharyngeal dysphagia within 72 hours of acute stroke. *Journal of Stroke and Cerebrovascular Disease, 21*(7), 569–576.

Lau, C., Fucille, S., & Gisel, E. G. (2012). Impact of nonnutritive oral motor stimulation and infant massage therapy on oral feeding skills of preterm infants. *Journal of Neonatal-Perinatal Medicine, 5*, 311–317.

Lau, C. (2014). Interventions to improve oral feeding performance of preterm infants. *SIG 13 Perspectives on Feeding and Swallowing (Dysphagia), 23*, 23–25.

Logemann, J. A., & Larsen, K. (2012). Oropharyngeal dysphagia: pathophysiology and diagnosis for the anniversary issue of diseases of the esophagus. *Diseases of the Esophagus, 25*(4), 299–304.

Matsui, T., Yamaya, M., Ohrui, T., et al. (2002). Sitting position to prevent aspiration in bed-bound patients. *Gerontology, 48*(3), 194.

Seckel, M. A., & Schulenburg, K. (2011). Eating while receiving mechanical ventilation. *Critical Care Nurse, 31*(4), 95–97.

Shaw, J. L., et al. (2004). Bronchial auscultation: an effective adjunct to speech and language therapy bedside assessment when detecting dysphagia and aspiration? *Dysphagia, 19*(4), 211.

Sura, L., Madhavan, A., Carnaby, G., et al. (2012). Dysphagia in the elderly: management and nutritional considerations. *Clinical Interventions in Aging, 7*, 287–298.

Tutor, J. D., & Gosa, M. M. (2012). Dysphagia and aspiration in children. *Pediatric Pulmonology, 47*(4), 321–337.

Tanner, D. (2013). CNA observations could save a resident: an interview. *Nursing Assistant. Cengage Learning, 18*(8).

Tanner, D. C., & Culbertson, W. R. (2014). Avoiding negative dysphagia outcomes. *OJIN: The Online Journal of Issues in Nursing, 19*(2).

van der Maarel-Wierink, C. D., Vanobbergen, J. N. O., Bronkhorst, E. M., et al. (2013). Oral healthcare and aspiration pneumonia in frail older people: a systematic literature review. *Gerodontology, 30*(1), 3–9.

Waito, A., Bailey, G. L., Molfenter, S. M., et al. (2011). Voice-quality abnormalities as a sign of dysphagia: validation against acoustic and videofluoroscopic data. *Dysphagia, 26*(2), 125.

Risk for imbalanced body Temperature

Betty J. Ackley, MSN, EdS, RN, and Mary Beth Flynn Makic, PhD, RN, CNS, CCNS, FAAN

NANDA-I

Definition

Vulnerable to failure to maintain body temperature within normal parameters, which may compromise health

Risk Factors

Acute brain injury; alteration in metabolic rate; condition affecting temperature regulation; decreased sweat response; dehydration; extremes of age; extremes of environmental temperature; extremes of weight; inactivity; inappropriate clothing for environmental temperature; increase in oxygen demand; increased body surface area to weight ratio; insufficient nonshivering thermogenesis; insufficient supply of subcutaneous fat; pharmaceutical agent; sedation; sepsis; vigorous activity

NOC, NIC, Client Outcomes, Nursing Interventions, *Rationales,* Client/Family Teaching and Discharge Planning, and References

Refer to care plans for Ineffective **Thermoregulation** (fever), **Hyperthermia,** or **Hypothermia.**

Risk for Thermal injury

Wendie A. Howland, MN, RN-BC, CRRN, CCM, CNLCP, LNCC

NANDA-I

Definition

Vulnerable to extreme temperature damage to skin and mucous membranes, which may compromise health

Risk Factors

Alteration in cognitive functioning; extremes of age; extremes of environmental temperature; fatigue; inadequate protective clothing (e.g., flame-retardant sleepwear, gloves, ear covering); inadequate supervision; inattentiveness; insufficient knowledge of safety precautions (client, caregiver); intoxication (alcohol, drug); neuromuscular impairment; neuropathy; smoking; treatment regimen; unsafe environment

T

NOC (Nursing Outcomes Classification)

Suggested NOC Outcomes

Safe Home Environment; Parenting: Early/Middle/Adolescent Physical Safety

Client Outcomes

Client Will (Specify Time Frame)

- Be free of thermal injury to skin or tissue
- Explain actions he or she can take to protect self and family from thermal injury
- Explain actions he or she can take to protect self and others in the work environment

NIC (Nursing Interventions Classification)

Suggested NIC Interventions

Environmental Management: Safety

Example NIC Activities—Environmental Management: Safety

Identify safety hazards in the environment; Modify the environment to minimize hazards and risk

Nursing Interventions and *Rationales*

- Teach the following interventions to prevent fires in the home, to handle any possible fire, and to have a readily available exit from the home:
  - Avoid plugging several appliance cords into the same electrical socket.
  - Do not use open candles or allow smoking in the home.
  - Keep a fire extinguisher within reach in case a fire should occur.
  - Install smoke alarms on every level of the home and in every sleeping area.
  - Keep furniture and other heavy objects out of the way of doors and windows.
  - Develop a fire escape plan that includes two ways out of every room and an outside meeting place. Practice the escape plan at least twice a year.
- Teach the following activities to homes with small children:
  - Lock up matches and lighters out of sight and reach.
  - Do not leave a hot stove unattended.
  - Do not allow small children to use the microwave until they are at least 7 or 8 years of age.
  - Keep all portable heaters out of children's reach and at least 3 feet away from anything that can burn.
  - Install thermostatic mixer valves in hot water system to prevent extreme hot water causing scalding burns. EB: *A study of the effects of the devices installed in public housing in Scotland identified a lower rate of scalding burns, which saved money (Phillips et al, 2011). Children ages 5 and younger are more than twice as likely to die in a fire as the rest of the population (Safe Kids USA, 2012). In the United States, burns are the third leading cause of unintentional injury death in children aged 1 to 14 years (Bowman et al, 2011).*
- Apply sunscreen as directed on the container when out in the sun. Use sun-blocking clothing, and stay in the shade if possible. *Sunburn predisposes to skin cancer development and premature skin aging. Up to 50% of children have at least one sunburn by the time they are 11 years of age and generally have another sunburn 3 years later (Dusza et al, 2012).*
- Teach the following to prevent fires in the home where medical oxygen is in use:
  - Never smoke in a home where medical oxygen is in use. "No smoking" signs should be posted inside and outside the home.
  - All ignition sources (e.g., matches, lighters, candles, gas stoves, appliances, electric razors, and hair dryers) should be kept at least 10 feet away from the point where the oxygen comes out.
  - Do not wear oxygen while cooking. Oils, grease, and petroleum products can spontaneously ignite when exposed to high levels of oxygen. Also, do not use oil-based lotions, lip balm, or aerosol sprays.
  - Homes with medical oxygen must have working smoke alarms that are tested monthly.
  - Keep a fire extinguisher within reach. If a fire occurs, turn off the oxygen and leave the home.

  - ❍ Develop a fire escape plan that includes two ways out of every room and an outside meeting place. Practice the escape plan at least twice a year. EB: *A study of people who smoked while having medical oxygen in the home found that many of the clients died, and most of them lost their independence following the burn accident augmented by the presence of oxygen (Murabit & Tredget, 2012; Joyner, 2012).*
- Be aware that thermal injury also includes injury from cold materials and environmental conditions, including freezing injury, nonfreezing injury, and hypothermia (Kiss, 2012).
- Provide adequate environmental temperatures. Older clients and others at risk for temperature dysregulation can easily become hypothermic in air-conditioned environments (e.g., a surgical suite) or with inadequate clothing (e.g., patient gowns). *Inadvertent hypothermia is common in surgical procedures (Moola & Lockwood, 2011).*
  - ❍ Monitor temperature in vulnerable clients. Core temperature is the best measure to assess for hypothermia. If a pulmonary artery catheter is not available, use a thermometer calibrated for lower body temperature (Moola & Lockwood, 2011).
  - ❍ Use active warming measures to help clients maintain body temperature (e.g., warming blankets, warm intravenous fluids, forced warm air warming devices, foil wraps, and radiant warmers) as indicated. *Passive devices such as socks or reflective blankets do not impart heat to body tissues (Moola & Lockwood, 2011).*
- Ensure that exposed skin is protected from cold with adequate clothing.
- Monitor for developing cold thermal injury by checking peripheral circulation, temperature, sensation, and fine motor coordination, which decreases as a very early sign of hypothermia. *Preventing progression of thermal injury is critical to client outcomes. Shivering is a late sign and consumes considerable metabolic energy (Soreide, 2014).*
- Check the temperature of all equipment and other materials before allowing them to contact client skin especially if client has increased risk factors for thermal injury.

REFERENCES

Bowman, S., et al. (2011). Trends in hospitalizations associated with pediatric burns. *Injury Prevention: Journal of the International Society for Child and Adolescent Injury Prevention, 17*(3), 166–170.

Dusza, S. W., et al. (2012). Prospective study of sunburn and sun behavior patterns during adolescence. *Pediatrics, 129*(2), 309–317.

Joyner, D. (2012). *Home oxygen can raise burn risk*. HealthDay News. Retrieved February 1, 20145, from: <http://consumer.healthday.com/Article.asp?AID=661193>.

Kiss, T. K. (2012). Critical care for frostbite. *Critical Care Nursing Clinics of North America, 24*, 581–591.

Moola, S., & Lockwood, C. (2011). Effectiveness of strategies for the management and/or prevention of hypothermia within the adult perioperative environment. *International Journal of Evidence-Based Healthcare, 9*, 337–345.

Murabit, A., & Tredget, E. E. (2012). Review of burn injuries secondary to home oxygen. *Journal of Burn Care and Research, 33*(2), 212–217.

Phillips, C., Humphreys, I., & Kendrick, D. (2011). Preventing bath water scalds: a cost-effectiveness analysis of introducing bath thermostatic mixer valves in social housing. *Injury Prevention: Journal of the International Society for Child and Adolescent Injury Prevention, 17*(4), 238–243.

Safe Kids USA. (2012). *Fire prevention for little kids at home*. Retrieved February 1, 2015 from: <http://www.safekids.org/safety-basics/little-kids/at-home/fire-prevention.html>.

Soreide, K. (2014). Clinical and translational aspects of hypothermia in major trauma patients: from pathophysiology to prevention, prognosis, and potential preservation. *Injury, 45*(4), 647–654.

T

Ineffective Thermoregulation

Mary Beth Flynn Makic, PhD, RN, CNS, CCRN, FAAN, and Betty J. Ackley, MSN, EdS, RN

NANDA-I

Definition

Temperature fluctuation between hypothermia and hyperthermia

Defining Characteristics

Cyanotic nail beds; fluctuations in body temperature above and below the normal range; flushed skin; hypertension; increase in body temperature above normal range; increase in respiratory rate; mild shivering; moderate pallor; piloerection; reduction in body temperature below normal range; seizures; skin cool to touch; skin warm to touch; slow capillary refill; tachycardia

Related Factors (r/t)

Extremes of age; fluctuating environmental temperature; illness; trauma

NOC (Nursing Outcomes Classification)

Suggested NOC Outcomes

Thermoregulation; Thermoregulation: Newborn

Example NOC Outcome with Indicators

Thermoregulation as evidenced by the following indicators: Body temperature/Skin temperature/Skin color changes/Hydration/Reported thermal comfort. (Rate the outcome and indicators of **Thermoregulation:** 1 = severely compromised, 2 = substantially compromised, 3 = moderately compromised, 4 = mildly compromised, 5 = not compromised [see Section I].)

Client Outcomes

Client Will (Specify Time Frame)

- Maintain temperature within normal range
- Explain measures needed to maintain normal temperature
- Describe two to four symptoms of hypothermia or hyperthermia
- List two or three self-care measures to treat hypothermia or hyperthermia

NIC (Nursing Interventions Classification)

Suggested NIC Interventions

Temperature Regulation; Temperature Regulation: Inoperative

Example NIC Activities—Temperature Regulation

Institute use of a continuous core temperature-monitoring device, as appropriate; Promote adequate fluid and nutritional intake

Nursing Interventions and *Rationales*

Temperature Measurement

T

- Measure and record the client's temperature using a consistent method of temperature measurement every 1 to 4 hours depending on severity of the situation or whenever a change in condition occurs (e.g., chills, change in mental status). CEB/EB: *Errors in accurate temperature measurement are most often associated with instrument related errors, choice of temperature site chosen for monitoring, and operator error (Barnason et al, 2012; Bridges & Thomas, 2009; Makic et al, 2011; Sessler, 2008).* EBN: *A consistent mode of temperature measurement for accurate trending of body temperature is important for accurate treatment decisions (Davie & Amoore, 2010; Barnason et al, 2012; Hooper et al, 2009). If different devices are used to obtain temperature measurements, the results should not vary more than 0.3° C to 0.5° C (Bridges & Thomas, 2009; Makic et al, 2011).*
- Select core, near core, or peripheral temperature monitoring mode based on ability to obtain an accurate temperature from that site and clinical situation dictating the need for mode of temperature monitoring required for clinical treatment decisions. CEB/EB: *Core temperature is obtained by pulmonary artery catheter and distal esophagus; near core temperature measurements include oral, bladder, rectal, and temporal artery; and peripheral measurements are obtained by skin surface measurements such as measurement in the axilla (Barnason et al, 2012; Jefferies et al, 2011; Davie & Amoore, 2010; Hooper et al, 2009; Sessler, 2008).*
- Caution should be taken in interpreting extreme values of temperature (less than 35° C or greater than 39° C) from a near core temperature site device. EB/EBN: *Accurate oral temperature measurement requires the probe to be placed in the posterior sublingual pocket to provide a reliable near core temperature measurement (Jefferies et al, 2011; Barnason et al, 2012; Ring et al, 2010; Hooper et al, 2009; Sessler, 2008; Torossian, 2008). Evidence is limited in testing the accuracy of temperature measurement devices outside of normal temperature ranges. Research has demonstrated the accuracy of temperature measurement from most*

accurate to least accurate are intravascular (pulmonary artery), distal esophageal, bladder thermistor, rectal, and oral. Research is limited on accuracy of temporal artery measurements outside normal ranges; axillary temperature is accurate in neonates but is not well supported in adults; tympanic membrane measurements and chemical dot thermometers are least accurate and should be avoided in caring for the acutely ill adult client (Barnason et al, 2012; Adam, 2013; Calonder et al, 2010; Davie & Amoore, 2010; Hooper et al, 2009; Makic et al, 2011; O'Grady et al, 2008; Wollerich et al, 2012).

- Evaluate the significance of a decreased or increased temperature. *Normal adult temperature is usually identified as 98.6° F (37°C), but in actuality the normal temperature fluctuates throughout the day. In the early morning it may be as low as 96.4° F (35.8° C) and in the late afternoon or evening as high as 99.1° F (37.3° C) (Becker & Wu, 2010). Disease, injury, or pharmacological agents may impair regulation of body temperature (Dinarello & Porat, 2011; Hooper et al, 2009; Sessler, 2008).*

▲ Notify the health care provider of temperature according to institutional standards or written orders, or when temperature reaches 100.5° F (38.3° C) and above (Saltzberg 2013; O'Grady et al, 2008). Also notify the health care provider of the presence of a change in mental status and temperature greater than 38.3° C or less than 36° C. *A change in mental status may indicate the onset of septic shock (Saltzberg 2013; Dellinger et al, 2013).*

Fever (Pyrexia)

- Recognize that fever is characterized as a temporary elevation in internal body temperature 1° C to 2° C higher than the client's normal body temperature. *A rise in body temperature is an innate immune response to a perceived threat and is regulated by the hypothalamus. Hyperthermia may occur when a client gains heat through either an increase in the body's heat production or is unable to effectively dissipate heat. Hypothermia occurs when a client loses heat or cannot generate heat (Rehman & deBoisblanc, 2013; Kenney et al, 2014; Pitoni et al, 2011; Scrase & Tranter, 2011).*
- Recognize that fever is a normal physiological response to a perceived threat by the body, frequently in response to an infection. EB: *Fever is a deliberate, active thermoregulatory defense action by the body (Kenney et al, 2014). Metabolic heat accelerates the body's antibody production to defend the body and assists the body's cellular repair processes (Scrase & Tranter, 2011). Nursing care should focus on supporting the body's normal physiological response (fever), locating the cause for the fever, and providing comfort (Rehman & deBoisblanc, 2013; Scrase & Tranter, 2011).*

▲ Review client history to include current medical diagnosis, medications, recent procedures/interventions, and review of laboratory analysis for cause of ineffective thermoregulation. EB: *Changes in body temperature, fever, should be explored for possible problems associated with a client's health status (Rehman & deBoisblanc, 2013).*

- Recognize that fever may be low grade (36° C to 38° C) in response to an inflammatory process such as infection, allergy, trauma, illness, or surgery. Moderate to high-grade fever (38° C to 40° C) indicates a more concerted inflammatory response from a systemic infection. Hyperpyrexia (40° C and higher) occurs as a result of damage of the hypothalamus, bacteremia, or an extremely overheated room (Scrase & Tranter, 2011; Kenney et al, 2014). EB: *Interventions to treat fever focus on client comfort, allowing the body to progress through the natural course of fever. Exceptions may exist with the client with hyperpyrexia (Carey, 2010; Scrase & Tranter, 2011).*
- Recognize that fever has a predictable physiological pattern. *The initial phase (cold or chill stage) presents with an increased heart rate, respiratory rate, shivering, pale, cold skin, absence of sweat, and piloerection. As the hypothalamus adjusts, the body temperature shivering ceases, skin becomes warm, and heart rate and respiratory rate remain elevated. The client may complain of thirst, poor appetite, painful muscles, exhaustion, and lethargy. The resolution phase presents with warm, flushed, sweaty skin, reduced shivering, and possible signs of dehydration (Kenney et al, 2014; Rehman & deBoisblanc, 2013; Carey, 2010; Pitoni, et al, 2011; Scrase et al, 2011).*
- Monitor and intervene to provide comfort during a fever by:
  - Obtaining vital signs and accurate intake and output
  - Checking laboratory analysis trends of white blood cell counts and other markers of infection
  - Providing blankets when the client complains of being cold, but removing surplus of blankets when the client is too warm
  - Encouraging fluid and nutrition
  - Limiting activity to conserve energy
  - Providing frequent oral care (Scrase et al, 2011)

T

▲ EBN/EB: *Current evidence that examined the evidence of antipyretic therapies used to treat fever such as administration of antipyretic medications, cooling blankets, and sponge baths found these therapies did not reduce the duration of illness and may even prolong it (Carey, 2010; Hammond & Boyle, 2011; Niven et al, 2013).*

Hypothermia

- Take vital signs frequently, noting changes associated with hypothermia: increased blood pressure, pulse, and respirations that then advance to decreased values as hypothermia progresses. *Mild hypothermia activates the sympathetic nervous system, which can increase the levels of vital signs; as hypothermia progresses, the heart becomes suppressed, with decreased cardiac output and lowering of vital sign readings (Dinarello et al, 2011).*
- Monitor the client for signs of hypothermia (e.g., shivering, cool skin, piloerection, pallor, slow capillary refill, cyanotic nailbeds, decreased mentation, dysrhythmias) (Pitoni et al, 2011).
- See the care plan for **Hypothermia** as appropriate.

Hyperthermia

- Note changes in vital signs associated with hyperthermia: rapid, bounding pulse; increased respiratory rate; and decreased blood pressure, accompanied by orthostatic hypotension, and signs and symptoms of dehydration (Rehman & deBoisblanc, 2013; Dinarello et al, 2011). *Consistent monitoring promotes prevention and early intervention in clients with altered cardiopulmonary status associated with hyperthermia. Hyperthermia is a different etiology than fever, and the cause of the elevated body temperature should be explored for definitive treatment (Rehman & deBoisblanc, 2013).*
- Monitor the client for signs of hyperthermia (e.g., headache, nausea and vomiting, weakness, extreme fatigue, delirium, and coma). *Monitoring for the defining characteristics of hyperthermia allows for early intervention.*
- Adjust clothing to facilitate passive warming or cooling as appropriate.
- See the care plan for **Hyperthermia** as appropriate.

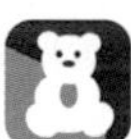

Pediatric

- For routine measurement of temperature, use an electronic thermometer in the axilla in infants younger than 4 weeks; for a child up to 5 years of age, use an electronic thermometer in the axilla or an infrared temporal artery thermometer. EB: *Oral and rectal routes should not be used routinely to measure the temperature of infants to children of 5 years of age (National Institute for Health and Clinical Excellence [NICE], 2013). Tympanic thermometers often provide inaccurate temperature from incorrect placement in the ear canal and presence of cerumen adversely affecting temperature reading (Adam, 2013). Fever strips and pacifier thermometers often provide inaccurate readings (Adam, 2013).*
- Recognize that pediatric clients have a decreased ability to adapt to temperature extremes. Take the following actions to maintain body temperature in the infant/child:
  - Keep the head covered.
  - Use blankets to keep the client warm.
  - Keep the client covered during procedures, transport, and diagnostic testing.
  - Keep the room temperature at 72° F (22.2° C).

The combination of a relatively smaller body surface area, smaller body fluid volume, less well-developed temperature control mechanisms, and smaller amount of protective body fat limits the infant's and child's ability to maintain normal temperatures (NICE, 2013).

- Recognize that the infant and small child are both vulnerable to develop heat stroke in hot weather; ensure that they receive sufficient fluids and are protected from hot environments. *Infants and young children are at risk for heat stroke for many reasons, including a decreased thermoregulatory ability in the young body and the inability to obtain their own fluids.*
- Antipyretic treatments typically are not indicated unless the child's temperature is higher than 38.3° C and may be given to provide comfort. EB: *The use of antipyretics in febrile children should be examined in light of the therapeutic goal for treatment, which may be primarily to improve the child's discomfort (Sullivan & Farrar, 2011; Adam, 2013). A systematic review found combination treatment with ibuprofen and acetaminophen in children older than 6 months may be beneficial in treatment of fever symptoms over one agent alone (Malya, 2013; Purssell, 2011).*

Geriatric

- Do not allow an older client to become chilled. Keep the client covered when giving a bath and offer socks to wear in bed. Be aware of factors such as room temperature (heating/air conditioning), clothing (layered/loose), and fluid intake. *Older adults have a decreased ability to adapt to temperature extremes and need protection from extreme environmental temperatures. The response to cold environment is also compromised with the cutaneous vasoconstrictor response, the shivering process being less effective, and decreased ability to feel cold (McLafferty et al, 2009; Outzen, 2009). Research indicates that this can be traced in part to medications used to treat chronic age-associated diseases and physiology of aging.*
- Recognize that the older client may have an infection without a significant rise in body temperature. *Febrile response to infection was found to be reduced with increasing age, and baseline temperatures were generally lower in older clients (Rehman & deBoisblanc, 2013; Barakzai & Fraser, 2008). This blunted febrile response may lead to delayed diagnosis and treatment; therefore, reviewing all data to include a change in temperature, rather than fever, is important in the care of older clients (Outzen, 2009).*
- Fever does not put the older adult at risk for long-term complications; thus, fever should not be treated with antipyretic agents or other external methods of cooling, unless there is serious heart disease present. CEB: *Exceptions in treating fever should be considered in some older clients with significant cardiovascular disease, because fever may increase metabolic rate by 10% and shivering may double the metabolic rate, greatly increasing the oxygen consumption requirements of the body and creating significant stress on the cardiovascular system (Outzen, 2009).*
- Ensure that older clients receive sufficient fluids during hot days and stay out of the sun. *Older adults may have trouble walking independently to obtain fluids, have decreased thirst sensation, and have chronic illnesses that predispose them to heat stroke, a hyperthermic condition (Wotton et al, 2008).*
- Assess the medication profile for the potential risk of drug-related altered body temperature. *Anesthetics, barbiturates, salicylates, nonsteroidal antiinflammatory drugs, diuretics, antihistamines, anticholinergics, beta-blockers, and thyroid hormones have been linked to decreased body temperature (American Geriatric Society, 2012).*

Home Care

Treating Fever

- Instruct client/parents on the physiological benefits of fever and provide interventions to treat fever symptoms, avoiding antipyretic agents and external cooling interventions.
- Ensure that client/parents know when to contact a health care provider for fever-related concerns.

Prevention of Hypothermia in Cold Weather

See the care plan **Hypothermia.**

Prevention of Hyperthermia in Hot Weather

See the care plan **Hyperthermia.**

Client/Family Teaching and Discharge Planning

- Teach the client and family the signs of fever, hypothermia, and hyperthermia and appropriate actions to take if either condition develops.
- Teach the client and family an age-appropriate method for taking the temperature.
- Teach the client to avoid alcohol and medications that depress cerebral function. *When the client is sedated or under the influence of alcohol, mentation is depressed, which results in decreased activities to maintain an adequate body temperature.*

T

REFERENCES

Adam, H. M. (2013). Fever: measuring and managing. *Pediatrics in Review, 34*, 368–370.

American Geriatrics Society. (2012). American geriatrics society updated beers criteria for potentially inappropriate medication use in older adults. *Journal of the American Geriatrics Society*, 1–16. <http://www.americangeriatrics.org/files/documents/beers/2012BeersCriteria_JAGS.pdf>.

Barakzai, M. D., & Fraser, D. (2008). Assessment of infection in older adults: signs and symptoms in four body systems. *Journal of Gerontological Nursing, 34*(1), 7–13.

Barnason, S., et al. (2012). Emergency nursing resource: non-invasive temperature measurement in the emergency department. *Journal of Emergency Nursing, 38*, 523–530.

Becker, J. H., & Wu, S. C. (2010). Fever: an update. *Journal of the American Podiatric Medical Association, 100*(4), 281–290.

Bridges, E., & Thomas, K. (2009). Noninvasive measurement of body temperature in critically ill patients. *Critical Care Nurse, 29*(3), 94–97.

Calonder, E. M., et al. (2010). Temperature measurement in patients undergoing colorectal surgery and gynecology surgery: a comparison of esophageal core, temporal artery, and oral methods. *Journal of Perianesthesia Nursing, 25*(2), 71–78.

Carey, J. V. (2010). Literature review: should antipyretic therapies routinely be administered to patient fever? *Journal of Clinical Nursing, 19*, 2377–2393.

Davie, A., & Amoore, J. (2010). Best practice in the measurement of body temperature. *Nursing Standard, 24*(42), 42–50.

Dellinger, R. P., et al. (2013). Surviving sepsis campaign: international guidelines for management of severe sepsis and septic shock, 2012. *Intensive Care Medicine, 39*, 165–228.

Dinarello, C. A., & Porat, R. (2011). Fever and hyperthermia. In D. L. Longo, et al. (Eds.), *Harrison's principles of internal medicine* (18th ed.). New York: McGraw-Hill.

Hammond, N. E., & Boyle, M. (2011). Pharmacological versus non-pharmacological antyipyretic treatments in febrile critically ill adult patients: a systematic review and meta-analysis. *Australian Critical Care, 24*, 4–17.

Hooper, V. D., et al. (2009). ASPAN's evidence-based clinical practice guideline for the promotion of perioperative normothermia. *Journal of Perianesthesia Nursing, 24*(5), 217–287.

Jefferies, S., et al. (2011). A systematic review of the accuracy of peripheral thermometry in estimating core temperatures among febrile critically ill patients. *Critical Care and Resuscitation: Journal of the Australasian Academy of Critical Care Medicine, 13*, 194–199.

Kenney, W. L., et al. (2014). Blood pressure regulation III: what happens when one system must serve two masters: temperature and pressure regulation? *European Journal of Applied Physiology, 114*, 467–479.

Makic, M. B. F., et al. (2011). Evidence-based practice habits: putting more sacred cows out to pasture. *Critical Care Nurse, 31*, 38–62.

Malya, R. R. (2013). Does combination treatment with ibuprofen and acetaminophen improve fever control? *Annals of Emergency Medicine, 61*(5), 569–570.

McLafferty, E., Farley, A., & Hendry, C. (2009). Prevention of hypothermia. *Nursing Older People, 21*(4), 34–38.

National Institute for Health and Clinical Excellence (NICE). (2013). *Feverish illness in children*, Clinical Guideline 47 London. <https://www.nice.org.uk/guidance/cg160>.

Niven, D. J., et al. (2013). Antipyretic therapy in febrile critically ill adults: a systematic review and meta-analysis. *Journal of Critical Care, 28*, 303–310.

O'Grady, N. P., et al. (2008). Guidelines for evaluation of new fever in critically ill adult patients: 2008 update from the American college of critical care medicine and the infectious diseases society of America. *Critical Care Medicine, 36*(4), 1330–1349.

Outzen, M. (2009). Management of fever in older adults. *Journal of Gerontological Nursing, 35*(5), 17–23.

Pitoni, S., Sinclair, H. L., & Andrews, P. J. D. (2011). Aspects of thermoregulation physiology. *Current Opinion in Critical Care, 17*, 115–121.

Purssell, E. (2011). Systematic review of studies comparing combine treatment with paracetamol and ibuprofen with either drug alone. *Archives of Disease in Childhood, 96*, 1175–1179.

Rehman, T., & deBoisblanc, B. P. (2013). Persistent fever in the ICU. *Chest, 145*(1), 158–165.

Ring, E. F. J., et al. (2010). New standards for devices used for the measurement of human body temperature. *Journal of Medical Engineering and Technology, 34*(4), 249–253.

Saltzberg, J. M. R. (2013). Fever and signs of shock: the essential dangerous fever. *Emergency Medicine Clinics of North America, 31*, 907–926.

Scrase, W., & Tranter, S. (2011). Improving evidence-based care for patients with pyrexia. *Nursing Standard, 25*(29), 37–41.

Sessler, D. L. (2008). Temperature monitoring and perioperative thermoregulation. *Anesthesiology, 109*(2), 318–338.

Sullivan, J. E., & Farrar, H. C. (2011). Clinical report: fever and antipyretic use in children. *Pediatrics, 127*, 580–587.

Torossian, A. (2008). Thermal management during anesthesia and thermoregulation standards for the prevention of inadvertent perioperative hypothermia. *Best Practice and Research. Clinical Anaesthesiology, 22*(4), 659–668.

Wollerich, H., et al. (2012). Comparison of temperature measurements in bladder, rectum, and pulmonary artery in patients after cardiac surgery. *Open Journal of Nursing, 2*, 307–310. <http://dx.doi.org/10.4236/ojn.2012.223045>.

Wotton, K., Crannitch, K., & Munt, R. (2008). Prevalence, risk factors and strategies to prevent dehydration in older adults. *Contemporary Nurse: A Journal for the Australian Nursing Profession, 31*(1), 44–56.

T

Impaired Tissue integrity *Karen Zulkowski, DNS, RN*

NANDA-I

Definition

Damage to the mucous membrane, cornea, integumentary system, muscular fascia, muscle, tendon, bone, cartilage, joint capsule, and/or ligament

Defining Characteristics

Damaged tissue; destroyed tissue

Related Factors

Alteration in metabolism; alteration in sensation; chemical injury agent (e.g., burn, capsaicin, methylene chloride, mustard agent); excess fluid volume; extremes of age; extremes of environmental temperature; high voltage power supply; humidity; imbalanced nutritional state (e.g., obesity, malnutrition); impaired circulation; impaired mobility; insufficient fluid volume; insufficient knowledge about maintain tissue integrity; insufficient knowledge about protecting tissue integrity; mechanical factor; peripheral neuropathy; pharmaceutical agent; radiation; surgical procedure

NOC (Nursing Outcomes Classification)

Suggested NOC Outcomes

Tissue Integrity: Skin and Mucous Membranes; Wound Healing: Primary Intention, Secondary Intention

Example NOC Outcome with Indicators

Intact **Tissue Integrity: Skin and Mucous Membranes** as evidenced by the following indicators: Skin intactness/Skin lesions absent/Tissue perfusion/Skin temperature. (Rate the outcome and indicators of **Tissue Integrity: Skin and Mucous Membranes:** 1 = severely compromised, 2 = substantially compromised, 3 = moderately compromised, 4 = mildly compromised, 5 = not compromised [see Section I].)

Client Outcomes

Client Will (Specify Time Frame)

- Report any altered sensation or pain at site of tissue impairment
- Demonstrate understanding of plan to heal tissue and prevent reinjury
- Describe measures to protect and heal the tissue, including wound care
- Experience a wound that decreases in size and has increased granulation tissue

NIC (Nursing Interventions Classification)

Suggested NIC Interventions

Incision Site Care; Pain Management; Pressure Ulcer Care; Risk Identification; Skin Care: Topical Treatments; Skin Surveillance; Wound Care; Wound Irrigation

Example NIC Activities—Pressure Ulcer Care

Monitor color of wound bed, temperature, edema, erythema, moisture, and appearance of surrounding skin; Note characteristics of any drainage

Nursing Interventions and *Rationales*

- • Assess the site of impaired tissue integrity and determine the cause and type of wound (e.g., acute or chronic wound, burn, dermatological lesion, pressure ulcer, leg ulcer, skin failure). EB: *The etiology or cause of the wound must be determined before appropriate interventions can be implemented. This provides the basis for additional testing and evaluation to start the treatment process (Baranoski & Ayello, 2012).*
- • Determine the size (length, width) and depth of the wound (e.g., full-thickness wound, deep tissue injury, stage III or IV pressure ulcer). *Consistency and accuracy in how the wound (tissue integrity) is measured are important for determining changes in the wound over time and for comparing effectiveness of various treatments (Baranoski & Ayello, 2012).*
- ▲ Classify pressure ulcers using national guidelines and definitions (http://www.npuap.org/resources/educational-and-clinical-resources/npuap-pressure-ulcer-stagescategories)
  - ❍ Pressure ulcer: localized injury to the skin and/or underlying tissue usually over a bony prominence, as a result of pressure, or pressure in combination with shear (note: friction is not included in the definition) (National Pressure Ulcer Advisory Panel [NPUAP] and European Pressure Ulcer Advisory Panel [EPUAP], 2014).
  - ❍ **Category/Stage III:** Full-thickness tissue loss. Subcutaneous fat may be visible but bone, tendon, or muscle is not exposed. Slough may be present but does not obscure the depth of tissue loss. May include undermining and tunneling. The depth of a category/stage III pressure ulcer varies by anatomical location. The bridge of the nose, ear, occiput and malleolus do not have (adipose) subcutaneous tissue and can be shallow. In contrast, areas of significant adiposity can develop extremely deep category/stage III pressure ulcers. Bone/tendon is not visible or directly palpable.

T

- **Category/Stage IV:** Full-thickness tissue loss with exposed bone, tendon, or muscle. Slough or eschar may be present on some parts of the wound bed. Often includes undermining and tunneling. The depth of a category/stage IV pressure ulcer varies by anatomical location. The bridge of the nose, ear, occiput, and malleolus do not have (adipose) subcutaneous tissue and can be shallow. Category IV ulcers can extend into muscle and/or supporting structures (e.g., fascia, tendon, or joint capsule), making osteomyelitis possible. Exposed bone/tendon is visible or directly palpable.
- **Suspected Deep Tissue Injury:** Purple or maroon localized area of discolored intact skin or blood-filled blister due to damage of underlying soft tissue from pressure and/or shear. The area may be preceded by tissue that is painful, firm, mushy, boggy, warmer, or cooler as compared to adjacent tissue. Suspected deep tissue injury may be difficult to detect in individuals with dark skin tones. Evolution may include a thin blister over a dark wound bed. The wound may further evolve and become covered by thin eschar. Evolution may be rapid, exposing additional layers of tissue even with optimal treatment.
- **Unstageable (Depth Unknown):** Full-thickness tissue loss in which the base of the ulcer is covered by slough (yellow, tan, gray, green, or brown) and/or eschar (tan, brown, or black) in the wound bed. Until enough slough and/or eschar is removed to expose the base of the wound, the true depth and, therefore, category/stage cannot be determined. Stable (dry, adherent, intact without erythema or fluctuance) eschar on the heels serves as a natural cover and should not be removed.

- Inspect and monitor the site of impaired tissue integrity at least once daily for color changes, redness, swelling, warmth, pain, or other signs of infection or per facility/agency policy. Determine whether the client is experiencing changes in sensation or pain. Pay special attention to all high-risk areas such as bony prominences, skin folds, sacrum, and heels. *Systematic inspection can identify impending problems early.* EB: *Pain secondary to dressing changes can be managed by interventions aimed at reducing trauma and other sources of wound pain (Wounds International, 2009).*
- Monitor the status of the skin around the wound. Monitor the client's skin care practices, noting type of soap or other cleansing agents used, temperature of water, and frequency of skin cleansing. *Individualize the plan according to the client's skin condition, needs, and preferences. Avoid harsh cleansing agents, hot water, extreme friction or force, or too-frequent cleansing (Baranoski & Ayello, 2012).*
- Monitor the client's continence status and minimize exposure of the skin impairment site and other areas to moisture from urine or stool, perspiration, or wound drainage. *If the client is incontinent, implement an incontinence management plan to prevent exposure to chemicals in urine and stool that can strip or erode the skin. Refer to a continence care specialist, urologist, or gastroenterologist for incontinence assessment (Borchert et al, 2010; Wound, Ostomy, and Continence Nurses Society [WOCN], 2010).* EB: *Implementing an incontinence prevention plan with the use of a skin or cleanser protectant can significantly decrease skin breakdown and pressure ulcer formation (Borchert et al, 2010).*
- Monitor for correct placement of tubes, catheters, and other devices. Assess the skin and tissue affected by the pressure of the devices and tape used to secures these devices. EB: *Mechanical damage to skin and tissues as a result of pressure, friction, or shear is often associated with external devices (NPUAP/EPUAP, 2014).* A medical device related pressure ulcer is defined as a localized injury to the skin or underlying tissue as a result of sustained pressure from a medical device and the skin/tissue injury will often have the same configuration as the device (NPUAP/EPUAP, 2014; Black et al, 2010).
- Assess frequently for correct placement of foot boards, restraints, traction, casts, or other devices, and assess skin and tissue integrity. Frequently assess for signs and symptoms of compartment syndrome (refer to the care plan for Risk for **Peripheral Neurovascular** dysfunction). *Mechanical damage to skin and tissues (pressure or shear) is often associated with external devices.*
- Implement and communicate a comprehensive treatment plan for the topical treatment of the skin impairment site. *A clearly stated treatment plan ensures consistency in care and documentation (Baranoski & Ayello, 2012).*

▲ Identify a plan for debridement if necrotic tissue (eschar or slough) is present and if consistent with overall client management goals. (i.e., curative vs. palliative care). EB: *Debride devitalized tissue within the wound bed or edge of pressure ulcers when appropriate to individual's condition and consistent with overall goals of care. Do not debride stable, hard, dry eschar in ischemic limbs or heels (NPUAP/EPUAP, 2014).*

- Select a topical treatment that maintains a moist, wound-healing environment and also allows absorption of exudate and filling of dead space. *No single wound care product provides the optimal environment for healing all wounds.* EB: *Choose dressings that provide a moist healing environment, keep periwound skin dry, and control exudate and eliminate dead space (Baranoski & Ayello, 2012; NPUAP/EPUAP, 2014; WOCN, 2010).*

- Avoid positioning the client on the site of impaired tissue integrity. EB: *If it is consistent with overall client management goals, reposition the client based on level of tissue tolerance and overall condition, and transfer or reposition the client carefully to avoid adverse effects of external mechanical forces (pressure, friction, and shear) (NPUAP/EPUAP, 2014; WOCN, 2010).*
- Evaluate for the use of support surfaces (specialty mattresses, beds) chair cushion, or devices as appropriate (Brienza et al, 2012; Lippoldt et al, 2014).
- If the goal of care is to keep the client comfortable (e.g., for a terminally ill client), repositioning may not be appropriate. *Position the client in position of optimal comfort (Horn et al, 2014). Maintain the head of the bed at the lowest degree of elevation possible to reduce shear and friction and use lift devices, pillows, foam wedges, and pressure-reducing devices in the bed (Baranoski & Ayello, 2012; NPUAP/EPUAP, 2014, WOCN, 2010).*

▲ Assess the client's nutritional status. Refer for a nutritional consult and/or institute dietary supplements as necessary. *Optimizing nutritional intake, including calories, fatty acids, protein, and vitamins, is needed to promote wound healing* (NPUAP/EPUAP, 2014; O'Hanlon et al, 2015).

▲ Develop a comprehensive plan of care that includes a thorough wound assessment, treatment interventions, support surfaces, nutritional products, adjunctive therapies, and evaluation of the outcome of care. *Documentation of these essential elements is paramount to establishing a framework for quality care.*

Home Care

- Some of the interventions previously described may be adapted for home care use.

▲ Assess the client's current phase of wound healing (inflammation, proliferation, maturation) and stage of injury; initiate appropriate wound management. EB: *Accurate understanding of tissue status combined with knowledge of underlying diagnoses and product validity provide a basis for determining appropriate treatment objectives (Baranoski & Ayello, 2012).*

- Instruct and assist the client and caregivers in understanding how to change dressings and in the importance of maintaining a clean environment. Provide written instructions and observe them completing the dressing change.

▲ Initiate a consultation in a case assignment with a wound specialist or wound, ostomy, and continence nurse to establish a comprehensive plan as soon as possible. Plan case conferencing to promote optimal wound care. *Case conferencing ensures that cases are regularly reviewed to discuss and implement the most effective wound care management to meet client needs.*

▲ Consult with other health care disciplines to provide a thorough, comprehensive assessment. *Consider referring to a dietitian, physical therapist, occupational therapist, and social worker/case manager as needed. Early engagement of wound care specialists can enhance overall care and reduce health care costs (Vrtis, 2013).*

T

Client/Family Teaching and Discharge Planning

- Teach skin and wound assessment and ways to monitor for signs and symptoms of infection, complications, and healing. *Early assessment and intervention help prevent serious problems from developing.*
- Teach the client why a topical treatment has been selected. Explain wound bed changes that the caregiver can expect to see. Instruct on when the dressing needs to be changed. EB: *The type of wound dressing needed may change over time as the wound heals and/or deteriorates (Baranoski & Ayello, 2012; NPUAP/EPUAP, 2014).*

▲ Teach the use of pillows, foam wedges, and pressure-reducing devices to prevent pressure injury. The use of effective pressure-reducing seat cushions for older wheelchair users significantly prevented sitting-acquired pressure ulcers (Brienza et al, 2012).

REFERENCES

Baranoski, S., & Ayello, E. A. (Eds.), (2012). *Wound care essentials: practice principles* (ed. 3). Ambler, PA: Lippincott Williams & Wilkins.

Black, J. M., Cuddigan, J. E., Walko, M. A., et al. (2010). Medical device related pressure ulcers in hospitalized patients. *International Wound Journal*, *7*(5), 358–365.

Borchert, K., et al. (2010). The incontinence-associated dermatitis and its severity instrument. *Journal of Wound, Ostomy, and Continence Nursing*, *37*(5), 527–535.

Brienza, D. M., et al. (2012). Pressure redistribution: seating, positioning, and support surfaces. In S. Baranoski & E. A. Ayello

(Eds.), *Wound care essentials: practice principles* (ed. 3). Ambler, PA: Lippincott, Williams & Wilkins.

Horn, J., & Iroin, G. L. (2014). The integument: current concepts in care at end of life. *Journal of Acute Care Physical Therapy*, *5*(1), 11–16.

Lippoldt, J., & Staudinger, T. (2014). Interface pressure at different degrees of backrest elevation with various types of pressure redistribution surfaces. *American Journal of Critical Care*, *23*(2), 119–126.

National Pressure Ulcer Advisory Panel (NPUAP) and European Pressure Ulcer Advisory Panel (EPUAP) (2014). *Prevention and treatment of pressure ulcers*. Emily Haesler (ed). Perth, Australia: Cambridge Media.

O'Hanlon, C., Dowsett, J., & Smyth, N. (2015). Nutrition assessment of the intensive care unit patient. *Topics in Clinical Nutrition*, *30*(1), 47–70.

Vrtis, M. C. (2013). The economic impact of complex wound care on home health agencies. *Journal of Wound, Ostomy, and Continence Nursing*, *40*(4), 360–363.

Wounds International. (2009). *Pain at wound dressing changes: EWMA Position Document*. Retrieved July 16, 2015. <http://www.woundsinternational.com/other-resources/view/pain-at-wound-dressing-changes>.

Wound, Ostomy, and Continence Nurses Society (WOCN). (2010). *Guideline for prevention and management of pressure ulcers*, WOCN Clinical Practice Guideline Series 2, Mount Laurel, NJ.

Risk for Impaired Tissue integrity

Mary Beth Flynn Makic, PhD, RN, CNS, CCNS, FAAN, and Karen Zulkowski, DNS, RN

NANDA-I

Definition

Vulnerable to damage to the mucous membrane, cornea, integumentary system, muscular fascia, muscle, tendon, bone, cartilage, joint capsule, and/or ligament, which may compromise health

Risk Factors

Alteration in metabolism; alteration in sensation; chemical injury agent (e.g., burn, capsaicin, methylene chloride, mustard agent); excessive fluid volume; extremes of age; extremes of environmental temperature; high voltage power supply; humidity; imbalanced nutritional state (e.g., obesity, malnutrition); impaired circulation; impaired mobility; insufficient fluid volume; insufficient knowledge about maintaining tissue integrity; insufficient knowledge about protecting tissue integrity; mechanical factor; peripheral neuropathy; pharmaceutical agent; radiation therapy; surgical procedure

NOC, NIC, Client Outcomes, Nursing Interventions, Client/Family Teaching and Discharge Planning, *Rationales*, and References

Refer to care plan for Impaired **Tissue** integrity.

Ineffective peripheral Tissue Perfusion

Lorraine Duggan, MSN, ACNP-BC

NANDA-I

Definition

Decrease in blood circulation to the periphery, which may compromise health

Defining Characteristics

Absence of peripheral pulses; alteration in motor function; altered skin characteristics (e.g., color, elasticity, hair, moisture, nails, sensation, temperature); ankle-brachial index (ABI) <0.90; capillary refill time >3 seconds; color does not return to lowered limb after 1 minute of leg elevation; decrease in blood pressure in extremities; decrease in pain-free distances achieved in the 6-minute walk test; decrease in peripheral pulses; delay in peripheral wound healing; distance in the 6-minute walk test below normal range (400 m to 700 m in adults); edema; extremity pain; femoral bruit; intermittent claudication; paresthesia; skin color pales with limb elevation

Related Factors

Diabetes mellitus; hypertension; insufficient knowledge of aggravating factors (e.g., smoking, sedentary lifestyle, trauma, obesity, salt intake, immobility); insufficient knowledge of disease process; sedentary lifestyle; smoking

NOC (Nursing Outcomes Classification)

Suggested NOC Outcomes

Circulation Status; Fluid Balance; Hydration; Tissue Perfusion: Peripheral

Example NOC Outcome with Indicators

Demonstrates adequate **Circulation Status** as evidenced by the following indicators: Peripheral pulses strong/Peripheral pulses symmetrical/Skin color and temperature/Peripheral edema not present. (Rate the outcome and indicators of **Circulation Status:** 1 = severely compromised, 2 = substantially compromised, 3 = moderately compromised, 4 = mildly compromised, 5 = not compromised [see Section I].)

Client Outcomes

Client Will (Specify Time Frame)

- Demonstrate adequate tissue perfusion as evidenced by palpable peripheral pulses, warm and dry skin, adequate urine output, and absence of respiratory distress
- Verbalize knowledge of treatment regimen, including appropriate exercise and medications and their actions and possible side effects
- Identify changes in lifestyle needed to increase tissue perfusion

NIC (Nursing Interventions Classification)

Suggested NIC Intervention

Circulatory Care: Arterial Insufficiency

Example NIC Activities—Circulatory Care: Arterial Insufficiency

Evaluate peripheral edema and pulses; Inspect skin for arterial ulcers and tissue breakdown

Nursing Interventions and *Rationales*

▲ Check the brachial, radial, dorsalis pedis, posterior tibial, and popliteal pulses bilaterally. If unable to find them, use a Doppler stethoscope and notify the health care provider immediately if new onset of absence of pulses along with a cold extremity. *Diminished or absent peripheral pulses indicate arterial insufficiency with resultant ischemia (White, 2011).*

- Note skin color and feel the temperature of the skin. *Skin pallor or mottling, cool or cold skin temperature, or an absent pulse can signal arterial obstruction, which is an emergency that requires immediate intervention (White, 2011). Rubor (reddish blue color accompanied by dependency) indicates dilated or damaged vessels. Brownish discoloration of the skin on the anterior tibia indicates chronic venous insufficiency (Jarvis, 2012).*
- Assess for pain in the extremities, noting severity, quality, timing, and exacerbating and alleviating factors. Differentiate venous from arterial disease. *In clients with venous insufficiency, the pain lessens with elevation of the legs and exercise. In clients with arterial insufficiency, the pain increases with elevation of the legs and exercise (Longo, 2011). Some clients have both arterial and venous insufficiency. Arterial insufficiency is associated with pain when walking (claudication) that is relieved by rest. Clients with severe arterial disease have pain while at rest, which keeps them awake at night. Venous insufficiency is associated with aching, cramping, and discomfort (White, 2011).*
- Check capillary refill. EBN: *Nail beds usually return to a pinkish color within 1 to 2 seconds after compression; a capillary refilling time greater than 3 seconds is abnormal (Jarvis, 2012).*
- Note skin texture and the presence of hair, ulcers, or gangrenous areas on the legs or feet. *Thin, shiny, dry skin with hair loss; brittle nails; and gangrene or ulcerations on toes and anterior surfaces of the feet are seen in clients with arterial insufficiency. If ulcerations are on the side of the leg, they are usually associated with venous insufficiency (Jarvis, 2012).*
- Note the presence of edema in the extremities and rate severity on a four-point scale. Measure the circumference of the ankle and calf at the same time each day in the early morning (White, 2011).

Arterial Insufficiency

▲ Monitor peripheral pulses. If there is new onset of loss of pulses with bluish, purple, or black areas and extreme pain, notify the health care provider immediately. *These are symptoms of arterial obstruction that can result in loss of a limb if not immediately reversed.* CEB: *A classic study concluded that (1) if pulses are palpable on both feet of a client, the prognosis for progression is relatively good regarding the client's peripheral arterial disease (PAD); (2) if pedal pulse is palpable, an arteriosclerotic ulcer on the foot will heal; (3) clients lacking palpable pulses in both feet actually suffer from PAD (Christensen, 1989).*

▲ Measure ABI via Doppler imaging. EB: *Automated ABI measurement using a professional blood pressure monitor allowing simultaneous arm-leg blood pressure measurements appears to be a reliable and faster alternative to Doppler measurement (Kollias et al, 2011).*

• Avoid elevating the legs above the level of the heart. With arterial insufficiency, leg elevation decreases arterial blood supply to the legs.

▲ For early arterial insufficiency, encourage exercise such as walking or riding an exercise bicycle from 30 to 60 minutes per day as ordered by the health care provider. EB: *Exercise was the most common nonpharmacological option recommended by health care providers for PAD (Bozkurk, 2011).*

• Keep the client warm and have the client wear socks and shoes or sheepskin-lined slippers when mobile. Do not apply heat. Clients with arterial insufficiency report being constantly cold; keep extremities warm to maintain vasodilation and blood supply. Heat application can easily damage ischemic tissues.

▲ Pay meticulous attention to foot care. Refer to a podiatrist if the client has a foot or nail abnormality. Ischemic feet are vulnerable to injury; meticulous foot care can prevent further injury. EBN: *Clients with diabetes and high risk for development of foot ulcer constitute a fragile group that needs special foot protective attention (Annersten Gershatner, 2011).*

• If the client has ischemic arterial ulcers, refer to the care plan for Impaired **Tissue** integrity.

▲ If the client smokes, aggressively counsel the client to stop smoking and refer to the health care provider for medications to support nicotine withdrawal and a smoking withdrawal program. EB: *Smoking cessation substantially reduces risk for PAD in women, but an increased occurrence of PAD persists even among former smokers who maintain abstinence (Conen, 2011).*

Venous Insufficiency

▲ Elevate edematous legs as ordered and ensure no pressure under the knee and heels to prevent pressure ulcers. *Elevation increases venous return, helps decrease edema, and can help heal venous leg ulcers (Longo et al, 2011). Pressure under the knee decreases venous circulation.* EBN: *Results indicate that leg elevation, compression hosiery, high levels of self-efficacy, and strong social support will help prevent recurrence (Finlayson et al, 2011).*

T

▲ Apply graduated compression stockings as ordered. Ensure proper fit by measuring accurately. Remove the stockings at least twice a day, in the morning with the bath and in the evening, to assess the condition of the extremity, then reapply. Knee length is preferred rather than thigh length. EB: *Hosiery is a dominant treatment—that is, on average it results in higher quality-adjusted life-years and lower costs than do bandages (Rebecca, 2014).*

• Encourage the client to walk with compression stockings on and perform toe-up and point-flex exercises. *Exercise helps increase venous return, builds up collateral circulation, and strengthens the calf muscles.* EBN: *Physical therapy modalities improves ABI, Doppler flow velocity, and blood parameters in clients with type 2 diabetes (Castro-Sanchez, 2013).*

• If the client is overweight, encourage weight loss to decrease venous disease. *Obesity is a risk factor for development of both deep vein thrombosis (DVT) and pulmonary embolism (PE) (Weitz, 2011).*

• If the client has venous leg ulcers, encourage the client to avoid prolonged sitting, standing, and elevation of the involved leg. Encourage proper use of compression stockings. Pain may prevent compliance. EBN: *A study shows a high incidence of ulcer pain, confirming that pain has a great impact on clients with venous leg ulcers (Akessonrut et al, 2014).*

• Discuss lifestyle with the client to determine if the client's occupation requires prolonged standing or sitting, which can result in chronic venous disease (Longo et al, 2011).

▲ If the client is mostly immobile, consult with the health care provider regarding use of a calf-high pneumatic compression device for prevention of DVT. EB: *Superficial venous surgery in addition to compression therapy is the most efficient treatment of venous leg ulcers. The compression therapy should be continued in both surgically and conservatively treated clients with healed ulcers (Taradaj et al, 2011).*

- Observe for signs of DVT, including pain, tenderness, swelling in the calf and thigh, and redness in the involved extremity. Take serial leg measurements of the thigh and calf circumferences. In some clients a tender venous cord can be felt in the popliteal fossa. Do not rely on Homan's sign. *Thrombosis with clot formation is usually first detected as swelling of the involved leg and then as pain. Symptoms of existing DVT are nonspecific and cannot be used alone to determine the presence of DVT (Ginsberg, 2011).*

▲ Note the results of a D-dimer test and ultrasounds. *High levels of D-dimer, a fibrin degradation fragment, are found in DVT and pulmonary embolism, but results should be confirmed with a duplex venous ultrasonogram (Ginsberg, 2011).*

- If DVT is present, observe for symptoms of a pulmonary embolism, including dyspnea, pleuritic chest pain, cough, and sometimes hemoptysis, especially with a history of trauma (Weitz, 2011).

▲ If the client develops DVT, after treatment and hospital discharge, recommend client wear below-the-knee elastic compression stockings during the day on the involved extremity. EBN: *Client education for post-thrombotic syndrome prevention compliance may be enhanced by specifically addressing individual risk factors and barriers to stocking application (Crumley, 2011).*

Geriatric

- Complete a thorough lower extremity assessment. Documenting the smallest change from previous assessment, and implement a plan immediately. EB: *Complete and accurate assessment is essential to guide health care providers in formulating efficacious plans of care. The prevalence of peripheral arterial disease increases with age. The elevated risk of ulcerations leading to amputation among older adults reflects not only increased rates of peripheral arterial disease and diabetic pathologies but also age-related changes of the integument (Hakim & Heitzman, 2013).*
- Change the client's position slowly when getting the client out of bed because of possible syncope. EB: *A study has confirmed a changing pattern in the etiology of syncope as a person ages. The burden of disease is greatest in older adults (Cooke et al, 2011).*
- Recognize that older adults have an increased risk for development of pulmonary embolism; if pulmonary embolism is present, the symptoms are nonspecific and often mimic those of heart failure or pneumonia (Weitz, 2011). EB: *A diagnostic review demonstrates an increase of prevalence of PE with age and a strong decrease of specificity and efficiency for clinical decision rules of VTE in older clients (Siccama et al, 2011).*

Home Care

- The interventions previously described may be adapted for home care use.
- If arterial disease is present and the client smokes, aggressively encourage smoking cessation.
- Examine the feet carefully at frequent intervals for changes and new ulcerations. CEB: *Lower Extremity Amputation Prevention (LEAP) Program documentation forms are available at* http://www.hrsa.gov/leap *(Health Resources and Service Administration, 2012).*

▲ Assess the client's nutritional status, paying special attention to obesity, hyperlipidemia, and malnutrition. Refer to a dietitian if appropriate. *Malnutrition contributes to anemia, which further compounds the lack of oxygenation to tissues. Obese clients have poor circulation in adipose tissue and increased coagulability (Weitz, 2011).*

- Monitor for development of gangrene, venous ulceration, and symptoms of cellulitis (redness, pain, and increased swelling in an extremity). *Cellulitis often accompanies peripheral vascular disease, especially with development of wounds on the leg (Longo et al, 2011).*

T

Client/Family Teaching and Discharge Planning

- Explain the importance of good foot care. Teach the client and family to wash and inspect the feet daily. Recommend that the diabetic client wear comfortable shoes and break them in slowly, watching for blisters (National Diabetes Information Clearing House, 2014).

▲ Teach the diabetic client that he or she should have a comprehensive foot examination at least annually (which includes an analysis for predicting foot ulceration risk), also including assessment of sensation using the Semmes-Weinstein monofilaments. If good sensation is not present, refer to a footwear professional for fitting of therapeutic shoes and inserts, the cost of which is covered by Medicare. EBN: *In a study, the strongest predictors of foot ulceration were prior ulcer, insulin treatment, absent monofilaments, structural abnormality, proteinuria, and retinopathy (Leese, 2011).*

- For arterial disease, stress the importance of not smoking, following a weight loss program (if the client is obese), carefully controlling a diabetic condition, controlling hyperlipidemia and hypertension, maintaining intake of antiplatelet therapy, and reducing stress. *All these risk factors for atherosclerosis can be modified (White, 2011).* EB: *Intermittent claudication due to PAD causes substantial impairment in quality of life and is strongly associated with increased cardiovascular morbidity and mortality. Management focuses on reducing cardiovascular events, preventing progression of underlying PAD (e.g., limb loss), and improving symptoms. Aggressive secondary prevention strategies (e.g., statins and smoking cessation) are of critical importance (Vodnala et al, 2011).*

- Teach the client to avoid exposure to cold; limit exposure to brief periods if going out in cold weather and wear warm clothing.
- For venous disease, teach the importance of wearing compression stockings as ordered, elevating the legs at intervals, and watching for skin breakdown on the legs. EB: *Difficulties regarding putting on and removal of the compression stockings remain significant but are counterbalanced by better comfort when they are on (Carpentier et al, 2011).*
- Teach the client to recognize the signs and symptoms that should be reported to a health care provider (e.g., change in skin temperature, color, or sensation or the presence of a new lesion on the foot).
- Provide clear, simple instructions about plan of care.
- Instruct and provide emotional support for client undergoing hyperoxygenation treatment. EB: *Hyperbaric oxygen may be associated with ulcer healing in selected diabetic foot ulcers (Oliveira et al, 2014).*

REFERENCES

Administration, H. R. (2012). *Lower Extremity Amputation Prevention.* Retrieved from HRSA: <http://www.hrsa.gov/leap>.

Akessonrut, N., ÖienHenrik, F., & Forssell, C. (2014). *Ulcer Pain in Patients with Venous Leg Ulcers Related to Antibiotic Treatment and Compression Therapy.* Retrieved from British Journal of Community Nursing: <http://dx.doi.org/10.12968/bjcn.2014.19.Sup9.S6>.

Annersten Gershatner, M. (2011). *Prevention of Foot Ulcers in Patients with Diabetes Mellitus.* Retrieved from: <http://hdl.handle.net>.

Bozkurk, A. (2011). Peripheral artery disease assessed by ankle-brachial index in patients with established cardiovascular disease or at least one risk factor for atherothrombosis-CAREFUL study: a national, multi-center, cross-section observational study. *BMC Cardiovascular Disorders, 11*, 4–15.

Carpentier, P., et al. (2011). Acceptability and practicability of elastic compression stockings in the elderly: a randomized controlled evaluation. *Phlebology, 26*(3), 107–113.

Castro-Sanchez, A. (2013). A program of 3 physical therapy modalities improves peripheral arterial disease in diabetes type 2 patients: a randomized controlled trial. *Journal of Cardiovascular Nursing, 28*(1), 74–82.

Christensen, H. (1989). Clinical relevance of pedal pulse palpation in patients suspected of peripheral arterial insufficiency. *Journal of Internal Medicine, 226*(2), 95–99.

Conen, D. (2011). Smoking, smoking cessation, and risk for symptomatic peripheral artery disease in women: a cohort study. *Annuls of Internal Medicine, 154*(11), 719–726.

Cooke, J., et al. (2011). The changing face of orthostatic and neurocardiogenic syncope with age. *QJM: Monthly Journal of the Association of Physicians, 104*(8), 689–695.

Crumley, C. (2011). Post-thrombotic syndrome patient education based on the health belief model: self reported intention to comply with recommendations. *Journal of Wound Ostomy Continence Nursing, 38*(6), 648–654.

Finlayson, K., et al. (2011). Relationships between preventive activities, psychosocial factors and recurrence of venous leg ulcers: a prospective study. *Journal of Advanced Nursing, 67*(10), 2180–2190.

Ginsberg, J. (2011). *Peripheral venous disease.* St. Louis: Saunders.

Hakim, E., & Heitzman, J. (2013). Wound management in the presence of peripheral arterial disease. *Topics in Geriatric Rehabilitation, 29*(3), 187–194.

Jarvis, C. (2012). *Physical examination & health assessment.* St. Louis: Saunders.

Kollias, A., et al. (2011). Automated determination of the ankle-brachial index using an oscillometric blood pressure monitor: validation vs. doppler measurement and cardiovascular risk factor profile. *Hypertension Research, 34*(7), 825–830.

Leese, G. (2011). Measuring the accuracy of different ways to identify the at-risk foot in routine clinical practice. *Diabetes Medicine, 28*(6), 747–754.

Longo, D., et al. (2011). *Harrison's principles of internal medicine* (18th ed.). New York: McGraw-Hill.

Oliveira, N., Rosa, P., Borqes, L., et al. (2014). Treatment of diabetic foot complications with hyperbaric oxygen therapy: a retrospective experience. *Foot and Ankle Surgery, 20*(2), 104–143.

Rebecca, L. (2014). Clinical and cost-effectiveness of compression hosiery verus compression bandages in treatment of venous leg ulcers (Venous Leg Ulcer Study IV, VenUS IV): a randomised controlled trial. *The Lancet, 383*(9920), 871–879.

Siccama, R. (2011). Systematic review: diagnostic accuracy of clinical decision rules for venous thromboembolism in elderly. *Ageing Research Reviews, 10*(2), 304–313.

Taradaj, J., et al. (2011). Early and long-term results of physical methods in the treatment of venous leg ulcers: a randomized control trial. *Phlebotomy, 26*(6), 237–245.

Vodnala, D., et al. (2011). Medical management of the patient with intermittent claudication. *Cardiology Clinics, 39*(3), 363–379.

Weitz, J. (2011). *Pulmonary embolism.* St. Louis: Saunders.

White, C. (2011). *Atherosclerotic peripheral arterial disease.* St. Louis: Saunders.

Risk for ineffective peripheral Tissue Perfusion

Betty J. Ackley, MSN, EdS, RN, and Mary Beth Flynn Makic, PhD, RN, CNS, CCNS, FAAN

NANDA-I

Definition

Vulnerable to a decrease in blood circulation to the periphery, which may compromise health

Risk Factors

Diabetes mellitus; endovascular procedure; excessive sodium intake; hypertension; insufficient knowledge of aggravating factors (e.g., smoking, sedentary lifestyle, trauma, obesity, salt intake, immobility); insufficient knowledge of disease process; insufficient knowledge of risk factors; sedentary lifestyle; smoking; trauma

NOC, NIC, Client Outcomes, Nursing Interventions, Client/Family Teaching and Discharge Planning, *Rationales*, and References

Refer to care plan for Ineffective peripheral **Tissue Perfusion.**

Impaired Transfer ability

Mary Beth Flynn Makic, PhD, RN, CNS, CCNS, FAAN

NANDA-I

Definition

Limitation of independent movement between two nearby surfaces

Defining Characteristics

Impaired ability to transfer between bed and chair; impaired ability to transfer between bed and standing position; impaired ability to transfer between car and chair; impaired ability to transfer between chair and floor; impaired ability to transfer between chair and standing position; impaired ability to transfer between floor and standing position; impaired ability to transfer between uneven levels; impaired ability to transfer in or out of bath tub; impaired ability to transfer in or out of shower; impaired ability to transfer on or off a commode; impaired ability to transfer on or off a toilet

T

Related Factors (r/t)

Alteration in cognitive functioning; environmental barrier (e.g., bed height, inadequate space, wheelchair type, treatment equipment, restraints); impaired balance; impaired vision; insufficient knowledge of transfer techniques; insufficient muscle strength; musculoskeletal impairment; neuromuscular impairment; obesity; pain; physical deconditioning

Note: Specify level of Independence using a standardized functional scale.

NOC (Nursing Outcomes Classification)

Suggested NOC Outcomes

Balance; Body Positioning: Self-Initiated; Transfer Performance

Example NOC Outcome with Indicators

Transfer Performance as evidenced by the following indicators: Transfers from bed to chair and back/Transfers from wheelchair to toilet and back/Transfers from wheelchair to vehicle and back. (Rate the outcome and indicators of **Transfer Performance:** 1 = severely compromised, 2 = substantially compromised, 3 = moderately compromised, 4 = mildly compromised, 5 = not compromised [see Section I].)

Client Outcomes

Client Will (Specify Time Frame)

- Transfer from bed to chair and back successfully
- Transfer from chair to chair successfully
- Transfer from wheelchair to toilet and back successfully
- Transfer from wheelchair to car and back successfully

NIC (Nursing Interventions Classification)

Suggested NIC Interventions

Exercise Promotion: Strength Training; Exercise Therapy: Muscle Control

Example NIC Activities—Exercise Promotion: Strength Training

Obtain medical clearance for initiating a strength-training program, as appropriate; Assist to set realistic short- and long-term goals and to take ownership of the exercise plan

Nursing Interventions and *Rationales*

▲ Request consult for a physical and/or occupational therapist (PT and OT) to develop exercise and strengthening program early in the client's recovery. *Leg/trunk strength is key for standing transfers; arm/trunk strength is key for slide-board transfers.* EB: *Progressive mobility earlier and more aggressively in the hospital stay, as early as in the ICU, decreases mechanical ventilation days and decreases complications such as weakness from disuse and contractures (Vollman, 2010; Kalisch et al, 2013).* EB: *Voet and colleagues (2010), via a Cochrane review, reported that strength training and aerobic exercise training for muscle disease may optimize function.*

▲ Obtain a consult for a PT, OT, or orthotist to evaluate and fit clients with proper orthoses, braces, collars, and walking aids before helping them stand. *Equipment helps clients move and function safely, comfortably, and independently (Hoeman et al, 2008).*

• Help client put on/take off collars, braces, prostheses in bed, as well as antiembolism stockings and abdominal binders. Applying antiembolism stockings while the client is in bed may reduce the risk of the client developing a deep vein thrombosis (DVT). EB: *A literature review reported knee-high stockings were as effective as above-the-knee stockings in preventing DVT in immobile medical/surgical inpatients, and compliance was better (Gordon et al, 2012).*

T

• Assess client's dependence, weight, strength, balance, tolerance to position change, cooperation, fatigue level, and cognition plus available equipment and staff ratio/experience to decide whether to do a manual or device-assisted transfer (Nelson et al, 2008; Cohen et al, 2010).

▲ Collaborate with PT and OT to use algorithms to identify technological aids to handle and transfer dependent and obese clients; do not use under-axilla method (Cohen et al, 2010). *Assess the client for appropriate use of assistive devices to include powered stand-assist devices, mechanical lifts, stretchers to chairs, and friction-reducing devices prevent musculoskeletal injuries of staff and allow safe client handling (Centers for Disease Control and Prevention, 2015).*

• Implement and document type of transfer (e.g., slide board, pivot), weight-bearing status (non–weight-bearing, partial), equipment (walker, sling lift), and level of assistance (standby, moderate) on care plan, white board in room, and/or electronic medical record.

• Apply a gait belt with handles before transferring clients with partial weight-bearing abilities; keep the belt and client close to provider during the transfer. *If used incorrectly, such as at arm's length, it prevents support of client and places staff at risk for back and arm injuries (Hallmark et al, 2015; Kalisch et al, 2013).*

• Help clients with wearing shoes with nonskid soles and socks/hose. *Proper shoes help prevent slips/pain/pressure and improve balance.* EB: *Suggest trying a running shoe that is comfortable and lightweight, because a recent study found that participants unable to see the type of shoe (control shoe, running shoe, or orthopedic shoe) chose the running shoe based on comfort and weight (Riskowski et al, 2011).*

- Remove or swivel wheelchair armrests, leg rests, and footplates to the side, especially with squat or slide board transfers. *This gives clients and nurses feet space to maneuver in and provides fewer obstacles to trip over.*
- Adjust transfer surfaces so they are similar in height. For example, lower a hospital bed to about an inch higher than commode height. **EB:** *Similar heights between seat surfaces require less upper extremity muscular effort during transfers (Hoeman et al, 2008; Cohen et al, 2010).*
- Place wheelchair and commode at a slight angle toward the surface onto which client will transfer. *The two surfaces are close together yet allow room for the caregiver to adjust the client's movements during the transfer (Hoeman et al, 2008).*
- Teach client to consistently lock brakes on wheelchair/commode/shower chair before transferring. *Wheels will roll if not locked, thus creating risk for falls. Pneumatic wheelchair tires must be adequately inflated for brakes to lock effectively (LaPlante et al, 2010).*
- Give clear, simple instructions, allow client time to process information, and let him/her do as much of the transfer as possible. *Over-assistance by staff and family may decrease client learning, independence, self-care, and self-esteem.*

▲ Remind clients to comply with weight-bearing restrictions ordered by their health care provider. *Weight bearing may retard healing in fractured bones.*

- Place client in set position before standing him or her—for example, sitting on edge of surface with bilateral weight bearing on buttocks and hips, with knees flexed, balls of feet aligned under knees, and head in midline. *This position prepares individuals for bearing weight and permits shifting of weight from pelvis to feet as the center of gravity changes while rising.*
- Support and stabilize client's weak knees by placing one or both of your knees next to or encircling client's knees, rather than blocking them. *This allows client to flex his/her knees and lean forward to stand and transfer.*
  - Squat transfer: client leans well forward, slightly raises flexed hips off the surface, pivots, and sits down on new surface. *This is beneficial for clients with slight weight-bearing ability.*
  - Standing pivot transfer: client leans forward with hips flexed and pushes up with hands from seat surface (or arms of chair), then stands erect, pivots, and sits down on new surface. *This is beneficial for clients who have fair weight-bearing ability.*
  - Slide board transfer: client should have on pants or have a pillowcase over the board. Remove arm and leg rest from wheelchair on one side, then slightly angle chair toward new surface. Help client lean sideways, thus shifting his/her weight so transfer board can be placed well under the upper thigh of the leg next to new surface. Make sure board is safely angled across both surfaces. Help client to sit upright and place one hand on board and the other hand on surface. Remind and help client perform a series of pushups with arms while leaning slightly forward and lifting (not sliding) hips in small increments across board with each pushup. *This benefits clients with little to no weight-bearing ability (Hoeman et al, 2008; Cohen et al, 2010; Hallmark et al, 2015).*
- Position walking aids appropriately so a standing client can grasp and use them once he/she is upright. *These aids help provide support, balance, and stability to help client stand and step safely (Kalisch et al, 2013; Mayeda-Letourneau, 2014).*
- Reinforce to clients who use walkers to place one hand on walker and push with opposite hand against chair arm or surface from which they are arising to stand up. *Placing both hands on the walker may cause it to tip and the client to lose balance and fall.*
- Use ceiling-mounted or bedside mechanical bariatric lifts to transfer dependent bariatric (extremely obese) clients. *Equipment prevents client/staff injury and is essential for clients who require a moderate/maximum assist transfer (Cohen et al, 2010).*
- Use bariatric devices and use available safe client handling equipment for lifting, transferring, positioning, and sliding client (Cohen et al, 2010).
- Place a mechanical lift sling in the wheelchair preventively. Place two transfer sheets or a slide board under bariatric client. Reinforce that head should be leaning forward and that knees should be level with hips; help hold wheelchair in place as therapist directs/helps client with a scoot transfer. *Client may be too fatigued to do a manual transfer back to bed after sitting, so sling/lift can be used.*
- Perform initial and subsequent fall risk assessment. *Use standardized tools for fall risk assessment and interdisciplinary multifactorial interventions to reduce falls and risk of falling in hospitals (Cameron et al, 2010).*

T

- ▲ Collaborate with PT, OT, and pharmacist for individualized preventive/postfall plans, for example, scheduled toileting, balance and strength training, removal of hazards, chair alarms, call system/phone in reach, and review of medications. EB: *Results from a study showed low-intensity exercise and incontinence care in residents in nursing homes reduced falls (Cameron et al, 2010). More than five drugs indicates polypharmacy and puts the client at risk for adverse drug reactions, drug-drug interactions, and overall low adherence to drug therapy due to taking too many drugs (Hovstadius et al, 2010).*
- • Encourage an exercise component such as tai chi, physical therapy, or other exercise for balance, gait, and strength training in group programs or at home.
- • Modify environment for safety; recommend vision assessment and consideration for cataract removal.
- • Recommend polypharmacy assessment with special consideration to sedatives, antidepressants, and drugs affecting the central nervous system; recommend evaluation for orthostatic hypotension and irregular heartbeats; and recommend vitamin D supplementation 800 IU per day (Barclay, 2011).

Home Care

- ▲ Obtain referral for OT and PT to teach home exercises and balance as well as fall prevention and recovery. They also evaluate for potential modifications such as an entry ramp, elevated toilet seat/toilevator (raised base under toilet), tub seat or shower chair, need for shower stall with built-in seat or wheel-in shower stall without a curb/threshold, handheld flexible shower head, lever-type facets, pull-out drawers with loop handles versus cupboards, standing lift, and so on. CEB: *Petersson et al (2008) reported study subjects self-ratings for everyday life, especially in terms of safety and less difficulty in the bathroom and transfers in/out of the home, increased after home modifications.*
- • Assess for adequate lighting and hazards such as throw/area rugs, clutter, cords, and unfitted bedspreads. Suggest safe floor surfaces, such as use of adhesive nonslip strips in tubs/thresholds/areas where floor height changes; removal of wax from slippery floors; and installing low-pile carpet/nonglazed or non-glossy tiles/wood/linoleum coverings. Stress relocating commonly used items to shelves/drawers in reach, applying remote controls to appliances, and optimizing furniture placement for function, maneuverability, and stability. *Barrier removal promotes safety and accessibility; steady furniture can be used to steady or pull oneself up with if a fall occurs (Petersson et al, 2008).*
- • Nurses can provide further safety assessments by suggesting installing hand rails in bathrooms and by stairs, ensuring client's slippers and clothes fit properly, and recommending repairing or discarding broken equipment in the home (Taylor et al, 2011).
- ▲ Involve social worker or case manager to educate clients about potential assistive technology, financial cost and benefits, regulations of payers, and local resources. *Information helps clients understand options and cost of services and aids to make informed decisions.*
- ▲ Implement approaches for home care staff and family to safely handle and transfer clients. *Risk of injury is high because people often work alone, without mechanical aids or adjustable beds and in crowded spaces while giving care (Mayeda-Letourneau, 2014).*
- • For further information, refer to care plans for Impaired physical **Mobility** and Impaired **Walking.**

T

Client/Family Teaching and Discharge Planning

- • Assess for readiness to learn and use teaching modalities conducive to personal learning styles, including written instructions for home use.
- • Supervise practice sessions in which client and family apply items such as gait belts, braces, and orthoses. Check skin once aids are removed. *Repetition reinforces motor learning for safety and sound skin integrity.*
- • Teach and monitor client/family for consistent use of safety precautions for transfers (e.g., nonskid shoes, correctly placed equipment/chairs, locked brakes, leg rests swiveled away) and for correct performance of transfer or use of lifts/slings. *Promotes safety.*
- • Teach client/family how to check brakes on chairs to ensure they engage and how to check tires for adequate air pressure; advise routine inspection and annual tune-up of devices. *Long-term use may loosen brakes or cause them to slip; brakes work only if they make sound contact with tire or wheel. Pneumatic tires must be adequately inflated.*
- • Offer information on safe use of shower and commode chairs to prevent discomfort, pressure, and falls during transfer, transport, care, and hygiene.
- • For further information, refer to the care plans for Impaired physical **Mobility,** Impaired **Walking,** and Impaired wheelchair **Mobility.**

REFERENCES

Barclay, L. (2011). *Updated guidelines to prevent falls in elderly*, Medscape Education Clinical Briefs. <http://www.medscape.com/viewarticle/735768> Retrieved July 16, 2015.

Cameron, I. D., et al. (2010). Interventions for preventing falls in older people in nursing care facilities and hospitals. *Cochrane Database of Systematic Reviews*, (1), CD005465.

Centers for Disease Control and Prevention. (2015). *Safe Patient Handling*. <http://www.cdc.gov/niosh/topics/safepatient/> Retrieved July 16, 2015.

Cohen, M. H., et al. (2010). *Patient handling and movement assessments: a white paper*, The Facility Guideline Institute <http://www.fgiguidelines.org/pdfs/FGI_PHAMA_whitepaper_042810.pdf> Retrieved July 16, 2015.

Gordon, et al. (2012). Executive summary: antithrombotic therapy and prevention of thrombosis, 9th ed: American college of chest physicians evidence-based clinical practice guidelines. *Chest*, *41*(2Supply), 7S–47S.

Hallmark, B., Mechan, P., & Shores, L. (2015). Ergonomics: safe patient handling and mobility. *The Nursing Clinics of North America*, *50*, 153–166.

Hoeman, S. P., Liszner, L., & Alverzo, J. (2008). Functional mobility with activities of daily living. In S. P. Hoeman (Ed.), *Rehabilitation nursing: process, application, and outcomes* (ed. 4). St Louis: Mosby.

Hovstadius, B., et al. (2010). Increasing polypharmacy—an individual based study of the Swedish population 2005-2008. *BMC Clinical Pharmacology*, *10*(16), 1–8.

Kalisch, B. J., Dabney, B. W., & Lee, S. (2013). Safety of mobilizing hospitalized adults: Review of the literature. *Journal of Nursing Care Quality*, *28*(2), 162–168.

LaPlante, M. P., & Kaye, H. S. (2010). Demographics and trends in wheeled mobility equipment use and accessibility in the community. *Assistive Technology*, *22*, 3–17.

Mayeda-Letourneau, J. (2014). Safe patient handling and movement: a literature review. *Rehabilitation Nursing*, *39*, 123–129.

Nelson, A., et al. (2008). Myths and facts about safe patient handling in rehabilitation. *Rehabilitation Nursing*, *33*(1), 10–17.

Petersson, I., et al. (2008). Impact of home modification services on ability in everyday life for people ageing with disabilities. *Journal of Rehabilitation Medicine*, *40*, 253–260.

Riskowski, J., Dufour, A. B., & Hannan, M. T. (2011). Arthritis, foot pain and shoe wear. *Current Opinion in Rheumatology*, *23*(2), 148–155.

Taylor, C. R., et al. (2011). Safety, security and emergency preparedness. In C. R. Taylor, et al. (Eds.), *Fundamentals of nursing, the art and science of nursing care* (ed. 7). Philadelphia: Lippincott Williams & Wilkins.

Voet, N., et al. (2010). Strength training and aerobic exercise training for muscle disease. *Cochrane Database of Systematic Reviews*, (1), CD003907.

Vollman, K. M. (2010). Progressive mobility in the critically ill. *Critical Care Nurse*, *30*(2), S3–S6.

Risk for Trauma

Julianne E. Doubet, BSN, RN, CEN, NREMT-P

NANDA-I

Definition

Vulnerable to accidental tissue injury (e.g., wound, burn, fracture), which may compromise health

Risk Factors

External

Absence of call for aid device; absence of stairway gate; absence of window guard; access to weapon; bathing in very hot water; bed in high position; children riding in front seat of car; defective appliance; delay in ignition of gas appliance; dysfunctional call for aid device; electrical hazard (e.g., faulty plug, frayed wire, overloaded outlet/fuse box; exposure to corrosive product; exposure to dangerous machinery; exposure to radiation; exposure to toxic chemical; extremes of environmental temperature; flammable object (e.g., clothing, toys); gas leak; grease on stove; high crime neighborhood; icicles hanging from roof; inadequate stair rails; inadequately stored combustible (e.g., matches, oily rags); inadequately stored corrosive (e.g., lye); insufficient lighting; insufficient protection from heat source; misuse of headgear (e.g., hard hat, motorcycle helmet); misuse of seat restraint; insufficient anti-slip material in bathroom; nonuse of seat restraints; obstructed passageway; playing with dangerous object; playing with explosive; pot handle facing front of stove; proximity to vehicle pathway (e.g., driveway, railroad track); slippery floor; smoking in bed; smoking near oxygen; struggling with restraints; unanchored electric wires; unsafe operation of heavy equipment (e.g., excessive speed while intoxicated with required eyewear); unsafe road; unsafe walkway; use of cracked dishware; use of throw rugs; use of unstable chair; use of unstable ladder; wearing loose clothing around open flame

Internal

Alteration in cognitive functioning; alteration in sensation (e.g., resulting from spinal cord injury, diabetes mellitus); decrease in eye-hand coordination; decrease in muscle coordination; economically disadvantaged; emotional disturbance; history of trauma (e.g., physical, psychological, sexual); impaired balance; insufficient knowledge of safety precautions; insufficient vision; weakness

T

NOC (Nursing Outcomes Classification)

Suggested NOC Outcomes

Risk Control; Fall Prevention Behavior

Example NOC Outcome with Indicators

Accomplishes **Risk Control** as evidenced by the following indicators: Acknowledges risk/Develops effective risk-control strategies/Follows selected risk control strategies. (Rate the outcome and indicators of **Risk Control:** 1 = never demonstrated; 2 = rarely demonstrated; 3 = sometimes demonstrated; 4 = often demonstrated; 5 = consistently demonstrated [see Section I].)

Client Outcomes

Client Will (Specify Time Frame)

- Remain free from trauma
- Explain actions that can be taken to prevent trauma

NIC (Nursing Interventions Classification)

Suggested NIC Interventions

Environmental Management: Safety; Skin Surveillance

Example NIC Activities—Environmental Management

Provide family/significant other with information about making home environment safe for client; Remove harmful objects from the environment

Nursing Interventions and *Rationales*

T

- Provide vision aids for visually impaired clients. EB: *Low-vision rehabilitation enables people to restart and/or maintain the capability of performing the tasks of daily living (Virgili et al, 2013).* EB: *This study proposes that a person with diagnosed visual impairments might again have enhanced independence and a better quality of life after rehabilitative efforts using visual aids and training, to restore reading abilities and improve orientation (Trauzettel-Klosinski, 2012).*
- Assist the client with ambulation. Encourage the client to use assistive devices in activities of daily living (ADLs) as needed. EB: *Studies reviewed by Edelstein (2013) have shown the advantages—if used correctly—of employing time-honored assistive devices (e.g., crutches, walker).*
- Evaluate client's risk for burn injury. EBN: *Grant (2013) states that the very young and the elderly are at an increased risk for burn injuries when compared with any other age group.* EBN: *It is apparent to Goodarzi et al (2014) in their research that there is a continuing need for further safety education and the utilization of environmental safety measures to reduce burn trauma.*
- Assess the client for causes of impaired cognition. EB: *Adults with intellectual disabilities are likely to have an elevated risk for traumatic injury in comparison to the general populace (Finlayson et al, 2014).*
- Provide assistive devices in the home. EB: *Those who are disabled should have access to assistive technology devices and services, so as to continue their inclusion and participation in society (Office of Special Education and Rehabilitative Service, Department of Education, 2014).* EBN: *According to Johnston et al (2014), shared conclusions between the health care giver and the client with disabilities allows the client to choose the best assistive devices and services that are vital to achieving their goals of education, community living, and employment, among others.*

▲ Question the client concerning his/her sense of safety. EB: *Future functional decline in older adults may have a basis in their observations of neighborhood safety (Sun et al, 2012).* EBN: *In their study, Edwards et al (2014) state that clients who wish to remain at home at the end of life are at increased risk for trauma due to declining cognitive and/or physical capabilities, environmental dangers, and concerns with caregivers.*

▲ Assess for a substance abuse problem and refer to appropriate resources for drug and alcohol education. EB: *According to Choi et al (2014), older adults who abuse alcohol and/or illicit drugs should be sent to the most appropriate service that meets his/her needs, both for rehabilitation and any mental health challenges that may be involved.* EB: *Although drinking and driving among student drivers has declined in recent years, driving after the use of marijuana has increased; therefore, O'Malley and Johnston (2013) believe that more attention should be focused on preventing those under the influence of illicit drugs from driving.*

- Review drug profile for potential side effects that may inhibit performance of ADLs. EB: *Health care providers should assess systemic (e.g., cognition) or drug-specific characteristics such as side effects on a regular basis when dealing with the client on multiple medications (Tsai et al, 2012).*
- See care plans for Risk for **Aspiration,** Risk for **Falls,** Impaired **Home** maintenance, Risk for **Injury,** Risk for **Poisoning,** and Risk for **Suffocation.**

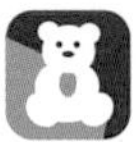

Pediatric

- Assess the client's socioeconomic status. CEB: *Pediatric clients living in poverty are at higher risk for injury (Shenessa et al, 2004).* EB: *The presently used evaluations that measure evidence of adverse childhood experiences (ACEs) may be insufficient to recognize the extent of adversity to which low-income urban children are exposed, so state Wade et al (2014).*
- Never leave young children unsupervised. EB: *According to van Beelen et al (2014), the death, disability, and loss of quality of life among young children is directly related to injuries that occur in the home.* EB: *"Drowning is a leading cause of child mortality globally," write Morrongiello et al (2013); to reduce this risk, more strategies are necessary to include increased parental awareness of children's drowning risk and their need for adult supervision when swimming.*
- Keep flammable and potentially flammable articles out of reach of young children. EB: *Infants and toddlers who scald themselves by spilling hot liquids on themselves or touching irons and hair straighteners are a main cause for concern for targeted prevention (Kemp et al, 2014).* EBN: *Hollywood and O'Neill (2014) maintain that nurses working with children in hospitals, schools, and the community can connect with parents, families, school staff, and children to offer professional advice, plus health and safety guidance for burn prevention.*
- Lock up harmful objects such as guns. EB: *Easy access to firearms in the home is responsible for injury to thousands of children in the United States (Barton & Kologi, 2014).* EB: *There is an increased risk for childhood injury when firearms are left loaded and unlocked (Schwebel et al, 2014).*

Geriatric

- Assess the geriatric client's cognitive level of functioning. EB: *Because some disease processes (e.g., Alzheimer's, Parkinson's) alter the integrity of that part of the brain that controls communication and cognitive ability, it is important to focus on a cognitive assessment that would include the evaluation of attention, memory, and executive functioning capabilities (Murray, 2012).* EB: *Patel et al (2014) agree that the occurrence of neurocognitive disorders can be an obstacle to the capability of older adults to carry out ADLs and this deficit will continue to escalate with age.*
- Assess for routine eye examinations. EBN: *The older client may find it difficult to adjust to vision loss and aging, due to the psychological, functional, social, and health implications that play a significant role in the process (Mac Cobb, 2013).* EB: *Addis et al (2013) maintain that vision loss in older adults due to cataracts, glaucoma, and/or stroke threaten their independence and may be a defining moment in their lives.*
- Perform a home safety assessment and recommend the following preventive measures: keep electrical cords out of the flow of traffic; remove small rugs or make sure they are slip resistant; increase lighting in hallways and other dark areas; place a light in the bathroom; keep towels, curtains, and other items that might catch fire away from the stove; store harmful products away from food products; provide at least one grab bar in tubs and showers; check prescribed medications for appropriate labels; store medications in original containers or in a dispenser of some type (e.g., egg carton, 7-day plastic dispenser). If the client cannot administer medications according to directions, secure someone to administer medications. Mark stove knobs with bright colors (yellow or red) and outline the borders of steps. EB: *The capability of older adults to use a home appliance depends on the client's comprehension of the appliance's operation (Soares et al, 2012b).* EBN: *As part of a person-centered, evidenced-based approach, a professional case manager/care coordinator is able to perform a thorough assessment of the client's needs and will design and put into operation an all-inclusive care plan to meet the clinical, psychosocial, and environmental requirements of the client (Johansson & Harkey, 2014).*

- Discourage driving at night. EB: *Driving is a complicated task, placing substantial demands on perceptual, cognitive, and motor capabilities, so it would seem that age-related decreases in these capabilities are negatively reflected in driving performance (Soares et al, 2012a).* EB: *Gruber et al (2013) suggest that there is an increasing number of older adults who continue to drive, and the population of drivers who are affected by deteriorating night vision is increasing.*
- Encourage the client to participate in resistance and impact exercise programs as tolerated. EB: *Graham and Connelly (2013) found that exercise plans for older adults were more successful if the exercise is enjoyable and familiar to them: the program is also more successful if the exercise is connected to training and strategies that relate to chronic conditions and offer potential health benefits.* EB: *In their review of current evidence, Carvalho et al (2014) suggest that physical activity may not only aid in improving cognitive function in older adults, but also could play a part in delaying the development of cognitive impairment in the older adult.*

Client/Family Teaching and Discharge Planning

- Educate the family regarding age-appropriate child safety precautions, environmental safety precautions, and intervention in an emergency. EB: *Safety education for parents of young children is essential in the prevention of accidental injuries in and/or around the home (van Beelen et al, 2013).* EB: *In their study, Morrongiello et al (2014) found that to decrease a child's risk of harm, the child must first understand the safety issue.*
- Teach the family to assess the child care provider's knowledge regarding child safety. EB: *Home safety interventions not only aid in reducing children's injuries, but also enhance the general safety of the home (Kendrick et al, 2013).*
- Educate the client and family regarding helmet use during recreation and sports activities. EB: *This study states that helmet use decreases bicycle-related head injuries, especially in single vehicle crashes and those in which the head strikes the ground (Owen et al, 2011).* EB: *It has been proven time and time again that wearing a bicycle helmet has averted or reduced the risk of serious head injuries (Basch et al, 2014).*
- Encourage the proper use of car seats and safety belts. EB: *Health care professionals who care for children must make every effort to impart to the child's caregiver the importance of using the size-appropriate restraint for every child on every trip (Macy et al, 2012).* EB: *Himle and Wright (2014) state that child passenger safety restraint, when used correctly, can diminish the risk of serious injury and/or death in motor vehicle crashes.*
- Teach parents to restrict driving for teens. EB: *Williams and Tefft (2013) found that in most fatal teen crashes, the passengers were the same sex and about the same age as the driver: risk factors include speeding, alcohol use, late-night driving, lack of a valid license, seat belt non-use, and multiple passengers.* EB: *According to Taubman et al (2014), research studies have shown that parents are the most important influence on young people's driving conduct.*
- Teach parents the importance of monitoring children after school. EB: *In a study by Freisthler et al (2014), children who are not supervised appropriately, either by inattentive parents and/or caregivers, could be considered neglected.* EB: *It is important to monitor teens' activities and behaviors, so that they have assistance in making important decisions (Cox et al, 2014).*
- Teach firearm safety. EB: *According to Schwebel et al (2014), firearms in the home that are loaded and unlocked are sources of increased risks for trauma.* EB: *Health care professionals must have knowledge and skills to address safe gun ownership in older adults (Pinholt et al, 2014).*
- For further information, refer to care plans for Risk for **Aspiration,** Risk for **Falls,** Impaired **Home** maintenance, Risk for **Injury,** Risk for **Poisoning,** and Risk for **Suffocation.**

T

REFERENCES

Addis, V. M., Devore, H. K., & Summeerfield, M. E. (2013). Acute visual changes in the elderly. *Clinics in Geriatric Medicine, 29*, 165–180.

Barton, B. K., & Kologi, S. M. (2014). Why do we keep them there? A qualitative assessment of firearms storage practices. *Journal of Pediatric Nursing, pii*, 14, 208–205.

Basch, C. H., Ethan, D., Rajan, S., et al. (2014). Helmet use among users of the Citi Bike bicycle-sharing program: a pilot study in New York City. *Journal of Community Health, 39*, 503–507.

Carvalho, A., Rea, I. M., Pariman, T., et al. (2014). Physical activity and cognitive function in individuals over 60 years of age: a systematic review. *Journal of Clinical Interventions in Aging, 12*, 661–682. eCollection 2014.

Choi, N. G., DiNitto, D. M., & Marti, C. N. (2014). Risk factors for self-reported driving under the influence of alcohol and illicit drugs among older adults. *The Gerontologist, 25*.

Cox, S., Pazol, K., Warner, L., et al., Centers for Disease Control and Prevention. (2014). Vital signs: births to teens age 15-17 years-United States, 1991-2012. *MMWR. Morbidity and Mortality Weekly Report*, *63*, 312–318.

Edelstein, J. E. (2013). Assistive devices for ambulation. *Physical Medicine and Rehabilitation Clinics of North America*, *29*, 291–303.

Edwards, S. B., Galanis, E., McGarvey, K., et al. (2014). Safety issues at the end of life in the home setting. *Home Health Nurse*, *22*, 398–401.

Finlayson, J., Jackson, A., Mantry, D., et al. (2014). The provision of aids and adaptions, risk assessments and incident reporting and recording procedures in relation to injury prevention in adults with intellectual disabilities: cohort study. *Journal of Intellectual Disability Research.*

Freisthler, B., Johnson-Motoyama, M., & Kepple, N. J. (2014). Inadequate child supervision: the role of alcohol outlet density, parent drinking behaviors, and social support. *Children and Youth Service Review*, *1*, 75–84.

Goodarzi, M., Reisi-Dehkordi, N., Darabeigi, R., et al. (2014). An epidemiologic study of burns: standards of care and patient education. *Iranian Journal of Nursing and Midwifery Research*, *19*, 385–389.

Graham, L. J., & Connelly, D. M. (2013). Any movement at all is exercise: a focused ethnograph of rural community-dwelling older adults' perceptions and experiences of exercise as self-care. *Physiotherapy Canada*, *65*, 333–341.

Grant, E. J. (2013). Preventing burns in the elderly. *Home Healthcare Nurse*, *31*, 561–575.

Gruber, R. M., Mosimann, U. P., Muri, R. M., et al. (2013). Vision and night driving abilities of elderly drivers. *Traffic Injury Prevention*, *14*, 477–485.

Himle, M. B., & Wright, K. A. (2014). Behavior skills training to improve installation and use of child passenger safety restraints. *Journal of Implied Behavior Analysis*, *47*, 549–559. [Epub 2014 Jun 3].

Hollywood, E., & O'Neill, T. (2014). Assessment and management of scalds and burns in children. *Nursing Children and Young People*, *26*, 28–33.

Johansson, B., & Harkey, J. (2014). Care coordination in long term home- and community-based care. *Home Healthcare Nurse*, *32*, 470–475.

Johnston, P., Currie, L. M., Drynan, D., et al. (2014). Getting it "right": how collaborative relationships between people with disabilities and professionals can lead to acquisition of needed assistive technology. *Disability and Rehabilitation: Assistive Technology*, *9*, 421–431.

Kemp, A. M., Jones, S., Lawson, Z., et al. (2014). Patterns of burns and scalds in children. *Archives of Diseases in Childhood*, *99*, 316–321. [Epub 2014 Feb 3].

Kendrick, D., Mulvaney, C. A., Yee, L., et al. (2013). Parenting interventions for the prevention of unintentional injuries in childhood. *Cochrane Database of Systematic Reviews*, *28*, 3.

Mac Cobb, S. (2013). Mobility restriction and co-morbidity in vision impaired individuals living in the community. *British Journal of Nursing*, *18*, 608–613.

Macy, M. L., Clark, S. J., Freed, G. L., et al. (2012). Carpooling and booster seats: a national survey of parents. *Pediatrics*, *129*, 290–298. [Epub 2012 Jan 30].

Morrongiello, B. A., McArthur, B. A., & Bell, M. (2014). Managing children's risk of injury in the home: does parental teaching about home safety reduce young children's hazard interactions? *Accident Analysis and Prevention*, *71*, 194–200.

Morrongiello, B. A., Sandomierski, M., Schwebel, D. C., et al. (2013). Are parents just treading water? The impact of participation on parents" judgements of children's drowning risk, swimming ability and supervision needs. *Accident Analysis and Prevention*, *50*, 1169–1175. [Epub 2012 Oct 6].

Murray, L. L. (2012). Assessing cognitive functioning in older patients: the why, who, what, and how. *Perspectives on Gerontology*, *17*, 17–26.

Office of Special Education and Rehabilitative Services, Department of Education. (2014). Final priority; rehabilitation services administration-assistive technology financing program. Final priority. *Federal Register*, *79*, 47575–47579.

O'Malley, P. M., & Johnson, L. D. (2013). Driving after drug or alcohol use bu US high school seniors, 2001-2011. *American Journal of Public Health*, *103*, 2027–2034.

Owen, R., Kendrick, D., Mulvaney, C., et al. (2011). Non-legislative interventions for the promotion of cycle helmet wearing by children. *Cochrane Database of Systematic Reviews*, (11).

Patel, D., Syed, Q., Messenger-Rapport, B. J., et al. (2014). Firearms in frail hands: an ADL or public health crisis. *American Journal of Alzheimer's Disease and Other Dementias*, pii: 1533317514545867.

Pinholt, G. M., Mitchell, J. D., Butler, J. H., et al. (2014). "Is there a gun in the home?"Assessing the risks of gun ownership in older adults. *Journal of the American Geriatric Society*, *62*, 1142–1146.

Schwebel, D. C., Lewis, T., Simon, S. R., et al. (2014). Prevalence and correlation of firearm ownership in the homes of fifth graders: Birmingham, Ala., Houston, Texas., and Los Angeles, Ca. *Health Education and Behavior*, *41*, 299–306.

Shenessa, E. D., Stubbendick, A., & Brown, M. J. (2004). Social disparities on housing and related pediatric injury: a multilevel study. *American Journal of Public Health*, *94*, 633–639.

Soares, M. M., Jacob, K., Gentzler, M. D., et al. (2012a). A literature review of major perceptual, cognitive, and/or physical test batteries for older drivers. *Work (Reading, Mass.)*, *41*, 5381–5383.

Soares, M. M., Jacobs, K., Higgins, P. G., et al. (2012b). Development of guidelines for designing appliances for older people. *Work (Reading, Mass.)*, *41*, 333–3339.

Sun, V. K., Stijacio, C. I., Kao, H., et al. (2012). How safe is your neighborhood? Perceived neighborhood safety and functional decline in older adults. *Journal of General Internal Medicine*, *27*, 541–547.

Taubman, B. A. O., Musicant, O., Lotan, T., et al. (2014). The contribution of parents' driving behavior, family climate for road safety, and parent-targeted intervention to young male driving behavior. *Accident Analysis and Prevention*, *2*, 296–301.

Trauzettel-Klosinski, S. (2012). Current methods of visual rehabilitation. *Deutsches Ärzteblatt International*, *108*, 871–878.

Tsai, K. T., Chen, J. H., Wen, C. J., et al. (2012). Medication adherence among geriatric outpatients prescribed multiple medications. *American Journal of Geriatric Pharmacotherapy*, *10*, 61–68. [Epub 2012 Jan 20].

van Beelen, M. E., Beirens, T. M., den Hartog, P., et al. (2014). Effectiveness of web-based tailored advice on parents' child safety behaviors randomized controlled trial. (2014). *Journal of Medical Internet Research*, *16*, e17.

van Beelen, M. E., Vogel, I., Bieriens, T. M., et al. (2013). Web-based e health to support counseling in routine well-child care: pilot study of E-health 4Uth home safety. *Journal of Medical Internet Research*, *2*, e9.

Virgili, G., Acosta, R., Grover, L. L., et al. (2013). Reading aids for adults with low vision. *Cochrane Database of Systematic Reviews*, (10).

Wade, R., Shea, J. A., Ruben, D., et al. (2014). Adverse childhood experiences of low-income, urban youth. *Pediatrics*, *134*, 13–20. [Epub 2014 Jun 16].

Williams, A. F., & Tefft, B. C. (2013). Characteristics of teens-with-teens fatal crashes in the United States, 2000-2010. *Journal of Safety Research*, *48*, 37–42.

T

Unilateral Neglect *Lori M. Rhudy, PhD, RN, CNRN, ACNS-BC*

NANDA-I

Definition

Impairment in sensory and motor response, mental representation, and spatial attention of the body and the corresponding environment characterized by inattention to one side and overattention to the opposite side; left-side neglect is more severe and persistent than right-side neglect

Defining Characteristics

Alteration in safety behavior on neglected side; disturbance of sound lateralization; failure to dress neglected side; failure to eat food from portion of plate on neglected side; failure to groom neglected side; failure to move eyes in the neglected hemisphere; failure to move head in the neglected hemisphere; failure to move limbs in the neglected hemisphere; failure to move trunk in the neglected hemisphere; failure to notice people approaching from the neglected side; hemianopia; impaired performance on line cancellation, line bisection, and target cancellation tests; left hemiplegia from cerebrovascular accident; marked deviation of the eyes to stimuli on the non-neglected side; marked deviation of the trunk to stimuli on the non-neglected side; omission of drawing on the neglected side; perseveration; representational neglect (e.g., distortion of drawing on the neglected side; substitution of letters to form alternative words when reading; transfer of pain sensation to the non-neglected side; unaware of positioning of neglected limb; unilateral visuospatial neglect; use of vertical half of page only when writing

Related Factors (r/t)

Brain injury (e.g., cerebrovascular impairment, neurological illness, trauma, tumor)

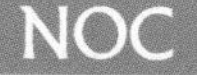

NOC (Nursing Outcomes Classification)

Suggested NOC Outcomes

Body Image; Body Positioning: Self-Initiated; Mobility; Self-Care: Activities of Daily Living (ADLs)

Example NOC Outcome with Indicators

Mobility as evidenced by the following indicators: Balance/Coordination/Gait/Muscle movement. (Rate the outcome and indicators of **Mobility:** 1 = severely compromised, 2 = substantially compromised, 3 = moderately compromised, 4 = mildly compromised, 5= not compromised [see Section I].)

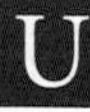

Client Outcomes

Client Will (Specify Time Frame)

- Use techniques that can be used to minimize unilateral neglect
- Care for both sides of the body appropriately and keep affected side free from harm
- Return to the highest functioning level possible based on personal goals and abilities
- Remain free from injury

NIC (Nursing Interventions Classification)

Suggested NIC Intervention

Unilateral Neglect Management

Example NIC Activities—Unilateral Neglect Management

Ensure that affected extremities are properly and safely and positioned; Rearrange the environment to use the right or left visual field

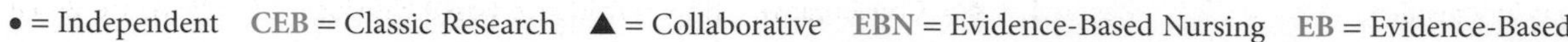

Nursing Interventions and *Rationales*

- Assess the client for signs of unilateral neglect (UN; e.g., not washing, shaving, or dressing one side of the body; sitting or lying inappropriately on affected arm or leg; failing to respond to environmental stimuli contralateral to the side of lesion; eating food on only one side of plate; or failing to look to one side of the body). *Many tests for UN exist, but there is no consensus about which is the most valid. Joint assessments of UN that include both clinical observation and precise testing perform better than either used alone (Jepson et al, 2008).* EB: *There is no difference in gender and UN in a sample of 155 women and 157 men with acute stroke (Kleinman et al, 2008).* EB: *UN was identified in 70 of 71 clients using National Institutes of Health Stroke Scale (NIHSS).*
- ▲ Collaborate with health care provider for referral to a rehabilitation team (including, but not limited to, rehabilitation clinical nurse specialist, physical medicine and rehabilitation health care provider, neuropsychologist, occupational therapist, physical therapist, and speech and language pathologist) for continued help in dealing with UN. EB: *There is some evidence that rehabilitation for unilateral spatial neglect using tools such as visual scanning and prism adaptation improves performance, but its effect on disability is not clear. Further studies are needed (Ting et al, 2011).*
- Use the principles of rehabilitation to progressively increase the client's ability to compensate for UN by using assistive devices, feedback, and support. EB: *Studies demonstrate that recovery from UN generally occurs in first 4 weeks after stroke with much more gradual recovery after that (Osawa & Maeshima, 2009).*
- Set up the environment so that essential activity is on the unaffected side:
  - Place the client's personal items within view and on the unaffected side.
  - Position the bed so that client is approached from the unaffected side.
  - Monitor and assist the client to achieve adequate food and fluid intake.

Helps in focusing attention and aids in maintenance of safety.

- Implement fall prevention interventions. Clients with right hemisphere brain damage are twice as likely to fall as those with left hemisphere damage (*Jepson et al, 2008*).
- Position affected extremity in a safe and functional manner. EB: *A study found that clients with UN had higher rates of shoulder-hand complications than those without UN (Wee & Hopman, 2008).* EB: *Clients with neglect had significantly lower FIM (functional independence measure) motor scores than those with aphasia (Gialanella & Ferlucci, 2010).*
- Teach the client to be aware of the problem and modify behavior and environment. EB: *Awareness of the environment decreases risk of injury. There is some evidence that use of scanning techniques may decrease visual neglect (Ting et al, 2011).*

Home Care

- Many of the previously listed interventions may be adapted for use in the home care setting.
- Position bed at home so that client gets out of bed on unaffected side. *Positioning the bed so that the client gets out on the unaffected side can increase safety.*

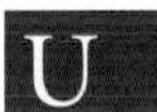

Client/Family Teaching and Discharge Planning

- Engage discharge planning specialists for comprehensive assessment and planning early in the client's stay. EB: *A study demonstrated that clients with UN have longer length of stay and less likelihood of discharge to home than subjects without UN (Cumming et al, 2009).*
- Encourage family participation in care and exercise. EB: *UN improved in clients who participated in exercise training with their family members (Osawa & Maeshima, 2009).*
- Explain pathology and symptoms of unilateral neglect to both the client and family.
- Teach the client how to scan regularly to check the position of body parts and to regularly turn head from side to side for safety when ambulating, using a wheelchair, or doing self-care tasks.
- Reinforce the client's use of adaptive devices such as prisms prescribed by rehabilitation professionals (Shiraishi et al, 2008).
- Teach caregivers to cue the client to the environment.

REFERENCES

Cumming, T. B., et al. (2009). Hemispatial neglect and rehabilitation in acute stroke. *Archives of Physical Medicine and Rehabilitation, 90*(11), 1931–1936.

Gialanella B, Ferlucci C. (2010). Functional outcome after stroke in patients with aphasia and neglect: assessment by the motor and cognitive functional independence measure instrument. *Cerebrovascular Diseases(Basel, Switzerland), 30*(5):440–447.

Jepson, R., Despain, K., & Keller, D. C. (2008). Unilateral neglect: assessment in nursing practice. *The Journal of Neuroscience Nursing: Journal of the American Association of Neuroscience Nurses, 40*(3), 142–149.

Kleinman, J. T., et al. (2008). Gender differences in unilateral spatial neglect within 24 hours of ischemic stroke. *Brain and Cognition, 68*, 49–52.

Osawa, A., & Maeshima, S. (2009). Family participation can improve unilateral spatial neglect in patients with acute right hemispheric stroke. *European Neurology, 63*, 170–175.

Shiraishi, H., et al. (2008). Long-term effects of prism adaptation on chronic neglect after stroke. *Neurorehabilitation, 23*(2), 137–151.

Ting, D. S. J., et al. (2011). Visual neglect following stroke: current concepts and future focus. *Survey of Ophthalmology, 56*(2), 114–134.

Wee, J. Y. M., & Hopman, W. M. (2008). Comparing consequences of right and left unilateral neglect in a stroke rehabilitation population. *American Journal of Physical Medicine and Rehabilitation, 87*(11), 910–920.

Impaired Urinary elimination

Michelle Acorn, DNP, NP PHC-Adult, BA, BScN/PHCNP, MN/ACNP, ENC(C), GNC(C), CAP, CGP, and Betty J. Ackley, MSN, EdS, RN

NANDA-I

Definition

Dysfunction in urine elimination

Defining Characteristics

Dysuria; frequent voiding; hesitancy; nocturia; urinary incontinence; urinary retention; urinary urgency

Related Factors

Anatomic obstruction; multiple causality; sensory motor impairment; urinary tract infection (UTI)

NOC (Nursing Outcomes Classification)

Suggested NOC Outcome

Urinary Elimination

Example NOC Outcome with Indicators

Urinary Elimination as evidenced by the following indicators: Urine clarity/urine odor, fluid intake, pain with urination. (Rate the outcome and indicators of **Urinary Elimination:** 1 = severely compromised 2 = substantially compromised, 3 = moderately compromised, 4 = mildly compromised, 5 = not compromised [see Section I].)

U

Client Outcomes

Client Will (Specify Time Frame)

- State absence of pain or excessive urgency during urination
- Demonstrate voiding frequency no more than every 2 hours

NIC (Nursing Interventions Classification)

Suggested NIC Intervention

Urinary Elimination Management

Example NIC Activities—Urinary Elimination Management

Monitor urinary elimination, including frequency, consistency, odor, volume, and color, as appropriate; Teach client signs and symptoms of UTI

Nursing Interventions and *Rationales*

- Ask the client about urinary elimination patterns and concerns. *Urinary elimination problems have many presenting signs and symptoms. Asking the client questions may help understand the subtle signs and symptoms associated with urinary elimination (Mayo Clinic, 2012).*
- Question the client regarding the following:
  - Presence of symptoms such as incontinence, dribbling, frequency, urgency, dysuria, and nocturia
  - Presence of pain in the area of the bladder
  - The pattern of urination and approximate amount
  - Possible aggravating and alleviating factors for urinary problems
- Ask the client to keep a bladder diary/bladder log. EB: *Use of a bladder diary may reduce client discrepancies in recall and is a valuable tool for assessment; short (24-hour) duration of the bladder diary may yield inadequate data, and excessive diary duration reduces compliance (Bright et al, 2011).*
- For interventions on urinary incontinence, refer to the following nursing diagnosis care plans as appropriate: Stress urinary **Incontinence,** Urge urinary **Incontinence,** Reflex urinary **Incontinence,** Overflow urinary **Incontinence,** or Functional urinary **Incontinence.**

▲ Perform a focused physical assessment including inspecting the perineal skin integrity, percussion, and palpation of the lower abdomen looking for obvious bladder distention or an enlarged kidney. *A palpable kidney or bladder provides direct evidence of a dilated urinary collection system (Policastro et al, 2014).* If signs of urinary obstruction are present, refer client to a urologist. *Unrelieved obstruction of urine can result in renal damage, and if severe, renal failure (Policastro et al, 2011). Refer to the nursing care plan for* ***Urinary Retention*** *if retention is present.*

▲ Check for costovertebral tenderness. *Costovertebral tenderness is seen with pyelonephritis and kidney stones (Gupta & Trautner, 2011).*

▲ Review results of urinalysis for the presence of urinary infection: white blood cells, red blood cells, bacteria, positive nitrites. If urinalysis results are not available, request a midstream specimen of urine (urine obtained during voiding, discarding the first and last portions) for a urinalysis (Norrby, 2011).

▲ If blood or protein is present in the urine, recognize that both hematuria and proteinuria are serious symptoms, and the client should be referred to a urologist to receive a workup to rule out pathology.

- Inquire about the client's history of smoking. EB: *Smoking and bladder symptoms in women found that urgency and frequency are three times more common among current than never smokers. Parallel associations suggest dose-related response associations. Nocturia and stress urinary incontinence (SUI) are not associated with smoking. Smoking cessation recommended (Tahtinen et al, 2011).*

Urinary Tract Infection

▲ Consult the provider for a culture and sensitivity testing and antibiotic treatment in the individual with evidence of a symptomatic UTI. *UTI is a transient, reversible condition that is usually associated with urgency or urge urinary incontinence (Norrby, 2011). Eradication of UTI will alleviate or reverse symptoms of suprapubic pressure and discomfort, urgency, daytime voiding frequency, and dysuria (Norrby, 2011).*

▲ Teach the client to recognize symptoms of UTI: dysuria that crescendos as the bladder nears complete evacuation; urgency to urinate followed by micturition of only a few drops; suprapubic aching discomfort; malaise; voiding frequency; sudden exacerbation of urinary incontinence with or without fever, chills, and flank pain. Recognize that a cloudy or malodorous urine, in the absence of other lower urinary tract symptoms, may not indicate the presence of a UTI and that asymptomatic bacteriuria in the older adult does not justify a course of antibiotics. *Asymptomatic bacteriuria may be associated with cloudy or malodorous urine, but these signs alone do not justify antimicrobial therapy when balanced against the potential adverse effects of treatment, including adverse side effects of the various antibiotics and encouragement of colonization of the urine with antibiotic-resistant bacterial strains (Ariathianto, 2011; Norrby, 2011).*

▲ Refer the individual with chronic lower urinary tract pain to a urologist or specialist in the management of pelvic pain. *Bladder pain and storage symptoms, in the absence of an acute urinary infection, may indicate the presence of interstitial cystitis, a chronic condition requiring ongoing treatment (Interstitial Cystitis Association, 2015).*

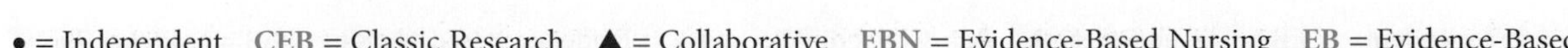

Geriatric

▲ Perform urinalysis in all older adults who experience a sudden change in urine elimination patterns such as new-onset incontinence, lower abdominal discomfort, acute confusion, or a fever of unclear origin. *Older adults often experience atypical symptoms with a UTI or pyelonephritis (Nazarko, 2009).*

- Encourage older women consume one to two servings of fresh blueberries and consider drinking at least 10 oz of cranberry juice daily or supplement the diet with cranberry concentrate capsules as ordered. EB: *While the evidence supporting the consumption of cranberry juice or tablets to reduce UTIs is inconclusive (Jepson et al, 2012), some evidence does suggest that the consumption of 8 to 10 oz of cranberry juice, ascorbic acid (vitamin C) supplement, or an equivalent portion of foods containing whole cranberries or blueberries exerts a bacteriostatic effect on* Escherichia coli, *the most common pathogen associated with urinary infection among community-dwelling adult women (Masson et al, 2009; Aydin et al, 2014).*

▲ Refer the older woman with recurrent UTIs to her health care provider for possible use of topical estrogen creams for treatment of atrophic vaginal mucosa from decreased hormonal stimulation, which can predispose to UTIs (Buhr et al, 2011; Norrby, 2011; Aydin et al, 2014).

▲ Recognize that UTIs in older men are typically associated with prostatic hyperplasia or strictures of the urethra. Refer to a urologist (Norrby, 2011).

Client/Family Teaching and Discharge Planning

- Teach the client/family methods to keep the urinary tract healthy. Refer to Client/Family Teaching in the care plan for Readiness for enhanced **Urinary** elimination.
- Teach the following measures to women to decrease the incidence of UTIs:
  - Urinate at appropriate intervals. Do not ignore need to void, which can result in stasis of urine.
  - Drink plenty of liquids, especially water. *Drinking water helps dilute the urine, allowing bacteria to be flushed from the urinary tract before an infection can begin (Norrby, 2011).*
  - Wipe from front to back. *This helps prevent bacteria in the anal region from spreading to the vagina and urethra.*
  - Wear underpants that have a cotton crotch. *This allows air to circulate in the area and decreases moisture in the area, which predisposes to infection.*
  - Avoid potentially irritating feminine products. *Using deodorant sprays, bubble baths, or other feminine products, such as douches and powders, in the genital area can irritate the urethra. There are multiple common sense measures that can be used to decrease the incidence of UTIs (Gupta & Trautner, 2011; Mayo Clinic, 2012).*
- Teach the sexually active woman with recurrent UTIs prevention measures including:
  - Void after intercourse to flush bacteria out of the urethra and bladder.
  - Use a lubricating agent as needed during intercourse to protect the vagina from trauma and decrease the incidence of vaginitis.
  - Watch for signs of vaginitis and seek treatment as needed.
  - Avoid use of diaphragms with spermicide.

Sexually active women have the highest incidence of UTIs (Norrby, 2011). The vagina and periurethral area can become colonized with organisms from the intestinal flora, such as E. coli, *and increase the risk for UTIs (Gupta & Trautner, 2011).*

- Teach clients with spinal cord injury and neurogenic bladder dysfunction to consider adding cranberry extract tablets or cranberry juice, or fruits containing D-mannose (e.g., apples, oranges, peaches, blueberries) on a daily basis, monitor fluid intake. The client is encouraged to discuss the use of probiotics and antibiotic therapy with the provider for frequent recurrent symptomatic UTIs. EB: *Limited evidence suggests that clients who regularly consume cranberry extract tablets experience fewer UTIs than clients who do not routinely consume cranberry extract tablets (Hess et al, 2008; Jepson et al, 2012; Keifer, 2013; Shmuely, 2012; Barbosa-Cesnik et al, 2011). Additionally, clients with spinal cord injury and neurogenic bladder dysfunction are at higher risk for UTI, and more frequent monitoring of symptomatic infection is necessary (Goetz & Klausner, 2014).*
- Teach all persons to recognize hematuria and to promptly seek care if this symptom occurs.

REFERENCES

Ariathianto, Y. (2011). Asymptomatic bacteriuria—prevalence in the elderly population. *Australian Family Physician, 40*(10), 805–809.

Aydin, A., Ahmed, K., Zaman, I., et al. (2014). Recurrent urinary tract infections in women. *International Urogynecology Journal, 26*(6), 795–804.

Barbosa-Cesnik, C., et al. (2011). Cranberry juice fails to prevent recurrent urinary tract infection: results from a randomized placebo-controlled trial. *Clinical Infectious Diseases: an Official Publication of the Infectious Diseases Society of America*, *52*(1), 23–30.

Bright, E., Drake, M. J., & Abrams, P. (2011). Urinary diaries: evidence for the development and validation of diary content, format, and duration. *Neurourology and Urodynamics*, *30*(3), 348–352.

Buhr, G. T., Genao, L., & White, H. I. (2011). Urinary tract infections in long-term care residents. *Clinics in Geriatric Medicine*, *27*(2), 229–239.

Goetz, L. L., & Klausner, A. P. (2014). Strategies for prevention of urinary tract infections in neurogenic bladder dysfunction. *Physical Medicine and Rehabilitation Clinics of North America*, *25*(3), 605–618, viii.

Gupta, K., & Trautner, B. (2011). Urinary tract infections, pyelonephritis, and prostatitis. In D. L. Longo, et al. (Eds.), *Harrison's principles of internal medicine* (18th ed.). New York: McGraw-Hill.

Hess, M. J., et al. (2008). Evaluation of cranberry tablets for the prevention of urinary tract infections in spinal cord injured patients with neurogenic bladder. *Spinal Cord*, *46*(9), 622–626.

Interstitial Cystitis Association: *Pain and IC.* (2015). From <http://www.ichelp.org/Page.aspx?pid=821>. Retrieved January 18, 2015.

Jepson, R. G., Williams, G., & Craig, J. C. (2012). Cranberries for preventing urinary tract infections. *Cochrane Database of Systematic Reviews*, (10), Art. No.: CD001321.

Keifer, D. (2013). *Vitamins and Supplements: D-Mannose. WebMD.* <http://www.webmd.com/vitamins-and-supplements/d-mannose-uses-and-risks>. Retrieved April 9, 2015.

Masson, P., et al. (2009). Meta-analyses in prevention and treatment of urinary tract infections. *Infectious Disease Clinics of North America*, *23*(2), 355–385.

Mayo Clinic. (2012). *Prevention of urinary tract infections.* From <http://www.mayoclinic.com/health/urinary-tract-infection/DS00286/DSECTION=prevention>. Retrieved January 18, 2015.

Nazarko, L. (2009). Urinary tract infection: diagnosis, treatment and prevention. *British Journal of Nursing (Mark Allen Publishing)*, *18*(19), 1170–1174.

Norrby, S. R. (2011). Approach to the patient with urinary tract infection. In L. Goldman & A. Schafer (Eds.), *Goldman's Cecil medicine* (24th ed.). St Louis: Saunders/Elsevier.

Policastro, M., Sinert, R. H., & Guerrero, P. (2014). *Urinary obstruction.* Medscape Reference <http://emedicine.medscape.com/article/778456-overview>. Retrieved January 18, 2015.

Shmuely, H., et al. (2012). Cranberry components for the therapy of infectious disease. *Current Opinion in Biotechnology*, *23*(2), 148–152.

Tahtinen, R. M., Auvinen, A., Cartwithgt, R., et al. (2011). Smoking and bladder symptoms in women. *Obstetrics and Gynecology*, *118*(3), 643–648.

Readiness for enhanced Urinary elimination

Michelle Acorn, DNP, NP PHC-Adult, BA, BScN/PHCNP, MN/ACNP, ENC(C), GNC(C), CAP, CGP, and Betty J. Ackley, MSN, EdS, RN

NANDA-I

Definition

A pattern of urinary functions for meeting eliminatory needs, which can be strengthened

Defining Characteristics

Expresses desire to enhance urinary elimination

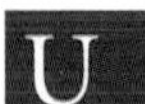

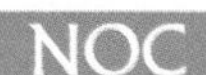

NOC (Nursing Outcomes Classification)

Suggested NOC Outcome

Urinary Elimination

Example NOC Outcome with Indicators

Urinary Elimination as evidenced by the following indicators: Urine clarity/urine odor, fluid intake, pain with urination. (Rate the outcome and indicators of **Urinary Elimination:** 1 = severely compromised, 2 = substantially compromised, 3 = moderately compromised, 4 = mildly compromised, 5 = not compromised [see Section I].)

Client Outcomes

Client Will (Specify Time Frame)

- Urinate every 3 to 4 hours while awake
- Remain free of undetected symptoms of a urinary tract infection (UTI) or cancer of the kidney or bladder
- Drink fluids at a sufficient level to have light yellow (e.g., straw-colored) urine

NIC (Nursing Interventions Classification)

Suggested NIC Intervention

Urinary Elimination Management

Example NIC Activities—Urinary Elimination Management

Monitor urinary elimination, including frequency, consistency, odor, volume, and color, as appropriate; Teach client signs and symptoms of UTI

Nursing Interventions and *Rationales*

- Ask the client questions regarding any bothersome or concerning urinary symptoms such as frequency, nocturia, urgency, dysuria, or retention of urine.
- Question the client regarding presence of incontinence. If incontinence is present, refer to the appropriate care plan: Stress urinary **Incontinence,** Urge urinary **Incontinence,** Functional urinary **Incontinence,** or Reflex urinary **Incontinence.**
- Question the client regarding history of urinary tract infections UTIs. If the client has had UTIs in the past, provide teaching for prevention as outlined in the care plan for Impaired **Urinary** elimination.
- Ask the client to complete a bladder diary of diurnal and nocturnal urine elimination patterns and patterns of urinary leakage. CEB: *A study demonstrated that women overestimated daytime urinary frequency from recall. Use of a bladder diary results in increased accuracy of reporting of bladder symptoms (Stay et al, 2009).*

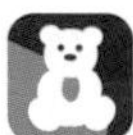

Pediatric

- Encourage children and adolescents to maintain normal weight because obesity has been related to cancers of the urinary tract. EB: *A large study found an increase in cancer of the bladder, ureter, and renal pelvis in adolescents who were obese at the age of 17 and developed cancer years later (Leiba et al, 2012). Refer to care plan for* ***Obesity*** *and* ***Overweight.***

Geriatric

- Encourage older women to consume one to two servings of fresh blueberries and consider drinking at least 10 oz of cranberry juice daily or supplement the diet with cranberry concentrate capsules as ordered. EB: *While the evidence supporting the consumption of cranberry juice or tablets to reduce UTIs is inconclusive (Jepson et al, 2012), some evidence does suggest that the consumption of 8 to 10 oz of cranberry juice, ascorbic acid (vitamin C) supplement, or an equivalent portion of foods containing whole cranberries or blueberries exerts a bacteriostatic effect on* Escherichia coli, *the most common pathogen associated with urinary infection among community-dwelling adult women (Masson et al, 2009; Aydin et al, 2014).*
- Older adults with toileting disability have increased care costs and dependency. *Prevention efforts include physical activity programs targeting impairments with walking, standing, sitting, stooping, reaching, and grasping. Therapy should improve dressing, bathing, and transferring skills (Tally et al, 2014).*

U

Client/Family Teaching and Discharge Planning

- Teach the client general guidelines for health of the urinary system:
- ▲ Ensure good hydration. Total daily fluid intake should be approximately 2.7 L per day for women and 3.7 L per day for men (Newman & Willson, 2011). *Adequate fluid helps wash out bacteria from the urethra to prevent UTIs, helps prevent kidney stones, and potentially protects the client from development of cancer of the bladder from exposure to carcinogens concentrated in the urine (Newman & Willson, 2011).*
- ▲ Recommend the client have a physical exam, a metabolic panel of laboratory tests, and a urinalysis done yearly. *A urinalysis includes tests for red blood cells and white blood cells, which can help identify cancer of the bladder and infection in the urinary tract, respectively. The urinalysis also includes testing for proteinuria, which can be found with damage to the kidney. The metabolic panel includes tests of blood urea nitrogen and serum creatinine, which, if elevated, indicate that the client has early kidney damage (Lin & Denker, 2011).*
- ▲ Recommend that the client not hold urine for long periods of time before emptying the bladder. It is normal to urinate every 3 to 4 hours. *Stasis of urine in the bladder leads to an increased chance of a UTI*

and may predispose to stone formation (Seifter, 2011). Note: *Health care professionals frequently are busy with clients and forget or ignore the urge to urinate. This can predispose individuals to UTIs.*

- ▲ Recommend that the client with frequency, urgency in the morning, or possible incontinence consider reducing or eliminating caffeine intake.
- • If the client has constipation at intervals, share measures to alleviate or prevent constipation, including adequate consumption of dietary fluids, dietary fiber, exercise, and regular bowel elimination patterns. *Constipation predisposes the individual to urinary retention and increases the risk for UTI. See care plan for* ***Constipation.***
- • Advise clients to stop smoking because of the association with damage to the kidney and bladder, including chronic kidney disease, bladder cancer, urinary incontinence, and bothersome lower urinary tract symptoms in men. *Smoking is a known risk factor for chronic kidney disease (Rezonzew et al, 2012).* CEB: *Smoking may increase the severity and risk of urinary incontinence, and it is clearly linked with an increased risk for bladder cancer (Lodovici & Bigagli, 2009).* EB: *Smoking and bladder symptoms in women found that urgency and frequency are three times more common among current smokers than never smokers. Parallel associations suggest dose-related response associations. Nocturia and symptomatic UTI are not associated with smoking. Smoking cessation recommended (Tahtinen et al, 2011).*
- ▲ Encourage the client to eat a healthy diet, avoiding processed meats, with sodium nitrate as a preservative, to decrease incidence of cancer of the bladder. EB: *A study demonstrated that people who ate more processed meats had an increased risk for development of cancer of the bladder (Wu et al, 2012).*

REFERENCES

Aydin, A., Ahmed, K., Zaman, I., et al. (2014). Recurrent urinary tract infections in women. *International Urogynecology Journal, 26*(6), 795–804.

Jepson, R. G., Williams, G., & Craig, J. C. (2012). Cranberries for preventing urinary tract infections. *Cochrane Database of Systematic Reviews*, (10), Art. No.: CD001321.

Leiba, A., et al. (2012). *Overweight in adolescence is related to increased risk of future urothelial cancer*, Apr 18, [Epub ahead of print].

Lin, J., & Denker, B. (2011). Azotemia and urinary abnormalities. In D. L. Longo, et al. (Eds.), *Harrison's principles of internal medicine* (18th ed.). New York: McGraw-Hill.

Lodovici, M., & Bigagli, E. (2009). Biomarkers of induced active and passive smoking damage. *International Journal of Environmental Research and Public Health, 6*(3), 874–888.

Masson, P., et al. (2009). Meta-analyses in prevention and treatment of urinary tract infections. *Infectious Disease Clinics of North America, 23*(2), 355–385.

Newman, D., & Willson, M. (2011). Review of intermittent catheterization and current best practices. *Urologic Nursing, 31*(1), 12–48.

Rezonzew, G., et al. (2012). Nicotine exposure and the progression of chronic kidney disease: role of the alpha7-nicotinic acetylcholine receptor. *American Journal of Physiology—Renal Physiology, 303*(2), F304–F312.

Seifter, J. (2011). Urinary tract obstruction. In D. L. Longo, et al. (Eds.), *Harrison's principles of internal medicine* (18th ed.). New York: McGraw-Hill.

Stay, K., Dwyer, P. L., & Rosamilia, A. (2009). Women overestimate daytime urinary frequency: the importance of the bladder diary. *The Journal of Urology, 181*(5), 2176–2180.

Tahtinen, R. M., Auvinen, A., Cartwithgt, R., et al. (2011). Smoking and bladder symptoms in women. *Obstetrics and Gynecology, 118*(3), 643–648.

Tally, K. M., Wyam, J. F., Bronas, U. G., et al. (2014). Factors associated with toileting disability in older adults. *Nursing Research, 63*(2), 94–104.

Wu, J. W., et al. (2012). Dietary intake of meat, fruits, vegetables, and selective micronutrients and risk of bladder cancer in the New England region of the United States. *British Journal of Cancer, 106*(11), 1891–1898.

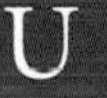

Urinary Retention

Michelle Acorn, DNP, NP PHC-Adult, BA, BScN/PHCNP, MN/ACNP, ENC(C), GNC(C), CAP, CGP, and Betty J. Ackley, MSN, EdS, RN

NANDA-I

Definition

Incomplete emptying of the bladder

Defining Characteristics

Absent urinary output; bladder distention; dribbling of urine; dysuria; frequent voiding; overflow incontinence; residual urine; sensation of bladder fullness; small voiding

Related Factors

Blockage in urinary tract; high urethral pressure; reflex arc inhibition; strong sphincter

NOC (Nursing Outcomes Classification)

Suggested NOC Outcome

Urinary Elimination

Example NOC Outcome with Indicators

Urinary Elimination as evidenced by the following indicators: Empties bladder completely/Absence of urinary leakage/Urine clarity. (Rate the outcome and indicators of **Urinary Elimination:** 1 = severely compromised, 2 = substantially compromised, 3 = moderately compromised, 4 = mildly compromised, 5 = not compromised [see Section I].)

Client Outcomes

Client Will (Specify Time Frame)

- Demonstrate consistent ability to urinate when desire to void is perceived
- Have measured urinary residual volume of less than 200 to 250 mL
- Experience correction or relief from dysuria, nocturia, postvoid dribbling, and voiding frequently
- Be free of a urinary tract infection

NIC (Nursing Interventions Classification)

Suggested NIC Interventions

Urinary Catheterization; Urinary Retention Care

Example NIC Activities—Urinary Retention Care

Perform a comprehensive urinary assessment focusing on incontinence (e.g., urinary output, urinary voiding pattern, cognitive function, and preexistent urinary problems); Use the power of suggestion by running water or flushing toilet

Nursing Interventions and *Rationales*

- Obtain a focused urinary history including questioning the client about episodes of acute urinary retention (complete inability to void) or chronic retention (documented elevated postvoid residual volumes), as well as symptoms such as dysuria, nocturia, postvoid dribbling, and voiding frequently. *A history of difficulty voiding, pain, infection, or decreased urine volume is common in clients with urinary obstruction (Seifter, 2012).*
- Question the client concerning specific risk factors for urinary retention including:
  - Spinal cord injuries
  - Ischemic stroke
  - Metabolic disorders such as diabetes mellitus, chronic alcoholism, and related conditions associated with polyuria and peripheral polyneuropathies
  - Herpetic infection
  - Heavy-metal poisoning (lead, mercury) causing peripheral polyneuropathies
  - Advanced stage human immunodeficiency virus (HIV) infection
  - Medications including antispasmodics/parasympatholytics, alpha-adrenergic agonists, antidepressants, sedatives, narcotics, psychotropic medications, illicit drugs
  - Recent surgery requiring general or spinal anesthesia
  - Vaginal delivery within the past 48 hours
  - Bowel elimination patterns, history of fecal impaction, encopresis
  - Recent surgical procedures
  - Recent prostatic biopsy

  Urinary retention is related to multiple factors affecting either detrusor contraction strength or urethral resistance to urinary outflow (Policastro et al, 2011).
- Complete a pain assessment including pain intensity using a self-report pain tool, such as the 0 to 10 numerical pain rating scale. Also determine location, quality, onset/duration, intensity, aggravating/

U

alleviating factors, and effects of pain on function and quality of life. *Acute onset of obstruction with inability to void is associated with significant pain; partial obstruction causes minimal pain, which may delay diagnosis (Policastro et al, 2011). Bladder distention is associated with pain overlying the bladder (Seifter, 2012).*

- Perform a focused physical assessment including perineal skin integrity and inspection, percussion, and palpation of the lower abdomen, looking for obvious bladder distention or an enlarged kidney. *A palpable kidney or bladder provides direct evidence of a dilated urinary collection system (Policastro et al, 2011).*
- Recognize that unrelieved obstruction of urine can result in kidney damage and, if severe, kidney failure. Urinary retention can be a medical emergency and should be reported to the primary provider as soon as possible. EB: *As urine backs up in the urinary tract, the pressure increases inside the ureters, which results in pressure on the nephrons, damaging the nephrons and decreasing glomerular blood flow (Policastro et al, 2011).*
- Review laboratory test results including serum electrolytes, blood urea nitrogen (BUN) and creatinine, along with calcium, phosphate, magnesium, uric acid, and albumin. *Serum electrolytes (sodium, potassium, chloride, bicarbonate, BUN, creatinine) as well as calcium, phosphate, magnesium, uric acid, and albumin should be measured. Elevations of BUN and creatinine and changes in electrolytes may be caused by kidney failure secondary to obstruction (Policastro et al, 2011).*
- Monitor for signs of dehydration, peripheral edema, elevating blood pressure, and heart failure. *The kidney can develop concentrating defects associated with partial obstruction of urine flow, resulting in symptoms that indicate kidney insufficiency (Policastro et al, 2011).*
- Ask the client to complete a bladder diary including patterns of urine elimination, urine loss (if present), nocturia, and volume and type of fluids consumed for a period of 3 to 7 days. CEB: *A study demonstrated that women overestimated daytime urinary frequency from recall. Use of a bladder diary results in increased accuracy of reporting of bladder symptoms (Stav et al, 2009).*
- Consult with the provider concerning eliminating or altering medications suspected of producing or exacerbating urinary retention. CEB: *Observational studies suggest that medications may play a role in approximately 10% of all cases of urinary retention. The most commonly implicated drug classes include antipsychotics, antidepressants, anticholinergic respiratory agents, opioid analgesics, alpha-adrenergic agonists, benzodiazepines, nonsteroidal antiinflammatory drugs, antimuscarinics, and calcium channel blockers (Verhamme et al, 2008).*
- Advise the male client with urinary retention related to benign prostatic hyperplasia (BPH) to avoid risk factors associated with acute urinary retention:
  - Avoid over-the-counter cold remedies containing a decongestant (alpha-adrenergic agonist) or antihistamine such as diphenhydramine that has anticholinergic effects.
  - Avoid taking over-the-counter dietary medications (frequently contain alpha-adrenergic agonists).
  - Discuss voiding problems with a health care provider before beginning new prescription medications.
  - After prolonged exposure to cool weather, warm the body before attempting to urinate.
  - Avoid overfilling the bladder by regular urination patterns and refrain from excessive intake of alcohol.

These modifiable factors predispose the client to acute urinary retention by overdistending the bladder and decreasing muscle contraction (Mayo Clinic, 2011).

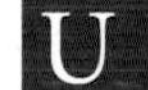

- Advise the client who is unable to void specific strategies to manage this potential medical emergency as follows:
  - Attempt urination in complete privacy.
  - Place the feet solidly on the floor.
  - If unable to void using these strategies, take a warm sitz bath or shower and void (if possible) while still in the tub or shower.
  - Drink a warm cup of caffeinated coffee or tea to stimulate the bladder, which may promote voiding.
- If unable to void within 6 hours or if bladder distention is producing significant pain, seek urgent or emergency care. *Attempting urination in complete privacy and placing the feet solidly on the floor help relax the pelvic muscles and may encourage voiding. Warm water also stimulates the bladder and may produce voiding; the cooling experienced by leaving the tub or shower may again inhibit the bladder (Joanna Briggs Institute, 2013).*

- Perform sterile (in acute care) or clean intermittent catheterization at home as ordered for clients with urinary retention. Refer to care plan for Reflex urinary **Incontinence** for more information about intermittent catheterization.

▲ Insert an indwelling catheter only as ordered by a health care provider. Catheter-associated urinary tract infections (CAUTI) are among the most common health care–associated infections. Each CAUTI episode is estimated to cost $600, rising to $2800 per episode when a CAUTI leads to a bloodstream infection. While certain conditions among hospitalized clients may require the use of a urinary catheter, limiting their use and decreasing the length of use are the most effective methods of reducing clients' exposure to CAUTIs (Choosing wisely.org, 2014).

- Nurse-led and computer-based reminders are both successful in reducing how long urinary catheters remain in place (Bernard et al, 2012).
- Nurse-driven practice recommendations to reduce CAUTI risk include securing catheters, maintaining drainage bags lower than level of bladder, and emptying drainage bags every 8 hours, when two-thirds full and before any transfer, daily evaluation of catheter indication/need to promote removal, and use of bladder scanner to prevent reinsertion. EB: *Incorporating nurse-driven catheter practices was found to reduce catheter days, decrease length of hospital stay, increase use of bladder scanners, and decrease reinsertions (Oman et al, 2012).*
- Current practice recommendations support aseptic catheter insertions, while the use of hydrophilic-coated catheters for clean intermittent catheters can reduce the rate of CAUTIs. Suprapubic catheterization is not more effective than urethral catheterization in reducing the incidence of catheter-related bacteremia. EB: *Evidence does not support routine use of antimicrobial-impregnated catheters to prevent CAUTIs (Tenke et al, 2014; Beattie et al, 2011).*
- For the individual with urinary retention who is not a suitable candidate for intermittent catheterization, recognize that the catheter can be a significant cause of harm to the client through development of a CAUTI or through genitourinary trauma when the catheter is pulled. *An indwelling catheter provides continuous drainage of urine; however, the risks for serious urinary complications, such as chronic CAUTIs, with prolonged use are significant.* EB: *One study found that the risk for genitourinary trauma was as common as symptomatic urinary tract infection when clients were repeatedly catheterized (Leuck et al, 2012).* EBN: *Indwelling urinary catheters are associated with up to 80% of hospital acquired CAUTIs. Appropriate use of bladder ultrasonography can reduce the rate of bladder damage as well as the need to use catheters. Incorporating bladder ultrasonography into the client's assessment can lead to decreased use of urinary catheter and rate of CAUTIs, lower risk for spread of multiresistant gram-negative bacteria, and lower hospital costs (Johansson et al, 2013).*
- Advise clients with indwelling catheters that bacteria in the urine is an almost universal finding after the catheter has remained in place for more than 1 week and that only symptomatic infections warrant treatment. *The long-term indwelling catheter is inevitably associated with bacterial colonization, with formation of biofilm on the catheter surfaces (Norrby, 2011).* CEB: *Most bacteriuria does not produce significant infection, and attempts to eradicate bacteriuria often produce subsequent morbidity because resistant bacteria are encouraged to reproduce while more easily managed strains are eradicated. Intermittent catheterization was preferred in a rehabilitation setting because it improves client quality of life and diminishes the time required to recover spontaneous voiding with a postvoid residual volume less than 150 mL (Tang et al, 2006).*
- Use the following strategies to reduce the risk for CAUTI whenever feasible:
  - Insert the indwelling catheter with sterile technique, only when insertion is indicated.
  - Remove the indwelling catheter as soon as possible; acute care facilities should institute a policy for regular review of the necessity of an indwelling catheter.
  - Maintain a closed drainage system whenever feasible.
  - Maintain unobstructed urine flow, avoiding kinks in the tubing and keeping the collecting bag below the level of the bladder at all times.
  - Regularly cleanse the urethral meatus with a gentle cleanser to remove apparent soiling.
  - Change the long-term catheter every 4 weeks; more frequent catheter changes should be reserved for clients who experience catheter encrustation and blockage.
- Educate staff about the risks for CAUTI development and specific strategies to reduce these risks. CEB: *These strategies are supported by sufficient evidence to recommend routine use (Gould et al, 2010). Numerous nursing studies have demonstrated that nurse-controlled methods to decrease the length of catheterization such as chart reminders and computerized interventions lead to decreased incidences of CAUTI (Andreessen et al, 2012).*

U

Postoperative Urinary Retention

- Urinary retention is a common complication of surgery, anesthesia, and advancing age. If conservative measures do not help the client pass urine, the bladder needs to be drained using either an intermittent catheter or indwelling urethral catheter, which places the client at risk for development of CAUTI (Steggall et al, 2013). CEB: *Factors associated with an increased risk for postoperative urinary retention included preoperative voiding difficulty, advanced age, total amount of fluid replacement during a 24-hour postoperative period, type of anesthesia, pain management medications, and route and length of medication administration (Baldini et al, 2009).* EBN: *A study demonstrated increased urinary retention after transurethral resection of the prostate in clients with preoperative increased prostate size, urinary tract infection, and clot retention (McKinnon et al, 2011).*
- Remove the indwelling urethral catheter at midnight in the hospitalized postoperative client to reduce the risk for acute urinary retention. CEB: *Removal of indwelling catheters at midnight in clients undergoing urologic surgery offers several advantages over morning removal, including a larger initial voided volume and earlier hospital discharge with no increased risk for readmission compared with those undergoing morning removal (Griffiths et al, 2004).*
- Perform a bladder scan before considering inserting a catheter to determine postvoid residual volume following surgery. EBN: *A study demonstrated a significant decrease in the number of catheterizations when ultrasonic bladder scanning was done to monitor postoperative urinary retention (Cutright, 2011).* CEB: *Another study found that in hip fracture clients, use of bladder scanning and intermittent catheterization resulted in less retention after surgery than in clients in whom a retention catheter was inserted (Johansson & Christensson, 2010).* CEB: *A meta-analysis found that performing bladder scanning was effective in decreasing urinary catheterization and development of urinary tract infection (Palese et al, 2010).*

Geriatric

- Aggressively assess older clients, particularly those with dribbling urinary incontinence, urinary tract infection, and related conditions for urinary retention. CEB: *Older women and men may experience urinary retention with few or no apparent symptoms; a urinary residual volume and related assessments are necessary to determine the presence of retention in this population (Johansson & Christensson, 2010).*
- Assess older clients for impaction when urinary retention is documented or suspected. CEB: *Fecal impaction and urinary retention frequently coexist in older clients and, unless reversed, may lead to acute delirium, urinary tract infection, or renal insufficiency (Waardenburg, 2008).*
- Monitor older male clients for retention related to BPH or prostate cancer. *Prostate enlargement in older men increases the risk for acute and chronic urinary retention.*

Home Care

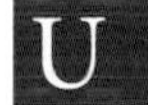

- Encourage the client to report any inability to void.
- Maintain an up-to-date medication list; evaluate side effect profiles for risk of urinary retention. *New medications or changes in dose may cause urinary retention.*
- Refer the client for health care provider evaluation if urinary retention occurs. *Identification of cause is important. Left untreated, urinary retention may lead to urinary tract infection or kidney failure.*

Client/Family Teaching and Discharge Planning

- Teach the client with mild to moderate obstructive symptoms to double void by urinating, resting in the bathroom for 3 to 5 minutes, and then trying again to urinate. *Double voiding promotes more efficient bladder evacuation by allowing the detrusor to contract initially and then rest and contract again (Mayo Clinic, 2011).*
- Teach the client with urinary retention and infrequent voiding to urinate by the clock. *Timed or scheduled voiding may reduce urinary retention by preventing bladder overdistention (Mayo Clinic, 2011).*
- Teach the client with an indwelling catheter to assess the tube for patency, maintain the drainage system below the level of the symphysis pubis, and routinely cleanse the bedside bag as directed.
- Teach the client with an indwelling catheter or undergoing intermittent catheterization the symptoms of a significant urinary infection, including hematuria, acute-onset incontinence, dysuria, flank pain, fever, or acute confusion.

REFERENCES

Andreessen, L., Wilde, M. H., & Herendeen, P. (2012). Preventing catheter-associated urinary tract infections in acute care: the bundle approach. *Journal of Nursing Care Quality, 27*(3), 209–217.

Baldini, G., et al. (2009). Postoperative urinary retention: anesthetic and perioperative considerations. *Anesthesiology, 110*(5), 1139–1157.

Beattie, M., & Taylor, J. (2011). Silver alloy vs. uncoated urinary catheters: a systematic review of the literature. *Journal of Clinical Nursing, 20*(15–16), 2098–2108.

Bernard, M. S., Hunger, K. F., & Moore, K. N. (2012). A review of strategies to decrease the duration of indwelling urethral catheters and potentially reduce the incidence of catheter-associated urinary tract infections. *Urologic Nursing, 32*(1), 29–37.

Choosing Wisely and the American Academy of Nursing. (2014). *Ten things nurses and patients should question*. <http://www.choosingwisely.org/wp-content/uploads/2015/02/AANursing-Choosing-Wisely-List.pdf>. Retrieved April 24, 2015.

Cutright, J. (2011). The effect of the bladder scanner policy on the number of urinary catheters inserted. *Journal of Wound, Ostomy, and Continence Nursing, 38*(1), 71–76.

Gould, C. V., et al. (2010). Guideline for prevention of catheter-associated urinary tract infections 2009. *Infection Control and Hospital Epidemiology, 31*(4), 319–326.

Griffiths, R. D., Fernandez, R. S., & Murie, P. (2004). Removal of short-term indwelling urethral catheters: the evidence. *Journal of Wound, Ostomy, and Continence Nursing, 31*(5), 299–308.

Joanna Briggs Institute. (2013). *Trial of Void: Post operative.*

Johansson, R. M., & Christensson, L. (2010). Urinary retention in older patients in connection with hip fracture surgery. *Journal of Clinical Nursing, 12*, 2110–2116.

Johansson, R. M., Malmmanvall, B. E., Andersson-Gare, B., et al. (2013). *Journal of Clinical Nursing, 22*(3), 346–355.

Leuck, A. M., et al. (2012). Complications of Foley catheters—is infection the greatest risk? *The Journal of Urology, 187*(5), 1662–1666.

Mayo Clinic. (2011). *Prostatic gland enlargement: lifestyle and home remedies*. From <http://www.mayoclinic.com/health/prostate-gland-enlargement/DS00027/DSECTION=lifestyle-and-home-remedies>. Retrieved October 14, 2012.

McKinnon, K., et al. (2011). Predictors of acute urinary retention after transurethral resection of the prostate: a retrospective chart audit. *Urologic Nursing, 31*(4), 207–213.

Norrby, S. R. (2011). Approach to the patient with urinary tract infection. In L. Goldman & A. Schafer (Eds.), *Goldman's Cecil medicine* (24th ed.). St Louis: Saunders/Elsevier.

Palese, A., et al. (2010). The effectiveness of the ultrasound bladder scanner in reducing urinary tract infections: a meta-analysis. *Journal of Clinical Nursing, 19*(21/22), 2970–2979.

Policastro, M., et al. (2011). *Urinary obstruction*, Medscape Reference <http://emedicine.medscape.com/article/778456-overview>. Retrieved April 9, 2015.

Oman, K. S., Makic, M. B. F., Fink, R., et al. (2012). Nurse-directed interventions to reduce catheter-associated urinary tract infections. *American Journal of Infection Control, 40*(6), 548–553.

Seifter, J. (2012). Urinary tract obstruction. In D. L. Longo, et al. (Eds.), *Harrison's principles of internal medicine* (18th ed.). New York: McGraw-Hill.

Stav, K., Dwyer, P. L., & Rosamilia, A. (2009). Women overestimate daytime urinary frequency: the importance of the bladder diary. *The Journal of Urology, 181*(5), 2176–2180.

Steggall, M., Treacy, C., & Jones, M. (2013). Post-operative urinary retention. *Nursing Standard, 28*(5), 43–48.

Tang, M. W., et al. (2006). Intermittent versus indwelling urinary catheterization in older female patients. *Maturitas, 53*(3), 274–281.

Tenke, P., Koves, B., & Johansen, T. E. B. (2014). An update on prevention and treatment of CAUTI. *Current Opinion in Infectious Diseases, 27*(1), 102–107.

Verhamme, K. M., et al. (2008). Drug-induced urinary retention: incidence, management, and prevention. *Drug Safety: An International Journal of Medical Toxicology and Drug Experience, 31*(5), 373–388.

Waardenburg, I. E. (2008). Delirium caused by urinary retention in elderly people: a case report and literature review on the "cystocerebral syndrome". *Journal of the American Geriatrics Society, 56*(12), 2371–2372.

Risk for Vascular Trauma

Mary Beth Flynn Makic, PhD, RN, CNS, CCNS, FAAN

NANDA-I

Definition

Vulnerable to damage to vein and its surrounding tissues related to the presence of a catheter and/or infusion solutions, which may compromise health

Risk Factors

Difficulty visualizing artery or vein; inadequate anchoring of catheter; inappropriate catheter type; inappropriate catheter width; insertion site; irritating solution (e.g., concentration, temperature, pH); length of time catheter is in place; rapid infusion rate

NOC (Nursing Outcomes Classification)

Suggested NOC Outcomes

Risk Control; Tissue Integrity: Skin and Mucous Membranes

Example NOC Outcome with Indicators

Accomplishes **Risk Control** as evidenced by the following indicators: Monitors environmental risk factors/Develops effective risk control strategies/Modifies lifestyle to reduce risk. (Rate the outcome and indicators of **Risk Control:** 1 = never demonstrated, 2 = rarely demonstrated, 3 = sometimes demonstrated, 4 = often demonstrated, 5 = consistently demonstrated [see Section I].)

Client Outcomes

Client Will (Specify Time Frame)

- Remain free from vascular trauma
- Remain free from signs and symptoms that indicate vascular trauma
- Remain free from impaired tissue and/or skin
- Maintain skin integrity, tissue perfusion, usual tissue temperature, color and pigment
- Report any altered sensation or pain
- State site is comfortable

NIC (Nursing Interventions Classification)

Suggested NIC Interventions

Intravenous (IV) Therapy; Medication Administration: Intravenous

Example NIC Activities—Intravenous (IV) Therapy

Monitor intravenous flow rate and IV site during infusion; Perform IV site care according to agency protocol

Nursing Interventions and *Rationales*

Client Preparation

▲ Verify objective and estimate duration of treatment. Check health care provider's order. *Verify if client will remain hospitalized during the whole treatment or will go home with the device (Phillips, 2014).*

- Assess client's clinical situation when venous infusion is indicated. *Consider possible clinical conditions that cause changes in temperature, color, and sensitivity of the possible venous access site. Verify situations that alter venous return (e.g., mastectomy, stroke) (Phillips, 2014). The site of catheter insertion influences the risk of infection and phlebitis, such as preexisting catheters, anatomic deformity, and bleeding diathesis (Xue, 2014).*
- Assess if client is prepared for an intravenous (IV) procedure. Explain the procedure if necessary to decrease stress. *Stress may cause vasoconstriction that can interfere in the visualization of the vein and flow of the infused solution (Xue, 2014).*
- Provide privacy and make the client comfortable during the intravenous insertion. *Privacy and comfort help decrease stress (Phillips, 2014). The nurse should minimize discomfort to the client and utilize measures to reduce the fear, pain, and anxiety associated with intravenous insertion (Royal College of Nursing [RCN], 2010).*
- Teach the client what symptoms of possible vascular trauma he should be alert to and to immediately inform staff if any of these symptoms are noticed. *Prompt attention to adverse changes decreases chance of adverse effects from complications.*

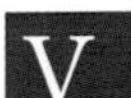

Insertion

- Wash hands before and after touching the client, as well as when inserting, replacing, accessing, repairing, or dressing an intravascular catheter (O'Grady et al, 2011; Society for Health Care Epidemiology of America, 2014).
- Maintain aseptic technique for the insertion and care of intravascular catheters. *Using an approved antiseptic solution, wearing gloves during insertion of an intravenous catheter, and immediately covering the insertion site with a transparent sterile semipermeable dressing are important interventions to reduce the risk of infection (Xue, 2014; McGowan, 2014).*

- Assess the condition of the client's veins, possible age-related influence, and previous intravenous site use. *To minimize the risk of complications, thorough client assessment and careful catheter management are essential (McCallum & Higgins, 2012).*
- In cases of hard-to-access veins, consider strategies such as the use of ultrasound to assist in vein localization and safe venipuncture. *Ultrasound-guided cannulations have a high success rate in clients with difficult venous access (Elia et al, 2012).*
- Avoid areas of joint flexion or bony prominences. *Movement in these sites can cause mechanical trauma in veins (RCN, 2010; McGowan 2014).*
- Choose an appropriate vascular access device (VAD) based on the types and characteristics of the devices and insertion site. Consider the following:
  - Peripheral cannulae: short devices that are placed into a peripheral vein; can be straight, winged, or ported and winged
  - Midline catheters or peripherally inserted central catheters (PICCs) with ranges from 7.5 to 20 cm
  - Central venous access devices (CVADs) are terminated in the central venous circulation and are available in a range of gauge sizes; they can be nontunneled catheters, skin-tunneled catheters, implantable injection ports, or PICCs.
  - Polyurethane venous devices and silicone rubber may cause less friction and consequently may reduce the risk of mechanical phlebitis (Phillips, 2014).

▲ Choose a device with consideration of the nature, volume, and flow of prescribed solution. **EBN:** *Choosing the right gauge size reduces the risk of vascular trauma (McGowan, 2014). Verify that the osmolarity of the solution to be infused is compatible with the available access site and device (Phillips, 2014; Loubani & Green, 2015).*

- If possible, choose the venous access site considering the client's preference. Engaging the client in choosing venous access site, when possible, may facilitate line patency.
- Select the gauge of the venous device according to the duration of treatment, purpose of the procedure, and size of the vein. *Emergency situations require short, large-bore cannulae. Hydration fluids and antibiotics can be delivered through much smaller cannulae (Loubani & Green, 2015). Select the smallest gauge necessary to achieve the prescribed flow rate (Infusion Nurses Society [INS], 2013). The time of infusion of the drug, especially chemotherapy and vasoactive agents, can contribute to the occurrence of phlebitis (Loubani & Green, 2015).*
- Verify whether client is allergic to fixation or device material.
- Disinfect the venipuncture site. Assess that skin is dry before puncturing to achieve maximal benefit of disinfection agent.
- Provide a comfortable, safe, hypoallergenic, easily removable stabilization dressing, allowing for visualization of the access site. *Catheter stabilization should be used to preserve the integrity of the access device, to minimize catheter movement at the hub, and to prevent catheter migration and loss of access (INS, 2013). Some peripheral cannulae have stabilization wings (which increase the external surface area) and/or ports (which are used to administer bolus medication) incorporated into their design.*
- Peripheral catheter intended dwell time is 72 to 96 hours and central catheters is 7 days (Helm et al, 2015).
- Use sterile, transparent, semipermeable dressing to cover catheter site. *Replace dressing with catheter change, or at a minimum every 7 days for transparent dressings (INS, 2013; O'Grady et al, 2011). The use of a transparent occlusive dressing can facilitate regular monitoring by visually inspecting the vascular access device (Xue, 2014; McGowan, 2014). If the client has local tenderness or signs of possible catheter-related bloodstream infection, the site should be visually inspected and the catheter removed (O'Grady et al, 2011). Use of gauze may be necessary if the client is diaphoretic, if the site is oozing or bleeding, or if it becomes damp; if gauze is used, it should be changed every 2 days (INS, 2013; O'Grady et al, 2011).*
- Document insertion date, site, type of VAD, number of punctures performed, other occurrences, and measures/arrangements.
- Always decontaminate the device before infusing medication or manipulating IV equipment (Xue, 2014; Helm et al, 2015).

▲ Verify the sequence of drugs to be administrated. Vesicants should always be administered first in a sequence of drugs (Loubani & Green, 2015).

Monitoring Infusion

- Monitor permeability and flow rate at regular intervals.
- Monitor catheter-skin junction and surrounding tissues at regular intervals, observing possible appearance of burning, pain, erythema, altered local temperature, infiltration, extravasation, edema, secretion, tenderness, or induration. Remove promptly. *The infusion should be discontinued at the first sign of infiltration or extravasation, the administration set disconnected, and all fluid aspirated from the catheter with a small syringe (INS, 2013).*
- ▲ Replace device according to institution protocol. EB: *There are variations regarding catheter permanence (dwell) time in the literature. Recommended catheter permanence time varies from 72 to 96 hours or less for peripheral catheters (O'Grady et al, 2011; Helm et al, 2015); catheter should be removed sooner if there are any clinical signs (Xue, 2014; McGowan, 2014).* EBN: *In a systematic review including five trials (3408 participants) on the replacement of peripheral venous catheters, authors did not identify evidence of the benefit of the replacement of catheters between 72 and 96 hours; thus, its authors recommended that catheters be replaced only in the presence of clinical signs (Webster et al, 2010).*
- ▲ Flush vascular access according to organizational policies and procedures, and as recommended by the manufacturer. *Vascular access devices should be flushed after each infusion to clear the infused medication from the catheter lumen, preventing contact between incompatible medications (INS, 2013). Sodium chloride 0.9% or heparinized sodium chloride has been studied to determine optimal solution for catheter patency. A recent Cochrane review found little difference in catheter patency between either solution; thus, given the cost and possible client risks to heparin exposure, sodium chloride flush solution is recommended (López-Briz et al, 2014).*
- Remove catheter on suspected contamination, if the client develops signs of phlebitis, infection, or a malfunctioning catheter, or when no longer required. *Vascular access devices should be removed on unresolved complication, therapy discontinuation, or if deemed unnecessary (INS, 2013). Replace any catheter inserted under emergency conditions within 24 hours because sterility of procedure may have been compromised.*
- Encourage clients to report any discomfort such as pain, burning, swelling, or bleeding (Xue, 2014).

Pediatric

- The preceding interventions may be adapted for the pediatric client. *Consider age, culture, development level, health literacy, and language preferences (INS, 2013; American Nurses Association, 2015). Consider the anatomic characteristics of the child or newborn in choice of VAD, equipment, and procedures for insertion and maintenance of infusion (Frey & Pettit, 2010). Consider the risk for dislodging the catheter when replacing the dressing in pediatric clients (O'Grady et al, 2011).*
- Inform the client and family about the IV procedure; obtain permissions, maintain client's comfort, and perform appropriate assessment prior to venipuncture. Assess the client for any allergies or sensitivities to tape, antiseptics, or latex. *Choose a healthy vein and appropriate site for insertion of selected device (Abolfotouh et al, 2014).*
- The use of an appropriate device to obtain blood samples reduces discomfort in the pediatric client. *Accessing a pediatric client's vein successfully can be difficult and measures to optimize the health care provider's skill is important to ensure successful venous cannulation (Goff et al, 2013; Frey, 2010).*
- Avoid areas of joint flexion or bony prominences. *Cannulae inserted away from joints remain patent for longer periods of time (McGowan, 2014).*
- ▲ Consider whether sedation or the use of local anesthetic is suitable for insertion of a catheter, taking into consideration the age of the pediatric client. *The use of effective local anesthetic methods and agents before each painful dermal procedure should be discussed with the health care provider (INS, 2013).*
- ▲ Use diversion while carrying out the procedure. *Diversion reduces anxiety (Goff et al, 2013).*

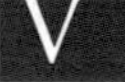

Geriatric

- The preceding interventions may be adapted for the geriatric client.
- Consider the physical, emotional, and cognitive changes related to older adults.
- Use strict aseptic technique for venipuncture of older clients. EB: *Older clients are at a higher risk for nosocomial and other health care–acquired complications due to defective host defenses that compromise their ability to ward off infectious agents (Laurent et al, 2012).*

Home Care

- Some devices may remain after discharge. Provide device-specific education to the client and family members about care of the selected device.
- Help in the choice of actions that support self-care. The nurse can provide valuable information that can be used to guide decision-making to maximize the self-care abilities of clients receiving home infusion therapy.
- Select, with the client, the insertion site most compatible with the development of activities of daily living (Xue, 2014; McGowan, 2014).
- Minimize the use of continuous IV therapy whenever possible. CEBN: *Clients who received intermittent IV therapy via a saline lock were more independent with regard to ability to perform self-care ADLs than those who received continuous IV therapy. The need for assistive mobility devices was also an independent predictor of ability to perform self-care ADLs (O'Halloran et al, 2008).*

REFERENCES

Abolfotouh, M. A., Salam, M., Bani-Mustafa, A., et al. (2014). Prospective study of incidence and predictors of peripheral intravenous catheter-induced complications. *Ther Clin Risk Management*, *10*, 993–1001.

American Nurses Association (ANA). *Pediatric nursing: scope and standards of practice, Silver Spring, MD*, 2015, Retrieved June 19, 2015. <http://www.nursingworld.org/scopeandstandardsofpractice>.

Elia, F., et al. (2012). Standard-length catheters vs. long catheters in ultrasound-guided peripheral vein cannulation. *The American Journal of Emergency Medicine*, *30*(5), 712–716.

Frey, A. M., et al. (2010). Infusion therapy in children. In M. Alexander (Ed.), *Infusion nursing: an evidence-based approach* (3rd ed.). St Louis: Saunders/Elsevier.

Goff, D. A., Larsen, P., Brinkley, J., et al. (2013). Resource utilization and cost of inserting peripheral intravenous catheters in hospitalized children. *Hosp Pediatr*, *3*(3), 185–191.

Helm, R. E., Klausner, J. D., Klemperer, J. D., et al. (2015). Accepted bu unacceptable: peripheral IV catheter failure. *J Infusion Nurs.*, *38*(3), 189–201.

Infusion Nurses Society (INS). (2013). *Recommendations for improving safety practices with short peripheral catheters.* Retrieved June 19, 2015. <http://www.ins1.org/i4a/pages/index.cfm?pageid=3412>.

Laurent, M., Bories, P. N., LeThuaut, A., et al. (2012). Impact of comorbidities on hospital-acquired infections in a geriatric rehabilitation unit: prospective study of 252 patients. *Journal of the American Medical Directors Association*, *13*(8), 760.e7–12.

López-Briz, E., Ruiz, G. V., Cabello, J. B., et al. (2014). Heparin versus 0.9% sodium chloride intermittent flushing for prevention of occlusion in central venous catheters in adults. *Cochrane Database of Systematic Reviews*, (10), Art. No.: CD008462.

Loubani, O. M., & Green, R. S. (2015). A systematic review of extravasation and local tissue injury from administration of vasopressors through peripheral intravenous catheters and central venous catheters. *J Cri Car*, *30*(3), 653–659.

McCallum, L., & Higgins, D. (2012). Care of peripheral venous cannula sites. *Nursing Times*, *108*(34–35), 12, 14–15.

McGowan, D. (2014). Peripheral intravenous cannulation: what is considered best practice? *British Journal of Nursing*, *23*(14), S26–S28.

O'Grady, N. P., et al. *Guidelines for the prevention of intravascular catheter-related infections*, 2011, Retrieved June 19, 2015, from <http://www.cdc.gov/hicpac/pdf/guidelines/bsi-guidelines-2011.pdf>.

O'Halloran, L., El-Masri, M. M., & Fox-Wasylyshyn, S. M. (2008). Home intravenous therapy and the ability to perform self-care activities of daily living. *Journal of Infusion Nursing*, *31*(6), 367–373.

Phillips, L. D. (2014). *Manual of IV therapeutics: evidence-based practice for infusion therapy* (6th ed.). Philadelphia: FA Davis.

Royal College of Nursing (RCN) (2010). *Standards for infusion therapy.* London: Author.

Society for Health Care Epidemiology of America (SHEA). (2014). *Expert CLABSI guidance adds real world implementation strategies.* Retrieved June 19, 2015 <http://www.shea-online.org/View/ArticleId/286/Expert-CLABSI-Guidance-Adds-Real-World-Implementation-Strategies.aspx>.

Webster, J., et al. (2010). Clinically-indicated replacement versus routine replacement of peripheral venous catheters. *Cochrane Database of Systematic Reviews*, (3), CD007798.

Xue, Y. (2014). Peripheral intravenous line: Insertion. *JoAnn Briggs Institute EBP Database.* JB11841.

Impaired spontaneous Ventilation

Debra Siela, PhD, RN, CCNS, ACNS-BC, CCRN-K, CNE, RRT

NANDA-I

Definition

Decreased energy reserves resulting in an inability to maintain independent breathing that is adequate to support life

Defining Characteristics

Alteration in metabolism; apprehensiveness; decrease in arterial oxygen saturation; decrease in cooperation; decrease in partial pressure of oxygen; decrease in tidal volume; dyspnea; increase in accessory muscle use; increase in heart rate; increase in partial pressure of carbon dioxide; restlessness

Related Factors

Alteration in metabolism; respiratory muscle fatigue

NOC (Nursing Outcomes Classification)

Suggested NOC Outcomes

Neurological Status: Central Motor Control; Respiratory Status: Gas Exchange, Ventilation

Example NOC Outcome with Indicators

Achieves appropriate **Respiratory Status: Ventilation** as evidenced by the following indicators: Respiratory rate/Respiratory rhythm/Depth of inspiration/Symmetrical chest expansion/Ease of breathing/Moves sputum out of airway/Accessory muscle use not present/Adventitious breath sounds not present/Chest retraction not present/Tidal volume/Vital capacity. (Rate the outcome and indicators of **Respiratory Status: Ventilation:** 1 = severe deviation from normal range, 2 = substantial deviation from normal range, 3 = moderate deviation from normal range, 4 = mild deviation from normal range, 5 = no deviation from normal range [see Section I].)

Client Outcomes

Client Will (Specify Time Frame)

- Maintain arterial blood gases within safe parameters
- Remain free of dyspnea or restlessness
- Effectively maintain airway
- Effectively mobilize secretions

NIC (Nursing Interventions Classification)

Suggested NIC Interventions

Artificial Airway Management; Mechanical Ventilation: Invasive; Respiratory Monitoring; Resuscitation: Neonate; Ventilation Assistance; Mechanical Ventilation Management: Noninvasive

Example NIC Activities—Mechanical Ventilation Management: Invasive

Monitor for conditions indicating a need for ventilation support (e.g., respiratory muscle fatigue, neurological dysfunction second to trauma, anesthesia, drug overdose, refractory respiratory acidosis); Consult with other health care personnel in selection of a ventilator mode

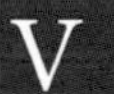

Nursing Interventions and *Rationales*

▲ Collaborate with the client, family, and health care provider regarding possible intubation and ventilation. Ask whether the client has advanced directives and, if so, integrate them into the plan of care with clinical data regarding overall health and reversibility of the medical condition. EB: *Client preferences and goals of care need to be acknowledged and discussed when planning care. Advanced directives protect client autonomy and help ensure that the client's wishes are respected (Siela, 2010; You et al, 2014).*

• Assess and respond to changes in the client's respiratory status. Monitor the client for dyspnea, increase in respiratory rate, use of accessory muscles, retraction of intercostal muscles, flaring of nostrils, decrease in O_2 saturation, cyanosis, and subjective complaints (Burns, 2011; Parshall et al, 2011).

• Have the client use a numerical scale (0-10) or visual analog scale to self-report dyspnea before and after interventions. *The numerical rating scale is a valid measure of dyspnea and has been found to be easiest for clients to use. Incorporating client self-report of dyspnea assists with assessment of symptom intensity, distress, progression, impact, and resolution of dyspnea (Grossbach et al, 2011; Mahler & O'Donnell, 2015).*

Determine intensity, unpleasantness, or distress of dyspnea using a rating scale such as an intensity-focused modified Borg scale or visual analog scale (Parshall et al, 2011).

- Assess for history of chronic respiratory disorders when administering oxygen. *When managing acute respiratory failure in clients with chronic obstructive pulmonary disease (COPD), continually assess the client's oxygenation needs. Long-term administration of oxygen (>15 hours per day) has been shown to increase survival in clients with severe, resting hypoxemia. (GOLD, 2015).*

▲ Collaborate with the health care provider and respiratory therapists in determining the appropriateness of noninvasive positive pressure ventilation (NPPV/NIV) for the decompensated client with COPD. Ventilatory support in a COPD exacerbation can be provided by either noninvasive or invasive ventilation (Burns, 2011; GOLD, 2015). NIV improves respiratory acidosis and decreases respiratory rate, severity of breathlessness, incidence of ventilator-associated pneumonia (VAP), and hospital length of stay (GOLD, 2015; Mas & Masip, 2014).

▲ Assist with implementation, client support, and monitoring if NPPV is used. EB/CEB: *In a client with exacerbation of COPD, NPPV can be as effective as intubation with use of a ventilator. NPPV has also been found to improve outcomes in clients with acute cardiogenic pulmonary edema (Mas et al, 2014). It can also be used if the client has other complications, such as hypotension or severely impaired mental status. The use of continuous positive airway pressure and bi-level positive airway pressure has been shown to improve oxygenation and decrease the rate of endotracheal intubation in clients with acute pulmonary edema (Burns, 2011; GOLD, 2015).*

- If the client has apnea, respiratory muscle fatigue, somnolence, hypoxemia, and/or acute respiratory acidosis prepare the client for possible intubation and mechanical ventilation. EB: *These indicators may predict the need for invasive mechanical ventilation to support the client's respiratory efforts (Burns, 2011; Stacy, 2013). The indications for initiating invasive mechanical ventilation during a COPD exacerbation include a failure of an initial trial of NIV (Burns, 2011; GOLD, 2015).*
- *If a client with acute respiratory failure (ARF) has a Rapid Shallow Breathing Index (RSBI) >105, endotracheal intubation is likely needed with invasive mechanical ventilation. A client with ARF with an RSBI of <105 may require only noninvasive ventilation (Berg et al, 2012).*

Ventilator Support

▲ Explain the endotracheal intubation and mechanical ventilation process to the client and family as appropriate, and during intubation administer sedation for client comfort according to the health care provider's orders. EBN: *Explanation of the procedure decreases anxiety and reinforces information; premedication allows for a more controlled intubation with decreased incidence of insertion problems (Burns, 2011; Joanna Briggs Institute, 2013).*

- Secure the endotracheal tube in place using either tape or a commercially available device, auscultate bilateral breath sounds, use a CO_2 detector, and obtain a chest radiograph to confirm endotracheal tube placement. CEBN: *Secure taping is needed to prevent inadvertent extubation. Nursing studies have shown conflicting results regarding the preferable way to secure the endotracheal tube (Goodrich, 2011a).* EB: *Auscultation alone is an unreliable method for checking endotracheal tube placement. A CO_2 detector can be used to confirm tube placement in the trachea (Goodrich, 2011; Stacy, 2013); however, correct position of the endotracheal tube in the trachea (3 to 5 cm above the carina) must be confirmed by chest radiograph (Goodrich, 2011b; Stacy, 2013). Calormetric CO_2 detectors have also been used successfully to detect inadvertent airway intubation during gastric tube placement (Goodrich, 2011a).*
- Review ventilator settings with the health care provider and respiratory therapy to ensure support is appropriate to meet the client's minute ventilation requirements (Grossbach, et al, 2011; Stacy, 2013; Chacko et al, 2015). *Ventilator settings should be adjusted to prevent hyperventilation or hypoventilation. A variety of new modes of ventilation are currently available that are responsive to client effort (pressure support).*

▲ Suction as needed and hyperoxygenate according to facility policy. Refer to the care plan for Ineffective **Airway** clearance for further information on suctioning.

- Check that monitor alarms are set appropriately at the start of each shift. *This action helps ensure client safety (Burns, 2011).*
- Respond to ventilator alarms promptly. If unable to immediately locate the source/cause of an alarm, use a manual self-inflating resuscitation bag to ventilate the client while waiting for assistance. *Common causes of a high-pressure alarm include secretions, condensation in the tubing, biting of the endotracheal tube, decreased compliance of the lungs, and compression of the tubing. Common causes of a low-pressure*

alarm are ventilator disconnection, leaks in the circuit, and changing compliance. Using a manual self-inflating resuscitation bag with supplemental oxygen, the nurse can provide immediate ventilation and oxygenation as needed (Burns, 2011; Goodrich, 2011; Grossbach et al, 2011).

- Prevent unplanned extubation by maintaining stability of endotracheal tube. EB: *Prevent unplanned extubation with use of weaning protocol (Jarachovic et al, 2011).*
- Drain collected fluid from condensation out of ventilator tubing as needed. *This action reduces the risk for infection by decreasing inhalation of contaminated water droplets (Burns, 2011).*
- Note ventilator settings of flow of inspired oxygen, peak inspiratory pressure, tidal volume, and alarm activation at intervals and when removing the client from the ventilator for any reason (Burns, 2011; Grossbach et al, 2011). *Checking the settings ensures that safety measures are taken and that the client is not left on 100% oxygen after suctioning (Burns, 2011).*

▲ Administer analgesics and sedatives as needed to facilitate client comfort and rest. Use behavioral and sedation scales for nonverbal clients to provide a consistent way of monitoring pain and sedation levels and ensuring that therapeutic outcomes are being met (Balas et al, 2012; Barr et al, 2013). Clients receiving mechanical ventilation frequently require sedation to help attenuate the anxiety, pain, and agitation associated with this intervention (Balas et al, 2012; Barr et al, 2013). The overall goal of sedation during mechanical ventilation is to provide physiological stability, ventilator synchrony, and comfort for clients.

- Tools such as the Riker Sedation-Agitation Scale, the Motor Activity Assessment Scale, the Ramsey Scale, or the Richmond Agitation-Sedation Scale may be useful in monitoring levels of sedation. *Each of these instruments has established reliability and validity and can be used to monitor the effect of sedative therapy (Balas et al, 2012; Barr et al, 2013).*
- Alternatives to medications for decreasing anxiety should be attempted, such as music therapy with selections of the client's choice played on headphones at intervals. EBN/EB: *Music therapy has been reported to decrease anxiety and reduce heart and respiratory rate in critically ill and intubated clients (Hunter et al, 2010; Tracy & Chlan, 2011; Gelinas et al, 2013).*
- Analyze and respond to arterial blood gas results, end-tidal CO_2 levels, and pulse oximetry values. *Ventilatory support must be closely monitored to ensure adequate oxygenation and acid-base balance.* EBN: *End-tidal CO_2 monitoring is best used as an adjunct to direct client observation and is used to monitor a client's ventilatory status and pulmonary blood flow (Burns, 2011; Rasera et al, 2011).*
- Use an effective means of verbal and nonverbal communication with the client. Barriers to communication include endotracheal tubes, sedation, and general weakness associated with a critical illness. Basic technologies should be readily available to the client, including eyeglasses and hearing aids (Grossbach et al, 2011; Khalaila et al, 2011). A variety of communication devices are available, including electronic voice output communication aids, alphabet boards, picture boards, computers, and writing slate. Ask the client for input into their care as appropriate (Grossbach et al, 2011; Khalaila et al, 2011). CEB: *Inadequate communication with the client and family may increase the risk for medical errors and adverse events (Kleinpell et al, 2008).*
- Move the endotracheal tube from side to side at least every 24 hours, and tape it or secure it with a commercially available device. Assess and document client's skin condition, and ensure correct tube placement at lip line (National Pressure Ulcer Advisory Panel, 2013).

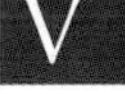

- Implement steps to prevent ventilator-associated events (VAE), such as ventilator-associated pneumonia (VAP), including continuous removal of subglottic secretions, elevation of the head of bed to 30 to 45 degrees (Siela, 2010; Hospital Quality Institute, 2015) unless medically contraindicated, change of the ventilator circuit no more than every 48 hours, and handwashing before and after contact with each client.
- *The accumulation of contaminated oropharyngeal secretions above the endotracheal tube may contribute to the risk of aspiration.* Use endotracheal tubes that allow for the continuous aspiration of subglottic secretions (Siela, 2010; Frost et al, 2013). EB: *Subglottic secretion drainage during mechanical ventilation results in a significant reduction in VAE, including late-onset VAP (Frost et al, 2013). Use of continuous subglottic suctioning endotracheal tubes for intubation in clients who are predicted to require more than 48 hours likely results in decreased incidence of VAP and costs of care (Speroni et al, 2011).*
- Position the client in a semirecumbent position with the head of the bed at a 30 to 45 degree angle to decrease the aspiration of gastric, oral, and nasal secretions (Siela, 2010; Bell, 2011; Hospital Quality Institute, 2015). Consider use of kinetic therapy, using a kinetic bed that slowly moves the client with 40 degree turns. *Rotational therapy may decrease the incidence of pulmonary complications in high-risk clients with increasing ventilator support requirements, at risk for ventilator-associated pneumonia, and clinical*

indications for acute lung injury or acute respiratory distress syndrome with worsening PaO_2:FIO_2 ratio, presence of fluffy infiltrates via chest radiograph concomitant with pulmonary edema, and refractory hypoxemia (Johnson, 2011; Bein et al, 2012; Joanna Briggs Institute, 2014).

- Perform handwashing using both soap and water and alcohol-based solution before and after all mechanically ventilated client contact to prevent spread of infections (Makic et al, 2013; Centers for Disease Control and Prevention, 2014).
- Provide routine oral care using tooth brushing and oral rinsing with an antimicrobial agent if needed (Siela, 2010; Martin, 2010; Joanna Briggs Institute, 2014; Ames, 2011). EB: *Reducing bacterial colonization of oral cavity includes interventions of daily oral assessment, deep suctioning every 4 hours, tooth brushing twice per day with a plaque reducer, oral tissue cleaning with peroxide every 4 hours. A Cochrane review found that routine oral care that included chlorhexidine mouthwash or gel resulted in a 40% reduction in development of VAP (Shi et al, 2013).*
- Maintain proper cuff inflation for both endotracheal tubes and cuffed tracheostomy tubes with minimal leak volume or minimal occlusion volume to decrease risk of aspiration and reduce incidence of VAP (Siela, 2010; Bell, 2011; Skillings & Curtis, 2011; Stacy, 2013).
- Reposition the client as needed. Use rotational bed or kinetic bed therapy in clients for whom side-to-side turning is contraindicated or difficult. EBN: *Changing position frequently decreases the incidence of atelectasis, pooling of secretions, and resultant VAP (Burns, 2011; Johnson, 2011).* EB/EBN: *Continuous, lateral rotational therapy has been shown to improve oxygenation and decrease the incidence of VAP (Burns, 2011; Johnson, 2011; Bein et al, 2012; Joanna Briggs Institute 2014).*

▲ If the client is intubated and is stable, consider getting the client up to sit at the edge of the bed, transfer to a chair, or walk as appropriate, if an effective interdisciplinary team is developed to keep the client safe (Gosselink et al, 2008; Balas et al, 2012). *For every week of bed rest, muscle strength can decrease 20%, early ambulation helped clients develop a positive outlook (Perme & Chandrashekar, 2009).*

- Assess bilateral anterior and posterior breath sounds every 2 to 4 hours and as needed; respond to any relevant changes (Burns, 2011).
- Assess responsiveness to ventilator support; monitor for subjective complaints and sensation of dyspnea (Burns, 2011).

▲ Collaborate with the interdisciplinary team in treating clients with acute respiratory failure (Grap, 2009, Balas et al, 2012). Collaborate with the health care team to meet the client's ventilator care needs and avoid complications (Grossbach et al, 2011). CEB: *A collaborative approach to caring for mechanically ventilated clients has been demonstrated to reduce length of time on the ventilator and length of stay in the intensive care unit (Grap, 2009).*

- *Document assessments and interventions according to policy.*

Geriatric

- Recognize that critically ill older adults have a high rate of morbidity when mechanically ventilated.

▲ NPPV may be used during acute treatment of older clients with impaired ventilation. EB: *A recent study found that older immunocompromised clients admitted with pneumonia had decreased morbidity and mortality when NPPV compared to mechanical ventilation was used to support impaired ventilation (Johnson et al, 2014).*

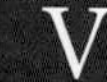

Home Care

▲ Some of the interventions listed previously may be adapted for home care use. Begin discharge planning as soon as possible with the case manager or social worker to assess the need for home support systems, assistive devices, and community or home health services.

▲ With help from a medical social worker, assist the client and family to determine the fiscal effect of care in the home versus an extended care facility.

- Assess the home setting during the discharge process to ensure the home can safely accommodate ventilator support (e.g., adequate space and electricity).
- Have the family contact the electric company and place the client residence on a high-risk list in case of a power outage. *Some home-based care requires special conditions for safe home administration.*
- Assess the caregivers for commitment to supporting a ventilator-dependent client in the home.
- Be sure that the client and family or caregivers are familiar with operation of all ventilation devices, know how to suction secretions if needed, are competent in doing tracheostomy care, and know schedules for

cleaning equipment. Have the designated caregiver or caregivers demonstrate care before discharge. *Some home-based care involves specialized technology and requires specific skills for safe and appropriate care.*

- Assess client and caregiver knowledge of the disease, client needs, and medications to be administered via ventilation-assistive devices. Avoid analgesics. Assess knowledge of how to use equipment. Teach as necessary. *A client receiving ventilation support may not be able to articulate needs. Respiratory medications can have side effects that change the client's respiration or level of consciousness.*
- Establish an emergency plan and criteria for use. Identify emergency procedures to be used until medical assistance arrives. Teach and role play emergency care. *A prepared emergency plan reassures the client and family and ensures client safety.*

Client/Family Teaching and Discharge Planning

- Explain to the client the potential sensations that will be experienced, including relief of dyspnea, the feeling of lung inflations, the noise of the ventilator, and the reality of alarms. EBN: *Knowledge of potential sensations and experiences before they are encountered can decrease anxiety. Administration of sedatives and/or narcotics may be needed to provide adequate oxygenation and ventilation in some clients (Barr et al, 2013).*
- Explain to the client and family about being unable to speak, and work out an alternative system of communication. See previously mentioned interventions.
- Demonstrate to the family how to perform simple procedures, such as suctioning secretions in the mouth with a tonsil-tip catheter, providing range-of-motion exercises, and reconnecting the ventilator immediately if it becomes disconnected. *Families are a critical part of the client's care, may be present at the bedside for prolonged periods of time, and need information about the plan of care (Burns, 2011).*
- Offer both the client and family explanations of how the ventilator works and answer any questions. *Having questions answered is often cited as an important need of clients and families when a client is on a ventilator (Burns, 2011).*

REFERENCES

Ames, N. J. (2011). Evidence to support tooth brushing in critically ill patients. *American Journal of Critical Care, 20*(3), 242–250.

Balas, M. C., Vasilevskis, E. E., Burke, W. J., et al. (2012). Critical care nurses' role in implementing the "ABCDE Bundle" into practice. *Critical Care Nurse, 32*(2), 35–38, 40–48.

Barr, J., Fraser, G. L., Puntillo, K., et al. (2013). Clinical practice guidelines for the management of pain, agitation, and delirium in adult patients in the intensive care unit. *Critical Care Medicine, 41*(1), 263–306.

Bein, T., Zimmermann, M., Schiewe-Laggartner, F., et al. (2012). Continuous lateral rotation therapy and systematic inflammatory response in posttraumatic acute lung injury: results from a prospective randomized study. *Injury, 43*, 1893–1897.

Bell, L. (2011). AACN Practice Alert-Prevention of Aspiration. *American Association of Critical Care Nurses.* Retrieved from: <http://www.aacn.org/wd/practice/docs/practicealerts/prevention-aspiration-practice-alert.pdf?menu=aboutus>.

Berg, K. M., Lang, G. R., Salciccioli, J. D., et al. (2012). The rapid shallow breathing index as a predictor of failure of noninvasive ventilation for patients with acute respiratory failure. *Respiratory Care, 57*(10), 1548–1554.

Burns, S. M. (2011). Invasive Mechanical Ventilation (Through an artificial airway): volume and pressure modes. In D. J. Lynn-McHale (Ed.), *AACN Procedure Manual for Critical Care* (6th ed.). Philadelphia: Saunders Elsevier.

Centers for Disease Control and Prevention. (2014). *Hand hygiene basics.* Retrieved April 23, 2015 <http://www.cdc.gov/handhygiene/Basics.html>.

Chacko, B., Peter, J. V., Tharyan, P. I., et al. (2015). Pressure-controlled versus volume-controlled ventilation for acute respiratory failure due to acute lung injury (ALI) or acute respiratory distress syndrome (ARDS). *Cochrane Database of Systematic Reviews*, (1), Art. No.: CD008807.

Frost, S. A., Azeem, A., Alexandrou, E., et al. (2013). Subglottic secretion drainage for preventing ventilator associated pneumonia: a meta-analysis. *Australian Critical Care, 26*(4), 180–188.

Gelinas, C., Arbour, C., Michaud, C., et al. (2013). Patients and ICU nurses' perspectives of non-pharmacological interventions for pain management. *Nursing in Care Nurse, 18*(6), 307–318.

GOLD: Global strategy for the diagnosis, management, and prevention of COPD (revised 2015), *Global Initiative for Chronic Obstructive Lung Disease.* Retrieved April 23, 2015 <http://www.goldcopd.org/uploads/users/files/GOLD_Report_2015_Apr2.pdf>.

Goodrich, C. (2011a). Endotracheal Intubation (assist). In D. J. Lynn-McHale (Ed.), *AACN Procedure Manual for Critical Care* (6th ed.). Philadelphia: Saunders Elsevier.

Goodrich, C. (2011b). Endotracheal Intubation (perform). In D. J. Lynn-McHale (Ed.), *AACN Procedure Manual for Critical Care* (6th ed.). Philadelphia: Saunders Elsevier.

Gosselink, R., Bott, J., Johnson, M., et al. (2008). Physiotherapy for adult patients with critical illness: recommendations of the European respiratory society and European society of critical care medicine task force on physiotherapy for critically ill patients. *Intensive Care Medicine, 34*, 1188–1199.

Grap, M. (2009). Not—so-trivial pursuit: Mechanical ventilation risk reduction. *American Journal of Critical Care, 18*(4), 299–309.

V

Grossbach, I., Stanberg, S., & Chlan, L. (2011). Promoting effective communication for patients receiving mechanical ventilation. *Critical Care Nurse*, *31*(3), 46–61.

Hospital Quality Institute. (2015). *Eliminating VAP/VAE. HQI Toolkit.* Retrieved April 23, 2015 <http://www.hqinstitute.org/hqi-toolkit/eliminating-vapvae>.

Hunter, B. C., Oliva, R., Sahler, O. J. Z., et al. (2010). Music therapy as an adjunctive treatment in the management of stress for patients being weaned from mechanical ventilation. *Journal of Music Therapy*, *17*(3), 198–219.

Jarachovic, M., Mason, M., Kerber, K., et al. (2011). The role of standardized protocol in unplanned extubations in a medical intensive care unit. *American Journal of Critical Care*, *20*(4), 304–312.

Joanna Briggs Institute (2013). *Endotracheal tube (ventilated patient) care.*

Joanna Briggs Institute (2014). *Ventilator-associated pneumonia prevention.*

Johnson, C. S., Frei, C. R., Metersky, M. L., et al. (2014). Non-invasive mechanical ventilation and mortality in elderly immunocompromised patients hospitalized with pneumonia: a retrospective cohort study. *BMC Pulmonary Medicine*, *14*(7), 1–10. Retrieved April 23, 2015 <http://www.biomedcentral.com/1471-2466/14/7>.

Johnson, S. (2011). Pressure Redistribution surfaces: continual lateral rotation therapy and Rotorest lateral rotations surface. In D. J. Lynn-McHale (Ed.), *AACN Procedure Manual for Critical Care* (6th ed.). Philadelphia: Saunders Elsevier.

Khalaila, R., Zbidat, W., Anwar, K., et al. (2011). Communication difficulties and psychoemotional distress in patients receiving mechanical ventilation. *American Journal of Critical Care*, *20*(6), 470–479.

Kleinpell, R. M., Patak, L., Wilson-Stronks, A., et al. (2008). *Communication in the ICU, Advance for Nurses.* <http://nursing.advanceweb.com/Article/Communication-in-the-ICU-2.aspx> Accessed April 27, 2015.

Mahler, D. A., & O'Donnell, D. E. (2015). Recent advances in dyspnea. *Chest*, *147*(1), 232–241.

Makic, M. B. F., Martin, S. A., Burns, S., et al. (2013). Putting evidence into nursing practice: four traditional practices not supported by the evidence. *Critical Care Nurse*, *33*(2), 28–42.

Martin, B. (2010). AACN practice alert-oral care for patients at risk for ventilator-associated pneumonia. *American Association of Critical Care Nurses.* Retrieved from: <http://www.aacn.org/wd/practice/docs/practicealerts/oral-care-patients-at-risk-vap.pdf?menu=aboutus> April 15, 2015.

Mas, A., & Masip, J. (2014). Noninvasive ventilation in acute respiratory failure. *International Journal of COPD*, *9*, 837–852.

National Pressure Ulcer Advisory Panel. (2013). *Best practices for prevention of medical device-related pressure ulcers in critical care.* Retrieved from: <http://www.npuap.org/wp-content/uploads/2013/04/BestPractices-CriticalCare1.pdf> April 15, 2015.

Parshall, M. B., Schwartzstein, R. M., Adams, L., et al. (2011). An official American thoracic society statement: update on the mechanisms, assessment, and management of dyspnea. *American Journal of Respiratory & Critical Care Medicine*, *185*(4), 435–452.

Perme, C., & Chandrashekar, R. (2009). Early mobility and walking program for patients in intensive care units: creating a standard of care. *American Journal of Critical Care*, *18*(3), 212–220.

Rasera, C. C., Gewehr, P. M., Domingues, A. M. T., et al. (2011). Measurement of end-tidal carbon dioxide in spontaneously breathing children after cardiac surgery. *American Journal of Critical Care*, *20*(5), 388–394.

Shi, Z., Xie, H., Wang, P., et al. (2013). Oral hygiene care for critically ill patients to prevent ventilator-associated pneumonia. *Cochrane Database of Systematic Reviews*, (8), Art. No.: CD008367.

Siela, D. (2010). Evaluation standards for management of artificial airways. *Critical Care Nurse*, *30*(4), 76–78.

Skillings, K., & Curtis, B. (2011). Tracheal tube cuff care. In D. J. Lynn-McHale (Ed.), *AACN procedure manual for critical care* (6th ed.). Philadelphia: Elsevier Saunders.

Speroni, K., O'Meara-Lett, M., Lucas, J., et al. (2011). Comparative effectiveness of standard endotracheal tubes vs. endotracheal tubes with continuous subglottic suctioning on ventilator-associated pneumonia rates. *Nursing Economics*, *29*(1), 15–20, 37.

Stacy, K. M. (2013). Pulmonary therapeutic Management. In L. D. Urden, K. M. Stacy, & M. E. Lough (Eds.), *Critical Care Nursing: Diagnosis and Management* (7th ed.). Maryland Heights, MO: Elsevier.

Tracy, M. F., & Chlan, L. (2011). Nonpharmacological interventions to manage common symptoms in patients receiving mechanical ventilation. *Critical Care Nurse*, *31*(3), 19–28.

You, J. J., Fowler, R. A., & Heyland, D. K. (2014). Just ask: discussing goals of care with patients in hospital with serious illness. *Canadian Medical Association Journal*, *186*(6), 425–432.

Dysfunctional Ventilatory weaning response

Debra Siela, PhD, RN, CCNS, ACNS-BC, CCRN-K, CNE, RRT

NANDA-I

Definition

Inability to adjust to lowered levels of mechanical ventilator support that interrupts and prolongs the weaning process

Defining Characteristics

Mild

Breathing discomfort; fatigue; fear of machine malfunction; increase in focus on breathing; mild increase of respiratory rate over baseline; perceived need for increased in oxygen; restlessness; warmth

Moderate

Abnormal skin color (e.g., pale, dusky, cyanosis); apprehensiveness; decrease in air entry on auscultation; diaphoresis; facial expression of fear; hyperfocused on activities; impaired ability to cooperate; impaired ability to respond to coaching; increase in blood pressure from baseline (<20 mm Hg); increase in heart rate from baseline (<20 beats/min); minimal use of respiratory accessory muscles; moderate increase in respiratory rate over baseline

Severe

Abnormal skin color (e.g., pale, dusky, cyanosis); adventitious breath sounds; agitation; asynchronized breathing with the ventilator; decrease in level of consciousness; deterioration in arterial blood gases from baseline; gasping breaths; increase in blood pressure from baseline (≥20 mm Hg); increase in heart rate from baseline (≥20 beats/min); paradoxical abdominal breathing; profuse diaphoresis; shallow breathing; significant increase in respiratory rate above baseline; use of significant respiratory accessory muscles

Related Factors (r/t)

Physiological

Alteration in sleep pattern; ineffective airway clearance; inadequate nutrition; pain

Psychological

Anxiety; decrease in motivation; fear; hopelessness; insufficient knowledge of weaning process; insufficient trust in health care professional; low self-esteem; powerlessness; uncertainty about ability to wean

Situational

Environmental barrier (e.g., distractions, low nurse to client ratio, unfamiliar health care staff); history of unsuccessful weaning attempt; history of ventilator dependence greater than 4 days; inappropriate pace of weaning process; insufficient social support; uncontrolled episodic energy demands

NOC (Nursing Outcomes Classification)

Suggested NOC Outcomes

Respiratory Status: Gas Exchange; Ventilation

Example NOC Outcome with Indicators

Achieves appropriate **Respiratory Status: Ventilation** as evidenced by the following indicators: Respiratory rate/Respiratory rhythm/Depth of inspiration/Symmetrical chest expansion/Ease of breathing/Moves sputum out of airway/Accessory muscle use not present/Adventitious breath sounds not present/Chest retraction not present/Tidal volume/Vital capacity. (Rate the outcome and indicators of **Respiratory Status: Ventilation:** 1 = severe deviation from normal range, 2 = substantial deviation from normal range, 3 = moderate deviation from normal range, 4 = mild deviation from normal range, 5 = no deviation from normal range [see Section I].)

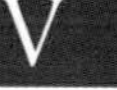

Client Outcomes

Client Will (Specify Time Frame)

- Wean from ventilator with adequate arterial blood gases
- Remain free of unresolved dyspnea or restlessness
- Effectively clear secretions

NIC (Nursing Interventions Classification)

Suggested NIC Interventions

Mechanical Ventilation Management: Invasive; Mechanical Ventilatory Weaning

Example NIC Activities—Mechanical Ventilatory Weaning

Monitor for optimal fluid and electrolyte status; Monitor to ensure client is free of significant infection before weaning

Nursing Interventions and *Rationales*

- Assess client's readiness for weaning as evidenced by the following:
  - Physiological and psychological readiness. There has been little research devoted to the study of psychological readiness to wean. EBN: *Assess fears and anxieties that can contribute to prolonged and repeated failure of ventilator weaning (Chen et al, 2011).* EBN: *Clinical assessment of comfort and anxiety are important predictors of ventilator weaning success (Grap, 2009).*
  - Resolution of initial medical problem that led to ventilator dependence
  - Hemodynamic stability
  - Normal hemoglobin levels
  - Absence of fever
  - Normal state of consciousness
  - Metabolic, fluid, and electrolyte balance
  - Adequate nutritional status with serum albumin levels >2.5 g/dL
  - Adequate sleep
  - Adequate pain management and minimal sedation

Adequate respiratory parameters historically include the following: adequate gas exchange ($Pa{O_2}/Fi{O_2}$ ratio >200), respiratory rate ≤35 breaths/min, a negative inspiratory pressure <20 cm, positive expiratory pressure >30 cm H_2O, spontaneous tidal volume >5 mL/kg, vital capacity >10 to 15 mL/kg (Burns, 2011a).

EB: *A spontaneous awakening trial in conjunction with a daily weaning assessment has a great impact on ventilator liberation outcomes (Haas & Loik, 2012; MacIntyre, 2012; Jones et al, 2014). Predictors of extubation failure include disease severity, secretion burden, higher minute ventilation, and lower oxygenation (Miu et al, 2014).* EBN: *Systematic tracking of weaning factors may be helpful in care planning and management and determining weaning potential (Burns et al, 2010; Grap, 2009).*

- For successful weaning, ensure that the client is in an optimal physiological and psychological state before introducing the stress of weaning (Burns, 2011a). *For more information on weaning assessment, please refer to the Burns Weaning Assessment Program (Burns et al, 2010; Burns, 2011d).*
- *An early mobility and walking program can promote weaning from ventilator support as a client's overall strength and endurance improve (Gosselink et al, 2008; Perme & Chandrashekar, 2009). If the client is intubated and is stable, consider getting the client up to sit at the edge of the bed, transfer to a chair, or walk as appropriate, if an effective interdisciplinary team is developed to keep the client safe. For every week of bed rest, muscle strength can decrease 20%, early ambulation also helped clients develop a positive outlook (Perme & Chandrashekar, 2009). Prolonged mechanical ventilation results in long periods of inactivity with deep sedation that results in disuse atrophy of skeletal and diaphragmatic muscles.*
- *Early mobility and physical rehabilitation can reduce muscle weakness, mechanical ventilation duration, ICU stay, and hospital stay (Mendez-Tellez & Needham, 2012, Spruit et al, 2013). The Awakening and Breathing Coordination, Delirium Monitoring and Management, and Early Mobility (ABCDE) bundle has criteria to determine when clients are candidates for early mobility (Balas, 2012).*
- Involve family as appropriate to help the client provide a maximal effort during weaning readiness measurements (Burns, 2011a).

- Provide adequate nutrition to ventilated clients, using enteral feeding when possible. EB: *Protein malnutrition results in decreased muscle strength, which impairs the weaning process. Enteral nutrition is preferred to total parenteral nutrition because it provides an equal number of calories at lower cost and with fewer complications, while preserving gut integrity (McClave et al, 2009). Parenteral nutrition should be initiated in any client in whom enteral nutrition cannot be used because of gut dysfunction (McClave et al, 2009).*
- Use evidence-based weaning and extubation protocols as appropriate. EBN/EB: *The duration of treatment with mechanical ventilation and ventilation utilization ratio (VUR) were reduced in clients who received a spontaneous breathing trial (SBT) protocol (Jones et al, 2014). Daily spontaneous breathing trials are superior to gradual ventilator-reduction strategies (Grap, 2009). Protocol-directed weaning has been demonstrated to be safe and effective but not superior to other weaning methods that used structured rounds and other processes that allow for timely and ongoing clinical decision-making by expert nurses and health care providers (Arias-Rivera et al, 2008; Burns, 2011a; Grap, 2009; Navalesi et al, 2008; Robertson et al, 2008, Balas et al, 2012).*
- Identify reasons for previous unsuccessful weaning attempts, and include that information in development of the weaning plan. EBN: *Analyzing client responses after each weaning attempt prevents repeated unsuccessful weaning trials (Burns, 2011d; Burns et al, 2010; Chen et al, 2011; Grap, 2009). Reducing the*

size of artificial airways can increase airway resistance and overly increase energy expenditures of the diaphragm (MacIntyre, 2012).

▲ Collaborate with an interdisciplinary team (health care provider, nurse, respiratory therapist, physical therapist, and dietitian) to develop a weaning plan with a timeline and goals; revise this plan throughout the weaning period. Use a communication device, such as a weaning board or flow sheet (Burns, 2011b; Grossbach et al, 2011). EBN: *Effective interdisciplinary collaboration can positively affect client outcomes (Grap, 2009). Decisions related to weaning trials should be made in conjunction with members of the interdisciplinary team (Grap, 2009; Haas & Loik, 2012, Balas et al, 2012; Rose et al, 2014).*

- In clients with chronic obstructive pulmonary disease who fail extubation, noninvasive ventilation (NIV) facilitates weaning, prevents reintubation, and reduces mortality. Early NIV after extubation reduces the risk for respiratory failure and lowers 90-day mortality in clients with hypercapnia during a spontaneous breathing trial (Epstein, 2009; Mas & Masip, 2014).
- Assist client to identify personal strategies that result in relaxation and comfort (e.g., music, visualization, relaxation techniques, reading, television, family visits). Support implementation of these strategies (Pattison & Watson, 2009). Music intervention can be used to allay anxiety and can be a powerful distractor from distressful sounds and thoughts in the intensive care unit (ICU) (Tracy & Chlan, 2011). EB: *Music therapy appears to reduce the physiologic signs of anxiety, which can be a major deterrent to successful liberation from mechanical ventilation (Hunter et al, 2010).* EBN: *A study found that use of music was beneficial as a relaxation technique for clients if they were willing to accept it and were able to choose the selection of music (Chan et al, 2009; Hunter et al, 2010).*
- Provide a safe and comfortable environment. EBN: *Stay with the client during weaning if possible (Pattison & Watson, 2009).*
- If unable to stay, make the call light button readily available and assure the client that needs will be met responsively. EBN: *Presence entails a focus by the nurse to engage attentively with the client (Tracy & Chlan, 2011).* EBN: *A client who feels safe and trusts the health care providers can focus on the immediate work of weaning; support from the nurse helps decrease anxiety (Burns et al, 2010). Knowing the client in association with objective clinical data helps individualize the weaning process (Rose et al, 2014).*

▲ Coordinate pain and sedation medications to minimize sedative effects. *Appropriate levels of sedation may be key to successful weaning.* EBN: *Nursing implemented sedation protocols have been used effectively to improve the probability of successful extubation (Arias-Rivera et al, 2008; Balas et al, 2012). Of note is that a recent study in Australia reported that sedation and analgesia scales did not reduce the duration of mechanical ventilation (Williams et al, 2008). This may be due, in part, to the nurse's autonomy in making decisions about the appropriate level of sedation for any given client. Wake up and breathe protocols that pair daily spontaneous awakening trials with daily spontaneous breathing trials result in better outcomes for mechanically ventilated clients in intensive care (Girad et al, 2008; Balas, 2012; Haas & Liok, 2012). Daily interruption of sedation (DIS) is safe in mechanically ventilated medical ICU clients. Further information is needed to determine benefits in other client populations. Current practice evidence suggests that sedation should be client specific to avoid overuse of sedating agents. DIS may not reduce the duration of mechanical ventilation (Makic et al, 2015).*

- Administer analgesics and sedatives as needed to facilitate client comfort and rest. Use behavioral and sedation scales for nonverbal clients to provide a consistent way of monitoring pain and sedation levels and ensuring that therapeutic outcomes are being met (Barr et al, 2013). *Clients receiving mechanical ventilation frequently require sedation to help attenuate the anxiety, pain, and agitation associated with this intervention (Barr et al, 2013; Balas, 2012). The overall goal of sedation during mechanical ventilation is to provide physiological stability, ventilator synchrony, and comfort for clients (Balas, 2012; Makic et al, 2015).*

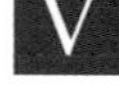

- Tools such as the Riker Sedation-Agitation Scale, the Motor Activity Assessment Scale, the Ramsey Scale, or the Richmond Agitation-Sedation Scale may be useful in monitoring levels of sedation (Balas et al, 2012; Barr et al, 2013).
- Schedule weaning periods for the time of day when the client is most rested. Cluster care activities to promote successful weaning. Avoid other procedures during weaning: keep the environment quiet and promote restful activities between weaning periods.
- Promote a normal sleep-wake cycle, allowing uninterrupted periods of nighttime sleep. *Limit visitors during weaning to close and supportive persons; ask visitors to leave if they are negatively affecting the weaning process.* EB: *Communication with a client and/or the client's family is important to assess the client's typical pattern of sleep (Tracy & Chlan, 2011).*

- During weaning, monitor the client's physiological and psychological responses; acknowledge and respond to fears and subjective complaints. Validate the client's efforts during the weaning process. EBN: *Weaning is a stressful experience that requires active participation by the client. The client's work needs to be understood and supported by health care providers to facilitate recovery from mechanical ventilation and weaning (Burns, 2011c; Grap, 2009).*
- Monitor subjective and objective data (breath sounds, respiratory pattern, respiratory effort, heart rate, blood pressure, oxygen saturation per oximetry, amount and type of secretions, anxiety, and energy level) throughout weaning to determine client tolerance and responses (Burns, 2011c; Grap, 2009).
- Involve the client and family in the weaning plan. Inform them of the weaning plan and possible client responses to the weaning process (e.g., potential feelings of dyspnea). Foster a partnership between clients and nurses in care planning for weaning (Pattison & Watson, 2009). EBN: *Consider the experience of client and client's family members to develop interventions for weaning success (Rose et al, 2014).*
- Coach the client through episodes of increased anxiety. Remain with the client or place a supportive and calm significant other in this role. Give positive reinforcement, and with permission use touch to communicate support and concern. *It is not unusual for a client with lung disease to experience self-limiting episodes of increased shortness of breath. Supporting and coaching a client through such episodes allows weaning to continue (Pattison & Watson, 2009; Tracy & Chlan, 2011).*
- Terminate weaning when the client demonstrates predetermined criteria or when the following signs of weaning intolerance occur:
  - Tachypnea, dyspnea, or chest and abdominal asynchrony
  - Agitation or mental status changes
  - Decreased oxygen saturation: Sao_2 <90%
  - Increased $PaCO_2$ or $ETCO_2$
  - Change in pulse rate or blood pressure or onset of new dysrhythmias

▲ If the dysfunctional weaning response is severe, consider slowing weaning to brief periods (e.g., 5 minutes). Continue to collaborate with the team to determine whether an untreated physiological cause for the dysfunctional weaning pattern remains. Consult with health care provider regarding use of noninvasive ventilation immediately after discontinuing ventilation. Consider an alternative care setting (subacute, rehabilitation facility, home) for clients with prolonged ventilator dependence as a strategy that can positively affect outcomes. *Use of noninvasive ventilation has been effective for the client who is difficult to wean from a ventilator (Epstein, 2009).*

Geriatric

- Recognize that older clients may require longer periods to wean.

Home Care

- Weaning from a ventilator at home should be based on client stability and comfort of the client and caregivers under an intermittent care plan. *Generally the client will be safer weaning in a hospital environment.*

REFERENCES

Arias-Rivera, S., del Mar Sanchez-Sanchez, M., Santos-Diaz, R., et al. (2008). Effect of a nursing-implemented sedation protocol on weaning outcome. *Critical Care Medicine, 36*(7), 2054–2060.

Balas, M. C., Vasilevskis, E. E., Burke, W. J., et al. (2012). Critical care nurses' role in implementing the "ABCDE Bundle" into practice. *Critical Care Nurse, 32*(2), 35–38, 40–48.

Barr, J., Fraser, G. L., Puntillo, K., et al. (2013). Clinical practice guidelines for the management of pain, agitation, and delirium in adult patients in the intensive care unit. *Critical Care Medicine, 41*(1), 263–306.

Burns, S. M. (2011a). Weaning process. In D. J. Lynn-McHale (Ed.), *AACN procedure manual for critical care* (6th ed.). Philadelphia: Elsevier Saunders.

Burns, S. M. (2011b). Noninvasive positive pressure ventilation: continuous positive airway pressure (CPAP) and Bilevel positive airway pressure (BiPAP). In D. J. Lynn-McHale (Ed.), *AACN procedure manual for critical care* (6th ed.). Philadelphia: Elsevier Saunders.

Burns, S. M. (2011c). Invasive mechanical ventilation (through an artificial airway): volume and pressure modes. In D. J. Lynn-McHale (Ed.), *AACN procedure manual for critical care* (6th ed.). Philadelphia: Elsevier Saunders.

Burns, S. M. (2011d). Standard weaning criteria: negative inspiratory force or pressure, positive inspiratory pressure, spontaneous tidal volume, vital capacity, and rapid shallow breathing index. In D. J. Lynn-McHale (Ed.), *AACN procedure manual for critical care* (6th ed.). Philadelphia: Elsevier Saunders.

Burns, S. M., Fisher, C., Tribble, S. S., et al. (2010). Multifactor clinical score and outcome of mechanical ventilation weaning trials: burns wean assessment program. *American Journal of Critical Care, 19*(5), 431–440.

Chan, M. F., Chung, Y. F. L., Chung, S. W. A., et al. (2009). Investigating the physiological responses of patients listening to music in the intensive care unit. *Journal of Clinical Nursing, 18*(9), 1250–1257.

Chen, Y. J., Jacobs, W. J., Quan, S. F., et al. (2011). Psychophysiological determinants of repeated ventilator weaning failure: an explanatory model. *American Journal of Critical Care, 20*(4), 292–302.

Epstein, S. K. (2009). Weaning from ventilatory support. *Current Opinion in Critical Care, 15*(1), 36–43.

Girad, T., Kress, J., Fuchs, B., et al. (2008). Efficacy and safety of a paired sedation and ventilator weaning protocol for mechanically ventilated patients in intensive care (Awakening and breathing controlled trial): a randomized controlled trial. *The Lancet, 371*, 26–134.

Gosselink, R., Bott, J., Johnson, M., et al. (2008). Physiotherapy for adult patients with critical illness: recommendations of the European respiratory society and European society of critical care medicine task force on physiotherapy for critically ill patients. *Intensive Care Medicine, 34*, 1188–1199.

Grap, M. (2009). Not—so-trivial pursuit: mechanical ventilation risk reduction. *American Journal of Critical Care, 18*(4), 299–309.

Grossbach, I., Chlan, L., & Tracy, M. F. (2011). Overview of mechanical ventilator support and management of patient- and ventilator-related responses. *Critical Care Nurse, 31*(3), 30–45.

Grossbach, I., Stranberg, S., & Chlan, L. (2011). Promoting effective communication for patients receiving mechanical ventilation. *Critical Care Nurse, 31*(3), 46–61.

Haas, C. F., & Loik, P. S. (2012). Ventilator discontinuation protocols. *Respiratory Care, 57*(10), 1649–1662.

Hunter, B. C., Oliva, R., Shaler, O. J. Z., et al. (2010). Music Therapy as an adjunctive treatment in the management of stress for patients being weaned from mechanical ventilation. *Journal of Music Therapy, 47*(3), 198–219.

Jones, K., Newhouse, R., Johnson, K., et al. (2014). Achieving quality health outcomes through the implementation of a spontaneous awakening and spontaneous breathing trial protocol. *AACN Advanced Critical Care, 25*(1), 33–42.

MacIntyre, N. R. (2012). Evidence-based assessments in the ventilator discontinuation process. *Respiratory Care, 57*(10), 1611–1618.

Makic, M. B. F., Rauen, C., Jones, K., et al. (2015). Continuing to challenge practice to be evidence based. *Critical Care Nurse, 35*(2), 39–50.

Mas, A., & Masip, J. (2014). Noninvasive ventilation in acute respiratory failure. *International Journal of COPD, 9*, 837–852.

McClave, S., Martindale, R., Vanek, V., et al. (2009). Guidelines for the provision and assessment of nutrition support therapy in the adult critically ill patient: Society of Critical Care Medicine (SCCM) and American Society for Parenteral and Enteral Nutrition (A.S.P.E.N.). *Journal of Parenteral Enteral Nutrition, 33*(3), 277–316.

Mendez-Tellez, P. A., & Needham, D. M. (2012). Early physical rehabilitation in the ICU and ventilator liberation. *Respiratory Care, 57*(10), 1663–1669.

Miu, T., Jofffe, A. M., Yanez, N. D., et al. (2014). Predictors of reintubation in critically ill patients. *Respiratory Care, 59*(2), 178–185.

Navalesi, P., Frigerio, P., Moretti, M. P., et al. (2008). Rate of reintubation in mechanically ventilated neurosurgical and neurologic patients: evaluation of a systematic approach to weaning and extubation. *Critical Care Medicine, 36*(11), 2986–2992.

Pattison, N., & Watson, J. (2009). Ventilatory weaning: a case study of protracted weaning. *Nursing in Critical Care, 14*(2), 75–85.

Perme, C., & Chandrashekar, R. (2009). Early mobility and walking program for patients in intensive care units: creating a standard of care. *American Journal of Critical Care, 18*(3), 212–220.

Robertson, T. E., Mann, H. J., Hyzy, R., et al. (2008). Multicenter implementation of a consensus-developed, evidence-based, spontaneous breathing trial protocol. *Critical Care Medicine, 36*(10), 2753–2762.

Rose, L., Dainty, K. N., Jordan, J., et al. (2014). Weaning from mechanical ventilation: a scoping review of qualitative studies. *American Journal of Critical Care, 23*(5), e54–e71.

Spruit, M. A., Singh, S. J., Garvey, C., et al. (2013). An official American thoracic society/European respiratory society statement: key concepts and advances in pulmonary rehabilitation. *American Journal of Respiratory and Critical Care Medicine, 188*(8), e13–e64.

Tracy, M. F., & Chlan, L. (2011). Nonpharmacological interventions to manage common symptoms in patients receiving mechanical ventilation. *Critical Care Nurse, 31*(3), 19–29.

Williams, T. A., Martin, S., Leslie, G., et al. (2008). Duration of mechanical ventilation in an adult intensive care unit after introduction of sedation and pain scales. *American Journal of Critical Care, 17*(4), 349–356.

V

Risk for other-directed Violence

Kathleen L. Patusky, MA, PhD, RN, CNS

NANDA-I

Definition

Vulnerable to behaviors in which an individual demonstrates that he or she can be physically, emotionally, and/or sexually harmful to others

Risk Factors

Access to weapon; alteration in cognitive functioning; cruelty to animals; fire setting; history of childhood abuse (e.g., physical, psychological, sexual); history of substance abuse; history of witnessing family violence; impulsiveness; motor vehicle offense (e.g., traffic violations, use of a motor vehicle to release anger); negative body language (e.g., rigid posture, clenching of fists/jaw, hyperactivity, pacing threatening stances); neurological impairment (e.g., positive electroencephalogram, head trauma, seizure disorders); pathological intoxication; pattern of indirect violence (e.g., tearing objects off walls, urinating/defecating on floor, stamping feet, temper tantrum, throwing objects, breaking a window, slamming doors, sexual advances); pattern of other directed violence (e.g., hitting/kicking/spitting/scratching others, throwing objects/biting someone, attempted rape, rape sexual molestation, urinating/defecating on a person); pattern of threatening violence (e.g., verbal threats against property/people, social threats cursing, threatening notes/gestures, sexual threats); pattern of violent anti-social behavior (e.g., stealing, insistent borrowing, insistent demands for privileges, insistent interrupting, refusal to eat/take medication, ignoring instructions); perinatal complications; prenatal complications; psychotic disorder; suicidal behavior.

NOC (Nursing Outcomes Classification)

Suggested NOC Outcomes

Abuse Cessation; Abusive Behavior Self-Restraint; Aggression Self-Restraint; Distorted Thought Self-Control; Impulse Self-Control; Risk Detection

Example NOC Outcome with Indicators

Aggression Self-Restraint as evidenced by the following indicators: Refrains from harming others/Expresses/Vents needs and negative feelings in a nondestructive manner/Identifies when angry. (Rate the outcome and indicators of **Aggression Self-Restraint:** 1 = never demonstrated, 2 = rarely demonstrated, 3 = sometimes demonstrated, 4 = often demonstrated, 5 = consistently demonstrated [see Section I].)

Client Outcomes

Client Will (Specify Time Frame)

- Stop all forms of abuse (physical, emotional, sexual; neglect; financial exploitation)
- Have cessation of abuse reported by victim
- Display no aggressive activity
- Refrain from verbal outbursts
- Refrain from violating others' personal space
- Refrain from antisocial behaviors
- Maintain relaxed body language and decreased motor activity
- Identify factors contributing to abusive/aggressive behavior
- Demonstrate impulse control or state feelings of control
- Identify impulsive behaviors
- Identify feelings/behaviors that lead to impulsive actions
- Identify consequences of impulsive actions to self or others
- Avoid high-risk environments and situations
- Identify and talk about feelings; express anger appropriately
- Express decreased anxiety and control of hallucinations as applicable
- Displace anger to meaningful activities
- Communicate needs appropriately
- Identify responsibility to maintain control
- Express empathy for victim
- Obtain no access or yield access to harmful objects
- Use alternative coping mechanisms for stress
- Obtain and follow through with counseling
- Demonstrate knowledge of correct role behaviors

Victim (and Children if Applicable) Will (Specify Time Frame)

- Have safe plan for leaving situation or avoiding abuse
- Resolve depression or traumatic response

Parent Will (Specify Time Frame)

- Monitor social/play contacts
- Provide supervision and nurturing environment
- Intervene to prevent high-risk social behaviors

NIC (Nursing Interventions Classification)

Suggested NIC Interventions

Abuse Protection Support; Anger Control Assistance; Behavior Management; Calming Technique; Coping Enhancement; Crisis Intervention; Delusion Management; Dementia Management; Distraction; Environmental Management: Violence Prevention; Mood Management; Physical Restraint; Seclusion; Substance Use Prevention

Example NIC Intervention—Environmental Management: Violence Prevention

Remove other individuals from the vicinity of a violent or potentially violent client; Provide ongoing surveillance of all client access areas to maintain client safety and therapeutically intervene as needed

Nursing Interventions and *Rationales*

Client Violence

- ▲ Monitor the environment, evaluate situations that could become violent, and intervene early to de-escalate the situation. Know and follow institutional policies and procedures concerning violence. Consider that family members or other staff may initiate violence in all settings. Enlist support from other staff rather than attempting to handle situations alone. EBN: *American Psychiatric Nurses Association (APNA) guidelines (2008) and workgroup report (Cafaro et al, 2012) warn that workplace violence can occur in all settings, from a variety of sources. Nurses need to be aware and informed of department policies and procedures. Policies should be developed and training programs should be provided in proper use and application of restraints. All nursing units should develop a proactive plan for dealing with violent situations.*
- • Assess causes of aggression: social versus biological. EB: *Knowing the client, having experience with similar clients, paying attention, and planning interventions are expert practices used by clinicians to predict and respond to aggressive behavior effectively. A nonconfrontational approach is the most effective (APA, 2014).*
- • Assess the client for risk factors of violence, including those in the following categories: personal history (e.g., past violent behavior, especially violent behavior in the community within 2 weeks of admission); psychiatric disorders (particularly psychoses, paranoid or bipolar disorders, substance abuse, posttraumatic stress disorder [PTSD], antisocial personality, or borderline personality disorder); neurological disorders (e.g., head injury, temporal lobe epilepsy, cardiovascular accident, dementia or senility), medical disorders (e.g., hypoxia, hypoglycemia, or hyperglycemia), psychological precursors (e.g., low tolerance for stress, impulsivity, hostility), coping difficulties (e.g., inability to plan solutions or see long-term consequences of behavior), younger age, risk of suicide, and childhood or adolescent disorders (e.g., conduct disorders, hyperactivity, autism, learning disability). EBN/EB: *All of these risk factors have been implicated in aggressive, agitated, or violent behavior, with prior history being a key indicator (American Psychiatric Association [APA], 2014; APNA, 2014a, b; Battaglini, 2014a).*
- • Measures of violence may be useful in predicting or tracking behavior, and serving as outcome measures. EBN: The Broset Violence Checklist (BVC) and the Kennedy Axis V have been shown to help identify clients at risk for seclusion (Sande et al, 2013). EB: *The Alert System identifies potential violent incidents (odds ratio = 7.74, 95% CI = 4.81-12.47), but should be combined with resources and procedures to prevent escalation of behavior (Kling et al, 2011).*
- • Assess the client with a history of previous assaults, especially violent behavior in the community within 2 weeks of admission. Listen to and acknowledge feelings of anger, observe for increased motor activity, and prepare to intervene if the client becomes aggressive. EBN/EB: *The most significant risk factor for physical violence is a past history of physically aggressive behavior (APA, 2014; Battaglini, 2014).*
- • Assess the client for physiological signs and external signs of anger. Internal signs of anger include increased pulse rate, respiration rate, and blood pressure; chills; prickly sensations; numbness; choking sensation; nausea; and vertigo. External signs include increased muscle tone, changes in body posture (clenched fists, set jaw), eye changes (eyebrows lower and drawn together, eyelids tense, eyes assuming a "hard" appearance), lips pressed together, flushing or pallor, goose bumps, twitching, and sweating. EBN/EB: *Anger is an early warning sign of possible violence (APA, 2014).*
- • Assess for the presence of hallucinations. EB: *Command hallucinations may direct the client to behave violently (APA, 2014).*

V

- Apply STAMPEDAR as an acronym for assessing the immediate potential for violence. CEBN: *A study of nurses experienced in workplace violence identified the following as factors and behaviors indicating the likelihood of a violent episode: staring, tone of voice, anxiety, mumbling, pacing, emotions, disease process, assertive/nonassertive behavior, and access to resources that might be used for violent behavior (Chapman et al, 2009).*
- Determine the presence and degree of homicidal or suicidal risk. A number of questions will elicit the necessary information: Have you been thinking about harming someone? If yes, who? How often do you have these thoughts, and how long do they last? Do you have a plan? What is it? Do you have access to the means to carry out that plan? What has kept you from hurting the person until now? Refer to the care plan for Risk for **Suicide.** Psychotherapists are required to report harm or threats of harm to another person, referred to as the "duty to warn." State laws and mental health codes should be checked to determine local mandates for threat reporting by specific health care professionals.
- Take action to minimize personal risk: use nonthreatening body language. Respect personal space and boundaries. Maintain at least an arm's length distance from the client; do not touch the client without permission (unless physical restraint is the goal). Do not allow the client to block access to an exit. If speaking with the client alone, keep the door to the room open. Be aware of where other staff is at all times. Notify other staff of where you are at all times. Take verbal threats seriously and notify other staff. Wear clothing and accessories that are not restricting and that will not be dangerous (e.g., sandals or shoes with heels can lead to twisted ankles; necklaces or dangling earrings could be grabbed). Ensure staff training to deal with violence. EBN/EB: *Aggression management training has been identified as a critical need (Battaglini, 2014a; Chu, 2014a). Programs for violence prevention have been implemented that reduce workplace violence. For OSHA guidelines, visit https://www.osha.gov/SLTC/workplaceviolence/index.html.*
- Remove potential weapons from the environment. Be prepared to remove obstructions to staff response from the environment. Search the client and his or her belongings for weapons or potential weapons on admission to the hospital as appropriate. EBN: *Preventive strategies are important (Chu, 2014a; Zhili, 2013). Clients prone to violence may use available weapons opportunistically. If client restraint becomes necessary, environmental hazards (e.g., chairs, wastebaskets) should be moved out of the way to prevent injuries.*
- Inform the client of unit expectations for appropriate behavior and the consequences of not meeting these expectations. Emphasize that the client must comply with the rules of the unit. Give positive reinforcement for compliance. Increase surveillance of the hospitalized client at smoking, meal, and medication times. CEB/EBN: *Clients benefit from clear guidance and positive reinforcement regarding behavioral expectations and consequences, providing much needed structure and emphasizing client responsibility for his/her own behavior (APNA, 2011; APNA, 2014a, b). The unit serves as a microcosm of the client's outside world, so adherence to social norms while on the unit models adherence on discharge and provides the client with staff support to learn appropriate coping skills and alternative behaviors.*
- Assign a single room to the client with a potential for violence toward others. The client will be able to take time away from unit stimulation to calm self as needed. Another client will not be placed at risk as a roommate.
- Maintain a calm attitude in response to the client. Provide a low level of stimulation in the client's environment; place the client in a safe, quiet place, and speak slowly and quietly. Anxiety is contagious. EBN/EB: *Maintenance of a calm environment contributes to the prevention of aggression (APA, 2011; APNA, 2014a, b). Harmony among staff can help prevent violence, in that disharmony transmits itself to clients' emotional state (Battaglini, 2014a). Music therapy may help (Chu, 2014b).*
- Redirect possible violent behaviors into physical activities (e.g., walking, jogging) if the client is physically able. Using a punching bag or hitting a pillow is not indicated, because these are not calming activities and they continue patterning violent behavior. However, activities that distract while draining excess energy help build a repertoire of alternative behaviors for stress reduction.
- Provide sufficient staff if a show of force is necessary to demonstrate control to the client. EBN: *When staff respond to an escalating or violent situation, it can reassure clients that they will not be allowed to lose control. On the other hand, leave immediately if the client becomes violent and you are not trained to handle it (APNA, 2011).*
- De-escalation is the first and most important action in response to anger, hostility. Constant special observation may be implemented. EBN: *Response to hostility should be appropriate, measured, and*

V

reasonable. Constant special observation should be used to prevent acutely disturbed clients from harming self or others (Battaglini, 2014a).

- Protect other clients in the environment from harm. Remove other individuals from the vicinity of a violent or potentially violent client. Follow safety protocols of the department. The risk of a violent client to others in the area (other clients, visitors) should be anticipated, even as efforts proceed to de-escalate the situation with the client. EBN: *Clients exposed to violence need timely support and assistance (Chu, 2014a).*
- Maintain a secluded area for the client to be placed when violent. Ensure that staff are continuously present and available to client during seclusion. EBN: *Staff presence is necessary to prevent the harmful effects of social isolation and to honor clients' motivation to connect with staff (APNA, 2014a, b). Seclusion should be short and should be reviewed at least every 2 hours (Zhili, 2013).*

▲ Recognize legal requirements that the least restrictive alternative of treatment should be used with aggressive clients. The hierarchy of intervention is as follows: promote a milieu that provides structure and calmness, with negotiation and collaboration taking precedence over control; maintain vigilance of the unit and respond to behavioral changes early; talk with client to calm and promote understanding of emotional state; use chemical restraints as ordered; increase to manual restraint if needed; increase to mechanical restraint and seclusion as a last resort. EBN: *APNA guidelines (2014a, b) support early assessment and intervention to prevent aggression, with nursing actions to reduce stimulation, divert client from aggressive thought patterns, set appropriate limits on behavior, and provide medications as needed. Chemical restraints are useful, but clients* must *be monitored for response, side effects (Chu, 2014b). Physical restraints should be avoided and used for short periods when necessary (Battaglini, 2014a; Chu, 2014b).*

▲ Use mechanical restraints if ordered and as necessary. Physical restraint can be therapeutic to keep the client and others safe. EBN: *Physical restraints should be avoided and used for short periods when necessary (Battaglini, 2014a; Chu, 2014b). Restraint skill training, audits of adverse events, and examination of the safe use of restraints and medications are important to safe restraint practices (APNA, 2014a, b).*

▲ Follow the institutional protocol for releasing restraints. Observe the client closely, remain calm, and provide positive feedback as the client's behavior becomes controlled. EBN: *The period during which restraints are removed can be dangerous for staff if they do not recognize that the client may choose to reinitiate violence. Protocols will specify safe procedures for removing restraints (APNA, 2014a, b).*

▲ After a violent event on a unit, debriefing and support of both staff and clients should be made available. *Allowing discussion of a violent episode, either individually or in a group, among other clients present reveals clients' responses to the event and provides the opportunity for staff to offer reassurance and support. Clients may have concerns that staff will attempt to restrain them without reason or may feel uncertain whether staff can keep them safe.* EBN: *A study of the impact of serious events on psychiatric units found that staff reported a variety of negative emotional responses, levels of containment increased, the provision of care could be affected, and client reactions were largely ignored (APNA, 2014a, b; Lim, 2011). Injury after violence has a strong negative influence on influence on staff and calls for treatment (Chu, 2014a).*

- Form a therapeutic alliance with the client, remaining calm, identifying the source of anger as external to both nurse and client, and using the therapeutic relationship to prevent the need for seclusion or restraint. The development of a therapeutic relationship before aggressive behavior occurs provides an alternative for working through anger and frustration. Assisting the client to identify a source of anger or frustration that is external to both the nurse and client prevents the need for defensiveness by both and directs energy at solving an external problem. EBN: *A therapeutic environment has a mitigating effect against violence (Zhili, 2013).*
- Allow, encourage, and assist the client to verbalize feelings appropriately either one-on-one or in a group setting. Actively listen to the client; explore the source of the client's anger, and negotiate resolution when possible. Teach healthy ways to express feelings/anger, appropriate gender roles, and how to communicate needs appropriately. CEBN: *When clients' feelings are not addressed, when an individual feels threatened, or when gratification is delayed or denied, violence may be used as a manifestation of the internal feeling state (APNA, 2008).*
- Identify with client the stimuli that initiate violence and the means of dealing with the stimuli. Have the client keep an anger diary and discuss alternative responses together. Teach cognitive behavioral techniques. Assisting the client to identify situations and people that upset him/her provides information needed for problem solving. The client may then identify alternative responses (e.g., leaving the stimulus; using relaxation techniques, such as deep breathing; initiating thought stopping; initiating a distracting activity; responding assertively rather than aggressively).

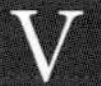

▲ Initiate and promote staff attendance at aggression management training programs. EBN: *Aggression management training programs have a positive influence on the ability and confidence of nurses in responding to aggressive or violent behavior (APNA, 2011).*

Intimate Partner Violence (IPV)/Domestic Violence

NOTE: Before implementation of interventions in the face of domestic violence, nurses should examine their own emotional responses to abuse, their knowledge base about abuse, and systemic elements within the emergency department (ED) to ensure that interventions will be compassionate and appropriate. EBN: *A metasynthesis of health care provider studies identified a strong therapeutic relationship and the ability to hear what the client is not saying as facilitators of IPV screening (LoGiudice, 2015).*

- Screen for possible abuse in women or children with a pattern of multiple injuries, particularly if any suspicion exists that the physical findings are inconsistent with the explanation of how the injuries were incurred. CEBN: *IPV/domestic violence is recognized as a nationwide public health issue. In one study, nurses cited insufficient evidence as a reason for not reporting IPV. Nurses with a personal history of IPV were more likely to report (Smith et al, 2008).*

▲ Report suspected child abuse to Child Protective Services. Refer women suspected of being in a spousal abuse situation to an area crisis center and provide phone number of area crisis hotline. *Rapid screening tools are helpful to identify IPV. All nurses are required by law to report suspected child abuse.* CEB: *Child and spouse maltreatment often occur together; all family members should be evaluated and provided with assistance as needed (Taylor et al, 2009).*

- Assess for physical and mental concerns of women, including risk of HIV. CEB: *Major health needs of women with a history of IPV were found to include chronic pain, chronic diseases, and mental illness, as well as concerns regarding risk of HIV. Barriers to health care created by the IPV may prevent these concerns from being addressed (Cole et al, 2008).*
- Assist the client in negotiating the health care system and overcoming barriers. CEBN: *Victims of IPV were found to experience barriers, including inappropriate responses from providers, when attempting to access health care services (Robinson & Spilsbury, 2008).*
- With women who repeatedly experience injuries from domestic violence, maintain a nonjudgmental approach and continue to offer resources/referrals. If the woman voices a willingness to leave her situation, assist with developing an emergency plan that will consider all contingencies possible (e.g., safe location, financial resources, care of children, when to leave safely). A woman in a domestic violence situation may change her mind several times before actually leaving. Proactive organization of an emergency plan helps increase the possibility that women will be able to leave safely. The most dangerous time of a domestic violence situation is when the spouse tries to leave.
- Maintain a nonjudgmental response when clients return to husbands or refuse to leave them. Women have many reasons for remaining in an abusive relationship, including economic concerns (especially with children), socialization about the woman's role, political or legal obstacles, powerlessness, and a realistic fear of retaliation or death. Refer to the care plan for **Powerlessness.** Experienced nurses working with abused women define success as client personal growth over time, rather than the woman leaving the relationship.
- Focus on providing support, ensuring safety, and promoting self-efficacy while encouraging disclosure about IPV events. CEB: *A review of evidence concluded that nursing care should focus on providing physical, psychological, and emotional support; ensuring safety of the client and family; and promoting the self-efficacy of the woman (Olive, 2007).*
- Screen pregnant women for the potential for domestic violence during pregnancy, especially in teenage pregnancies. CEBN: *In a study of high-risk teen mothers, IPV was reported by 61% of the participants, with 37.5% reporting IPV during pregnancy (Mylant & Mann, 2008). Psychological health was found to be predicted by a history of abuse among women in a high-risk prenatal care clinic (Svavarsdottir & Orlygsdottir, 2008).* CEB: *Pregnant women will remain in an abusive relationship if they perceive it to be in the best interest of the child, part of a process of "double-binding" with child and abusive spouse (Lutz et al, 2006). Systematic screening of pregnant women is recommended, and choking is a danger that should be added to routine screening (Jeanjot et al, 2008). Screen women and children for effects of domestic violence during the postpartum period.* CEB: *Less educated women, women who reported substance abuse by spouse, and women who reported unwanted pregnancies were at risk for IPV both during and after pregnancy. Violence during pregnancy predicted postpartum violence. U.S. women employed during pregnancy were most likely to leave an abusive partner at 1 year postpartum (Charles & Perreira,*

V

2007). *In cases of high IPV, less than optimal infant health and difficult temperament were found (Burke et al, 2008).*

- Women with physical or mental disabilities require extended assessment, including a comprehensive functional assessment, with attention to cultural issues, the nature of the disability, and needed resources. Women with disabilities may experience abuse from multiple sources, and particular attention should be paid to the additional emotional stressors present. Difficulties leaving home, physical needs that shelter may not be able to accommodate, and the undesirability of nursing home placement are just a few stressors. Personal assistance providers may be abusive or take advantage financially. CEB: *Women with disabilities may follow a unique model of IPV progression, requiring adaptation of the usual interventions, and may be slower in returning to usual routines (Copel, 2006; Focht-New et al, 2008). Women with schizophrenia are especially vulnerable and have complex needs (Bengtsson-Tops & Tops, 2007; Rice, 2006).*
- ▲ Referral for spiritual counseling may be considered, but be aware that clergy vary in their helpfulness. CEBN: *Survivors of sexual violence described being able to cope with their situation through spiritual connection, spiritual journey, and spiritual transformation (Knapik et al, 2008). A study of women in abusive relationships who sought spiritual guidance from male clergy revealed themes of spiritual suffering, devaluation, loss, and powerlessness consistent with old societal biases. The authors noted that conclusions could not be drawn regarding the helpfulness of female clergy (Copel, 2008).*
- Identify risk factors such as ongoing mental illness of a parent, and monitor family closely. CEB: *Concern for the children of parents with a mental illness has been identified in light of the potential for family dysfunction and violence among the mentally ill (Copeland, 2007; Mason et al, 2007).*
- Be aware that IPV may arise or continue under circumstances of medical illness. EBN: *Older women with breast cancer reported they experienced negative relationship changes and IPV (Sawin & Parker, 2011).*
- Consider risk versus benefit when deciding if, when, and in how great a depth to explore client responses to abuse or violence. EB: *A systematic review of research on violence and abuse concluded that risks as well as benefits may derive from clients talking about such experiences (Appollis et al, 2015).*
- ▲ When spouse or child abuse accompanies substance abuse, refer the abusive client to a substance abuse treatment program. Refer the spouse receiving abuse to Al-Anon and the children to Alateen. CEB: *Use of drugs or alcohol may decrease impulse control and aggravate abusive behavior, depending on specific drug used and culture (Caetano et al, 2008; Stalans & Ritchie, 2008).*
- ▲ When an adult reveals a history of unresolved/untreated sexual abuse as a child, referral to a local Adults Molested as Children (AMAC) group may be helpful. CEB: *Childhood sexual abuse has been associated with adult depression, attempted suicide, self-harm, and higher risk for later interpersonal violence (Murrell et al, 2007). Interventions tailored to the AMAC experience may be helpful.* Refer to the care plans for Risk for **Suicide, Self-Mutilation,** and Risk for **Self-Mutilation.**
- ▲ Referral of women for psychiatric/psychological treatment or parenting classes should be considered as an appropriate intervention. CEB: *Overcoming shame, building a stable sense of identity, and becoming less dependent on others' approval should be addressed, along with physical health and PTSD symptoms (Woods et al, 2008).* EB: *In a study of 3429 women enrolled in an HMO, 46% reported a lifetime history and 14.7% reported a history within the previous 5 years of physical, sexual, and/or nonphysical abuse, with PTSD being a potential outcome (Dutton, 2009). Self-blame was associated with all factors involved in IPV, with outcomes of PTSD, depression, suicidality, and substance abuse (Campbell et al, 2009).*

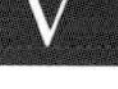

- ▲ Referral of children for psychiatric/psychological treatment should be considered as an appropriate intervention. CEB: *Children living with domestic violence were found to express fear and anxiety, self-esteem issues, ambivalent relationships with the abuser, and a sense of a lost childhood (Buckley et al, 2007).*
- ▲ Refer to batterer intervention programs that are often available and may be court mandated. CEB: *Batterers believe behaviors toward them are not justified, and their behaviors toward others are justified and minimized. Treatment should include emotional skills training that addresses these areas (Smith, 2007).*

Social Violence

- Assess for acute stress disorder (ASD) and PTSD among victims of violence. CEB: *In the acute phase following an assault, women reported high rates of ASD symptoms. Four months after an attack, dissatisfaction with previous life, prior mental health problems, recent life events, and earlier abuse were risk factors for PTSD (Renck, 2006).*
- ▲ Assess the support network of women who become victims of violent crime and refer for appropriate levels of assistance. Of particular concern would be women who do not have family or friends to provide support or who have difficulty accessing other types of assistance.

- Be aware that hate crime is increasing, particularly toward gay and transgendered individuals, and it requires support and advocacy for victims. CEB: *Gay men who experienced antigay abuse reported that the events affected their self-image. In addition to verbal and physical abuse, spiritual abuse emerged as the men internalized schemas of outcast and sinner (Lucies & Yick, 2007).*

▲ Victims of violence seen in the ED should receive an assessment for needed services and assignment to case management. *Establishment of linkages with social service agencies can provide important services for referral.*

Rape-Trauma Syndrome

- Assist client to cope with potential stalking activity. EBN: *The usual coping of college students in response to stalking was found to include ignoring or minimizing the problem; distancing or depersonalizing; using verbal escape strategies, attempting to end the relationship; and restricting availability (Amar & Alexy, 2010). Emphasizing the need to take stalking behavior seriously and problem-solving interventions may prevent a rape situation.*
- Approach client with sensitivity. CEBN: *Using Peplau's theory of nursing roles, researchers found that the roles of counselor and technical expert were most helpful, with interpersonal sensitivity important to clients (Courey et al, 2008).*

▲ Monitor for paradoxical drug reactions, and report any to the health care provider. Violent behavior can be stimulated by a medication intended to calm the client.

- Assess for brain insults, such as recent falls or injuries, strokes, or transient ischemic attacks. Clients with brain injuries may respond to stimulus control, problem solving, social skills training, relaxation training, and anger management to reduce aggressive behaviors. Brain injuries, lowered impulse control, and reduced coping can cause violent reactions to self or others. Brain injury symptoms may be mistaken for mental illness.
- Decrease environmental stimuli if violence is directed at others. Removal of the client to a quiet area can reduce violent impulses. Use a calm voice to "talk down" the client.
- Assess holistic needs of the client. CEBN: *Risk factors for negative mental health outcomes following sexual violence were found to be low income, low education level, lack of social support, and poor health promotion (Vandemark & Mueller, 2008).*
- Discuss with client her wishes regarding use of an emergency contraceptive. CEBN: *If emergency contraception was offered to every female victim of sexual assault, researchers concluded that unintended pregnancies would decline. However, the findings are limited, in that only 15% of women who are raped seek health care promptly (Womack, 2008).*

▲ If abuse or neglect of an older client is suspected, report the suspicion to an adult protective services agency with jurisdiction over the geographical area where the client lives.

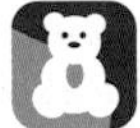

Pediatric

- Assess for predictors of anger that can lead to violent behavior. EBN: *A meta-analysis of adolescent anger predictors identified trait anger, anxiety, depression, stress, and exposure to violence as moderate to substantial predictors of anger; victim of violence, hostility, self-esteem, and social support were low to moderate predictors (Mahon et al, 2010).*
- Be alert for both shaken baby syndrome and exposure of children to violence. *In homes where domestic violence exists, children are involved as either witnesses or victims. Such children tend not to seek help and need care providers to elicit actively the need for assistance (Lepisto et al, 2010).*
- Pregnant teens should be assessed for abuse, particularly if they are with an older partner. CEB: *In a study of predominantly African American pregnant teens, 13% reported domestic violence during pregnancy. Teens with adult partners (4 or more years older) were twice as likely to report abuse as teens with similar-age partners (Harner, 2004).*

▲ In the case of child abuse or neglect, refer for early childhood home visitation. CEB: *Home visits during a child's first 2 years of life have been found to be effective in preventing child abuse and neglect (Hahn et al, 2003).*

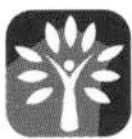

Geriatric

- Be alert to the potential for elder abuse in clients, including the possibility of psychological abuse. EBN: *Abuse may be physical, sexual, psychological, financial, or may appear as neglect. Look for signs of bruising, malnutrition, and fearful responses to or around caregivers (Battaglini, 2014b). Cognitive impairment, behavioral problems, and psychiatric illness in the client are risk factors for becoming recipients of abuse (Battaglini, 2014c). Assess for changes in physiological functions (e.g., constipation, dehydration) or impairment of the ability to meet basic needs (e.g., inadequate toileting, decreased mobility). Observe for signs of fear, anxiety, anger, and agitation, and intervene immediately. In older adults, subtle physiological changes, interruptions of or changes in routine, or fears about medical disorders or potential loss of independence can be transformed into anger, irritability, or agitation.* EBN: *A comprehensive physical exam should include a neurological exam and x-rays as needed (Battaglini, 2014b).*

- Assess for presence or client history of mental illness or treatment. EBN: *There is a high likelihood of elder abuse in the presence of mental illness, even if receiving psychiatric treatment (Battaglini, 2014c).*
- Assess and observe for aggressive behavior in older clients at long-term care facilities. EBN: *Between 25% and 50% of clients with dementia have demonstrated aggressive behavior. Knowledge of the client's history and risk factors is important. Treatment with antipsychotics should be individualized and carefully monitored. Use of restraints should be avoided, used for a short time, and removed at the earliest possible time. Staff should receive training in aggression management (Battaglini, 2014d).*
- Observe clients for dementia and delirium. EBN: *Between 25% and 50% of clients with dementia have demonstrated aggressive behavior. Clients with dementia or delirium may strike out if they are frustrated or if they have the sense that their personal space is being violated. The competency of the client should be assessed to determine if he/she possesses a cognitive capacity that permits discussion of the behavior (Battaglini, 2014c, d).*
- Be aware of laws and regulations in the appropriate jurisdiction where client is located. EBN: *Confidentiality, consent, and information sharing are sensitive issues that are determined by federal as well as local regulation (Battaglini, 2014b; Goh, 2014a).*
- Document and record suspected elder abuse according to mandatory regulations. EBN: *Incidents of abuse should be recorded with date, time, chronology of abuse, family history, potential indicators of abuse, details regarding care planning and decision-making process, and actual care provided. Photographic evidence of abuse should be obtained. The police may be requested to take forensic pictures (Goh, 2014b).*
- Apart from mandated requirements, abide by the older client's wishes regarding action to be taken in response to abuse. Avoid interventions that increase the risk of abuse. EBN: *Discuss with client their reasons for refusing to disclose abuse. There may be a fear that the only available caregiver will withdraw, leaving the client helpless. Allow adequate time for the discussion; respect the client's pace and need for a sense of control. Corroborate events as possible (Battaglini, 2014b). Avoid the use of antidepressants or sedatives without a thorough abuse assessment; the recommendation of family counseling without intervention for the abuser; blaming the victim; colluding with the abuser; or minimizing the possible danger (Goh, 2014c).*
- Develop a safety plan and provide referrals to all relevant agencies or services. EBN: *Discuss safety options for both client and provider. Contact police if there is a concern regarding the availability of a gun. RN should debrief with manager as necessary (Battaglini, 2014c). Multidisciplinary and interagency collaboration is important to meet client needs (Goh, 2014c).*

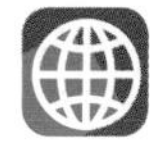

Multicultural

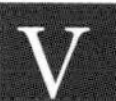

- Exercise cultural competence when dealing with domestic violence. CEBN: *Battered Latina women reported protecting their partner, preventing their mother from worrying, and fear of losing their children as barriers to disclosing IPV (Montalvo-Liendo et al, 2009).*
- Identify and respond to unique needs of immigrant women who experience IPV. EBN: *A study of Sri Lankan immigrants to Canada revealed that violence prior to the immigration, gender inequity in the marriage, changes in social networks and supports, and changes in socioeconomic status were identified by the women as factors involved in IPV (Guruge et al, 2010). Filipina women focused on keeping their family together and did not realize that IPV has a negative influence on the mental health of the women and their children (Shoultz et al, 2010).*
- Assist with acculturation and activating social support. CEB: *Type of support and acculturation helped promote resiliency and improved mood among Hispanic women in IPV situations (Shoultz, et al, 2009).*

Home Care

- Be alert to the potential for violent behavior in the home setting. Respond to verbal aggression with interventions to deescalate negative emotional states. Violence is a process that can be recognized early. Deescalation involves reducing client stressors, responding to the client with respect, acknowledging the

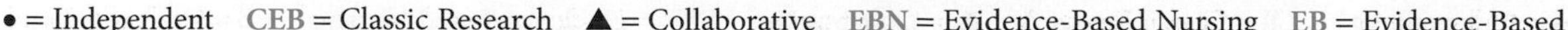

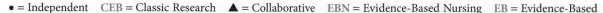

client's feeling state, and assisting the client to regain control. If deescalation does not work, the nurse should leave the home.

- • Assess family members or caregivers for their ability to protect the client and themselves. The safety of the client between home visits is a nursing priority. Caregivers often need assistance with recognizing or admitting fear of or danger from a loved one.
- • Include an initial and ongoing assessment and evaluation of potential abuse and neglect. Photograph evidence of abuse or neglect when possible. *Victims of abuse perceive themselves to be powerless to change the situation. Indeed, the abuser fosters this perception and may threaten violence or death if the victim attempts to leave. Chronic abuse and neglect by a spouse or other family among older adults is often hidden until home care is actively involved.* Refer to the care plan for **Powerlessness.**
- ▲ If neglect or abuse is suspected, identify an emergency plan that addresses the problem immediately, ensures client safety, and includes a report to the appropriate authorities. Discuss when to use hotlines and 911. Role-play access to emergency resources with the client and caregivers. *Client safety is a nursing priority. An emergency plan should address either immediate removal to a safe environment or identification of appropriate steps to take in the event of abuse and the securing of resources for the anticipated action (e.g., available phone, packed bag, alternative living arrangements). Reporting is a legal requirement for health care workers.*
- • Encourage appropriate safety behaviors in abused women; call the client at intervals during a 6-month period to determine whether safety behaviors are being carried out. CEB: *A study of telephone contacts to women who sought help through the district attorney's office demonstrated that safety behaviors increased dramatically. Safety behaviors included hiding money; hiding an extra set of house and car keys; establishing a code for abuse occurrence with family or friends; asking neighbors to call police if violence occurs; removing weapons; keeping available family social security numbers, rent and utility receipts, family birth certificates, identification or driver licenses, bank account numbers, insurance policies and numbers, marriage license, valuable jewelry, important phone numbers, and a hidden bag with extra clothing (McFarlane et al, 2002).*
- • Assess the home environment for harmful objects. Have the family remove or lock objects as able. *The safety of the client and caregivers is a nursing priority.*
- ▲ Refer for homemaker or psychiatric home health care services for respite, client reassurance, and implementation of a therapeutic regimen. Responsibility for a person who may become violent provides high caregiver stress. Respite decreases caregiver stress. The presence of caring individuals is reassuring to both the client and caregivers, especially during periods of client anxiety. Individuals exhibiting violent behaviors can respond to the interventions described previously, modified for the home setting.
- ▲ If the client is taking psychotropic medications, assess client and family knowledge of medication and its administration and side effects. Teach as necessary. Knowledge of the medical regimen supports compliance.
- ▲ Evaluate effectiveness and side effects of medications. Accurate clinical feedback improves the health care provider's ability to prescribe an effective medical regimen specific to a client's needs.
- • If client displays mildly intensifying aggressive behavior, attempt to diffuse anger or violence (e.g., ask for a glass of water to distract client). Later in the visit, explain that aggressive behavior is not acceptable and present consequences of continued aggressive behavior (i.e., right of agency to discontinue services). *Mild aggression can be defused safely. Confronting the client before severe aggression is evident places responsibility on the client and family for respectful partnership in care.*
- • Document all acts or verbalizations of aggression. Safety of the staff is a primary responsibility of home health agencies. Law enforcement intervention may be necessary.
- ▲ If client verbalizes or displays threatening behavior, notify your supervisor and plan to make joint visits with another staff person or a security escort. *Having a second person at the visit is a show of power and control used to subdue aggressive behavior.*
- • If the client's behavior is not overtly threatening but makes the nurse uncomfortable, a meeting may be held outside the home in sight of others (e.g., front porch). *The nurse should trust a "gut" reaction that prompts concern regarding the client's potential for aggressive or violent behavior. Such intuitive reactions are often the result of subliminal cues that are not readily voiced.*
- • Never enter a home or remain in a home if aggression threatens your well-being.
- ▲ Never challenge a show of force, such as a gun threat. Leave and notify your supervisor and the appropriate authorities. Document the incident. *Safety of the staff is a primary responsibility of home health agencies. Law enforcement intervention may be necessary.*

▲ If client behaviors intensify, refer for immediate mental health intervention. The degree of disturbance and ability to manage care safely at home determines the level of services needed to protect the client.

Client/Family Teaching and Discharge Planning

- Instruct victims of IPV in the dynamics and prognosis of domestic violence behavior, as well as the effect on children who witness or are victims of domestic violence. *Victims of IPV feel alone and isolated. They can begin to take back control of their circumstances once they better understand what is happening within the interpersonal relationship, what their options are, and what the consequences of inaction may be. Do not expect an immediate change in the victim's behavior.*
- Teach relaxation and exercise as ways to release anger and deal with stress. CEB: *IPV and parenting stress were found to be risk factors for child maltreatment (Taylor et al, 2009).*
- Teach cognitive behavioral activities, such as active problem solving, reframing (reappraising the situation from a different perspective), or thought stopping (in response to a negative thought, picture a large stop sign and replace the image with a prearranged positive alternative). Teach the client to confront his or her own negative thought patterns (or cognitive distortions), such as catastrophizing (expecting the very worst), dichotomous thinking (perceiving events in only one of two opposite categories), magnification (placing distorted emphasis on a single event), or unrealistic expectations (e.g., "should get what I want when I want it"). *Cognitive behavioral activities address clients' assumptions, beliefs, and attitudes about their situations, fostering modification of these elements to be as realistic as possible. Through cognitive behavioral interventions, clients become more aware of their cognitive choices in adopting and maintaining their belief systems, thereby exercising greater control over their own reactions (Hagerty & Patusky, 2011).*

▲ Refer to individual or group therapy.

- Teach the adolescent client violence prevention, and encourage him/her to become involved in community service activities. School programs that couple community service with classroom health instruction can have a measurable effect on violent behaviors of young adolescents at high risk for being both the perpetrators and victims of peer violence. Community service programs may be a valuable part of multicomponent violence prevention programs.
- Teach the use of appropriate community resources in emergency situations (e.g., hotline, community mental health agency, ED, 911 in most places in the United States, the toll-free National Domestic Violence Hotline [1-800-799-SAFE]). Internet resources are increasing and should be made available to clients. It is necessary to get immediate help when violence occurs.
- Encourage the use of self-help groups in nonemergency situations.
- Inform the client and family about any applicable medication actions, side effects, target symptoms, and toxic reactions.

REFERENCES

Amar, A. F., & Alexy, E. M. (2010). Coping with stalking. *Issues in Mental Health Nursing, 31*, 8.

American Psychiatric Association (APA): *American Psychiatric Association Practice Guidelines*. Retrieved December 30, 2014, from <http://psychiatryonline.org/guidelines>.

American Psychiatric Nurses Association (APNA). *Position statement on seclusion and restraint*, 2014a, Retrieved December 30, 2014, from <http://www.apna.org/i4a/pages/index.cfm?pageid=3728>.

American Psychiatric Nurses Association (APNA). *Seclusion and restraints standards of practice*, 2014b, Retrieved December 30, 2014, from <http://www.apna.org/i4a/pages/index.cfm?pageid=3730>.

American Psychiatric Nurses Association (APNA). *Position statement on workplace violence*, 2008, Retrieved July 6, 2009, from <http://www.apna.org/i4a/pages/index.cfm?pageid=3786>.

American Psychiatric Nurses Association (APNA). *Position statement on staffing inpatient psychiatric units*, 2011, Retrieved December 30, 2014, from <http://www.apna.org/i4a/pages/index.cfm?pageid=4662>.

Appollis, T. M., Lund, C., de Vries, P., et al. (2015). Adolescents' and adults' experiences of being surveyed about violence and abuse: a systematic review of harms, benefits, and regrets. *American Journal of Public Health, 105*(2), e31–e45.

Battaglini, E. (2014a). *Violence management: Acute psychiatric acilities [Evidence Based Recommended Practice]*. Retrieved from <http://0-connect.jbiconnectplus.org.library.newcastle.edu.au>.

Battaglini, E. (2014b). *Domestic elder abuse (Persons with mental health problems): Clinical management: Screening, detection/assessment (Nurses; Rural and Remote Areas) [Evidence Based Recommended Practice]*. Retrieved from <http://0-connect.jbiconnectplus.org.library.newcastle.edu.au>.

Battaglini, E. (2014c). *Domestic elder abuse (Persons with mental health problems): Clinical management: Competency of the elderly and safety issues (Nurses; Rural and Remote Areas) [Evidence Based Recommended Practice]*. Retrieved from <http://0-connect.jbiconnectplus.org.library.newcastle.edu.au>.

Battaglini, E. (2014d). *Aggression in the elderly: Risk factors and management [Evidence Based Recommended Practice]*. Retrieved from <http://0-connect.jbiconnectplus.org.library.newcastle.edu.au>.

Bengtsson-Tops, A., & Tops, D. (2007). Self-reported consequences and needs for support associated with abuse in female users of

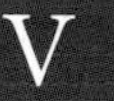

psychiatric care. *International Journal of Mental Health Nursing, 16*, 35.
Buckley, H., et al. (2007). Listen to me! Children's experiences of domestic violence. *Child Abuse Rev, 16*, 296.
Burke, J., et al. (2008). An exploration of maternal intimate partner violence experiences and infant general health and temperament. *Maternal and Child Health Journal, 12*, 172.
Caetano, R., et al. (2008). Drinking, alcohol problems and intimate partner violence among White and Hispanic couples in the U.S.: longitudinal associations. *Journal of Family Violence, 23*, 37.
Cafaro, T., Jolley, C., LaValla, A., et al. (2012). *Workplace violence workgroup report*. Retrieved January 20, 2015 from <http://www.apna.org/i4a/pages/index.cfm?pageID=4912>.
Campbell, R., et al. (2009). An ecological model of the impact of sexual assault on women's mental health. *Trauma, Violence and Abuse, 10*, 225.
Chapman, R., et al. (2009). Predicting patient aggression against nurses in all hospital areas. *British Journal of Nursing (Mark Allen Publishing), 18*, 476.
Charles, P., & Perreira, K. M. (2007). Intimate partner violence during pregnancy and 1-year postpartum. *Journal of Family Violence, 22*, 609.
Chu, V. (2014a). *Healthcare facilities: Patient aggression/violence [Evidence Based Recommended Practice]*. Retrieved from <http://0-connect.jbiconnectplus.org.library.newcastle.edu.au>.
Chu, V. (2014b). *Aggressive behavior management: Acute care [Evidence Based Recommended Practice]*. Retrieved from <http://0-connect.jbiconnectplus.org.library.newcastle.edu.au>.
Cole, J., et al. (2008). Self-perceived risk of HIV among women with protective orders against male partners. *Health and Social Work, 33*, 287.
Copel, L. C. (2006). Partner abuse in physically disabled women: a proposed model for understanding intimate partner violence. *Perspectives in Psychiatric Care, 42*, 114.
Copel, L. C. (2008). The lived experience of women in abusive relationships who sought spiritual guidance. *Issues in Mental Health Nursing, 29*, 115.
Copeland, D. A. (2007). Conceptualizing family members of violent mentally ill individuals as a vulnerable population. *Issues in Mental Health Nursing, 28*, 943.
Courey, T. J., et al. (2008). Hildegard Peplau's theory and the health care encounters of survivors of sexual violence. *Journal of the American Psychiatric Nurses Association, 14*, 136.
Dutton, M. (2009). Pathways linking intimate partner violence and posttraumatic stress disorder. *Trauma, Violence and Abuse, 10*, 211.
Focht-New, G., et al. (2008). Persons with developmental disability exposed to interpersonal violence and crime: Approaches for intervention. *Perspectives in Psychiatric Care, 44*, 89.
Goh, C. (2014a). *Domestic elder abuse (Persons with mental health problems): Clinical management: Confidentiality, consent, information sharing, consultation and supervision (Nurses; Rural and Remote Areas) [Evidence Based Recommended Practice]*. Retrieved from <http://0-connect.jbiconnectplus.org.library.newcastle.edu.au>.
Goh, C. (2014b). *Domestic elder abuse (Persons with mental health problems): Clinical management: Documentation, reporting, and referral (Nurses; Rural and Remote Areas) [Evidence Based Recommended Practice]*. Retrieved from <http://0-connect.jbiconnectplus.org.library.newcastle.edu.au>.
Goh, C. (2014c). *Domestic elder abuse (Persons with mental health problems): Clinical management: Planning, interventions and follow-up (Nurses; Rural and Remote Areas) [Evidence Based Recommended Practice]*. Retrieved from <http://0-connect.jbiconnectplus.org.library.newcastle.edu.au>.
Guruge, S., et al. (2010). Intimate male partner violence in the immigration process: intersections of gender, race, and class. *Journal of Advanced Nursing, 66*, 103.
Hagerty, B., & Patusky, K. (2011). Mood disorders: depression and mania. In K. M. Fortinash & P. A. Holoday-Worret (Eds.), *Psychiatric mental health nursing* (5th ed.). St Louis: Mosby.
Hahn, R. A., et al. (2003). First reports evaluating the effectiveness of strategies for preventing violence: early childhood home visitation. *MMWR. Recommendations and Reports: Morbidity and Mortality Weekly Report. Recommendations and Reports, 52*(RR–14), 1.
Harner, H. M. (2004). Domestic violence and trauma care in teenage pregnancy: does paternal age make a difference? *Journal of Obstetric, Gynecologic, and Neonatal Nursing, 33*(3), 312.
Jeanjot, I., et al. (2008). Domestic violence during pregnancy: survey of patients and healthcare providers. *Journal of Women's Health, 17*, 557.
Kling, R. N., Yassi, A., Smailes, E., et al. (2011). Evaluation of a violence risk assessment system (the Alert System) for reducing violence in an acute hospital: a before and after study. *International Journal of Nursing Studies, 48*(5), 534–539.
Knapik, G. P., et al. (2008). Being delivered: spirituality in survivors of sexual violence. *Issues in Mental Health Nursing, 29*, 335.
Lepisto, S., et al. (2010). Adolescents' experiences of coping with domestic violence. *Journal of Advanced Nursing, 66*, 1232.
Lim, B. C. E. (2011). A systematic literature review: managing the aftermath effects of patient's aggression and violence towards nurses. *Singapore Nurs J, 38*, 6.
LoGiudice, J. (2015). Prenatal screening for intimate partner violence: a qualitative metasynthesis. *Applied Nursing Research, 28, 2–9.*
Lucies, C., & Yick, A. G. (2007). Images of gay men's experiences with antigay abuse: object relations theory reconceptualized. *J Theory Construct Test, 11*, 55.
Lutz, K. E., et al. (2006). Double binding, abusive intimate partner relationships, and pregnancy. *The Canadian Journal of Nursing Research, 38*(4), 118–134.
Macy, R. J., Ferron, J., & Crosby, C. (2009). Partner violence and survivors' chronic health problems: informing social work practice. *Social Work, 54*, 29.
Mahon, N. E., et al. (2010). A meta-analytic study of predictors of anger in adolescents. *Nursing Research, 59*(3), 178.
Mason, C., et al. (2007). Clients with mental illness and their children: implications for clinical practice. *Issues in Mental Health Nursing, 28*, 1105.
McFarlane, J., et al. (2002). An intervention to increase safety behaviors of abused women: results of a randomized clinical trial. *Nursing Research, 51*, 347.
Montalvo-Liendo, N., et al. (2009). Factors influencing disclosure of abuse by women of Mexican descent. *Journal of Nursing Scholarship, 41*, 359.
Murrell, A. R., et al. (2007). Characteristics of domestic violence offenders: associations with childhood exposure to violence. *Journal of Family Violence, 22*, 523.
Mylant, M., & Mann, C. (2008). Current sexual trauma among high-risk teen mothers. *J Child Adol Psychiatr Nurs, 21*, 164.
Olive, P. (2007). Care for emergency department patients who have experienced domestic violence: a review of the evidence base. *Journal of Clinical Nursing, 16*, 1736.
Renck, B. (2006). Psychological stress reactions of women in Sweden who have been assaulted: acute response and four-month follow-up. *Nursing Outlook, 54*, 312.
Rice, E. (2006). Schizophrenia and violence: the perspective of women. *Issues in Mental Health Nursing, 27*, 961.
Robinson, L., & Spilsbury, K. (2008). Systematic review of the perceptions and experiences of accessing health services by adult

V

victims of domestic violence. *Health and Social Care in the Community, 16*, 16.
Sande, R., Noothroon, E., Wierdsma, A., et al. (2013). Association between short-term structured risk assessment outcomes and seclusion. *International Journal of Mental Health Nursing, 22*(6), 475–484.
Sawin, E. M., & Parker, B. (2011). If looks would kill then I would be dead": intimate partner abuse and breast cancer in older women. *Journal of Gerontological Nursing, 37*(7), 26.
Shoultz, J., & Magnussen, L. (2009). Understanding cultural perceptions: foundation for IPV interventions. *Comm Nurs Res, 42*, 288.
Shoultz, J., et al. (2010). Listening to Filipina women: perceptions, responses and needs regarding intimate partner violence. *Issues in Mental Health Nursing, 31*, 54.
Smith, J. S., et al. (2008). Barriers to the mandatory reporting of domestic violence encountered by nursing professionals. *Journal of Trauma Nursing, 15*, 9.
Smith, M. E. (2007). Self-deception among men who are mandated to attend a batterer intervention program. *Perspectives in Psychiatric Care, 43*, 193.
Stalans, L. J., & Ritchie, J. (2008). Relationship of substance use/abuse with psychological and physical intimate partner violence: variations across living situations. *Journal of Family Violence, 23*, 9.
Svavarsdottir, E. K., & Orlygsdottir, B. (2008). Effect of abuse by a close family member on health. *J Nurs Scholarsh, 40*, 311.
Taylor, C. A., et al. (2009). Intimate partner violence, maternal stress, nativity, and risk for maternal maltreatment of young children. *American Journal of Public Health, 99*, 175.
Vandemark, L. M., & Mueller, M. (2008). Mental health after sexual violence: the role of behavioral and demographic risk factors. *Nursing Research, 57*, 175.
Womack, K. A. (2008). Emergency contraception to avoid unintended pregnancy following sexual assault. *Womens Health Care, 7*, 10.
Woods, S. J., et al. (2008). Physical health and posttraumatic stress disorder symptoms in women experiencing intimate partner violence. *Journal of Midwifery and Women's Health, 53*, 538.
Zhili, C. (2013). *Violence: Short-term management [Evidence Based Recommended Practice]*. Retrieved from <http://0-connect.jbiconnectplus.org.library.newcastle.edu.au>.

Risk for self-directed Violence

Kathleen L. Patusky, MA, PhD, RN, CNS

NANDA-I

Definition

Vulnerable to behaviors in which an individual demonstrates that he or she can be physically, emotionally and/or sexually harmful to self

Risk Factors

Age ≥45 years; age 15 to 19 years; behavioral cues (e.g., writing forlorn love notes, directing angry messages at a significant other who has rejected the person, giving away personal items, taking out a large life insurance policy); conflict about sexual orientation; conflict in interpersonal relationships; employment concern (e.g., unemployed, recent job loss/failure); engagement in autoerotic sexual acts; history of multiple suicide attempts; insufficient personal resources (e.g., achievement, insight, affect unavailable and poorly controlled); marital status (e.g., single, widowed, divorced); mental health issue (e.g., depression, psychosis, personality disorder, substance abuse); occupation (e.g., executive, administrator/owner of business, professional, semi-skilled worker); pattern of difficulties in family background (e.g., chaotic or conflictual, history of suicide); physical health issue; psychological disorder; social isolation; suicidal ideation; suicidal plan; verbal cues (e.g., talking about death, "better off without me," asking about lethal dosage of medication)

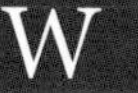

NOC, NIC, Client Outcomes, Nursing Interventions and *Rationales,* Client/Family Teaching and Discharge Planning, and References

Refer to care plans for Risk for **Suicide, Self-Mutilation,** and Risk for **Self-Mutilation.**

Impaired Walking

Wendie A. Howland, MN, RN-BC, CRRN, CCM, CNLCP, LNCC

NANDA-I

Definition

Limitation of independent movement within the environment on foot

Defining Characteristics

Impaired ability to climb stairs; impaired ability to navigate curbs; impaired ability to walk on decline; impaired ability to walk on incline; impaired ability to walk on uneven surface; impaired ability to walk required distance

Related Factors

Alteration in cognitive functioning; alteration in mood; decrease in endurance; environmental barriers (e.g., stairs, inclines, uneven surfaces, obstacles, distances, lack of assistive device); fear of falling; impaired balance; impaired vision; insufficient knowledge of mobility strategies; insufficient muscle strength; musculoskeletal impairment; neuromuscular impairment; obesity; pain; physical deconditioning

NOC (Nursing Outcomes Classification)

Suggested NOC Outcomes

Ambulation; Mobility

Example NOC Outcome with Indicators

Ambulation as evidenced by the following indicators: Walks with effective gait/Walks at moderate pace/Walks up and down steps/Walks moderate distance. (Rate the outcome and indicators of **Ambulation:** 1 = severely compromised, 2 = substantially compromised, 3 = moderately compromised, 4 = mildly compromised, 5 = not compromised [see Section I].)

Client Outcomes

Client Will (Specify Time Frame)

- Demonstrate optimal independence and safety in walking
- Demonstrate the ability to direct others on how to assist with walking
- Demonstrate the ability to properly and safely use and care for assistive walking devices

NIC (Nursing Interventions Classification)

Suggested NIC Intervention

Exercise Therapy: Ambulation

Example NIC Activities—Exercise Therapy: Ambulation

Assist client to use footwear that facilitates walking and prevents injury; Encourage to sit in bed, on side of bed ("dangle"), or in chair, as tolerated

Nursing Interventions and *Rationales*

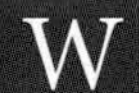

- Progressively mobilize clients (e.g., gradual elevation of head of bed [HOB], sitting in reclined chair, standing). *Limited mobility is an independent predictor of negative outcomes for hospitalized older clients (Doherty-King et al, 2014).*
- Assist clients to apply orthosis, immobilizers, splints, and braces as prescribed before walking. EB: *Assistive devices are prescribed for specific reasons and should be used correctly to help prevent falls (Boelens et al, 2013).*
- Apply thromboembolic deterrent stockings (TEDs) and/or elastic leg wraps; raise HOB slowly in small increments to sitting, have clients move feet/legs up and down then stand slowly; avoid prolonged standing. *Movement promotes venous return and decreases edema.* EB: *Sleeping with the HOB elevated produces minor improvement in postural hypotension; compression bandages have been found to improve postural drop by more than 10 mm Hg (Logan & Witham, 2012; Anthony, 2013).*
- Carefully monitor blood pressure of older adults at least from 30 to 90 minutes after meals before walking. There are significant differences in systolic and diastolic pressure over time, with the biggest drop in systolic and diastolic blood pressure occurring at 45 minutes after a meal (Son & Lee, 2012; Lee, 2013).
- Maintain partial head elevation when resting in bed to help decrease orthostatic hypotension. *HOB elevation stimulates baroreceptors and decreases nocturnal diuresis (Feldstein & Weder, 2012).*

- Compare morning lying/sitting/standing blood pressures. If systolic pressure falls 20 mm Hg or diastolic pressure falls 10 mm Hg from lying to standing within 3 minutes, and/or if lightheadedness, dizziness, syncope, or unexplained falls occur, consult a health care provider (Lee, 2013).
- Detection of orthostatic hypotension is key to fall prevention. EB: *Review medication for possible contributing factors. Give prescribed hydration and medications to treat orthostatic hypotension. Consider leg wraps. Client should perform warm-up bed exercises (Lee, 2013). Cerebral hypoperfusion is a common cause of orthostatic intolerance and hypotension (Lee, 2013). Severe spinal cord injury above T6-8 is a risk factor for orthostatic hypotension due to reduced efferent sympathetic nervous activity and loss of reflex vasoconstriction at arterial baroreceptors below the level of injury (Phillips et al, 2012).*
- *Use a formalized screening tool to identify persons at high risk for thromboembolism (deep venous thrombosis). Best clinical practice is supported by use of a clinical decision model that determines risk based on predisposing factors and certain clinical signs and symptoms (Anthony, 2013).*

▲ Implement thromboembolism prophylaxis/treatment as prescribed (e.g., anticoagulants, antiembolic stockings, elastic leg wraps, sequential compression devices, feet/ankle exercises, and hydration). Refer to care plan for Ineffective peripheral **Tissue Perfusion.**

- Reinforce correct use of prescribed mobility devices and remind clients of weight-bearing restrictions. Canes provide stability in persons with hemiparesis; canes are prescribed to improve gait, balance and alleviate joint pain and are usually used on the contralateral side of the affected limb.
  - Teach clients with leg amputations to correctly don stump socks, liner, immediate postoperative prostheses or traditional prosthesis before standing/walking.
  - Teach client importance of avoiding prolonged hip and knee flexion. If contractures occur, the client may have difficulty with prosthesis fit and use. *Limit amount of time the client is permitted to sit to no more than 40 minutes of each hour, ensure when client sits, stands or is recumbent, the hip and knee are in extension and periodic prone lying is recommended (Pierson & Fairchild, 2008).*
- Emphasize the importance of wearing properly fitting, low-heeled shoes with nonskid soles, and socks/hose, and of seeking medical care for foot pain or problems with abnormal toenails, corns, calluses, or diabetes. *Suggest trying a running shoe that is comfortable and lightweight, in that a recent study found participants unable to see the type of shoe (control shoe, running shoe, or orthopedic shoe) chose the running shoe based on comfort and weight (Ambrosea et al, 2013).*
- Use a snug gait belt with handles and assistive devices while walking clients, as recommended by the physical therapist (PT). *A gait belt must be applied before and during all ambulation and functional gait activities. It should be applied securely around the waist. Do not use client's clothing, upper extremity, or personal belt for control because these items are not strong or secure to provide a safe grasp (Pierson & Fairchild, 2008).*
- Walk clients frequently with an appropriate number of people; have one team member state short, simple motor instructions. *Standing/weight bearing benefits gut motility, spasticity, and respiratory/bowel/bladder function, and promotes muscle stretching (Doherty-King et al, 2014).*
- Cue and manually guide clients with unilateral neglect to prevent clients from bumping into objects/people. EB: *Research subjects with left neglect veered left when driving a powered wheelchair, whereas when walking, they veered right (Turton et al, 2009).*
- Document the number of helpers, level of assistance (e.g., maximum, standby), type of assistance, and devices needed on the care plan and room white board (if used). *Communication and consistency promote client learning/safety, help prevent staff injury, and use all client handling and movement equipment as possible (Cohen et al, 2010).*

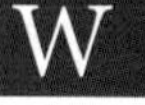

- Take pulse rate/rhythm and pulse oximetry before walking clients, and reassess within 5 minutes of walking, then ongoing as needed. If either is abnormal, have the client sit 5 minutes, then reassess. If still abnormal, walk clients more slowly and with more help, or for a shorter time or notify the health care provider.
- If uncontrolled diabetes/angina/arrhythmias/tachycardia (≥100 bpm) or resting systolic blood pressure ≥200 mm Hg or diastolic blood pressure ≥110 mm Hg occur, do not initiate walking exercise without consulting the health care prescriber. *Pulse rate and arterial blood oxygenation indicate cardiac/exercise tolerance. Tachycardia and low pulse oximetry readings, generally <88%, are indicators of unstable hemodynamic status; rest the client and apply oxygen (Ambrosea et al, 2013).*

Refer to the care plan for **Activity** intolerance.

- Perform initial/ongoing screening for risk of falling and perform postfall assessments including medications and lab results to prevent further falls. *Nurses must assess fall risk; in a Medicare review, fewer than*

60% of older adults who reported falls talked to a health care provider about the problem (Matsuda et al, 2011).

- Individualize interventions to prevent falls, e.g., scheduled toileting, monitored rooms, bed alarms, wheelchair alarms, balance/strength training, sleep hygiene, education on risk of medication/alcohol use, removal of hazards and attention to safe handling during any transfers, wound care, toileting, showering/bathing (Cohen et al, 2010). EB: *Root cause analysis can be an effective tool to decrease rate of falls in facilities with challenge to keep personnel trained in the process. The fall prevention program should include fall prevention interventions as well as assessment of risk and assessment of a fall (Boelens et al, 2013).*

Geriatric

▲ Assess for swaying, poor balance, weakness, and fear of falling while older adults stand/walk. If present, refer to PT. *Fear of falling and repeat fallers are common. Balance rehabilitation provides individualized treatment for persons with various diseases/deficits (Ambrosea et al, 2013). Assess all geriatric clients and have heightened awareness for risk of fall in clients with chronic diseases such as multiple sclerosis, Parkinson's disease or parkinsonism, or stroke (Matsuda et al, 2011).*

▲ Review medications for polypharmacy and those that place older adults at risk for falls; consult with pharmacy as needed. More than five drugs indicates polypharmacy and puts the client at risk for adverse drug reactions, drug-drug interactions, and overall low adherence to drug therapy due to too many drugs to take (Hovstadius et al, 2010).

▲ Encourage an exercise component such as tai chi, physical therapy, or other exercise for balance, gait, and strength training in group programs or at home; modify environment for safety; recommend vision assessment for corrective lenses and consideration for cataract removal; conduct polypharmacy assessment with special consideration to sedatives, antidepressants, and drugs affecting the central nervous system; evaluate for orthostatic hypotension and dysrhythmia; recommend vitamin D supplementation 800 IU per day (National Institutes of Health, 2014).

- Assess fall risk, then implement fall precautions, such as clearing obstacles, reviewing medications, and using a visual identifier on clients starting exercise/education programs. *Previous falls, physiological changes, and adverse effects from multiple medications put older adults at risk for falls (Ambrosea et al, 2013).*

Home Care

▲ Establish a support system for emergency and contingency care (e.g., remote monitoring, emergency call system, alert local EMS). *Impaired walking may pose a life threat during a crisis (e.g., fall, fire, orthostatic episode).*

▲ Assess for and modify any barriers to walking in the home environment to promote safety. EB: *Effective precautions for ambulation safety in the home are removal of small rugs or mats that may slip or slide, use of extreme caution when using a bath mat, avoidance of waxing floors or use of nonskid wax, and immediate clearance of spills from non-carpeted floors (Ambrosea et al, 2013).*

▲ Obtain prescription for PT home visits for individualized strength, balance retraining, and an exercise plan. EB: *Original research shows the use of simple stretching program for older clients counteracts age-related decline in gait function (Watt et al, 2011).*

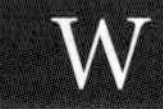

▲ Make referrals for home health services for support and assistance with activities of daily living (ADLs). *This is a key component of discharge planning.* Listen to and support client/caregivers; refer to support groups that meet or are online. Refer to care plan for **Caregiver Role Strain.**

Client/Family Teaching and Discharge Planning

- Teach clients to check ambulation devices weekly for cracks, loose nuts, or worn tips; clean dust and dirt on tips; remove all items from stairways; be certain hand rails are strong and secure; position furniture to allow a 36-inch wide unobstructed pathway when possible, and remove electrical cords or loose objects from walking paths (Boelens et al, 2013).
- Teach clients with diabetes that they are at risk for foot ulcers and train them in preventive interventions. EB: *Literature continues to address risk factors for foot ulcers, previous amputation, foot ulcer history, peripheral neuropathy, foot deformity, peripheral vascular disease, visual impairment, diabetic nephropathy, poor glycemic control, and cigarette smoking; clients with diabetes need education on these risk factors (National Diabetes Information Clearing House, 2014).*

- Instruct anyone at risk for osteoporosis or hip fractures to bear weight, walk, engage in resistance exercise (with appropriate adjustments for conditions), take good nutrition, especially adequate intake of calcium and vitamin D, stop smoking, monitor alcohol intake, and consult a health care provider for antiresorptive therapy. EB: *Supplementation with vitamin D3 (cholecalciferol) and calcium reduced the risk of hip fracture by 43%. The National Osteoporosis Foundation recommends daily calcium intake of at least 1200 mg with diet plus supplements, if needed, for postmenopausal women and men aged 50 years and older intake of vitamin D3 800 to 1000 IU per day (Cotton D, 2011).*
- For more information, refer to the care plans for Impaired **Transfer** ability and Impaired wheelchair **Mobility.**

REFERENCES

Ambrosea, A. F., Geet, P., & Hausdorff, J. M. (2013). Risk factors for falls among older adults: a review of the literature. *Maturitas, 75*, 511–521.

Anthony, M. (2013). Nursing assessment of deep vein thrombosis. *Medsurg Nursing, 22*(2), 95–98.

Boelens, C., Hekman, E. E. G., & Verkerke, G. J. (2013). Risk factors for falls of older citizens. *Technology and Health Care, 21*, 521–533.

Cohen, M. H., et al. *Patient handling and movement assessments: a white paper.* (2010). The Facility Guideline Institute. From <http://www.fgiguidelines.org/pdfs/FGI_PHAMA_whitepaper_042810.pdf> Retrieved July 29, 2015.

Cotton, D., et al. (2011). In the clinic: osteoporosis. *Annals of Internal Medicine, 5*, ITCI-1–ITCI-16.

Doherty-King, B., Yoon, J. Y., Pekanac, K., et al. (2014). Frequency and duration of nursing care related to older patient mobility. *Journal of Nursing Scholarship, 46*(1), 20–27.

Feldstein, C., & Weder, A. B. (2012). Orthostatic hypotension: a common, serious, and underrecognized problem in hospitalized patients. *J Am Soc Hypertens, 6*(1), 27–39.

Hovstadius, B., et al. (2010). Increasing polypharmacy—an individual based study of the Swedish population 2005-2008. *BMC Clinical Pharmacology, 10*(16), 1–8.

Lee, Y. (2013). Orthostatic hypertension in older people. *J Am Assoc Nurse Pract, 25*, 451–458.

Logan, I. C., & Witham, M. D. (2012). Efficacy of treatments for orthostatic hypotension: a systematic review. *Age and Ageing, 41*, 587–594.

Matsuda, P. N., et al. (2011). Falls in multiple sclerosis. *PM R, 3*(7), 624–632.

National Diabetes Information Clearing House. (2014). *Prevent diabetes problems: keep your feet healthy.* Available at: <http://www.niddk.nih.gov/health-information/health-topics/Diabetes/prevent-diabetes-problems/Pages/index.aspx>.

National Institutes of Health, Office of Dietary Supplements. (2014). *Vitamin D fact sheet for health professionals.* <https://ods.od.nih.gov/factsheets/VitaminD-HealthProfessional/>.

Phillips, A. A., Krassioukov, A. V., Ainslie, P. N., et al. (2012). Baroreflex function after spinal cord injury. *Journal of Neurotrauma, 29*(15), 2431–2445.

Pierson, F. M., & Fairchild, S. L. (2008). Ambulation aids, patterns, and activities. In F. M. Pierson & S. L. Fairchild (Eds.), *Principles & techniques of patient care* (4th ed.). St Louis: Saunders.

Son, J. T., & Lee, E. (2012). Postprandial hypotension among older residents of a nursing home in Korea. *Journal of Clinical Nursing, 21*(23–24), 3565–3573.

Turton, A. J., et al. (2009). Walking and wheelchair navigation in patients with left visual neglect. *Neuropsychological Rehabilitation, 19*(2), 274–290.

Watt, J. R., et al. (2011). Effect of a supervised hip flexor stretching program on gait in elderly individuals. *PM R, 3*(4), 324–329.

Wandering

Laura May Struble, PhD, GNP-BC

NANDA-I

Definition

Meandering; aimless or repetitive locomotion that exposes the individual to harm; frequently incongruent with boundaries, limits, or obstacles

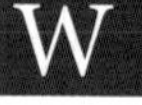

Defining Characteristics

Continuous movement from place to place; eloping behavior; frequent movement from place to place; fretful locomotion; haphazard locomotion; hyperactivity; impaired ability to locate landmarks in a familiar setting; locomotion into unauthorized spaces; locomotion resulting in getting lost; locomotion that cannot be easily dissuaded; long periods of locomotion without an apparent destination; pacing; periods of locomotion interspersed with periods of non-locomotion (e.g., sitting, standing, sleeping); persistent locomotion in search of something; scanning behavior; searching behavior; shadowing a caregiver's locomotion; trespassing

Related Factors (r/t)

Alteration in cognitive functioning; cortical atrophy; overstimulating environment; physiological state (e.g., hunger, thirst, pain, need to urinate); premorbid behavior (e.g., outgoing, sociable personality); psychological disorder; sedation; separation from familiar environment; time of day

NOC (Nursing Outcomes Classification)

Suggested NOC Outcomes

Safe Wandering; Caregiver Home Care Readiness; Fall Prevention Behavior; Falls Occurrence

Example NOC Outcome with Indicators

Safe Wandering as evidenced by the following indicators: Moves about without harming self or others/Sits for more than 5 minutes at a time/Paces a given route/Appears content in environment/Distracts easily/Can be redirected from unsafe activities. (Rate the outcome and indicators of **Safe Wandering:** 1 = never demonstrated, 2 = rarely demonstrated, 3 = sometimes demonstrated, 4 = often demonstrated, 5 = consistently demonstrated [see Section I].)

Client Outcomes

Client Will (Specify Time Frame)

- Maintain psychological well-being and reduce any felt need to wander
- Decrease the amount of time getting lost
- Engage in meaningful activities daily
- Remain safe and free from falls and elopement
- Maintain physical activity and remain comfortable and free of pain
- Maintain appropriate body weight and be well nourished and well hydrated
- Be physically well rested and demonstrate absence of fatigue

Caregiver Will (Specify Time Frame)

- Be able to explain interventions he/she can use to provide a safe environment for a care receiver who displays wandering behavior
- Develop strategies to reduce caregiver stress levels

NIC (Nursing Interventions Classification)

Suggested NIC Intervention

Dementia Management

Example NIC Activities—Dementia Management

Place identification bracelet on the client; Provide space for safe pacing and wandering

Nursing Interventions and *Rationales*

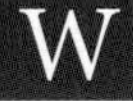

Acute Care Hospital: Wandering

- Screen clients with cognitive impairment at the time of admission and when the client is transferred to another unit in the hospital. Assess for concerns that the client will wander from family members and other health professionals. In addition, assess for the client's ability to walk independently or with minimal assistance. EB: *A two-question assessment tool was developed by a multidisciplinary team that identified clients at risk for wandering. The tool used electronic health records and initiated a list of wandering interventions required once a client was identified as a wandering risk (Sheth et al, 2014).*
- If the client is at risk for wandering in the hospital setting, the following interventions may be implemented: dress the client in a brightly colored hospital gown that is easily identifiable, provide appropriate supervision and surveillance of the at risk client, identify in the chart (electronic record) the client's risk for wandering, discuss with the client and family the risks of wandering, set up appropriate alarm systems, consult with geriatric or mental health advanced practice nurse regarding wandering risks and individualized interventions, and have a current client photograph on file to help with identification in case the client leaves unattended. EBN: *The suggested interventions may reduce the risk of clients getting injured or lost, or wandering into restricted areas in the hospital setting (Sheth et al, 2014).*

Nursing Care Facilities: Wandering

- Assess and document the amount (frequency and duration), percentage of hours with wandering, and 24-hour distribution of wandering behavior over 3 days. EBN: *Assessment over time provides a baseline against which behavioral change can be evaluated and targets the time of day when behavioral interventions are most necessary (Algase et al, 2009).*
- Assess and document the quantity and qualities of wandering behaviors (e.g., persistent walking, repetitive walking, eloping behaviors, spatial disorientation, goal directed, negative outcomes). CEB: *Instruments such as the Revised Algase Wandering Scale indicate whether the behavior is persistent or spatially disordered, or if the client is prone to elopement. A recent review of 34 wandering instruments concluded that the Algase tool had the most in-depth description of wandering behaviors (White & Montgomery, 2014).*
- Obtain a history of personality characteristics and behavioral responses to stress. EBN: *Premorbid personality traits (e.g., history of a physically active job or leisure activities) and behavioral responses to stress (e.g., history of responding to stress with psychomotor activity) may reveal circumstances under which wandering will occur and can aid in interpreting both positive and negative meanings of wandering behavior (Song & Algase, 2008).*
- Evaluate for neurocognitive strengths and limitations, particularly language, attention, and visuospatial skills. CEB: *Wanderers may have expressive language deficits that hamper their ability to communicate needs (Algase, 1992).* CEB: *Knowledge of attentional and visuospatial deficits, which may account for certain patterns of wandering or way-finding deficits, can lead to identification of appropriate environmental modifications that could enhance functional ambulation, such as elimination of distractions and enhancement of cues marking desired destinations (Chiu et al, 2004).*
- Assess for level of cognitive and emotional status and age. CEB: *In a secondary analysis of a multisite study, higher rates of wandering were related to younger age and severe cognitive impairment. In addition, positive emotional expressions were related to higher rates of wandering and should be considered a positive result of wandering behavior (Lee et al, 2014).*
- Assess for changes in cognition and signs and symptoms of medical illness such as pneumonia or cardiovascular disease. EB: *A large longitudinal study found advancing dementia and/or an undiagnosed medical event that affects cognition but spares mobility are associated with the onset of wandering (King-Kallimanis et al, 2010).*
- Assess and monitor for drug-induced akathisia (motor restlessness). CEB: *Although wandering has not been specifically linked to akathisia, medications such as antipsychotics, selective serotonin reuptake inhibitors, antiemetics, and dopamine antagonist drugs may increase restlessness, pacing, and the urge to move (Molinari et al, 2008; Schneider et al, 2006).* CEB: *The occurrence of akathisia can be assessed with the Barnes Akathisia Rating Scale (Barnes, 1989).*
- Discontinue use of medications and physical restraints that are used for the sole purpose of controlling wandering behavior. CEB: *The Omnibus Budget Reconciliation Act (OBRA) of 1978 requirements specify that wandering behavior is not an appropriate target symptom for the use of psychotropic medications or physical restraints. In addition, there is no evidence that psychotropic medications should be used to treat any type of wandering behavior (Sink et al, 2005; Rosenberg et al, 2012).*
- Assess for emotional or psychological distress, such as anxiety, fear, or feeling lost. EB: *Anxiety, loneliness, and separation may be related to restlessness and wandering (Ata et al, 2010).*
- Assess for physical distress or unmet needs (e.g., hunger, thirst, pain discomfort, elimination) with the Need-Driven Dementia-Compromised Behaviors (NBD) model. EBN: *The NBD model may help explain reasons for wandering and offers direction in the development of management strategies (Futrell et al, 2010; Miranda-Castillo et al, 2010).*
- Observe wandering episodes for antecedents and consequences. CEB: *Triggers for wanderers include being placed in an unfamiliar environment, seeing a coat and hat, experiencing an argumentative or confrontational situation, a change in schedule or routine, and recent relocation to a care facility (Silverstein & Flaherty, 2003).*
- Observe the location where and environmental conditions in which wandering is occurring and modify those that appear to induce wandering. EBN: *In a recent observational study, wanderers were less likely to wander from where the likelihood of social interaction was greater (i.e., activities room, dayroom, staff area); where the environment was more soothing (i.e., their own room); or where rooms had a designated purpose (e.g., dayrooms, the wanderer's own room, activities and staff areas), and wandering was less likely when lighting was low and variation in sound levels was small (Algase et al, 2010).*

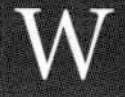

- Assess regularly for the presence of or potential for negative outcomes of wandering (e.g., elopement, declining social skills, onset of falls, becoming lost, and injuries). CEB: *Wanderers are at great risk for falls and other adverse events (Nelson & Algase, 2007).*
- Weigh the client at defined intervals to detect onset of weight loss, and watch for symptoms associated with inadequate food intake, including constipation, dehydration, muscle wasting, and starvation. CEB: *Wandering behavior can affect the client's ability to eat, when the client is unable to sit at a table for the time needed to eat a meal (Beattie & Algase, 2002).*
- For the client who displays wandering behavior during mealtimes, use behavioral interventions to shape behavior, including verbal statements, nonverbal social behavior, and systematic extinguishing of undesirable client behavior. CEB: *Results of a study using behavior interventions demonstrated that they were effective in increasing the time the client sat at the table and the amount of food the client ate (Beattie et al, 2004).*
- Provide for safe ambulation with comfortable and well-fitting clothes, shoes with nonskid soles and foot support, and any necessary walking aids (e.g., a cane or walker). CEB: *Wanderers are at increased risk for falls (Katz et al, 2004).*
- Refer to physical therapy for core therapeutic exercise, balance, gait, and assistive device training. EB: *In a case study, physical therapy demonstrated positive functional outcomes using fall prevention interventions modified for the client's cognition, communication deficits, and behavior problems (Mirolsky-Scala & Kraemer, 2009).*
- Provide safe and secure surroundings that deter accidental elopements, using perimeter control devices or electronic tracking systems. CEB: *A review of technology identified boundary alarms activated by wrist bands, alarms alerting caregivers of wandering behavior, and electronic monitoring and tracking systems, such as global positioning systems (GPS), as effective in improving client safety (Lauriks et al, 2007).*
- There are ethical concerns in the use of tracking technologies. EB: *Qualitative and quantitative results from a large study recommend that clients with dementia should be part of the decision process related to the use of monitoring systems as early as possible in the dementia disease process (Landau & Werner, 2012). In an ethnographic field study, the themes that emerged suggested that technology may contribute to the client's autonomy if a person-centered approach is used and the client's experience with devices is evaluated (Niemeijer et al, 2014).*
- During periods of inactivity, position the wanderer so that desirable destinations (e.g., bathroom) are within the client's line of vision and undesirable destinations (e.g., exits or stairwells) are out of sight. CEB: *Functional, nonwandering ambulation is possible even into late-stage dementia and may be facilitated by keeping appropriate visual cues accessible (Passini et al, 2000).*
- Facilitate way-finding through therapeutic environmental design. EB: *Thirty nursing homes were analyzed for architectural characteristics, and the significant characteristics that impact spatial orientation included limiting the number of people with dementia per living area, providing straight layouts without changes in direction to important locations, and providing only one living/dining room (Marquardt & Schmieg, 2009).*
- Enhance the physical environment by increasing visual appeal and provide interesting views and opportunities to sit. CEB: *In a cross-sectional study, environmental ambience influenced walking frequencies, walking duration, and sitting duration (Yao & Algase, 2006).*
- Engage wanderers in social interaction and structured activity such as painting or coloring, especially when wanderers appear distressed or otherwise uncomfortable, or their wandering presents a challenge to others in the setting. EB: *In a case study, simple leisure activities such as picture coloring significantly reduced wandering behavior (Giulio et al, 2011).*

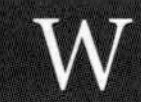

- Provide headphones and iPod with individualized preferred music while the person with dementia is wandering, or encourage the person to participate in a music group. EBN: *In an intervention nursing home study in Taiwan, researchers found preferred music listening had a positive impact by reducing the level of anxiety in older residents with dementia (Sung et al, 2010).*
- If wandering has a pacing quality, attempt to identify and address any underlying problems or concerns. Offer stress-reducing approaches, such as music, massage, or rocking. Attempts to distract or redirect the pacing wanderer may worsen wandering. EB: *In a field study, the researchers found a close relationship between wandering and restlessness (Ata et al, 2010).*
- Provide a regularly scheduled and supervised exercise or walking program, particularly if wandering occurs excessively during the night or at times that are inconvenient in the setting. CEB: *Although exercise or walking programs do not reduce daytime wandering, they have been shown to reduce or eliminate nighttime wandering (Carillon Nursing and Rehabilitation Center, 2000).*

- Use soft tactile hand massage before the times of day or events that induce wandering. EB: *In an intervention study, soft hand message for 20 minutes reduced aggressiveness and stress in clients with dementia (Suzuki et al, 2010).*

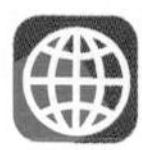

Multicultural

- Recognize that wandering occurs with little variation in expression among individuals with dementia regardless of culture or ethnicity. CEB/EB: *Wandering has been reported in multiple populations and varies little by cultural group (Greiner et al, 2007; Young et al, 2008).*
- Assess for the influence of cultural beliefs, norms, and values on the family's understanding of wandering behavior. CEB: *Latina caregivers of people with dementia delay institutionalization significantly longer than female Caucasian caregivers because of Latino cultural values and positive views of the caregiving role (Mausbach et al, 2004; Sink et al, 2004).*
- ▲ Refer the family to social services or other supportive services to assist with the impact of caregiving for the wandering client.
- Encourage the family to use support groups or other service programs.

Home Care

- Help the caregiver set up a plan to deal with wandering behavior using the interventions mentioned earlier.
- Assess the home environment for modifications that will protect the client and prevent elopement. *Security devices are available to notify the caregiver of the client's movements such as alarms at doors, bed alarms, and ongoing surveillance (McKenzie et al, 2013).*
- Assist the family to set up a plan of exercise for the client, including safe walking. *Walking is a valuable source of exercise, even for clients with dementia.*
- Enroll wanderers in the Safe Return Program of the Alzheimer's Association, and help the caregiver develop a plan of action to use if the client elopes. CEB: *The Safe Return Program has assisted in locating numerous persons who have eloped from their homes or other residential care settings. Mortality rates are high if there is failure to locate elopers within the first 24 hours (Rowe & Glover, 2001).*
- Help the caregiver develop a plan of action to use if the client elopes.
- Refer for homemaker or psychiatric home health care services for respite, client reassurance, and implementation of a therapeutic regimen. Refer to the care plan for **Caregiver Role Strain.** *Responsibility for a person at high risk for wandering provides high caregiver stress. Respite care decreases caregiver stress. The presence of caring individuals is reassuring to both the client and caregivers, especially during periods of client anxiety. Wandering behavior can make use of the interventions described previously, modified for the home setting.*

Client/Family Teaching and Discharge Planning

- Use a broad range of descriptions for the term "wandering" to enhance caregivers' understanding. EB: *In structured interviews, it was found that informal caregivers rarely used the term "wandering," which could lead to miscommunication with health care providers (Houston et al, 2011).*
- Inform the client and family of the meaning of and reasons for wandering behavior. An understanding of wandering behavior will enable the client and family to provide the client with a safe environment.
- Teach the caregiver/family methods to deal with wandering behavior using the interventions mentioned in Nursing Interventions and *Rationales*.

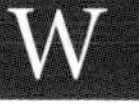

REFERENCES

Algase, D. L. (1992). Cognitive discriminants of wandering among nursing home residents. *Nursing Research, 41*(2), 78–81.

Algase, D. L., Beattie, E., & Antonakos, C. (2010). Wandering and the physical environment. *American Journal of Alzheimer's Disease and Other Dementias, 25*(4), 340–346.

Algase, D. L., et al. (2009). New parameters for daytime wandering. *Res Gerontol Nurs, 2*(1), 58–68.

Ata, T., et al. (2010). Wandering and fecal smearing in people with dementia. *International Psychogeriatrics, 22*(3), 493–500.

Barnes, T. R. E. (1989). A rating scale for drug-induced akathisia. *The British Journal of Psychiatry: The Journal of Mental Science, 154*, 672–676.

Beattie, E. R. A., & Algase, D. L. (2002). Improving table-sitting behavior of wanderers via theoretic substruction. *Journal of Gerontological Nursing, 28*(10), 6–11.

Beattie, E. R. A., et al. (2004). Keeping wandering nursing home residents at the table: improving food intake using a behavior communication intervention. *Aging and Mental Health, 8*(2), 109–116.

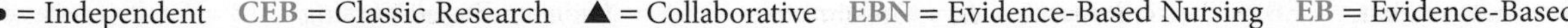

Carillon Nursing and Rehabilitation Center. (2000). Nature walk: from aimless wandering to purposeful walking. *Nurs Homes Long Term Care Manage, 49*(11), 50–55.

Chiu, Y. C., Algase, D., & Whall, A. (2004). Getting lost: directed attention and executive functions in early Alzheimer's disease patients. *Dementia and Geriatric Cognitive Disorders, 17*(3), 174–180.

Futrell, M., et al. (2010). Evidence-based guideline. Wandering. *Journal of Gerontological Nursing, 36*(2), 6–16.

Giulio, L., et al. (2011). A man with severe Alzheimer's disease stops wandering during a picture colouring activity. *Dev Neurorehabil, 14*(4), 242–246.

Greiner, C., et al. (2007). Feasibility study of the integrated circuit tag monitoring system for dementia residents in Japan. *American Journal of Alzheimer's Disease and Other Dementias, 22*(2), 129–136.

Houston, A. M., Brown, L. M., Rowe, M. A., et al. (2011). The informal caregivers' perception of wandering. *American Journal of Alzheimer's Disease and Other Dementias, 26*(8), 616–622.

Katz, I. R., et al. (2004). Risperidone and falls in ambulatory nursing home residents with dementia and psychosis or agitation: secondary analysis of a double-blind, placebo-controlled trial. *The American Journal of Geriatric Psychiatry, 12*(5), 499–508.

King-Kallimanis, B., et al. (2010). Longitudinal investigation of wandering behavior in department of veterans affairs nursing home care units. *International Journal of Geriatric Psychiatry, 25*, 166–174.

Landau, R., & Werner, S. (2012). Ethical aspects of using GPS for tracking people with dementia: recommendations for practice. *International Psychogeriatrics, 24*(3), 358–366.

Lauriks, S., et al. (2007). Review of ICT-based services for identified unmet needs in people with dementia. *Ageing Research Reviews, 6*(3), 223–246.

Lee, K. H., Algase, D. L., & McConnell, E. S. (2014). Relationship between observable emotional expression and wandering behavior of people with dementia who wander. *International Journal of Geriatric Psychiatry, 29*(1), 85–92.

Marquardt, G., & Schmieg, P. (2009). Dementia-friendly architecture: environments that facilitate wayfinding in nursing homes. *American Journal of Alzheimer's Disease and Other Dementias, 24*(4), 333–340.

Mausbach, B. T., et al. (2004). Ethnicity and time to institutionalization of dementia patients: a comparison of Latina and Caucasian female family caregivers. *Journal of the American Geriatrics Society, 52*(7), 1077–1084.

McKenzie, B., Bowen, M. E., Keys, K., et al. (2013). Safe home program: a suite of technologies to support extended home care of persons with dementia. *Am J Alzheimer's Dis Other Demen, 28*(4), 348–354.

Miranda-Castillo, C., et al. (2010). Unmet needs, quality of life and support networks of people with dementia living at home. *Health and Quality of Life Outcomes, 8*, 132.

Mirolsky-Scala, G., & Kraemer, T. (2009). Fall management in Alzheimer-related dementia: a case study. *Journal of Geriatric Physical Therapy (2001), 32*(4), 181–189.

Molinari, V., et al. (2008). Wandering behavior in veterans with psychiatric diagnoses residing in nursing homes. *International Journal of Geriatric Psychiatry, 23*(7), 748–753.

Nelson, A. L., & Algase, A. (Eds.), (2007). *Evidence-based protocols for managing wandering behaviors*. New York: Springer.

Niemeijer, A. R., Depla, M., Frederiks, B., et al. (2015). The experience of people with dementia and intellectual disabilities with surveillance technologies in residential care. *Nursing Ethics, 22*(3), 307–320.

Omnibus Budget Reconciliation Act of 1978 (Public law #100-203). amendments 1990, 1991, 1992, 1993, 1994, Rockville, Md). Health Care Financing Administration, U.S. Department of Health and Human Services.

Passini, R., et al. (2000). Wayfinding in a nursing home for advanced dementia of the Alzheimer's type. *Environment and Behavior, 32*(5), 684–710.

Rosenberg, P. B., et al. (2012). The association of psychotropic medication use with the cognitive, functional, and neuropsychiatric trajectory of Alzheimer's disease. *In J Geriatr Psychiatry, 27*(12), 1248–1257.

Rowe, M. A., & Glover, J. C. (2001). Antecedents, descriptions and consequences of wandering in cognitively-impaired adults and the Safe Return (SR) program. *Am J Alzheimers Dis, 16*(6), 344–352.

Schneider, L. S., et al. (2006). Efficacy and adverse effects of atypical antipsychotics for dementia: meta-analysis of randomized, placebo-controlled trials. *The American Journal of Geriatric Psychiatry, 14*, 191–210.

Sheth, H. S., Krueger, D., Bourdon, S., et al. (2014). A new tool to asses risk of wandering in hospitalized patients. *Journal of Gerontological Nursing, 40*(3), 28–33, quiz 34-5. [Epub 2014 Feb 5].

Silverstein, N. M., & Flaherty, G. (2003). Dementia and wandering behaviour in long-term care facilities. *Geriatr Aging, 6*, 47–52.

Sink, K. M., et al. (2005). Pharmacological treatment of neuropsychiatric symptoms of dementia: a review of the evidence. *JAMA: The Journal of the American Medical Association, 293*, 596–608.

Sink, K. M., et al. (2004). Ethnic differences in the prevalence and pattern of dementia-related behaviors. *Journal of the American Geriatrics Society, 52*(8), 1277–1283.

Song, J. A., & Algase, D. L. (2008). Premorbid characteristics and wandering behavior in persons with dementia. *J Psychosoc Nurs, 22*(6), 318–327.

Sung, H. C., et al. (2010). A preferred music listening intervention to reduce anxiety in older adults with dementia in nursing homes. *Journal of Clinical Nursing, 19*(7–8), 1056–1064.

Suzuki, M., et al. (2010). Physical and psychological effects of 6-week tactile massage on elderly patient with severe dementia. *American Journal of Alzheimer's Disease and Other Dementias, 25*(8), 680–686.

White, E. B., & Montgomery, P. (2014). A review of "wandering" instruments for people with dementia who get lost. *Research on Social Work Practice, 24*(4), 400–413.

Yao, L., & Algase, D. (2006). Environmental ambiance as a new window on wandering. *Western Journal of Nursing Research, 28*, 89–104.

Young, M. L., et al. (2008). Factors affecting burden of family caregivers of community-dwelling ambulatory elders with dementia in Korea. *Archives of Psychiatric Nursing, 22*(4), 226–234.

APPENDIX A

Nursing Diagnoses Arranged by Maslow's Hierarchy of N

Because human beings adapt in many ways to establish and maintain the self, health problems are much more than simple physical matters. Maslow's Hierarchy of Needs (see diagram below) is a system of classifying human needs. Maslow's hierarchy is based on the idea that lower-level physiological needs must be met before higher-level, abstract needs can be met.

For nurses, Maslow's hierarchy has special significance in decision-making and planning for care. By considering need categories as you identify client problems, you will be able to provide more holistic care. For example, a client who demands frequent attention for a seemingly trivial matter may require help with self-esteem needs. Need levels vary from client to client. If a client is short of breath, the client is probably not interested in or capable of discussing spirituality. In addition, a client's need level may change throughout planning and intervention, so you will need to be vigilant in your assessment.

All needs are relevant. Too many times, physiological problems are caused by unmet ps example, po needs for lov as a source of and resultant heart disease.

Read the descriptions of each category in the diagram and see how you would relate them to nursing diagnoses. Compare your evaluation with how the authors categorized the nursing diagnoses according to this hierarchy. Be sure to assess clients for potential problems at all levels of the pyramid, regardless of their initial complaint.

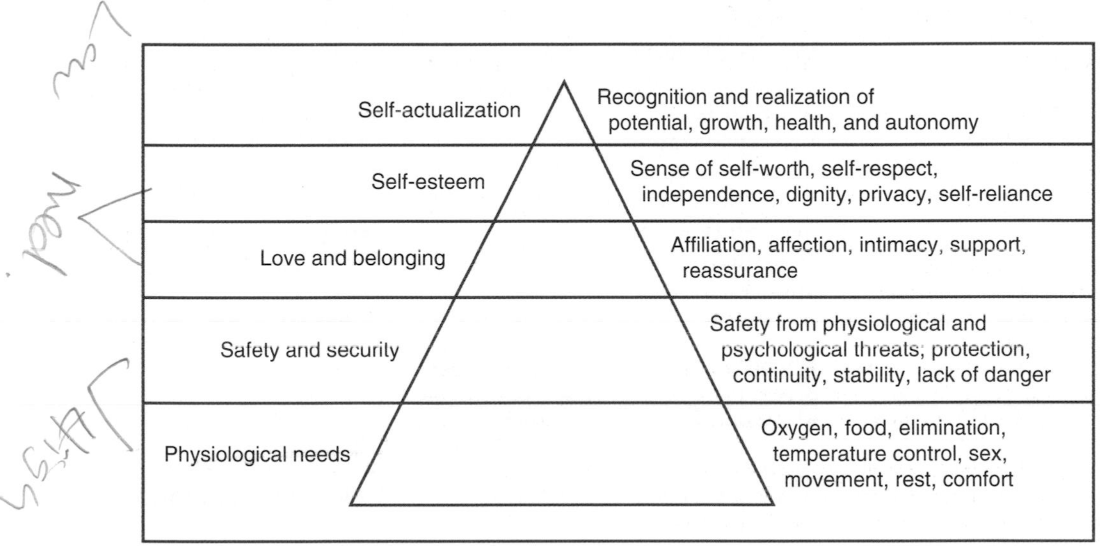

Reprinted with permission from *Nursing diagnosis referred manual,* copyright 1991, Springhouse Corp. All rights reserved.

PHYSIOLOGICAL NEEDS

Activity intolerance
Activity intolerance, risk for
Airway clearance, ineffective
Aspiration, risk for
Autonomic Dysreflexia
Bleeding, risk for
Breastfeeding, ineffective
Breastfeeding, interrupted
Breastfeeding, readiness for enhanced
Breast Milk, insufficient
Breathing pattern, ineffective
Cardiac output, decreased
Cardiac output, risk for decreased
Cardiac tissue perfusion, risk for decreased
Cardiovascular function, risk for impaired
Cerebral tissue perfusion, risk for ineffective
Comfort, impaired
Comfort, readiness for enhanced
Constipation
Constipation, chronic functional
Constipation, perceived
Constipation, risk for
Constipation, risk for chronic functional
Dentition, impaired
Diarrhea
Electrolyte imbalance, risk for
Eye, risk for dry
Fatigue
Feeding pattern, ineffective infant
Fluid balance, readiness for enhanced
Fluid volume, deficient
Fluid volume, excess
Fluid volume, risk for deficient

me, risk for imbalanced
hange, impaired
rointestinal motility, dysfunctional
astrointestinal motility, risk for dysfunctional
Gastrointestinal perfusion, risk for ineffective
Glucose level, risk for unstable blood
Hyperthermia
Hypothermia
Hypothermia, risk for
Hypothermia, risk for **Perioperative**
Incontinence, bowel
Incontinence, functional urinary
Incontinence, overflow urinary
Incontinence, reflex urinary
Incontinence, risk for urge urinary
Incontinence, stress urinary
Incontinence, urge urinary
Infant behavior, disorganized
Infant behavior, readiness for enhanced organized
Infant behavior, risk for disorganized
Injury, risk for corneal
Injury, risk for urinary tract
Insomnia
Intracranial adaptive capacity, decreased
Jaundice, neonatal
Jaundice, risk for neonatal
Latex Allergy response
Liver function, risk for impaired
Mobility, impaired bed
Mobility, impaired physical
Mobility, impaired wheelchair
Nausea
Nutrition: less than body requirements, imbalanced
Obesity
Oral Mucous Membrane, impaired
Oral Mucous Membrane, risk for impaired
Overweight
Overweight, risk for
Pain, acute
Pain, chronic
Pain syndrome, chronic
Pain, labor
Pressure ulcer, risk for
Protection, ineffective
Renal perfusion, risk for ineffective
Self-Care deficit, bathing
Self-Care deficit, dressing
Self-Care deficit, feeding
Self-Care deficit, toileting
Sexual dysfunction
Sexuality pattern, ineffective
Shock, risk for
Sitting, impaired
Skin integrity, impaired
Skin integrity, risk for impaired
Sleep deprivation
Sleep pattern, disturbed
Sleep, readiness for enhanced
Standing, impaired
Surgical recovery, delayed
Surgical recovery, risk for delayed
Swallowing, impaired
Temperature, risk for imbalanced body
Thermoregulation, ineffective
Tissue integrity, impaired
Tissue integrity, risk for impaired
Tissue Perfusion, ineffective peripheral
Tissue Perfusion, risk for ineffective peripheral
Transfer ability, impaired
Urinary elimination, impaired
Urinary elimination, readiness for enhanced
Urinary Retention
Vascular Trauma, risk for
Ventilation, impaired spontaneous
Ventilatory weaning response, dysfunctional
Walking, impaired

SAFETY AND SECURITY NEEDS

Anxiety
Anxiety, death
Autonomic Dysreflexia
Autonomic Dysreflexia, risk for
Communication, impaired verbal
Communication, readiness for enhanced
Confusion, acute
Confusion, chronic
Confusion, risk for acute
Contamination
Contamination, risk for
Contrast Media, risk for adverse reaction to iodinated
Coping, ineffective community
Coping, readiness for enhanced community
Decision-Making, impaired emancipated
Decision-Making, risk for impaired emancipated
Disuse syndrome, risk for
Emotional Control, labile
Falls, risk for
Family processes, dysfunctional
Fear
Frail Elderly syndrome
Frail Elderly syndrome, risk for
Grieving
Grieving, complicated
Grieving, risk for complicated
Growth, risk for disproportionate
Health, deficient community
Health behavior, risk-prone
Health maintenance, ineffective
Health management, ineffective
Health management, ineffective family
Home maintenance, impaired
Identity, risk for disturbed personal
Impulse control, ineffective
Infection, risk for
Injury, risk for
Knowledge, deficient
Knowledge, readiness for enhanced
Latex Allergy response, risk for
Memory, impaired
Mood regulation, impaired
Perioperative Positioning injury, risk for
Peripheral Neurovascular dysfunction, risk for
Poisoning, risk for
Resilience, risk for impaired
Sedentary lifestyle
Self-Neglect
Sorrow, chronic
Sudden Infant Death syndrome, risk for
Suffocation, risk for
Thermal injury, risk for
Trauma, risk for
Unilateral Neglect
Vascular Trauma, risk for
Wandering

LOVE AND BELONGING NEEDS

Anxiety
Attachment, risk for impaired
Caregiver Role Strain
Caregiver Role Strain, risk for
Childbearing process, ineffective
Childbearing process, readiness for enhanced

Childbearing process, risk for ineffective
Coping, compromised family
Coping, disabled family
Coping, readiness for enhanced
Coping, readiness for enhanced family
Family processes, dysfunctional
Family processes, interrupted
Family processes, readiness for enhanced
Grieving
Loneliness, risk for
Maternal–Fetal dyad, risk for disturbed
Moral Distress
Parenting, impaired
Parenting, readiness for enhanced
Parenting, risk for impaired
Relationship, ineffective
Relationship, readiness for enhanced
Relationship, risk for ineffective
Religiosity, impaired
Religiosity, risk for impaired
Relocation stress syndrome
Relocation stress syndrome, risk for
Role conflict, parental
Social interaction, impaired
Social isolation
Sorrow, chronic
Spiritual distress
Spiritual distress, risk for

SELF-ESTEEM NEEDS

Activity planning, ineffective
Activity planning, risk for ineffective
Body Image, disturbed
Coping, defensive
Coping, ineffective
Decision-Making, readiness for enhanced
Decisional Conflict
Denial, ineffective
Diversional activity, deficient
Health behavior, risk-prone
Hope, readiness for enhanced
Hopelessness
Human Dignity, risk for compromised
Identity, disturbed personal
Noncompliance
Post-Trauma syndrome
Post-Trauma syndrome, risk for
Power, readiness for enhanced
Powerlessness
Powerlessness, risk for
Rape-Trauma syndrome
Resilience, impaired
Resilience, risk for impaired
Role performance, ineffective
Self-Esteem, chronic low
Self-Esteem, risk for chronic low
Self-Esteem, risk for situational low
Self-Esteem, situational low
Self-Mutilation
Self-Mutilation, risk for
Social interaction, impaired
Stress overload
Suicide, risk for
Violence, risk for other-directed
Violence, risk for self-directed

SELF-ACTUALIZATION NEEDS

Childbearing process, readiness for enhanced
Decision-Making, readiness for enhanced
Decision-Making, readiness for enhanced emancipated
Development, risk for delayed
Health management, readiness for enhanced
Knowledge, readiness for enhanced
Nutrition, readiness for enhanced
Power, readiness for enhanced
Religiosity, readiness for enhanced
Resilience, readiness for enhanced
Self-Care, readiness for enhanced
Self-Concept, readiness for enhanced
Spiritual well-being, readiness for enhanced

APPENDIX B

Nursing Diagnoses Arranged by Gordon's Functional Health Patterns

Diagnoses currently accepted by NANDA-I (North American Nursing Diagnosis Association—International).

HEALTH-PERCEPTION—HEALTH-MANAGEMENT PATTERN

Ineffective **Airway** clearance
Risk for **Allergy** response
Risk for **Aspiration**
Autonomic Dysreflexia
Risk for **Autonomic Dysreflexia**
Risk for **Bleeding**
Contamination
Risk for **Contamination**
Risk for adverse reaction to iodinated **Contrast Media**
Risk for dry **Eye**
Risk for **Falls**
Frail Elderly syndrome
Risk for **Frail Elderly** syndrome
Deficient community **Health**
Ineffective **Health** maintenance
Ineffective **Health** management
Risk-prone **Health** behavior
Readiness for enhanced **Health** management
Risk for **Infection**
Risk for **Injury**
Risk for corneal **Injury**
Risk for urinary tract **Injury**
Latex Allergy Response
Risk for **Latex Allergy** Response
Noncompliance
Risk for **Perioperative Positioning** injury
Risk for **Poisoning**
Ineffective **Protection**
Self-Neglect
Risk for **Shock**
Impaired **Skin** integrity
Risk for impaired **Skin** integrity
Risk for **Suffocation**
Risk for **Thermal** injury
Impaired **Tissue** integrity
Risk for impaired **Tissue** integrity
Risk for **Trauma**
Risk for **Vascular Trauma**
Impaired spontaneous **Ventilation**
Dysfunctional **Ventilatory** weaning response

NUTRITIONAL-METABOLIC PATTERN

Risk for **Aspiration**
Insufficient **Breast Milk**
Ineffective **Breastfeeding**
Interrupted **Breastfeeding**
Readiness for enhanced **Breastfeeding**
Impaired **Dentition**
Risk for **Electrolyte** imbalance
Ineffective infant **Feeding** pattern
Deficient **Fluid** volume
Excess **Fluid** volume
Readiness for enhanced **Fluid** balance
Risk for deficient **Fluid** volume
Risk for imbalanced **Fluid** volume
Dysfunctional **Gastrointestinal** motility
Risk for dysfunctional **Gastrointestinal** motility
Risk for ineffective **Gastrointestinal** perfusion
Risk for unstable blood **Glucose** level
Hyperthermia
Hypothermia
Risk for **Hypothermia**
Neonatal **Jaundice**
Risk for neonatal **Jaundice**
Latex Allergy response
Risk for impaired **Liver** function
Nausea
Imbalanced **Nutrition:** less than body requirements
Readiness for enhanced **Nutrition**
Obesity
Overweight
Risk for **Overweight**
Impaired **Oral Mucous Membrane**
Risk for **Perioperative Hypothermia**
Risk for **Pressure** ulcer
Impaired **Skin** integrity
Risk for impaired **Skin** integrity
Risk for **Sudden Infant Death** syndrome
Impaired **Swallowing**
Risk for imbalanced body **Temperature**
Ineffective **Thermoregulation**
Impaired **Tissue** integrity
Risk for impaired **Tissue** integrity

ELIMINATION PATTERN

Chronic functional **Constipation**
Perceived **Constipation**
Risk for chronic functional **Constipation**
Diarrhea
Bowel **Incontinence**
Functional urinary **Incontinence**
Overflow urinary **Incontinence**
Reflex urinary **Incontinence**

Risk for urge urinary **Incontinence**
Stress urinary **Incontinence**
Urge urinary **Incontinence**
Risk for ineffective **Renal** perfusion
Impaired **Urinary** elimination
Readiness for enhanced **Urinary** elimination
Urinary Retention

ACTIVITY-EXERCISE PATTERN

Activity intolerance
Risk for **Activity** intolerance
Ineffective **Breathing** pattern
Risk for decreased **Cardiac** tissue perfusion
Decreased **Cardiac** output
Risk for decreased **Cardiac** output
Risk for impaired **Cardiovascular** function
Risk for delayed **Development**
Risk for **Disuse** syndrome
Deficient **Diversional** activity
Fatigue
Impaired **Gas** exchange
Risk for disproportionate **Growth**
Impaired **Home** maintenance
Disorganized **Infant** behavior
Readiness for enhanced organized **Infant** behavior
Risk for disorganized **Infant** behavior
Impaired bed **Mobility**
Impaired physical **Mobility**
Impaired wheelchair **Mobility**
Risk for **Peripheral Neurovascular** dysfunction
Sedentary lifestyle
Bathing **Self-Care** deficit
Dressing **Self-Care** deficit
Feeding **Self-Care** deficit
Readiness for enhanced **Self-Care**
Toileting **Self-Care** deficit
Impaired **Sitting**
Impaired **Standing**
Delayed **Surgical** recovery
Risk for delayed **Surgical** recovery
Ineffective peripheral **Tissue Perfusion**
Risk for ineffective peripheral **Tissue Perfusion**
Impaired **Transfer** ability
Unilateral Neglect
Risk for **Unilateral Neglect**
Impaired **Walking**
Wandering

SLEEP-REST PATTERN

Insomnia
Disturbed **Sleep** pattern
Readiness for enhanced **Sleep**
Sleep deprivation

COGNITIVE-PERCEPTUAL PATTERN

Ineffective **Activity** planning
Risk for ineffective **Activity** planning
Risk for ineffective **Cerebral** tissue perfusion
Impaired **Comfort**
Readiness for enhanced **Comfort**
Acute **Confusion**
Chronic **Confusion**
Risk for acute **Confusion**
Readiness for enhanced **Decision-Making**
Decisional Conflict
Labile **Emotional Control**
Ineffective **Impulse** control
Decreased **Intracranial** adaptive capacity
Deficient **Knowledge**
Readiness for enhanced **Knowledge**
Impaired **Memory**
Acute **Pain**
Chronic **Pain**
Chronic **Pain** syndrome
Labor **Pain**
Unilateral Neglect

SELF-PERCEPTION—SELF-CONCEPT PATTERN

Anxiety
Death **Anxiety**
Disturbed **Body Image**
Fear
Readiness for enhanced **Hope**
Hopelessness
Risk for compromised **Human Dignity**
Disturbed personal **Identity**
Risk for disturbed personal **Identity**
Risk for **Loneliness**
Readiness for enhanced **Power**
Powerlessness
Risk for **Powerlessness**
Readiness for enhanced **Self-Concept**
Chronic low **Self-Esteem**
Risk for chronic low **Self-Esteem**
Situational low **Self-Esteem**
Risk for situational low **Self-Esteem**
Risk for self-directed **Violence**

ROLE-RELATIONSHIP PATTERN

Risk for impaired **Attachment**
Caregiver Role Strain
Risk for **Caregiver Role Strain**
Impaired verbal **Communication**

Readiness for enhanced **Communication**
Dysfunctional **Family** processes
Ineffective Family **Health** management
Interrupted **Family** processes
Readiness for enhanced **Family** processes
Grieving
Complicated **Grieving**
Risk for complicated **Grieving**
Risk for disturbed **Maternal–Fetal** dyad
Impaired **Parenting**
Readiness for enhanced **Parenting**
Risk for impaired **Parenting**
Ineffective **Relationship**
Risk for ineffective **Relationship**
Readiness for enhanced **Relationship**
Ineffective **Role** performance
Parental **Role** conflict
Impaired **Social** interaction
Social isolation
Chronic **Sorrow**

SEXUALITY-REPRODUCTIVE PATTERN

Ineffective **Childbearing** process
Readiness for enhanced **Childbearing** process
Risk for ineffective **Childbearing** process
Risk for disturbed **Maternal–Fetal** dyad
Sexual dysfunction
Ineffective **Sexuality** pattern

COPING—STRESS-TOLERANCE PATTERN

Compromised family **Coping**
Defensive **Coping**
Disabled family **Coping**
Ineffective community **Coping**
Ineffective **Coping**
Readiness for enhanced community **Coping**
Readiness for enhanced **Coping**
Readiness for enhanced family **Coping**
Ineffective **Denial**
Risk-prone **Health** behavior
Impaired **Mood** regulation
Post-Trauma syndrome
Risk for **Post-Trauma** syndrome
Rape-Trauma syndrome
Relocation stress syndrome
Risk for **Relocation** stress syndrome
Impaired **Resilience**
Readiness for enhanced **Resilience**
Risk for impaired **Resilience**
Self-Mutilation
Risk for **Self-Mutilation**
Stress overload
Risk for **Suicide**
Risk for other-directed **Violence**

VALUE-BELIEF PATTERN

Impaired emancipated **Decision-Making**
Readiness for enhanced emancipated **Decision-Making**
Risk for impaired emancipated **Decision-Making**
Moral Distress
Impaired **Religiosity**
Readiness for enhanced **Religiosity**
Risk for impaired **Religiosity**
Spiritual distress
Risk for **Spiritual** distress
Readiness for enhanced **Spiritual** well-being

APPENDIX C

Motivational Interviewing for Nurses

Mary P. Mancuso, MA

Motivational interviewing (MI) is an evidenced-based interpersonal style used with individuals who would benefit from changes in their behaviors. Nurses may find this approach helpful in guiding clients toward making positive lifestyle changes and adhering to recommended treatment regimens. Unlike other aspects of nursing, MI does not involve *directing* clients to engage in certain behaviors. Rather, it involves *guiding* clients to take steps toward making a behavioral change through collaboration, support, and inspiration (Miller & Rollnick, 2013).

The origins of MI are in the field of psychology, but this technique has been applied in a variety of settings including health care. A recent systematic review and meta-analysis found MI to be effective in helping clients make a number of behavioral changes leading to positive health outcomes including body weight, cholesterol level, blood pressure, reduction in alcohol consumption, smoking cessation, and lowering HIV viral load (Lundahl et al, 2013). These studies took place in medical care settings and involved brief consultations with a variety of clients with different characteristics demonstrating that MI can be a successful approach for health care providers working with clients. Further evidence is being compiled, but single studies demonstrate promising findings that MI can be effective in helping clients adhere to treatment regimens, particularly clients with chronic disease (Moral et al, 2015).

As individuals begin to take steps toward making a behavioral change, they often experience ambivalence; individuals both want to change and do not want to change at the same time. Clients may express agreement about the benefits of changing *(change talk)* as well as argue against making a change *(sustain talk)* (Miller & Rollnick, 2013). The central concept of MI is an approach to communication that motivates the client to change by resolving ambivalence and unresolved feelings. The nurse who uses MI does not directly confront the client's ambivalence or resort to using methods that try to coerce the client into changing behaviors. Rather, the nurse recognizes the client's autonomy and understands that clients will only make a change when they are ready. Ideally, the client will voice his/her own reasons to change; if the nurse provides the client with reasons to change (e.g., "You will be more healthy if you exercise more"), the client may argue against it. People are more convinced to change when they formulate their own arguments (Miller & Rollnick, 2013).

At the heart of MI are four interrelated elements: collaboration, acceptance, compassion, and evocation. The nurse and client collaborate to move toward change; the nurse accepts where the client is in the process of change, feels and demonstrates compassion for the client, and helps call forth change from within the client himself (Miller & Rollnick, 2013). The nurse, over time, helps the client focus on the hope of success in making a change as well as recognizing and using the resources the client already has supporting change (Csillik, 2015). Four principles of MI help the nurse accomplish collaboration with the client to achieve positive change: (1) expressing empathy, (2) supporting self-efficacy, (3) allowing for resistance, and (4) developing discrepancy. Expressing empathy involves reflecting what the client is feeling and experiencing. Supporting self-efficacy encompasses the understanding that clients are the experts on their own lives and facilitating hope for change. Allowing for resistance involves seeking to understand the client while not arguing for change or offering solutions for change. Developing discrepancy entails cultivating the client's perception of the gap between current behaviors and the values he/she holds deeply (Miller & Rollnick, 2013).

Case example: A female client is admitted to an inpatient unit; she is experiencing multiple medical conditions secondary to obesity. Her provider has ordered a low-calorie diet while she is in the hospital. The client makes angry comments during meal times and refuses to adhere to the diet, asking friends and family to sneak in prohibited snacks. Nurses not educated about MI may use logical expressions when communicating with this client. An example of this approach would be, "Eating foods high in calories will increase your risk for continued weight gain, resulting in further medical problems." In contrast, MI requires that a therapeutic rapport be established between the nurse and the client and that logical expressions that confront the client be avoided. The nurse using MI uses empathy statements, expressing an understanding of the client's ambivalence, for example, "You are frustrated about being on a low-calorie diet." Establishing rapport facilitates trust in the nurse-client relationship and allows for future collaboration.

After developing a collaborative relationship, the nurse uses the process of evocation to expose the client's own thoughts and ideas. The client may exhibit varying levels of resistance to change. During these periods, the nurse must not confront the resistance; rather, the nurse should allow the client to express himself or herself freely. Allowing for this resistance prevents a power struggle between the nurse and the client. The client may say, "I know I'm fat and unhealthy. I see myself in the mirror every day, but that doesn't mean I need to be on a diet." Instead of presenting the low-calorie diet as the recommended strategy, the nurse reflects back the client's statements and encourages his or her own ideas for change (e.g., "It sounds like being overweight frustrates you; what are some weight loss strategies that might work for you?"). Although not all of the client's suggestions may be appropriate, recognizing the client's own motivation for change by using reflective listening is important. The nurse must refrain from instructing the client, using persuasion, or minimizing feelings by saying, for example, "You just have to try the diet; it won't be that bad." During this phase of MI, the nurse continues with open-ended statements and positive affirmations in an attempt to get the client to recognize the need for a change: "I am impressed that you realize it takes a lot of work to get healthy; tell me how that makes you feel."

Last, when MI is consistently used, the client begins to examine discrepancies between his or her future goals and his or her current patterns of behavior. During this phase of MI, the nurse uses the technique of exploration and clarification in an attempt to get the client to recognize the need for a change. "In what ways do you feel like being overweight affects your health?" As the client begins to expose discrepancies between his or her current behavior and future goals, the impetus for change will emerge. The nurse then provides positive affirmations to empower the client to make changes: "You seem very determined to get healthy. I think your plan is definitely achievable."

When the client begins to make statements that express the intent to change, the nurse uses an MI summary to reinforce what has been discussed. The summary communicates a mutual interest and understanding of the significant elements that were addressed. This summary serves as a platform to move the client toward implementing change and typically reveals the client's ambivalence, discrepancy, and self-empowerment; however, it is up to the nurse to recognize what aspects should be included to encourage the client to move forward. An example summary statement is, "You get frustrated and sad about being overweight but realize that change is a hard thing. You have decided to increase your exercise once a week to help you get healthier. You have made changes like that in the past with much success. Your plan is very doable and a step in the right direction."

Motivating clients to make behavioral changes is an important nursing task and requires diligence and patience. Motivational Interviewing is a fluid method that does not always follow a direct formula, so it is essential for nurses to be flexible and allow the principles of MI to evolve differently, depending on the individual and the situation.

HELPFUL WEBSITES

www.motivationalinterviewing.org
www.motivationalinterview.net
www.nrepp.samhsa.gov/MotivationalInterviewing.aspx
www.2sft.com/resources.php
www.healthsciences.org/Motivational-Interviewing-Health-Coach-Training
www.gp-training.net/training/communication_skills/consultation/motivational_interviewing.htm
www.recoverytoday.net/archive/19-june/45-motivational-interviewing-listening-for-change-talk
www.adultmeducation.com/FacilitatingBehaviorChange_2.html

BIBLIOGRAPHY

Anstiss, T. (2009). Motivational interviewing in primary care. *Journal of Clinical Psychology in Medical Settings, 16*(1), 87–93.

Brobeck, E., Bergh, H., Odencrants, S., et al. (2011). Primary healthcare nurses' experiences with motivational interviewing in health promotion practice. *Journal of Clinical Nursing, 20*(23–24), 3322–3330.

Csillik, A. (2015). Positive motivational interviewing: activating clients' strengths and intrinsic motivation to change. *Journal of Contemporary Psychotherapy, 45*, 119–128.

Levensky, E. R., Forcehimes, A., O'Donahue, W. T., et al. (2007). Motivational interviewing: an evidence-based approach to counseling helps patients follow treatment recommendations. *The American Journal of Nursing, 107*(10), 50–58.

Lundahl, B., Moleni, T., Lurke, B. L., et al. (2013). Motivational interviewing in medical care settings: a systematic review and meta-analysis of randomized controlled trials. *Patient Education and Counseling, 93*, 157–168.

Mesters, I. (2009). Motivational interviewing: hype or hope? *Chronic Illness, 5*(1), 3–6.

Miller, W. R., & Rollnick, S. (2013). *Motivational interviewing: helping people change* (3rd ed.). New York, NY: Guilford Press.

Miller, W. R., & Rollnick, S. (2009). Ten things that motivational interviewing is not. *Behavioural and Cognitive Psychotherapy, 37*(2), 129–140.

Moral, R. R., Torres, L. A., Ortega, L. P., et al. (2015). Effectiveness of motivational interviewing to improve therapeutic adherence in patients over 65 years old with chronic diseases: a cluster randomized clinical trial in primary care. *Patient Education and Counseling, 98*, 977–983.

APPENDIX D

Wellness-Oriented Diagnostic Categories

This is a list of NANDA-I diagnoses in a wellness format. When available, readiness diagnoses are listed first in each category. Risk diagnoses are listed next. The goal is to support wellness, prevent illness, and intervene when illness is present.

Diagnoses are arranged first by priority according to the ABCs (airway, breathing, circulation). They are then arranged according to possible priority physiological needs and then psychosocial needs. Diagnoses dealing with family, infant, and child are grouped together. It is the responsibility of the nurse to individualize and reorder based on the client's assessment data.

This list refers to adult care plans. Asterisked diagnoses have pediatric interventions in the care plans.

PHYSIOLOGICAL

Airway/Breathing

- Risk for **Aspiration**
- Risk for **Suffocation**
- Impaired **Swallowing**
- Ineffective **Airway** clearance
- Ineffective **Breathing** pattern
- Impaired **Gas** exchange
- Impaired spontaneous **Ventilation**
- Dysfunctional **Ventilatory** weaning response

Circulation

- Risk for **Bleeding**
- Risk for decreased **Cardiac** output
- Risk for impaired **Cardiovascular** function
- Risk for decreased **Cardiac** tissue perfusion
- Risk for ineffective **Cerebral** tissue perfusion
- Risk for ineffective **Gastrointestinal** tissue perfusion
- Risk for **Peripheral Neurovascular** dysfunction
- Risk for ineffective **Renal** perfusion
- Risk for **Shock**
- Decreased **Cardiac** output
- Ineffective peripheral **Tissue Perfusion**

COGNITION/SENSORY PERCEPTION

- Risk for acute **Confusion**
- Risk for **Autonomic Dysreflexia**
- Ineffective **Activity** planning
- **Autonomic Dysreflexia**
- Decreased **Intracranial** adaptive capacity
- Acute **Confusion**
- Chronic **Confusion**
- Impaired **Memory**

INJURY: FALLS/ INFECTION/POISONING/ TRAUMA

- Readiness for Enhanced **Health** management
- Risk for **Contamination**
- Risk for corneal **Injury**
- Risk for **Falls**
- Risk for **Injury***
- Risk for **Infection***
- Risk for **Latex Allergy** response
- Risk for **Perioperative Positioning** injury
- Risk for **Poisoning***
- Risk for delayed **Surgical** recovery
- Risk for **Trauma**
- Risk for urinary tract **Injury**
- Risk for **Vascular Trauma***
- Acute **Pain*** (psychosocial)
- Chronic **Pain*** (psychosocial)
- **Contamination**
- Delayed **Surgical** recovery
- Ineffective **Protection**
- **Latex Allergy** response
- **Rape-Trauma** syndrome

HOMEOSTASIS

- Risk for **Hypothermia**
- Risk for impaired **Liver** function
- Risk for unstable blood **Glucose** level
- Risk for imbalanced body **Temperature***
- Risk for **Electrolyte** imbalance
- Risk for **Perioperative Hypothermia**
- **Hyperthermia**
- **Hypothermia***
- Ineffective **Thermoregulation**

FLUID/NUTRITION/ GASTROINTESTINAL/ ORAL/DENTAL MANAGEMENT

- Readiness for enhanced **Fluid** balance
- Readiness for enhanced **Nutrition**
- Risk for dysfunctional **Gastrointestinal** motility
- Risk for **Overweight**
- Risk for impaired **Oral Mucous Membrane**
- Risk for imbalanced **Fluid** volume
- Risk for deficient **Fluid** volume
- Dysfunctional **Gastrointestinal** motility
- **Nausea**
- Imbalanced **Nutrition**: less than body requirements
- Deficient **Fluid** volume*
- Excess **Fluid** volume
- **Obesity**
- **Overweight**
- Impaired **Oral Mucous Membrane**
- Impaired **Dentition**

ELIMINATION

Urinary Elimination

- Readiness for enhanced **Urinary** elimination

- Impaired **Urinary** elimination
- **Urinary Retention**

INCONTINENCE, BOWEL

- Bowel **Incontinence**

INCONTINENCE, BLADDER

- Risk for urge urinary **Incontinence**
- Functional urinary **Incontinence**
- Overflow urinary **Incontinence**
- Reflex urinary **Incontinence**
- Stress urinary **Incontinence**
- Urge urinary **Incontinence**

BOWEL ELIMINATION

Constipation

- Risk for chronic functional **Constipation**
- Risk for **Constipation**
- Perceived **Constipation**
- Chronic functional **Constipation**
- **Constipation**

Diarrhea

- Diarrhea*

ACTIVITY/MOVEMENT/ SELF-CARE

- Readiness for enhanced **Self-Care**
- Risk for **Activity** intolerance
- Risk for **Disuse** syndrome
- **Sedentary** lifestyle*
- Deficient **Diversional** activity*
- **Activity** intolerance
- **Fatigue**
- Impaired physical **Mobility**
- Bathing **Self-Care** deficit
- Dressing **Self-Care** deficit
- Feeding **Self-Care** deficit
- Toileting **Self-Care** deficit
- **Self-Neglect**
- Impaired **Sitting**
- Impaired **Standing**
- Impaired **Walking**
- Impaired **Transfer** ability
- Impaired bed **Mobility**
- Impaired wheelchair **Mobility**
- **Unilateral Neglect**
- **Wandering**

SKIN/TISSUE

- Risk for **Pressure** ulcer
- Risk for impaired **Skin** integrity
- Risk for impaired **Tissue** integrity
- Impaired **Skin** integrity
- Impaired **Tissue** integrity

SLEEP

- Readiness for enhanced **Sleep**
- Disturbed **Sleep** pattern
- **Insomnia**
- **Sleep** deprivation

PSYCHOSOCIAL

Comfort

- Readiness for enhanced **Comfort**
- Impaired **Comfort**
- Acute **Pain*** (physiological)
- Chronic **Pain*** (physiological)
- Chronic **Pain** syndrome
- Labor **Pain**

COMMUNICATION/ HEALTHY BEHAVIORS/ THERAPEUTIC REGIMEN/ KNOWLEDGE

Individual

- Readiness for enhanced **Communication***
- Readiness for enhanced **Health** management
- Readiness for enhanced **Knowledge***
- Risk-prone **Health** behavior
- Impaired verbal **Communication***
- Ineffective **Health** management
- Deficient **Knowledge***
- Ineffective **Health** maintenance

Family

- Ineffective Family **Health** management

SPIRITUALITY/ RELIGIOUS BELIEFS

- Readiness for enhanced **Spiritual** well-being
- Readiness for enhanced **Religiosity***
- Readiness for enhanced **Hope**
- Risk for **Spiritual** distress
- Risk for impaired **Religiosity**
- Impaired **Religiosity**
- **Spiritual** distress
- **Hopelessness**

HARM: SELF AND OTHERS

- Risk for **Suicide**
- Risk for **Self-Mutilation**
- Risk for other-directed **Violence**
- Risk for self-directed **Violence**
- **Self-Mutilation**

ANXIETY/STRESS

- Readiness for enhanced **Decision-Making**
- Risk for **Relocation** stress syndrome
- Risk for compromised **Human Dignity**
- **Anxiety**
- Death **Anxiety**
- Ineffective **Denial**
- **Decisional Conflict**
- Dysfunctional **Family** processes*
- **Fear***
- **Noncompliance**
- **Relocation** stress syndrome*
- **Stress** overload

COPING

Individual

- Readiness for enhanced **Coping***
- Readiness for enhanced emancipated **Decision-Making**
- Readiness for enhanced **Power**
- Readiness for enhanced **Resilience**
- Risk for impaired emancipated **Decision-Making**
- Risk for **Caregiver Role Strain**
- Risk for impaired **Resilience**
- Risk for **Powerlessness**

- Risk for **Loneliness***
- Risk for **Post-Trauma** syndrome*
- Ineffective **Activity** planning
- Defensive **Coping**
- Ineffective **Coping**
- **Caregiver Role Strain**
- Impaired emancipated **Decision-Making**
- Labile **Emotional Control**
- Impaired **Mood** regulation
- Impaired **Resilience**
- Impaired **Social** interaction
- **Post-Trauma** syndrome
- **Powerlessness**
- Ineffective **Role** performance*
- **Social** isolation

Community

- Readiness for enhanced community **Coping**
- Ineffective community **Coping**

SEXUALITY/BODY IMAGE

- Disturbed **Body Image**
- **Sexual** dysfunction
- Ineffective **Sexuality** pattern*

GRIEF/SORROW

- Risk for complicated **Grieving***
- **Grieving***
- Complicated **Grieving***
- Chronic **Sorrow**

SELF-CONCEPT/SELF-ESTEEM/PERSONAL IDENTITY

- Readiness for enhanced **Self-Concept***
- Risk for situational low **Self-Esteem**
- Disturbed personal **Identity**
- Situational low **Self-Esteem**
- Chronic low **Self-Esteem**

ELDERLY

- Risk for **Frail Elderly** syndrome
- **Frail Elderly** syndrome

FAMILY/INFANT/CHILD

Sudden Infant Death

- Risk for **Sudden Infant Death** syndrome

Development/Growth

- Risk for delayed **Development**
- Risk for disproportionate **Growth**

Neonate

- Neonatal **Jaundice**

Infant Care

- Readiness for enhanced organized **Infant** behavior
- Risk for disorganized **Infant** behavior
- Risk for impaired **Attachment**
- Disorganized **Infant** behavior
- Ineffective infant **Feeding** pattern

Parenting

- Readiness for enhanced **Parenting**
- Risk for impaired **Parenting**
- Impaired **Parenting**
- Parental **Role** conflict

Breastfeeding

- Readiness for enhanced **Breastfeeding**
- Interrupted **Breastfeeding**
- Ineffective **Breastfeeding**

Coping/Family

- Readiness for enhanced family **Coping**
- Readiness for enhanced **Relationship**
- Risk for disturbed **Maternal–Fetal** dyad
- Compromised family **Coping**
- Disabled family **Coping**
- Ineffective Family **Health** management

Family Processes

- Readiness for enhanced **Childbearing** process
- Readiness for enhanced **Family** processes
- Interrupted **Family** processes
- Dysfunctional **Family** processes

APPENDIX E

Nursing Care Plans for Hearing Loss and Vision Loss

Hearing Loss

Betty J. Ackley, MSN, EdS, RN, and Mary Beth Flynn Makic, PhD, RN, CNS, CCNS, FAAN

NANDA-I

Definition

A condition where there is the inability to detect some or all frequencies of sound and may involve complete or partial impairment of the ability to hear.

NOTE: **Hearing Loss** is not a NANDA-I accepted diagnosis, but is included here because of the frequency of occurrence of hearing loss, especially in the geriatric population.

Defining Characteristics

Inability to hear in noisy environments, difficulty following conversations with more than one person, change in speech, change in usual response to stimuli; disorientation; impaired communication; irritability; poor concentration; restlessness; sensory distortions

Related Factors (r/t)

Altered sensory integration; altered sensory reception; altered sensory transmission; biochemical imbalance; electrolyte imbalance; excessive noise exposure; psychological stress

NOC (Nursing Outcomes Classification)

Suggested NOC Outcomes (Auditory)

Cognitive Orientation; Communication: Receptive; Distorted Thought Self-Control; Hearing Compensation Behavior

Example NOC Outcome with Indicators

Hearing Compensation Behavior as evidenced by the following indicators: Monitors symptoms of hearing deterioration/Positions self to advantage hearing/Reminds others to use techniques that advantage hearing/Eliminates background noise/Uses sign language/Uses lip reading/Uses closed captioning for television viewing/Uses hearing assistive devices/Uses hearing aid(s) correctly. (Rate the outcome and indicators of **Hearing Compensation Behavior:** 1 = never demonstrated, 2 = rarely demonstrated, 3 = sometimes demonstrated, 4 = often demonstrated, 5 = consistently demonstrated [see Section I].)

Client Outcomes

Client Will (Specify Time Frame)

- Demonstrate understanding by a verbal, written, or signed response
- Demonstrate relaxed body movements and facial expressions
- Explain plan to modify lifestyle to accommodate hearing impairment
- Demonstrate familiarity with hearing assistive devices

NIC (Nursing Interventions Classification)

Suggested NIC Interventions

Cognitive Stimulation; Communication Enhancement: Hearing Deficit, Visual Deficit; Environmental Management

Example NIC Activities—Communication Enhancement: Visual Deficit

Identify yourself when you enter the client's space; Build on client's remaining vision, as appropriate

Nursing Interventions and *Rationales*

- Observe for signs of a hearing loss, especially in people exposed to loud noise and people older than 60 years of age. *Signs include the following: miscommunication, difficulty understanding words in a noisy environment or when in a crowd of people, frequently asking others to speak more slowly, clearly, or loudly, listening to the television or radio at a loud volume, withdrawal from conversations, and social isolation (Mayo Clinic, 2014).*
- Use the National Institutes of Health (NIH) Toolbox to test hearing as available. *The toolbox is an automated procedure that allows nonspecialists to administer the hearing test reliably. In addition, conductive hearing loss can be differentiated from sensorineural loss, the ability to hear in a noisy environment is tested, and the effects of a hearing loss on the emotional and social life of a hearing impaired person can be determined (Zecker et al, 2013).*
- Recognize that certain populations are especially vulnerable to noise-induced hearing loss, including farmers, industrial workers, firefighters, construction workers, musicians, and music lovers using personal listening devices.

▲ Refer to otolaryngologist and/or audiologist. *Conductive hearing loss can be ameliorated by treatment such as removal of ear wax or surgical treatment for hearing disorders. Sensorineural hearing loss is generally permanent; hearing aids can be helpful (Baloh & Jen, 2011).*

- Keep background noise to a minimum. Turn off the television and radio when communicating with the client. If in a noisy environment, take the client to a private room and shut the door. *Background noise significantly interferes with hearing in the hearing impaired client (Harkin & Kelleher, 2011).*
- Stand or sit directly in front of the client when communicating. Make sure adequate light is on the nurse's face, avoid chewing gum or covering mouth or face with hands while speaking, establish eye contact, and use nonverbal gestures. *Clients with hearing impairment read lips and also interpret nonverbal communication, which is a significant part of communication. To increase communication, it is important that the client be able to clearly see the face of the person speaking (Harkin & Kelleher, 2011; Spyridakou, 2012).*
- Speak clearly in lower voice tones if possible. Do not overenunciate or shout at the client. *In many kinds of hearing loss, clients lose the ability to hear higher-pitched tones but can still hear lower-pitched tones. Overenunciating makes it difficult to read lips. Shouting makes the words less clear and is seen as aggressive (Harkin & Kelleher, 2011; Spyridakou, 2012).*
- Verify that the client understands critical information by asking the client to repeat the information. *Hearing impaired clients will often smile or nod when asked if they understand to avoid embarrassment; asking them to repeat the information is the best way to verify they understand what is being said.*
- If necessary, provide a communication board, personnel who know sign language, or any method helpful to increase understanding for the hearing impaired client. *Health care institutions are required to provide and pay for qualified interpreters under the Americans with Disabilities Act.*
- Prepare pictures or diagrams depicting tests or procedures; have books with relevant pictures available for more detailed discussions. *The use of visual aids can improve communication when hearing is impaired.*
- Watch for signs of depression such as withdrawal, impaired sleep, flat affect, and refer for treatment if needed. **EB:** *A large study found that hearing loss was significantly associated with depression, especially in women (Li et al, 2014).*
- Encourage the client to wear a hearing aid if available. **EB:** *A study demonstrated that use of a hearing aid was associated with a reduced chance of developing a major depressive disorder in older adults (Mener et al, 2013).*
- Recognize that clients with a hearing aid may choose to wear a hearing aid intermittently because hearing aids can create distortion of speech and extraneous noise that is bothersome (Shah & Lotke, 2013).

Critical Care

- Develop a communication cart to foster communication with hearing impaired clients. Contents can include spiral notebooks, felt tip markers, clipboards, communication boards (picture, word, whole phrases, alphabet), hearing aid batteries, and electronic speech generators.
- Develop good communication skills to interact with hearing impaired clients. It is unfair to expect critically ill older adults to understand what is being said to them only through auditory means. **EBN:** *A study of nurses receiving training in basic communication skills found them to be helpful, but also found advanced communication skills utilizing electronic speech generating devices time consuming (Radtke et al, 2012).*

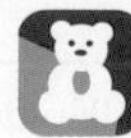

Pediatric

- ▲ Refer infants or children for hearing tests as indicated so that treatment/therapy begins early as needed. *Early treatment of a hearing loss can decrease the effects of a hearing loss on social, emotional, and academic development of a child (Shah & Lotke, 2013).*
- In the child, recommend parents watch for signs of hearing loss including worsening speech or school performance, withdrawal from social activities, playing alone, and playing the television and music increasingly louder (Shah & Lotke, 2013).
- Refer the child to the use of a language wizard player with Baldi, a computer-animated tutor for teaching vocabulary. CEB: *A study demonstrated that use of the computer system resulted in excellent retention of learned words 4 weeks after the end of the experiment (Massaro & Light, 2004).*
- Recognize that children who are deaf or hard of hearing are particularly vulnerable to abuse, both by parents/caregivers and by sexual predators. *Parental abuse may be caused by frustration dealing with the child; sexual abuse may be associated with increased isolation of the child and decreased ability to report abuse to others* (Shah & Lotke, 2013).
- Recommend that teenagers avoid use of personal listening devices, or try to keep the volume down. Use culturally appropriate teaching materials. *There is an increased rate of hearing loss in teenagers 12 to 19 years of age (Shah & Lakte, 2013).* EB: *A study found that more than half of young people using personal listening devices had the volume at a level that could damage hearing. In addition, African American participants listened to music at the highest volume (Fligor et al, 2014).*

Geriatric

- ▲ Routinely screen geriatric clients for presence of hearing loss because up to two thirds of all people 70 or older have a hearing loss (Bainbridge & Wallhagen, 2014).
- ▲ Inspect the ear canal for wax buildup in the ears. *Older adults have drier wax and slower than normal movement of skin and debris out of the ear. Ear hairs at the entrance can sometimes block the movement of wax out of the ear (Harkin & Kelleher, 2011).* EB: *Removal of wax from the ear was found to significantly improve the well-being of older clients (Oron et al, 2011).*
- Work with the client to ensure contact with others and maintenance of meaningful activities to strengthen the social network and maintain cognitive abilities. EB: *A large observational study found that hearing loss predicted loss of cognition in older adults (Lin et al, 2013).*

Home Care

- The previously listed interventions are applicable in the home care setting.
- Recommend that the client change the home environment if needed for better acoustics. Avoid glossy walls, high and reflective ceilings, reflective glass counters, and tiled floors. Use acoustic paneling if needed. *The goal is to reduce noise reverberating off the walls, floors, and surfaces of the home.*
- Suggest installation of devices such as strobe lights for the telephone, alarm clock, fire alarms, and doorbell; sensors that detect an infant's cry; alarm clocks that vibrate the bed; and closed caption decoders for television sets. Other helpful devices include telephone amplifiers, speakerphones, cell phones with text messaging or instant messaging, pocket talker personal listening systems, and FM and infrared amplification systems that connect directly to a TV or audio output jack. Also available is a telecommunication device, a typewriter keyboard with an alphanumeric display that allows the hearing impaired person to send typed messages over the telephone line. Use of hearing ear dogs (dogs specially trained to alert their owners to specific sounds) may also be helpful. *These methods can be helpful to increase communication and safety for the hearing impaired client (Shah & Lotke, 2013).*

Client/Family Teaching and Discharge Planning

- Teach client to avoid excessive noise at work or at home and to wear hearing protection when necessary. *Any noise that hurts the ears or is above 90 decibels is excessive. Sources of noise that can cause hearing loss include motorcycles, firecrackers, and small firearms, all emitting sounds from 120 to 150 decibels. Long or repeated exposure to sounds at or above 85 decibels can cause hearing loss; music, lawnmowers, leaf blowers, and shop tools may contribute to hearing loss (NIH, 2011).*
- Teach the client to avoid inserting objects such as cotton-tipped swabs or bobby pins into the ears. *The ear is self cleaning, and using devices can interfere with the process and also damage the ear structures (Harkin & Kelleher, 2011).*

REFERENCES

Bainbridge, K. E., & Wallhagen, M. I. (2014). Hearing loss in an aging American population: extent, impact and management. *Annual Review of Public Health*, *35*, 139–152.

Baloh, R. W., & Jen, J. (2011). Hearing and equilibrium. In L. Goldman & A. Schafer (Eds.), *Goldman's cecil medicine* (24th ed.). Philadelphia: Saunders Elsevier.

Fligor, B. J., Levey, S., & Levey, T. (2014). Cultural and demographic factors influencing noise exposure estimates from use of portable listening devices in an urban environment. *Journal of Speech, Language, and Hearing Research*.

Harkin, H., & Kelleher, C. (2011). Caring for older adults with hearing loss. *Nursing Older People*, *23*(9), 22–28.

Li, C. M., et al. (2014). Hearing impairment associated with depression in US adults, national health and nutrition examination survey 2005–2010. *JAMA Otolaryngol Head Neck Surg*, *140*(4), 293–302.

Lin, F. R., et al. (2013). Hearing loss and cognitive decline in older adults. *JAMA Intern Med*, *173*(4), 293–299.

Massaro, D. W., & Light, J. (2004). Improving the vocabulary of children with hearing loss. *Volta Rev*, *104*(3), 141.

Mayo Clinic. (2014). *Hearing Loss*. Retrieved from: <http://www.mayoclinic.org/diseases-conditions/hearing-loss/basics/coping-support/con-20027684>.

Mener, D. J. (2013). Hearing loss and depression in older adults. *Journal of the American Geriatrics Society*, *61*(9), 1627–1629.

National Institutes of Health (NIH). (2011). *Interactive Sound Ruler: How Loud is Too Loud?* Retrieved from: <http://www.nidcd.nih.gov/health/hearing/pages/sound-ruler.aspx>.

Oron, Y., et al. (2011). Cerumen removal: comparison of cerumenolytic agents and effect on cognition among the elderly. *Archives of Gerontology and Geriatrics*, *52*(2), 228–232.

Radtke, V., Tate, J., & Happ, M. B. (2012). Nurses' perceptions of communication training in the ICU. *Intensive and Critical Care Nursing*, *28*(1), 16–25.

Shah, R., & Lotke, M. (2013). *Hearing impairment*. Medscape, Retrieved from: <http://emedicine.medscape.com/article/994159-overview#a0199>.

Spyridakou, C. (2012). Hearing loss: a health problem for all ages. *Primary Health Care*, *22*(4), 16–20.

Zecker, S. G., Hoffman, H. J., Frisina, R., et al. (2013). Audition assessment using the NIH Toolbox. *Neurology*, *80*(11 Suppl. 3), S45–S48.

Vision Loss

Michelle Acorn, DNP, NP PHC-Adult, BA, BScN/PHCNP, MN/ACNP, ENC(C), GNC(C), CAP, CGP, and Betty J. Ackley, MSN, EdS, RN

Definition

Decreased or absence of vision when it existed previously; vision loss can be either acute in onset or occur as a slow progressive chronic visual loss

NOTE: This is not a NANDA-I nursing diagnosis. The authors have identified this health problem because vision loss is commonly seen in nursing practice.

Defining Characteristics

Change in behavior pattern; change in problem-solving abilities; disorientation; decreased visual acuity; loss of vision; visual hallucinations

Related Factors

Aging; diabetes mellitus; exposure to UV light; impaired visual function; impaired visual integration; impaired visual reception; impaired visual transmission; nutritional deficiency

(Adapted from the work of NANDA-I)

NOC (Nursing Outcomes Classification)

Suggested NOC Outcomes (Visual)

Sensory Function: Vision; Vision Compensation Behavior

Example NOC Outcome with Indicators

Vision Compensation Behavior as evidenced by the following indicators: Uses adequate light for activity being performed/Wears eyeglasses correctly/Uses vision assistive devices/Uses computer assistive devices/Uses support services for low vision. (Rate each indicator of **Vision Compensation Behavior:** 1 = never demonstrated, 2 = rarely demonstrated, 3 = sometimes demonstrated, 4 = often demonstrated, 5 = consistently demonstrated [see Section I].)

Client Outcomes

Client Will (Specify Time Frame)

- Demonstrate relaxed body movements and facial expressions
- Remain as independent as possible

- Explain plan to modify lifestyle to accommodate visual impairment
- Incorporate use of lighting to maximize visual abilities
- Demonstrate familiarity with vision assistive devices
- Remain free of physical harm resulting from loss of vision

NIC (Nursing Interventions Classification)

Suggested NIC Interventions

Cognitive Stimulation; Visual Deficit; Environmental Management

Example NIC Activities—Communication Enhancement: Visual Deficit

Identify yourself when you enter the client's space; Build on client's remaining vision, as appropriate

Nursing Interventions and *Rationales*

- Identify yourself immediately whenever you enter the client's area. *Effective communication assists in the development of trust and decreases fear (Lawrence, 2011).*
- Provide environmental predictability. Consistently remind staff, family members, and visitors to tell the client when something is added or removed from the environment. *Consistency in placement of furniture and personal items aids in location detection and independence, and decreases chances of injury (Cattan, 2011; Lawrence, 2011).*
- Assist with feeding at mealtimes if blindness is temporary.
- Keep side rails up using half rails; maintain bed in a low position.
- Converse with and touch the client frequently during care if frequent touch is within the client's cultural norm. *Appropriate touch can decrease social isolation.*
- Walk the client by having the client grasp nurse's elbow or shoulder and walk partially behind nurse.
- Walk a frightened or confused client by having the client place both hands on the nurse's shoulders or waist. Then the nurse backs up in the desired direction while holding the client around the waist. This method helps the client feel secure and ensures safety.
- Keep the call light within the client's reach; check location of call light before leaving the room. **CEB:** *A study demonstrated that a large percentage of hospitalized clients are unable to use the call light button and feel vulnerable as a result (Duffy et al, 2005).*
- Provide good lighting in rooms, task lights, and night lights. **CEB:** *Good overall lighting is essential for safety, and task lighting makes everyday activities easier. Night lights allow safer navigation in the dark (Lighthouse International, 2015).*
- Make doorframes and light switches a contrasting color to the walls. **CEB:** *Contrast increases the likelihood of identifying them during navigation (Lighthouse International, 2015).*
- Ensure access to eyeglasses or magnifying devices as needed. Vision aid devices include readers, microscopes, handheld magnifiers, and stand magnifiers (Ventocilla, 2013).
- Encourage expression of feelings and expect grieving behavior if onset of blindness is new. Blind people grieve the loss of vision and experience a loss of identity and control over their lives. **CEB:** *Anxiety and depression are common in people with decreased vision (Watkinson, 2010).* **CEB:** *A study of clients with age-related macular degeneration found that a problem-focused group was effective in helping clients (Wahl et al, 2006).*
- Recommend client have vision evaluated by an optometrist or ophthalmologist as appropriate to determine whether an improvement in visual acuity is possible. *Clients may not have the correct prescription for their visual acuity; for some clients, the correct prescription of glasses may restore visual acuity (Goldman & Schafer, 2011).*
- Question the client regarding the presence of visual hallucinations. If present, reassure the client that the experience is common and does not mean he or she has a mental illness. It is helpful for the client to know that this is common and usually does not require treatment. **CEB:** *Up to half of all severely visually impaired persons have visual hallucinations, that is, fully formed images in their mind (Ricard, 2009; Watkinson, 2010).*
- Provide a CD player, radio, or books on tape as desired. These provide sensory stimulation and can help deal with the boredom of hospitalization.

- Take protective measures to prevent falls. Refer to the care plan for Risk for **Falls.**
- Explore and enhance available support systems to ensure a safe discharge. Caregivers and/or family may not have the ability to assist the client after discharge. See care plan for Risk for **Injury** or Risk for **Falls.**
- Assess the client's visual and other sensory loss using valid and reliable tools. EB: *The Severe Dual Sensory Loss Screening Tool for hearing and visual impairment is a valid and reliable tool, enabling nurses to identify impairment among older adults (Roets-Merken, 2014).* EB: *The vision-target HRQOL measure provides a comprehensive assessment of the impact of eye disease on daily functioning and well-being in adults (Paz et al, 2013).*
- Encourage the client to implement lifestyle strategies that promote avoidance of cardiovascular disease and diabetes to prevent vision loss. CEB: *Lifestyle strategies for the prevention of vision loss are important by promoting the avoidance of cardiovascular disease and diabetes (Sharts-Hopko, 2010).*

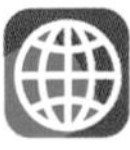

Multicultural

- Consider race/ethnicity as a possible related factor to vision loss. EB: *African Americans are at higher risk for rapid worsening of glaucoma than Caucasians (Lee et al, 2014).*

Geriatric

- Keep environment quiet, soothing, and familiar. Use consistent caregivers. These measures are comforting to older adults with a sensory loss and help decrease confusion (Lawrence, 2011).
- Increase the amount of light in the environment for older eyes; ensure it is nonglare lighting. CEB: *Increased lighting can help compensate for some of the visual changes of aging, including reduced visual acuity, reduced contrast sensitivity, and reduced color discrimination (Boyce, 2003).*

▲ Determine origin of vision loss if possible. *There are five main causes of vision loss in older adults: macular degeneration, cataracts, glaucoma, diabetic retinopathy, and refractive error (Horton, 2012).*

- Cataract is a leading cause of reversible vision impairment and may increase the risk for falls in older adults. *Use appropriate refractive management between timely surgeries (Meulers et al, 2014).*
- Hearing and vision rehabilitation services need to screen for dual sensory impairment. EB: *If audiologists are made aware of visual conditions affecting their clients, they can facilitate access to technologies for aid retention and benefit (Schneider et al, 2014).*

▲ Refer to a comprehensive vision rehabilitation center early in the disease process of macular degeneration to prevent some of the negative consequences of vision loss (Maturi, 2011).

- Teach the client methods to preserve remaining vision as much as possible, including not smoking or breathing second-hand smoke, protecting the eyes from sunlight, and including fish and leafy green vegetables in the diet (Maturi, 2011).
- Vision impairment is independently associated with malnutrition. EB: *Older assisted living residents with visual impairment were more often female, had lower body mass index, suffered more dementia, and had more chewing problems (Murrinen et al, 2014).*
- Monitor for signs of new onset of increased vision loss, such as not recognizing familiar people, difficulty seeing in bright light or low light, new problems with reading, the client complains of tired eyes, and/or verbalizes vision problems with current glasses facilitating effective vision (Ventocilla, 2013).
- Age-related visual problems can also occur with stroke (Pollock et al, 2011). If vision loss is from a stroke, watch for hemianopia, an ability to see to one side only. Encourage clients to scan environment by turning head from side to side. Also assess for visual spatial misconception.

▲ EB: *A Cochrane study found that there was evidence supporting scanning to improve reading ability, but scanning techniques were not helpful for improved visual field outcomes, and there was insufficient evidence to demonstrate effectiveness in improving activities of daily living ability (Pollock et al, 2011).*

▲ Refer client to low-vision clinics or independent living programs, which are designed for individuals who are vision impaired or blind to help maintain independence. *Clients with vision loss should be referred to clinics early, preferably before vision is gone, for help dealing with the loss (Kalinowski, 2008).* EB: *A study demonstrated that mobility function improved after blind rehabilitation training for a group of older veterans (Kuyk & Elliot, 2004).*

- Work with the client to ensure contact with others, to maintain meaningful activities, and to strengthen the social network. CEB: *Severe loneliness can accompany sensory loss in older adults as a result of self-imposed isolation (Girdler et al, 2008).*

- Watch for signs of depression: decreased appetite, withdrawal from usual life activities, flat affect, excessive time in bed, and somatization. CEB: *In one study, clients with severe vision loss identified their reality as a cause for feelings of despair (Girdler et al, 2008).*
- For the client with both vision loss and dementia, provide nursing care including:
  - Recognize that vision loss can increase problems for the client with dementia, including decreased orientation, decreased recognition of others, less recall, impaired judgment, and possibly aggression (Barrand, 2011).
  - Use one-to one conversations to maintain socialization. *These clients often cannot process conversations with a group; communication is enhanced with one-to-one communication (Lawrence, 2011).*
  - Obtain and use visual aids to help maintain orientation and contact with the environment, including such things as talking clocks, speaking Freeview digital boxes to give an auditory version of what is on the television, and use of memory photo dial pads so that clients can use the telephone to maintain contact with others (Barrand, 2011).

Home Care

- Most of the listed interventions are applicable in the home care setting.
- Monitor home care clients for recent visual loss and resulting decrease in social activity. CEB: *A study found that recent visual loss commonly resulted in decreased socialization and decrease in outdoor activities due to a fear of falling (Grue et al, 2010).*
- Enable the visually impaired client to do things for himself/herself to maintain independence as long as possible (Cattan, 2011).

Client/Family Teaching and Discharge Planning

Low Vision

- Use contrast to increase visibility of items; for example, place a dark background around the light switch so that it can be located more easily. *Improving the contrast between images results in better visual recognition (Ventocilla et al, 2013).*
- Place red, yellow, or orange identifiers on important items that need to be seen, such as a red strip at the edge of steps, red behind a light switch, or a red dot on a stove or washing machine to indicate how far to turn knob, or use a dial marker that will offer a tactile cue to the client to turn on ovens, stoves, and washing machines. *Color cues can improve the legibility of the environment and increase the ability to target objects quickly.*
- Use a watch or clock that verbally tells time, and a phone with large numerals and emergency numbers programmed into it (Ventocilla et al, 2013).
- Teach blind clients how to feed self; associate food on plate with hours on a clock so that the client can identify location of food.
- Use low-vision aids including magnifying devices for near vision and telescopes for seeing objects at a distance, a closed-circuit television that magnifies print, and guides for writing checks and envelopes. *Low vision aids can improve vision in clients with limited sight (Ventocilla et al, 2013).*
- Teach the client with vision loss to do the following:
  - Use a magnifying mirror to shave or apply makeup. Use an electric razor only.
  - Put personal care products in brightly colored pump containers (red, yellow, or orange) for identification.
  - Use tactile clues such as safety pins or buttons placed in hems to help client match clothing. Or place matching outfits of clothing in separate plastic bags.
  - Use a prefilled medication organizer with large lettering or three-dimensional (3D) markers.

These methods can help maintain the independence of the client (Ventocilla et al, 2013).

- Increase lighting in the home to help vision in the following ways:
  - Ensure adequate illumination of the entire home, adding light fixtures and increasing wattage of existing bulbs as needed.
  - Decrease glare; where light reflects on shiny surfaces, move or cover object.
  - Use nonglare wax on the floor.
  - Use motion lights that turn on automatically when a person enters the room for nighttime use.
  - Add indoor strip or "runway"-type lighting to baseboards.

Visual acuity can be improved by taking steps to overcome age-related changes in vision (American Federation for the Blind, 2011).

- ▲ Refer the client to an occupational therapist for assistance in dealing with vision loss and learning how to meet personal needs to maintain maximum independence.

Occupational therapists can help with a large number of problems for the visually impaired client, including safety, independence, quality of life, and agencies for support (Ventocilla et al, 2013).

- Encourage the client to wear a hat and sunglasses when out in the sun. *Direct sunlight and glare have been associated with vision loss.*
- Work with the client to find rewarding recreational pursuits. *Recognize that advancing vision loss can often discourage people from participating in the recreational pursuits they enjoyed in the past. When an activity becomes too much of a struggle, it simply is no longer fun. However, vision loss does not erase the basic need for the physical and mental rewards of play and relaxation.*

REFERENCES

American Federation for the Blind. (2011). *Website.* From: <http://www.afb.org> Retrieved October 13, 2014.

Barrand, J. *Supporting sight loss and dementia 2013.* From: <http://www.magonlinelibrary.com/doi/abs/10.12968/nrec.2011.13.9.448> Retrieved October 13, 2014.

Boyce, P. R. (2003). Lighting for the elderly. *Technology Disability, 15*(3), 165.

Cattan, M. (2011). How to assist residents with sight loss in your home. *Nursing Residential Care, 13*(2), 91–93.

Duffy, S., et al. (2005). Ability of hospitalized older adults to use their call bell: a pilot study in a tertiary care teaching hospital. *Aging Clinical Experience Residence, 17*(5), 390–393.

Goldman, L., & Schafer, A. I. (Eds.), (2011). *Goldman's Cecil medicine* (24th ed.). Philadelphia: Saunders Elsevier.

Girdler, S., Packer, T., & Boldy, D. (2008). The impact of age-related vision loss. *OTJR: Occupation, Participation and Health, 28*(3), 110–120.

Grue, E. V., et al. (2010). Recent visual decline: a health hazard with consequences for social life: a study of home care clients in 12 countries. *Curriculum Gerontology Geriatrics Research*, pii:503817.

Horton, J. (2012). Disorders of the eye. In D. Longo, et al. (Eds.), *Harrison's principles of internal medicine* (18th ed.). New York: McGraw Hill Medical.

Kalinowski, M. A. (2008). "Eye" dentifying vision impairment in the geriatric patient. *Geriatric Nursing (New York, N.Y.), 29*(2), 125–132.

Kuyk, T., & Elliot, J. L. (2004). Mobility function in older veterans improves after blind rehabilitation. *Journal of Rehabilitation Residential Development, 41*(3), 337.

Lawrence, V. (2011). Caring for older people with dementia and sight loss. *Nursing Residential Care, 13*(4), 186–188.

Lee, J. M., et al. (2014). Baseline prognostic factors predict rapid visual field deteriorations in glaucoma. *Investigative Ophthalmology Science, 55*(4), 2228–2236.

Lighthouse International: *Tips for confident living at home.* (2015). <http://li129-107.members.linode.com/services-and-assistance/lifestyle-independence/living-better-at-home/tips-for-confident-living-at-home/>. Accessed October 22, 2015.

Maturi, R. K. (2011). *Nonexudative ARMD. Medscape Review.* From: <http://emedicine.medscape.com/article/1223154-overview> Retrieved October 11, 2014.

Meulers, L., et al. (2014). The impact of first and second eye cataract surgery on injurious falls that require hospitalization: a whole population study. *Age and Ageing, 43*(3), 341–346.

Murrinen, S. M., et al. (2014). Vision impairment and nutritional status among older assisted living residents. *Archives of Gerontology Geriatrics, 58*(3), 384–387.

Paz, S., et al. (2013). Development of a vision-targeted health-related quality of life measure. *Quality Life Research, 22*(9), 2477–2487.

Pollock, A., et al. (2011). Interventions for visual field defects in patients with stroke. *Cochrane Database Systematic Review*, (10), CD008388.

Ricard, P. (2009). Vision loss and visual hallucinations: the Charles Bonnet syndrome. *Community Eye Health, 22*(69), 14.

Roets-Merken, L., et al. (2014). Screening for hearing, visual and dual sensory impairment in older adults using behavioral cues: a validation study. *International Journal of Nursing Studies, 51*(11), 1434–1440.

Schneider, J., et al. (2014). Improving access to hearing services for people with low vision: piloting a hearing screening and education model of intervention. *Ear and Hearing, 35*(4), e153–e161.

Sharts-Hopko, N. C. (2010). Lifestyle strategies for the prevention of vision loss. *Holistic Nursing Practice, 24*(5), 284–291.

Ventocilla, M. (2013). Low vision therapy. *Medscape.* <http://emedicine.medscape.com/article/1832033-overview>. Accessed October 22, 2015.

Wahl, H., et al. (2006). Psychosocial intervention for age-related macular degeneration: a pilot project. *Journal of Visual Impairment Blind, 100*(9), 533–545.

Watkinson, S. (2010). Management of older people with dry and wet age-related macular degeneration. *Nursing Older People, 22*(5), 21–26.

Index

Boldface entries indicate care plan titles; page numbers in *italics* indicate care plan locations.

B

C

D

E

J

K

L

M

O

P